Inside back cover: Measurement Conversion Guides

Procedures written by Jennifer Burton, Karen Stevens, Kim Jones McKillips, and Paula Delmore
Nursing Care Planning Guides written by Karen Stevens

Maternal-Newborn Nursing

THEORY AND PRACTICE

Francine H. Nichols, PhD, RNC
Elaine Zwelling, PhD, RN

Maternal-Newborn Nursing

THEORY AND PRACTICE

W.B. SAUNDERS COMPANY
A Division of Harcourt Brace & Company
Philadelphia London Toronto Montreal Sydney Tokyo

W.B. SAUNDERS COMPANY
A Division of Harcourt Brace & Company

The Curtis Center
Independence Square West
Philadelphia, Pennsylvania 19106

Library of Congress Cataloging-in-Publication Data

Nichols, Francine H.
Maternal-newborn nursing: theory and practice / Francine H. Nichols, Elaine Zwelling.—1st ed.

p. cm.

ISBN 0-7216-6777-5

1. Maternity nursing. I. Zwelling, Elaine. II. Title.
[DNLM: 1. Maternal-Child Nursing. WY 157.3 N618m 1997]

RG951.N527 1997 610.73′678—dc20

DNLM/DLC 96-15371

NOTICE

Nursing is an ever-changing field. Standard safety precautions must be followed, but as new research and clinical experience broaden our knowledge, changes in treatment and drug therapy become necessary or appropriate. The editors of this work have carefully checked the generic and trade drug names and verified drug dosages to ensure that the dosage information in this work is accurate and in accord with the standards accepted at the time of publication. Readers are advised, however, to check the product information currently provided by the manufacturer of each drug to be administered to be certain that changes have not been made in the recommended dose or in the contraindications for administration. This is of particular importance in regard to new or infrequently used drugs. It is the responsibility of the treating physician, relying on experience and knowledge of the patient, to determine dosages and the best treatment for the patient. The editors cannot be responsible for misuse or misapplication of the material in this work.

THE PUBLISHER

MATERNAL-NEWBORN NURSING: Theory and Practice ISBN 0-7216-6777-5

Printed in the United States of America

Last digit is the print number: 9 8 7 6 5 4 3 2 1

This book is dedicated to

---

the students and nurses who care for childbearing families,
the educators who teach maternal-newborn nursing, and
the researchers who contribute to the scientific basis
of maternal-newborn nursing
and with love to our families

---

the memory of my father, Eugene Hensley,
my mother, Marjorie Hensley,
and my sons, David and Gary Nichols

FRANCINE H. NICHOLS

---

my husband, David Zwelling,
my son and daughter-in-law, Mark and Melissa Schroeder,
and my first grandchild, Madeline Schroeder

ELAINE ZWELLING

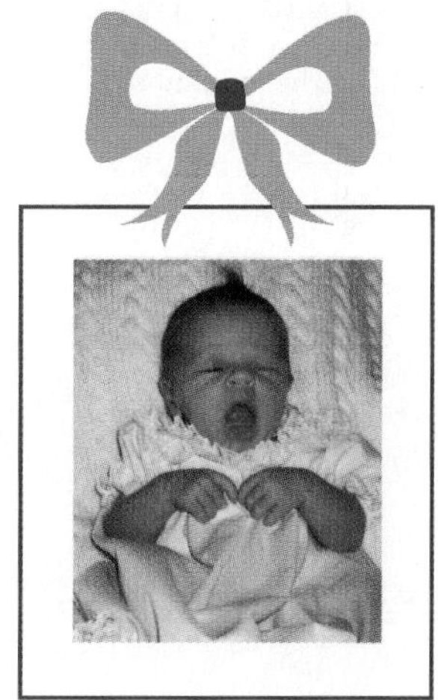

Contributors

MARY K. BARGER, CNM, MPH, FACNM
Assistant Professor,
Boston University School of Public Health,
Nurse-Midwifery Education Program,
Boston;
Nurse-Midwife,
Harvard Pilgrim Health Care,
Brigham and Women's Hospital,
Boston, Massachusetts
High-Risk Pregnancy

MARY C. BRUCKER, CNM, DNSc
Director,
Parkland School of Nurse-Midwifery,
Dallas, Texas
The Reproductive System; Fetal Development; The Physiology of Childbirth; Pain Management During Childbirth; High-Risk Childbirth

JENNIFER W. BURTON, RNC, MSN
Clinical Nurse Specialist, Perinatal,
The Arlington Hospital,
Arlington, Virginia
Procedures

LYNN CLARK CALLISTER, RN, PhD
Associate Dean of Curriculum,
Associate Professor of Nursing,
College of Nursing,
Brigham Young University,
Provo, Utah
Social Issues and Childbearing Women

PAULA M. DELMORE, RN, MSN
Nursing and Research Coordinator,
Department of Neonatology,
Columbia Wesley Medical Center,
Wichita, Kansas
Alterations in Health Status of Newborns

KATHLEEN M. DRISCOLL, RN, JD, MS
Associate Professor,
University of Cincinnati,
College of Nursing and Health,
Cincinnati, Ohio
Legal Aspects of Maternal-Newborn Nursing

SHARON L. DuMENIL, RN, MSN
Nurse Manager,
Mother-Baby Units,
Methodist Hospital,
Methodist Women's and Children's Hospital,
San Antonio, Texas
Alterations in the Health Status of Postpartum Mothers

MARGARET R. EDWARDS, RN, DSN
Professor,
Northeast Louisiana University,
Monroe, Louisiana
Maternal-Newborn Nursing in the Community

ELIZABETH FEIN, CNM, MPH
Certified Nurse-Midwife,
Harvard Pilgrim Health Care,
Boston, Massachusetts
High-Risk Pregnancy

BOBBIE S. FRYE, RN, MS
Formerly Clinical Nurse Specialist, Women's Health,
University of North Carolina Hospitals,
Chapel Hill, North Carolina
Termination of Pregnancy

CATHERINE H. GARNER, RNC, MSN, DrPH, FAAN
President, Innovative Health Strategies, Inc.,
Tucson, Arizona
Infertility

KATHY GILL, ARNP, MSN
Assistant Professor,
Kansas Newman College,
Wichita, Kansas
Nursing Care of Mothers

LINDA GOODWIN, RNC, MEd
Manager,
Family Birthplace,
Group Health Eastside Hospital,
Redmond, Washington
Roles of the Maternal-Newborn Nurse

BETTY GLENN HARRIS, RN, MSN, PhD
Dean,
Health Education Division,
Wake Technical Community College,
Raleigh, North Carolina
Postpartum Adaptation

LYNDA L. HARRISON, RN, MSN, PhD
Professor and Director of Research,
The University of Alabama Capstone College of Nursing,
Tuscaloosa, Alabama
Parenting the Healthy Infant; Parenting the High-Risk Neonate

SUSAN GOTHARD HUFFMAN, ARNP, CNM, MN
Private Practice,
Fullscope Nurse-Midwifery,
PrimeCare,
Pensacola, Florida
Perinatal Infections

LINDA CORSON JONES, RN, PhD, FACCE, FAAN
Professor and Coordinator, Research,
Louisiana State University Medical Center,
Graduate Program,
New Orleans, Louisiana
Maternal-Newborn Nursing Practice

JAN L. KABLER, RN, MSN, FACCE, IBCLC
Education Coordinator,
Maternal-Child Nursing,
Via Christi Regional Medical Center,
Wichita, Kansas
Alterations in the Health Status of Postpartum Mothers; Alterations in Health Status of Newborns

SUSAN F. KRUGER, RN, MN, PhD
Associate Professor, Parent-Child Nursing,
School of Nursing,
Wichita State University,
Wichita, Kansas
Family Dynamics

MIRA L. LESSICK, RN, PhD
Associate Professor,
Rush University College of Nursing, Chicago;
Practitioner-Teacher,
Rush-Presbyterian-St. Luke's Medical Center,
Chicago, Illinois
Genetics

MARGARET A. LYNCH, RN, MSN, FNP
Adjunct Faculty,
Massachusetts General School of Health Professions,
Boston;
Family Nurse Practitioner,
The Zinberg Clinic,
The Cambridge Hospital,
Cambridge, Massachusetts
HIV in *Perinatal Infections*

KIM JONES McKILLIPS, RNC, MSN
Procedures

NANCY J. MacMULLEN, RN, MSN, PhD
Associate Professor,
Maternal-Child Nursing,
Rush University College of Nursing,
Chicago, Illinois
High-Risk Childbirth

BONNIE O'BRIEN MAESTRI, RNC, MN, FACCE
Instructor,
Loyola University,
School of Nursing,
New Orleans, Louisiana
Maternal-Newborn Nursing Practice

MARY LOU MOORE, RN, PhD, FACCE, FAAN
Research Assistant Professor,
Department of Obstetrics and Gynecology,
Bowman Gray School of Medicine of Wake Forest University,
Winston-Salem, North Carolina
Newborn Adaptation; Neonatal Assessment; Perinatal Loss and Grief

FRANCINE H. NICHOLS, RNC, PhD, FACCE
President,
MCH Consultants,
Washington, District of Columbia
Maternal-Newborn Nursing Science; Roles of the Maternal-Newborn Nurse; Family Dynamics; Legal Aspects of Maternal-Newborn Nursing; Ethical Issues in Maternal-Newborn Nursing; Perinatal Education; Principles of Family-Centered Maternity Care; Postpartum Adaptation; Newborn Adaptation; Neonatal Assessment; Adolescent Pregnancy and Parenthood

MARY JO PODGURSKI, RNC, MA, FACCE
Director,
Washington Hospital Team Outreach:
Postpone Prevent Prepare,
Washington, Pennsylvania;

Member, ASPO/Lamaze National Faculty,
Member, Board of Directors, Pennsylvania Coalition for Teenage Pregnancy Prevention,
Lemoyne, Pennsylvania
Adolescent Pregnancy and Parenthood

CATHERINE E. RUHL, RN, CNM, MSN
Clinical Adjunct Faculty,
University of Illinois at Chicago College of Nursing,
Chicago;
Director,
Nurse Midwifery Service,
Illinois Masonic Medical Center,
Chicago, Illinois
Promoting a Normal Childbirth

ROSEMARIE DiMAURO SATYSHUR, RN, DNSc
Assistant Professor,
Maternal-Child Health Nursing,
The Catholic University of America,
Washington, DC
Ethical Issues in Maternal-Newborn Nursing

KAREN STEVENS, RN, PhD
Graduate Coordinator,
Associate Professor,
Bowie State University,
Department of Nursing,
Bowie, Maryland
Nursing Care of Newborns

DONNA FREDE VINAL, RN, CNM, PhD, FACCE
Adjunct Professor CNEP,
The Frontier School of Nurse-Midwifery,
Hyden, Kentucky;
Adjunct Professor,
University of Virginia School of Nursing,
Charlottesville, Virginia;
Private Practice,
Fullscope Nurse-Midwifery,
Charlottesville, Virginia
Perinatal Infections

LORRAINE O. WALKER, RN, EdD, FAAN
Luci B. Johnson Centennial Professor in Nursing,
The University of Texas at Austin,
Austin, Texas
Maternal-Newborn Nursing Science

MARSHA WALKER, RN, IBCLC
President,
Lactation Associates,
Weston;
Executive Director,
National Alliance for Breastfeeding Advocacy,
Weston, Massachusetts
Breastfeeding

MARJORY K. WATERMAN, MN
Clinical Instructor,
University of Texas Health Science Center at San Antonio,
San Antonio;
Chief Nursing Officer,
Methodist Women's and Children's Hospital,
San Antonio, Texas
Alterations in the Health Status of Postpartum Mothers

DEBORAH WOOLLEY, RN, CNM, PhD, FACCE
Assistant Professor and Director,
Nurse-Midwifery Obstetrics-Gynecology,
Nurse Practitioner Program,
University of Illinois College of Nursing,
Chicago, Illinois
Fetal Monitoring

ELAINE ZWELLING, RN, PhD, FACCE
Director and Faculty,
ASPO/Lamaze Childbirth Educator Program,
College of Public Health,
University of South Florida,
Tampa;
Consultant: Maternal-Newborn Care,
Sarasota;
Childbirth Educator,
Columbia HCA Doctors Hospital,
Sarasota, Florida
Sexuality During Pregnancy; Family Planning; Physiologic Changes of Pregnancy; Psychological Responses to Pregnancy; Sociocultural Aspects of Pregnancy; Promoting a Healthy Pregnancy; Perinatal Education; The Physiology of Childbirth; Promoting a Normal Childbirth; Pain Management During Childbirth; High-Risk Childbirth; Principles of Family-Centered Maternity Care

Preface

Childbirth is a unique and powerful human experience that has physiologic, psychological, and social importance. Birth represents a new beginning in every parent's life and forever influences the way an individual sees the self, the world, and the future. Maternal-newborn nurses have the distinct privilege of helping families respond positively to the major life transition of childbearing. They also have the responsibility to ensure that childbirth is as safe as possible and, equally important, as psychologically positive as possible. Regardless of age, students in maternal-newborn nursing have the opportunity to participate in the excitement, wonder, and mystery of birth, as well as to examine the information from a personal perspective and to explore their beliefs and values about childbirth and parenting.

PHILOSOPHICAL BASE

The following philosophical beliefs related to maternal-newborn nursing provided the foundation for this text:

- Childbearing is a family affair and maternal-newborn services are best provided in a family-centered approach, while maintaining the physical safety of the individual family members.
- The reproductive health of the total family is important to the health of society and of the infant, and maternal mortality rates indicate both the health status of the population and the quality of health services for a population.
- Childbirth is a normal physiologic process that generally requires few medical interventions. While advancements in technology have improved outcomes for high-risk women and infants, technology for low-risk women should be used judiciously.
- Parenting is learned and nurses can play a critical role in assisting families as they navigate the critical passages to parenthood.

FEATURES

Research and Theory Based

A scientific base of research and theory is essential to provide a firm foundation for the practice of maternal-newborn nursing. Research and theory are also the basis for the knowledge that is a key factor in advancing maternal-newborn nursing. Such knowledge forms the cornerstone of maternal-newborn nursing's power: professionally, politically, and socially.

This text provides students and nurses with a comprehensive guide to maternal-newborn care and the scientific research and theoretical basis that promote consistent approaches to specific situations while fostering insight that is essential in providing individualized care for maternal-newborn clients. Throughout the text, conclusions from the research are presented as opposed to emphasis on one or two isolated studies. The "Trends in Research" unit openers were developed to emphasize the importance of looking at the **total body of research** related to a specific situation in order to evaluate the validity of findings, draw conclusions, and determine implications for practice. The "Implications for Research" section in each chapter provides information on research that is needed in maternal-newborn nursing practice. A summary of research from the *Cochrane Pregnancy and Childbirth Database* on effective care in pregnancy and childbirth based on an analysis of controlled research trials is included in Appendix IX. As students and nurses study and provide maternal-newborn nursing care, we encourage them to refer to this information and determine what the research indicates about specific practices.

Nursing Process

Maternal-newborn nursing practice encompasses promoting wellness, preventing potential health problems, and caring for actual health problems of childbearing women, their infants, and their families. The nursing process is a critical decision-making tool that enables nurses to plan individualized research- and diagnosis-based nursing care for clients. The approved NANDA system of nursing diagnosis (problem-oriented diagnosis) is used throughout this text. Information is also presented on how to develop wellness-oriented diagnoses for maternal-newborn nursing by modifying the NANDA system.

Nursing Care Planning Guides

Six comprehensive Nursing Care Planning Guides that cover the major areas of maternal-newborn nursing care are included. Nursing care is presented in steps with rationales for both usual and potential nursing diagnoses, with appropriate interventions and expected outcomes for the typical client. While there are common client problems, each individual's response to a situation is unique and the nurse needs to adapt the plan of care to each client's needs. Students will find the Nursing Care Planning Guides helpful in preparing for clinical experiences, during the process of providing nursing care, and when reviewing for examinations over the content. The Nursing Care Planning Guides include assessment tools currently used in clinical practice. We believe that incorporating actual assessment tools used in practice will help the student make the transition from the classroom to the practice setting more easily.

Procedures

Thirty illustrated detailed Procedures are presented. These Procedures will increase learning and help students prepare for clinical experiences. Students can also refer to them as needed during clinical practice and in reviewing content.

Community and Home Care

The advances and challenges of community and home care during pregnancy, postpartum, and neonatal periods are discussed. In addition to the usual information on community and home care, detailed guidelines are included on planning and accomplishing the home visit, documenting the home visit, communicating with the primary health care provider, safety precautions within the community, and essential risk management practices.

Social and Political Issues

We have strived to provide balanced coverage of social and political issues. Our goal is to encourage informed decision making and a higher level of practice through a straightforward discussion of sensitive and controversial issues in health care and politics related to maternal-newborn nursing. We believe that an individual needs to be knowledgeable about all aspects of the problem in order to make appropriate decisions related to situations that are enmeshed in ethical, political, and legal issues as well as influenced by one's personal beliefs.

Critical Thinking Boxes

Examples of ethical, legal, and practice dilemmas from actual case histories are presented and questions that focus on the stark reality of "real world" situations are included. The practice in values clarification and decision making that results from these exercises will increase a person's ability to deal with the complex problems faced in clinical practice.

Teaching Guides

Appropriate chapters provide a Teaching Guide that covers related content for client teaching in maternal-newborn practice. Tips for improving teaching effectiveness and teaching aids are included in one convenient table.

Improving Your Practice Boxes

These boxes promote values clarification, critical thinking, and cultural sensitivity. Discussing the relationships between your values, beliefs, and attitudes and their impact on providing nursing care will promote self-analysis and self-awareness, which are crucial components of critical thinking.

Historical Perspectives Boxes

The historical perspectives and time lines in this book provide the reader with a context for understanding today's practice, ethical, legal, and political issues. This historical information is helpful in evaluating current maternal-newborn care practices.

Illustrations

This text contains nearly 500 original full-color drawings and photographs that have been developed specifically to promote understanding of often complex material. Where appropriate, text entitled "Understanding . . . " and highlighting key points is included with the illustrations. Photographs are included that depict specific situations commonly encountered in maternal-newborn nursing.

Definitions and Key Concepts

Definitions and Key Concepts are included in each chapter to promote learning and emphasize major concepts in the chapter. These features will also aid the student in studying or reviewing content.

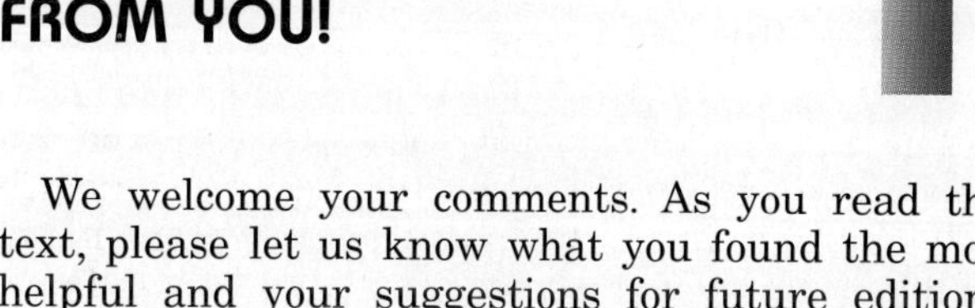

WE WANT TO HEAR FROM YOU!

We welcome your comments. As you read this text, please let us know what you found the most helpful and your suggestions for future editions. Our goal is to provide in-depth coverage of content in a readable and understandable format. You can contact us at:

FRANCINE H. NICHOLS, RNC, PhD
E-mail: fnichols@dgs.dgsys.com
ELAINE ZWELLING, RN, PhD
E-mail: zwelling@gate.net

Acknowledgments

This book is the result of the contributions and expertise of many, many individuals. A special thank you goes to the contributing authors of chapters, Nursing Care Planning Guides, and Procedures for their critical analysis of the literature and for presenting the scientific basis for the practice of maternal-newborn nursing. Many clinical experts gave us constructive feedback on the manuscript throughout the development of this text and provided assessment forms, collaborative care plans, and other information that has been included in the book. Reviewers provided us with valuable feedback on the manuscript related to teaching maternal-newborn nursing and student needs. We are deeply indebted to each of them.

We are also most appreciative of the research consultants: Dr. Lorraine Walker, who reviewed the "Trends in Research" unit openers and assisted with the integration of research in the text; and Dr. Sharron Humenick and Dr. Susan Gennaro, who reviewed selected "Trends in Research" unit openers. Dr. Kay Avant reviewed and refined the use of nursing process throughout the text as well as its presentation in the Nursing Care Planning Guides. Linda Goodwin, RNC, MEd, served as clinical consultant for the text and provided valuable recommendations.

Special acknowledgments go to Anne Ford Doyle and Deborah McKeown, photographers, and all of the staff at Fairfax Hospital and INOVA Health System who assisted in obtaining the wonderful photographs for this text. Sincere appreciation is also extended to the parents who allowed us to take these pictures. Other individuals shared specific photographs with us that are included throughout the text and we thank each of them for this.

We also thank our editorial assistants, Frances Wood and Connie Reed, for their excellent organizational and project management skills, which were vital to a project of this complexity. We thank Catherine Dally, MS, RNC, Thelma Patrick, PhD, RN, and Linda Goodwin, RNC, MEd, for undertaking the writing of the Instructor's Manual, Study Guide, and Testbank.

Finally, this book became a reality because of the efforts of the following individuals: Ilze Rader, acquisitions editor, for her continued belief in this project, her vision for the final product, and her guidance throughout; Sue Bredensteiner, developmental editor, for her overall coordination of the project and for her creativeness in developing our ideas for art; Martha Tanner, developmental editor, for her meticulous work on the Nursing Care Planning Guides and Procedures; Marie Thomas, editorial assistant, for keeping communications flowing; David Harvey, senior manuscript editor, for his precise attention to detail and superb editing of the manuscript; Ellen Zanolle, senior book designer, for her elegant design for the book; Peg Shaw, illustration coordinator; DesignPointe Communications, Inc., especially Vicky Heim and Richard A. Fritzler, artists, for the excellent drawings; and Linda R. Garber, senior production manager, and all of the other members of the production team for the work necessary to achieve the splendid metamorphosis from manuscript to book.

FRANCINE H. NICHOLS
ELAINE ZWELLING

REVIEWERS

BERNARDINE ADAMS, RN, MN
School of Nursing
Northeast Louisiana University
Monroe, Louisiana

KAY AVANT, RN, PhD, FAAN
School of Nursing
The University of Texas at Austin
Austin, Texas

PAMELA A. BACHMEYER, RN, PhD, CPNP
College of Nursing
Chicago State University
Chicago, Illinois

JUDY F. BARNES, RN, MSN
School of Nursing
East Carolina University
Greenville, North Carolina

JOANNE H. BARTER, RN, MS
College of Nursing
Montana State University
Billings, Montana

JO ELLEN BRANNAN, RN, MSN
School of Nursing
MacMurray College
Jacksonville, Illinois

GAIL J. BRICELAND, RN, MSN, CPNP
School of Nursing
Lynchburg College
Lynchburg, Virginia

SANDRA GODMAN BROWN, RN, DSN
College of Nursing
Medical University of South Carolina
Charleston, South Carolina

ALFREDA BURBLIS, CNM, EdD
School of Nursing
Southern Connecticut State University
New Haven, Connecticut

VIRGINIA DAVIDSAVER, RNC, MS
School of Nursing
Bishop Clarkson College
Omaha, Nebraska

PERSEVERANDA DELA CRUZ, RN, MEd, MSN
College of Nursing
Chicago State University
Chicago, Illinois

SHARON E. DELANEY, RN, MPH
College of Nursing
Montana State University
Missoula, Montana

BARBARA ENGELHARDT, RN, MN, PhD
School of Nursing
Youngstown State University
Youngstown, Ohio

SUSAN GENNARO, RN, DSN, FAAN
Associate Professor, School of Nursing
University of Pennsylvania
Philadelphia, Pennsylvania

RITA S. GLAZEBROOK, RNC, PhD
School of Nursing
St. Olaf College
Northfield, Minnesota

CHERRY A. GUINN, RN, MSN, EdD
School of Nursing
University of Tennessee
Chattanooga, Tennessee

MARCIA HILTABIDLE, BS, PT
Mariner Health Care
Bethesda, Maryland

JACQUELYN HOWELL, RN, PhD
School of Nursing
Augustana College
Sioux Falls, South Dakota

BARBARA KEMP HUBERMAN, RN, BSN, MEd
Advocates for Youth
Washington, District of Columbia

SHARRON S. HUMENICK, RN, PhD, FAAN
Professor
School of Nursing
University of Wyoming
Laramie, Wyoming

MARIANNE H. HUTTI, RN, DNS, OGNP
School of Nursing
University of Louisville
Louisville, Kentucky

BARBARA HYDE-ROBERTSON, RN, EdD
School of Nursing
Southeastern Louisiana University
Baton Rouge, Louisiana

CHERYL POPE KISH, RN, MSN, EdD
School of Nursing
Georgia College
Milledgeville, Georgia

PHYLLIS M. KLEIN, RN, MSN
Clinical Specialist/Consultant
Maternal-Infant Nursing
Fairfax, Virginia

JEANNETTE A. LANDA, RN, MS
Lienhard School of Nursing
Pace University
Pleasantville, New York

DONNA M. LAWRENCE, RNC, MSN
College of Nursing
Marquette University
Milwaukee, Wisconsin

JANICE C. LEGGETT, RN, MSN
School of Nursing
East Carolina University
Greenville, North Carolina

JUDITH A. LOTHIAN, RN, PhD, FACCE
Maternal and Child Health Consultant
Brooklyn, New York

TERESA W. MARCHESE, RN, MSN, CNM
School of Nursing
Georgetown University
Washington, District of Columbia

KATHLEEN A. MARTIN, RN, MS
School of Nursing
Boise State University
Boise, Idaho

ROMONA B. MAYEUX, RNC, MS, FNP
School of Nursing
University of Southwestern Louisiana
Lafayette, Louisiana

CAROLYN MERCER-BOWERS, PT, BS
Holy Cross Hospital
Silver Spring, Maryland

BARBARA MORAN, CNM, MS, MPH
Center for Clinical Education and Development
Fairfax Hospital
Falls Church, Virginia

IRENE C. MORELLI, RN, MSN
School of Nursing
Georgetown University
Washington, District of Columbia

JUDITH THOMAS MYERS, RNC, MS
School of Nursing
Bishop Clarkson College
Omaha, Nebraska

JUDITH PETERS, RN, MS
School of Nursing
Loma Linda University
Loma Linda, California

LONA RATCLIFFE, RN, MN
School of Nursing
East Carolina University
Greenville, North Carolina

MARY M. REEVE, RN, EdD
School of Nursing
San Jose State University
San Jose, California

JACQUELYN D. REID, RNC, EdD
School of Nursing
University of Louisville
Louisville, Kentucky

JACQUELINE W. RILEY, RN, MSN, EdD
School of Nursing
West Virginia University
Morgantown, West Virginia

JANICE M. RIORDAN, RN, EdD, FAAN
School of Nursing
Wichita State University
Wichita, Kansas

KATHLEEN ROBBINS, RNC, MSN
School of Nursing
University of Louisville
Louisville, Kentucky

CATHY ROZMUS, RN, DSN, FACCE
School of Nursing
Belmont University
Nashville, Tennessee

SUSAN L. RUSH, RN, EdD
School of Nursing
Fairleigh Dickinson University
Teaneck, New Jersey

ALLISON D. SADR, CNM, MPH
School of Nursing
Georgetown University
Washington, District of Columbia

BARBARA J. SHELTON, RN, PhD
School of Nursing
University of Missouri
Columbia, Missouri

ANN L. SILVONEK, RN, MS, CNM
School of Nursing
Georgetown University
Washington, District of Columbia

KATHLEEN V. SMITH, RNC, MSN
School of Nursing
Bishop Clarkson College
Omaha, Nebraska

TERRY TOBIN, RN, MSN, MPH
School of Nursing
Marquette University
Milwaukee, Wisconsin

LOIS TSCHETTER, RN, MS
College of Nursing
South Dakota State University
Brookings, South Dakota

JULIA VAN MUISWINKEL, RN, PhD, CNM
School of Nursing
University of Pittsburgh
Pittsburgh, Pennsylvania

LUANNE WIELICHOWSKI, RN, MSN
School of Nursing
Alverno College
Milwaukee, Wisconsin

AMY MUR WORTH, MSN, ARNP
School of Nursing
University of Miami
Miami, Florida

PATRICIA E. ZANDER, RNC, MSN
School of Nursing
Viterbo College
LaCrosse, Wisconsin

Contents

Chapter 10

Chapter 11

Chapter 12

Chapter 15

Chapter 16

Unit 4

Nursing Care During Childbirth 701

Chapter 22

Chapter 23

Chapter 28

Chapter 29

Chapter 30

Chapter 37

Chapter 38

Chapter 39

Chapter 40

Appendix I

Appendix II

Appendix III

Appendix IV

Appendix V

Unit 1

Perspectives on Maternal-Newborn Nursing

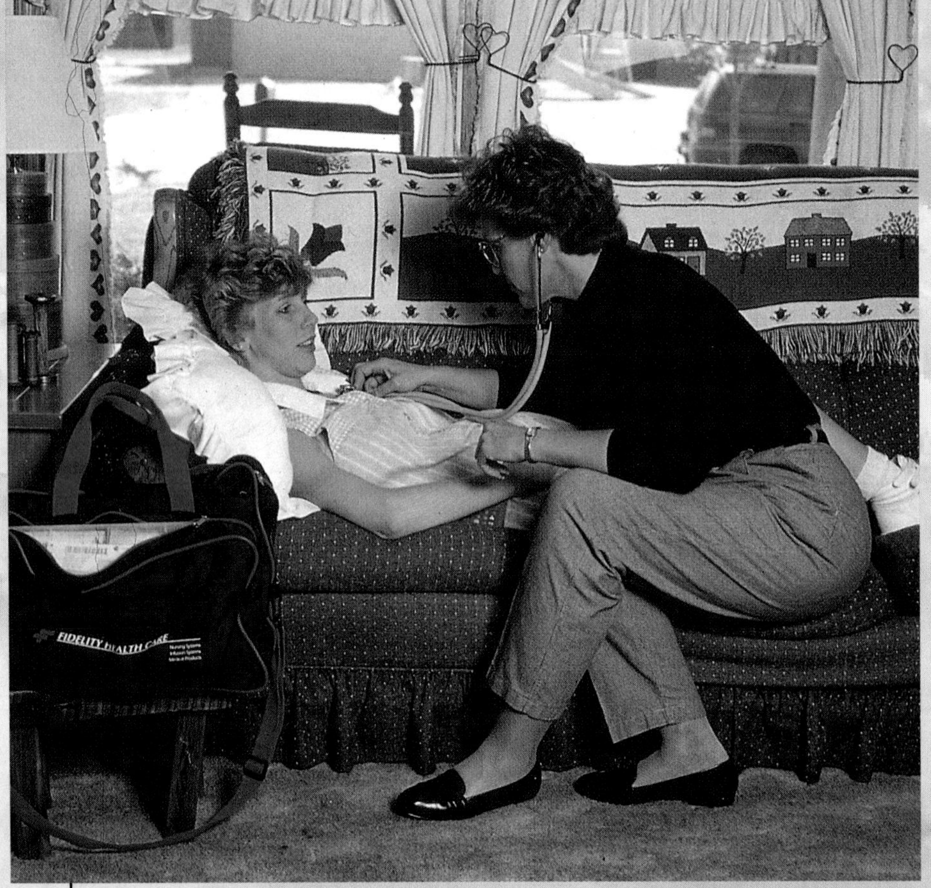

A home health nurse examines a pregnant client at 33 weeks' gestation who had been hospitalized with an episode of preterm labor that began when she had the flu. While in the hospital, the client was treated with continuous intravenous magnesium sulfate and intermittent subcutaneous injections of terbutaline to stop labor. After discharge, her treatment continued at home with subcutaneous terbutaline administered by continuous pump infusion, and she remained on bed rest. She was monitored for preterm labor with a home uterine activity monitor. From the time of her discharge from the hospital until 36 completed weeks of gestation, her care was managed by a home health nurse, who visited frequently at first, and then as needed once the woman's ability to handle her own care increased. Throughout the care period, the home health nurse talked with the expectant mother twice every day at the same time, once in the morning and once at night, to determine whether she had experienced any signs of preterm labor. Labor was successfully delayed until 40 weeks' gestation, when she gave birth to a healthy 6-pound 9-ounce infant. (Photo courtesy of Fidelity Health Care, Antepartum Home Care Services, Dayton, OH.)

Trends in Research

EFFECTIVENESS OF HOME CARE

The most effective home visiting programs are those that include a comprehensive focus with multiple goals, have frequent visits over an extended period, are staffed by well-trained and committed professionals, and serve high-risk families.

Home visiting has existed since Elizabethan times in England and the 1890s in the United States. The effectiveness of the program elements of home visiting programs for pregnant women and families with newborns has been evaluated extensively. However, the diversity of the program elements, goals, and families served limit to some extent the conclusions that can be drawn from the research.[1]

CONCLUSIONS FROM RESEARCH

- Research that supports the effectiveness of home visiting programs is as good as or better than research that supports the effectiveness of many other programs that exist to serve children and families.[1]
- The most effective home visiting programs are those that include a comprehensive focus with multiple goals, have frequent visits over an extended period, are staffed by well-trained and committed professionals, and serve high-risk families.[2]
- Not all families will benefit from the same home visiting program. High-risk families benefit the most, but there are still many questions regarding specifically which families are likely to be helped by different types of home visiting programs.[1]
- Prenatal outreach and home visiting programs have been shown to be effective in helping African-American pregnant women and other minority groups to reach and participate in prenatal care.[3]
- Early discharge of newborns and mothers with repeated follow-up postpartum home visits by a nurse may be safe for newborns in populations that are medically, psychosocially, and economically at low risk and that have been prepared for early discharge.[4]
- Home visiting programs, evaluated by the most rigorous research designs, have proved both effective in promoting the health and development of low-birth-weight infants and cost effective.[5]
- Planning and implementing effective home visiting programs is not an easy task; it requires careful thought and appropriate goals for the community served and the outcomes desired.[2]
- While some studies have documented the economic effectiveness of home visiting programs,[5] most studies do not include an essential evaluation of the economic component: cost effectiveness and cost benefit.[6]

IMPLICATIONS FOR PRACTICE

Home visiting programs provide nurses with a unique opportunity to improve the health and well-being of pregnant women, infants, and families through continued contact and interventions specific to the population served. Continued research is needed to determine how home visiting services are best provided, to ascertain which populations are best served and by which interventions, and to establish the cost effectiveness of the programs.

---

[1]Gomby, D. S., Larson, C. S., Lewit, E. M., and Behrman, R. E. (1993). Home visiting: Analysis and recommendations. *The Future of Children,* 3(3), 6–22.

[2]Olds, D. L., and Kitzman, H. (1993). Review of research on home visiting for pregnant women and parents of young children. *The Future of Children,* 3(3), 53–92.

[3]Fowler, B. A. (1995). Prenatal outreach: An approach to reduce infant mortality of African American infants. *ABNF Journal,* 6(1), 15–18.

[4]Braverman, P., Egerter, S., Pearl, M., Marchi, K., Miller, C. (1995). Early discharge of newborns and mothers: A critical review of the literature. *Pediatrics,* 96(4), 716–726.

[5]Brooten, D., Kumar, S., Brown, L. P., et al. (1986). A randomized clinical trial of early hospital discharge and follow-up of very low-birth-weight infants. *New England Journal of Medicine,* 315, 924–939.

[6]Barnett, W. S. (1993). Economic evaluation of home visiting programs. *The Future of Children,* 3(3), 93–112.

–Francine H. Nichols

1 Chapter

> When nurses' sensitivity to human needs (their intuition) is joined with the ability to find and use expert opinion, with the ability to find reported research and apply it to their practice, and when they themselves use the scientific method of investigation, there is no limit to the influence they might have on health care worldwide.
>
> VIRGINIA HENDERSON (1987)

Maternal-Newborn Nursing Science

Lorraine O. Walker
Francine H. Nichols

HIGHLIGHTS

- The Basis of Maternal-Newborn Nursing Science
- The Importance of Theory to Nursing Science
- The Relationship Between Theory and Practice
- Maternal-Newborn Theories
- Use of Theoretic Approaches in Nursing Practice
- Maternal-Newborn Nursing Research
- Nursing Assessment Research
- Future Research Priorities
- Implications for Research

A scientific base of theory and research is essential to provide a firm foundation for the practice of maternal-newborn nursing. Theory and research are also the foundation of knowledge that is a key factor in advancing maternal-newborn nursing. This knowledge forms the basis of maternal-newborn nursing's power: professionally, politically, and socially (Walker 1992).

THE BASIS OF MATERNAL-NEWBORN NURSING SCIENCE

Donnelly (1986) describes theory as "a window on the world, constructed out of the stuff of observation, the rigor of experience, and the power of imagination." Theory provides a guide for practice, in much the same way

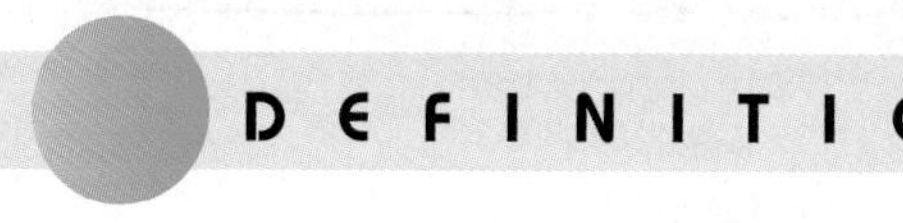

Applied research—The scientific investigation of techniques to directly improve patient care.

Basic research—The scientific investigation of fundamental processes that are usually not directly observable. Such processes, when explained, provide understanding of observed events.

Bonding theory—A theory by Klaus and Kennell that used the concept of a "sensitive period" to explain mothers' attachment to their infants as well as disruptions in attachment.

Child health assessment model—A model developed by Barnard that explains how perinatal, parental, and child characteristics and parent-child interaction factors may interact in complex ways to shape the development of children.

Concept—A mental picture of an event or object.

Maternal-newborn nursing science—An organization of tested theories and research findings related to the field of maternal-newborn nursing.

Maternal-newborn theories—Abstract descriptions and explanations of phenomena that pertain to pregnancy, childbirth, and parenting.

Maternal-role attainment theory—A theory that describes the psychological aspects that accompany pregnancy and the postpartum period and the factors that hinder or facilitate women's successful development of the maternal role. Rubin and Mercer have both contributed to the development of the maternal-role attainment theory.

Paradigm—An abstract pattern, example, or model of a family of related theories.

Phenomenon—An event that actually occurs and can be observed.

Research-based nursing intervention—A scientifically tested method or approach to a health-related need of mothers or infants that has been shown to be effective.

Theory—An interrelated set of abstract concepts and statements that gives a systematic picture of phenomena in a field of study. A theory can describe, explain, predict, provide the potential for control, or give a sense of understanding about what is happening.

that a road map gives direction from your starting point to the desired destination. Theory is a tool that makes the practice of maternal-newborn nursing more efficient and effective because nursing actions are goal directed.

Research is "diligent, systematic inquiry or investigation to validate and refine existing knowledge and generate new knowledge" (Burns and Grove 1993, p. 3). Research is used to validate, refute, or modify theory. Through research, problems and phenomena in the area of maternal-newborn nursing are investigated and solutions and approaches for practice are identified.

Research is a continuous, evolving process. During the investigation of one question, new questions that require answers will emerge. Thus, science does not once and forever provide the answers for practice. Nursing practice requires constant evaluation. As new knowledge emerges, it should be integrated into nursing practice, and nursing practice revised accordingly.

An example of a research study used to develop theory that also provides a guide for practice is seen in the work of Jones and Flaherty (1992). These maternal-newborn researchers investigated

- The stressors that preeclamptic mothers who remained in the delivery suite at least 24 hours after birth experienced during a period of intensive care, and
- The nursing care that the women described to be helpful in decreasing stress

Jones and Flaherty identified three general themes that reflected the women's responses to the situation. On the basis of these themes, they were able to recommend successful nursing care actions for women who experienced intensive care after delivery. The findings of this study can improve maternal-newborn nursing practice because it offers a scientific base for practice.

The Importance of Theory to Nursing Science

The term *theory* often sparks responses such as: "difficult to understand" and "hard to use." Students may question theory's relevance to practice and prefer a "just give me the facts" approach that specifies what they should do in any given situation. However, discrete technical information does not provide a complete knowledge base for the practice of maternal-newborn nursing. There are very few black and white situations in nursing. Rather, the broad viewpoints, values, and sense of understanding concerning what is happening that are provided by theory are essential for the nurse to make *accurate expert judgments* about appropri-

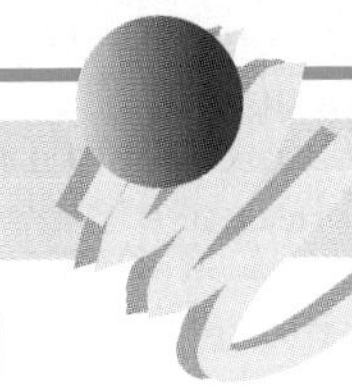

CRITICAL THINKING CASE HISTORY

YOU CAN NEVER PROVE A THEORY TRUE

Science makes progress not by proving that theories are true but by testing them rigorously and being unable to prove them false. That's a crucial distinction to keep in mind when evaluating the claims and counterclaims that are hurled about so often on almost any issue.

. . . There are very few things in science that can be stated honestly with absolute certainty. The closest that researchers usually get is to express a high degree of confidence that something is true. But they can reach that level of confidence only after rigorously testing the hypothesis.

For example, there is no strictly logical way to prove unequivocally that the sun will come up tomorrow. But it is possible to test that theory. You can do it by looking for the sun on repeated mornings. After enough testing, you gain confidence that the theory is true. But you can't be certain it will happen the next time.

Let's study this issue with a trickier example: What are the chances that any given birth will produce a boy or a girl?

You might simply observe your own family. You might record that it has two boys and one girl. That might lead you to propose a hypothesis that nature is built so that twice as many boys are born as girls. That's fine. It's a perfectly valid hypothesis, based on real world observation.

Should you believe it? Not yet. If you want to reduce your chance of being fooled, you should first follow the standard scientific approach and test your hypothesis.

How? One simple rule is to make many observations and examine them as a group.

So you look at another family and find that it has three girls. A third family has one boy and one girl. Gradually, as you widen your sample, you find the boy-girl ratio approaches 50-50. Then, a strange thing starts to happen—once your sample approaches a certain number of families, the ratio never again varies much. You may feel satisfied that you have looked far enough.

Now you have produced a piece of scientific information—the chances of any birth producing a boy, you might conclude, are about 50 percent, and the same goes for girls. For now, let's say you are satisfied with your data.

You are now entitled to take the next step and ask why the sexes should be evenly matched.

The usual practice in science when faced with a "why" question is to think up a "because" answer. You can search your memory for something that you already know. Or you can make up something. It's okay; scientists make up explanations all the time. That's what a hypothesis is. Scientists just try not to believe them without testing them. "The sexes are equally matched," you might hypothesize, "because everybody needs somebody to love and a 50-50 ratio would make this possible."

One of the rules of the scientific method is that the only good hypothesis is one that can be tested. The "somebody to love" hypothesis is not very testable. It's the kind of hypothesis that was popular among the ancient Greeks. Objects fell downward, Aristotle taught, because the ground was their rightful place.

Since ancient times, science has developed a very different approach—testing and careful observation. In the 1930s, the late philosopher Karl Popper recognized this tradition in science, analyzed its logic and named it "critical rationalism."

"The work of the scientist," Popper wrote in a 1934 essay, "consists in putting forward and testing theories."

It was Popper who formalized the idea that theories can only be proven wrong, never right.

A hypothesis for our birth-ratio research project might be as follows: "The sexes are equally matched because parents can bequeath only two combinations of sex-determining chromosomes, and the odds that an embryo gets one or the other must be 50-50." This could be tested by looking at other species with the same chromosome situation to see whether they produce half males and half females.

Now imagine that it is a year or so later and that we have had a wonderful time on our field trips checking up on the sex ratios of lions and hummingbirds and termites and tuna. And we have looked up the reports of other scientists

Continued on facing page

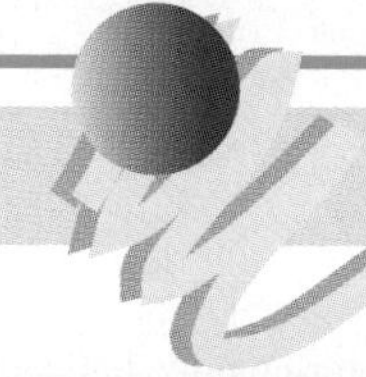

CRITICAL THINKING CASE HISTORY Continued

YOU CAN NEVER PROVE A THEORY TRUE

who have studied sex ratios for other species. We would find that not all of the ratios are 50-50. Some are but others are not. Our hypothesis needs work. It isn't as simple as we thought. We can't count on the Nobel Prize this year.

In the meantime, one of our graduate students has been examining the human birth ratio more closely and has made a surprising finding. If you look at the number of males and females at each age of life, the ratios change over time. Among newborns, boys predominate. As we move through older age groups, the ratio edges closer to 50-50. Among older people, there are more women than men. And among the elderly, there are many more women than men.

Our grad student—clearly a promising candidate—has also gotten death rates. They fit the pattern. At every age, males are more likely to die than females. He has even dug up reports showing that although more male embryos are conceived than female embryos, they are more likely to die. Females are clearly the stronger sex.

A deeper analysis of the data has revealed a phenomenon far more profound than it seemed at the outset. We can now refine our hypothesis: "Nature has arranged things so that the number of males who die before the age of parenthood is offset by the larger number of males conceived and born in the first place."

. . . rigorous testing of our hypothesis has led us to a far more complex problem. The arithmetic of sex-determining chromosomes would seem to dictate a 50-50 ratio. The fact that nature doesn't work that way shows that a more subtle phenomenon must be at work.

We need another grant.

Editor's Note: The original study led the researchers to the discovery of another more subtle phenomenon that needed to be investigated. They "need another grant" so they can do further research to explore the new phenomenon they uncovered. This article shows, by example, why research is a continuous process. During the investigation of one question, new questions requiring answers emerge. Thus, science doesn't once and forever provide the answers for practice. Science is a perpetual, cyclic process which constantly provides new knowledge on which nursing practice should be based.

From Rensberger, B. (December 14, 1994). How to think: You can never prove a theory true. © *The Washington Post.* Reprinted with permission.

ate care in a specific situation (Carveth 1987). Thus, theory becomes relevant to daily practice—in both clinical and research orientations—as a building block for critical assessments and evaluation.

Theory is useful to maternal-newborn nurses in a number of different ways as they provide care for clients. Theory can *describe* a phenomenon, it can *explain* what is happening, it can *predict* what will happen in a given situation, and it provides the *potential for control* because if the practitioner knows what will happen in a given situation, the nurse can take steps to modify or control the situation. Theory gives the practitioner a *sense of understanding* as events unfold that allows for greater flexibility and more effective nursing care for clients (Reynolds 1971).

The use of theory is a very practical and precise way to individualize care for mothers and newborns. The inclusion of theory offers a more complete picture for practice than factual knowledge alone. Also, the use of theory helps organize existing knowledge into larger categories called *concepts.* Just as you organize your closet by putting similar items together—slacks, shirts, skirts, dresses—applying theory makes retrieval of information in practice easier. At the same time, it aids new and important discoveries to advance practice (Walker and Avant 1995).

The Relationship Between Theory and Practice

The relationship between theory and practice is a cyclic, ongoing, and continual evolution. Theory stems from practice through observations, insights, and research by maternal-newborn nurses. This *theory development phase* is an inductive process in which generalizations about a phenom-

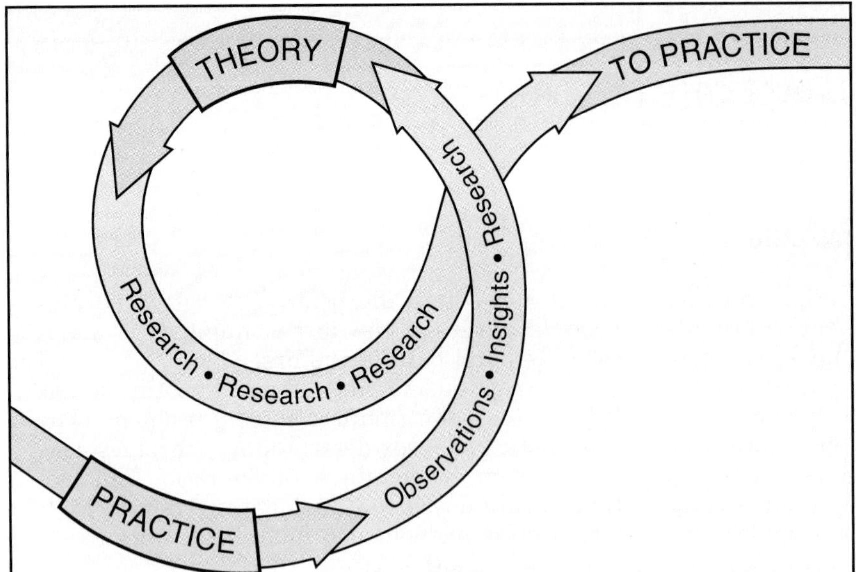

Figure 1–1
There is a cyclic relationship between theory and nursing practice • a development phase consisting of observations, insights, and research leads to a theory about a phenomenon • a theory testing phase with research, research, and more research tests existing hypotheses • and the research findings are used in practice, which includes both application of theory to practice and the generation of new problems.

enon are developed based on information about the phenomenon that occurred in specific situations. When a theory has been developed, the *theory testing phase* or deductive process begins in which research studies are developed to test the theory. In this case, generalizations about a phenomenon are tested to see if they apply in specific situations. The results of the theory testing phase can be that the theory is supported, refuted, or modified if there is a need to make changes and refine the theory. Theories that are verified or refined can then be applied in practice (Fig. 1–1).

The cyclic, continually evolving nature of the relationship between theory and practice is demonstrated by a research study in which Nichols (1992) examined the adolescent childbirth experience. The investigator's original intent was to determine the effect of prepared childbirth on teens based on the literature on prepared childbirth. However, during the study, Nichols noted that adolescents' responses to childbirth were markedly different from those of adults in studies on prepared childbirth in the literature. In addition to presenting findings about the effect of prepared childbirth on teens (theory testing phase), the researcher developed a model to describe the adolescent childbirth experience (theory development phase) and presented research questions that need to be investigated about this phenomenon (this leads back to the theory testing phase).

Maternal-Newborn Theories

A number of theories have influenced maternal-newborn nursing. Some theories have come from other fields, such as medicine; others have been developed by nurses. The writings of Rubin (1984) and Mercer (1981) on maternal role attainment and maternal identity and the Barnard Child Health Assessment Interaction Model (Barnard and Douglas 1974; Barnard 1978) are examples of theories developed from nursing research. The theoretical writings of Klaus and Kennell (1976) on bonding of parents to their infants is an example of theory from another field. Each of these theories has been important in shaping maternal-newborn nursing research and practice. They are presented here because of the interest they have generated among researchers as well as for their historical significance in the development of maternal-newborn nursing.

MATERNAL ROLE ATTAINMENT

A nurse theorist, Reva Rubin, approached the explanation of mothers' relationship to their infants from the standpoint of taking on the maternal role. Rejecting the idea that the maternal role is learned in childhood play, Rubin (1967a, 1967b) used information from interviews with and observations of pregnant women and new mothers to formulate her theory. Rubin proposed that the maternal role is attained through use of several psychological operations such as mimicry, role play, and fantasy that begin prenatally. Women's own mothers as well as their peers serve as models for women's evolving ideas of themselves as mothers. Although Rubin further refined her ideas in 1984, she retained an emphasis on the internal psychological experience of women during pregnancy and the postpartum period as central to an understanding of motherhood (Rubin 1984). Rubin's theory was important in highlighting the psychological aspects that accompany pregnancy and the postpartum period.

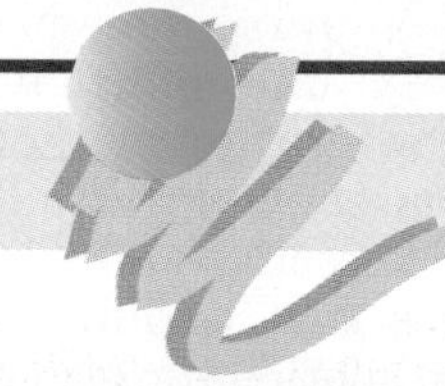

HISTORICAL PERSPECTIVES

THE DEVELOPMENT OF MATERNAL-NEWBORN NURSING SCIENCE

1967 Reva Rubin's theory on maternal role attainment published.

1971 *Journal of Obstetric, Gynecologic, and Neonatal Nursing published by NAACOG.*

1972 *Maternal-Child Nursing Journal* published by the University of Pittsburgh.

1974 Kathryn Barnard's review of the research literature on child health assessment, which led to the development of her Child Health Assessment Model, published.

1978 Nursing Child Assessment Satellite Training Project (NCAST) established by Kathryn Barnard at the University of Washington to train nurses to use research-based child health assessment strategies.

1980 Committee on Research established by NAACOG.

1981 Ramona Mercer's theory on maternal role attainment published.

1984 NAACOG sponsors first Invitational Research Conference.

1988 NAACOG establishes first priorities for research.

1992 *Parent-Infant Nursing Science: Paradigms, Phenomena, Methods* by Lorraine Walker published.

Acknowledging Rubin's tenet that the maternal role is learned and not intuitive, another nurse theorist, Ramona Mercer (1981), sought to explain what factors hinder or facilitate women's successful attainment of the maternal role. Mercer's theory assumes that for an individual the maternal role develops as a complex interaction of her perceptions of her experience, others' responses to her role performance, and her relatively stable "self." Further, an infant is seen as having behaviors that also influence the mother's developing maternal role. Finally, Mercer identified a number of key variables that may influence the maternal role, such as maternal age, perceptions of the birth experience, early maternal-infant separation, social stress, support systems, self-concept, and maternal and infant illness. Mercer's theory continues to be an important framework guiding research in maternal-newborn nursing.

CHILD HEALTH ASSESSMENT INTERACTION MODEL

Kathryn Barnard began her theoretical work in order to "identify children in adverse situations so that preventive services" might be provided to promote optimal health (Barnard and Douglas, 1974, p. 1). Review of the literature led Barnard to reject simplistic models in which early biologic risks such as prematurity directly predict the later development of children. Instead, Barnard drew on emerging research that indicated that biologic risk and environmental factors may interact in complex ways to shape the development of children. From this assumption, Barnard (1978) proposed that four general factors are needed to assess children's potential for healthy development: (1) perinatal factors, (2) parental factors, (3) child characteristics, and (4) parent-child interaction. This theory was important in broadening nursing assessment of young children so that it included the family environment and the interaction between parents and children, not simply biologic risks.

BONDING THEORY

Bonding theory, proposed by the physicians Klaus and Kennell in 1976, was an attempt to explain mothers' attachments to their infants as well as disruptions in attachment. One of the key principles of bonding theory specified the existence of a "sensitive period in the first minutes and hours of life" during which parents must have contact with their babies for optimal attachment to occur (Klaus & Kennell 1976, p. 14). In 1982, partially in response to criticism that their bonding theory lacked strong evidence, Klaus and Kennell modified their view that early contact was essential for attachment. Instead, they acknowledged that multiple factors shape the developing parent-infant relationship, and stated, "The human is highly adaptive, and there are many fail-safe routes to attachment" (Klaus and Kennell 1982, p. 55). Despite its tenuous scientific support, these authors' theory on the essential nature of early mother-infant contact has dramatically altered hospital birthing practices.

SELF-CARE THEORY

At a more abstract level, nurses have also proposed general theories that can apply to any nursing practice situation. One such theory, Orem's theory of self-care (Orem 1985), is especially useful in maternal-newborn nursing. Self-care refers to actions that are necessary to maintain human integrity, functioning, and development. Self-care theory can be used as a basis for evaluating a new mother's capability to care for herself and her infant. Because Orem views self-care as learned through social interaction, nurses assess the mother's self-care abilities (called *self-care agency*) as well as family members' needs and capabilities. Thus, this self-care theory also includes the infant's needs.

When using Orem's self-care theory, the nurse both supports the self-care abilities of the new mother and counsels and teaches her about actions that promote her own functioning and the development of her infant. Orem's theory of self-care provides a means of pulling together knowledge from many areas, including nursing, medicine, psychology, physiology, and sociology, and for providing patient-focused nursing care.

APPLICATION OF MATERNAL-NEWBORN NURSING SCIENCE

Theoretic information is an essential part of the research process in maternal-newborn nursing because it provides a structure for the research study. The inclusion of theory is also useful in practice. The work of theorists such as Barnard and Mercer gives the beginning student a more complete picture of the mother and infant within a context of their larger environment.

Use of Theoretic Approaches in Nursing Practice

In the delivery of nursing care, the inclusion of theory establishes a perspective based on knowledge rather than a routine "cookbook" approach. Numerous methods may achieve the same clinical outcome, and selecting the one most suitable for a specific patient requires more than knowledge of routines. For example, suppose a nurse has noticed that a new mother is very uncomfortable feeding her new baby. After showing the mother proper feeding technique, the nurse notices that the mother still seems unsure of herself.

At this point the nurse decides that perhaps a more thorough assessment of the mother's psychological preparation for motherhood may be useful. She takes the time to ask the mother about her pregnancy and how she felt throughout it. She listens to the mother's concern about knowing how to care for her baby because she will be at home alone after she leaves the hospital. Neither her husband who works out of town, nor her mother who had a stroke a year ago, will be able to help the new mother during the first few days at home.

Drawing on Rubin's 1984 theory, the nurse decides that this new mother is struggling to develop a clear model of herself in the maternal role. The nurse informs the mother about the home care program available through the hospital and also gives her the name of the contact person for a mothers' group that meets each month in the community. The nurse selected both of these resources for this particular mother because they are ones that offer both information and affirmation to new mothers. She also knew that the home care nurse and the contact person for the new mothers' group were themselves mothers who could serve as supportive role models for the new mother. The nurse realized that although information might help this new mother with specific needs, her more fundamental need was for temporary supportive resources who could help her develop a clear model of herself as a mother.

In this example, Rubin's theory helped the nurse interpret her observations about the new mother with greater insight and plan supportive follow-up care suited to the new mother's needs. While nurses may practice without using theoretical frameworks, their nursing care is usually more insightful, flexible, individualized, and effective if they do. With the use of theory, their practice will become richer, more rewarding, and more challenging.

Maternal-Newborn Nursing Research

Maternal-newborn nursing research explores *basic* and *applied* problems related to maternal and newborn care. In basic research, nurses investigate processes that enlighten us about matters such as stress and coping during pregnancy, newborn sleep and response patterns, maternal health patterns, family changes associated with a new baby, attachment and loss experiences of parents and young children, and the influence of stimulation and family environment on infant development (Walker 1992). Also, maternal-newborn nurses have been interested particularly in studying how mothers develop the maternal role and their relationship to their infants. In contrast, applied nursing research focuses on solving patient care problems that occur in day-to-day nursing practice. One key aspect of applied nursing research is to compare the effectiveness of different nursing approaches in achieving a desired clinical outcome.

BASIC RESEARCH

Basic research is the empirical study of fundamental processes that are usually not directly observable. These processes, when explained, provide understanding of observed events. As in other scientific fields, basic research in maternal-newborn nursing requires the use of a variety of approaches. Some nurses rely on their careful *clinical observations* to build theories about how basic processes occur. The qualitative research of Rubin (1967a, 1967b) describing maternal role attainment followed this pattern.

Nurses may also draw heavily on *research from related fields,* such as the social sciences and child development. Demonstrating this second pattern, Barnard drew from a variety of disciplines to formulate her scientific study of predictors of early child development for nursing (Bee et al. 1982). Nurses may also use *nursing theories* as the structure within which they develop their specific research questions. For example, Fawcett (1989) used Rogers' Life Process Theory (1970) to study spouses' pregnancy-related experiences.

The variety of theoretic and research approaches used by nurses permits the same situation to be studied from *multiple viewpoints.* For example, nurses may study a wide variety of aspects associated with the birth of a preterm infant: family stresses that precede or follow preterm birth, the organization of preterm infant wake-sleep cycles, the influence of environmental stimulation on preterm infant growth, or alterations in maternal role attainment when birth is premature. Each approach is valid and provides nurses with different kinds of information about preterm birth.

In an in-depth review of maternal-newborn nursing research, Beck (1989) analyzed maternal-newborn research published from 1977 to 1986. Basing her analysis on articles appearing in three refereed nursing research journals, Beck reported that the largest number of studies were in the area of the postpartum period, followed in order by the antepartum, newborn, and intrapartum periods. In the antepartum period the three most researched topics were social support, stress, and anxiety. For the postpartum period the three most studied areas covered maternal role attainment, social support, and mother-infant interaction. Both full-term and premature infants were the focus of nursing studies in the newborn period. The most frequently used research designs were observational (descriptive versus experimental) methods and longitudinal follow-up of mothers or infants.

Maternal-newborn nursing is developing a rich and increasing research base that can serve as a firm foundation for practice. It has contributed, along with research in other fields, to an increased understanding of factors that affect the health and development of mothers and infants. For example, maternal-newborn nursing research has led, in part, to an appreciation of the *impact of stress* on pregnant women and new mothers (Norbeck and Tilden 1983; Walker 1989). Maternal-newborn nursing research has also aided the identification of relationships of *social support* to maternal health, parenting behaviors, and infant development (Norbeck and Tilden 1983; Bee et al. 1982; Kaufman and Hall 1989). While these are important findings, maternal-newborn research is a continual process in which new findings will lead to even more in-depth investigations and sometimes a complete rethinking of the phenomenon being studied.

A prime example of such a reevaluation based on current research is the dramatic change in beliefs and practice concerning the importance of nipple preparation for breastfeeding that has occurred over the past 10 years. Prenatal nipple preparation had been thought essential to successful breastfeeding. However, current research does not support this recommendation and in fact indi-

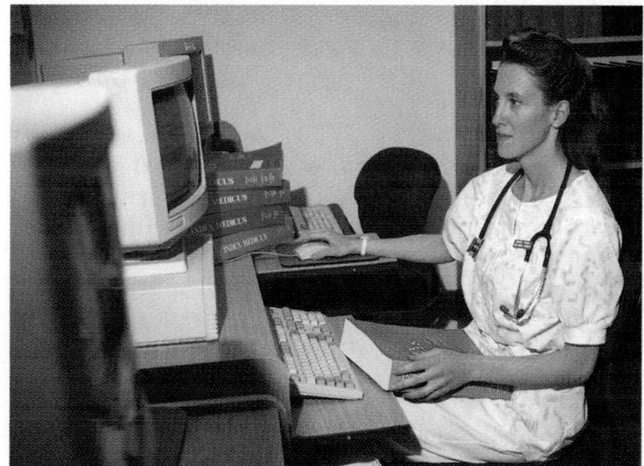

Figure 1–2

There is a rich and increasing body of knowledge in the area of maternal-newborn nursing that nurses can use as a basis for nursing practice. This literature is available on-line via computer and in the traditional print forms of monographs, journals, and books. An increasing number of health care agencies have computers on nursing units designated for literature searches and internet access so that nurses can retrieve research and clinical information more easily.

Table 1–1

REVIEWS CITING MATERNAL-NEWBORN RESEARCH LITERATURE

TOPIC	SOURCE
Obstetric nursing	Mercer, R. T. (1985). Obstetrical nursing research: Past, present, and future. NAACOG invitational research conference. *Birth Defects Original Article Series,* 21 (3), 29–70.
Parenting	McBride, A. B. (1984). The experience of being a parent. *Annual Review of Nursing Research,* 2, 63–81.
Anxiety and fears as related to delivery and infant outcome	Lederman, R. P. (1986). Maternal anxiety in pregnancy: Relationship to fetal and newborn health status. *Annual Review of Nursing Research,* 4, 3–19.
Positions for childbirth	Roberts, J., Mendez-Bauer, C., Woodell, D. (1983). The effects of maternal position on uterine contractility and efficiency. *Birth,* 10, 243.
Social support and its effect on pregnancy and childbirth outcomes	Jones, L. C. (1988). Support systems. In F. H. Nichols, and S. S. Humenick (Eds.). *Childbirth education: Practice, research, and theory* (pp. 362–375). Philadelphia: W. B. Saunders.
Childbirth preparation outcomes	Gennaro, S. (1988). The childbirth experience. In F. H. Nichols, and S. S. Humenick (Eds.). *Childbirth education: Practice, research, and theory* (pp. 52–68). Philadelphia: W. B. Saunders.
Fatigue related to childbearing	Milligan, R., and Pugh, L. C. (1994). Fatigue during the childbearing period. *Annual Review of Nursing Research,* 12, 33–49.
Maternal role attainment	Mercer, R. T. (1995). *Becoming a mother: Research on maternal identity from Rubin to the present.* New York: Springer.

cates that the practice can be detrimental to the mother (Riordan and Auerbach 1993). It is important to remember that *the findings from one research study do not prove a scientific hypothesis conclusively. For this reason, careful review of a number of studies on a given topic is more important than considering one study in isolation.*

Reviews of the research on a particular topic are becoming increasingly common as the amount of nursing research grows. They can be found in nursing research journals, clinical nursing journals, or the *Annual Review of Nursing Research.* Review articles are extremely helpful in identifying the state of the art on a particular topic, determining areas of needed research, and finding research instruments that can be used in conducting a study (Table 1–1).

APPLIED RESEARCH

Applied research is the scientific investigation of techniques to directly improve patient care. Applied maternal-newborn research is focused on the direct care of women during pregnancy, childbirth, and early parenting; on the direct care of infants in hospital or home settings; and on the supportive care of families (fathers or partners, siblings and grandparents) of mothers and infants. Applied research contributes to the development of valid and useful nursing interventions for practice. In contrast to basic research, applied research typically involves comparing two or more approaches of patient care to determine which is most effective in reaching desired maternal or infant goals or outcomes. Examples of the variety of topics investigated in applied maternal-newborn nursing research are presented in Table 1–2. Occasionally, when a topic has been studied extensively, nurses carry out reviews of the available research in order to make recommendations for practice.

For example, Blackburn (1983) reviewed studies of extrauterine stimulation of preterm infants, and Hampson (1989) reviewed studies of postpartum nursing interventions. Such reviews are often hampered by lack of clear-cut findings across studies and differences in methods, which raise additional questions for further research.

Especially noteworthy are innovations in nurs-

Table 1–2

EXAMPLES OF APPLIED RESEARCH ON MATERNAL-NEWBORN PRACTICE

TOPIC	STUDY	DESIGN	MAJOR FINDINGS
Aerobic exercise during pregnancy	Koniak-Griffin, D. (1994). Aerobic exercise, psychological well-being, and physical discomfort during adolescent pregnancy. *Research in Nursing and Health,* 17, 253–263.	Quasi-experimental pretest-posttest design	Depression symptoms decreased while self-esteem increased in exercising group; physical discomforts increased in comparison group
Hygienic care before breast pumping in mothers with infants in a neonatal intensive care unit	Costa, K. M. (1989). A comparison of colony counts of breast milk using two methods of cleansing. *Journal of Obstetric, Gynecologic, and Neonatal Nursing,* 18, 231–236.	Experimental design	Bacterial colony counts were lower in breast milk of women using a special breast cleansing method compared with control group
Comprehensive health care for adolescent mothers and their infants	O'Sullivan, A. L., and Jacobsen, B. S. (1992). A randomized trial of a health care program for first-time adolescent mothers and their infants. *Nursing Research,* 41, 210–215.	Experimental design	Comprehensive care was more effective than routine well-baby care in reducing repeat pregnancy and increasing full immunization of infants
Nonnutritive sucking for preterm infants	Pickler, R. H., Higgins, K. E., Crummette, B. D. (1993). The effect of non-nutritive sucking on bottle-feeding stress in preterm infants. *Journal of Obstetric, Gynecologic, and Neonatal Nursing,* 22, 230–234.	Quasi-experimental design	Nonnutritive sucking for 5 minutes before and after bottle feeding resulted in a greater amount of quiescent behavior after feedings and better feeding performance compared with control condition
Method of administering meperidine to women in labor	Isenor, L., and Penny-Mac Gillivray, T. (1993). Intravenous meperidine infusion for obstetric analgesia. *Journal of Obstetric, Gynecologic, and Neonatal Nursing,* 22, 349–356.	Experimental design	Intravenous administration of meperidine was more effective in pain control than intramuscular, but higher doses were given intravenously; with dosage equated, intravenous administration remained more effective in controlling pain
Methods to relieve nipple soreness in breastfeeding mothers	Buchko, B. L., Pugh, L. C., Bishop, B. A., Cochran, J. F., Smith, L. R., Lerew, D. J. (1994). Comfort measures in breastfeeding, primiparous women. *Journal of Obstetric, Gynecologic, and Neonatal Nursing,* 23, 46–52.	Experimental design	Warm water compresses were more effective than tea compresses, expressed milk massage, or education in managing nipple soreness

Table 1–3

RESEARCH TOOLS DEVELOPED FOR MATERNAL-NEWBORN NURSING

CONCEPT MEASURED	TOOL	RESEARCH SOURCE
Prenatal attachment	Maternal-Fetal Attachment	Cranley, M. S. (1981). Development of a tool for the measurement of maternal attachment during pregnancy. *Nursing Research,* 30, 281–284.
Transition to parenthood	Transition to Parenthood Concerns Scale	Imle, M. A., Atwood, J. R. (1988). Retaining qualitative validity while gaining quantitative reliability and validity: Development of the transition to parenthood concerns scale. *Advances in Nursing Science,* 11 (1), 61–75.
Postpartum functional status	Inventory of Functional Status After Childbirth	Fawcett, J., Tulman, L., Myers, S. T. (1988). Development of the inventory of functional status after childbirth. *Journal of Nurse-Midwifery,* 33, 252–260.
Personal control during labor	Labour Agentry Scale	Hodnett, E. D., Simmons-Tropea, D. A. (1987). The labour agentry scale: Psychometric properties of an instrument measuring control during childbirth. *Research in Nursing and Health*, 10, 301–310.
Parents' involvement in child care	Child Care Activities Scale	Cronenwett, L. R., Sampselle, C. M., Wilson, W. R. (1988). The child care activities scale and parental role preference scale. *Research in Nursing and Health,* 11, 301–308.
Infant-adult interaction	Dyadic Mini Code	Censullo, M., Bowler, R., Lester, B., Brazelton, T. B. (1987). An instrument for the measurement of infant-adult synchrony. *Nursing Research,* 36, 244–248.
Infant pain	Photogrammetric Techniques	Franck, L. S. (1986). A new method to quantitatively describe pain behavior in infants. *Nursing Research,* 35, 28–31.
Stressful life events	Revised Life Event Questionnaire	Norbeck, J. S. (1984). Modification of life event questionnaire for use with female respondents. *Research in Nursing and Health,* 7, 61–71.
Coping	Coping Responses Inventory	Collins, C., Post, L. (1986). An instrument to measure coping responses in employed mothers: Preliminary results. *Research in Nursing and Health,* 9, 309–316.
Neuromuscular relaxation	Neuromuscular Dissociation Relaxation Scale	Humenick, S., Marchbanks, P. (1981). Validation of a scale to measure relaxation in childbirth education classes. *Birth and Family Journal,* 8:3.
Postpartum biopsychosocial adjustment	Postpartum Adaptation Scale	Nichols, F. H. (1989). The use of an assessment tool to measure postpartum adaptation [Abstract]. *MCN, The American Journal of Maternal/Child Nursing,* 14, 273.
Maternal adaptation	Postpartum self-evaluation questionnaire	Lederman, R. P., Weingarten, C. T., Lederman, E. (1981). Postpartum self-evaluation questionnaire: Measures of maternal adaptation. *Birth Defects: Original Article Series,* 17 (6), 201–231.

ing care that may enhance the development of infants and reduce health care costs. For example, Brooten and colleagues (1986) studied the impact of early discharge with nurse specialist follow-up on the development and health care costs for low-birth-weight infants. These researchers compared the effects of early discharge on preterm infants within an experimental protocol that included follow-up home care by a clinical nurse specialist with infants who remained in the hospital longer and were discharged at the routine time (weight of 2200 g). The two groups did not differ in rehospitalizations, acute care episodes, or physical and mental development, but the cost of care averaged $18,560 less for each infant in the early discharge group. The findings from this study make a convincing case for follow-up home care by a clinical nurse specialist for the preterm infant.

NURSING ASSESSMENT RESEARCH

Finally, before conducting either basic or applied research, nurses must develop and refine tools or instruments to measure the patient outcome or process in which they are interested. Maternal-newborn nursing science is still developing and, as in any field of research, significant energy needs to focus on the development of the scientific tools needed for that research, and afterward, to be used in clinical practice. Examples of nurse-developed tools useful to maternal-newborn nursing research and practice are presented in Table 1–3.

The development of tools for maternal-newborn nursing research is important to the advancement of scientific study of nursing care of mothers and infants. Often, tools developed for research purposes later lead to new assessment approaches in nursing practice. Sometimes, however, observations made in clinical practice can lead to the development of tools for research.

FUTURE RESEARCH PRIORITIES

Specific research priorities for maternal-newborn nursing are established by the Research Committee of the Association of Women's Health, Obstetric, and Neonatal Nurses (AWHONN) (Table 1–4). The Bureau of Maternal and Child Health establishes research priorities in this area, and the National Institute for Nursing Research (NINR) sets research priorities for nursing that are applicable to all specialty areas. The nurse who is seeking funding for a research project should check with each of these organizations to determine current research priorities (see Appendix VIII).

Table 1–4

AWHONN RESEARCH PRIORITIES IN PERINATAL AND WOMEN'S HEALTH NURSING

The Association of Women's Health, Obstetric, and Neonatal Nurses (AWHONN) has established the following research priorities, which identify areas of particular significance to the specialty:

1. Research in perinatal and women's health nursing, especially studies of nursing process, interventions and outcomes of care. Areas of high priority are:

Maternal-Newborn

- Prenatal Care
  - Access
  - Utilization
  - Content
- Low-birth-weight prevention
- Adolescent pregnancy and motherhood
- Preconceptual health
- Perinatal substance use
- Family planning

Neonatal

- Low-birth-weight infants
- Promotion of infant growth and development
- Short and long-term consequences of care and parenting

Women's Health

- Sexually transmitted diseases (STDs)
- Health of women in midlife and beyond
- Neoplastic disease in women
- Women's adaptation to multiple roles and related health outcomes
- Impact of reproductive technology

In All Specialty Areas

- Care needed by vulnerable populations
- Depression
- Family violence
- HIV/AIDS prevention and care

2. Research on professional role of maternal-newborn, neonatal, and women's health nurses in delivery of care:
   - Context of nursing practice: constraints and support in professional environment
   - Factors affecting recruiting, retention, and attrition
   - Changing models of nursing practice (e.g., cross training, LDRPs, evolving models of transitional care and home care)

From the Committee on Research, Association of Women's Health, Obstetric and Neonatal Nurses (1994). (Unpublished.)

Implications for Research

Today, research directly affects all nursing professionals. Synthesized research findings that are consistently incorporated into practice link maternal-newborn science with clinical application.

Nurses should view research as lifelong participants and consumers. This includes the graduates of nursing programs who practice in the clinical arena and clinical nurse specialists generating critical research questions in conjunction with medical clinicians or seeking new information from ongoing studies. The nurse scientist who pursues a doctorate degree and acquires the knowledge and skills specific to the conduct, implementation, and dissemination of research will be responsible for generating and testing the body of nursing knowledge that is needed for practice.

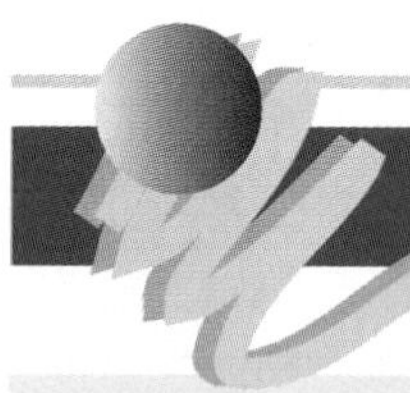

IMPROVING YOUR PRACTICE

HOW TO START YOUR RESEARCH PROJECT

Planning a research project and writing a research proposal may seem overwhelming. Using a five-step process, taking one step at a time, will make the task easier. The five steps consist of the following questions: What is the research question? What does the literature say about the clinical problem? What is the most appropriate research design? How should I collect the data? How should I analyze the data?

- WHAT IS THE RESEARCH QUESTION? Brainstorming sessions with fellow students and nurses in the maternal-newborn areas are an effective way to identify clinical problems that need to be examined. After deciding on a clinical problem, write down what it is you want to find out. Don't worry about stating the answer in proper research format. Just try to capture the essence of what it is that you want to know about the particular clinical problem. Now take this information and put it into a research format. For example, single room maternity care (care in which the mother labors, delivers, and in some agencies stays during the postpartum period) is being implemented at the agency where you are working. From a nursing care perspective, you could ask the following questions: How satisfied are new parents with single room maternity care? What do new parents say about specific aspects of single room maternity care? You will need to identify the specific aspects of care that you want to investigate, such as laboring and giving birth in the same room or having the baby stay in the room with the mother.
  From a marketing perspective, you could ask: What influence has single room maternity care had on the number of births at the agency? What are the characteristics of expectant parents who choose to give birth at the agency? Has there been a change in the type of expectant parents who give birth at the agency since single room maternity care was implemented? From an administrative perspective you could ask: What are the attitudes of nursing staff and medical staff toward single room maternity care? What changes in nursing practice occur when single room maternity care is implemented? Is single room maternity care a cost-effective approach to maternity care?
- WHAT DOES THE LITERATURE SAY ABOUT THE CLINICAL PROBLEM? Carefully examine the research literature related to your topic. What is known about the clinical problem? Are there gaps in the literature? What conflicting views are there? The amount of research on a topic and the findings will help determine the type of research design you should select.
- WHAT IS THE MOST APPROPRIATE RESEARCH DESIGN? After you have decided on the research question that you want to study, your next step is to select the most appropriate research design. The nature of your research question dictates to some extent the type of design that you should use. For example, if you want to know "What is . . . ," you will want to use a descriptive design. If you are looking at "What the effects are . . . ," an experimental or quasi-experimental design is

Continued on facing page

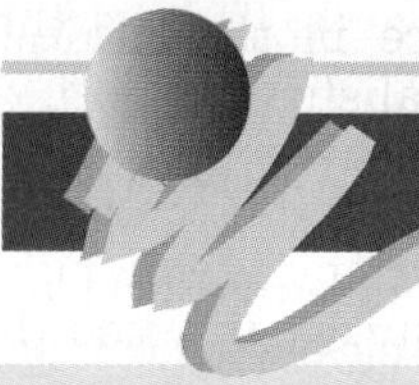

IMPROVING YOUR PRACTICE Continued

the most appropriate. If you are examining "What changes occur . . . ," a longitudinal design is indicated. Within a particular design category, such as descriptive designs, there is usually considerable flexibility. At this point, you may want to refer to your research resources for information on the most useful design format. Next, you need to plan the data collection phase of your study.

- HOW SHOULD I COLLECT THE DATA? The method of data collection will depend on the object, characteristic, or element that you want to measure. For concrete concepts, measurement strategies are usually simple and straightforward: for example, a subject's age, education, or parity. Such information can be obtained during an interview or from a patient's hospital chart. The measurement of abstract attributes is more complex. For example, stress, pain, or satisfaction are often measured in different ways. When you choose a tool to use in your study, you need to make sure it matches the conceptual definition you have selected for the specific attribute. Also, you will need to determine the most appropriate data collection approach. In some situations, you may be able to obtain the information through an interview, a questionnaire, or some other established tool. However, in other situations, direct observation may be the only suitable way to measure an attribute. Your major task is first to gather information about all the different approaches and the various tools that can be used. Your review of the literature will be very helpful. Make a chart of the different approaches and the various tools that have been used to measure the specific attribute(s) that you want to study. Also, note the researcher's comments about the approach or tool that was used. Finally, you will need to make a decision about the most useful data collection measures for your research study.
- HOW SHOULD I ANALYZE THE DATA? The method of data analysis is determined by your research question and the type of data that you collect. Your knowledge of statistical tests comes into play here. A good research text or statistical consultant will be most helpful in determining the correct way to analyze the data.

Summary

Systematically approach the development of a research project using the five questions above. Add your creativity and thoughtful reflections about what you see happening in the clinical area. Critically review the literature on the topic you have chosen. Then, structure a plan that will enable you to answer the questions you have asked. The end result: you will have developed a valuable research project from a clinical problem.

Bibliography

Burns, N., and Grove, S. (1993). *The practice of nursing research: Conduct, critique and utilization* (2nd ed.). Philadelphia: W. B. Saunders.

Polit, D., and Hungler, B. (1995). *Nursing research: Principles and methods* (5th ed.). Philadelphia: J. B. Lippincott.

Woods, N., and Catanzaro, M. (1988). *Nursing research: Theory and practice.* St. Louis: C. V. Mosby.

Adapted from Nichols, F. H. (1989). Translating clinical problems into research projects. *NAACOG Newsletter,* 16 (3), 9, 11.

However, all professionals play an important part in the research process.

Nurses have become skillful in developing and conducting research studies. Previous theoretic and research work provides the basis for future research. Walker's 1992 identification of parent-infant nursing research, which was published in eight nursing journals over a 10-year period, provides a strong example. In a careful analysis, Walker compiled the research, organizing studies into five paradigms that reflected the state of knowledge in parent-infant nursing—Stress, coping and social support; Health; Parental development; Behavioral organization and behavioral interaction; and Person-environment interaction and development. For each of these paradigms, Walker then recommended numerous avenues for new research.

Questions that need to be asked about existing research are:

- What is the most effective approach for increasing the integration of research into practice?
- Which nursing interventions are research based?
- What are the gaps in nursing intervention research?
- Where are the weak links between theoretic knowledge and research-based interventions?

Where possible, the information in this book is based on research findings. Enkin and colleagues (1995) published an analysis of controlled research trials that lists clinical practices during pregnancy and childbirth according to their effectiveness (beneficial, likely to be beneficial, of unknown effectiveness, unlikely to be beneficial, and ineffective or harmful). Across the health care continuum, there are still many clinical problems that lack definitive research answers. Nurses, however, are making great strides in linking solid scientific findings into maternal-newborn nursing practice. As a result, the cycle of research-based knowledge from new findings to student to practitioner to more new research will continue to increase.

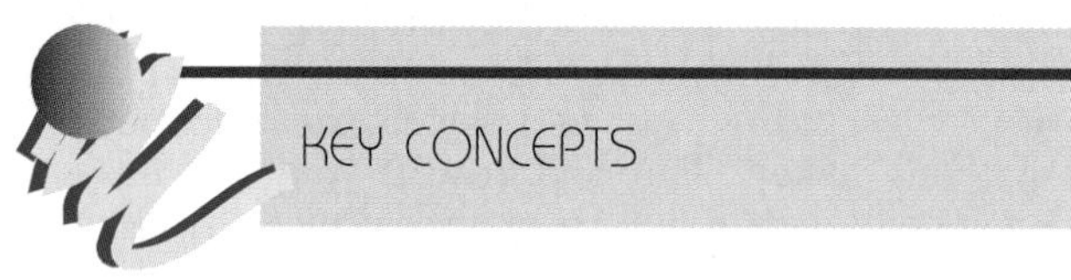

KEY CONCEPTS

- ▼ A scientific base of theory and research is essential to provide a firm foundation for the practice of maternal-newborn nursing. Theory and research also provide the knowledge that is a key factor in advancing maternal-newborn nursing.
- ▼ Scientific knowledge is a cumulative process and the findings from no one research study prove a point conclusively.
- ▼ Theory is useful to maternal-newborn nurses because it can describe a phenomenon, it can explain what is happening, it can predict what will happen in a given situation, it provides the potential for control, and it provides a sense of understanding about what is happening in a given situation.
- ▼ The relationship between theory and practice is a cyclic, ongoing, and continual evolving relationship.
- ▼ Theory stems from practice through observations, insights, and research. This is the theory development phase in which generalizations about a phenomenon are developed on the basis of information about what occurred in a specific situation.
- ▼ Theory is tested through research. This is the theory testing phase in which, on the basis of research findings, a theory can be supported, refuted, or refined.
- ▼ Rubin developed a theory of maternal role attainment that describes the psychological aspects that accompany pregnancy and the postpartum period.
- ▼ Mercer developed a theory of maternal role attainment that explains what factors hinder or facilitate women's successful development of the maternal role.
- ▼ Barnard developed a Child Health Assessment Model that explains how perinatal, parental, and child characteristics and parent-child interaction factors may interact in complex ways to shape the development of children.
- ▼ Klaus and Kennell proposed a theory on bonding that used the concept of a "sensitive period" to explain a mother's attachment to her infant as well as disruptions in attachment.
- ▼ Basic research and applied research are used in maternal-newborn nursing to examine problems related to maternal and newborn care.
- ▼ Basic research describes fundamental, psychosocial, biobehavioral, or human-environmental processes that underlie the health and development of mother and infants.
- ▼ Applied research contributes to patient care by testing different methods of giving care.
- ▼ Nursing research tools facilitate measurement in nursing science and can sometimes be adopted for use in actual practice.
- ▼ Although a young field, maternal-newborn research has already made major contributions to health sciences and the care of mothers and infants.

References

Barnard, K. E. (1978). *NCAST instructor's learning resource manual.* Seattle, WA: University of Washington.

Barnard, K. E., and Douglas, H. B. (1974). *Child health assessment.* Part 1: *A literature review.* Washington, D.C.: U.S. Government Printing Office, DHEW Publications No. (HRA) 75-30.

Beck, C. T. (1989). Maternal-newborn nursing research published from 1977 to 1986. *Western Journal of Nursing Research,* 11 (5), 621–626.

Bee, H. L., Barnard, K. E., Eyres, S. J., Gray, C. A., Hammond, M. A., Spietz, A. L., Snyder, C., Clark, B. (1982). Prediction of IQ and language skill from perinatal status, child performance, family characteristics, and mother-infant interaction. *Child Development,* 53, 1134–1156.

Blackburn, S. (1983). Fostering behavioral development of high-risk infants. *Journal of Obstetric, Gynecologic, and Neonatal Nursing,* 12 (Supplement), 76s–86s.

Brooten, D., Kumar, S., Brown, L. P., Butts, P., Finkler, S. A., Bakewell-Sachs, S., Gibbons, A., Delivoria-Papadopoulos, M. (1986). A randomized clinical trial of early hospital discharge and home follow-up of very-low-birth-weight infants. *New England Journal of Medicine,* 315 (Oct), 934–939.

Burns, N., and Grove, S. K. (1993). *The practice of nursing research: Conduct, critiques and utilization* (2nd ed.). Philadelphia: W. B. Saunders.

Carveth, J. A. (1987). Conceptual models in nurse-midwifery. *Journal of Nurse-Midwifery,* 32 (1), 20–25.

Donnelly, G. F. (1986). Nursing theory: Evolution of a sacred cow. *Holistic Nursing practice,* 1 (1), 1–7.

Enkin, M., Keirse, M. J. N. C., Refrew, M., Neilson, J. (1995). *A guide to effective care in pregnancy and childbirth* (2nd ed.). Oxford: Oxford University Press.

Fawcett, J. (1989). Spouses' experiences during pregnancy and the postpartum: A program of research and theory development. *Image,* 21, 149–152.

Hampson, S. J. (1989). Nursing interventions for the first three postpartum months. *Journal of Obstetric, Gynecologic, and Neonatal Nursing,* 18, 116–122.

Henderson, V. (1987). Keynote speech at Clinical Excellence in Nursing: International Networking Conference, Edinburgh, Scotland, July 1987. Indianapolis: Sigma Theta Tau International.

Jones, K., and Flaherty, M. J. (1992). Preeclamptic mothers' perceptions of the early postpartum period. *Journal of Perinatal Education,* 1 (3), 5–12.

Kaufman, K. J., and Hall, L. A. (1989). Influences of the social network on choice and duration of breast-feeding in mothers of preterm infants. *Research in Nursing and Health,* 12, 149–159.

Klaus, M. H., and Kennell, J. H. (1976). *Maternal-infant bonding.* St. Louis: Mosby.

Klaus, M. H., and Kennell, J. H. (1982). *Parent-infant bonding* (2nd ed.). St. Louis: Mosby.

Mercer, R. T. (1981). A theoretical framework for studying factors that impact on the maternal role. *Nursing Research,* 30, 73–77.

Nichols, F. H. (1992). The psychological effects of prepared childbirth on single adolescent mothers. *Journal of Perinatal Education,* 1 (1), 41–49.

Norbeck, J. S., and Tilden, V. P. (1983). Life stress, social support and emotional disequilibrium in complications of pregnancy: A prospective, multivariate study. *Journal of Health and Social Behavior,* 24 (Mar), 30–46.

Orem, D. E. (1985). *Nursing: Concepts of practice* (3rd ed.). New York: McGraw-Hill.

Reynolds, P. D. (1971). *A primer in theory construction.* Indianapolis: Bobbs-Merrill.

Riordan, J., and Auerbach, K. G. (1993). *Breastfeeding and human lactation.* Boston: Jones & Bartlett Publishers.

Rogers, M. E. (1970). *An introduction to the theoretical basis of nursing.* Philadelphia: F. A. Davis.

Rubin, R. (1967a). Attainment of the maternal role. Part I. Processes. *Nursing Research,* 16, 237–245.

Rubin, R. (1967b). Attainment of the maternal role. Part II. Models and referrants. *Nursing Research,* 16, 342–346.

Rubin, R. (1984). *Maternal identity and the maternal experience.* New York: Springer.

Walker, L. O. (1989). Stress process among mothers of infants: Preliminary model testing. *Nursing Research,* 38, 10–16.

Walker, L. O. (1992). *Parent-infant nursing science: Paradigms, phenomena, methods.* Philadelphia: F. A. Davis.

Walker, L. O., and Avant, K. K. (1995). *Strategies for theory construction in nursing* (3rd ed.). Norwalk, CT: Appleton & Lange.

2 Chapter

> Of all of life choices, none are more important to society, none has more far reaching consequences, none represents a more complete blending of social, biological, and emotional forces than bringing another life into the world.
>
> VICTOR FUCHS (1983)

Maternal-Newborn Nursing Practice

Linda Corson Jones
Bonnie O'Brien Maestri

HIGHLIGHTS

- A Definition of Maternal-Newborn Nursing
- The Philosophy of Maternal-Newborn Nursing
- Legal and Professional Regulation of Nursing Practice
- The Tools of Nursing Practice
- The Importance of Critical Thinking Skills
- Indicators of Maternal and Infant Health
- Initiatives to Improve Maternal and Infant Health
- Changes in the Maternal-Newborn Health Care System
- Social, Scientific, and Economic Issues in Maternal-Newborn Health Care
- Implications For Research

Childbirth is a unique and powerful human experience that has physiologic, psychological, spiritual, and social importance. Throughout history, birth has been viewed as a significant event surrounded by rituals and filled with meaning. Humenick (1994) describes childbirth as one of those rare events in life in which women have the opportunity to find inner resources and strength they didn't know they had and therefore emerge changed forever with increased self-esteem and increased competence. A new mother's reflection on how she felt after giving birth describes the powerful impact of the birth experience on a woman: "As I lay awake the night he was born, watching his eyes wide open, exploring his new world, I had a strong feeling of now I know I can do anything" (Kitzinger 1994).

Birth represents a new beginning in every parent's life. It is a learning experience that will forever influence the way one sees the self, the world, and the future. Maternal-newborn nurses have the distinct privilege of helping families respond positively to this major life transition of childbearing. They also have a responsibility to ensure that the childbirth is as safe

DEFINITIONS

Birth rate—The number of births per 1000 population.

Critical thinking—The examination and analysis of ideas, assumptions, beliefs, arguments, conclusions, and actions to determine their validity and credibility using scientific reasoning, problem-solving, and decision-making skills.

Collaborative care map—A multidisciplinary plan of care for a client that includes the key interventions necessary to promote desired client outcomes and efficient use of resources according to a timeline. A collaborative care map may also be called a case management plan, critical pathway, or care map.

Family-centered maternity care (FCMC)—Maternity care that is family oriented and views childbirth as a vital, natural life event rather than an illness.

Infant—A baby born alive; also from 28 days of age until the first birthday.

Infant mortality rate—Number of deaths of infants under 1 year of age per 1000 live births.

Live birth—An infant who after birth demonstrates evidence of life, including heartbeat, pulsation of the umbilical cord, and movement of voluntary muscles.

Low birth weight—Weight less than 2500 g at birth; very low birth weight is less than 1500 g at birth.

Maternal mortality rate—The number of deaths of women from complications of pregnancy, childbirth, and the postpartum period per 100,000 live births.

Neonatal—The period from birth to 28 days of life.

Neonatal mortality rate—The number of deaths for infants under 28 days per 1000 live births.

Nursing process—A critical decision-making tool used to plan individualized, theory-based nursing care.

Nursing care planning guide—A written form of the nursing process that specifies the nursing care needed for an individual client.

Preterm birth—Birth of less than 37 completed weeks of gestation.

Standards of care—A written description of a competent level of nursing care.

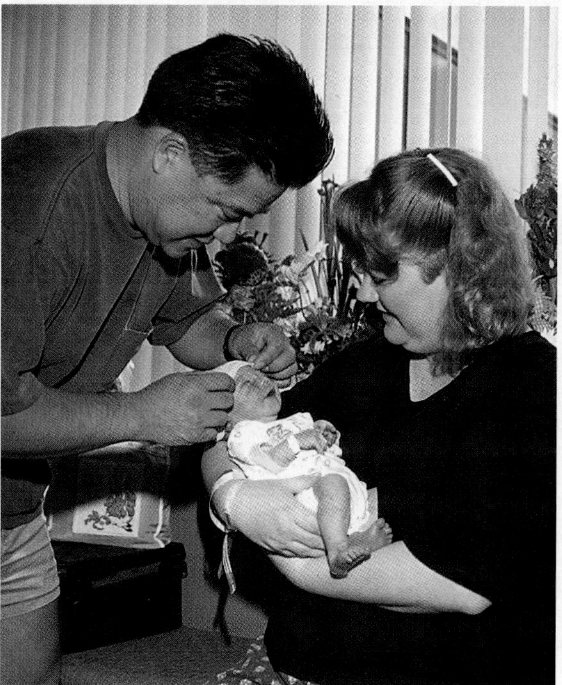

Figure 2–1
For parents, the birth of a baby heralds the beginning of new learning experiences • The wonder and mystery of birth, the delight and pride in the unique capabilities of their baby, and the responsibility of caring for their newborn infant produce a whirlwind of joyous feelings and concerns for parents.

as possible and (equally important) as emotionally positive as can be. Students, regardless of age, who are learning about maternal-newborn nursing not only have the opportunity to participate in the excitement, wonder, and mystery of birth, they also have the opportunity to examine the information from a personal perspective and to explore their beliefs and values about childbirth and parenting.

WHAT IS MATERNAL-NEWBORN NURSING?

Maternal-newborn nursing is a specialized area of maternal-child nursing practice that focuses on the health needs and responses of women, their partners, and their families. Thus, maternal-newborn nursing is the diagnosis and treatment of the responses of childbearing women, their infants, and their families to health and illness (ANA, 1995).

The practice of maternal-newborn nursing is directed toward improving the quality of life for infants and the adults who assume primary responsibility for the infants' well-being. Nursing not only involves direct care to the childbearing family, but also includes health teaching and counseling.

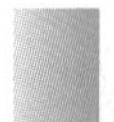

Levels of Care

Nursing practice includes the provision of primary, secondary, and tertiary levels of care (ANA 1985). Each level of care will be discussed separately. In actual practice, however, nursing actions may overlap as nurses provide care for any individual.

PRIMARY CARE

Primary care involves actions directed toward the prevention of illness and promotion of optimal health. Nurses may work with healthy individuals or those at risk for developing behaviors that could jeopardize their health (Lindberg et al. 1990). Primary care can occur in a variety of settings. Many nursing actions in primary care represent nurses' independent functions. Areas of concern to maternal-newborn nursing include such things as prenatal education, anticipatory guidance, prevention of risk factors, and family planning services.

SECONDARY CARE

Secondary or intermediate care involves actions directed toward treatment of common complications. Nursing actions within the secondary care domain include treatment, education, and counseling. Areas of concern to maternal-newborn nursing include, for example, working with a woman who is experiencing increased pain during labor, assessing an infant with poor temperature regulation, and counseling a breastfeeding mother with sore nipples.

TERTIARY CARE

Tertiary care involves care of women and newborns with complex diseases and disabilities. Use of specialized knowledge and reliance on technology is essential. Interdisciplinary collaboration among health care providers is vital to ensure quality health care. Areas of concern to maternal-newborn nursing include care of a diabetic woman in preterm labor as well as care of the newborn in a neonatal intensive care unit.

Independent and Interdependent Functions

The independent and interdependent functions of maternal-child nurses were defined in *A Statement on the Scope of Maternal and Child Health Nursing Practice* (ANA 1985). Interdependent functions of maternal-child nursing are performed in collaboration with other health care professionals. On the other hand, independent functions of maternal-child nursing are those actions that can be initiated because the specialty encompasses unique knowledge and skills. The number and nature of independent functions of the nurse change with the practice setting and agency policies (Mechanic 1988). For example, maternal-newborn nurses may have many independent functions in a community setting, a lesser number in a well-maternity health care setting, and an even lesser amount while working in an acute care practice area (Fig. 2–2).

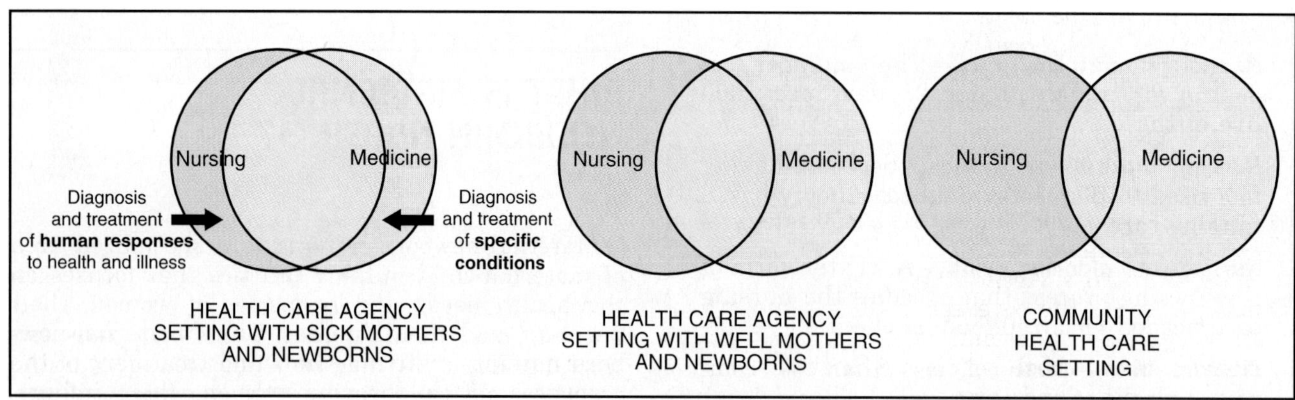

Figure 2–2

The independent and interdependent roles of the nurse change with the practice setting • The green areas in the diagrams indicate nurses' large interdependent role in the obstetric and neonatal intensive care settings, moving to an increasingly independent role with well mothers and babies in the health care agency, and a largely independent role in the community health care setting.

PHILOSOPHY OF MATERNAL-NEWBORN NURSING

Maternal-newborn nursing is an exciting field. Nurses work in many different settings with a variety of client populations. These include services, such as gynecologic care, family planning, prenatal care, neonatal care, prenatal education, intrapartum and postpartum care, and home care.

Regardless of the practice setting, a number of beliefs are widely accepted by maternal-newborn nursing leaders and provide a philosophical foundation for practice. In addition, such beliefs challenge maternal-newborn nurses to refine the care they provide to the childbearing family. Among the most important are the following:

1. *Childbearing is a family affair.* Maternal-newborn services are best provided in a family-centered approach, while maintaining the physical safety of the individual members. Members of the family need to be included in all aspects of care. Closely tied to this belief is the view that family members are capable of making decisions about childbearing care. What these individuals often need is education, support, and advocacy.

   A vast array of maternal-newborn services for the complete family is now offered for the low-risk population. These services include expectant prenatal classes for siblings and grandparents, breastfeeding support services, and family inpatient care. Family-centered care is still inadequate, though, for women at risk for developing complications or women who are poor, single, and nonwhite. More work needs to be done in this area.
2. *The reproductive health of the total family is important to the health of society.* Infant and maternal mortality rates are frequently cited statistics to indicate both the health status of a population and the quality of health services for a population (Lederman 1990). Moreover, infant mortality rate is cited as an index of the status of economic and social development of a country (Wallace 1988). A publication from ANA, *Nursing's Agenda for Health Care Reform,* calls for the coverage of essential services for pregnant women and children. The publication describes these services as critical "in the future health and prosperity of the nation" (1991, p. 3).
3. *Childbirth is a normal physiologic process that generally requires few medical interventions.* The advancement of health science has resulted in tremendous advances in the development of technologic interventions. In most cases, however, childbirth remains a noncomplicated, joyful event in the lives of families. Therefore, the goal of maternal-newborn nursing is to safeguard the health of individual family members by providing direct care, education, and support. Nurses must understand the social and psychological factors related to childbirth and parenting in order to provide care that is satisfying and meaningful to families.
4. *Parenting is learned.* Childbearing families encounter many physical, psychological, and social changes as they negotiate the transition to parenthood. Individuals do not automatically have the appropriate expectations, knowledge, and skills for good parenting. Nurses can play a critical role in assisting families as they navigate the critical passage to parenthood.

REGULATION OF NURSING PRACTICE

The scope of nursing practice refers to the area of professional responsibility that is considered to be the domain of nursing (ANA 1987).This is governed by two parallel forces: legal and professional regulation (Fig. 2–3). Legal regulation includes practice acts and rules and regulations about licensure. Professional regulation includes recognition of standards of practice and self-regulation through involvement in professional organizations. It is important that maternal-newborn nurses keep abreast of the professional and legal regulations that govern their practice area.

Legal Regulation

The limits of nursing practice are specified in state practice acts. These statutes legally define the nature, purpose, and scope of professional nursing. In a survey of 51 state and territorial practice acts, ANA (1984–1985) found that three core components of nursing practice were common to state statutes: nursing functions that are clearly nursing practice (monitoring, observing, assessing, and providing direct care to patients); teaching, supervision, and delegation of nursing practice; and carrying out the medical regimen (administering prescribed treatments).

Most state practice acts also delineate functions that are appropriate for nurses functioning in expanded roles. These include a variety of maternal-

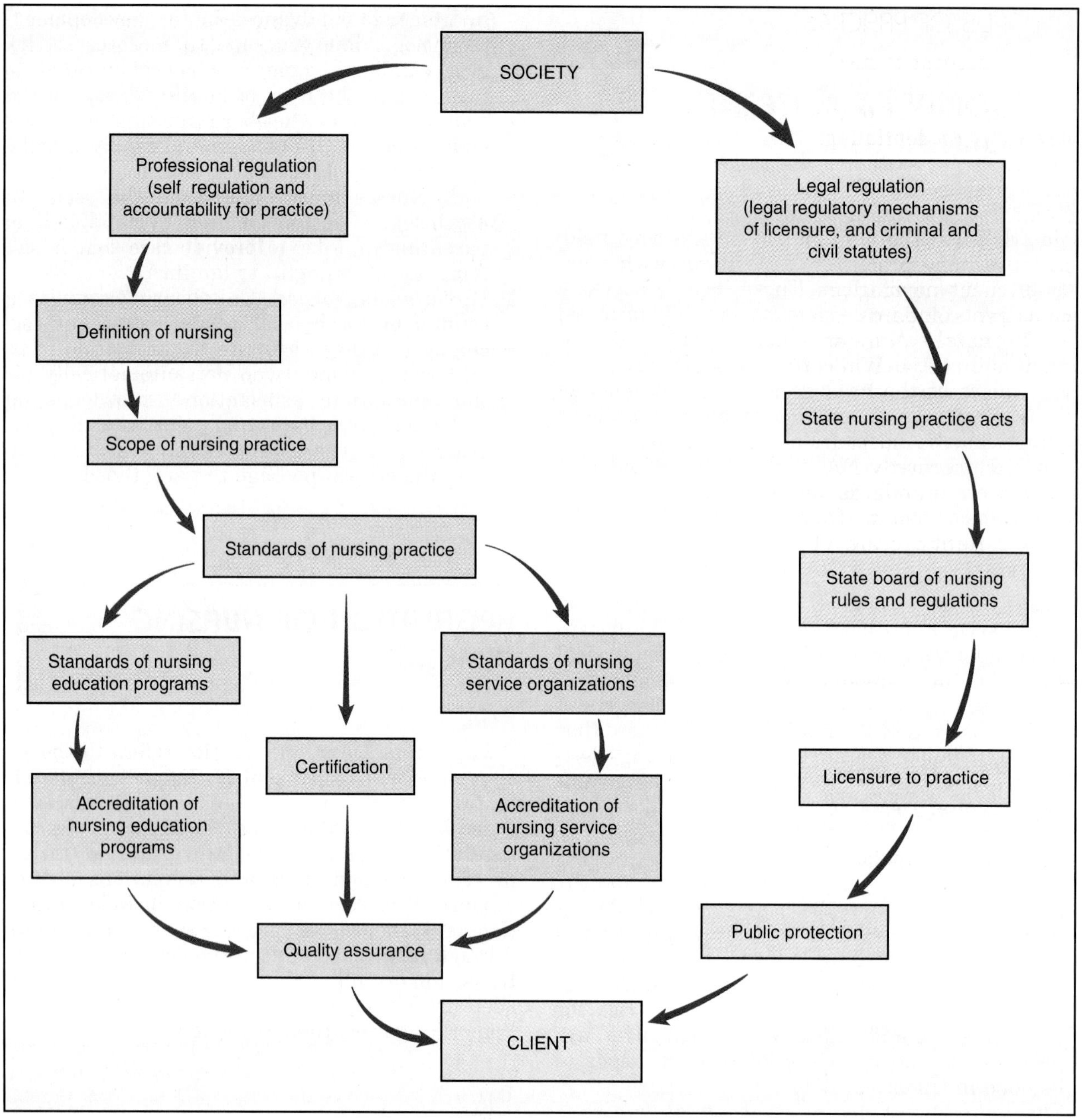

Figure 2–3

Regulation of nursing practice. (Data from the American Nurses Association [1995]. *Nursing's social policy statement.* Washington, D.C.: Author, and State Nursing Practice Acts.)

newborn nursing specialists, including midwives, neonatal nurse practitioners, and perinatal clinical nurse specialists.

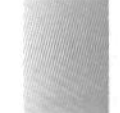

Professional Regulation

Nursing has a professional obligation to society to provide high-quality nursing care. To ensure this accountability, the profession has developed a number of strategies to regulate the practice of nursing. These include defining its practice base, encouraging research, establishing a system of professional education, establishing structures for the delivery of nursing services, and providing quality assurance mechanisms.

The process of professional regulation is dynamic and evolutionary. It is responsive to societal and health care delivery changes. Moreover, advances in health sciences and technology influence nursing practice and professional regulation.

STANDARDS OF PRACTICE

Quality assurance mechanisms have been developed since the mid 1970s and include a code of ethics, standards of practice, a structure for peer review, and credentialing. A nursing standard is an authoritative statement by which the quality of nursing practice can be judged. Standards are important; they provide a common base for the profession. In 1973 the ANA published the first standards of nursing practice, which were general and focused on the nursing process.

The first standards for Obstetric, Gynecologic and Neonatal Nursing were published by NAACOG in 1974. While the ANA standards focused on process, the NAACOG standards addressed professional performance and nursing functions in the specialty area. Both ANA and AWHONN* (formerly NAACOG) have refined and revised their standards for practice periodically, and the major points from the AWHONN standards for nursing care of women and newborns are listed in Table 2–1 (NAACOG 1991).

Standards of care describe a competent level of nursing care using the nursing process, including assessment, diagnosis, outcome identification, planning, intervention, and evaluation.

Standards of professional performance describe a component level of behavior in the professional nurse, including activities such as quality of care, education, performance appraisal, collegiality, ethics, collaboration, research, and resource utilization.

ANA (1983) identified the essential knowledge and skills required to practice maternal-child nursing. Two categories of nurses who provide care to the maternal-child population were differentiated. The nurse generalist has completed a generic nursing education program and has addi-

*AWHONN became the organization's name in 1993. Before that time, publications are referenced to NAACOG, The Nurses Association of the American College of Obstetricians and Gynecologists.

Table 2–1

MAJOR POINTS FROM AWHONN STANDARDS FOR THE NURSING CARE OF WOMEN AND NEWBORNS

Standard I: Nursing Practice

Comprehensive nursing care for women and newborns focuses on helping individuals, families, and communities achieve their optimum health potential. This is best achieved within the framework of the nursing process.

Standard II: Health Education and Counseling

Health education for the individual, family, and community is an integral part of comprehensive nursing care. Such education encourages participation in and shared responsibility for health promotion, maintenance, and restoration.

Standard III: Policies, Procedures, and Protocols

Written policies, procedures, and protocols clarify the scope of nursing practice and delineate the qualifications of personnel authorized to provide care to women and newborns within the health care setting.

Standard IV: Professional Responsibility and Accountability

Comprehensive nursing care for women and newborns is provided by nurses who are clinically competent and accountable for professional actions and legal responsibilities inherent in the nursing role.

Standard V: Utilization of Nursing Personnel

Nursing care for women and newborns is conducted in practice settings that have qualified nursing staff in sufficient numbers to meet patient care needs.

Standard VI: Ethics

Ethical principles guide the process of decision making for nurses caring for women and newborns at all times and especially when personal or professional values conflict with those of the patient, family, colleagues, or practice setting.

Standard VII: Research

Nurses caring for women and newborns utilize research findings, conduct nursing research, and evaluate nursing practice to improve the outcomes of care.

Standard VIII: Quality Assurance

Quality and appropriateness of patient care are evaluated through a planned assessment program using specific, identified clinical indicators.

From NAACOG Standards for the Nursing Care of Women and Newborns. (1991). (4th ed.). Reprinted with permission. NAACOG is now AWHONN, The Association of Women's Health, Obstetric and Neonatal Nurses.

tional continuing education in the specialized area of maternal-newborn nursing. The nurse specialist has educational preparation at least at the graduate level. Also, the specialist has expertise in the field.

CERTIFICATION

An increasing number of health care agencies encourage and in some cases require maternal-newborn nurses to be certified by a national organization in their area of expertise. Also, it is not unusual that third-party reimbursement programs for health care services require an individual to be certified by a national organization to be eligible to receive payment. Thus, it is most likely that there will be an increasing number of maternal-newborn nurses who seek certification in the coming years.

Certification indicates to the public and health care agencies that an individual has demonstrated competence in a specific area of study (Jacobs 1992). Since national certification programs usually require evidence of continued competence, such as continuing education, to maintain certification, health care agencies also view continued certification as an indicator of competence in the area.

Nationally recognized organizations that provide certification by examination in a variety of areas for maternal-newborn nurses are American Nurses Association, National Certification Corporation (NCC), ASPO/Lamaze, and the International Board of Lactation Consultant Examiners (see Appendix VIII). Numerous other programs exist, many of which provide continuing education programs leading to a certification credential. It is essential that the maternal-newborn nurse select a certification program carefully. The nurse needs first to ask the employer which certification programs the employer recognizes, and then to evaluate the available programs carefully.

Nichols (1993) identified the following questions that individuals seeking certification can use to evaluate a program:

- By whom is the program sponsored?
- What are the entry requirements?
- How long has the program been established?
- How many individuals have been certified since the program began?
- How is certification determined? (Certification should be separate from a program to prepare an individual in a specific area.)
- What materials are needed or provided, such as textbooks or a study guide?
- What are the total costs of the certification program? Are there any hidden costs?
- What are the requirements to maintain the certification credentials?
- What is the reputation of the certification program among the health care community?
- Is the certification credential recognized nationally? Internationally?

Nurses should choose the program that best meets their needs and resources, recognizing the program's strengths and limitations.

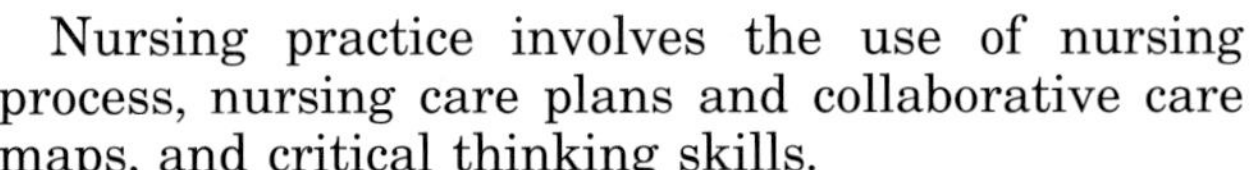

NURSING PRACTICE

Nursing practice involves the use of nursing process, nursing care plans and collaborative care maps, and critical thinking skills.

Nursing Process

Maternal-newborn nursing practice is accountable for three domains: "promoting wellness; preventing potential health problems; and caring for actual health problems of childbearing women, their infants, and their families" (Popkess-Vawter 1991). Because this nursing specialty requires its nurses to function at both independent and collaborative levels, maternal-newborn nurses must possess a broad knowledge base. Maternal-newborn education imparts a multidisciplinary focus that enables nurses to recognize and treat the unique physiologic, psychological, and social responses of childbearing clients.

The nursing process provides maternal-newborn nurses with an organized system to define and guide the independent aspects of their practice: "the art of nursing that distinguishes the nurse from other members of the health-care team" (NAACOG 1989, p. 3). For example, the teaching actions of maternal-newborn nurses promote healthy behaviors throughout the entire childbearing cycle. Learning about the normal discomforts of late pregnancy helps expectant parents cope more effectively with the physical and emotional challenges of this period. Likewise, nurses facilitate confidence in the parenting role by preparing new parents to respond to the unique needs of the newborn.

Thus, the nursing process is a critical decision-making tool that maternal-newborn nurses use to plan individualized research- and theory-based nursing care. Caring without knowledge lacks direction, and a number of theoretic models exist that can guide nursing practice. Lindberg and associates (1990) emphasize that learning about and understanding a client's life experiences require use of a holistic, person-centered approach.

The ANA views the nursing process as the basis for all significant nursing actions and considers it the framework for professional nursing practice. The relationship between nursing practice, nursing process, and standards of nursing practice is diagrammed in Figure 2–4. This scientific problem-solving method is characterized by "cognition, client-centeredness, and goal direction" (Clark 1996, p. 8). It is cognitive because it requires formalized thought and not routinized action. More importantly, it is client centered because nurses work *with* clients, not *on* them. The nursing process manifests the essence of nursing practice: caring. It promotes working with clients in identifying their perceptions of personal needs, and helping them devise individual goals to meet their health care needs. Most nurse scholars identify five distinct components of the nursing process: assessment, diagnosis, planning, intervention, and evaluation. Although these components are designed to occur in sequence, with each phase dependent on the work accomplished in the previous phase, the nursing process itself is circular and dynamic. "The process is one in which the results at any point are constantly being evaluated" (Spradley 1991, p. 203). As new information is learned, the nurse modifies the process, as needed, to assist the client in achieving his or her highest level of functioning.

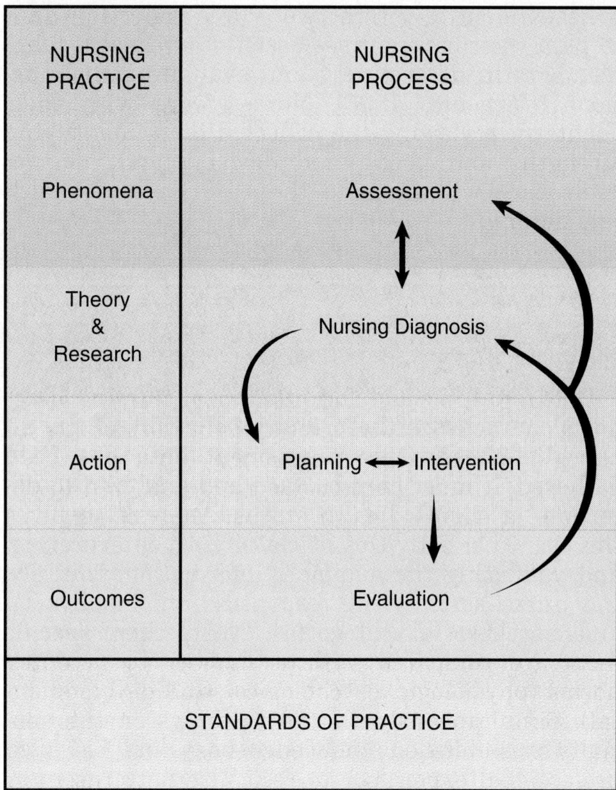

Figure 2–4

The interrelationships between nursing practice, nursing process, and the standards of practice are integral to nursing practice • Both practice and process are based on the standards of practice for maternal-newborn nursing.

ASSESSMENT

Yura and Walsh (1988) describe assessment as "the act of reviewing" information for the purpose of determining the strengths (i.e., wellness state) and diagnosing the actual or potential health problems of a particular human situation. Consequently, the main activity of this initial phase is data collection. The nurse obtains relevant facts and information about the client (individual, family) from various sources (Table 2–2) in order to better understand the client's feelings, thoughts, and biophysical responses.

Table 2–2

SAMPLE DATA COLLECTION SOURCES

PRIMARY	SECONDARY	TERTIARY
Data collected from client responses: • Formal or informal interview • Standardized biophysical measures • Standardized psychological measures	Data collected from family and friends • Formal or informal interview • Standardized or informal measures of environment • Nurse observations	Data collected from health-team members: • Formal or informal interview • Clients' records

Assessment is interactive. While collecting data to plan their care, nurses assist other health team members in determining and evaluating their actions (Carpenito 1995). Nurses work with their clients in reviewing the collected data, identifying strengths and needs, and devising and revising goals that will promote the best level of health functioning.

DIAGNOSIS

Data analysis and formulation of nursing diagnosis characterize the primary behaviors of the diagnostic phase. Once assessment data has been gathered, it must be processed and analyzed to determine a client's health status. Analysis involves the cognitive activities of classifying, interpreting, and validating the available information. Initially, the nurse sorts client responses into biophysical and psychosocial categories. Next, client-specific facts are compared with a number of accepted norms (physiologic, psychological, and developmental). Simultaneously, the nurse draws on the specialty's established knowledge base and her own professional experience to recognize patterns in or relationships among the data (Lindberg et al. 1990; Clark 1996). The nurse then validates her conclusions with the client. Like assessment, analysis is a continual process. Frequently, the nurse must collect additional information before identifying valid diagnoses.

Nursing diagnoses emerge from the assessment analysis. They represent the nurse's conclusions regarding the client's strengths and needs, and identify those activities that fall within nursing's domain of independent practice as well as those that require collaborative management with medicine. The ANA incorporated the term nursing diagnosis into the nursing practice standards in 1973. That same year the North American Nursing Diagnosis Association (NANDA), the official authority for sanctioning nursing diagnosis, had their first meeting to develop a classification system that would provide nursing with a common language base. This group continually works to refine the system and has formulated a list of over 125 diagnostic categories; Appendix IV gives the current list of approved categories (NANDA 1994). The ninth NANDA conference of March 1990 adopted the following as the official working definition of nursing diagnosis: "It is a clinical judgment about individual, family, or community responses to actual or potential health problems/life processes. Nursing diagnoses provide the basis for selection of nursing interventions to achieve outcomes for which the nurse is accountable" (Carroll-Johnson 1990, p. 50; Lindberg et al. 1990).

Although the standardization of nursing diagnoses has helped to define the scope of nursing practice, the NANDA system has not been without controversy (Stolte 1986; Stevens 1988; Popkess-Vawter 1991). Nurse-scholars have expressed concern that the use of "prefabricated labels" may deter individual care and keep nurses from exploring the client experience that does not fit the mold or the label. Also, the dominant illness framework of most nursing diagnoses has limited the use of the NANDA system in wellness settings.

Since childbearing is typically a normal, healthy event for most families, experts advocate a dual approach to nursing diagnoses for maternity clients. This holistic model utilizes both problem- and wellness-based nursing diagnoses that address the assets as well as the problems encountered in maternal-newborn nursing (Stolte 1986; Stevens 1988; Starn and Niederhauser 1990).

Stevens (1988) shows that, despite previous difficulties, the current NANDA system is flexible and can be modified to include both problem and wellness diagnoses. The typical diagnostic statement consists of three phrases: problem, etiology, and signs and symptoms. The statement identifies the problem from the approved NANDA list and relates the contributing factors with objective or subjective evidence. To formulate wellness diagnosis in the childbearing setting, Stevens (1988) recommended substituting a positive word for the negative word in the NANDA system. Note the following:

- *Adequate sleep pattern* instead of sleep pattern disturbance
- *Improved physical mobility* instead of impaired physical mobility
- *Progressive positive social interaction* instead of impaired social interaction

When using a dual approach to develop nursing diagnoses, the nurse should consider

▼ Problem-Oriented Diagnosis

Problem: Fear

Related to (etiology): Caring for new baby correctly

Manifested by (symptoms): Expression of concern

Nursing diagnosis: Fear related to ability to care for new baby correctly as manifested by client's statement of concern

▼ Wellness-Oriented Diagnosis

Strength: Effective family coping

Related to (etiology): Adequate support resources

Manifested by (symptoms): Parents have secured assistance of others to help at home during first week after birth

Nursing diagnosis: Effective family coping related to adequate support resources as manifested by parents' securing assistance of others to help at home during first week after birth

PLANNING

Once the nursing diagnoses have been established, the nurse begins developing the action component of the nursing process, the plan of care (Lederer et al. 1990). This third phase involves designing strategies that will utilize the client's assets to prevent, correct, and/or diminish the needs identified in the nursing diagnoses. Planning challenges the critical thinking skills of maternal-newborn nurses. It involves working with the client in prioritizing needs and strengths, setting both short- and long-term goals, determining the best methods to achieve those goals, and documenting the actual progress made toward goal attainment.

INTERVENTION

The fourth phase of the nursing process encompasses implementation. The nurse coordinates those actions, both independent and collaborative, that are deemed necessary to achieve the client goals set in the planning phase.

Although the intervention phase has a "doing" focus, the intellectual action required during this period cannot be underestimated. Providing care to childbearing families is a rewarding but complex experience that draws heavily on the intellectual, interpersonal, and technical skills of the maternal-newborn nurse (Yura and Walsh 1988).

EVALUATION

The final phase of the nursing process should always be measured in terms of how the client responded to the plan of care (Yura and Walsh 1988). Since evaluation is considered in terms of short- and long-term goals, appraisal of actual outcomes at one point in the process may result in modifying and refocusing the plan of care.

Nursing Care Planning Guides

The nursing care planning guide is a written form of the nursing process that specifies the nursing care needed for an individual client. Although the purpose of the nursing care planning guide is the same, the structure may differ from agency to agency and nursing unit to nursing unit. A variety of formats can be used for care plans, such as a computer printout, Kardex, or care planning guide form, but Watson and Mayers emphasize that regardless of the format used, the nursing care plan should be organized so that "anyone can quickly visualize what care is needed and why" (Mayers 1993).

The purposes of nursing care plans in health care agencies and in nursing education differ. In health care agencies, the purpose of the nursing care plan is to communicate relevant data, care needed, and expected outcomes for a specific client "rapidly and efficiently (Mayers 1993). In contrast, in an educational setting, the nursing care planning guide serves as a detailed tool for learning about a particular client problem or condition, and (most important) for learning how to plan individual-ized nursing care in a scientific and systematic manner.

STANDARDIZED NURSING CARE PLANS

A standardized care plan is a protocol developed and written for clients with a specific condition. It includes the usual and potential nursing diagnoses with appropriate nursing actions and expected outcomes in a typical situation for a client who is expecting the condition or disease process. Standardized nursing care plans aid in improving the care planning process and in making it more efficient (Mayers 1993).

The standardized care plan represents the standard of nursing care for the particular condition or disease process. While there are common client problems that can be expected, each client's response to a given situation is unique. The standardized nursing care plan must be adapted to each individual client's needs. The Improving Your Practice box provides a guide that is helpful in adapting and individualizing a standardized nursing care planning guide for a specific client.

COLLABORATIVE CARE MAPS

A collaborative care map, also called a case management plan, critical pathway, or care map, is a multidisciplinary plan of care for a client that includes the key interventions necessary to promote desired client outcomes and efficient use of resources according to a timeline (see Appendix I for examples). In essence, a collaborative care map reflects the typical care for the average client with a specific condition or disease process according to an expected timetable. A collaborative care map aids in the evaluation of care because client outcomes are measured against the timeline, and deviations are readily apparent (Zander 1991, 1992).

The use of collaborative care maps (critical

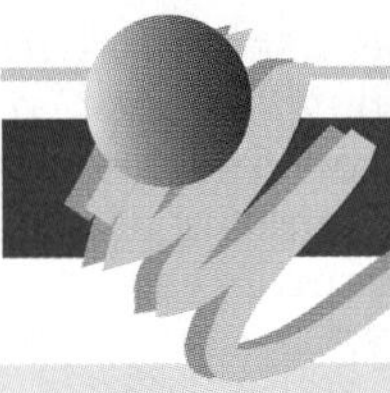

IMPROVING YOUR PRACTICE

INDIVIDUALIZING A STANDARDIZED NURSING CARE PLAN

A standardized nursing care plan is a protocol developed and written for clients with a specific condition. It includes the usual and potential nursing diagnoses with appropriate nursing actions and expected outcomes in a typical situation for a client who is experiencing the condition or disease process.

The standardized care plan represents the standard of nursing care for that particular condition or disease process. While there are common client problems that can be expected, each client's response to a given situation is unique. The standardized nursing care plan must be adapted to each individual client's needs. The following guide is helpful in adapting and individualizing a standardized nursing care plan for a client:

- Read the client's chart and related records, Kardex, medication administration record, records of previous hospital admission, etc.
- Carefully review the client's admitting history and physical examination, current medical diagnosis, results of diagnostic and laboratory tests, any consultation records, and nursing notes and physician's progress notes for the past 2 days. Your aim is to develop a snapshot picture of the client and his or her condition.
- Interview the client and complete a physical assessment, noting any abnormal data obtained.
- Read about the client's condition in a maternal-newborn nursing text and other related literature.
- Select the appropriate standardized nursing care plan.
- Select the nursing diagnoses, expected outcomes, and nursing actions that are appropriate for the client based on the information you have obtained, modifying them as needed.
- Add nursing diagnoses with related expected outcomes and nursing actions according to the client's unique needs.
- Prioritize nursing diagnoses according to the client's needs.
- Prioritize nursing actions for each nursing diagnosis according to the client's needs.

When you have finished this process, you should have a comprehensive and individualized nursing care plan for the client.

pathways) in the Intensive Care and Intermediate Care Nurseries has been found to improve the quality of care and reduce the length of time that infants need to remain in the hospital, which represented a 23 percent decrease in costs (Thompson 1994). The collaborative care map was developed and implemented in response to the increasing emphasis on managed care in the health care environment. Managed care is a system of organizing care that increases coordination of care and communication among the health care team members and focuses on achieving quality patient outcomes in the most cost-effective manner (Etheredge 1989).

Any health care team member involved in the care of aclient can document outcomes on the collaborative care map. However, the nurse is the ultimate coordinator of care and has the responsibility to record any negative variance from the expected outcome on this document (Hampton 1993).

CRITICAL THINKING

Critical thinking is an important and integral aspect of nursing practice. To think critically means to examine and analyze ideas, assumptions, beliefs, arguments, conclusions, and actions to determine their validity and credibility using scientific reasoning, problem-solving and decision-making skills. Thinking critically involves choosing a course of action from the options available. The end point of critical thinking is making a decision (Bandman and Bandman 1988). Nurses use critical thinking skills daily in nursing practice.

Using critical thinking demands that the nurse take a comprehensive look at the problem (Grant

Critical Thinking Skills for Nursing Practice

- Assess and interpret client behaviors
- Identify and formulate nursing diagnoses
- Gather and interpret data and clues accurately
- Analyze and clarify arguments and beliefs
- Evaluate approaches to nursing care
- Justify decisions and actions
- Analyze and evaluate client outcomes

1994). It increases the nurse's awareness and helps the individual focus and evaluate all potential solutions to a problem in a systematic manner. The problem-solving process is an indispensable and crucial part of critical thinking (Burns and Grove 1993) and involves

- Gathering and evaluating data
- Defining the problem
- Determining and evaluating potential options
- Choosing an approach and taking action
- Evaluating the outcomes of the action

Critical thinking and problem solving are learned skills that are polished and refined through practice. The ability to think critically is one of the key differences that distinguishes the expert nurse from the novice.

IMPROVING MATERNAL AND INFANT HEALTH

During the twentieth century, great strides in science and technology advances have resulted in significant reductions in illnesses and deaths of infants and women during childbirth. The definition of terms used in reporting statistics that are indicators of maternal and infant health, the efforts that have been made in the past to improve maternal and infant health, and current developments and goals that have been developed to improve maternal and infant health are important to an understanding of these improved outcomes.

Indicators of Maternal and Infant Health

Vital statistics on birth rate, birth weight, infant mortality rate, maternal mortality rate, and neonatal mortality rate are valuable indications of maternal and infant health. The primary source of data on these indicators of maternal and infant health is the *Monthly Vital Statistics Report* published by the National Center for Health Statistics (NCHS).

BIRTH RATE

Birth rate is the number of births per 1000 population. Birth rates have generally declined for all ages and races from a high in the 1950s to a low in 1975 (Fig. 2–5). From 1985 until 1990, birth rates increased slightly each year and then began to drop steadily. The birth rate in 1993 was 15.5, the lowest point in 15 years (15.0 in 1978) (NCHS 1995). Birth rates for women over 30 started to increase in 1976 and are continuing to rise as more women are delaying childbearing. Birth rates for black and Hispanic women tend to be higher than those for white women (NCHS 1995) (see also Chapter 4).

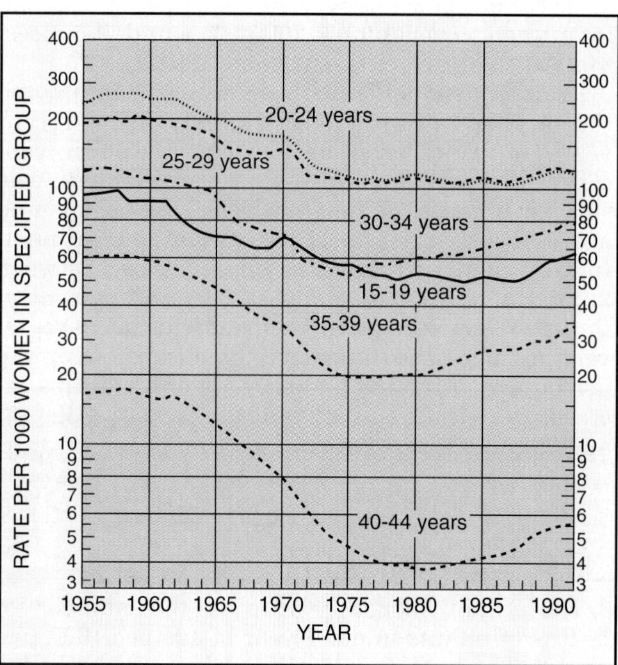

Figure 2–5

Birth rates by age of mother: United States, 1955 to 1991. Note: Beginning with 1959, trend lines are based on registered live births; trend lines for 1955 to 1959 are based on live births adjusted for underregistration. (Data from National Center for Health Statistics [September 9, 1993]. Advance report of final natality statistics, 1991. *Monthly Vital Statistics Report,* 42 [Suppl. 3].)

BIRTH WEIGHT

Higher infant mortality is associated with low birth weight, and thus birth weight is an important indicator of infant health. In 1991 the average weight of infants born in the United States was 3360 g (7 pounds, 7 ounces). Low birth weight is defined as less than 2500 g (5 pounds, 8 ounces) at birth; very low birth weight is less than 1500 g (3 pounds, 5 ounces).

Traditionally, adolescents, black women, and women over 40 have been more likely to have a low-birth-weight infant. In 1993 the incidence of low birth weight increased to 7.2 percent, the highest rate observed since 1976 (7.3 percent). Low birth weight for black births remained unchanged at 13.3 percent; the most substantial increases were seen in births to white mothers. However, this rise was influenced by an increase in the multiple birth ratio, and low-birth-weight data for singleton white births declined slightly. Statistics continue to show that the risk of low birth weight is greatest for the youngest and oldest mothers (NCHS 1995).

Before the 1950s, an infant under 1000 g (2 pounds, 3 ounces) rarely survived. With the increase of technology in newborn intensive care units and sophisticated transport systems, the survival rate of low-birth-weight infants has increased dramatically (Fig. 2–6). In 1938 an infant who weighed 1800 g (3 pounds, 15 ounces) had a 50 percent chance of survival, whereas in 1987 an infant had to weigh only 700 g (1 pound, 9 ounces) to have the same outlook (Avery 1994).

Dramatic strides have been made in improving the survival rates of preterm infants during recent years, but another issue has emerged. This concerns the quality of life of preterm infants who survive because of new obstetric technology and aggressive resuscitation and neonatal treatment. In very immature preterm infants, those between 22 and 25 weeks, as many as 60 to 80 percent of those who survive have been reported to have severe to moderate functional handicaps, with the percentage of infants and severity of handicaps increasing as the gestational age decreases (Allen et al. 1993; Hack and Fanaroff 1993).

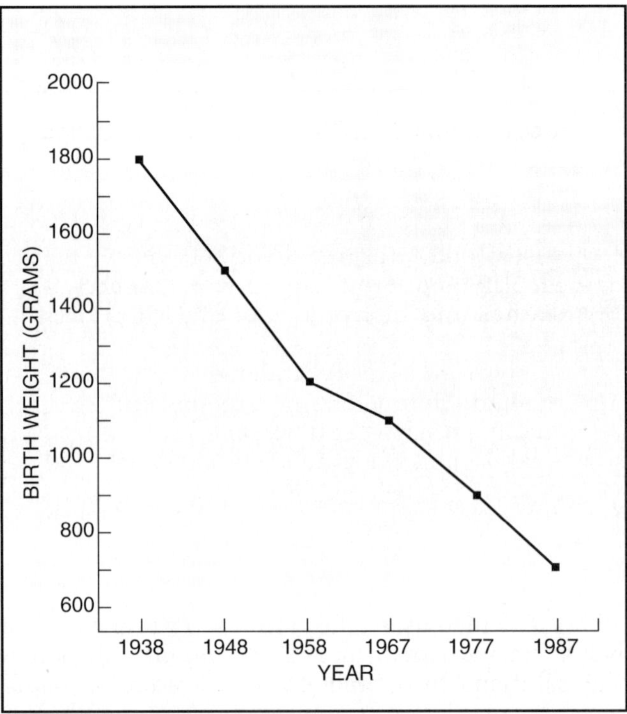

Figure 2–6

Neonatal mortality of low-birth-weight infants from 1938 to 1987 (approximately 50 percent survival at 28 days). (Adapted from Avery, M. E. [1994]. Changes in care of the newborn: Personal reflections over forty years. *Neonatal Network,* 13 [6], 13–14. Reprinted by permission.)

INFANT MORTALITY RATE

The infant mortality rate is the number of deaths of infants under 1 year of age per 1000 live births. The infant mortality rate in the United States for 1993 was 8.3. This represents a decline in infant mortality from 1992 and is the lowest rate ever recorded for this country (Wegman 1994). In 1993 the United States ranked eighteenth, with 20 countries reporting lower mortality rates than this country (Table 2–3).

The infant mortality rate for black infants has consistently been higher than for white infants; black infants are 2.4 times more likely to die during their first year of life than white infants. Since the mid-1970s the infant mortality rate for black infants has declined more slowly than that for white infants. Figure 2–7 shows the increasing differences between infant mortality rates for black and white infants since that time (NCHS 1993).

MATERNAL MORTALITY RATE

The maternal mortality rate is the number of deaths per 100,000 live births. It includes only those pregnant women whose deaths were attributed to complications of pregnancy, childbirth, and puerperium listed in the *International classification of diseases* (9th revision) (ICD-9), nos. 630 to 676. From 1960 to 1982 the maternal mortality rate declined nearly fivefold, from 37.1 in 1960 to 7.9 in 1982. Since 1982, the maternal mortality rate has fluctuated, with no clear trend apparent (NCHS 1992).

Black women have a higher risk of death during childbirth than white women. In 1991 the maternal mortality rate for white women was 5.8, while that for black women was 18.3, over three times higher (Fig. 2–8).

Table 2–3

INFANT MORTALITY RATES FOR INDUSTRIALIZED COUNTRIES, 1993

RANK	COUNTRY	RATE
1	Japan	4.4
1	Finland	4.4§
2	Singapore	4.7§
3	Sweden	4.8§
4	Denmark	5.7
5	Norway	5.9¶
6	Ireland	6.0
7	Canada	6.1¶
8	France	6.2
8	Germany	6.2¶
8	Switzerland	6.2§
9	Netherlands	6.3§
10	Hong Kong	6.4¶
11	Austria	6.5§
12	United Kingdom	6.6
13	Australia	7.0¶
14	New Zealand	7.2§
15	Italy	7.4§
16	Spain	7.2§
17	Belgium	8.0§
18	United States	8.3§
19	Greece	8.5§

Infant mortality rates per 1,000 live births for countries with population greater than 2,500,000.
§ provisional;
¶ 1992. (Adapted from Wegman, M. E. [1994]. Annual summary of vital statistics—1993. *Pediatrics,* 94 [6], 792–803. Reproduced by permission of PEDIATRICS, Vol 94, page 792–803, Copyright 1994.)

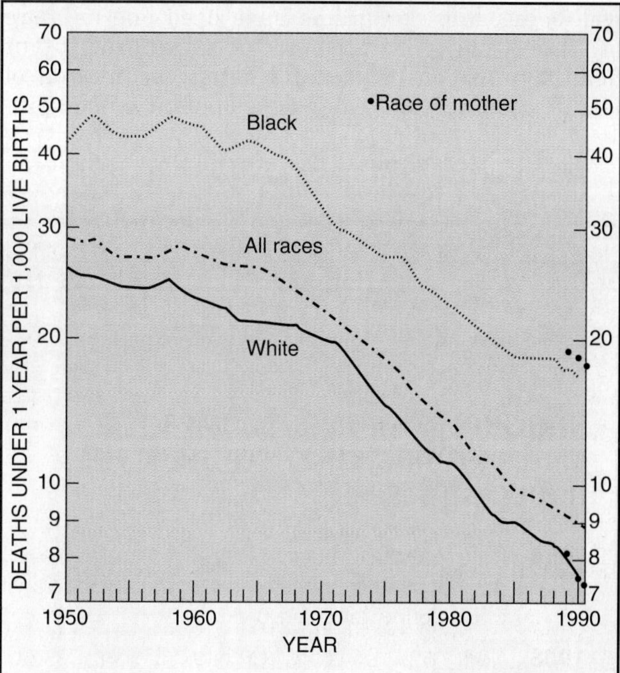

Figure 2–7

Infant mortality rates by race: United States, 1950 to 1991. Note: Infant mortality rates are classified by race of descendant. Beginning in 1989, live births are classified by race of mother; from 1950 to 1989, by race of child. (Data from National Center for Health Statistics. [August 31, 1993]. Advance report of final mortality statistics, 1991. *Monthly Vital Statistics Report,* 42 [Suppl. 2].)

NEONATAL MORTALITY RATE

The neonatal mortality rate is the number of deaths per 1000 live births under 28 days of age. Between 1990 and 1991, the neonatal mortality rate declined 3.4 percent, from 5.8 to 5.6 percent. For white infants the rate declined from 4.8 to 4.5 percent, and for black infants from 11.6 to 11.2 percent. Since 1980, neonatal mortality rates have declined for both races. However, the rates for the white population have declined faster than for the black population (NCHS 1993).

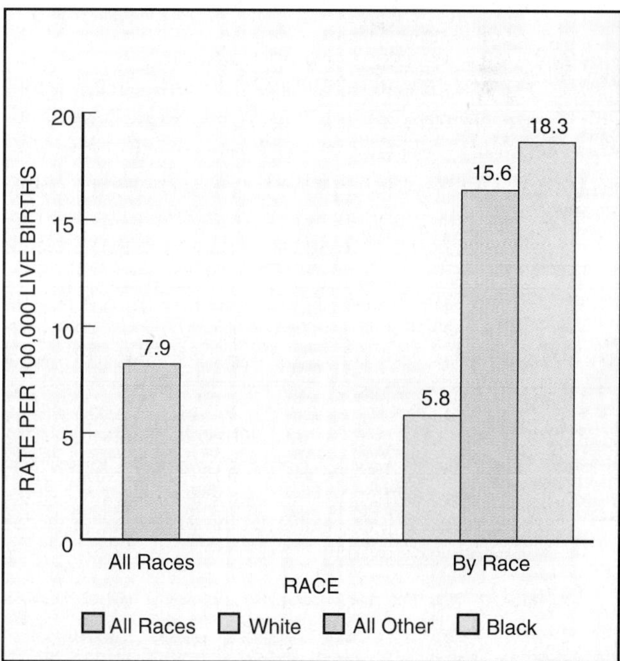

Figure 2–8

Maternal mortality rates by race: United States, 1991. (Data from National Center for Health Statistics [August 31, 1993]. Advance report of final mortality statistics, 1991. *Monthly Vital Statistics Report,* 42 [Suppl. 2].)

Initiatives to Improve Maternal and Infant Health

Since the early 1900s, a number of federal programs have been established to improve infant well-being. Most programs have used one or more of three major strategies to safeguard infant health: provision of prenatal care: coordination of health care services; and development of comprehensive services, including medical care, social support, nutrition programs, and health education. The Historical Perspectives timeline highlights important related events.

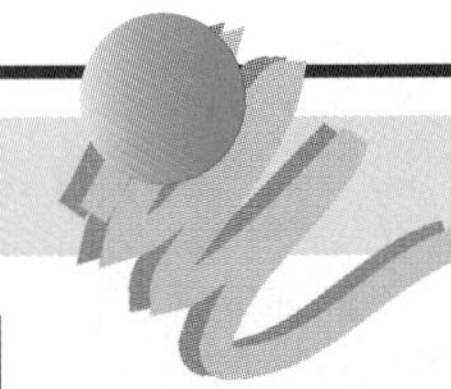

HISTORICAL PERSPECTIVES

NATIONAL INITIATIVES TO IMPROVE MATERNAL AND CHILD HEALTH IN THE UNITED STATES

1906 First prenatal nursing care program developed. Women visited by a nurse at least once during pregnancy.

1908 New York Division of Child Hygiene established by Lillian Wald, a nurse, and a physician to consolidate efforts to reduce infant mortality.

1909 Prenatal care program for women with special health care needs developed. Women visited every 10 days by nurse.

The first White House Conference on Children was convened by President Theodore Roosevelt to examine the health and welfare of children and focus national attention on children's issues and their solutions.

1912 U.S. Children's Bureau established. Its purpose was to coordinate federal child health initiatives, particularly in investigations of infant mortality.

1921 Sheppard-Towner Act passed. First public health program that provided grants for development of maternal-infant health services. Established a precedent for federal responsibility for maternal and child health. Was hotly opposed by the American Medical Association on the grounds that it would introduce socialized medicine.

1924 Children's Bureau published a prenatal care booklet. Over 42 percent of babies died during the first month of life. Poor prenatal nutrition and maternal health identified as the causes of many of the deaths.

1930s During the Depression, services for mothers and infants were reduced.

1935 Title V of the Social Security Act signed into law. Authorized federal money to states for the provision of prenatal care, well-baby clinics, and school health services.

1937 First report on infant mortality published by the Children's Bureau, "Infant Mortality Among Negroes." Described disparity in infant death rates among the black population compared with the white population.

1943 Emergency Maternity and Infant Care Act passed to deal with the overtaxing of maternity services in military hospitals by servicemen's wives. Provided for free maternity care and well-baby care to wives of servicemen in the four lowest pay grades.

1950s Programs to treat premature infants and children with mental retardation developed.

1956 Dependents Medical Care Act restored the program of the Emergency Maternity and Infant Care Act.

1961 President's Panel on Mental Retardation prepared plan to reduce mental retardation. Reported that mental retardation was most closely associated with inadequate prenatal care and preterm birth.

1963 Title V of the Social Security Act amended to provide comprehensive maternity and infant care for low-income, high-risk patients.

1965 Medicare and Medicaid programs established.

1966 Civilian Health Medical Program for dependents of military personnel established.

1967 Early and Periodic Screening Diagnosis and Treatment (EPSDT) program established to provide children who are Medicaid recipients with periodic physical and developmental examinations and treatment of certain illnesses.

1969 Department of Health, Education, and Welfare reorganized. The Children's Bureau was dissolved. The bureau's health grants were taken over by the Public Health Service. Other services of the bureau were transferred to the new Office of Child Development.

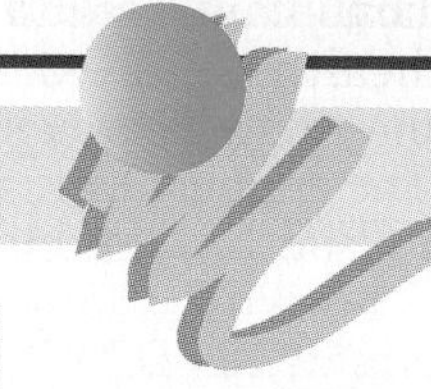

HISTORICAL PERSPECTIVES Continued

1972 Special Supplemental Food Program for Women, Infants, and Children (WIC), which provides food and nutrition education to pregnant and nursing women, and to children under 5 years old, initiated.

1979 U.S. Department of Health, Education, and Welfare released *Healthy People*. The report established 1990 goals to improve health services. Emphasized preventive health services and health promotion. Fifteen targeted areas, including all age groups, were identified. Many objectives involved mothers and children.

1980 Last White House Conference on Children held.

1986 National Commission to Prevent Infant Mortality chartered by Congress. Its purpose was to develop solutions to the nation's infant mortality problem.

1986 Public Health Service completed a mid-decade evaluation of the achievement of the 1990 health objectives. Published in *The 1990 Health Objectives for the Nation: A Midcourse Review*. Half of the 226 objectives were projected to be achieved by 1990. One fourth were projected not to be achieved and another fourth could not be measured or there were insufficient data.

1987 The National Commission on Children created by Congress and the President on December 22, 1987. The task of the Commission was to assess the status of children and families in the United States and propose new directions for policy and program development.

1988 National Commission to Prevent Infant Mortality published *Death Before Life: The Tragedy of Infant Mortality*. The report concluded that although progress has been made in improving infant health, much work remains in lowering infant mortality. The solutions identified by the commission primarily focused on ensuring universal access to prenatal and well-baby care.

1991 The National Commission on Children unanimously approved a blueprint of a national policy for America's children and families: *Beyond Rhetoric: A New American Agenda for Children and Families*. The recommendations focused on strengthening families and promoting healthy development of all the nation's children. It included ensuring income security, improving health, increasing educational achievement, preparing adolescents for adulthood, and protecting vulnerable children and their families.

1994 The United States "signed on" to the International Code of Marketing on Breastmilk Substitutes in May 1994, reversing its earlier position of nonsupport. The Code provides guidelines for marketing of breast milk substitutes that forbid the advertisement of artificial infant formula directly to consumers. It also includes guidelines for educational information that is to accompany breast milk substitutes.

In 1981, the Code was approved by a vote of 118 to one. The United States was the only country that voted not to support the Code. Critics suggested that the U.S. decision had been based on economic concerns. The United States is the world's largest producer of infant formula.

Data from Arnold, Brecht, Hockett, Amspacher, Grad, 1989; Cohen, 1990; and Lederman, 1990.

Several phases characterize past federal efforts to improve infant health. During the first part of the twentieth century, awareness of the shocking rates of infant mortality resulted in initial efforts to establish basic programs of prenatal care. After the Great Depression, attention to infant mortality resurfaced, and federal initiatives to provide comprehensive maternity services gained favor. During this time, programs to enhance the general health care, nutritional status, and developmental outcomes of infants and young children were launched. This phase continued through the 1960s. In the 1960s the federally funded developmental screening programs began, and enhancement programs both for the prevention of mental retardation and for early intervention for retarded children were funded. However, by the 1970s, few new federal maternal-child enhancement programs were initiated, and the trend to severely curtail federal programs or slash funding continued throughout the 1980s.

Current Status of Maternal and Infant Health

In the early 1900s the infant mortality rate was 150; in 1993 it was 8.3 in the United States (Wegman 1994). Although infant mortality has dropped drastically since the early 1900s, the United States continues to rank much lower than many other industrialized nations. The *Healthy People 2000: National Health Promotion and Disease Prevention Objectives on Infant Mortality* are shown in Table 2–4 (U.S. Department of Health and Human Services, 1995).

Differences in infant mortality exist between different regions of the country. The highest rates of mortality are reported in the south. Similar rates are also reported by large cities with a large low socioeconomic population (Wegman 1994).

Prenatal care is strongly associated with infant mortality. For example, black mothers are twice as likely as white mothers to receive either no or substantially inadequate prenatal care. Consistent with this fact, the mortality rate among black infants is more than double that of white infants (Wegman 1994).

A number of barriers exist in women seeking prenatal care. They are often hesitant to seek early care because of the cost. Over 9.5 million women of childbearing age carry no health insurance. Of the women who have health insurance, 5 million do not have maternity insurance benefits

Table 2–4

HEALTHY PEOPLE 2000—REVISED HEALTH STATUS OBJECTIVE ON INFANT MORTALITY

HEALTHY PEOPLE 2000 GOAL

Reduce infant mortality rate to no more than 7 per 1000 live births (baseline: 10.1 per 1000 live births in 1987)

SPECIAL POPULATION TARGETS

Infant Mortality (per 1000 live births)	1987 Baseline	2000 Target
Blacks	18.8	11.0
American Indians/Alaska Natives	13.4*	8.5
Puerto Ricans	12.9*	8.0

TYPE-SPECIFIC TARGETS

Neonatal and Postnatal Mortality (per 1000 live births)	1987 Baseline	2000 Target
Neonatal mortality	6.5	4.5
Neonatal mortality among blacks	12.3	7.0
Neonatal mortality among Puerto Ricans	8.6*	5.2
Postneonatal mortality	3.6	2.5
Postneonatal mortality among blacks	6.4	4.0
Postneonatal mortality among American Indians/Alaska Natives	7.0*	4.0
Postneonatal mortality among Puerto Ricans	4.3*	2.8

Note: Infant mortality is deaths of infants under 1 year; neonatal mortality is deaths of infants under 28 days; postneonatal mortality is deaths of infants aged 28 days up to 1 year.

*1984 baseline.

Adapted from U. S. Department of Health and Human Services. (1995). *Healthy people 2000: Midcourse review and 1995 revisions.* Washington, D.C.: Author.

(National Commission to Prevent Infant Mortality 1988). Many women lack transportation and must travel great distances to seek care. Often clinics are crowded; the waiting time is long. Moreover, most clinics do not offer child care services.

The neonatal mortality rate, which occurs in about 7 percent of all live births, is closely related to low birth weight. Forty percent of all infant deaths occur in infants with very low birthweight and very-low-weight infants are twice as likely to experience severe developmental delays or congenital anomalies (Public Health Service 1990).

A number of risk factors have been associated with low birth weight, including low maternal education status, low income, limited prenatal care, poor housing, poor nutrition, teen pregnancy, smoking, substance and alcohol abuse, unmarried status, and low social support (Miller 1985; Lederman 1990).

Another factor that some experts believe contributes to high infant mortality may be that U.S. social policy dictates few supports for childbearing families (Grad 1989; Miller 1985). This is in direct contrast to most other industrialized countries. European countries, with infant mortality rates below those of the United States, provide all mothers with early adequate prenatal care. Moreover, Japanese pregnant women can ride free on city buses. In England, health visitors visit all new mothers. France has developed an elaborate cash payment program for women engaged in prenatal care.

Most industrialized countries have established policies that protect not only the mother and infant but the family. Among these countries, only the United States and South Africa do not have a charter stating that the health and well-being of families is a national priority (Grad 1989). The United States is also one of the few industrialized countries without a central administrative office to coordinate policies and initiatives for maternal-child health (Cohen 1990).

The U.S. Department of Health and Human Services (1990) released a report to succeed *Healthy People* (1979). The new report, *Healthy People 2000,* describes the national public health goals and objectives for the year 2000. It outlines three goals for public health over the next decade: to increase the span of healthy life, to reduce disparities in health status among different populations, and to provide access to preventive health care for all persons. In 1995, the *Healthy People 2000* objectives were reviewed and revised (U.S.D.H.H.S., 1995).

Objectives of *Healthy People 2000* differ from the earlier 1990 objectives. The objectives for the year 2000 emphasize quality of life and also target high-risk groups. Separate targets have been identified for population groups at risk.

A number of the objectives for the year 2000 address maternal and infant health. These include increasing prenatal care, reducing complications of pregnancy, and decreasing low birth weight and infant mortality. Risk screening objectives include increasing preconceptional counseling and prenatal and newborn screening.

Since 1990, many groups have recommended actions that the U.S. needs to take to reduce infant mortality, including:

- Providing family planning services for all women who wish to use them
- Encouraging women to attend preconceptional counseling
- Providing maternity benefits for all pregnant women
- Ensuring accessibility of health care services for pregnant women by providing an adequate number of strategically located clinics and transportation and child care facilities
- Removing barriers to prenatal care, including negative provider attitudes, lack of continuity in care, and unnecessary waiting for care
- Protecting childbearing women from occupational hazards
- Extending the Special Supplemental Food Program for Women, Infants and Children (WIC) to all pregnant and breastfeeding women
- Encouraging pregnant women to decrease smoking and use of drugs and alcohol
- Providing special follow-up of all high-risk women after delivery
- Granting parental leave for employed parents
- Strengthening the interdisciplinary approach for the provision of maternity, perinatal, and infancy programs

MATERNITY HEALTH CARE SYSTEM CHANGES

A review of the current trends in maternity care shows that this area of the American health care system is in a period of dramatic change. This transition reflects years of debate between two conflicting approaches that direct the way maternity health care is organized and delivered: the medical model and the family-centered maternity care (FCMC) model.

Experts in women's health care affirm that childbearing does not occur in a vacuum; it is a sociocultural experience as much as a biologic one (McBride 1976; Leavitt 1986; Andrist 1988). Thus, the evolution of maternity care in the United States has been shaped by the social context (economic, interpersonal, political, temporal) in which it occurred (Leavitt 1986).

Historical Perspectives

In learning about the present practice of maternity care, it is essential to understand the vital impact that female influence has had and continues to have on the practice of childbirth. For over 200 years (1700 to 1930), childbirth was a women-centered event, an experience in which women not only decided the circumstances of the birth environment (the home), but also provided comfort for each other during the childbearing process. The childbearing women of this era played a significant role in determining the practice of maternity care. Because of their continued efforts to make childbirth safer, they slowly incorporated changing medical advances into their home-based practice and eventually helped to change the birth process from a woman-centered home event to a hospital-centered medical event during the second and third decades of the twentieth century (Leavitt 1986). However, the women who participated in these decisions did not realize that this shift in location would also mean a shift in their ability to control their environment of birth. Although these women gained confidence in achieving healthier outcomes for themselves and their infants, they lost the control to participate in planning how this significant life event would occur (Leavitt 1986). Inspired by the writings of the prepared childbirth movement in the 1950s and 1960s childbearing women began to question the safety and rationale of the hospital routine: (1) drugged births, (2) complete obstetric enema preparations and perineal shaves, (3) forceps deliveries, (4) scheduled inductions, (5) episiotomies, and (6) separation from family and friends. Concern with the impersonal, sterile hospital setting was common: "The worst feature is the lonesomeness; the cruelest part is being alone among strangers" (Leavitt 1986, pp. 182, 190). Leavitt's analysis of childbirth history describes three forms of women's responses to hospitalized childbirth: (1) total rejection of current medical practice, (2) negotiation with the medical community to transform care to meet their needs, and (3) passive acceptance of the status quo. Not surprisingly, a growing segment of women started voicing their disillusionment with the invasiveness and isolation of the hospital environment. They began to demand the best of both worlds: "the confidence in a healthy outcome with the freedom to make choices about how to conduct the important event" (Leavitt 1986, p. 196).

While women were reclaiming their legacy as active agents of change, economic conditions during this period also played a major role in transforming the practice of maternity care. "When increased yearly costs of 15 percent or more for hospital care became routine in the late 1960s, efforts began to deal with shrinking resources for payment of these costs" (Phillips 1989, p. 233). The implementation of Medicare's prospective reimbursement system in 1983 forced the entire health care system to switch the focus from the unconscious spending of health care dollars to one of cost containment. Medicare is based on the prepayment of set fees according to diagnosis-related groupings (DRGs). If a client's hospital stay exceeds the prescribed amount, the hospital must absorb the cost (Edwardson 1985). On the other hand, if the costs of the client's stay are less than the set fee, the hospital may keep the difference.

Many third-party payers followed Medicare's lead and established their own prospective payment system (PPS). Alternative health care delivery systems, including Health Maintenance Organizations (HMOs), Preferred Provider Organizations (PPOs), and Independent Practice Organizations (IPOs), that manage health care for groups by contracting physician and hospital services at lower prices were also introduced to help curtail the spiraling costs of health care. These new delivery systems further challenged the traditional functioning of the health care system by adding services that emphasize preventive maintenance, in addition to the treatment of illness. To survive the financial constraints of prospective reimbursement and to secure HMO and PPO contracts, hospitals have responded by reducing operating costs, decreasing the average length of stay (ALOS), and implementing market strategies that target the health care needs of women. Thus, the interaction of consumer demand and economic constraints mandated that hospitals replace outmoded obstetric systems with maternity services that are high in quality, cost efficient, and consumer sensitive.

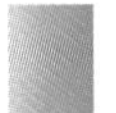

Traditional Care

Traditional care describes the practice of maternity care that dominated throughout most of the twentieth century. In 1900, less than 5 percent of women in the United States gave birth in hospitals. Childbirth moved to the hospital during the 1920s and 1930s for two major reasons. First, the introduction of various drugs and obstetric techniques to control pain and combat puerperal fever (infection) convinced both physicians and women that advances in medical science superseded giving birth in the home environment. Second, the increasing mobility and urbanization created by the Industrial Revolution of the nineteenth century finally robbed the twentieth century childbearing woman of her social network of female support (Leavitt 1986; Lindell 1988). Consequently, by 1975, over 90 percent of women in the United States gave birth in hospitals.

Childbirth was viewed as a pathophysiologic, physician-centered process (Wilkerson and Barrows 1988). Once under the realm of medicine, traditional maternity care was organized into subspecialties (i.e., labor and delivery, postpartum, and newborn nursery), and its functioning was based on the surgical multitransfer system (Phillips 1988). Maternity nursing care followed the same pattern. In the traditional setting, mothers labored in one room, delivered in another, recovered in yet another, and spent the remainder of their hospital stay on a postpartal unit. Infants were immediately separated from their mothers at birth, placed in a separate nursery, and transported to their mothers only at uniformly set feeding times (e.g., 9:00 AM, 1:00 PM, 5:00 PM). Scheduling was based on institutional needs, rather than the individual needs of mothers and infants.

Rapid advances in perinatal technology and treatment for high-risk conditions such as diabetes, threatened preterm labor, and pregnancy-induced hypertension (PIH) further promoted the medicalization of childbirth (Gennaro 1988). Consequently, physicians and nurses were trained to treat childbirth as a high-risk event. To prevent such outcomes as preterm labor, stillbirth, postpartal hemorrhage, and neonatal infection, intrusive perinatal care became the norm for management of childbearing women. In fact, traditional care in the 1970s became a time of convenience owing to the common practice of scheduled inductions, fetal monitoring, and cesarean births. By 1980, the cesarean birth rate had nearly doubled from that of the previous decade (McBride 1982). Concerned with the assumption that every pregnant woman was a disaster waiting to happen, some professionals and consumers began to argue that traditional hospital care detracted from the biopsychosocial development of the new family unit. They maintained that the oppressive and sterile routines of traditional hospital care must be changed to promote the health and well-being of the family unit (Fenwick 1984; Wilkerson and Barrows 1988).

Family-Centered Maternity Care

In response to consumer demand for family-oriented maternity care and to balance the use of technology in obstetrics, ANA, NAACOG, the American Academy of Pediatrics, and the American College of Nurse-Midwives published the *Joint Position Statement on the Development of Family-Centered Maternity/Newborn Care in Hospitals* in 1978. This statement was later endorsed by the American Hospital Association and subsequently influenced hospitals throughout the country to implement FCMC.

Within a decade, FCMC made significant progress in putting the "family" back into the childbearing process, and forever changed the practice of traditional care in hospitals. It is estimated that over 70 percent of hospitals throughout the country have revamped their traditional care system to include some type of alternative childbirth service (birthing room, mother-baby care, labor-delivery-recovery [LDR] rooms). The philosophy of FCMC views childbirth as a vital, natural life event rather than an illness. The primary goals of FCMC are to assist expectant parents to make informed decisions about their own health care and to foster family unity while providing safe, quality, cost-effective care. Leaders in contemporary maternity care predict, "By the turn of the century, what we know now as traditional maternity care will be history" (Phillips 1988, p. 6).

Environments for Birth

SINGLE-ROOM MATERNITY CARE

Single-room maternity care (SRMC) is viewed as the logical replacement for the antiquated multitransfer system that characterizes the traditional care of childbirth. Visionaries in the childbirth field contend that SRMC is the most viable approach for holistic, dynamic, cost-effective maternity practice in the twenty-first century. This contemporary system is based on the philosophy of FCMC and modeled on the efficient design of coronary intensive care units. In this comprehensive approach, childbearing women will labor, deliver, recover, and (in some settings) spend the remainder of their postpartum stay in one room. Unlike the traditional care system, staff and equipment are brought to women on the basis of their individual needs and the different stages of the childbearing process. Also, normal newborns are not routinely separated from their mother after birth. Infants may remain in the room with mothers under the care of a maternal-newborn nurse who is proficient in both maternal and neonatal nursing, or families may choose to have their babies taken to a holding nursery for care. Preterm and ill infants are cared for in a Level II or Level III nursery.

The primary functioning unit of the SRMC system is known as the labor-delivery-recovery and/or postpartum (LDR, LDRP) room. These private rooms are designed and equipped to accommodate the entire birthing process, including complicated vaginal deliveries. There are no screening criteria, and whatever equipment may be necessary for a high-risk patient can be brought into the room. Cesarean births occur in delivery/operating rooms located on the unit, and (depending on the hospital) the mother recovers in an LDR room, an LDRP room, or a designated recovery room. A wide array of SRMC units exist in the United States because of the physical and budgetary constraints of many hospitals. However, the ideal SRMC facility is patterned on the cluster system, in which LDR/LDRP rooms are clustered around a central area containing a nurses' station, a holding nursery, and ancillary services. Each system has at least one, if not two, delivery/operating rooms to accommodate cesarean births. Depending on the institution's level of care, a Level II or Level III nursery may be included in the system.

Phillips (1988) cited three categories of advantages that are a result of the comprehensive design of SRMC (Table 2–5). Proponents of SRMC (Gerlach and Schmid 1986; Phillips 1988) advise that there are three risks to be aware of when planning to implement a SRMC: inability to change culture, staff attrition, and loss of commitment. Converting to SRMC is a complex process that involves internal (attitudinal) as well as exterior changes. Phillips (1988) maintains that hospitals can expect to lose those staff who are unwilling to change. The key to retaining loyal staff is to provide them with a comprehensive cross-training program that promotes ownership of the new system and provides all staff (labor and delivery, postpartum, newborn nursery) with sufficient time and learning resources to function competently. Hospitals that are planning their services toward early discharge for uncomplicated births (vaginal or cesarean) and structuring the practice of SRMC according to the humanistic values of FCMC will emerge as the leaders of maternity care in the twenty-first century.

Interestingly, a 1991 household survey of women who had given birth within the previous 12 months indicates that 53.2 percent had used either a labor-delivery room, an LDR room, or an LDRP room. Only 41 percent had given birth in separate labor and delivery rooms. Figure 2–9 shows the change from 1988 to 1991 in the type of settings, traditional medical childbirth (separate labor and delivery rooms) versus family-centered childbirth (some combination of labor, delivery, recovery, and postpartum rooms), in hospitals in which women gave birth.

Table 2–5

ADVANTAGES OF SINGLE-ROOM MATERNITY CARE (SRMC)

Clinical safety	• Increased effectiveness in responding to emergencies • Improved communication and continuity of care • Decreased risk of patient exposure to many different areas and departmental staff
Marketability	• Noninstitutional environment increases market share by attracting parents-to-be and promotes their using facility for future family needs • Continuity of care and comprehensive cross-training promote recruitment and retention of staff
Cost efficiency	• Space is more efficient since SRMC eliminates need for duplication of support areas (i.e., utility and linen rooms) • Staffing for one area rather than three combined with increased flexibility of staff through cross-training reduces labor costs • Nontransfer care and smaller space decreases cleaning and maintenance costs • Combined practices of physiologic labor management with mother-baby nursing help to decrease use of technology and provide support needed for early discharge, thereby reducing operational costs

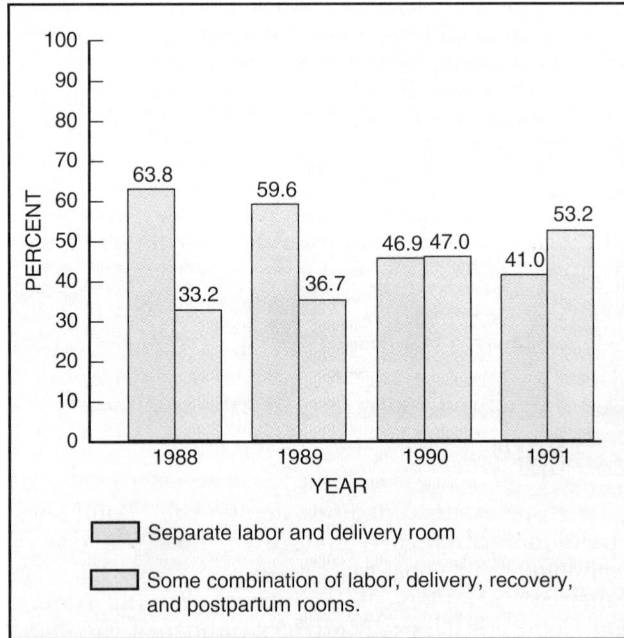

Figure 2–9

Changes from 1988 to 1991 in the type of settings in hospitals in which women gave birth. Totals do not add up to 100. (Adapted from More women using new birth site options [1991]. *Hospitals,* 65 [20], 14. With permission from American Hospital Publishing, Inc.)

BIRTH CENTERS

In response to family requests for increased decision making and participation in childbirth, birth centers (originally called alternative birth centers [ABCs]) emerged in the United States during the technologic era of the 1970s (Jones 1989). Ideally, a birth center is a maternity unit that provides low-technology care in a homelike setting from which women return home shortly after giving birth (Kitzinger 1991).

Since the establishment of the first birth center, the Maternity Center Association, in New York in 1975, the growth and recognition of these centers in the United States continue to gain momentum. Although only a tiny percentage of childbearing women (0.5 percent) use birth centers, most out-of-hospital births occur in this setting (Jones 1989).

Birth centers are classified as freestanding or in-hospital centers. The freestanding birth center is separate from the acute care hospital setting and has more autonomy in formulating policies and procedures for the operations of the center and the programs of care for clients (Ernst 1988). Most freestanding centers provide comprehensive maternity services that include prenatal care, education and counseling, and intrapartum and postpartum care with home visiting and family planning. Jones (1989) reported that there are over 170 freestanding birth centers operating in the United States. In-hospital birth centers are located in hospital grounds or inside a hospital building and typically provide only intrapartum and early postpartum care. Both types of centers are designed with the capability of initiating emergency procedures and have developed contingency plans for access to in-hospital obstetric and newborn services. The caregivers in both of these settings generally consist of certified nurse-midwives (CNMs), obstetricians, pediatricians, and registered nurses. However, some centers are run by midwives with no nursing background (Kitzinger 1991).

The literature shows that the major distinction between the freestanding and in-hospital centers is philosophical. Many birth centers genuinely direct their practice according to the physiologic and psychosocial aspects of childbirth.

In the Garden of Life Birth Center in Dearborn, Michigan, where the focus is on cultural sensitivity to the needs of the Muslim, Italian, Hispanic, Polish, and Anglo parents using the center, the sole machinery is a coffeemaker. Staff wear ordinary clothing, not uniforms. Women can move around in labor and adopt any position they like for birth. Childbirth education is an integral part of the program, and other members of the family can be present at the birth. The bed is king-sized, low, and comfortable, so that mother, father, and new baby can cuddle together.

(KITZINGER 1991, p. 58)

Owing to profit and marketing incentives, there is an increasing trend toward physician-owned birth centers, both in-hospital and freestanding. As physicians gain access to this alternative setting, they also impart their philosophy of birth as a medical event and of the high technology practices it embraces. Kitzinger (1991, p. 60) describes "the typical California center as physician-owned in a commercial building, with a couple of birth rooms, and births are attended by the obstetricians."

A review of research on birth centers (Jones 1989) shows that, in contrast with freestanding centers, in-hospital centers had an increased rate of episiotomies and maternal transfers because of the need for analgesia. Also, in-hospital centers experienced more maternal-newborn postpartum transfers. However, intrapartum transfer, complications, cesarean, and forceps rates were similar for both centers. Overall, the research affirms that both types of birth centers practice safe and cost-effective maternity care. Compared with traditional care facilities, birth center financial reports show a 30 to 40 percent decrease in operating costs, savings that are passed on to the consumer (Jones 1989). A study of the outcomes of 11,814 women admitted to 84 freestanding centers throughout the United States reported the perinatal mortality rate to be as low as 1.3 per 1000 births compared with 8 per 1000 for all hospital births (Eakins 1986). Jones (1989) concludes that birth center research has had a positive influence on the practice of contemporary maternity care. The results support the view of pregnancy and birth as healthy events, and show that the invasive obstetric routines of traditional care are unnecessary for most childbearing women.

HOME BIRTHS

Birth certificate data document the occurrence of 82,210 home births in the United States from 1989 to 1991 (Declercq et al. 1995). Although this represents a tiny percentage (less than 0.8 percent) of the total births in this country during this time, it is significant that many of these women choose to give birth in their homes rather than in the hospital setting. Leavitt (1986) maintains that this segment of mostly middle- and upper-class women are voicing an outright rejection of physician-directed and hospital-based rituals. "It's the difference between nurses rushing past you in the corridor, in a place where you don't belong, and inviting people into your home, the place that belongs to you" (Kitzinger 1991, p. 8).

On the other hand, a large group of women give birth at home because of lack of choice. Through poverty and neglect, women in this group are twice as likely to have a baby who dies shortly after birth as middle-class women (Kitzinger 1991; Leavitt 1986).

The following information taken from birth certificates in 1989 showed that different patterns of birth attendance emerged in different settings. In home births, midwives (certified and lay-midwives) attended 66 percent of all births. In freestanding birth centers, physicians and certified nurse-midwives (CNMs) attended 75.1 percent of all births (Declercq 1993). Thirty states reported home births, and most took place in California, Florida, and Pennsylvania. CNMs are registered nurses who have successfully completed an advanced accredited university program in pregnancy, childbirth, gynecology, and family planning. After passing national boards, administered by the American College of Nurse-Midwives, the RN becomes a CNM. A CNM always has a contingency arrangement with a backup physician in case complications should arise.

McCartney and van der Meer (1991) defined the term "other midwives" as lay-midwives who are licensed after attending a state approved training program, but they are not nurses. Some licensed lay-midwives have collaborative arrangements with backup physicians. Unlicensed lay-midwives come from a variety of apprenticeship backgrounds and in most states practice outside the law (Leavitt 1986).

Because of the difficulty in retrieving accurate data on home births, statistics reported on home births must be interpreted cautiously. For instance, unplanned births that occur outside a hospital setting, such as in a taxi, a shopping mall, or an ambulance, are often recorded as home births. Also, women who have out-of-hospital births include those individuals who deliver prematurely, teenagers attempting to hide a birth, or those who have had no access to prenatal care. Documentation of these births as "home births" gives a false impression of the comparative risks of home and hospital birth (Kitzinger 1991). Kitzinger defends planned home birth as a safe alternative to hospital birth in low-risk populations that utilize skilled birth attendants. Separate studies conducted in Australia and the Netherlands, where a large amount of planned births occur at home, report a concomitant perinatal mortality rate as low as 3 to 5.9 per 1000 births as compared with 9 to 10 per 1000 hospital births (Kitzinger 1991).

Despite the recognized safety of planned home births, the fear of litigation, the problem of adequate health care backup services, and the expense of securing malpractice coverage for the home setting are forcing even the most approachable health care providers to relocate their home birth practice to the birth center environment. Those women desiring home birth in the United States will probably have to rely increasingly on lay-midwives to attend their births (Hafner-Eaton and Pearce 1994). As long as home births remain an option for childbearing women, nurses must be knowledgeable of the criteria that promote the best outcomes for both mother and baby: comprehensive assessments throughout the prenatal period; prepared childbirth education; and a skilled, experienced birth attendant who is relaxed working in a home environment.

A number of questions can be used to help childbearing women make decisions about home birth (McCartney and van der Meer 1991, pp. 25–27):

- In the event of complications, who is my backup physician?
- How close is the nearest hospital to my home?
- How would I be transported there? By ambulance or by car?
- How receptive is the hospital to handling an emergency that arises for a delivery begun at home?
- Does my midwife have privileges at this hospital?
- If I am moved to a hospital, will my midwife stay with me even if she cannot do deliveries there?
- Who assists the midwife at a home birth?
- What supplies and equipment do I need to have at home?
- What supplies and equipment will the midwife bring?
- What types of emergencies can be handled at home and what would prompt a move to the hospital?
- Do I have to preregister at a particular hospital just in case I need to go there?
- Who will examine the baby after birth? Who will administer the necessary eyedrops, injections? Do I need to contact a pediatrician?
- Who fills out the birth certificate?

ISSUES IN MATERNAL-NEWBORN NURSING

A number of contemporary issues challenge maternal-newborn nursing and can be divided into three major areas: social, scientific advancement, and economic. Each area is briefly discussed in this section. Because these issues are critically important to maternal-newborn nursing, they are addressed throughout the text.

Social Issues

Maternal-newborn health care is confronted with very serious problems that stem from larger social issues. Drug abuse by pregnant women and their addicted infants has reached astounding numbers. Childbearing by unmarried women has dramatically increased. The prevalence of human immunodeficiency virus (HIV) infection in childbearing women and their infants continues to grow. Compounding these problems is the fact that the women and their infants who experience drug abuse, HIV infection, and single parenting often live in poverty and have few resources.

Maternal-newborn health care is also affected by the state of women's health care. Although the importance of women's health began gaining national recognition during the last two decades, questions continue to be raised about the health and well-being of American women.

While progress has been made in treating women, who make up 52 percent of the total population, there are continuing issues related to women's health. These include questions related to areas of health care neglect, shortcomings of health services available to women, and the need to continue studying key health problems of women.

Women's problems related to breast cancer, heart disease, depression, and family violence are serious but are not well understood. For example, the rate of breast cancer deaths has increased 24 percent, yet no one knows why (Sharp 1990). Heart disease is a major killer of women, but virtually all research has been conducted on men. Women are the fastest growing high-risk group for developing acquired immunodeficiency syndrome (AIDS), yet few investigations have included women. Most types of depression are twice as common in women as in men (McGrath 1991). The gender difference in rates of depression persists in all races and at all levels of education and income (Russo 1990). Sexual and physical violence remain significant health problems (McGrath 1991; Sampselle 1991). Rape of women continues to rise (Chiarelli and Nadon 1985; Sampselle 1991). Tragically, one in ten American women is abused each year by the man with whom she lives (Sampselle 1991). It has been estimated that one third of women will experience sexual violence during their lifetime (Sampselle 1991).

Scientific Advancement

Maternal-newborn health care has been blessed with remarkable scientific breakthroughs and technologic advances (Phillips 1988). These advances include electronic fetal monitoring, tocolytic medications to arrest preterm labor, sophisticated biochemical and cytologic techniques for early detection of fetal disorders, techniques to assess fetal gestational age, reproductive technologies to assist infertile women, and technology to increase the survival rate of low-birth-weight infants.

Scientific advancements have affected the lives of many childbearing families. Women who had little hope of ever becoming pregnant have given birth. In addition, the outcome of pregnancy for many high-risk women, such as those at risk for preterm labor, has improved. Many more infants have survived who would have died only a few years ago.

With the advancement of scientific progress, new problems and questions have emerged. Women with low-risk pregnancies are being exposed to more specialized technology. The increased use of such technology is contributing to the rising high cost of maternal-newborn care.

Many questions related to scientific advancements in maternal-newborn care need to be addressed, including

- What guidelines should be used to determine the judicious and cost-effective use of health care technology?
- How does technology change the human components of childbirth and nursing care? Does technology actually save money, lead to better patient outcomes, and provide greater job satisfaction for nurses?
- What is quality survival for high-risk infants?
- How will the enormous costs of highly sophisticated treatment of high-risk mothers and infants be subsidized?

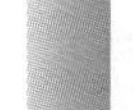

Obstetric Interventions

Childbirth has increasingly become a technical event filled with interventions that often do not support the normal physiologic labor process or are invasive. As early as 1933, the White House Conference on Child Health and Protection report entitled *Fetal, New Born, and Maternal Mortality and Morbidity* stated that "excessive intervention" was the principal cause of increased maternal and infant mortality (Brackbill et al. 1984).

A report from the Hastings Center (Steinfels 1978) on the value of childbirth technology pointed out: "Pain-killing drugs, anesthesia, induced labors, and restricted diets are often introduced for well-defined therapeutic ends and quickly become routine practice, even in normal pregnancies." While childbirth technology has proved beneficial in high-risk pregnancies, current evidence does not support the benefit of this technology in low-risk pregnancies. The following questions need to be answered for each childbirth intervention:

- Is it beneficial for the woman and her baby? If so, what are the beneficial outcomes?
- Has it been adequately tested?
- Is it cost effective?

Another cause for concern is that the use of an intervention often leads to the need for other interventions. An example of this, called the "intervention daisy chain" by Brackbill and colleagues (1984), is putting a woman in active labor to bed *(first intervention)* upon admission to the Labor and Delivery Unit. This procedure hinders the process of physiologic labor, and labor contractions usually decrease in strength and frequency. Because of ineffective labor contractions, intravenous fluids are started *(second intervention).* This procedure further inhibits the labor process and decreases the effectiveness of contractions. To stimulate contractions, an oxytocic drug (oxytocin [Pitocin]) is started *(third intervention).* Since oxytocin causes strong and often painful contractions, it is not unusual for the woman to use medication *(fourth intervention)* earlier in labor. And so it goes.

It is most interesting that the two most common interventions used for women in normal labor, bed rest and intravenous fluids, are also the same two primary interventions used for women in preterm labor to decrease contractions. The practice question here is: Why are bed rest and intravenous fluids used when women are in normal labor? The research question that needs to be examined is: Do women who are active (e.g., walking) during normal labor and who are not receiving intravenous fluids have more effective labor contractions than women in normal labor who have bed rest and intravenous fluids?

Advocates of routine obstetric interventions claim that they are beneficial and promote improved outcomes. Opponents of routine obstetric interventions during labor assert that there is overuse and misuse of obstetric interventions in normal labor that can lead to dysfunctional labor and the increased need for cesarean section. The question of the use of obstetric technology must be answered on the basis of research related to this area.

The Agency for Health Care Policy and Research (1994), based on a research study conducted by Lemrow and colleagues (1990) stated: "Hospital statistics raise questions about obstetrical care" (Fig. 2–10). The findings of the study were as follows:

- National statistics based on U.S. hospitalizations in 1986 (in all areas of practice, e.g., obstetrics, pediatrics, medical-surgical) indicate that four of the top seven principal procedures being performed were related to birth: circumcision, episiotomy, low cervical cesarean section, and manually assisted delivery.
- Pay source (private insurance versus Medicaid) and race/ethnicity (white versus black or Hispanic) appeared to be related to whether interventions were used. White women with private insurance were more likely to have interventions.
- Blacks and Hispanics accounted for a disproportionately high percentage of hospitalizations for problem pregnancies related to fetal distress, preterm labor, and spontaneous abortions, which may reflect inadequate care.

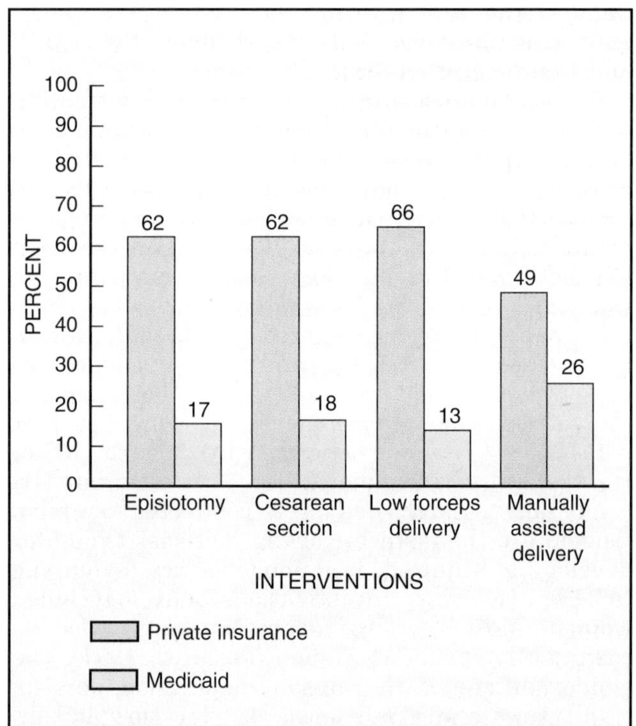

Figure 2–10

Percentage of common obstetric procedures performed by pay source in 1986 in hospitals in the HCUP-2 60 parcel sample. Women with Medicaid were less likely to receive interventions than were women with private insurance. (Adapted from Lemrow, N., Adams, D., Coffey, R., Farley, D. [1990]. *The 50 most frequent diagnosis-related groups (DRGs), diagnoses, and procedures: Statistics by hospital size and location.* [DHHS Publication No. (PHS) 90-3465]. Hospital Studies Program Research Note 13, Agency for Health Care Policy and Research. Rockville, MD: Public Health Service.)

These research findings raise serious policy and research questions about how obstetric services are provided in the hospital setting. These descriptive statistics cannot explain the appropriateness of the interventions. Only in-depth examination of each intervention and the different patterns of obstetric care can determine whether the intervention is beneficial and appropriate. The findings do stimulate thought and discussion on the role of childbirth interventions and also provide a starting point for research.

Economic Issues

Health care services for childbearing families continue to change. Many changes have been initiated because the cost of health care continues to increase. Cost containment, the closure of services, and redefinition of the patient population are strategies that have been employed to deal with cost increases.

Health care professionals are urged to identify costly and often unnecessary procedures. In recent years, the high rate of cesarean births has come under close scrutiny. Programs to decrease cesarean births have gained acceptance in many parts of the United States.

Across America, a great deal of competition exists regarding the delivery of maternal-newborn health care services. Women's health care is an area that is often launched as a marketing strategy, with the intention of recruiting new patients as a primary goal. Many times these programs are short-lived. Moreover, programs that have been developed in one part of the country are adopted by other agencies without much thought to tailoring the program for a particular clientele.

Experts in this field recommend developing maternity programs that focus on high-touch rather than just high-tech. Provision of comprehensive services that address preventive health care and promotion of healthy behaviors will counterbalance the routine and unnecessary use of expensive technology in the low-risk childbearing population. It is essential that maternal-newborn nurses become aware of the economic inequalities of the childbearing population. As family advocates, maternal-newborn nurses must work to shift some of this nation's wealth to its most vulnerable citizens: indigent mothers and their babies.

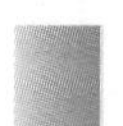

Health Care Reform

While almost everyone agrees that the health care system needs to be reformed, there is little agreement over how it should be changed.

In August 1993, nursing leaders from 63 major nursing organizations, representing nearly 1 million registered nurses, met for a National Nursing Summit (1993) to discuss nursing's role in the future reformed health care system. The recommendations for *Nursing's Agenda for Health Care Reform* contained goals and strategies to position nursing in a reformed health care system.

The goals for national health care reform were as follows:

- Assure universal health care coverage that is portable and unrestricted by preexisting conditions.
- Assure involvement of nurses and consumers in health care planning and policy development.
- Remove barriers to nurses to practice to the full extent of their education and receive payment for services.
- Allocate resources to redesign the nursing workforce to deliver services in a restructured health care system.

For each of the above goals, specific strategies were presented. Goals and strategies for state health care reform, nursing education, advanced nursing practice, and the workforce were also developed.

In 1994, Congress and the Clinton Administration grappled with health care reform. Much of the debate focused on the 37 million Americans without health insurance and the spiraling cost of health care. Many strategies were examined, often in heated debate. Unable to reach a decision on health care reform, Congress finally closed without taking any action on the issue. Health care reform will continue to be addressed in future sessions of Congress. While the outcome is unknown, it is certain that health care reform will happen in the future and that every American will be affected in some manner (League of Women Voters Education Fund et al. 1994).

It is also clear that health care reform will place increasing emphasis on primary, preventive, and community care. The opportunities for maternal-newborn nurses in a reformed health care system are great as barriers are removed to practice (especially advanced practice), new and expanded roles are created for nurses in the hospital, and increasing emphasis is placed on preventive and community care.

IMPLICATIONS FOR RESEARCH

In-depth specialized knowledge is required for the practice of maternal-newborn nursing. Our knowledge in the area of maternal-newborn nursing is incomplete; there are questions that remain unanswered and problems that need solutions. Research provides a method to increase our knowledge through study using the scientific method and the careful framing of questions.

Walker (1992) identified a number of problems in research related to maternal-newborn nursing. She recommended the following approaches for strengthening research in the area:

- Use larger sample sizes
- Conduct longitudinal investigations
- Carefully select the way in which to best measure a variable (instrument, interview)
- Design studies to ensure that the method selected for studying the problem is appropriate for the problem
- Test a variety of nursing interventions
- Increase the quality of research design (design, measurement, statistics)
- Strengthen sampling procedures; use random assignment for intervention research
- Use power analysis as a basis for determining sample size
- Locate and examine previous research studies to ensure the cumulative building of a scientific base for practice; changes in clinical practice and new discoveries will emerge through the findings of well-designed research studies

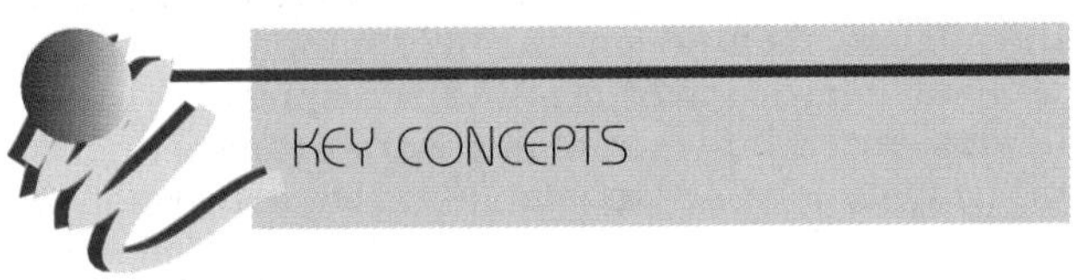

KEY CONCEPTS

- ▼ Childbirth is a unique and powerful human experience that has physiologic, psychological, spiritual, and social importance.
- ▼ Maternal-newborn nursing consists of diagnosis and treatment of the responses of childbearing women, their infants, and their families to health and illness.
- ▼ The independent role of the maternal-newborn nurse changes with the practice setting from many independent functions in the community setting, to a lesser number in a well maternity care setting, and to an even lesser amount in an acute care practice setting.
- ▼ The philosophy (beliefs and values) of maternal-newborn nursing provides a foundation for practice and gives direction for the care the nurse provides for childbearing women, their infants, and their families.
- ▼ Childbirth is a normal physiologic process that generally requires few medical interventions, it is a family affair, and the reproductive health of the total family is important to the health of society.
- ▼ Parenting is learned; individuals do not automatically have the appropriate expectations, knowledge, and skills for good parenting.
- ▼ The nursing process provides maternal-newborn nurses with an organized system to define and guide the independent aspect of their practice.
- ▼ The components of the nursing process are assessment, nursing diagnosis, planning, intervention, and evaluation.
- ▼ Nursing care planning guides are written forms of the nursing process that specify the nursing care needed for an individual client. Although the purpose of the nursing care plan is the same, its structure may differ from agency to agency, and from nursing unit to nursing unit within the same agency.
- ▼ A standardized nursing care plan is a prewritten protocol developed for clients with a specific condition or disease process.
- ▼ A collaborative care map is a multidisciplinary plan of care for a client that includes the key interventions necessary to promote desired client outcomes according to a timeline and efficient uses of resources. A collaborative care map is also called a case management plan, critical pathway, or care map.
- ▼ Critical thinking is an important and integral aspect of nursing practice. To think critically means to examine and analyze ideas, assumptions, beliefs, arguments, conclusions, and actions to determine their validity and credibility using scientific reasoning, problem-solving, and decision-making skills.
- ▼ Since childbearing is a normal healthy event, a dual approach, both problem-oriented diagnoses and wellness-oriented diagnoses, is helpful.
- ▼ Vital statistics are important indicators of maternal and infant health.
- ▼ Low birth weight is the leading cause of infant mortality. Adolescents, black women, and women over 40 are more likely to have a low-birth-weight infant.
- ▼ Black infants are twice as likely to die during their first year of life as white infants.
- ▼ Black women have a higher risk of death during childbirth than white women.
- ▼ Numerous national initiatives have been undertaken to improve maternal and infant health in the United States, yet in 1993 this country ranked eighteenth in infant mortality compared with other industrialized countries.
- ▼ Family-centered maternity care is important because it fosters a wellness orientation to childbirth, it is family focused, and it balances the use of technology in childbirth.

- ▼ Scientific discoveries and technologic advancement have led to improvement in maternal-newborn care for high-risk women.
- ▼ Current evidence does not support the routine use of technology for women with low-risk pregnancies.
- ▼ Health care reform will place increasing emphasis on primary, preventive, and community care.

References

Agency for Health Care Policy and Research. (May 1994). Women's health: Hospital statistics raise questions about obstetrical care. *Intramural Research Highlights.* No. 35. Hospital Cost and Utilization Project, Agency for Health Care Policy and Research. Rockville, MD: Public Health Service.

Allen, M. C., Donohue, P. K., Dusman, A. E. (1993). The limit of viability—neonatal outcome of infants born at 22 to 25 weeks' gestation. *New England Journal of Medicine,* 329 (22), 1597–1601.

American Nurses Association. (1983). *Standards of maternal and child health nursing practice.* Kansas City, MO: Author.

American Nurses Association. (1984–1985). *Issues in professional nursing practice: Legal authority for practice.* Kansas City, MO: Author.

American Nurses Association. (1985). *A statement on the scope of maternal and child health nursing practice.* Kansas City, MO: Author.

American Nurses Association. (1987). *The scope of nursing practice.* Kansas City, MO: Author.

American Nurses Association. (1991). *Nursing's agenda for health care reform.* Washington, D.C.: Author.

American Nurses Association. (1995). Nursing's social policy statement. Washington, D.C.: Author.

Andrist, L. (1988). Feminist framework for graduate education in women's health. *Journal of Nursing Education,* 27 (2), 66–70.

Arnold, L. S., Brecht, M. C., Hockett, A. B., Amspacher, K. A., Grad, R. K. (1989). Lessons from the past: A historical account of infant mortality in the United States provides useful background for judging current initiatives. *MCN,* 14, 75–82.

Avery, M. E. (1994). Changes in care of the newborn: Personal reflections over forty years. *Neonatal Network,* 13 (6), 13–14.

Bandman, E. L., and Bandman, B. (1988). *Critical thinking in nursing.* Norwalk, CT: Appleton & Lange.

Brackbill, Y., Rice, J., Young, D. (1984). *Birth trap: The legal low-down on high-tech obstetrics.* St. Louis: C. V. Mosby.

Burns, N., and Grove, S. K. (1993). *The practice of nursing research: Conduct, critique and utilization.* Philadelphia: W. B. Saunders.

Carpenito, L. J. (1995). *Nursing diagnosis: Application to clinical practice* (6th ed.). Philadelphia: J. B. Lippincott.

Carroll-Johnson, R. M. (1990). *Classification of nursing diagnoses: Proceedings of the eighth conference.* Philadelphia: J. B. Lippincott.

Chiarelli, M., and Nadon, F. (1985). Women and mental health: A feminist view. *Canadian Nurse,* 23–28.

Clark, M. J. (1996). *Nursing in the community* (2nd ed.). Norwalk, CT: Appleton & Lange.

Cohen, S. S. (1990). Overview of maternal-child health policies. In J. N. Natapoff, and R. R. Wieczorek (Eds.). *Maternal-child health policy: A nursing perspective* (pp. 17–56). New York: Springer.

Declercq, E. R. (1993). Where babies are born and who attends their births: Findings from the revised 1989 United States Standard Certificate of Live Birth. Merrimack College, North Andover, Massachusetts. *Obstetrics and Gynecology,* 81 (6), 997–1004.

Declercq, E. R., Paine, L. L., Winter, M. R. (1995). Home birth in the United States, 1989–1992. A longitudinal descriptive report of national birth certificate data. *Journal of Nurse-Midwifery,* 40 (6), 474–482.

Eakins, P. S. (1986). *Freestanding birth centers in California: Structure, cost, medical outcome, and issues.* California Department of Health Services.

Edwardson, S. R. (1985). Shedding light on a shifting marketplace: Competition in maternity care. *Nursing and Health Care,* 6, 73.

Ernst, E. (1988). Alternate site provider report: An update. *Health Industry Manufacturing Association.*

Etheredge, M. L. (1989). *Collaborative care: Nursing case management.* Chicago: American Hospital Publishing, Inc.

Fenwick, L. (1984). Birthing: Techniques for managing the physiologic and psychologic aspects of childbirth. *Perinatology-Neonatology,* 8 (3), 51–52, 55, 58–60.

Fuchs, Victor. (1983). *How we live.* Cambridge, MA: Harvard University Press.

Gennaro, S. (1988). The childbirth experience. In F. H. Nichols, and S. S. Humenick (Eds.). *Childbirth education: Practice, research and theory* (pp. 52–68). Philadelphia: W. B. Saunders.

Gerlach, C., and Schmid, M. (1986). Staffing a single-room maternity system. *Nurse Management,* 17 (8), 36–40.

Grad, R. K. (1989). National commission acts on behalf of children. *MCN,* 14, 237–242.

Grant, A. B. (1994). *The professional nurse.* Springhouse, PA: Springhouse Corporation.

Hack, M. A., and Fanaroff, A. A. (1993). Outcomes of extremely immature infants: A perinatal dilemma [Editorial]. *New England Journal of Medicine,* 329 (22), 1649–1650.

Hafner-Eaton, C., and Pearce, L. K. (1994). Birth choices, the law, and medicine: Balancing individual freedoms and protection of the public's health. *Journal of Health Politics, Policy and Law,* 19 (4), 813–835.

Hampton, D. C. (1993). Implementing a managed care framework through care maps. *Journal of Nursing Administration,* 23 (5), 21–27.

Humenick, S. (1994). Choice, the joy of childbirth, and epidurals. *The Journal of Perinatal Education,* 3 (4), 63–65.

International Task Force on Health Care of Women and Children. (1978). *Joint position statement on the development of family centered maternal-newborn care in hospitals.* Chicago: AACOG.

Jacobs, A. (1992). *Certification and accreditation law handbook.* Washington, D. C.: American Society of Association Executives.

Jones, L. C. (1989). Birth centers. *International Childbirth Education Association,* 13 (3), 1–6.

Kitzinger, S. (1991). *Homebirth: The essential guide to giving birth outside of the hospital.* New York: Kindersley.

Kitzinger, S. (1994). *The year after childbirth: Surviving and enjoying the first year of motherhood.* New York: Charles Scribner & Sons.

League of Women Voters Education Fund, The Henry J. Kaiser Family Foundation, and The Robert Woods Johnson Foundation. (September 1994). *Critical choices in health reform.* Washington, D. C.: Author.

Leavitt, J. W. (1986). *Brought to bed: Childbearing in America 1750–1950.* New York: Oxford University Press.

Lederer, J., Marculescu, G., Mocnik, B., Seaby, N. (1990). *Care planning pocket guide: A nursing diagnosis approach* (3rd ed.). Menlo Park, CA: Addison-Wesley.

Lederman, R. (1990). Infant mortality and prenatal care. In J. N. Natapoff, and R. R. Wieczorek (Eds.). *Maternal-child health policy: A nursing perspective* (pp. 99–130). New York: Springer.

Lemrow, N., Adams, D., Coffey, R., Farley, D. (September 1990). *The 50 most frequent diagnosis-related groups (DRGs), diagnoses and procedures: Statistics by hospital size and location.* (DHHS Publication No [PHS] 90-3465). Hospital Studies Program Research Note 13, Agency for Health Care Policy and Research. Rockville, MD: Public Health Service.

Lindberg, J. B., Hunter, M. L., Kruszewski, A. Z. (1990). *Introduction to nursing: Concepts, issues and opportunities.* Philadelphia: J. B. Lippincott.

Lindell, S. G. (1988). Education for childbirth: A time for change. *Journal of Obstetric, Gynecologic, and Neonatal Nursing,* 17 (2), 108–112.

Mayers, M. G. (1993). *A systematic approach to the nursing care plan.* Norwalk, CT: Appleton-Century-Crofts.

McBride, A. (1976). *Living with contraindications. A married feminist.* New York: Harper.

McBride, A. (1982). The American way of birth. In M. Kay (Ed.). *An anthropology of human birth* (pp. 413–429). Philadelphia: F. A. Davis.

McCartney, M., and van der Meer, A. (1991). *The midwife's pregnancy and childbirth book: Having your baby your way.* New York: Harper Perennial.

McGrath, E. (1991). Women and depression: Report of the national task force. *Harvard Mental Health Letter,* 8 (5), 4–6.

Mechanic, H. F. (1988). Redefining the expanded role. *Nursing Outlook,* 36 (6), 280–284.

Miller, C. A. (1985). Infant mortality in the U.S. *Scientific American,* 253 (1), 31–37.

Nurses Association of the American College of Obstetricians and Gynecologists (NAACOG), and Neonatal Nurses Committee on Practice. (1989). *OGN nursing practice resources: Nursing diagnosis.* Washington, D.C.: Author.

Nurses Association of the American College of Obstetricians and Gynecologists (NAACOG). (1991). *Standards for the nursing care of women and newborns* (4th ed.). Washington, D.C.: Author.

National Center for Health Statistics (NCHS). (January 1992). *Monthly Vital Statistics Report,* Supplement, 40 (8), S2.

National Center for Health Statistics (NCHS). (August 31, 1993). Advance report of final mortality statistics, 1991. *Monthly Vital Statistics Report,* 42 (Suppl. 2), S11, S12.

National Center for Health Statistics. (September 21, 1995). Advance report of final natality statistics, 1993. *Monthly Vital Statistics Report,* 44 (Suppl. 3), S1–S88.

National Commission to Prevent Infant Mortality. (1988). *Death before life: The tragedy of infant mortality.* Washington, D.C.: Author.

National Nursing Summit. (October 1993). National nursing summit unites organizations and targets key issues for health care reform. *The American Nurse,* 25, 8.

Nichols, F. (1993). Issues in perinatal education. *AWHONN's Clinical Issues in Perinatal and Women's Health Nursing: Perinatal Education,* 4 (1), 55–59.

North American Nursing Diagnosis Association. (1994). *NANDA nursing diagnoses: Definitions and classification 1995–1996.* Philadelphia: Author.

Phillips, C. R. (1988). Rehumanizing maternal-child nursing. *MCN,* 13, 313–318.

Phillips, C. R. (1989). Contemporary approaches to the labor process. In J. S. Malinowski, C. G. Pedigo, C. R. Phillips (Eds.). *Nursing care during the labor process* (3rd ed.)(pp. 232–271). St. Louis, C. V. Mosby.

Popkess-Vawter, S. (1991). Wellness nursing diagnosis: To be or not to be. *Journal of the North American Nursing Diagnosis Association,* 2 (1), 19–25.

Public Health Service. (1979). *Healthy people: The surgeon general's report on health promotion and disease prevention.* Washington, D.C.: U.S. Department of Health and Human Services.

Public Health Service. (1990). *Healthy people 2000: National health promotion and disease prevention objectives.* Washington, D.C.: U.S. Department of Health and Human Services.

Russo, N. F. (1990). Overview: Forging research priorities for women's mental health. *American Psychologist,* 45 (3), 368–373.

Sampselle, C. M. (1991). The role of nursing in preventing violence against women. *Journal of Obstetric, Gynecologic, and Neonatal Nursing,* 20 (6), 481–487.

Sharp, N. (1990). Women's health equity act of 1990. *Nursing Management,* 21 (12), 21–22.

Spradley, B. (1991). Readings in community health nursing (4th ed.). Philadelphia: J. B. Lippincott.

Starn, J., and Niederhauser, V. (1990). An MCN model for nursing diagnosis to focus intervention. *American Journal of Maternal-Child Nursing,* 15, 180–183.

Steinfels, M. O. (February 1978). New childbirth technology: A clash of values. *Hastings Center Report,* 8, 9.

Stevens, K. (1988). Nursing diagnosis in wellness childbearing settings. *Journal of Obstetric, Gynecologic and Neonatal Nursing,* 17 (5), 329–336.

Stolte, K. M. (1986). Nursing diagnosis and the childbearing woman. *American Journal of Maternal-Child Nursing,* 11, 13–15.

Thompson, D. G. (1994). Critical pathways in the intensive care and intermediate care nurseries. *MSN,* 19 (January/February), 29–32.

U. S. Department of Health and Human Services. (1995). *Healthy people 2000: Midcourse review and 1995 revisions.* Washington, D.C.: Author.

Walker, L. O. (1992). *Parent-infant nursing science: Paradigms, phenomena, methods.* Philadelphia: F. A. Davis.

Wallace, H. M. (1988). Infant Mortality. In H. M. Wallace, G. Ryan, A. C. Oglesby (Eds.). *Maternal and child health practice* (3rd ed.)(pp. 411–426). Oakland, CA: Third Party Publishers.

Wegman, M. E. (1992). Annual summary of vital statistics—1991. *Pediatrics,* 90 (6), 835–845.

Wegman, M. E. (1994). Annual summary of vital statistics—1993. *Pediatrics,* 94 (6), 792–803.

Wilkerson, N., and Barrows, T. L. (1988). Reuniting mothers and babies: Synchronizing care with mother-baby rhythms. *The American Journal of Maternal-Child Nursing,* 13, 264–268.

Yura, H., and Walsh, M. (1988). *The nursing process: Assessing, planning, implementing, evaluating* (5th ed.). Norwalk, CT: Appleton & Lange.

Zander, K. (1991). CareMaps: The core of cost/quality-care. *The New Definition,* 6 (3), 1–3.

Zander, K. (1992). Quantifying, managing, and improving quality: How CareMaps link CQI to the patient. *The New Definition,* 7 (2), 1–3.

Chapter 3

Roles of the Maternal-Newborn Nurse

Linda Goodwin
Francine H. Nichols

> This is a dynamic time. Rapid changes present new challenges—and new career opportunities—for nurses. Now is the time when we can recapture the art and science of nursing and can improve and enrich the lives of our patients.
>
> LORNA M. FACTEAU (1996)

HIGHLIGHTS

- Today's Health Care Environment
- Careers in Maternal-Newborn Nursing
- Role Dimensions
- Implications for Research

Today's health care environment is distinctively different from that of the past. The increasing emphasis on health care reform, cost-effective treatment, shorter or eliminated hospital stays, and improved quality of care has changed *where* health care is delivered, *how* it is delivered, and *by whom* it is delivered (Cassetta 1994; Ketter 1994; Mattera 1994). Changes in health care delivery in the 1990s have resulted in significant alterations in the traditional approach to career pathways for nurses. Nurses in maternal-newborn nursing are faced with a rapidly changing work environment and a limited number of positions in the acute care hospital setting—the predominant work setting for maternal-newborn nurses of the past. However, today, there are many new and challenging opportunities in community, clinic, and outpatient settings for maternal-newborn nurses.

In a study during 1990–1991 to determine maternal-newborn nurses' perceptions about changes in maternity care and the impact of these changes on practice, Stolte and colleagues (1994) found eight most frequently reported changes. As ordered by the report, these were increased use of technology, increased emphasis on the legal aspects of care, shorter patient stays, increased emphasis on cost containment, increased involvement of the family in the birth process, cross-training so that the nurse could function in multiple maternal-newborn areas (labor and delivery, nursery, postpartum period), increased consumer demand for childbirth education and childbirth options, and implementation of single-room maternity care (Fig. 3–1).

DEFINITIONS

Acute care—Health care services provided within the hospital setting.

Advanced practice—Nurses with advanced education in specialty areas within maternal-newborn nursing: nurse-midwife, nurse practitioner, and clinical nurse specialist.

Ambulatory care—Health care services provided within clinics and outpatient settings.

Case management—Health care management that uses individuals to determine the necessity of services for clients and then to authorize necessary services.

Certified nurse-midwife—A registered nurse who has specialized training to care for women during pregnancy and childbirth and who is certified by the American College of Nurse-Midwives.

Consultant—An individual with expertise in a specialized area who provides advice and recommendations.

Entrepreneur—An individual who undertakes a business venture.

Executive—A manager or administrator.

Home care—Health care services that are provided within the client's home.

Role dimensions—The components of a role. Core dimensions are those components that are always present in the maternal-newborn nursing role. Functional dimensions may be present, depending on a specific role of the maternal-newborn nurse.

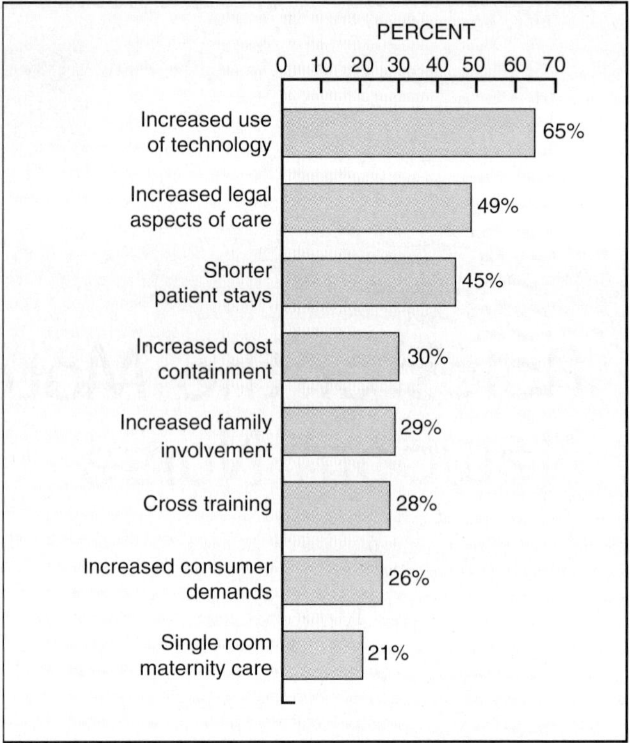

Figure 3–1

The eight most frequently mentioned changes in maternity care as reported in a survey of maternal-newborn nurses, 1990–1991. (Data from Stolte, K., Myers, S. T., Owen, W. L. [1994]. Changes in maternity care and the impact on nurses and nursing practice. *Journal of Obstetric, Gynecologic, and Neonatal Nursing,* 23 [7], 603–608.)

CAREERS IN MATERNAL-NEWBORN NURSING

Change will continue to be a constant factor in maternal-newborn nursing. Nursing practice will be altered as maternal-newborn nurses and other health care providers find new and improved methods of delivering care. Nursing practice must also respond to initiatives in the health care system as well as to consumer demands. Nurses can choose among maternal-newborn nursing careers in acute care hospital, ambulatory care, home care, or advanced practice settings; they may serve as case managers, executives in health care agencies or businesses, consultants, nursing educators, scientists, and entrepreneurs; or they may work in international health-related positions (Fig. 3–2).

Acute Care

Registered nurses have traditionally practiced almost exclusively in the acute care hospital setting, especially as new graduates. This acute care experience has been considered an essential basis for practice in alternative settings, such as outpatient clinics, schools, and business. Extended orientation and internship programs have been provided by hospitals to promote the success of the novice nurse, and employment opportunities have always been abundant for new graduates in the acute care hospital setting. In the past, a lifelong career as a hospital nurse was a realistic expectation (Fig. 3–3); choosing an alternative setting for career development as a nurse was considered innovative and, perhaps, risky.

Today, opportunities in the acute care setting are decreasing, and registered nurses must look to

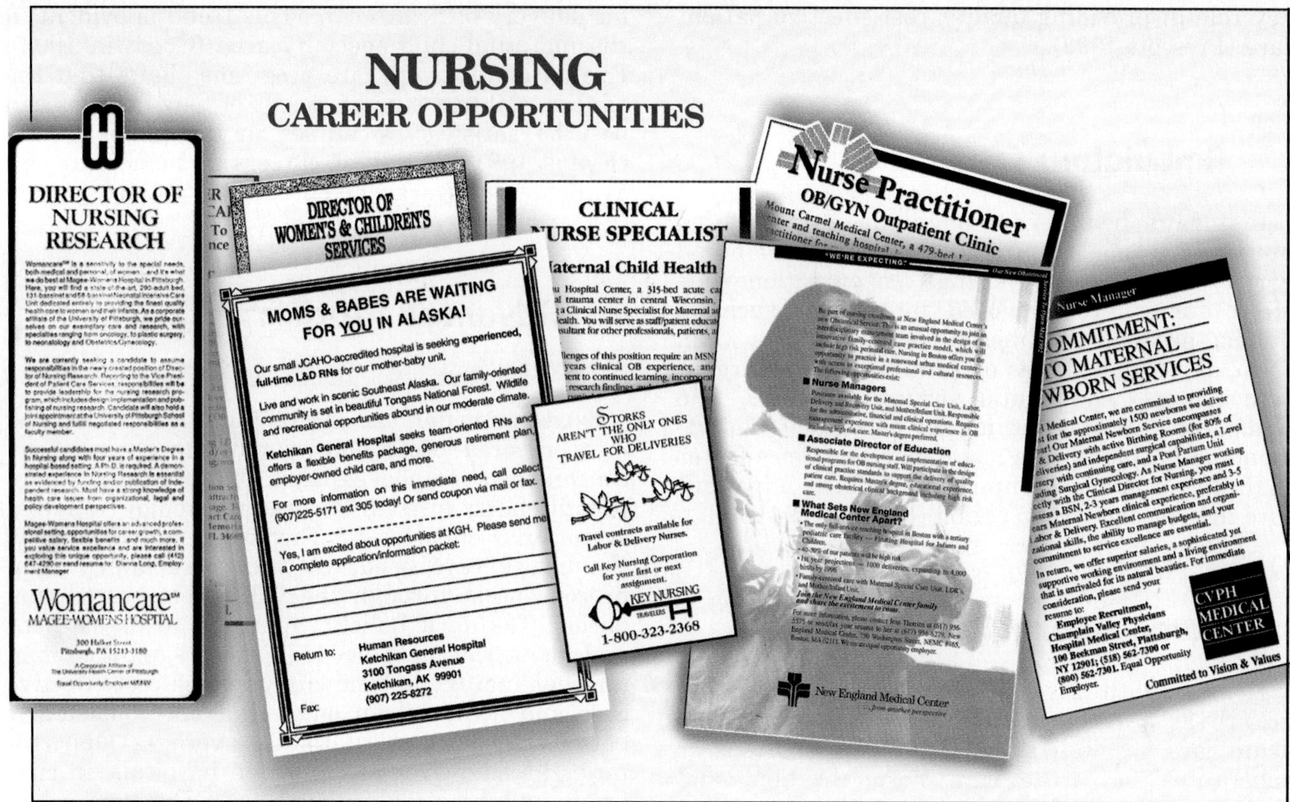

Figure 3–2

Myriad career opportunities are available in maternal-newborn nursing.

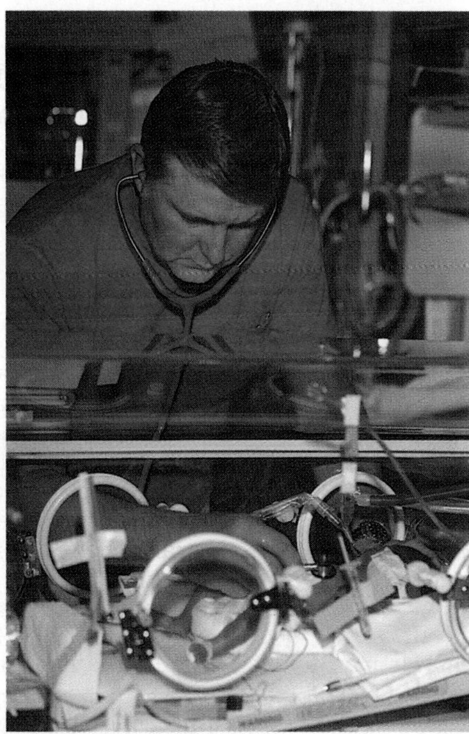

Figure 3–3

Maternal-newborn nurses will continue to play important roles in providing nursing care in vital acute care areas, such as neonatal intensive care units.

alternative career choices. A 1994 survey of 640 nurses revealed that only 12 percent of their hospitals hired new graduates in the usual numbers during the previous year, 54 percent hired fewer than usual, and 32 percent hired no new graduates (Meissner and Carey 1994). New graduates and practicing nurses may choose to view this trend as a problem or as an opportunity.

Because of cost reduction mandates, insurance providers demonstrate increasing unwillingness to pay for prolonged hospitalization; they promote outpatient, short stay, and home care and other alternative services through case management and reimbursement plans. The acute care hospitals will not continue to be the primary employers of registered nurses. Predictions are that acute care admissions will continue to decrease and that one in ten U.S. hospitals will close its doors by the year 2000 (Hurley 1994). Outpatient staff numbers increased by 66 percent in a recent year while hospital staff increased by only 6 percent (Division of Nursing 1992). Nurses who do remain in the inpatient setting will be cross-trained to provide care in at least one additional clinical area and will increase job security by being able to move throughout the hospital, thus enabling hospitals to accommodate patient census fluctuations. In the acute care setting, nurses will play a key role in providing quality, cost-effective patient care (Prescott 1993).

Ambulatory Care

In today's health care environment, registered nurses have opportunities for careers in a broad variety of outpatient settings. In outpatient services, nurses are employed in settings such as public, private, and hospital-based clinics (Fig. 3–4); day surgery units or surgical centers; urgent care centers; and dental surgery practices. The number of nurses working in outpatient departments of hospitals rose more than ten times faster than the number of nurses delivering inpatient care in a recent 4-year period (Hurley 1994).

Home Health Care

Home health care is experiencing significant growth as a result of the movement away from acute care hospitalization. Home care shortens or substitutes for acute care hospitalization, and there is a clear trend toward use of home services for delivery of health care. This trend is evident in the maternal-child specialty area (Goodwin 1992). Evaluation of home care programs shows that the educational and support needs of new families can best be satisfied by nurses in the home setting (Evans 1991). Excellent careers in home care are available to nurses who choose this option.

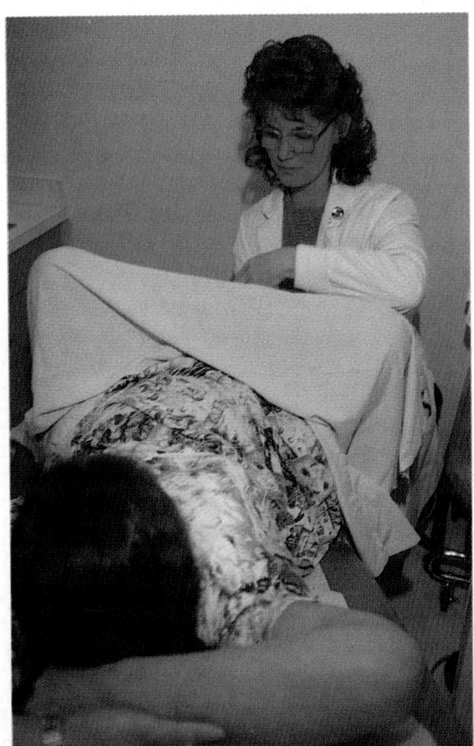

Figure 3–4
An increasing number of maternal-newborn nurses will work in ambulatory care settings and provide prenatal care and other outpatient services. This nurse practitioner is doing a vaginal examination of a prenatal client.

Advanced Practice

NURSE-MIDWIFERY

Nurse-midwifery is one of nursing's oldest and most revered professions. As health care reform continues to emphasize the role of primary care practitioners, nurse-midwives will enjoy renewed status and opportunity. The nurse-midwife meets the health care needs of the entire family from preconception through the vulnerable postpartum period. Taking a holistic approach to assessment and identification of needs of the pregnant woman and her family, the midwife provides cost-effective care and achieves outcomes that are consistently better than national statistical averages. Opportunities for midwives are found in hospitals, in clinics, in collaborative practices with obstetrician-gynecologists, and in independent practice in some states.

NURSE PRACTITIONER

The nurse practitioner role has enjoyed new status as a result of health care reform in the 1990s. There is substantial evidence that when nurses provide primary care to appropriate clients, money is saved (Finkler and Kovner 1993). As primary care providers, family nurse practitioners and neonatal nurse practitioners will be in demand in this new world of wellness-focused, cost-effective care. Increased funding for the education of nurse practitioners will most likely become available as a result of health care reform. Those advanced practice nurses who agree to work in underserved rural and urban areas after graduation may receive tax benefits and other incentives (Hurley 1994).

CLINICAL NURSE SPECIALIST

The clinical nurse specialist (CNS) is a master's-prepared nurse who is an expert in a specific clinical area (Hamric and Spross 1989). The primary focus of the CNS is on improving nursing practice in a particular area of clinical practice through evaluating nursing practice, making recommendations to improve nursing practice, establishing standards of care, and conducting research studies (Mitchell and Grippando 1993). The CNS has

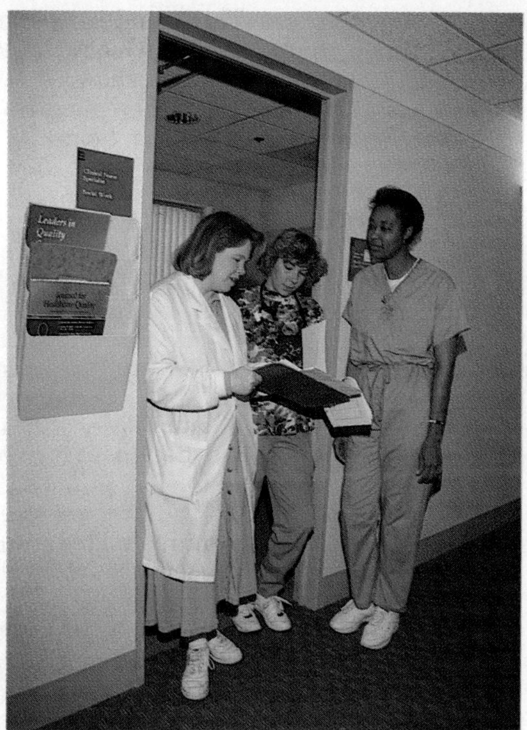

Figure 3–5
The clinical nurse specialist focuses on evaluating and improving nursing practice in the clinical area. Here a clinical nurse specialist and two staff nurses are discussing the plan of care for a new mother.

played an important role in improving nursing practice and implementing changes in maternal-newborn nursing (Fig. 3–5).

Case Manager

In managed care, a designated person, usually called a case manager, acts as an intermediary between patients and providers of services. Providers are people and organizations that perform health care services. Traditional providers include physicians, nurses, and hospitals. The case manager is employed by the payer (the individual or organization that will pay for the services). The case manager functions as a gatekeeper by determining necessity of services for patients and then authorizing the services considered to be indicated. Reimbursement, or payment for the services, usually depends on prior authorization by the case manager. The major goal of managed care is to decrease cost by eliminating unnecessary services; however, case managers also ensure that patients receive appropriate and timely care (Finkler and Kovner 1993). Managed care will continue to expand as an integral part of cost containment in health care. The future will bring excellent career opportunities for registered nurses in this new role of case manager.

Executive in Health Care Management

A career as an executive in health care is a traditional nursing role and will continue to exist. Nurse executives will practice as supervisors of units; vice-presidents and presidents of nursing in health care agencies will provide administrative leadership and supervision for nursing and other services. Because of today's health care climate, nurse executives in health care settings will increasingly be challenged to balance quality and cost toward achieving the ultimate goal of cost-effective care—a difficult task at best.

Nurses today also find opportunities for executive careers outside traditional health care in corporations or businesses. Examples of such business practice settings are positions with medical equipment and supply companies, advertising and media agencies, sales and marketing departments for medical equipment and pharmaceutical vendors, and nurse recruiter agencies; maternal-newborn education for nonprofit agencies and corporations that make products in the maternal-newborn area; and clinical application specialists for medical equipment companies.

Educator

Maternal-newborn nurses are educators in all practice venues. They may specialize in this area as clinical educators for staff, as perinatal educators focusing on childbirth education, as lactation consultants, and as academics. The role of educator in the area of maternal-newborn nursing can be expected to increase in response to the increasing emphasis on preventive health care and health education.

Scientist

Increasingly, nurses are assuming roles as scientists in departments of research at health care agencies and corporations that produce health care products. Nurses working as scientists in health care agencies provide leadership and direction in developing and conducting research studies in the clinical area. In corporations, nurses practicing as scientists are usually involved in evaluating the design and effectiveness of products.

They may also be involved in product development.

Consultant

Nurses who develop expertise in a selected area of nursing may choose the consultant's role as a career option. As a consultant, the nurse uses specific expertise to make observations and assessments and then provide problem identification and recommendations. The ultimate choice for action and implementation of the selected plan remains the responsibility of the individual or organization that employs that consultant. A nurse may choose a full-time career as a consultant or may supplement both income and interest by working on short-term projects that complement other commitments. Examples of consultant roles include technical review of patient instruction materials to accompany a medical product; review of medical records to provide expert opinions for legal purposes; product design and development for corporations that develop products in the maternal-newborn area; and work with a health care agency to evaluate the current status of nursing practice, then planning and recommending approaches to improve it. Indeed, maternal-newborn nurse consultants have played a pivotal role in assisting agencies to implement the single-room maternity care concept.

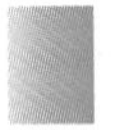

Entrepreneur

An entrepreneur is someone who undertakes a business venture. Nurse entrepreneurs have found small business opportunities as independent nurse practitioners who see patients on a fee-for-service basis; nurse owners of home health, temporary employment agencies or equipment rental companies; continuing education providers; and independent nurse consultants. A well-conceived and detailed business plan is essential for success in any business venture. The entrepreneur with sufficient business management skill to create and implement a business plan can achieve financial success and job satisfaction; however, an uninformed approach to any business venture may result in financial misfortune or entanglement in regulatory red tape leading to unwelcome litigation. Knowledge and skills necessary for entrepreneurship can be gained in college or private classes and seminars, through self-study, by employing a consultant, and through experience as an employee or supervisor in a successful small business. Nurses who accept this challenge will realize long hours, hard work, and other sobering realities of the business world, but success can be achieved through prudent business management (Goodwin 1994).

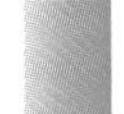

International Health Care

International health care is an exciting and challenging area in which highly skilled nurses are vitally needed and greatly valued. The maternal-newborn nurse who chooses to work in a developing country encounters daily challenges in determining how to provide quality health care to underserved populations with scarce resources and primitive facilities. A number of organizations have short- and long-term international health care opportunities for the maternal-newborn nurse.

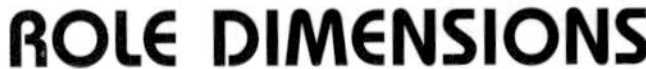

ROLE DIMENSIONS

The role of the maternal-newborn nurse has several dimensions. Three core dimensions run through every role of the nurse regardless of the setting in which a nurse practices: expertise, critical thinking, and problem solving. Seven functional dimensions of the maternal-newborn nursing role vary in degree, depending on the setting and position in which the nurse practices. These are advocate, caregiver, educator, manager, change agent, political activist, and researcher (Walker, L., and Nichols, F. H., 1994, unpublished manuscript). The core and functional dimensions of the maternal-newborn nursing role are described in Table 3–1.

Implications for Research

Nursing is in the midst of a transition as health care moves out of the acute care hospital and into the community, clinic, surgical center, home, and school. Research in the following areas will assist nursing to skillfully navigate through this transition, improve client care, and turn challenges into opportunities:

- What are the biggest problems that nurses face in the changing health care environment?

Table 3–1

DIMENSIONS OF THE MATERNAL-NEWBORN NURSE'S ROLE

The role of the maternal-newborn nurse has three core dimensions that are always present and seven functional dimensions.

CORE DIMENSIONS

Core dimensions are those elements that are always present in the maternal-newborn nurse's role. The three core dimensions are expertise, critical thinking, and problem solving.

Dimension	Characteristic
Expertise	The ability to intuitively understand the situation and make accurate diagnoses and decisions rapidly; expertise develops through experiential and theoretical knowledge in a specific area of practice
Critical thinking	The ability to analyze a situation, belief, or argument using scientific reasoning and to choose a course of action from alternatives available
Problem solving	The ability to accurately identify and evaluate a problem, select an approach and take action, and evaluate the outcome

FUNCTIONAL DIMENSIONS

Functional dimensions are those elements of the maternal-newborn nurse's role that may or may not be present and vary in degreee, depending on the setting and position in which the maternal-newborn nurse practices. The seven functional dimensions are advocate, caregiver, educator, manager, change agent, political activist, and researcher.

Dimension	Characteristic
Advocate	The act of defending or pleading for the cause of another; the nurse is an advocate for the patient, in the area of health and social policy, and for the profession of nursing
Caregiver	The act of providing physical or psychological nursing care, comfort, and support to promote optimal health for clients and their families
Educator	The act of providing information and teaching skills based on needs of the clients and their families
Manager	The act of controlling, directing, or guiding nursing care
Change agent	The act of bringing about desired change in a positive manner using planned approaches based on theories of change
Political activist	The act of influencing political and legislative activities in the area of health and social policy related to improving health of clients and their families
Researcher	The act of being involved in research related to improving nursing care in the area of maternal-newborn nursing

From Walker, L., and Nichols, F. H. (1994). Dimensions of the maternal-newborn nursing role. Unpublished manuscript.

- What solutions have nurses used effectively to solve problems?
- What are the most important skills that nurses need to practice effectively in alternative settings in the community?

The findings from well-designed research studies will provide nurses with information that can be used to design nursing's future.

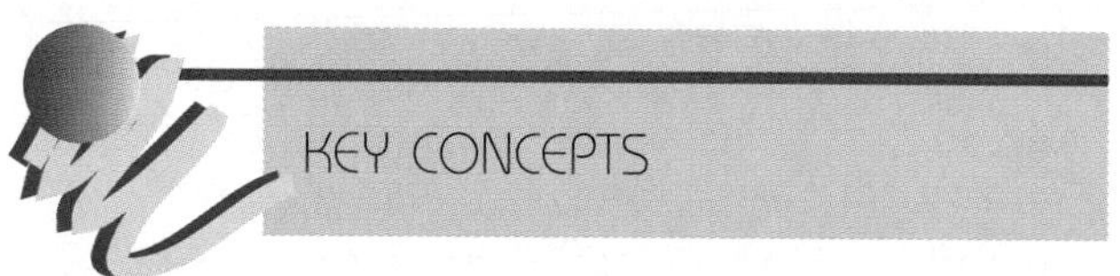

▼ Changes in health care delivery in the 1990s have resulted in significant alterations in the traditional career pathways for registered nurses.

- Nursing practice must change in response to health care system changes and consumer demands. Nursing practice will also change as maternal-newborn nurses find new and improved methods for providing nursing care.
- Acute care hospitals will not continue to be the primary employers of registered nurses. Today, registered nurses must look to alternative career choices.
- In today's health care environment, registered nurses have opportunities for careers in a broad variety of ambulatory care settings.
- Home health care in the maternal-child specialty area is an expanding practice environment.
- Careers for advanced practice nurses, such as nurse-midwives and nurse practitioners, will continue to increase.
- The future will bring excellent career opportunities for registered nurses in the role of case manager in this era of managed care.
- Traditional careers as executives, administrators, and managers in health care agencies will continue to exist. Nurses will find opportunities for careers outside the traditional acute care setting as executives for corporations and businesses.
- Nurses who develop expertise in a specialized area of nursing may choose the consultant's role as a career option.
- An increasing number of nurses are becoming entrepreneurs and are setting up their own business ventures.
- International health care is an exciting and challenging area in which highly skilled nurses are vitally needed and greatly valued.

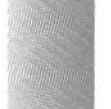

References

Cassetta, R. A. (1994). The future holds open doors for nursing opportunities. *Directions: A Supplement to the American Nurse,* October, 4.

Division of Nursing. (1992). *National sample survey of registered nurses.* Washington, D.C.: Bureau of Health Professions, U.S. Department of Health and Human Services.

Evans, C. (1991). Description of a home follow-up program for childbearing families. *Journal of Obstetric, Gynecologic, and Neonatal Nursing,* 20 (2), 113–118.

Facteau, L. M. (1996). Director, Center for Clinical Education and Development, Fairfax Hospital, Falls Church, VA.

Finkler, S. A., and Kovner, C. T. (1993). *Financial management for nurse managers and executives.* Philadelphia: W. B. Saunders.

Goodwin, L. (1992). Home fetal assessment. *Journal of Perinatal and Neonatal Nursing,* 5 (4), 33–45.

Goodwin, L. (1994). Essential program components for perinatal home care. *Journal of Obstetric, Gynecologic, and Neonatal Nursing,* 23 (8), 667–673.

Hamric, A. B., and Spross, J. A. (1989). *The clinical nurse specialist in theory and practice.* Philadelphia: W. B. Saunders.

Hurley, M. L. (1994). Where will you work tomorrow? *RN,* 57 (8), 31–35.

Ketter, J. (1994). Restructuring: Affecting the workforce and workplace for new grads. *Directions: A Supplement to the American Nurse,* October, 4.

Mattera, M. D. (1994). Editor's memo: On options. *RN,* 57 (8), 7.

Meissner, J. E., and Carey, K. W. (1994). How's your job security? *Nursing 94,* 24 (7), 33–38.

Mitchell, P. R., and Grippando, G. M. (1993). *Nursing perspectives and issues* (5th ed.). Albany, NY: Delmar Publishers.

Prescott, P. A. (1993). Nursing: An important component of hospital survival under a reformed health care system. *Nursing Economics,* 11 (4), 192.

Stolte, K., Myers, S. T., Owen, W. L. (1994). Changes in maternity care and the impact on nurses and nursing practice. *Journal of Obstetric, Gynecologic, and Neonatal Nursing,* 23 (7), 603–608.

Chapter 4

Family Dynamics

Susan F. Kruger
Francine H. Nichols

> The childbearing year is a psychosocial transition that involves changes in role and status for each member of the family. The change is perhaps most significant in the transition that occurs with the birth of the first child. . . . This time is an opportunity to strengthen family systems through anticipatory guidance and skill building that family members may use throughout the life cycle.
>
> JANE STARN (1993)

HIGHLIGHTS

- Changes in the American Family
- Types of Families
- The Childbearing Family
- The Adoptive Family
- Selected Family Theories
- Factors Influencing Families
- The Family's Influence on Health
- The Family as Caregiver
- Family Assessment
- Families with Special Needs
- Nursing Practice
- National Family Policy
- Implications for Research

Since Florence Nightingale's time, the family has been a focus of nursing practice (Whall and Fawcett 1991). A family is the basic economic and social unit for the care of children, and the health and welfare of individual family members are significantly influenced by this unit. Within families, bloodlines are neither necessary nor sufficient. What matters is that individuals assume responsibility for the nurturing of children's intellectual, moral, emotional, and physical development (Mahoney 1986).

During the perinatal period, multiple roles and relationship changes within the family emerge that place stressors on the family unit. These stressors may lead to a socioemotional crisis in some families, but most families perceive these same stressors as a life transition. The maternal-newborn nurse provides family-centered care to promote optimal functioning for the individual and for the family as a unit. Interventions are designed to address needs at the individual level, interpersonal level, family system level, and environmental level (Cooley 1995). The pregnant woman and her family will benefit from support and guidance while coping with life's challenges encountered during the perinatal period.

DEFINITIONS

Boundary—Filters both the kind and rate of inputs and outputs to and from the system.

Closed family system—A family system with strong boundaries that is mostly resistant to inputs from the environment. There is minimal processing of information by the family and minimal feedback to the environment.

Executive subsystem—The governing family members, usually the parents.

Extended family—A family group that includes at least three generations of individuals related by blood or marriage.

Family—A group of individuals related by blood, marriage, or mutual goals.

Family Systems Theory—Within this theory, the family is viewed as an open, ongoing interaction system in which every member influences the family system and is influenced by it.

Input—Products, events, or series of events that are brought into the system.

Open family system—A family system with permeable boundaries that allows information to enter the system; the family is open to information from the environment. The information is processed (throughput) by the family and then provided as feedback (output) to the environment.

Output—The product of throughput, given off the system; feedback.

Random or weak family system—A family system with diffuse boundaries. Any and all information enters into this system. The family fails to process the information adequately, and the information may easily or may not at all influence the family system.

Social Exchange Theory—This theory is derived from economic theories and is based on the premise that the interaction between persons in the family is an exchange of goods, material and nonmaterial.

Subsystem—Each family member belongs to a subsystem within the family system.

Symbolic Interaction Theory—A family theory based on the broader interactionist perspective that uses concepts to illustrate the internal processes that occur within individuals and families. The basic concepts include mind, self, and society.

System—A set of elements (family members) interacting with each other within a boundary.

Throughput—Input is processed, organized, and transformed.

THE AMERICAN FAMILY

The changes that have occurred in family units throughout the years have influenced the definition of families. The traditional view of the family composed of father, mother, and children, with the father assuming the role of breadwinner and the mother the role of homemaker, no longer characterizes the majority of American families. A more relevant definition in today's society is the family as a group of individuals related by blood, marriage, or mutual goals. There are numerous definitions of family in the literature. Feetham (1984) states that it is not essential to have a single definition of family. However, in reading a research report, it is important to understand how family is defined in that particular study.

Current statistics show a decline in births in the United States. In 1993, just more than 4 million babies were born (a 4 percent decrease from the most recent high in 1990); provisional data for 1994 indicate a continued decline of about 1 percent (National Center for Health Statistics [NCHS] 1995). A continued decline in birth rates for women in the peak childbearing years (represented by those aged 20 to 24 and 25 to 29 years) as well as for older teenagers (18 to 19 years) is projected. Also, increases in births to young teens (15 to 17 years) and Hispanic teens (15 to 19 years) due to the growing proportion of these groups in the population are expected. The projected continued increase in births to women aged 40 to 44 years (6 percent between 1992 and 1993) reflects the combined effect of a 3 percent increase in the birth rate and a 2 percent increase in the number of women in this age group (NCHS 1995) (see also Chapter 2).

Data on marital status are reported on birth certificates in 44 states and the District of Columbia. In the six states that do not track marital status directly, such statistics are inferred from comparison of the mother and child's surname—not an exact method today when mothers often retain their maiden name. The number of babies born to unmarried women in 1993 has been reported as approximately 31 percent (1,240,172) (NCHS 1995). Of that number, approximately 30 percent (357,432) were born to teens (15 to 19 years), approximately 54 percent (672,314) to women in the peak childbearing years (20 to 29 years), and approximately 16 percent (198,959) to women older than 30 years (Table 4–1) (see also Chapter 39).

The period of gestation and low birth weight have been closely linked with poor outcomes in newborns. Eleven percent of all births were preterm (less than 37 weeks of gestation completed) in 1993, a 3 percent increase above the level in 1992. Low birth weight (less than 2500 g), while at its highest reported level since 1976, increased only slightly above 1992 rates to 7.2 percent. Interestingly, the level for singleton births was virtually unchanged from 1980 to 1993 (5.96 compared with 6.01 percent), while the overall low birth weight rose from 6.8 to 7.2 percent (NCHS 1995). Abnormal conditions and congenital anomalies are closely associated with prematurity and low birth weight. In 1993, approximately 4 percent of births (149,499) had abnormal conditions including anemia, birth injury, fetal alcohol syndrome, hyaline membrane disease, and others; reporting states recorded 1 percent of births (40,749) with congenital anomalies ranging from anencephaly to Down syndrome to cleft lip-palate (see also Chapters 36 and 37).

Changes in the American Family

In the past four decades, the structure of the American family has changed radically. Some sociologists now claim that there is no such thing as a "typical" American family ("The Changing American Family" 1991).

Major changes in today's family include the rapid increase of single-parent families; blended families when remarriage occurs; and other nontraditional family forms, such as lesbian and gay families. The number of mothers working outside the home has soared and is expected to continue to increase. There has been a dramatic decrease in the size of families and a sharp increase in annual divorce rates.

Etzioni (1977) projected that if the reported decline in the traditional family continued, traditional families would cease to exist within a generation. He encouraged the study of the effects of divorce, remarriage, societal attitudes, public policy, and educational efforts on the future of the family. Gaylin (1980), however, discouraged viewing the family as a decaying institution and advocated evaluating emerging family structures so that strategies could be developed to enable all families to meet their potential. According to researchers at the University of Minnesota's Humphrey Institute for Public Policy, the possibility for new changes in family structure to occur at the same spiraling rate as during the past 30 years is low (Ahlburg and DeVita 1993).

Table 4–1

BIRTHS TO UNMARRIED WOMEN IN THE UNITED STATES, 1993

	RATE PER 1000 UNMARRIED WOMEN IN SPECIFIED GROUP			
AGE OF MOTHER	All Races	White	Black	Hispanic
All ages	45.3	35.9	84.0	95.2
15–19	44.5	33.6	102.4	74.7
20–24	69.2	54.2	142.2	140.5
25–29	57.1	46.7	94.5	137.7
30–34	38.5	32.2	57.3	90.9
35–39	19.0	16.4	25.9	47.8
40 and older	4.4	3.9	5.8	14.1

Adapted from National Center for Health Statistics. (1995). Advanced report of final natality statistics, 1993. *Monthly Vital Statistics Report,* 44 (Suppl. 3, Sep 21, Table 14, S47).

INCREASE IN WORKING MOTHERS

One of the most dramatic changes in families during the past 20 years is the steady increase of mothers in the paid labor force. In 1991, 60 percent of all mothers worked outside the home, and the number of mothers in the workforce continues to climb each year ("The Changing American Family" 1991).

The percentage of mothers with children younger than 6 years in the paid workforce increased from 32 percent in 1970 to 58 percent in 1990 (Fig. 4–1). Mothers whose youngest child was between 6 and 17 years were even more likely (65 percent) to be in the paid labor force in 1990. In that same year, among employed mothers, 74 percent of mothers whose youngest child was between 6 and 17 years were employed full-time, while 70 percent of mothers whose youngest child was younger than 6 years were also employed full-time. Those women who are most likely to be employed in the paid labor force after they become mothers are women who wait until after 25 years of age to have their first baby and women with 4 years or more of college (National Commission on Children 1991).

Because mothers have been the traditional caregivers for their children, the increasing employment of mothers has critical implications for the care of children. Resources from outside the home are needed and must be drawn into the family constellation to care for the children and supplement the ability to meet family needs as a result of the decreased time resources and available energy of the working mother. In this situation, the family can be viewed as consisting of important outside persons, such as the babysitter who may be a grandmother, neighbor, or daycare worker (Harris et al. 1981). While society's ability to adjust and meet the changing needs of working mother, working father, and their children is crucial to the health and well-being of families and children, needed changes in the workplace and communities have to date been slow to occur (National Commission on Children 1991).

DECREASING FAMILY SIZE

Today, on the average, families are smaller than they were in the 1950s. Women are having fewer children, and the fertility rate (the number of live births per 1000 women 15 to 44 years old) has decreased from the mid-1950s to 1992 by close to half, from 122.7 to 68.9. "The total fertility rate is a measure that indicates how many births 1,000 women would have if they experienced throughout their childbearing years the set of age-specific birth rates observed in a given calendar year. It is a hypothetical measure that shows the implications of current fertility levels for completed family size. The total fertility rate is age adjusted because it is computed from age-specific birth rates; it assumes the same number of women in each age group" (National Center for Health Statistics 1993, p. 6).

Indeed, the total fertility rate has not exceeded replacement level—the level considered necessary for a given generation to replace itself exactly in population in the long run—since 1971 (NCHS 1993). The decreasing size of families is partially attributed to economic conditions. Because of the economy, families cannot afford to support a large number of children. The new family profile has

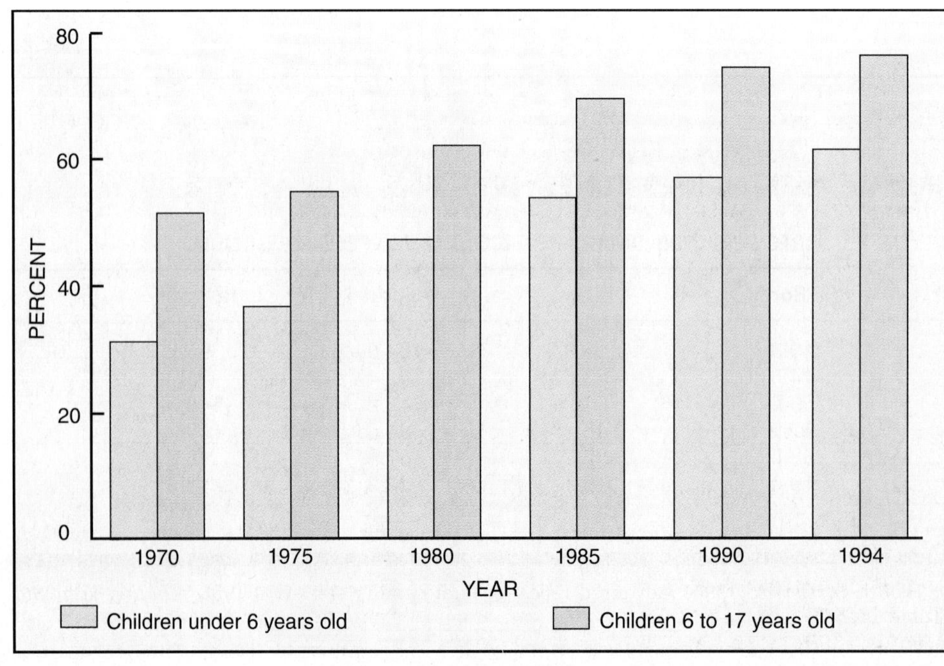

Figure 4–1

Mothers in the paid labor force, 1970–1990. (Data from U. S. Department of Labor, Bureau of Labor Statistics. [1989]. *Handbook of labor statistics* [Bull. 2340] [p. 244, Tables 56 and 57]). Washington, D.C.: Government Printing Office; U. S. Department of Labor, Bureau of Labor Statistics [March 1994]. *Current Population Survey* [Unpublished data].)

also been attributed to changing human priorities as more individuals choose to have fewer children and the family planning methods available that allow women to control their fertility and seek careers.

Types of Families

TRADITIONAL FAMILY FORMS

Family Functions. Historically, the family served five major functions: ensuring economic survival, providing protection, passing on values and beliefs, educating children, and conferring status (Curran 1983). The family also serves as a fundamental support system for the following activities (Caplan 1982):

- Collecting and sharing information about the outside world with the children in the family
- Providing feedback to individual members regarding their behavior and providing a training ground for members to learn how to make adjustments in behavior based on feedback
- Serving as a source of belief systems, value systems, and codes of behavior that enable members to determine the nature and meaning of the universe, their place in it, and their future goals and aspirations
- Providing guidance and assistance with problem solving
- Serving as a source of practice help, concrete aid, and resources especially during times of crises or life transitions
- Providing a safe haven for rest and recuperation
- Serving as a reference and control group for determining behavior
- Serving as the primary source of ingredients that mold an individual's self-image and identity
- Contributing to the emotional mastery of individual members through support and feedback

The structural form of families has changed through the years and now varies widely (see Box). However, the functions of the family that are essential for healthy families and healthy children are the same, regardless of structural form.

Nuclear Family. The concept of the nuclear family refers to a specific family form that came into being with industrialization in the nineteenth century and peaked in the post–World War II era in the 1950s. This family form was historically composed of a male breadwinner, his wife as the full-time homemaker, and their dependent children. The children were viewed as requiring nurturing and protection through adolescence; their task was to learn about their societal roles. In the

Family Forms

Nuclear: A father, mother, and child living together but apart from both sets of their parents

Extended: Three generations, including married brothers and sisters and their families

Three-generational: Any combination of first-, second-, and third-generation members living within a household

Dyad: Husband and wife or other couple living alone without children

Single-parent: Divorced, never married, separated, or widowed man or woman and at least one child. Most single-parent families are headed by women

Stepparent: One or both spouses have been divorced or widowed and have remarried into a family with at least one child

Blended or reconstituted: A combination of two families with children from one or both families and sometimes children of the newly married couple

Single adult living alone: An increasingly common occurrence for the never married, divorced, or widowed

Cohabiting: An unmarried couple living together

No-kin: A group of at least two people sharing a relationship and exchanging support who have no legalized or blood tie to each other

Compound: One man (or woman) with several spouses

Gay: A homosexual couple living together with or without children; children may be adopted, from previous relationships, or artificially conceived

Commune: More than one monogamous couple sharing resources

Group marriage: All individuals are married to each other and are considered parents of all the children

From Cooley, M. (1995). A family perspective in community health nursing. In C. M. Smith and F. A. Maurer (Eds.). *Community health nursing: Theory and practice* (p. 209). Philadelphia: W. B. Saunders.

1990s, the dual-earner model of the nuclear family has replaced the breadwinner model (Walsh 1993).

Extended Family. The extended family has been defined as three generations of family members related by blood, adoption, or remarriage who live together as a group. Today, this definition has been expanded to include other significant persons who have emotional ties to a family. These multigenerational kinships can provide support and aid to burdened parents as well as serve as a rich source of cultural heritage for the children (Boyd-Franklin 1993).

NONTRADITIONAL FAMILY FORMS

The contemporary family consists of several different forms in addition to the traditional nuclear and extended families (Fig. 4–2). A single culturally dominant family form no longer exists in our society. Instead, there are numerous coexisting and evolving family forms (Walsh 1993).

Single-Parent Family. In the past, most single-parent families resulted from the death of a spouse. Today, this family form is more often the result of divorce, separation, or out-of-wedlock childbearing. For whites, the increase in single-parent families is primarily due to divorce or separation; for blacks, it results from childbearing outside of marriage (National Commission on Children 1991). Regardless of cause, in 1970, about 12 percent of children lived in a single-parent family (National Commission on Children 1991); the number had increased to 26 percent by the early 1990s ("The Changing American Family" 1991).

The annual divorce rate rose from 9.2 per 1000 women in the 1950s to 20.7 per 1000 women in 1988. Half of all marriages now end in divorce ("The Changing American Family" 1991). Marriage and childbearing are increasingly becoming separate events. In 1960, approximately 5 percent of all births in the United States were to unmarried women. In 1991, more than 25 percent of all births (1,213,769) were to unmarried women. The birth rate for single women increased by 54 percent between 1980 and 1991 (NCHS 1993). An increasing number of women in their 30s and 40s are choosing to become single parents through either adoption or artificial insemination. Although most single-parent families are headed by women, the number of single fathers increased 65 percent from 1970 to 1979 (U. S. Department of Labor 1980).

Both single mothers and single fathers face similar problems: inadequate family income and resources and an overabundance of problems related to child care and parenting responsibilities. Children living with only their mothers are more likely to be poor. Forty-three percent of single-parent families headed by mothers are poor compared with 7 percent of two-parent families. Children in minority single-parent families are more likely to be poor than are children in white families. While poverty in two-parent families fluctuates according to the economy, the poverty of single-parent families headed by women is constant (National Commission on Children 1991).

Single-parent families are a diverse group whose characteristics and circumstances vary widely, depending on family functioning, capabilities of the parent, socioeconomic and income level, employment, and amount of extended family support. Boyd-Franklin (1993) emphasized that "the fact of single parenthood does not automatically make a family dysfunctional."

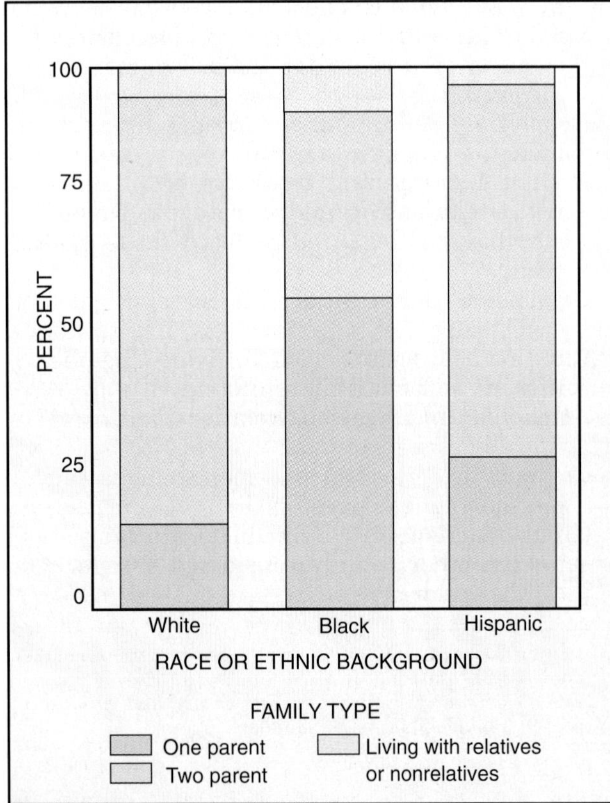

Figure 4–2

Family type by race or ethnic background of children under 18 years in 1993. (Data from Marital status and living arrangements, March 1994. *Current population study* [Table 74]. Washington, D.C.: Government Printing Office.)

Blended Families. Blended families, a household containing a child who is biologically related to only one of the adults (Visher and Visher 1993), have increased dramatically. In 1987, 33 percent of the entire population was a part of a blended family (Glick 1991). Glick and Lin (1986) have predicted that by the year 2000, there will be more blended families than any other type of family form in our society.

The blended family system is more complex than the nuclear family because it has a larger number of built-in subsystems and greater ambiguity in which boundaries are less clear. It is also subject to fluctuating stability because of constant changes and transitions in the family system (Visher and Visher 1993). The blended family must deal with six major dynamic issues: helping "outsiders" to become "insiders"; resolving "turf" and boundary problems; resolving power issues; coping with conflicting loyalties; preventing rigid, unproductive triangles of relationship within the family system; and achieving unity as opposed to fragmentation in the new couple's relationship.

Family reorganization, reidentification, and the highly charged role of stepparenting are the major issues of concern to blended families (Engebretson 1982). Wymore (1989) has described adjustment phases of stepfamilies. During the honeymoon phase, parents are described as having high hopes for promoting strong relationships with their stepchildren. True feelings and frustrations will usually be repressed during this phase. The regret phase is described as a vulnerable period when stepparent-child issues become obvious and the stepparent will want to look back to the past when life was easier. Confrontation of family issues, letting go of the past, and focusing on positive aspects of the future are considered the major tasks of this period. The acceptance phase involves the transition from the old to the new lifestyle. The working phase focuses on interpersonal conflict resolution and problem solving of family issues (Wymore 1989). Reutter and Strang (1986) have stated that the integration of blended families may take as long as 7 years. It is important to understand the process blended families go through to become integrated in endeavoring to provide them the support needed during this time.

Researchers have identified several characteristics of successful blended families in which both children and adult members have warm personal relationships and are satisfied with their lives (Visher and Visher 1993). These are:

- Individual family members do not attempt to force their blended family into the traditional nuclear family mold. They have realistic expectations about blended family life and recognize that there will be challenges and problems that need to be resolved.
- Adult family members are sensitive to the sadness and mourning of children (often exhibited as anger, depression, and acting out) over the major changes resulting from the blended family environment. Since the blended family is usually a result of loss, either through death or divorce, the adults in successful families allowed themselves and their children to mourn their loss.
- Couples work together and are a strong team. This provides the atmosphere of stability, vital to all families, that is especially important in blended families.
- Stepparents form positive satisfactory relationships with their stepchildren. This is often a long process and fraught with difficulties in which tolerance and respect for each individual are paramount.
- New families establish satisfying family rituals, which are important in creating a sense of family and ways of doing things.
- Parents work out satisfactory arrangements that promote cooperation between the two households of children rather than competition between the two groups.

To become a successful blended family, the adults must first recognize that time is needed to accomplish the tasks for successful integration and allow the time for these tasks to be completed. Blended families are uniquely different from nuclear families and have additional tasks that must be accomplished. Professional counseling and education are often helpful during the process of reorganizing two families into one successful blended family.

▼ **Lesbian and Gay Families.** During the last 10 years, the number of lesbian and gay families, those families having same-sex couples or single-parent families headed by a lesbian woman or gay man, has increased (Laird 1993). However, the normality of lesbian and gay families and the acceptability of children being raised in this family type are still controversial. In the past, the existence of lesbian and gay families basically has been ignored, and research on which to base practice is scarce.

Lesbian and gay families, like heterosexual families, vary tremendously in values, beliefs, and lifestyle. In most respects, lesbian and gay families are similar to all other family types. They must negotiate their relationships with their family of origin and their community, forge social networks, establish boundaries for outside and inside the family, develop problem-solving strategies, and mediate conflict (Laird 1993). Lesbian and gay families differ from other family forms in two ways. First, they are usually, although not always, headed by same-sex couples. Some lesbian and gay families are headed by a single-parent individual. Second, these families must function in a world that may not recognize or accept their family structure; many lesbian and gay families are stigmatized. However, current research indicates that children in lesbian and gay families appear to grow and thrive as well as children in heterosexual families (Laird 1993).

Wismont and Reame (1989) have outlined developmental tasks for pregnancy, adapted from the psychosocial tasks described by Rubin (1984), that a lesbian couple will need to confront. These tasks have been described as acceptance of the pregnancy by themselves and by others (family, friends); assurance of an environment that will provide optimal health care during the childbearing period, which may be hindered by bias found among health care professionals; "binding into the child" or emotional investment from the self to the well-being of the child, which may be hampered by the absence of a father image; assurance of support during the pregnancy from the partner, which is thought to be met on a higher level by a lesbian partner than by a male partner; and parental role development of the co-parents. Research is needed to better understand the implications of pregnancy and the birth of a child for lesbian couples as well as the impact of adoption of children and parenting on gay couple families.

The Childbearing Family

The childbearing family is typically thought to consist of a mother, a father, and siblings. However, a broader concept is better since both nuclear and extended family members are important influences on the childbearing family (Stainton 1989). The influence of both internal and external family members is critically important in the assessment and nursing care of the childbearing family. Although this concept has become widely accepted, the central focus of care usually continues to be the pregnant woman; other family members are included only in the woman's care for support or problem resolution (Stainton 1989).

CHILDBEARING FAMILY LIFE CYCLE

The dynamics within the childbearing family as it evolves from one family life cycle to another become increasingly complex as relationships change (Peterson and Peterson 1993). The couple's relationship is affected by their new role as parents. Also, the role as parent differs for each child, depending on the child's age, temperament, and gender (Peterson and Peterson 1993). These changing relationships and interactions influence each family member. On the basis of Duvall's work, Stainton (1989) proposed that satisfactory developmental progression of the childbearing family involves three major changes:

- Making adjustments in the marital system to make space for a child or additional children
- Assuming the role as parent
- Realigning relationships with extended family members as parenting and grandparenting roles are assumed

A discussion of the psychological and developmental tasks of the childbearing family during pregnancy is presented in Chapter 17. A review of these tasks during parenting is included in Chapter 34.

EDUCATIONAL NEEDS

Comprehensive perinatal education for the childbearing family should focus on the multiple roles of individual family members, the transition from one developmental stage to another, and the programs designed to include all family members (Peterson and Peterson 1993). The essential components of such a curriculum include classes about early pregnancy, pregnancy exercise, childbirth preparation, breastfeeding preparation, sibling preparation, grandparenting, parenting, and infant care (Biasella 1993). Numerous other classes as well as follow-up support would also be of benefit to the childbearing family (see Chapter 20).

The Adoptive Family

Adoptive families encounter many of the same experiences as childbearing families do and progress through the same developmental stages. In addition to the typical experiences and tasks of the childbearing family, adoptive families face complex experiences inherent in the process of adoption and being an adoptive family (Anderson et al. 1993). The underlying feeling of loss from being unable to produce a child that most adoptive families have experienced is primarily responsible for the differences and problems that they encounter (Brodzinsky and Schechter 1990). The background of loss influences how the adoptive family interprets developmental events, creates their family structure, and responds to developmental life cycle transitions (Anderson et al. 1993).

In addition to the developmental tasks of the childbearing family, the adoptive family must also complete six critical tasks related to adoption. These tasks are reaching the decision to adopt; pursuing adoption; claiming the new child, which involves committing themselves emotionally to the new child, seeing the child as a full and equal member of the family, and seeing themselves as entitled to parent the child, which involves providing the structure and discipline necessary for the child's development; forging a sense of family; telling the child about his or her adopted status; and supporting the child—usually during adolescence—as the child searches for identity and belonging and seeks information about his or her "real" parents (Anderson et al. 1993).

ADOPTION OPTIONS

Adoption terminology can be confusing. Learning the common adoption terms and their meaning is essential in understanding the language of adoption (Alexander-Roberts 1994). In an agency adoption, both public and private agencies provide various services that usually include both preadoption and postadoption counseling. The requirements with which adoptive parents must comply vary from agency to agency. Both international and domestic agencies provide adoption programs.

In an independent or private adoption, the adoptive parents work to find a birth parent or child directly through a physician, lawyer, or nonagency adoption source. Usually no other services are provided, and the fees can be high. When adoptive parents and birth parents find each other and go to an agency or attorney to complete the adoption, the proceedings are called an identified adoption.

International or intercountry adoption, in which a child is adopted from another country, is increasingly being selected by adoptive parents today. Since the mid-1950s, when international adoptions began, more that 100,000 children have been placed in adoptive families; an average of 9000 children have been placed each year since 1983 (Adoptive Families of America 1994). Adoptive families choose international adoption for a number of reasons: the family may not meet the stringent guidelines, particularly for parent age, for domestic adoption but can qualify for international adoption; the waiting time is usually less; some adoptive parents prefer the distance and separation from the birth parents; and adoptive parents often want a child of their family's specific ethnic origin.

When there is communication between the adoptive and birth families, the process is called open adoption. An adoption without contact between adoptive and birth parents is called traditional, closed, or confidential adoption. Special needs adoption is usually handled by an agency and involves children who have severe medical or emotional problems or siblings who need to be placed together with one family. An adoption in which adoptive parents and the adoptive child are from the same country but of different racial or ethnic backgrounds is called transracial domestic adoption.

EDUCATIONAL NEEDS

An adoptive family's educational needs are similar to those of the typical childbearing family, with the addition of information about the adoption process. Their unique needs relate to the six developmental tasks of the adoptive family cited previously. Much of the information about planning and preparation for an adoptive child can be provided by a resource person who is knowledgeable about adoption; other developmental and emotional issues are best handled by a therapist skilled in working with adoptive families. The role of the nurse is to provide education about becoming a successful family; the nurse refers the adoptive family as needed to professionals skilled in counseling related to the developmental and emotional tasks.

FAMILY THEORIES

In the last 50 years, various groups of scholars have studied the concept of family. No one theory has been considered right or wrong; indeed, all information has been viewed as helpful in understanding the concept of the family (Table 4–2). Because the prenatal period requires continued adjustment to physical and psychological change, the maternal-newborn nurse must understand the interpersonal dynamics of the family unit. Sociologists, family therapists, developmentalists, and family life educators have made major contributions to the understanding of family dynamics. Although these perspectives sometimes differ in approach, similarities, particularly in the characteristics of functional families, are also evident (see Box).

Concept of Family

The study of the family is generally approached by seeking descriptive information, such as structure, functions, development, and expected social behavior. In addition, expected roles of family members and interactions have been major areas for examination.

THE SOCIOLOGIST'S PERSPECTIVE

Sociologists have studied families for several decades and described the family as a social institution, a unity of interacting personalities having historical and cultural influences (Hill and Hansen 1960). Christensen (1964) stated that marriage is customarily viewed as a precondition of family organization, and a family signifies a set of roles acquired through marriage and procreation. Therefore, from a sociological standpoint,

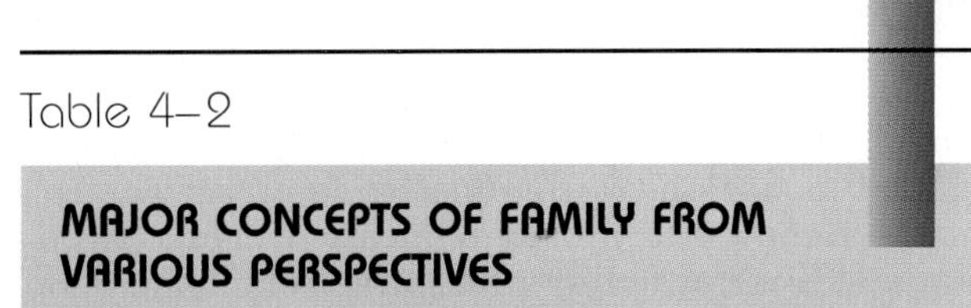

Table 4–2

MAJOR CONCEPTS OF FAMILY FROM VARIOUS PERSPECTIVES

CLASSIFICATION	STRUCTURE	FUNCTION
Traditional	Basic unit of society:	
	Father	Breadwinner
	Mother	Homemaker and nurturer
	Children	Learners of traditional societal roles
Sociological	Social institution; marriage (usually prerequisite) and progeny	Procreation Protection Socialization
Family Theory	Relationship system: open, dynamic	Develop mature persons
Developmental	Described according to stages	Achieve developmental tasks, re: stages, socialization
Contemporary	Changing system, network of relationships	Support, nurture to achieve individual and family goals

families are described as having structure within a larger social system with functions, such as procreation, socialization, and protection of children. Each of these functions is influenced by family history and culture. The interactional functions of families focus primarily on the development of roles of family members through transmission of role expectations (Hill and Hansen 1960; Broderick and Smith 1979; Burr et al. 1979).

THE FAMILY THERAPIST'S PERSPECTIVE

Family therapists have studied families from the standpoint of pathology. Bowen (1971) described the family as an emotional relationship system made up of interlocking systems and subsystems. The definition of families, according to family therapists, has focused on their dynamic natures, which have changing needs at physical, emotional, and cultural levels. The impact of roles, power, and interactional patterns within the family system is used to describe the open, ongoing nature of a family system (Haley 1963; Jackson 1968; Satir 1971).

THE DEVELOPMENTAL PERSPECTIVE

Families have also been described from a developmental approach (Duvall 1977; Smith 1983). With use of the traditional family as the point of reference, norms of role behavior are described according to the changes that usually occur within the family (Fig. 4–3). As transitions occur within the family, a growth responsibility arises in the life of the family. Successful achievement of this growth responsibility leads to satisfaction and success with later tasks. When failure occurs, there is dissatisfaction, and difficulty will probably be apparent in later family developmental tasks.

Considering the many changes that are occurring in the traditional family, Murphy and Stapels (1979) developed a modernized family life cycle (Fig. 4–4). Their approach includes the adult who never marries, the couple who does not have children, the divorced or single parent, and remarried families. This view of family recognizes the need to move away from the traditional view of the family to a more contemporary framework.

THE PERSPECTIVE OF CHANGE

Kennedy (1980), a family life educator, has described the family by attempting to encompass the changes in American families. The family system is viewed as part of a larger system of other social organizations. The family system is seen as a group of individuals who have a commitment to a network of relationships that offer a sense of identity, support, and opportunity for socialization. This network is described as usually having ties of blood or adoptive relationships. The family is further viewed as a vital nurturing organism that strives to assist its members in meeting their goals throughout the life span (Kennedy 1980). The continuous process of change within the family structure necessitates the view that family dynamism influences family function.

Selected Family Theories

Throughout the years, anthropologists, historians, psychologists, and sociologists have established various views on the family unit and its interaction. Three perspectives for study are pre-

Characteristics of Functional Families

Developmental stages and tasks: A family goes through predictable stages according to the age and development of its members. Tasks must be achieved at the stage-appropriate time or they may never be achieved. Maturational crises are predictable. Some crises are unpredictable and interfere with achievement of tasks.

Roles: Define certain patterns of expected behavior. Often are male/female linked. Need to be appropriate for age and sex. Also need to be flexible, not rigid, and able to support family functioning.

Boundaries: Exist around the system to handle exchange between the family and the environment. Also exist between subsystems to differentiate members belonging to each subsystem. Need to be permeable to allow information and resources in and out. Boundaries between subsystems should have clear generational lines and support a strong parental coalition. Should be neither too rigid nor diffuse.

Subsystems: Each member of the family belongs to several simultaneously: spouse, parent/child, sibling, grandparents. Subsystems should include all (and only) age-appropriate members.

Patterns of interaction: Repeat themselves. Are healthier when one member does not end up blamed, left out, or put down in the interaction. Should be somewhere between enmeshed and disengaged. Communication theorists describe how people communicate (e.g., placator, blamer, superresponsible one). Bowen talks about four ways of handling fusion: distance, conflict, projection, dysfunction.

Power: Results from clear role definition and appropriate rules. Should be somewhat shared, appropriate to age, and within the parental subsystem until the children are independent.

External stressors: Usually present at some point. If they vary, are not very intense, and are spread out in time, the family has a chance to adapt. Illness brings its own set of demands to the family.

Open/closed system: As the system closes, all variables and patterns become fixed and less adaptable. Energy is used in dysfunctional ways. Open systems can adapt and change as feedback is received from within and outside the system. This is related to permeability of boundaries.

Communication: Healthier when it is clear, honest, direct, congruent, and specific and when the family is able to use it as a mechanism to resolve conflict.

Values: Related to cultural, socioeconomic groups. Provide some stability, rules, and guidelines. Need to be able to change with changing times.

Encouragement of autonomy/acceptance of difference: A balance needs to exist between autonomy of members and the need to be a cohesive group.

Level of anxiety: When the family is calm, people in the family can think and problem solve better. The family tends to do better during calm periods than in times of stress. Anxiety can be transitional or long-term. Long-term anxiety tends to wear down the ability of the family to function well.

Resources/social support: Available to most families from within and outside the family, but the family must be able to use them. Extended family is often used. Socioeconomic status and geographic location tend to influence these. All families have some strengths.

Meaning, perception, and paradigm: The way a family perceives a situation, the meaning it attaches to the events, and its typical way of relating to the outside environment influence the ways families react.

Adaptability: Flexibility, adaptability, and resilience are necessary for a family to be able to cope with changing demands. A family needs to maintain a certain degree of flexibility and yet a certain degree of cohesiveness and predictability.

From Cooley, M. (1995). A family perspective in community health nursing. In C. M. Smith and F. A. Maurer (Eds.). *Community health nursing: Theory and practice* (p. 217). Philadelphia: W. B. Saunders.

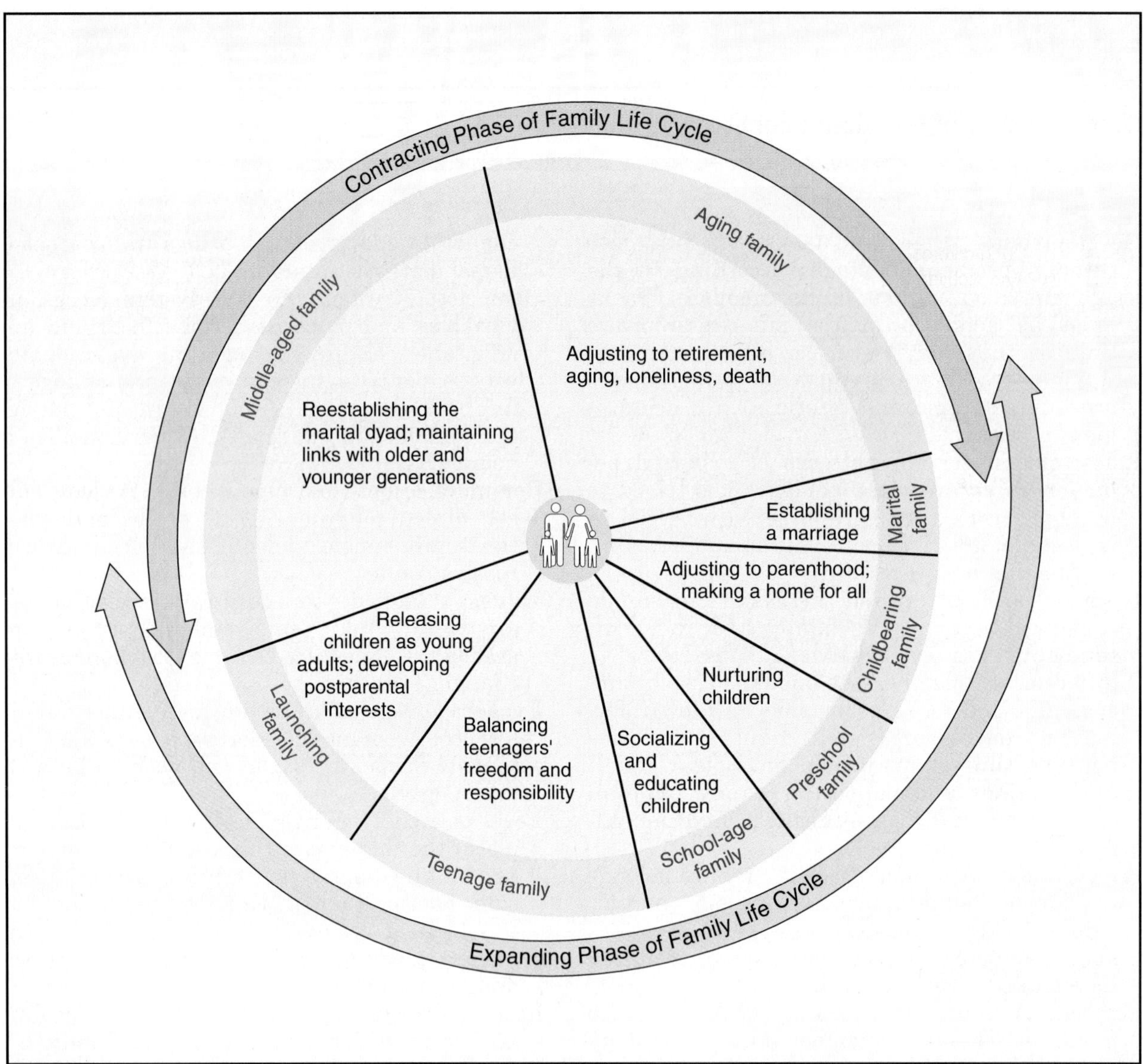

Figure 4–3

Duvall's Developmental Family Life Cycle. Duvall has developed a family life cycle model with eight stages of developmental family transitions that are chronologic and segmental. (Adapted from Janosik, E., and Green, E. [1992]. *Family life: Process and practice.* Boston: Jones & Bartlett. Reprinted with permission.)

sented here and include symbolic interaction, social exchange, and the systems approach. Table 4–3 includes the major concepts of each.

SYMBOLIC INTERACTION THEORY

The beginnings of symbolic interactionism have been credited to Mead (1934), who used concepts from the broader interactionist perspective to illustrate the internal processes that occur within individuals and families. Basic concepts include mind, self, and society. The mind is viewed as being capable of organizing and managing responses to symbols and gestures from others in society. Therefore, this internal process of assigning meaning to symbols and gestures is important in determining and understanding behaviors of individuals and families. The self is developed through the process of the experience the individual has within society. It may follow, then, that an individual's behavior is a result of one's perception of experiences with society. Society is viewed as the organized interaction patterns from which the individual develops the self. Thus, society depends

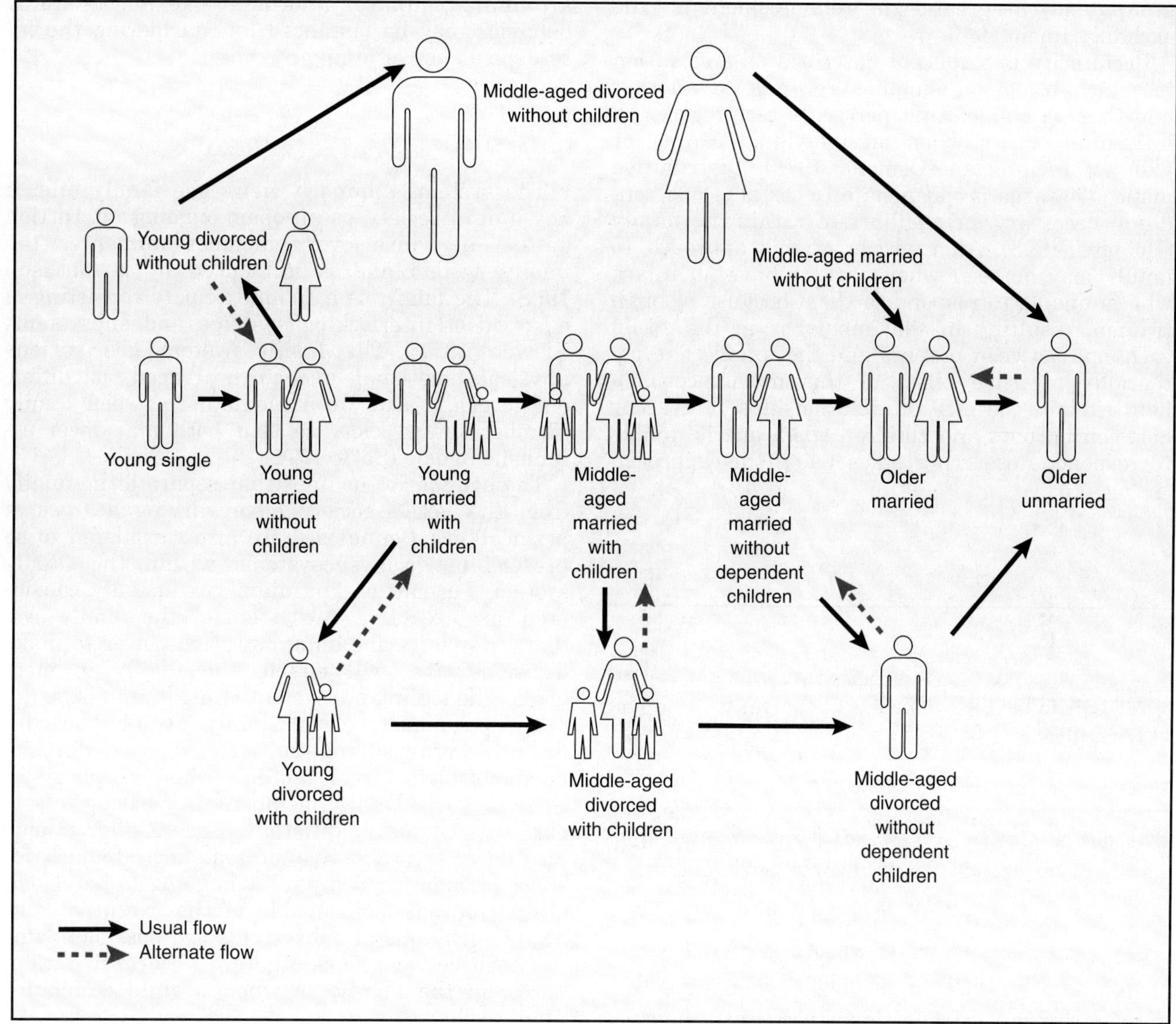

Figure 4–4

A contemporary family life cycle including all types of families, never married individual, couple without children, divorced or single parent, remarried family, and traditional family. (Adapted from Murphy, P. E., and Staples, W. A. [1979]. A modernized family life cycle. *Journal of Consumer Research,* 6 [6], 12–22. Publisher: The University of Chicago Press. Copyright © Journal of Consumer Research, Inc., 1979.)

on the organizing and managing responses of individuals (Turner 1978; Nye 1979).

To describe family dynamics from a symbolic interactionist approach, various internal processes have been studied. Mercer (1981, 1985, 1986) used role theory to study maternal role attainment during the first year of motherhood. The study of infant behavior and mothers' perceptions of their experience have added information to the development of the maternal role.

Symbolic interaction theory is a helpful approach to examining family phenomena. A major constraint in the further development of this theory is the limited research in the use of this approach.

SOCIAL EXCHANGE THEORY

The social exchange perspective is derived primarily from economic theories. This perspective is based on the premise that "interaction between persons is an exchange of goods, material and non-material" (Homans 1958, p. 597). Individuals are perceived as making choices to result in the greatest reward and least cost regarding material and nonmaterial concerns, as in status and relationships. The more the individual conforms to the group, the more choices the individual will have. Further, the more cohesive a group, the more valuable the exchange between individuals in the groups and the greater the reinforcement for the exchanged behavior.

Reciprocity is a concept described as a situation in which a person supplies rewards to another and thereby obliges that person to reciprocate. An imbalance occurs when an individual cannot or will not reciprocate (Osmond 1978). Distributive justice (rewards proportionate to costs) is one condition necessary for equilibrium within the family (Homans 1958). An example of this approach to family may be seen when parents have an infant who is unable to respond to them because of birth trauma, resulting in the imbalance in the social exchange between parents and the infant. The potentially negative effect of this imbalance may help explain the difficult relationships that occur between parents and children when one is unable to respond. Research studies using this approach are limited; however, information related to family behavior may be enhanced by considering the interdependency of family members.

Table 4–3

MAJOR CONCEPTS OF SELECTED FAMILY THEORIES

THEORY	CONCEPT
Symbolic interaction	*Mind:* Derives meaning from symbols and gestures in interaction with others *Self:* Symbolic object in the mind's eye *Society:* Provides attitudes assimilated as part of self
Social exchange	*Group cohesiveness:* Interaction between persons is an exchange of material and non-material goods *Choices:* Individuals make choices to result in the greatest reward and least cost *Reciprocity:* A reward obligates return or payback *Distributive justice:* A balanced relationship equals rewards that are proportionate to costs
Family systems	*Family system:* Includes subsystems, boundaries, input, throughput, and output communication *Cohesion:* Refers to the emotional bonds between family members *Adaptability:* Ability to change

FAMILY SYSTEMS THEORY

The systems approach views the family unit, a key unit of society, as an open, ongoing interaction system in which every member influences the family system and is influenced by it (Jackson 1968). The family is a complex entity consisting of a series of interlocking systems and subsystems (Bowen 1971). The family system has various physical, emotional, and cultural needs on different levels. It acts as a mediator between family members and society so that both may meet established goals (Satir 1971).

The boundaries or lines that separate the family from the larger society have varying degrees of permeability. Boundaries are also considered to be present between subsystems within the family system. Parents or guardians are usually considered the executive subsystem of the family system. They have the administrative power to make decisions that will enable the family to meet goals. The sibling subsystem is made up of the dependent members of the family, usually the children. Several sibling subsystems may develop, particularly in larger families where responsibilities may vary. Family members may belong to several subsystems at different times. Children may also enter the executive subsystem by request for short periods when a parent is going to be absent or if a parent is incapable of the executive role. Many variations of subsystems are possible. Some are positive variations; others have negative influences on the family, as when a child dominates family behavior.

There are three general types of family systems (Fig. 4–5). Families will usually fall into one of these systems, although they may move from one type to another, depending on the issue under consideration. The open family system has permeable boundaries that allow information to enter the system. The family is open to information from the environment. The information is processed (throughput) and provides feedback to the environment (outputs). Kantor and Lehr (1975, p. 27) described the open family system as one in which ". . . a visitor, upon gaining access to the family space, is invited to enter the interpersonal system as well . . . the family says, 'Come in. Here we are. Know us.' Such families virtually eliminate the social interspace."

The closed family system experiences boundaries that are mostly resistant to inputs from the environment. Throughputs, therefore, are minimal, and feedback to the environment is limited (Kantor and Lehr 1975, p. 27): "Upon entering such a family, the visitor may very quickly locate the in-

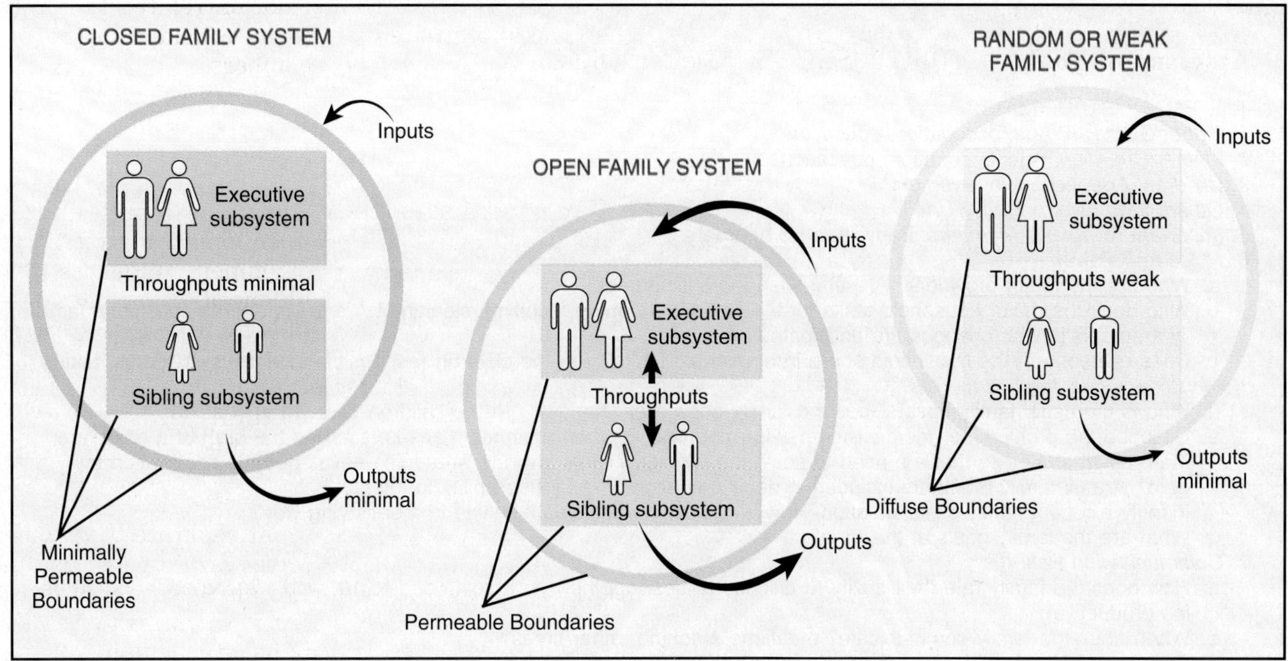

Figure 4–5

Types of family systems. Families usually fall into one of three systems, although they may move from one type to another, depending on the situation or issue.

terpersonal subsystem's walls, which he recognizes as thick and initially impregnable. The family's signals can be interpreted as, 'Here we are. There you are. You may enter by invitation only.'" The closed system is considered to be isolated from the environment and to have a tendency to maximal disorder (Bertalanffy 1968).

The random or weak family system exhibits diffuse boundaries. Any and all information enters this system, easily influencing or not influencing the family system and subsystems because the family fails to function adequately in processing information from the environment (throughputs). The feedback from this family is therefore ineffectual and weak (Kantor and Lehr 1975, p. 27): "The metaphorical outside wall of this kind of interpersonal subsystem is difficult to find. In effect, the family says, 'Since you happen to be here, find us. If you can.'" Members of a random system move around a lot and may be absent at strategic times. Relationships may often be unclear (Kantor and Lehr 1975, p. 27): ". . . the visitor may not be sure whether he is occupying the social interspace or whether he has stumbled into the family's interspace subsystem. Such a space without walls, where walls are culturally expected, can be highly disorienting to the outsider." The family subsystems may be easily swayed by inputs and may switch from one course to another. Behavior is not coordinated, and the family system tends to give nothing back to their sources of input.

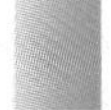

Factors Influencing Families

Family theorists have used the systems approach to describe how a family functions or behaves relative to power and roles, interactional patterns, and culture and values.

POWER

Power is usually described according to family roles. As already discussed, the family system is viewed as being structured with executive and sibling subsystems. The executive subsystem usually has the most power in the family system. Parents are traditionally charged with the responsibility for the welfare of the total family and therefore are assigned the roles within the executive subsystems. One can immediately see that the power within the family will shift as the sibling subsystem matures and assumes more responsibility for decision making within the family. Family therapists have found the concept of power helpful in assisting families having difficulties because of role conflict. An example may be the newly formed single-parent family, where assignment of roles has been inadequate or inappropriate. More relevant to the topic of this text is the role conflict that may arise after the birth of a child when decisions have not been made regard-

Assessment Tool: Family Assessment Guide

THE FAMILY STRUCTURE:

1. *Father/Guardian:* Age, occupation, education
2. *Mother/Guardian:* Age, occupation, education
3. *Children:* Age, school involvement
4. *Others Who Live in Family Unit*
5. *Important Nonfamily Members:* Babysitters or boarders
6. *Roles and Power*
   a. Who are the major providers? Are any changes anticipated?
   b. Who does the major household tasks for the family? shopping, cooking, cleaning? Are tasks alternated among family members? What changes are anticipated?
   c. Does everyone in the household share in household tasks? Are the children responsible for their own rooms, taking garbage out, tending to pets?
   d. Who is the usual family boss? Does the family boss ever change? Are the children ever left in charge?
   e. Describe the problem-solving/decision-making approach? When a situation arises, such as the birth of a child, are there usual strategies that are used to solve the problem? How are new strategies developed? Is negotiation evident? Are all family members included in decisions according to their ability to interact?
   f. Identify a recent family crisis situation. How was it resolved? Was it solved in a satisfying way?
   g. What are the family goals at this time?
7. *Communication Patterns*
   a. How does the family rate their ability to discuss issues together (on a scale of 1 to 10, with 1 being poor and 10 being productive).
   b. When does the family communicate? mealtime, bedtime, other times?
   c. Does the family consider their family to be an affectionate family? How is this displayed? Is affection withheld as punishment?
   d. Observe the family interaction.
      i. Is the atmosphere relaxed or tense? Give examples.
      ii. Who answers most of the questions? Are all family members allowed to speak for themselves?
      iii. Do family members speak to one another? Do family members maintain eye contact with one another?

THE FAMILY SYSTEM'S RELATIONSHIP WITH THE SUPRASYSTEM

1. Identify clubs, church, sports activities, school, and other organizations the family attends together or alone.
2. Identify activities the family plans together: trips to the zoo? bowling?
3. Identify people who enter the house on a regular basis: babysitter, grandparents, friends of children or parents, others?
4. Who can you count on to give assistance when needed?

CULTURE AND VALUES

1. *Language*
   What is the first language of the family?
   If English is not spoken, is there someone who can speak for the family? Should language cards be used to communicate with the family? (These cards have pictures that depict statements or questions for the family.)
2. *Diet*
   Does the family have any food preferences?
   Are any foods forbidden because of cultural or religious beliefs?
   Are special foods required for a childbearing woman?
   Are there special practices of feeding a newborn infant?
   Is there special preparation of foods during a childbearing experience?
   Are there special practices surrounding eating, for example, is privacy expected?
3. *Health and Illness Beliefs*
   How are health and illness described in the family's culture? Do all family members hold these beliefs?
   How is childbirth viewed in this culture? Is it illness or wellness oriented? Is it women's work? Are men involved in the childbearing experience?
   Who does the family member respect as the health practitioner? the physician? the public health nurse? the grandmother? the curandero?
   What are the family's customs and beliefs related to birth? childbearing? death? Are there religious practices surrounding birth, illness, and death? Describe.
4. *Family Values*
   What are the major values of the family? education, work, wealth, spiritual life, sports, other?
5. *Family Relationships*
   What health care practices for the child's welfare does the family value? Are there cultural objections to any practices? circumcision? Are there practices the family wishes to follow? bellybands?
   What are the family goals for the child? What approach does the family take to help the child reach those goals?
   Are there specific practices that the family wishes the new mother to follow? avoidance of bathing?
   From what source does the family derive its greatest support? extended family? religion? friends?
   What role does the extended family play?

ing new tasks, new roles, and redistribution of previous tasks and roles.

The assignment and appropriation of power within a family is considered a major factor influencing all the members of the family. A healthy family with children is considered to be an open family system with a strong executive subsystem. Within such a family system, the adults of the family (parents or other adults they have designated for this role, such as a babysitter) make the necessary decisions for the welfare of the family. The members of the sibling subsystem are included in the process of decision making (throughput), allowing interaction to occur. If one member of the family system is allowed excessive power, the family system will function less openly. An excessively controlling parent or child will not allow the family to interact dynamically (Jackson 1968).

INTERACTIONAL PATTERNS

The family system is also greatly influenced by interactional patterns. Satir (1971), a noted family therapist, has emphasized the importance of observing and assessing family interactional patterns. Using the family systems approach, one needs to observe the inputs, throughputs, and outputs of each family member; the subsystems; and the family system within the larger suprasystem (community). Who is the major spokesperson in the family? Are the children allowed to speak for themselves? Do children dominate the conversation? Who is listened to? Are extended family members involved in decision making (grandmothers and grandfathers)? Interactional patterns allow nurses to add to their understanding of the structure and function of the family they are assessing.

CULTURE AND VALUES

The culture and values the family holds are other factors that influence family functioning. The culture is viewed as the combination of those behaviors and expectations that have been transmitted to us by our extended family and caregivers. Values and beliefs are the practices that are handed down to instruct us in areas of role expectations, power structure, rights, and responsibilities. Society at large also influences family values and beliefs. Indeed, television has become particularly significant in the lives of today's families. The media are reported to influence children's thoughts and activities, including the foods they wish to eat and perhaps even their value of life and death.

The health care professional should pay close attention to the elements of culture and values that concern everyday living, including language, diet, concepts of health and illness, and practices at life cycle events such as birth and death. Practitioners of parent and child nursing will find views about the birth of a new child of particular interest.

Other important observations include noting how the roles are allocated for family members during a childbirth experience. Is the father expected to play a part in the childbirth experience? In our society, we encourage and often insist that the father be present during the birth experience. Is this in conflict with the family's cultural beliefs? What special specific culture practice is used during and after a childbirth experience? The Family Assessment Guide outlines specific questions regarding culture and values. A nurse's knowledge of a family's particular beliefs can help in communication and planning nursing care for the family.

THE FAMILY'S INFLUENCE ON HEALTH

The family has a powerful influence on health and illness. Families establish health-promoting behaviors, define illness, confirm the validity of the sick role, and initiate treatment for sick members (Diamond and Jones 1983). An individual's compliance with health care treatment is significantly affected by the family unit (Gilliss 1989). Thus, the family can influence the health outcomes of family members. To achieve the best health outcomes for family members, the interactions, beliefs, and values of the total family unit as well as of the specific individual family member must be recognized and considered.

The Family as Caregiver

In addition to establishing the belief system and values about health and illness, the family is also the caregiver and can promote healthy behaviors as well as provide appropriate care during illness (Cigoll and Binda 1993). While the importance of the family unit on the health status of individuals within it is acknowledged, the focus of health care providers many times unfortunately remains on the individual's problems and needs. To evaluate a family's functioning and its effect on health and illness, the nurse can assess each of the areas relevant to the family health and illness cycle described by Doherty and McCubbin (1985). These are:

- What family health promotion and risk reduction behaviors does the family use?
- Is the family vulnerable to specific illnesses?
- How does the family respond to the onset of illness?
- How does the family view health and illness?
- How does the family make the critical choice to seek health care?
- How does the family adapt to the illness of a member?
- How does the family respond in times of acute illness?
- How does the family interact with the health care system: in a positive or negative manner? in an open and assertive, submissive, or hostile manner?
- How does the family view its interaction with the health care community: positive and supportive? negative, threatening, and confusing?

Viewing the family unit as both the recipient of nursing care and the provider of health care rather than focusing only on the individual will provide the nurse with valuable additional data that can be used to increase the effectiveness of nursing care.

FAMILY ASSESSMENT

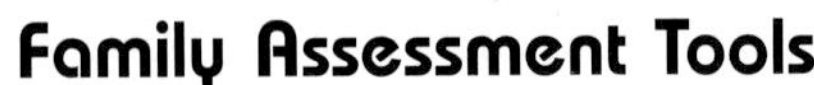

Family Assessment Tools

Assessment tools provide the link between theory, research, and practice. The use of family assessment tools furnishes a framework for the nurse to gather information about family dynamics, which can be used to interpret interactions and patterns of behavior. On the basis of this assessment, the nurse can then develop a more effective plan of nursing care. Two commonly used family assessment tools, the Circumplex Model and the Family Apgar Questionnaire, are discussed.

CIRCUMPLEX MODEL

Olson and associates (1985) developed a model to describe concepts from family theory and family therapy. From their study, three primary dimensions have been derived and provide a framework for the Circumplex Model (Fig. 4–6). The primary dimensions are described as cohesion, adaptability (change), and communication.

Family cohesion is defined as the emotional bonding that family members have for one another. Besides family bonding, the dimension of cohesion encompasses family issues, such as the strength or weakness of the boundaries between the family members (distance or closeness allowed) and the boundaries between the family system and larger systems outside of the family.

Family adaptability (change) is described as the ability of the family system to be flexible when a situation arises in which family function may require change such as the birth of a child into the family system. Family communication is considered the facilitator of the dimensions of family cohesion and adaptability.

As the result of numerous studies, the Circumplex Model has demonstrated a range of family systems from balanced family systems to family systems with low or excessive levels of cohesion or emotional bonding. Levels of adaptability within family systems range from structured and flexible to extremes of chaotic or rigid. More than 300 studies of family systems using the Circumplex Model have been conducted. Family assessment tools using the Circumplex Model may be found in the manual *Family Inventories* by Olson and colleagues (1985).

FAMILY APGAR QUESTIONNAIRE

The Family Apgar Questionnaire is designed to provide an overview of an individual's perception of his or her family's level of function. This screening tool was initially developed to assist physicians by providing information concerning the family as a resource or a source of stress (Smilkstein 1978; Smilkstein et al. 1982). The tool was formulated because of professional awareness of the role of the family on health outcomes.

Five areas of family function are assessed: adaptation, partnership, growth, affection, and resolve. Adaptation is defined as the use of family resources in problem solving; partnership is the sharing of decision making and nurturing responsibilities of families; growth is the potential for self-fulfillment that is achieved through the support of the family; affection is the caring relationship within the family; and resolve is the commitment to spending time with other members of the family. Each of the five items is rated on a 5-point scale: 0 = never, 1 = hardly ever, 2 = some of the time, 3 = almost always, and 4 = always. The final rating for each respondent is the sum of the five items with a range of 0 to 10. The sum of each respondent's ratings indicates that she or he perceives the family's functioning in one of three categories: a rating of 18 to 20 suggests a highly functional family; 12 to 17, a moderately functional family; and ratings below 12, a severely dysfunctional family. In addition, respondents provide demographic data regarding family members

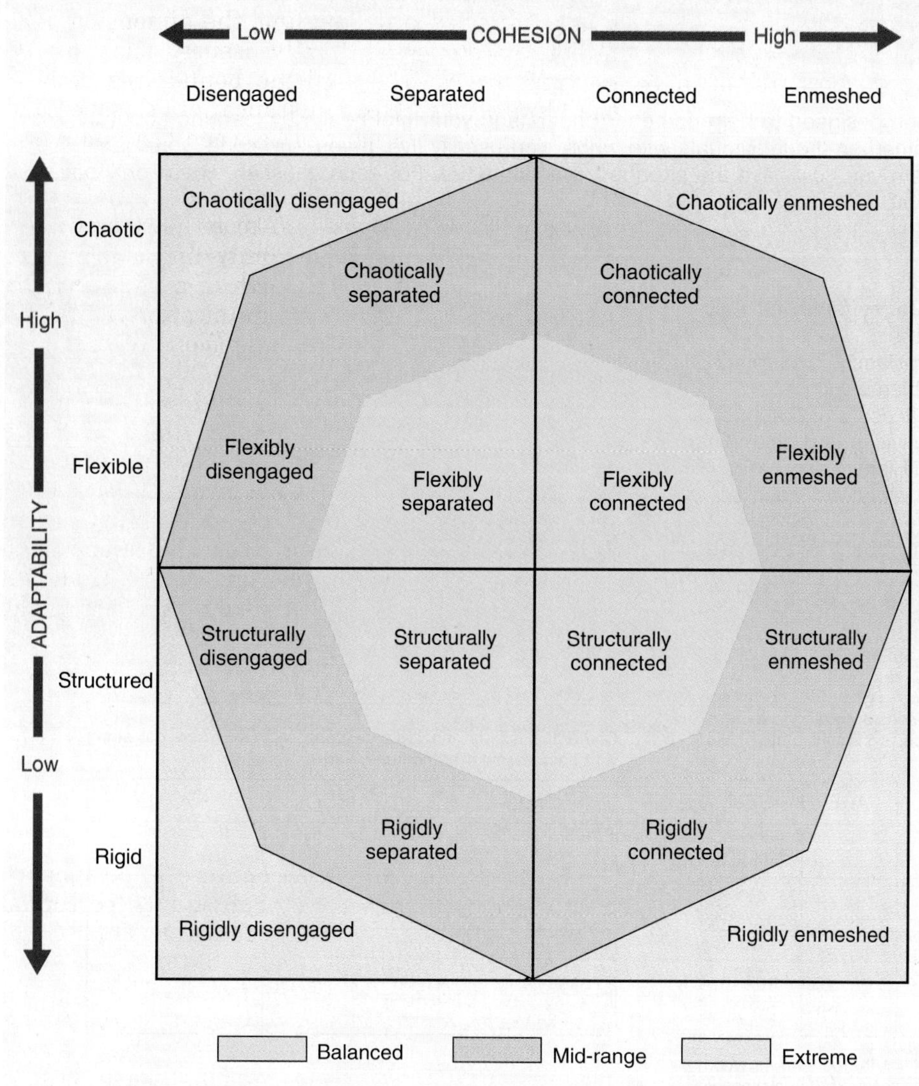

Figure 4–6

Circumplex Model of 16 family typologies. (From Olson, D. H., Russell, C. S., Sprenkle, D. H. [1983]. Circumplex model VI: Theoretical update. *Family Process,* 22, 69–83.)

and describe how well they perceive their interaction with each family member, rating their relationship as getting along well, fairly, and poorly. Reliability and validity of the Family Apgar Questionnaire have been reported from 0.80 to 0.86 on Cronbach's alpha scale (Smilkstein et al. 1982).

Families with Special Needs

Among today's special challenges in maternal-newborn nursing, there is a need to work with families whose structure differs from the two-parent nuclear family and help families with other special needs during the childbearing years. Families of single childbearing women, lesbian childbearing women, women with human immunodeficiency virus (HIV) infection, women with communication difficulties, women with physical disabilities, mentally impaired women, women of low socioeconomic status, women in prison, and homeless women are included in these groups.

Specialized care should be available during pregnancy, birth, and early parenting periods to families in which the mother-to-be has

- Visual impairment, including partial or total loss of vision (Cheatham et al. 1994)
- Hearing impairment that disrupts her ability to utilize hearing for communication purposes (Cheatham et al. 1994)
- Physical disabilities such as rheumatoid arthritis, spinal cord injury, and cerebral palsy (Bertosa et al. 1993)
- Physical illnesses, including systemic lupus erythematosus, HIV infection, and acquired immunodeficiency syndrome (AIDS) (Acosta et al. 1992; Bastin et al. 1992)
- Mental retardation that substantially limits her

Assessment Tool: Family Apgar Questionnaire

PART I

The following questions have been designed to help us better understand your total health by learning about the support in your life. Family is defined as the individuals with whom you usually live. If you live alone, your "family" consists of the persons with whom you now have the strongest emotional ties. For each question, check only one column that seems to apply to you.

	Never	Hardly Ever	Some of the Time	Almost Always	Always
1. I am satisfied that I can turn to my family for help when something is troubling me.					
2. I am satisfied with the way my family talks things over with me and shares problems with me.					
3. I am satisfied that my family accepts and supports my wishes to take on new activities and directions.					
4. I am satisfied with the way my family expresses affection and responds to my emotions, such as anger, sorrow, and love.					
5. I am satisfied with the way my family and I share time together.					

Comments:

PART II

Who lives in your home?* List the persons according to their relationship to you (for example, spouse, significant other,[†] child, or friend).

RELATIONSHIP	AGE	SEX

Check the column that best describes how you now get along with each member of the family listed.

WELL	FAIRLY	POORLY

If you don't live with your own family, list the persons to whom you turn for help most frequently. List according to relationship (for example, family member, friend, associate at work, or neighbor).

RELATIONSHIP	AGE	SEX

Check the column that best describes how you now get along with each person listed.

WELL	FAIRLY	POORLY

*If you have established your own family, consider your "home" the place where you live with your spouse, children, or significant other (see next footnote for definition); otherwise, consider home your place of origin, for example, the place where your parents or those who raised you live.

[†]Significant other is the partner you live with in a physically and emotionally nurturing relationship but to whom you are not married.

Adapted from Smilkstein, G. (1978). The family APGAR: A proposal for a family function test and its use by physicians. *The Journal of Family Practice,* 6, 1231–1239.

functioning as related to communication, self-care, home living, social skills, self-direction, health and safety, functional academics, leisure, and work (Keltner and Tymchuk 1992)
- Homelessness that may result from poverty, lack of low-income housing, mental illness, alcohol or drug addiction, or lack of social support (Damrosch et al. 1988)

All women and their families, with or without a special need, have the right to weigh the consequences of childbearing and to make decisions regarding the risks they wish to take (Cheatham et al. 1994). Likewise, women with disabilities or difficult social situations have the right to the same quality of care in the maternity care system as other populations. Families with special needs express the desire to be treated as normally as possible by their caregivers. It is important that nurses strive to be nonjudgmental about the special needs of families during the childbearing experience and provide the additional support required.

The family is the unit that society believes to be responsible for providing children with an environment that meets their physical and emotional needs. However, a great number of pregnant women and new parents today are challenged with enormous problems—parental unemployment, divorce, drug abuse, loss of family housing, prison confinement, and stigmatization by society. Nurses are in a pivotal position to provide support to these families, assisting them to maximize their strengths and mobilize resources that may not be familiar to them. It is important to have some understanding of the complex dynamics these families face.

RESILIENCY MODEL OF FAMILY STRESS, ADJUSTMENT, AND ADAPTATION

While families with special needs face many stressors, they may also demonstrate great strengths and adaptive abilities. The Resiliency Model of Family Stress, Adjustment, and Adaptation is a useful framework for working with families with special needs (McCubbin and McCubbin 1993). This model represents many years of family theory building and is based on the research of Hill ABCX Model (Hill 1949, 1958) and McCubbin and Patterson Double ABCX Model (McCubbin and Patterson 1983). It identifies key components of families that affect their functioning.

There are several advantages to using this model to provide care for special families. First, it shows important relationships among family variables, helping nurses systematically organize knowledge and ideas about families (Artinian 1994). Second, the model identifies potential family strengths and capabilities as well as stressors (McCubbin and McCubbin 1993). Third, a great deal of research from a variety of disciplines has helped to shape and validate the ABCX models (Failla and Jones 1991; McCubbin 1993).

A diagram of the adjustment phase of the Resiliency Model of Family Stress, Adjustment, and Adaptation is shown in Figure 4–7. The major components of the model are as follows.

▼ **Demands or Illness Stressor (A Factor).** Stressors are defined as events or transitions (for example, pregnancy, death, illness) that influence the family or could potentially affect the family. Demands include not only the initial stressors but also the changes and events in families as a *result* of the stressors. Demands differ in their severity, the degree to which the demands threaten or disrupt the family stability.

▼ **Vulnerability (V Factor).** Vulnerability is the interpersonal condition of the family system. This is influenced by the pileup of demands within the family and the family's life cycle stage with its normative demands. The impact of stressors, such as loss of family housing or a family member's being diagnosed with HIV, is likely to be greater during a family transition time, such as the birth of an infant, than in a period of less turmoil.

▼ **Family Type (T Factor).** Family typologies characterize families' typical manners of perceiving, processing, and coping with stress and transitions. Predictable patterns of family behavior, including rules and routines, play an important role in explaining differences in families. Families who share a sense of purpose and value regular, meaningful family activities demonstrate great strength. This explains why some families, when faced with a great crisis, endure and appear to be resilient to disruptions. These families are characterized by their hardiness and their sense of coherence. Conversely, other families may be vulnerable to hardships and changes.

▼ **Resistance Resources (B Factor).** Resistance resources describe the family's capabilities and strengths in dealing with the stressors. In addition, families can develop or reinforce their ability to solve problems, cope, and adjust in response to the stressor. These developed resources then become part of a family's capabilities in resisting disruption and in adapting. A variety of family resistance resources have been described, including economic resources, stability, cohesiveness, and organization (Curran 1983; McCubbin et al. 1988).

▼ **Family Appraisal (C Factor).** As families confront stressors, they determine the seriousness of each situation, forming a subjective definition.

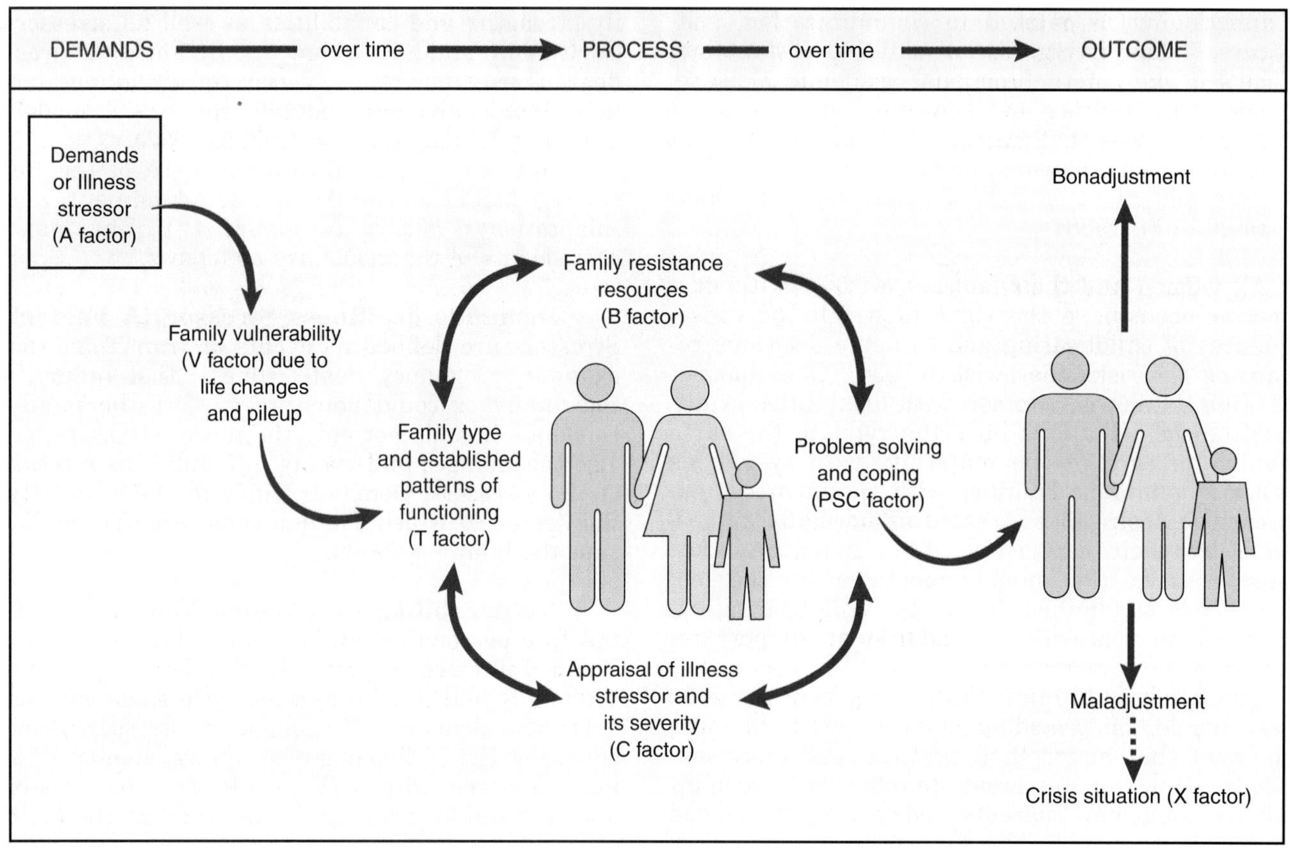

Figure 4–7

The adjustment phase of the Resiliency Model of Family Stress, Adjustment, and Adaptation. This model identifies key components that affect family functioning: demands or illness stressor (A factor); family vulnerability (V factor); family type and established patterns of functioning (T factor); family resistance resources (B factor); appraisal of illness stressor and its severity (C factor); problem solving and coping (PSC factor); bonadjustment, maladjustment, and crisis situation (X factor). (Adapted from Danielson, C. B., Hamel-Bissell, B., Winstead-Fry, P. [1993]. *Families, health, and illness: Perspectives on coping and intervention* [p. 27]. St. Louis: Mosby.)

Families appraise not only the stressor but also the hardships and the resulting effects on them. Several families could be faced with the same stressor. Whereas one family may interpret the stressor as a challenge, others may perceive the same stressor as devastating to the family.

▼ **Family Problem Solving and Coping (PSC Factor).** This factor represents the family's management of the situation. This includes problem solving and coping.

▼ **Family Adjustment.** The family attempts to achieve balance at the individual-family and the family-community level of functioning through the interplay of a number of components that include family vulnerability, family type and established patterns of functioning, family resistance resources, family appraisal of the stressor, and problem-solving and coping strategies. These components of the model help explain the nature of the outcome—why some families move through stressful situations with ease (bonadjustment) and other families, faced with the same stressor, experience numerous threats to their stability (maladjustment) and must make great changes in the family system. The X factor represents the crisis situation that may develop when the family does not have the resources to resolve maladjustment.

The Resiliency Model of Family Stress, Adjustment, and Adaptation dispels the notion that a stressor (A factor) automatically determines an outcome (X factor). Each of the components of this model can be considered when nursing care is being provided to families with special needs. By assessing a number of different aspects of the family system's response to stressors, a more realistic picture of the family can be drawn. For example, it is as important to consider the sense of coherence demonstrated by these families as it is to identify their stressors. The model underscores the importance of obtaining the family's perspective of their situation. A situation that a nurse might consider insurmountable might simply be judged a minor annoyance by a particular family. The Resiliency Model of Family Stress, Adjustment, and Adaptation emphasizes the complex interplay of family factors contributing to a family's adjustment to stressors (see also Chapter 17).

Evaluating Family Strengths

The issue of family strengths has become an important area of study in recent years. Families are usually described from the standpoint of problems and weaknesses. The focus on family strengths helps everyone recognize what a family may strive for and analyze how the family has developed these strengths. The identification and recognition of a family strength may be of more help to a troubled family than emphasizing their problems.

Stinnett (1979) and Stinnett and associates (1981), family researchers, have studied family strengths. Families who had a high degree of marital satisfaction, had a high degree of happiness with their children, and were supportive of one another's emotional needs were identified from a broad spectrum of communities. When these families were surveyed, six characteristics were identified as strengths critical for the growth and development of each family member.

Text continued on page 81

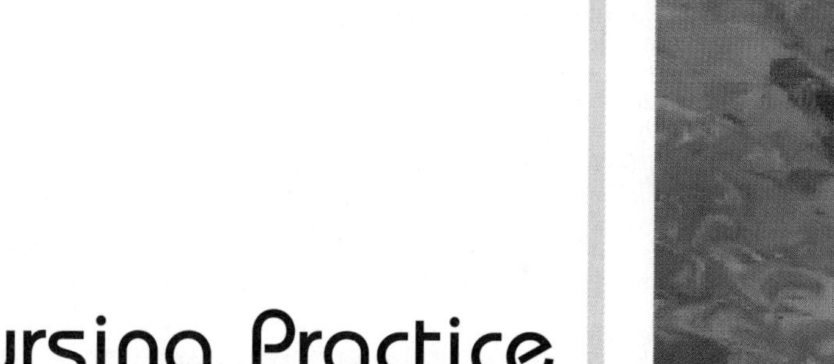

Nursing Practice

Nursing Process

▼ Assessment

The assessment of the childbearing family can be done by use of a number of different approaches, such as the Symbolic Interaction Theory or Social Exchange Theory. Using a family system framework is an effective and efficient way to determine family structure and function in terms of roles and power, communication patterns, the family's relationship with the suprastructure, cultural values, health and illness beliefs, family values, and family relationships (see Family Assessment Guide, p. 72). The Family Apgar Questionnaire (p. 76) or other assessment tools can also provide the nurse with additional information. After the family assessment is completed, the next step is to interpret the data and determine the appropriate nursing diagnoses.

▼ Diagnosis

Nursing diagnoses are formulated on the basis of findings from the assessment data and then validated with the family. Together, the nurse and the family prioritize the nursing diagnoses according to importance and urgency.

Possible nursing diagnoses for the typical childbearing family include

- Altered family processes
- Family coping: potential for growth
- Knowledge deficit: *specify* . . . related to

Possible nursing diagnoses for the high-risk childbearing family include

- Ineffective family coping: compromised
- Risk for altered parenting
- Knowledge deficit: *specify* . . . related to

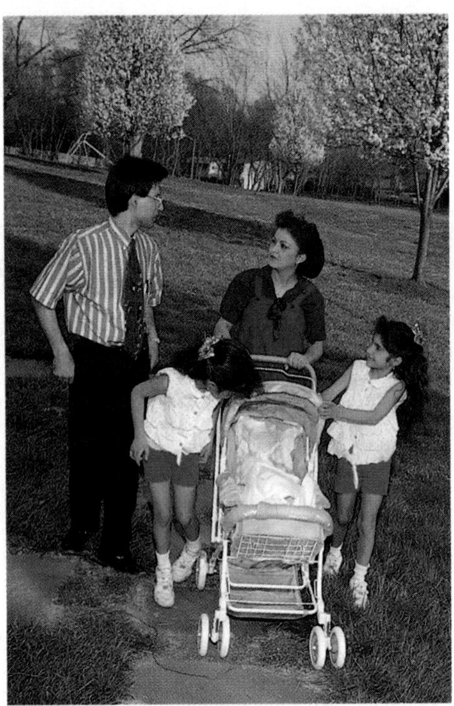

Figure 4–8
Each member of the childbearing family experiences stressors as a new baby is integrated into the family system. The nurse can provide valuable support, education, and guidance to ease the adjustment of each family member during this time of transition. While these two siblings are obviously proud of "their" new baby, both they and their parents will experience stress and may have negative feelings at times as the demands of the new baby take center stage.

▼ Planning

The first step is to plan expected family outcomes or goals and then to select appropriate nursing interventions (Fig. 4–8). While family outcomes will depend on the individual family, some possible outcome behaviors appropriate for most childbearing families are

- The family will acknowledge changes in family roles and structure
- The family will identify and use effective coping patterns
- The family will participate in the decision-making process related to pregnancy, childbirth, and postbirth care

▼ Intervention

Nursing interventions for the family are based on the interviewing and counseling techniques of listening, clarifying, reflecting, and reinforcing those behaviors that will assist the family in making the needed adjustments. Developing an open, trusting relationship with the family will enhance the potential for achieving the desired family outcomes. Nursing interventions appropriate for most childbearing families are

PROVIDING SPECIAL NEEDS FAMILIES WITH QUALITY CARE

Working with families who have special needs can be a new, challenging, and therefore intimidating experience. The following steps can help you to increase your awareness of women and their families who have special needs and provide the quality care necessary throughout the pregnancy, birth, and early parenting experience.

- ANALYZE YOUR FEELINGS ABOUT PREGNANCY AND PARENTHOOD IN SPECIAL NEEDS POPULATIONS. Some professionals may be judgmental about decisions to have children by mothers who are disabled or have other special needs. It is important to identify whether you have these feelings, and if so, to explore the reasons they exist so that your care of pregnant women with special needs will not be compromised.
- UPDATE YOUR KNOWLEDGE BASE. Learn all you can about women who are visually or hearing impaired, physically or mentally disabled, or homeless. Read professional journal articles and attend continuing education seminars to identify how care should be altered to meet their needs.
- NETWORK WITH OTHER NURSES. Talk with your colleagues to get helpful, creative ideas about ways to provide the education and care that special needs families have during pregnancy and childbirth.
- BE OPEN AND HONEST WITH SPECIAL NEEDS CLIENTS. If you are uncertain, ask them how you can best care for them. Your honesty will be appreciated and they will probably be pleased to share with you approaches to care that will be helpful.
- BE FLEXIBLE. Have alternative strategies for teaching or providing care for special needs families.

- Assess family interaction, being alert for potential destructive behaviors (see Family Assessment Guide, p. 72)
- Encourage family members to verbalize feelings, for example, "It's often helpful to talk about any concerns that you have for . . ."
- Encourage family members to interact, providing privacy when possible. "Why don't you discuss this concern?" "I'll leave you alone for a while so you can talk more freely." "Why don't you discuss it together? I'll be back in a half-hour or so and we can talk more at that time."
- Assist family members to identify personal strengths. "Your family discusses things so well together. You must find that very helpful."
- Provide positive reinforcement for effective use of coping mechanisms. "It is so helpful that you can share your fears about . . . ; it is the first step to finding a way to deal with this problem."
- Encourage family members to express concern and to help plan postbirth care
- Explore available hospital and community resources with the family

For the high-risk childbearing family, an intervention that is extremely helpful in addition to the specific interventions needed for the family's situation is

- Request a social service consultation to assist with determining the family's needs, identify community support resources, and provide follow-up care

Nursing interventions for the family with special needs related to a physical, mental, or social challenge depend on each individual family's unique situation. An individualized assessment of each special needs family is essential to identify goals and interventions; each family's needs will vary widely because of the particular circumstances. Providing quality care for families with special needs can be an opportunity for professional growth (see Improving Your Practice).

▼ Evaluation

The effectiveness of nursing care is determined by comparing the current status of the family with the stated desired outcomes of care. The major sources of data for evaluating family outcomes are direct observation of family interactions and discussions about progress toward the set goals with the family. The plan for nursing care is revised according to the results of evaluation.

---

1. Family members expressed a great deal of appreciation for one another. In the identified strong families, family members made efforts to affirm another family member with expressions of appreciation.
2. Family members spent a lot of time together, in work and in play. They enjoyed being together. They made time to spend together.
3. The family members expressed a high degree of commitment to the family group. The active involvement of the family members was directed toward the welfare of one another and also toward developing a sense of unity.
4. The family members demonstrated direct communication patterns. The family members did not always agree, but they got their conflicts out in the open and discussed them.
5. A large number of the identified strong families held a high degree of religious orientation. Although no definite religions were mentioned, the families mentioned activities such as attending church, praying, or studying their beliefs together as usual practice. A spiritual lifestyle was a commitment among these families.
6. The families also stated that they were able to cope with crisis situations. They reported that they were able to demonstrate support to one another during difficult times (Stinnett 1979; Stinnett et al. 1981).

Curran (1983) has also studied family strengths. She queried professionals for their view of characteristics of a healthy family. In compiling the responses, she developed 15 descriptors of family behaviors. The family communicates and listens; affirms and supports; teaches respect for others; develops a sense of trust; has a sense of play and humor; exhibits a sense of shared respect; teaches a sense of right and wrong; has rituals and traditions; demonstrates a balance of interaction; shares religious beliefs; respects privacy; values service to others; fosters table time and conversation; shares leisure time; and admits to and seeks help for problems.

The characteristics of families described as strong by the professionals and the characteristics of families who described themselves as strong are similar.

FAMILY STRENGTHS INVENTORY

Stinnett (1979) developed a Family Strengths Inventory that assesses major family strengths, marital relationships, and parent-child relationships. In 1981, the Family Strengths Inventory

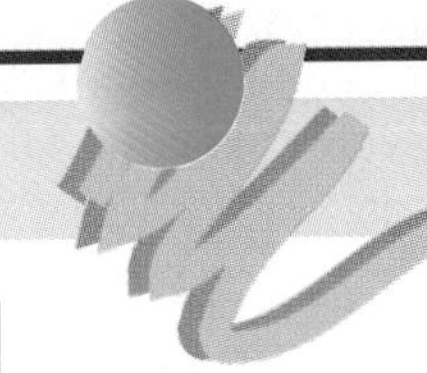

HISTORICAL PERSPECTIVES

NATIONAL FAMILY POLICY FOR 25 YEARS

The Nixon Administration (1969–1974)

During the Nixon Administration, improvements to the modern welfare system were greater in size and scope than the initiatives of Johnson's "Great Society" in the 1960s. Changes during the Nixon Administration included extensive expansion of the food stamp program, development of affirmative action policies, establishment of the Occupational Safety and Health Administration (OSHA), addition of family planning programs to the Public Health Act, and approval of the Child Abuse Prevention Act of 1973.

Nixon also attempted to establish a Family Assistance Plan that included the provision of a guaranteed income for all families, daycare for young children, and other family benefits. The Plan, which would have meant a major overhaul of the welfare system, was defeated in 1972. Liberals thought the Plan went too far; conservatives claimed it did not do enough.

Nixon, although a conservative, supported these family policy changes because he was an astute politician. He was responding to the cries for social changes that still echoed from the 1960s. He supported the Family Assistance Plan because he was assured that if it was implemented, it would make possible the reduction of the massive numbers of social workers in the social welfare system. While there was significant change for the betterment of the American family during his tenure, Nixon was in general against social service programs of all kinds and vetoed most child development legislation during his administration.

The Ford Administration (1974–1976)

During the Ford Administration, there was little progress in the area of family policy. President Ford's main contribution was to preside over a debate between conservatives and liberals on the future of the welfare state. The debate ended in a stalemate. The Democratic majority in both houses generated many bills for proposed social programs, all of which President Ford vetoed.

The Carter Administration (1977–1980)

The American family was the cornerstone of Carter's campaign for President. In spite of his political rhetoric, there were few successes in developing policy that would help the American family. The family President Carter wanted to preserve and support was the traditional nuclear family of the 1950s. He wavered when it came to providing services for different types of American families, such as daycare for children of working mothers and shelters for battered women. President Carter was violently opposed to abortion and supported the legislation that prohibited the use of federal Medicaid funds for abortion. The primary contribution to family policy during the Carter Administration was the passage of the Adoption Assistance and Child Welfare Reform Act of 1980. This legislation refined good child welfare practice and laid the foundation for dramatic changes in adoption practice and home-based services to families.

The Reagan Administration (1981–1988)

The conservatism on family policy that began during President Nixon's second term continued throughout the Ford and Carter Administrations and became even stronger during the Reagan years. By the end of the Reagan Administration, the average income for the 10 percent of families with the lowest incomes had dropped 18 percent from 1977 to $3504. In contrast, the average income for the 10 percent of families with the highest incomes had increased 16.5

Continued on facing page

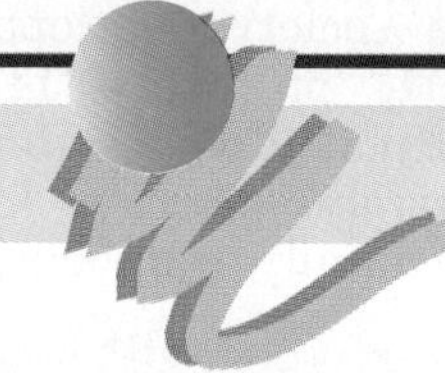

HISTORICAL PERSPECTIVES Continued

percent for the same period to $166,000. During Reagan's tenure, the total expenditures for social programs were drastically cut, and 57 federal programs were eliminated or included in block grants. In 1987, the National Commission on Children was formed by the President and Congress to evaluate the status of children and families and propose an action plan for policy and program development.

The Bush Administration (1989–1992)

The Bush Administration has frequently been referred to as the third Reagan term. During the Bush tenure, a steady decrease in funding for social programs continued. There were cutbacks in Medicare, Medicaid, and Aid to Families with Dependent Children (AFDC) benefits, all of which influenced the welfare of families. In 1991, a comprehensive and bold blueprint of a national policy for America's families and children was unanimously approved by the National Commission on Children and submitted to the President and Congress.

The Clinton Administration (1993–)

The Clinton Administration inherited problems—troubled families in poverty, violence, hopelessness—caused by the nation's neglect of family policy. While President Clinton's promises to improve the welfare of families raised hopes and expectations, little progress has been made to date.

Adapted from Hartman, A. (1993). Challenges for family policy. In F. Walsh (Ed.). *Normal family processes* (2nd ed.). New York: Guilford Press; National Commission on Children. (1991). *Beyond rhetoric: A new American agenda for children and families.* Washington, D.C.: Author.

was used to study 283 families from 25 states who identified themselves as strong families. The findings from this study described these family characteristics: love, commitment, communication, religion, understanding, doing things together, compliments/appreciates, builds ego/supports, trust, and individuality (Stinnett et al. 1981). Stinnett has shown that many of these characteristics can be learned, and therefore he supports education for families to learn to develop these strengths. He recommends workshops, seminars, and secondary and college family education courses (Stinnett 1979; Stinnett et al. 1981).

NATIONAL FAMILY POLICY

Debate and decisions related to the family touch the very core of Americans' cultural beliefs and values. Family policy has continued to be one of the hottest political issues in America. Hartman (1993, p. 474) captures the essence of the controversy: "Some have claimed the field of family policy doesn't exist, some say it does, but shouldn't, whereas still others argue for a clear and coherent national family policy."

The first national public discussion on family policy was held by Jimmy Carter during his campaign. Although America does not have an official stated position on family policy, the federal government has enacted policy through the years that has affected family welfare and influenced family life (Hartman 1993).

An American Family Policy Agenda

In 1987, the National Commission on Children was created by Congress and the President to "serve as a forum on behalf of the children of the Nation." The Commission unanimously approved a comprehensive and bold blueprint for a national family policy in 1991 and submitted it to the President and Congress. The policy action agenda was based on the following principles concerning family roles and responsibilities, children's basic needs, and society's obligation (National Commission on Children 1991).

- Every American child should have the opportunity to develop to his or her potential.
- Parents bear primary responsibility for meeting their children's physical, emotional, and intellectual needs and for providing moral guidance and direction. It is in society's best interests to support parents in their childbearing roles, to enable them to fulfill their obligations, and to hold them responsible for the care and support of their children.
- Children do best when they have the personal involvement and material support of a father and a mother and when both parents fulfill their responsibility to be loving providers.
- The family is and should remain society's primary institution for bringing children into the world and supporting their growth and development throughout childhood.
- Cultural diversity is one of America's greatest riches; it must be represented and preserved, while at the same time ensuring that all children have an equal opportunity to enter the social and economic mainstream.
- Community institutions—schools, religious organizations, service and charitable organizations, and employers—have an important role in creating an environment that is supportive of parents and children.
- Communities have a responsibility to provide safe, secure environments for families with children.
- Society has a legitimate interest in childbearing and a moral obligation to intervene when parents fail to meet their responsibilities and put their children at risk.
- Preventing problems before they become crises is the most effective and cost-effective way to address the needs of troubled families and vulnerable children.
- Basic moral values are part of our national heritage and should guide society in its actions toward children and families.
- Effectively addressing the needs of America's children and families will require a significant commitment of time, leadership, and financial resources by individuals, the private sector, and government at all levels.

The Commission pointed out that the most critical factor influencing a child's development and welfare was the child's family and the circumstances in which the child lived. An explicit, clear, and coherent family policy is fundamental in supporting and rebuilding American families. Adaptable and flexible programs are needed to meet the needs of our diverse American society (National Commission on Children 1991, pp. 311–314). Nurses need to be sensitive to policy issues that can affect the family and actively advocate for health policy that will improve family well-being.

Implications for Research

Numerous areas related to the study of the health of families need to be examined. A significant area for research includes the attitudes and beliefs of the American society about the value of children as a national resource and society's responsibility for the satisfactory rearing of these children. The impact of pregnancy and childbirth in emerging nontraditional family forms (such as the single mother, lesbian or gay couples, and blended families) requires careful study.

Specific research questions that need to be examined are:

- What are the most effective approaches for strengthening families?
- What approaches do families use to incorporate siblings into the childbearing experience and prepare them for the new baby?
- What are the most effective strategies for helping families meet the demands and responsibilities of childbearing?

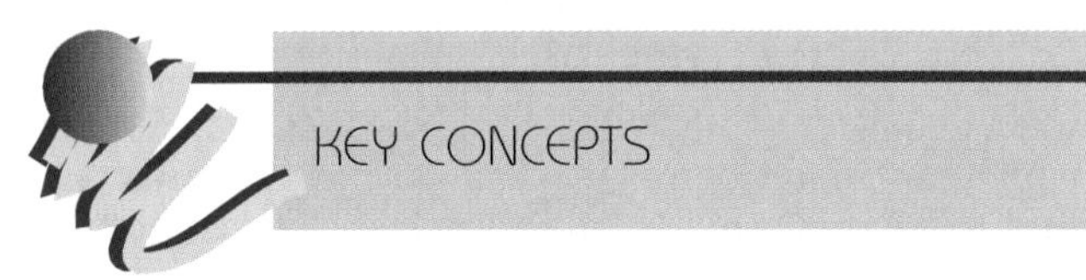

KEY CONCEPTS

▼ The health and welfare of individual family members are significantly influenced by the family unit.

▼ During the perinatal period, the family encounters numerous stressors from relationship and role changes. Some families perceive these stressors as a socioemotional crisis; most families perceive these same stressors as a life transition.

▼ In 1993, just more than 4 million babies were born, approximately 31 percent (1,240,172) to unmarried women.

▼ Abnormal conditions and congenital anomalies are closely associated with prematurity and low birth weight. In 1993, approximately 4 percent of births (149,499) showed abnormal conditions; reporting states recorded 1 percent of births (40,749) with congenital anomalies.

▼ The structure of the American family has changed radically in the past four decades. Major changes include the rapid increase of single-parent families; blended families resulting from remarriage; and other nontraditional family forms, such as lesbian and gay families.

- Other changes that have occurred in the family are the dramatic increase in working mothers and the sharp decreases in size of families.
- The family serves five major functions: ensuring economic survival, providing protection, passing on beliefs and values, educating children, and conferring status.
- The nuclear family consisting of a male breadwinner, his wife as full-time homemaker, and their dependent children came into being with industrialization in the nineteenth century and peaked in the post–World War II era in the 1950s.
- The contemporary family consists of several different forms in addition to the traditional nuclear and extended families. A single culturally dominant form no longer exists in our society. Instead, there are numerous coexisting and evolving family forms.
- Symbolic Interaction Theory, Social Exchange Theory, and Systems Theory are all useful in assessing and understanding family dynamics.
- The assignment and appropriation of power, interactional patterns, and culture and values all influence family functioning.
- Family assessment tools provide the link between theory, research, and practice and furnish a framework for the nurse to gather information about family dynamics, which can be used to interpret interactions and patterns of behavior and plan nursing care.
- An explicit, clear, and coherent national family policy is needed and is fundamental in supporting and rebuilding American families.

References

Acosta, Y., Goodwin, C., Alvarez, A., Tinkle, M., Acosta, E., Jaquez, I. (1992). HIV disease and pregnancy: Part 2. Antepartum and intrapartum care. *Journal of Obstetric, Gynecologic, and Neonatal Nursing,* 21 (2), 97–104.

Adoptive Families of America. (1994). *Adoption: How to begin.* Minneapolis: Author.

Ahlburg, D., and DeVita, C. (1993). New families, old values? *The Futurist,* 27 (Jan–Feb), 45–46.

Alexander-Roberts, C. (1994). Know your options. In Adoptive Families of America. *Adoptions: How to begin.* Minneapolis: Adoptive Families of America.

Anderson, S., Plantanida, M., Anderson, C. (1993). Normal processes in adoptive families. In F. Walsh (Ed.). *Normal family processes* (2nd ed.) (pp. 254–281). New York: Guilford Press.

Artinian, N. T. (1994). Selecting a model to guide family assessment. *Dimensions of Critical Care Nursing,* 14 (1), 4–12.

Bastin, N., Tamayo, O., Tinkle, M., Alvarez, A., Trejo, L., Herrea, C. (1992). HIV disease and pregnancy: Part 3. Postpartum care of the HIV-positive woman and her newborn. *Journal of Obstetric, Gynecologic, and Neonatal Nursing,* 21 (2), 105–113.

Bertalanffy, L. V. (1968). *General system theory.* New York: George Braziller.

Bertosa, H., Cellura, M., Pierce, L., Rothacker, C. (1993). Women with spinal cord injuries require sensitive reproductive care. *MCN,* 18 (5), 254–257.

Biasella, S. (1993). A comprehensive perinatal education program. *AWHONN's Clinical Issues in Perinatal and Women's Health Nursing: Perinatal Education,* 4 (1), 5–19.

Bowen, M. (1971). The use of family theory in clinical practice. In J. Haley (Ed.). *Changing families.* New York: Grune & Stratton.

Boyd-Franklin, M. (1993). Race, class, and poverty. In F. Walsh (Ed.). *Normal family processes* (2nd ed.) (pp. 361–376). New York: Guilford Press.

Broderick, C., and Smith, J. (1979). The general systems approach to the family. In E. R. Burr, R. Hill, F. I. Nye, I. Reiss (Eds.). *Contemporary theories about the family* (Vol. 2). New York: Free Press.

Brodzinsky, D., and Schechter, M. (1990). *The psychology of adoption.* New York: Oxford University Press.

Burr, E. R., Hill, R., Nye, F. I., Reiss, I. (1979). *Contemporary theories about the family* (Vol. 2). New York: Free Press.

Caplan, G. (1982). The family as a support system. In H. McCubbin, A. E. Cauble, J. Patterson (Eds.). *Family stress, coping, and social support* (pp. 200–220). Springfield, IL: Charles C Thomas, Publisher.

Cheatham, D., King, E., Bartz, A. (1994). *Childbirth education for women with disabilities and their partners.* Columbus, OH: The Ohio State University Nisonger Center.

Christensen, H. T. (1964). *Handbook of marriage and the family.* Chicago: Rand McNally.

Cigoll, U., and Binda, W. (1993). Health and the family. *World Health,* 6 (Nov-Dec), 7.

Cooley, M. (1995). A family perspective in community health nursing. In C. M. Smith and F. A. Maurer (Eds.). *Community health nursing: Theory and practice.* Philadelphia: W. B. Saunders.

Curran, D. (1983). *Traits of a healthy family.* Minneapolis: Winston Press.

Damrosch, S., Sullivan, P., Scholler, A., Gaines, J. (1988). On behalf of homeless families. *MCN,* 13 (4), 259–263.

Diamond, M., and Jones, S. L. (1983). *Chronic illness across the life span.* Norwalk, CT: Appleton-Century-Crofts.

Doherty, W., and McCubbin, H. (1985). Families and health care: An emerging area of theory, research and clinical intervention. *Family Relations,* 34 (1), 5–11.

Duvall, E. M. (1977). *Marriage and family development* (5th ed.). Philadelphia: J. B. Lippincott.

Engebretson, J. C. (1982). Stepmothers as first-time parents: Their needs and problems. *Pediatric Nurse,* 8 (Nov-Dec), 387–390.

Etzioni, A. (1977). Science and the future of the family. *Science,* 196, (4289), 487.

Failla, S., and Jones, L. C. (1991). Families with children with developmental disabilities: Relationship between family hardiness and family functioning. *Research in Nursing and Health,* 14, 41–50.

Feetham, S. L. (1984). Family research: Issues and directions for nursing. *Annual Review of Nursing Research,* 3, 3–25.

Gaylin, N. L. (1980). Rediscovering the family. In N. L. Gaylin. *Family strengths* (Vol. 2) (pp. 5–15). Lincoln, NB: University of Nebraska Press.

Gilliss, C. (1989). Why family health care? In C. L. Gilliss, B. L. Highley, B. M. Roberts, I. M. Martinson (Eds.). *Toward a science of family nursing* (pp. 3–8). Menlo Park, CA: Addison-Wesley.

Glick, P. C. (1991 Oct). *Address to annual conference.* Lincoln, NB: Stepfamily Association of America.

Glick, P., and Lin, S. (1986). Recent changes in divorce and remarriage. *Journal of Marriage and the Family,* 48, 737–747.

Haley, J. (1963). *Strategies of psychotherapy,* New York: Grune & Stratton.

Harris, L., et al. (1981). *Families at work: General Mills American family report, 1980–81.* Minneapolis: Author.

Hartman, A. (1993). Challenges for family policy. In F. Walsh (Ed.). *Normal family processes* (2nd ed.) (pp. 474–502). New York: Guilford Press.

Hill, R. (1949). *Families under stress.* New York: Harper & Row.

Hill, R. (1958). Generic features of families under stress. *Social Casework,* 49, 139–150.

Hill, R., and Hansen, D. A. (1960). The identification of conceptual frameworks utilized in family study. *Marriage and Family Living,* 22, 299–311.

Homans, G. C. (1958). Social behavior as exchange. *American Journal of Sociology,* 63, 597–606.

Jackson, D. (1968). The question of family homeostasis. In D. Jackson (Ed.). *Communication, family, and marriage.* Palo Alto, California: Science and Behavior.

Kantor, D., and Lehr, W. (1975). *Inside the family.* San Francisco: Jossey-Bass.

Keltner, B., and Tymchuk, A. (1992). Reaching out to mothers with mental retardation. *MCN,* 17 (3), 136–140.

Kennedy, C. (1980). The case for family life education. In E. E. Kennedy (Ed.). *Readings in family life education and consultation.* Manhattan, KS: Kansas State University.

Laird, J. (1993). Lesbian and gay families. In F. Walsh (Ed.). *Normal family processes* (2nd ed.) (pp. 282–330). New York: Guilford Press.

Mahoney, M. E. (1986). *The President's report: Families.* New York: Harkness House.

McCubbin, M. A. (1993). Family stress theory and the development of nursing knowledge about family adaptation. In Feetham, S., et al. (Eds.). *The nursing of families: Theory, research, administration, practice* (pp. 546–558). Newbury Park, CA: Sage.

McCubbin, M., and McCubbin, H. (1993). Families coping with illness. In C. B. Danielson, B. Hamel-Bissell, P. Winstead-Fry (Eds.). *Families, health, & illness: Perspectives on coping and intervention.* St. Louis: Mosby.

McCubbin, H. I., and Patterson, J. M. (1983). The family stress process: The double ABCX model of adjustment and adaptation. In H. McCubbin, M. Sussman, J. Patterson (Eds.). *Advances and development in family stress theory and research* (pp. 7–37). New York: Haworth.

McCubbin, H. I., Thompson, A., Pirner, P., McCubbin, M. A. (1988). *Family types and strengths: A life cycle and ecological perspective.* Edina, MN: Burgess International Group.

Mead, G. H. (1934). *Mind, self, and society.* Chicago: Chicago University Press.

Mercer, R. T. (1981). A theoretical framework for studying factors that impact on the maternal role. *Nursing Research,* 30, 73–77.

Mercer, R. T. (1985). The process of maternal role attainment over the first year. *Nursing Research,* 34, 198–204.

Mercer, R. T. (1986). *First-time motherhood: Experiences from teens to forties.* New York: Springer-Verlag.

Murphy, P. E., and Staples, W. A. (1979). A modernized family life cycle. *Journal of Consumer Research,* 6 (6), 12–22.

National Center for Health Statistics. (1993). Advanced report of final natality statistics, 1991. *Monthly Vital Statistics Report,* 42 (Suppl. 3, Sep 9), S1–S13.

National Center for Health Statistics. (1995). Advanced report of final natality statistics, 1993. *Monthly Vital Statistics Report,* 44 (Suppl. 3, Sep 21), S1–S88.

National Commission on Children. (1991). *Beyond rhetoric: A new American agenda for children and families.* Washington, D.C.: U. S. Government Printing Office.

Nye, F. I. (1979). Choice, exchange, and the family. In E. R. Burr, R. Hill, F. I. Nye, I. Reiss (Eds.). *Contemporary theories about the family* (Vol. 2). New York: Free Press.

Olson, H., McCubbin, H. I., Barnes, H., Larsen, A., Muxen, M., Wilson, M. (1985). *Family inventories.* University of Minnesota: Family Social Science.

Osmond, M. W. (1978). Reciprocity: A dynamic model and a method to study family power. *Journal of Marriage and the Family,* 40, 49–61.

Peterson, K., and Peterson, F. (1993). Family-centered perinatal education. *AWHONN's Clinical Issues in Perinatal and Women's Health Nursing: Perinatal Education,* 4 (1), 1–4.

Rubin, R. (1984). *Maternal identity and the maternal experience.* New York: Springer.

Reutter, L., and Strang, V. (1986). Yours, mine and ours: Stepparents and their children. *Maternal Child Nursing,* 11 (4), 264–266.

Satir, V. (1971). *Peoplemaking,* Palo Alto, CA: Science and Behavior.

Smilkstein, G. (1978). The family Apgar: A proposal for a family function test and its use by physicians. *The Journal of Family Practice,* 6, 1231–1239.

Smilkstein, G., Ashworth, C., Montano, D. (1982). Validity and reliability of the family Apgar as a test of family function. *The Journal of Family Practice,* 15 (2), 303–311.

Smith, L. (1983). A conceptual model of families incorporating an adolescent mother and child into the household. *Advances in Nursing Science,* 6, 45–60.

Stainton, M. C. (1989). The perinatal family. In C. Gillis, B. Highley, B. Roberts, I. Martinson (Eds.). *Toward a science of family nursing* (pp. 199–215). Menlo Park, CA: Addison-Wesley.

Starn, J. (1993). Strengthening family systems. In F. Nichols (Ed.). *AWHONN's clinical issues in perinatal and women's health nursing: Perinatal education* (pp. 35–41). Philadelphia: J. B. Lippincott.

Stinnett, N. (1979). In search of families. In N. Stinnett, J. DeFrain, K. King, P. Knaut, G. Rowe (Eds.). *Building family strengths: Blueprints for action.* Lincoln, NB: University of Nebraska Press.

Stinnett, N., Sanders, G., DeFrain, J. (1981). Strong families: A national study. In N. Stinnett, J. DeFrain, K. King, P. Knaut, G. Rowe (Eds.). *Family strengths 3.* Lincoln, NB: University of Nebraska Press.

The changing American family. (1991). *Scholastic Update,* 124 (Sep 6, Teachers' edition), 2–23.

Turner, J. H. (1978). *The structure of sociological theory.* Homewood, IL: Dorsey.

U. S. Department of Labor, Bureau of Labor Statistics. (1980). *U. S. working women: A data book.* Washington, D.C.: U. S. Government Printing Office.

Visher, E., and Visher, J. (1993). Remarriage, families, and stepparenting. In F. Walsh (Ed.). *Normal family processes* (2nd ed.) (pp. 235–253). New York: Guilford Press.

Walsh, F. (1993). Conceptualization of normal family processes. In F. Walsh (Ed.). *Normal family processes* (2nd ed.) (pp. 3–72). New York: Guilford Press.

Whall, A. L., and Fawcett, J. (1991). *Family theory development in nursing: State of the science and art.* Philadelphia: F. A. Davis.

Wismont, J. F., and Reame, N. E. (1989). The lesbian childbearing experience: Assessing development tasks. *Image,* 21 (3), 137–141.

Wymore, J. D. (1989). Stepfamily integration through development phases of adjustment. *Kansas Nurse,* 64 (10), 1–10.

Chapter 5

Maternal-Newborn Nursing in the Community

Margaret R. Edwards

> Home care in the perinatal nursing area has experienced dramatic growth during the recent years . . . Services spanning the trimesters of pregnancy and the postpartum-newborn period have developed and grown. Programs that facilitate early postpartum discharge of mothers and neonates have not only successfully demonstrated cost savings and improved outcome, but have also shown that the education and support needs of new families can best be satisfied by nurses in the home setting.
>
> LINDA GOODWIN (1994)

HIGHLIGHTS

- Scope of Maternal-Newborn Nursing in the Community
- The Family as Client
- Planning and Accomplishing the Home Visit
- Documenting the Home Visit
- Communicating with the Primary Health Care Provider
- Safety Precautions within the Community
- Defining and Assessing the Client's Community
- Linking Clients with Community Resources
- Referring Clients to Other Agencies and Professionals
- Risk Management
- Implications For Research

Maternal-newborn nursing in the community provides the nurse with a unique opportunity to influence the health of the pregnant woman, the new mother, the newborn, and all members of the family. Home visits are an ideal way to provide care that is truly holistic. By making home visits, the nurse is able to assess clients in their own natural setting. During a home visit the nurse can assess the entire family unit and the impact of the family on the health of the mother and newborn. In addition, the influences of the home environment on health and well-being can be assessed. A unique rapport can be developed that enhances the nurse-client relationship. The nurse can link clients with community resources that augment nursing care and improve the well-being of the pregnant woman or mother and newborn.

DEFINITIONS

Childbearing family—An intimate social unit of persons living together in a household, going through the developmental processes of conceiving, bearing, and raising children.

Closing phase—The final portion of a home visit, in which the content of the visit is summarized, goal accomplishment is evaluated, and plans are made for future visits.

Community resources—Organizations or services available in the community to meet a variety of client needs.

Community—Variously defined to mean the group of persons with whom the client interacts or shares common characteristics, or more commonly, a geographic area, from a neighborhood to a large city, consisting of persons, organizations, and services for independent and interdependent living.

Home visit—A goal-directed nurse-client interaction that takes place in the client's residence.

Home health agency—An organization through which nurses work under physicians' orders to provide direct skilled nursing care to clients in their homes.

Primary health care provider—The physician or other health care professional who assumes basic responsibility for the client's health care.

Referral—The process of connecting a client with another professional, organization, or service for the purpose of meeting client needs.

Social phase—The brief opening portion of a home visit, in which friendly conversation paves the way for the concentrated work of the visit.

Third-party payer—An entity other than the client or the health care provider that assumes responsibility for the cost of the health care; most commonly a health insurance company, the client's employer, Medicare, or Medicaid.

Working phase—The goal-directed portion of a home visit, in which the nursing process is employed to meet the client's needs.

SCOPE OF MATERNAL-NEWBORN NURSING IN THE COMMUNITY

Maternal-newborn nursing in the home offers new challenges to the nurse. The knowledge and skills needed to provide successful home visits include more than just competency in the care of antepartum, postpartum, and newborn clients. In addition, the nurse must understand basic principles of providing care in the home setting, and must follow certain procedures to ensure safe and effective home visits. This chapter offers guidance to nurses as they begin the challenging and rewarding experience of providing maternal-newborn nursing in the community.

Health Care of Maternal-Newborn Clients

When asked to form a mental picture of maternal-newborn care, many people think of the obstetric unit in a hospital setting. Acute care during labor, delivery, and the immediate postpartum period is important to the well-being of mother and newborn. It is not, however, the only care needed by maternal-newborn clients. In fact, in the time continuum, acute care in the hospital represents a relatively small portion of the total package of maternal-newborn care.

ACUTE AND COMMUNITY CARE SETTINGS

The hospital experience for a healthy mother and healthy baby with an uncomplicated delivery is usually limited to the time of labor, delivery, and 1 or 2 days post partum. To promote a healthy pregnancy and facilitate successful postpartum adaptation for the new mother and newborn, health care should be provided over a much longer period. Prenatal care should begin in the first trimester and continue throughout the pregnancy. Most prenatal care occurs in ambulatory care settings. This prenatal care can be significantly enhanced by the care and teaching that are provided through home visits.

Hospitalization usually occurs for labor and delivery, but today's health care economics and insurance limitations dictate that clients are discharged as soon as they are physically able. Such early discharge severely limits hospital time for helping the new mother to work through emotional changes or learn about child care (Evans

1991). New mothers are full of questions about themselves and their babies. Therefore, after delivery and discharge from the hospital, follow-up care in the home should be provided to help the mother, the newborn, and others in the family adapt successfully to the new experiences facing them (Bull 1981; Bull and Lawrence 1985; Rush and Valaitis 1992). In fact, nurses traditionally have performed an important role for pregnant women, new mothers, and newborns in community settings (Donaldson 1981; Mercer 1981).

Research has demonstrated the critical importance of prenatal care to the health of mother and newborn (Merkatz et al. 1990). Inadequate prenatal care is the single greatest cause of low birth weight, and low birth weight is the single greatest cause of infant mortality (Institute of Medicine 1985; Hogue et al. 1987; Kramer 1987). Unfortunately, not all women obtain adequate prenatal care, and women living in poverty and members of minority groups have the highest incidence of inadequate prenatal care, as well as the highest infant mortality rates (Kramer 1987; Institute of Medicine 1988; McClanahan 1992).

Home visits may be used as a means of providing direct nursing care and health education to pregnant women, new mothers, and newborns. In addition, home visits may be used to encourage the client to seek adequate prenatal care, facilitate the process of obtaining adequate prenatal care, and reinforce the teaching and health care that occurs during the client's visits to prenatal care services.

IMPLICATIONS FOR NURSING CARE

Even clients who do obtain adequate prenatal care may have questions or concerns that are not answered during their regular visits to the prenatal clinic or physician's office. In addition, problems may be discovered and addressed in the

Table 5–1

SUMMARY OF KEY DIFFERENCES ACROSS HOME VISITING PROGRAMS

DIMENSION	PROGRAM VARIATIONS
Goals	Primary focus on child outcomes *versus* parent outcomes. Emphasis on child competence *versus* equal emphasis on different child and adult outcomes (e.g., child health and parent literacy)
Assumptions	
Family resourcefulness	All families need support *versus* some families have insufficient resources for childrearing
Determinants of behavior	Primary emphasis on parent *versus* environment as determinant of parenting competence
Strategy for change	Emphasis on home visitor–parent interpersonal relationship as primary vehicle of individual change *versus* dissemination of information as key to individual change
Host agency	Technical expertise and approach to professional helping or sponsorship agency Loose *versus* close connection between program and sponsoring agency
Content	On basis of program goals, program content can be single- *versus* multiple-focus (attention to child and parent-child relationship *versus* attention to broader ecology of family functioning)
Intensity of services	Length of home visit (30–90 min) Frequency of visits (typically, weekly or monthly) Length of program (typically, 9 months or longer) Inclusion of home visiting in combination with other program services
Program adaptiveness to child and family needs	Use of formal assesment tools Methods for securing parent input
Staffing pattern	Professional *versus* paraprofessional home visitors

From Powell, D. R. (1993). Inside home visiting programs. *The future of children,* 3 (3), 23–37. [*The Future of Children,* The David and Lucile Packard Foundation, 300 Second Street, Suite 102, Los Altos, CA 94022.]

home setting that would not be evident during the brief, structured interaction of a clinic or office visit. Home visits to maternal-newborn clients allow the nurse to perform a comprehensive assessment of client needs, with the opportunity to develop insight into the many factors in the family, the environment, and the community that influence the client's well-being (Combs-Orme et al. 1985).

Providing nursing care in community settings is a rewarding experience for the nurse, for many reasons. One important reason is the relative autonomy of the nursing role in the community. Decisions are made and interventions provided in settings where the nurse is the only health care professional present. Because of this autonomy, community-based nursing care during the pregnancy and postpartum period demands a broad knowledge base and a high level of skill. The role requires critical thinking and independent nursing judgments.

Hand in hand with the need for nursing competency in community-based maternal-newborn nursing comes an opportunity to develop a deep

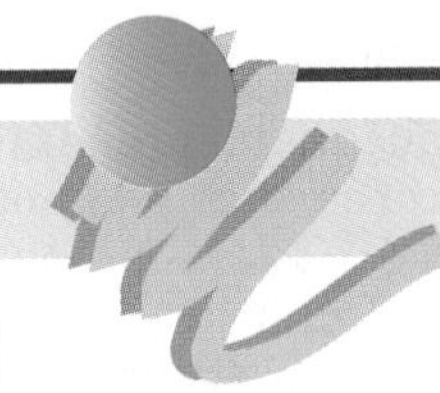

HISTORICAL PERSPECTIVES

HOME VISITS CONTINUE TO BENEFIT MATERNAL-INFANT HEALTH

Home visiting to provide health care began in France, near the beginning of the seventeenth century, with the activities of St. Francis de Sales. St. Vincent de Paul took home care a step further when he organized the Sisterhood of the Dames de Charité in 1617. This Paris-based Sisterhood introduced a basic principle of contemporary maternal-infant nursing in the home: By teaching during home visits, we can help people learn to help themselves.

In England in the nineteenth century, Florence Nightingale influenced the evolution of maternal-infant nursing in the home through her endorsement of the concept of district nursing. Nightingale encouraged home visits that included not only care of the sick but also teaching about health and wellness.

In the United States, Lillian Wald pioneered taking health care and health teaching to people in their homes. In 1893, she established a visiting nurse service in New York City. A major focus of Wald's nursing care was the health of mothers and children.

In 1918, Mary Breckinridge established the famous Frontier Nursing Service in the mountains of Kentucky. Traveling through Appalachia on horseback, she brought health care and health education to poor, isolated families, many of whom had no other source of health care. Breckinridge felt a special commitment to improving the health of disadvantaged mothers and children. The impact of this commitment was clear, as maternal and infant mortality rates decreased after the establishment of the Frontier Nursing Service, which included midwifery. In 1939, Breckinridge established the Frontier Nursing Service School of Nurse Midwifery.

As a result of efforts to focus government attention and support on the needs of mothers and infants, Congress established the Children's Bureau in 1912. The *Shepherd-Towner Act* of 1921, administered by the Children's Bureau, provided grants with which states could develop programs for mothers and infants at risk. Many programs in which nurses provided care to mothers and infants grew out of programs that had begun with the *Shepherd-Towner Act.*

It soon became clear that education for mothers in their homes could improve maternal-infant health and prevent many maternal and infant deaths. Thus, home health nurses and public health nurses began to focus on preventive education. This role in home visits grew to encompass not only education but also assessment of needs and referral to appropriate resources. Home visits often supplemented traditional office or clinic visits for perinatal care, especially for women who were at high risk owing to medical, environmental, or social circumstances.

During the 1970s and most of the 1980s, economic constraints led to a decrease in home visitation to childbearing families. Instead, many

continued on facing page

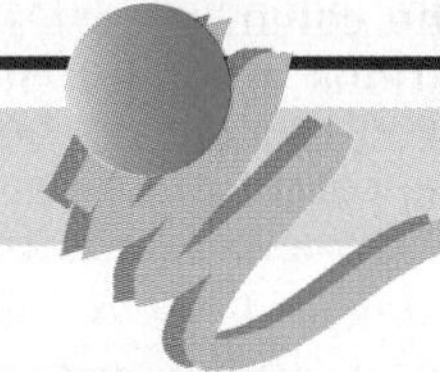

HISTORICAL PERSPECTIVES Continued

agencies began providing care exclusively in clinic settings, without the supplemental home visits of the past. This change was influenced by a dramatic decline in the infant mortality rate, which led some health planners to view home visits as an expensive and unnecessary luxury. By the end of the 1980s, however, the infant mortality rate had begun to stabilize and was still particularly high among the poor and minority populations. In addition, there was new evidence that home visits could help to prevent low birth weight and infant mortality by promoting good nutrition and prenatal care and by teaching about the negative influences of smoking and alcohol use.

Thus, in the 1990s, home visits have again become a valued method of influencing perinatal outcomes. Childbearing families at risk now may receive home visits from nurses through a variety of sponsoring agencies, including public health departments, home health agencies, and various clinics. In addition, home visits have become an effective and satisfying vehicle for student nurses to learn a holistic approach to nursing care of the childbearing family.

Data from Brainard, A. M. (1985). *The evolution of public health nursing.* Philadelphia: W. B. Saunders; Browne, H. (1966). A tribute to Mary Breckinridge. *Nursing Outlook,* 14 (5), 54–55; Coss, C. (1989). *Lillian Wald: A progressive activist.* New York: Feminist Press; Dolan, J. (1978). *History of nursing* (14th ed.). Philadelphia: W. B. Saunders; Fitzpatrick, M. L. (1975). *The National Organization of Public Health Nursing, 1912–1952: Development of a practice field.* New York: National League of Nursing; Maynard, T. (1939). *The apostle of charity: The life of St. Vincent de Paul.* New York: Dial Press; Peoples-Sheps, M. D. (1990). Perinatal home visiting returns. *Nursing Outlook,* 38, 54–55; Salmon, M. E., and Peoples-Sheps, M. (1989). Infant mortality and public health nursing: A history of accomplishments, a future of challenges. *Nursing Outlook,* 37, 6–7, 51; Tirpak, H. (1975). The Frontier Nursing Service: Fifty years in the mountains. *Nursing Outlook,* 33 (5), 308–310; Williams, L. R., and Cooper, M. K. (1993). Nurse-managed postpartum home care. *Journal of Obstetric, Gynecologic, and Neonatal Nursing,* 22, 25–31.

and lasting rapport with the client and family. The family is included in the care. All aspects of the client's life are considered when planning and implementing care. Thus, the nurse has the opportunity to provide nursing care that is truly holistic.

In addition, the nurse is able to assess the client's home environment as well as the constraints with which the client must deal on a daily basis. The client is more at ease than she would be in agency settings and thus displays more of her true behaviors, attitudes, and concerns. Therefore, the nurse is able to tailor nursing care to fit the client's unique needs. This can offer the nurse a high level of professional satisfaction.

Roles of the Maternal-Newborn Nurse in the Community

In addition to the role of caregiver, the community nurse acts as case manager, patient advocate, teacher, and researcher. Nurse-managed postpartum home care has provided early identification and treatment of complications, thereby preventing readmissions (Williams and Cooper 1993). Indeed, nurses acting as case managers facilitate continuity of care and speed referrals for testing when problems or developmental delays are evidenced.

The nurse in the community gains a unique perspective on the client's strengths and needs. This allows the nurse to communicate effectively with professionals and services in the community as the patient's advocate.

The maternal-newborn nurse as political activist and change agent in the community has a unique opportunity to influence health policy. Maternal-newborn clients are among those who benefit the most if health care delivery systems change in positive ways. Therefore, it is important for maternal-newborn nurses to take an active role in the development of new policy and make sure changes benefit and improve the health status of pregnant women, mothers, and newborns throughout the nation.

Maternal-Newborn Nursing Agencies in the Community

Nurses work through a variety of agencies to provide nursing care to pregnant women, mothers, and newborns in the community. Health departments are official agencies, funded and controlled by government funds. Maternal-child health is a high priority for health departments, which employ many nurses to provide clinic services for pregnant women, mothers, and newborns as well as older children. In addition, health departments may provide maternal-newborn care through home visits, especially to high-risk clients.

Nurses also work through home health agencies. The latter provide direct nursing care under a physician's orders. This care might include home uterine monitoring for a pregnant woman at high risk for preterm labor (Freda 1991), apnea monitoring for a newborn at risk, supervising the use of a home bilirubin light, or other nursing interventions that require physician's orders (Fig. 5–1). Home health agencies may be hospital based or freestanding. They operate on a fee-for-service basis, with the cost of nursing care often covered by insurance or Medicaid.

Nurses also work through public and private ambulatory clinics and out of physicians' offices. Home visits from nurses based in clinics, health departments, and home health agencies occur more frequently than do home visits from nurses who are based in a physician's office. Nevertheless, all these agencies have the potential to provide maternal-newborn nursing in the community.

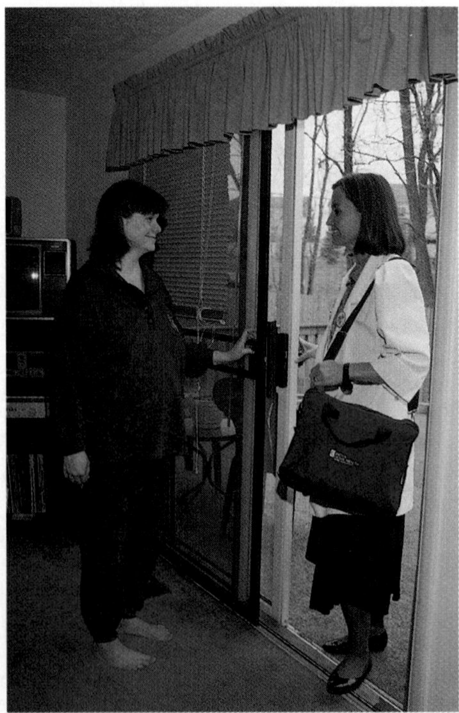

Figure 5–1

An increasing number of nurses provide care for pregnant women, mothers, and newborns in the community through community health care departments and home care agencies.

THE FAMILY AS CLIENT

Maternal-newborn nursing in the community offers the nurse an opportunity to provide care to entire family units. Although the pregnant woman and her fetus, or the new mother and her newborn, may be the primary focus of care during home visits, the entire family should be considered. Family members and other members of the household may influence the health status, the health care, and the health decisions of the primary client. In addition, family members and others in the household may have needs that the nurse could address. Therefore, the entire household is considered in assessing and planning care for maternal-newborn clients.

Families as the Unit of Service

Families and households vary a great deal, and it is important for the nurse who makes home visits to recognize and accept this. One client may be part of a typical nuclear family that consists of a husband, a wife, and children. Another client may live alone and be unmarried. Often, childbearing adolescents live with their own parents and siblings. The client may be part of an extended family household in which it is difficult to determine the relationships involved. Still other maternal-newborn clients live with a partner to whom they are not married.

The nurse working in the community may experience discomfort if the families being visited do not fit within the nurse's own value system. When this occurs, it is important for the nurse to examine and work through his or her feelings. Clients have a right to make their own decisions and lifestyle choices. The nurse's role is to assist them in terms of health status, health knowledge, and health behaviors. Judgmental approaches are inappropriate in nursing care.

Assessing the Family

Assessment of the family or household is important for two reasons. First, it is important because of the family's influence on the health of the pregnant woman, new mother, and newborn. The attitudes of others in the home, as well as relationships within the household, can have a positive or negative impact on the health and health behaviors of the primary client. Chapter 4, Family Dynamics, provides guidance in assessment and care of the family.

The second reason for assessing the family or household is to address nursing needs in other household members. As the nurse interacts with members of the household, any indication of health problems will lead to further exploration, a health history, and possibly some physical assessment. In this way, the nurse may discover health problems among household members that require intervention. In such situations the nurse may intervene or may refer the person to an appropriate resource for care. For example, on the basis of information that has been gathered, the nurse may decide to check the blood pressure of another member of the family, may discover uncontrolled hypertension, and may refer the person to a physician or clinic for follow-up. Health problems may also be discovered in other children in the household, such as a preschooler who is behind on immunizations. The nurse would make a diagnosis of altered health maintenance, work out a plan with the mother to include appropriate health teaching, refer the child for the needed immunizations, and follow through with evaluation. Holistic nursing care that views the family as the client offers a challenge as well as a great deal of satisfaction to the maternal-newborn nurse in the community.

THE HOME VISIT

The home visit is a unique vehicle for providing nursing care to antepartum and postpartum clients and families. During a visit to the client's home, the nurse is able to assess and intervene in many areas that otherwise would remain unknown. These include such things as the physical environment, the emotional climate in the home, family interaction, and personal behaviors. In addition, the client usually feels more at ease at home than in an agency health care setting. Her comfort in her own home setting may help her to be more open in talking with the nurse, thereby making it easier to establish a trusting relationship. The nurse is able to individualize care on the basis of resources, constraints, and other factors that are best discovered through a home visit. Thus, nursing assessment, diagnosis, planning, intervention, and evaluation that may not have been possible in a health care setting may be successful in the home environment.

Planning the Home Visit

Making a successful home visit requires systematic planning. All available assessment data are studied, including data from other health care providers and data from previous home visits. Tentative goals are established, including short-term goals to be accomplished on this visit as well as long-term goals for the client family.

To make the visit a productive, professional nurse-client interaction, it is important to clarify the difference between a social visit and a professional visit. In our daily lives, most of the visits that one person makes to the home of another person are made for social purposes. Conversation centers on social amenities, and the more personal discussions that are part of quality nursing care are not acceptable topics for conversation. The visit of a nurse to a maternal-newborn family in the community, however, is not a social visit. Instead, it is a professional visit, made to accomplish specific goals through professional nursing care. It is the goal-directed character of the visit that distinguishes the professional nursing visit from a social visit. Therefore, the visit must be planned with a clear focus on goal accomplishment.

To focus the visit on goals does not mean that the visit is all business from start to finish. An effective visit is made up of three phases: the social phase, the working phase, and the closing phase. In the social phase the nurse exchanges social pleasantries with the client and other household members, thereby beginning to establish rapport and a trusting relationship. The visit then moves on to the working phase, where the nurse and client work together to establish and accomplish health-related goals. Finally, the visit ends with the closing phase, which consists of evaluation, new goal setting and planning, and the social interaction that is appropriate for leaving the home. Thus, planning an effective visit includes attention to all three phases of the home visit.

Preparing for the Visit

A few simple steps of preparation can make the visit safer and more productive. Whenever possible, it is wise to make sure that the client is home and is expecting the visit. This may be accomplished in two ways. First, each visit should end with an agreement as to the date and time of the next visit. Thus, unless this is the first visit to this client, she will know that the nurse is coming. Second, if the client has a telephone, it is wise to make a quick phone call to be sure that she is home. This simple act can help avoid wasting a significant amount of time and effort on a fruitless trip.

When leaving to travel to the client's home, the nurse checks for all needed information and supplies. Important information for a successful home visit includes the client's name, address, and phone number; clear directions to the home (and a map, if needed); phone numbers of health care providers involved with the care of this client; the nursing care plan (including goals for this visit); and background information about the client and family. Supplies needed for a home visit include pencil and paper, resource materials for teaching, and all equipment that may be required for health assessment and nursing care. In addition, the nurse should carry money (correct change) for a phone call as well as identification. Nurses should always leave word with someone about where they are going and when they expect to return. Purses, backpacks, and other valuables should be left at the agency or school or placed in the trunk of the car *before* leaving for the visit.

Entering the Home

On the first home visit, a nurse may experience some anxiety when approaching the house. There are many unknowns waiting beyond the door. How will the client respond? Will the nurse be welcomed? What kind of problems will the family present? Will the nurse be able to provide the nursing care needed? What will the environment be like? Even expert nurses experience these uncertainties when initiating home visits with a new client, and the feelings are likely to be stronger in the nurse who is learning how to conduct a home visit. A quick review of the "Checklist for Effective Home Visits" can help the nurse feel well prepared.

The very act of calling a resident to the front door may take some persistence. If there is a doorbell, try ringing it. If there is no answer after two or three attempts, the bell may not be loud enough to be heard over other noises in the house, or it may not be in working order. Knocking on the door is the next approach. Begin with a series of firm, sharp knocks. If there is no response, try knocking louder. It is possible that no one is home, but it is also possible that the knocks have not been heard. In homes where there are children or where music or a television set is playing loudly, knocking may not be heard over the other noises. A technique that is often effective in these situations is to rap sharply on glass with the large end of a key. This can be done on a window pane in or near the door. The sound created by a key striking glass is higher pitched and more piercing than the sound created by knocking; it can often be heard over the general noise in a house and catch the attention of persons in the household who had not heard the doorbell or the knocking.

If these techniques do not arouse anyone in the house, the nurse may decide to try another entrance. Some people routinely use a side or back

Assessment Checklist for Effective Home Visits

PREPARING FOR THE HOME VISIT

- Do you let the client know to expect you (through prior arrangements and a quick phone call now if feasible)?
- Do you obtain and assess all available background information in order to plan the visit effectively?
- Do you gather all needed supplies for health assessment, patient education, and other nursing care?
- Do you place your purse or backpack and other valuables in a safe place, out of sight, before leaving for the visit?

MAKING THE HOME VISIT

- Do you try a variety of techniques to call someone to the door?
- Do you begin the visit with a brief social phase, to establish rapport?
- Do you make an effective transition to the working phase?
- Do you focus the visit on accomplishing goals that are mutually established?
- Do you close the visit with evaluation and mutual goal setting for the next visit?

DOCUMENTATION AND FOLLOW-UP

- Do you document the visit promptly and thoroughly?
- Do you follow through with information, referrals, and other interventions that were promised to the client?
- Do you communicate with the primary health care provider?

entrance or stay in another part of the house and do not hear visitors at the front door. It can be dangerous, however, to go into back yards or alleys or to go down dark hallways when looking for another entrance to the client's residence. Nurses must keep their own safety in mind at all times and avoid taking unnecessary risks.

When the door is answered, the nurse begins by introducing herself or himself by name and as a nurse and asking for the client by name. The reason for the visit is explained to the client in brief terms. For example, "I am Mary Jones, a student nurse with the Washington County Health Department. I'm here to see how you are doing with your pregnancy and to help you prepare for the birth of your baby." For most clients, this is a sufficient introduction, and the nurse will be invited into the home. If the client seems skeptical, a more detailed explanation may be needed.

If this is the first home visit to this client, the nurse does not enter if the client is not at home. Information can be requested about when the client will be home, and arrangements can be made to return at a later time. On repeat visits, the absence of the client may not completely cancel the visit. Occasionally there are other household members with whom the nurse can interact productively on a professional level. The nurse must always be careful, however, not to enter a home where there is any question about safety or comfort with those who are present.

Social Phase of the Home Visit

The visit begins with a social phase. Upon entering the home, the nurse greets not only the primary client but also the other persons present. Although the nursing care may focus on the pregnant woman or the new mother and infant, the nurse should make a point to acknowledge and consider the entire family. Children, other adults, and even pets are important to the client. Therefore, it helps establish rapport if all members of the household are greeted, respected, and valued by the nurse.

To make a successful visit, the nurse initially focuses on establishing rapport and conveying a caring attitude. Goal accomplishment is difficult at best, and perhaps impossible, without establishing a trusting relationship between nurse and client. Keep in mind that the nurse is a guest in the client's home. A brief period of polite, friendly conversation helps put both the nurse and the client at ease and helps begin establishing rapport with the client and family. Be careful, however, to keep this social phase of the visit short. A visit that spends too much time on the social phase can easily deteriorate into a purely social visit. When this happens, it may be difficult to switch the focus to the accomplishment of professional goals.

Transition to the working phase of the visit is accomplished by determining the place where the professional interaction with the client will take place. In some situations the nurse may ask the client where she would like to sit to talk about her own and her baby's health. In other situations the nurse may prefer to make the suggestion. In addition, if there are other persons in the home, it is best to find a place where the client and the nurse will have some quiet and privacy. The client may sit where she is comfortable, and the nurse can sit nearby so that they may look at materials together and have good eye contact. Allow for the client's personal space, but stay close enough to discuss sensitive issues comfortably. The kitchen table is often a good place for the working phase of the visit.

Working Phase of the Home Visit

CONTROLLING DISTRACTIONS

Distractions are often encountered in the home setting and may interfere with an effective nurse-client interaction. Thus, the working phase begins by attempting to ensure an environment free of distractions. Distractions may originate in the environment, in the behaviors of those present, or in nurses themselves (Pruitt et al. 1987). One example of an environmental distraction is the television. If the television is distracting during the visit, it is appropriate for the nurse to request, politely, that it be turned off during the visit to allow for better concentration on the business at hand. If the client does not want to turn if off, the nurse may ask when would be a better time of day for the visit, and schedule the next visit to avoid conflicting with a favorite program. Disruptive children may also constitute a distraction and may be given a toy or a task to keep them busy during the visit.

Behavioral distractions include actions taken by the client to distract from the purpose of the visit (Pruitt et al. 1987). Suppose, for example, the client does not stay focused on the purpose of the visit and changes the subject frequently. The nurse would be wise to encourage the client's discussion of her feelings and to undertake therapeutic interaction to deal with the client's discomfort, guilt, or embarrassment before proceeding with the focus of the visit.

There may also be distractions that originate in the nurse. A nurse who is uncomfortable in the setting may be distracted from providing the best possible nursing care. Such distractions might stem from a negative reaction to the home environment. When conditions in the home differ from the nurse's view of how a home should be kept, the nurse must evaluate the extent to which those conditions have an impact on health. Only when health is endangered by the conditions in the home should the nurse intervene with teaching and counseling.

Differences between the lifestyle or values of the client and those of the nurse may also be distracting to the nurse. Concerns about personal safety are distracting as well. In addition, the nurse may be distracted by feelings of uncertainty when first learning the role of the maternal-newborn nurse in the community. It is important to recognize any distractions that the nurse may be experiencing. By examining their own feelings, nurses can decide how to deal with them. If fears for safety are well founded, the nurse may need to change the situation or leave. If distractions relate to the characteristics of the home environment or the client's lifestyle or values, the nurse must remember that the client has a right to make choices that differ from those that the nurse would make. Finally, if the nurse feels anxious in the new role, thorough preparation for the visit will help alleviate the anxiety, and continued experience in conducting home visits will increase the nurse's comfort level (Pruitt et al. 1987).

NURSING PRACTICE

Nursing care in the home, as in other settings, begins with assessment. The nurse takes a health history and conducts those portions of the physical assessment that are appropriate. The assessment will vary in its comprehensiveness according to whether this is a first or repeat visit. The assessment also varies according to any changes that have occurred in the client's status. On the basis of this assessment, nursing diagnoses are generated to guide interventions. The client should be involved in goal setting and planning. Interventions are then tailored to meet identified client needs. The client is involved in evaluation as well. This complete use of nursing process should occur during every home visit.

Nursing interventions are most effective when a positive approach is taken. Although it is important to address problems and negative factors, progress toward improved health is greatest if the nurse can also identify strengths and positive factors in the home and help the client build upon them. When discussing prenatal nutrition, for example, an effective strategy is to focus on the healthy foods in the home and help the client develop eating plans built around those nutritious foods, rather than focusing exclusively on inappropriate foods. Similarly, if there is a toy in the home that is safe and age appropriate, parents can be taught to use it to stimulate the child, to build motor skills, and to improve hand-eye coordination.

NURSING CARE OF THE ANTEPARTUM CLIENT

Many factors should be assessed when providing nursing care to an antepartum client in the home (Fig. 5–2). A health history should be taken and an appropriate physical assessment conducted. Any discomforts the client is experiencing, as well as other client concerns, should be discussed. Nutritional status and eating patterns should be examined (Bowles and Williamson 1990; Ausman 1993). For example, the client should be questioned about pica, the practice of consuming materials not meant for human consumption. Eating laundry starch during pregnancy is a common practice among some groups and may impair the

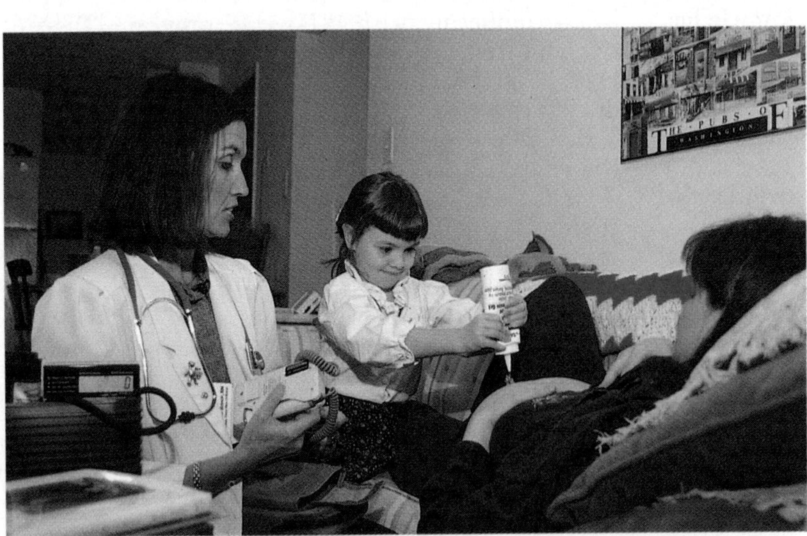

Figure 5–2
Nursing care of the high-risk pregnant woman at home includes taking fetal heart tones and involving other family members in the client's care.

client's nutritional status. If it is determined that the amount of starch being consumed may be leading to inadequate intake of nutritional foods, the nurse makes a diagnosis of altered nutrition: less than body requirements. A plan is then made for nutritional counseling and appropriate follow-up. Other behaviors that have an impact on pregnancy should also be assessed, including exercise and rest (Kemp and Hatmaker 1992), smoking, use of alcohol, and use of illicit drugs (Campinha-Bacote and Bragg 1993).

The client's utilization of prenatal care should be assessed. Research has demonstrated that many factors may influence a client's likelihood of obtaining adequate prenatal care. These include such diverse areas as insurance and financial status (Petitti et al. 1990) and self-esteem (Edwards 1993). Therefore, it is important to be thorough, both in assessment and in follow-up care, to ensure that the client obtains adequate prenatal care.

The nurse also assesses the client's knowledge of and preparedness for labor and delivery, as well as her knowledge of newborn care and the preparations being made for the newborn. This assessment may lead to a discussion of prepared childbirth classes that are available in the community, with referral if appropriate. See Chapter 20, Perinatal Education, for guidance in this aspect of antepartum care.

The pregnant woman's attitude toward the pregnancy is another important piece of information. In addition, attitudes toward the pregnancy should be assessed in her significant other, in children in the family, and in other members of the household. Research has shown that attitudes may influence health behaviors (Giblin et al. 1990) and may have an impact on the pregnancy outcome.

The home environment should also be assessed. Sleeping arrangements, food preparation and storage facilities, water supply, and the condition of the kitchen and bathrooms are but a few of the home environment factors that may influence the client's health. Excessive or steep stairs may lead to a nursing diagnosis of risk for injury for the late antepartum woman or the infant or newborn. In some instances, pets in the home may pose a threat to the health or safety of family members, especially a newborn. The conditions found in some homes may be distressing to the nurse. It is important to avoid being judgmental about the client's home; however, those factors that may pose a threat to the client or family's health or safety should be addressed.

Assessment data are used to develop nursing diagnoses that in turn guide nursing interventions. Nursing interventions include health teaching, psychological interventions, direct nursing care, and referral to community services and other agencies or professionals as needed. See Unit Three, Nursing Care During Pregnancy, for more detailed guidance.

NURSING CARE OF THE POSTPARTUM CLIENT

For the postpartum health assessment to be appropriate, it must be adapted according to the length of time between delivery and the home visit. Assessment may include collection of data about lochia, episiotomy and perineal discomfort, breast tenderness, bowel and bladder function, and nutrition. Physical and psychological adaptation to the new mother role should be discussed and assessed. Patterns of rest and physical activity should be addressed. The mother's handling of infant feeding and other newborn care is considered. Her knowledge about newborn care should be assessed and her comfort level in caring for the newborn noted. Mother-newborn interaction should also be assessed to determine whether effective attachment is taking place. Any assistance she is receiving from others, or problems related to these others, should also be assessed in regard to both her own care and care of the newborn. Nursing diagnoses are formulated, and nursing care is directed toward those areas in which actual or potential problems are detected. Unit Five, Nursing Care of Healthy Mothers and Newborns, and Unit Six, Nursing Care of Mother and Newborns with Special Needs, provide additional guidance in the care of the postpartum client.

NURSING CARE OF THE NEWBORN CLIENT

An appropriate newborn assessment should be conducted, adapted to the age of the infant. Healing of the umbilicus, circumcision, length and weight, head circumference, nutritional status, feeding patterns, and bowel and bladder function are but a few of the parameters to be assessed (Fig. 5–3). In addition, a Brazelton Neonatal Behavioral Assessment may be conducted. Assessment leads to nursing diagnoses, the planning of appropriate interventions, and evaluation.

CONTRACTING WITH CLIENTS

The client should be involved in goal setting, planning, and activities to promote her health and the health of her fetus or newborn. A very effective way to do this is through the development of a contract between client and nurse. The contract makes clear both the goals and the activities that will be undertaken to accomplish the goals. Furthermore, the contract makes clear which activi-

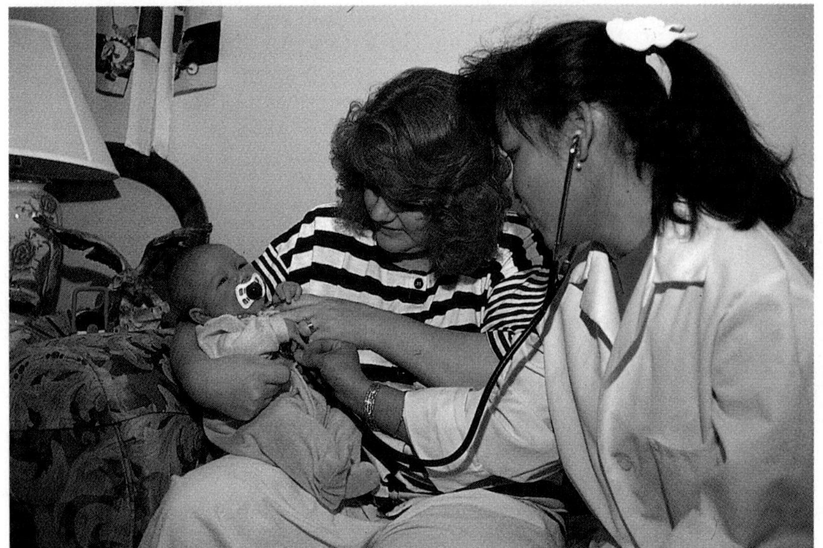

Figure 5–3

Nursing students often make postpartum home visits to mothers with newborn infants • During this experience, a student can provide information and support to the new mother and assess the status of the infant • Such visits allow students to gain insight into differences between a mother's and an infant's needs in hospital compared with their needs at home.

ties will be carried out by the nurse and which are the responsibility of the client. Timelines are also included in the contract. Thus, the contract between client and nurse serves as a guide for carrying out activities to accomplish mutually agreed goals. When the client is involved in goal setting, she feels more responsible for her own health and is more likely to follow through with the plan of care. Chapter 19, Promoting a Healthy Pregnancy, provides guidance in the development and implementation of nurse-client contracts.

Closing Phase of the Home Visit

To bring the home visit to a close, several actions are required. The nurse begins by indicating that the visit is coming to an end. The goals of the visit are restated. The nurse and client then work together to summarize what has occurred during the visit; this should include a content summary of any teaching as well as other activities. The nurse and client jointly evaluate their goal attainment for this visit, as well as the progress they have made toward achieving their long-term goals. Goals are set for the next visit. Both the client's and the nurse's responsibilities are made clear, so that each knows what is expected of them in the interim before the next visit.

The date and time are set for the next visit. If this visit has appeared to be inconvenient for the client, or if environmental distractions were a problem, it may be wise to discuss the possibility of changing the time for the next visit. Timing the visit during a young child's nap, at a time other than that of a favorite television program, or at some other time that avoids conflicts and distractions can enhance the effectiveness of the home visit. Finally, the visit ends with very brief social conversation.

Documenting the Home Visit

The home visit is not completed until it has been documented in the client's chart. The chart provides an ongoing record of the application of the nursing process, services rendered, changes in client status, involvement of other professionals, and other pertinent information about the client. Documentation therefore serves three major purposes. First, it helps nurses and other caregivers to provide continuity of care. Second, it serves as justification for reimbursement where third-party payers are involved. Finally, it is an important legal record. For all these reasons, documentation of the home visit is an important part of maternal-newborn nursing in the community.

Documentation must be accurate, complete, and concise. Assessment findings are included, as well as any changes in health status since the last visit. Nursing diagnoses are presented and form the basis for planning and intervention. Goals are stated and progress toward their attainment is discussed. Nursing interventions are described. It is also important to document the client's response to the home visit and to the various nursing interventions that occurred during this visit. Contracts established between nurse and client are described and copies of the contracts added to the chart. Evaluation of the visit and plans for future visits are also entered in the chart. Finally, any

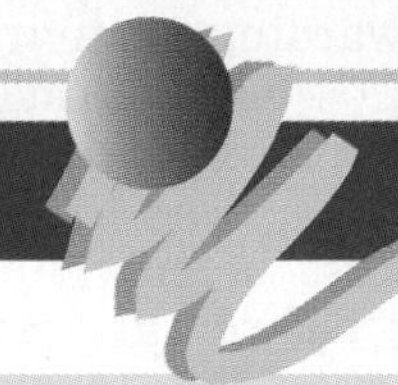

IMPROVING YOUR PRACTICE

BETTER SKILLS FOR HOME VISITS

The nurse who provides home visits for childbearing families has a unique opportunity to influence the well-being of both mother and infant. The most effective home visits use the nursing process to provide professional, goal-directed interactions with the client family. The following steps will help you improve your nursing practice in home visits to childbearing families:

- IDENTIFY YOUR OWN ATTITUDES ABOUT MAKING HOME VISITS. Clarify your feelings about providing nursing care in the home. Recognize the influence your own culture and social experiences have on your attitudes. Know that the professional nurse discusses personal matters and conducts physical assessments in the home setting. If this feels uncomfortable to you at first, think it through and consider the client's need for nursing care. Work to become comfortable with your new role as a professional nurse in the home.
- AVOID VALUE JUDGMENTS. Keep in mind that everyone has a right to his or her own opinions and values. Remember your professional responsibility to accept others as they are, regardless of differences between their ideas and values and your own. Do not let your own prejudices interfere with providing the best possible nursing care to all clients.
- CONDUCT THE VISIT AS A PROFESSIONAL, GOAL-DIRECTED NURSING ENCOUNTER. Follow the nursing process. Conduct a thorough assessment and plan each visit carefully. Generate nursing diagnoses to guide your interventions. Maintain a friendly but professional approach in which both the nurse and the family focus on the goals for the visit. Evaluate each visit in terms of goal attainment and seek ways to make each encounter as productive as possible.
- ALLOW FOR PHASES OF THE VISIT. Begin with the introductory phase, establishing rapport and clarifying the purpose of the visit. During the working phase, keep the activities goal directed. Continue to involve the client when you move to the evaluation phase of the visit. Close with a discussion of what is to happen after the visit ends. Clarify the responsibilities of both the nurse and the client for follow-through from this visit and preparation for the next visit.
- FOLLOW THROUGH AFTER EVERY VISIT. Be sure that you have documented the visit appropriately and have communicated with the primary health care provider. If the client will need additional services, seek them out and follow through with appropriate referrals.
- EVALUATE EACH HOME VISIT THAT YOU MAKE. Identify your strengths and look for ways to build on them. Identify the areas in which you could improve and seek ways to strengthen these areas. Continue to seek professional growth in your ability to conduct effective home visits to maternal-newborn clients.

formal or informal referrals to community resources or to other professionals should be clearly described. The description of referrals should include the process followed, persons contacted, dates and times established for future service, and the responsibilities of the nurse and the client for follow-through.

It is important that telephone calls, as well as home visits, be documented in the client's chart. The telephone can be a valuable tool for follow-up communication with the client after a home visit. The nurse always records the date and purpose of the call, the information exchanged, and the nurse's analysis and plans. As with the documentation of home visits, the charted documentation of telephone calls provides important information about the care of the client in the community.

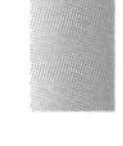

Communicating with the Primary Health Care Provider

The final step in completing the home visit is communication with the primary health care provider. The frequency of such communication may vary with the responsibilities and agreements that exist between nurse and primary provider. In some situations, this communication occurs after every home visit. In other situations, communication is expected monthly or according to another regular schedule. It may also be understood that communication will occur whenever it seems appropriate to the nurse. It is the nurse's responsibility to find out what the expectations are for routine communication and to follow through with this. The nurse must be certain to communicate significant changes in the client's status whenever they occur.

When communicating with the primary health care provider, it is important to be clear, complete, and concise. A systematic approach will help the nurse to provide pertinent data in a concise format. Sample steps that may be helpful to guide the communication follow:

- State the nurse's name and agency
- State the client's name, age, and diagnosis
- If this is a first visit, report all pertinent assessment data (be selective and concise); if this is a repeat visit, report changes in status since the last report to this provider
- Briefly describe nursing diagnoses and plans for nursing care
- State nursing interventions that have been implemented and the client's response to those interventions
- Provide a brief evaluation
- List any referrals that have been made and any community services that are being utilized
- Request input from the primary health care provider

With the above format, communication can be systematic and complete while remaining concise. This kind of regular communication is an important component of comprehensive care. It can help limit the fragmentation of services that has become a serious problem in our health care delivery system.

SAFETY

An important consideration when providing maternal-newborn nursing through home visits is the safety of the nurse. Safety problems are infrequent, and a nurse may make home visits throughout an entire career without ever encountering a potentially dangerous situation. In fact, maternal-newborn nursing in the community is a particularly satisfying and rewarding activity. Nevertheless, circumstances can occur that may jeopardize the nurse's well-being. Prevention is essential to avoid such a situation. Safety can be addressed at every step of the process of providing nursing care, from the planning before the visit through the visit itself and the return to the school or agency.

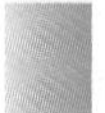

Planning a Safe Visit

Provision for the nurse's safety begins during planning for the home visit. The first step is to seek out any information that may indicate a potential safety problem. The wise nurse is alert to cues that something may be amiss and takes precautions.

Two principal sources of preliminary information are available to the nurse for background information on the client and family: formal written documentation and informal feedback from colleagues. It is appropriate to consult all available sources, both formal and informal. Formal documentation may include records of the client's visits to the health agency as well as records of previous home visits. Informal feedback may be obtained through talking with providers who are familiar with the client. In addition, when the neighborhood in which the client lives is known to be a high crime area, it may be appropriate to consult the police department for information and safety guidelines.

When consulting resources for background information, it is important to be alert to both stated and implied impressions from previous health care providers. Pay attention to descriptions of the client's affect, as well as to any concerns expressed about inappropriate or disturbing behavior of the client or other members of the household. Be aware of the variety of factors that can influence behavior, such as substance abuse and psychiatric disorders. Such disorders may be formally diagnosed or simply suspected. They may be preexisting or may be a new development (including postpartum psychosis). Be aware also that family violence is a major concern in society today. Pregnancy and/or childbirth may constitute stressors that precipitate or exacerbate family violence. It is the nurse's responsibility not only to be alert to possible dangers to clients, but also to recognize the potential threat this may pose to the nurse.

If background information indicates that a safety hazard may exist, the nurse consults superiors and experts for guidance. Sometimes visiting in pairs is recommended, or an escort may be provided. Occasionally it is decided to suspend home visits to a particular client until the safety problem is rectified.

Traveling Safely to the Client's Home

Before leaving to drive to the client's home, it is important that basic data about the visit be given to a contact person, usually the student's professor or the nurse's supervisor. These data should include the name, address, and phone number of the client to be visited; the time of expected arrival at the client's home; and the expected time of return. If any problems are anticipated on the visit, they should also be discussed. Specific arrangements are made for the nurse to check back with the contact person immediately upon returning to the school or agency.

As stated earlier, purses, backpacks, and other valuables should be locked in a safe place at the work station or in the trunk of the car *before* leaving for the visit. The client's neighborhood, and even the house itself, could contain unexpected hazards, so it is best not to invite trouble. Leaving valuables in view in the car, or being seen moving them to the trunk before leaving the car, may invite break-ins. A nurse walking on the street becomes vulnerable to thievery if carrying a purse or backpack in addition to health care supplies and materials. Furthermore, it is distracting to have to keep track of personal belongings during a home visit. Concentration needs to be on the nurse-client interaction without having to worry about what may be happening to one's purse. Problems arising from leaving a purse or backpack unattended during a home visit may include thievery by adults, accidental poisoning or other injury in curious children, or damage to the nurse's belongings by children or pets. For all these reasons, the best approach is to move the purse or backpack to the trunk before starting out for the client's home.

Obtain clear directions for locating the client's home. Plan the route carefully, considering not only the most direct route but also the safety of the streets and areas to be traveled. Knowledge of potentially dangerous parts of town may lead the wise nurse to select a less direct but safer route. All car doors should be kept locked while traveling. Wear the car's safety belt. Always check the fuel level in the car before starting out for a home visit; never risk running out of gas in an unfamiliar or unsafe neighborhood.

When arriving at the destination, the selection of a parking place can affect the nurse's safety. Be alert to the surroundings. Are there potentially dangerous people or places that must be walked past to get from the car to the client's residence? Are there loose dogs that may not be friendly? If any of these concerns are present, it may be best to look for another parking place, wait until a closer place becomes available, or wait until the unsavory condition clears, rather than confront a potentially dangerous situation. When leaving the car, be sure the doors are locked.

When in doubt or in danger, the nurse should use other means of providing contact with the client. In some areas, nurses visit in pairs. In other situations, an escort, possibly even a police officer, accompanies the nurse. There are situations in which the home visit simply is not appropriate as a means of contact. Sometimes the client must be required to come to the clinic or other setting to meet with the nurse because of the dangers inherent in the nurse's visit to the neighborhood or home. Whatever the situation, the nurse must keep safety in mind at all times.

Maintaining Safety During the Visit

The nurse must continue to keep safety precautions in mind when approaching and entering the home. Note dogs or other animals that may appear to be guarding the home. Animals that are territorial may threaten a stranger who invades their terrain. If someone other than the primary client answers the door, the nurse asks for the client. Sometimes, in the absence of the primary client, a brief but productive interaction can be held with other family members. If, however, the primary client is not there and the nurse is uncomfortable with any of the persons in the house, the nurse does not enter the home. Rather, a polite inquiry is made about when the client will return and arrangements are made to conduct the visit at a later time.

Once the nurse is in the home, it is best to select a hard chair to sit on, if possible. Hard surfaces are less likely than soft fabric or deep upholstery to harbor pests, parasites, sharp objects, or other potential threats to the nurse's health. Lice and roaches are particular concerns in upholstered furniture and are usually unseen.

During the home visit, the nurse's focus is the nursing care being provided to the client and family. Nevertheless, it is important to remain alert to potential safety problems. Keep in mind that the home includes not only the client but also other members of the household and visitors. Clues to problems include such things as a disturbing affect, verbal abuse, or threatening behavior in someone in the home that leads the nurse to suspect that violence might follow. A general rule of thumb is "When in doubt, get out." Do not argue against verbal attacks or belligerent behavior. Do not attempt to become a mediator or get involved in any way in domestic disputes.

Assessment Checklist for Ensuring Your Own Safety During Home Visits

PREPARING FOR THE HOME VISIT

- Do you check the client's record for any suggestion of concerns about safety?
- Do you lock up your purse or valuables *before* leaving for the visit (in a safe place at your work station or in the trunk of your car)?
- Does your car have more than enough gasoline for the round trip?
- Do you keep your car doors locked?
- Do you have clear directions and a safe route for getting to your destination?
- Does someone know where you are going (client's name, address, and phone number) and when you expect to return?

MAKING THE HOME VISIT

- Do you assess the path from your car to the client's home, to avoid walking into situations where people or animals may threaten your safety?
- Do you lock your car upon leaving it?
- If your client is not home, do you decline to enter the home if you are uncomfortable with the person inviting you in?
- Do you select a hard chair to sit on, if possible?
- Are you alert to the emotional climate in the home and the neighborhood? Are you prepared to leave if tensions or unexpected circumstances represent any potential threat to your safety?
- Do you reassess the pathway from the home to your car before leaving the home?
- Do you check back in with your contact person as soon as you return from the home visit?

Returning Safely to the Home Base

After the visit is concluded, the return to the school or agency requires the same precautions taken in traveling to the home. Note any potential risks that may be encountered when leaving the house to return to the car, and wait rather than confront a problem. Once inside the car, lock the doors. Do not remove purses, backpacks or other valuables from the trunk until after arriving back at the school or health care agency. The first thing the nurse does upon returning to the agency is to check back in with the contact person.

It is important to emphasize that home visits are not generally considered to be dangerous or risky activities. A discussion of safety precautions is meant to serve as primary prevention. It is most unlikely that the maternal-newborn nurse in the community will encounter any difficulties. Nevertheless, a review of the precautions outlined in the Assessment Checklist for Ensuring Your Own Safety During Home Visits can serve as an important reminder. A preventive approach, begun during the planning phase and continued throughout the home visit and the return to the agency, will allow the visit to be focused on client needs and make it a satisfying interaction for both nurse and client.

ASSESSING THE CLIENT'S COMMUNITY

To provide comprehensive care to maternal-newborn clients in the community, it is important for the nurse to have some knowledge about the community in which the client lives. This knowledge can help the nurse gain a better understanding of the issues the client faces. Such knowledge includes information about the characteristics of the community, factors that may influence the client's health either positively or negatively, and services available in the community to meet the needs of maternal-newborn clients.

Defining the Community

One way to define the community in which the client lives is to view it as the physical place where the client's residence is located. This is perhaps the most common definition of a community. When looking at a community as a place, many factors can be discovered that may affect the client's health status.

Another useful way to define a community is as a collection of people with common characteristics or common interests. Looking at the client's community in this way may help the nurse to discover interpersonal support systems as well as interpersonal conflicts that may have some bearing on the client's health and health behaviors. In addition, knowledge about the characteristics and health problems that are common in a particular group of people may direct the nurse to assess those characteristics or health problems in the individual client.

Assessing the Community

Knowledge of the community can be gained in several ways. A general look at the community, often accomplished simply by driving around, can provide a beginning impression of the environment. Information about the people in the community can be gained by talking to formal and informal community leaders. The client and family are also good resources for information about the people in the area. Finally, other health care professionals can be consulted for information about community resources, and directories of community services are sometimes available.

In looking at the community as a place, several factors are important to the health of the client. Environmental characteristics are assessed in relation to both the client's immediate environment and the larger community. Air, water, and noise pollution are pertinent to the health of the pregnant woman and fetus as well as of the new mother and newborn. Potential teratogens should be considered. Water hazards, trash and litter, and other hazardous conditions in the environment can create a threat to the well-being of the client. Rats and other pests in the community can create problems for the client. The condition of housing in the area may also be important. For example, older homes may have lead-based paint, which presents a health hazard to families with young children. Assessment may lead to a nursing diagnosis of high risk for poisoning. Appropriate plans and interventions would then include both education and referral for medical testing and follow-up if needed.

Safety is another aspect of the environment that should be assessed. In urban areas, the nurse notes whether the neighborhood feels safe. Is it a high crime area in which the client fears for her safety? Traffic in the area may also pose a danger. In rural areas, health hazards may include farm chemicals, pesticides, or well water contaminants such as nitrates or coliform bacteria. Whether rural or urban, older homes may contain fire hazards such as old wiring, space heaters, or other problems. The nurse conducting a home visit is alert to all factors that may pose potential threats to the client's safety.

Resources in the community should be assessed to determine how effectively the client's needs can be met. In urban areas, is public transportation

Understanding the Childbearing Family's Community

Age distribution	Are there other people the age of your client in the neighborhood? These people may be able to share experiences and offer advice and support.
Culture	Is the community accepting of your client's cultural and religious activities and beliefs? Is your client able to interact with others who share the same orientation?
Environment	Are there environmental hazards that may pose a problem for your client, such as rodents, heavy traffic, air pollution, excessive noise, water hazards, temperature extremes, trash and litter, or other hazards?
Housing	Are homes in the area in good repair, free of lead-based paint, well-spaced, and free of overcrowding?
Safety	Is your client's home in a neighborhood that feels relatively safe, or is it a high crime area? What about fire safety? Can you identify other threats to safety in the area?
Transportation	Does your client have access to transportation, public or private, that is adequate for getting to places of employment, grocery shopping, recreation, social interaction, and health care (including emergency needs)?
Resources	Are there resources and services in the community to meet the needs of antepartum, postpartum, and newborn clients?

available for getting to work, to the grocery store, to recreational and spiritual resources and to health care? Are there health care services such as prenatal care, well-baby care, and sick child care that are accessible and affordable for the client? What is the distance to these services for clients living in rural areas? What about the availability of emergency services, especially to rural areas? Are there services to meet other needs of maternal-newborn clients?

Finally, it is useful to find out something about the people in the client's community. How are they similar to or different from her? Are there people in the community whose age and interests are similar to those of the client? Are there people who can provide a support system for her? Is she part of the mainstream or the minority within the community? Is the community accepting of her religious and cultural beliefs and her lifestyle? Are there others in the community who share her orientation, or does she feel like an outcast in the community?

Implications of Community Assessment Findings

Maternal-newborn nursing in the community does not require a complete community assessment in order to provide effective care. It is important, however, to have a sense of the community in which the client lives (see Understanding the Childbearing Family's Community). Characteristics of the community can influence the client's health in positive or negative ways. Therefore, the nurse must understand the community and its actual and potential contributions to the client's well-being. In this way, nursing care can be provided that addresses all potential problems and utilizes all possible resources to maximize the well-being of the client.

LINKING CLIENTS WITH COMMUNITY RESOURCES

When working with the client and family in the home, the nurse conducts many assessments, both formally and informally. Through this process of ongoing assessment, the nurse may become aware of client needs that might be met by resources in the community. Linking clients with appropriate community programs or services is a satisfying experience for the nurse. It provides a unique opportunity to see clients benefit from outside sources as a result of the nurse's skill in community assessment, client assessment, interpretation of services, and linking clients with resources.

Assessing Community Services

The nurse who provides care to mothers and newborns in the community must have a good working knowledge of the community services that may benefit those clients. Therefore, in addition to conducting appropriate client assessments, it is important to discover the programs and services that the community offers to the maternal-newborn population.

Information that will provide the maternal-newborn nurse with a beginning knowledge base about community resources includes

- Programs in the community that address the needs of the maternal-newborn client and family
- Purposes and goals of the programs
- Eligibility criteria for program participants
- Fees or other requirements for participation
- Logistic details of the program functions (e.g., time, place, transportation)
- The process for enrolling a client in the program
- The contact person for further information

To learn all these characteristics about every relevant resource in the community would be a formidable task for the nurse who is just learning to provide maternal-newborn nursing care in the community. Fortunately, nurses employed in the field and other professionals make excellent resource people. By consulting them, the new maternal-newborn nurse can develop a beginning awareness of programs designed for childbearing families.

A great variety of local services may be available. Some offer health education, support groups, individual counseling, or even home visits in which a lay person provides individual support and role modeling. Others provide direct health care or material goods such as emergency food and formula supplies. It is the nurse's responsibility to assess the client's need for resources and then seek out services that best meet those needs.

Some communities are rich in services and programs that support the material-newborn client and family, while other communities are less well equipped. Local health department nurses are among the excellent resource persons for such information. Social workers in local hospitals and health departments may also be extremely helpful. Welfare agencies and professional organizations can provide useful information, and telephone book yellow pages should not be overlooked. Many communities have printed resource directories.

Assessing the Client's Need for Community Services

While the nurse conducts the initial client assessment, and as an ongoing process throughout each home visit, the nurse becomes aware of a variety of client needs. Some needs are obvious; others are more subtle, with evidence emerging gradually. Whenever a clue appears about a need that may not be met through the nurse's home visits, a more thorough assessment of the need is in order. Questions that should be answered include the following:

- What are the indications that the need exists?
- Are there overt signs of the problem or is the evidence more subtle?
- Does the client openly discuss the problem or seem totally unaware of it?
- Is the client's attitude toward the problem one of acceptance, ambivalence, guilt, or denial?
- How does the need affect the well-being of the mother, the fetus or newborn, or other members of the household?
- How serious is the problem or need?
- Does the client accept the need for change? (This is essential for the nursing intervention to be effective.)

To obtain the answers to these questions, the nurse observes closely, encourages the client to explore her feelings about the problem, and asks probing questions.

For example, during a home visit to a postpartum client who is breastfeeding, assessments are performed and appropriate teaching is provided as described in Chapter 33, Breastfeeding. If assessment findings lead to a nursing diagnosis of ineffective breastfeeding, open-ended questions can be used to explore the client's feelings about breastfeeding and to determine whether she might be a candidate for additional assistance. It is important for the nurse to develop a trusting relationship with the client so that communication can be open and the client will be able to speak openly about her concerns. After working with her, the nurse may decide that she could benefit from more counseling and support for breastfeeding than can be provided during the relatively brief period of a home visit. The nurse would then discuss this perception with the client. This is an important step, because a mutual understanding of the problem or need is vital to successful resource utilization. The client may not be aware of the need, may disagree that the need exists, or may recognize the need but resist acting to meet it. Often the greatest challenge in the process of linking clients with community resources lies in helping the client to acknowledge the need and accept help. Therefore, communication skills are used carefully to help the client recognize that she may benefit from further assistance.

Interpreting Community Services for the Client

The next step is to describe to the client the services that may be available to assist her. Here the nurse's professional judgment is used in determining whether to have the client choose from all possible services or whether to discuss only the one that the nurse believes would be most appropriate for the client. Some clients respond well to being given more than one choice, while others focus best on a single option. In either case, the nurse interprets to the client the possible benefits that she may experience from the program(s) or service(s).

It is important to make clear to the client that she alone will decide whether or not to utilize the community resource. The nurse's role is to help the client explore the need and to interpret to her the services available to meet the need. Therefore, the nurse should describe not only the services available but also the logistics such as enrollment procedures, time, place, and other details about the service. In addition, it is important to make clear what responsibilities, if any, the client would have to assume. These might include such things as transportation, regular attendance, cooperation with the service provider, fees, or other requirements. To provide all this information, the nurse may have to consult resource directories, make telephone calls from the client's home for additional information, or bring back more information at a later visit. Achieving a fit between client and service is a skill that may take some practice but is very rewarding.

Returning to the example of the postpartum client who is having trouble breastfeeding, the nurse may decide that the La Leche League might be of benefit to the client. Since the client has acknowledged that she may need some help, it would now be appropriate to discuss the La Leche League and its services with her. Help her to explore her feelings about receiving a consultant from the organization or attending one of their support group meetings. Make it clear that the decision is hers. The nurse's responsibility is to help the client recognize and accept her need for help and to interpret for her the ways in which she could benefit from the available resources. If the nurse needs more information about the La Leche League, it is appropriate to telephone from the client's home to obtain this. Alternately, the nurse can make arrangements to return with more information in the near future. It is important to follow through quickly with this, however, since unresolved difficulties can lead to a decision to discontinue breastfeeding.

After the nurse has described the services to the client and assisted her in exploring her feelings about the referral, the client makes the decision whether to make use of the service. If she declines to take advantage of the service, the nurse will explore her reasons for this decision. If the decision is based on misunderstandings, incomplete information, or fear of the unknown, the nurse may be able to help her work it through. It is important to remember, however, that it is the client's decision, and her right to make her own decision must be respected. Nonetheless, the nurse's responsibility does not end with the client's refusal to use the suggested community resource. The nurse should address the need in the plan of care and do everything possible to assist the client to meet the need. If, on the other hand, the client accepts the idea of using the community resource to meet her need, the nurse facilitates her link with the resource.

Facilitating the Link Between Clients and Community Services

The nurse and client share responsibility for seeing that the client is successful in making use of services to which the nurse has directed her. The nurse's actions vary according to the characteristics of both the client and the resource.

The individuality of clients dictates that the nurse assess the client's ability to follow through with utilization of the resource. On the basis of this assessment, the nurse provides whatever assistance is indicated. For some clients, all that may be necessary is to provide the name of the person or place to contact, the address and telephone number, dates and times, and any other pertinent information. The client then follows through with the arrangements and develops a sense of independence and pride in having handled the situation. For other clients, follow-through will be more likely if the nurse initiates the contact with the resource and makes the initial arrangements. In either case, the nurse must follow through with additional information as needed, provide emotional support to the client as she takes this new step, and undertake troubleshooting as needed.

The nurse must document the client's use of community resources in the client's chart. Documentation should include a description of the client problem or need that prompted the use of a community resource. The service used and the client's response to it should also be made clear in the chart.

It is important to keep the client's primary care provider informed when the client begins to use a resource or service in the community. In addition, the primary provider should be notified of the outcome of the client's use of those services. To this end, the nurse must stay in contact with the primary care provider throughout the process of home visits.

Follow-up to Complete the Link Between Clients and Community Services

The nurse's responsibility may not be over once the client is linked with the resource. Some clients need ongoing support if they are to continue their use of outside services. To accomplish this, the nurse might telephone or visit the client after her first scheduled encounter with the resource to assess her reactions and offer support and encouragement. Any misgivings can be addressed at this time. In this way the nurse can help promote the client's continued use of the resource.

The referral requirements of community resources are as varied as the resources themselves. For some, a simple telephone call from a client in need is all that is necessary. Others may require the name of the nurse who refers the client, details about the client, or even a formal referral form. It is the nurse's responsibility to find out the resource's referral procedure and to carry out all nursing responsibilities for the referral in order to achieve a successful link of client with resource.

REFERRING CLIENTS TO OTHER AGENCIES AND PROFESSIONALS

Some say that a mark of true wisdom is the ability to know one's own limitations. The wise nurse is able to recognize when the client's needs exceed the nurse's own abilities or go beyond the scope of nursing practice. In those situations it becomes appropriate to refer the client to other agencies or other professionals. In this way the client can benefit not only from the nurse's expertise but also from the expertise of disciplines other than nursing.

Formal Referral Process

Much of the formal referral process follows the principles and steps described in the preceding discussion of linking clients with community services. The nurse seeks to become knowledgeable about other disciplines and professionals in the community. A careful assessment is conducted to clarify the client's need for other professional help. An attempt is made to create the best possible match of client, need, and caregiver. The nurse carefully interprets to the client the services that are available to help meet her need. The advantages of accepting the referral are discussed with the client. Again, it is the client who makes the ultimate decision whether to accept the referral. Finally, the referral is made and the nurse follows up to ensure successful completion of the process.

Nursing can meet many needs for maternal-newborn clients. There are other disciplines and other professionals, however, that are more appropriate for meeting some client needs. For referral to some of these resources, the referral process is more formal than just linking the client with a local service by giving a name or making a telephone call. Resources that might require a formal referral process include such professionals as physicians or dentists, or such agencies as those providing mental health services and social services, among others.

For example, the nurse may be making home visits to a postpartum mother who exhibits signs of depression. The client is encouraged to express her feelings. The nurse conducts appropriate assessments that confirm the nursing diagnosis of ineffective individual coping. The nurse's perceptions are shared with the client when this is appropriate. The evidence indicates that her need for help goes beyond the scope of nursing practice. Therefore, the nurse decides that the most appropriate nursing intervention for this problem is to refer the client for psychiatric help.

Involving the Client in the Referral Process

There are two important components in the success of a referral: the effectiveness with which the nurse helps the client to accept the need for help, and the clarity with which the nurse interprets the available resources to the client. Therefore, the nurse carefully helps the client work through her feelings about her problems and her need for further care. In addition, the nurse helps to clarify for her the professional resources available.

If the nurse has not already done so, it will be necessary to assess the available resources. For example, in this community the nurse finds that there are several psychiatrists in private practice as well as a mental health center. Because this client lives on a limited income, the nurse may believe that the mental health center provides the best fit for her needs. Nevertheless, all viable alternatives are presented to the client, and she makes a choice among the available options. The nurse suggests a referral to the mental health center or a private psychiatrist as a way to help her cope with the feelings she is experiencing.

Initiating the Referral

Once the client agrees to use the service, the formal referral process begins. To do this, the nurse must first discover the referral system preferred by the professional or agency to which the client is being referred. In some instances, the first contact is made verbally, either on the telephone or through face-to-face contact. Alternatively, a formal written referral provides the first contact. If the original referral is verbal, it is important to follow up with a written communication. Written follow-up ensures that all information has been transmitted clearly and completely, and provides a permanent record of the referral.

The written referral, and the verbal referral if that occurs, should provide objective patient assessment data. The reason(s) for the referral and comprehensive information about the presenting problem should be clearly stated. Include the name of the nurse making the referral, as well as a suggested mechanism for providing feedback to that nurse.

Just as the nurse facilitates informal referrals to services in the community, so the nurse also facilitates more formal referrals to professionals. The client should receive whatever help she needs to obtain an initial appointment at a time that suits her needs. If transportation, fees, or other situational constraints might threaten the success of the referral, the nurse intercedes to ensure effective utilization of the new resource. A telephone call or visit before the first appointment can help to answer any last-minute questions or concerns the client may have. In addition, this added contact may provide the encouragement that the client needs to follow through with the referral.

Documenting and Evaluating the Referral

Documentation of the referral becomes part of the client's record. A copy of the referral form should be inserted in the chart. All communication about the referral should also be documented. Names, dates, and other pertinent data should be included.

Evaluation of the referral is an important component of the referral process. Both process and outcome are evaluated. In terms of outcome, did the client keep the appointment? What was her reaction to the service? If continued interaction with the new care provider was appropriate, did the client stay with the service? How has the referral changed the status of her problem? Did she benefit from the service in the ways that she and the nurse hoped?

To evaluate the referral process, one should ask if the referral process itself was appropriate for the client and her needs. Was the process efficient? Was it effective in making the connection between client in need and new provider of care? Are there things to be learned from this experience that will make future referrals more successful?

The results or outcome of the referral should be documented in the chart. The client's response to the referral provides important data that can help in future referrals. In addition, it is important to document changes in the status of her problem under the care of the new provider. Finally, the results of the referral may lead to new plans for the client's care. These should also be documented in the client's chart, making clear the connection between the referral and the new plans for care.

Risk Management

The first step in risk management for maternal-newborn nursing in the community is careful preparation for each home visit. When the nurse is visiting in the home, other health care experts are not as easily accessible for feedback as they are in clinical facilities. Clinical decision making thus becomes a very independent nursing function. Therefore, when preparing for the home visit, it is wise to review developmental stages, normal assessment parameters, and health problems that the client and family may be at risk for at this stage in the childbearing experience. A thorough knowledge base in antepartum, postpartum, and newborn nursing is essential.

The second step in risk management is careful assessment of the client for risk factors. At the time of the home visit, the nurse is the only health care provider interacting with the client, and the client is totally dependent on the nurse for quality care. Therefore, the nurse must be prepared to make careful, thoughtful decisions. An awareness of common risk factors will help the nurse avoid overlooking an important sign or symptom that should have been addressed.

A third factor in risk management is to ensure that nursing interventions are thorough, that health teaching and other nursing care are grounded in a sound theory base, and that teaching is appropriate to the needs and level of the client. Part of the visit should involve checking on the outcomes of previous visits to ensure that the client is following earlier nursing recommendations appropriately. Referrals must always be considered when the client has needs outside the scope of nursing practice.

The last important step in risk management is follow-up after the home visit. This includes thorough documentation of the visit in the client's chart, including assessment data, interventions, evaluations, and plans for future visits. Communication with the primary health care provider is important here as well as follow-up on any referrals made.

Each of these steps in risk management is important. With thorough preparation before the visit, careful assessment for risk factors, nursing interventions grounded in a sound knowledge base, and careful follow-up, the nurse can help to ensure safe and appropriate nursing care to maternal-newborn clients during home visits.

Implications for Research

Nurses have been using home visits as a mode of health care delivery to antepartum and postpartum families for many years. Anecdotal reports in the literature indicate that home visits by nurses to childbearing families at risk can improve maternal-newborn outcomes. However, nursing research about home visits to childbearing families has been sparse (Combs-Orme et al. 1985). Therefore, nursing research is needed to establish a scientific base for maternal-newborn nursing practice in the community. Questions that might be answered through systematic nursing research include the following:

- What nursing interventions are most effective in home visits to the childbearing family?
- What timing is most effective for antepartum and postpartum home visits?
- What are the effects of home visits by the nurse on maternal outcomes?
- What are the effects of home visits by the nurse on newborn and infant outcomes?
- What is the cost-benefit ratio of providing professional nursing care to childbearing families through home visits?
- What community-based programs are most ef-

fective for improving maternal-newborn outcomes?

Nursing research on maternal-newborn nursing in the community is an important component of nursing research for the future. Society has an increasing concern about health care costs and a critical need to decrease the infant mortality rate. Therefore, nurses have both the opportunity and the obligation to develop innovative, cost-effective methods of health care delivery that improve maternal-newborn outcomes. Through research, nurses can play an important and exciting role in the development of the future in health care for childbearing families.

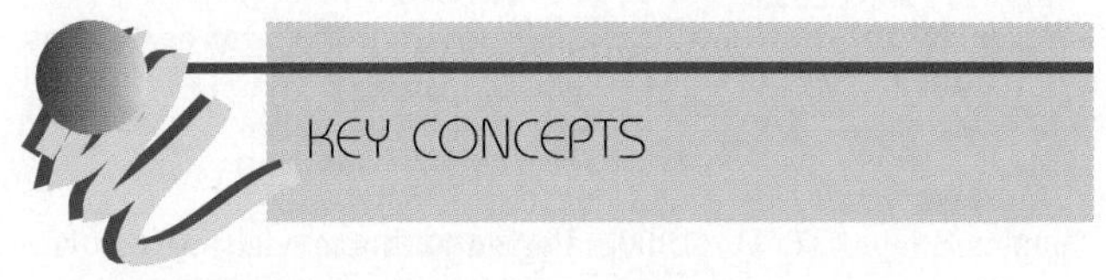

KEY CONCEPTS

- Most health care for maternal-newborn clients takes place outside the hospital.
- Nurses are in a unique position to provide comprehensive, sensitive, and cost-effective care to antepartum, postpartum, and newborn clients in the community.
- Prenatal care is one of the most important determinants of infant birth weight and survival. Through home visits, nurses can monitor and encourage adequate prenatal care.
- The trend toward early discharge after delivery leaves the postpartum mother in need of information and nursing care that can be effectively provided through home visits.
- The roles of the maternal-newborn nurse in the community are many and varied, including caregiver, case manager, client advocate, teacher, researcher, and political activist and change agent.
- The maternal-newborn nurse in the community approaches the entire family as the client, because of the influence the family may have on the health of the identified client, and because other family members may also have needs that the nurse can address.
- The home visit is a unique vehicle for providing nursing care to childbearing families. The nurse is able to assess and work with factors that would not be apparent outside the client's home. In addition, the client may be more open and at ease in this setting.
- The professional visit is goal directed. The nurse reviews available information and plans the visit to achieve the goals. Any needed supplies are prepared and arrangements are made, if possible, for the client to expect the visit.
- A home visit consists of three phases. The social phase is a brief introductory phase in which social amenities are exchanged and rapport is developed. The working phase takes up most of the visit and is focused on goal attainment. In the closing phase the visit is summarized, progress toward goal attainment is evaluated, and plans are made for the next visit.
- Nursing process provides the framework for the home visit. Whenever possible, the client participates in her care, including involvement in goal setting as well as in the interventions and evaluation. A contract between nurse and client is one effective way to involve the client in her own care.
- Complete and concise documentation of the home visit is important to facilitate continuity of care, to provide justification for reimbursement, and to serve as a legal record.
- The maternal-newborn nurse in the community must maintain communication with the client's primary care provider. Both written and verbal exchanges of information and ideas are important and should occur on a regular basis.
- The nurse's own safety is a vital consideration that must be addressed when planning the visit, traveling to the client's home, conducting the visit, and returning to the home base after the visit.
- To make effective home visits, the nurse assesses the client's community. This assessment will reveal characteristics about the community's people, environment, and services and will provide information about safety issues.
- The nurse must be familiar with services in the community that address the needs of childbearing families. When the nurse determines that the client could benefit from a community resource, this is discussed with the client. The nurse facilitates the link between client and resource, and follows up to promote a satisfactory outcome.
- Through a formal referral process, the nurse refers the client to other professionals or agencies for the meeting of needs outside the realm of nursing care. The nurse seeks to involve the client in decision making about referrals.
- Risk management for home visits involves comprehensive previsit planning, careful assessment for risk factors, nursing interventions grounded in a sound theory base, and follow-up after the home visit.

References

Ausman, L. F. (1993). Toxoplasmosis and pregnancy. *The Canadian Nurse,* 89 (4), 31–32.

Bowles, B. C., and Williamson, B. P. (1990). Pregnancy and lactation following anorexia and bulimia. *Journal of Obstetric, Gynecologic, and Neonatal Nursing,* 19, 233–238.

Brainard, A. M. (1985). *The evolution of public health nursing.* New York: Garland: Reprinted from A. M. Brainard. (1922). *The evolution of public health nursing.* Philadelphia, W. B. Saunders.

Browne, H. (1966). A tribute to Mary Breckinridge. *Nursing Outlook,* 14 (5), 54–55.

Bull, M. (1981). Change in concerns of first-time mothers after one week at home. *Journal of Obstetric, Gynecologic, and Neonatal Nursing,* 10 (5), 391–394.

Bull. M., and Lawrence, D. (1985). Mothers' use of knowledge during the first postpartum weeks. *Journal of Obstetric, Gynecologic, and Neonatal Nursing,* 14 (4), 315–319.

Campinha-Bacote, J., and Bragg, E. J. (1993). Chemical assessment in maternity care. *MCN,* 18 (1), 24–28.

Combs-Orme, T., Reis, J., Ward, L. O. (1985). Effectiveness of home visits by public health nurses in maternal and child health: An empirical review. *Public Health Reports,* 100, 490–499.

Coss, C. (1989). *Lillian Wald: A progressive activist.* New York: Feminist Press.

Dolan, J. (1978). *History of nursing* (14th ed.). Philadelphia: W. B. Saunders.

Donaldson, N. (1981). The postpartum follow-up nurse clinician. *Journal of Obstetric, Gynecologic, and Neonatal Nursing,* 10 (4), 249–253.

Edwards, M. R. (1993). Self-esteem, sense of mastery, and adequacy of prenatal care [Doctoral dissertation, University of Alabama at Birmingham, 1991]. *Dissertation Abstracts International,* 53/02-B, 768.

Evans, C. J. (1991). Description of a home follow-up program for childbearing families. *Journal of Obstetric, Gynecologic, and Neonatal Nursing,* 20, 113–118.

Fitzpatrick, M. L. (1975). *The National Organization of Public Health Nursing, 1912–1952: Development of a practice field.* New York: National League of Nursing.

Freda, M. C. (1991). Home care for preterm birth prevention: Is nursing monitoring the interventions? *MCN,* 16 (1), 9–14.

Giblin, P. T., Poland, M. L., Ager, J. W. (1990). Effects of social supports on attitudes, health behaviors and obtaining prenatal care. *Journal of Community Health,* 15, 357–368.

Goodwin, L. (1994). Essential program components for perinatal home care. *Journal of Obstetric, Gynecologic, and Neonatal Nursing,* 23 (8), 667.

Hogue, C. J. R., Buehler, J. W., Strauss, L. T., Smith, J. C. (1987). Overview of the National Infant Mortality Surveillance (NIMS) project: Design, methods, results. *Public Health Reports,* 102, 126–138.

Institute of Medicine. (1985). *Preventing low birth weight.* Washington, D.C.: National Academy Press.

Institute of Medicine. (1988). *Prenatal care: Reaching mothers, reaching infants.* Washington, D.C.: National Academy Press.

Kemp, V. H., and Hatmaker, D. D. (1992). Health practice and anxiety in low-income, high- and low-risk pregnant women. *Journal of Obstetric, Gynecologic, and Neonatal Nursing,* 22, 266–272.

Kramer, M. S. (1987). Determinants of low birth weight: Methodological assessment and meta-analysis. *Bulletin of the World Health Organization,* 65, 663–737.

Maynard, T. (1939). *The apostle of charity: The life of St. Vincent de Paul.* New York: Dial Press.

McClanahan, P. (1992). Improving access to and use of prenatal care. *Journal of Obstetric, Gynecologic, and Neonatal Nursing,* 21, 280–284.

Mercer, R. (1981). The nurse and maternal tasks of early postpartum. *MCN,* 6 (5), 341–345.

Merkatz, I. R., Thompson, J. E., Mullen, P. D., Goldenberg, R. L. (1990). *New perspectives on prenatal care.* New York: Elsevier.

Peoples-Sheps, M. D. (1990). Perinatal home visiting returns. *Nursing Outlook,* 38, 54–55.

Petitti, D., Coleman, C., Binsacca, D., Allen, B. (1990). Early prenatal care in urban black and white women. *Birth,* 17 (1), 1–5.

Powell, D. R. (1993). Inside home visiting programs. *The future of children,* 3 (3), 23–37. [*The Future of Children,* The David and Lucile Packard Foundation, 300 Second Street, Suite 102, Los Altos, CA 94022.]

Pruitt, R. H., Keller, L. S., Hale, S. L. (1987). Mastering distractions that mar home visits. *Nursing & Health Care,* 8, 344–347.

Rush, J. P., and Valaitis, R. K. (1992). Postpartum care: Home or hospital? *The Canadian Nurse,* 88 (5), 29–31.

Salmon, M. E., and Peoples-Sheps, M. (1989). Infant mortality and public health nursing: A history of accomplishments, a future of challenges. *Nursing Outlook,* 37, 6–7, 51.

Tirpak, H. (1975). The Frontier Nursing Service: Fifty years in the mountains. *Nursing Outlook,* 33 (5), 308–310.

Williams, L. R., and Cooper, M. K. (1993). Nurse-managed postpartum home care. *Journal of Obstetric, Gynecologic, and Neonatal Nursing,* 22, 25–31.

Chapter 6

Social Issues and Childbearing Women

Lynn Clark Callister

> It's not just prenatal care . . . it's total mothering . . . Before I can go in there and say, "Well, Ms. Susan, why don't you come on and make this appointment?" I have to first address Ms. Susan's problem of feeding these other babies that she already has, because otherwise, she doesn't want to hear anything I have to say, because it's not important at that point, not to her . . . If I can't get Mom a roof over her head, then I'm never going to get her to that clinic.
>
> Vivian Louis-Burnett
> Casefinder, Chicago, Illinois
> (National Commission on Children 1991)

HIGHLIGHTS

- ▼ Poverty and Childbearing Women
- ▼ Access to Health Care
- ▼ Violence Against Women and Children
- ▼ Perinatal Substance Abuse
- ▼ Employment Concerns of Childbearing Women
- ▼ Breastfeeding and the Employed Mother
- ▼ Child Care
- ▼ Occupational Health Hazards
- ▼ Influencing Policy Related to Health and Social Issues
- ▼ Political Activism
- ▼ Implications for Research

Women's health problems, their biopsychosocial status, and their environment are closely related, and each one influences the others. Contemporary women's health means redefining the very nature of health care so that physical and psychological well-being are always presumed to be intertwined, as well as determined by the context (interpersonal, socioeconomic, political, environmental) in which the individual operates (Fogel and Woods 1995).

Because of these linkages, the Public Health Service Task Force on Women's Health Issues recommends (Burst 1987):

- Promoting a safe, healthful physical and social environment
- Providing services for health promotion and disease prevention
- Coordinating research and evaluation
- Educating and informing the public
- Disseminating research information
- Influencing public policy related to women's health issues

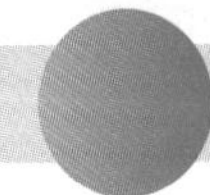

DEFINITIONS

Child abuse—The physical abuse or neglect, emotional abuse or mistreatment, or sexual abuse of a child.

Childhood sexual abuse—The use, persuasion, or coercion of a child to engage in sexually explicit conduct or any simulation of such conduct.

Early prenatal care—The first prenatal care visit to a health provider is within 3 months of conception (first trimester).

Occupational health hazards—Workplace exposure to potential reproductive toxins, physical hazards (e.g., ionizing radiation), chemical agents, and biologic hazards.

Political activism—Acting as a maternal-newborn advocate through the political process, support for candidate's campaigns for public office, recruitment of voters, work for change through political parties and nonpartisan groups, and involvement in advocacy activities of professional nursing associations.

Poverty—The lack of money and material goods (visible poverty) and/or social and cultural deprivation (invisible poverty).

Prenatal care—Prenatal care consists of health promotion, risk assessment, and intervention activities carried out by prenatal health care providers, women, and families during pregnancy to promote healthy outcomes for women and their infants.

Rape—A sexual act with a nonconsenting victim, including the use of physical force, intimidation, deception, threat, and coitus or vaginal penetration.

Role stress—A situation in which an individual encounters role overload (excessive demands), role conflict (contradictory role expectations), role ambiguity (norms for the role are vague or ill defined), and/or role incongruity (role expectations are different from the individual's self-perception, attitudes, or values).

Substance abuse—The use of any mind-altering drug or agent in such a way that it interferes with the individual's ability to function, either physiologically, emotionally, or socioculturally.

Violence—The use of physical force to injure or harm, which is a major social problem threatening the physical health as well as spiritual and emotional well-being of women and children.

Social issues, the implications for nursing, and strategies for influencing public policy in relation to social and political issues play an important role in nursing in America today.

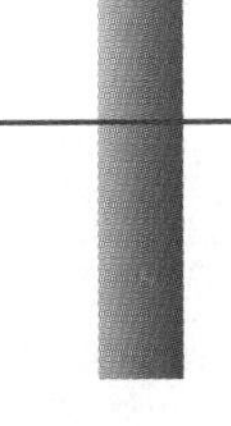

SOCIAL ISSUES INFLUENCING THE HEALTH OF WOMEN AND CHILDREN

The social issues of poverty, access to care, violence against women and children, perinatal substance abuse, and employment need to be understood and considered in the context of their influences on the health of childbearing women and their infants.

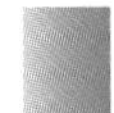

Poverty and Childbearing Women

Those families consistently living at or below the poverty level are in a perpetual state of despair. Poverty may be either visible or invisible. Visible poverty refers to a lack of money or material resources, including insufficient clothing, poor sanitation, and inadequate housing. Poverty may also be invisible, referring to social and cultural deprivation, such as limited employment opportunities and health care services, lack of educational opportunities, and an absence of community services.

No single indicator of health status makes the connection between poverty and less than optimal health more clear than does infant mortality. Poor pregnancy outcomes, including prematurity, low birth weight, birth defects, and infant mortality, are linked to low income, low educational level, low occupational status, and other indicators of social and economic disadvantage (Alexander and Korenbrot 1995).

Feminization of poverty has occurred as a result of increased female-headed households, homelessness, and labor market inequities (Fig. 6–1). Government cuts in maternal-child welfare have been made at a time when the benefits of adequate nutrition and prenatal care have been documented to improve health outcomes as well as being cost effective (Alexander and Korenbrot 1995).

Those who live in poverty face stressors, including frustration over insecure employment, repeated exposure to violence and crime, inadequate child care assistance, and the insensitive and judgmental attitudes of social service and health care agencies. Sometimes there is a perception that caregivers blame victims for their life circum-

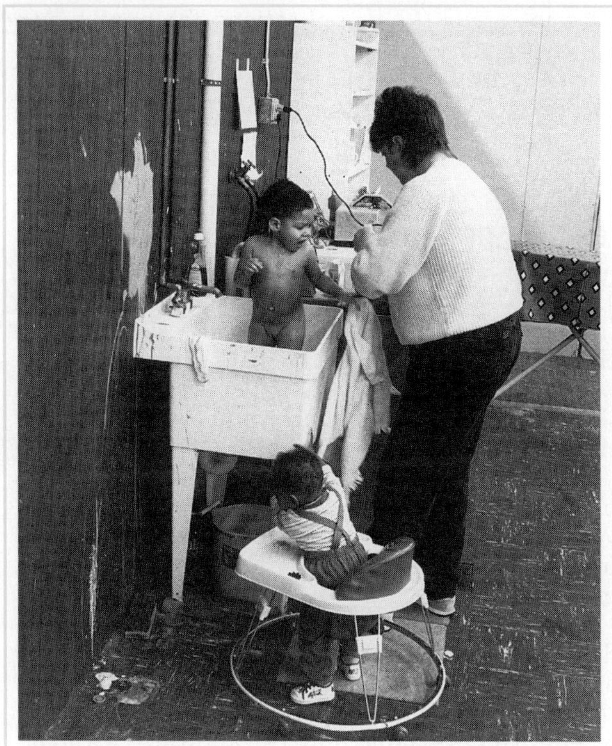

Figure 6–1

A mother gives her toddler a bath in a sink in the basement of the homeless shelter where they live. In addition to the need for safety and shelter, women with children who live in such shelters need caretaking and nurturing parenting skills, together with information on children's growth and development, the proper use of discipline, and injury prevention techniques. (Photograph copyright Jim Hubbard from Hubbard, J. [1991]. *American refugees* [p. 94]. Minneapolis, MN: University of Minnesota Press.)

stances. Coping proves difficult in the face of unpredictable and unrelenting cumulative stressors. Those childbearing families engulfed in the cycle of poverty and despair may feel helpless and hopeless, contributing to a lack of motivation (Pesznecker 1984).

Rae K. Grad, a nurse who served as the executive director of the National Commission to Prevent Infant Mortality, shared her experience of volunteering in a community prenatal clinic serving disadvantaged women:

I have learned more there than in most of my years of formal and political education . . . Scratch the surface and you will find women filled with dignity and honor. They want to do right for themselves and their children but honestly don't know how or can't get the help they need. They have been stripped of their history and culture, deprived of jobs and decent living conditions, and then asked to act with character and self-esteem (Grad 1991, p. 168).

Homelessness is a major social problem for those who live in poverty, directly affecting an estimated 3 million persons, including families headed by single mothers, many of whom are minority women (National Center for Health Statistics 1994). Female-headed families are the fastest growing element of the homeless in the United States. There are profound effects on the physical and emotional morbidity in homeless children as well as their mothers (Wright and Weber 1987; Schlosstein 1990). Berne and colleagues (1990) portray the sense of despair that may be experienced by a single homeless mother and her children (see the Critical Thinking Case History about homeless mothers and children).

It is vital that the nurse develop a personal awareness and understanding of the impact of poverty in the lives of the childbearing family. It is important to identify women at risk so that support, counseling, and referral can be provided. Assistance should be both tangible and intangible. These women should be approached with caring and respect, in contrast to the dehumanizing attitudes often faced by those who live in poverty. Homeless families can best be assisted through strategies that empower women to develop confidence and increased self-esteem, to pursue opportunities for moving out of homelessness and poverty, and to gain positive coping skills (Hodnick 1990).

Nursing care should focus on working with community leaders to provide affordable housing, quality child care, education and job training, employment options, and adequate levels of public assistance for disadvantaged women and their children. Access should be provided to comprehensive health promotion and disease prevention services, including family planning, substance abuse prevention and treatment, and support groups.

Access to Health Care

The Expert Panel on the Content of Prenatal Care has specified that the major objective of prenatal care is to "promote the health and well-being of the pregnant woman, the fetus, the infant and the family" (USDHHS 1989, p. 4). Prenatal care is the cornerstone of health care delivery. The overwhelming general recommendation of health care professionals is that all pregnant women should be assured access to timely, comprehensive, high-quality prenatal care (Machala and Miner 1991). However, fewer than half of adolescents seek prenatal care during the first trimester (Scholl et al. 1994). In 1993, 21 percent of expectant mothers did not receive early or adequate prenatal care (USDHHS 1995). Younger women as well as black and Hispanic women are more likely to have either no or only third-trimester prenatal care (Horton 1995).

The United States and South Africa are the

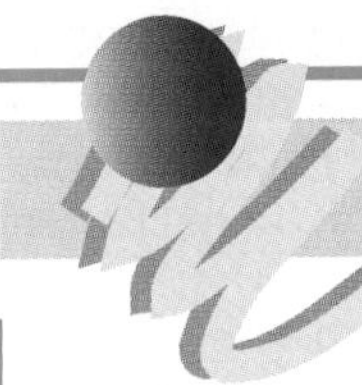

CRITICAL THINKING CASE HISTORY

SOCIAL ISSUES: HOW DOES THE REALITY OF HOMELESSNESS AFFECT THE DAILY LIFE OF A MOTHER AND HER CHILDREN?

Imagine you are a 33-year-old woman with three children. Your apartment burned down 6 months ago. You and your children have been living with your sister in her cramped apartment until she had another baby, and now there simply is not enough room for everyone.

You sleep in your car at night. During the day you walk the streets with your children, trying to find an apartment you can afford. Finally, you go to the department of social services to try to find shelter for the night, and are told that your children may have to be placed in foster care if a place cannot be found for all of you. Knowing that the foster care system in this city is unreliable and sometimes unsafe, you agree to spend the first night in an overcrowded warehouse-type shelter, where you end up sleeping on the floor.

You and your children have no privacy here. Many of the other children and adults have colds, and you hear that tuberculosis has been an increasing problem among the homeless. When the opportunity arises, you agree to move into one of the single-room occupancy hotels that the city is using to house homeless families "temporarily." That temporary shelter becomes your home for 13 months. The temporary shelter consists of one 10 × 10 foot room. You have no kitchen, refrigerator, stove, or cooking facilities. There is one bed for you and your three children.

You pull the mattress off the bed at night to make room for all of you to sleep, and then pull the sheets off the bed in the day to use as a cloth for eating on the floor. You use running water to keep your baby's milk cool, and you do the dishes in the tub where you bathe and store things.

There is no place for your children to play, no place to sit, no place to do their homework. When they try to play in the hall, they are approached by drug dealers and sometimes even pimps.

This is what life is like for you and your children. Imagine the gradual dissipation of your own and your children's self-esteem, and the isolation and depression that eventually overwhelm you. Imagine having a future without space, without privacy, without hope.

Society's Responsibility

What moral and social responsibilities does a community have for its members, particularly families with children? What kinds of support should be available for single parents, the impoverished, children in need? What constitutes a healthy and safe environment? How do we keep families together? At what point should cost be considered?

Adapted from Berne, A. S., Dato, C., Mason, D. J., Rafferty, M. (1990). A nursing model for addressing the health needs of homeless families. *Image: Journal of Nursing Scholarship,* 22 (1), 8–13. Reprinted with permission.

only industrialized nations that do not ensure the provision of a basic package of childbearing and pediatric health care services (Inglis 1991). Care is provided within a complex framework of social, financial, and health care policies (Kotch et al. 1992). For some childbearing women, particularly those who live in poverty, maternal and infant outcomes are tenuous at best, as in the case of the women described in the Critical Thinking Case History about access to health care (p. 116).

The percentage of pregnant women receiving first-trimester care has changed dramatically from the figures for 1970 to 1989 as noted by the statistics (National Center for Health Statistics 1990). Between 1970 and 1980 there was a significant trend toward increasing early prenatal care, but the trend has since leveled off. It is estimated that 14 million women of reproductive age lack medical insurance coverage for prenatal care in the United States (Richardson 1994).

Pregnant women who do not receive prenatal care are three times as likely to have a low-birth-weight infant (Kogan et al. 1995). In a study of births to urban disadvantaged black adolescent

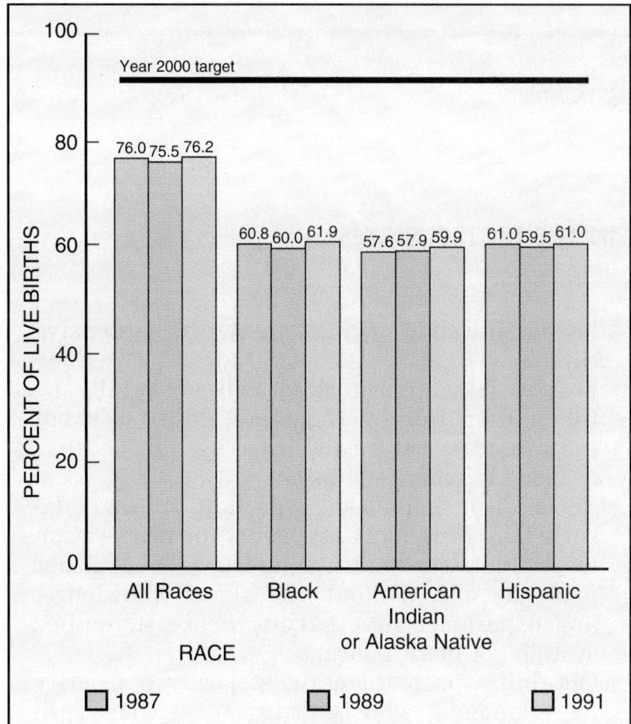

Figure 6–2

Proportion of mothers of live births who received prenatal care in the first trimester: United States, 1987–1991, and the year 2000 targets. (From National Center for Health Statistics [1994]. *Healthy people 2000 review 1993* (p. 87). Hyattsville, MD: United States Public Health Service.)

mothers, 23 percent of the newborns were of low birth weight (Scott 1988).

High correlations have been demonstrated between adequate prenatal care and positive pregnancy outcomes (Alexander and Korenbrot 1995). It is estimated that comprehensive prenatal care for all women would reduce the incidence of low birth weight nationally by 20 percent, and one in eight infant deaths could be prevented (Alexander and Korenbrot 1995).

The cost of prenatal care as compared with the cost of caring for low-birth-weight infants requiring critical care demonstrates the efficacy of providing prenatal care. Research findings indicate that for every instance of low birth weight averted by prenatal care, the health care system saves between $14,000 and $30,000 in health care costs (Alexander and Korenbrot 1995). A meta-analysis of studies on the effectiveness of the Special Supplemental Food Program for Women, Infants, and Children (WIC) shows that providing WIC benefits to pregnant women is estimated to reduce the incidence of low birth weight by 25 percent and the incidence of very low birthweight by 44 percent. Because of the estimated program cost savings, the U.S. General Accounting Office recommended that all pregnant women at or below 185 percent of the Federal poverty level be eligible for the WIC program (Avruch and Cackley 1995). Besides the financial cost, there are tremendous human costs that cannot be calculated in terms of negative emotional and physical outcomes.

There is strong research evidence that adequate prenatal care reduces low birth weight—strong enough to support a broad, national commitment to ensure that *all* pregnant women in the United States, especially those at medical or socioeconomic risk, receive high-quality prenatal care (Buekens et al. 1993; Netapoff and Wieczorek 1990).

One national public health objective of the year 2000 is to increase to at least 90 percent the proportion of all pregnant women who begin prenatal care in the first trimester (National Center for Health Statistics 1994). Low birth weight and other perinatal complications can be prevented by early and regular prenatal visits to qualified health care providers, including certified nurse midwives and nurse practitioners (Buekens et al. 1993).

Prenatal health care services can also serve as a resource and a reinforcer of health promotion efforts that are also important to positive perinatal outcomes. Preconceptional and prenatal health care services also provide education and counseling related to health-promoting behaviors such as nutrition, regular exercise, and avoidance of toxic exposure (e.g., lead and radiation); and avoidance of risk-taking behaviors related to substance use and transmission of sexually transmitted diseases, including human immunodeficiency virus (HIV) infection (Moos 1989; Stotland 1990).

BARRIERS TO ACCESS TO PRENATAL CARE

Despite recommendations that all childbearing women receive health care as well as the definitive research findings that prenatal care is logical, economical, and practical, there are many continuing barriers to care. The current system of prenatal care is based on the premise that such services are important and that all pregnant women will seek prenatal care as their "maternal responsibility" as long as it is available to them. However, although prenatal care services for the poor may be available, there may be significant barriers to the receipt of that care (Curry 1989).

Barriers to accessing prenatal care are variables that either increase the perceived costs of such care or decrease its perceived value. They include financial barriers, public policy barriers, provider barriers, and client barriers (ANA 1984; Lia-Hoagberg et al. 1990). Nonfinancial barriers are summarized in Table 6–1. When barriers to prenatal care, including bureaucratic ones, are removed, low-income women will seek care earlier and more frequently (Piper et al. 1994).

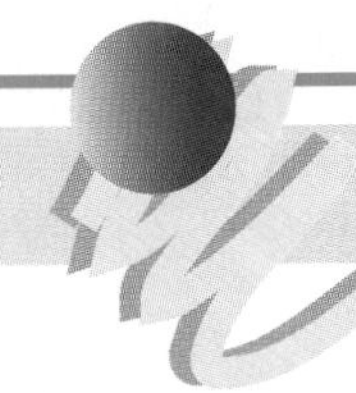

CRITICAL THINKING CASE HISTORY

SOCIAL ISSUES: ACCESS TO PRENATAL HEALTH CARE IN THE UNITED STATES DURING THE 1990S

Many citizens, health care providers, and politicians say that our health care system is broken. This assessment is based on recent statistics that show differences in health care outcomes among the various population groups: white, black, Hispanic, and Native American. Infant mortality is the most significant of these health care outcomes, and although it continues to decline, "measures of increased risk of infant death, such as incidence of low birthweight and receipt of prenatal care, show little or no recent improvement. A black infant is over twice as likely to die as a white infant, while mortality rates for Hispanic and American Indian babies is considerably higher than for white infants" (National Center for Health Statistics 1994).

Indeed, if health care is too expensive or if access is unavailable, the most sophisticated knowledge and expert clinical care in the world does little good. The National Commission on Children (1991) points out that "the neglect [caused by unavailable preventive care] is most troubling in the case of pregnant women and children, who cannot get care on their own, and for whom the lack of access to health care can lead to unnecessary illness, disability, and death, as well as unnecessary financial costs."

The following vignettes illustrate some of the circumstances faced by pregnant women in the United States:

- Twenty-five-year-old Maria, expecting her third child and having had no prenatal care, arrives in active labor at the emergency room of a charitable nonprofit Catholic hospital, knowing she will not be refused care.
- Jeanne, a 16-year-old estranged from her family, delays seeking prenatal care at a medical center clinic until the third trimester. "I just couldn't be pregnant because I'm not sick—and all pregnant women I knew were always sick," she explains. A few days later she goes into premature labor, delivering a low-birth-weight infant requiring intensive care.
- Fearful her unborn child will eventually be taken from her by the state, Julie does not try to access the health care system because of her addiction to cocaine.
- Rebecca, a homeless expectant mother deserted by her husband, comes in desperation to a midtown health clinic, swallowing her pride as one without the skills, knowledge, and experience necessary to deal with public systems of health care.
- Obtaining prenatal care is hardly a priority for Lashonda, who is facing the harsh realities of the December cold with no heat in a tiny frame house and four young children to feed and keep warm. Pregnancy is considered just another life event over which she has no control.

Questions for Discussion

- What moral and social responsibility does society or a community have to protect the health of its members, particularly pregnant women, infants, and children?
- What individual responsibility do women and families have to be informed and make sure they obtain prenatal care?
- Research shows that early prenatal care is very cost effective. How can access to early prenatal health care be made available to all pregnant women?
- What role should educational or other community institutions play in providing accurate information on health and family planning to women of childbearing age?

Data from the National Center for Health Statistics. (1994). *Healthy people 2000 review* 1993. Hyattsville, MD: U. S. Public Health Service, and the National Commission on Children. (1991). *Beyond Rhetoric A new American agenda for children and families.* Washington, D.C.: U. S. Government Printing Office.

Nursing Practice

Strategies for change are based on recommendations made by the Institute of Medicine (1985) study and the ANA Consensus Conferences on Access to Prenatal Care and Low Birth Weight (1984) (Table 6–2). Nurses may more effectively serve as advocates to actively improve the delivery

Table 6–1

NONFINANCIAL BARRIERS TO PRENATAL CARE

Public Policy

- Uncoordinated care
- Inefficient use of time and resources
- Inconvenient location and hours of service
- Inadequate outreach and follow-up programs
- Poor distribution of providers
- Inadequate support for and use of nurse practitioners and certified nurse midwives

Provider

- Negative behavioral characteristics
- Insensitivity to psychosocial and cultural aspects of care
- Inadequate awareness and use of community resources
- Poor communication between providers

Client

- Inadequate knowledge about importance of care
- Lack of incentive to seek and remain in care
- Ambivalence and denial of pregnancy
- Fear of system
- Competing life demands

of maternal-newborn care by assessing the experiences of childbearing women in relation to prenatal health care services. Attempts to meet the identified needs of childbearing women may communicate an understanding of their social environment and lifestyles, as well as professional concern for their health status (Clancy and Massion 1992).

On the basis of this assessment, the nurse should work to alter the health care delivery system. This may include outreach programs for women who are at risk for not receiving adequate prenatal care. Women perceive that nurses are caring and concerned professionals (Callister 1993, 1995). A woman's perception of caring influences the time when she registers for health care, whether she continues in prenatal care, how well she communicates with her provider, and the perinatal outcomes (Callister 1994). An example of innovative nursing care is an urban program at the Maternity Center Association in New York City. Women are triaged to appropriate levels of care in neighborhood birthing centers managed by certified nurse midwives. The cost of care is about that estimated by insurance companies for normal childbirth. In Utah the "Baby Your Baby" program provides prenatal care for women with incomes at or below the poverty level and has been credited with a significant decrease in the infant mortality rate in the state.

Nurses should support legislative initiatives, including provision of state funds for maternal and infant care programs and the expansion of Medicaid funds for pregnant women and children. Two years of consensus building by major nursing organizations produced *Nursing's Agenda for Health Care Reform* (National League of Nursing 1991), which builds on the existing health care system. The essential package of health care includes the provision of maternal-newborn services through an integration of public and private sources (Fig. 6–3). Childbearing women would be empowered by lateral relationships with their health care providers (such as certified nurse midwives) who encourage active participation in decision making, self-care measures, and personal responsibility for health and wellness (Callister 1994).

Improving access to prenatal care has important and long-range implications for improving the quality of life for children as well as for women. Since the first prenatal visit is also essentially the first pediatric visit, the health of the mother and her child are virtually inseparable. Linkages have been demonstrated between the use of health care services during pregnancy and subsequent interactions with the health care delivery system by the entire family (USDHHS 1989; Meister and Nichols 1991; Richardson 1994).

Violence Against Women and Children

Violence against women and children is a major social problem threatening physical health, as well as spiritual and emotional well-being. It is associated with chronic pain, suicide, addictive behaviors, and high-risk pregnancy (King and Ryan 1989; Plichta 1992). Physical abuse accounts for the greatest portion of abuse, followed by emotional and then sexual abuse. Violence within the family, such as fetal abuse, child abuse, and spousal abuse, are increasingly recognized as an important community health problem (National Center for Health Statistics 1992). Fetal abuse is associated with perinatal substance use and is discussed later in this chapter.

BATTERED WOMEN

The battering and abuse of women is a serious and life-threatening problem that adversely affects

Table 6–2

STRATEGIES TO OVERCOME NONFINANCIAL BARRIERS TO PRENATAL CARE

BARRIERS	STRATEGIES
Systems barriers	Coordinated care Convenient place and time Reduced waiting time Prompt initial scheduling Uniform eligibility system System stress reduction Provider incentives Social support and community services Client involvement in care Free and confidential pregnancy tests Outreach and follow-up Transportation and child care assistance Group programs Low birth weight and access to care research funding Study of what constitutes adequate prenatal care Quality assurance
Provider barriers	Improved provider attitudes and communication skills Realistic patient loads Prevention and reduction of stress and burnout Failure to use certified nurse midwives and nurse practitioners Equitable distribution of providers
Client barriers	Promotion of early prenatal care Retention in prenatal care with a primary care provider or case manager (continuity of care) Meeting competing survival needs
Policy barriers	Extension of Medicaid coverage to all pregnant women and infants at or below 200 percent of poverty level Adequate reimbursement system Malpractice and professional liability reform Family life education Marketing of contraceptive services Increased funding for maternal and child health block grants, community and migrant health center programs, Women-Infant-Children (WIC) Supplemental Food Program, federal Family Planning Program (Title X), and National Service Corporations

the lives and health of an estimated 2 to 4 million women each year. More than 1 million women seek medical assistance for injuries related to battering incidents every year (Campbell and Oliver 1993).

Extreme isolation may characterize battering victims. A significant number of battered women were themselves abused as children or were witnesses to abuse. The woman who is being battered may fear greater physical danger to herself and her children if she attempts to leave and may maintain the abusive relationship conceptualized as "traumatic bonding" (Benton 1986).

Some myths about battering are (1) that battering is more common in lower socioeconomic groups; (2) that battered women must enjoy abuse (otherwise they would take the children and leave); and (3) that battered women provoke men by pushing them beyond the breaking point, thereby inciting physical violence. Other myths are that substance abuse causes battering and that battered women can easily leave the situation (ACOG 1989; King and Ryan 1989). The reasons why a battered woman stays in the relationship are based on multiple, complex, and highly varied factors. An abused woman may feel inhibited by economic, social, and emotional factors. Victimization of the battered woman may be economic in nature, since many lack job skills or may be unemployed. In addition, cultural attitudes toward

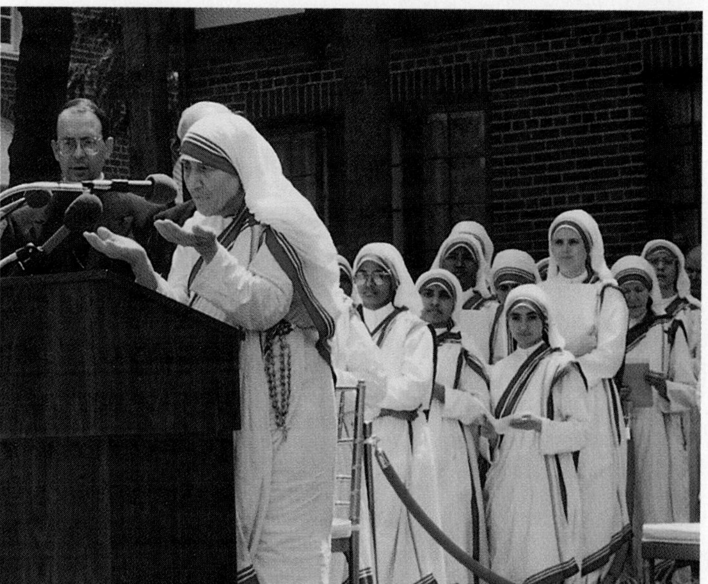

Figure 6–3
Adequate maternal-newborn care for all women can only become possible through the joint efforts of public and private agencies • Mother Teresa dedicates the "Mother Teresa Home for Infants" in Washington, D.C., a home for pregnant women and homeless babies, in June 1995. (Courtesy of Mary Lee O'Connell.)

gender roles affects a woman's self-image (Slaght et al. 1996; Stenchever and Stenchever 1991).

Abused women may present with physical symptoms such as headaches; sleep disorders; choking sensations; hyperventilation; gastrointestinal symptoms; chest, back, or pelvic pain; and physical injuries. Emotional symptoms may include shyness, fright, embarrassment, evasiveness, jumpiness, passivity, frequent crying, and substance use (including drug overdose) (Lichtman and Papera 1990). The physical and emotional sequelae associated with battering often fit the profile of a person suffering from posttraumatic stress disorder.

Carrying an unborn child does not provide immunity against violence. It is estimated that abuse occurs in at least one out of ten women beginning in or escalating during pregnancy (King and Ryan 1989). It may result in pregnancy loss, preterm labor, low-birth-weight infants, fetal injury, and fetal death (Bohn 1990; Campbell and Oliver 1993; McFarlane 1993). A woman who was 6 months pregnant described a battering incident: "He yelled at me to prepare dinner. He ate one bite then threw the plate on the floor. He grabbed me, threatened me with a knife then punched me in the stomach. He said if I told anyone, he would kill me" (McFarlane 1989, p. 69).

Nursing Practice

Violence against women is of special concern to nurses because it can lead to serious injury or death. Battered women and their children may suffer long-term emotional effects and continue the multigenerational cycle of abuse (King and Ryan 1989). Nursing interventions should focus on (1) prevention; (2) treatment of acute physical injuries; (3) counseling regarding available options, including leaving the violent situation; and (4) helping women to obtain long-term help (McBride 1990).

Prevention includes community education programs providing information on battering, the cycle of violence, and the effects of battering on women, children, men, and society (Lichtman and Papera 1990). Nurses can identify women at risk for battering through use of questions that assess abuse, and provide counseling to prevent violence from occurring (see Identifying the Abused Woman).

Battering should be carefully documented to provide legal evidence of violence. Nurses should assist battered women in accessing resources for emergency care in shelters such as women's crisis centers, which are available in many communities, and provide ongoing support such as counseling and peer support groups. The Domestic Violence Hotline (1-800-333-5723) provides women with information about available community resources, including legal rights and resources. Nurses should encourage the empowerment of women rather than emphasizing pathology and victimization (Stenchever and Stenchever 1991; King et al. 1993). Recent federal legislation is the Violence Against Women Act, which provides assistance for victims of sexual assault and domestic violence, as well as resources for prevention and public education, rape crisis centers, and battered women's shelters.

RAPE

Rape is defined as a nonconsensual sexual act, including the use of physical force, intimidation, deception, or threat; nonconsent of the victim; and

Identifying the Abused Woman

- Do you feel emotionally abused by your partner?
- Has your partner ever hit, slapped, kicked, or otherwise physically hurt you?
- Are you afraid of your partner?
- Do you feel your partner tries to control you?
- Has your partner ever forced you into sex in which you did not wish to participate?

From King, M. C., Campbell, D., Ryan, J., Sheridan, D., Ulrich, Y., McKenna, L. S. (1993). Violence and abuse of women: A perinatal health care issue. *AWHONN's Clinical Issues in Perinatal and Women's Health Nursing,* 4 (2), 163–172. Reprinted with permission from the Association of Women's Health, Obstetric and Neonatal Nurses.

coitus or vaginal penetration. One perpetuated myth is that women provoke rape. The reality is that a woman can be abused sexually anywhere, anytime, regardless of her physical characteristics. Often, rape is not perceived as rape by the legal system or social services agencies when the perpetrator is the victim's spouse, if there has been a previous sexual relationship, if the victim is a prostitute, if the victim is drunk, or if the rape occurred during conditions of war.

Three phases of the rape experience have been identified: the acute phase, the outward adjustment phase, and the reorganization phase. The acute phase is characterized by fear, shock, disbelief, desire for revenge, anger, denial, anxiety, guilt, embarrassment, humiliation, helplessness, and dependency. The woman may seek help, or in many instances the rape may go unreported. In the outward adjustment phase the victim may appear outwardly composed, denying and repressing her feelings. During the reorganizational phase the victim may experience sexual dysfunction, fears, sleep disorders, anxiety, and a strong urge to talk about and/or resolve her feelings (Atkeson et al. 1989).

Nursing Practice

In the acute phase the woman may present at medical center emergency rooms, rape crisis centers, women's resource centers, or health care providers' offices. The woman may respond to this devastating personal crisis in different ways. She may openly express fear, anger, or anxiety or she may appear calm, subdued, stoic, or composed. Some women may even laugh or smile as a defense mechanism. Whatever the woman's response, she requires nonjudgmental support, respect, privacy, and physical care. Perhaps the most important nursing intervention is empathy, encouraging the woman to talk about her feelings about the rape and helping her to regain a sense of control of her life (Atkeson et al. 1989). Guidelines for counseling the rape victim are summarized in Table 6–3.

Data collection should include a thorough history and physical assessment by the nurse. Physical evidence should be collected, documented, and preserved, including clothing; swabs of oral, vaginal, rectal, and body stains; scrapings from under fingernails; combings of pubic hair; and photographs. Sexually transmitted disease testing and prevention, as well as pregnancy testing and counseling, should be performed. It is estimated that 1 to 5 percent of sexual assault victims become pregnant. Two tablets of Ovral (ethinyl estradiol and norgestrel) can be administered within 72 hours after unprotected coitus and repeated 12 hours later to prevent pregnancy (Hampton 1995; Ledray and Arndt 1994).

Written aftercare instructions and information on community resources should be provided. Rape

Table 6–3

COUNSELING THE RAPE VICTIM

1. Initiate a supportive relationship. Reassure the victim about her safety and personal integrity. Listen with empathy and communicate an understanding of her pain.
2. Identify the victim's major concerns (psychological, medical, legal) and her perception of the help she needs.
3. Educate about health care, legal issues, and police investigation.
4. Encourage the victim to use social supports available to her. Offer to call or meet with friends or family.
5. Educate about feelings and responses to be anticipated and counseling services available.
6. Explore and support existing coping skills.
7. Plan with the victim for safety (e.g., alternative shelter) and support needs, for health care and counseling services, and for nurse advocacy availability.

Data from Ledray, L. (1990). Counseling rape victims: The nursing challenge. *Perspectives in Psychiatric Care,* 26 (2), 21–27.

crisis centers often serve the needs of sexual assault victims by providing escort services, information, and long-term counseling.

The woman who has been raped may have recurring thoughts about the assault. She may have difficulty falling asleep or may experience early-morning awakenings or recurrent dreams. Some women report a sense of numbness, with a lack of interest in life and daily activities. Other women feel jumpy and easily startled. There may be feelings of guilt, that she should or could have done something to prevent the attack or deter the attacker, or that she may somehow have been responsible for the assault. The woman should be given information about the signs and symptoms of posttraumatic stress disorder and depression, which may occur weeks or months after the rape (Stenchever and Stenchever 1991).

Although they represent a serious violent crime with significant trauma for the victimized woman, most sexual assaults are unreported. Major life disruptions can be prevented, and satisfactory resolution of the crisis of rape facilitated, if rape victims are identified and interventions begun to promote the best possible outcome. By gaining an understanding and awareness of the scope and impact of rape, nurses can better identify victims and prevent unnecessary trauma by providing appropriate care to these women and their families at critical stages in the rape crisis (Golding 1996).

CHILD ABUSE

Child abuse may involve physical abuse or neglect, emotional abuse, or sexual abuse. These categories are not mutually exclusive, and all of them are devastating to the child's well-being (Newman and Buka 1991). The true incidence of child abuse and maltreatment is unknown and frequently unreported, but it is estimated that 23 of every 1000 children yearly are reported victims of child abuse (Devlin and Reynolds 1994). Although the cause is unknown, there are three indicators related to predispositions for child abuse; these are summarized in Table 6–4.

Child abuse and maltreatment is said to have occurred if the child has

- Suffered physical harm, either inflicted by the person responsible for the child or caused by that person's failure to adequately care for, provide for, supervise, or protect that child
- Been sexually molested or sexually exploited by the person responsible for the child, or by another individual
- Needed health care to prevent or alleviate physical harm or suffering because the person responsible for the child does not provide or consent to treatment
- Suffered emotional harm, demonstrated by severe anxiety, depression, or withdrawal or severe self-destructive or aggressive behavior, and if the person responsible for the child does not provide services or treatment to remedy or alleviate the harm, refuses to provide such services or treatment, or is unavailable to consent for care
- A mental, emotional, or developmental condition that, if not remedied, could seriously impair the child's development, and if the person responsible for the child does not provide or consent to treatment to alleviate the condition (Thomas 1983)

Nursing Practice

Since child abuse is an emotionally loaded issue, it is important for nurses to clarify their personal values and attitudes toward the abused and the abuser. In assessing the child, a knowledge base about normal physical, social, emotional, and cognitive development of children is essential to effectively assess the child as well as the family unit. It is important to document physical injuries, behavioral-developmental symptoms, observations of parent-child interactions, and the history of the injury or complaint. Since treatment of the effects of child abuse is complex and often long term, the nurse should maintain a nonjudgmental approach to ensure that the family seeks therapy. The nurse can assist the family to access community resources, including health and social services agencies.

CHILDHOOD SEXUAL ABUSE

Sexual abuse is one of the most damaging kinds of abuse. It has been defined in the Child Abuse and Prevention Act (Public Law 100-294) as "the use, persuasion, or coercion of any child to engage in sexually explicit conduct (or any simulation of such conduct) for producing any visual depiction of such conduct, or rape, molestation, prostitution, or incest with children". Conservative estimates are that one in three women and one in ten men are childhood sexual abuse victims (Becker and Coleman 1990).

Incest is sexual activity that occurs between family members who are not spouses. Risk factors related to families at risk for incest have been identified (Lesniak 1993). Incest represents the betrayal of trust that should exist between family members, which increases the devastation experienced by the child. One survivor of childhood sexual abuse wept as she poignantly reflected on the terror of her experience as a 4-year-old girl, "Mommy's gone and there's no place in the house to hide from Daddy." Incest often results in shame and guilt when the needs of the perpetrator are met through sexual molestation of an innocent child (Peterson 1991; Ridley 1993).

Table 6–4

INDICATORS OF HIGH-RISK FAMILIES FOR CHILD ABUSE

Prenatal Indicators

- Unplanned or unwanted pregnancy
- Short interpregnancy interval
- Denial or depression related to pregnancy
- Desire to either abort pregnancy or relinquish baby
- Women who have marked concerns about body changes (body image concerns)
- Adolescent or single mothers
- Mother does not seek prenatal care or follow health care recommendations
- Parents overconcerned about sex of fetus
- Parents with unrealistic expectations of infant or parenting
- Parents who make no or few preparations for infant
- Parents who have poor social network or who are isolated (physically and emotionally)

Perinatal Indicators

- Pregnancy or birth complications
- Separation of mother and infant for health reasons after birth
- Parents who avoid touching or looking at infant
- Parents who voice disappointment over sex or appearance of infant
- Lack of mutual support by parents
- Sick or deformed infant requiring long-term care
- Parents who do not visit neonatal intensive care unit or inquire about infant's condition
- Parents who are very irritated by infant's crying and make little or no attempt to comfort infant
- Parents with limited parenting skills and knowledge

Neonatal Indicators

- Preterm infant
- Infant with congenital anomalies
- Infant with physical or developmental problems
- Parents who have unreal expectation of infant
- Parents who believe baby is too demanding
- Parents who become unduly tense and irritable when caring for infant
- Parents who are unduly anxious about minor health problems
- Father jealous of time mother spends with infant
- Parents who change health care providers and agencies frequently
- Parents whose focus is on themselves versus infant
- Parents who are unable to identify any support system during times of stress

Times of Crisis

- Lifestyle changes such as marital separation or moving, or loss of support systems
- Sudden unemployment or other family financial difficulties
- Death of spouse
- Diagnosis of serious illness in family or extended family members
- Very ill infant or child
- Birth of another child within short interpregnancy interval
- Parental substance abuse
- Multiple stressors

A victim of childhood sexual abuse may manifest symptoms of depression, anger, and low self-esteem; feelings of worthlessness; a poor sense of his or her right to set limits; a sense of abandonment and inability to trust; social isolation; and suicidal tendencies (Hau et al. 1993; Holz 1994). The individual may experience a sense of confusion between expressions of love, affection, and nurturance and sexual relations, power, and issues of control. Posttraumatic stress syndrome (PTSS), frequently seen in women who have been victims of childhood sexual abuse, is repressed horror that the mind brings to consciousness through flashbacks and nightmares. This syndrome may begin to occur when triggered by a life event such as childbirth or when the psyche feels "safe," which in many instances may be decades after the abuse has occurred (Loftus et al. 1994; Blume 1989; Horton et al. 1993).

Women may present with vague physical complaints such as abdominal pain for which no definitive diagnosis may be made, have an aversion to a male caregiver, or have difficulty submitting to a pelvic examination or having sexual intercourse. They may manifest symptoms of depression that seem largely unexplained (Forest et al. 1996). Flashbacks may be precipitated by the intensity of the childbirth experience itself, or by having a child the same age as they were when the abuse occurred (Rhodes and Hutchinson 1994; Rose 1992). In all such instances, childhood sexual abuse should be explored as a possible cause.

Nursing Practice

Nursing practice focuses on the prevention and treatment of childhood sexual abuse. In terms of prevention, nurses can assist parents in cultivating open communication in the home, encouraging them to use the word "secret" very carefully. Children should be taught that no one should touch them in certain ways or on certain parts of their bodies, and that it is appropriate to say no, even to an adult authority figure. They should be encouraged to trust and communicate their feelings. Books are available for children that describe sexual abuse and its prevention, such as *A Very Touching Book* (Hindman) and *Private Zone* (Dayee) for young children, and *Sexual Abuse: Let's Talk About It* (Hyde) for children 10 years of age and older.

In the treatment of childhood sexual abuse, nurses, particularly those working in community settings, should identify the abuse by careful attention to indications of such activity occurring. It should be reported immediately to child protective services, and the child should be protected from further abuse. The best interests of the child should be foremost, emotional support being essential. Appropriate referrals should be made for individual and family therapy, which should be characterized by ongoing communication between providers (Gil 1992; Hooper 1992).

There are important implications for nurses working with women across the lifespan. The nurse should become educated about the long-term effects of childhood sexual abuse. In communication with the adult survivor of childhood sexual abuse, the survivor's feelings of anger and pain should be validated through empathetic listening and genuine expressions of concern. The nurse should clearly convey the sense that the survivor was not responsible for the abuse. The nurse should respect the time and space it takes to heal and encourage the survivor to get professional counseling, particularly essential if he or she is suicidal (Bass and Davis 1993; Holz 1994).

The adult female survivor of childhood sexual abuse should be seen not as a victim but as a strong, courageous woman who is reclaiming her own life by overcoming the effects of her trauma:

> *She is a "survivor" because a "victim" is characterized by passive helplessness and is seen with pity. But in survivors of the Holocaust, prisoner of war camps, or natural disasters, as well as incest, there is strength, dignity, resilience, and entitlement of respect . . . She can go beyond surviving and work for the quality of life she deserves (Lichtman and Papera 1990, p. 96).*

Perinatal Substance Abuse

Substance abuse is the use of any mind-altering agent in such a way that it interferes with the individual's abilities to function, either physiologically, emotionally, or socioculturally (Sullivan et al. 1993). While there is growing concern about substance abuse, little is known about factors that produce or cause chemical dependency in women, what causes women to seek help, or what treatment is most effective. Women's experiences with substance abuse differ from men's, and thus assumptions about substance abuse in men cannot necessarily be made about women, and treatment programs effective for men may be ineffective for women. Research findings from studies with samples that are only male or white may have limited applicability to women, particularly childbearing women (Hughes 1990). Theories that attempt to explain substance use include the genetic and biologic model, the abusing patterns, psychological theories, family theory, social psychologic models, and interactive models (Naegle 1988).

In substance abuse among women, biologic and psychosocial antecedents interact in a complex fashion. Wilsnack and Beckman (1984) postulate that differences exist in both causes and consequences in a cross section of substance-abusing women. They feel that social factors contribute in significant ways, including gender-specific behavior of partners and characteristics of substance abuse treatment programs.

Substance abuse by women may be influenced by the social context of their lives, which is characterized by complex and conflicting role expectations to meet seemingly impossible demands achieved only by a superwoman: homemaker, caretaker, nurturer, professional, wage earner, wife, mother, daughter. Paradoxically, the societal belief still exists that women are dependent on men and less able to cope with the complex and harsh realities of life.

Patterns of substance abuse were examined in a study that included 1176 women who were in substance abuse treatment programs. Women over 30 years of age showed a strong preference for alcohol; they were often solitary, daily drinkers, and 25 percent also used prescribed tranquilizers. Women in the younger age group were four to six times as likely to have used marijuana, cocaine and other stimulants, and hallucinogens (Hughes and Fox 1993).

For a variety of reasons, the effects of maternal substance use on perinatal outcomes have not been fully explored (Free et al. 1990). There are ethical issues related to maternal-fetal research. Substance abuse during pregnancy is often unreported or underreported, since denial of substance abuse or its consequences is common. Polydrug or concomitant substance abuse also confounds conclusions on the effects of a single substance. Illicit drugs may be contaminated, containing impurities such as lead oxide and cyanide, which also may be teratogenic. It is also difficult to separate the effects of substance use from other social issues, including inadequate prenatal care, low socioeconomic status, or less than ideal maternal health and nutrition. It has been documented that low birth weight and preterm births are the most serious known consequences of maternal illicit drug use (National Center for Health Statistics 1994). More research is needed on long-term outcomes in substance-using mothers and their neonates.

Risks due to maternal substance use are heightened by lack of prenatal care. It is estimated that 75 percent of pregnant women who are substance dependent do not seek prenatal care until the onset of labor (Keith et al. 1988). Reliable data on the prevalence of substance use in childbearing women are difficult to obtain, but it is estimated to be as much as 20 percent (Chasnoff 1989). In 1988, 425,000 infants were estimated to be exposed to harmful substances, with a cost of $63,000 for treatment of each drug-affected neonate (National Center for Health Statistics 1992).

A 1994 study, the National Pregnancy and Health Survey, sponsored by the National Institute on Drug Abuse (NIDA), National Institutes of Health, provides the first nationally representative data on drug use during pregnancy. The findings of the study indicate that substance abuse during pregnancy is widespread and that one in four babies born each year has been exposed to harmful legal or illegal drugs. The findings are as follows:

- 5.5 percent of pregnant women used an illegal drug, primarily marijuana or cocaine
- 18.8 percent of pregnant women used alcohol
- 32 percent of pregnant women smoked cigarettes
- 32 percent of those women who reported the use of one drug also used alcohol and smoked cigarettes
- In general, the rate of drug use declined during pregnancy, but there was no total discontinuation of drug use
- Illegal drug use was higher in women who were not married, had less than 16 years of formal education, were not working, and relied on some public source of funding to pay their childbirth hospital stay
- Illegal drug use by women who did not use alcohol or smoke cigarettes was very low; 0.2 percent used marijuana and 0.1 percent used cocaine
- African-American women had a higher rate of cocaine use (4.5%) than white women (0.4%) or Hispanic women (0.7%)
- White women had the highest rate of alcohol use (22.7%), compared with 15.8 percent among African-American women and 8.7 percent among Hispanic women

Another serious concern is the transmission of the HIV virus to the fetus. Infected childbearing women are frequently intravenous drug users or partners of men who are bisexual or intravenous drug users. The infection can be contracted through contaminated drug paraphernalia or sexual intercourse. Between 1978 and 1993 in the United States, approximately 14,920 infants born to HIV-infected women acquired HIV infection (Davis et al. 1995).

ALCOHOL

Alcohol consumption during pregnancy is associated with increased risk for fetal alcohol syndrome or fetal alcohol effects, such as (1) central nervous system dysfunction, including mental retardation; (2) facial malformations; (3) growth deficiency; and (4) hepatic and renal abnormalities. A safe level of alcohol consumption during pregnancy has not been established, but most adverse effects are associated with consumption during the early months of pregnancy (National Center for Health Statistics 1994). It is estimated that 40,000 babies yearly are born with fetal alcohol syndrome resulting from maternal perinatal consumption of alcohol (Newman and Buka 1991).

ILLICIT DRUGS

Commonly used illicit "street" drugs include heroin, marijuana, and cocaine. Heroin use is associated with intrauterine growth retardation, respiratory depression, decreased mental and neurologic abilities, neonatal withdrawal syndrome, and neonatal death (Lee and Chiang 1985). The use of methadone for heroin withdrawal is controversial since it crosses the placenta and its usage is associated with pregnancy-induced hypertension, hepatitis, fetal distress, and neonatal withdrawal syndrome (Hans 1989). However, "cold turkey" withdrawal during pregnancy is not recommended because of potential adverse effects on the fetus.

Marijuana usage is estimated to be as high as 37 percent in childbearing women and is associated with low birth weight, intrauterine growth retardation, and preterm labor. The major ingredient in marijuana, THC (tetrahydrocannabinol), crosses the placenta, and the concentration of THC in breast milk has been found to be higher than in the mother's plasma (Lee and Chiang 1985). Therefore, it is recommended that mothers using marijuana do not breastfeed their infants.

Cocaine use brings social problems, including family dysfunction, employment problems, financial difficulties, emotional stress, guilt, and anger. Compounding the problem is the frequent concurrent use of a central nervous system depressant such as alcohol to mediate the side effects of cocaine (Landry and Smith 1987).

When cocaine is ingested by the expectant mother, it remains in the body longer than in a normal adult because of a decreased ability to metabolize the drug, contributing to more detrimental effects for the childbearing woman and her fetus (Peters and Theorell 1991).

Research in recent years has identified the following effects of cocaine:

- Teratogenic effects, including fetal skull abnormalities and genitourinary malformations
- Increased uterine contractibility, fetal activity, increased incidence of spontaneous abortions, premature labor, precipitous labor, and abruptio placentae
- Low-birth-weight infants, small-for-gestational-age infants, shorter lengths, smaller head circumferences, and prune-belly syndrome
- Classic neonatal drug withdrawal (neurologic and physiologic alterations, including depressed interactive abilities and impaired organizational ability, orientation, and state control)
- Increased incidence of sudden infant death syndrome (SIDS) (Hadeed and Siefel 1989; Lynch and McKeon 1990)

Cocaine exposure can also occur in neonates after childbirth, because it is highly lipid soluble and remains in breast milk for as long as 36 hours after maternal cocaine use (Lynch and McKeon 1990).

PRESCRIPTION MEDICATIONS

More than 200 million prescriptions are written annually for tranquilizers, analgesics, barbiturates, and amphetamines. Most of these are for women (Vener et al. 1982), which may be related to the fact the women seek health care for symptoms more readily and express their feelings more openly than men. Consequently health care providers may be more likely to prescribe medication to women (Fogel and Woods 1995). Problems associated with prescription drug abuse include addiction, concomitant or polydrug use, and teratogenic effects. Prescription medications frequently abused include barbiturates (sedatives such as Amytal Sodium, Tuinal, Nembutal, Luminal Sodium), amphetamines (stimulants such as Benzedrine, Methedrine, Dexedrine), and tranquilizers (benzodiazepines such as Valium, Librium, Serax, Ativan).

OVER-THE-COUNTER MEDICATIONS

A high proportion of women use over-the-counter medications, including vitamins, analgesics, antacids, laxatives, and sleep-promoting medications. Women are often unaware of the properties of ingredients in such medications. For example, Midol, a popular drug for the relief of menstrual symptoms, contains the muscle relaxant cinnamedrine. Combining over-the-counter medications with prescription drugs and alcohol can be dangerous, particularly for childbearing women. Any childbearing woman or woman using oral contraceptives should be encouraged to discuss the use of over-the-counter medications with her health care provider (Vener et al. 1982).

CAFFEINE

Caffeine is a stimulant affecting many parts of the nervous system; however, most women consider caffeine harmless. It is found in soft drinks, cocoa and chocolate, and over-the-counter medications such as NoDoz, Excedrin, and Anacin. Women concerned with weight maintenance or loss often consume excessive quantities of coffee, tea, and diet soft drinks. Caffeine is physically addictive, a central nervous system stimulant that may be associated with maternal irritability, anxiety, and insomnia (Campinha-Bacote and Bragg 1993). Withdrawal symptoms include severe headache, drowsiness, inability to concentrate, lethargy, irritability, and depression (Cunningham et al. 1993). There is no evidence that caffeine increases reproductive or teratogenic risks in childbearing women (Cunningham et al. 1993).

TOBACCO

It is estimated that 25 percent of childbearing women smoke throughout their pregnancies (Schoenborn 1988). Maternal cigarette smoking has been linked with 20 to 30 percent of all low-birth-weight births in the United States (Chomitz et al. 1995). The adverse effects of smoking are due to carbon dioxide, which reduces the amount of oxygen delivered to the fetus by inactivating fetal and maternal hemoglobin. The vasoconstrictive action of nicotine also reduces placental perfusion. There may be a reduction in caloric intake due to decreased maternal appetite related to smoking (Kleinman and Kopstein 1987).

One *Healthy People 2000* public health objective is the reduction in the number of childbearing women who smoke from 25 to 10 percent. It is estimated that if all pregnant women refrained from smoking, fetal and infant deaths would be reduced by 10 percent, saving the lives of about 4000 infants per year (National Center for Health Statistics 1994).

FETAL ABUSE

Substance abuse during pregnancy raises difficult ethical and legal questions (Macklin 1990). How can a safe intrauterine environment be provided for the fetus while at the same time demonstrating respect for the mother's right for privacy, personal freedom, and bodily integrity? Is legal intervention appropriate to safeguard the fetus? Do maternal substance abuse, poor nutrition, refusal of health care, and an unhealthy lifestyle during pregnancy require legal intervention? Under what circumstances should a newborn be sent home with a mother who is a known substance abuser?

Although parents have a constitutional right to the custody and care of their children, this right is limited in cases of abuse or neglect, according to the U.S. Supreme Court. "Parens patriae" or "state as a parent" describes action taken to protect the fetus (Rhodes 1990). Court cases in Illinois illustrate that the recent judicial trend has been to protect the neonate and hold the mother accountable for her substance abuse. In one instance a mother who tested positive for cocaine in her system had a newborn who died 2 days after birth. An autopsy showed that the newborn's death was caused by oxygen deprivation before birth because of maternal cocaine use. The mother was charged with involuntary manslaughter and delivery of a controlled substance to a minor. In another case the juvenile court judge found a mother who used cocaine during her pregnancy guilty of child abuse and neglect, and the infant was temporarily removed from the mother's custody.

While these judicial cases uphold fetal and neonatal rights, the rights of the mother to make decisions about her fetus have been upheld in other cases. These issues are current, emotionally charged, and subject to review on an individual case-by-case basis (Chavkin 1990; Rhodes 1990).

Nursing Practice

Many ethical and legal issues need to be addressed when dealing with the childbearing substance user. The question whether substance use is a health problem or willful criminal behavior is a significant policy issue. There is a growing trend to report fetal exposure to harmful substances to social service agencies. Some women in the United States who exposed their fetuses to harmful substances have been arrested, criminally prosecuted, and incarcerated rather than receiving treatment for their addiction. While the cost of treatment is great, the costs of prosecuting these women and caring for substance-dependent children is bound to be socially and economically higher.

The negative consequences of substance use during pregnancy should be identified through communication and education, targeting women of childbearing age. Women should be encouraged to exercise caution in relation to use of harmful substances during pregnancy and to seek treatment for addictive behaviors (Blume et al. 1993). Because of the high incidence of cocaine use, it may be helpful to display the hot-line number, 1-800-COCAINE, in the waiting room of health care providers offices and on other community bulletin boards.

All childbearing women should be screened for substance use, including the type and amount of substances used, the duration of use and most recent use, the usual symptoms of withdrawal, current physiologic and psychological status, previous treatment, negative consequences, and motivating factors. Physical appearance and demeanor, along with health and obstetric histories, can help identify the substance-using woman (see Identifying the Substance User).

A nonjudgmental attitude by the nurse is very important, and it is suggested that the nurse "view her as a woman who is pregnant and currently using or abusing drugs" rather than a substance-abusing pregnant woman (Campinha-Bacote and Bragg 1993, p. 26; Sullivan et al. 1993).

Treatment for substance use should include stabilizing the physiologic status and treating the

Identifying the Substance User

PHYSICAL APPEARANCE AND DEMEANOR

- Looks physically exhausted
- Pupils are extremely dilated or constricted
- Appearance of pregnancy fails to coincide with stated gestational age
- Track marks, abscesses, or edema are visible in extremities
- Nasal mucosae are inflamed or indurated
- Is not well oriented

HEALTH HISTORY

- Acquired immunodeficiency syndrome
- Cellulitis
- Cirrhosis
- Endocarditis
- Hepatitis
- Pancreatitis
- Pneumonia

OBSTETRIC HISTORY IN PREVIOUS PREGNANCIES

- Abruptio placentae
- Fetal death
- Low-birth-weight infant
- Meconium staining
- Preterm labor
- Premature rupture of membranes
- Sexually transmitted diseases
- Spontaneous abortion

OBSTETRIC HISTORY IN CURRENT PREGNANCY

- Early contractions
- Inactive or hyperactive fetus
- Poor weight gain
- Sexually transmitted diseases
- Spotting or vaginal bleeding

From Chasnoff, I. J. (1989). Drug use and women: Establishing a standard of care. *Annals of the New York Academy of Sciences,* 562, 208. Reprinted with permission.

woman for intoxication or withdrawal symptoms, malnutrition, dehydration, infections, and injuries. Other interventions may include support groups, education, personal and family counseling, and transitional living programs, to assist both mother and child to develop their full potential (Chomitz et al. 1995). An example is Hawaii's Baby SAFE (Substance Abuse Free Environment), which is making important differences for women and their infants who are exposed to drugs (Starn et al. 1993).

Research is needed to document women's experience with substance use and chemical dependency and which behaviors contribute to their seeking treatment (Hughes and Fox 1993). Treatment models specifically for women should be developed and their effectiveness evaluated. Research on substance use in ethnic minorities is needed, as well as in other areas such as lesbians, elderly women, and women in specific occupations. For example, health professionals such as female physicians and nurses seem especially vulnerable to substance use. Research interest in substance use by women is increasing. In 1984, women were added as a priority population for the Alcohol, Drug Abuse, and Mental Health Administration. In 1987, only 13.5 percent of the budget for the National Institutes of Health (NIH) was spent on research related to women's health. In response to growing criticism, NIH recently developed the Office of Research on Women's Health, which will monitor research efforts at the NIH in an effort to further the prevention, diagnosis, and treatment of women's health problems. It is hoped that this initiative will narrow the knowledge gap related to research on substance use in women (Hughes 1990).

EMPLOYMENT CONCERNS OF CHILDBEARING WOMEN

Over 63 percent of women are employed outside the home either full or part time. This may be related to the rising educational level of women (who now constitute 50 percent of the student body in colleges and universities), which has led to improved job opportunities. In addition, the women's movement has heightened awareness of alternatives for women. In recent years, women have entered employment considered exclusively the domain of men. Economic constraints have also contributed to women working outside the home.

Maternal Employment

In 1977, 32 percent of women with a child under 1 year of age worked outside the home compared with 10 years later when most women with infants (52 percent) were in the labor force (USDL, WB 1989). By 1990, 70 percent of women with school-age children worked outside the home (Tager 1990).

Despite the growing numbers of women in the workplace, there has been no significant improvement in the earnings gap between men and women. Women of color account for a disproportionate share of the women in low-status, low-paying occupational categories and are plagued by higher unemployment rates (USDL, WB 1989; Aburdene and Naisbitt 1992).

Maternal Employment During Pregnancy

Maternal employment during pregnancy may be viewed from two different perspectives: the *role stress perspective,* whose premise is that work is a source of stress because of role overload and conflict between competing demands of multiple roles; and the *health benefits perspective,* whose premise is that work is beneficial to maternal well-being because it offers social support, information, and personal gratification (Killien 1990).

A number of studies have demonstrated that as a mother's satisfaction with her role increases, so does her effectiveness as a parent. Decisions regarding maternal employment can be evaluated only when they reflect an individual woman's underlying values and wishes. Ideally, the mother would have a 4-month leave, then work part time until the infant is 6 months old. Reality may differ greatly from this ideal. First-time mothers should be encouraged to maintain an open mind about combining work and motherhood in light of changing life circumstances.

The number of women working during pregnancy, and especially through its last months, has increased dramatically. There are conflicting studies on the affects of occupational activity during pregnancy. In general, studies comparing pregnant with nonpregnant women have not found occupational activity to be a risk factor. However, studies have shown that preterm birth was more likely in pregnant women employed in situations that involved strenuous work, prolonged standing, and long hours (Luke et al. 1995). These authors recommended three measures to reduce the incidence of preterm birth associated with occupational activity: reducing the number of hours worked per day and per week, changing to a less strenuous work area during pregnancy, and granting work leave for pregnant women with complications.

Role stress is part of the dilemma encountered by employed mothers. This includes *role overload,* or confrontation with excessive demands; *role conflict,* when there are contradictory role expectations or expectations that are mutually exclusive; *role ambiguity,* a condition in which norms for position are vague or ill defined; and *role incongruity,* a condition in which role expectations counter self-perception, attitudes, or values. Role strain may be related to conflicts between personal needs and career and family obligations. In addition, strain may be due to childbearing problems associated with maternal fatigue and guilt, concerns about adequacy of role performance, strains related to insufficient time to fulfill home and work responsibilities, and a sense of emotional depletion (Brown 1987; McBride 1988).

Maternity Leave

The Pregnancy Discrimination Act has been added to Title VII of the Civil Rights Act to prohibit discrimination on the basis of pregnancy, childbirth, or related conditions. According to this act, childbearing women must be treated in the same manner as other applicants and employees who are not pregnant but who are similarly able or unable to work. This legislation can be summarized as follows:

- *Hiring.* An employer cannot refuse to hire a woman because of her pregnancy-related condition as long as she is able to perform the major functions necessary for the job.
- *Health insurance.* An employer who provides health insurance must cover expenses for pregnancy on the same basis as expenses for other medical conditions.
- *Pregnancy and maternity leave.* An employee must be permitted to work at all times during pregnancy when she is able to perform her job. If she is temporarily absent as a result of pregnancy, she must not be required to remain on leave until after the baby is born. An employee cannot be prohibited from returning to work for a predetermined length of time after childbirth. Her job must be held open on the same basis as other employees on sick or disability leave for other reasons. Leave for child care purposes is not covered by this act.

Congress enacted the Family and Medical Leave Act of 1993, providing up to 12 weeks of unpaid leave for parents, to be used for birth or adoption of a child or for the serious illness of the employee or of a child, spouse, or parent.

Planning for maternity leaves is at best tentative, depending on the physical ability of the pregnant woman to work until a specified date, an uneventful postpartum course, and a healthy infant. Therefore, childbearing women should consider the possibility of later or earlier delivery dates in making plans for coverage during absence and return to work.

Breastfeeding and the Employed Mother

Breastfeeding mothers who are employed need information, counseling, and anticipatory guidance in planning for the breastfeeding experience. There are several alternatives. The nursing mother can manually express breast milk, express milk with a breast pump, supplement with formula during working hours, or make arrangements to breastfeed the infant at intervals during the day. However, of necessity, many women resume employment during a period that conflicts with the need for considerable mother-infant contact in breastfeeding. Expressing breast milk is possible but may be challenging in many work settings.

In a prospective survey of 1179 first-time mothers employed outside the home, women returning to professional occupations had a longer duration of breastfeeding than women returning to sales or technical positions. The researchers concluded that until employers develop a maternity policy that does not discourage breastfeeding, 6 months of breastfeeding will be difficult to achieve for most employed women (Kurinij et al. 1989). Another study suggested that 64 percent of women who worked 20 hours or fewer per week were still breastfeeding at 3 months compared with only 36 percent of women working more hours (Gielen et al. 1991). One innovative workplace benefit consists of corporate lactation programs that offer worksite pumping stations for lactating mothers as well as counseling by lactation specialists and referrals to community resources.

The health needs of working women, related both to their occupations and to their multiple roles, must be addressed by those concerned with employee health. Employee programs range from on-site prenatal health care services to breastfeeding education for mothers working outside the home (Gates and O'Neill 1990).

Child Care

It is ironic that the child care "policy vacuum" means that quality child care is difficult to obtain, while the virtual lack of adequate government policies governing maternity and child care leave makes early return to employment necessary for many childbearing women. Child care arrangements include in-home care by a family member or housekeeper/child caretaker/nanny, family day care in a home environment by a caregiver who may care simultaneously for her own and other children, and the institutional setting of daycare centers in which a group of children are cared for by one or more adults (Fig. 6–4). Some government-subsidized child care programs are available, but generally these efforts have proved inadequate.

Currently, research is being generated on the

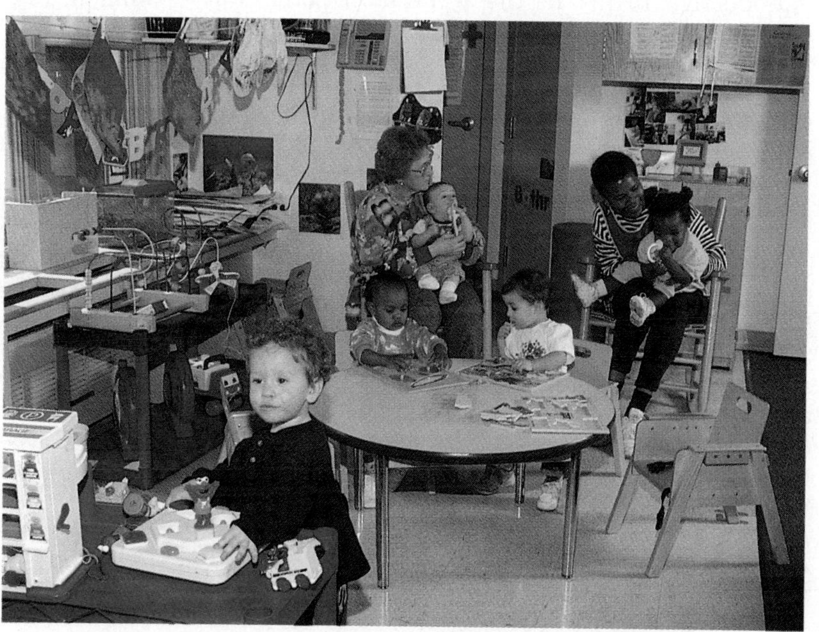

Figure 6–4

An increasing number of corporations are providing on-site child care centers for children of their employees. Research has shown that everyone benefits: the children, their parents, and the corporation. (Courtesy of Fairfax Hospital, Falls Church, VA.)

level of adjustment of infants and children receiving child care, and the effects of maternal employment on the health of the family system. Older children are also of concern, since as many as 3.4 million children are without adult supervision for a significant portion of the day because of maternal employment (Hofferth 1990).

NURSING PRACTICE

Nurses should be involved in education and counseling of employed women, assisting them with decision making and coping strategies. Nurses should assist women in time management skills and problem solving such as planning ahead, delegating tasks effectively, and tailoring household chores to the needs and personalities of individuals within the families. Health promotion should be encouraged through self-care, which is often of low priority for women. For these reasons, maternal employment has been called a "balancing act." Excessive fatigue, lack of time for self-care such as proper nutrition and exercise, and failure to find even temporary escapes are associated with maternal employment. Findings indicate that the use of health-promoting strategies is associated with positive health outcomes for working mothers (McKivergin et al. 1996).

OCCUPATIONAL HEALTH HAZARDS

Childbearing women risk exposure to potential reproductive toxins in the workplace, potentially affecting the approximately 2 million employed women who become pregnant each year (AMA 1984). It is estimated that 85 percent of women workers will become pregnant at some time during their working career, and 62 percent of women will work during their pregnancy (Griffith-Kenney 1986).

Negative reproductive outcomes from workplace exposure to toxic substances include sexual dysfunction, infertility, spontaneous abortion, congenital anomalies, and transplacental carcinogenesis. Sexual dysfunction may include loss of libido or an altered menstrual cycle. Infertility in both men and women may be due to high but nonlethal doses of ionizing radiation (Bernhardt 1990). The role of paternal exposure to noxious chemical should not be ignored (Kristensen et al. 1993).

Spontaneous abortion may be related to exposure to radiation, viruses, and chemicals (Ricci 1990). Some diagnosed congenital anomalies have no identifiable cause, but other anomalies have been associated with environmental factors such as viruses, chemicals, and radiation. Toxins can directly affect the fetus through maternal exposure, or indirectly affect it by altering both maternal and paternal germ cell chromosomes. Carcinogenesis is associated with either prezygotic exposure, transplacental exposure, ingestion of contaminated breast milk, or inhalation of workplace toxins (Bloom and Brenner 1993).

How injurious the effects of workplace exposure are depends on the specific hazard, the gestational age of the fetus at the time of exposure, and the dosage or duration of exposure (AMA 1984). Hazards may be physical, chemical, or biologic. Table 6–5 summarizes these risks and the potential effects, and lists those workers at risk.

Physical Hazards

Ionizing radiation is a workplace hazard for health care workers. The American Medical Association's Council on Scientific Affairs (1984) recommends that gonadal exposure of any employee to radiation or of the developing fetus to radiation is contraindicated unless clinical indications point to an unavoidable need to perform an x-ray examination. Childbearing health care workers should wear film badges for dose monitoring to make certain that radiation exposure remains within safe limits. Research findings related to the use of video display terminals and an increased incidence of spontaneous abortion and cardiac anomalies are inconclusive (Schorr 1990).

Hyperthermia is another physical hazard. Sustained elevation of body temperature from occupational exposure should be avoided by pregnant women and also by men during the reproductive years.

Chemical Hazards

Only a small portion of the chemicals used in industry have been tested for toxic effects on the unborn child. One chemical studied extensively is lead. Transplacental transfer and the teratogenic effects of lead are well documented (Brown et al. 1990; Scialli 1989). Such exposure is associated with increased rates of spontaneous abortions, stillbirth, and prematurity. Children exposed to lead in utero may exhibit neurologic damage and growth retardation (Brown et al. 1990). It was estimated by the Agency for Toxic Substances and Disease Registry (1988) that 4 million fetuses would be at risk for toxic effects from in utero exposure to lead over the next 10 years.

Table 6–5

OCCUPATIONAL HAZARDS THAT MAY AFFECT REPRODUCTION

PHYSICAL HAZARDS

Hazard	Potential Effect(s)	Workers at Risk
Extreme heat	Male infertility Female infertility Congenital anomalies Decreased sperm count	Bakery workers Laundry workers Nuclear industry workers Firefighters Steel workers Auto workers Dry cleaning workers
Ionizing radiation	Transplacental carcinogenesis	X-ray technicians Health care workers Dental office workers

CHEMICAL HAZARDS

Hazard	Potential Effect(s)	Workers at Risk
Anesthetic gases	Spontaneous abortion Minor congenital anomalies from male exposure	Health care workers Dental office workers Veterinary workers
Antineoplastic drugs	Spontaneous abortion	Female health care workers Female pharmaceutical workers
Dibromochloropropane (DBCP)	Decreased sperm count Spontaneous abortion from male exposure	Agricultural workers Pesticide makers Chemical workers
Ethylene oxide	Spontaneous abortion	Workers involved in sterilizing surgical instruments
Lead	Defects in spermatogenesis Spontaneous abortion Minor congenital anomalies Decreased mental development in first year of life	Electronics assemblers Painters Ceramic workers Battery workers Transportation operatives Plumbers Miners Welders
Methyl mercury	Central nervous system effects on infant	Agricultural workers Pharmaceutical workers Dye workers
Polychlorinated biphenyls (PCBs)	Dermatologic abnormalities and fever in children exposed postnatally	Communication workers Utilities workers Electric machinery workers
Vinyl chloride	Spontaneous abortion Stillbirth from male exposure	Plastic fabrication workers

Table continued on following page

Table 6–5

OCCUPATIONAL HAZARDS THAT MAY AFFECT REPRODUCTION Continued

BIOLOGIC HAZARDS

Hazard	Potential Effect(s)	Workers at Risk
Infection	Spontaneous abortion Premature rupture of membranes Preterm birth Stillbirth Intrauterine growth retardation Congenital anomalies	Women with other children at home Daycare workers Teachers Health care workers Laboratory workers
Physical work	Preterm birth Intrauterine growth retardation	Construction workers Electricians Pipe fitters Plumbers Firefighters Carpenters Moving company workers Health care providers

From Ricci, E. S. (1990). Reproductive hazards in the workplace. *NAACOG's Clinical Issues in Perinatal and Women's Health Nursing,* 1 (2), 226–239. Reprinted with permission from the Association of Women's Health, Obstetric and Neonatal Nurses.

Recently, there have been legal challenges to the denial of the right to work to women of childbearing age in specific industries, such as the lead industry, or in specific jobs. Exclusionary policies were designed to protect the health of future children of female workers exposed to toxic chemicals. Women's activists contend that industries' reasons for protecting the unborn are not only economic but discriminatory, because such policies fail to consider the effect of male exposure. Corporations may fear that women will sue for injuries to a deformed fetus. A 1991 Supreme Court decision upheld the rights of women in this regard.

Assessment Tool: Reproductive Health Hazards

- Are you planning pregnancy?
- Do you have any history of menstrual irregularities or changes in your menstrual cycle?
- Do you or your partner have any history of changes in sexual function (e.g., decreased libido)?
- Do you or your partner have any history of infertility?
- Do you have any history of spontaneous abortion, stillbirth, an infant born smaller than average at term, preterm birth, an infant with congenital anomalies, or children who developed cancer? Has your partner ever been involved in a relationship in which any of these outcomes occurred?
- Have you ever been told by a health care provider that the outcome of pregnancy was related to an exposure to a harmful substance at work?
- Where do you and your partner work outside the home? Note the nature of your work, how long employed at the current job, any site changes or shift changes that occur on the job.
- Where were you and your partner last employed and for how long?
- Are you aware of any potential hazards, such as chemicals, metals, pesticides, radiation, excess heat, anesthetic gases, chemotherapeutic drugs, or infections, that are not properly controlled in your workplace?
- Are you planning to breastfeed your infant?

From Ricci, E. S. (1990). Reproductive hazards in the workplace. *NAACOG's Clinical Issues in Perinatal and Women's Health Nursing,* 1 (2), 226–239. Reprinted with permission from the Association of Women's Health, Obstetric and Neonatal Nurses.

Biologic Hazards

Infections may be acquired in the workplace by direct contact with infected persons or through exposure to contaminated articles. Strenuous physical effort, standing, continuous tension, and commuting time longer than 1½ hours are related to preterm birth and low birth weight (Gates and O'Neill 1990; Ricci 1990). The childbearing woman and her fetus constitute a high-risk population in the workplace. The public is becoming increasingly intolerant to adverse reproductive outcomes that are preventable, such as work-related health and safety violations by corporations.

The importance of preconceptual counseling to individuals of childbearing age is becoming increasingly emphasized. Education on the potential effects of male and female exposure to hazards should be made available so that the individual can protect his or her reproductive health and decrease the incidence of infertility and poor pregnancy outcomes arising from hazards in the workplace.

NURSING PRACTICE

It is important for the nurse to make an assessment, obtaining a thorough database on the client's medical, surgical, gynecologic, obstetric, and family history and her employment and exposure history. A structured assessment tool may facilitate obtaining a comprehensive database (see Assessment Tool: Reproductive Health Hazards).

INFLUENCING POLICY RELATED TO HEALTH AND SOCIAL ISSUES

Influencing public policy related to health and social issues is a vital role for the maternal-newborn nurse. It can be categorized into educational strategies, research strategies, community consultation, legislative resource, and political activism.

Educational Strategies

Nurses should be involved in providing gender-specific educational material in community education programs and education of other health care professionals related to social issues that affect the lives of childbearing women. Course content in nursing education should serve to promote awareness of social issues related to women's health, as well as promoting political awareness and skills for nurses.

Research Strategies

Current requests for research proposals from the NIH stress the importance of including women in all clinical research, except in instances in which males are affected exclusively or when involvement of pregnant women would expose the fetus to undue risk. Federal grant applications criteria emphasize that gender differences should be noted and evaluated in research reports, and the rationale should be stated whenever less women are excluded from a research study (Pinn 1992). Previous research has determined the number of women affected by a specific situation, such as poverty. Research is now needed to examine the woman's experience in a given situation so that health care providers have an increased understanding of the condition and can design more comprehensive and effective approaches to nursing care (Callister 1994).

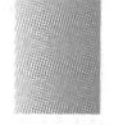

Community Consultation

It is important to work with civic leaders within the context of the community to develop strategies for primary, secondary, and tertiary prevention related to social issues concerning the childbearing woman and her family.

Legislative Resource

The maternal-newborn nurse can perform an important function by monitoring legislation that affects women's health, employment, and economic status. Serving as a resource person for legislators regarding women's issues is an important professional role.

Political Activism

Political strategies for maternal-newborn nurses include becoming knowledgeable about the political process, actively supporting women running for public office, recruiting voters, running for public office, and becoming active in political parties and campaigns (Styles 1992). Active involvement in nursing organizations that have a political program is vital. These include the American Nurses

Association (ANA) and its member state organizations, which focus on strategies to improve the political climate for women and health care. AWHONN, the Association of Women's Health, Obstetric, and Neonatal Nurses, is also politically active in maternal-newborn and women's health issues. Another strong organization for public activism is the American Public Health Association (APHA). The National Women's Health Network (NWHN) focuses on issues affecting women's health by monitoring and supporting legislation conducive to women's health.

Healthy People 2000 has identified health as an improved quality of life attained through personal choices made in a social context (National Center for Health Statistics 1994). Nurses who are sensitive to the complex interplay of women's lives and social issues can make an important difference in the health and well-being of women across the lifespan (Natapoff and Wieczorek 1990).

Implications for Research

The questions that remain unanswered related to the effect of social issues on the health of women and children are unlimited. There is an increasing number of such questions on the magnitude of the problems that women encounter and the impact on fetal health. However, there is minimal research on the impact of social issues on women's health, and the effectiveness of interventions and treatment programs for problems associated with social issues. A continued emphasis on documenting the impact of social issues on women and children is needed. However, before the many very specific questions that remain unanswered are examined, some general research questions that require answers are:

- Which of the current interventions and treatment programs are effective?
- What is the most effective approach to providing nursing care to women and children who are affected by a specific condition or situation?
- What political approaches are most effective in improving health policies for women and children?

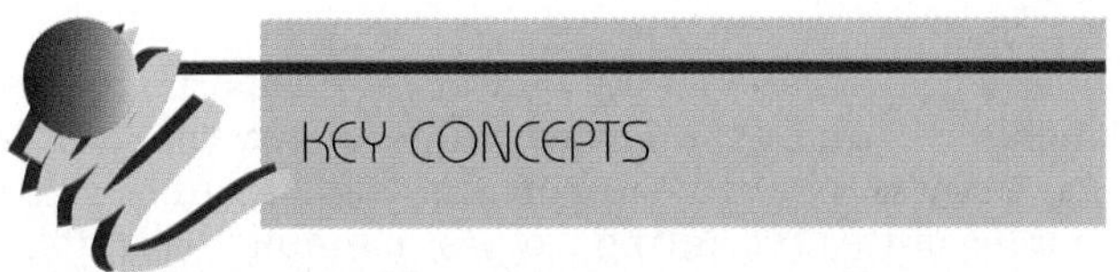

KEY CONCEPTS

- ▼ Women's health problems, their biopsychosocial status, and their social environment are closely related and each one influences the others.
- ▼ Women and children in poverty is a serious social issue that affects physical and emotional health status.
- ▼ Nurses need to work with community leaders in the implementation of social policies such as affordable housing; education and job training; employment options; adequate levels of public assistance, including shelter, child care, and access to health care; and the provision of treatment for substance use.
- ▼ All childbearing women should be assured access to timely, comprehensive, high-quality prenatal care, since adequate prenatal care is associated with positive pregnancy outcomes.
- ▼ Violence against women and children, including rape, is a major social problem threatening physical health and emotional and spiritual well-being.
- ▼ Nursing interventions for violence against women and children should focus on prevention, treatment of acute physical injuries, counseling regarding available options, and helping women to obtain long-term therapy.
- ▼ Substance abuse may interfere with a woman's abilities to function, either physiologically, emotionally, or socioculturally.
- ▼ The effects of maternal substance abuse on perinatal outcomes have not been fully explored but may profoundly affect the fetus. Substance use during pregnancy raises difficult and ethical questions related to fetal abuse.
- ▼ Increasing numbers of mothers are in the workplace. Issues related to maternal health and well-being, including occupational health hazards, family leave policies, support of breastfeeding, and the facilitation of appropriate child care, are important nursing considerations.
- ▼ Nurses should work to promote a safe and healthy social environment for women across the lifespan, provide services on health promotion and disease prevention, coordinate research and program evaluation, educate and inform the public, and disseminate research findings.
- ▼ Nurses can influence public policy related to social and political issues that affect women's lives through educational strategies, research activities, community consultation, and political activism, and as a legislative resource.

References

Aburdene, P., and Naisbitt, J. (1992). *Megatrends for women.* New York: Villard Books.

Agency for Toxic Substances and Disease Registry. (1988). *The nature and extent of lead poisoning prevention in children in the United States.* Washington, D. C.: United States Department of Health and Human Services.

Alexander, G. R., and Korenbrot, C. C. (1995). The role of prenatal care in preventing low birth weight. *The Future of Children: Low Birth Weight,* 5 (1), 103–120.

American College of Obstetricians and Gynecologists. (1989). The battered woman. *ACOG Technical Bulletin,* 124, 1–7.

American Medical Association. (1984). Council on Scientific Affairs. Effects of physical forces on the reproductive cycle. *Journal of the American Medical Association,* 251, 247–250.

American Nurses Association, Division on Maternal Child Health Nursing. (1984). *Access to prenatal care: Key to preventing low birth weight.* Kansas City, MO: Author.

Atkeson, B., Calhoun, K., Resick, P., et al. (1989). Victims of rape: Repeated assessment of depression symptoms. *Journal of Consulting and Clinical Psychology,* 50 (1), 96–102.

Avruch, S., and Cackley, A. P. (1995). Savings achieved by giving WIC benefits to women prenatally. *Public Health Reports,* 110 (1), 24–34.

Bass, E., and Davis, L. (1993). *Beginning to heal.* New York: HarperCollins.

Becker, J. V., and Coleman, E. (1990). Sexual abuse. In R. Litchman, and S. Papera (Eds.). *Gynecology: Well-woman care.* Norwalk, CT: Appleton-Lange.

Benton, D. A. (1986). Battered women: Why do they stay? *Health Care for Women International,* 7, 403–411.

Berne, A. S., Dato, C., Mason, D. J., Rafferty, M. (1990). A nursing model for addressing the health needs of homeless families. *Image: Journal of Nursing Scholarship,* 22 (1), 8–13.

Bernhardt, J. H. (1990). Potential workplace hazards to reproductive health. *Journal of Obstetric, Gynecologic, and Neonatal Nursing,* 19 (1), 53–62.

Bloom, A. D., and Brenner, D. D. (1993). Occupational exposures and reproductive risks. *Environment in Practice,* 1 (2), 2–3.

Blume, E. S. (1989). *Secret survivors: Uncovering incest and its after effects in women.* New York: John Wiley & Sons.

Blume, S. B., Counts, S. J., Turnball, J. M. (1993). When you first suspect substance abuse. *Contemporary Obstetrics-Gynecology,* 38 (3), 74–94.

Bohn, D. K. (1990). Domestic violence and pregnancy: Implications for practice. *Journal of Nurse-Midwifery,* 35 (2), 86–98.

Brown, M. J., Bellinger, D., Matthews, J. (1990). In utero lead exposure. *Maternal Child Nursing,* 15 (2), 94–96.

Buekens, P., Kotelchuck, K. M., Blondel, B., et al. (1993). A comparison of prenatal care use in the United States and Europe. *American Journal of Public Health,* 83 (1), 31–36.

Burst, H. V (1987). Issues and concerns of healthy pregnant women. School of Nursing, New Haven, CT. *Public Health Reports* July/August (4), Suppl., 57–61

Callister, L. C. (1993). The role of the nurse in childbirth: Perceptions of the childbearing woman. *Clinical Nurse Specialist, 7* (6), 288–293.

Callister, L. C. (1994). Finding a fit: Choice of a health care provider by childbearing women. *Clinical Consultations in Obstetrics, 6* (4), 252–257.

Callister, L. C. (1995). Beliefs and perceptions of childbearing women choosing different primary health care providers. *Clinical Nursing Research, 4* (2), 72–73.

Campbell, J. C., and Oliver, C. (1993). Why battering during pregnancy? *AWHONN's Clinical Issues in Perinatal and Women's Health Nursing, 86* (5), 343–349.

Campinha-Bacote, J., and Bragg, E. (1993). Chemical assessment in maternity care. *Maternal Child Nursing,* 18 (1), 24–28.

Chasnoff, I. J. (1989). Drug use and women: Establishing a standard of care. *Annals of the New York Academy of Sciences,* 562, 208–210.

Chavkin, W. (1990). Drug addiction and pregnancy: Policy crossroads. *American Journal of Public Health,* 80 (4), 483–487.

Chomitz, V. R., Cheung, L. W. Y., Lieberman, E. (1995). The role of lifestyle in preventing low birth weight. *The Future of Children: Low Birth Weight, 5* (1), 121–138.

Clancy, C. M., and Massion, C. T. (1992). American women's health care: A patchwork quilt with gaps. *Journal of the American Medical Association,* 268 (14), 1918–1919.

Cunningham, F. G., MacDonald, P. C., Gant, N. F., Leveno, K. J., Gilstrap, L. C. (1993). *Williams obstetrics* (19th ed.). Norwalk, CT: Appleton & Lange.

Curry, M. A. (1989). Nonfinancial barriers to prenatal care. *Women and Health,* 15 (3), 85–89.

Davis, S. F., Byers, R. H. Jr., Lindegren, M. L., et al. (1995). Prevalence and incidence of vertically acquired HIV infection in the United States. *Journal of the American Medical Association,* 274 (12), 952–955.

Devlin, B. K., and Reynolds, E. (1994). Child abuse: How to recognize it, how to intervene. *American Journal of Nursing, 94,* 26–32.

Fogel, C. I., and Woods, N. F. (1995). *Women's health care.* Thousand Oaks, CA: Sage.

Forest, K. B., Moen, P., Dempster-McClain, D. (1996). The effects of childhood family stress on women's depressive symptoms. *Psychology of Women Quarterly,* 20, 81–100.

Free, T., Russell, F., Mills, B., et al. (1990). A descriptive study of infants and toddlers exposed prenatally to substance abuse. *Maternal Child Nursing,* 15 (4), 245–249.

Gates, D., and O'Neill, N. (1990). Promoting maternal-child wellness in the work place. *American Association of Occupational Health Nurses,* 38 (6), 258–263.

Gielen, A. C., Faden, R. R., O'Campto, P. (1991). Maternal employment during the early postpartum period: Effects on initiation and continuation of breastfeeding. *Pediatrics,* 87, 298–305.

Gil, E. (1992). *Outgrowing the pain together.* New York: Bantam Doubleday Dell Publishing.

Golding, J. M. (1996). Sexual assault history and women's reproductive and sexual health. *Psychology of Women Quarterly, 20,* 101–121.

Grad, R. K. (1991). Making a difference for mothers and children. *Women's Health Issues,* 1 (4), 166–171.

Hadeed, A., and Siefel, S. (1989). Maternal cocaine use during pregnancy: Effect on the newborn infant. *Pediatrics,* 84, 205–210.

Hall, L. A., Sachs, B., Ravens, M. K., Lutenbacher, M. (1993). Childhood physical and sexual abuse: Their relationship with depressive symptoms in adulthood. *Image,* 25 (4), 317–323.

Hampton, H. L. (1995). Care of the woman who has been raped. *New England Journal of Medicine,* 332, 234–237.

Hans, S. L. (1989). Developmental consequences of prenatal exposure to methadone. *Annals of the New York Academy of Science,* 562, 195.

Heinrich, L. B. (1987). Care of the female rape victim. *Nurse Practitioner,* 12 (110), 9–27.

Hodnick, D. R. (1990). Homelessness: Health-care implications. *Journal of Community Health Nursing,* 7 (2), 59–67.

Hofferth, S. (1990). *National childcare survey of all children 5–12.* Urban Institute Study 91–5. Washington, D. C.: Urban Institute.

Holz, R. A. (1994). A practical approach to clients who are survivors of childhood sexual abuse. *Journal of Nurse Midwifery,* 39 (1), 13–18.

Hooper, C. A. (1992). *Mothers surviving sexual abuse.* New York: Routledge.

Horton, A. L., Harrison, B. K., Johnson, B. L. (1993). *Confronting abuse.* Salt Lake City, UT: Deseret Book.

Horton, J. A. (1995). *The women's health data book: A profile of women's health in the United States.* Washington, D.C.: Elsevier.

Hughes, T. (1990). Evaluating research on chemical dependency among women: A women's health perspective. *Family and Community Health,* 13 (3), 35–46.

Hughes, T., and Fox, M. L. (1993). Patterns of alcohol and drug use among women. *AWHONN's Clinical Issues in Perinatal and Women's Health Nursing* 4 (2), 203–212.

Inglis, A. D. (1991). United States maternal and child health services: Right or privilege? *Neonatal Network,* 9 (8), 35–43.

Keith, L. G., McGregor, S. N., Sciarra, J. J. (1988). Drug abuse in pregnancy. In I. J. Chasnoff (Ed.) *Drugs, alcohol, pregnancy and parenting.* Hingham, MD: Kluwer Academic Publishers.

Killien, M. G. (1990). Working during pregnancy: Psychological stressor or asset? *Clinical Issues in Perinatal and Women's Health,* 1 (3), 325–332.

King, M. C., Campbell, D., Ryan, J., et al. (1993). Violence and abuse of women: A perinatal health care issue. *AWONN's Clinical Issues in Perinatal and Women's Health Nursing,* 4 (2), 163–172.

King, M. C., and Ryan, J. (1989). Abused women: Dispelling myths and encouraging intervention. *Nurse Practitioner,* 14 (5), 47–58.

Kogan, M. D. (1995). Social causes of low birth weight. *Journal of the Royal Society of Medicine,* 88 (11), 611–615.

Kotch, J. B., Blakely, C. H., Brown, S. S., et al. (1992). *A pound of prevention: The case for universal maternity care in the United States.* Washington, D.C.: American Public Health Association.

Kristensen, P., Irgens, L., Kjersti Daltveit, A., et al. (1993). Perinatal outcome among children of men exposed to lead and organic solvents in the printing industry. *American Journal of Epidemiology,* 137 (2), 134–144.

Kurinij, N., Shiono, P. H., Ezrine, S. F., et al. (1989). Does maternal employment affect breast-feeding? *American Journal of Public Health,* 79 (9), 1247–1250.

Landry, M., and Smith, D. E. (1987). Crack: Anatomy of an addiction. *California Nursing Review,* 10 (3), 28–32.

Ledray, L. E., and Arndt, S. (1994). Sexual assault victim: A new model for nursing care. *Journal of Psychosocial Nursing,* 32 (2), 4–12.

Lee, C. C., and Chiang, C. N. (1985). Maternal-fetal transfer of abused substances. *National Institute of Drug Abuse Research Monograph,* 60, 110–147.

Lesniak, L. P. (1993). Penetrating the conspiracy of silence: Identifying the family at risk for incest. *Family and Community Health,* 16 (2), 66–76.

Lia-Hoagberg, B., Rode, P., Skovholt, C. J., et al. (1990). Barriers and motivators to prenatal care among low-income women. *Social Science and Medicine,* 30 (4), 487–495.

Lichtman, R., and Papera, S. (1990). *Gynecology: Well-woman care.* Norwalk, CT: Appleton & Lange.

Loftus, E. F., Polonsky, S., Fulilove, M. T. (1994). Memories of childhood sexual abuse: Remembering and repressing. *Psychology of Women Quarterly,* 18, 67–84.

Luke, B., Mamelle, N., Keith, L., et al. (1995). The association between occupational factors and preterm birth: A United States nurses' study. *American Journal of Obstetrics and Gynecology,* 173 (3), 849–862.

Lynch, M., and McKeon, V. A. (1990). Cocaine use during pregnancy: Research findings and clinical implications. *Journal of Obstetric, Gynecologic, and Neonatal Nursing,* 19 (4), 285–292.

Machala, M., and Miner, M. W. (1991). Piecing together the crazy quilt of prenatal care. *Public Health Reports,* 106 (4), 353–360.

Macklin, R. (1990). Maternal-fetal conflict: An ethical analysis. *Women's Health Issues,* 1 (1), 28–30.

McBride, A. B. (1988). Mental health effects of women's multiple roles. *Image,* 20 (1), 41–47.

McBride, A. B. (1990). Violence against women: Implications for research and practice. *Reflections,* Fall, 10–12.

McFarlane, J. (1989). Battering during pregnancy: Tip of an iceberg revealed. *Women and Health,* 15 (3), 69–84.

McFarlane, J. (1993). Abuse during pregnancy: The horror and the hope. *AWHONN's Clinical Issues in Perinatal and Women's Health,* 4 (3), 350–362.

McKivergin, M., Wimberly, T., Loversidge, J. M., Fortman, R. H. (1996). Creating a work environment that supports self-care. *Holistic Nursing Practice,* 10 (2), 78–88.

Meister, S. B., and Nichols, B. L. (1991). Health care and our communities: Defining the American Academy of Nursing's Agenda for Policy Action. In P. L. Chinn (Ed.). *Health policy: Who cares?* Kansas City, MO: American Academy of Nursing.

Moos, M. K. (1989). Preconceptional health promotion: A health education opportunity for all women. *Women and Health,* 15 (3), 55–68.

Naegle, M. A. (1988). Theoretical perspectives on the etiology of substance abuse. *Holistic Nursing Practice,* 2, 1–13.

Natapoff, J. N., and Wieczorek, R. R. (1990). *Maternal-child health policy: A nursing perspective.* New York: Springer.

National Center for Health Statistics. (1994). *Healthy people 2000 review, 1993.* Hyattsville, MD: U.S. Public Health Service.

National Commission on Children. (1991). *Beyond rhetoric: A new American agenda for children and families.* Washington, D.C.: U. S. Government Printing Office.

National Institute on Drug Abuse (NIDA). (1994). *Release of findings from NIDA national pregnancy and health survey.* Press Briefing, Sept 12, 1994. Sheraton Premiere, Tysons Corner, VA: National Institute of Health.

National League for Nursing. (1991). *Nursing's agenda for health care reform.* New York: Author.

Newman, L., and Buka, S. L. (1991). *Every child a learner: Reducing risks of learning impairment during pregnancy and infancy.* Denver, CO: Education Commission of the States.

Peters, H., and Theorell, C. J. (1991). Fetal and neonatal effects of maternal cocaine use. *Journal of Obstetric, Gynecologic, and Neonatal Nursing,* 20 (2), 121–126.

Peterson, B. (1991). *Dancing with daddy: A childhood lost and a life regained.* New York: Bantam Books.

Pinn, Y. N. (1992). Women's health research: Prescribing change and addressing the issues. *Journal of the American Medical Association,* 268 (14), 1921–1922.

Piper, J. M., Mitchell, E. F. Jr., Ray, W. A. (1994). Presumptive eligibility for pregnant Medicaid enrollees: Its effects on prenatal care and perinatal outcome. *American Journal of Public Health,* 84 (10), 1626–1630.

Plichta, S. (1992). The effects of woman abuse on health care utilization and health status. *Women's Health Issues,* 2 (3), 154–163.

Rhodes, A. M. (1990). Maternal liability for fetal injury. *Maternal Child Nursing,* 15 (1), 41.

Rhodes, W., and Hutchinson, S. (1994). Labor experiences of childhood sexual abuse survivors. *Birth,* 21 (4), 213–220.

Ricci, E. S. (1990). Reproductive hazards in the workplace. *NAACOG's Clinical Issues in Perinatal and Women's Health Nursing,* 1 (2) 226–239.

Richardson, G. (1994). *A welcome for every child.* Arlington, VA: National Center for Education in Maternal and Child Health.

Ridley, P. J. (1993). Kaufman's theory of shame and identity in treating childhood sexual abuse. *Journal of Psychosocial Nursing,* 31 (6), 13–17.

Rose, A. (1992). Effects of childhood sexual abuse on childbirth. *Birth,* 19 (4), 214–218.

Schnorr, T. M. (1990). The NIOSH study of reproductive outcomes among video display terminal operators. *Reproductive Toxicology,* 4 (1), 61–65.

Schoenborn, C. A. (1988). Health promotion and disease prevention: United States, 1985. *Vital and Health Statistics,* Series 10, Number 163. DHHS Publication Number (PHA) 88–1591. Hyattsville, MD: United States Department of Health and Human Services.

Scholl, T. O., Hediger, M. L., Belsky, D. H. (1994). Prenatal care and maternal health during adolescent pregnancy. *Journal of Adolescent Health,* 15, 444–456.

Scialli, A. R. (1989). Who should paint the nursery? *Reproductive Toxicology,* 3 (3), 159.

Scott, L. C. (1988). *The health and development of infants of black adolescent mothers.* Unpublished master's thesis, Wichita State University, Wichita, KS.

Slaght, E., Malloy, C., Zambrang, R. E. (1996). Women in the context of their family and community. In J. A. Lewis, and J. Bernstein (Eds.). *Women's health.* Boston: Jones & Bartlett.

Starn, J., Patterson, K., Bemis, G., et al. (1993). Can we encourage pregnant substance abusers to seek prenatal care? *Maternal Child Nursing,* 18 (3), 148–152.

Stenchever, M. A., and Stenchever, D. H. (1991). Abuse of women: An overview. *Women's Health Issues,* 1 (4), 187–192.

Stotland, N. L. (1990). Social change and women's reproductive health care. *Women's Health Issues,* 1 (1), 4–11.

Styles, M. M. (1992). Challenges for nursing in this new decade. *Maternal Child Nursing,* 15 (6), 347–352.

Sullivan, J., Boudreaux, M., Keller, P. (1993). Can we help the substance abusing mother and infant? *Maternal Child Nursing,* 18 (3), 153–157.

Tager, M. J. (1990). Work and family issues: A new frontier for health promotion. *American Journal of Health Promotion,* 4 (1), 237.

United States Department of Health and Human Services, Public Health Service, National Center for Health Statistics. (1995). *Monthly Vital Statistics Report,* 44 (3), 1–88.

United States Department of Health and Human Services. (1989). *Caring for our future: The content of prenatal care.* Rockville, MD: U. S. Government Printing Office.

United States Department of Labor, Women's Bureau. (1989). *Twenty facts on women workers.* Washington, D.C.: U. S. Government Printing Office.

Vener, A. M., Krupka, L. R., Climo, J. J. (1982). Drugs (prescription, over the counter, social) and the young adult: Use and attitudes. *International Journal of Addiction,* 17 (3), 399–415.

Wilsnack, S. C., and Beckman, L. J. (1984). *Alcoholic problems in women: Antecedents, consequences and intervention.* New York: Guilford Press.

Zigler, E., and Muenhow, S. (1983). Infant care and infant care leaves—a policy vacuum. *American Psychologist,* 38 (1), 91–95.

7 Chapter

> Ignorance of the law excuses no man; not that all men know the law, but because 'tis an excuse every man will plead, and no man can tell how to confute (disprove) him.
>
> JOHN SELDEN (1892)

Legal Aspects of Maternal-Newborn Nursing

Kathleen M. Driscoll
Francine H. Nichols

HIGHLIGHTS

- ▼ Negligence
- ▼ Malpractice
- ▼ Determining Liability
- ▼ Types of Insurance
- ▼ The Standard of Care
- ▼ Principles of Risk Management
- ▼ Consent to Research
- ▼ Confidentiality
- ▼ Licensure—Basic and Advanced Practice
- ▼ Implications for Research

Law is a societal institution that governs relationships among members of that society. Health care law governs relationships among health care providers, third-party payers, and consumers of health care. The chief focus of this chapter is the law as it affects the relationship of the maternal-newborn nurse to the consumer of care. Other legal relationships of concern to the maternal-newborn nurse are those with licensure boards and malpractice insurers.

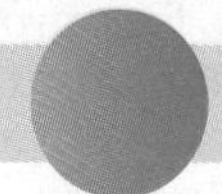

DEFINITIONS

Amicus brief—A concise written statement from some person or group not a party to the case presented to the court with the court's permission that presents argument of information or law relevant to the case.

Captain-of-the-ship doctrine—The concept that as "captain," the physician was held responsible for the "crew," including nurses.

Charitable immunity—The concept that hospitals as charitable organizations should not be sued for negligence.

Claims made insurance—Insurance coverage occurs only when a policy is currently in force.

Incident—An event outside that expected in the ordinary course of business of health care.

Indemnity—An assurance by one person to another that the other will be free from loss or damage.

Malpractice—A specialized form of negligence based on breach of a standard of care known to a person because of education in a professional field.

Negligence—An unintentional action or inaction that breaches a duty of care owed another person and foreseeably causes harm to that person.

Occurrence insurance—Coverage by a carrier if a policy was in force at the time of occurrence of the events leading to a lawsuit.

Ordinary negligence—Breach of a standard of care known to a layperson resulting in harm to the person.

Respondeat superior—The concept that the employer is responsible for the actions of the employees.

Risk management—Activities undertaken by any organization to identify, prevent, provide for risk coverage for, and respond to adverse events that do occur.

Specific informed consent—The person understands (1) the nature and purpose of the treatment or procedure; (2) the alternatives, including no treatment or procedure; and (3) the expected outcomes, that is, the material risks, benefits, and probabilities of success.

Tail policy—Negligence and malpractice insurance coverage for persons who have stopped working or retired and who previously carried claims made insurance.

Unlicensed assistive personnel—Persons trained to perform nursing tasks under the supervision of a licensed nurse.

TORT LAW

In our society, competent adults are responsible and accountable for their behavior. When others may be at risk of harm, adults are expected to meet certain standards of behavior that ordinary reasonable prudent persons would use under similar circumstances. For example, suppose someone is cleaning out the attic and tossing unwanted articles from a window into a city-approved trash container in the yard below. Inadvertently, the person throws a large article toward the container but misses. Another person walking on the public sidewalk located near the container is struck by the flying object.

The walker is injured and sues the homeowner for negligence. Probably no criminal law was violated and the homeowner had no malice toward the walker. It was simply an accident. Now a court has to determine whether an ordinary reasonable prudent person should have foreseen the possibility of injury to the person walking on the public walkway. The question arises whether the ordinary reasonable prudent person under similar circumstances would have looked for persons below and avoided throwing articles out when persons were present. If a court proceeding determines negligence, the homeowner is held responsible for the injuries to the walker and pays compensation for harm suffered.

Negligence

Four legal elements constituting negligence must be present for a court to award compensation. These are (1) a duty of care because of the foreseeability of harm, (2) breach of that duty of care, (3) causal relation of breach to harm, and (4) actual harm (Jeffers v. Olexo 1989). An example of negligence in an obstetric setting would be a nurse turning away from the scale while weighing a newborn. An ordinary reasonable prudent layperson would foresee that a wriggling infant could fall from the scale. Therefore the elements of negligence would be fulfilled if the infant fell and was injured when the nurse turned away. The nurse had a duty of care as harm was foreseeable, turning away breached that duty, a causal relationship existed between the turning away and the fall, and actual harm occurred. If any of these four elements is missing, there is no negligence under the law. Note that harm may include physical injury or, in some cases, emotional trauma. If the mother of the newborn saw the infant's fall, the mother might suffer emotional harm.

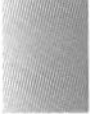

Malpractice

Malpractice is a specialized form of negligence. It is an extension of the ordinary reasonable prudent person standard to behaviors for professionals. Professionals including physicians, nurses, lawyers, teachers, social workers, and physical therapists have, through specialized education and experience, gained knowledge and skills that are unique. For this reason witnesses expert in the profession must provide testimony in malpractice cases as to whether the standard of care was met. The public recognizes these specialized skills and trusts the professional to apply them reasonably and prudently for the benefit of clients. Malpractice is a breach of professional duty to a client brought about by an unintentional but unreasonable action or inaction that foreseeably results in harm to the client.

Failure to monitor a small-for-gestational-age infant for signs of hypoglycemia with resultant brain damage is an example of malpractice. On the basis of educational preparation, the nurse should foresee that damage to the infant could occur with low blood sugar levels. A nurse who failed to monitor the infant would not be acting as an ordinary reasonable prudent nurse.

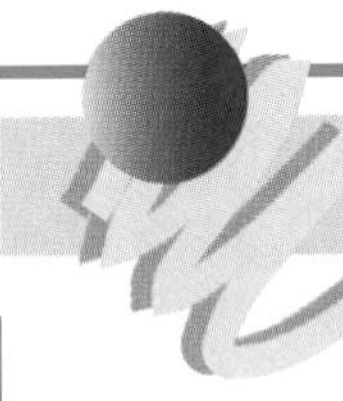

CRITICAL THINKING CASE HISTORY

LEGAL ACCOUNTABILITY: THE NURSE IS RESPONSIBLE FOR SKILLFUL ASSESSMENT AND ACCURATE INTERPRETATION OF ASSESSMENT DATA

The following report of a legal case describes the failure of the labor and delivery nurse to determine that the fetus was breech presentation, which led to difficult vaginal delivery and caused damage to the baby (Calfee 1994).

Alvis v. Henderson Obstetrics, 592 N.E.2d 678 (Illinois, 1992)

Two sonograms were used to establish a due date of December 25, 1983, for Martha Alvis, gravida 2. The second sonogram showed that the fetus was in a breech presentation. Ms. Alvis' physician told her that if the baby was still breech 3 weeks before her December due date, he would deliver the baby by cesarean section.

On November 14, the physician examined Ms. Alvis vaginally twice in his office. Both times, he found her cervix thick, 2 cm dilated, and the fetal presenting part as vertex. Ms. Alvis was admitted at 1:15 AM on November 15 to Brokaw Hospital. The admitting nurse performed a vaginal examination and determined that Ms. Alvis was 3 to 4 cm dilated, 60 to 70 percent effaced, and in a vertex presentation. She reported these findings to the physician by telephone at 1:50 AM and also called him with a report on Ms. Alvis at 6:30 AM. Oxytocin (Pitocin) was started to augment labor per the physician's orders.

The day shift nurse, MK, caring for Ms. Alvis testified that she had been uncertain about the fetal presentation when she did a vaginal examination at 6:30 AM. However, she made no mention of this in the patient's chart. Ms. Alvis' physician examined her at 9:00 AM, found the baby to be "vertex," and performed an amniotomy.

During the 8 hours that Nurse MK cared for Ms. Alvis, she monitored the Pitocin infusion,

Continued on facing page

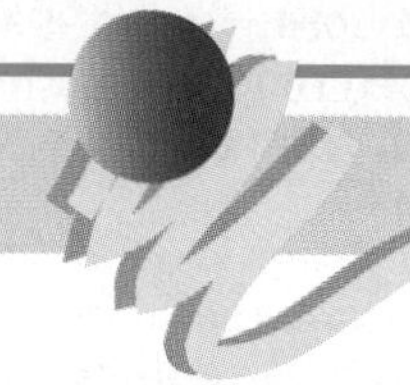

CRITICAL THINKING CASE HISTORY Continued

performed nine vaginal examinations, and reported to the physician at regular intervals. At 2:35 PM, Nurse MK called the physician to tell him that Ms. Alvis was 7 to 8 cm dilated and was "making good progress."

The second shift nurse, LT, assigned to care for Ms. Alvis performed her first vaginal examination at 2:55 PM. She found Ms. Alvis completely dilated and the fetus in frank breech presentation. The fetal monitor strip indicated decelerations of the fetal heart rate. Ms. Alvis' physician was called and arrived 3 minutes later. The baby's buttocks were visible at the vaginal opening and the physician determined that it was too late for a cesarean section.

The vaginal delivery was difficult. Nurses testified that the physician "had his hands around the baby's body with his thumbs in the small of the back and fingers gripping the abdomen and upper thighs." The umbilical cord was wrapped around the baby's neck. When the baby was finally delivered, baby girl Alvis was "blue and not breathing." Resuscitation was started and in a short time the baby started to breathe on her own.

Baby girl Alvis suffered kidney damage as a result of the difficult delivery. The prognosis was that by the time she was 12 to 15 years old, she would need a kidney transplant. If the donor was a relative, the kidney transplant could be expected to be effective for 10 to 15 years.

The Court's Decision

The court determined that the physician's and nurse's actions violated the standards of care. Failure to determine that the fetus was in breech presentation resulted in a difficult vaginal delivery, which caused damage to the baby. The expert for the plaintiff (baby girl Alvis) testified that a "competent obstetrical and delivery nurse should be able to determine" when a baby is in breech presentation prior to delivery. The hospital also had a written policy requiring that labor and delivery nurses be able to determine fetal presentation by vaginal examination.

The jury awarded the plaintiffs $2.9 million. The verdict was apportioned 75 percent against the physician and 25 percent against the hospital (because the nurse was an employee of the hospital).

Questions for Discussion

- What approaches could be used to prevent such an incident happening again?
- What are the indications of a breech presentation? Findings of vaginal examination? Position of fetal heart tones? Labor pattern?
- What have you learned from this legal case that you can use to improve your practice?
- What assessment techniques and procedures are the maternal-newborn nurse expected to perform skillfully and accurately in the following areas: prenatal clinic, labor and delivery unit, newborn nursery, postpartum unit, and neonatal intensive care unit?

Adapted from Calfee, B. E. (1994). Nurses in the courtroom. Huntsburg, OH: ARC Publishing.

Determining Liability

Staff nurses are seldom sued as individuals. The reason for lack of suits against individual nurses is that plaintiffs—persons who bring lawsuits—generally view the nurse's employer as having greater assets than the nurse to compensate the consumer of care or the consumer's family for injury.

RESPONDEAT SUPERIOR

As employees, nurses fall under the legal doctrine of respondeat superior. This term means the master—here, the hospital or other health care facility employer—is legally responsible for the nurse's acts or failures to act within the scope of the nurse's employment. When might this not be the case? A nurse who on his or her own makes a home visit and gives poor advice that results in harm to an infant or mother is not acting within the scope of employment. Neither is a self-employed nurse.

The nurse acted or failed to act. The employer is liable. Why so? In effect the nurse acts as agent for the employer, carrying out the employer's responsibility. The law views the employer as responsible for hiring nurses capable of making reasonable and prudent judgments in the care of clients. The law also views the employer as responsible for creating a workplace climate that supports reasonable and prudent nursing judgments about care. When the nurse is negligent or malpractices, the law says the employer is accountable because of the responsibility to clients in making judgments about hiring and in creating the workplace climate.

CAPTAIN OF THE SHIP

In the past nurses were often seen as acting at the direction of physicians. In maternal-newborn nursing this could occur during cesarean deliveries. If an event occurred that resulted in harm to the infant or the mother, the physician often had full legal accountability for the adverse consequences. The captain of the ship doctrine viewed the physician, rather than the hospital that employed the nurse, as in control of the actions of the nurse. This is infrequently the case today. Courts see nurses as educated professionals who are often responsible for foreseeing the same potential harm as a physician and thus have overlapping responsibility for client care: "the fact that a particular act is within a physician's duty of care does not necessarily exclude it from the duty of care owed to the patient by the nurse" (Berdyck v. Shinde 1993, p. 583).

CHARITABLE IMMUNITY

For over half of the 20th century the law provided immunity from negligence lawsuits for health care facilities. Today only some government facilities retain this immunity. The rationale for the immunity was that an institution that often provided care without remuneration should not have to compensate victims of its negligent acts. However, by the 1960s third-party payers began to pay for increasing percentages of care. Hospitals thus began to look more like businesses. In addition, the 1960s saw the rise of consumer rights. Consumers viewed safe products and services, including health care services, as their right.

In 1965 a landmark lawsuit, Darling v. Charleston Community Hospital, established a legal precedent for abolishing the doctrine of charitable immunity. The law held health care facilities responsible for setting standards of care. Gradually those standards became nationally rather than simply geographically based. In Berdyck v. Shinde (1993) the court identified standards as belonging to "the community of persons engaged in the practice of professional nursing" (p. 582).

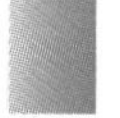

Types of Insurance

There are two types of negligence and malpractice insurance. These are occurrence and claims made. Occurrence insurance covers any monetary damages that may stem from a point in time during which a policy was in force *whether or not the defendant currently has a policy.* Claims made insurance covers a defendant *only when a policy is currently in force.*

Occurrence insurance benefits the health care provider. Insurance companies may suffer financially when they remain potentially at risk for long periods. The nurse may no longer carry insurance but the company remains liable to defend any claims. This is particularly true when harm occurs to infants, and the statute of limitations extends until the child reaches 18 *plus* the period of time for bringing a lawsuit in negligence. On the other hand, claims made insurance benefits the insurance company. Claims made insurance limits the length of time the company is at risk to the period when the health care provider is covered. Health care providers who stop working for a period or retire can remain covered by purchasing what is known as a tail policy.

No form of insurance protects the nurse from action or inaction that intentionally rather than carelessly causes harm to a person. Intention in the eyes of the law involves reckless or dangerous action or inaction. Deliberately choosing to omit timely assessment of a newborn might be viewed as an intentional act.

Is it important to carry malpractice insurance? Conservative legal advisors say yes. This is so because back fence nursing guidance to a neighbor can constitute the practice of nursing outside the scope of employment. A personal insurance policy covers such an instance. Health care facility employers may tell nurses they need not carry malpractice insurance because their negligent actions or inactions would be covered by the facility's policy. The term used to describe this promise of freedom from monetary damages in the event of a lawsuit is *indemnity.* The nurse can be secure in this advice only if the nurse confines practice to the employment setting promising indemnity.

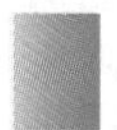

The Standard of Care

To begin to establish the elements of a negligence or malpractice lawsuit, a breach of the duty of care—also termed the standard of care—must occur. The standard of care changes as health care and nursing research determine the effectiveness or ineffectiveness of approaches to care.

SOURCES OF THE STANDARD OF CARE

From what sources can the nurse determine the standard of care? There are several.

One source is the state nurse practice act. Authority for setting standards can be found in the nurse practice act of the state. For example, Ohio's Board of Nursing authority is set forth in Section 4723.08 of the Ohio Revised Code.

Another important source is current professional literature. Regularly reading articles in one's field of practice is expected. The professional nurse is expected to apply results of research in practice.

Another source is professional association standards. These standards tend to reflect the nursing process of assessment, diagnosis, planning, implementation, and evaluation. The American Nurses' Association (ANA), the Association of Women's Health, Obstetric, and Neonatal Nurses (AWHONN), and the National Association of Neonatal Nursing (NANN) publish standards for nursing practice. When seeking to establish negligence, expert witnesses review records to see that the nurse has provided care that incorporates each step. Professional associations also often develop position statements that more specifically identify current standards of care. Nurses in a field should be aware of these.

Regulatory law—also called administrative law—often sets standards in obstetric care. Licensing laws in various states may dictate the structure of an obstetric unit, for example, the location of bassinets in relation to precautions against infection. State regulations may also support regionalization in health care. An example is having regional rather than local centers for neonatal intensive care. The federal standards for blood-borne pathogens originally promulgated by the Occupational Safety and Health Administration in 1991 (29 CFR Part 1910 S 1030) are federal regulatory law. Regulations can spring from Medicaid as a payer source. For instance, different states may have different regulations with respect to length of stay on maternity units.

Hospital policy and procedure set standards of care. However, these are expected to be based on the professional literature and reviewed at regular intervals so that they remain current. Accrediting bodies like the Joint Commission on Accreditation of Healthcare Organizations (JCAHO) also set standards of care. Often these standards identify the policies and procedures as well as quality measurements that should be in place and used to benefit the health care client (JCAHO 1995).

The professional nurse reflects the standard of care through documentation in the client's record. Figure 7–1 shows the relationship of documentation to professional and legal accountability. Professional accountability occurs when the nursing process is complete. Legal accountability occurs when duty to the client is fulfilled and results in benefit to the client.

MEETING THE STANDARD OF CARE

Shortened acute care stays have affected the practice of maternal-newborn nursing. Most important, they have raised awareness of the need to appreciate and plan for delivery of care to the client across a continuum of care. Nurses must not only hone their personal monitoring skills but also support clients by providing knowledge and skills related to the care that they will need to carry out on discharge. Health care professionals need to regard clients as members of the health care team. Without client empowerment, health care can fail to achieve its goals.

Monitoring and Reporting Client Resources

The Ohio case of Berdyck v. Shinde (1993) illustrates the importance of monitoring and reporting clients' responses. In the case of Donna Berdyck, a woman in her 38th week of pregnancy who had a history of preeclampsia, drove herself to the hospital when a called-in prescription for analgesic medication failed to relieve the abdominal pains she was experiencing for the second time in several days. During her pregnancy visits the obstetrician had noted an elevated blood pressure and trace protein in her urine. The client arrived at the hospital at 3:00 AM and was admitted directly to the obstetric unit at the order of her obstetrician.

On her admission to the obstetric unit she told the nurse she had severe upper abdominal pain and was experiencing nausea and headache. She was unable to provide a urine sample for testing. At 3:20 AM the nurse noted the client's elevated blood pressure. A reading at 3:40 AM was also elevated. At 4:00 AM the nurse notified the obstetrician of the elevated blood pressure, the client's inability to void, and abdominal pain. The obstetrician did not recall being told of a headache.

On the basis of the information from the nurse, including results of laboratory tests, the obstetrician believed Donna Berdyck had a gastric disturbance resulting from flu and dehydration. He told the nurse to keep the patient quiet and to closely monitor the blood pressure. Five minutes after the termination of the conversation between the obstetrician and nurse the client's blood pressure was 192/112, but the nurse did not report this informa-

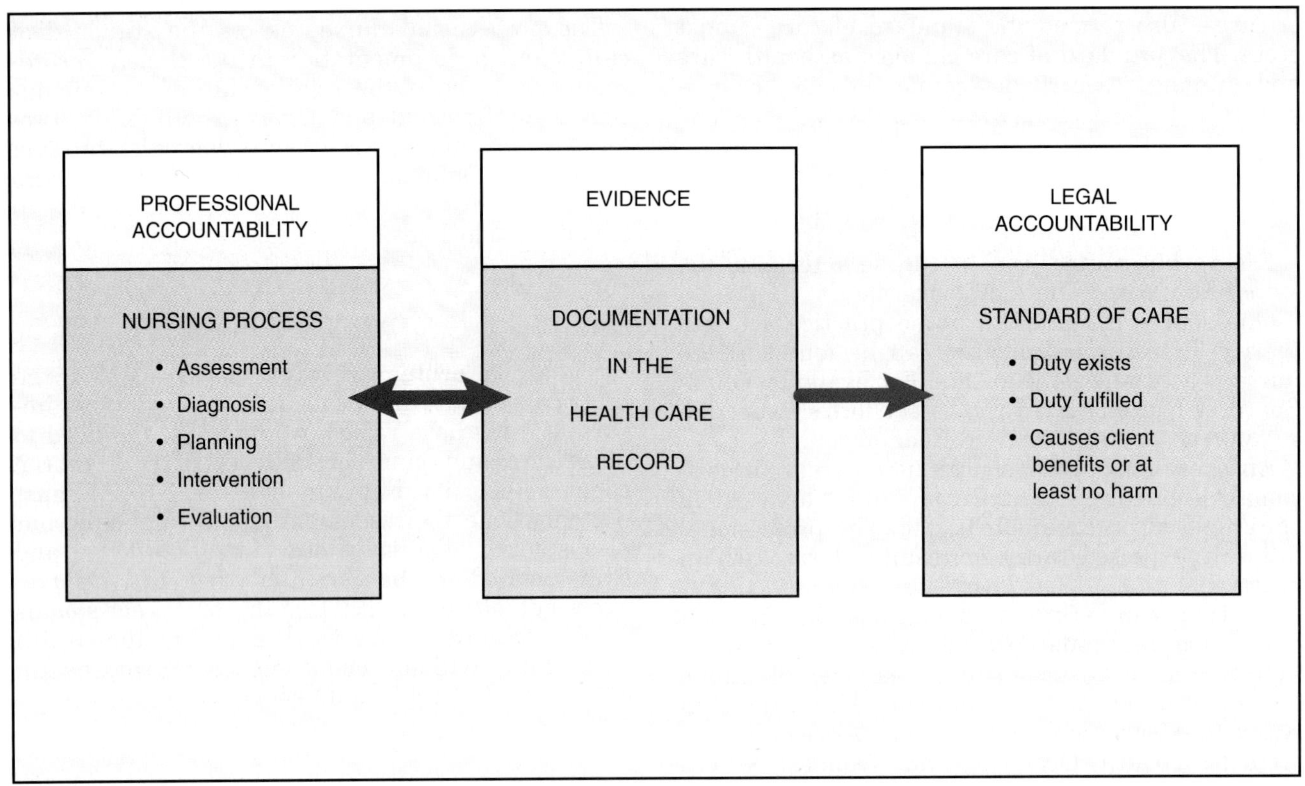

Figure 7–1
The relationship of professional and legal accountability.

tion to the obstetrician. The nurse did not take another blood pressure reading and at 5:15 AM found the client having a grand mal seizure. Donna Berdyck delivered a healthy child by cesarean section but suffered left-sided paralysis as a result of the seizure. She did not make a complete neurologic and muscular recovery. The court found both physician and nurses (as employees of the hospital) in violation of the standard of care.

What lessons about monitoring and reporting are to be learned from this scenario? First, a complete picture of the client should be reported to

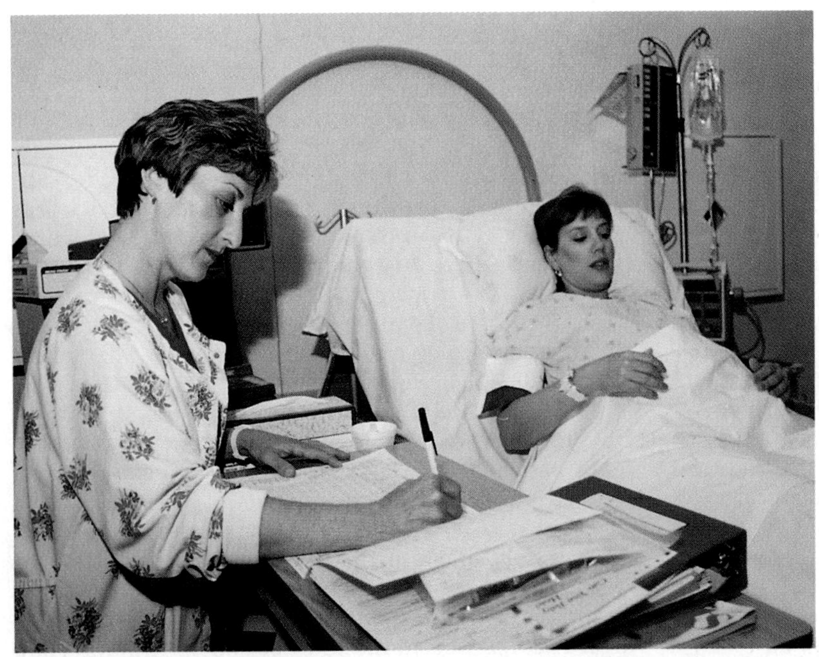

Figure 7–2
Clear, concise, accurate, and complete charting is essential to document changes in the patient's condition over time and to provide continuity of care. Documentation of appropriate care is also a risk management activity that provides the first line of defense in lawsuits.

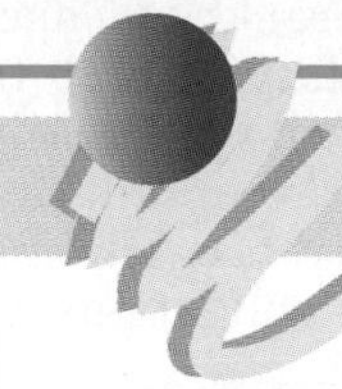

CRITICAL THINKING CASE HISTORY

LEGAL ACCOUNTABILITY: THE NURSE HAS THE RESPONSIBILITY TO MONITOR THE PATIENT CORRECTLY

The following report of a legal case describes the failure of the nurse to use a fetal monitor during labor to monitor the patient as ordered by the patient's physician (Calfee, 1994).

Nelson v. Trinity Medical Center, 419 N.W.2d 886 (North Dakota, 1988)

Diane Nelson was admitted in active labor to the Labor Unit at Trinity Medical Center on November 20, 1982 at 4:00 PM. Her physician had standing orders that continuous fetal monitoring be used for all patients. The physician also discussed the use of the fetal monitor with the nurse caring for Ms. Nelson.

The nurse did not place a fetal monitor on Ms. Nelson until 5:07 PM. At that time, the fetal monitor strip indicated that the infant was in fetal distress and an emergency cesarean section was performed. Baby girl Nelson was born "severely brain-damaged" and will require "extensive treatment and nursing-home care" as long as she lives.

The nurse who took care of Ms. Nelson during labor testified that she did not place a fetal monitor on Ms. Nelson, as ordered by the physician, because she believed that both of the fetal monitors in the Labor Unit were in use. The nurse admitted that she did not look for a monitor. Evidence presented during the trial indicated that a fetal monitor was available for use in the unit and could have been used for Ms. Nelson.

The Court's Decision

The court determined the "captain-of-the-ship" doctrine was not applicable in this case and held the nurse responsible for not monitoring the patient properly. The nurse should have checked to see if a fetal monitor was available. Perhaps, if a fetal monitor had been used, "the infant's injuries could have been mitigated or avoided altogether."

Principles for Practice

- The nurse is responsible for his or her own personal actions. The attending physician is not responsible for the actions of health care workers caring for his or her patient.
- The nurse should carry out the physician's orders for accepted and appropriate care and document them in the patient's chart.
- If for some reason, the nurse cannot carry out the physician's orders or if the orders are questionable or inappropriate, the nurse has a responsibility to notify his or her superior.

Questions for Discussion

- What strategies can be used to prevent a similar incident from happening in a labor and delivery unit?
- What are examples of documentation that should appear in a patient's chart when fetal monitoring is used? When signs of possible fetal distress are noted?
- What level of skill in fetal monitoring is required for a nurse working in a labor and delivery unit?

Adapted from Calfee, B. E. (1994). Nurses in the courtroom. Huntsburg, OH: ARC Publishing.

the physician. In this case the nurse did not report the symptom of headache, which would have heightened the concern of the obstetrician. Although the physician admitted the elevated blood pressure should have caused him to go to the hospital, additional information in the call from the nurse would have helped him to make a sound differential diagnosis. Additional information would probably have resulted in magnesium sulfate being ordered and the grand mal seizure avoided. The court noted that nurses in this situation must report not only specific information gained but also the full range of information that can be derived from an assessment that meets nursing standards in a given situation. Thus, failure to provide complete information to the obstetrician resulted in misjudgment that harmed the client.

The malpractice escalated when the nurse failed to report the elevated blood pressure reading after the conversation with the obstetrician. This report was particularly relevant in light of the obstetrician's admonition to monitor the client's blood pressure closely. The court noted that an earlier case had established that

> *accepted standards of nursing practice include a duty to keep the attending physician informed of a patient's condition so as to permit the physician to make a proper diagnosis of and devise a plan of treatment for the patient.*
>
> (Albain v. Flower Hospital 1990, p. 265)

Recognizing the signs of preeclampsia is an accepted standard of maternal-newborn nursing practice. The admitting nurse stated that she did not know the signs of preeclampsia, and the nurse on the obstetric unit admitted that she "lacked an appropriate level of nursing information about that condition and its symptoms" (Berdyck v. Shinde 1993, p. 581).

Second, the hospital failed in its duty of care by failing to provide competent staff on its obstetric unit. This became evident when the nurses admitted their lack of knowledge of the signs and symptoms of preeclampsia.

In Berdyck, both the plaintiff and the Ohio Nurses Association in an amicus brief, a written statement presented to the court that argues the information or law relevant to the case, argued that (when the physician did not attend to the signs of preeclampsia) the nurses should have sought care through other available routes. The court agreed that both medicine and nursing had the duty to recognize the signs and symptoms of preeclampsia. However, since the nurses involved in this particular case did not know those signs and symptoms, the court found this not an issue. The court noted that had the nurses been aware of the signs of preeclampsia they could have fulfilled their duty of care by seeking the assistance of others. Other states have recognized this duty (Campbell v. Pitt County Memorial Hospital, Inc. 1987).

Nurses learn early in their education that they are responsible for questioning the appropriateness of care when they believe harm to a client may occur. This includes raising concerns with nursing supervisors and, absent a satisfactory response, carrying their concerns to the hospital physician chief of staff. The ANA's *Code for Nurses* (1985) supports this stance in Standard 3, which states: "The nurse acts to safeguard the client and the public when health care and safety are affected by the incompetent, unethical, or illegal practice of any person."

Monitoring and reporting client responses require that health care facilities hire knowledgeable nurses willing to fulfill their duty of care to the client. The facts of *Berdyck* could as easily have included failure to monitor the infant for signs of fetal distress. Maternal-newborn nursing carries the extra burden of having obligations to the welfare of both mother and child.

Berdyck emphasizes the responsibility of the nurse to communicate verbally adequate information about the client to the responsible physician. The entire nursing process, including physician notification, needs to be reflected in the client's record. The guidelines for written communication in the Improving Your Practice box reflect charting standards.

The Nurse and Informed Consent

Clients give consent to routine hospital care including nursing care when they are admitted. Procedures that are outside the realm of routine care require specific consent. Surgery, imaging procedures requiring insertion of catheters into the cardiovascular system, and medications with potentially seriously harmful side effects are examples that fall in this category. Nurses frequently become involved in specific informed consent on an obstetric unit with respect to consent to a cesarean section.

Specific informed consent is legally the responsibility of the physician. Legal requirements of informed consent include explanation of (1) the nature and purpose of the treatment or procedure; (2) the alternatives, including no treatment or procedure; and (3) the expected outcomes, that is, the material risks, benefits, and probabilities of success.

What is the nurse's role? Ideally, the nurse should be present during the physician's conversation with the client about informed consent. Should the woman have questions later, the nurse can often help her understand what the physician said. The nurse may reiterate or explain what a physician has said but should not attempt to expand on the physician's explanation in the areas of diagnosis and prognosis. These are areas of care reserved to the practice of medicine. The nurse needs to notify the physician when the mother has questions in these areas or the mother is refusing consent.

Cesarean sections are one example of procedures for which specific informed consent is required. Another example is nonroutine ultrasonography. A nurse doing an ultrasound examination would describe the procedure to the woman. The nurse would not discuss anomalies found on the ultrasonogram that the nurse can recognize because of experience (diagnosis) or the health impact on fetus and mother of the anomaly (prognosis). Working with both parents to cope with

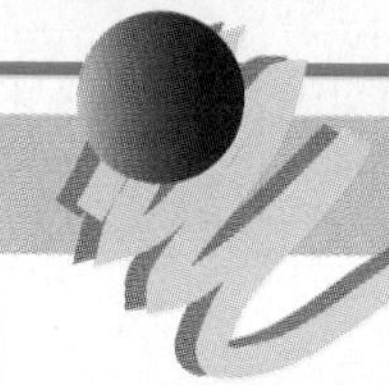

CRITICAL THINKING CASE HISTORY

LEGAL ACCOUNTABILITY: THE NURSE IS RESPONSIBLE TO REPORT THE SITUATION TO THE NURSE'S SUPERIOR WHEN THE PHYSICIAN DOES NOT ACT ON INFORMATION FROM THE NURSE REGARDING CONCERNS ABOUT PATIENT SAFETY

The following report of a legal case describes the failure of the nurse to take proper action when the physician does not act on the nurse's concerns regarding fetal distress (Calfee, 1994).

Campbell v. Pitt County Memorial Hospital, Inc., 352 S.E.2d 902 (North Carolina, 1987)

Margaret Campbell was admitted to Pitt County Memorial Hospital (defendant) for the delivery of a child (plaintiff, Jennifer Campbell) on April 30, 1979. Ms. Campbell's baby was determined, by the attending obstetrician, to be in a footling breech (feet first) presentation.

For several hours before the delivery, the nurse noted signs of fetal distress and expressed concern to Ms. Campbell's physician. The physician failed to take any action. The nurse did not notify her supervisor of the situation when the physician did not take action. The physician delivered the baby vaginally and the umbilical cord was wrapped around the baby's legs.

The infant suffered brain damage from "severe asphyxia from the entangled cord" and requires constant care and supervision.

The Court's Decision

The court held the nurse responsible for not notifying her superior of the situation when she could not get the physician to respond. The court also held the hospital responsible because it did not have a procedure in place for the prompt reporting of such situations.

Principles for Practice

- Nurses have a responsibility to notify their superiors promptly if they are concerned about a client and the physician fails to take the proper action.
- Nurses should know the proper reporting procedures that are to be followed if such situations of compromised patient safety occur.
- All agencies should have a clear, well-defined, written reporting procedure that specifies the steps to be followed in situations in which a patient's safety is compromised.

Questions for Discussion

- What actions should the nurse take if a physician fails to respond to concerns about the patient's safety?
- What is the reporting procedure in such a situation in the hospital in which you study or practice?
- What type of documentation should the nurse include in the patient's chart in such situations?

Adapted from Calfee, B. E. (1994). *Nurses in the courtroom.* Huntsburg, OH: ARC Publishing.

adverse findings would be appropriate once the physician informed parents abut the diagnosis and prognosis. Helping persons to cope is within the realm of nursing practice.

What about the nurse signing the consent form? A nurse who does this is simply acting as a witness to the signature. This means the nurse can attest that the client agreeing to the surgery was the person who signed the informed consent form. In fact, many risk managers prefer that the physician witness the client's signature. There is a good reason for this. If a question regarding the informed consent process arises later, evidence then exists that the physician and the woman were together at a point in time.

Can a woman refuse surgical intervention when the welfare of her fetus is apparently at risk? In general, when a woman refuses, courts order a cesarean section because of the threat to the health of the fetus. However, there have been instances in which courts have ordered surgical intervention and prior to the surgical intervention healthy in-

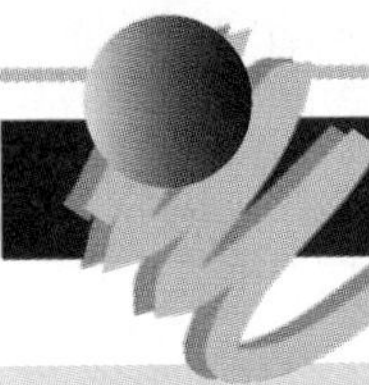

IMPROVING YOUR PRACTICE

WRITTEN COMMUNICATION: DEFENSE THROUGH DOCUMENTATION

The nurse's clear, accurate, and complete essential written communication in the patient's chart can be a valuable defense tool if a lawsuit is filed. Failures in documentation can be damaging in determining liability in a legal issue.

Guiding Principles

- Documentation should be clear, accurate, comprehensive, descriptive, and factual.
- Documentation should reflect the standards of nursing care.
- Documentation should include nursing assessment, patient's needs or problems, interventions, outcomes of care, and discharge planning.
- Documentation should be done according to the agency's policies.
- Documentation or corrections can be entered into the patient's chart as a "late entry," but they must be clearly marked as an addendum and the reason for the late entry noted.

What to Include in the Patient's Chart

- A careful, concise, and accurate account of the nurse's activities with the patient
- A record of each major task such as administering medications and carrying out procedures
- A record of all the patient's reactions and responses to the health care condition or problem
- A record of all the patient's reactions and responses to the care provided
- Documentation of each verbal order

What *Not* to Include in the Patient's Chart

- Critical comments of any kind, such as comments about another health care provider, the patient, or her family
- Commentary on what you believe is happening or should be happening
- Opinions and judgments about the situation

Adapted from Blackwell, M. K. (1993). Documentation serves as invaluable defense tool. *The American Nurse,* 25 (7), 40–41.

fants have been delivered vaginally (Field 1989). To arrive at court-ordered intervention courts must weigh and balance the rights of the unborn child against the rights of an existing person, the mother.

Do fathers have rights with respect to surgical intervention? The answer is no. To consent or not consent to reproductive procedures is reserved to the mother (Planned Parenthood v. Casey 1992).

Instructing Clients

The occurrence of adverse events following less than or only a 24-hour hospital stay after birth has raised questions about this insurer-driven practice as an appropriate standard of care. Cases of infant dehydration with harmful consequences, including loss of limbs and even death, have been reported. This can occur when first-time mothers have not mastered breastfeeding before discharge. Mothers may also not recognize signs of jaundice that may lead to brain damage (Bonfield 1995). The practice has led to several states passing laws that require longer stays.

Eager to assure parents and children at risk that reported catastrophic consequences to infants linked to early discharge were of national concern, the 104th Congress passed Senate Bill 969, the "Newborns' and Mothers' Health Protection Act of 1996." The Act sets a national standard requiring that health insurance plans and employer-provided benefit plans that include maternity benefits provide a minimum of 48 hours of inpatient care after a vaginal delivery and 96 hours of care after delivery by cesarean section. States may more strictly regulate discharge practices but must minimally meet the national standard.

Exceptions to this standard occur only when the physician writes an early discharge order after consulting with the mother *and* the health plan provides postdelivery follow-up care, including home care. Follow-up care must occur within 24 to 72 hours of discharge. The Act also requires the Department of Health and Human Services to conduct a series of three studies over a 5-year period examining maternal and child health care. The studies will address (1) changes in obstetric practice over time, (2) outcomes of childbirth, (3) factors determining length of hospital stay, (4) diversity of outcomes affecting not only mothers and infants but also families, and (5) financial incentives that may affect newborn and maternal health and the clinical decision making of health care providers. An advisory panel composed of representatives from the Department and all sectors of the health care industry will guide the studies.

Does the federal law ensure avoidance of adverse consequences of early discharge for mothers and infants? The law does help *if* the nurse takes responsibility for recommending timely follow-up care, perhaps a home visit, when a mother seems at risk after a longer stay. An example is a mother discharged at 48 hours after childbirth who is experiencing difficulty breastfeeding. Nurses will still need to take responsibility to instruct mothers to promptly report changes in skin color to their physician to ensure treatment for kernicterus. Since parents may forget or misunderstand instructions, verbal instructions should be accompanied by written instructions. The nurse should keep in mind that the duty of care related to instruction may not be fulfilled if the reading level of parents is not kept in mind when preparing written instructions.

The legal protection provided by laws protecting against the so-called "drive-through" delivery does not nullify the nurse's duty of care with respect to instruction of parents. The new laws do give the nurse the advantage of 48 rather than 24 hours to carry out the plan of instruction, including evaluation of the parents' learning. The nurse will still have to put on an advocate hat for follow-up care or longer stay when mothers and infants discharged within the new statutory parameters are at risk.

Delegating Care

In addition to the adverse outcomes created by early discharge there are potential adverse outcomes to be avoided with increased use of unlicensed assistive personnel (UAPs) on obstetric units. Nurses must remember that *judgments about client status cannot be delegated* to UAPs. Portions of assessment such as taking vital signs may be delegated but always with the understanding that measurements are accurate and documented and deviations from normal parameters are reported to nursing staff.

Distinctions between levels of personnel must be clear to clients. The teaching function of the professional nurse should be delegated only with great discretion. At a minimum the professional nurse should evaluate the client's understanding of what has been taught.

To ensure appropriate delegation—delegation that is reasonable and prudent—both nursing staff and UAPs must appreciate the capabilities and limitations of UAPs. Client care is best when teams composed of nurses and UAPs work together consistently. Like concerns about risks for clients with early discharge, concerns about the potential for inappropriate use of UAPs are leading to regulation. Ohio is one state that has recently adopted rules for delegation of nursing care under the authority of the state nurse practice act (ORC S 4723.28 [B] [18] 1995).

Principles of Risk Management

Overall, the goal of risk management is "to reduce unplanned or unexpected financial loss to an organization" (Krauss 1986, p. 1). Steps taken to achieve this goal include (1) identifying risk, (2) preventing or reducing risk by creating awareness of risk and risk management strategies, (3) providing for coverage of loss through self-insurance or use of outside insurance carriers, and (4) engaging in early investigation and appropriate response to adverse events when they occur. Risk managers set in place procedures for managing risk (Cohen 1990).

Emphasis should be placed on assessment accuracy, documentation, paying attention to clients' needs, knowing personal professional limitations, and knowing institution policy and procedures. These measures are risk preventive measures (see Measures to Diminish the Risk of a Lawsuit).

INCIDENT REPORTS

Incident reporting is also a risk preventive measure. Events outside those expected in the ordinary course of health care facility business are termed incidents. When these occur they require documentation.

A report should be made when there is a medication error or when a fall occurs even though no harm results. Why so? Because incident reports are a management tool that help a health care fa-

Measures to Diminish the Risk of a Lawsuit

- Do an accurate comprehensive nursing assessment—know your client.
- Follow up on laboratory reports.
- Document timely and thoroughly during the course of care—DOCUMENT, DOCUMENT, DOCUMENT.
- Do not alter the chart.
- Read the nurse's notes, the laboratory reports, and the physician's progress notes.
- Do not promise the impossible to clients.
- Do not ignore a dissatisfied client—maintain communication, exercise courtesy, and make sure you maintain good relations with patients.
- Do not point fingers when something goes wrong. State the facts—incident report facts should match those in the client's record.
- Do not go beyond your educational training and ability—practice within the limits of your educational preparation and experience.
- Know and follow your facility's policies and procedures.

cility determine where it might make efforts to reduce risk. For example, a particular postpartum analgesic medication may be associated with a series of falls. Even though no mother or infant has been injured, the pharmacy review committee may wish to substitute another analgesic in its drug formulary rather than continue to supply the drug associated with falls.

Incident reports are not part of the clients' records. Therefore, they are considered confidential to management and are generally not discoverable in lawsuits. However, the contents of the incident report should match the part of the client's record that leads to the suit. For example, the client's record should contain the facts as known when a client is found on the floor, such as date, time, witnesses, personnel involved, and what was done to mitigate any potential or actual injury. This last would include total client assessment incorporating taking vital signs and observation for injury followed by increased subsequent monitoring of the client. As blame is not assigned in the client's record, blame should also not be assigned in the incident report. Incident reports should not be limited to caregiving situations. Situations that put employees and visitors at risk should also be reported.

For the individual staff nurse, remaining current in areas of practice is the most important risk management strategy. Remaining current applies to all steps of the nursing process.

EQUIPMENT USE

Remaining current also means being familiar with new equipment. Nurses should know that tampering with equipment to make it work may void the manufacturer's warranty and make the facility rather than the manufacturer liable for any harm that occurs to a client.

OTHER AREAS OF LAW AFFECTING THE NURSE IN MATERNAL-NEWBORN PRACTICE

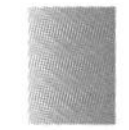

Consent to Research

Maternal-newborn nurses may become involved in research studies. Consent to research on human subjects, including pregnant women and fetuses that is funded by government funds must adhere to strict federal regulations (45 CFR Part 46 SS 2.01–2.11 [1993]). Researchers cannot be compelled in legal procedures to disclose identifying characteristics of research subjects (42 CFR Part 2a [1993]). However, research related to alcohol and drug abuse by policy requires notification of participants that child abuse and neglect are exceptions to the protection of confidentiality (personal communication, Lura Abbott, NIAAA, October 24, 1995). Many facilities regard these regulations as standards for research even though research may not be federally funded.

Just as consent is critical to procedures or treatments that put the client at a higher level of risk, so too is the consent process important in research. Of foremost importance is that the potential subject understand the consent process. Thus, nurses working on units where research is being done should become familiar with both the purposes of the research and consent processes.

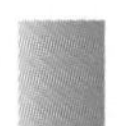

Confidentiality

Confidentiality is both a legal and an ethical concept. Confidentiality protects information provided by the client for the purposes of receiving care. Legally the nurse is not required to reveal information to another person if the law of a state regards information provided to the nurse as privileged. Some state statutes specifically mention nurses. Others mention only physicians. By case law some states protect nurses from revealing information when there is a close working relationship with physicians.

Persons bringing lawsuits in negligence waive their legal right to patient privilege. When admitted to a health care facility clients consent to care and agree that information regarding their care may be shared with hospital peer review committees and for other quality measures. Consent of the client is specifically required for release of records for treatment of alcohol and drug abuse (42 CFR Part 2) to any persons other than those holding the records. States may also have statutes requiring specific consent for release of mental health as well as alcohol and drug abuse records.

The ANA *Code* (1985) calls for the nurse to recognize her ethical responsibility to safeguard privacy rights of the client with the exception of situations where innocent persons are in danger. The advent of computerized data has potential for threatening the privacy of client records. Therefore, the professional nurse must carefully protect her personal password for entry of data. Nurse managers must participate with other administrative staff in assuring that computer networks are accessed only by designated personnel. Printed records should not be accessed by uninvolved health care personnel. Workplace verbal communication should carefully protect client information. Visitors should not overhear patient data or concerns.

CONFIDENTIALITY IN THE ELECTRONIC AGE

Paper health care records are usually relatively secure because of limited access. With the increasing use of computers and facsimile machines, electronic health care records are more readily available to health care providers and at the same time are more vulnerable to loss of patient confidentiality if the information is handled or transmitted improperly. Every health care agency should have information security policies in place that apply for all employees, medical staff members, students, volunteers, and others in the health care agency (AHIMA 1996).

To protect your patients from invasion of privacy as well as yourself from legal problems, know how to restrict access to on-line data and what information you are authorized to disclose. Also, never tell anyone your password or let anyone else use your password. This is for your protection as well as for your patients' protection. Many computer information systems keep a record of who accesses the database and when it is accessed. If someone uses your password to change a record or obtain information that is used inappropriately, you could be suspected of wrongdoing (Frawley 1994).

Procedures of Facsimile Transmission of Health Information

- Place fax machines in a secure, limited access area.
- Assign one individual to monitor all incoming faxes, which includes determining that all pages are included and are legible, sealing fax in an envelope, and sending them to the designated individual.
- Include a confidentiality notice on the cover sheet and the phone and fax numbers of the sender.
- Ask individuals to call to verify the fax was received, or call them to verify their receipt of the document.
- Establish the procedures to be followed if the fax is misdirected.

From American Health Information Management Association. (May 1994). Issue: Facsimile transmission of health information (position statement). Washington, D.C.: Author.

Facsimile transmission of health care records has great potential for breach of patient confidentiality either through a transmission error or if the information is available to unauthorized persons. The agency should have specific policies and procedures for transmitting and receiving faxes (see Procedures of Facsimile Transmission of Health Information). Facsimile transmission of an individual's health care records should be done only in situations where they are urgently needed for patient care or when required by a third-party payer for on-going certification for a hospitalized patient (AHIMA 1994).

If you receive facsimile transmission of physicians' orders for a patient or other information that should be a part of the patient's chart, always make a photocopy of documents that are on thermal paper before including the information in the patient's chart, because these faxes will fade with time. You should then destroy the original thermal paper document.

State law and institutional policies vary widely. Check with your supervisor or the agency's medical records department for guidelines on information disclosure (Frawley 1994). Also, the American Health Information Management Association in

Washington, D.C. has developed position papers and guidelines for electronic health care records (Frawley 1996).

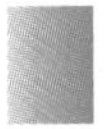

Licensure—Basic and Advanced Practice

Maternal-newborn care is an evolving area. Midwives are more frequently used. For normal pregnancies their outcomes are similar to obstetricians. At least one study has shown that with similar clients costs are less, interventions are fewer, and complications are fewer (Oakley 1994). These results have implications for changing the field of obstetrics in the future. Professional nurses on obstetrical units may find themselves collaborating with more midwives and fewer physicians. Already changes are occurring in nursing licensure laws.

In contrast to the practice of medicine where board certification recognizes specialty practice, state licensure laws are the legal vehicle for recognizing advanced practice in nursing care. Generally states accomplish distinction for this level of practice through title recognition or separate licensure. Midwifery is maternal-newborn nursing's advanced practice. Education, often coupled with certification, in midwifery leads to state recognition of advanced practice status (Pearson 1994).

Midwives who seek appointments and clinical privileges in health care facilities come under the purview of the Health Care Quality Improvement Act of 1986. Malpractice payments by them or on their behalf or actions against their licenses are placed in the National Practitioner Data Bank. Facilities must query this data base before granting privileges (Denega 1993).

In contrast to nurses licensed at the basic or generalist level, midwives conduct as well as monitor deliveries. Midwives would also be more skilled at identifying problems during labor. Thus, they are held to a higher standard of care. Unlike the nurses in the Berdyck case cited earlier, nurses licensed at the basic level must recognize the well known and major complications of pregnancy and delivery.

Maternal-newborn nurses should anticipate more professional accountability to clients across the continuum of care, increasing need to learn to maintain capability to deliver the current standard of care, and increasing delegation of care with concurrent responsibility for assuring maintenance of quality maternal-newborn nursing care.

Implications for Research

Risk management is a growing concern and an increasing area of practice for nurses. The best approach to legal and liability problems is prevention and expert clinical practice, which is the goal of risk management. Some of the questions that should be examined in this area include:

- What is the most effective risk-management program?
- What components of a risk management program are the most effective?
- What are the environmental, psychological, interactional, and physical factors that increase the risk of liability problems in the clinical setting?
- What modifications are effective in the clinical setting during time of high-risk in decreasing the incidence of liability problems?

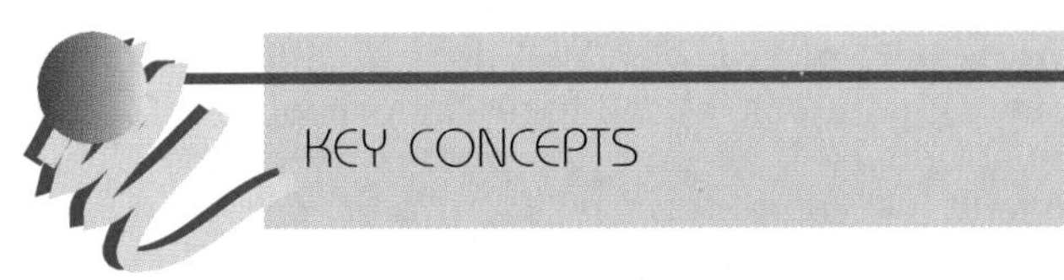

- ▼ The standard use for determining malpractice is what the ordinary, reasonable, prudent, professional nurse of similar education and experience would have done under similar circumstances.
- ▼ Expert witnesses must testify in malpractice cases as to whether the nursing standard of care was met.
- ▼ When the practice of a professional nurse is questioned in a lawsuit it is usually through a suit against his or her employer. Nurses may, however, also be sued individually.
- ▼ Hospitals are no longer covered under the concept of "charitable immunity" today in most states.
- ▼ Health care facilities are held legally accountable for the action of their employees under the concept of "respondeat superior" today.
- ▼ There are five elements of a case that must be documented before malpractice can be determined; existence of a duty, foreseeability of harm, breach of duty, causation, and injury or harm.
- ▼ The best prevention for malpractice is risk management, which includes staff education, development of procedures and policies, and continual review of standards of care.
- ▼ When the professional nurse expands her base of knowledge by becoming an advanced practice nurse, the nurse is held to a higher standard of care.

References

Albain v. Flower Hospital, 50 Ohio St.3d 251, 553 N.E.2d 1038 (1990).

Alvis v. Henderson, 592 N.E.2d 678 (Illinois, 1992).

American Health Information Management Association. (June 1996). Issue: Information security—an overview (practice brief). Washington, D.C.: Author.

American Health Information Management Association. (May 1994). Issue: Facsimile transmission of health information (position statement). Washington, D.C.: Author.

American Nurses Association. (1985). *Code for nurses with interpretive statements.* Washington, DC: Author.

Berdyck v. Shinde, 66 Ohio St.3d 573 (1993).

Blackwell, M. K. (1993). Documentation serves as invaluable defense tool. *The American Nurse,* July/August, 40–41.

Bonfield, T. (1995). Bill targets quickie deliveries: Tragedy, lawsuit follow one day hospital stay. *Cincinnati Enquirer,* November 15, Metro B-1.

Calfee, B. E. (1994). *Nurses in the courtroom.* Huntsburg, OH: ARC Publishing.

Campbell v. Pitt County Memory Hospital, Inc., 352 S.E.2d 902 (North Carolina, 1987).

29 CFR Part 1910 S 1910.30. Bloodborne pathogens (1995).

42 CFR Part 2 SS 2.1–2.67. Confidentiality of alcohol and drug abuse patient records (1993).

42 CFR Part 2a SS 2a.1–2a.8. Protection of identity of research subjects (1993).

45 CFR Part 46 Subpart B SS 46.201–211. Additional protections pertaining to research, development, and related activities involving fetuses, pregnant women, and human in vitro fertilization (1993).

Cohen, S. D. (1990). *Malpractice and liability in clinical obstetrical nursing.* Rockville, MD: Aspen.

Darling v. Charleston Community Memorial Hospital, 33 Ill.2d 326, 211 N.E.2d 253 (1965), cert. denied 383 U. S. 246 (1966).

Denega, D. (1993). National practitioner data bank impacts nursing practice, *The American Nurse,* July/August, 10.

Field, M. A. (1989). Controlling the woman to protect the fetus. *Law, Medicine & Health Care,* 17 (2), 114–129.

Frawley, K. A. (1994). Confidentiality in the computer age. *RN,* 57 (7), 59–60.

Frawley, K. A. (1996). Personal communication, Director, American Health Information Management Association, 1225 I Street. NW, Ste 500, Washington, DC 20005. Phone: (202) 218-3535, Fax (202) 682-0078.

Jeffers v. Olexo, 43 Ohio St.3d 140 (1989).

Joint Commission on Accreditation of Healthcare Organizations. (1995). *Accreditation manual for hospitals.* Chicago: Author.

Krauss, G. P. (1986). *Health care risk management: Organization and claims administration.* Owings Mills, MD: National Health Publishing.

Law Regulating the Practice of Nursing, Ohio Revised Code S 4723.28 (B) (18); Ohio Administrative Code SS 4723-4-01-05, 4723-13-01-10 (1995).

Nelson v. Trinity Medical Center, 419 N.W.2d 886 (North Dakota, 1988).

Newborns' and Mothers' Health Protection Act of 1996, S.969, 104th Cong., 2d Sess.

Oakley, D. (1994). Pathways to linking nursing research and health policy. Presentation at Health Policy Section Preconference of the Midwest Nursing Research Society, Milwaukee, WI.

Pearson, L. J. (1994). Annual update of how each state stands on legal issues affecting advanced nurse practice. *Nurse Practitioner,* 19 (1), 11–13, 17, 18, 21, 22, 24–27, 31–34, 39–40, 42–44, 50.

Planned Parenthood v. Casey, 505 U.S. 833, 112 S.Ct. 2791 (1992).

Selden, J. (1892). *Table talk* (p. 99). In *The Oxford Dictionary of Quotations* (2nd Ed.), 1955 (p 422). London, University Press.

8 Chapter

Ethical Issues in Maternal-Newborn Nursing

Rosemarie DiMauro Satyshur
Francine H. Nichols

> My heart ached and my mind questioned, "Why" as I watched the doctors working feverishly over the tiny limp, lifeless bit of humanity that was hardly bigger than my hand. His eyes were still fused. There were tubes coming from every part of his body. His heart rate was irregular. The ventilator breathed for him. An overwhelming feeling of anguish and anger welled up inside of me. I wanted to scream, "Let him go. Let him die in peace!"
>
> Anonymous Neonatal Nurse

HIGHLIGHTS

- ▼ Values Clarification for Ethical Decision Making
- ▼ Framework for Ethics
- ▼ Impact of Ethics on Maternal-Newborn Nursing Practice
- ▼ Ethical Considerations in Assisted Reproduction
- ▼ Ethical Considerations in Amniocentesis and Chorionic Villus Sampling
- ▼ Ethical Considerations in Abortion
- ▼ Ethical Considerations in Embryo Research
- ▼ Ethical Considerations for the Fetus and Neonate
- ▼ Implications for Research

Ethical foundations underlie all of nursing practice. Nurses as client advocates have an obligation to act in a morally appropriate manner and to avoid harm to those they care for. Maternal-newborn nurses are confronted regularly by ethical decision making and the prevention and resolution of ethical dilemmas in clinical practice. Conflict arises in the independent and collaborative domains of practice as nurses consider their professional commitment and responsibility to the physician, client, and the family. Maternal-newborn nurses are more likely to be challenged by situations in which the interests of one family member are in opposition to those of another. Genetic engineering, artificial insemination, in vitro fertilization, abortion, fetal experimentation, fetal surgery, neonatal intensive care, and care of the mother or infant with acquired immunodeficiency syndrome (AIDS) are just a few areas that maternal-newborn nurses encounter in their practice. Nurses must clarify their personal values and religious beliefs in order to assist clients in reaching decisions through listening supportively, providing accurate and up-to-date information, and helping the family to clarify their personal values.

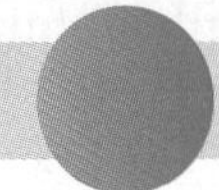

DEFINITIONS

Aggressive treatment—Using all means of treatment available when the outcome of the individual appears hopeless.

Amniocentesis—The process in which amniotic fluid is removed through a needle inserted into the amniotic sac. The fluid can be used to determine fetal maturity and fetal health.

Anencephalic—The condition of having no encephalon or brain.

Artificial insemination—Placement of one or more semen samples, produced by the husband or a donor, in the vagina, cervical canal, or uterus of a woman by artificial means such as a syringe.

Chorionic villus sampling (CVS)—A technique for the diagnosis of genetic disorders in which chorionic villi from the placenta are aspirated and examined.

Code of ethics—An ethical document that contains general principles of appropriate behavior.

Ethics—A philosophy of moral behavior that deals with basic questions of meaning and value.

Ethical decision making—The process of resolving an ethical dilemma through critical and systematic analyses, using the principles of ethics to reach a decision about what it is morally right to do in the situation.

Ethical dilemma—A difficult situation in which there are conflicting values, obligations, or principles about resolution.

Morals—A code of behavior established by traditions or societal norms.

Patient's rights—The rights of the patient to informed, safe, competent, confidential, and considerate care.

Principles of ethics—A set of rules that can be universally applied to all situations. They provide a framework by which values, morals, beliefs, and attitudes may be identified, ethical dilemmas examined and clarified, and obligations ordered in terms of their precedence.

Surrogate parenthood—The contractual hiring of a woman by a couple to bear their child for a fee.

Values clarification—The process of examining and clarifying one's values.

BUILDING BLOCKS FOR ETHICAL DECISION MAKING

Values Clarification

In order to coexist in a helping relationship with clients, nurses need to develop a high level of self-awareness. They should be in touch with their own values and act in accord. Values are developed as part of one's self-identity early on. Value systems represent one's attitudes, beliefs, and moral judgments and are influenced by families, religions, educators, peers, and society as a whole. Uustal (1978) defined "values [as] general guides to behavior, standards of conduct that one endorses and tries to live up to or maintain." Values are freely and thoughtfully chosen and are prized and acted on (Uustal 1985).

Values held by nurses often have a profound effect on the care given to clients. Nurses need to recognize their feelings regarding alternatives in client care. Values clarification is the intense and ongoing process that allows nurses to identify and analyze their personal and professional values, leading to a better understanding of self (Steele and Harmon 1983). Values clarification exercises are a beginning exploration in ethical decision making. Nurses learn to rank and prioritize their values and can discuss and compare them with the values of colleagues. The group can then reach an understanding of each other's beliefs. Peer discussions concerning professional values are essential to nurses as they face ethical dilemmas in practice.

Framework for Ethics

Ethics is defined as a philosophy of moral behavior (Mappes and Zembaty 1986) that deals with basic questions of meaning and value (Veatch 1989). While the term ethics is often used interchangeably with the term morals, they are distinctly different. Ethics is a broad, general term that denotes an area of intellectual contemplation and reflection about a situation beyond what may be acceptable by society. Morals refer to codes of behavior established by traditions or societal norms (Beauchamp and Walters 1982).

PRINCIPLE OF ETHICS

The foundation of ethical decision making is provided by the principles of ethics, a set of rules

ETHICAL DECISION MAKING

Nurses employed in a maternal-newborn setting find many situations that embody the need to resolve conflicting values. A regular part of this special practice involves ethical dilemmas and ethical decision making. In order to fully consider ethical issues in light of their practice and to facilitate an environment in which clients and peers can participate in the decision process, nurses need to engage in the following:

- IDENTIFY ATTITUDES, VALUES, AND BELIEFS ABOUT ETHICAL DILEMMAS IN MATERNAL-NEWBORN NURSING, recognizing the influence of cultural, religious, and social considerations on the development of values.
- ENGAGE IN SELF-VALUES CLARIFICATION ACTIVITIES WITH PEERS. Recognize the influence your values have on the care you provide for clients.
- REVIEW AND UPDATE THEORETIC BASES; gather current information on technologic advances in maternal-newborn nursing and changing trends; review ethical principles and practice codes in regard to new technology; read lay literature related to maternal-newborn advances to be familiar with the client's knowledge base.
- ATTEND CONTINUING EDUCATION PROGRAMS related to ethical issues and decision making; participate in ethics committees with other health care professionals and inservice peers.
- REVIEW RESEARCH JOURNALS regarding current trends in ethical decision making by parents and nurses as well as other health professionals; compare and contrast the results of these studies with what is occurring in clinical practice.
- EVALUATE CURRENT SOCIAL NORMS; follow up on current social, legal, religious, and political debates that may influence clinical decision making and quality care for clients experiencing dilemmas.
- AVOID JUDGMENTS ABOUT THE LIFE DECISIONS OF OTHERS; aim to be accepting of the values of others and their decisions regarding issues and provisions of care; do not allow your personal beliefs and values to interfere with the provision of quality care.

that can be universally applied to all situations. Various ethical principles are defined in Table 8–1. They provide a framework in which values, morals, beliefs, and attitudes may be identified; ethical dilemmas examined and clarified; and obligations ordered in terms of precedence (Penticuff 1992).

Table 8–1

DEFINITIONS OF THE PRINCIPLES OF ETHICS

ETHICAL PRINCIPLE	DEFINITION
Beneficence	Duty to do good
Nonmaleficence	Duty to do no harm
Veracity	Duty to tell the truth
Justice	Equitable distribution of risks and benefits
Fidelity	Duty to keep one's promise or word
Reparation	Duty to make up for a wrong
Gratitude	Duty to make up for a good
Autonomy	Being one's own person without constraints by another's action or psychological and physical limitations
Informed consent	Contains four elements: Disclosure of information, comprehension, voluntary agreement, competency to make decision
Confidentiality	Holding information entrusted in context of special relationships as private
Utility	Greatest good or least harm for the greatest number
Universality	Same principle must hold for everyone, regardless of time, place, or persons involved
Generality	Must not refer to specific people or situations
Finality	May override demands of law or custom
Publicity	Principles must be known and recognized by all
Ordering	Ethical principles must be prioritized even though they may be conflicting

From Gilbert, E., and Harmon, J. (1993). *Manual of high risk pregnancy* (p. 154). St. Louis: Mosby-Year Book.

NURSING CODES OF ETHICS

Since the beginning of nursing, ethical principles have formed a foundation for nursing practice. The principles of doing good, avoiding harm, respecting the rights of others, and treating all people fairly underlie the tradition of nursing through the ages. The Florence Nightingale pledge, written in 1893, clearly points out the obligations of the nurse to the patient and to the profession of nursing (Gretter 1956) (Table 8–2).

In 1903 Isabel Hampton Robb's textbook, *Nursing Ethics,* was published (Robb 1903). In her textbook, Robb, an eloquent advocate for the profession of nursing, examined the beliefs, values, and obligations or duties of the nurse along with the ethical conflicts that are inherent in nursing practice. The International Council of Nurses Pledge; *Nursing: A Social Policy Statement,* first published in 1980 by the American Nurses Association; and the American Nurses Association Code for Nurses (Table 8–3) all identify ethical nursing behaviors.

PATIENTS' RIGHTS

The professional nurse's responsibility is to help ensure that the basic rights of clients are protected. The National League of Nursing first discussed patients' rights in a 1959 position statement. Fourteen years later, patients' rights were given serious thought by other health professionals (Ellis and Hartley 1989). The American Hospital Association published its official statement, "A Patient's Bill of Rights," in 1973. This statement identified ethical commitment to informed, safe, competent, confidential, and considerate care for all patients.

In 1975, the International Childbirth Education Association adapted "A Patient's Bill of Rights" and presented "The Pregnant Patient's Bill of Rights." This document ensures the pregnant patient of the right to all information about decisions that affect her health, the health of the unborn, or both. The pregnant patient also has the right to participate in all decision making unless medical emergency prevents her from doing so. Appendix IV contains a complete copy of

Table 8–2

THE FLORENCE NIGHTINGALE PLEDGE

I solemnly pledge myself before and in the presence of this assembly, to pass my life in purity and to practice my profession faithfully.

I will abstain from whatever is deleterious and mischievous, and will not take or knowingly administer any harmful drug.

I will do all in my power to maintain and elevate the standard of my profession; and will hold in confidence all personal matters committed to my keeping, and all family affairs coming to my knowledge in the practice of my calling.

With loyalty will I endeavor to aid the physician in this work and devote myself to the welfare of those committed to my care.

From Gretter, L. (1956). The Florence Nightingale pledge. In L. R. Seymer (Ed.). *A general history of nursing* (4th ed., p. 317). New York: MacMillan.

Table 8–3

AMERICAN NURSES ASSOCIATION CODE FOR NURSES

1. The nurse provides services with respect for human dignity and the uniqueness of the client, unrestricted by considerations of social or economic status, personal attributes, or the nature of health problems.
2. The nurse safeguards the client's right to privacy by judiciously protecting information of a confidential nature.
3. The nurse acts to safeguard the client and public when health care and safety are affected by the incompetent, unethical, or illegal practices of any person.
4. The nurse assumes responsibility and accountability for individual nursing judgments and actions.
5. The nurse maintains competence in nursing.
6. The nurse exercises informed judgment and uses individual competence and qualifications as criteria in seeking consultation, accepting responsibilities, and delegating nursing activities to others.
7. The nurse participates in activities that contribute to the ongoing development of the professional body of knowledge.
8. The nurse participates in the profession's efforts to implement and improve standards of nursing.
9. The nurse participates in the profession's efforts to establish and maintain conditions of employment conducive to high-quality nursing care.
10. The nurse participates in the profession's effort to protect the public from misinformation and misrepresentation and to maintain the integrity of nursing.
11. The nurse collaborates with members of the health professions and other citizens in promoting community and national efforts to meet the health needs of the public.

From American Nurses Association. (1985). *Code for Nurses with Interpretive Statements.* Washington, DC: Author.

"The Pregnant Patient's Bill of Rights and Responsibilities."

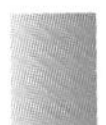

Ethical Decision Making

Maternal-newborn nurses are faced with ethical dilemmas as part of daily practice. The nurse needs to learn to recognize ethical dilemmas that interfere with clients' rights and participation in decision making.

An ethical dilemma can be defined as an inherently difficult situation in which there exist conflicting values, obligations, or principles related to the "right" course of action (Davis and Aroskar 1985). In an ethical dilemma there is no solution; a choice exists between equally unfavorable options (Nosek 1988; Uustal 1985). Ethical decision making is the process of resolving dilemmas through critical and systematic analyses that assist in leading to a decision that will be in the best interest of the client or clients (Fig. 8–1).

Many models exist for ethical decision making based on problem solving (Omery 1989). Thompson and Thompson (1985) and Pellegrino (1987) present a ten-step clinical ethical framework to guide nurses in the process of making ethical decisions in perinatal care (Fig. 8–2). This is a flexible framework, including all relevant medical and nursing care information, knowledge of the pregnant patient's and family's ethical beliefs, treatment preferences, and legal factors, which facilitates a morally justifiable and ethical decision.

ETHICAL ADVISORY COMMITTEES

Over the past two decades, hospital-wide deliberation on ethical decision making regarding complexities in care has become common. Committees examine and clarify moral and ethical concerns. They do not relieve the nurse of the responsibility for moral and ethical reflection. However, they can assist in educating staff, clients, and families about ethical care aspects and values clarification. These committees should consist of representatives with a variety of backgrounds and expertise who are educated and/or have broad experience in ethical decision making. Nursing input is critical, since the nurse spends more time with the client and family than any other health care profes-

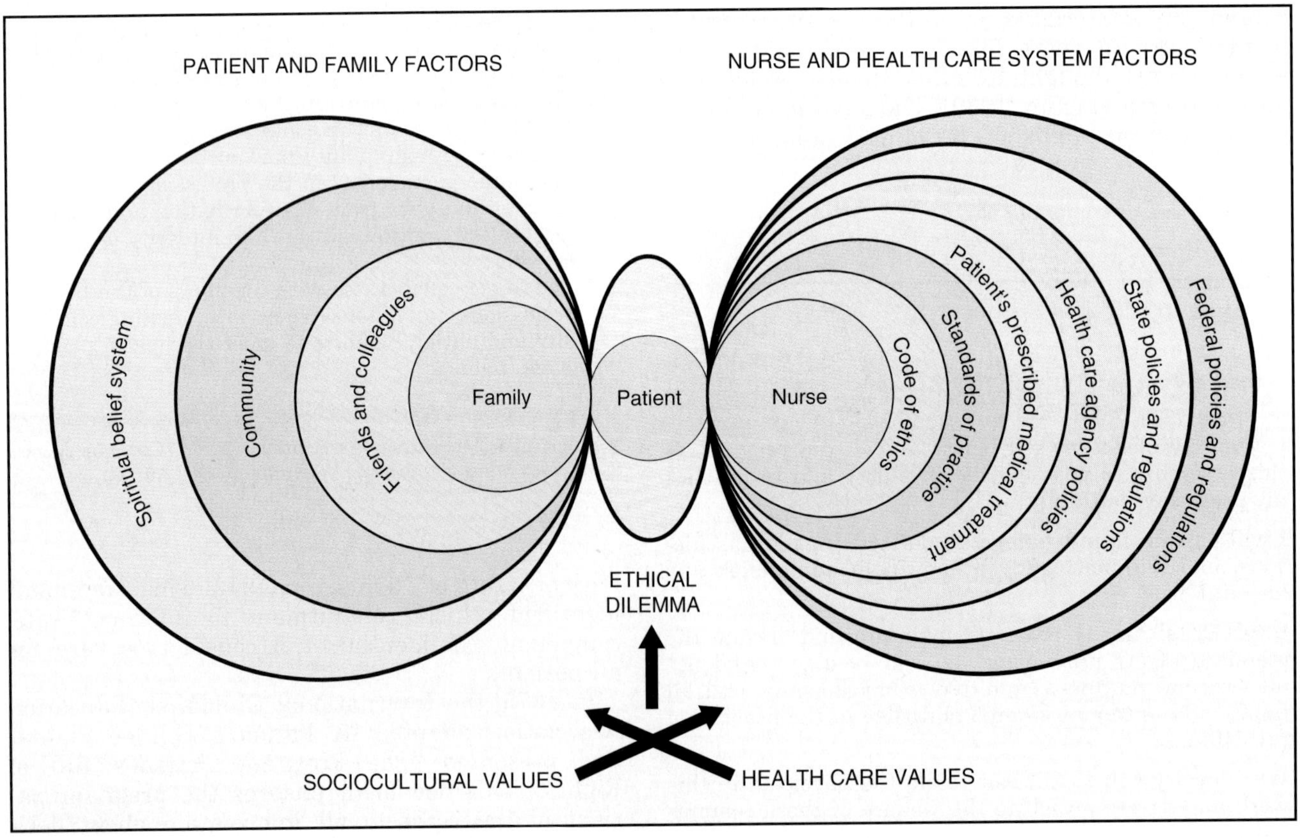

Figure 8–1

An ethical dilemma exists when there are conflicting values, obligations, or principles about the "right" course of action • When sociocultural values of the patient and family and health care values of the nurse and health care system conflict, there is an ethical dilemma. (Zaner, R. M. *Ethics and the Clinical Encounter,* © 1988, p. 35. Adapted by permission of Prentice Hall, Upper Saddle River, New Jersey.)

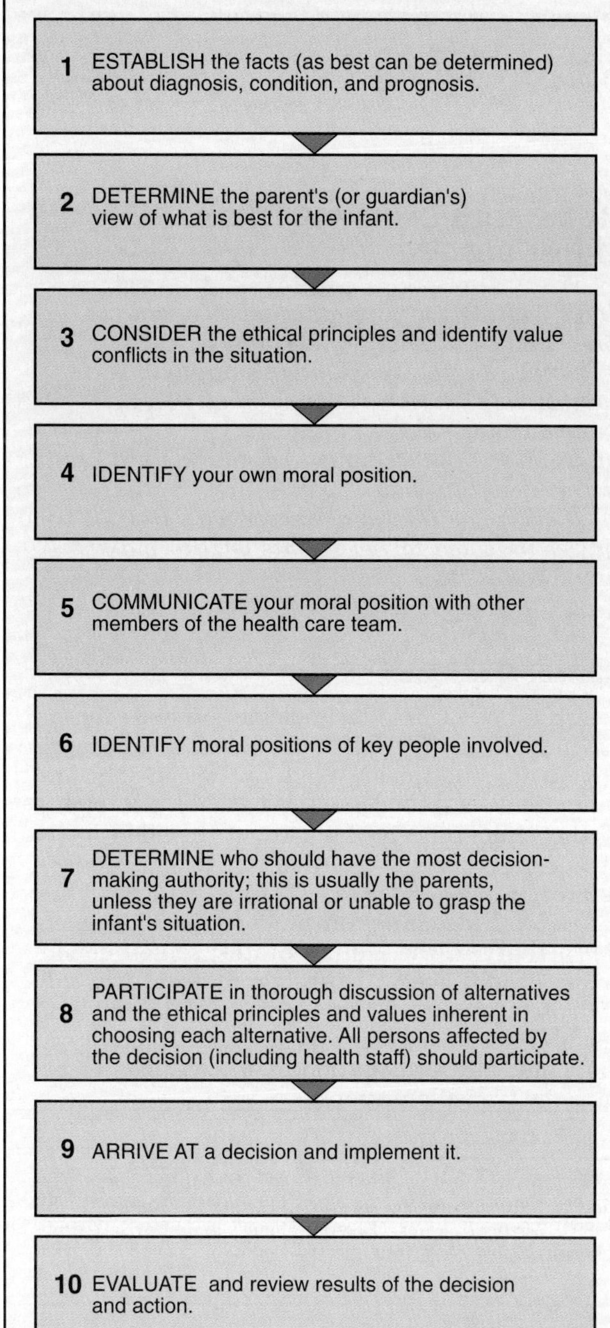

Figure 8–2

Perinatal-bioethical model for ethical decision making. (Adapted from Penticuff, J. H. [1992]. Ethical issues. In P. Beachy and J. Deacon [Eds.]. *Core curriculum for neonatal intensive care nursing* [p. 666]. Philadelphia: W. B. Saunders.)

sional. The nurse, as a member of the ethics committee, can communicate valuable information regarding the views and beliefs of the client and family (Murphy 1989).

ETHICAL CONSIDERATIONS THAT IMPACT MATERNAL-NEWBORN NURSING PRACTICE

Ethical Considerations in Assisted Reproduction

Today, for a variety of reasons, many couples are unable to achieve pregnancy. Advances in biomedical technology offer infertile couples methods of reproduction without intercourse. These methods include artificial insemination (with husband or donor sperm), in vitro fertilization, and embryo transfer. There has been limited success with these methods of assisted reproduction over the past decade, with attendant ethical controversy (Annas 1984; Williams 1988). Proponents defend assisted reproduction as life offering; it is denounced as unnatural by its detractors (Annas 1984).

Additional concern has been raised about assisted reproduction because it may extend to include third-party donors and surrogate mothers and because it has the potential for use in eugenics research (Abramowitz 1984; Gersz 1984).

ARTIFICIAL INSEMINATION

Artificial insemination is performed by one of two methods. The wife may be inseminated with her husband's sperm through a mechanical procedure (i.e., use of a syringe) within her vagina, cervical os, or uterus. This method generally does not raise serious ethical inquiry.

However, in cases in which the husband has a serious genetic disease or absence of sperm, insemination can be accomplished by the use of donor sperm. This method raises various ethical questions, since the donor or genetic father is not the husband and legal father of the offspring.

IN VITRO FERTILIZATION

In vitro fertilization is a method of medically assisted reproduction for women with nonpatent, diseased, or missing fallopian tubes or with infertility of an unknown etiology. Donor semen can also be employed in cases of male sterility, low sperm count, or genetic defect (Holmes 1988).

Ova and sperm are collected from potential parents or donors, placed in a nutrient medium, and allowed to incubate, and then the fertilized ovum is transferred into the woman's uterus. The

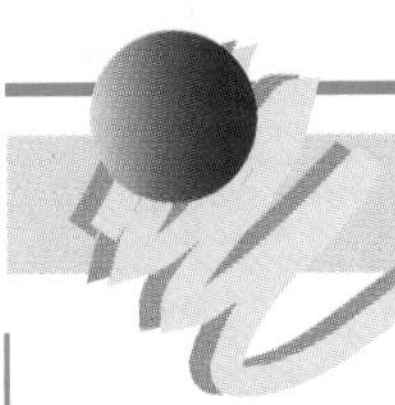

CRITICAL THINKING CASE HISTORY

ETHICAL DILEMMA: IS THE USE OF NEW TECHNOLOGIC METHODS OF REPRODUCTION JUSTIFIABLE?—THE CASE OF HANNAH AND HER "TEST-TUBE DADDY"

Hannah's mother had always planned on getting married and having children some day. Suddenly, it was her 35th birthday, and marriage seemed a remote possibility. She felt that "giving up on the idea of a loving husband was painful, but possible; considering a life without a child was impossible." After considering her options, Hannah's mother, who was financially secure and well established in a satisfying career, opted for artificial insemination by a donor.

Hannah's mother carefully studied the list of sperm donors at the fertility clinic. She finally decided that she "wanted a donor who could give my child all the physical characteristics I could not—long legs, a tall slender body, and good eyesight."

After five unsuccessful attempts, Hannah's mother became pregnant and Hannah, a healthy baby girl, was born. Hannah and her mother live in a brick house with a large, fenced backyard, and Hannah is part of a neighborhood play group for toddlers. Hannah's mother declares, "My baby might not have a father, but she will have all the trappings of a traditional home." Hannah and her mother are surrounded by loving family and caring friends. Hannah's mother expresses her feelings about having a baby by donor artificial insemination as follows:

'Da' was Hannah's first and favorite sound. When she said it at 9 months in the pediatrician's waiting room, another mother told me, 'She must be thinking of her daddy.'

Frankly, I doubt it. Hannah's daddy has a number, not a name. He is number 741, an anonymous Los Angeles law student who was paid $50 to produce the sperm that helped create my beautiful baby.

I don't know him and I never will. But I'll be forever indebted to 741 for his part in making Hannah possible.

Ethical Questions

Is the use of new technologic methods for reproduction justified? If it is, are they appropriate in all situations? What are the rights and obligations of the donor? What are the rights of the child conceived to know the identity of his or her biological father or to the donor's estate?

Artificial insemination by donor is a commercial activity in the United States; semen donors are paid and sperm banks profit from the sale of frozen semen. Should semen donation and distribution be a voluntary, nonprofit activity in the same way as donation of whole blood or organs for transplantation?

Data from Abrams, T. (1994). My test-tube daddy. *The Washingtonian,* March, 44–48, 114, and Veatch, R. M. (1989). *Medical ethics.* Boston: Jones and Bartlett Publishers.

woman houses the pregnancy throughout gestation and gives birth. Ethical questions concern the moral status of the fetus, allocation of funds and cost, and long-term complications and risks. Ethical concerns regarding in vitro fertilization and embryo transfer continue to increase as the demands for the procedure grow.

SURROGATE PARENTHOOD

The contractual hiring of a woman by a couple to bear their child for a fee is controversial. It is considered dehumanizing to the child and exploitative of the woman by opponents (Annas 1984). It is viewed as a technologic miracle by others who support this method of having a baby. Other ethical problems can arise in the event that the child is born with a defect and is unwanted by both the adoptive parents and the surrogate mother (Furrow 1984). The use of a surrogate mother involves a highly complex process and may involve a stressful relationship with potentially negative effects. This has been documented when things did not go as planned or the parties were emotionally unstable.

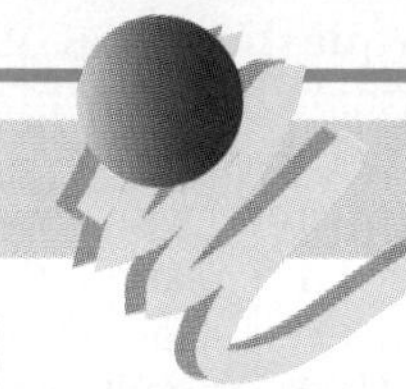

CRITICAL THINKING CASE HISTORY

ETHICAL DILEMMA: WHOSE CHILD IS IT?—THE CASE OF BABY M

William Stern, a biochemist, and Elizabeth Stern, a physician with a Ph.D. in genetics, were well-educated, financially secure professionals. Married in 1974, they had delayed having children while they established their careers. Later, when Elizabeth Stern was diagnosed with multiple sclerosis, they feared that pregnancy would be too risky for her and they asked the Infertility Center of New York (ICNY) about a surrogate mother.

In 1985, William Stern signed an agreement for surrogate motherhood through the ICNY with Mary Beth Whitehead and Richard Whitehead. The surrogate mother would relinquish all rights to the child after birth, and Elizabeth Stern would adopt the child. The ICNY received a fee of $7500 for recruiting the surrogate mother and facilitating the contracts. All of Mary Beth Whitehead's expenses related to the pregnancy were paid by the Sterns, and she also received $10,000 from them.

After nine artificial insemination attempts using Mr. Stern's sperm, Ms. Whitehead became pregnant and delivered a healthy baby girl on March 27, 1986. Shortly after the baby's birth, Ms. Whitehead decided that she could not give the baby up.

Mary Beth Whitehead left the hospital with the infant on March 30, 1986. The Sterns went to the Whiteheads' home later that day, recovered the baby, and took her to their home. From that time on, for nearly 2 years, the Sterns and Whiteheads battled in court over who should have custody of "Baby M." In April 1987, four days after Baby M's first birthday, the New Jersey Superior Court for Bergen County awarded Mr. Stern permanent custody of Baby M, severed all of Mary Beth Whitehead's parental rights, and processed Baby M's adoption, in which Elizabeth Stern became the child's legal mother. The Whiteheads appealed the court's decision.

In February 1988, the New Jersey Supreme Court reversed the lower court's decision to sever all of Mary Beth Whitehead's parental rights to Baby M. While Mr. Stern was allowed to retain custody of Baby M, her birth mother remained her legal mother and was allowed weekly visitation rights.

In 1996 Baby M was 10 years old. Called "Melissa" by the Sterns and "Sara" by her legal mother, Mary Beth Gould (formerly Whitehead), the child refers to herself as "Sassy." She lives with the Sterns in New Jersey most of the year. She spends every other weekend and 2 weeks in the summer with Mary Beth Gould and her four children on Long Island.

Ethical Questions

Integral to the surrogate parenthood relationship: when a contract is not honored as agreed on, who should have parental rights? In addition, should the adopting couple be able to control the lifestyle of the surrogate mother during pregnancy? If they should, to what extent? Should the adoptive parents be obligated to accept the child if he or she is born with a physical or mental handicap?

Data from Alpern, K. D. (1992). *The ethics of reproductive technology* (pp. 317–334). New York: Oxford University Press; Butzel, H. M. (1987). The essential facts of the Baby M case. In H. Richardson (Ed.). *On the problem of surrogate parenthood* (pp. 7–20). Lewiston, NY: The Edwin Mellen Press; Colen, B. D. (1994). Whatever happened to baby Jane Doe? *Neonatal Intensive Care,* 7 (5), 40; Walters, L. (1989). Genetics and reproductive technologies. In R. M. Veatch (Ed.). *Medical ethics* (pp. 201–228). Boston: Jones and Bartlett Publishers.

Amniocentesis and Chorionic Villus Sampling

Mothers at high risk for fetal disorders that can be identified by amniocentesis or chorionic villus sampling (CVS) must be informed of the availability of these tests along with their risks and benefits. Amniocentesis is most commonly performed near the 16th week of gestation. In cases in which the mother might be considering early termination of pregnancy, this test enables her to consider whether to do so before the age of viability

(22 weeks of gestation). Chorionic villus sampling can establish the existence of some congenital conditions at approximately 8 to 10 weeks of gestation.

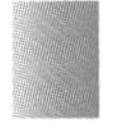

Ethical Considerations in Abortion

Nurses are involved in counseling or caring for clients experiencing abortion. They may care for the client before and after the procedure even if they have refused an assignment to provide care for the client during the procedure. It is of utmost importance that nurses engage in values clarification activities and determine their ethical position on abortion in order to ensure the delivery of quality care for these clients (Cohen 1988).

Heated opposition based on ethical considerations remains between groups that support and groups that oppose abortion in the United States. Abortion removes the fetus from the woman's uterus and results in termination of the fetal life. Supporters believe that a woman has freedom of choice and the right to privacy. She has the ultimate responsibility for making decisions regarding her body. This does not necessarily mean that supporters are pro-abortion. Many proponents profess the use of abortion as a last resort with the responsible use of contraception, amniocentesis, and adoption to be considered whenever possible.

Groups that oppose abortion believe that the fetus is human from the point of conception and should be protected. Other ethical questions are raised by technologic advances in contraception (Norplant) and agents that prevent implantation (RU 486). The issue of abortion forces the nurse to consider many unsolved ethical dilemmas encountered in maternal-newborn nursing practice.

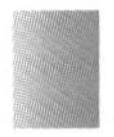

Embryo Research

Embryo research was forbidden by the pro-life Reagan and Bush administrations. During those years, scientists could only marvel at the complex drama of conception and development. In 1993, President Clinton asked the National Institutes of Health (NIH) to develop guidelines for research in this area.

Proponents argue that the findings of such research could lead to new treatments for infertility, disease, and aging. Opponents claim that embryo research raises the same ethical question that is at the center of the abortion debate: "When do life and human rights begin?" (Gorman 1994).

An expert NIH advisory committee was appointed in early 1994 and debated the issues related to and details of embryo research. Sensitive to the ethical concerns involved, their report, *Final Report of the NIH Human Embryo Research Panel,* released in September 1994, recommended "stringent guidelines" for embryo research (NIH Expert Panel 1994). The panel concluded that certain areas of research, approved on a case-by-case basis, involving the "preimplantation human embryo" were acceptable. The panel defined the preimplantation human embryo as "a fertilized ovum in vitro that has never been transferred or implanted in a uterus." With one exception, for research specifically conducted to identify the appearance of the primitive streak, the panel recommended that embryo research not be permitted beyond 14 days, which is the time of the usual appearance of the primitive streak in vivo. The report also includes examples of "acceptable" and "unacceptable" research. One can expect debate on this issue by both supporters and opponents of the NIH recommendations to be loud and continuing.

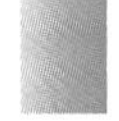

Ethical Consideration for the Fetus

It has been determined that the fetus has rights from the moment of conception. With technologic advances, professionals are maintaining fetuses at earlier and earlier gestational ages. Nurses, parents, and other health care providers are faced with the question of whether aggressive treatment is appropriate for the fetus and what kind of treatment is in the best interest of the fetus and the family.

FETAL TISSUE TRANSPLANTATION

Technical advances and current research have led to the suggestion that transplantation of fetal tissue into adults with neurologic or metabolic disease holds the promise of rehabilitation and recovery. The ethics of fetal tissue transplantation has fueled several heated questions for debate (Fine 1988). Who has the right to determine what is done with fetal remains? Does the mother who anticipates an abortion have the right to allow experimentation in vitro? Can an aborted fetus be kept alive for experimental use? It is important that no mother who is weighing the decision to have an abortion be pressured for the use of fetal tissue (Council on Scientific Affairs 1990).

FETAL RIGHTS VERSUS MATERNAL RIGHTS

Fetuses that would have died while in utero or shortly after birth are now being treated with medical and surgical interventions in utero (Harrison et al. 1981). Interventions during childbirth to improve outcomes for the mother and her infant are also commonplace today. Ethical conflicts can emerge in situations in which the mother refuses to consent to medical or surgical intervention for the fetus or herself. Is this fetal abuse by the mother? What is the mother's right to make decisions concerning her body and her right to autonomy? As technology and expertise continue to develop in fetal and maternal treatment, ethical issues will continue to increase in maternal-newborn nursing practice.

Ethical Consideration for the Neonate

Neonatal intensive care nurses uphold the values of "preserving life, decreasing morbidity, and relieving pain and suffering" for the infant (Sandling et al. 1993). The neonate has no choice in deciding for or against treatment or the continuation of treatment. Deciding on treatment or continuation of treatment for the neonate may be difficult, especially when the benefit is unclear or the situation appears hopeless. What role does the health professional have in decision making? How much and what type of care should the nurse provide to ensure the infant has a comfortable and dignified death? Society as a whole must make further provision for the neonate who survives aggressive technology with disability or impairment and for respite measures for their families (Fig. 8–3). It is particularly important that nurses understand that their values as well as the medical data influence clinical decision making in the care of compromised neonates.

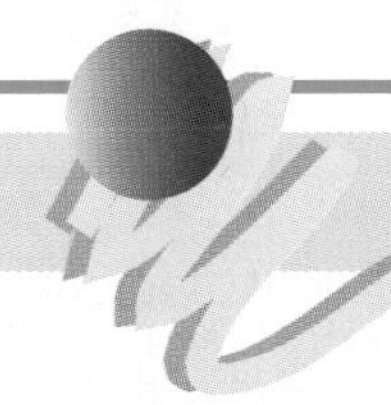

CRITICAL THINKING CASE HISTORY

ETHICAL DILEMMA: DOES A WOMAN HAVE THE RIGHT TO REFUSE A "LIFESAVING" CESAREAN? —THE CASE OF MARYAM

Maryam, a 34-year-old Iranian woman, gravida 6, para 4, was 39 weeks pregnant when she was admitted to the labor and delivery unit in active labor. Late decelerations indicating fetal distress were noted on the fetal monitor strip. A vaginal examination revealed that Maryam was 7 cm dilated and the presenting part of the fetus was an elbow. A transverse lie was confirmed by ultrasonography. The obstetrician advised Maryam and her husband that an immediate cesarean section was necessary for the baby's safety. The couple was also informed that delaying cesarean would result in the baby having increased distress and Maryam having uterine rupture and maternal hemorrhage.

Maryam and her husband "adamantly refused" the cesarean and insisted that the obstetrician "reach up and turn the baby around." Maryam kept crying, "No C-section, no C-section." The physician explained to the couple that he could not turn the baby and emphasized the need for an immediate cesarean section; then he ordered the nurse to take Maryam to the surgical suite for the operation. As Maryam was taken in her bed to the operating room, her cries of "No C-section, no C-section, please, no C-section" echoed through the halls.

Ethical Questions

Does a pregnant woman have the right to refuse treatment that may benefit her fetus or herself? Which is more important, maternal autonomy or fetal welfare? How much risk should the mother be asked to assume in order to benefit her fetus? Does the health care practitioner have the right to override maternal decisions regarding refusal of health care?

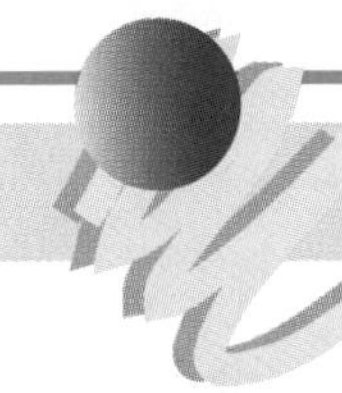

CRITICAL THINKING CASE HISTORY

ETHICAL DILEMMA: SHOULD LIFE SUPPORT TREATMENT BE USED FOR ANENCEPHALIC NEWBORNS?—THE CASE OF BABY K

In October 1992, Baby K, an anencephalic infant, was born to a single mother in a Virginia hospital. Because of her religious convictions, Baby K's mother had refused an abortion when she was informed of the diagnosis of anencephaly. The mother believed that "her daughter's life had value and that God, not humans, should decide the moment of the infant's death." Before Baby K's birth, the mother requested that the baby be treated aggressively. Baby K's father showed little interest in the child; his preference was not to use aggressive treatment and to allow the child to die.

Baby K was delivered by cesarean section and intubated at birth. Her mother consistently refused to agree to a do-not-resuscitate (DNR) order or the provision of only palliative care in response to repeated urging to do so from those treating the baby. The bioethics committee of the hospital recommended that aggressive treatment be discontinued and that if Baby K's mother would not agree, a court order be obtained.

Baby K's mother contacted Rights of Virginians with Disabilities, a state agency. The agency informed the hospital of its concerns that "the hospital might be violating state or federal antidiscrimination statutes or medical neglect statutes."

Baby K was eventually weaned from the ventilator and transferred to a nursing home, with her mother's permission. However, her mother insisted that if the infant had problems, she be readmitted for emergency treatment. In April 1993, during the infant's third readmission to the hospital for respiratory problems, a tracheostomy was performed and she was transferred back to the nursing home.

Soon after Baby K's return to the nursing home, the hospital filed a request in federal court that a guardian be appointed for Baby K and that the hospital be allowed to refuse to provide anything but "comfort" care. The court appointed a guardian for Baby K, and he agreed to the termination of aggressive treatment.

In response, both the U. S. District Court for the Eastern District of Virginia and the U. S. Court of Appeals for the Fourth Circuit found that a refusal to treat Baby K aggressively would be a violation of the Federal Medical Treatment and Active Labor Act of 1992. Also, the lower court informed the hospital that, based on the Federal Rehabilitation Act of 1973 and the Americans with Disabilities Act of 1990, the hospital was obligated to provide the infant with "full medical care as long as such care was requested by her mother." In the spring of 1995 Baby K was rushed to the hospital for the sixth—and final—time. She died 30 minutes later as a result of cardiac arrest.

Ethical Questions

What is the appropriate treatment for an anencephalic newborn? What constitutes a living person? Should terminating human life be based on the individual's capacity for achieving conscious thought? Is an anencephalic newborn clinically "dead" or an impaired newborn? Who has the right to decide whether Baby K should be kept alive? Her mother? Her physician and the hospital? Or the courts and society?

The role of a bioethics committee is to examine the moral and ethical concerns in a case and to encourage discussion and value clarification. In Baby K's case, the bioethics committee recommended court action to force the mother to comply with the treatment approach that the hospital thought was best. Was that action appropriate?

Adapted from Fry-Revere, S. (1994). Anencephalic newborns: Legal and ethical comments regarding the matter of baby "K." *Neonatal Intensive Care,* 7 (5), 36–39. Data from Tousignant, M. and Miller, B. Death of 'Baby K' leaves a legacy of legal precedents. *The Washington Post,* April 7, 1995, p. B3.

Continued on facing page

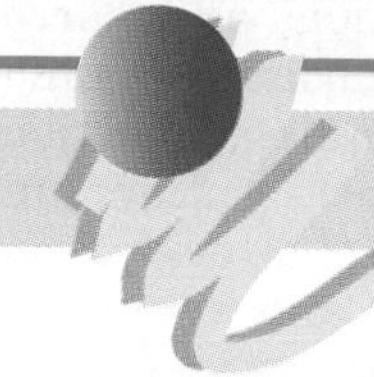

CRITICAL THINKING CASE HISTORY Continued

ETHICAL DILEMMA: SHOULD SOCIETY SPEND LARGE SUMS OF MONEY TO TREAT INFANTS WHEN THE OUTCOME APPEARS HOPELESS?—THE CASE OF THE LAKEBERG CONJOINED TWINS

Amy and Angela Lakeberg, conjoined twins (commonly called Siamese twins), were born joined together from the lower chest to midabdomen. They shared a six-chambered heart and a fused liver. Although the twins' shared liver could be divided, their heart had major defects. The physicians' initial recommendation to the twins' parents was that the babies be taken off the ventilators and allowed to die. While the father seemed willing to accept that recommendation, the mother could not.

When the babies were 7 weeks old, they were transferred to Children's Hospital in Philadelphia for surgery to separate them. Angela, the stronger twin, was viewed by the surgeons as having the best chances for survival. Even then, the odds were less than 1 in 100 that the operation would be successful.

Amy died during the surgery, as was expected. Angela lived until June 9, 1994 (11 months). She required intensive medical treatment in the hospital throughout her short life. The twins' parents did not have medical insurance. Amy and Angela's medical bills totaled over $1 million.

Ethical Questions

As in the Lakeberg case, should society spend thousands of dollars for medical treatment when the outcome appears futile? Is it morally and ethically right to use extraordinary means to try to save an individual's life no matter how slim the chances of success? "Does duty demand that doctors always intervene, or should they set limits? . . . Where do love, responsibility, and justice lie?" (Toufexis 1993). What is the balance between love (in this case, the mother's love), responsibility (in this case, the physician's), and justice (in this case, society's obligation)?

Data from Rosenthal, E. (1993). One Siamese twin survives an extraordinary separation. *The New York Times,* August 21, Section I, p. 1; Toufexis, A. (1993). The ultimate choice. *Time,* August 30, 43–44; Toufexis, A. (1994). The brief life of Angela Lakeberg. *Time,* June 27, 61–62.

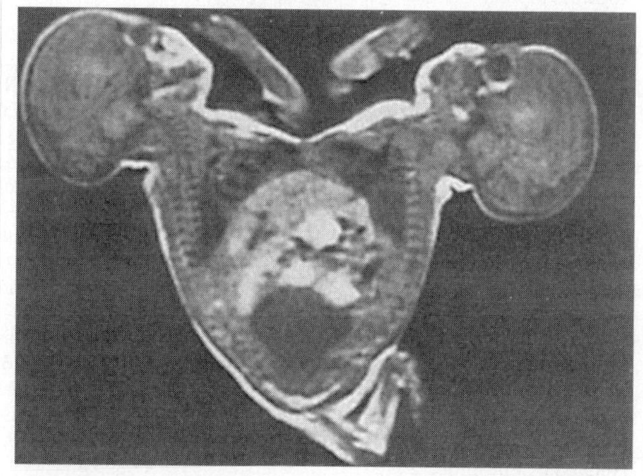

Figure 8–3

This postnatal magnetic resonance image demonstrates the extensive degree of conjunction of twins joined at the xiphoid process of the sternum through the pelvis • There were two normally formed legs and a hypoplastic leg • There were two normal and two nonfunctional kidneys • Portions of the intestinal tract were shared • The twins were successfully separated at about 1 year of age. (From Callen, P. W. [1994]. *Ultrasonography in obstetrics and gynecology* [p. 122]. Philadelphia: W. B. Saunders.)

IMPLICATIONS FOR RESEARCH

Reproductive, maternal, and neonatal issues are noted daily by our society's chroniclers: the newspapers, television, and broadcast news. It is essential that maternal-newborn nurses concern themselves with issues of ethics and acknowledge that their clinical decisions have far-reaching implications. Nursing is an essential and responsible part of society, committed to caring for all. Advanced nursing practice coupled with continual technologic and scientific developments will continue to confront nursing care with even more unimaginable dilemmas. It is through caring, coordination, advocacy, and research that nursing can assist society in reassessing and resolving ethical dilemmas.

Numerous areas related to ethics in maternal-newborn nursing require research. The following queries need to be examined to enable maternal-newborn nurses to handle ethical dilemmas more effectively:

- What are the most common ethical dilemmas that maternal-newborn nurses encounter?
- What are the most difficult ethical dilemmas that maternal-newborn nurses encounter?
- What are the most effective approaches that maternal-newborn nurses have used in resolving ethical dilemmas in clinical situations and when the situation is in conflict with their own personal values?
- What is the impact of education in clinical ethics on the maternal-newborn nurse's ability and comfort level in ethical decision making?

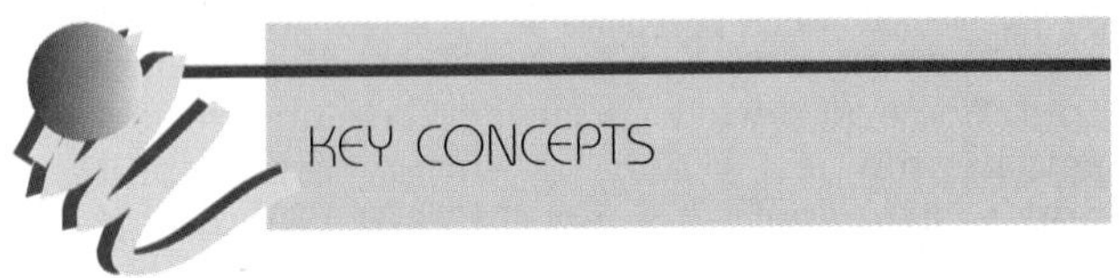

KEY CONCEPTS

▼ Nurses as client advocates have an obligation to act in a morally appropriate manner and to avoid harm to those they care for.

▼ In order to coexist in a helping relationship with clients, nurses must develop a high level of self-awareness.

▼ Ethics is a broad, general term that denotes an area of intellectual contemplation and reflection about a situation beyond what may be acceptable to society.

▼ The principles of ethics provide the foundation for ethical decision making. They serve as a framework in which values, morals, beliefs, and attitudes may be identified; ethical dilemmas examined and clarified; and obligations ordered in terms of their precedence.

▼ The professional nurse has the responsibility to help ensure that the basic rights of the client are protected.

▼ Nurses need to be involved in the ethical decision-making process.

▼ Using a perinatal-bioethical model for ethical decision making assists the nurse in reaching a decision about the morally "right" thing to do in a given situation.

▼ The role of the ethical advisory committee in an agency is to examine and clarify moral and ethical concerns about a situation.

▼ Ethical dilemmas in maternal-newborn nursing arise in assisted reproduction through artificial insemination, in vitro fertilization, and surrogate parenthood; prenatal diagnosis by amniocentesis or chorionic villus sampling; abortion; new technologic advances in contraception; embryo research; fetal tissue transplantation; maternal rights versus fetal rights; and aggressive treatment for defective neonates.

References

Abramowitz, S. (1984). A stalemate on (test-tube) baby research. *Hastings Center Report,* 14 (1), 5–9.

American Nurses Association. (1985). *Code for nurses with interpretive statements.* Washington, DC: Author.

Annas, G. J. (1984). Redefining parenthood and protecting embryos: Why we need new laws. *Hastings Center Report,* 14 (5), 50–52.

Beauchamp, T. R., and Walters, L. R. (1982). *Contemporary issues in bioethics.* Belmont, CA: Wadsworth.

Cohen, L. (1988). Professionally speaking: Whose right to life? *MCN: American Journal of Maternal Child Nursing,* 13 (2), 83.

Council on Scientific Affairs and Council on Ethical and Judicial Affairs. (1990). Medical applications of fetal tissue transplantation. *Journal of the American Medical Association,* 263 (4), 565–570.

Davis, A. J., and Aroskar, M. A. (1985). *Ethical dilemmas and nursing practice.* Norwalk, CT: Appleton & Lange.

Ellis, J., and Hartley, C. (1989). *Nursing in today's world: Challenges, issues, and trends* (3rd ed.). Philadelphia: J. B. Lippincott.

Fine, A. (1988). The ethics of fetal tissue transplants. *Hastings Center Report,* 18 (3), 5–8.

Furrow, B. (1984). Surrogate motherhood: A new option for parenting? *Law Medicine and Health Care,* 12 (3), 106.

Gersz, G. (1984). The contract in surrogate motherhood: A review of the issues. *Law Medicine and Health Care,* 12 (3), 107–113.

Gilbert, E., and Harmon, J. (1993). *Manual of high risk pregnancy and delivery.* St. Louis: C. V. Mosby.

Gorman, C. (1994). Brave new embryos. *Time,* August 29, 60–61.

Gretter, L. (1956). The Florence Nightingale pledge. In L. R. Seymer (Ed.). *A general history of nursing* (4th ed., p. 317). New York: Macmillan.

Harrison, M. R., Golbus, M. S., Filly, R. A. (1981). Management of the fetus with a correctable congenital defect. *Journal of the American Medical Association,* 246 (7), 774–777.

Holmes, H. B. (1988). In vitro fertilization: Reflections on the state of the art. *Birth,* 15, 134–145.

Mappes, T., and Zembaty, J. S. (1986). *Biomedical ethics* (2nd ed.). New York: McGraw-Hill.

Murphy, P. (1989). The role of the nurse on hospital ethics committees. *Nursing Clinics of North America,* 24 (2), 551–556.

National Institutes of Health Expert Panel. (1994). *Final report of the NIH human embryo research panel.* Bethesda, MD: NIH, Office of Communication, Public Information Branch, released September 27.

Nosek, J. (1988). Ethics. *Journal of Perinatal and Neonatal Nursing,* 1 (3), 1–87.

Omery, A. (1989). Values, moral reasoning, and ethics. *Nursing Clinics of North America,* 24 (2), 499–508.

Pellegrino, E. D. (1987). The anatomy of clinical-ethical judgments in perinatology: A substantive and procedural framework. *Seminar in Perinatology,* 11, 202–210.

Penticuff, J. H. (1992). Ethical issues. In P. Beachy and J. Deacon (Eds.). *Core curriculum for neonatal intensive care nursing.* Philadelphia: W. B. Saunders.

Robb, I. H. (1903; reprint 1926). *Nursing ethics: For hospital and private use.* Cleveland: E. C. Koeckert.

Sandling, J., Carter, B., Moore, C., Sparks, J. (1993). Ethics in neonatal intensive care. In G. B. Merenstein and S. L. Gardner (Eds.). *Handbook of neonatal intensive care* (3rd ed., p. 609). St. Louis: Mosby Year Book.

Steele, S. M., and Harmon, V. M. (1983). *Values clarification in nursing* (2nd ed.). Norwalk, CT: Appleton-Century-Crofts.

Thompson, J. E., and Thompson, H. O. (1985). *Bioethical decision making for nurses.* Norwalk, CT: Appleton-Century-Crofts.

Uustal, D. B. (1978). Values clarification in nursing: Application to practice. *American Journal of Nursing,* 78 (2), 2058–2063.

Uustal, D. B. (1985). *Values and ethics in nursing: From theory to practice.* East Greenwich, RI: Educational Resources in Nursing and Holistic Health.

Veatch, R. M. (1989). *Medical ethics.* Boston: Jones and Bartlett Publishers.

Williams, L. S. (1988). It's going to work for me: Response to failures of SVF. *Birth,* 15, 154–156.

Unit 2

Human Reproduction

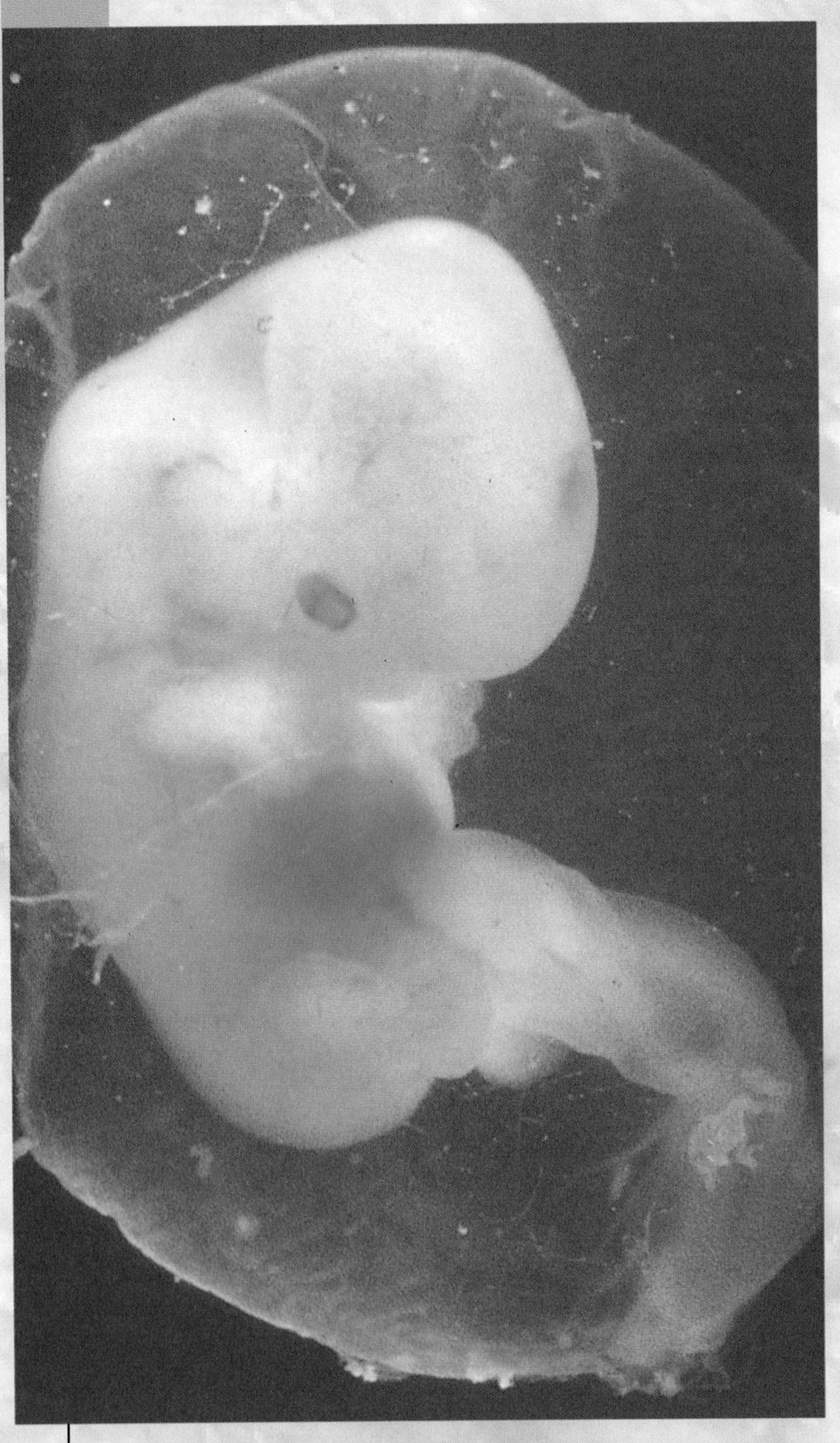

By the eighth week, the embryo measures approximately 1¼ inches in length and has distinctly human characteristics. The head is round but still large in comparison to the rest of the body. The fingers and toes are well defined and elongated. Sheltered in the warmth and security of the uterus, the fetus is very protected, but the placenta cannot block all toxic agents that are capable of interfering with the vulnerable yet resilient process of fetal development. (© Petit-Format/Nestle/Science Source/Photo Researchers.)

Trends in Research

PROTECTING THE FETUS FROM HAZARDOUS ENVIRONMENTAL AGENTS

The effect of toxic environmental agents on the fetus depends on the dose of the agent, the timing of the exposure during gestation, the presence or absence of other teratogens, and the individual biochemical enzyme levels of the mother or fetus.

Exposure of the fetus to hazardous environmental agents including drugs, chemicals, intrauterine infection, radiation, nutritional deficiency, and maternal disease causes 5 to 10 percent of all birth malformations and developmental problems.[1]

CONCLUSIONS FROM RESEARCH

Key research findings on the impact of hazardous environmental agents on the fetus provide information that can be used to protect the fetus:

- The effects of hazardous environmental agents on the fetus are different depending on the stage of gestation. The most critical period for the fetus is between the second and eighth weeks of gestation, when environmental agents can cause major structural malformations. However, toxic environmental agents are able to produce fetal abnormalities at any stage of gestation, from preconception through birth.[2]
- The effect of toxic environmental agents on the fetus depends on the dose of the agent, the timing of the exposure during gestation, the presence or absence of other teratogens,[3] and the individual biochemical enzyme levels of the mother or fetus.[1]
- There is a characteristic response of the fetus to each specific environmental teratogenic agent.[4]
- All teratogens have a typical toxic dose level that, once reached, causes malformations or developmental problems; lower dose levels produce no effect.[4]
- Drugs and chemical agents that have fetal teratogenic effects include anticonvulsants, folic acid antagonists, alcohol, diethylstilbestrol, thalidomide, chemotherapeutic agents, radioactive iodine, lead, organic mercury compounds, carbon monoxide, iodine-containing medicines, and tetracycline.[1]
- Physical factors such as radiation (x-rays) and radioactive materials can cause fetal malformations.[1]
- Intrauterine infections that can cause fetal damage include rubella, cytomegalovirus (CMV), varicella-zoster virus, toxoplasmosis, and syphilis.[1]
- Nutritional deficiencies of both folic acid and zinc can have a teratogenic effect on the fetus.[3]
- Diabetes mellitus is the most important maternal disease that can cause fetal malformation. The incidence of fetal malformations is in direct relation to the severity of the disease.[1]
- While caffeine does not appear to pose a teratogenic risk, it potentiates the teratogenic effects of other substances such as tobacco, alcohol, and vasoconstrictive medication. The combined effect can induce maternal-fetal vasoconstrictions and cause malformations as a result of ischemia.[5]

IMPLICATIONS FOR PRACTICE

The nurse, as educator, plays a key role in decreasing the incidence of fetal damage by toxic environmental agents. Educating parents before conception and throughout pregnancy helps them detect hazards, evaluate risks, and prevent to minimize the exposure of the fetus to harmful agents.

---

[1] Ornoy, A., and Arnon, J. (1993). Clinical teratology. In Fetal Medicine (Special Issue). *Western Journal of Medicine,* 159 (3), 382–390.

[2] Kimmel, C. A., Generoso, W. M., Thomas, R. D., Bakshi, K. S. (1993). Contemporary issues in toxicology: A new frontier in understanding the mechanisms of developmental abnormalities. *Toxicology and Applied Pharmacology,* 119 (2), 159–165.

[3] Glantz, J. C. (1994). Reproductive toxicology of alkylating agents. *Obstetrical and Gynecological Survey,* 49 (10), 709–715.

[4] Brent, R. L., Beckman, D. A., Landel, C. P. (1993). Clinical teratology. *Current Opinions in Pediatrics,* 5 (2), 201–211.

[5] Nehlig, A., and Debry, G. (1994). Potential teratogenic and neurodevelopmental consequences of coffee and caffeine exposure: A review of human and animal data. *Neurotoxicology and Teratology,* 16 (6), 531–543.

—FRANCINE H. NICHOLS

9 Chapter

We talk of hormonal cycles, ovulation, tell how the sperm rush, cells fuse, segment, multiply, travel, embed themselves in the lining of the womb. Yet how did the union of this particular egg and sperm urge life forward to make this child and no other? The more we learn, greater the wonder, more the mystery.

SHEILA KITZINGER (JOHNSTON 1994)

The Reproductive System

Mary C. Brucker

HIGHLIGHTS

- ▼ Intrauterine Development
- ▼ Female Reproductive System
- ▼ Endocrinologic Aspects of the Female Reproductive System
- ▼ Male Reproductive System
- ▼ Life Cycle for Reproduction
- ▼ Implications for Research

A nurse in the field of maternity nursing needs a firm foundation in the science of reproduction. Clinical practice does not require a sophisticated degree of knowledge of gynecologic endocrinology or biochemistry. However, a clear understanding of reproductive anatomy and physiology is necessary in order to form competent clinical assessments and plans for the childbearing family. The focus of this chapter is a basic review of reproductive anatomy and physiology for both the female and the male. Anatomic structures and functions are discussed and reproductive endocrinology is reviewed.

INTRAUTERINE DEVELOPMENT

The gender of the intrauterine conceptus is determined by the sperm of the male at the time of conception. However, the gonads (gamete-producing glands) do not develop male or female morphologic characteristics until approximately 9 weeks of gestational age (Sadler 1995). The gonads arise initially as a pair of ridges formed by coelomic epithelial proliferation and condensation of the underlying mesenchyme (Fig. 9–1). Primordial germ cells appear among the endoderm cells in the wall of the yolk sac and eventually invade the genital ridges. While the primordial cells are developing, the

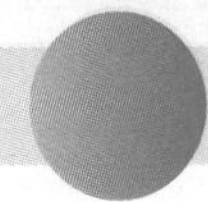

DEFINITIONS

Cervix—Lowermost portion of uterus that extends into the vagina; the opening of the uterus that dilates during labor.

Clitoris—Female organ composed of erectile tissue located at the top of the vulva; the homolog of the male penis.

Corpus luteum—Remnant of the ruptured ovarian follicle that facilitates production of progesterone in the second half of the menstrual cycle.

Endometrium—Mucous membrane lining of the uterus.

Fallopian tubes—Oviduct.

Labia majora—The larger folds of skin that form the overall architecture of the vulva.

Labia minora—Thin folds of skin under the labia majora; contain sebaceous and sweat glands.

Penis—Male external reproductive organ composed of erectile tissue; the homolog of the female clitoris.

Perineum—Tissues posterior to the labia and anterior to the anus.

Pubis—Bony part of the innominate pelvic bone found where the rami merge.

Scrotum—Sac of tissue posterior to the penis containing the male testes.

Symphysis pubis—Fibrocartilaginous joint found in the midline of the bony pelvis that lacks a capsule or synovial membranes.

Testes—Male gonads containing seminiferous tubules and Leydig cells, where sperm and testosterone are produced.

Uterus—Female reproductive organ composed of inner lining (endometrium) that sheds during menstruation; composed of the fundus, corpus (body) isthmus, and cervix.

Vagina—Fibromuscular canal linking the female external genitalia and the internal reproductive organs.

coelomic epithelium of the genital ridge penetrates the mesenchyme and forms the irregularly shaped primitive sex cords. The gonad becomes known as an indifferent gonad, since gross differentiation between male and female gonads is impossible at this stage (see Fig. 9–1).

If the fetus is male, a testis-determining effect is associated with the XY chromosomes and the primitive sex cords continue to proliferate and penetrate deep into the medulla, forming the medullary cords or testes. As they lose contact with the surface epithelium, a dense layer of fibrous connective tissue is formed, the tunica albuginea (see Fig. 9–1).

If the fetus is female, the XX chromosomes influence the process of development of the primitive sex cords. The cords break into the irregular cell clusters that later form the ovarian medulla. A second generation of cords, the cortical cords, arise from the surface epithelium of the female gonad. By 4 months after conception, these cords are split into cell clusters each surrounding one or more primitive germ cells that eventually develop into the oogonia. The surface epithelium that surrounds the epithelial cells forms the follicular cells (see Fig. 9–1).

The genital duct systems are directly influenced by the sex glands themselves. The Sertoli cells in the fetal testes produce a nonsteroidal substance, müllerian inhibiting substance (MIS), that causes regression of the paramesonephric ducts and stimulates the mesonephric ducts so that the typical external genitalia of the male develop. Conversely, under the influence of estrogens, the paramesonephric ducts are stimulated and the uterus and upper third of the vagina develop. Estrogens also stimulate development of the female external genitalia (Fig. 9–2).

FEMALE REPRODUCTIVE SYSTEM

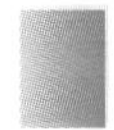

The Bony Pelvis

In contrast to those of the male, the pelvic bones of the female are designed for childbearing (Fig. 9–3). The purposes of the pelvis during pregnancy are to protect the pelvic organs, support the growing fetus and enlarging uterus, and direct the passage of the fetus during birth. The pelvis consists of four bones: two innominate bones, the sacrum, and the coccyx. These four bones are united by four joints. Figure 9–3 illustrates the bones and joints of the pelvis.

INNOMINATE BONES

The large innominate bones are anterior and lateral and consist of three bones that are fused around the acetabulum:

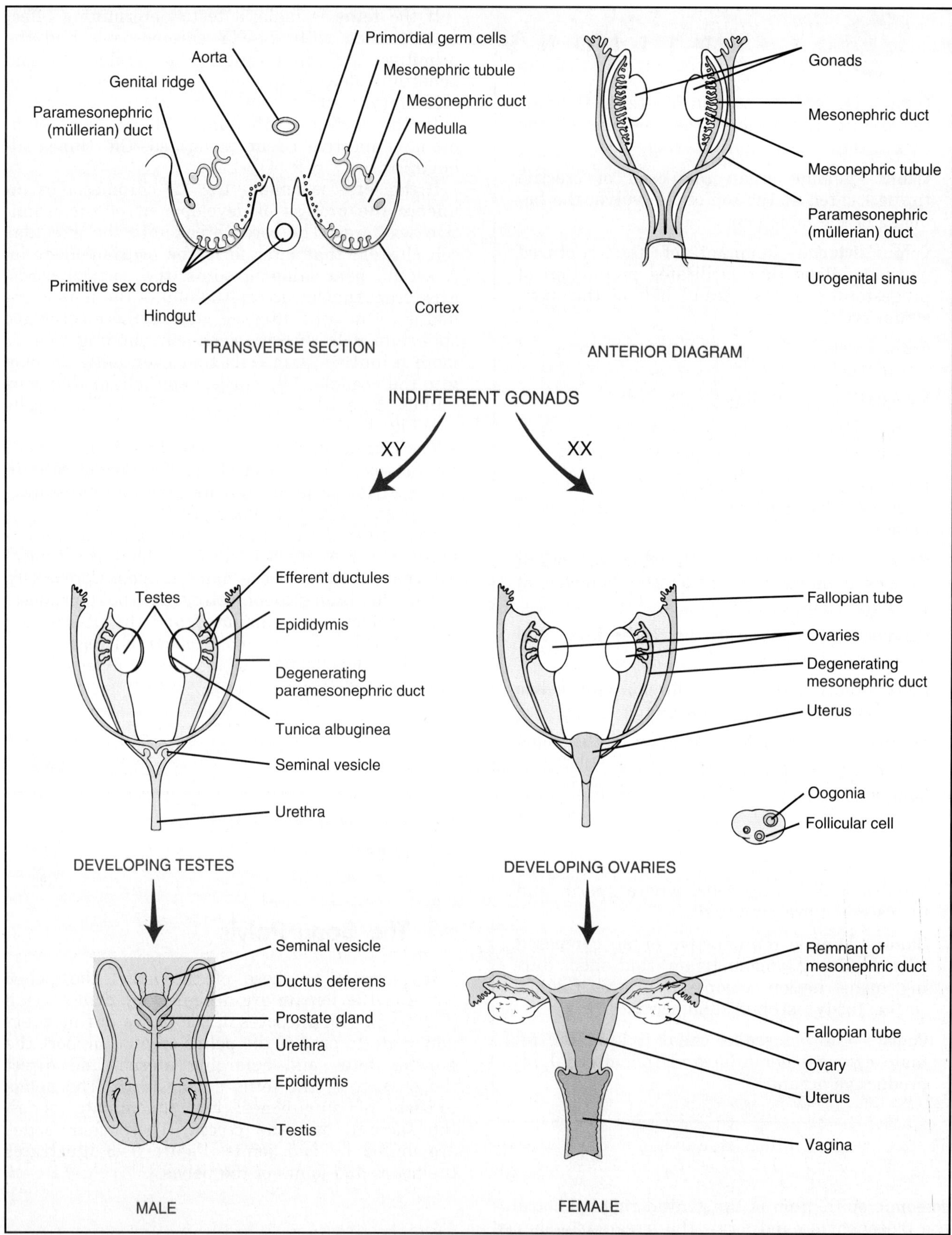

Figure 9–1

Embryonic differentiation of internal male and female reproductive organs from the indifferent gonads through developing testes and ovaries to the male and female organs.

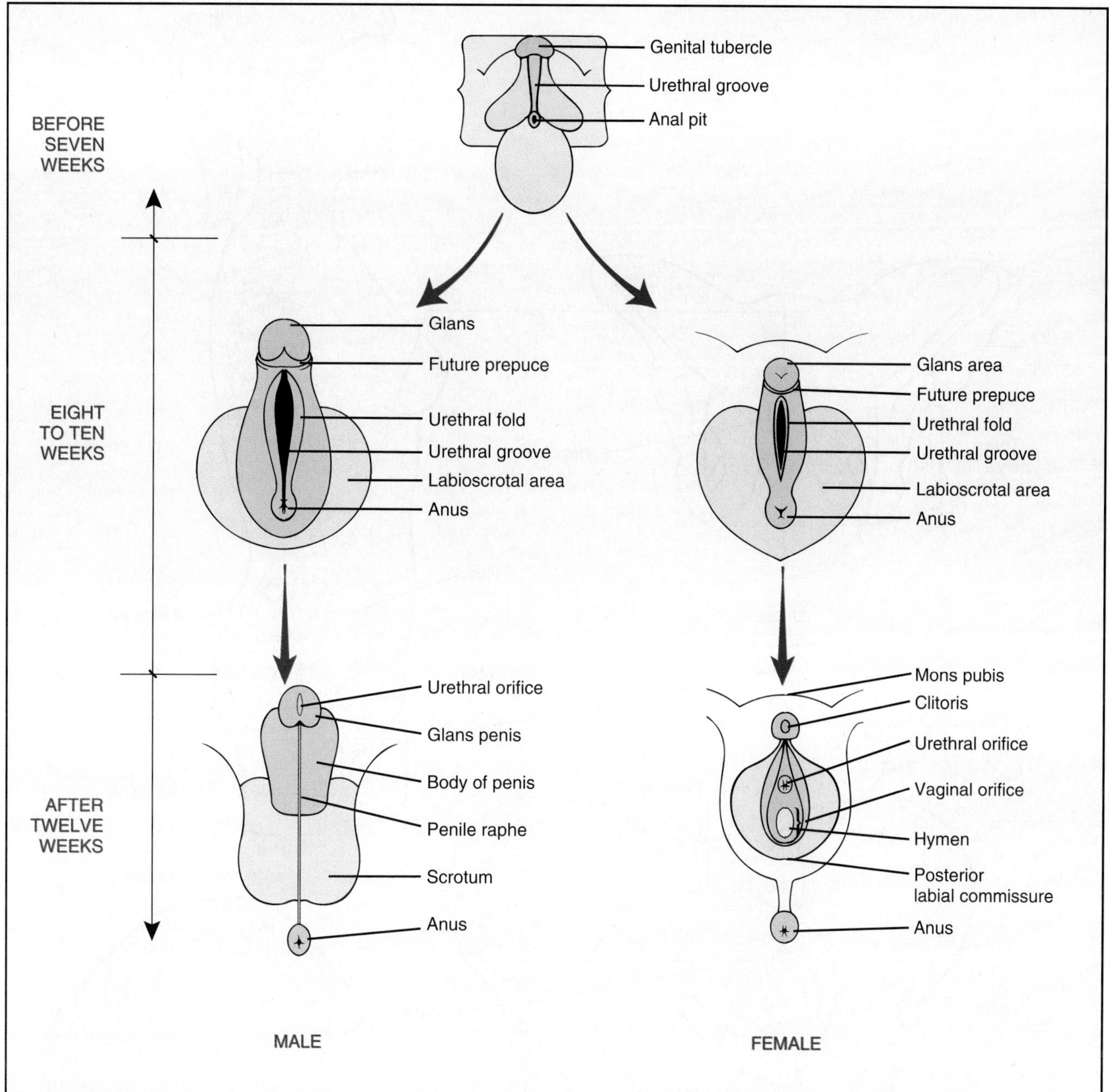

Figure 9–2

Even though gender is predetermined by genetics, gross identification of external genitalia is impossible until approximately 9 weeks of gestational age • Before that point, the gonad is often termed indifferent since there is no visual difference between *male* and *female.*

1. The upper bone, known as the ilium, and its ridge, the iliac crest, which forms the hips.
2. The ischium, which is under the ilium. At its base is the ischial tuberosity, the bony prominence that can be palpated when sitting. On its internal planes are the ischial spines, which separate the greater sciatic from the lesser sciatic notch. The spines are at the level of the midplane of the pelvis, project into the pelvic cavity, and are often used in labor by a health care professional to determine how far down in the pelvis the presenting part of the fetus has descended.
3. The pubis, which is the front portion of the pelvis. The rounded area under the pubis is called the pubic arch.

SACRUM AND COCCYX

The sacrum is a triangular bone that usually consists of five fused vertebrae and articulates with the lower surface of the fifth lumbar verte-

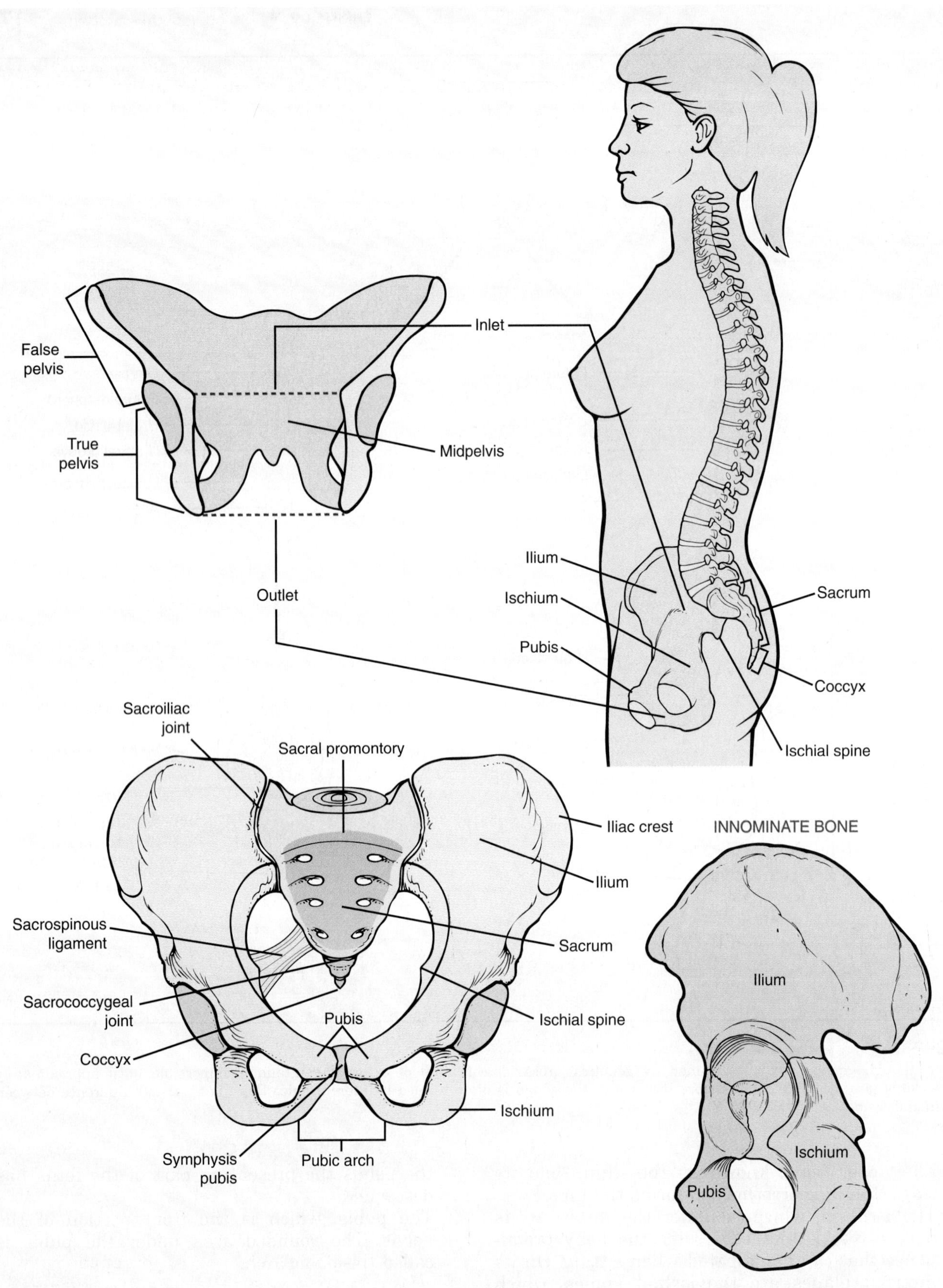

Figure 9–3

The normal female pelvis has a bowl-shaped cavity, encouraging the fetus to assume a well-flexed occiput anterior position and enhancing the normal progress of labor • These views show the relationship between the vertebral column and bony pelvis • Enlargements clarify how the bones work together to provide support for the fetus yet allow for birth.

bra. The sacral promontory is an area of the sacrum on the upper anterior surface that juts into the pelvic cavity. The sacrum meets posteriorly with the coccyx, which is commonly known as a tailbone and consists of four rudimentary vertebrae. During pregnancy the sacrum is somewhat flexible because of hormonal influences, and it can move backward during labor to allow easier passage of the fetus through the pelvis (Oxorn 1996).

JOINTS

Four joints link the sacrum, coccyx, and innominate bones. These are the symphysis pubis, the sacrococcygeal, and the two sacroiliac synchondroses. It should be noted that although some clinicians use the terms pubis and symphysis pubis interchangeably, the former refers specially to the bone and the latter to a cartilaginous joint that lacks both capsule and synovial membrane.

DIVISIONS OF THE PELVIS

The female pelvis is divided into two areas—the true and the false pelvis (see Fig. 9–3). The false pelvis is the upper portion of the pelvis, between the ilia. It is called false because from an obstetric point of view, it has little clinical significance related to the passage of the fetus during labor and birth. During pregnancy it supports the uterus and directs the fetus into the true pelvis. The true pelvis is the area bordered by the sacrum in the back, the innominate bones on the side, and the pubis in the front, and it forms the bony passage through which the fetus must pass during labor and birth. The false pelvis is separated from the true pelvis by the inlet, also called the brim, or linea terminalis. The true pelvis consists of three planes—the inlet, the midpelvis, and the outlet. These planes greatly influence the process of labor and birth. Since these dimensions of the pelvis have direct clinical applications, they are discussed in further detail in Chapter 22.

PELVIC TYPES

There are four classic types of pelves: gynecoid, android, anthropoid, and platypelloid (Fig. 9–4). However, because variations of these types exist from one plane of the pelvis to another, the pure classic types are often not seen.

▼ **Gynecoid Pelvis.** Although the average woman has a gynecoid, or normal female pelvis, some variations in shape exist. The inlet of this type is usually rounded, with a smaller anteroposterior diameter than transverse diameter. The midpelvis is adequate, having nonprominent ischial spines, straight and parallel side walls, and a sacrum that is short, slopes backward, and has a wide, deep sacral curve. The outlet is marked by a round and wide pubic arch and a long anteroposterior diameter. The gynecoid pelvis is most favorable for successful labor and birth. This pelvic type is seen in 50 percent of women.

▼ **Android Pelvis.** The android pelvis is seen in males. In contrast to the gynecoid pelvis, the inlet is heart shaped. Although the diameters of the inlet might be adequate, the posterior segment of the inlet is shallow because of an indented sacral promontory. The midpelvis is narrow, having prominent ischial spines, convergent side walls, and a long sacrum that inclines forward. The outlet is marked by a narrow, deep, and sharp pubic arch. Its anteroposterior diameter is short and the transverse diameter is narrow, reducing the capacity of the outlet. The android pelvis would not be favorable for labor; slow descent and midpelvis arrest can be caused by the narrow pelvic planes. This pelvic type is seen in 20 percent of women.

▼ **Anthropoid Pelvis.** The anthropoid pelvis has an inlet that is oval in shape because of a long anteroposterior diameter and an adequate but short transverse diameter. The midpelvis has adequate diameters because it has variable ischial spines, straight side walls, and a sacrum that is long and narrow and inclines backward. The outlet is also adequate, with a normal or moderately narrow pubic arch. This pelvic type is seen in 25 percent of women.

▼ **Platypelloid Pelvis.** The platypelloid pelvis has a flat shape. The inlet is oval with a short anteroposterior diameter and even shorter transverse diameter. The midpelvis is not usually adequate, having variable ischial spines, parallel side walls, and a wide sacrum with a deep inward curve. Only the transverse diameter is adequate. The outlet is marked by an extremely wide pubic arch. The transverse diameter is wide but the anteroposterior diameter is short, making the outlet inadequate. This pelvic type is seen in 5 percent of women.

External Genitalia

ANATOMIC LANDMARKS OF THE VULVA AND PERINEUM

In many cultures, clothing of the upper body is almost optional. A woman may expose her breasts with few, if any, sanctions. However, in almost all cultures, a woman's external genitalia are covered. Even in a modern society, the nurse may find taboos, embarrassment, and ignorance expressed by women about their own external genitalia. Just

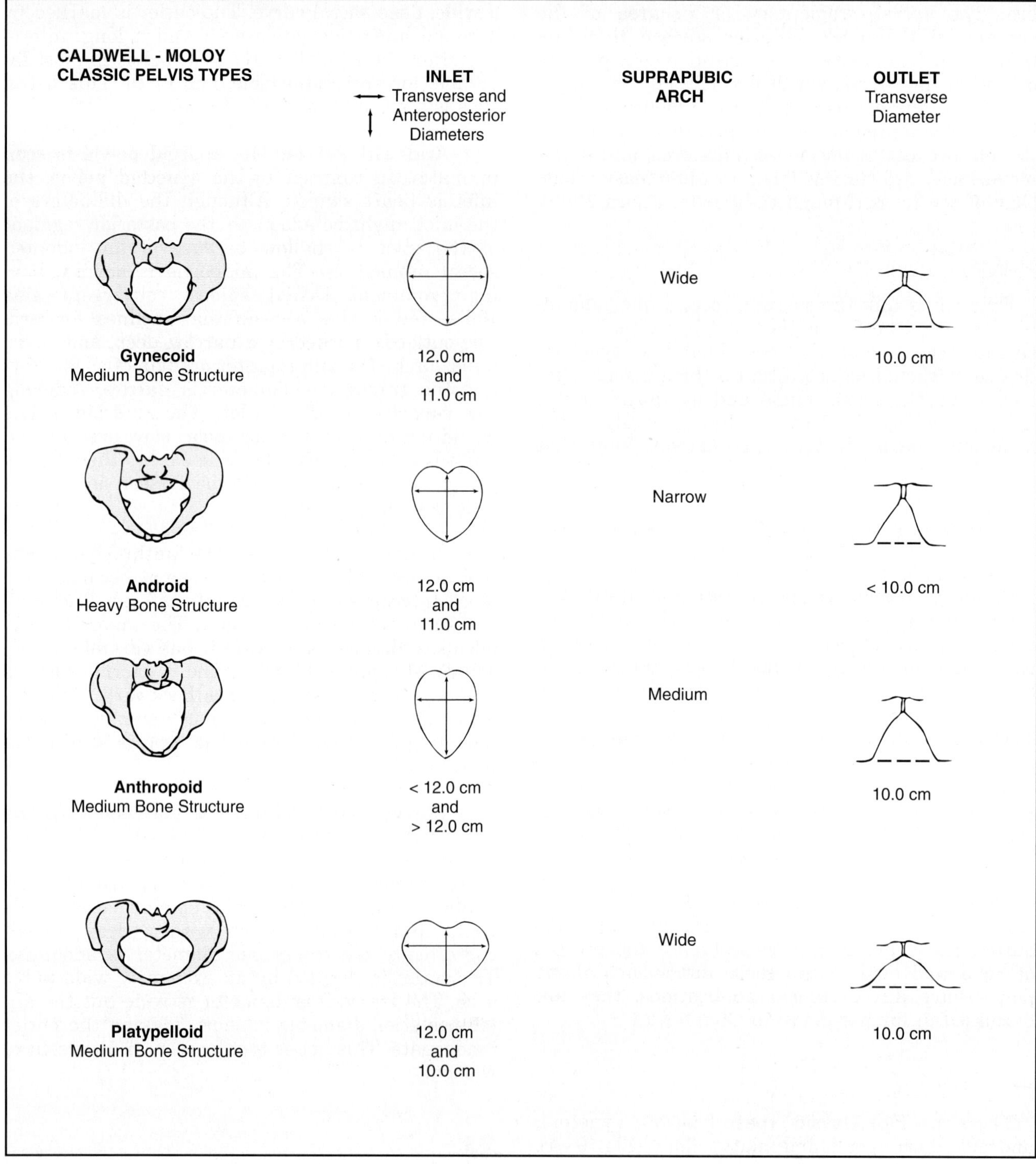

Figure 9–4

Four classic types of pelves have been identified • The average woman has a gynecoid pelvis • Many others may have some degree of variation or a mixture of types • Few women have pure android, anthropoid, or platypelloid types.

as women are now encouraged to perform breast self-examinations, it is becoming common to encourage regular self-examination of the external genitalia to observe for lesions, growths, or color changes. Yet for many women this is an exercise in futility, for they have no knowledge of the normal parameters. It is important that a nurse caring for childbearing women knows the anatomy of the external genitalia, not only in order to provide appropriate care but also to use the opportunity to educate the woman about her own body. For the discussion of the external genitalia, it is best for the professional to envision the woman in a dorsal position with her legs relaxed, allowing exposure of the area (Fig. 9–5).

▼ **Vulva.** The entire external genitalia from the pubis to the perineum are called the vulva or pudendum. The vulva includes the mons pubis, labia majora and minora, clitoris, urethral meatus, vaginal vestibule, and perineal body.

▼ **Mons Pubis.** The mons pubis (or mons veneris) may be the first area noted visually. It is the hair-covered fat pad overlying the symphysis pubis. The hair is usually in a triangular pattern and is coarser than hair elsewhere on the woman's body. The amount and coarseness of the pubic hair vary with ethnic background. The mons pubis is actually the anterior fusion of the labia majora. It serves to cushion the pubic bone during sexual intercourse. As a woman ages, the amount of pubic hair and fatty tissue decreases.

▼ **Labia Majora.** The labia majora are the folds of skin that form the overall architecture of the vulva and serve to protect the structures lying underneath them. These protruding skin folds cover a varying amount of adipose tissue. As with most anatomic structures that have two distinct sides, one labium majus may be slightly smaller than the other. This is a normal variation. The skin of the labia majora has hair follicles and large numbers of sebaceous glands and sweat glands. The hair is most concentrated on the mons pubis and gradually becomes more scant toward the posterior aspect so that little is visible at the posterior fusion of the labia majora. The labia majora merge with the thighs laterally and with the labia minora medially. In girls and nulliparous women the labia majora are approximated, covering the structures underneath. After childbirth, the labia majora usually remain separated. After menopause, the labia majora may shrink considerably (Jones et al. 1988; Lichtman and Papera 1990).

▼ **Labia Minora.** The labia minora are thin folds of hairless skin containing only sebaceous and sweat glands. Posteriorly, the labia minora blend with the labia majora and perineum, forming the fourchette. Anteriorly the labia minora form the prepuce and frenulum of the clitoris. The rich vascularity of the labia minora gives them a pink color and allows them to swell during sexual excitement, while the rich innervation of the area makes them very sensitive to stimulation. The glands in the labia minora serve to lubricate the vulva. The labia minora also decrease in size after menopause.

▼ **Clitoris.** The clitoris is an erectile organ that is the female homolog of the penis. It lies under the symphysis pubis and is supported by the suspensory ligament and frenulum. The clitoris is covered by the prepuce and is composed of the glans and the corpus. Because of its rich blood and nerve supplies, the clitoris is the most sensitive part of the female genitalia and its stimulation can result in orgasm. The sebaceous glands of the clitoris secrete a cheeselike substance called smegma, which has an odor that is sexually exciting to the male (Jones et al. 1988; Lichtman and Papera 1990).

In visualizing the external genitalia of a woman, the labia majora, labia minora, clitoris, and perineum are the structures most easily seen. However, the labia minora generally cover other anatomic structures of importance. Figure 9–5 illustrates the separation of the labia minora for discussion of additional external structures.

▼ **Vestibule.** The vestibule is a fossa that lies between the labia minora and extends anteriorly to the clitoris. Posteriorly, the vestibule extends to the perineum. The junction with the perineum is also called the posterior fourchette. Within the vestibule lie the urethra, ducts from the paraurethral glands (Skene glands), ducts from the greater vestibular glands (Bartholin glands), and the vaginal orifice. The urethral meatus is the terminal end of the urethra and is located about 1 inch below the clitoris. It has a puckered appearance that may be difficult to see without separation of the mucosal folds. The Skene glands are found posteriorly on either side of the urethra and secrete small amounts of mucus that serve for lubrication. The Bartholin glands are lateral and immediately posterior to the vagina and also secrete a clear mucus during sexual intercourse. The vaginal orifice is the external opening to the female internal reproductive organs. The outer orifice of the vagina may be ringed by an extra fold of connective tissue in the child or adolescent. This is called the hymen, and it is gradually replaced with irregular tissue tags called hymenal remnants after sexual activity and childbearing. An intact hymen is not an indication of virginity, for women who are virgins may have torn the hymen through vigorous exercise or use of tampons, and sexually active women may have intact hymens (Jones et al. 1988; Lichtman and Papera 1990).

MUSCLES OF THE PERINEUM

Perineum is a commonly used term that refers to the tissues posterior to the labia and anterior to the anus. If the musculature of the region is visualized for a woman in the dorsal position as in the previous figures, it appears as in Figure 9–6. The major muscles of obstetric significance are the bulbocavernosus, superficial transverse perineal

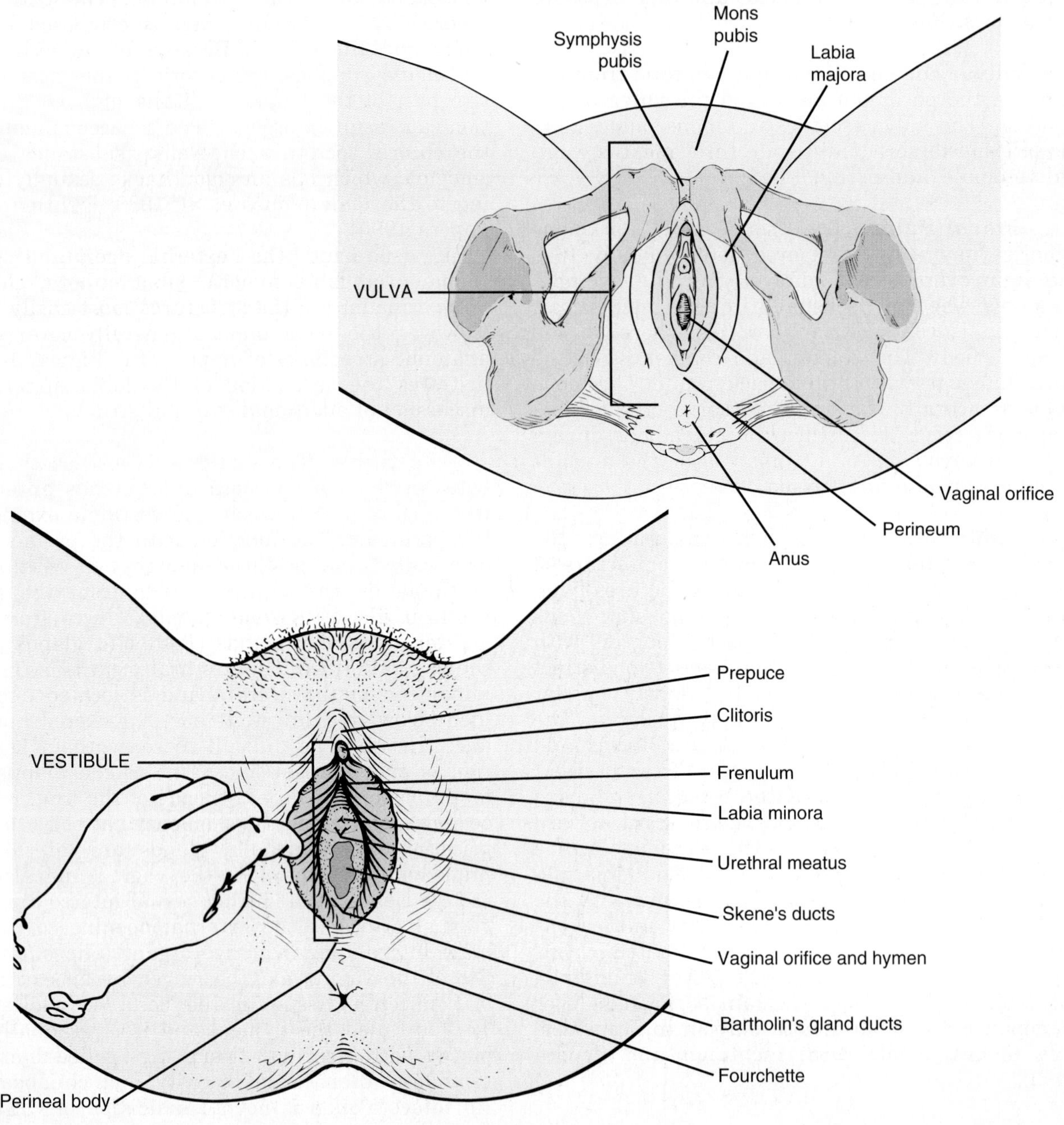

Figure 9–5

During a pelvic examination, the external female genitalia are carefully inspected • Several important structures can be visualized only after the labia are gently spread by the examiner's fingers.

muscle, and levator ani, which includes the pubococcygeus, puborectalis, and iliococcygeus muscles. Strength, elasticity, and a woman's control over these muscles are directly related to the integrity of the perineum at the time of birth, as well as muscular strength associated with retarding urinary incontinence (Oxorn 1986; Jones et al. 1988; Lichtman and Papera 1990) (Table 9–1). Several exercises have been suggested to increase perineal strength. Many programs are described as Kegel exercises in recognition of Arnold Kegel, an early advocate of perineal exercise in his work on urinary incontinence (Doress et al. 1987) (see the Teaching Guide in Chapter 19).

Two additional terms are sometimes used to describe the muscles and anatomic structures of the

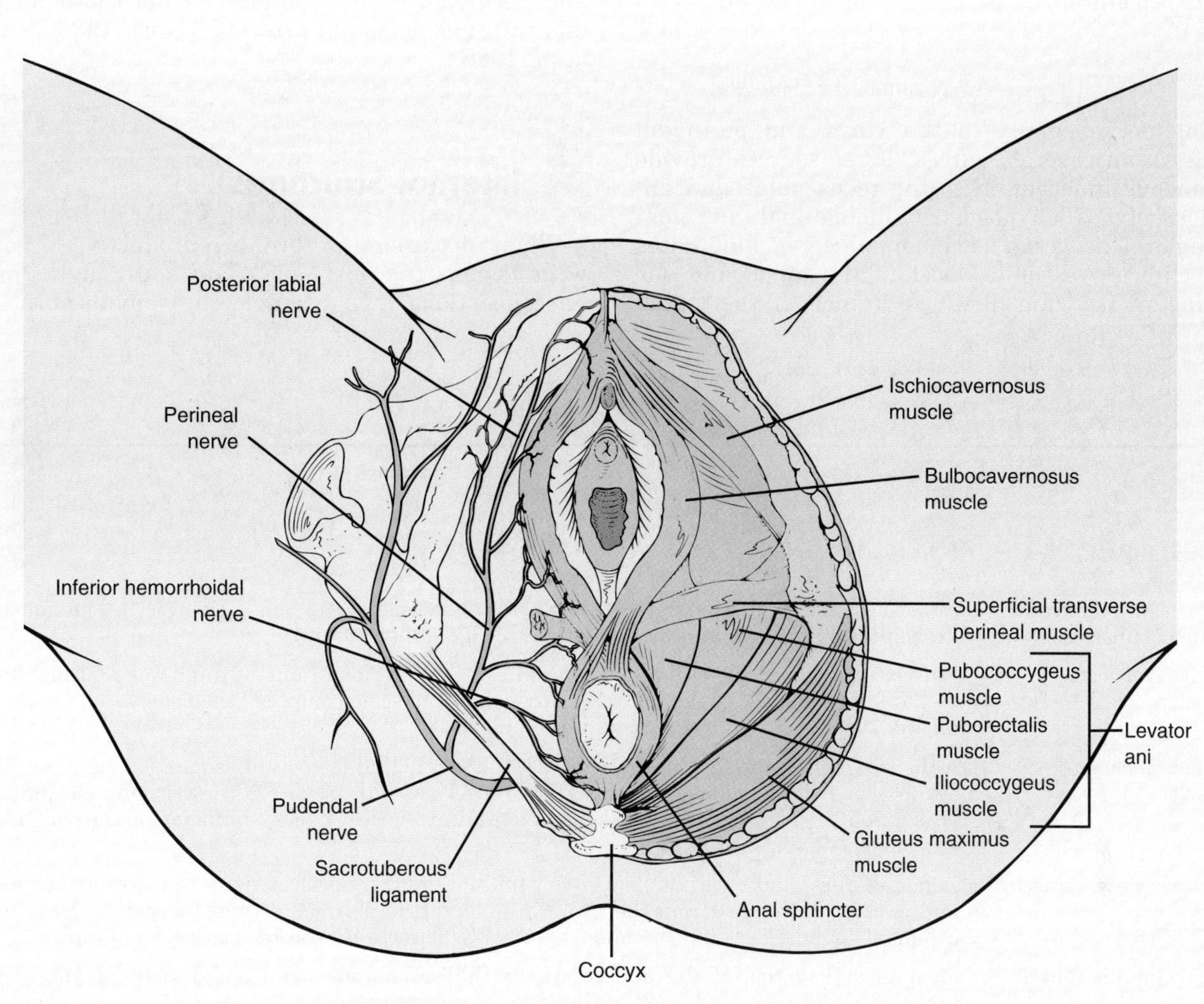

Figure 9–6

The pudendal nerve and vessels are of great importance, especially during labor and birth • They provide the major innervation and blood supply to the area.

pelvic floor. The urogenital triangle is the anatomic sector that is bounded by the pubic angle in the front, the ischiopubic rami and ischial tuberosities laterally, and the transverse perineal muscle and the base of the urogenital diaphragm in the back. It is composed of the vaginal open-ing, urethral meatus, clitoris and ischiocavernosus muscles, vestibular bulbs covered by bulbocavernosus muscles, Bartholin glands and ducts, urogenital diaphragm, blood vessels, nerves, and lymphatics. The urogenital diaphragm is the muscular tissue that lies in the anterior triangle of the perineum and is surrounded by fascia. It includes the deep transverse perineal muscles and urethral sphincter. Although the superior layer of fascia is weak, the inferior fascial layer is fibrous and strong.

This fascial layer extends from a short distance beneath the pubic ligament to the ischial tuberosities. Superiorly it is fused and forms the transverse perineal ligament; inferiorly it joins in the central point of the perineum (Oxorn 1986).

NERVE SUPPLY TO VULVA AND PERINEUM

The nerve supply to the vulva and perineum comes from several sources. Three sources provide cutaneous innervation to the mons pubis and anterior vulva: iliohypogastric, ilioinguinal, and genitofemoral nerves. The pudendal nerve innervates the clitoris, vestibule, most of the labia, and the perineum (see Fig. 9–6). A branch of the sacral plexus provides innervation for the lateral perineum, the posterior vulva, and the perianal area (see also Chapter 24, Pain Management During Childbirth). The arterial blood supply to the vulva and perineum is predominantly from the external and internal pudendal arteries (Oxorn 1986; Jones et al. 1988).

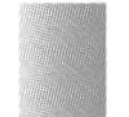

Internal Structures

When discussing internal reproductive organs with women, the nurse may find many myths and misconceptions. For example, a woman may in-

Table 9–1

DESCRIPTIONS OF THE PERINEAL MUSCLES

Superficial transverse perineal muscles	Superficial parts of deep muscles with the same origin and insertion; occur outside the urogenital diaphragm and are sometimes congenitally absent.
Ischiocavernosus muscles	Muscles that cover the clitoris, with origin in the inferior ramus of the pubis and insertion at the lateral aspect of the clitoral crura. These muscles compress the crura and, by blocking venous return, cause erection of the clitoris.
Bulbocavernosus muscle	A figure eight muscle that surrounds the vagina and rectum; some sources use the synonymous term bulbospongiosus. This muscle assists in clitoral erection by closing the dorsal vein; it can act as a weak vaginal sphincter (the major sphincter of the vagina is the pubovaginalis section of the levator ani).
Pubococcygeus muscle	Major perineal muscle that lies in the midline and is perforated by the urethra, vagina, and rectum; originates from the posterior side of the pubis and from the pelvic fascia and commonly subdivides into the pubovaginalis, puborectalis, and pubococcygeus proper.
Pubovaginalis muscle	Most medial section of the pubococcygeus that surrounds the vaginal opening; the fibers insert into the sides and back of the vagina and into the central point of the perineum. It is the major sphincter of the vagina.
Puborectalis muscle	Intermediate part of the pubococcygeus and forms a loop around the anal canal and rectum; it inserts into the lateral and posterior walls of the anal canal between the sphincter ani internus and externus and into the anococcygeal body. It supports the rectum by suspending it, but has little other perineal supportive function.
Pubococcygeus proper	The most lateral fibers of the pubococcygeus muscle that insert into the lateral margins of the coccyx. During muscle contractions, it propels the coccyx forward, so that the anorectal junction is increased and, in conjunction with the external sphincter, helps control passage of feces.
Iliococcygeus muscles	Muscles that arise from the pelvic fascia behind the obturator canal and insert into the lateral margins of the coccyx, essentially acting as a musculofascial layer.
Ischiococcygeus muscles	Also known as the coccygeus muscles, these muscles originate from the ischial spines and insert into the lateral borders of the coccyx and the fifth sacral vertebra. They supplement the levator ani and lie mostly on the posterior portion of the pelvic floor.
Levator ani	Composed of the pubococcygeus, puborectalis, pubovaginalis, and iliococcygeus muscles, the levator ani originates from the posterior side of the pubis, the pelvic fascia, and pelvic aspect of the ischial spine. It inserts into the vaginal walls, central point of the perineum, anal canal, anoccoccygeal body, and lateral border of the coccyx.

Adapted from Oxorn, H. (1986). *Human labor and birth* (5th ed.). Norwalk, CT: Appleton & Lange.

stinctively conceptualize her nonpregnant uterus as being located immediately posterior to the umbilicus. The sharing of accurate information is an important facet of women's education. Figure 9–7 illustrates the relationship of the reproductive organs within the pelvic cavity. The accompanying magnification of the organs is designed to allow easy identification.

VAGINA

The vagina is a fibromuscular canal with a visible orifice from the view of the external genitalia. It is lined with mucous membranes and covered by a stratified squamous epithelium. The vagina provides the conduit to link the vestibule to the cervix of the uterus. The posterior wall is 8 to 10 cm in length and the anterior wall is approximately 6 cm in length as the cervix enters its upper third in the average woman. The upper end of the vagina is often referred to as the vault. The vagina is a highly elastic structure. When a woman is in an upright position, it essentially folds in upon itself. Yet it can be distended to admit examining fingers for assessment, an engorged penis for sexual pleasure; or the head of a 7-pound (or larger) infant for delivery.

The vagina is lined with stratified epithelium arranged in ridges or rugae. This mucosa is normally continuous and usually covered with a transparent secretion that is odorless. No glands exist in the vagina; the secretion is the result of transudation of lymph and cast-off epithelial cells. Certain changes occur in the vagina in relation to developmental changes: in the nonpregnant reproductive woman, the mucosa is usually pink; during pregnancy it is frequently cyanotic as a result of increased venous congestion and secretions are increased; during lactation the rugae may be diminished; and postmenopausally, the mucosa may be pale with few rugations.

The acid medium of the vagina tends to prevent inhabitation by pathologic organisms. The acidity is maintained by the Döderlein bacillus, which is part of the normal flora of the vagina. Different conditions can be reflected not only in the visual assessment of the vagina but also in changes in the vaginal flora, making pathology more apparent. For example, the use of antibiotics changes the vaginal milieu, resulting in an overgrowth of the normal inhabitant *Candida albicans.* This can result in a symptomatic yeast infection.

Anatomically, the lower half of the anterior wall is proximate to the urethra. The upper half is in close contact with the bladder. The lower third of the posterior wall is next to the perineal body, the middle part proximate to the rectum, and the upper part next to the peritoneum at the base of the pouch of Douglas. The vagina is laterally located in relation to the levator ani muscles. The anterior aspect of the vagina leads to the uterus, specifically to the lowermost portion of the uterus, the cervix.

During pregnancy, the increased vascularity of the vagina results in softening of the connective tissues. In early pregnancy, the hyperemia results in a bluish or violet color change of both cervix and vagina, called the Chadwick sign. Smooth muscles appear to hypertrophy as pregnancy continues and the vagina prepares for the distention that accompanies birth (Cunningham et al. 1993). During pregnancy, cervical secretions and vaginal secretions increase in amount. Many women report a white thick discharge that has no odor or itching associated with it. The pH of the discharge is acidic, usually between 3.5 and 6. The acidic pH is probably a protective factor against vaginitis during pregnancy (Cunningham et al. 1993).

UTERUS

▼ **Cervix.** The cervix, or neck, of the uterus is found in the vault of the vagina. Its diameter is usually approximately 3 to 5 cm and it protrudes into the vagina approximately 1 to 3 cm. The cervix has an opening, or os, leading to a cervical canal that allows a connection with the isthmus of the uterus. This then leads to the corpus or body of the uterus (Fig. 9–8).

The cervical canal is lined with mucous membranes that secrete alkaline mucus. The external opening of the cervical canal is known as the external cervical os. The external os of a nulliparous woman usually appears as a small dot. After a vaginal birth, this commonly changes to a slitlike appearance, as illustrated in Figure 9–8. The exterior of the cervix, or ectocervix, is usually covered with epithelial cells that are smooth and pink in appearance. When the epithelial cells adjoin the external cervical os, it is common in the reproductive woman to visualize some of the columnar cells, which are prolific in the internal cervical canal or the endocervix. The ectocervix and endocervix meet in the transformation zone, an area of rapid change or metaplasia. The endocervix is the best area from which to obtain cells for assessment of dysplasia or neoplasia. Thus, a Papanicolaou (Pap) smear is frequently obtained to detect changes suggestive of cervical carcinoma. Pap smears are most accurate for women of reproductive age and especially pregnant women, since after menopause the endocervix recedes, making it more difficult to obtain endocervical cells.

Table 9–2 summarizes the most common interpretations of a cytology reading or Pap smear of the cervix. During pregnancy, because of the ease of access to the transformation zone, most Pap smears have adequate numbers of the squamocolumnar cells that are necessary for appropriate interpretation. Should a Pap smear not be normal,

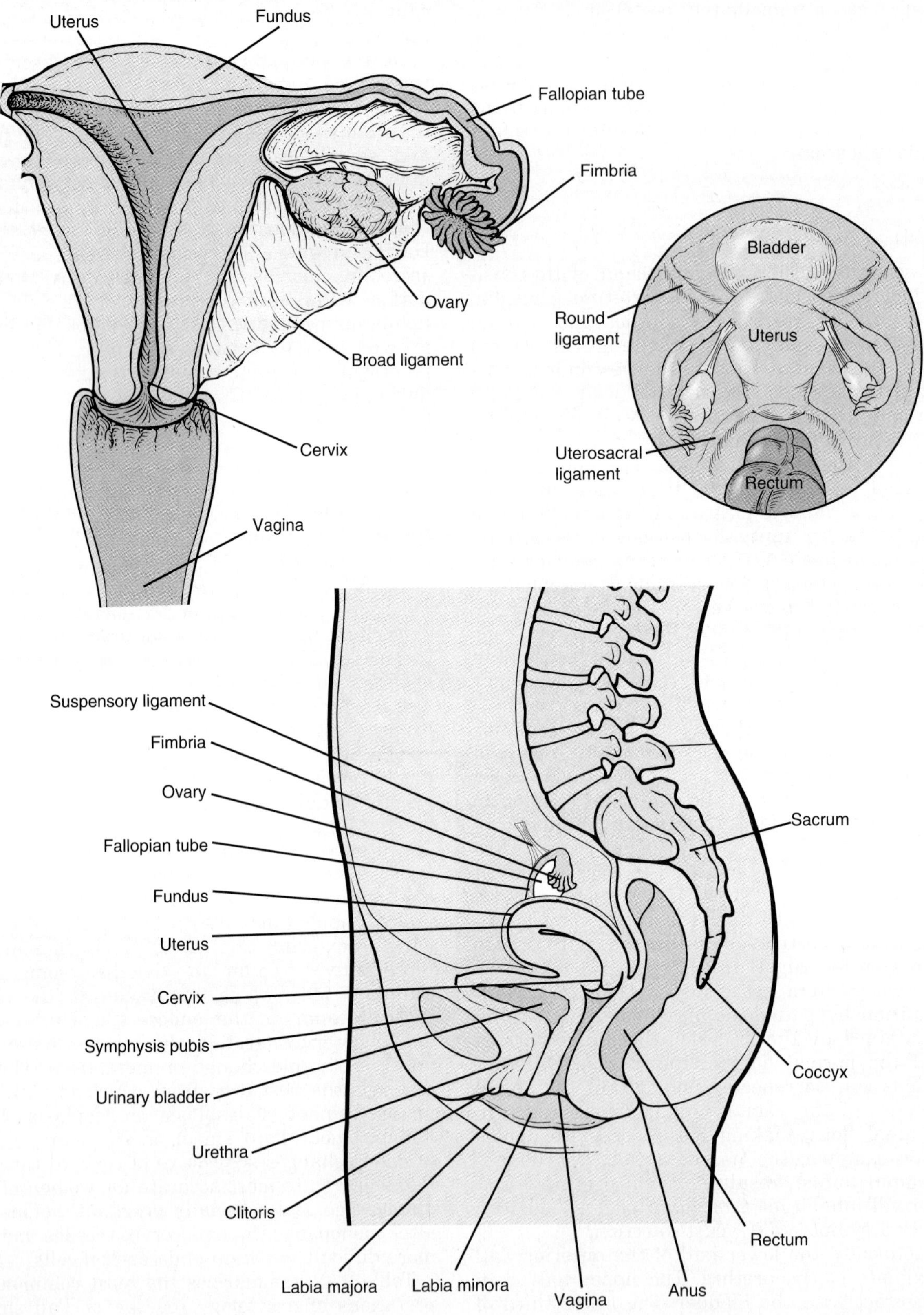

Figure 9–7

The placement and design of the female reproductive organs provide for great flexibility that accommodates both the nonpregnant state and a growing fetus.

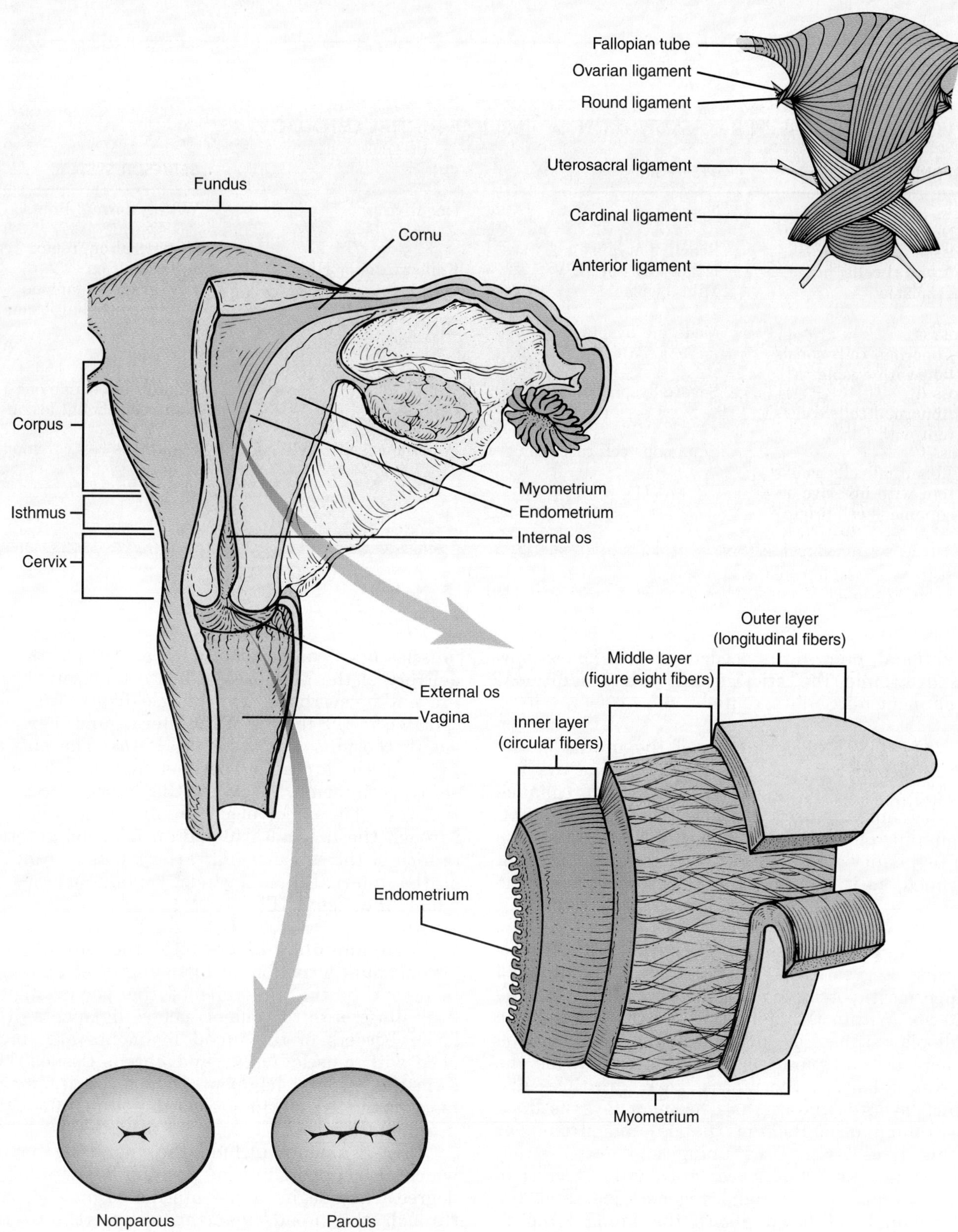

Figure 9–8

The uterus is a unique muscular organ supported by a complex pattern of ligaments • Its size can increase by 16 times (70 g to 1100 g) during pregnancy • After vaginal delivery the appearance of the external cervical os shows marked change.

Table 9–2

VARIOUS SYSTEMS FOR CLASSIFICATION OF CERVICOVAGINAL CYTOLOGY

PAPANICOLAOU CLASS	DYSPLASIA	CIN*	BETHESDA SYSTEM
Class I Normal smear	Negative	Negative	Within normal limits
Class II Atypical cells, no dysplasia	Reactive atypia Koilocytosis or HPV Mild dysplasia	 Koilocytosis or HPV CIN 1	Regeneration, repair Inflammation Low-grade squamous intraepithelial lesion
Class III Abnormal cells consistent with dysplasia	Moderate dysplasia	CIN 2	
Class IV Abnormal cells consistent with CIS	Severe dysplasia, CIS	CIN 2 CIN 3	High-grade squamous intraepithelial lesion
Class V Abnormal cells consistent with invasive or squamous cell origin	Squamous cell carcinoma	Squamous cell carcinoma	Squamous cell carcinoma

*CIN = cervical intraepithelial neoplasia.
From Stenchever, M. (1992). *Office gynecology* (p. 339). St. Louis: C. V. Mosby.

additional follow-up is needed, such as colposcopy, to determine the etiology and what additional treatment may be warranted.

▼ **Isthmus.** The isthmus of the uterus is the area of connection between the cervix and the corpus or body of the uterus (Fig. 9–8). In pregnancy it distends to form the lower uterine segment. Softening of the isthmus is one of the earlier signs of pregnancy. Anatomically, the isthmus is not well defined, as it is immediately continuous with the corpus.

▼ **Corpus.** The corpus or body of the uterus forms the greatest part of the uterus. The rounded uppermost portion is termed the fundus of the uterus. Within the fundus is the insertion of the fallopian tubes or oviducts. The specific area where the fallopian tubes insert is known as the cornu or horn of the uterus. There are three distinct layers of the uterus. The inner layer is lined by columnar epithelium, glands, and stroma, or connective tissue. This lining is known as endometrium and it produces an alkaline secretion. The stroma allows rapid regeneration, and the rich supply of blood allows the lining often to reach a thickness of 1 to 2 mm. The muscular level of the uterus, or myometrium, consists of several layers of interconnected muscles as illustrated in Figure 9–8. Many of these muscles are in such proximity that their fibers interconnect in a figure eight design. This configuration allows the muscles upon constriction (such as after birth and delivery of the placenta) to ligate themselves and prevent hemorrhage. The muscle fibers are most common in the fundus of the uterus, and they also act in the efforts to expel the fetus. The outside lining of the uterus, or perimetrium, is a layer of shiny peritoneum. It covers the uterus except at the sides. The major blood supply to the uterus is through the uterine artery branch of the anterior branch of the internal iliac artery. Other branches of the internal iliac include vaginal arteries to supply the vagina (Fig. 9–9).

▼ **Ligaments.** Lateral to the uterus the perimetrium forms broad ligaments that allow attachment to the sidewalls of the pelvis. Figure 9–8 illustrates the major pelvic ligaments. The lower borders of the broad ligaments are thickened with muscle, fascia, and fibrous tissue. They form the cardinal ligaments, which are the single most important uterine supports and maintain the uterine position.

Other ligaments include the round ligaments, which also support uterine position but to a lesser degree. They begin at the uterine cornu and pass through the broad ligament to insert into the labia majora. The uterosacral ligaments form the base of the pouch of Douglas and consist of folds of peritoneum that connect the sacrum to the sides of the isthmus. They also promote uterine position by pulling the cervix backward, encouraging the uterine position of anteversion.

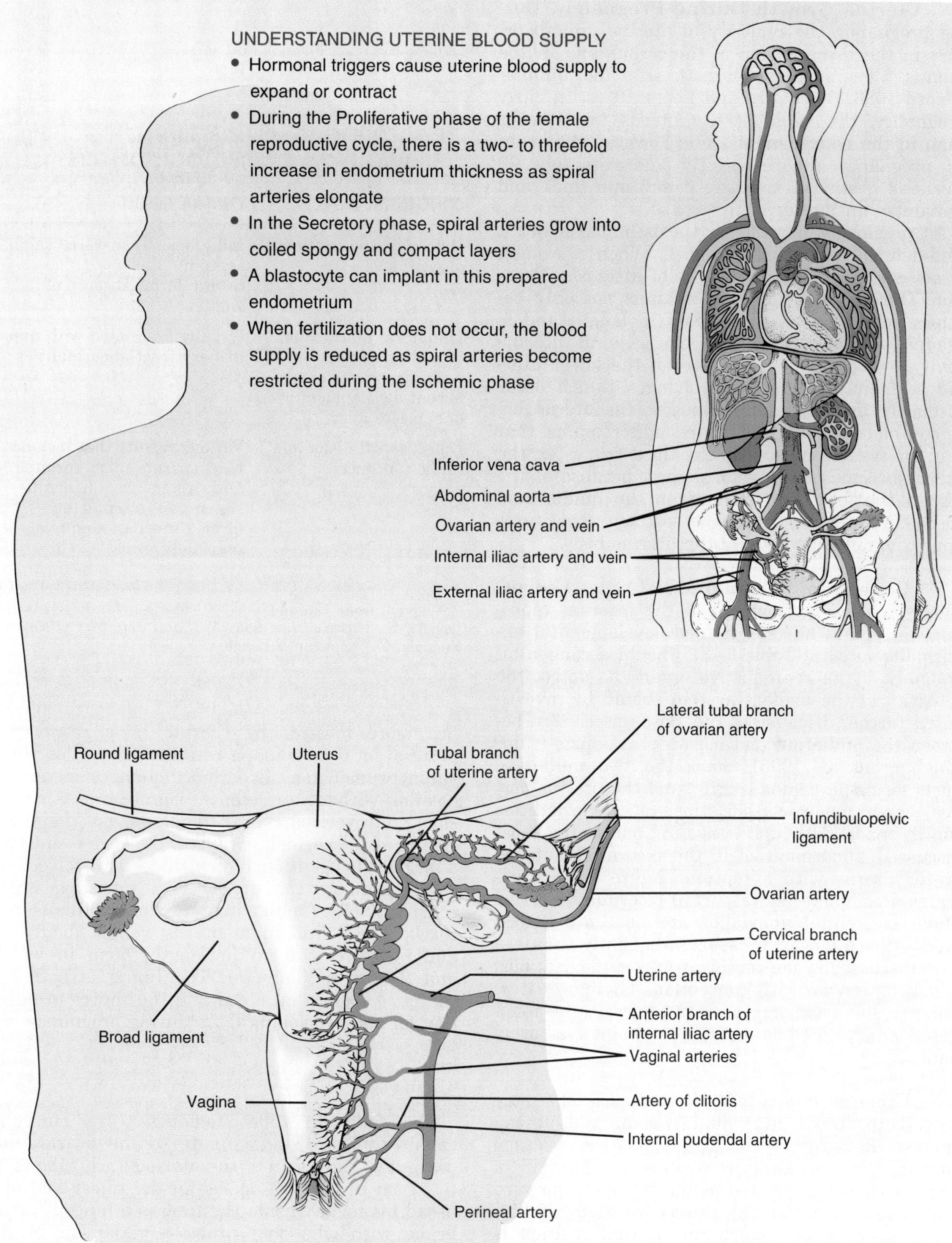

Figure 9–9
Pelvic and uterine blood supply in relation to the circulatory system.

Uterine Growth During Pregnancy. During pregnancy, the majority of uterine growth occurs in the myometrium of the corpus and in the fundus. Cells increase in both size and number (Oxorn 1986; Blackburn and Loper 1992). In early pregnancy, the walls of the uterus are thicker than in the nonpregnant state; however, they thin as pregnancy progresses. By approximately 20 weeks of gestation, they are 3 to 5 mm thick and remain so until after birth.

As previously mentioned, the isthmus is not a well-defined anatomic landmark. When a woman is not pregnant, the isthmus is of little consideration. During pregnancy the isthmus not only becomes softer but also increases in length and is gradually incorporated into the general uterine cavity, eventually forming part of the lower uterine segment. During these changes, which occur primarily in the second trimester, the uterus becomes more globular in shape and remains that way for several weeks. By the third trimester, the uterus becomes more pear shaped, because of the size of the fetus and changes in the fundus and corpus. Yet the lower uterine segment constitutes approximately one third of the uterine body.

Congenital Anomalies of the Uterus. Rarely in the development of the internal reproductive organs, an unexplained developmental abnormality occurs (Table 9–3). Should a congenital anomaly of the reproductive organs be noted, the integrity of the urinary system should be investigated further, because of the close association between the müllerian and mesonephric ducts (Cunningham et al. 1993). Since the two müllerian ducts form the vagina, cervix, and the uterine corpus, three major classifications of abnormalities can be made. Although it is rare, one of the most discussed abnormalities is the bicornuate uterus or the uterus with a septum. Figure 9–10 illustrates a complete and a partial bicornuate uterus. Major congenital anomalies are not only associated with childbearing issues; frequently they are first discussed when a woman has difficulty with menstruation or with conception. Therefore, it is common for a major congenital defect to be diagnosed and treated long before a woman is pregnant.

Uterine Positions. Uterine positions may vary, both in an individual woman and among women. Because of the ligaments, the average woman has an anteverted uterus. Thus, in a woman standing erect, the uterus leans forward and is almost horizontal as seen in Figure 9–11. However, in some women the uterine position is not as horizontal. Variations of uterine position are also illustrated in Figure 9–11. The uterus may be in a midline position. In some women the uterus is forward but bent upon the corpus or in an anteflexed position. In other women, the uterus lies more toward the sacrum in a retroverted position or, if extreme, a retroflexed position. Individual women may experience changes in uterine position without any clinical significance. Anteversion, retroversion, and midplane positions are variations of normal, except in the rare event that a pathologic agent such as a tumor is involved.

In summary, the uterus is a muscular organ consisting of a fundus, cornu, corpus, isthmus, and cervix. The nonpregnant uterus weighs about 60 g and measures 7.5 cm in length, 5 cm in width, and 2.5 cm in diameter. The lining is both the source of menstrual blood and the source of nutrition for the developing fetus during pregnancy.

Table 9–3

DEVELOPMENTAL ABNORMALITIES ARISING FROM EMBRYOLOGIC DEFECTS

CONGENITAL DEFECT	CLINICAL RESULT
Defective canalization of vagina	Mild form: Transverse vaginal septum Severe form: Absence of vagina
Unilateral maturation of müllerian duct with incomplete or absent development of opposite duct	Usually associated with upper urinary tract abnormalities
Defects with fusion of müllerian ducts	Various results that include two separate uteri, cervices, and vaginas, or a fusion between two incompletely formed uteri, or simply a uterine septum

Adapted from Cunningham, F., MacDonald, P., Gant, N., Leveno, K., Gilstrap, L. (1993). *Williams obstetrics* (19th ed.). Norwalk, CT: Appleton & Lange.

FALLOPIAN TUBES

The fallopian tubes (oviducts) are muscular canals that are approximate to the ovaries and connect to the cornu of the uterus. Each tube is 10 to 12 cm in length and lies in the upper fold of a broad ligament. Inside the tube is a mucous membrane with cilia that promote peristalsis of the ovum from the ovary along the tube to the uterus. Fallopian tubes are frequently divided into four anatomic areas as illustrated in Figure 9–12. The interstitial area is the area that passes into the uterine cavity. The lumen of the interstitial part is

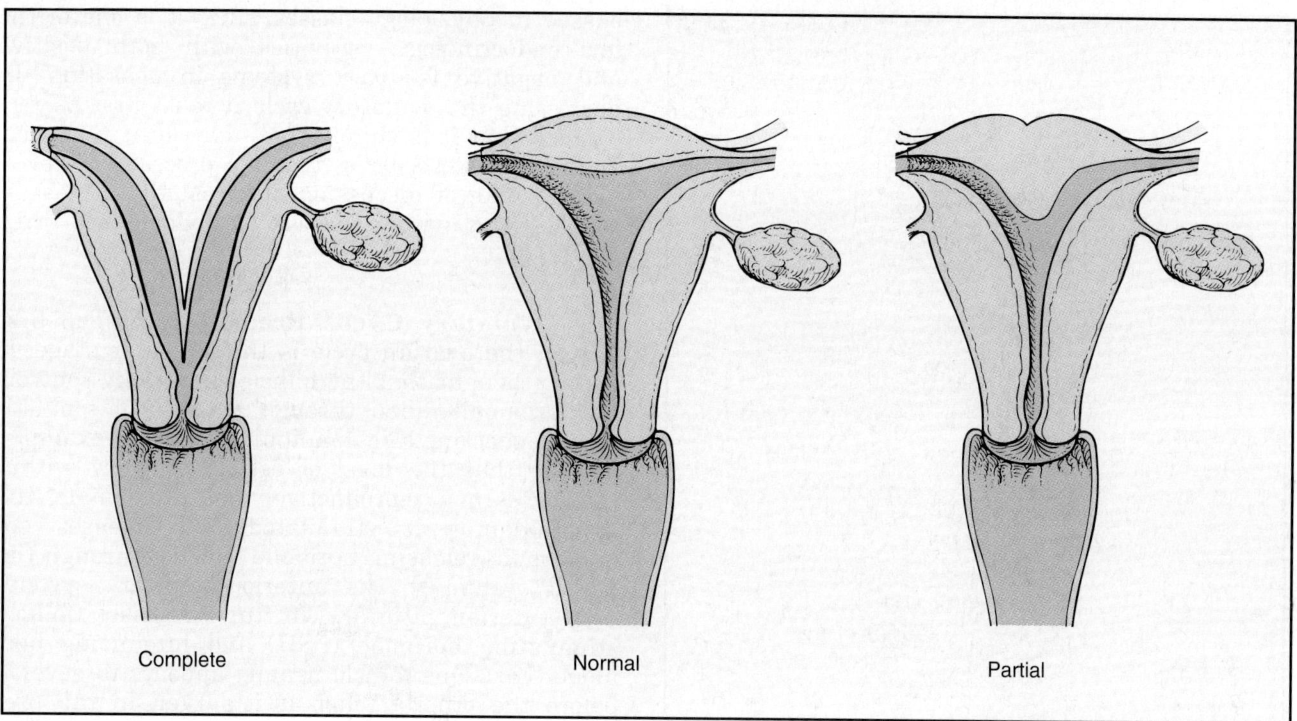

Figure 9–10

Uterine abnormalities are usually congenital • Often they are minor enough not to be clinically recognized.

about 1 mm in diameter. The isthmus connects the uterus to the larger portion of the oviduct, or the ampulla, in which fertilization usually occurs. The infundibulum is the area of the fallopian tube that is funnel shaped and terminates in a fimbriated margin that is proximate to the ovary. Clinically, fallopian tubes are rarely palpable except on very thin women. In that situation, they may be palpated as a tubular mass that is mobile and without tenderness. Enlargement, fixation or discomfort upon palpation suggests pathology, usually infection.

OVARIES

The two ovaries, although small, are of great reproductive and endocrinologic importance (see Fig. 9–12). They usually measure 4 cm in length, 2 cm in width, and 1.25 cm in diameter. The mesovarium attaches them to the broad ligaments. A hilum or stalklike structure on the anterior edge allows vascularization and nerve innervation. The ovarian ligament allows the ovary to be attached to the uterus at the cornu, and the longest fimbria of the fallopian tube, the fimbria ovarica, allows contact between the fallopian tube and the ovary. Laterally the ovary is suspended to the side of the pelvis by the lateral margin of the broad ligament or suspensory ligament of the ovary. The major blood supply to the ovary is from the ovarian artery (Oxorn 1996; Lichtman and Paper 1990).

The ovary has both a medulla and a cortex. The medulla is a supporting framework for the ovary. It consists of connective tissue, blood vessels, and nerves. The cortex is the active area. Follicles are contained in the cortex as shown in Figure 9–12. These follicles include the primordial follicles, which precede the development of oocytes. At birth, the average female has approximately 100,000 primordial follicles. During the ovarian cycles that occur during her reproductive life span, she has less than 500 mature or graafian follicles. The majority are victims of atresia during the menopausal period. The mature graafian follicle is approximately 10 mm in diameter. The theca externa is the outer layer and the theca interna the innermost lining. Inside the theca interna is an inner layer (antrum) of granulosa membranes with a clear fluid, or liquor folliculi. Granulosa cells surround the ovum contained within the graafian follicle (Oxorn 1986).

Endocrinologic Aspects of the Female Reproductive System

HYPOTHALAMUS-PITUITARY-OVARIAN AXIS

Ovulation is one of the major results of an interaction between the hypothalamus, pituitary, and ovaries. The ovulatory cycle is frequently dis-

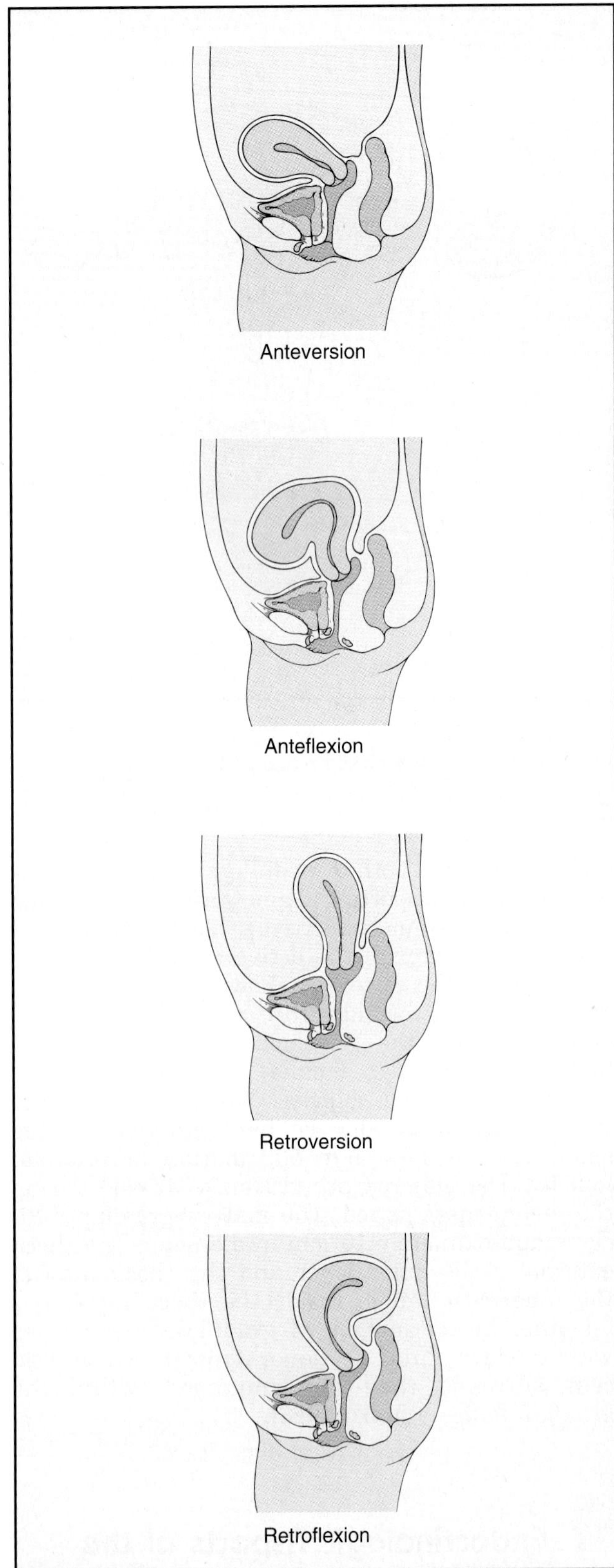

Figure 9–11

An anteverted uterine position is the most common one, although the others are not necessarily clinically significant.

cussed in physiology classes, since it is one of the few endocrinologic activities with both positive and negative feedback systems in operation. In discussing the ovulatory cycle it must first be recognized that it is simply that, a cycle. It is always artificial to describe a dynamic process. However, for the sake of discussion, it is usually easiest to consider the ovulatory cycle as divided into three parts.

▼ **Ovulatory Cycle: Preovulation.** The first part of the ovarian cycle is the follicular stage. It is now thought that the follicle essentially controls its hormonal milieu through a series of sophisticated endocrinologic manipulations. For example, assume that the level of estrogen is low within the body. In a reproductively mature female, the hypothalamus is stimulated and releases gonadotropin releasing hormone (GnRH) through the portal system to the anterior pituitary system. The anterior pituitary in turn releases follicle stimulating hormone (FSH) and luteinizing hormone (LH). One follicle usually appears to develop before the others. When it is larger, in the preantral phase, a granulosa layer grows and another layer is formed beneath it, the theca. Under the influence of FSH these cells produce an estrogenic environment. Estrogen and progesterone are the two major female reproductive hormones. Table 9–4 illustrates some of the effects they can have on the reproductive system. As high levels of estrogen are produced during the preovulatory period, a positive feedback occurs; specifically, the high estrogen levels influence increased production of GnRH, FHS, and especially LH. During this period progesterone is also being produced, albeit slowly. However, it too seems to be essential for the cycle as it appears to be necessary for a midcycle rise in FSH (Speroff et al. 1994).

▼ **Ovulatory Cycle: Ovulation.** At a certain point, usually after about 2 weeks of increasing levels of estrogen, the sensitivity of the anterior pituitary is such that an outpouring of LH occurs, the LH surge. The LH surge is an essential event in ovulation. It is the single event that marks the cyclic nature of the female pituitary secretion pattern. Primed by the increasing levels of estrogen in the follicle, FSH causes the development of LH receptors on the granulosa cells and production of small amounts of progesterone (Lichtman and Papera 1990). LH causes ovulation by stimulating the ovarian membrane to dissolve at the bulge of the mature follicle (Fig. 9–13). The ovum then erupts and escapes into the fimbriated end of the fallopian tube.

▼ **Ovulatory Cycle: Postovulation.** After ovulation, the granulosa cells continue to enlarge for

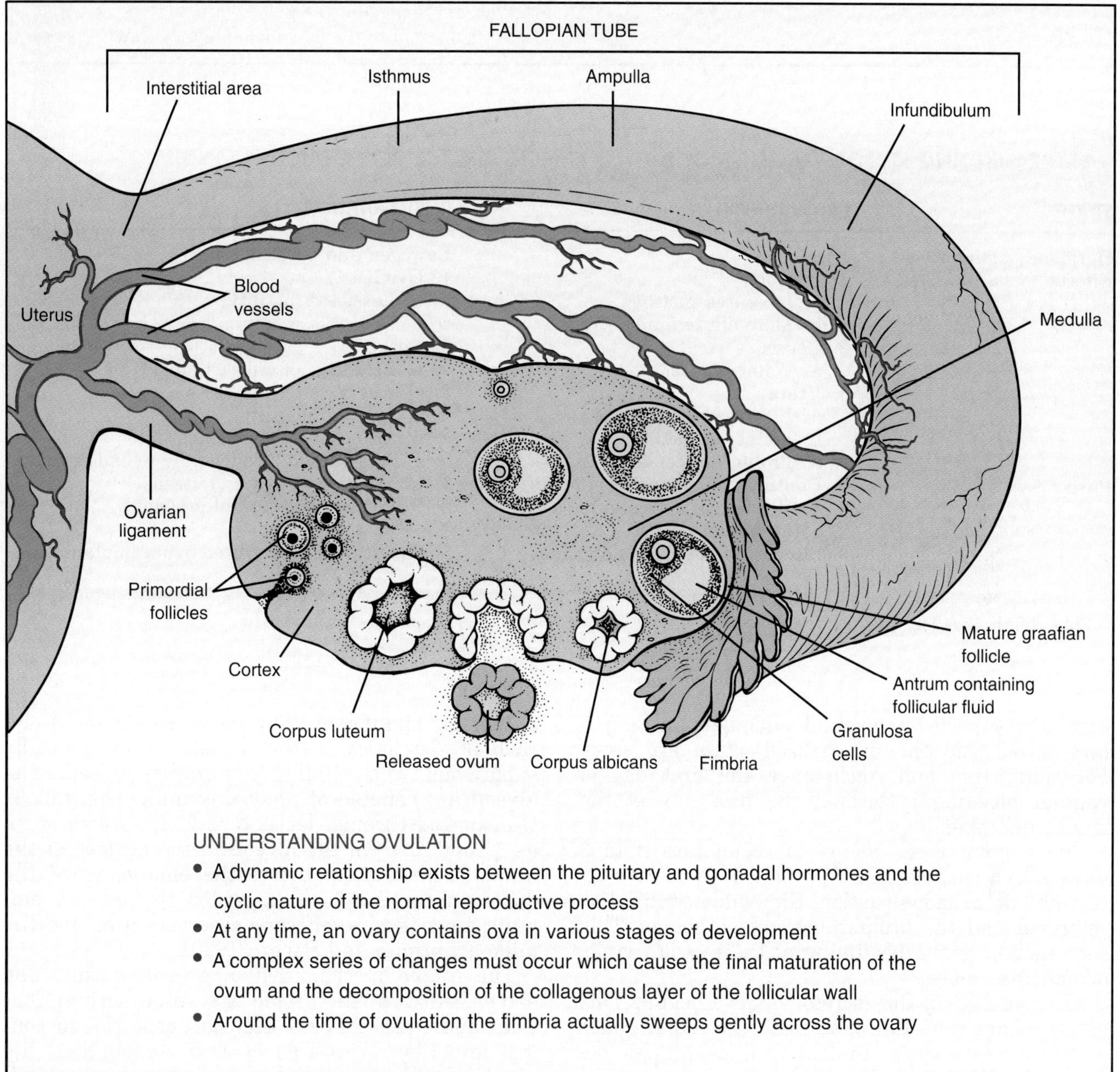

Figure 9–12

Cross section of the human ovary shown in relation to the uterus and fallopian tubes.

2 to 3 days. These cells accumulate a yellow pigment (lutein), and peak vascularization of the area occurs after 8 or 9 days (Lichtman and Papera 1990). The remains of the ruptured follicle are known as the corpus luteum, or yellow body. Progesterone is manufactured from the cholesterol delivered to the site from the low-density lipoproteins carried in the increased vascular network. Failure of fertilization is associated with eventual degeneration of the corpus luteum and diminishing production of estrogen and progesterone. As the blood concentrations of the hormones fall, it is assumed that the hypothalamus is able to assess that the level of estrogen is low. Thus, the cycle begins anew.

▼ **Menstrual Cycle and Ovulatory Cycle.** The menstrual cycle is intimately intertwined with the ovulatory cycle. As the blood concentrations of the gonadotropins drop (see Fig. 9–13), the menstrual phase of the menstrual cycle begins. This phase is characterized by vaginal bleed-

Table 9–4

ESTROGEN AND PROGESTERONE-MODULATED EFFECTS ON THE REPRODUCTIVE SYSTEM

STAGE	PREOVULATION	POSTOVULATION
Hormone dominance	Estrogen	Estrogen and progesterone
Effects	1. Oviducts a. Increased motility b. More dilute fluid secretion 2. Cervix a. Watery mucous secretion 3. Uterus a. Increased energy stores b. Increased motility c. Proliferated endometrium	1. Oviducts a. Lessened motility 2. Cervix a. Secretion of mucous plug 3. Uterus a. Quieted motility b. Secretion of nourishing fluid c. Augmented blood supply to endometrium
Purposes	1. Capture and retention of ovum 2. Facilitation of sperm entry and ascension to oviduct 3. Support of potential pregnancy	1. Conduction of ovum to uterus 2. Protection of potential pregnancy 3. Facilitation of fertilized ovum implantation

From Smith, E. (1982). *Abortion: Health care perspectives*. East Norwalk, CT: Appleton-Century-Crofts.

ing as a superficial layer of endometrium, capillary blood, and the unfertilized ovum are shed. For convention and consistency, the first day of vaginal bleeding is termed the first day of the menstrual cycle.

The endometrium begins to regenerate 2 to 3 days after menstruation. Approximately 5 days after the end of menstruation, the endometrium has reformed and the proliferative phase begins. This corresponds to the beginning of the ovarian cycle, or follicular phase.

After ovulation, the secretory phase begins. This phase occurs simultaneously with the luteal phase of the ovarian cycle. Endometrial capillaries become distended with blood and the endometrium itself has a thick, softened vascular bed that promotes implantation of a fertilized ovum. Should implantation not occur, as the corpus luteum degenerates, the endometrium begins changes that result in menstruation. It is the cyclic nature of the female reproductive system that distinguishes it from the male system.

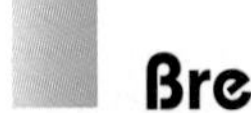

Breasts

The female mammary glands are compound secreting glands that have approximately 20 lobes of glandular tissue each. As with other organs that develop embryologically as two, one breast is often somewhat larger than the other without any pathologic significance. As shown in Figure 9–14, each of the lobes in the breasts is anatomically subdivided into lobules containing alveoli. The alveoli are capable of producing milk. The milk is transported through lactiferous ducts, which serve as a conduit from the alveoli to the surface of the nipple. Immediately before the emergence of the ducts on the nipple, they widen to form an ampulla that is a temporary reservoir area for the milk (Lichtman and Papera 1990).

The nipple is composed of erectile tissue. The external area of the nipple is covered with epithelium and muscle fibers that can constrict to control milk flow. The area of skin surrounding the nipple is pigmented and termed the areola. Small Montgomery glands can be found on the areola, as well as an occasional hair follicle. The major lymphatic vessels of the breast lie in the spaces around the breast lobes. These vessels drain primarily into two groups of nodes: the axillary nodes and the internal mammary nodes along the sternum. The vascular supply to the breast includes branches of the internal thoracic artery and lateral thoracic artery.

The major influences on breast development include estrogen, progesterone, lactogen, prolactin, growth hormone, thyroid hormone, and insulin. During pregnancy, the breasts tend to experience glandular proliferation. After delivery, the low levels of estrogen and progesterone appear to have a negative effect on prolactin inhibition, and lactation begins. Lactation is discussed in Chapter 33.

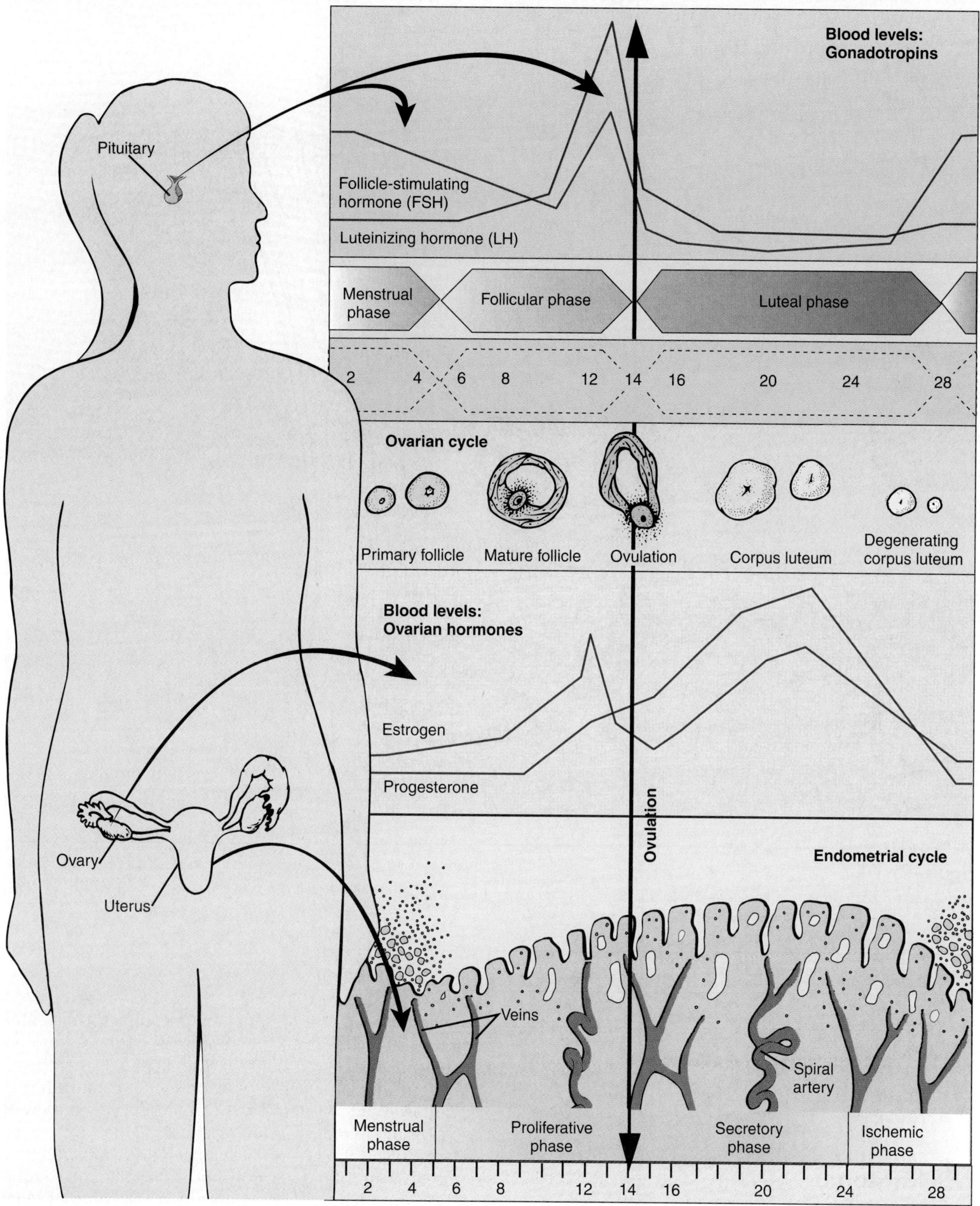

Figure 9–13

The female ovulatory cycle is directed by complex interrelationships between levels of hormone secretion, development of follicles, and changes in uterine endometrium. (Data from Speroff, L., Glass, R., Kase, N. [1994]. *Clinical gynecologic endocrinology and infertility* (5th ed.). Baltimore: Williams & Wilkins.)

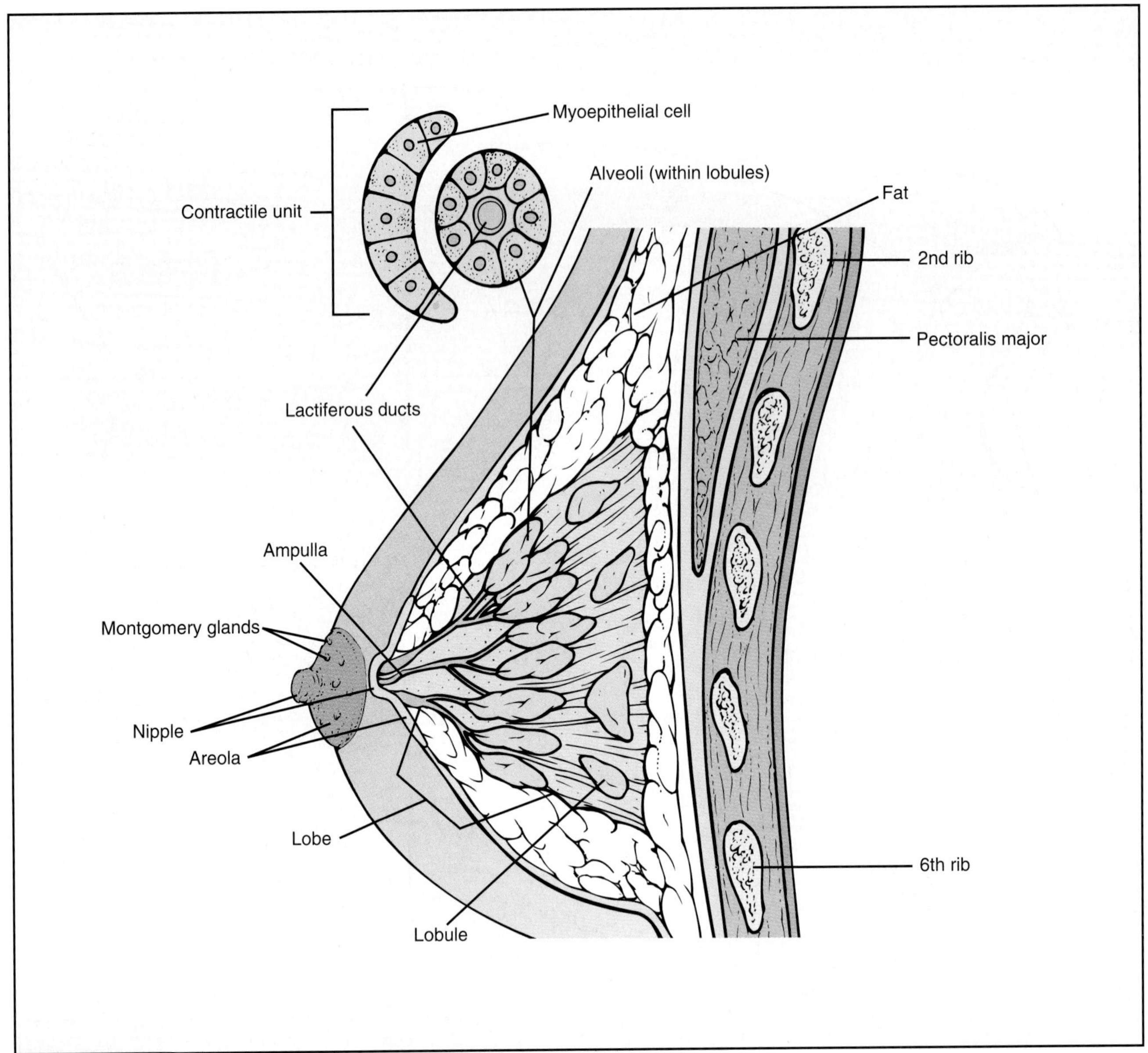

Figure 9–14

The breast, or mammary gland, has 15 to 25 lobes • Lobes radiate from the areola like a wheel, cushioned by varying amounts of fat • Under hormonal influence the alveoli secrete milk.

MALE REPRODUCTIVE SYSTEM

Anatomy

Anatomically, the male testes are usually located in the scrotum, a loose sac of tissue with a fairly constant milieu below body core temperature (Fig. 9–15). Each testis is approximately 4.5 cm in length and weighs 40 g. The spermatic arteries provide the major blood supply to the testes, carrying blood from the aorta. In the testes, approximately 80 percent of the space is composed of seminiferous tubules and the remainder is composed of supportive connective tissue with scattered Leydig cells. Leydig cells are pure steroid-secreting cells. Their major product is testosterone. The seminiferous tubules are coiled masses of loops. The beginning and end of each loop is the tubulus rectus. The tubuli recti eventually drain through the ducti efferentes into the epididymis. The epididymis is connected to the penis through the vas deferens and ejaculatory duct.

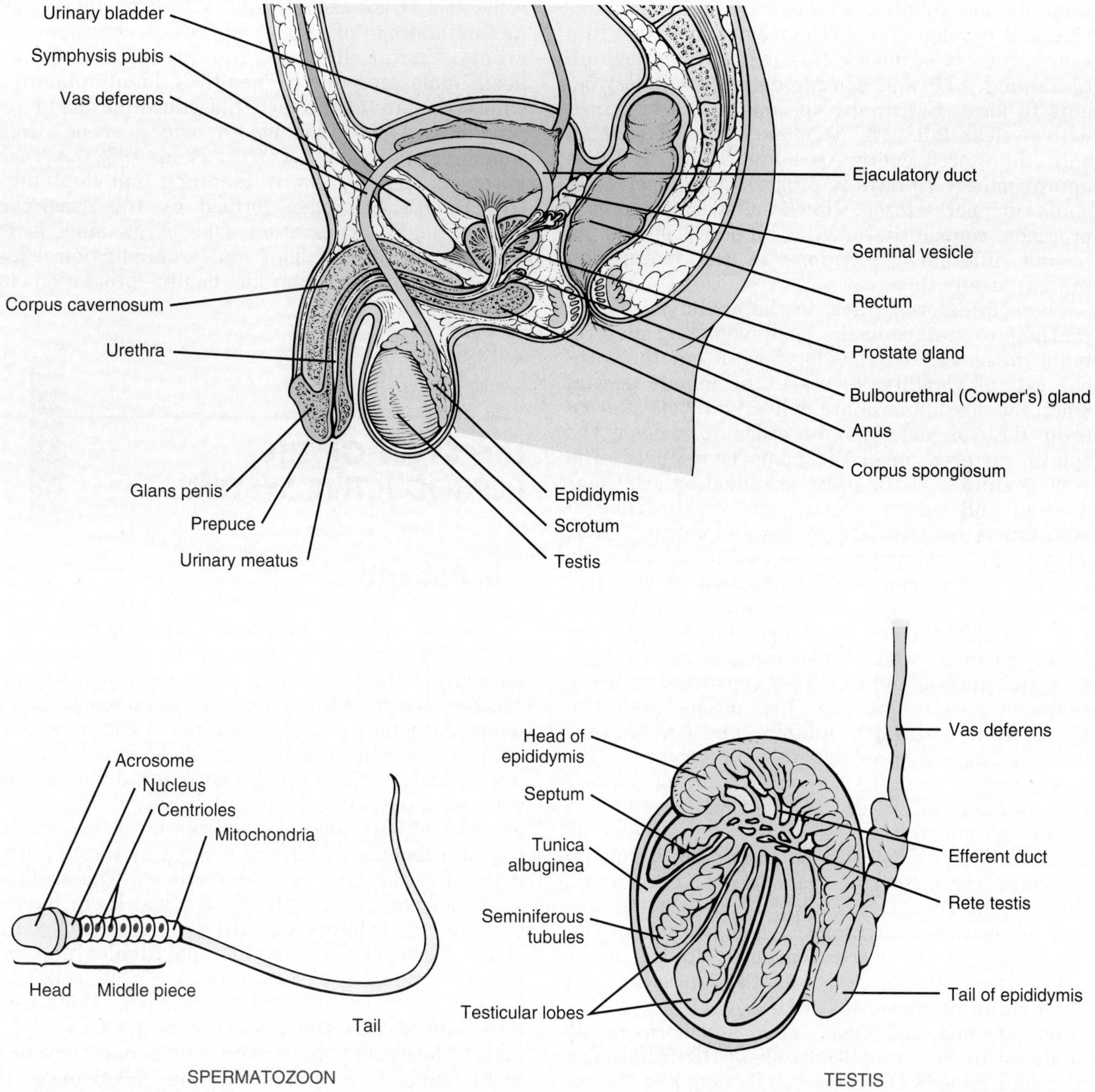

Figure 9–15
Male reproductive organs with enlargements of a spermatozoon and testis.

Every seminiferous tubule is separated from the connective tissue and Leydig cells by a basement membrane. Immediately proximate to the basement membrane are Sertoli cells and spermatogonia. Each tubule is bathed in locally generated testosterone from the Sertoli cells. The seminiferous tubules are the functional units for spermatogenesis.

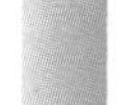

Spermatogenesis

In contrast to the female reproductive system, the male reproductive system is neither cyclic nor of an amount predetermined at birth. A female infant is born with a fixed number of oocytes, which decrease throughout life. However, a male can produce sperm continuously throughout his reproductive life. He usually produces 100 to 200 million sperm daily. Sperm production takes place in the seminiferous tubules, wherein spermatogonia divide and develop into spermatocytes and then into spermatids. It is during this period that the tail, containing ATP and contractile microtubules, begins to form. Eventually spermatozoa are formed with a clear tail with flagellar motion associated with the stored energy (see Fig. 9–15). It takes approximately 70 days to progress from spermatogonia to spermatozoa. However, spermatogenesis proceeds constantly but in different stages by having different generations in the maturation process at any time.

The spermatozoa travel to the epididymis. They continue to mature in the epididymis and may remain in the vas deferens for several months without loss of viability. To reach the female genital tract, the spermatozoa are delivered by ejaculation from the vas deferens. In order to deliver the sperm, an erection of the penis is required. The venous sinuses of the penis are filled by arteriolar dilation and venous constriction. At the time of ejaculation, the prostate glands add calcium, zinc, citrate, and acid phosphatase, which provides alkalinity and promotes neutralization of the acid medium of the vagina. The seminal vesicles provide extra fluid in the form of the terminal portion of the ejaculate, whose major components are fructose and prostaglandins. Other constituents of the seminal vesicles include LH, FSH, prolactin, testosterone, estradiol, inhibin, and endorphins, whose exact role is not yet well understood. A typical ejaculate contains 200 million to 400 million spermatozoa in a volume of 3 to 4 mL.

The hormonal control of spermatogenesis is probably less well understood than the hormonal control of the menstrual cycle (Vander et al. 1989; Wilson and Foster 1992). FSH, LH, testosterone, and an estrogen (estradiol) appear to coordinate the regulation of spermatogenesis. In the male, LH is frequently referred to as the interstitial cell stimulating hormone, or ICSH.

Testosterone, the major male sex hormone, is produced in the interstitial cells of the testes. The hormonal control of male reproduction, like that of female reproduction, involves the hypothalamus-pituitary axis. Testosterone causes a negative feedback for LH secretion by both the hypothalamus and anterior pituitary. When testosterone is low, the hypothalamus releases a gonadotropin releasing hormone to cause the anterior pituitary to release FSH and LH. FSH directly influences spermatogenesis by stimulation of the Sertoli cells. LH influences testosterone secretion in the testes. Stimulation of the Sertoli cells results in release of another hormone, inhibin, which is similar to testosterone in its negative feedback to the hypothalamus and anterior pituitary. The hormonally complex event of spermatogenesis is still under exploration by basic scientists.

The lack of adequate educational materials is a reflection of the complexity as well as the recent understanding of male hormonal reproductive events. Forrest discussed the lack of information about male reproductive health in family planning clinics in spite of the fact that education about reproduction must include a wider scope than women's health only (Forrest et al. 1989). A Task Force on Men in Family Planning and Reproductive Health has been formed by the American Public Health Association. One of its aims is to promote education about male reproduction. This area is another focus for health promotion in nursing.

LIFE CYCLE OF THE REPRODUCTIVE SYSTEM

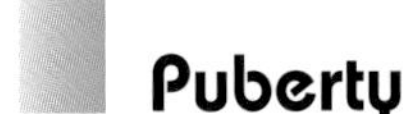

Puberty

Puberty and the initiation of the functional reproductive systems warrant a brief discussion. Sex maturity ratings (SMRs) were proposed several decades ago by Tanner and are in common usage today. Although puberty does not occur at a constant age in males or females, there appears to be a constant sequence for the normal individual. Development of pubic hair and breast development are two of the major landmarks of sexual maturity of a female. Puberty is defined by the development of secondary sex characteristics. The earliest stages of puberty are the SMR stage II. In males, as noted in Table 9–5, SMR II is marked by increased size of the seminiferous tubules and increased numbers of Leydig and Sertoli cells accompanied by secretion of testosterone. Table 9–5 also summarizes the Tanner classification of female adolescent breast and pubic hair development. Table 9–6 summarizes the mean onset of female pubertal changes in the United States.

The events of puberty are linked theoretically with the beginning of maturation of the hypothalamus. It has been hypothesized that maturation of the hypothalamus leads to an increase in production of gonadotropin releasing hormones in both females and males. The pulsatile nature of the production of FSH and LH is less well explained. It appears that the cyclic nature of the female reproductive system is secondary to both the pulsatile nature of the early production of these hormones and intricate negative and positive feedback systems.

Table 9–5

TANNER CLASSIFICATION OF ADOLESCENT DEVELOPMENT

FEMALE

Stage	Breasts	Pubic Hair
I	Papillae elevated, preadolescent	None
II	Breasts and papillae, small mounds	Sparse, long, slightly pigmented
III	Breasts and areolae confluent, elevated	Darker, coarser, curly
IV	Areolae and papillae projected above breast	Adult type—pubic only
V	Papillae projected, mature	Lateral distribution

MALE

Stage	Penis	Testes	Pubic Hair
I	Preadolescent	Preadolescent	None
II	Slight enlargement	Enlarged scrotum, pink texture altered	Scanty, long, slightly pigmented
III	Longer	Larger	Darker, starts to curl, small amount
IV	Larger; glans and breadth increase in size	Larger, scrotum dark	Resembles adult type but less in quantity; coarse, curly
V	Adult size	Adult size	Adult distribution, spread to medial surface of thighs

Adapted from Lichtman, R., and Papera, S. (1990). *Gynecology* (p. 16). Norwalk, CT: Appleton & Lange.

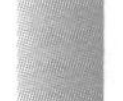

Menarche

Menarche marks the first menstrual period. Strictly speaking, it is incorrect to refer to it as the first menstrual cycle, since menarche signals maturation of the uterus, but not reproductive maturity. The first few periods are frequently noncyclic in nature because of anovulation. Often, menstruation occurs several times before menses are regular and predictable. Controversy remains over the triggers for menarche; the most common theories include skeletal growth and accumulation of body fat (Golub 1992).

Today, the average female in the United States experiences menarche at slightly less than 13 years of age.

It is important to realize that for many women the process of menstruation is fraught with taboos and colored by cultural norms. Less than two decades ago, a large survey of American residents was conducted. Eight percent of these individuals, who represented all ethnic, gender, and socioeconomic categories, felt that menstruating women should limit contact with others. More than one third of those surveyed felt that menstruating women should conceal the fact, even among family members at home (Golub 1992). The respondents with the least bias toward menstruation and the most openness toward the event were the most educated and affluent of the survey participants. Thus, the nurse can help influence a woman's perspective on her own biology by educating her during professional interactions.

Menopause

Menopause indicates the cessation of menses permanently. For the average woman in the United States, this occurs at approximately 50 years of age. As with menarche, there are some suggested influences on the timing of menopause. Women who are smokers or heavy drinkers appear to experience menopause slightly earlier than their cohorts. Menopause is the result of follicular atresia. Circulating levels of FSH and LH begin to rise almost a decade before menopause. Eventually the cyclic nature of the hypothalamic-pituitary-ovarian axis is severely disrupted. Ovulation ceases and follicular atresia increases. Production

Table 9–6

MEAN ONSET OF FEMALE PUBERTAL CHANGES IN THE UNITED STATES

AGE	CHARACTERISTIC
9–10	Beginning of height spurt
	Growth of bony pelvis
	Female contour fat deposition
	Budding of nipples
10–11	Budding of breasts
	Appearance of pubic hair (may precede breast budding in 10%)
11–12	Appearance of vaginal secretions
	Growth of internal and external genitalia
	Increase in vaginal glycogen content; lowering of pH
12–13	Pigmentation of areolae
	Growth of breasts
13–14	Appearance of axillary hair
	Increase in amount of pubic hair
	Acne (in 75%–90%)
	Menarche
15–16	Arrest of skeletal growth

From Goldfarb, A. (1977). Puberty and menarche. *Clinical Obstetrics and Gynecology,* 20 (3), 629.

of estrogen and progesterone moves from inside the ovary to the other sites, including the adrenals. The woman's endocrine milieu moves from a dependence on estradiol to estrone, a less potent estrogen.

As with menarche, cultural influences are major factors in how a woman views menopause. Some women are extremely uncomfortable discussing menopause as they view it as an ending rather than a beginning. Denial is used as a method of coping with this biologic event. As older women are entering the childbirth arena, it is important that nurses share information about menopause as another life development. Recent lay literature has focused on menopause, helping women to understand that it should not be the taboo that it once was, and nurses can provide an opportunity to discuss this phenomenon.

Implications for Research

Research related to many aspects of the reproductive system has increased dramatically in the past two decades. The area that has been of particular interest is that of the ovulatory and menstrual cycles and factors influencing conception. With technologic advances resulting in the clini-

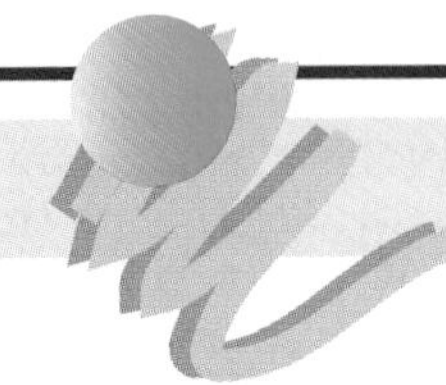

HISTORICAL PERSPECTIVES

KNOWLEDGE OF REPRODUCTION

Knowledge of the menstrual cycle is of relatively recent vintage. Although the ovary had been described as early as 1668 by Stensen, it was not until 1827 that the human ovum was discovered by Von Baer. Later in that century, in 1871, Sigismund found that there was mucosal destruction when menstruation occurred. With this information, he deduced that menstruation was the result of lack of fertilization.

Two years later, Kundrat and Engelmann were the first to discuss cyclic endometrial changes. In 1893, Regis demonstrated that the ovary produced some "internal secretions" by injecting ovarian extracts subcutaneously and observing clinical changes. However, it was not until 1929 that Doisy and Butenandt were able to isolate a human estrogenic substance, later to be named estrone. Thus, the ovarian hormones that influence the menstrual cycle were unheard of until approximately 60 years ago. That basic discovery, combined with technologic improvements and increased assay capabilities, promoted the rapid advancement of knowledge.

Within the next decade syntheses of estrogens and progesterones were introduced. After three decades, these hormones began to be used to influence artificially and manipulate the menstrual cycle and, in turn, female reproductive processes for therapeutic or contraceptive purposes.

From Grollman, A. (1962). *Clinical endocrinology.* Philadelphia: J. B. Lippincott.

cal identification and management of infertility, nurses in many areas of the country have had an opportunity to become involved in medical research studies related to the reproductive system. However, nursing research also has a place in this field of inquiry. The following are examples of research questions that would provide helpful information for nurses or childbirth educators working with pregnant women and families:

- What is the knowledge level of expectant parents regarding the anatomy and physiology of pregnancy and childbirth?
- What is the essential information that pregnant women need about the anatomy and physiology of pregnancy and childbirth?
- What is the most effective method of teaching expectant parents about the anatomy and physiology of pregnancy and childbirth?

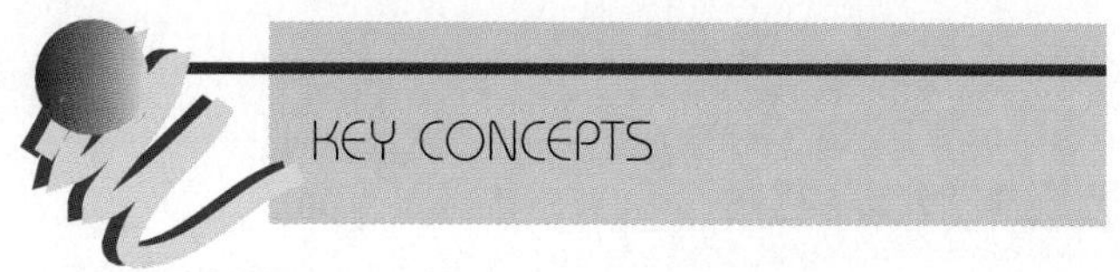

KEY CONCEPTS

- ▼ The gonads initially arise in the embryo as a pair of ridges that are grossly identical in males and females; differentiation depends upon genetic constitution.
- ▼ The female genital tract is developed primarily from the müllerian ductal system.
- ▼ The female bony pelvis is gynecoid in design, which facilitates childbearing.
- ▼ Major external female genitalia include the mons pubis, labia majora, labia minora, clitoris, urethral meatus, vagina, perineum, and fourchette.
- ▼ The major internal female reproductive structures include the vagina, uterus, oviducts, and ovaries.
- ▼ The usual uterine position is anteverted, although variations of version and flexion are frequently found.
- ▼ Ovaries are composed of follicles in different stages of maturation.
- ▼ The hypothalamic-pituitary-ovarian axis reflects the dynamic changes in the endocrine milieu of a woman that are necessary for the biologic events of ovulation and menstruation.
- ▼ In contrast to the pulsatile and cyclic nature of the female reproductive system, male spermatogenesis can occur at any time and usually proceeds constantly. At any point different stages of sperm maturation may be found in a healthy male adult.
- ▼ The female reproductive life cycle proceeds from puberty (maturation) through menstruation until at approximately the sixth decade of life menstruation ceases (menopause).

References

Berek, J. S., Adashi, E. Y., Hillard, P. A. (1996). *Novak's textbook of gynecology* (12th ed.). Baltimore: Williams & Wilkins.

Blackburn, S., and Loper, D. (1992). *Maternal, fetal and neonatal physiology: A clinical perspective.* Philadelphia: W. B. Saunders.

Cunningham, F., MacDonald, P., Gant, N., Leveno, K., Gilstrap, L. (1993). *Williams obstetrics* (19th ed.). Norwalk: Appleton & Lange.

Doress, P., Siegal, D., the Midlife and Older Women Book Project in cooperation with the Boston Women's Health Book Collective. (1987). *Ourselves, growing older.* New York: Simon & Schuster.

Forrest, K., Swanson, J., Beckstein, D. (1989). The availability of educational and training materials on men's reproductive health. *Family Planning Perspectives,* 21 (3), 120–122.

Goldfarb, A. (1977). Puberty and menarche. *Clinical Obstetrics and Gynecology,* 20 (3), 629.

Golub, S. (1992). *Periods: From menarche to menopause.* Newbury Park, CA: Sage.

Grollman, A. (1962). *Clinical endocrinology.* Philadelphia: J. B. Lippincott.

Johnston, G. P. (1994). *The wish, the wait, the wonder* (p. 15). New York: Harper Collins.

Lichtman, R., and Papera, S. (1990). *Gynecology.* Norwalk, CT: Appleton & Lange.

Oxorn, H. (1986). *Human labor and birth* (5th ed.). Norwalk, CT: Appleton & Lange.

Sadler, T. (1995). *Langman's medical embryology* (5th ed.). Baltimore: Williams & Wilkins.

Smith, E. (1982). *Abortion: Health care perspectives.* Norwalk, CT: Appleton-Century-Crofts.

Speroff, L., Glass, R., Kase, N. (1994). *Clinical gynecologic endocrinology and infertility* (5th ed.). Baltimore: Williams & Wilkins.

Stenchever, M. (1992). *Office gynecology* (p. 339). St. Louis: C. V. Mosby.

Vander, S., Sherman, J., Luciano, D. (1989). *Human physiology: The mechanism of body function.* New York: McGraw-Hill.

Wilson, J. D., and Foster, D. W. (1992). *Textbook of endocrinology* (8th ed.). Philadelphia: W. B. Saunders.

10 Chapter

> For women, pregnancy often creates an increased need for physical affection—a craving that may be greater than the desire for sexual satisfaction. . . . Finding pleasure in each other's body by cuddling, holding, and discovering new positions and new ways of pleasuring each other are also part of sexuality, and pregnancy is a wonderful time to explore these other aspects of making love.
>
> Elizabeth Bing (1994)

Sexuality During Pregnancy

Elaine Zwelling

HIGHLIGHTS

- Sexual Development from the Fetal Period Through Adulthood
- Physical Aspects of Sexuality
- Masters and Johnson's Sexual Response Cycle
- Kaplan's Triphasic Theory
- Sexual Adaptation in Pregnancy
- Sexual Adaptation in the Postpartum Period
- Psychological Aspects of Sexuality
- Sociocultural Aspects of Sexuality
- Cognitive Aspects of Sexuality
- Nursing Practice
- Risk Management
- Implications for Research

Sexuality is an integral component of the human experience. As humans, we are sexual beings from the moment of our conception until our death. Our sexuality is one factor that shapes our physical, emotional, social, and cognitive being, and each of these elements in turn shapes our sexuality. Awareness of one's sexuality can be a celebration of the self, a voyage into the body, mind, and spirit. Sexuality encompasses the whole person and all his or her traits. Because sexuality involves each facet of an individual, it can have many meanings.

The subject of sexuality is capable of triggering strong emotional reactions along with a wide variety of rigid opinions, dogmatic religious beliefs, or strict legal sanctions. Our life experiences are therefore likely to dictate how we express our sexuality. For some people, sexuality can mean feeling good about oneself and having a positive body image. For others, sexuality may mean intimacy, love, security, comfort, joy, or status. Sexual desires are inborn and instinctive, but sexual attitudes and behavior are learned. Thus,

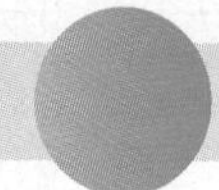

DEFINITIONS

Anal stage—The stage of development identified by Freud during which the young child's interest revolves around the processes of elimination.

Chorioamnionitis—Infection of the fetal membranes.

Coitus—Sexual intercourse.

Cunnilingus—Oral sexual stimulation of the female genitals.

Dyspareunia—Painful intercourse.

Electra complex—The jealousy experienced by a young girl of her mother's relationship with her father.

Genital stage—The adolescent stage of development identified by Freud during which the oral, anal, and genital sexual urges fuse together.

Latent stage—The stage of development identified by Freud during which the school-age child experiences decreased interest in sexuality.

Masturbation—Self-stimulation of the genitals or other body parts to achieve sexual excitement or orgasm.

Myotonia—Increase in muscle tension experienced during sexual excitement.

Oedipus complex—The jealousy experienced by a young boy of his father's relationship with his mother.

Oral stage—The stage of development identified by Freud during which the infant receives pleasure and gratification through sucking.

Phallic stage—The stage of development identified by Freud during which the preschool child demonstrates an increased focus on sex play and masturbation.

Vasocongestion—Primary response to sexual stimulation in which veins in the genital area fill with blood.

the same sexual activity can hold different meanings for different people or a different meaning for the same person from one time to the next. Since sexual behavior can find expression in many ways, people who equate sex only with sexual intercourse narrow the range of possibilities for satisfying sexual needs.

Pregnancy and early parenthood most certainly influence the sexuality of the couple. Physical, emotional, social, and cognitive factors all contribute to the overall impact of the childbearing year. Other influences include the couple's sexual experiences before the pregnancy, whether the pregnancy was planned or wanted, and how the couple has accommodated past sexual experiences into their life together. The demands of the childbearing year can prompt a period of personal growth for expectant parents, motivating them to take the opportunity to learn new intimacy and sexual skills.

Unfortunately, there is little research about sexuality during pregnancy on which to build a knowledge base. The information that is available is not always communicated to the expectant couple. Sexuality in pregnancy and the early postpartum period is often ignored, and the scant information available is likely to be inconsistent and outdated, based on tradition rather than scientific research, and imparted with embarrassment.

The nurse can be an important source of information about sexuality during pregnancy for expectant parents because the nurse is the health team member who has the opportunity to provide regular assessment and counseling. A sound knowledge base of sexuality through the physiologic theory of the sexual response, knowledge of the influence of pregnancy on sexuality, and identification of psychological, sociocultural, and cognitive aspects of sexuality prepare the nurse to understand and discuss the nursing process as it relates to sexuality in pregnancy.

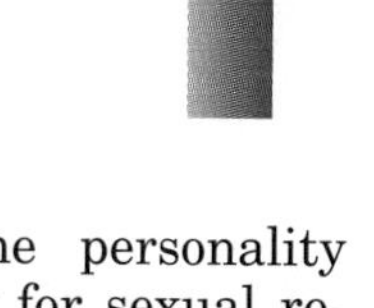

SEXUAL DEVELOPMENT

Sexuality is a dimension of the personality rather than just a person's capacity for sexual response (Masters et al. 1995). As such, it is an integral part of all developmental processes.

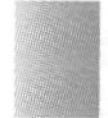

Fetal Period

Each stage of the life cycle presents new aspects of sexual growth and behavior (Table 10–1). An individual's gender is determined by chance at the time of conception. The man's sperm provides either an X or Y sex chromosome to the woman's egg, which is always an X chromosome. The development of the embryo as female (XX) or male (XY) during the fetal stage begins the life process of sexual identity.

Table 10–1

SEXUAL DEVELOPMENT THROUGHOUT THE LIFE SPAN

DEVELOPMENTAL STAGE	DEVELOPMENTAL MILESTONES AND BEHAVIORS	INFLUENCING FACTORS
Embryonic period to birth	Male infant: Larger, more muscle mass; more active Female: More sensitive to tactile stimulation and pain	Sex chromosome assignment: male—XY female—XX Development of testes at 6–7 wk, ovaries at 12 wk Secretion of androgens in male embryo Gender assignment at birth
Infancy (birth–1 yr)	Oral exploration Sucking Tactile responsiveness Erection or vaginal lubrication Genital exploration and masturbation Orgasmic potential	Caressing and touching by caretakers Feeding Social sex-typing behaviors Reinforcement of gender identity by society
Toddler period (1–3 yr)	Development of pride in gender identity Control of bladder and bowel functions Genital exploration and masturbation Use of vocabulary re: genital anatomy and elimination	Sex role modeling of parents Parental attitudes re: genital exploration and toilet training
Preschool child (4–6 yr)	Identity with same-sex parent Oedipal attachments to opposite-sex parent Masturbation Heterosexual play Increased display of affection	Peer play opportunities Adult acceptance of genital exploration
School-age child (7–12 yr)	Socialization with same-gender peers Beginning of sexual awakening and development Increased self-consciousness and self-awareness Masturbation Sexual fears or fantasies and curiosity Use of "dirty words"	Information provided to child Reactions of parents and adults to sexual behavior Self-esteem

During the period of embryonic development, fetal hormones influence sexual development. In the male embryo, the testes form after the seventh week of gestation and begin to produce androgen testosterone. Primary female sexual differentiation does not depend on hormones (Moore and Persaud 1993). By the time of birth, the physiologic structures of the male and female sexual organs are complete, and gender assignment may be confirmed. Physical sexual differences, in addition to the external genitalia, can be observed even at birth. Male infants are usually larger, have more muscle mass, and are more active than female infants. Female infants tend to be more passive in motor responses and more sensitive to tactile stimulation and pain (Woods 1984).

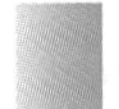

Infancy

From the time of birth, learning is a stronger influence on sexual development than biology. While both play an integral role in final development, physical and hormonal influences take a subordinate role until adolescence (Masters et al. 1995). During infancy, from birth through the first year of life, sexual expression is evidenced through oral exploration. Freud identified this period as the oral stage and believed that the infant received pleasure from sucking. This oral drive is easily observed during feeding and when babies examine new objects by placing them in their mouths.

Table 10–1

SEXUAL DEVELOPMENT THROUGHOUT THE LIFE SPAN Continued

DEVELOPMENTAL STAGE	DEVELOPMENTAL MILESTONES AND BEHAVIORS	INFLUENCING FACTORS
Adolescence Early (12–15 yr)	Increased concern re: body image Masturbation with orgasm Development of heterosexual relationships Menarche Nocturnal emissions	Parental attitudes Peer relationships Peer pressure Information provided Popular music; media
Late (16–19 yr)	Heterosexual sexual activity Development of intimacy Development of sex role behaviors Development of morals and ethics	Peer attitudes and pressures Peer relationships Parental influence Information provided Popular music; media
Adulthood Young (20–40 yr)	Experimentation with sexual relationships Development of commitment Marriage Childbearing decisions	Peer attitudes and pressures Peer relationships Education Financial and career status Religious views
Middle (40–60 yr)	Responses to influence of aging on sexuality Increase in intimacy and sexual satisfaction Extramarital sexual activity	Decreased hormone production Health status Stress levels Career and financial status
Late (older than 60 yr)	Continued interest in sexual activity Decreased physical responsiveness	Illness or loss of partner Attitudes of society

Infants also enjoy sexual expression through their sense of touch. Tactile stimulation is known to be important to infants as a means of communication and security, and their sense of touch is highly developed. Indeed, infants who do not receive frequent touching and holding may show evidence of alterations in physical, emotional, or social development.

Signs of physiologic sexual response are also present in infancy. Male infants have frequent penile erections and may experience orgasm, although ejaculation is not possible until puberty. Female infants show evidence of vaginal lubrication and may also experience orgasm. Both female and male infants explore and stimulate the external genitalia during the first year of life. This behavior is a normal part of development and does not represent a pathologic or deviant response (Rice 1995).

External social factors may already influence the sexual development of the infant. Even though parents may make a concerted effort to avoid sex-typing behavior with their infant, research has shown that adults do subconsciously respond to an infant of a given sex with certain behaviors. For example, mothers look at and talk to girls more and respond to a girl's irritability more quickly. Boys are touched, held, rocked, and kissed more as infants (Woods 1984). Male and female infants are dressed differently, their rooms are decorated differently, and different toys are selected for their play. These parental behaviors play a significant role in the development of gender identity.

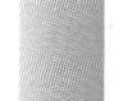

Toddler Period

In the toddler period, defined as the first through third year, children begin to learn and show pride in their gender identity. They observe female and male role models and begin to notice sex role differences.

Freud called this period the anal stage of development because the child's interest is centered around the processes of elimination. Toilet training has usually begun and focuses the child on the process of elimination. In addition, the act of releasing the contents of the bowel or bladder may actually be a source of enjoyment both physically and psychologically since the child can exercise a good measure of control over the process. As they become interested in excretory function, toddlers begin to notice the difference in male and female genitals. Exploration of their own as well as a sibling's or playmate's genitals continues as a part of learning about all parts of the body.

Preschool Period

The preschool child, age 4 to 6 years, continues to learn about sex roles and now begins to identify with the same-sex parent. According to Freud, strong fantasy attachments to the opposite parent also occur. Little boys experience jealousy of their father's relationship with the mother (Oedipus complex). The process with little girls is more complex; their discovery that they do not have a penis leads to envy; there is a desire to possess the father accompanied by hostility and jealousy toward the mother (Electra complex). Freud termed this the phallic stage because there is an increased interest in sex play and masturbation.

Heterosexual sexual interest begins as children become more social and is expressed as children mimic their parents by hugging or holding hands. Children of this age additionally develop a concept of marriage and can be observed "playing house." Preschoolers also become more affectionate with their parents and enjoy hugging and kissing. They are also more modest and private, and now genital exploration or masturbation is done in private. Interest in the process and function of elimination continues, and parents are often dismayed by the child's love of bathroom vocabulary and jokes (Rice 1995).

School-Age Period

School-age children, 7 to 12 years, have traditionally been described as entering a period of decreased sexual interest and activity. Freud called this the latency stage. Today it is believed that this is a misconception; school-age children do continue to show interest in and curiosity about their sexuality (Masters et al. 1995). Perhaps the fact that older children are not as open about sex as are younger children contributed to the belief about the existence of a latent period. Children are now more interested in socializing with peers of their own gender, but they continue to be observant of the opposite sex. The school-age period may actually be a period when sexual awakening occurs. In some children, the physical body changes of puberty can be seen as early as 9 or 10 years of age. An increasing self-consciousness and self-awareness begins, and children may be embarrassed to be seen nude by their parent of the opposite sex.

School-age children do engage in masturbation, and the frequency may increase during this period. "By ages eight or nine, there is little question that children have awareness of the erotic element of such activities, and it is no longer accurate to think of these as 'play' only. Sexual arousal is more than a by-product of these deliberate activities and is willfully sought, not just an accidental happening" (Masters et al. 1995, p. 219). Boys usually begin earlier than girls and learn from their peers or from reading. Girls are more likely to learn to masturbate by accidental self-discovery. Homosexual sexual exploration may take place through mutual masturbation and is a normal part of growing up. Children also begin to share their sexual fears and fantasies with peers and show interest in approaching sexual changes such as secondary sex characteristics, menstruation, and nocturnal emissions. Interestingly, when children learn about sexual intercourse for the first time, they often find the physical aspects of the sexual act shocking (Wilkerson and Bing 1988).

SEX EDUCATION

Although most people agree that children need to be educated about sex, there is much controversy about where the education should take place, what should be taught, and who should teach it. From the time of birth, parents provide the primary sex education for their children, either consciously or unconsciously. The parents' own attitudes about sex and the way in which sexuality is manifested in the home form the basis of the child's impressions. Unfortunately, many parents, uncomfortable in dealing with sex education, avoid the issue altogether, give negative or frightening messages about sex, or are too liberal in their views and thus place too much emphasis on sex. Ideally, sex education should be presented in a balanced way within family life, children's questions should be answered matter-of-factly when they arise, and reasonable limits on sexual behavior should be set.

Unfortunately, many parents are uncomfortable in providing sex education. For this reason, the issue of sex education in the schools has come to the forefront in the past decade. Many schools now offer courses called Family Life Education that are included as a component of the curriculum from the elementary through high-school years. These courses not only deal with the basic anatomy and physiology of reproduction but also address attitudes and emotions related to sexuality, current issues related to sex, and personal responsibility (Masters et al. 1995).

AIDS EDUCATION

Because of the prevalence of media attention regarding the human immunodeficiency virus (HIV) and acquired immunodeficiency syndrome (AIDS), children will hear about the disease and its relationship to sex. Parents today are thus presented with a dilemma of how to balance children's need to have correct information about the disease without frightening them or giving them "dirty" or negative attitudes about sex. Obviously, the information given depends on the age of the child. Preschool children may not understand an abstract concept such as AIDS but can be taught general good health habits and shown that any question they have about their bodies will be answered comfortably. School-age children may begin to ask questions about AIDS as a result of what they have heard from the media or friends. They need to know that they will not get AIDS from being bad or from general contact with someone who might have HIV infection. Preteens need more specific information about HIV and AIDS because of the pressures they begin to face as they go through puberty. They need to understand the relationship between HIV transmission and sexual intercourse and drug use. They also need to be given information about prevention of HIV transmission (Masters et al. 1995).

Adolescence

Adolescence, age 12 to 19 years, is a period of rapid physical changes, stressful psychosocial demands, and exciting new challenges and discoveries. Freud called adolescence the genital stage and viewed this period as a time when oral, anal, and genital urges fuse together. Teens are faced with the task of achieving independence, learning to interact with their peers, gaining intellectual and emotional maturity, developing ethical principles, and learning social and personal responsibility (Masters et al. 1995).

According to Masters and colleagues (1995), the development of adolescent sexuality is centered around five primary factors:

1. The physical changes of puberty and their relationship to body image and self-esteem. Physical appearance is of primary importance to adolescents, and concern about physical attractiveness can be a major stressor. It is of extreme importance to teens that their appearance be similar to that of their peers and meet an accepted standard. Any deviation from what is considered acceptable by the peer group can be devastating.
2. The task of learning about normal body functioning and its sensual and sexual responses and needs. Physical changes may begin to occur for both girls and boys that can be disturbing if they are not explained. Physical inspection and exploration are the primary ways that teens learn about their sexual development. Masturbation continues in both sexes; however, there is a sharp increase in frequency in boys between 12 and 15 years. Boys now have the capacity to ejaculate, and both boys and girls can experience their first orgasm. Masturbation is often accompanied by sexual fantasies (Masters et al. 1994, 1995).
3. Developing a gender role identity and comfort with one's sexual orientation. Rigid cultural stereotypes about "acceptable" behaviors of men and women greatly affect teens. Any deviation from what is considered appropriate behavior or activity for a woman or man is unfortunately strongly criticized by the peer group.
4. Learning about sexual and romantic relationships begins with group dating and then proceeds to heterosexual pairing. By the end of adolescence, most teens will have experienced some form of heterosexual sex. This usually begins with kissing and hugging, may progress to mutual masturbation ("petting"), or may involve sexual intercourse. Throughout all ages of adolescence, more boys than girls report having had sexual intercourse (Masters et al. 1995).
5. Developing a personal sexual value system. This task is closely related to the task of developing a personal identity and is influenced by parents, religious beliefs, and peers.

PREGNANCY PREVENTION

Today's adolescents are more sexually active than they have ever been in the past, and sexual activity is beginning at an earlier age. When pregnancy occurs during the adolescent period, it is most often unplanned and unwanted. Because of that fact, the pregnancy thrusts the teenage girl and her partner into having to make major adult decisions (e.g., abort the pregnancy, consider adoption, raise the baby), face potential health risks, deal with psychological stress, and consider serious economic consequences. For these reasons, it is imperative that teens be given early education about methods of pregnancy prevention. This education should include factual information about all methods of family planning, how each method is used, and how each can be obtained. An honest, accepting, and open approach will make teens comfortable in asking questions and encourage them to seek further help if needed. Further discussion of adolescent pregnancy can be found in Chapter 39.

SAFER-SEX GUIDELINES

Education about pregnancy prevention is only one component of teaching safe sex to teens. Despite the fact that adolescents are very much aware of the HIV epidemic, they are often uninformed about other sexually transmitted diseases (STDs) and misinformed about how to prevent any of them. Even if cognitive understanding is achieved, unfortunately many teens have a feeling of omnipotence, believing that they could never contract any of these diseases. As a result, even though adolescents often know about "safer sex" practices, the majority of them rarely use condoms regularly. A greater effort must be made to make teens aware of how easily all STDs are spread. Adolescent boys need to take greater responsibility for contraceptive use. Educational programs can target teens through schools, churches, community-based programs, and the media. Safer sex practices can be seen in Table 10–2; further discussion of STDs is in Chapter 40.

Adulthood

Young adulthood, 20 to 40 years, is the time when important personal and career decisions are made, increasing responsibilities are assumed, and maturity is achieved. Young adults face the personal choices of living a single life, cohabitating in a heterosexual (or homosexual) relationship, marrying, or perhaps even becoming divorced (Masters et al. 1995). According to Erikson's developmental theory, the task of adulthood is to develop intimacy with another individual.

Young adults may experiment with multiple sexual relationships for a time. There may still be unresolved issues from adolescence left to complete, such as the achievement of comfort or confidence about sexuality or the development of a positive self-concept. Factors such as accessibility of birth control methods and the disappearance of the "double standard" of sexual behavior have allowed many young adults to be more sexually active than in years past. Because young adults are postponing marriage for much longer periods than in the past, the delay in a long-term monogamous relationship causes them to face the same sexual concerns regarding pregnancy and STDs as those faced by teens in late adolescence. The young adult must also continue to develop a sexual value system and learn to be tolerant of the sexual values of others.

Once a monogamous relationship or marriage occurs, young people begin to learn about a long-term commitment to a sexual relationship. The security and confidence that can develop in such a relationship can allow people to begin to experiment with their sexual expression together. For example, the discovery of alternative pleasuring techniques or sexual positions can enhance the sexual relationship. At some point during early adulthood, people usually face the decision about childbearing (Masters et al. 1995; Wilkerson and Bing 1988). As time passes, some couples may find

Table 10–2

RISK ESTIMATES OF HIV TRANSMISSION FROM VARIOUS SEXUAL PRACTICES

Safer Sex: Extremely Low- or No-Risk Practices

- Abstention from sexual contact
- Self-masturbation
- Touching, massaging, hugging, caressing
- Social (dry) kissing

Probably Safe: Very-Low-Risk Practices (Small Theoretic Risk)

- French (wet) kissing
- Mutual masturbation (if no cuts on hands, or ulcers or lesions on genitals of either partner)
- Vaginal sex with a male or female condom (put latex or polyurethane condom in place before any penetration)
- Fellatio with condom (place latex condom on partner's penis before oral contact)
- Cunnilingus with dental dam (place latex dam over partner's vaginal area before oral contact)
- Anilingus (rimming) with dental dam (place latex dam over anus before oral contact)
- Contact with urine (water sports; only with intact skin; avoid contact with mouth)
- Using one's own sex toys (no sharing of any toys that contact body fluids)
- Anal sex with condom (place latex condom on penis prior to penetration; probably safer with use of ample water-based lubrication)
- Mutually monogamous sex between two persons who have no HIV risk factors and who are known to be uninfected

Possibly Unsafe: No Strong Proof But Some Evidence That Transmission Can Occur

- Fellatio (sucking partner's penis and swallowing semen)
- Cunnilingus (oral contact with partner's genital area and vaginal secretions)
- Anilingus without a latex dam

Unsafe Sex: High Risk of Transmitting HIV

- Anal intercourse without a latex condom (highest risk is to the receptive partner)
- Anal penetration with the hand (fisting) or other rectal trauma without a latex glove or fisting followed by anal intercourse
- Anal douching in combination with anal sex
- Vaginal intercourse without a male or female condom
- Sex with numerous partners

that sex becomes less exciting and gratifying, and the frequency of sexual activity declines.

By middle adulthood, 40 to 60 years, people may begin to face a midlife crisis as they realize that youth is in the past and they face for the first time the reality of their own mortality. People may become disillusioned when they see their physical body changing and realize that all goals and dreams have not been met. New sexual issues surface during these middle years. Physical changes caused by aging may begin to affect the sexual relationship. The lower hormone production in both women and men may influence sexual functioning. With menopause, women may notice vaginal atrophy and decreased vaginal lubrication. With the male climacteric, men may experience slower erections. The influence of these changes on body image determines the adjustment of the individual. If middle adults feel good about themselves, they will see these changes in the context of normal development and not allow them to be a detrimental influence on the relationship with their partner or on their lives. Maturity can allow an increase in intimacy and sexual satisfaction. On the other hand, if these physical changes are viewed in a negative light and adversely affect self-concept, midlife behaviors may manifest themselves in an attempt to prove or confirm masculinity or femininity. Extramarital affairs are most likely to occur in people of this age group.

During late adulthood, older than 60 years, people continue to be sexual and enjoy sexual activity. This activity may decrease in frequency but is no less satisfying. The psychological need for intimacy, excitement, and pleasure does not disappear in old age (Masters et al. 1995). The challenge for older adults may be to find new ways to achieve sexual intimacy and sexual satisfaction, particularly after the illness or loss of the partner. It is unfortunate that our society has in the past held somewhat negative attitudes regarding sexuality in the elderly. It is to be hoped that as we become more knowledgeable about sexuality across the life span, we will understand that older adults also enjoy sex and need to continue to express the sexual aspects of their being (Masters et al. 1994, 1995; Wilkerson and Bing 1988).

PHYSICAL ASPECTS OF SEXUALITY

Human sexuality is a complex dimension of each individual's being. Physical, psychological, and social components are intertwined to affect each sexual response. Understanding the physiologic process helps establish a comfortable familiarity with the body's responses during sexual arousal.

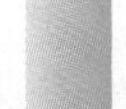

Research

Compared with other aspects of human physiology, less research has been conducted on the physiology of the sexual response than on any other area. This is unfortunate in view of the importance of sexuality throughout our lives. One reason that research has been minimal has been the social taboo existing for centuries regarding public attention to or discussion of sex. Another factor has been the difficulties encountered in doing research about sexuality. Problems such as sampling bias (nonrandom or small samples) and erroneous or inaccurate answers have plagued researchers in this field for decades.

Sex research can be conducted in several different ways. None of the methods is ideal or suited for every research question (Masters et al. 1995).

SURVEY RESEARCH

Most of the early pioneering work done on sexuality is based on interview or questionnaire data. The survey method has been the one most commonly used and is by far the easiest. The best known of these studies were the Kinsey reports, which were done by face-to-face interviews (Kinsey 1948, 1953). Many major national magazines have conducted questionnaire surveys in the past decade. While data from these studies have provided some valuable information, many of the studies are poorly designed, and the information from this research has the possible limitation of being biased by the subjective responses of subjects. The findings of these studies cannot be used to reach broad conclusions about human sexuality.

OBSERVATIONAL RESEARCH

Observational research is done with a human observer or an instrument that actually records the biophysical aspects of the sexual response taking place during sexual activity, either in the laboratory or in the subject's natural environment. The benefits of this type of research are that it avoids the bias of subjects' self-reports. However, conducting observational research has not been easy. Obtaining approval and funding for such research, as well as recruiting subjects, has been a difficult challenge. The best known studies done by this research method are those of Masters and Johnson (1966).

CASE STUDIES

Case studies are in-depth examinations of a particular aspect of sexuality, such as the effect of recreational drugs on sexual activity, done with one or more individuals for a period of time. Case studies require a long-term commitment from the researcher because data may be collected for many months or years. The findings from case studies cannot be generalized to a larger population. However, case studies can examine problems in depth and can provide the basis for designing larger descriptive or prospective studies.

CLINICAL RESEARCH

Clinical research is research done to study a specific clinical problem. It may be done to compare two groups of subjects, one group that receives a particular treatment for a sexual problem (experimental group) and one group that does not (control group). It may also include epidemiologic studies that focus on the pattern of distribution of a particular phenomenon related to sexuality and descriptive studies that examine various aspects of a problem. Examples of clinical research are the work by Masters and Johnson (1970) and Helen Singer Kaplan (1974, 1979, 1993) related to various forms of sex therapy provided for people with sexual dysfunctions.

EXPERIMENTAL RESEARCH

Experimental research is a tightly controlled method that is designed by the researcher to test the effect of a particular factor (the independent variable) and study the outcome (the dependent variable). For example, experimental research has been used to study the effects of viewing erotic materials on sexual arousal and the effects of sex education on teenage pregnancy rates (Masters et al. 1995). Experimental research related to sexuality often has the limitation of involving artificial situations, so the findings cannot always be applied to general populations. It is also difficult for the researcher to control volunteer subject bias and to control all possible variables in the study.

Sexual Response

No accurate explanation of sexual physiology and response existed before the 1960s. On the basis of observational and clinical research, Masters and Johnson (1966) identified a specific four-stage pattern of sexual response that is widely accepted today. Others, including Kaplan (1974, 1979), have modified this model for use in their clinical practice as sex therapists.

MASTERS AND JOHNSON'S SEXUAL RESPONSE CYCLE

The most widely accepted clinical research on sexual response that has been done to date is the work of Masters and Johnson. Their research began in 1954 with the publication of a book that for the first time in history described physiologic changes that occur in response to sexual stimulation. The original study included "direct laboratory observation of more than 10,000 episodes of sexual activity in 382 female and 312 male subjects" (Masters and Johnson 1966; Masters et al. 1995).

Basic Physiologic Reactions

As arousal increases during sexual activity, many body systems become involved and changes occur in their functioning. The neurologic system acts as the central coordinator of these systemic changes and influences the progression of the sexual response. Masters and Johnson (1966) identified two basic physiologic reactions that occur throughout the four stages of the sexual response cycle. These are vasocongestion and neuromuscular tension.

▼ **Vasocongestion.** Vasocongestion is the primary reaction to sexual stimulation in which veins in the genital area of both women and men fill with blood. In women, there is also congestion in breast tissue and swelling in the glans of the clitoris, which increases in diameter. Lubrication of the vagina results from seepage of fluid through semipermeable membranes in the vaginal walls; this reaction is sometimes called vaginal sweating. In men, erection of the penis is due to the filling of the corpus cavernosum and corpus spongiosum with blood. For both women and men, vasocongestion can result from direct stimulation of the genitals or other body parts or from erotic thoughts.

▼ **Neuromuscular Tension (Myotonia).** The second basic physiologic reaction that occurs with sexual stimulation is increased neuromuscular tension. This is a buildup of energy in the nerves and muscles that is associated with involuntary contraction of muscles, or myotonia, throughout the body. As the phases of sexual response progress, this muscle tension gradually increases until it reaches a peak and is followed by a sudden release after orgasm.

Four-Stage Cycle

The four-stage sexual response cycle includes excitement, plateau, orgasm, and resolution. These phases reflect levels of sexual arousal as well as typical responses. Masters and colleagues (1995, p. 75) warn that one should not "equate the speed, size, and strength of sexual responses (such as erection, vaginal lubrication, or muscular contractions during orgasm) with the gratification a person experiences or with his or her proficiency as a lover."

▼ **Excitement.** During the excitement stage, erotic arousal begins. This can result from a number of sources, such as merely thinking about sex, seeing an erotic movie, or expressing love to one's partner. The initiation of the physiologic processes of vasocongestion and neuromuscular tension takes place. Vasocongestion usually occurs rapidly (in 10 to 60 seconds) in both women and men but can be altered by fatigue, alcohol or drugs, and age. The excitement phase may be prolonged if desired by the sexual partners, or it can be interrupted or ended by distracting stimuli.

Women begin to show physical signs of sexual excitement with vaginal lubrication. This is the direct result of vasocongestion in the walls of the vagina, which causes fluid to seep through the permeable tissue lining. The amount of lubrication varies in women from being small to copious in amount. The inner two thirds of the vagina begin to expand in both width and depth, and a color change (from the ordinary purplish red to a darker purple) takes place as a result of vasocongestion. As this "ballooning" response of the upper vagina occurs, the uterus and cervix are pulled up into the pelvis (Fig. 10–1). The labia minora and majora swell and begin to separate from the vaginal orifice, the clitoris enlarges, and the Bartholin glands increase in size. Swelling of the breasts and nipple erection are due to pooling of blood in the breast tissues and contraction of muscle fibers around the nipple. Increases in blood pressure, pulse, and respirations are seen. A sex flush that looks like a fine rash may appear over the abdomen and chest (Masters et al. 1994, 1995).

For men, the first visible sign of sexual excitement is the erection of the penis. This occurs from increased blood flow into the penis, resulting in increased fluid pressure. The increased pressure causes the penis to increase in size and angle with the body. As vasocongestion increases, the skin of the scrotum begins to thicken, and the testes are drawn up closer to the body (Fig. 10–2). The testes also increase slightly in size as a result of vasocongestion. The urinary meatus dilates, and the urethra is moistened with mucus. The Cowper gland may secrete fluid. Some men may also show signs of breast swelling and nipple erection. Men also demonstrate increases in blood pressure, pulse, and respirations and a sex flush over the abdomen and chest (Masters et al. 1994, 1995).

▼ **Plateau.** During this second stage, vasocongestion and muscle tension intensify. Although the plateau stage can be affected by distracting stimuli, by the time the physical changes in this phase have occurred, orgasm is near.

In the woman, the formation of the orgasmic platform occurs during the plateau phase. This is the marked vasocongestive swelling or thickening of the tissues surrounding the outer third of the vagina, forming a cufflike region. As a result, the size of the vaginal entrance actually becomes smaller to grip the penis. The uterus enlarges slightly and elevates to a higher position; the cervical os opens slightly; and the inner two thirds of the vagina expands further in width and depth, creating a "tenting" effect (see Fig. 10–1). The clitoris enlarges further as a result of increasing vasocongestion, but it elevates by retracting and drawing into the clitoral hood. The Bartholin glands produce a few drops of fluid. The color of the labia minora changes from bright red to deep wine in multiparous women and from pink to bright red in nulliparous women. The breasts continue to swell, and the areolae become prominently swollen. The sex flush intensifies in color and spreads more widely over the breasts and chest. The blood pressure, pulse, and respirations remain elevated (Masters et al. 1994, 1995).

In the man, the penis completes its erection, the coronal ridge at the edge of the glans swells, and the glans enlarges in diameter and develops a deeper color due to greater pooling of blood. The scrotum further thickens, and the testes become so engorged with blood that they may become 25 to 50 percent larger. They are pulled up even higher and closer to the body, rotating in position until their back surfaces are pressed against the perineum. The urethral bulb increases twofold in size, and seminal fluid collects in the prostatic urethra. A few drops of preejaculatory fluid, which may contain sperm, are secreted by bulbourethral (Cowper) glands, two pea-sized structures just below the prostate gland that drain into the urethra and reach the tip of the penis (see Fig. 10–2). Elevations in blood pressure, pulse, and respirations continue (Masters et al. 1994, 1995).

▼ **Orgasm.** At orgasm, vasocongestion and neuromuscular tension reach their peak and then are released. Once this stage is reached, the physiologic responses that have occurred cannot be interrupted by distracting stimuli. Both women and men show intense muscle tension (myotonia) at orgasm before muscle relaxation. There may be a contraction of all body muscles. Muscles of the neck, arms, and legs may contract in a spasm. Gluteal and abdominal muscles contract, and carpopedal spasms of the hands and feet may occur. The face may be contorted with a grimace. Blood pressure, pulse, and respirations reach their peak. These responses to physiologic and psychological stimulation are highly personal experiences and

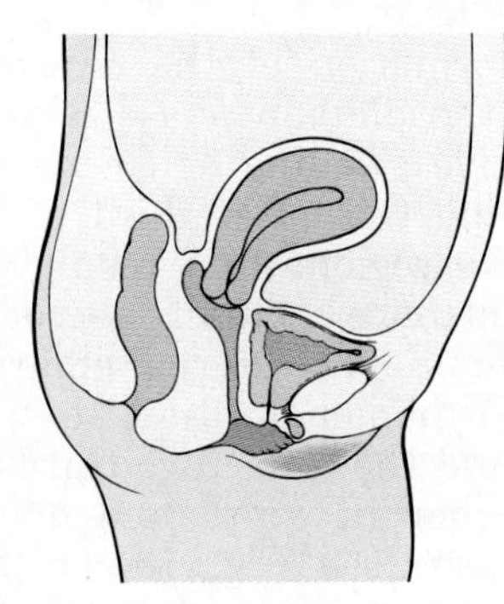

EXCITEMENT

- Vasocongestion begins
- Vaginal lubrication appears
- Vagina lengthens and uterus pulls up
- Labia swell
- Clitoris enlarges
- Breasts swell and nipple erection occurs
- Sex flush may appear late during excitement
- Blood pressure, pulse, respirations, and neuromuscular tension increase

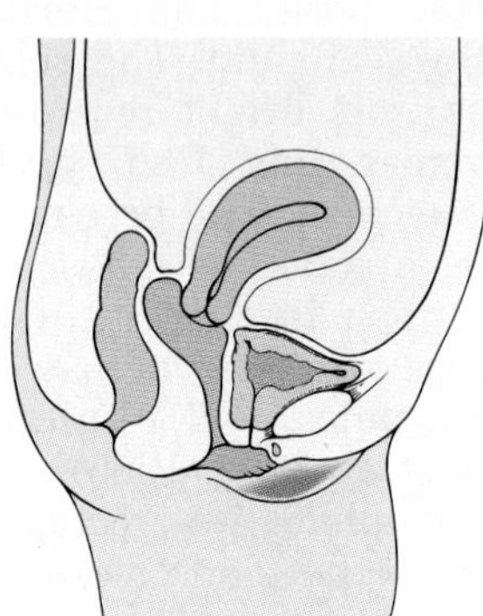

PLATEAU

- Vasocongestion intensifies
- Outer one third of vagina forms orgasmic platform
- Cervix elevates and enlarges
- Inner two thirds of vagina expands as uterus elevates ("tenting")
- Clitoris pulls back against pubic bone
- Labia change color
- Breast engorgement continues
- Blood pressure, pulse, respirations, and neuromuscular tension continue to increase

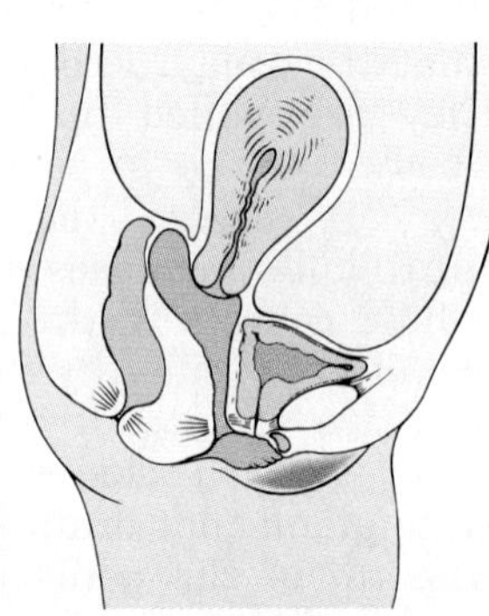

ORGASM

- Vasocongestion and neuromuscular tension peak and release
- Intense myotonia occurs throughout body
- Orgasmic platform contracts rhythmically
- Uterine contractions begin at fundus and move down cervix
- Anal sphincter contracts
- Blood pressure, pulse, and respirations peak

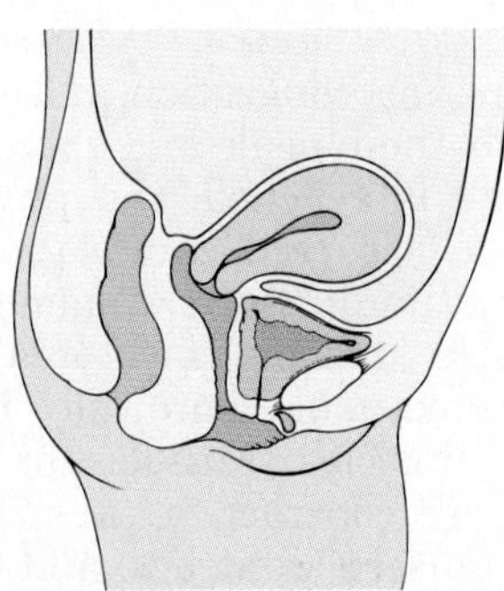

RESOLUTION

- Following orgasm, vasocongestion subsides quickly and body returns to an unaroused state
- Clitoris returns to normal position
- Orgasmic platform relaxes and shrinks
- Labia return to normal
- Vagina shortens
- Uterus decreases in size and descends
- Cervix drops into seminal pool
- Breast size decreases
- Sex flush disappears
- Blood pressure, pulse, and respirations return to normal
- Light perspiration may cover body

Figure 10–1

The female sexual response cycle.

EXCITEMENT

- Vasocongestion begins
- Penis increases in size and angle from unstimulated state to erection
- Testes partially elevate
- Breasts swell and nipple erection occurs
- Sex flush may appear late during excitement
- Blood pressure, pulse, respirations, and neuromuscular

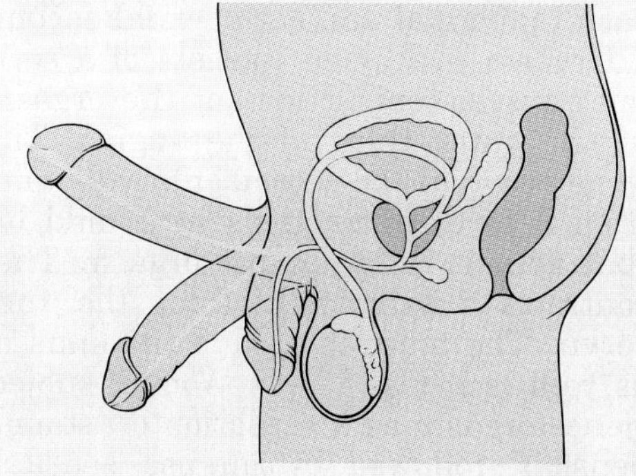

PLATEAU

- Vasocongestion intensifies
- Erection is full and stable
- Head of penis enlarges and color deepens
- Testes increase markedly in size, pull closer to body, and rotate
- Scrotum thickens and folds disappear
- Prostate enlarges
- Cowper's glands usually secrete fluid
- Blood pressure, pulse, respirations, and neuromuscular

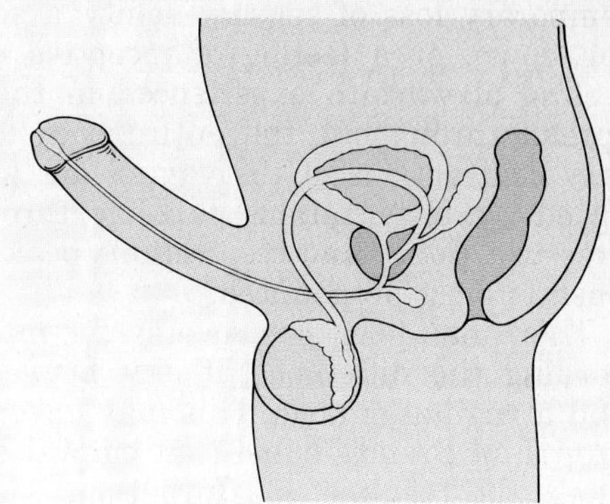

ORGASM

- Vasocongestion and neuromuscular tension peak and release
- Intense myotonia occurs throughout body
- Internal sphincter of bladder closes
- Emission stage: vas deferens, prostate, and seminal vesicles contract forcing ejaculate into prostatic urethra
- Ejaculation stage: urethral bulb and penis contract rhythmically expelling semen from penis
- Anal sphincter contracts
- Blood pressure, pulse, and respirations peak

RESOLUTION

- Following orgasm, vasocongestion subsides quickly and the body returns to an unaroused state
- Penis decreases rapidly in size and angle
- Testes descend and return to normal size
- Scrotum loosens and folds return
- Refractory period occurs
- Sex flush disappears
- Blood pressure, pulse, and respirations return to normal
- Light perspiration may cover body

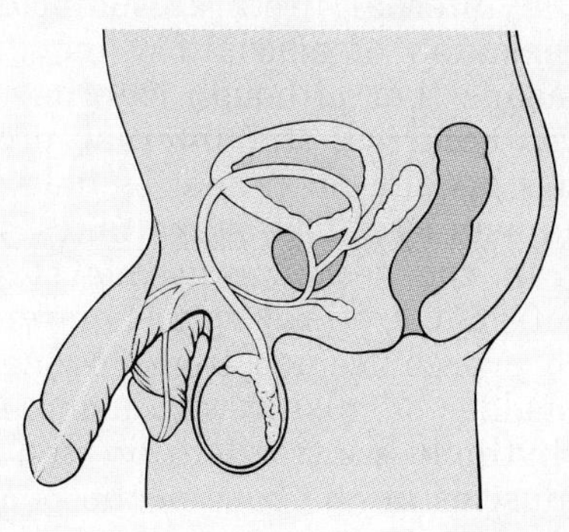

Figure 10–2

The male sexual response cycle.

vary not only from person to person but also for each individual and each sexual encounter.

Orgasm in women consists of a series of rhythmic muscle contractions of the orgasmic platform at the outer third of the vagina. These contractions occur at 0.8-second intervals and may range from 3 to 5 contractions in a mild orgasm to 15 contractions in an intense orgasm. The uterus also contracts rhythmically from the fundus to the cervix. The muscles around the anus may contract as well (see Fig. 10–1). Women subjectively experience orgasm as a sensation of "stoppage" or "suspension" followed by intense sensual awareness centered in the clitoris, which remains retracted. The anal sphincter also contracts. There may be temporary loss of sensory acuity, a sense of bearing down, or a feeling of receptive opening. The feeling of warmth experienced in the pelvis may spread throughout the entire body. The involuntary contractions of the vagina are perceived, followed by a sensation of pelvic throbbing. Blood pressure, pulse, and respirations peak, and the sex flush is most pronounced.

There has been controversy for many years regarding the difference, if any, between a clitoral and a vaginal orgasm. This may have been an outgrowth of Freud's belief that clitoral orgasm, most likely the result of masturbation, is an immature type of orgasm, whereas a vaginal orgasm occurring as a result of sexual intercourse is a more "mature" orgasm. Unfortunately, many women continue to have this belief today. One type of orgasm is no better than the other, and both cause the same physiologic responses (Masters et al. 1994, 1995).

Men also experience orgasm as a series of rhythmic contractions of the pelvic organs at 0.8-second intervals. However, in men, orgasm occurs in two distinct stages. The preliminary stage, or emission, is started by a series of rhythmic reflex contractions in the prostate gland, seminal vesicles, and vas deferens, forcing ejaculate into the bulb at the base of the prostatic urethra. The semen collects in a pool, the urethral bulb expands, the internal urethral sphincter contracts, and a sensation of ejaculatory inevitability occurs. This means that although external ejaculation has not yet occurred, the internal process of ejaculation has begun and cannot be held back under any circumstances. This stage takes only 2 to 3 seconds.

In the second orgasmic stage, ejaculation, the internal urethral sphincter remains tightly closed to prevent semen from flowing backward into the bladder or mixing with urine. A series of powerful rhythmic contractions in the urethral bulb, the muscles at the base of the penis, and the shaft of the penis occur, forcing semen out of the penis with great force (see Fig. 10–2). The anal sphincter also contracts. Although these contractions begin at regular 0.8-second intervals, after the first 3 or 4 contractions the rate and intensity begin to fade. Blood pressure, pulse, and respirations peak, and the sex flush is most pronounced. The subjective experience of orgasm for the man is a sensation of deep internal warmth or throbbing pressure, quickly leading to contraction of the urethral sphincter and a perception of the volume of seminal fluid being expelled through the urethra (Masters et al. 1994, 1995).

▼ **Resolution.** The final stage, or resolution, is the physiologic return to an unaroused baseline state, and a general state of relaxation occurs. The anatomic changes seen in the excitement and plateau phases are reversed. Orgasm triggers a massive release of muscle tension (myotonia) and release of blood from engorged vessels (vasocongestion). The length of this phase is parallel to the length of the excitement phase, usually 15 to 30 minutes.

In women, the clitoris returns to its normal position within 5 to 10 seconds after orgasm; however, it takes longer to return to normal size. The labia minora and majora return to normal size, position, and color. The orgasmic platform relaxes and shrinks rapidly after orgasm. The ballooning of the vagina decreases; the size of the uterus decreases; and the uterus descends to its normal position, allowing the cervix to drop into the seminal pool (see Fig. 10–1). Breast size decreases, temporarily making the nipples look more erect (Masters et al. 1994, 1995).

During the resolution phase, the man loses his erection in two stages. First, there is a rapid decrease in the size and angle of the erection, resulting from the emptying of blood from the corpus cavernosum. However, the penis still remains somewhat enlarged. In the second stage, the continued decrease in penis size occurs more slowly as a result of the slower emptying of the corpus spongiosum and glans. The scrotum thins, and the testes return to normal size and position (see Fig. 10–2). During this stage, the man experiences a refractory period and is incapable of further arousal or ejaculation for a time. Depending on age, fatigue, stress, and other variables, this period may last from a few minutes to 24 hours.

Both women and men experience a decrease in the sex flush, and blood pressure, pulse, and respirations return to normal. A light perspiration may cover the body. This is a distinct response to the resolution phase and not the result of physical exertion (Masters et al. 1994, 1995).

Even if orgasm does not occur, the interruption of sexual stimulation will lead to a resolution phase. However, vasocongestion in the pelvic region does not resolve as quickly, particularly if the plateau phase of sexual arousal was prolonged. The orgasmic platform in women and erection in men still disappear quickly; however, there may be a lingering sensation of pelvic heaviness or aching because of continued vasocongestion that was not released with orgasm. These symptoms may be relieved by orgasms that occur during sleep or by masturbation (Masters et al. 1994).

KAPLAN'S TRIPHASIC THEORY

Masters and Johnson's theory of the sexual response cycle is the best known and most widely accepted today. However, another theory explaining sexual physiologic response is useful because of its helpfulness in identifying possible causes of alterations in sexual responses and for employing differential treatment procedures. Helen Kaplan (1974, 1979, 1993), a psychiatrist, proposes that the human sexual response cycle results from changes occurring in three phases: desire, excitement, and orgasm.

Desire

Sexual desire is not included in the stages of the sexual response cycle described by Masters and Johnson, for they describe only the genital phases of the sexual response. In contrast, Kaplan's desire phase recognizes the emotional or psychological components of sexual behavior as well. Sexual desire is experienced by individuals as specific sensations that cause them to seek out, or become receptive to, sexual experiences. These sensations are produced by the physical activation of the limbic system of the brain, causing the person to feel restless and sexy and have an increased desire for sex. When this system is inhibited or inactive, a person has no interest in sex. Inhibition of sexual desire can occur in both women and men and is evidenced by low libido in both genders. Kaplan (1979) believes that desire-phase disorders are the most difficult to treat, for they tend to be associated with deep-seated psychological difficulties.

Sexual Excitement

Kaplan's phase of excitement corresponds to the excitement and plateau stages described by Masters and Johnson. During this phase, female vaginal lubrication and swelling and male penile erection occur as a result of vasodilation and increased blood supply to genital vessels. Kaplan points out that this phase is under the influence of the parasympathetic division of the autonomic nervous system. When the excitement phase is inhibited, it produces impotence in men (difficulty in attaining or maintaining an erection) and "general sexual dysfunction" in women (the woman does not become excited and does not lubricate adequately during sexual activity).

Orgasm

The orgasm phase discussed by Kaplan corresponds to that described by Masters and Johnson. It is under the influence of the sympathetic nervous system and results in smooth muscle contractions and release of tension. When the orgasm phase is disrupted, the clinical syndromes seen are premature or retarded ejaculation in men and orgasmic inhibition in women.

The strength of the triphasic theory is that it allows clear comprehension of the differential effects of such variables as disease, trauma, medications, or age on the three separate functions of the sexual response (i.e., desire, excitement, and orgasm). For example, impairment of vaginal lubrication has a different origin and treatment than impairment of orgasm in the woman; in like manner, inability to achieve an erection has a different origin and treatment than an impairment of ejaculation in the man. According to this theory, one component of the sexual response may be impaired while the others may remain functional (Kaplan 1974, 1979, 1993).

Differences in Women and Men

Although the sexual response cycle is similar for women and men, there are slight differences between the sexes. Women do not experience a refractory period in the resolution phase and as a result are capable of experiencing multiple orgasms. While multiple orgasms are possible in women, not all women experience them, and they should not be seen as an ultimate sexual goal. Some women may experience a multiple orgasm for the first time during pregnancy because of the increased vasocongestion; other women may experience a multiple orgasm for the first time in middle adulthood. Female sexual response patterns are also more varied than the male sexual response pattern in regard to the sensations experienced and the length of each of the phases. For women, the excitement phase may vary in length, the plateau phase may occur in several peaks or not at all, there may or may not be orgasm, and the resolution phase may vary in length. For men, one sexual response pattern is common. Excitement usually proceeds rapidly, leading to a short plateau period, orgasm, and resolution (Masters et al. 1994, 1995).

Because of these differences in the sexual response pattern of men and women, partners may reach orgasm at different times. This can create problems and concerns for a couple if they believe it is desirable to reach orgasm simultaneously. This may be an unrealistic goal. It is important for a couple to learn about the sexual response cycle, to communicate with one another regarding sexual desires and feelings, and to strive to please one another through sensitivity and attention to the other's needs.

Sexual Adaptation in Pregnancy

HEALTH STATUS

There are a number of factors that may occur before and during pregnancy that alter the physiologic sexual response cycle. The physical aspects of the couple's sexual relationship before the pregnancy will influence their physical adaptation during the pregnancy. Preexisting health problems in either partner or concurrent health problems that the woman experiences during the pregnancy will also influence sexual adaptation. If the woman is healthy and feels well, she is less likely to find pregnancy a deterrent to her continued enjoyment of sex with her partner. Many women do find that the normal discomforts of pregnancy have some effect on their sexual desire and on their ability to respond sexually.

SYMPTOMS OF PREGNANCY

During the first trimester, fatigue, nausea and vomiting, and breast tenderness are the symptoms most likely to deter the woman's sexual interest. The male partner may find that the increase that occurs in the woman's vaginal discharge is a deterrent to his enjoyment of oral sex. On the other hand, some couples find that confirmation of the pregnancy releases them from the fear of conception and from the need to use birth control. These couples may find sex during pregnancy even more rewarding as a result.

CHANGES IN DESIRE

By the second trimester, the woman is usually feeling better, and the couple may begin to experience a time of stability and well-being in regard to their sexual relationship. For some men, the woman's enlarging abdomen denotes increased femininity and fulfillment and is seen as being erotic. The woman's sexual desire may increase during this time as the physical discomforts of the first trimester subside. Fear of harming the fetus or loss of the pregnancy subside with confirmation of the fetal heartbeat and the experience of fetal movement. During the third trimester, physical discomforts experienced by the woman are related to her size and may decrease her interest in sexual intercourse. Difficulty in finding a comfortable position, pain or vaginal spotting with deep penile penetration, and uterine contractions occurring after orgasm all may contribute to her waning sexual interest (Miller and Friedman 1988; Bing and Colman 1989; Fogel and Lauver 1990; Bogren 1991; Hart et al. 1991; Barclay et al. 1994). Discouragement by health care providers regarding sexual intercourse in the last weeks of pregnancy may also be a contributing factor in the woman's reluctance to have sex at that time.

Changes in the positions used for sexual intercourse are often necessary during pregnancy. The most common missionary or man-astride position becomes awkward and uncomfortable as the woman's abdominal girth increases. Simple movements such as turning from side to side, lifting the legs, or moving the body to get in or out of bed become awkward and difficult for the pregnant woman. Frequently, the woman-astride position, side-lying position, or rear entry position offer the pregnant woman more comfort and control. A number of variations in position are possible (Fig. 10–3), and the couple should be encouraged to experiment and find which positions are most comfortable and satisfying for them (Wilkerson and Bing 1988; Bing and Colman 1989; Fogel and Lauver 1990).

PATTERNS OF INTEREST

Four patterns of sexual interest during pregnancy have been described (Bing and Colman 1989; Fogel and Lauver 1990; Bogren 1991). One pattern is that of a decrease in sexual interest and performance in the first trimester, followed by a significant increase in eroticism and performance in the second trimester, and then a decrease again in the third trimester. Other women report a continual increase in sexual interest throughout the pregnancy, a continual decrease throughout the pregnancy, or no change at all. Even though interest in sexual intercourse may decrease during pregnancy, many women report an increased need for other expressions of affection, such as kissing, holding, cuddling, or fondling. Couples can show their affection by giving back rubs, body massages, or just lying in each other's arms.

CHANGES IN SEXUAL RESPONSE CYCLE

The physiologic changes that occur during pregnancy contribute to changes in the pregnant woman's physical responses during the sexual response cycle (Wilkerson and Bing 1988; Fogel and Lauver 1990; Masters et al. 1995).

▼ **Excitement Phase.** The excitement phase may be shortened because of the increased vascularity of the genital area, which leads to increased

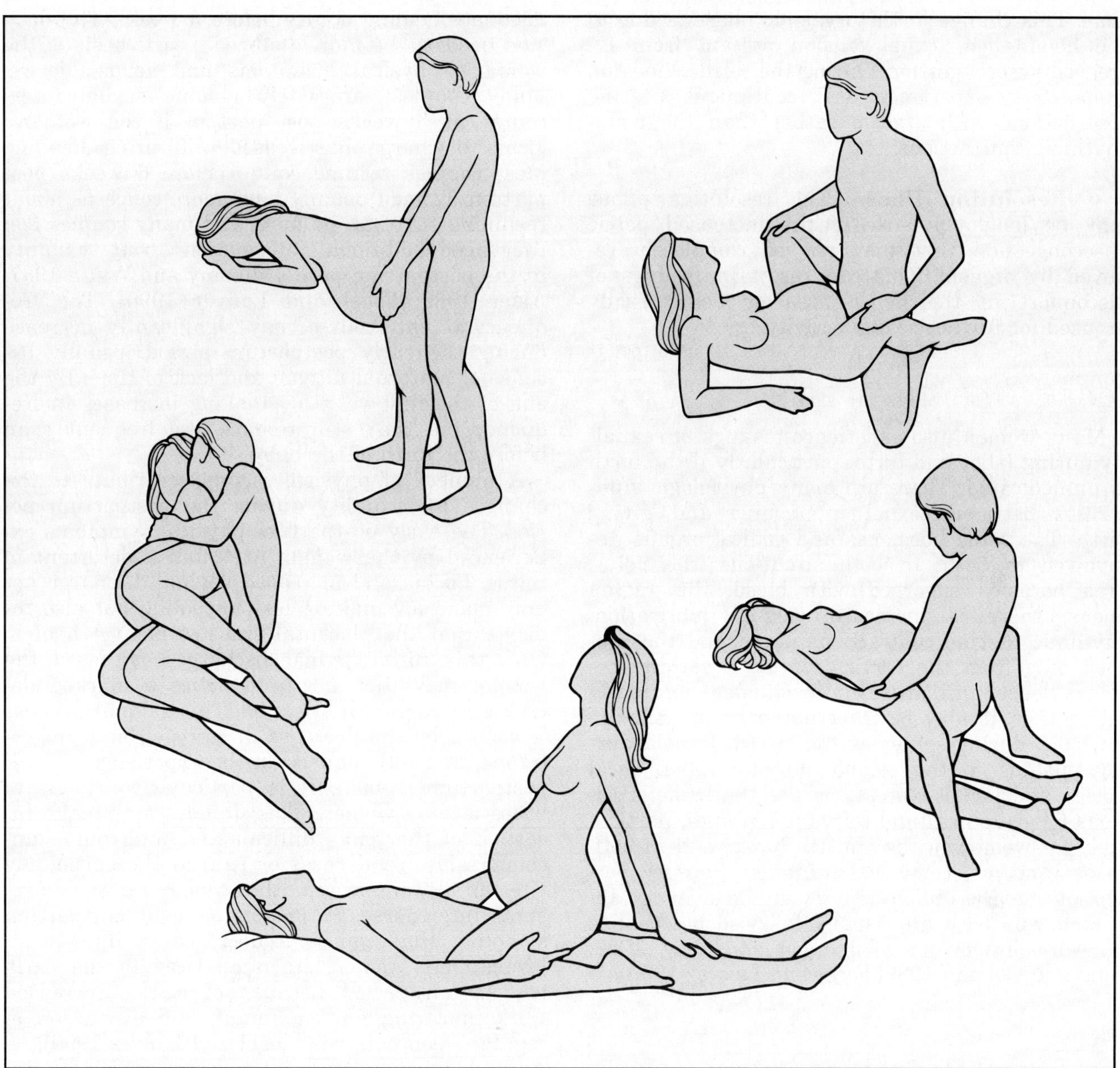

Figure 10–3

Couples may need to try different positions for intercourse during pregnancy. These positions facilitate comfort for the woman, as the man's weight is not placed on the pregnant abdomen.

sexual tension. Generalized vasocongestion of the pelvic viscera and increased amounts of vaginal lubrication occur by the end of the first trimester and persist throughout the remainder of the pregnancy. Vaginal lubrication develops more rapidly and extensively during the excitement phase in pregnant women than in nonpregnant women. The labia increase in size. Breast size also increases during sexual excitement, often as much as 20 to 25 percent, because of the vasocongestion of pregnancy. Venous drainage patterns develop in the breasts, and nipple erection and areolar engorgement become more visible. These breast changes can increase sexual excitement or be painful and uncomfortable. There are physiologic changes during the plateau phase of the sex cycle also. Normally, a marked venous engorgement of the outer third of the vagina develops to form the orgasmic platform. As pregnancy advances, this venous engorgement becomes more severe, causing greater engorgement of the vaginal barrel. Muscle tension and vasocongestion increase substantially; as a result, some women become more easily aroused and responsive.

▼ **Orgasmic Phase.** During pregnancy, some women experience orgasm for the first time or may experience multiple orgasms for the first time. This change in the orgasmic phase is due to the heightened sexual tension present from increased vasocongestion. During the third trimester, women may experience tonic (continuous) uterine contractions with orgasm rather than the usual rhythmic contractions.

Resolution Phase. The resolution phase may be longer because of the increased pelvic vasocongestion that may not be completely relieved by orgasm. This can result in feelings of discomfort in the pelvic area or being easily aroused for further sexual activity.

SEXUAL SENSATIONS AT BIRTH

Many women also experience feelings of sexuality during labor and birth, particularly if the birth is unmedicated. There are many physiologic similarities between sexual intercourse and giving birth. The same hormones and genital organs are involved in both. In both situations, the pelvic area becomes engorged with blood, the vagina opens, there is increased vaginal lubrication, rhythmic uterine contractions occur, and the mucous plug from the cervix loosens. Breathing becomes deeper in both sexual excitement and early labor; then it may be interrupted as orgasm approaches during sex or as the breath is held during pushing in the second stage of labor. Vocal noises and facial expressions are the same. Positions for childbirth and coitus are similar, particularly for women in the United States, and in both cases women become less inhibited. Sensory perception may be dulled as orgasm and delivery approach, and both are usually followed by feelings of well-being or joy (Wilkerson and Bing 1988; Bing and Colman 1989; Fogel and Lauver 1990).

Sexual Adaptation in the Postpartum Period

RESUMING SEXUAL INTERCOURSE

Unfortunately, little attention is paid to the sexual adjustment of parents during the postpartum period. For many years, the common practice has been to ask women to wait until after the first postpartum examination, usually 6 weeks post partum, before resuming intercourse. This is a long period of abstinence for any couple, particularly if it follows a few weeks of abstinence at the end of pregnancy. The theory behind this practice has been the desire for completion of the involutional process and healing of the genital tract before the resumption of intercourse. Although the process of involution does take approximately 6 weeks, it is probably not necessary for the couple to wait that entire time to resume lovemaking, for adequate healing occurs before 6 weeks. The decision needs to be individualized on the basis of the woman's physical symptoms and sexual desire. Many couples can safely resume sexual intercourse at 3 weeks post partum if the woman's lochia discharge has ceased, indicating healing. Most couples resume coitus before 6 weeks post partum. Women usually have more concerns about resuming sex than do men, and many couples feel they need additional information about sexuality in the postpartum period (Reamy and White 1987; Alder 1989; Fogel and Lauver 1990). The frequency of intercourse may significantly decrease during the early postpartum period, usually because of maternal fatigue and lack of time. By the end of the first year, lovemaking increases in frequency but may still remain less frequent than before the birth of the baby.

A number of physical factors contribute to the changes in sexuality during the postpartum period. The early postpartum physical symptoms experienced by the woman are often a deterrent to coitus. Lochia and increased vaginal discharge not only make lovemaking less appealing but also indicate that the placental site has not yet healed. Once this initial vaginal discharge has ceased, the woman may then begin to notice a marked decrease in vaginal lubrication. This vaginal dryness is caused by the decrease in estrogen and progesterone, and although it can be experienced by all postpartum women, it is particularly evident in breastfeeding women. This dryness may make insertion of the penis difficult and intercourse uncomfortable. Tenderness or pain at the episiotomy site can also interfere with a woman's desire to resume intercourse. Fatigue is a major postpartum symptom that causes a decrease in interest in lovemaking. Women are often tired in the early postpartum period because of stress, increased work in caring for the infant, and disruption of regular sleep patterns (Fogel and Lauver 1990).

BREASTFEEDING

If the woman is breastfeeding, she may experience leaking or even spurting of milk during sexual excitement. This symptom, particularly if it is not expected or understood by the couple, can also have a negative effect on sexuality for the woman or her partner. Breastfeeding the baby just before having sex decreases the problem of milk ejection. Finally, the postpartum couple may need to once again consider using birth control. In the early postpartum period, the couple's choices of birth control methods are somewhat limited, particularly if the woman is breastfeeding, has not experienced her first menstrual cycle, or has not yet had her first postpartum examination. A condom with spermicide can be used safely during this time before other birth control methods can be initiated (Wilkerson and Bing 1988; Alder 1989).

CHANGES IN SEXUAL RESPONSE CYCLE

The physiologic reactions that occur in the sexual response cycle are once again altered in the postpartum period, showing changes from both the nonpregnant and the pregnant pattern. The excitement and plateau phases are lengthened, with a decrease in the rapidity and intensity of physical response to sexual stimulation. This decreased responsiveness results from decreased vaginal vasocongestion and lubrication due to hormonal changes. The vaginal walls are thinner, and there is a decrease in the wine-colored hue of the labia minora with impending orgasm. In the orgasmic phase, the orgasmic platform is not nearly as vasocongested as before or during pregnancy. Orgasms are therefore shorter and weaker. By the third month postpartum, vaginal rugae return, the uterus descends into the pelvis, the labia minora and majora respond more readily, vaginal lubrication returns to prepregnancy levels, and expansion of the vaginal barrel returns to prepregnancy dimensions (Fogel and Lauver 1990; Masters et al. 1995).

PSYCHOLOGICAL ASPECTS OF SEXUALITY

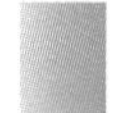

Emotions

The sexual experience is as much an emotional experience as it is a physical experience. In fact, the psyche of both the woman and the man can have a direct influence on their ability to be sexually responsive physically. The emotional state of an individual can either block or enhance sexual performance. Olfactory, visual, and auditory stimuli are each capable of either initiating and facilitating or blocking the progression of the human sexual response cycle. From an emotional perspective, women and men may view their sexuality differently and approach a sexual experience differently.

Differences Between Women and Men

Women seem to be more likely to associate sex with love and commitment, whereas men are more able to view sex as independent of such emotions. Masters and colleagues (1994, 1995) found that a woman's subjective perception of sexual pleasure was influenced by her perception of her relationship with her partner. Women reported that their most pleasurable sexual feelings were in response to intercourse with their partner, even though the most profound physiologic responses occurred through masturbation. The woman's experience of orgasm seems to be the area of most concern regarding her sexual performance and tends to be dependent on her perception and acceptance of her own sexuality and on her perception of her partner as being dependable and trustworthy. Changes in a woman's social situation or role demands can cause a woman to reevaluate or reorient her sexual behavior. For example, a woman may feel differently about her sexuality if she is single, if she is married, or if she is a mother.

Masters and Johnson (1970) stated that historically the man's ejaculatory necessity has relieved him of the psychological pressures that limit the woman's orgasmic experience. Sexual behavior has traditionally been more easily accepted by the man and by others, and men tend to be more aggressive in regard to sexuality. Fears of performance (i.e., being able to establish and maintain an erection) are the aspect of sexuality of most concern to men. For both men and women, guilt and anxiety about sexual performance are capable of interfering with the progression of the sexual response cycle. Fear of failure may perpetuate failure, and guilt may lead to sexual dysfunction. Because of these differences between women and men, communication regarding their sexual experiences is extremely important. Couples need to be able to talk to one another about sex, just as they talk about other aspects of their lives, if the sexual relationship is to grow and improve.

Adaptations in Pregnancy

CHANGES IN THE COUPLE RELATIONSHIP

During pregnancy, the emotional component of the sexual experience becomes even more important as the couple begins to make changes in their relationship and in their roles. During this time, couples change from being lovers to being parents. Their identity changes from that of a couple to that of a family. The existing sexual patterns that they have developed can be tried and tested by a pregnancy. If the couple had an emotionally satisfying sexual relationship before the pregnancy, along with an ability to openly communicate about sexual issues, their emotional adaptation to the sexual changes of pregnancy will be easier.

PLANNED VERSUS UNPLANNED PREGNANCY

Among the psychological factors that can influence the sexual relationship during pregnancy, whether the pregnancy was planned or unplanned can be a major factor in the couple's emotional responses. If the pregnancy is unwanted, the partners may begin to view their sexual relationship in a negative light and draw away from one another. On the other hand, if the pregnancy was wanted and planned, sex during pregnancy can be a continued celebration of the life already created.

WOMAN'S BODY IMAGE

The woman's body image can influence her comfort in an intimate relationship with her partner. If she feels unattractive because of the physiologic changes of pregnancy or "fat" because of her increasing size, she may be reluctant to be seen by her partner or to enjoy sexual encounters. If she finds herself unappealing, she may believe that her partner does also and that he does not desire her sexually. If, however, she sees her pregnant body as being beautiful, her changing body image will not negatively influence her sexual relationship with her partner (Wilkerson and Bing 1988). Men respond differently to the woman's changing body image. Some men may be repelled or distressed by their partner's new appearance and begin to view her as a maternal figure rather than a sexual partner. Other men may find the pregnant woman to be more appealing and attractive. The pregnant female body can actually be erotic to men who view it as being the expression of ultimate femininity. As the pregnancy progresses, the woman may begin to focus on her growing baby and become more introverted and passive. The male partner may interpret these emotional changes in the woman as disinterest or rejection of him and feel jealous or isolated.

FEAR OF HARMING THE FETUS

Both the woman and the man may experience fears that sex during pregnancy might harm the infant. During the first trimester, those fears usually relate to the concern that intercourse might contribute to the loss of the pregnancy by causing a miscarriage. By the third trimester, fears may again surface regarding the influence that coitus might have on the initiation of preterm labor. Men may also worry that the thrusting of the penis against the cervix during intercourse could cause direct harm to the infant. Although all of these fears are understandable, unless the woman is high risk or is experiencing a particular problem during pregnancy, sexual intercourse is not usually a cause of fetal loss or injury or of preterm labor. As the baby becomes larger, couples may also express the feeling that the baby is a third person in the bed with them, watching them as they make love. Although the partners know logically that this is not the case, they often cannot shake the feeling that the baby is an intruder and they are being observed during lovemaking. These feelings can interfere with spontaneous sexual responsiveness. It is important that expectant parents communicate with one another about their feelings during pregnancy. If the couple knows and understands how each other feels about the woman's changing body image, about fears they may have regarding the baby's safety, or about the feelings they have for the developing baby, the psychological influences of pregnancy will have minimal impact on their sexual relationship.

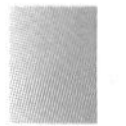

Adaptations in the Postpartum Period

EMOTIONAL EQUILIBRIUM

The woman experiences a number of emotional changes during the postpartum period that may affect her interest in sex. The first few weeks after delivery often feel like a psychological letdown after the emotional high that built throughout pregnancy and peaked with birth. Feelings of depression and guilt may develop as the woman compares her emotional state with society's image of a blissful new mother. These feelings, known as the baby blues, can interfere with a woman's desire to reestablish an intimate relationship with her partner.

CONCERN ABOUT INVOLUTIONAL HEALING

The new mother may also worry about her physical recovery and whether the process of involutional healing is progressing as it should. Fatigue contributes to her emotional lability at this time. The partner, on the other hand, may be on a different track. He may experience a resurgence of feelings of role accomplishment, affirmation of his manhood, and increased self-esteem. The man may expect sex to be precisely as it was before pregnancy, while the woman regards this as impossible. She may want and need caring and loving from her partner, but not as a prelude to intercourse. She may want only to be hugged and caressed. The new mother often feels as though she herself needs mothering. As during pregnancy, the man may experience conflicting feelings about his partner as he struggles between viewing her as a mother and as his sexual partner. For example, he may have problems with the feelings he has regarding her breasts. He may find it difficult to view the woman's breasts in an erotic way because they now represent the source of nourishment for the baby (Wilkerson and Bing 1988).

CONCERN ABOUT THE BABY

The new baby has a psychological influence on the sexuality of the parents as well. The baby may be awake and fussy when the parents are trying to make love. Parents may fear that the baby will see or hear their lovemaking. The rigid scheduling that may be necessary to plan for intimate time together within the baby's schedule does away with any spontaneity that might have existed before the baby's birth and reminds the couple of the loss of privacy and independence they once had. The woman may begin to feel that she is being forced to choose between her own needs, her partner's needs, and the needs of her infant. The increased attachment she feels for the baby may leave her little need for other emotional ties, and the father must struggle with feelings of jealousy. New mothers describe feeling "touched out" as a result of the constant physical contact they experience with the baby and therefore may not feel a strong desire for sexual contact (Wilkerson and Bing 1988).

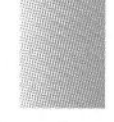

SOCIOCULTURAL ASPECTS OF SEXUALITY

Sexual Attitudes

The development of sexuality is also influenced by sociocultural factors. Family, culture, law, socioeconomic status, and religion all shape an individual's attitudes and behavior regarding sex. Sex is as much a product of society and culture as it is a biologic and psychological function.

Social influences on a person's sexuality begin first in the home within the structure of the family. As the institution responsible for the socialization of an individual, the family is important in conveying its own sexual attitudes and behaviors as well as those of the society. It is within the family that a young child first learns the gender role behaviors expected of women and men, accepted ways of expressing affection, and sexual mores.

The larger structure of the society and its culture also influence sexual development. The society defines what a sexual behavior is and sets norms or rules for that behavior that are understood and guide the behavior of the people in the culture. A given sexual behavior may be defined as evil by one cultural group or desirable by another. There may be differences in regard to views on marital versus extramarital or premarital sex, appropriate positions for sex, accepted foreplay activities, or duration of the act of coitus. In nearly all societies, sexual modesty is valued and incest is a taboo. Laws are usually made in a society to regulate and control unacceptable sexual behaviors. It is possible that sexual norms may differ for women and men or for different social classes. For example, lower socioeconomic groups are more often associated with more restricted, inhibited sexual expression. Foreplay is less elaborate in this group, fewer women have orgasms, and oral sex is seldom practiced. A sexual behavior is usually considered to be acceptable if it has positive meaning to the individual, if it enriches rather than impoverishes the life of the individual and partner, and if it is tolerable to the society. Social issues or public health concerns may also influence sexual practices. For example, the increase in STDs and HIV has altered sexual behavior in many groups.

Religion also influences sexual attitudes and behavior. The ethical and moral influences of a religion can be strong and can shape a person's sexuality throughout life. Viewing sexual intercourse as acceptable for procreation or for pleasure, accepting or rejecting premarital sex, and condoning or condemning homosexuality are all examples of the influence that religion can have on our sexuality.

Adaptation in Pregnancy and the Postpartum Period

Social norms for sexual behavior may be altered during pregnancy and the postpartum period. The view that the society has of pregnancy can shape the cultural expectations of sexuality during that time. In some cultures, what was acceptable sexual behavior before pregnancy may no longer be accepted once pregnancy occurs or once the baby is born. Among some cultural groups, pregnancy may be seen as evidence of the sexual adequacy of both the woman and the man, or it may be seen as a time for shame because of the recognition that the woman must have had coitus to become pregnant. In some societies, the pregnant woman must hide from evil spirits that will harm the baby if the pregnancy is publicized. In other societies, the marriage may not be finalized until the woman proves her fertility by becoming pregnant. In Western society, pregnancy may be used in an attempt to get married, to solidify a marriage, or to ward off divorce.

Pregnancy may be viewed as a time of debilitation, with the woman seen as being particularly vulnerable. This view no doubt has contributed to the belief of health care professionals that sexual intercourse may be dangerous for the pregnant woman. The attitudes of nurses and physicians are a major sociocultural influence on the sexual

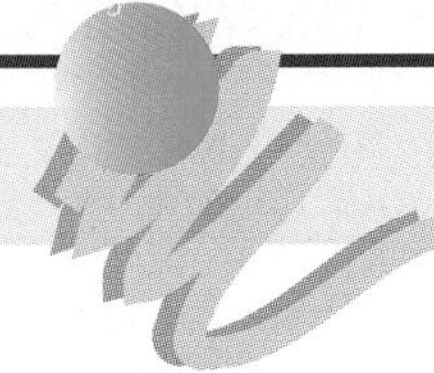

HISTORICAL PERSPECTIVES

CHANGING ATTITUDES ABOUT SEXUALITY AND SEXUAL BEHAVIORS

Early Nineteenth Century

The attitudes regarding sexuality, sexual behavior, and sexual practices have changed throughout history. In the first half of the nineteenth century, an early sexual revolution occurred along with the scientific and industrial revolution. For the first time, women began to protest for equal rights, marital reform, and birth control. The traditional "double standard" of accepted sexual behavior for men and women began to be questioned. Books about sexual physiology and marriage were published and made available to the general public, although they were filled with a great deal of misinformation. This period of early sexual reform was short-lived since the sexual and economic freedom being sought by women was thought to be a threat to the social stability of the family structure. By 1820, the taste of freedom experienced by women was replaced by the Victorian sexual ethic of purity.

Victorian Era

The Victorian era was repressive in all aspects of sexuality. For men, late marriage was encouraged to allow successful career development. Virility was measured by the ability to have rigid control over all sexual impulses and activities and to delay sexual gratification. The woman's sexuality was totally denied. She was expected to have no sexual interest other than a desire to be pure and to fulfill her duty to her husband and her duty of reproduction. Sexual practices were looked on with a great deal of reproach. Men were told that masturbation would cause baldness, impotence, insanity, mental decay, acne, or even death. Devices known as penile rings were made to prevent masturbation or nocturnal emissions. Physicians advocated such practices as castration of sexually active children, clitoridectomy, cauterization of the genitals and prostate, and application of leeches to the base of the penis to begin bleeding. Hot poultices to the genitals, hot mustard hip baths, and protective devices such as chastity belts were used to make sexual arousal difficult and painful for both women and men.

Turn of the Century: 1900–1930s

By 1900, values changed from the rigid Victorian principles to a more relaxed view of life. The man of the early twentieth century became an individual who enjoyed himself and left his inhibitions behind. Women, however, continued to experience a number of personal and social inhibitions related to sexuality. The double standard of sexual behavior for men and women did still exist. Advertising began to use sex as a selling device, and it became evident that sex and sexuality were enjoyable and could no longer be controlled or remain invisible as in the Victorian era. The influence of jazz, flappers, and rising hemlines was seen in the 1920s and 1930s. During this time, the 19th Amendment gave women the right to vote. Birth control methods became more readily available, and penicillin proved an effective treatment for venereal disease. These factors all served to relax the previous rigid sexual standards.

Post–World War II: The Kinsey Report

After World War II, the first large sex survey was published by Alfred Kinsey and his colleagues. Not only did it offer the most explicit information about sexual practices to date, it showed a discrepancy in male and female sexual practices. In contrast to men, women continued to be restricted by social and religious views as to what was acceptable sexual behavior. However, women were viewed as objects of sexual interest for the enjoyment of the

Continued on facing page

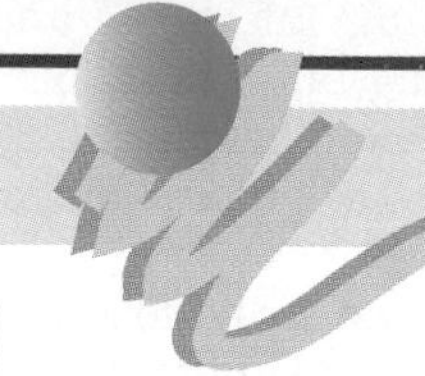

HISTORICAL PERSPECTIVES Continued

man. The first issue of *Playboy* magazine was published in 1953. The birth control pill became available in 1956 and enabled both women and men to have intercourse without the fear of pregnancy.

The 1960s and 1970s: The Sexual Revolution

The 1960s and 1970s ushered in the sexual revolution, a period of liberation and awareness for women and men. This era paralleled a general social relaxation of all moral codes. The women's movement began. Masters and Johnson published their clinical research, and for the first time the general public learned about the sexual response cycle. An explosion of information on human sexual activity was seen in literature and the media. There was a lifting of sanctions on sexually explicit descriptions of behavior. People began to experiment with such alternative sexual lifestyles as communal living, group marriages, swinging, open marriage, and premarital cohabitation. The American Psychiatric Association declared in 1973 that homosexuality was no longer considered to be a mental disorder. Abortion was also made legal in 1973, and birth control methods were improved and made more easily available.

Conservative Values Return

The return of a more conservative view of sexual behavior has occurred during the 1980s and 1990s as a result of such social influences as rising teenage pregnancy rates, increased awareness of sexual abuse, sexually transmitted diseases, and AIDS. Because society's view of sexuality seems to parallel the social history of a given time, sexuality in the future is likely to be influenced by greater knowledge, technology, and the moral standards of the day.

behavior of the woman and her partner during pregnancy and the early postpartum period. Cultural beliefs can link the parent's sexual behavior to the health and welfare of the infant, thus providing grounds for parental guilt if the baby is sick or abnormal at birth. The role conflicts of the pregnant couple as they try to sort through their identities as husband, wife, partner, lover, or parent can also influence their sexual relationship.

COGNITIVE ASPECTS OF SEXUALITY

Sources of Knowledge Versus Misinformation

The information and cognitive understanding that a person has regarding sexuality is the final component that influences sexual behavior. As with other areas of life, increased knowledge usually relates to more positive attitudes and increased comfort with selected behaviors. If an individual is given correct and honest information throughout life about the physical and emotional aspects of sex, that person is more likely to be comfortable with his or her sexuality and to enjoy sexual relationships. On the other hand, if an individual has no knowledge, is given misinformation, or relies on old wives' tales, sex may be a frightening or negative life experience. Information beneficial to all individuals includes sexual changes throughout the life cycle, the physiology of both female and male sexuality, the sexual response cycle, techniques of intimacy and lovemaking, alternative sexual lifestyles, and moral and ethical aspects of sexuality.

Information about sex usually emanates first from the family. This information may be presented within the family in the form of formal sex education, or it may be imparted in less formal ways through behaviors and attitudes. Additional sources of information about sex are peers, formal educational programs within the society, reading materials, the media, and the church. No matter what the source of the sexual education, the information given is shaped by the personal attitudes and beliefs of the individual, the family, the church, and the cultural institution.

Adaptation in Pregnancy and the Postpartum Period

Information about sex during pregnancy and the early postpartum period is often not readily available to couples. Nurses and physicians may be uncomfortable discussing sex or may have difficulty finding the time to do so. Childbirth educators may feel ill at ease about including the topic of sexuality in a group class and may also find that time does not allow complete discussion of the topic. Couples may be reluctant to raise issues or questions about sexuality in a group. The result is that women and their partners may experience the entire childbearing year with little, if any, information about what changes they might experience in their sexual relationship. Without this cognitive understanding, the sexual changes experienced during pregnancy and in the early postpartum period can be surprising at best and frightening and anxiety-producing at worst. The couple's intimate relationship can be seriously threatened during this time because of a lack of knowledge.

Health care professionals who can provide information about sex during the childbearing year are nurses and physicians who see women during pregnancy in prenatal clinics, health departments, or physician's offices; childbirth educators; nurses and physicians who see women post partum; and nurses who make antepartum or postpartum home visits (Fig. 10–4). Parents can also be referred to a number of excellent lay publications available in most bookstores or libraries. Expectant couples identify a strong desire for more information regarding sexual intercourse and sexual feelings and behavior during pregnancy. Other information that is important includes changing sexual desires, physiological changes influencing the sexual response cycle, emotional influences on sexuality, the safety of sex during the childbearing year, and alternative techniques and positions for lovemaking. The sexual experience is a physical, psychological, sociocultural, and cognitive experience. An understanding of all these aspects and how they interrelate will form the basis for a satisfying sexual relationship during the childbearing year and throughout life.

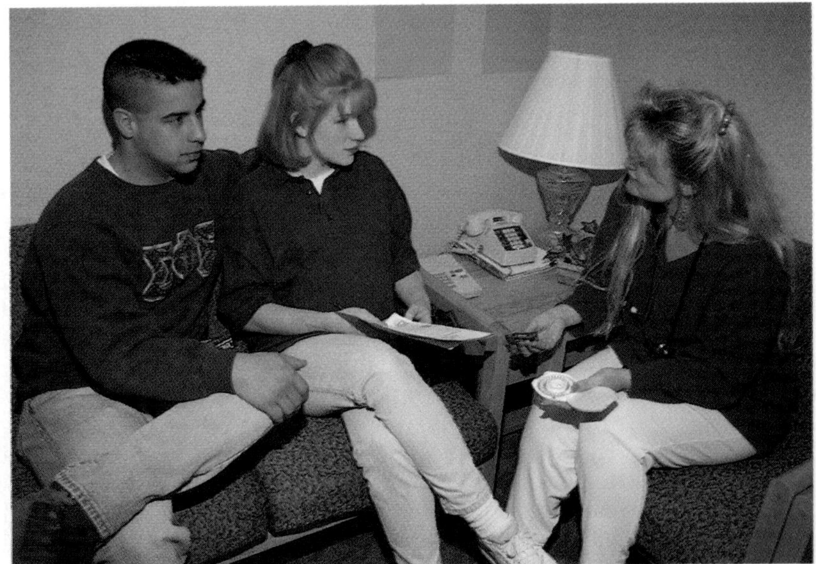

Figure 10–4

Throughout pregnancy, expectant parents need information regarding sexual changes that occur. Counseling from the nurse during late pregnancy should also include information on family planning based on the cultural beliefs and needs of the couple.

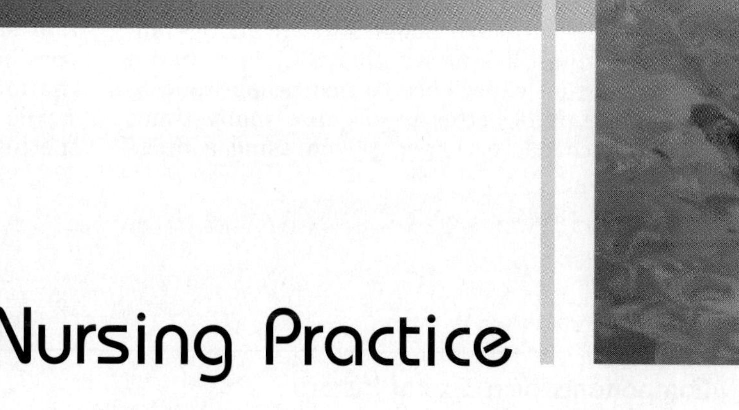

Nursing Practice

Nursing Process

▼ Assessment

All components of the nursing process can be applied in regard to the sexuality of the pregnant woman and her partner. Assessment of the couple's sexual relationship and the effects of pregnancy on that relationship should be a part of the overall initial antepartum assessment. Obtaining information about the couple's sexuality and their sexual relationship during pregnancy should be done early, for it will form a basis for planning and providing more holistic physical care and emotional support throughout pregnancy.

Sexual History. The most important aspect of the assessment process in relation to sexuality is the sexual history. Taking a sexual history should be done in a professional manner and should enable the woman and her partner to maintain a sense of personal privacy and dignity. The value of the information gathered to the planning of prenatal care must be balanced against the risk of encouraging unnecessary embarrassment or self-disclosure. There are a number of reasons that a sexual history is appropriate and necessary. These include the need to understand the relationship of sexuality to the pregnancy experience; the provision of an opportunity for communication and discussion of sex; a basis for the provision of sex education; and the demonstration that sex counseling is an appropriate component of prenatal care.

As with any interview, it is important to set a positive tone before beginning a sexual history. The nurse needs to develop rapport and trust with the woman and her partner. By informing the couple at the beginning of the antepartum assessment that a sexual history will be included, the nurse establishes this as being an important component of the total history and alerts the woman and her partner so that they will not be surprised at its inclusion. A leisurely, relaxed approach is helpful.

Although some type of assessment guide is helpful, provides direction, and prevents omission of data, it is often desirable to allow the couple to direct the discussion, with gentle guidance from the nurse. If the interview is kept too formal and structured, the nurse may miss the direction the woman or her partner wish to go. The sexual history should be taken only in privacy; therefore, it is the nurse's responsibility to provide an environment that is comfortable, quiet, without interruptions, and removed from the eyes or ears of others. It is important to sit as close to the couple as possible, rather than behind a desk. The sexual history should not be rushed, so scheduling should allow enough time for assessment and discussion. The nurse needs to be sensitive to the language used by the couple, use terms that are familiar to them, and avoid medical jargon. The attitude and approach of the nurse during the sexual history is important. If the nurse appears nervous, embarrassed, shocked, or judgmental, these responses will block communication. The nurse should avoid talking too much, a response that can occur from discomfort or nervousness. By allowing occasional silences, the nurse encourages the couple to talk. If the nurse conveys comfort talking about sex, the couple will feel more comfortable as well. The process of the interview is as important as the information gathered. The nurse should at all times be aware of the nonverbal responses of the couple, clarify perceptions, and adapt the interview accordingly. Direct eye contact is important and conveys sincere interest and honesty.

A complete sexual history contains both subjective and objective information about the sexuality of the partners before the pregnancy as well as the current influence of the pregnancy on their sexual identities and sexual relationship. Questions should be open ended and move from simple (i.e., How did you learn about sex?) to more complex. Rather than asking whether they have had a particular sexual experience (which people tend to always deny), it is better to ask how many times the experience has occurred. By phrasing a question in this way, the experience is viewed as being normal. A life cycle chronology is a useful framework for gathering data.

After the data have been gathered, the information should be recorded on the woman's chart. If possible, the nurse should not take notes during the interview, for this can be distracting and awkward. If it is difficult to remember the content of the history, a few words could be written down on

Components of a Sexual History

DEVELOPMENTAL DATA

A developmental history; any other historical information

- When you were a child and adolescent, what were you told about sex? How were your questions answered?
- How did you first find out about sexual intercourse?
- What sexual experiences did you have as a child or adolescent?

PHYSICAL DATA

Current sexual practices; health status; influence of physical changes of pregnancy; sexual dysfunction

- Describe your current sexual activity.
- What problems do you have related to sexual functioning? How has the pregnancy affected your sexuality?
- What health problems do you have that affect your sexual functioning?

PSYCHOLOGICAL DATA

Current attitudes, feelings, and beliefs; sexual self-concept; concerns or fears about sex during pregnancy

- How important is a sexual relationship to you?
- Are you satisfied with your current sexual activity? What would you change?
- Do you believe you are sexually appealing?
- What concerns do you have about sex during pregnancy?
- What concerns do you have about birth control?

SOCIOCULTURAL DATA

Family values; religious influences; socioeconomic influences; and cultural influences

- Tell me about your family's attitudes regarding sex.
- Does your religion influence your feelings about sex?
- How does your cultural background influence your sexuality? Do you know of any old wives' tales about sex?

COGNITIVE DATA

Sex education; current knowledge and understanding; language used; commonly held myths regarding sex in pregnancy; goals; and expectations

- How did you receive your education about sex?
- What things about sex would you still like to learn?
- How do you think pregnancy will affect your sexual activity?
- What terms do you usually use for the following: sexual intercourse, penis, vagina, breasts, oral sex?

occasion as reminders of information covered, or the interview could be taped with the couple's permission. The information recorded should be such that it will assist health care providers in working with the woman and her partner toward their goals. Comments recorded need to be phrased so they could be read by the woman or her partner. In addition to the information gathered from the interview, data from the physical examination and from laboratory tests are also recorded.

▼ Diagnosis

Once an assessment has been completed, nursing diagnoses should be identified. These diagnoses are based on the data gathered from the physical examination, the laboratory work, and the sexual history and should reflect the areas identified by the nurse as needing interventions during the pregnancy or early postpartum period. Examples of nursing diagnoses related to sexuality in pregnancy might be

- Knowledge deficit: lack of information related to sexual changes during pregnancy
- Pain related to sexual intercourse
- Fear: lack of information related to concern for well-being of the fetus as a result of sexual activity

▼ Planning

Once the nursing diagnoses have been formulated, a plan of care can be developed. The plan should include both the woman and her partner. Three primary areas might be involved in the care plan relating to sexuality in pregnancy: teaching, counseling, and referral. Goals or measurable behavioral objectives should be developed. Examples of objectives for teaching and counseling are as follows.

Teaching. The expectant woman and her partner will

1. Ask questions regarding sex in pregnancy
2. Discuss facts regarding physical and psychological effects of pregnancy on sexuality
3. Describe methods of modifying sexual activity in pregnancy
4. List risks and potential effects of sex in pregnancy
5. Discuss techniques to enhance sex in pregnancy
6. Name risk factors for HIV transmission and list four ways to practice safer sex

Counseling. The expectant woman and her partner will

1. Discuss sexual feelings with each other
2. Express concerns, fears, or worries about sexuality in general or during pregnancy
3. Discuss perceptions and expectations of sexual functioning

▼ Intervention

Nursing interventions should incorporate the physical, emotional, sociocultural, and cognitive components of nursing care for the woman and her partner. Interventions will probably include teaching, counseling, or referral.

Teaching. Teaching should be an ongoing process throughout the pregnancy. Many women today are more aware of their bodies and are interested in the influence of the pregnancy on their sexual relationship. Because sexuality is a sensitive issue, offering too much information at one time may be overwhelming. For example, information presented to a woman in her first trimester about sexual changes that might occur in the third trimester is likely to be forgotten. If possible, both the woman and her partner should be present when information is presented. Although information about sex in pregnancy can be presented in groups of expectant parents, it is more ideally presented individually, so that the couple can feel comfortable in asking questions and expressing concerns. The nurse needs to be comfortable with a variety of communication styles and not become offended by a style different from her own. For example, sex can be discussed in professional and anatomical terms or in private, public, childhood, biblical, or street language. Visual aids and handouts that can be taken home are helpful in supplementing the information being presented.

Parents also need information regarding sex during the early postpartum period. From an ideal learning perspective, this information would best be presented after delivery in the first few postpartum days. Waiting until the first postpartum examination, which is often not until 4 to 6 weeks post partum, is too late. The practice of early discharge after birth makes it difficult to meet teaching needs; therefore, it might also be advisable to include information about postpartum sexuality during the last few weeks of the pregnancy. Couples should be advised to plan ahead and have condoms and lubricant available if they do not normally use them.

Counseling. The second area for nursing intervention is that of counseling. The nurse's background

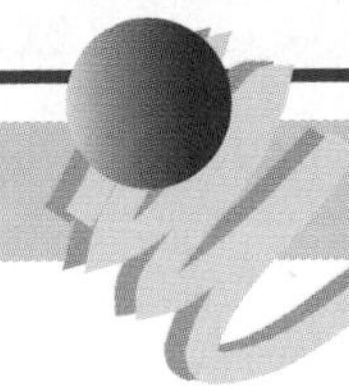

TEACHING GUIDE

SEX DURING PREGNANCY AND THE POSTPARTUM PERIOD

TOPIC	*MAJOR CONCEPTS*
Physical changes in pregnancy	Some physical changes may alter sexual desire and responsiveness: fatigue; nausea and vomiting; breast tenderness; increased pelvic vasocongestion; and longer or multiple orgasms.
Emotional changes in pregnancy	Emotional changes that may alter sexual desire and responsiveness include changes in libido and fears regarding fetal well-being. Communication between partners is important.
Sociocultural and religious influences in pregnancy	Other factors may influence comfort with sex in pregnancy: family; friends; culture; church.
Alternative positions for sexual intercourse in pregnancy	Couples may need to try new positions during pregnancy to keep the weight of the man off the abdomen of the woman: man behind; woman superior; woman on edge of bed; side by side.
Alternative methods of sexual pleasuring in pregnancy	Sexual pleasure can be shared in ways other than intercourse during pregnancy: massage; mutual masturbation; orogenital sex.
Safety of sexual intercourse in pregnancy	Sexual activity continues to be appropriate if the pregnancy is not high risk. Potential influences of sexual intercourse include uterine contractions and decreased fetal heart rate. The risks to avoid are blowing into the vagina during orogenital sex play; sexual intercourse if there is risk for preterm labor; and sexual intercourse if there is bleeding or membranes have ruptured.
Techniques to enhance sex in pregnancy	Several exercises can enhance sexual comfort: Kegel exercise; pelvic rock exercise; tailor sitting exercise; progressive relaxation technique.
Physical changes in postpartum period	Physical changes that may alter sexual desire and responsiveness after birth include fatigue; pain from episiotomy; lochia; decreased vaginal lubrication; and breast tenderness and leaking.
Emotional changes in postpartum period	Sexual desire may also be altered by baby blues and fear regarding physical healing. Communication between partners is important.
Sociocultural and religious influences in postpartum period	Other factors may influence sex after birth: family; friends; culture; church teachings.
Alternative methods of sexual pleasuring in postpartum period	As during pregnancy, other ways of showing affection can be used until intercourse is comfortable: bathing; massage; music and candles; "honeymoon" weekend away from home and baby.

Continued on facing page

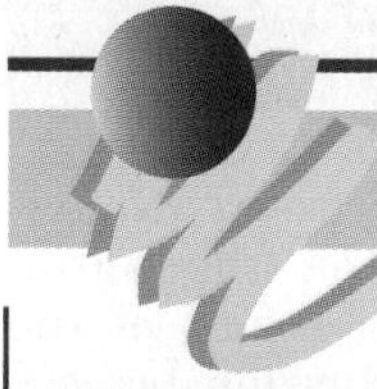

TEACHING GUIDE Continued

SEX DURING PREGNANCY AND THE POSTPARTUM PERIOD

TOPIC	*MAJOR CONCEPTS*
Safety of sexual intercourse in postpartum period	Sharing and comforting one another are important. Intercourse is safe when bleeding is gone, there is no perineal discomfort, and parents are psychologically ready. Contraception concerns should be met before first postpartum intercourse.
Techniques to enhance sex in postpartum period	Techniques to enhance sexual comfort include the Kegel exercise to relax the pubococcygeal muscle; spermicide or K-Y jelly for lubrication; sitz baths to decrease tenderness and promote comfort; digital foreplay with two fingers to help the woman relax the pubococcygeal muscle; side by side position or woman-superior position; nursing the baby before lovemaking or wearing a bra with pads for leaking milk; and planning for sexual time in advance.
Birth control information	See Chapter 11.

Teaching Aids

1. Pictures or posters illustrating physical changes of pregnancy
2. Drawings illustrating alternative positions for sexual intercourse that can be used during pregnancy
3. Pamphlets or booklets about prenatal care that include information about sex during pregnancy
4. Pamphlets or booklets about prenatal care that include information about prenatal exercise that would enhance sex in pregnancy
5. Pamphlets or booklets about postnatal care that include information about sex in the early weeks after birth
6. Pamphlets or booklets about methods of family planning that can be used in the immediate postpartum period (i.e., condoms, spermicides)

Increasing Your Teaching Effectiveness

Your teaching about sex during pregnancy and in the postpartum period will be more effective by using the following approaches.

1. Assess whether sexuality issues are of interest or concern to parents by
   - Including questions about sexual concerns along with other data collected from the expectant woman on a prenatal questionnaire
   - Verbally asking the woman about sexual concerns during the initial interview and succeeding prenatal visits
2. Demonstrate your willingness to discuss sexual concerns by
   - Showing sincere interest and comfort when talking with expectant parents
   - Using a positive, professional, and unembarrassed approach
3. Allow time for the woman to become comfortable enough to discuss sexual issues or to ask questions.
4. Use visual aids and teaching materials.
5. Follow up initial discussions several times during the pregnancy or in the postpartum period.

in physical, social, and behavioral sciences, as well as preparation in interview and communication techniques, makes the nurse an ideal member of the health care team to provide counseling in sexuality. The female nurse may find her gender to be an advantage in counseling pregnant women about sex; however, male nurses can also be effective counselors, particularly when the male partner is involved. Although there are many opportunities for sexuality counseling within the field of maternity care, unless the nurse feels prepared and comfortable with this role, an attempt should not be made to implement it.

Counseling differs from teaching in that it implies more than the presentation of information. With counseling, the nurse seeks to help the pregnant woman and her partner improve their current sexual relationship or work to solve a particular problem that they have expressed. As with teaching, the attitude and approach of the nurse are crucial factors in the effectiveness of counseling interventions. A nonjudgmental atmosphere is essential. The nurse should not moralize in regard to the sexual behavior of the couple but should be sensitive to their needs.

Counseling is a three-step process: (1) identification of what has occurred in the sexual relationship in the past; (2) assessment of what is happening currently in regard to the effects of the pregnancy on the couple's sexual relationship; and (3) planning an appropriate course of action for the future. It is important to encourage the verbalization of feelings to facilitate communication and understanding between partners. Reassurance that feelings expressed are normal and acceptable is helpful.

The sexual problems most likely to be identified during pregnancy are painful intercourse (dyspareunia), differing sexual drives, and impotence. Dyspareunia is usually caused by pressure on the woman's pregnant abdomen from the man's superior position, deep penile thrusting, backache, breast tenderness, or postcoital cramping. The first four situations can usually be corrected with a change in position during intercourse. Facilitation of mutual understanding and communication are strategies that help couples deal with different sexual desires during pregnancy. Male impotence can occur if the man has a negative view of pregnancy or conflicts regarding his partner's maternal versus sexual image. Factual information, an opportunity to express fears and concerns, and communication with the partner may help to alleviate this problem. If the nurse is not comfortable in assuming the role of sexual counselor, or if the initial counseling indicates that further expertise is needed, referral to other sources of sexual counseling should be initiated.

▼ Evaluation

The final step in the nursing process is evaluation. Evaluation should be based on the initial goals and objectives identified as a result of the assessment and diagnoses. The evaluation process should be ongoing throughout the prenatal period and serve as a means for the nurse's continual reassessment of the woman's sexual adaptation, formulation of new diagnoses, and implementation of interventions.

Collaborative Process

The team members involved in sexuality teaching and counseling may vary from one setting to another but may include the nurse, the nurse-midwife, the childbirth educator, the physician, a psychologist, or a trained sexual counselor. With so many professionals able to provide assessment, teaching, and counseling, it is important to guard against the belief on the part of team members that someone else on the team is being responsible for seeing that it takes place, when in fact no one is doing it and the service is falling through the cracks. Communication among team members, the development of protocols for sexuality teaching and counseling, and a commitment to the importance of its inclusion in antepartum care are all important factors that will ensure that attention to sexuality does occur.

▼ NURSE'S ROLE

The nurse who includes sexuality in her plan for the pregnant woman's care should assume the responsibility of becoming as comfortable and well prepared for that role as possible. A beginning point is to develop an awareness of personal attitudes, feelings, values, and biases about sex. This is important, for the nurse's attitudes and values must be separated from those of the woman and her partner. The nurse should strive to develop a balanced viewpoint that recognizes one's personal value system while at the same time accepting and supporting (or at least being nonjudgmental about) the values of others. This balance can be achieved by first clarifying one's own values through reading, talking with peers, objective evaluation of personal experiences, introspection, and self-assessment. Attendance at courses or workshops in human sexuality allows desensitization through films, group discussion, and additional factual information. A reexamination of feelings about masturbation, premarital sex, extramarital sex, orogenital sex, and sex in pregnancy and the postpartum period will help the nurse identify the extent to which these feel-

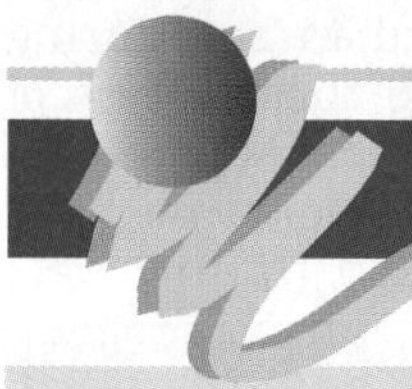

IMPROVING YOUR PRACTICE

HOW TO HELP EXPECTANT COUPLES MAINTAIN A POSITIVE SEXUAL RELATIONSHIP

Helping expectant couples deal with their sexuality and maintain a positive sexual relationship during pregnancy can be challenging and rewarding. The following steps will help nurses strengthen their skills so that they can better meet the needs of expectant parents related to sexuality in the childbearing year.

- ANALYZE YOURSELF AS A SEXUAL BEING. Evaluate your own body image, sexual feelings, values, and attitudes. Discuss sexuality issues with friends and colleagues. Identify how you personally feel about sexual issues and how your feelings could affect your nursing care. Be open to growth and change in this area so that outdated or immature beliefs and values can be shed to allow maturing and emotional growth.
- UPDATE YOUR THEORETICAL BASE. Obtain accurate information regarding the physical, emotional, sociocultural, and cognitive aspects of sexuality. Read current lay and professional literature. Attend a college course on sexuality or sexual issues.
- REVIEW THE PROFESSIONAL LITERATURE AND STANDARDS OF PRACTICE regarding sexuality during pregnancy and the postpartum period. Contrast what you are seeing done in clinical practice with what the current research shows about sex in pregnancy and the early postpartum period.
- EVALUATE CURRENT SOCIAL NORMS. Identify the influences of today's society on sexual attitudes and behavior. Recognize the gaps between personal and public sexual standards. Become aware of how social norms influence you in your beliefs.
- AVOID VALUE JUDGMENTS. Be clear about your own beliefs so that you understand your feelings and can incorporate your values into a practice discipline. Try not to impose your personal biases or preferences on others. Become aware of any prejudices you may have and do not allow prejudice to influence your nursing care.
- ATTEND CONTINUING EDUCATION SEMINARS. Obtain instruction and practice to improve your skills in interviewing, teaching, and counseling techniques. Practice using sexual terminology. Role play with friends or colleagues or in front of a mirror.

ings may affect the ability to assist the expectant couple.

▼ OTHER ROLES

The physical assessment is usually the responsibility of the physician, although nurses with additional training in assessment skills may be involved in that process. A sexual history as part of the assessment process might be completed by any one of the members of the health care team, although it is most likely to be done by the nurse or physician who is completing the general antepartum history. The development of nursing diagnoses and client goals should be done by the nurse. The interventions that are carried out to meet those goals might be initiated by one or a combination of the members of the team. Care should be taken, however, to ensure that the provision of teaching and counseling about sexuality is not fragmented among several people. Continuity of care is important in dealing with an area as sensitive as that of sexuality. Complete documentation and evaluation of the interventions should be the responsibility of the team member who initiated them. The inclusion of sexuality in the management of care for women and their partners during pregnancy is an important and essential aspect of health care and one that is often overlooked. The nurse should be one member of the health care team who insists that it be an integral component of prenatal care.

Risk Management

The safety of sexual intercourse during pregnancy, particularly during the last trimester, has been debated in the medical literature for a number of years. There is still no complete consensus among health care providers as to whether sexual activity should stop during pregnancy. Four potential problems form the primary cause of concern about the safety of sex in pregnancy: (1) the risk of premature rupture of membranes (PROM) or preterm labor; (2) the risk of chorioamnionitis or infection of the fetal membranes; (3) the risk of a maternal air embolism; (4) the risk of HIV transmission.

A number of studies have been done to identify whether PROM or preterm labor occurs more frequently in women who continue to have intercourse in the later weeks of pregnancy compared with women who do not (Brustman et al. 1989; Cunningham et al. 1993; Read and Klebanoff 1993). This concern results from the knowledge that the pregnant woman's orgasm does trigger uterine contractions, which could have the effect of causing cervical dilation or stimulating labor to begin. It is also known that semen contains prostaglandins, which could also stimulate uterine contractions. To date, there has not been conclusive evidence that there is a significant difference in the occurrence of preterm labor between women who do and women who do not continue intercourse, particularly for women who have experienced uncomplicated pregnancies. However, until further information is obtained as to the relationship between orgasm and preterm labor, it seems advisable to caution women who have experienced preterm labor during the current pregnancy or those who are at risk for the development of preterm labor to abstain from intercourse.

Another risk factor that has been discussed in the literature is the development of chorioamnionitis, infection of the fetal membranes (Naeye and Ross 1982; Cunningham et al. 1993). Several studies have shown that preterm delivery due to PROM was more frequent when chorioamnionitis was present and recent sexual intercourse had occurred. Whether the infection of the fetal membranes had occurred as a result of intercourse or from some other cause is not clear. Despite the cause of the chorioamnionitis, the concern of some researchers is that intercourse may cause membranes weakened by infection to rupture. However, consensus has not been reached among physicians regarding this potential risk (Cunningham et al. 1993), and the research to date has shown a potential relationship between chorioamnionitis and preterm labor, not a definite cause and effect occurrence.

A third risk identified in regard to sex during pregnancy is specifically related to the practice of orogenital sex (cunnilingus). There have been several cases reported of pregnant women who have died of a fatal air embolism caused by the male partner's blowing into the vagina during orogenital sex play (Fyke et al. 1985; Bernhardt et al. 1988; Eckert 1991). Air blown into the vagina can be rapidly absorbed by the highly vascular uterine lining, transported to all areas of the body, and result in sudden death. The pregnant woman and her partner do not have to refrain from the practice of cunnilingus during pregnancy, but they should be informed that the forceful blowing of air into the vagina is associated with serious risks and should not be a part of orogenital sex. The position of the woman seems to also have some relationship to the occurrence of air embolism, and the knee-chest position is contraindicated.

The prevention of the transmission of HIV is of as much concern during pregnancy as in any other period of life. Surveys suggest that approximately 1.5 per 1000 pregnant women are HIV positive; higher rates occur in inner-city populations (Cunningham et al. 1993). The rate of perinatal transmission of HIV is uncertain. The virus is transmitted to the infant either through transplacental infection during pregnancy or at the time of birth. If the mother is HIV positive at the time of delivery, the infant will also be HIV positive at birth. However, not all infants will actually have the HIV infection. The initial positive results of some newborns are due to passive maternal antibodies that can persist for up to 18 months. At some later point, the infant may have a negative test response as maternal antibodies are no longer present. Postnatal HIV transmission from mother to infant may also occur. Further discussion of HIV can be found in Chapters 21 and 40. All women and their sexual partners must be informed about the sexual practices that pose the greatest risks of HIV transmission and be given the guidelines for safer sex (Cohen et al. 1990). Table 10–2 outlines the important information to share with pregnant women.

Although these potential risks of sex during pregnancy do exist, the majority of health care providers today agree that sexual expression is an important part of the couple's relationship throughout the entire pregnancy. Unless the woman is identified as being at high risk, there should be no restrictions placed on the continuation of sexual activity. Prevention of risk should be ensured by educating women regarding symptoms that indicate a potential problem (i.e., bleeding, leaking amniotic fluid, signs of preterm labor), informing them of sexual positions or practices to avoid (i.e., knee-chest positions; blowing into vagina during orogenital sex), and teaching safer sex practices for the prevention of HIV transmission.

Implications for Research

The majority of the research that has been done to date regarding sexuality has related to the biophysical aspects of the sexual response cycle and to the physical aspects of sex during pregnancy. Little research has been done regarding the psychological, sociocultural, and cognitive aspects of sexuality or the application of the nursing process regarding sexuality during pregnancy.

Research that could be conducted by nurses within the framework of their clinical practice should be designed to answer the following questions:

- What is the best method for obtaining a sexual history?
- What teaching strategies are most effective in regard to comfort and recall when teaching expectant women and their partners about sex?
- What counseling strategies are successful in helping expectant couples communicate their sexual needs to each other?
- How can nurses incorporate sexual assessment and teaching into the already rushed system of antepartum and postpartum care?

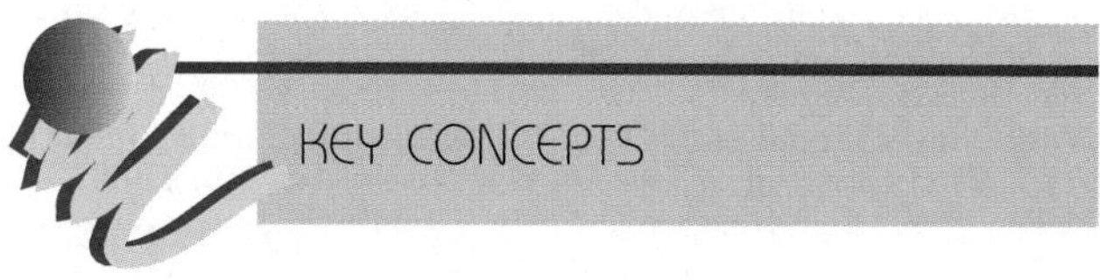

KEY CONCEPTS

- ▼ Humans are sexual beings from the moment of conception until death. Each stage of the life cycle presents new aspects of sexual growth and behavior.
- ▼ During embryonic development, the testes form at 6 to 7 weeks' gestation and the ovaries form at 12 weeks' gestation. By the time of birth, the physiologic structures of the male and female sexual organs are complete.
- ▼ During infancy, sexual expression is evidenced through oral exploration and touch.
- ▼ In the toddler period, gender identity begins through observation of the male and female role models in the toddler's life. The focus is on the external genitalia and excretory functions.
- ▼ According to Freud, during the preschool years, boys experience jealousy of the father's relationship with the mother (Oedipus complex) and girls experience jealousy of the mother's relationship with the father (Electra complex).
- ▼ School-age children become increasingly aware of their bodies. Masturbation as well as mutual sexual exploration may begin in both boys and girls.
- ▼ Body image is a primary concern of adolescents as the physical changes of puberty become evident. Heterosexual sexual activity is experienced by most teens by late adolescence.
- ▼ Because young adults are delaying marriage longer, concerns about STDs and pregnancy must be faced. A sexual value system develops, and issues of monogamous commitment arise.
- ▼ By middle adulthood, sexual issues related to aging occur; however, maturity allows an increase in intimacy and sexual satisfaction.
- ▼ Sexuality is still important to people in late adulthood. Sexual activity may decrease in frequency but is no less satisfying.
- ▼ Masters and Johnson's theory of sexual response describes a four-stage cycle: (1) excitement, (2) plateau, (3) orgasm, and (4) resolution.
- ▼ Two basic physiologic responses take place during Masters and Johnson's four-stage cycle: vasocongestion (an increase in blood concentration to genitals and breasts) and neuromuscular tension (myotonia).
- ▼ According to Kaplan's triphasic theory of sexual response (desire, excitement, and orgasm), two physiologic processes occur during sexual activity: vasocongestive reaction (parasympathetic nervous system) and reflex clonic muscle contraction (sympathetic nervous system).
- ▼ Sexual adaptation during pregnancy is influenced by the woman's health status or medical problems, her pregnancy symptoms, changing sexual desires of either partner, changes in the woman's sexual response cycle, and necessary position changes.
- ▼ Pregnancy and the early postpartum period may alter the physiologic responses that occur during the phases of the sexual response.
- ▼ Women may experience sexual sensations during labor and birth that are similar to those felt during intercourse.
- ▼ Sexual activity during the postpartum period can begin when the woman's postpartum physical symptoms subside and her sexual desire returns. For most women, this occurs between 3 and 6 weeks post partum.
- ▼ Sex is an emotional as well as a physical experience and may be viewed differently by women and men. Factors that influence the emotional experience of sex during pregnancy include the nature of the intimate relationship already established, whether the pregnancy was planned or unplanned, fears regarding harm to the

pregnancy or fetus, and the woman's body image.

- ▼ During the postpartum period, emotional factors such as baby blues, concerns about physical healing, or concerns about the baby may affect sexual interest.
- ▼ The cultural influences on sexuality include the home environment, society's cultural influences, and religion.
- ▼ Taking a sexual history is an important component of the prenatal assessment.
- ▼ Teaching, counseling, and referral should be the areas incorporated into the nurse's plan related to sexuality in pregnancy.
- ▼ Risk management should include an assessment for four potential problems related to the safety of sex during pregnancy: PROM, chorioamnionitis, maternal air embolism, and HIV transmission.

References

Alder, E. M. (1989). Sexual behavior in pregnancy, after childbirth, and during breast feeding. *Baillieres Clinical Obstetrics and Gynaecology,* 3 (4), 805–821.

Barclay, L. M., McDonald, P., O'Loughlin, J. A. (1994). Sexuality and pregnancy: An interview study. *Australian and New Zealand Journal of Obstetrics and Gynecology,* 34 (1), 1–7.

Bernhardt, T. L., Goldman, R. W., Thombs, P. A., Kindwell, E. P. (1988). Hyperbaric oxygen treatment of cerebral air embolism. *Critical Care Medicine,* 16 (7), 729–730.

Bing, E. (1996). Is it safe to have sex during pregnancy? *Lamaze Parents Magazine,* Spring/Summer, 16–19.

Bing, E., and Colman, L. (1989). *Making love during pregnancy.* New York: Farrar, Straus, & Giroux.

Bogren, L. Y. (1991). Changes in sexuality in women and men during pregnancy. *Archives of Sexual Behavior,* 20 (1), 35–45.

Brustman, L., Raptoulis, M., Langer, O., Anyaegbunam, A., Merkatz, I. (1989). Changes in the pattern of uterine contractility in relationship to coitus during pregnancies at low and high risk for preterm labor. *Obstetrics and Gynecology,* 73 (2), 166–168.

Cohen, P. T., Sande, M. A., Volberding, P. A. (1990). *The AIDS knowledge base.* Waltham, MA: The Medical Publishing Group.

Cunningham, F. G., MacDonald, P. C., Gant, N. F., Leveno, K. J., Gilstrap, L. C. (1993). *Williams obstetrics* (19th ed.). Norwalk, CT: Appleton & Lange.

Eckert, W. G. (1991). The unusual accidental death of a pregnant woman by sexual foreplay. *American Journal of Forensic Medicine and Pathology,* 12 (3), 247–249.

Fogel, C. I., and Lauver, D. (1990). *Sexual health promotion.* Philadelphia: W. B. Saunders.

Fyke, F. E., Kazmier, F. J., and Harms, R. W. (1985). Venous air embolism: Life threatening complication of orogenital sex during pregnancy. *American Journal of Medicine,* 78 (2), 333–336.

Hart, J., Cohen, E., Gingold, A., Homburg, R. (1991). Sexual behavior in pregnancy: A study of 219 women. *Journal of Sex Education and Therapy,* 17 (2), 86–90.

Kaplan, H. S. (1974). *The new sex therapy.* New York: Brunner/Mazel Publications.

Kaplan, H. S. (1979). *Disorders of sexual desire.* New York: Simon & Schuster.

Kaplan, H. S. (1993). *The new injection treatment for impotence.* New York: Brunner/Mazel Publications.

Kinsey, A. C. (1948). *Sexual behavior in human male.* Philadelphia: W. B. Saunders.

Kinsey, A. C. (1953). *Sexual behavior in human female.* Philadelphia: W. B. Saunders.

Masters, W. H., and Johnson, V. E. (1966). *Human sexual response.* Boston: Little, Brown.

Masters, W. H., and Johnson, V. E. (1970). *Human sexual inadequacy.* Boston: Little, Brown.

Masters, W. H., Johnson, V. E., Kolodny, R. C. (1994). *Heterosexuality.* New York: Harper Collins.

Masters, W. H., Johnson, V. E., Kolodny, R. C. (1995). *Human sexuality* (5th ed.). New York: Harper Collins.

Miller, W. E., and Friedman, S. (1988). Male and female sexuality during pregnancy: Behavior and attitudes. *Journal of Psychology and Human Sexuality,* 1 (2), 17–37.

Moore, K. L., and Persaud, T. V. N. (1993). *The developing human: Clinically oriented embryology* (5th ed.). Philadelphia: W. B. Saunders.

Naeye, R. L., and Ross, S. (1982). Coitus and chorioamnionitis, a prospective study. *Early Human Development,* 6, 91–97.

Read, J. S., and Klebanoff, M. A. (1993). Sexual intercourse during pregnancy and preterm delivery: Effects of vaginal microorganisms. *American Journal of Obstetrics and Gynecology,* 168 (2), 514–519.

Reamy, K., and White, S. E. (1987). Sexuality in the puerperium: A review. *Archives of Sexual Behavior,* 16 (2), 165–186.

Rice, F. P. (1995). *Human development: A life span approach* (2nd ed.). Englewood Cliffs, NJ: Prentice-Hall.

Wilkerson, N., and Bing, E. (1988). Sexuality. In F. Nichols and S. Humenick (Eds.). *Childbirth education: Practice, research, and theory.* Philadelphia: W. B. Saunders.

Woods, N. F. (1984). *Human sexuality in health and illness* (2nd ed.). St. Louis: C. V. Mosby.

Chapter 11

Family Planning

Elaine Zwelling

> An individual's or couple's decisions about birth control depend on many factors including age, future plans, marital or relationship status (including trust and cooperation), finances, religious beliefs, sexual attitudes, health, and prior experiences . . . choosing to use birth control, whatever the reason, is a personal decision.
>
> William H. Masters, Virginia E. Johnson, Robert C. Kolodny (1995)

HIGHLIGHTS

- Family Planning and Pregnancy
- Methods of Family Planning
- Ideal Contraceptive Method
- Theoretic Versus Use Effectiveness
- Birth Control Methods of the Future
- Nursing Practice
- Role of Team Members
- Risk Management
- Implications for Research

The decision to become a parent is no doubt one of the most important decisions that an individual makes in a lifetime, yet many people today continue to enter the role of parenthood inadvertently, with little thought or planning for the addition of a child to the family unit. The ideal situation might be one in which parents are able to have discussions and make decisions about their desired family before the first pregnancy occurs. Preconception counseling and preconception planning classes are now available in many areas to help couples contemplating parenthood have the opportunity to talk with others and consider in advance all aspects of pregnancy, childbirth, and parenting.

PLANNED VERSUS UNPLANNED PREGNANCY

Planning a family enables parents to feel ready physically, emotionally, and financially for the roles and tasks of parenthood. Having children in an unplanned manner may contribute to frustrations, resentments, health

DEFINITIONS

Abstinence—Refraining from sexual intercourse completely for a period of time; can be used as a method of birth control.

Basal body temperature—A method of natural family planning based on identification of the shift in the woman's body temperature that takes place after ovulation.

Coitus interruptus—The practice of the male withdrawing the penis when ejaculation seems imminent to prevent the deposit of sperm in the vaginal tract.

Condom—A rubber or animal skin sheath placed on the erect penis before sexual intercourse to prevent deposition of semen in the vagina.

Contraception—Prevention of conception.

Diaphragm—A barrier method of birth control; a shallow, dome-shaped device with a flexible metal rim that fits into the vagina against the cervix to block sperm from entering the uterus; used with a spermicidal agent.

Intrauterine device—A small plastic device inserted into the uterus for an extended period to prevent pregnancy by causing cellular and biochemical changes in the endometrium.

Natural family planning—A fertility awareness form of birth control that consists of a group of methods based on an understanding and awareness of the woman's reproductive cycle and its associated symptoms; includes the calendar method, basal body temperature method, cervical mucus method, and symptothermal method.

Oral contraceptive—"The pill"; a hormonal contraceptive that combines estrogen and progestin to prevent pregnancy by suppressing ovulation and altering cervical mucus production, tubal mobility, and endometrial lining development.

Prophylaxis—Prevention.

Spinnbarkeit—The characteristic viscosity or elasticity of cervical mucus seen as ovulation approaches.

Thermal shift—The rise in basal body temperature that occurs after a woman has ovulated.

Tubal ligation—A sterilization procedure for females in which the fallopian tubes are cut, tied, cauterized, plugged, capped, coagulated, or clipped to prevent the passage of the ovum through the tubes.

Vasectomy—A sterilization procedure for males in which the vasa deferentia are severed, tied, clipped, or coagulated to prevent the passage of sperm.

100 Women Years—The effectiveness of a contraceptive for 1 year's use in a group of 100 women.

strains, or financial strains that can interfere with the parent-child bond, with quality parenting, or with family needs. Nevertheless, more than half of all pregnancies in the United States are unplanned (NAACOG 1991). Eighty-five percent of teenage pregnancies are unintended, and 55 percent of pregnancies among older women are unintended (AGI 1994).

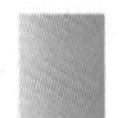

Health Considerations

Consideration of the prospective parent's health status before conception is ideal, because often women who intend to improve their health habits once they are pregnant are not aware of their pregnancy until a number of weeks of gestation have passed. Improving nutritional status before the pregnancy will allow the mother to best nourish her developing embryo in the early weeks of pregnancy. Eliminating habits such as smoking and taking alcohol or drugs, and assessing any potential home or job-related health risks before pregnancy, is certainly advantageous. Beginning a program of regular exercise also contributes to overall health status. If the parents have been using a method of family planning, it is wise to identify whether that method poses any risks should pregnancy occur.

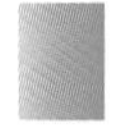

Benefits of Family Planning

A World Health Organization Expert Committee has defined family planning as those practices that help individuals or couples avoid unwanted births, bring about wanted births, regulate the intervals between pregnancies, control the time at which births occur in relation to the ages of the parents, and determine the number of children in the family (Kurtzman and Block 1986). Fertility control has long-range implications for the health of women in a society and for the society as a whole. The effects of frequent pregnancies and short birth intervals are avoided, thus decreasing maternal morbidity and infant mortality. With reproductive freedom, women realize opportunities within their families and their communities that otherwise might be closed to them.

Influences on Family Planning

Many fertile American couples practice some form of family planning today, but too often the choice of a contraceptive method is based on emotional factors such as fear, prejudice, or rumor rather than fact. Physical risks and health problems, and social and religious factors, also influence family planning choices. The selection of a contraceptive method is a complex decision that involves social, cultural, religious, educational, psychological, and monetary factors, as well as medical considerations. It is important for nurses and nurse counselors to be knowledgeable about each of the contraceptive methods available today so that they can provide factual information about family planning options and support clients in the use of their method of choice.

METHODS OF FAMILY PLANNING

Ideal Contraceptive Method

If a perfect and ideal contraceptive method existed, it would need to meet a series of criteria that include effectiveness, safety, ease of understanding and use, a low degree of interference with sexual pleasure, reversibility, affordability, and availability. First, and probably most important, it would be 100 percent effective. It would also have to be completely safe, causing no risk to the user's health or reproductive status.

In addition, a perfect contraceptive would have few, if any, side effects. It would be easy to understand and use as well as being acceptable to both partners. A characteristic that would make a contraceptive particularly ideal is for its use not to be directly related to sexual intercourse, i.e., not to disrupt lovemaking in any way. Neither would it interfere with sexual pleasure. Such a contraceptive would be totally reversible, enabling the couple to conceive immediately after discontinuing use of the method. It would also be inexpensive and easy to obtain.

Unfortunately, the perfect contraceptive does not exist. Therefore, sexually active individuals must weigh all these factors in their consideration of the contraceptive method they wish to use, and decide which factors are most important to them.

Theoretic Versus Use Effectiveness

Each of the methods of family planning available today are discussed in this chapter. A description of the method will be provided, followed by a discussion of its effectiveness and the advantages, disadvantages, and risks. In discussing the effectiveness of a contraceptive method, two aspects of its potential can be reported. "Theoretic effectiveness" refers to the maximal possible effectiveness of a particular contraceptive method when it is used precisely as advised by the manufacturer. This rate is approximated by the lowest observed failure (i.e., pregnancy) rates, and reflects what the potential effectiveness of a method should be without the variable of human error. The second and clinically more valid effectiveness rate reported is "use effectiveness." This rate refers to the success of a sample of individuals actually using the method to prevent pregnancy, and it does reflect possible human error or lack of compliance. In this chapter the effectiveness rates are reported according to "100 women years," i.e., 1 year of use in a sample of 100 women. In counseling clients, the use effectiveness rate is the more advisable one (Mishell 1989) and is the one reported in this text (Table 11–1).

Natural Family Planning

Natural family planning, or fertility awareness, consists of a group of methods that can be used to plan, space, or prevent pregnancy on the basis of an understanding and continual awareness of the woman's reproductive cycle and its associated symptoms. These methods enable couples to time sexual intercourse in relation to the fertile and infertile phases of the menstrual cycle. Natural family planning methods are particularly attractive to individuals who are unable to use other contraceptive methods because of medical contraindications or religious or cultural beliefs. Natural family planning is also useful to women who wish to learn more about their body's responses throughout the reproductive cycle, and it can assist couples who wish to conceive (Queenan et al. 1991a, 1991b). The four methods of natural family planning discussed in this chapter are the calendar, basal body temperature, cervical mucus, and

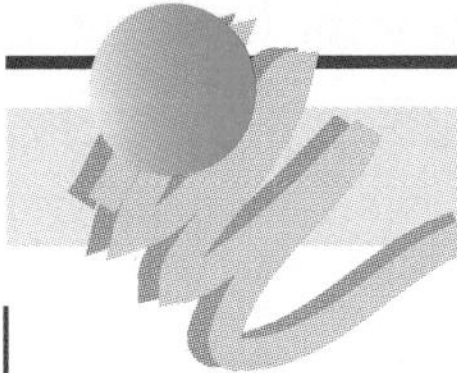

HISTORICAL PERSPECTIVES

FAMILY PLANNING

The use of vaginal barriers to prevent pregnancy has been attempted for many centuries. An Egyptian named Petri Papyrus recorded the use of vaginal plugs made out of honey and crocodile dung in 1850 BC. In India and Asia, small balls of feathers were used as vaginal plugs, while the Hebrews advocated the use of moistened sponges to act as a barrier to sperm. Cervical caps date back to ancient Eastern cultures before Christ. In China and Japan, prostitutes placed small disks of silky, oiled bamboo tissue over the cervix. A common practice in the sixth century was to cut open a pomegranate and insert the hollow cup into the vagina before intercourse. Later, Casanova in the mid-1700s recommended the use of half a lemon, with the skin acting as a cervical cap or diaphragm and the juice as the spermicide.

In some parts of the world, women are still using homemade pessaries, instruments inserted into the vagina as a contraceptive device, to block the cervix. These are often prepared from materials such as rags or chopped grass. The modern cervical cap was devised by a German physician, F. A. Wilde, who began taking impressions of patients' cervices and molding rubber caps from the impressions in 1838. During the late nineteenth century, German and Dutch women used these cervical caps. When their use spread to England, they became known as "Dutch caps."

Diaphragms were first made by a German physician, C. Hasse, who described them in an 1880 article. Using the pseudonym Wilhelm P. J. Mensinga, "Mensinga's pessary" quickly became popular among some physicians in Germany and Holland. The diaphragm became readily available around the world in the 1920s when advances in the rubber industry allowed the manufacture of better-quality, long-lasting, less expensive rubber products. In the United States, Margaret Sanger, the early family planning nurse, popularized the diaphragm and fitted them in her clinic in New York City during the 1920s.

Contraceptive penile sheaths for men have also been used since Egyptian times, initially for protection against disease. The use of animal intestines as condoms became popular in England during the reign of Charles II from 1630 to 1685. It is thought that condoms derived their name from a physician of the court during this period.

The use of intrauterine devices (IUDs) for contraception can be traced back to the early 1900s. Known as cervicouterine pessaries, these early IUDs had intravaginal stems of wood, bone, or glass. Although the stated purpose of these pessaries was to support the uterus, prevent delayed or irregular menstruation, or cure dysmenorrhea and infertility, the devices were also used to prevent conception and sometimes were even used to stimulate abortion. These early IUDs often caused serious and fatal infections, and as a result cervicouterine devices were condemned by the medical community. The first published evidence of the modern IUD was a report of Richard Richter's silkworm gut ring in 1909. Later, Ernst Graffenberg presented a report of a silver intrauterine ring at a 1929 International Sexual Reform Congress in London, giving the first scientific identity, exposure, and credibility to the IUD. In 1934, Tenres Ota of Japan replaced the Graffenberg ring with gold-plated silver, gold, or plastic IUDs.

Data from Eichhorst, B. (1989). Contraception. *Primary Care,* 15 (3), 437–459; Hutchings, J., Benson, P., Perkin, G., Soderstrom, R. (1985). The IUD after 20 years: A review. *Family Planning Perspectives,* 17 (6), 244–255; Kovacs, G. T., Jarman, H., Dunn, K., Dip, M. W., Baker, H. W. (1986). The contraceptive diaphragm: Is it an acceptable method in the 1980s? *Australian and New Zealand Journal of Obstetrics and Gynecology,* 26, 76–77.

symptothermal methods. In addition, high-risk methods of natural family planning such as abstinence, coitus interruptus, douching, and breastfeeding are addressed. Because all of the natural family planning methods have very similar advantages, disadvantages, and risks or contraindications, these aspects of the methods are discussed collectively after a description of each method.

Table 11–1

REPORTED PREGNANCY RATES OF CONTRACEPTIVE METHODS

METHOD OF CONTRACEPTION	NO. OF PREGNANCIES PER 100 WOMEN YEARS	EFFECTIVENESS (%)
Male sterilization (vasectomy)	0.15–0.4	99.6–99.85
Hormonal implant (Norplant)	0.2–0.6	99.4–99.8
Female sterilization (tubal ligation)	0.04–5	95–99.96
Combined oral contraceptives	1–10	90–99
Intrauterine device	3–5	95–97
Condom with spermicide	5	95
Hormonal injection (Depo-Provera)	5–10	90–95
Female condom	2.6–12.4	87.6–97.4
Cervical cap with spermicide	4–20	80–96
Symptothermal method	6–19	81–94
Basal body temperature	6–20	80–94
Condom alone	10–20	80–90
Diaphragm with spermicide	2–23	77–98
Coitus interruptus (withdrawal)	20–25	75–80
Ovulation/cervical mucus method	15–28	72–85
Spermicides alone	11–31	69–89
Calendar method	14–47	53–86

CALENDAR METHOD

Description

The calendar method, also known as the "rhythm" method of natural family planning, is based on mathematical calculations to predict the probable time of ovulation, and thus the fertile period, as determined from knowledge of the length of previous menstrual cycles. Before using this method, the woman should have a record of at least six to 12 of her previous consecutive menstrual cycles. She must then identify from that information the length of her shortest and longest cycles. The first day of the menstrual period is always used as the first day of the cycle when making calculations. The fertile period during the cycle is considered to be the time from the eighteenth day before the end of the shortest cycle through the eleventh day before the end of the longest cycle (Mishell 1989; NAACOG 1991). For example, if the woman's shortest cycle was 21 days and her longest cycle 30 days, she would use the above rule regarding the fertile period to make the following calculation:

Shortest = 21 days	Longest = 30 days
− 18	− 11
3	19

Therefore, the woman's fertile period (and the time she should abstain from sexual intercourse) would be from day 3 of her menstrual cycle through day 19 of the cycle. Her safe period would be from day 20 of this cycle through day 2 of the next cycle.

Effectiveness

The use effectiveness of the calendar method when used alone is reported as ranging from 14 to 47 pregnancies per 100 women years (Mishell 1989; Fehring 1990, 1991). This means that this form of natural family planning is between 53 and 86 percent effective in actual use. The risks that occur with the method include that of ovulation occurring unexpectedly early or late in the cycle. This method is contraindicated for women who do not have regular cycles: e.g., women who are anovulatory, women approaching menopause, adolescents, and women who have recently given birth.

BASAL BODY TEMPERATURE

Description

Another method of natural family planning uses the basal body temperature (BBT). The BBT method is based on identification of the shift in the woman's body temperature (thermal shift) that occurs after ovulation has taken place. The practice of observing temperature changes can be traced back almost 100 years. It was first described by a Dutch gynecologist and sexologist, Theodor Henry van de Velde, in 1904. A German Catholic priest, Wilhelm Hillebrand, was the first person to use fluctuations of the woman's body temperature to determine infertile days (Fehring 1991; Foxwell 1994).

In a healthy woman, the basal body temperature ranges from 96.6° to 98.2°F during the follicular phase of the menstrual cycle, and from 97.6° to 99.2°F during the luteal phase. These sequential temperature changes occur because of the presence of estrogen and progesterone. To use this method, the woman should purchase a special basal thermometer, which is calibrated from 96° to 100°F in tenths of a degree. A regular fever thermometer is calibrated in two tenths of a degree and is therefore not as accurate in denoting minute basal temperature changes. The temperature should be taken orally and recorded on a graph at the same time daily, usually upon waking after 5 to 6 hours of uninterrupted sleep. The temperature graph is then used to identify the safe and unsafe periods of the cycle (see Symptothermal Method, p. 240). The woman assumes she has ovulated when there is a slight rise (at least 0.2°C) over the last six readings.

Many women also observe a definite drop in BBT just before the temperature rise. The elevation must last at least 3 days before it can be assumed that it indicates ovulation. To avoid pregnancy, the couple should abstain from intercourse until the third consecutive day of the temperature rise. The infertile or safe time is thus identified as being from the period after ovulation has occurred until the end of the cycle. It is important to remember that BBT method recordings do not allow for a prediction of ovulation, only identification that ovulation has occurred (Fehring 1990; NAACOG 1991; Foxwell 1994).

Effectiveness

The use effectiveness of the basal body temperature method when used alone is six to 20 pregnancies per 100 women years, or 80 to 94 percent effective. The risks of using this method relate to the fact that temperature elevations may not always be a reliable indicator of ovulation, and temperature graphs may be difficult to interpret. Other factors such as fatigue, illness, or exertion can also cause temperature elevations (Fehring 1990, 1991).

CERVICAL MUCUS METHOD

Description

The ovulation or cervical mucus method is a third component of natural family planning. This method bases recognition of the fertile and infertile periods of the menstrual cycle on recognition of changes in cervical mucus. The method was first described in 1952 by Drs. John and Evelyn Billings of Australia and therefore may also be called the "Billings method." Women who use this method are taught to focus on sensations of vaginal "wetness" or "dryness," indicating the type of cervical mucus being secreted, and should record their observations at the end of each day.

When the ovulatory phase of the menstrual cycle is about to begin, cervical mucus begins to increase in amount; usually about 20 to 60 mg of mucus is produced. At the time of ovulation the amount increases to about 600 mg. This mucus is necessary for the viability and motility of sperm (Fehring 1990; Davis 1992; Foxwell 1994). Near the time of ovulation the appearance of the mucus begins to change from being thick, yellow or cloudy, and tacky to becoming clear, watery, and slippery. The thick, "dry" mucus (Type G) predominates during the luteal phase of the menstrual cycle and prevents the passage of sperm into the cervix. The mucin of the thick, dry mucus cross-links the cervical canal to form a net that entraps the sperm (Fig. 11–1). Progesterone is responsible for the production of this dry mucus. During the follicular phase of the menstrual cycle, the clear "wet" mucus (Type E) allows increased permeability of the mucus to sperm and facilitates the passage of sperm into the cervix. The mucin fibers of this wet mucus lay almost parallel to each other and to the cervical canal by channels formed by the mucin. Estrogen is responsible for this wet mucus (Mishell 1989; NAACOG 1991; Foxwell 1994).

As ovulation approaches, the mucus also becomes stretchable and can be drawn into long threads with considerable elastic recoil. This characteristic viscosity is called spinnbarkeit and signals the peak day of the ovulatory phase (Fig. 11–1). The sodium chloride content increases in cervical mucus near ovulation and causes the appearance of a fern pattern due to crystallization when the mucus dries on a glass slide (Fig. 11–2). Women are taught to assess the cervical mucus changes by sight and by the degree of "wetness" felt in the vaginal area (Fehring 1990; NAACOG 1991; Foxwell 1994). It is important that assessment of cervical mucus be made without the influence of semen, vaginal discharges that might be related to infections, or spermicidal creams or jellies.

To avoid pregnancy, sexual contact must be avoided on all "wet" days, especially 3 days following the peak mucus day. Menstrual days are also considered possibly fertile in the event of an unexpected short cycle. Therefore, sexual abstinence is advised during the menstrual days, every other night on "dry" preovulatory days, and from the beginning of the wet cervical mucus symptoms until

CERVICAL MUCUS METHOD OF CONTRACEPTION		
	INFERTILE PERIOD	FERTILE PERIOD
Menstrual cycle phase	Luteal phase	Follicular phase (ovulation)
Cervical mucus characteristics	Amount: 20 to 60 mg (vaginal dryness) Appearance: thick, yellow, cloudy Type: G Hormonal influence: progesterone Viscosity: none	Amount: 600 mg (vaginal wetness) Appearance: clear, watery, slippery Type: E Hormonal influence: estrogen Viscosity: spinnbarkeit 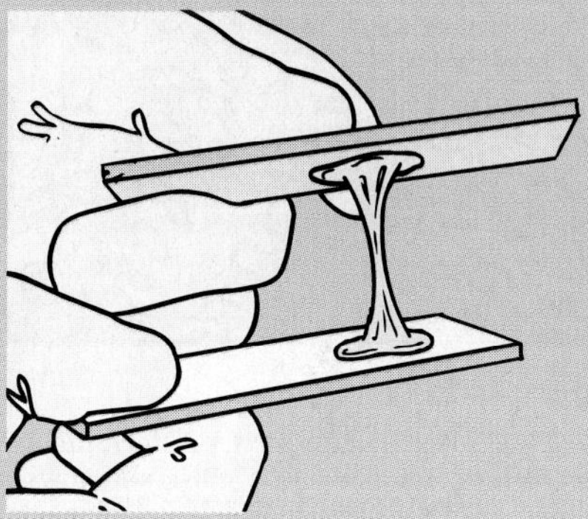
Sperm permeability	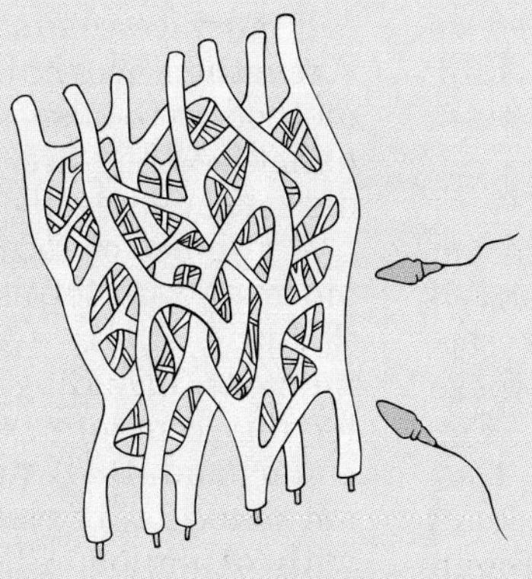	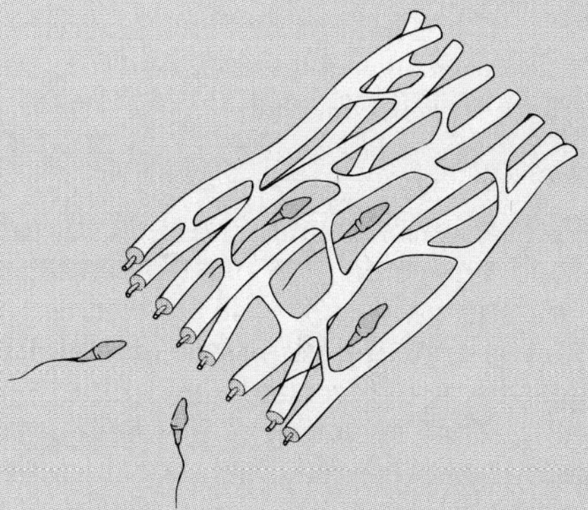
Microscopic appearance	No ferning	Fern pattern

Figure 11–1

The appearance and viscosity of cervical mucus changes dramatically between the infertile and fertile periods, resulting in an environment that favors sperm permeability.

the fourth day after peak mucus is observed (Mishell 1989; Fehring 1990; NAACOG 1991).

The Creighton model is another form of ovulation method available to women. Like the Billings method, it is based on the presence or absence of cervical mucus as the determinant of fertility. However, the Creighton model has a standard teaching format and language for classifying cervical mucus that differs from the Billings method. It is taught only by natural family planning practitioners who have been trained in a year-long program accredited by the American Academy of Natural Family Planning (AANFP) (Hilgers et al. 1992; Fehring et al. 1994).

Effectiveness

The use effectiveness of the ovulation method is reported as ranging between 15 and 28 pregnancies per 100 women years, or 72 to 85 percent. The risks of the ovulation method relate to difficulty in identifying cervical mucus changes. Vaginal discharge due to infection, sexual arousal, semen, or use of lubricants can give false readings.

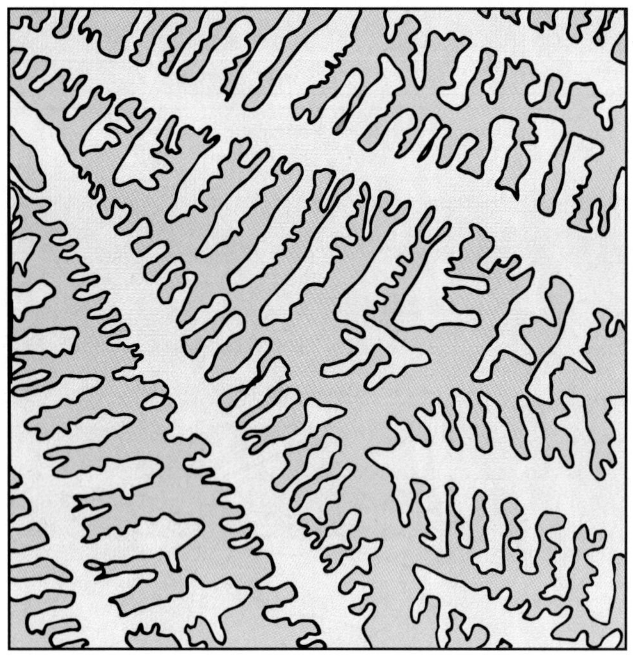

Figure 11–2

Ferning of cervical mucus • A fernlike pattern can be seen as cervical mucus dries on a glass slide owing to crystallization from increased sodium chloride content near ovulation.

SYMPTOTHERMAL METHOD

Description

The symptothermal method is a combination method based on the multiple indicators of cervical mucus patterns, BBT patterns, and other secondary physical symptoms of ovulation. All these indicators are recorded on a chart each day (Fig. 11–3). The secondary physical symptoms that should be recorded include mittelschmerz (pain from the rupturing ovarian follicle), breakthrough bleeding from high estrogen levels before ovulation, bearing-down pains, general tenderness in the pelvic region, abdominal bloating, breast tenderness, and increased sexual interest. These symptoms are helpful in confirming the major ovulatory signs for some women. In addition, many symptothermal method programs offer instruction in how to detect changes in the cervix that occur throughout the menstrual cycle. When the symptothermal method is used to prevent pregnancy, abstinence starts from the beginning of the cervical mucus symptom and ends on either the third night of temperature rise or the fourth day of mucus, whichever sign appears later (Fehring 1990; Foxwell 1994).

Effectiveness

The combination of natural family planning methods that make up the symptothermal method may be more difficult to learn, but the effectiveness when combining methods is increased. Reported use effectiveness ranges from six to 19 pregnancies per 100 women years, or 81 to 94 percent (Mishell 1989; NAACOG 1991).

ADVANTAGES AND DISADVANTAGES

The advantages and disadvantages of all four of the natural family planning methods discussed are very similar. One advantage of any of these methods is that they are safe in regard to their effects on the woman's body. They require no mechanical or pharmacologic intervention. This may appeal to women who favor a lifestyle characterized by avoidance of unnatural interventions. Use of these methods develops a keen awareness of the menstrual cycle and the body's response to it. The natural family planning methods are either free or very inexpensive, and they are usually acceptable to all religious and cultural groups (Queenan et al. 1991b). They are easily taught and can be easily reversed when pregnancy is desired. Many couples favor natural family planning methods because they require shared responsibility for fertility control between the woman and the man. Some couples feel that these methods can enhance communication between partners and strengthen marital ties. Natural family planning methods are also as useful for planning a pregnancy as they are for preventing one, and can be discontinued easily at any time.

A number of recently developed devices can now aid in the use of natural family planning methods (Fehring 1991; Queenan 1991a). Computerized methods, including the Bioself 110 and the Rabbit fertility computer, can assist in the use of the calendar and BBT methods. Electronic devices can aid detection of electrochemical charges associated with ovulation. Chemical and hormonal test kits are being developed to help detect the luteinizing hormone (LH) surge that occurs in the urine about 12 to 24 hours before ovulation. Although these new devices can help couples to monitor fertility, they should not be used without an understanding of the menstrual cycle and the changes that can be observed indicating periods of fertility.

The primary disadvantage of natural family planning methods are that they may require extended periods of abstinence from sexual intercourse during each menstrual cycle. The methods require a highly motivated couple for most effective use. No protection against sexually transmitted diseases (STDs) is offered, unless a spermicidal agent is used along with the natural methods. There have been reports in the literature of an increased risk of a fetal anomaly when natural family planning is used, owing to an increased chance of an overripe ovum being fertilized. However, the data regarding this potential occurrence are incon-

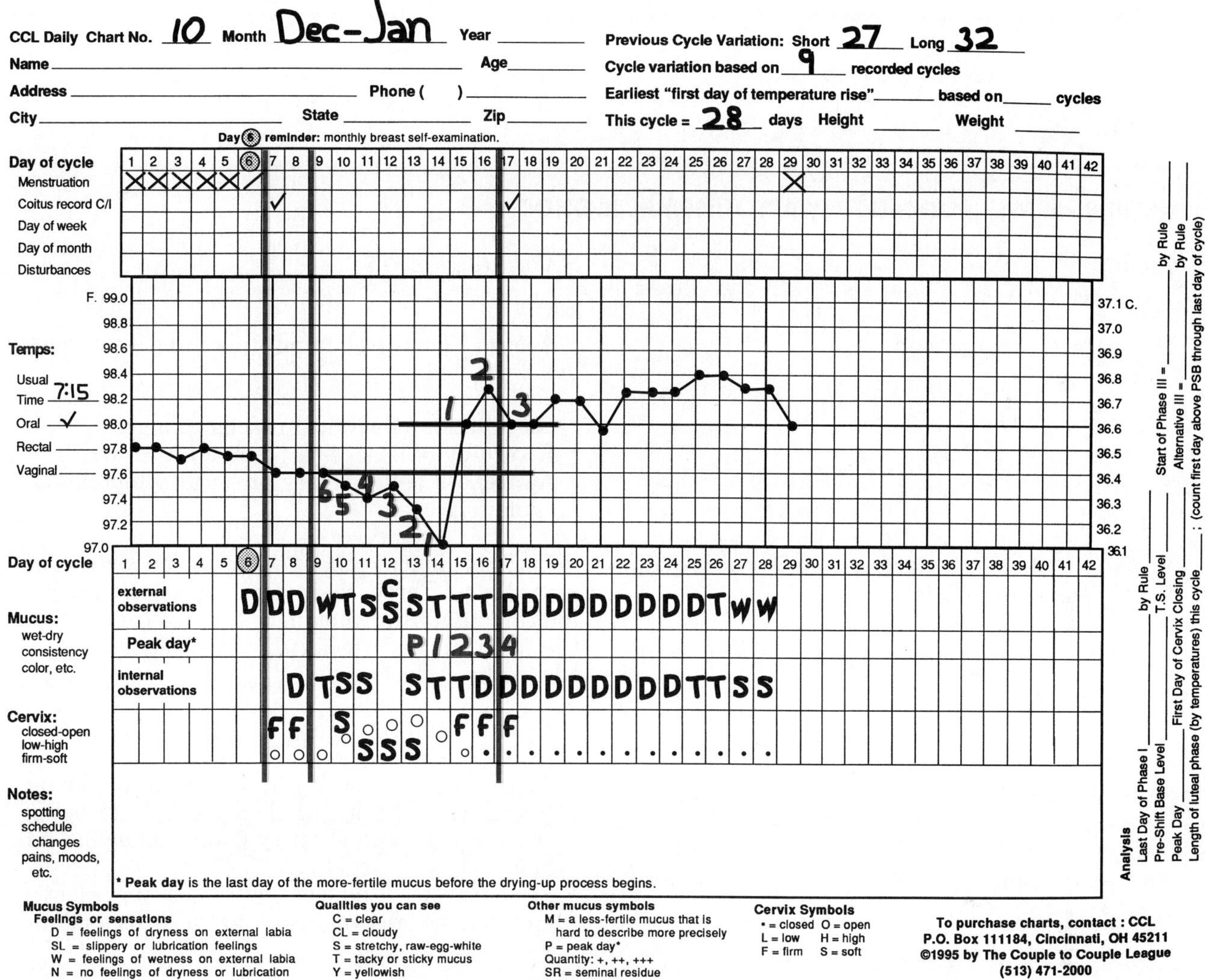

Figure 11–3

The symptothermal chart is used to record basal body temperature, cervical mucus, and coitus and help the client be aware of the fertile and unfertile periods during her menstrual cycle. (Copyright © The Couple to Couple League, Box 111184, Cincinnati, OH 45211. Used with permission.)

clusive, and any increase in risk is thought to be very small (Queenan 1991a).

ADDITIONAL NATURAL FAMILY PLANNING METHODS

In addition to the primary methods of natural family planning just discussed, there are additional methods that couples may attempt to use to prevent conception. These can be labeled high-risk natural methods.

▼ **Abstinence.** The first of these methods is abstinence, or total abstention from sexual intercourse. Although abstinence is 100 percent effective in the prevention of pregnancy, it is obviously a radical and very difficult form of family planning to maintain. The high-risk aspect of using abstinence is the likelihood that adherence to it will be difficult and that it will not be possible to use it for extended periods.

▼ **Coitus Interruptus.** Another high-risk natural family planning method is coitus interruptus, the practice of the male withdrawing the penis when ejaculation seems imminent. Withdrawal can then be followed by mutual masturbation or "outercourse," movement of the penis against an external part of the woman's body to achieve orgasm. The use effectiveness of coitus interruptus

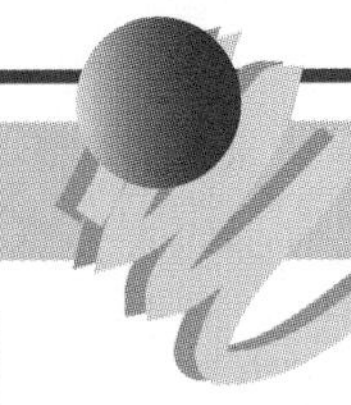

TEACHING GUIDE

NATURAL FAMILY PLANNING: SYMPTOTHERMAL METHOD

TOPIC	*MAJOR CONCEPTS*
Description of method	A form of natural family planning that combines the following: • Observation of cervical mucus changes • Recording of basal body temperature (BBT) • Awareness of secondary physical symptoms of ovulation
Physical changes during menstrual cycle that indicate ovulation	Cervical mucus changes occur as ovulation approaches. Three characteristics of the mucus indicate that the woman is moving from infertile ("dry mucus") to fertile ("wet mucus") periods in the cycle: • Amount—an increase in amount of mucus will be noted to signal ovulation • Appearance—mucus will change from being thick, yellow, tacky, or cloudy ("dry") to being clear, watery, and slippery ("wet") as ovulation approaches • Stretchability—mucus will become elastic and can be drawn into long threads (spinnbarkeit) BBT (i.e., temperature at rest) increases slightly as ovulation approaches (thermal shift). A rise of at least 0.2° over previous readings and lasting at least 3 days indicates that the ovary has released an egg. This rise in temperature occurs after, not before, ovulation. Secondary physical symptoms occur for many women as ovulation approaches. These may include the following: • Pain, tenderness, or soreness in lower pelvic area (mittelschmerz) • Breakthrough bleeding • Abdominal bloating • Breast tenderness • Increased sexual interest
Recording cervical mucus changes	Observe the characteristics of the day. Record the consistency ("wet" vs. "dry") and characteristics (color, elasticity) of the mucus on a symptothermal chart each day.

Continued on facing page

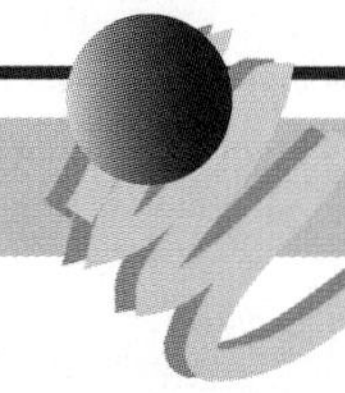

TEACHING GUIDE Continued

NATURAL FAMILY PLANNING: SYMPTOTHERMAL METHOD

TOPIC	*MAJOR CONCEPTS*
Recording basal body temperature (BBT)	With a special basal thermometer the woman should take her temperature orally immediately upon awakening every morning and before moving about or ingesting food or beverages. The temperature should be recorded on the symptothermal chart.
Recording secondary physical symptoms	Any observed symptoms throughout the cycle should be recorded on the symptothermal chart. In addition, the woman should record the days of the menstrual cycle and the days when coitus occurred.
Identification of fertile period and abstinence from coitus	The woman should refrain from having sexual intercourse from the beginning of the cervical mucus symptoms until either the third night of BBT rise *or* the fourth day of "wet" mucus, whichever sign appears *later.*
Advantages of symptothermal method	The combination of the three components of natural family planning that comprise the symptothermal method increase the effectiveness. Other advantages include • Safety • No mechanical or pharmacologic intervention • Development of awareness of menstrual cycle changes • Is acceptable to all religious groups • Is inexpensive • Is easily reversible • Requires shared responsibility for fertility control; enhances couple communication
Disadvantages of symptothermal method	The primary disadvantage of the symptothermal method is the required abstinence from sexual intercourse during extended periods of the menstrual cycle. The method also offers no protection against sexually transmitted diseases.

Continued on following page

is reported as ranging from 20 to 25 pregnancies per 100 women years, or 75 to 80 percent. The problems with coitus interruptus relate to difficulty in withdrawing the penis in time, or with the withdrawal not being complete before semen is deposited on the external female genitalia. It is also possible that, without the male's knowledge, a small amount of seminal fluid containing sperm can escape from the penis before ejaculation. This method demands a great deal of self-control.

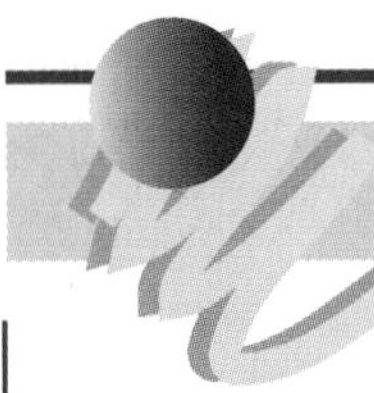

TEACHING GUIDE Continued

NATURAL FAMILY PLANNING: SYMPTOTHERMAL METHOD

Teaching Aids

1. Pamphlets or booklets explaining natural family planning
2. Pictures or posters illustrating the phases of the menstrual cycle and changes in cervical mucus
3. A raw egg white to illustrate the characteristics of "wet" cervical mucus
4. A basal body thermometer
5. Movies or filmstrips to explain natural family planning
6. Symptothermal charts for recording cycle changes

Increasing Your Teaching Effectiveness

Your teaching about natural family planning will be more effective by using the following approaches:

1. Identify whether the woman is a good candidate for using natural family planning by assessing
   - Her understanding of the menstrual cycle and the physical changes that accompany it
   - Her motivation to make daily observations and recordings and to periodically abstain from sexual intercourse
   - The willingness of her sexual partner to comply with the method

   Spend time talking with the woman about these aspects before teaching her about the method.
2. Ask for frequent feedback and clarification from the woman as the method is described. Allow ample time for her questions.
3. Use visual aids and teaching materials.
4. Have the woman practice reading a basal body thermometer and record temperature on a symptothermal chart.
5. Plan for follow-up counseling after the woman's first cycle using the method.

The advantages of coitus interruptus as a natural family planning method are that it is always available, there is no cost involved, no supplies are needed, and there is no medical risk to either partner. It is a valid method if no other form of contraception is available at the time. The obvious disadvantages are the worry it may cause the couple regarding whether it has been effective and the interruption of the excitement phase of sexual arousal, decreasing pleasure for both partners. This method requires considerable control of the man's sexual response, and so should be contraindicated for a male who has problems with ejaculatory control or for couples who make love frequently (Lethbridge 1991; NAACOG 1991).

▼ **Vaginal Douching.** Many sexually active couples today still believe that the practice of female vaginal douching immediately after intercourse is a valid method of natural family planning. The use effectiveness of douching has not been reported in the literature, but most health care professionals agree that douching is not effective and in fact is probably very risky. It is likely that the action of the solution used in douching may increase, rather than decrease, the chance of pregnancy, by forcing sperm farther up the vagina toward the cervical os.

▼ **Breastfeeding.** A final method of natural family planning that can be labeled high risk is breastfeeding. Although for centuries breastfeeding provided natural spacing of births for many women and is a method still being used successfully today in other cultures, the typical breastfeeding practices of women today in our culture do not usually provide the necessary hormonal influence needed to inhibit ovulation. The release of prolactin during breastfeeding discourages the release of LH by the anterior pituitary gland. High levels of prolactin may also directly affect ovarian response to LH and follicle stimulating hormone (FSH), preventing the induction of ovulation. Through neural stimulation of the nipples caused by the infant's sucking, beta endorphins are released to suppress hypothalamic gonadotropin releasing hormone (GnRH). It is also thought that gonadotropins may have a decreased response to

GnRH during lactation (Lethbridge 1989). However, for this hormonal response to be sufficient to inhibit ovulation, nursing must be frequent and regular over a 24-hour period.

In non-Western cultures the baby is with the mother at all times and nurses for brief periods, as often as every 15 to 20 minutes. The breast is used for pacification, breastfeeding is on demand, and night feedings continue for many months. Solid foods are not introduced until the baby is close to 1 year of age. In Western cultures the breastfeeding experience is usually somewhat different. It is more common that the baby nurses no more than eight times a day, and the goal is to encourage the baby to sleep through the night as soon as possible. Solid foods are introduced much sooner, often as early as 6 weeks of age. As a result, the prolactin level is not maintained at a consistent high level, and ovulation is more likely to occur.

The use effectiveness of breastfeeding as a natural family planning method has not been reported in the literature, but 80 percent of lactating women in Western cultures ovulate before their first menstrual period, and 3 to 7 percent become pregnant before the first menstrual period. The advantages of using breastfeeding as a natural family planning method are that it may delay ovulation for a time, it bears no medical risk to the woman, there is no associated cost, and it is accepted by all religious groups. The disadvantages are that the woman has no way of knowing when ovulation has begun, and other natural family planning methods such as the BBT and cervical mucus methods are not good predictors of ovulation during breastfeeding (Lethbridge 1989; NAACOG 1991; Queenan 1991a). Although these high-risk natural family planning methods are probably better than giving no consideration to contraception at all, they are not recommended if prevention of pregnancy is a primary concern.

Vaginal Spermicidal Methods

DESCRIPTION

Vaginal spermicides consist of two basic components: the active spermicidal agent and a carrier substance. The spermicidal agent is a compound that destroys the sperm cell membrane through a chemical action and makes the sperm incapable of fertilizing the ovum. In the United States the spermicidal agent used in most products is either nonoxynol 9 or octoxynol 9. Seven basic spermicidal carriers are available. These carriers are an inert base and include jellies, creams, foam, melting suppositories, foaming tablets, foaming suppositories, and a soluble film. In addition to the chemical action of the spermicidal agent, the carrier substance also helps prevent pregnancy by forming a physical barrier over the cervix to prevent sperm from entering. For this reason, a spermicidal agent should be inserted as high up in the vagina, near the cervix, as possible. Most spermicidal products are sold with some type of an inserter for this purpose (Fig. 11–4). The woman should be instructed to wait the recommended time (usually 5 to 20 minutes) after inserting the spermicide before having intercourse. This allows the spermicide to become adequately distributed. Every time intercourse is repeated after the initial application, an additional application of the spermicidal agent should be used. The woman should not douche for at least 6 hours after the last intercourse (Mishell 1989; NAACOG 1991; Woolley 1991).

EFFECTIVENESS

The reported use effectiveness of spermicidal agents used alone ranges from 11 to 31 pregnancies per 100 women years, or 69 to 89 percent. The greatest effectiveness has been seen with women who are well educated, are highly motivated, and use spermicidal agents consistently. Failures with this method occur as a result of inconsistent use or failure to use the spermicidal agent properly (e.g., not applying before each intercourse, not placing the substance high enough in the vagina, not waiting the specified time, using too little spermicidal agent, or douching earlier than 6 hours after intercourse).

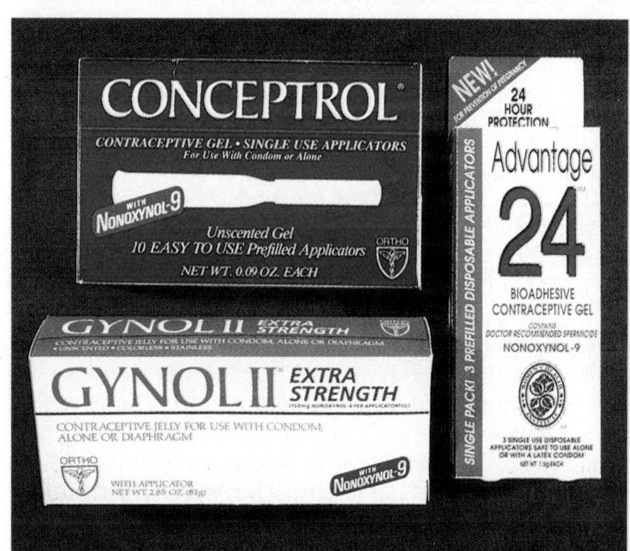

Figure 11–4

Spermicidal agents work by destroying sperm • Creams, gels, and vaginal suppositories are available, some with prefilled disposable applicators.

ADVANTAGES AND DISADVANTAGES

The advantages of spermicidal agents are that they are relatively inexpensive, are available over the counter without prescription, are easy to use, enhance the effectiveness of the barrier methods, provide additional vaginal lubrication, have few side effects, and have an antiviral action that helps to protect against venereal disease (particularly human immunodeficiency virus [HIV], gonorrhea, and trichomoniasis). Some studies have also shown that they may decrease the incidence of cervical cancer.

The disadvantages of spermicidal agents include the possibility of a local irritation of the vagina or penis, although in the more than 60 years that commercial spermicides have been sold, no cases of serious side effects or safety problems have been reported. Other disadvantages might include the messiness of the substance, too much lubrication, an unpleasant odor or taste, having to wait the 5 to 30 minutes after inserting before having intercourse, and having to interrupt lovemaking to insert the spermicidal agent. For most spermicides, effectiveness is limited to 1 hour and additional spermicide must be added before each act of intercourse. A few studies have raised the question whether spermicides used early in pregnancy might be absorbed through the vaginal walls into the bloodstream and have an adverse effect on the developing fetus. These fears have not been confirmed by further research, however, and the studies that did show this possibility have been criticized in regard to the research methods used (Mishell 1989; NAACOG 1991; Woolley 1991).

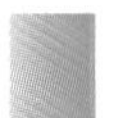

Barrier Methods

MALE CONDOM

Description

The condom is a rubber or animal-skin sheath that prevents deposition of semen in the vagina. It is the only birth control method other than sterilization that is currently available for men (Fig. 11–5). The condom is placed on the penis as soon as the penis becomes erect during sexual excitement. This can be done by either the man or the woman as part of sexual foreplay. A half-inch of space should be left at the top of the condom to collect semen and prevent leakage and tearing. If necessary, a water-soluble lubricant (e.g., K-Y jelly, any spermicidal jelly or cream) can be used to ease entry of the penis into the vagina. Promptly after intercourse has ended, the penis should be carefully withdrawn from the vagina before the erection is lost, with the condom rim held firmly against the base of the penis.

All condoms are approximately the same size, but they are available in different textures and shapes, with or without lubricants, and with or without spermicides. Latex condom brands vary widely in strength. If condoms are purchased from a vending machine, the expiration date, which is stamped on the package, should be checked. If the expiration date has passed, the condom should not be used. An oil-containing vaginal lubricant (e.g., Vaseline, body or hand cream, baby oil, mineral oil) should never be used with a condom, as it will erode the latex and make the condom leak. Attempts to develop new male condom designs, such as the "microcondom," which covers only the tip of the penis, have as yet been unsuccessful (Hatcher and Warner 1992; Libbus 1992; Faundes et al. 1994).

Effectiveness

The reported use effectiveness of male condoms when used alone is ten to 20 pregnancies per 100 women years, or 80 to 90 percent. When condoms are used along with a spermicidal agent, the effectiveness has been reported to rise to as high as five pregnancies per 100 women years, or 95 percent. The primary reason that condoms fail to prevent pregnancy is inconsistent and careless use. This includes touching the penis to the vagina before putting the condom on, using an oil-based lubricant, or not withdrawing the penis promptly and removing the condom before losing the erection (Hatcher and Warner 1992; Libbus 1992; Faundes et al. 1994).

Advantages and Disadvantages

The advantages of male condoms are that they are safe, easy to use, readily available without prescription, and inexpensive. Perhaps an even more important advantage is that condoms can play an important part in the prevention of venereal disease, particularly the transmission of herpes, chlamydial infection, and the HIV virus. Some studies have indicated that condoms may play some part in preventing cancer of the cervix in the female partner by preventing the transmission of the human papillomavirus. This finding is not proved, however, and further studies are needed. Condoms also permit male participation in the prevention of pregnancy.

One disadvantage of the condom is the possibility of an occasional allergic reaction to the rubber or latex. The prevalence of latex sensitivity is increasing, particularly among people who have repeated exposure to latex medical devices or latex consumer products. Reactions to latex in a sensitive individual can vary between mild local reactions and severe systemic reactions. While lambskin condoms may be used for pregnancy prevention, their use is probably contraindicated for the prevention of STDs. A new condom, called the Avanti, has been cleared by the U.S. Food and

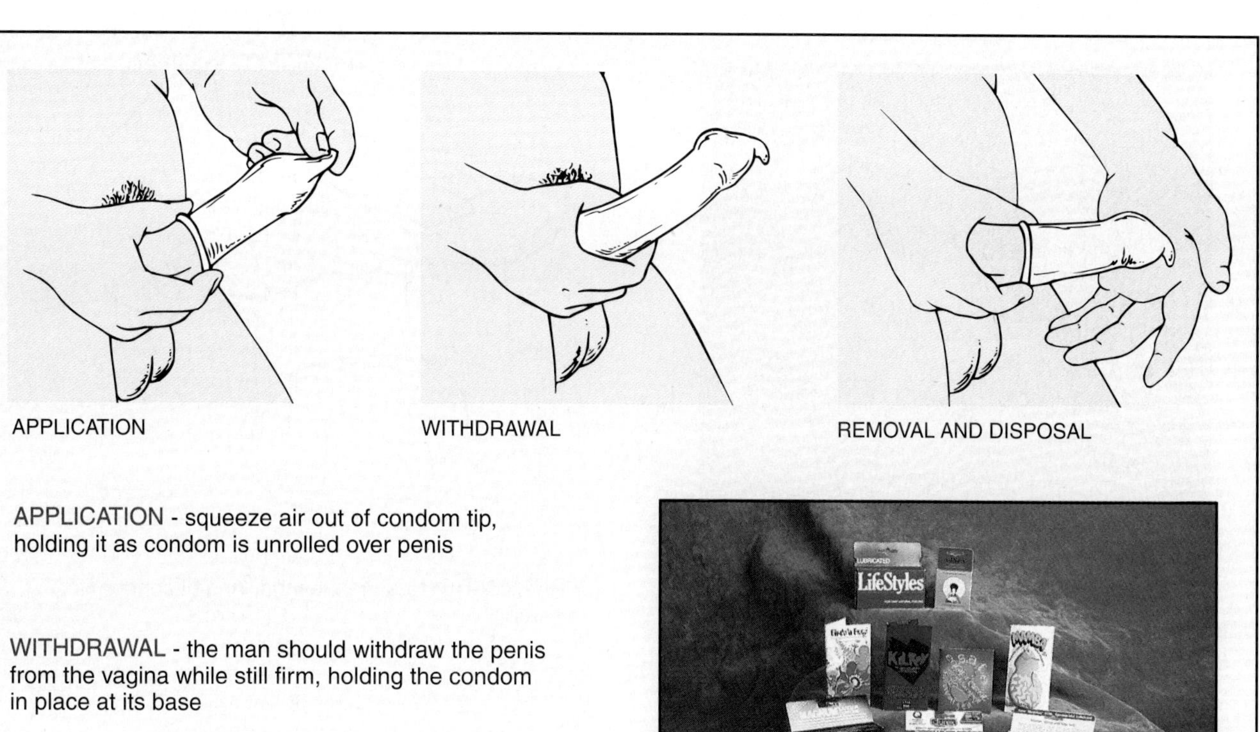

Figure 11–5

Male condoms prevent the deposit of sperm in the vagina • There are many types of condoms, and packaging becomes an important part of marketing • The male condom is a sheer rubber sheath before use.

Drug Administration (FDA). It is now available specifically for people who are allergic to latex. Two other condoms, one made of polyurethane and the other of a synthetic rubber, have also been cleared by the FDA for latex-sensitive people but are not as yet available to the public. Additional disadvantages include decreased sensation in the glans of the penis, the interruption of sexual foreplay to apply the condom, and the need to quickly remove the penis from the vagina after ejaculation to remove the condom (NAACOG 1991; Libbus 1992).

FEMALE CONDOM

Description

The new female condom, approved by the FDA in 1993, combines traits of the male condom and the female diaphragm. Invented in Denmark, it is a prelubricated, 7-inch, transparent polyurethane sheath with two soft, flexible rings. One ring forms the edge of the open end, and the other ring, which is not attached, rests inside the closed end as an internal anchor. To insert the female condom, the woman grasps the condom at the closed end and squeezes the inner ring so that it becomes narrow (about the size of a tampon). She gently pushes the ring, with the sheath on the outside, up inside the vagina as far as it will go, pushing the inner ring toward the cervix. Once the inner ring is behind the pubic bone and cannot be felt, the condom is in place. The sheath follows it in and adheres to the vaginal wall, fitting like a second skin. The woman should check to make sure the condom is not twisted. The ring at the open end remains outside the body, protecting the outer labia (Fig. 11–6).

The female condom protects the entire vaginal and urethral area from contact with the shaft and base of the penis, reducing the risk of pregnancy and STDs. Although the female condom can be put in place up to 8 hours before intercourse, most women insert it anytime from an hour to several minutes before intercourse.

To remove the condom, the woman grasps the

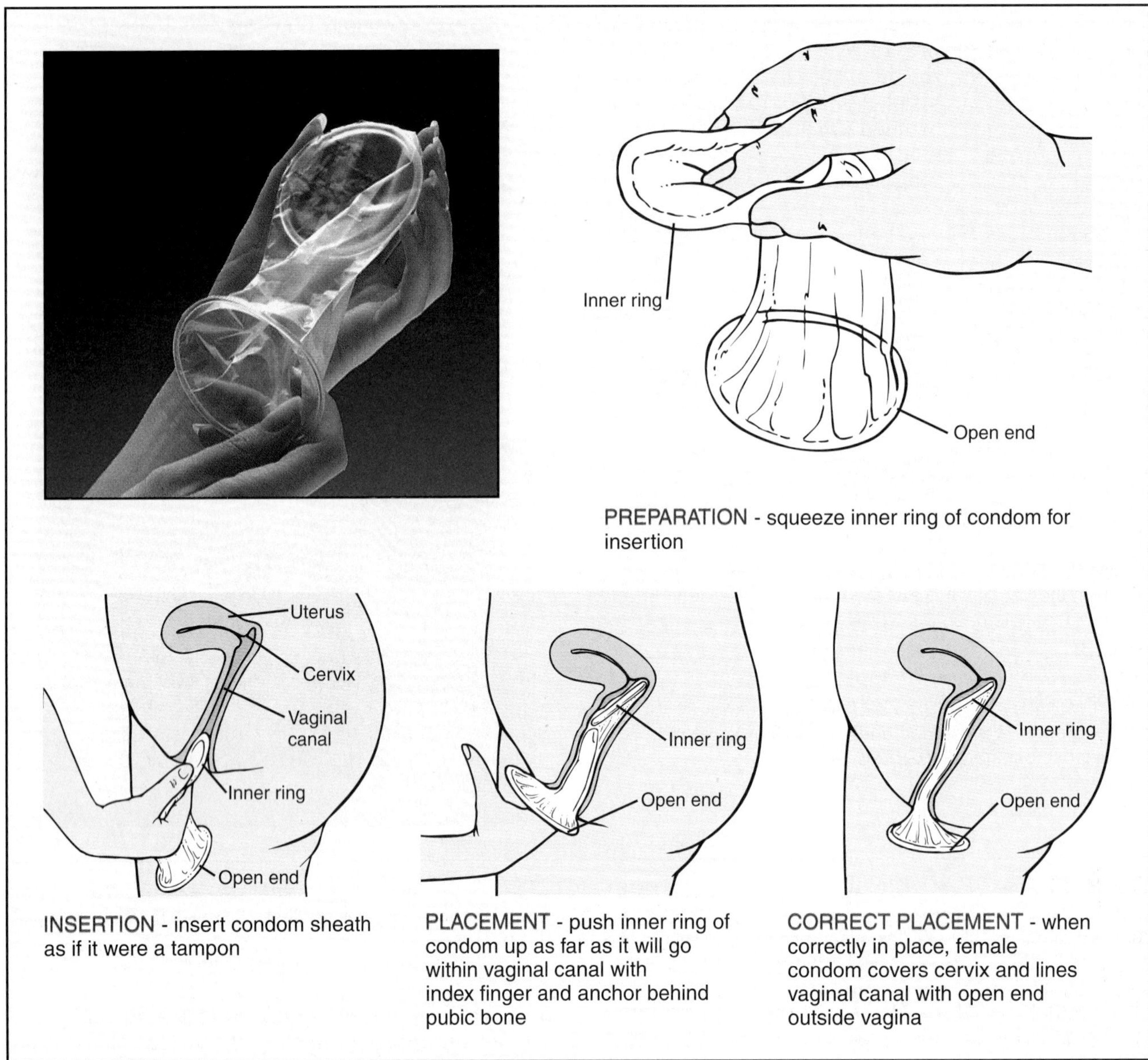

Figure 11–6

The female condom is a prelubricated transparent sheath that forms a second skin inside the vagina when inserted properly • It shields the vaginal and urethral areas from contact with the penis while capturing semen during intercourse. (Photo © Joel Gordon 1988.)

open outer edge of the sheath and twists it closed, capturing the fluids inside. She then gently pulls, and the condom slips out for disposal. Like all condoms, the female condom is used one time only.

Effectiveness

More than 7 years of clinical trials for the female condom show that it is as effective as the diaphragm in preventing pregnancy. In typical use, the use effectiveness is 12.4 pregnancies per 100 women years, or 87.6 percent after 6 months. When the female condom is used correctly every time, use effectiveness improves, with 2.6 pregnancies per 100 women years, or 97.4 percent after 6 months (Farr et al. 1994).

Advantages and Disadvantages

One advantage of the female condom is that it offers the woman control over condom use. Because it can be inserted in advance of the sexual encounter, it is less disruptive than some barrier methods. Another advantage is that it does not require fitting by a health care professional. For many, the sheath does not seem to interfere with sexual enjoyment, since the material transmits heat between partners. In clinical studies, 56 to 80 percent of women and men found sex when using the female condom as pleasurable as sex when not using one. Some women even experienced increased clitoral sensation because of the movement of the outer ring against the vaginal opening.

Men found little reduction of sensation, since the female condom is less constricting than the male condom. Because the female condom is made of polyurethane, which is stronger than the latex used in male condoms, and because it does not have to stretch, causing less stress during use, it is not as likely to rip or tear (Soper et al. 1991). In addition, the female condom provides a new option for people with latex allergy and can be used with spermicide or oil-based lubricant, if desired.

Disadvantages might include the necessity for manual insertion of the female condom. Women who are uncomfortable with birth control methods that require them to touch themselves might not like this aspect of the female condom. Also, the new and unusual look may put people off at first because of aesthetics. Although it is comfortable and easy to use, some couples might perceive it as awkward. The outer ring outside the body takes some getting used to for some people.

DIAPHRAGM

Description

The diaphragm is a shallow, dome-shaped rubber device with a flexible metal rim that fits into the vagina to block sperm from entering the cervix (Fig. 11–7). It rests anteriorly against the soft tissues behind the symphysis pubis, posteriorly within the posterior vaginal fornix, and laterally against the vaginal walls. The diaphragm is used along with a spermicidal agent such as a cream or jelly to increase its effectiveness.

Three types of diaphragms are available: an arcing spring, a flat or wide-seal spring, or a coil spring. The arcing spring assumes an arc-shaped form when compressed in the woman's hand and may be easier to insert for women who have a posteriorly pointed cervix; it can also be used by women with poor pelvic muscle tone. It is the most popular of the three designs in the United States. The flat spring and coil spring diaphragms fold on a single plane when compressed and can be used with a plastic inserter. The flat spring has a flat metal band within the rim, while the coil spring has a wire spiral within the rim.

A study conducted to compare consumer satisfaction with these three types of diaphragms found that none was significantly more comfortable or easier to insert than the other (Loucks 1989). The diaphragm must be fitted by a trained health care provider and can be obtained only through prescription. Use of the diaphragm has increased in popularity in past years owing to increased consumer concerns regarding oral contraceptives and the prevention of STDs (Ferreira et al. 1993; Faundes et al. 1994).

The diaphragm can be inserted up to 6 hours before sexual intercourse. However, if it is inserted more than 2 hours before, it is wise to add an additional application of a spermicidal agent. After sexual intercourse, the diaphragm must remain in place 6 to 8 hours. If intercourse is repeated during that time, an additional application of the spermicidal agent should be inserted, or the male partner should wear a condom. The diaphragm can be inserted best in one of four positions: sitting on the edge of a chair, lying on the back with knees bent, squatting, or standing with one leg up on a chair. The woman should be taught to pinch the rim of the diaphragm together with one hand while spreading the labia with the other hand. The diaphragm is inserted along the posterior wall of the vagina as far as it will go. The rim is pressed behind the ridge of the pubic bone in the front and the vaginal fornix in the back. The woman should feel her cervix through the dome of the diaphragm to ensure that it is in place. To remove the diaphragm, the woman places her index or middle finger behind the front rim and pulls the diaphragm down and out.

Effectiveness

The reported use effectiveness of the diaphragm when used along with a spermicidal agent ranges from two to 23 pregnancies per 100 women years, or 77 to 98 percent (Loucks 1989; Ferreira et al. 1993; Faundes et al. 1994). Most failures occurring with the diaphragm are due to improper use, e.g., not using a spermicidal agent along with the diaphragm, not using a backup method with repeated sexual intercourse, removing the diaphragm earlier than 6 to 8 hours after the last intercourse, or douching immediately after intercourse. One study has suggested that it may not be necessary to use a spermicide with the diaphragm, since the findings did not conclusively demonstrate that pregnancy rates were lower when a spermicide was used with the diaphragm than when the diaphragm was used alone (Mishell 1989).

Proper fit of the diaphragm is also essential to its effectiveness. It is recommended that it be refitted every year or so; with increased sexual activity; or after a pregnancy, an abortion, or pelvic surgery. There is controversy in the literature about the effect of weight loss or gain on the fit of a diaphragm. It has been traditionally recommended that the diaphragm be refitted after a change in weight, but one study showed no signifi-

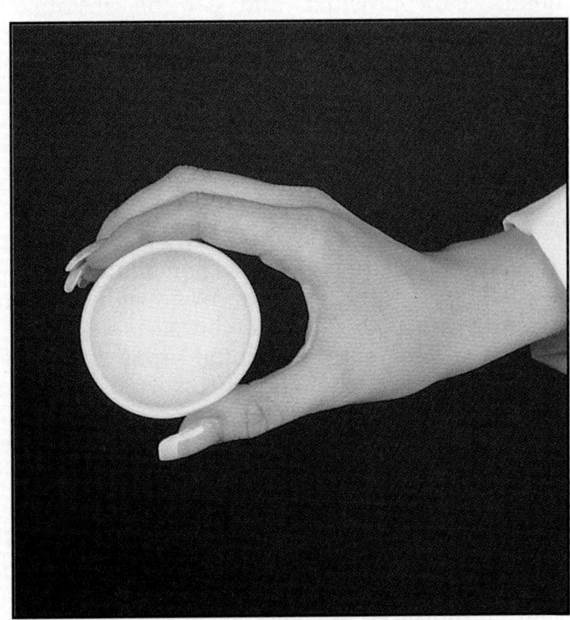

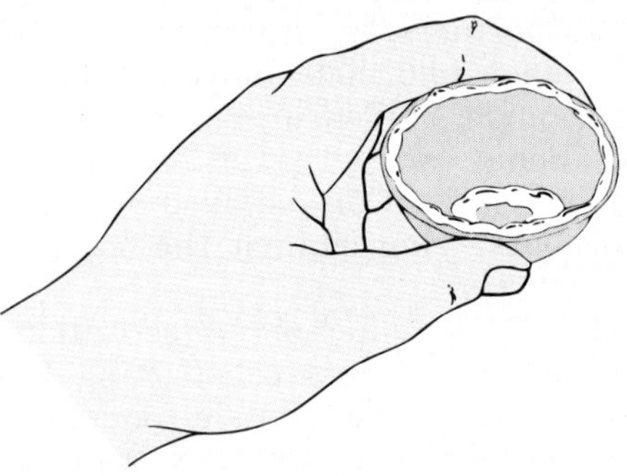

PREPARATION - spread about a tablespoon of spermicidal cream or jelly inside dome and around rim

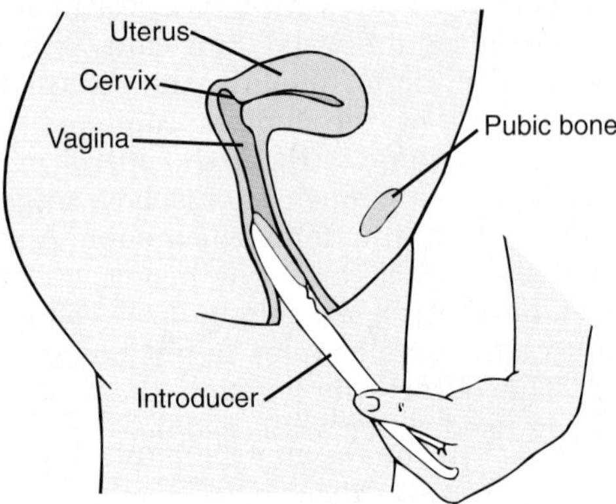

INSERTION WITH INTRODUCER - place one end of rim over grooved end of introducer and fit other rim at appropriately sized notch • carefully insert introducer into vagina as far as it will go • gently twist introducer to disengage diaphragm and remove from vagina • wash, rinse, and dry introducer thoroughly

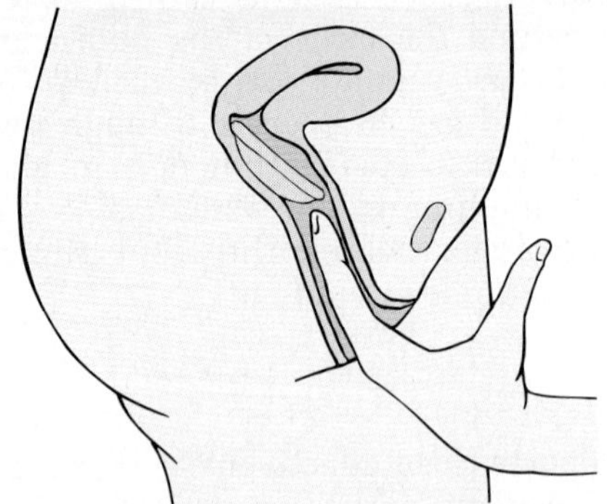

INSERTION BY HAND - fold diaphragm and insert it into vagina with spermicide toward cervix

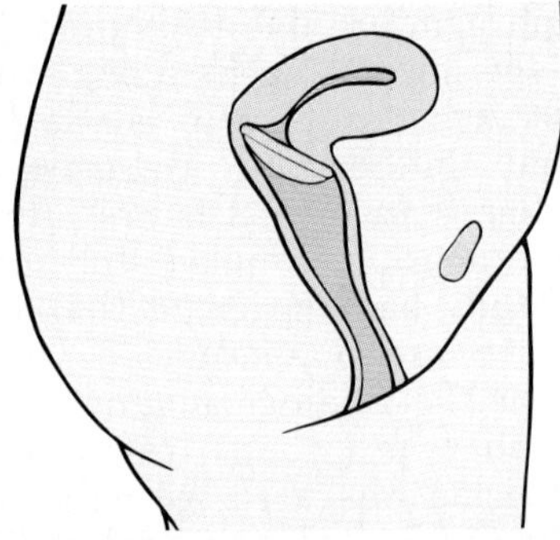

CHECKING PLACEMENT - diaphragm should fit between upper edge of pubic bone and posterior vaginal wall; if correctly placed, it should not be felt by either partner

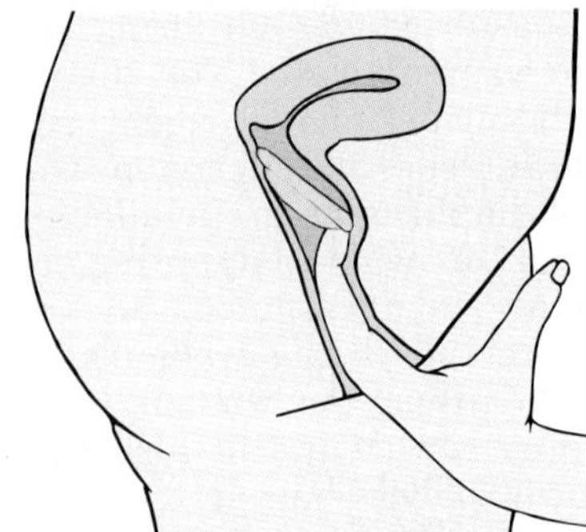

REMOVAL - remove diaphragm by grasping rim with forefinger and pulling down and out • diaphragm should be washed with mild soap and water and dried thoroughly before storage

Figure 11–7

The diaphragm is a barrier contraceptive that blocks sperm from entering the cervix • This palm-sized cup is easily inserted by hand or introducer • It is designed to be used with spermicidal cream or gel.

cant relationship between a weight change of 20 pounds and diaphragm size (Kugel and Verson 1986). The diaphragm should be replaced every 2 years and should be checked regularly for holes or puckering.

Advantages and Disadvantages

The advantages of the diaphragm are that it is easy to use, does not dull sexual sensation for either partner, is not expensive, helps prevent STDs and pelvic inflammatory disease (PID), can be inserted before lovemaking and is effective immediately upon insertion, and can be used by lactating women and in the immediate postpartal period. The diaphragm can also be used during the woman's menstrual period for the purpose of blocking blood flow when having sexual intercourse. It is also thought that it may protect against cervical cancer by preventing sexual transmission of the herpesvirus or papillomavirus (NAACOG 1991).

Since the diaphragm is to be used with a spermicidal agent, it shares the risks and disadvantages of these agents. An allergic reaction to the rubber or latex diaphragm can occur, and in this event a plastic diaphragm can be used. The diaphragm can become dislodged during intercourse, particularly when the woman assumes the superior position. It may also contribute to frequent bladder infections (cystitis) due to upward pressure of the rim of the diaphragm against the urethra. Women should be instructed to void before and after sexual intercourse in order to decrease this risk. Some women may experience pain, bleeding, vaginal discharge, or constipation with diaphragm use, particularly if it is too large.

There has been some concern about the relationship of the diaphragm to toxic shock syndrome. Symptoms of toxic shock have been reported in a few women, but studies have found no definite relationship. In most cases, when toxic shock symptoms occur, the diaphragm has been left in place for 24 hours. Leaving the diaphragm in place longer than the recommended 6 to 8 hours after intercourse may increase *Staphylococcus aureus* colonization in the lower genital tract. A final disadvantage of the diaphragm can be difficulty with learning or executing its proper insertion and care. If a woman is uncomfortable touching her genitalia, she may be unable to insert or remove the diaphragm successfully.

CERVICAL CAP

Description

The cervical cap was used in the United States until the late 1950s, when its popularity declined owing to favoritism toward the diaphragm, intrauterine devices (IUDs), and oral contraceptives. It was even eliminated from the market for a number of years, but it has now regained popularity and been approved for use in the United States. The cervical cap is a small, thimble-shaped cup that fits over the cervix to mechanically block sperm from entering the cervical canal (Fig. 11–8). As with the diaphragm, the cervical cap is also filled with a spermicidal agent to increase its effectiveness, and it can be inserted 6 to 8 hours before sexual intercourse. The cervical cap is made of a flexible rubber or plastic material and must be fitted by a trained health care provider. It fits deeper and is smaller in diameter than the diaphragm. It is approximately 1¼ to 1½ inches long and comes in 22-mm, 25-mm, 28-mm, and 31-mm sizes. It remains in place by suction against the cervix, rather than spring tension within the vaginal walls as with the diaphragm.

When inserting the cervical cap, the woman must be careful not to misplace the cap against the wall of the vagina where it may become lodged by suction. When the cap is inserted, a small space should be felt between the dome of the cap and the cervical os. This space serves as a pocket for the spermicidal agent. The woman should feel a suction or resistance with gentle tugging on the cap. The cap is removed by running the index finger up to the cap's rim, hooking the edge, and pulling the cap away and downward from the cervix to break the suction. The cap is then pulled down the vaginal canal and grasped with the thumb and forefinger at the vaginal introitus for removal. The woman should not pull on the dome portion of the cap, as this may harm the cervical tissue or the cap itself. There are differing opinions over how long the cervical cap can be left on the cervix, ranging from 24 hours to 1 month. The general consensus regarding the ideal time for the cap to be left in place seems to be 3 days (Mishell 1989; Monier and Laird 1989; Hatcher and Warner 1992).

Effectiveness

The reported use effectiveness of the cervical cap ranges between 4 and 20 pregnancies per 100 women years, or 80 to 96 percent. Reasons for failure of the cervical cap parallel those for the diaphragm and relate primarily to improper use.

Advantages and Disadvantages

The advantages of the cervical cap are that insertion is not related to the time of intercourse; it is more comfortable and less messy than the diaphragm; it can be left in place longer than the diaphragm without the additional application of a spermicidal agent; there are minimal side effects; less of the vagina is covered, which may increase

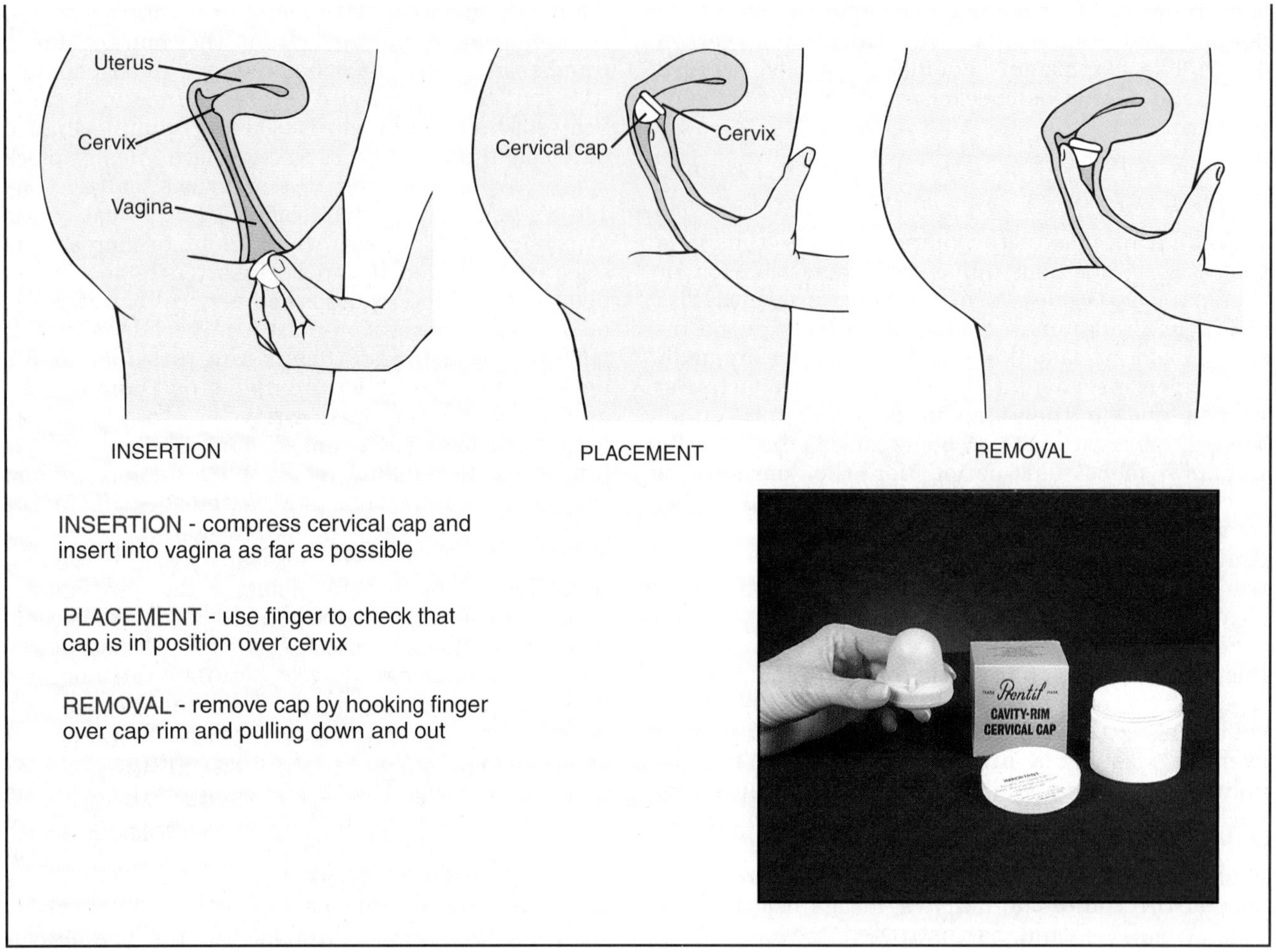

Uterus
Cervix
Vagina
Cervical cap
Cervix

INSERTION PLACEMENT REMOVAL

INSERTION - compress cervical cap and insert into vagina as far as possible

PLACEMENT - use finger to check that cap is in position over cervix

REMOVAL - remove cap by hooking finger over cap rim and pulling down and out

Prentif CAVITY-RIM CERVICAL CAP

Figure 11–8

Another barrier method of contraception, the cervical cap blocks sperm from entering the cervical canal • A small, thimble-shaped cup, the cap is designed to fit snugly over the cervix when correctly inserted.

sexual pleasure; it can be used in women who have poor pelvic floor muscle tone; there is no bladder pressure; and, like the diaphragm, it may protect the woman against STDs, PID, and cervical cancer.

The disadvantages of the cervical cap are that the woman may have an allergic reaction to the spermicide or the rubber cap, insertion and removal of the cap is more difficult than the diaphragm, more professional time may be required to teach proper insertion and removal of the cap, and it is possible to dislodge the cap during intercourse. Vaginal odor can occur with use of the cap; this can be prevented by removing it every 2 or 3 days for cleansing. The cervical cap should not be used in women who have cervical lacerations, cervical malformations, cervicitis, or an abnormal Papanicolaou (Pap) smear. Successful cap use requires a highly motivated, persistent woman who will correctly insert and remove the cap (NAACOG 1991).

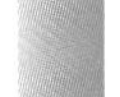

Intrauterine Device

DESCRIPTION

Although the concept of an IUD to prevent pregnancy has been recognized for centuries (see Historical Perspectives), IUDs were not mass produced in the United States for contraceptive use until the 1960s. IUDs are small plastic devices that are inserted into the uterus and remain in place for varying lengths of time, depending on the type used (Fig. 11–9). They can be made in varying shapes and are composed of either an inert substance or a medicated substance such as copper or progestogen. The IUD has a tail positioned so that it protrudes through the cervical os 1 to 2 inches; it should be checked periodically by the woman to ensure that the IUD is in place. The IUD can be inserted into the uterus at any time during the woman's menstrual cycle, but insertion

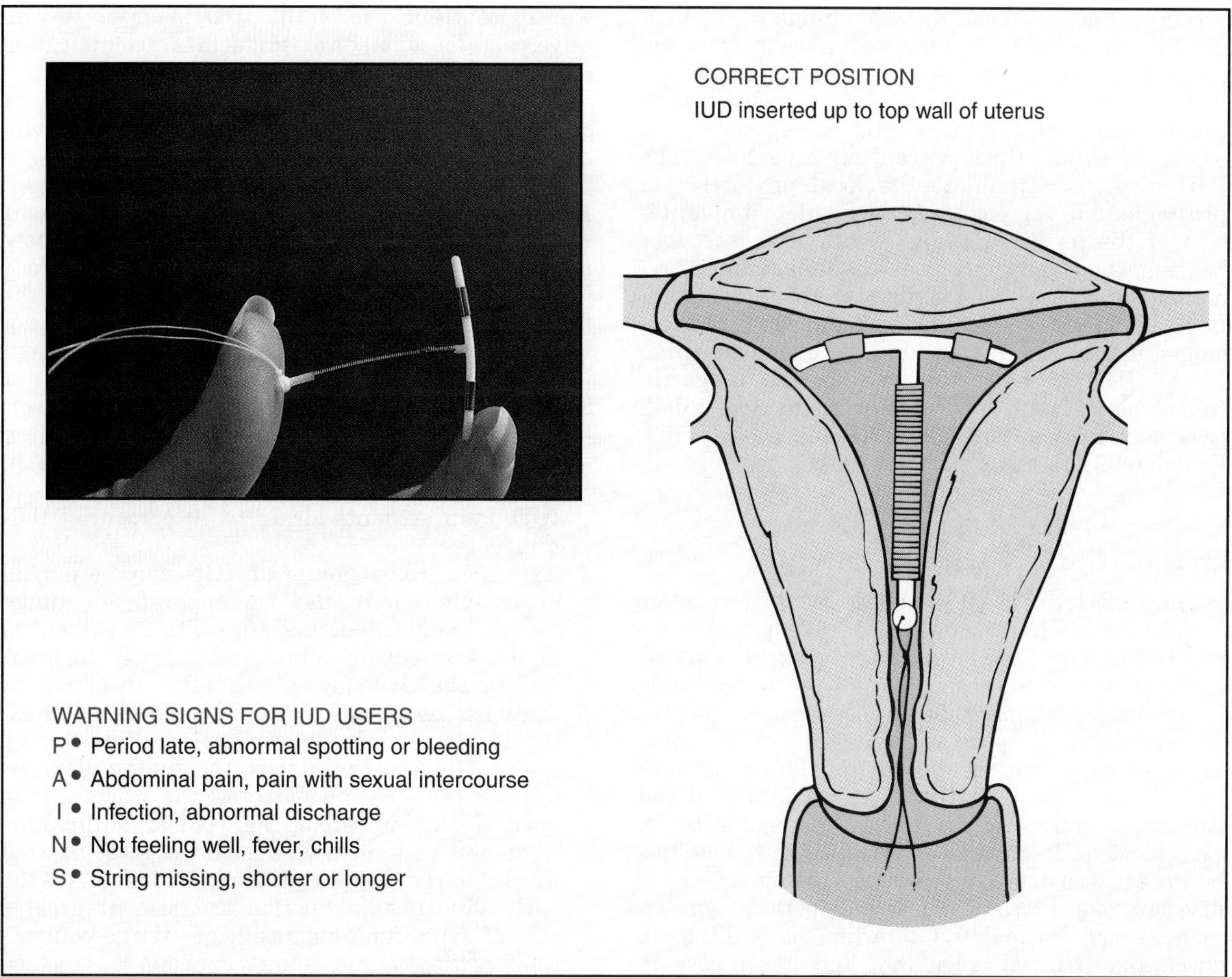

Figure 11–9

The intrauterine device (IUD) causes an inflammatory reaction in the uterus, preventing implantation of the fertilized ovum. ("Pains" from Treiman, K., and Liskin, L. IUDs—a new look. Population Reports, Series B, No. 5. Baltimore: Johns Hopkins School of Public Health, Population Information Program, March 1988.)

is usually made during menstruation because it is easier at that time and the woman and her caregiver can be assured that she is not pregnant. Insertion can be made without anesthesia in a clinic or physician's office. If the IUD is made of an inert substance, it can theoretically stay in place indefinitely. If it is medicated with copper, it should be replaced every 4 years, because, as the copper corrodes, mineral deposits that build up on the IUD affect the release of the copper ions. If the IUD is medicated with progestogen, it must be replaced annually, because the hormonal supply is depleted over a 12-month period (Chi 1993; Rivera et al. 1993).

Several types of IUDs have been used since they were introduced, but only two types are currently available in the United States: the Progestasert and the CU 380 T (ParaGard). The Progestasert has a T shape and releases $65 \mu g$ of progesterone daily through the permeable wall of the vertical stem. The hormonal supply is depleted over a 12-month period, so annual replacement is necessary. The CU 380 T is also shaped like a T but has a copper collar on each horizontal arm, as well as copper wire that is wound on the vertical stem. It is approved for 6 years of continuous use. The IUDs no longer available are the Dalkon shield, Lippes loop, and Copper-7. These were removed from the market because of economic or liability factors or because of serious complications and problems (Mishell 1989; Rivera et al. 1993).

The precise mechanisms by which the IUD prevents pregnancy remain unclear, but several theories are currently accepted as the probable cause of effectiveness. Because the IUD is a foreign body, it stimulates an inflammatory reaction in the uterus, causing both cellular and biochemical changes in the endometrium and uterine fluids. In response, an increase in the number of neutrophils, mononuclear cells, and plasma cells appears to cause an attack on the invading foreign body. However, while these cells are powerless to remove the IUD, they do engulf the sperm or the fertilized ovum, thus preventing pregnancy. The IUD may also stimulate the local production of prostaglandin compounds, which affect implantation of the fertilized ovum. If the IUD is copper bearing, the copper increases the inflammatory reaction, decreases the viability of the sperm, impairs ovum transport, and may interfere with estrogen uptake and utilization by the endometrium. If the IUD is progestin bearing, the progestin causes changes in cervical mucus, making it less easy to penetrate by sperm (Reinprayoon 1992; Bromham 1993; Rivera et al. 1993).

EFFECTIVENESS

The reported use effectiveness of the intrauterine device ranges from three to five pregnancies per 100 women years, or 95 to 97 percent. This effectiveness rate is second only to the implantable contraceptives. When failure does occur, it is usually contingent on such variables as lack of expert insertion technique on the part of the health care provider, expulsion of the IUD, or failure of the woman to check for the tail on a regular basis. The ideal IUD candidate is a woman who has borne at least one child, has no history of pelvic disease, has normal menstrual periods, has a monogamous sexual relationship, is willing to check the IUD tail regularly, and has access to continuing medical assessment. The IUD should never be used by women with a history of PID, blood coagulation problems, heart disease, any gynecologic malignancy, a history of ectopic pregnancy, menstrual problems, an abnormal Pap smear, uterine abnormalities, fibroids, or anemia (Reinprayoon 1992; Chi 1993; Cunningham et al. 1993).

ADVANTAGES AND DISADVANTAGES

The primary advantage of the IUD is that it makes the fewest demands on the user. Once it is inserted, the woman assumes very little responsibility other than to periodically check for the tail or to have the IUD checked or replaced at recommended intervals. The IUD is not related in any way to the time of sexual intercourse and does not require partner cooperation. It has no general systemic effects and does not interfere with lactation. The woman's subsequent ability to conceive after using an IUD is not significantly affected, and return to fertility is usually rapid. However, the data on post-IUD fertility are based on women who discontinue use of the IUD in order to conceive, not for a medical problem or complication resulting from the IUD.

Six potential disadvantages of the IUD must be considered before its selection as a family planning method:

1. Bleeding and heavy menstrual blood loss. Some women using an IUD experience longer menstrual periods and a greater amount of blood loss during menstruation than before using the IUD. Midcycle bleeding may also occur. This increase in bleeding accounts for 10 to 20 percent of IUD discontinuation.
2. Pain. Women may experience pain during insertion of the IUD or for a few days thereafter. Some women also complain of an increase in cramping during the menstrual cycle with an IUD. Pain accounts for 15 to 40 percent of IUD removals.
3. Expulsion. Expulsion of an IUD may be partial or complete and may be apparent or undetected. Expulsion occurs after 5 to 24 percent of all IUD insertions and is most likely to occur during the first few weeks after insertion or during a menstrual period. The likelihood of expulsion is influenced by clinician skill in placing the IUD in the uterus, the timing of insertion, or the age and parity of the woman. It is most likely to occur in young, nulliparous women or in women who have the IUD inserted in the early postpartal period. Women in the early breastfeeding period are also at greater risk of expulsion as a result of uterine contractions caused by the infant's sucking.
4. Perforation. Perforation of the uterus is a rare but potentially serious complication that can occur as a result of an IUD. In the United States an estimated 40 per 100,000 IUD users are hospitalized each year because an IUD has perforated the uterine wall or migrated into the peritoneal cavity. Perforation can lead to infection, intestinal obstruction, or bowel strangulation. Most perforations occur during insertion. If perforation occurs at a time after insertion, it is not usually accompanied by bleeding, pain, or other symptoms.
5. Pelvic inflammatory disease. PID has been reported to occur at an incidence two to four times greater than for non-IUD users, or in 90 percent of the 9600 IUD-associated hospitalizations in the United States every year. Pelvic infection results from the ascent of microbes through the uterus into the upper genital tract. The bacteria causing such infections may enter the uterus at the time of insertion of the IUD or by ascending the IUD tail. The increased volume and duration of menstrual bleeding may also enhance bacterial growth by creating an easy access to the endometrium and by provid-

ing a hospitable environment for bacterial growth. PID can lead to sterility due to tubal occlusion from the infectious process. Factors that influence the risk of developing PID are the technique of insertion, the type of IUD used, exposure to STDs, age under 25 years, and the duration of IUD use (the risk decreases with time).

6. Ectopic pregnancy. Data have shown that if an IUD user becomes pregnant with the IUD still in place, her risk of an ectopic pregnancy is greater (3 to 4 percent) than that for a non-IUD user (0.8 percent). This relative risk varies among IUD users, depending on the woman's fecundity, any history of ectopic pregnancy, any history of PID, and age. It is theorized, however, that the higher ratio of ectopic to intrauterine pregnancies among IUD users may reflect a decrease in intrauterine pregnancies, rather than an increase in extrauterine gestations (NAACOG 1991; Chi 1993; Cunningham et al. 1993; Chi 1994).

Regular counseling and follow-up with the woman using an IUD is crucial. The woman must be given clear information regarding the possible side effects. If she understands that mild cramping and bleeding in the days after IUD insertion are to be expected and that heavier menstrual periods while the IUD is used are common, she will be less likely to have the IUD removed unnecessarily. On the other hand, she must also be informed of possible symptoms that would not be considered normal but that could indicate infection, expulsion, or pregnancy (Fig. 11–9). It is important that a woman understand that the IUD offers no protection against STDs. She must be taught to check for the IUD tail, informed of the length of time the IUD can be worn before replacement is needed, and scheduled for a follow-up visit for assessment (Rivera et al. 1993).

Hormonal Contraception

The idea that ovulation, and thus conception, could be inhibited by hormones was suggested as early as 1940. However, this theory remained untested until 1950 when new classes of hormones were discovered and large quantities of synthetic hormones became available. Several forms of hormonal contraception are currently available, including oral contraception, injectable contraception, and implant therapy. Today, hormonal contraception remains the second most popular method of birth control, next to sterilization.

Hormonal contraceptives have more than one site of action. Their effectiveness depends on a number of simultaneously occurring factors. The most important event is the suppression of ovulation, caused by the suppression of the FSH-LH sequence from the anterior pituitary gland. In addition, hormonal contraceptives alter the production of cervical mucus, making it less acceptable to sperm. They also alter tubal mobility, and finally they alter the endometrial lining of the uterus, making it inhospitable to implantation (Cunningham et al. 1993).

ORAL CONTRACEPTIVE

Description

Oral contraception, or the "pill," is the most common and widely available form of hormonal contraception today. The pill was developed by Gregory Pincus and gynecologist John Rock during the 1950s, and by 1965 it was the leading contraceptive. Seventy percent of all women of reproductive age in the United States have, at some time, taken oral contraceptives. Although use of oral contraceptives declined during the 1970s and 1980s after reports of side effects, they are still used by over 10 million women in the United States and 60 to 80 million women around the world. Oral contraceptives remain popular and are particularly effective among sexually active teenagers and young married couples. Two types are on the market today: a combined oral formulation and a progestin only formulation. Combined oral contraceptives contain both estrogen and progestin. The dosage of both estrogen and progestin has decreased markedly since the original oral contraceptives. Early birth control pills contained 100 to 150 μg of estrogen and 1 to 10 mg of progestin. Most pills on the market today range in estrogen (either ethinyl estradiol or mestranol) dosage from 30 to 35 μg and in progestin dosage from 0.15 to 1.0 mg. This reduction in dosage has decreased many of the side effects of oral contraceptives (Moore 1994).

The combined pills are taken in a monthly series, usually for 21 days, followed by a week with no pills before beginning the next 21-day series. The pills are often dispensed in packets of 28 pills, the first 21 containing the hormones and the last seven consisting of an inert substance or an iron supplement (Fig. 11–10). Two types of combined oral contraceptives are available today: fixed dose regimens containing an identical low dose of both estrogen and progestin in each of the 21 active pills, and incremental regimens (either biphasic or triphasic) that alter the hormone dosage (usually the progestin) throughout the cycle to reflect normal hormonal variations. The advantage of the phasic formulations is a reduction in the metabolic changes and adverse effects that can be caused by progestin (Cunningham et al. 1993; Moore 1994).

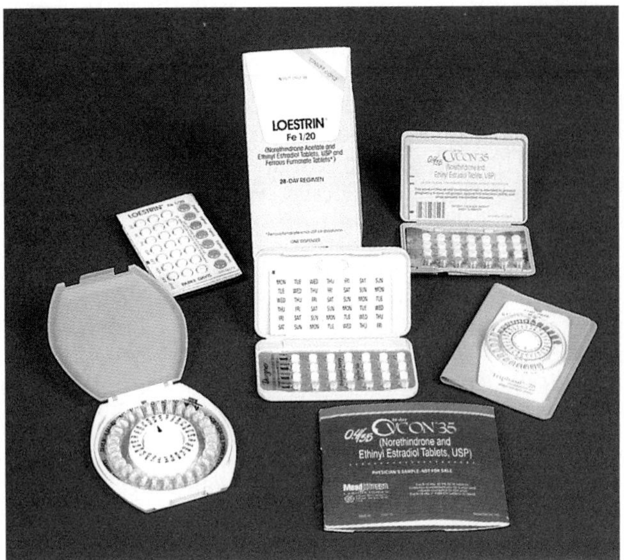

Figure 11–10

Oral contraceptives suppress ovulation and alter the production of cervical mucus, tubal mobility, and the endometrial lining of the uterus.

Effectiveness

The reported use effectiveness of combination oral contraceptives ranges from one to ten pregnancies per 100 women years or 90 to 99 percent. The primary cause of ineffectiveness of oral contraceptives is failure to take them at a regular daily time. If a pill is forgotten, it is best to use a backup method of birth control until the 21-day pill cycle is completed (see Guidelines for Oral Contraceptive Use). Failure with oral contraceptives can also be the result of interactions from concurrent use of other medications (Monier and Laird 1989; Cunningham et al. 1993; Kubba and Guillebaud 1993). Since the introduction of low-dose estrogen pills, the importance of the potential reduction in the effectiveness of combined oral contraceptives (COCs) when used simultaneously with other medications has come to light. Hormonal contraceptives affect many organ systems, and the metabolism of oral contraceptive compounds may be influenced by various drugs. Interactions between oral contraceptives and other drugs may be divided into three categories: (1) those in which oral contraceptive effectiveness is impaired by other drugs, causing breakthrough bleeding or pregnancy; (2) those in which oral contraceptive activity is enhanced by other drugs; and (3) those in which oral contraceptives interfere with the metabolism or activity of other therapeutic agents. For example, barbiturates may induce enzymes that are responsible for degradation of estrogens, and broad-spectrum antibiotics may change bowel flora, reducing enterohepatic recirculation of estrogen (Table 11–2). Although women do show enormous variability in the degree of interaction between oral contraceptives and other drugs, it is wise to assume reduced protection in every case when a woman is taking other medications. Drug interactions are less of a problem for progestogen users than combined oral contraceptive users, although women using low-dose progestogen only pills, Norplant implants, or vaginal rings may run some risk of interaction with certain drugs. When taking a drug history, it is important to identify whether there is a possibility of drug interactions. All women taking oral contraceptives should be informed of the possible effect of drug interactions when placed on a medication that may decrease contraceptive effectiveness. Women should be instructed to use a backup contraceptive, such as condoms (Hatcher et al. 1994; Loudon et al. 1995).

Advantages and Disadvantages

A primary advantage of combined oral contraceptives is their convenience. No action to prevent pregnancy is needed at the time of sexual intercourse, which allows for complete sexual spontaneity. Additional social benefits may include freedom and confidence in the ability to postpone pregnancy with a high degree of effectiveness and subsequent reversibility. The ability of the woman to be totally self-reliant in regard to her birth control may also be viewed as an advantage.

There may also be a number of physical advantages resulting from oral contraceptives. Studies have shown that women taking the pill experience a decrease in premenstrual syndrome (PMS), less menstrual flow and cramping, and less iron deficiency anemia. There seems to be some protection against benign breast disease with oral contraceptive use. Researchers believe that one half to three quarters of all cases of benign breast disease that would ordinarily occur are prevented by the use of birth control pills.

Women using the pill have a decreased incidence of ovarian, endometrial, and uterine cancer. There is a 40 to 60 percent reduction of risk for ovarian cancer that persists for as long as 10 to 15 years after oral contraceptive use ceases. The risk of endometrial cancer is one half that for non–pill users. Oral contraceptive use for 5 or more years decreases the risk of endometrial cancer to one third that of nonusers. This protective effect also lasts at least 10 to 15 years after pill use has been discontinued.

Pill users develop fewer ovarian cysts, have fewer ectopic pregnancies, and develop less PID. When oral contraceptives are used for longer than 12 months, oral contraceptive users with no history of PID have only half the risk of developing PID of women using no contraception. It is believed that an estimated 50,000 initial cases of

Table 11–2

THE MORE IMPORTANT DRUG INTERACTIONS WITH COMBINED ORAL CONTRACEPTIVES (COCs)*

CLASS OF DRUG	APPROVED NAMES OF IMPORTANT EXAMPLES	MAIN ACTION	CLINICAL IMPLICATIONS FOR COC USE
Drug That May Reduce COC Efficacy			
Anticonvulsants	Barbiturates (esp. phenobarbitone) Phenytoin Primidone Carbamazepine	Induction of liver enzymes increasing their ability to metabolize *both* COC steroids.	Preferably tricycling with shortened pill-free interval. One can use 50-μg estrogen COCs, increasing to 90 μg if BTB occurs. Sodium valproate, clonazepam, and all the newly introduced anticonvulsants are not enzyme inducers.
Antibiotics			
Antitubercle	Rifampicin	Marked induction of liver enzymes.	Use of alternative contraception is preferred (e.g., DMPA with 8-week injection interval).
Antifungal	Griseofulvin	Induction of liver enzymes.	Short courses—additional contraception during treatment and for 7 days after treatment. Long courses—same as for anticonvulsants.
Broad spectrum	Ampicillin and relatives Tetracyclines	Change in bowel flora, reducing enterohepatic recirculation of EE only, after hydrolysis of its conjugates.	Short courses—wisest to use additional contraception during treatment up to 14 days plus an additional 7 days. POP is unaffected.
Hypnotics/tranquilizers	Meprobamate Glutethimide Dichloralphenazone	Induction of liver enzymes.	Avoid these drugs in COC users (alternatives available).
Drugs That May Increase COC Efficacy			
	Ascorbic acid	Theoretically, drug competes in bowel wall for conjugation to sulphate. Hence more EE is available for absorption.	Recent research suggests that this effect is immeasurable and can be disregarded.
	Co-trimoxazole	Inhibits EE metabolism.	None, if short course given to low-dose COC user.

* Drug interactions are less of a problem with progesterone only oral contraceptives. However, women using low-dose methods are at risk when using certain drugs. Additional contraception should be used during treatment and for 7 days after treatment.

BTB, breakthrough bleeding; DMPA, depomedroxyprogesterone acetate; EE, ethinyl estradiol; POP, progestin only pill.

Modified from Loudon, N., Glasier, A., Gebbie, A. (1995). Handbook of Family Planning and Reproductive Health Care (3rd ed.). Edinburgh: Churchill Livingstone.

Guidelines for Oral Contraceptive Use

- Take one pill daily; do not miss a day
- Take pill at same time every day
- Use a second birth control method during first pill cycle
- If you miss one pill, take it as soon as remembered and take next pill at usual time
- If you miss two pills, take both as soon as remembered; take two pills the next day also; use another birth control method for remainder of cycle
- If you miss three pills, discontinue use for that cycle and use another birth control method

PID are prevented each year by oral contraceptive use. There is also a decreased risk of rheumatoid arthritis, and women may experience an improvement in acne while using the pill (Brown and Hammond 1989; Mishell 1989; NAACOG 1991).

The disadvantages of combined oral contraceptives include the possible side effects and the potential health risk that have been identified. The birth control pill carries the highest "risk-to-life" of any birth control method. The risk increases with age, duration of use, smoking, and any predisposing health factors. Most of the complications are associated with estrogen, but progestin is also linked to risks (Cunningham et al. 1993). Side effects of the birth control pill can be classified as minor or potentially serious. Minor effects that women may experience while using oral contraceptives may range from breakthrough bleeding to weight gain and bloating.

▼ **Breakthrough Bleeding.** Bleeding at any time during the midcycle is seen most commonly with very-low-dose formulations and often resolves over time. If it persists for three full cycles, a higher dose formulation is required. A common cause of breakthrough bleeding is missed or late pills.

▼ **Amenorrhea.** Absence of menstrual bleeding is seen in 1 percent of cycles with combined oral contraceptives, but up to 20 percent of women using hormonal therapy may experience amenorrhea at some time. Persistent amenorrhea is due to endometrial atrophy. If it is bothersome, the woman can change to a preparation with a higher estrogen content or an incremental progestin formulation.

▼ **Dysmenorrhea.** Painful menstruation usually disappears or is decreased with combined oral contraceptives. If it does continue, an increased progestin component can be useful. If the dysmenorrhea is not relieved, a menstrual disorder such as endometriosis should be suspected.

▼ **Breast Symptoms.** Fullness or tenderness of the breasts can be relieved by decreasing the estrogen dose or increasing the progestin dose of the pill.

▼ **Nausea.** If nausea occurs, the pill should be taken at night. If it persists for more than two cycles, decreasing the estrogen dose or changing to a progestin only pill may be necessary.

▼ **Chloasma.** The darkened pigmentation of the cheeks is caused by an increased production of melanocyte stimulating hormone triggered by estrogen and progestin. The client may need to discontinue the combined oral contraceptive and try a progestin only pill. If chloasma occurs, she should use a sunscreen lotion and wear a hat when in the sun, as chloasma is aggravated by sunlight.

▼ **Depression.** Six percent of women using combined oral contraceptives complain of fatigue, loss of libido, or depression. It is theorized that estrogen use produces a relative deficiency of vitamin B_6, leading to a reduction in the synthesis of transmitter amines in the brain, which may be responsible for the mood changes. The client can be given a supplement of vitamin B_6, can be changed to a more estrogenic formulation of the combined oral contraceptive or an incremental progestin pill, or can discontinue hormonal contraception and use another birth control method.

▼ **Acne.** Acne is usually improved by taking combined oral contraceptives, since estrogens decrease sebaceous secretions in the skin. However, 3 percent of women find that acne worsens. If this occurs, the client should change to a more estrogenic formulation of the combined oral contraceptive.

▼ **Migraine Headaches.** Migraine headaches may occur because of fluid retention. The client should be advised to discontinue use of the oral contraceptive.

▼ **Weight Gain or Bloating.** The progestin component of the pill may increase the appetite and facilitate fat deposition. Weight gain can be controlled either by careful selection of a healthy diet, including vegetables and fruits, or by changing to a pill with a lower estrogen component to reduce bloating caused by water retention (Brown and Hammond 1989; NAACOG 1991; Cunningham et al. 1993).

Risks and Safety

Potentially serious and more long-term effects that women may experience as a result of taking combined oral contraceptives are associated with a variety of risk factors.

▼ **Cardiovascular Risks.** Women who smoke and are over 35 years of age have the greatest risk of developing cardiovascular disease. The risk seems to be related to the effects of various progestins on lipid and lipoprotein metabolism. There is an increase in total plasma triglyceride concentration and high-density lipoprotein (HDL), and a decrease in low-density lipoprotein (LDL). Data regarding the cardiovascular risks of oral contraceptive use have been conflicting, and many studies have been poorly designed. Further research is needed (Brown and Hammond 1989; Mishell 1989; Cunningham et al. 1993).

▼ **Thromboembolic Disease.** The risk of an increased tendency toward clotting and resultant venous thromboembolism has been reported as being three to 11 times higher in women using oral contraceptives, but the risk is also influenced by smoking. Deep vein and pulmonary embolisms account for over 7000 hospitalizations among oral contraceptive users every year. The occurrence of superficial venous thrombosis, which seldom requires hospitalization and almost never causes death, affects approximately 11,800 oral contraceptive users every year. The mechanisms causing a change in the clotting mechanism are not known with certainty. Although it appears that estrogen is the primary culprit, there is also some evidence to suggest a contributory role for some progestins (Brown and Hammond 1989; Cunningham et al. 1993; Bagshaw 1995).

▼ **Hypertension.** Hypertension is a commonly accepted side effect of oral contraceptive use; preexisting hypertension is a contraindication to their use. An increase in blood pressure may be caused by either the estrogen ethinyl estradiol or the progestin component of the pill, which can affect the renin-angiotensin-aldosterone system. Older users are more likely to be diagnosed as having hypertension, and continued use of the pill seems to increase the risk. Vigilant blood pressure monitoring is important for women using oral contraceptives. Both acute and chronic hypertension should be resolved by discontinuing the oral contraceptive agent. Hypertension caused by the pill usually dissipates, with rare exceptions, on discontinuation of the drug (Mishell 1989; Cunningham et al. 1993; Bagshaw 1995).

▼ **Cerebrovascular Accident.** Few well-controlled studies have been conducted on the relationship of stroke and oral contraceptive use, and findings have been inconsistent. One U. S. multicenter investigative study found a high relative risk for thrombotic stroke, a low relative risk for hemorrhagic stroke, and no risk for other kinds of stroke in oral contraceptive users. The risk of stroke may be five times greater for oral contraceptive users, and stroke may account for 5 to 10 percent of deaths among users. However, age, hypertension, and smoking contribute to this risk. The risk of stroke may continue after stopping the pill (Mishell 1989; Cunningham et al. 1993; Bagshaw 1995).

▼ **Myocardial Infarction.** The risk of heart attack in young women taking oral contraceptives is less than the risk from pregnancy and delivery. Most myocardial infarctions occur in women who have additional risk factors, primarily smoking and increased age. The risk of heart attack in oral contraceptive users aged 41 to 45 who are also smokers is 350 to 800 times higher than in nonsmokers aged 27 to 37. The mortality from heart attack associated with oral contraceptive use increases with advancing age and with the length of pill usage. The risk of myocardial infarction persists beyond the discontinuation of the oral contraceptive, particularly in older women who used the pill for more than 5 years and were heavy smokers (Brown and Hammond 1989; Cunningham et al. 1993; Bagshaw 1995).

▼ **Breast Cancer.** Data on the relationship between oral contraceptives and breast cancer have been conflicting and not definitive. Several studies have found some relationship between breast cancer and use of the pill among women under 45 years of age. However, most studies have not shown this relationship. The results of studies are contradictory, and none found an increased risk in the same subgroup of women. Therefore, a committee advising the FDA concluded that the existing data do not support a change in the use of oral contraceptives. It must be recognized that possible very late effects of hormonal contraceptive agents may yet become evident, and the final weighing of risks and benefits is yet to take place (Brown and Hammond 1989; Cunningham et al. 1993).

▼ **Cervical Cancer.** The findings of an increased risk of cervical cancer for women on the pill have been questionable and inconclusive, and more evidence is needed before a definite association can be made. The mechanisms by which an increased risk of cervical cancer is effected are not clear, but there is some preliminary evidence that contraceptive steroids act as promoters for such risk factors as herpesvirus or human papillomavirus, or may accelerate the progression of preinvasive lesions. One confounding factor is the fact that women on the pill tend to have more sexual partners, which adds to the risk of cervical cancer. Other variables that may influence the development of cervical cancer are young age at first intercourse, exposure to human papillomavirus, multiparity, high frequency of intercourse, and low socioeconomic status (Brown and Hammond 1989; Mishell 1989; Cunningham et al. 1993).

▼ **Liver Tumors.** Benign hepatic adenomas occur at a rate of three per 100,000 women using oral contraceptives, a rate that has remained unchanged for 30 years. The incidence increases over age 30, with high-potency oral contraceptives, and with long-term use of the pill. The risk inherent in these tumors is their potential for spontaneous rupture and life-threatening hemorrhage. Usually, spontaneous regression of these tumors occurs with cessation of oral contraceptive use. The relationship of extremely rare malignant liver tumors with oral contraceptive use is difficult to verify, but some data have supported such an association. However, owing to the methodologic problems with these studies and the small number of cases, it is too early to incriminate the pill as a causative factor in the development of malignant liver tumors (Brown and Hammond 1989; Mishell 1989; Cunningham et al. 1993).

▼ **Gallbladder Disease.** The risk of gallbladder disease is greatest in the first year of oral contraceptive use. The pill may precipitate clinical symptoms in women at risk for developing gallbladder disease or in women who have the disease already (Cunningham et al. 1993).

▼ **Malignant Melanoma.** The link between oral contraceptive use and malignant melanoma reported in early studies has not been confirmed by later investigations (Brown and Hammond 1989).

Women who have the greatest risk for developing complications with oral contraceptive use are over age 35; have a clotting or circulation problem, varicose veins or thrombophlebitis, heart disease or heart defects, or a history of stroke; have a history of breast or reproductive organ cancer; have undiagnosed vaginal bleeding; have liver disease; have diabetes; are obese; or smoke more than 15 cigarettes a day. Table 11–3 lists absolute, strong relative, and other relative contraindications to oral contraceptive use. It is important to note that research has shown the combined oral contraceptive to be safe for most healthy, nonsmoking women under the age of 35.

Table 11–3

CONTRAINDICATIONS TO ORAL CONTRACEPTIVES

Absolute Contraindications
Thromboembolic disease or history of same
Cerebrovascular disease or history of same
Myocardial infarction or known coronary artery disease
Liver tumors, benign or malignant
Carcinoma of breast
Estrogen-dependent neoplasia
Known or suspected pregnancy
Liver disease
Strong Relative Contraindications
Smokers over age 35
Nonsmokers over age 40 with second risk factor
Nonsmokers over age 45
Hypertension (systolic >140, diastolic >90)
Undiagnosed abnormal vaginal bleeding
Diabetes mellitus
Hyperlipidemia
Severe vascular headaches, migraine headaches
Gallbladder disease
Cervical dysplasia
Surgery injury, or casting requiring immobilization
Sickle cell disease
Other Relative Contraindications
Gestational diabetes
Coagulopathies
Systemic lupus erythematosus
Porphyria
Cholestatic jaundice of pregnancy
Irregular menses, oligomenorrhea
Family history of breast disease
Urinary tract infections
Epilepsy
Depression
Asthma
Marked varicosities
Cardiac or renal disease
Conditions likely in woman who is unreliable with pill usage
Family history of myocardial infarction before age 50
Breastfeeding

From Eichhorst, B. (1989). Contraception. *Primary Care,* 15 (3), 437–459.

In fact, for this group, taking the pill is safer than the risk of driving a car. The benefits are the greatest and the risks the least for young women who have the highest fertility rates. Therefore, a balance must be made between the advantages and the risks of oral contraceptives (Mishell 1989; NAACOG 1991; Bagshaw 1995).

When a woman using the pill decides to become pregnant, she should stop the oral contraceptive several months before attempting to conceive, to allow the ovaries to begin functioning normally again. Some women may experience a longer time before conception occurs after using the pill. The mean time for conception to occur has been reported to be 13 months. The rate of spontaneous abortion or chromosomal abnormalities is no higher in women using the pill than in women using other methods. Women who wish to breastfeed should not use combined oral contraceptives as a birth control method, because the estrogen component of the pill reduces the quantity of breast milk and may also pass into the milk. These women may be able to use the progestin only pill, which has less effect on milk production (Erwin 1994).

PROGESTIN ONLY PILL

Description

Another form of oral contraceptive is the progestin only pill (POP), also known as the "mini" pill. This form of oral contraception has been available since 1973. It contains no estrogen and less than 0.5 mg of progestin. It is therefore particularly beneficial for women who experience extreme estrogen-related side effects while using the combination oral contraceptive. The mini pill works primarily by changing the cervical mucus so that sperm are unable to penetrate, by altering ovum transport, and by inhibiting endometrial lining development so that implantation cannot occur. Unlike combination oral contraceptives, the mini pill is taken every day for a 28-day cycle, followed the next day by a new 28-day cycle (Cunningham et al. 1993; Moore 1994).

Effectiveness

The progestin only pill is reported to be slightly less effective than combination oral contraceptives. The reported use effectiveness ranges from five to ten pregnancies per 100 women years, or 90 to 95 percent. The highest failure rate with the progestin only pill occurs in the first 6 months of use. As with the combination oral contraceptives, if a pill is forgotten or taken late, another birth control method should also be used for the remainder of the cycle. Women may ovulate while using the progestin only pill. The mini pill inhibits total ovarian function in only 10 percent of women using it; 40 percent of mini pill users ovulate regularly and another 50 percent occasionally ovulate (Cunningham et al. 1993).

Advantages and Disadvantages

Since the mini pill contains no estrogen and the progestin dose is so low, the advantages are very few side effects or risks, other than occasional amenorrhea or irregular bleeding and menstrual cramping. The mini pill has not been shown to increase cardiovascular complications and is less likely to cause headaches, blood pressure elevation, and other estrogen-related side effects. When used by the breastfeeding woman, the progestin only pill is 100 percent effective and has less effect on milk production (Cunningham et al. 1993).

The disadvantages are that the mini pill is infrequently prescribed in the United States and clinicians are less familiar with managing side effects. Pills taken as little as 3 hours late require a backup method of contraception. Menstrual irregularities may occur and ectopic pregnancies and functional ovarian cysts can occur because ovulation is not inhibited completely (NAACOG 1991).

POSTCOITAL PILL

Description

A third type of oral contraceptive is the postcoital or "morning after" pill. This hormonal therapy is either a high-dose combination estrogen and progestin pill (100 μg of ethinyl estradiol and 500 μg of levonorgestrel) or an estrogen compound (diethylstilbestrol). It must be given within 72 hours of unprotected sexual intercourse to prevent implantation and pregnancy. It is given initially after intercourse, repeated in 12 hours, and then taken twice a day for 5 days (Cunningham et al. 1993; Hatcher et al. 1994). The estrogen suppresses the hypothalamic-pituitary axis to prevent ovulation and alter the endometrial lining of the uterus. Menstruation usually begins 5 days after the final pill is taken. Nausea and vomiting may be possible side effects. Postcoital therapy is most commonly used to prevent pregnancy in women who have been raped, but it is not yet available for general use.

INJECTABLE HORMONAL THERAPY

Description

Other types of hormonal contraceptives are injectable and implant hormonal therapy. Injectable hormonal therapy has been used by 30 million women worldwide since it was introduced in the late 1960s, but it was not approved for use in the United States until 1991. This form of hormonal therapy is administered every 3 months and contains progestin only (Depo-Provera). It works by suppressing the function of the hypothalamic-pituitary axis and inhibiting the production of

LH, which inhibits the development of the graafian follicle, and by interfering with sperm and ovum transport and the development of the endometrium.

Effectiveness

The reported use effectiveness is slightly better than that of oral contraceptives and is between five and ten pregnancies per 100 women years, or 90 to 95 percent.

Advantages and Disadvantages

There are no additional and possibly fewer side effects with injectable than with other hormonal methods of contraception. The injectable form of hormonal therapy may cause amenorrhea, bleeding irregularities, occasional heavy bleeding in the first few months of use, or a 3- to 5-pound weight gain. After 1 year of use, up to 50 percent of women stop menstruation, often for as long as they take the drug. It is possible that reestablishment of regular ovulation and menstruation may be delayed 1 year or longer after injectable hormonal therapy is discontinued. Injectable therapy may protect against endometrial, ovarian, and breast cancer and decrease the risk of PID (Monier and Laird 1989; Cunningham et al. 1993; Moore 1994).

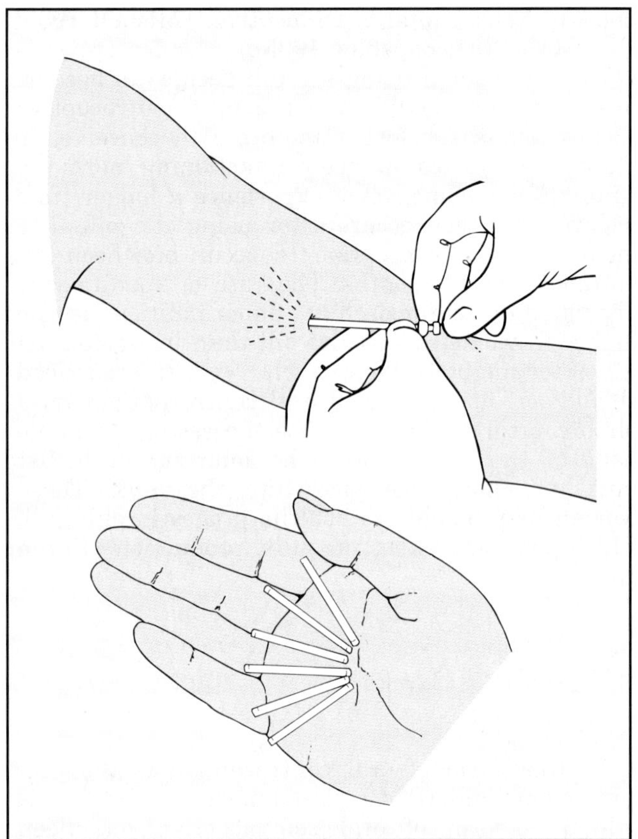

Figure 11–11

Norplant hormonal inserts work by suppressing ovulation, causing cervical mucus changes, and suppressing the endometrium. Norplant consists of six matchstick-size capsules that are implanted in a fan-shaped pattern on the client's inner arm.

IMPLANT HORMONAL THERAPY

Description

Implant therapy consists of a system of subdermal implants that release a steady dose of a progestin (levonorgestrel) for long-term, reversible contraception. These implants, known as Norplant, are matchstick-size, permeable, removable silicon rods or capsules. They are implanted under the skin in the upper arm or the scapular area in a fan-shaped pattern (Fig. 11–11) and provide effective contraception for approximately 5 to 7 years. Norplant has several mechanisms of action. It suppresses ovulation, causes cervical mucus changes, suppresses the growth and development of the endometrium, and prevents conception by depressing progesterone in the luteal phase of the menstrual cycle. When the implants are removed, fertility returns within 48 hours.

Effectiveness

The use effectiveness of Norplant is reported to be 0.2 to 0.6 pregnancies per 100 women years, or 99.4 to 99.8 percent effective in the first year of use. The rate of pregnancy may rise with continued years of use. The high effectiveness is probably related to the fact that levonorgestrel is released continuously and serum levels remain consistently adequate to prevent pregnancy.

Advantages and Disadvantages

The primary advantage of Norplant is that it is not user dependent, thus eliminating failures that might result from noncompliance. It becomes effective within 24 hours of insertion and remains effective for up to 5 years. It contains no estrogen and low daily amounts of progestin. Because the progestin is released continuously and directly into the blood, a lower dose can be given with continued high effectiveness. Norplant may help menstrual cycle problems by suppressing ovulatory pain and decreasing bleeding. It may also reduce the risk of endometrial cancer.

Disadvantages include the side effects of irregular menstrual bleeding, prolonged menses, spotting between periods, amenorrhea, and slight weight gain. Norplant does not offer protection against STDs. The cost may be prohibitive for some women. Insertion and removal of the implants require a minor surgical procedure by a trained provider. The implants remain slightly visible (Shoupe and Mishell 1989; NAACOG 1991; Hinkle 1994).

Sterilization

Twenty-seven percent of all women now rely on sterilization as a birth control method. It has become the most common and popular birth control method among married women age 30 and over. It is estimated that one quarter of all American couples will use sterilization within 2 years of the birth of their last child, and more than one half will use sterilization by 10 years after the last child. Two types of sterilization procedures are possible; both render the individual infertile by occluding the passageways for ova or sperm. Tubal ligation is the procedure used for women; vasectomy is the procedure used for men (Horton 1995).

TUBAL LIGATION

Description

Tubal ligation, also known as bilateral partial salpingectomy, is a procedure in which the fallopian tubes are either cut, tied, cauterized, plugged, capped, coagulated, or clipped. The surgical procedure can be performed on an outpatient basis, most commonly through a small abdominal incision just below the umbilicus (laparoscopy) (Fig. 11–12). It is also possible to perform the procedure through a vaginal incision. Preoperative sedation and local anesthesia are customary; on occasion a general anesthetic may be used. The procedure can be completed in 20 to 30 minutes. Tubal sterilization renders the woman immediately infertile by preventing the passage of the ovum from the ovary to the uterus. Tubal sterilization can be carried out immediately after birth, after an abortion, or at any other time. Although the procedure is most often performed immediately after childbirth when it may be most convenient, the lowest failure and morbidity rates occur when it is done at a time other than immediately after pregnancy.

Effectiveness

The reported effectiveness of tubal sterilization is 0.04 to five pregnancies per 100 women years, or 95 to 99.96 percent. Failure with this method would not be user dependent but would occur only as a result of spontaneous rejoining of the tubes. This risk is related to the method used and seems to be greater with ligation and crushing than with ligation and resection.

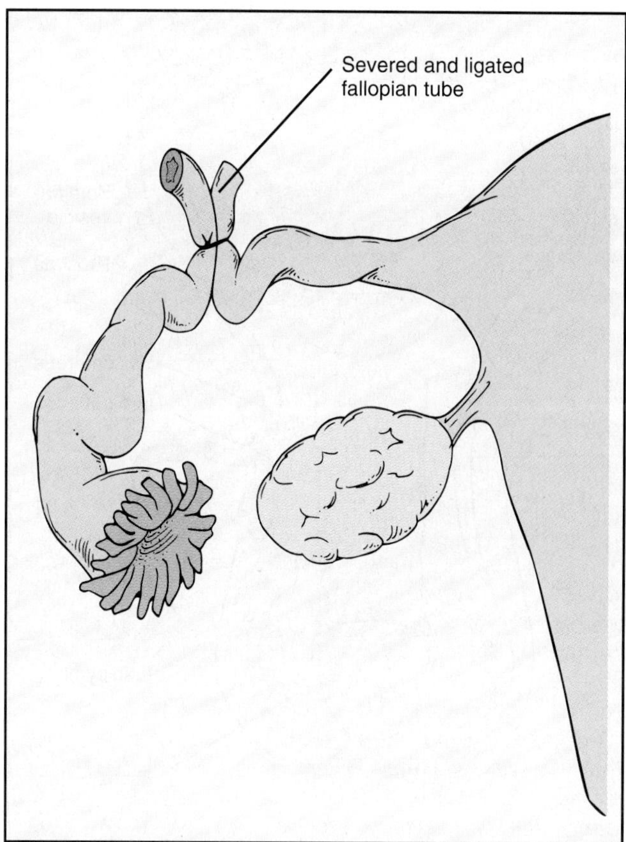

Figure 11–12

Tubal ligation is a surgical procedure during which the fallopian tubes are ligated and severed, cauterized, plugged, capped, coagulated, or clipped to prevent the passage of the ovum from the ovary to the uterus.

Risks and Safety

The potential risks of tubal ligation include infection, hemorrhage, bowel or bladder trauma, and uterine perforation. The reported fatality rate is 3.8 per 100,000 women (Cunningham et al. 1993).

VASECTOMY

Description

Vasectomy is a surgical procedure in which the vasa deferentia are severed, tied, clipped, or coagulated, preventing sperm from entering the semen. The procedure can take place in a physician's office with local anesthesia and is done through a small incision in the scrotum (Fig. 11–13). Each vas deferens is ligated with nonabsorbable sutures and then incised between the ligatures. The cut ends of the vas deferens may be buried into scrotal fascia or cauterized to decrease the chance of reunion. To reduce swelling and relieve discomfort, ice packs may be applied to the scrotum postoperatively. A dressing to support the scrotum is also helpful. After a vasectomy, the man is not immediately infertile and will need to

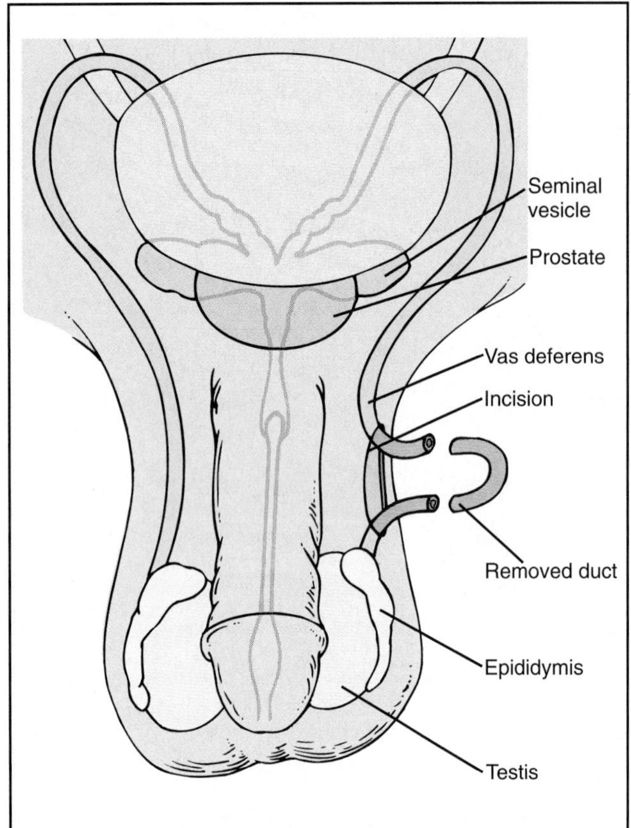

Figure 11–13

Vasectomy is a surgical procedure during which the vasa deferentia are severed and ligated, clipped, or coagulated to prevent sperm from entering the semen.

use another method of birth control until two consecutive tests show no sperm in the semen. It usually takes approximately 15 to 20 ejaculations, or 4 to 6 weeks, before all sperm are removed from the proximal portions of the sperm ducts. The vasectomy does not render the man impotent and has no effect on his ability to have an erection or to ejaculate.

Effectiveness

The reported effectiveness of vasectomy is 99.6 to 99.85 percent. Failure with this method of sterilization would occur only as a result of no other birth control method being used after the vasectomy until two negative sperm tests have occurred. There are no identified long-term risks of vasectomy. The immediate potential risks of infection, hematoma, epididymitis, or sperm granuloma are less than 5 percent (Cunningham et al. 1993; Farley et al. 1993).

ADVANTAGES AND DISADVANTAGES

There are a number of advantages of both tubal ligation and vasectomy. The one-time decision that allows permanent freedom from worry about pregnancy, and the fact that no other methods of birth control are needed, are the primary advantages. Although the initial cost of both surgical procedures is high, sterilization becomes inexpensive when prorated over the remainder of the person's lifetime. An additional advantage is that both methods have no influence on sexual desire and allow for spontaneous lovemaking.

There are also disadvantages of both methods of sterilization. Failures can occur or couples can change their mind about wanting more children. In most cases the methods are irreversible. It is possible to perform a reanastomosis of both the fallopian tubes and the vas deferens, but the incidence of successful pregnancy after reanastomosis of the fallopian tubes is only about 15 percent and after reanastomosis of the vas deferens only about 40 to 60 percent. The rate of success decreases with the passage of time. Because reanastomosis in an elective procedure, it is not usually covered by insurance. Complications from the surgery can occur, including bleeding, pain, and infections. Vasectomy is generally a safer, simpler procedure than tubal ligation (NAACOG 1991).

Birth Control Methods of the Future

FEMALE METHODS

Research continues in an attempt to find birth control methods that meet all the criteria identified at the beginning of this chapter. The following methods are those currently under investigation for use by women (Hatcher et al. 1994; Loudon et al. 1995):

▼ **Cervical Test.** This is an at-home test of cervical mucus that would tell women with certainty the 5 critical days before ovulation. It will detect the rapid drop of cervical enzymes before ovulation.

▼ **Injectable Microscopic Capsules.** These will contain hormones to inhibit pregnancy and could be 30-, 90-, or 180-day capsules. Use effectiveness is projected to be 98 percent. Clinical trials are currently going on in Mexico and the United States.

▼ **GnRH.** GnRH, or gonadotropin releasing hormone, administered by a nasal spray pump or as an implant is being studied. It inhibits ovulation by affecting the pituitary gland to block the LH surge.

▼ **Tubal Occlusion Without Surgery.** This will be accomplished with the chemical methylcyanoacrylate applied to the lumina of the fallopian tubes through the cervix. The chemical causes the tubes to close by stimulating the development of adhesions.

▼ **Disposable Diaphragms.** These will be similar to cervical caps in that one size will fit all and the diaphragm will contain a spermicidal agent. These diaphragms will be sold over the counter.

▼ **Lea's Shield.** Lea's Shield combines the features of a diaphragm and cervical cap and is made of flexible silicone rubber. It is a one-size-fits-all device with a one-way "flutter" valve to allow air to escape during placement, thus creating better retention against the cervix. The valve also allows uterine and cervical fluids to escape (so the risk of bacterial growth during long-term placement is reduced), yet it prevents sperm from getting into the cervix.

▼ **FemCap.** The FemCap is a cervical cap–like barrier made of silicone and shaped like a U. S. sailor's cap. It comes in three sizes, depending on the user's parity. It is claimed to fit the cervix better than current cervical caps and to adapt more easily to changes in cervical shape and size during the menstrual cycle. The FemCap should be approved by the end of the 1990s.

▼ **Vaginal Rings.** These are silicon rubber rings that are donut shaped and secrete contraceptive hormones (levonorgestrel and estradiol). They can remain in place for as long as 3 to 4 weeks and are removed to facilitate menstruation. The same ring can then be reinserted after menses has ended. One ring will be good for about 6 months. Potential disadvantages include discomfort during sexual intercourse, the risk of being expelled, vaginal discharge, and irregular bleeding. These rings will be available in the future.

▼ **Silicone Plugs.** Silicone plugs, made of silicone rubber to block the fallopian tubes, are being studied at this time. These plugs could be removed when pregnancy is desired.

▼ **Norplant II.** Norplant II will be an improved version of the Norplant system already in use; however, it will contain two rods instead of six. It will achieve similar drug levels of levonorgestrel and duration of action. Norplant II should be available for routine use in several years.

MALE METHODS

New birth control methods are also being studied for men. At present, none are available for general use, but these are possibilities for the future:

▼ **Gossypol.** Gossypol is a substance found in cottonseeds that has been found to suppress sperm production and motility. It would be administered in the form of an oral tablet. Unfortunately, gossypol can cause a number of side effects, such as nausea, fatigue, hypokalemia, and decreased libido. The infertility it causes can persist after the medication is no longer taken.

▼ **LHRH-A.** LHRH-A is a synthetic copy of the naturally occurring luteinizing releasing hormone that suppresses sperm production. Problems identified to date include a decrease in testosterone and libido. It may also increase the risk of heart disease.

▼ **Testosterone Enanthate.** This is a synthetic form of testosterone given by injection to suppress sperm production. Early studies seem to show that it is safer than gossypol, but it takes a number of months to cause infertility and may take some months after discontinuation of injections to restore fertility. To date, there are insufficient data regarding possible long-term health risks.

▼ **Removable Vas Deferens Plugs.** These are intraluminal devices that could be inserted to block the vas deferens and then removed when fertility is desired. Clinical trials have not yet begun in the United States.

▼ **Electrically Induced Coagulation of Vas Deferens.** This would provide another form of male sterilization (Monier and Laird 1989).

No doubt research will always be ongoing to develop contraceptive methods that will be safe and effective and will meet the needs of couples who desire to practice family planning. These methods currently being studied in clinical trials will become available only if their safety and efficacy are confirmed and FDA approval is granted.

Nursing Practice

Nursing Process

The application of the nursing process provides direction for the nurse working with women and their partners who desire to use a method of family planning. Essential skills needed in the implementation of the nursing process related to family planning include interviewing, history taking, teaching, and counseling.

▼ Assessment

As in any therapeutic situation, assessment is an essential first step to identify the needs and desires of the woman and her partner. The initial assessment should be conducted in an unhurried and private atmosphere to make the woman and her partner feel comfortable. They should be greeted warmly and treated with respect. It is important to be accepting of the couple's feelings and beliefs, even if those beliefs are different from the nurse's. The assessment should include the gathering of physical, emotional, sociocultural, and cognitive data that relate to family planning.

Physical. Physical assessment can be carried out by a physician or by a nurse with advanced skills in physical assessment or family planning. The physical assessment should include a medical, reproductive, and contraceptive history; a complete gynecologic examination; and routine laboratory tests. These data will help identify the existence of any contraindications to a particular birth control method. It is helpful to know about the couple's previous experiences with contraception, what they liked or disliked, problems they encountered, and factors that led to discontinuing a previous method. A record of all assessment data should be started and important information recorded.

Emotional. The emotional, sociocultural, and cognitive assessments are often made by the nurse or by a family planning counselor during an interview. The emotional assessment should include data regarding the couple's feelings about their sexuality, family planning in general, and specific contraceptive methods. Discussion of the couple's goals for family planning is helpful in identifying a long-range plan. It is important to know the number of children they want and the spacing of those children. If they have concerns or strong feelings about a particular birth control method, this needs to be noted. An assessment of the couple's motivation and an estimation of their compliance with a particular method are important. Studies have shown that a woman's partner has a great impact on her use or nonuse of a contraceptive method. A woman's perception of her partner's support is a major predictor of her compliance with the method. An evaluation of the woman's comfort with her body, her self-image, and her willingness to touch her genitals all provide information that is helpful in identifying the best method of contraception for her. Assessment of the couple's nonverbal, as well as verbal, behavior is an important component of the emotional assessment.

Sociocultural. Sociocultural data are important, for the couple's compliance with a particular birth control method may be strongly influenced by their family backgrounds, religious beliefs, or cultural taboos. Myths or sexual practices that are culture related must be identified. Social information such as the nature of the woman's sexual activity, the number of sexual partners, and her desire for partner involvement in birth control are important. The relationship she has with her sexual partner(s) and the type of communication they share will influence her use of a contraceptive. The woman's or man's financial situation may also

FAMILY PLANNING

The nurse in most family planning settings provides a major portion of the care the woman receives. To apply the nursing process in the most effective way to help women with their family planning needs, the following steps will help the nurse to improve her practice:

- IDENTIFY YOUR OWN ATTITUDES ABOUT FAMILY PLANNING. Clarify your feelings about the prevention of pregnancy and child spacing. Recognize the influence your own culture, religion, and social group have on your attitudes.
- UPDATE YOUR THEORETIC BASE. Obtain accurate information regarding all contraceptive methods currently available, as well as new and changing trends in family planning. Be certain you understand the mode of action and risks and contraindications of each method. Read the lay literature relating to contraception so that you are aware of the information your clients are receiving.
- ATTEND CONTINUING EDUCATION SEMINARS related to family planning issues. Discuss with your colleagues ways in which you can provide more effective services to your clients. Continually refine your skills in interviewing, teaching, and counseling.
- REVIEW THE PROFESSIONAL LITERATURE AND STANDARDS OF PRACTICE regarding family planning. Contrast what you see done in clinical practice with current research findings.
- EVALUATE CURRENT SOCIAL NORMS. Keep abreast of the current social, religious, or political issues that might influence the provision of comprehensive family planning services.
- AVOID VALUE JUDGMENTS. Strive to be open-minded and accepting of the opinions and values of others, even if they do not agree with your own. Do not allow your own prejudices to influence your nursing care.

influence their choice of a method of family planning.

Cognitive. An assessment of the couple's cognitive understanding of the reproductive cycle and of various birth control methods is essential. Many people today know a great deal about family planning from other sources in their lives. New information regarding contraception is rapidly disseminated by the lay media, sometimes even before it is published in professional journals. When the couple's specific educational needs are identified through individualized assessment, these needs can be better met and health care providers can better utilize their time with them.

Assessment of educational needs can be made as part of an interview or through the use of paper and pencil assessment questionnaires. The Educational Needs Assessment Tool can be given to a couple to complete when they arrive at a family planning clinic and will help the nurse to quickly measure knowledge of birth control methods, assess educational needs, and identify personal preferences regarding family planning methods. The Contraceptive Knowledge Assessment Tool measures whether the couple have a basic knowledge of all methods of birth control as well as an adequate knowledge of the specifics of their particular method. The form reproduced here is designed for those using oral contraceptives; a different form should be available for each method of birth control (Johnson 1985).

▼ Diagnosis

Nursing diagnoses should be identified on the basis of the data gathered during the initial assessment. They should further reflect identified needs in all four components of the assessment, i.e., physical, emotional, sociocultural, and cognitive aspects. Examples of nursing diagnoses related to family planning include

- Risk for infection related to multiple sexual partners and unprotected sexual intercourse
- Knowledge deficit: lack of information related to reproductive cycle and birth control methods
- Situational low self-esteem related to discomfort in touching genital area
- Noncompliance: unwillingness of sexual partner related to participation in use of birth control method

▼ Planning

A plan of care can be developed once the nursing diagnoses have been identified. Because most family planning methods currently in use relate to the female partner, it is common for the plan to be developed for her. However, if both sexual partners are interested and involved, the plan should re-

Assessment Tool: Educational Needs Assessment

It is important that you make your own choice about your method of contraception (birth control). Please complete this form so that we can help you.

Have you received instruction about contraception before? _____Yes. _____No.
If yes, where? ______________________ When? ______________

Have you already decided what method of contraception you want? _____Yes. _____No.
If yes, what method? ______________________

Do you want a birth control method that (check all that apply)

_____Will allow you to have spontaneous or uninterrupted sex.
_____Will keep you absolutely safe from getting pregnant.
_____You use only when you have sex (because you don't have sex often).
_____Doesn't have any side effects.
_____Your partner likes.
_____You can keep secret.

If you are not sure about what method of contraception to use, would you like to

_____Hear about the methods with a small group class, then have a chance to ask questions in private.
_____See a filmstrip and/or read about the methods, then have a chance to ask questions in private.
_____Have a counselor show and explain the methods to you in private.

Check the methods you have questions about:

_____Abstinence
_____Withdrawal
_____Natural family planning
_____Vaginal suppositories
_____Foam, jellies, creams
_____Male condom
_____Female condom
_____Vaginal sponge
_____Diaphragm
_____Cervical cap
_____IUD
_____Pill
_____Injections
_____Norplant
_____Sterilization

See if you can match the birth control methods below with their description:

_____Abstinence	a. Hormone shots given every 3 months to prevent ovulation.
_____Oral contraceptive pill	b. Mushroom-shaped cap inserted into vagina to block and inactivate sperm and absorb semen.
_____IUD	c. Contains chemicals that kill sperm or stop their movement.
_____Withdrawal	d. Prevents release of eggs from ovaries.
_____Male condom (rubber)	e. Placed inside vagina to cover cervix and prevent sperm from entering uterus.
_____Diaphragm	f. Matchstick-size rods implanted under skin in upper arm to release hormones to prevent ovulation.
_____Natural family planning	g. Permanent method of contraception.
_____Female condom	h. Used to determine times in a woman's menstrual cycle when she is fertile or able to become pregnant.
_____Norplant	i. Placed inside uterus to prevent fertilized egg from settling into wall of uterus.
_____Sterilization	j. When a man removes his penis from woman's vagina just before he ejaculates (comes).
_____Depo-Provera	k. Rolled onto a man's penis to catch semen as he has an orgasm (comes).
_____Foam, jellies, creams	l. Thimble-shaped cup that fits over cervix to block sperm.
_____Cervical cap	m. Thin plastic sheath that fits into vagina to prevent direct contact with penis.
_____Vaginal sponge	n. Not having intercourse.

Assessment Tool: Contraceptive Knowledge Assessment for Oral Contraceptive Patients

We want to be sure you know about your options concerning birth control and how your chosen method works. Please fill out this form so we can see whether you have any further questions.

CIRCLE TRUE OR FALSE:

T F Vasectomies and tubal ligations should be considered permanent methods of contraception.
T F The pill stops a woman's ovaries from releasing eggs.
T F IUDs are put in and out each time a couple has intercourse.
T F Condoms help prevent the spread of some types of sexually transmittable diseases.
T F Diaphragms and cervical caps have many serious side effects.
T F Natural family planning requires a couple to abstain from intercourse at certain times during the month.
T F Vaginal sponges must be prescribed and fitted by a physician.
T F Once Norplant rods are implanted under the skin of the arm, they cannot be removed.
T F Smoking increases the risk of someone on the pill developing serious side effects.
T F Not taking your pills at the same time every day can cause bleeding between periods.
T F When starting a new pack of pills, you should start with the seven reminder pills first and then the 21 hormone pills.
T F Foam and condoms used together are nearly as effective as the pill.

ANSWER EACH OF THE QUESTIONS BELOW:

A woman is not considered safe from getting pregnant until she has taken how many birth control pills from her first package?

What should you do if you forget to take one pill?

What should you do if you forget to take two pills?

List two common minor side effects from the pill.

List two serious side effects from the pill.

List two danger signals to watch for when taking the pill.

Reproduced with the permission of The Alan Guttmacher Institute from Jeanette H. Johnson, "Individual vs. Group Education in Family Planning Clinics," *Family Planning Perspectives,* Volume 17, Number 6, November/December 1985.

flect both woman and man. Developing measurable objectives will assist the nurse in implementing and evaluating her interventions. These objectives should include the physical, emotional, sociocultural, and cognitive components of family planning. For example, the woman (and her sexual partner) will

- Describe physical signs that indicate the fertile and infertile periods of the woman's menstrual cycle
- Correctly explain the mode of action of the selected birth control method and, if applicable, demonstrate its use
- Discuss attitudes and feelings regarding family planning in general and the selected birth control method in specific terms
- Ask questions and express concerns regarding the implementation of the selected birth control method
- Return for follow-up care and demonstrate through prevention of pregnancy the successful use of the selected birth control method

▼ Intervention

Physical. Nursing interventions are based on the assessment data and the identified plan of care. Physical interventions related to family planning are usually minimal once the physical assessment is completed. The physical interventions to be implemented may include the fitting of a diaphragm or cervical cap, inserting an IUD, or performing a surgical tubal ligation. In most clinical settings, these interventions are performed by a physician, although advanced practice nurses (nurse practitioners or clinical nurse specialists in family planning) also fit diaphragms, cervical caps, and IUDs.

Cognitive. Interventions that relate to the emotional, sociocultural, and cognitive needs of the woman and her partner are most often carried out by the nurse or family planning counselor through teaching and counseling (Fig. 11–14). This can be accomplished through group sessions or individual counseling. The format chosen to meet the client's needs will depend on the type of family planning service, the staff available, and the desires of the clients who use the service. To meet cognitive needs, education about the various contraceptive methods can be effective in group or individual settings. However, if the client has already decided on a contraceptive method, a group class that discusses all methods may not be appropriate (Johnson 1985). It is essential to provide complete, accurate, and timely contraceptive information, no matter what the format of the class. The following information is important to any discussion (NAACOG 1991):

- Description of method, including the type of method and an example or illustration
- Mode of action to show how the method works to prevent pregnancy
- Effectiveness, including the theoretic versus use failure rate and the cause of method failure
- Requirements for use, including how to obtain, implementation, and necessary compliance
- Influence on lovemaking, including when implemented in relationship to coitus and effects on coitus
- Advantages, medical and emotional
- Disadvantages, medical and emotional
- Risks and contraindications, including possible side effects, drug interactions, and factors that prevent safe use
- Cost of initial and long-term use
- Reversibility, including how to discontinue and when fertility will return

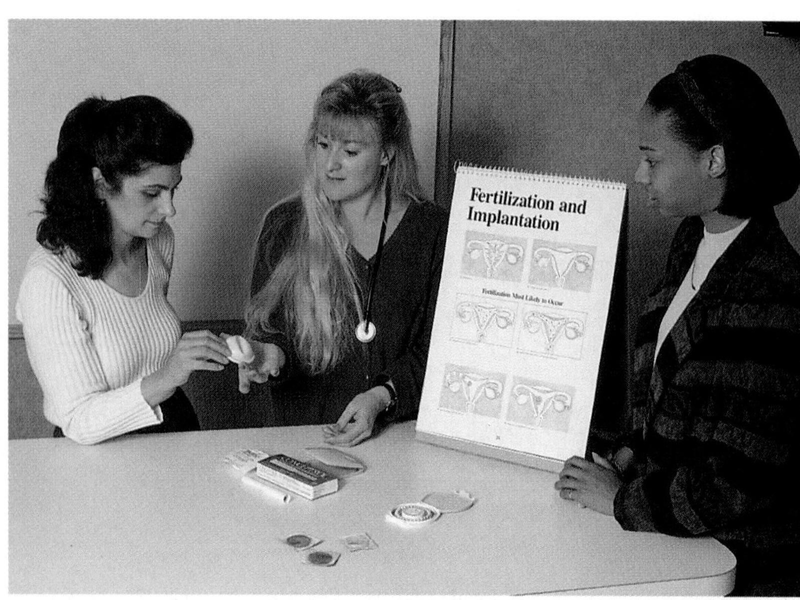

Figure 11–14

Family planning counseling can be done individually or in a group setting. Establishing a comfortable relationship with clients is extremely important.

Emotional and Sociocultural. Individual counseling sessions are more desirable than group classes to meet the emotional and sociocultural needs of clients because they offer the privacy needed to express feelings, opinions, and concerns as well as to ask personal questions about intimate aspects of their lives. Religious and cultural influences can be explored and social and financial factors identified. Individual counseling also offers the nurse an opportunity to evaluate interventions and reassess clients' understanding, acceptance, and likely compliance. The nurse's thorough preparation in interview and communication techniques enables her to provide therapeutic, individualized counseling in family planning. It is important that the nurse establish a warm and accepting atmosphere for both partners and be sensitive to their needs and concerns.

▼ Evaluation

Evaluation is an essential step in the nursing process as applied to family planning, for if the established plan and interventions are not evaluated, the couple may experience contraceptive failure. Evaluation is usually carried out by scheduling follow-up visits with the couple to reassess their physical adaptation to the chosen method, and also to discuss their cognitive understanding and emotional adaptation. An initial evaluation appointment may be scheduled for the couple after they have used the chosen contraceptive method for one complete menstrual cycle. Additional appointments are then made according to personal needs and the type of method being used.

Collaborative Process

A variety of health care personnel may be part of the family planning team, depending on the type of service, the setting, the type of clients being served, or the funding of the service. The nurse might find herself working with a physician or certified nurse midwife, a nurse practitioner, a family planning educator or counselor, a social worker, or lay counselors. The roles of these team members are also likely to vary from one setting to another, or to overlap within a given setting (Table 11–4). Because of the differences in educational preparation and the potential overlapping of roles, it is important that team members clarify

Table 11–4

TYPICAL ROLES OF FAMILY PLANNING TEAM MEMBERS

LAY COUNSELOR	NURSE	NURSE MIDWIFE/PRACTITIONER OR PHYSICIAN
History Taking	**History Taking**	**History Taking**
• Demographic • Family	• Demograpic • Health • Reproductive • Contraceptive • Family	• Demographic • Health • Reproductive • Contraceptive • Family
	Physical Examination (Assist)	**Physical Examination (Perform)**
	• Weight • Blood pressure • Laboratory	• General Systems • Gynecologic • Pap
Teaching	**Teaching**	
• Menstrual cycle • Contraception (selected methods)	• Menstrual cycle • Contraception (all methods)	
	Counseling	**Counseling**
	• Attitudes/values • Concerns • Problems	• Attitudes/values • Concerns • Problems

among themselves the role each is to play in delivering quality family planning care to clients. Communication among team members and the development of protocols for physical assessment, education, and counseling will ensure that quality services are provided.

The initial client history may be taken by the nurse, the physician, or a trained family planning counselor. The physical assessment is often made by a physician, although nurses with advanced preparation, such as certified nurse midwives or family planning nurse practitioners, may also conduct the physical examination. The development of nursing diagnoses and client goals should be handled by the nurse. The interventions carried out to meet these goals may be initiated by one or more of the members of the family planning team. It is ideal if the couple can interact with the same team member each time they come to the health care setting so that they can establish rapport and trust and the care is not fragmented. The documentation and evaluation of the interventions should be the responsibility of the team member who initiated them. The quality of family planning services depends on the ability of the health care team to work together effectively.

Risk Management

Clinical observation and research have provided a body of knowledge about each contraceptive method that should serve as a basis for safe practice in the field of family planning. Research is ongoing to obtain additional data about the safety and efficacy of current and future contraceptive methods. The first step in risk management for any professional working in the field of family planning is to become an informed provider, maintaining current knowledge about each method. The second step is to carefully assess and screen every couple to identify potential risk factors before recommending or prescribing a particular contraceptive method. For example, an IUD should never be prescribed for a woman with a history of ectopic pregnancy or PID. Oral contraceptives are proven to have a high degree of safety for young, nonsmoking women who have no history of cardiovascular disease, but would be risky for a 35-year-old woman who smokes a pack of cigarettes a day and has a history of thrombophlebitis. A final step in risk management is to provide adequate teaching, counseling, and follow-up supervision to ensure that the couple is using the selected method in a safe and effective manner.

Implications for Research

A great deal of medical research has been done and is ongoing in regard to each of the methods of contraception. This research focuses on the physical aspects of family planning. However, there is little research dealing with the emotional, sociocultural, or cognitive components of family planning. Nursing research could contribute valuable information in these areas. Research questions that could be answered by nurses might include the following:

- What factors influence the couple's choice of contraceptive method?
- What is the relationship between partner support and involvement with contraception and contraception success?
- What teaching and counseling strategies are most effective in regard to contraception selection and effective use?
- Is there a relationship between type of contraception education and patient compliance?

Research regarding family planning will continue to be important for many years to come. The development and refinement of safe, effective contraceptive methods is essential to the well-being of families. Research relating to the provision of family planning services that meet the needs of women and their partners will supply the information needed to make contraception accessible to all who want it.

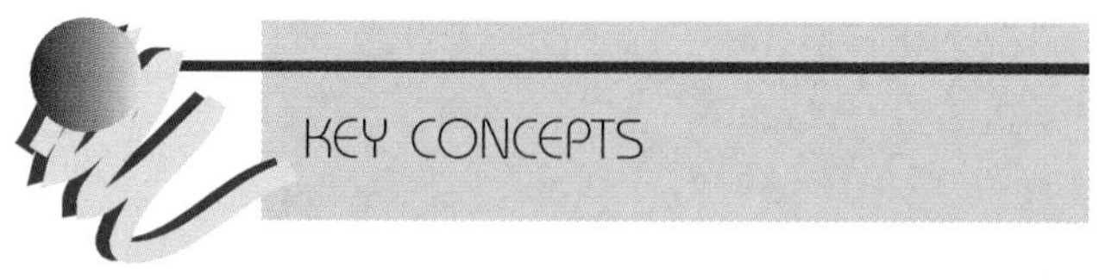

KEY CONCEPTS

- ▼ Family planning helps couples avoid unwanted births, bring about wanted births, regulate the intervals between pregnancies, control the time when births occur in relation to the ages of the parents, and determine the number of children in the family.
- ▼ An ideal contraceptive method should be effective, safe, low risk, associated with few side effects, easy to understand and use, acceptable to both partners, and not directly related to lovemaking; cause no interference with sexual pleasure; be totally reversible; enable the couple to conceive immediately after discontinuing use of the method; and be inexpensive and easy to obtain.

- ▼ Natural family planning consists of the following methods: (1) the calendar method (rhythm method), based on mathematical calculations to predict the probable time of ovulation and the fertile period; (2) the basal body temperature method, based on identification of the shift in the woman's body temperature that occurs after ovulation; (3) the cervical mucus method, based on recognition of the fertile and infertile periods of the menstrual cycle through the recognition of changes in cervical mucus; and (4) the symptothermal method, based on a combination of the indicators of cervical mucus, basal body temperature, and other secondary symptoms of ovulation.
- ▼ Vaginal spermicides include jellies, creams, foam, melting suppositories, foaming tablets, foaming suppositories, and a soluble film. They avoid pregnancy by forming a physical barrier over the cervix to prevent sperm from entering and by destroying sperm through a chemical action.
- ▼ The male condom is a rubber or animal-skin sheath placed on the erect penis to prevent deposition of semen in the vagina; it can be used along with a spermicidal agent.
- ▼ The female condom is a soft, transparent polyurethane sheath with two flexible rings. One ring forms the edge of the open end, and the other ring, which is not attached, rests inside the closed end as an internal anchor; it protects the entire vaginal and urethral area from contact with the shaft and base of the penis.
- ▼ A diaphragm is a shallow, dome-shaped rubber device with a flexible metal rim that fits into the vagina, where it rests anteriorly against the soft tissues behind the symphysis pubis, posteriorly within the vaginal fornix, and laterally against the vaginal walls. It blocks sperm from entering the cervix and is used along with a spermicidal agent to increase its effectiveness.
- ▼ The cervical cap is a small, thimble-shaped rubber or plastic cup that fits over the cervix to mechanically block sperm from entering the cervical canal; it is filled with a spermicidal agent to increase its effectiveness.
- ▼ The IUD is a small plastic device that is inserted into the uterus and remains in place for an extended period. It prevents pregnancy by causing an inflammatory reaction in the uterus in an attempt to attack the foreign body, and as a result engulfs the sperm or fertilized ovum.
- ▼ Hormonal contraception consists of oral contraceptives (the pill), injectable contraceptives (Depo-Provera), and implant therapy (Norplant). All of these forms suppress ovulation by suppressing the FSH-LH sequence from the anterior pituitary gland. Hormonal contraceptives also alter the production of cervical mucus, making it less acceptable to sperm; alter tubal mobility; and alter the endometrial lining of the uterus, making it inhospitable to implantation.
- ▼ Sterilization includes tubal ligation for women and vasectomy for men. With tubal ligation the fallopian tubes are cut, tied, cauterized, plugged, capped, coagulated, or clipped to prevent the passage of ovum from the ovary to the uterus. With vasectomy the vasa deferentia are severed, tied, clipped, or coagulated to prevent sperm from entering the sperm ducts.
- ▼ Nurses involved in family planning use the nursing process to implement interviewing, history taking, teaching, and counseling strategies. Nurses in advanced practice roles may be involved in physical assessment, fitting, and prescription of various birth control methods.

References

Alan Guttmacher Institute (1994). *Sex and America's Teenagers.* New York: Author.

Bagshaw, S. (1995). The combined oral contraceptive. Risks and adverse effects in perspective. *Drug Safety,* 12 (2), 91–96.

Bromham, D. (1993). Intrauterine contraceptive devices—a reappraisal. *British Medical Bulletin,* 49 (1), 100–123.

Brown, K., and Hammond, C. (1989). The risks and benefits of oral contraceptives. *Advances in Internal Medicine,* 34, 285–306.

Chi, I. (1993). What we have learned from recent IUD studies: A researcher's perspective. *Contraception,* 48 (2), 81–108.

Chi, I. (1994). A bill of health for the IUD: Where do we go from here? *Advances in Contraception,* 10 (2), 121–131.

Cunningham, F., MacDonald, P., Gant, N., Leveno, K., Gilstrap, L. (1993). *Williams Obstetrics (19th ed.).* Norwalk, CT: Appleton & Lange.

Davis, M. (1992). Natural family planning. *Clinical Issues in Perinatal and Women's Health Nursing,* 3 (2), 280–290.

Eichhorst, B. (1989). Contraception. *Primary Care,* 15 (3), 437–459.

Erwin, P. (1994). To use or not use combined hormonal oral contraceptives during lactation. *Family Planning Perspectives,* 26 (1), 26–30, 33.

Farley, T., Meirik, O., Mehta, J. S., Waites, G. (1993). The safety of vasectomy: Recent concerns. *Bulletin of the World Health Organization,* 71 (3–4), 413–419.

Farr, G., Gabelnick, H., Sturgen, K., Dorflinger, L. (1994). Contraceptive efficacy and acceptability of the female condom. *American Journal of Public Health,* 84 (12), 1960–1964.

Faundes, A., Elias, C., Coggins, C. (1994). Spermicides and barrier contraception. *Current Opinion in Obstetrics and Gynecology,* 6 (6), 552–558.

Fehring, R. J. (1990). Methods used to self-predict ovulation: A comparative study. *Journal of Obstetric, Gynecologic, and Neonatal Nursing,* 19 (3), 233–237.

Fehring, R. J. (1991). New technology in natural family planning. *Journal of Obstetric, Gynecologic, and Neonatal Nursing,* 20 (3), 199–205.

Fehring, R., Dawrence, D., Philpot, C. (1994). Use effectiveness of the Creighton model ovulation method of natural family planning. *Journal of Obstetric, Gynecologic, and Neonatal Nursing,* 23 (4), 303–309.

Ferreira, A., Araujo, M., Regina, C., Diniz, S., Faundes, A. (1993). Effectiveness of the diaphragm, used continuously, without spermicide. *Contraception,* 48 (1), 29–35.

Foxwell, M. (1994). Natural family planning. *Modern Midwife,* 4 (3), 21–24.

Hatcher, R., and Warner, D. (1992). New condoms for men and women, diaphragms, cervical caps, and spermicides: Overcoming barriers to barriers and spermicides. *Current Opinion in Obstetrics and Gynecology,* 4 (4), 513–521.

Hatcher, R., Trussell, J., Stewart, F., Stewart, G., Kowal, D., Guest, F., Cates, W., Policar, M. (1994). *Contraceptive Technology* (16th ed.). New York: Irvington Publishers, Inc.

Hilgers, T., Daly, K., Prebil, A., Hilgers, S. (1992). Cumulative pregnancy rates in patients with apparently normal fertility and fertility-focused intercourse. *Journal of Reproductive Medicine,* 37 (10), 864–866.

Hinkle, L. (1994). Education and counseling for Norplant users. *Journal of Obstetric, Gynecologic, and Neonatal Nursing,* 23 (5), 387–392.

Horton, J. (1995). *The Women's Health Data Book* (2nd ed.). Washington, D.C.: The Jacobs Institute of Women's Health.

Hutchings, J., Benson, P., Perkin, G., Soderstrom, R. (1985). The IUD after 20 years: A review. *Family Planning Perspectives,* 17 (6), 244–255.

Johnson, J. (1985). Individual versus group education in family planning clinics. *Family Planning Perspectives,* 17 (6), 244–255.

Kovacs, G., Jarman, H., Dunn, K., Dip, M., Baker, H. W. (1986). The contraceptive diaphragm: Is it an acceptable method in the 1980s? *Australian and New Zealand Journal of Obstetrics and Gynecology,* 26, 76–77.

Kubba, A., and Guillebaud, J. (1993). Combined oral contraceptives: Acceptability and effective use. *British Medical Bulletin,* 49 (1), 140–157.

Kugel, C., and Verson, H. (1986). Relationship between weight change and diaphragm size change. *Journal of Obstetric, Gynecologic, and Neonatal Nursing,* 15 (2), 123–129.

Kurtzman, C., and Block, D. (1986). Family planning: Beyond contraception. *MCN,* 11 (5), 340–343.

Lethbridge, D. (1989). The use of breastfeeding as a contraceptive. *Journal of Obstetric, Gynecologic, and Neonatal Nursing,* 18 (1), 31–37.

Lethbridge, D. (1991). Coitus interruptus: Considerations as a method of birth control. *Journal of Obstetric, Gynecologic, and Neonatal Nursing,* 20 (1), 80–85.

Libbus, M. K. (1992). Condoms as primary prevention in sexually active women. *MCN,* 17 (5), 256–260.

Loucks, A. (1989). A comparison of satisfaction with types of diaphragms among women in a college population. *Journal of Obstetric, Gynecologic, and Neonatal Nursing,* 18 (3), 194–200.

Loudon, N., Glasier, A., Gebbie, A. (1995). *Handbook of Family Planing and Reproductive Health Care* (3rd ed.). New York: Churchill Livingstone.

Mishell, D. (1989). Contraception. *New England Journal of Medicine,* 320 (12), 777–787.

Monier, M., and Laird, M. (1989). Contraception: A look at the future. *American Journal of Nursing,* 89 (4), 496–499.

Moore, R. (1994). Contraception issues and options for young women. *AWHONN's Contemporary Studies in Women's Health.* Fair Lawn, NJ: MPE Communications, Inc.

NAACOG. (1991). Contraceptive options. *OGN Nursing Practice Resources.* Washington, D.C.: Author.

Queenan, J. T., Jennings, V. H., Spieler, J. M., von Hertzen, H. (1991a). Natural family planning: Current knowledge and new strategies for the 1990s. Part I. *American Journal of Obstetrics and Gynecology,* [Supplement], 165 (6), 1979–2078.

Queenan, J. T., Jennings, V. H., Spieler, J. M., von Hertzen, H. (1991b). *Natural family planning: Current knowledge and new strategies for the 1990s. Part II.* Washington, D.C.: WHO and Institute for International Studies in Natural Family Planning, Georgetown University.

Reinprayoon, D. (1992). Intrauterine contraception. *Current Opinion in Obstetrics and Gynecology,* 4 (4), 527–530.

Rivera, R., Chi, I., Farr, G. (1993). The intrauterine device in the present and future. *Current Opinion in Obstetrics and Gynecology,* 5 (6), 829–832.

Shoupe, D., and Mishell, D. R. (1989). Norplant: Subdermal implant system for long-term contraception. *American Journal of Obstetrics and Gynecology,* 160 (5), 1286–1292.

Soper, D. E., Brockwell, N. J., Dalton, H. P. (1991). Evaluation of the effects of a female condom on the female lower genital tract. *Contraception,* 44, 21–29.

Woolley, R. (1991). Contraception—a look forward. Part I: New spermicides and natural family planning. *Journal of American Board of Family Practice,* 4 (1), 33–46.

Chapter 12

Infertility

Catherine H. Garner

> How do we, the infertile, . . . explain the yearning that drives couples to subject themselves over the course of years to all sorts of drugs and surgeries, to torture themselves through four, five, and six attempts at in vitro fertilization (IVF)? . . . All we are saying to those who do not understand our feelings, our efforts, our obsession, is we want a child of our own to love. . . . We want only to hold a child in our arms.
>
> D. Clements (1988)

HIGHLIGHTS

- Demographics and Incidence of Infertility
- Essential Conditions for Conception
- Ovulation Disorders
- Male Infertility Factors
- Cervical, Tubal, and Pelvic Infertility Factors
- Endometrial Development Infertility Factors
- Unexplained Infertility
- Common Infertility Conditions
- Assisted Reproductive Technologies
- Nursing Practice
- Risk Management
- Implications for Research

Infertility is a condition affecting many couples in their childbearing years. In 1988, of the nearly 58 million women of childbearing age in the United States, approximately 1 in 12, or 4.9 million, reported difficulty in becoming pregnant. About half of these women were childless, while slightly more than half had one or more births before they experienced difficulty in conceiving further pregnancies (Mosher and Pratt 1990). There has been a tremendous explosion of the knowledge base regarding human reproduction in the last decade, with significant advances in medical therapies. Yet, with expert diagnosis and care, only 50 percent to 60 percent of these couples can expect to achieve a pregnancy. This presents a tremendous challenge to nurses who care for couples who are infertile. As many as 20 percent of couples delivering babies may have had infertility problems and have unique needs for nursing care during the maternity cycle (Garner 1991).

Approximately 1.35 million women (23 percent of women of reproductive age) reported using infertility services in 1987, about 264,000 more than in 1982 (Office of Technology Assessment [OTA] 1988; Pratt et al. 1984). The number of women seeking infertility services in 1988 was 25 percent higher

DEFINITIONS

Artificial insemination—A procedure in which an ejaculated semen sample is collected and placed directly into a woman's vagina or cervix by use of a catheter and a cervical cap. The sperm may be from the woman's partner or from a donor.

Endometriosis—A condition in which tissue containing typical endometrial elements grows outside of the uterus in the pelvic cavity or some other area of the body.

Gamete intrafallopian transfer (GIFT)—A variation of the IVF procedure in which oocytes are removed, identified, and then placed with sperm into the end of a fallopian tube by laparoscopic surgery. Fertilization is allowed to occur naturally within the body.

Infertility—The inability to conceive a child after a year or more of regular unprotected intercourse or the inability to carry a pregnancy to live birth (recurrent miscarriages).

Intrauterine insemination—This procedure is one of the simplest fertility treatments and is often performed in conjunction with drug therapy. Sperm from the partner or a donor is shuttled with a catheter into the uterus, where fertilization may occur.

In vitro fertilization (IVF)—A procedure in which mature oocytes are removed from the ovaries and placed together with sperm in a Petri dish to aid fertilization. After fertilization occurs, embryos are transferred by a small catheter into the uterus, where they may implant.

Laparoscopy—The insertion of a telescope-like instrument through a small umbilical incision. A second incision at the pubic hairline is made to allow the insertion of a probe for manipulation of the pelvic organs.

Pelvic inflammatory disease (PID)—A general term for inflammation of the female genital tract. PID is caused by a number of microorganisms, most often gonococcal or chlamydial infections, and can produce irreparable damage to fallopian tubes, resulting in infertility and ectopic (tubal) pregnancies.

Postcoital test—A microscopic examination of mucus taken from the cervix within 24 hours of intercourse to evaluate sperm-mucus interaction.

Primary infertility—Occurs when the female partner has no history of pregnancy.

Secondary infertility—A condition when previous pregnancy has occurred regardless of the outcome.

Selective reduction—A procedure sometimes used during pregnancy when there are multiple fetuses to reduce the number of fetuses.

Surrogacy—A woman is paid, or volunteers, to have an embryo implanted and to carry the child to term. The egg may come from the legal or surrogate mother, the sperm from the legal father or a donor.

Therapeutic donor insemination—Insemination with donor semen.

Zygote intrafallopian transfer (ZIFT)—A variation of the IVF or GIFT procedure in which eggs fertilized in a Petri dish (zygotes) are placed in the woman's fallopian tubes, where they may move on their own to the uterus.

than in 1982 (Mosher and Pratt 1990). However, an analysis of the use of infertility services in 1988 revealed that only 43 percent of the women who reported impaired fertility had obtained some type of infertility service (Wilcox and Mosher 1993).

Since the early 1970s, the number of babies available for adoption has steadily declined because of increased availability of effective methods of birth control, legalized abortion, and a trend for single women to keep their babies (Kabanitz et al. 1987). As a result of this change in the number of babies available for adoption, consumer demand for medical care to treat infertility has increased. The need for medical infertility services is expected to continue to rise owing to the number of women seeking treatment, the availability of new drugs and treatments, and the growing number of physicians specializing in infertility.

THE INFERTILITY PROBLEM

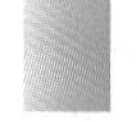

Demographics

Infertility is defined as the inability to conceive a child after a year or more of regular unprotected intercourse or the inability to carry a pregnancy

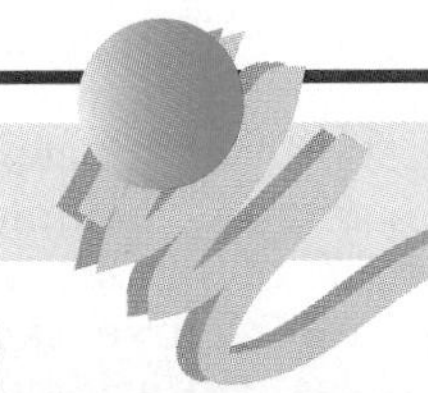

HISTORICAL PERSPECTIVES

ASSISTED REPRODUCTION

1799 First pregnancy reported from artificial insemination

1935 Animal research on in vitro fertilization begins

1944 First attempt at in vitro fertilization

1949 Researchers discover that glycerol can be used to freeze sperm for later use

1951 First successful transfer of an embryo from one cow to another

1952 First calf produced with use of frozen semen
Frogs cloned from the cells of tadpoles

1953 Frozen sperm used for human artificial insemination

1959 Live rabbit offspring from in vitro fertilization

1970 Mice embryos are cloned

1972 Live offspring from frozen mouse embryos

1973 First calf produced from a frozen embryo

1978 First test-tube baby, Louise Brown, born in Britain
First National Commission convened by the U.S. Secretary of Health, Education, and Welfare to address the ethical aspects of in vitro fertilization

1979 Sheep embryos cloned

1980 Cattle embryos cloned

1981 First test-tube baby, Elizabeth Carr, born in the United States

1983 A baby is born to a mother from an embryo formed by her husband's sperm and a donor's egg

1984 Australian girl, named Zoe, born from a frozen embryo

1986 Surrogate mother Mary Beth Whitehead of New Jersey refuses to relinquish her daughter, sparking landmark court case

1993 George Washington University researchers clone human embryos

1994 Guidelines on Human Embryo Research released by the National Institutes of Health

Excerpted from Elmer-Dewitt, P. (1993). Cloning: Where do we draw the line? *Time*, November 8, 142 (19), 64–70.

to live birth (recurrent miscarriages). Primary infertility occurs when the female partner has no history of pregnancy. Secondary infertility is a condition when previous pregnancy has occurred regardless of the outcome.

Data from the National Survey of Family Growth on infertility among married women have been collected since 1965. Data from the 1988 survey indicate that there has been virtually no change in the proportion of infertile couples reported since the prior survey in 1982 (Mosher and Pratt 1990). Despite these findings, there is a public perception of increasing infertility. Although the proportion of couples who are considered infertile has remained stable, the number of childless women aged 25 to 44 years is increasing because of the aging of the baby boom cohort and the tendency of this group to delay marriage and childbearing (Mosher and Pratt 1990; OTA 1988). Infertility increases with age, as shown in the 1988 data (Table 12–1). Infertility increases from 4.1 percent at ages 15 to 24 years to 21.4 percent at ages 35 to 44 years.

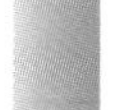

Incidence

The evaluation of an infertile couple should include both partners. The conditions necessary for normal conception to occur include female factors, male factors, and the interaction of both female and male factors (Table 12–2). Forty percent of infertility can be expected to be due to a male factor, 40 percent to a female factor, and 20 percent to both. Even in situations in which the problem seems apparent, evaluating only one partner is inappropriate because of the high incidence of multiple problems.

A couple attempting pregnancy should seek medical help if pregnancy is not achieved after 1 year of regular, unprotected intercourse. In a nor-

Table 12–1

PERCENTAGE OF WOMEN WITH IMPAIRED FECUNDITY IN THE UNITED STATES

PARITY AND AGE (YEARS)	ALL WOMEN		CURRENTLY MARRIED WOMEN	
	1982	1988	1982	1988
All parities				
15–44	8	8	11	11
15–24	4	5	9	8
25–34	10	10	10	11
35–44	12	11	13	11
Parity 0				
15–44	8	9	22	20
15–24	4	4	11	8
25–34	15	13	21	20
35–44	26	21	48	36
Parity 1 or more				
15–44	8	8	8	8
15–24	5	8	7*	7
25–34	8	8	7	8
35–44	10	8	10	9

*Statistic does not meet standard of reliability or precision.

Reprinted with permission from the Jacobs Institute of Women's Health. Horton, J. A., editor: The Women's Health Data Book, Second Edition. WOMEN'S HEALTH ISSUES, Vol. No. 5, Copyright 1995—Spring Supplement.

mal couple, conception is expected to be 60 percent at 6 months, 90 percent at 12 months, and 95 percent at 24 months (Garner 1991).

The frequency of intercourse can have a significant impact on fertility rates. If a couple has intercourse once a week for 6 months, there is only about a 15 percent chance of pregnancy. If a couple increases intercourse to four times per week around the time of ovulation, the rate of conception increases to 83 percent for 6 months. Simple counseling about the expected time of ovulation and the timing and frequency of intercourse can often resolve the problem, and couples will achieve a pregnancy (Garner 1991).

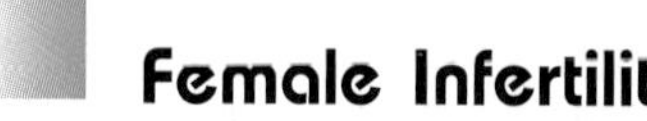

Female Infertility

The most significant contributor to the increase in female infertility is delayed childbearing. Although fertility rates in the United States are at historically low levels, one age group is having more babies—those women 30 to 34 years old. This is occurring as women delay childbearing to pursue advanced education and careers. This is significant because the age of maximal fertility in both men and women is 24 years. Women older than 30 years have a higher incidence of ovulation problems and of endometriosis, and a greater length of time to be exposed to sexually transmitted diseases, all of which can cause infertility.

The second major factor for female infertility is the sequela of pelvic inflammatory disease (PID). Women are at higher risk for sexually transmitted diseases when they become sexually active at a younger age, have more than one sex partner, and change partners more frequently. The most important sexually transmitted disease among American women today is PID, a general term for inflammation of the female genital tract. PID is caused by a number of microorganisms and can produce irreparable damage to fallopian tubes, resulting in infertility and ectopic (tubal) pregnancies. PID is most often caused by gonococcal or chlamydial infection. About 10 percent to 20 percent of these infections will develop into acute

Table 12–2

ESSENTIAL CONDITIONS NECESSARY FOR NORMAL CONCEPTION

FEMALE FACTORS	MALE FACTORS	FEMALE AND MALE INTERACTION FACTORS
• Regular ovulation • Open, anatomically normal fallopian tubes • Endometrium capable of fostering implantation • Pelvic cavity free of disease	• Normal sperm count, motility, and morphology	• Normal sperm–cervical mucus interaction

PID. The incidence of ectopic pregnancy and sterility rises greatly with each episode of PID. The most common female problems related to infertility are ovulation disorders, tubal disease, and endometriosis.

There is no evidence that the use of the birth control pill or abortion contributes to infertility (Fraser and Weisberg 1982). Women who use the intrauterine device (IUD) as a method of contraception and who are at high risk for PID because of sexual behaviors do have a higher incidence of tubal infertility. Several studies of women seeking treatment for infertility suggest that caffeine consumption is linked to reduced fertility (Amar 1994). While the association between caffeine and infertility requires further investigation, it is clear that a healthy lifestyle includes a well-balanced diet, exercise, and avoidance of drugs and substances such as caffeine. A healthy lifestyle is important for individuals seeking to achieve pregnancy.

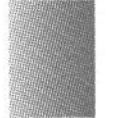

Male Infertility

Male infertility has been thought to be increasing, although much of this documented increase may be due to more sophisticated testing. The common causes of male infertility are shown in Table 12–3. Male fertility declines much more slowly than female fertility, with no real significant change in sperm count until after age 55 years. Even then, men can father children throughout their life span.

Table 12–3

COMMON CAUSES OF MALE INFERTILITY

LIFESTYLE HABITS	OTHER
Smoking	Testicular damage
Medications	Infections (systemic)
Thermal exposure	Prostate infection
Steroids	Testicular torsion
Marijuana use	Sexually transmitted diseases
	Mumps (after adolescence)
	Radiation
	Pelvic surgery
	Undescended testicles
	Cystic fibrosis
	Varicocele
	Antisperm antibodies
	Ejaculatory failure
	Hypospadias

INFERTILITY EVALUATION

The purpose of the infertility evaluation is to document the normal or abnormal functioning of the man and woman. Diagnostic tests with the purpose and timing of each test are shown in Table 12–4.

Essential Conditions for Conception

The infertility evaluation should proceed in a logical fashion, starting with the basics. First, a women must ovulate on a regular basis for conception to occur. A woman who experiences menstrual periods at regular intervals (every 26 to 38 days) is presumed to be ovulating. Menstrual periods often vary by a few days from month to month. It is rare that a woman menstruates every 28 days month after month.

The male partner must ejaculate a sufficient number of normal, motile sperm to achieve conception. The semen analysis is the fundamental first test for evaluating the man. Once ejaculation occurs with intercourse, spermatozoa are nourished by mucus secreted from the cervical mucous glands. Sperm are housed in cervical crypts and are intermittently released into the uterus as long as the cervical mucus remains receptive, a condition created by high estrogen levels in the middle of the menstrual cycle. Cervical mucus is generally receptive to sperm for 48 to 72 hours, around the time of ovulation. At other times, the cervical mucus is hostile and blocks sperm transport and survival. A postcoital test is a microscopic examination of mucus taken from the cervix within 24 hours of intercourse. Mucus is examined for clarity, consistency, and spinbarkeit (a stretchy characteristic), properties that are consistent with sperm transport and survival. The presence of motile sperm in the mucus is indicative of normal sperm-mucus interaction.

Fallopian tubes must be open and anatomically normal for conception to occur in the outer third of the fallopian tube. Assessment of the tubes and of the uterine contour is accomplished with an x-ray examination or hysterosalpingography.

The developing embryo enters the uterine cavity and begins implantation into the endometrial lining. Endometrial development is a systematic process subject to disruption by hormonal insufficiency. Failure of implantation may be due to fail-

Table 12–4

INFERTILITY EVALUATION

TEST	PURPOSE	TIMING
Basal body temperature	Document ovulation	Chart entire cycle
Postcoital test	Evaluate sperm survival in cervical mucus	1 to 2 days before ovulation
Hysterosalpingography	X-ray study of the uterus and tubes	After menses, before ovulation
Endometrial biopsy	Evaluate maturity of the uterine lining for implantation	1 to 2 days before expected menses
Laparoscopy	Visualize the pelvis	Before ovulation
Semen analysis	Evaluate sperm count, motility, morphology, volume, and pH	After 2 days, but no longer than 1 wk of abstinence
Antisperm antibodies	Document presence of antibodies in male serum and semen, female serum and cervical mucus	Variable
Sperm penetration assay	Evaluate ability of sperm to penetrate egg	After 2 days, but no longer than 1 wk of abstinence

ure of the embryo or abnormal development of the endometrium. Failure of the endometrial development, called a luteal phase defect, is a factor in as many as a third of first-trimester spontaneous abortions. An endometrial biopsy is the test performed to assess the development of the endometrium.

Diseases of the pelvis, such as endometriosis or multiple pelvic adhesions from PID, can also cause infertility by distorting the normal ovarian-tubal anatomy. A woman may or may not have a history of pelvic pain or pelvic infections. After these factors have been evaluated, the pelvic organs should be evaluated surgically for endometriosis, adhesions, and other abnormalities by use of laparoscopy.

Phases of the Infertility Evaluation

The infertility evaluation starts with a detailed history of the woman and man (see Assessment Tool) and can then be divided into phases looking at six areas: (1) ovulation; (2) male factors; (3) sperm-mucus interaction; (4) tubal and uterine anatomy; (5) endometrial sufficiency; and (6) pelvic factors. Testing can be organized to evaluate these factors according to the menstrual cycle in a women who is menstruating regularly (Fig. 12–1). A semen analysis can be obtained at any time that can be coordinated with the laboratory. A postcoital test is done to evaluate sperm-mucus interaction at midcycle around the time of ovulation. Hysterosalpingography, or x-ray examination of the tubes, is performed after menstruation but before ovulation. Biopsy of the uterine lining to assess endometrial development is accomplished 1 to 2 days before expected menses. Five sixths of the infertility evaluation can thus be accomplished in one menstrual cycle in the ovulatory woman. Once these factors have been evaluated, a diagnostic laparoscopy is performed to assess whether factors such as pelvic adhesions or endometriosis are present in the pelvis. This testing should be done in an efficient and logical sequence to minimize the stress and cost to the couple.

When a woman is anovulatory, a hysterosalpingogram and a sperm count of the man are done first. The next step is to induce ovulation so that the woman has the opportunity to become pregnant. Once ovulation has been induced, the clinician performs a postcoital test and endometrial biopsy. If pregnancy does not occur in 6 to 12 months of ovulation, laparoscopy should be performed.

At the start of the infertility evaluation, the nurse should explain the components of the infertility investigation, their purpose, and the reasons for exact timing. The rigid scheduling is often difficult for the couple, particularly if they have to travel some distance or arrange time away from the workplace. Where slight variations in time or date of appointment are reasonable, allowing a couple to choose the day and the time of the appointment provides some measure of control.

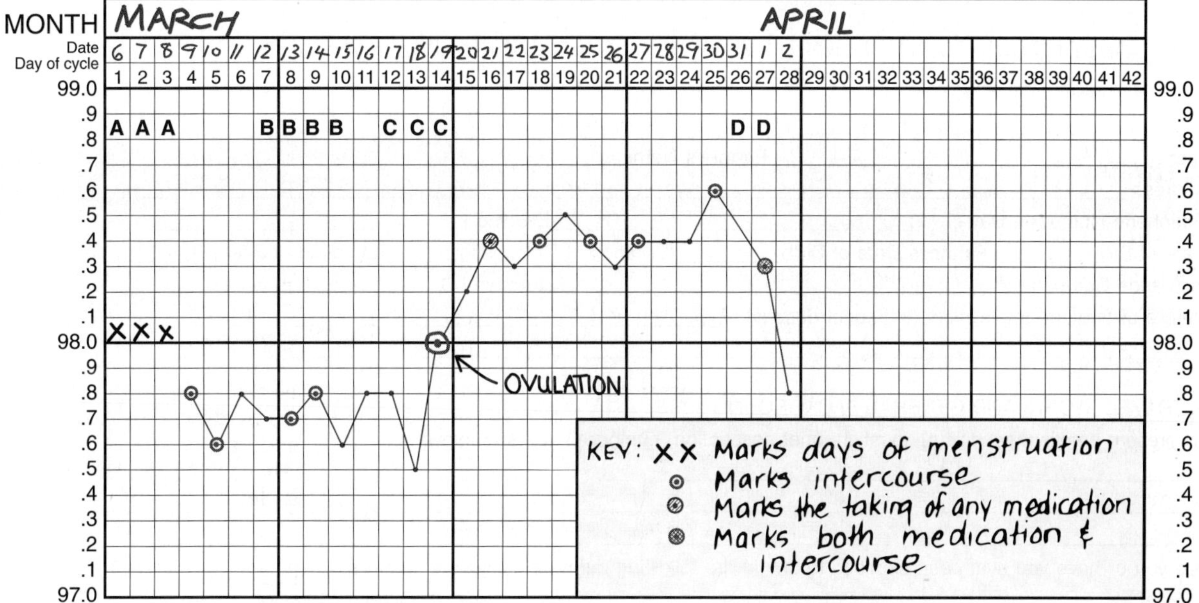

Figure 12–1

The basal body temperature graph charts infertility testing intervals. Testing intervals are represented by A, semen analysis; B, hysterosalpingography; C, postcoital test; and D, endometrial biopsy. (From Garner, C., *An Overview of Infertility,* 4, in *Principles of Infertility Nursing,* Garner, C., Ed., CRC Press, Boca Raton, FL, ©1991. With permission.)

Ovulation Disorders

Disorders of ovulation account for 20 percent to 30 percent of factors affecting women. Documentation of regular menstrual cycles (every 24 to 38 days) with premenstrual symptoms can be considered presumptive evidence of ovulation. Another way to document ovulation is with the use of a temperature chart. A woman takes her temperature every morning before any activity and records this on the chart. During the first half of the cycle, because of the influence of estrogen, the temperature is usually below 98°F. Within 24 hours after ovulation, because of the influence of progesterone, the temperature rises approximately 1°F. This is called a biphasic temperature chart (see Chapter 9). Ovulation can be documented only in retrospect; therefore, it cannot be used to time intercourse.

Extensive evaluation is necessary if the woman has had episodes of irregular bleeding, a time lapse of more than 40 days between periods, significant weight loss or gain, excessive facial or body hair, or history of discharge from the breast.

DESCRIPTION

Disorders may originate in the hypothalamus, ovary, or pituitary, or they may be due to congenital anomalies of the reproductive tract. In rare cases, a chromosomal anomaly may first manifest as absence of menses. An evaluation of pituitary function should include determination of follicle stimulating hormone (FSH), luteinizing hormone (LH), and prolactin levels and thyroid function tests. Physical examination is necessary to ascertain normal development of secondary sexual characteristics (breast, pubic hair, and ancillary hair). Since estrogen produced by the ovary is necessary for development of breasts and pubic hair, this implies a normally functioning ovary. Physical examination of the vaginal opening and pelvic palpation of the uterus and ovaries are necessary to document a normal reproductive tract. If a girl has not started development of secondary sexual characteristics by age 14 years, she should be evaluated by a pediatric or reproductive endocrinologist. Precocious puberty, or puberty before 8 years of age, should also be evaluated by a specialist.

The most common cause of amenorrhea is pregnancy. Pregnancy must be ruled out first, even in a young woman who has not started menstruation, as pregnancy can occur with the first ovulation. Stress, excessive exercise, and eating disorders such as anorexia nervosa can cause a disruption in the release of gonadotropin releasing hormone (Gn-RH) from the hypothalamus. In this case, the normal stimulus to the pituitary is disrupted, and FSH levels drop. Without the stimulus from FSH, the ovary stops estrogen secretion. Thus, the woman who desires pregnancy may need medication to start the cycle leading to ovulation. The woman who does not desire pregnancy immediately will need estrogen replacement with a low-dose oral contraceptive to protect her bones from osteoporosis (Flynn 1991).

Text continued on page 286

Assessment Tool: Combined Female and Male Patient History

I. IDENTIFYING INFORMATION

Date_______________

Name_______________ Partner's Name_______________

Address _______________

Telephone Number—Day ( )_______________Evening ( ) _______________

Date of Birth________ Partner's Date of Birth_________ Duration of Relationship_____ Duration of Infertility _____

Insurance Company_______________ Insurance I.D. # _______________

Nature of present employment (title, brief description) _______________

II. TRAVEL, WORK, AND GENERAL BACKGROUND

All present employment: title(s), location, brief description, number of years employed

Are you or have you ever been exposed to any of the following during employment or military service:

☐ Heat ☐ Toxic fumes ☐ Other—Specify:_______________

☐ Chemicals ☐ Nuclear radiation

III. MEDICAL HISTORY

	YES	NO
Weight__________ Height__________ Blood Type (if known) __________		
Have you lost greater than 20 pounds of weight in the last year?	☐	☐
Do you follow a particular food diet or have any special dietary habits?	☐	☐
If yes, specify: __________		
List the forms and frequency of regular vigorous exercise (swimming, cycling, running) and age you began:		
Exercise:__________ hr/wk__________ age__________ Exercise:__________ hr/wk__________ age __________		
Have you ever had pelvic surgery?	☐	☐
If yes, specify date and type: __________		

Do you have or have you ever had (check all that apply):

☐ Anemia
☐ Appendicitis
☐ Arthritis
☐ Blood transfusions
☐ Breast milky discharge
☐ Breast soreness
☐ Breast tenderness
☐ Cancer? Specify _______________
☐ Chlamydia
☐ Chronic bronchitis
☐ Chronic headaches
☐ Colitis
☐ Color blindness
☐ Cystic fibrosis
☐ Diabetes
☐ Dizziness
☐ Endometriosis
☐ Epilepsy
☐ Gallbladder problems
☐ Gonorrhea
☐ Heart disease
☐ Hepatitis
☐ Herpes
☐ High blood pressure
☐ Hirsutism (excess hair growth)
☐ Immunization: German measles
☐ Kidney infection
☐ Liver problems
☐ Loss of balance
☐ Measles: German
☐ Measles: regular
☐ Mumps
☐ Mumps with testes involved
☐ Neurological problems
☐ Nongonococcal urethritis
☐ Ovarian cysts
☐ Parasitic infection
☐ Pelvic infection
☐ Pneumonia
☐ Poor sense of smell
☐ Prostatitis
☐ Rheumatic fever
☐ Scarlet fever
☐ Seizures
☐ Syphilis
☐ Testes infection
☐ Testes injury
☐ Testes tumor
☐ Thyroid problems
☐ Tuberculosis
☐ Ulcers
☐ Vaginitis (trichomoniasis, yeast) # of episodes_______________
☐ Visual disturbances
☐ Any allergies: List_______________

	YES	NO
Have you ever been treated for cancer?.	☐	☐
If yes, explain therapy:__________		
Have you ever received x-rays to the pelvic area for therapy or diagnosis?	☐	☐
If yes, specify: __________		

Continued on facing page

Assessment Tool: Combined Female and Male Patient History **Continued**

Within the last year, have you taken any prescription medications? . . . . ☐ ☐

If yes, list all prescriptions and problems for which you were taking them: ______________________________

____

Are you taking any over-the-counter medications on a regular basis? . . . . ☐ ☐

If yes, list all medications and diagnoses: ______________________________________

____

Do you use or have you ever used (check all that apply):

☐ Alcohol—How many glasses per week do you usually drink? Wine________ Beer________ Cocktails _______

☐ Cigarettes—Number of packs per day_________

☐ Illicit or Recreational Drugs (marijuana, cocaine, etc.) If you would feel more comfortable not writing anything down, please discuss this directly with your physician. Specify: ______________________________

____

IV. MENSTRUAL AND PREGNANCY HISTORY — YES NO

Age at first period?____________ When was your last period?______________________________

Are your periods regular? . . . . ☐ ☐

If yes, what is the usual number of days between periods? ______________________________

If no, how many times per year do you menstruate?______________________________

What is the usual duration of your period?______________________________ Use: ☐ Tampons? ☐ Pads?

Are cramps present before, during, or after your period? ______________________________

Are cramps: ☐ Mild ☐ Moderate ☐ Severe

Do you have to take pain medication for cramps? . . . . ☐ ☐

If yes, specify medication: ______________________________

Do you bleed or spot between periods? . . . . ☐ ☐

How many pregnancies (including abortions) have you had? ______________________________

	When? (year)	End in abortion?	End in miscarriage?	Ectopic pregnancy?	Infertility therapy required to conceive?	How long to conceive?	Baby born alive?	Is current partner the father?
1st Pregnancy								
2nd Pregnancy								
3rd Pregnancy								
4th Pregnancy								
5th Pregnancy								

Were there any complications during or after your pregnancies? . . . . ☐ ☐

If yes, explain: ______________________________

Did your mother have any difficulty with conception or pregnancy? . . . . ☐ ☐

If yes, explain: ______________________________

How long have you now been trying to get pregnant? ______________________________

Did your mother take diethylstilbestrol (DES) when she was pregnant with you? . . . . ☐ ☐

V. CONTRACEPTIVE AND SEXUAL HISTORY (Female) — YES NO

What form of contraception do you use now or have you used in the past? Check all that apply:

☐ Pill's Name______________ ☐ IUD Name:__________ ☐ Diaphragm ☐ Withdrawal ☐ Foams/Jellies

☐ Condom ☐ Rhythm ☐ None ☐ Other: ______________________________

For each contraceptive method used, specify length of use and reason for discontinuation:

Method	Length of Use	Reason for Discontinuation

If you've ever been on oral contraceptives (pills), were your periods regular after stopping the pills? . . . . ☐ ☐

Continued on following page

Assessment Tool: Combined Female and Male Patient History Continued

	YES	NO
How many times per week do you and your partner have sexual intercourse? ______		
How many times do you have intercourse around ovulation? ______		
Is intercourse painful or difficult for you?	☐	☐
Do you use lubricants for intercourse?	☐	☐
If yes, which one? ______		
Do you douche before or after intercourse?	☐	☐

SEXUAL HISTORY (Male)	YES	NO
Are you circumcised?	☐	☐
When you were a child, were both testes descended into the scrotum?	☐	☐
At what age did you begin shaving regularly or start to grow a beard? ______		
How many times have you been married? ______		
Have you ever produced a child with another partner?	☐	☐
If yes, how long did it take to produce a child? ______ When was this (dates)? ______		
Have you ever *tried* to produce a child with another partner?	☐	☐
Do you have trouble getting an erection?	☐	☐
Maintaining an erection?	☐	☐
Do you have trouble with ejaculations?	☐	☐
If yes: ☐ premature ejaculations? ☐ retrograde ejaculations?		
Do you feel that some of your ejaculate is deposited in the vagina?	☐	☐
Do you ever have orgasms without ejaculation during masturbation?	☐	☐
Do you have any discharge from the penis?	☐	☐
How many times per week do you and your partner now have intercourse? ______		
How many times do you have intercourse around ovulation? ______		
Have you noticed a change in your sexual drive recently?	☐	☐

VI. FAMILY HISTORY	YES	NO
Is there a family history of infertility?	☐	☐
If yes, who (list all members and relationship to you): ______		
Is there a history of hormonal disorders in your family?	☐	☐
If yes, who and what type: ______		

VII. HISTORY OF FERTILITY THERAPY	YES	NO
Have you been treated for infertility before?	☐	☐
If yes, who was your physician? ______		
What cause of infertility was diagnosed? ______		

What drugs have you taken for infertility? Check all that apply:

☐ clomiphene citrate (Serophene, Clomid)	☐ Gn-RH or LH-RH (Factrel)
☐ hMG (Pergonal)	☐ hCG (Profasi, A.P.L.)
☐ estrogens	☐ bromocriptine (Parlodel)
☐ progesterone	☐ fluoxymesterone (Halotestin)
☐ prednisone (or cortisone-like drugs)	☐ danazol (Danocrine)
☐ antibiotics	☐ urofollitropin or FSH (Metrodin)
☐ tamoxifen	☐ Other—Specify: ______
☐ testolactone	☐ None

Female

Which of the following tests have you had performed? Check all that apply and the results if known:

☐ Basal body temperature	When? ______	Results: ______
☐ Postcoital test	When? ______	Results: ______

Continued on facing page

Assessment Tool: Combined Female and Male Patient History **Continued**

			YES	NO
☐ Hormonal assays (FSH, LH, prolactin, estrogen, DHEA-S, testosterone, progesterone)	When?______	Results: ______		
☐ Endometrial biopsy	When?______	Results: ______		
☐ Hysterosalpingography	When?______	Results: ______		
☐ Ultrasound	When?______	Results: ______		
☐ Antibodies	When?______	Results: ______		
☐ Laparoscopy, hysteroscopy	When?______	Results: ______		
☐ Mycoplasma and chlamydia cultures	When?______	Results: ______		
☐ Thyroid tests	When?______	Results: ______		
☐ Other—Specify:______	When?______	Results: ______		

Have you ever had surgery for tubal reversal? . . . . ☐ ☐

If yes, specify dates: ______

Have you ever had surgery for lysis of adhesions? . . . . ☐ ☐

Have you ever had cervical conization or cautery? . . . . ☐ ☐

Have you ever had any other surgery (D&C, ovarian, appendectomy, thyroid)? . . . . ☐ ☐

If yes, please specify: ______

Have you ever undergone artificial insemination or in vitro fertilization? . . . . ☐ ☐

If yes, using partner or donor sperm? ______

Is your partner seeing a doctor for evaluation of infertility? . . . . ☐ ☐

If yes, specify physician name and location: ______

Does the doctor feel that your partner has an infertility problem? . . . . ☐ ☐

If yes, what is the diagnosis and how is he being treated?______

Has he ever fathered a child with another woman? . . . . ☐ ☐

If yes, when? ______

Male

Have you ever had varicocele repair? . . . . ☐ ☐

If yes, when? ______

Have you ever had vasectomy reversal or repair? . . . . ☐ ☐

If yes, when? ______

Have you and your partner ever tried artificial insemination? . . . . ☐ ☐

If yes: using ☐ your sperm? ☐ donor sperm?

Have you and your partner ever tried in vitro fertilization? . . . . ☐ ☐

If yes, when and explain: ______

Which of the following tests have you had performed? Check all that apply and the results if known:

☐ Semen analysis	When?______	Results: ______
☐ Chlamydia test	When?______	Results: ______
☐ Mycoplasma test	When?______	Results: ______
☐ Antibody test	When?______	Results: ______
☐ Hamster egg test	When?______	Results: ______
☐ Chromosome test	When?______	Results: ______
☐ Testicular biopsy	When?______	Results: ______
☐ X-ray or ultrasound of testes	When?______	Results: ______
☐ Hormonal tests (FSH, LH, prolactin, testosterone)	When?______	Results: ______
☐ Thyroid tests	When?______	Results: ______
☐ Other—Specify:	When?______	Results: ______

Is your partner currently seeing a doctor for evaluation of infertility? . . . . ☐ ☐

If yes, specify physician name and location: ______

Does the doctor feel that your partner has an infertility problem? . . . . ☐ ☐

If yes, what is the diagnosis and how is she being treated?______

______

Has she ever had children with another man? . . . . ☐ ☐

If yes, when? ______

Galactorrhea, or secretions from the breast in the absence of pregnancy or lactation, may signal an elevated serum prolactin level. This often suppresses normal ovulation. An elevated serum prolactin level in reproductive-age women is commonly caused by a pituitary adenoma or by hypothyroidism. More serious disorders must be ruled out with a computed tomographic scan of the pituitary before treatment. Treatment of a benign pituitary adenoma with bromocriptine (Parlodel) usually corrects the anovulation.

An elevated level of FSH may indicate ovarian failure (menopause). Premature ovarian failure may occur in women younger than 40 years and is sometimes related to other autoimmune disorders. Ovarian failure before age 30 years is often correlated with genetic defects and should be evaluated by a reproductive endocrinologist. A low FSH level indicates either a problem with hypothalamic release of Gn-RH or an unresponsive pituitary. This condition is usually easily treated.

Polycystic ovarian disease is a condition associated with hirsutism (male pattern hair growth), obesity, and amenorrhea. The laboratory evaluation will reveal that these women frequently have an elevated LH:FSH ratio (at least 2:1) and increased testosterone or dehydroepiandrosterone (DHEA-S) levels. Treatment involves weight loss, suppression of the ovary with oral contraceptives or Gn-RH agonists, and use of spironolactone (aldosterone) to treat the hirsutism. If the woman desires pregnancy immediately, the choice of therapy is clomiphene citrate. Excessive facial and body hair is greatly disturbing to a woman of any age and should be evaluated to rule out a testosterone-secreting tumor of the ovary or adrenal glands. Hirsutism is readily treated.

MANAGEMENT

Once a diagnosis of the ovulation disorder is made, proper treatment can be started. In cases of imbalance in the hypothalamus-pituitary-ovarian response, ovulation is induced with medication. Ovulation induction medications are often mistakenly referred to as fertility drugs. These medications simply induce ovulation; they do not enhance fertility. In some cases when a woman is already ovulating normally, these drugs can actually decrease fertility. There is a higher incidence of ovulation of multiple oocytes and of multiple births when these drugs are used.

Clomiphene citrate (Clomid, Serophene) is the drug of choice for inducing ovulation. In a normally ovulating woman, a lack of circulating estrogen signals the hypothalamus to release Gn-RH and stimulate the pituitary to release FSH to initiate the menstrual cycle. It is thought that clomiphene citrate binds to estrogen receptors in the pituitary to block them from detecting circulating Gn-RH. The hypothalamus then releases more Gn-RH, stimulating pituitary release of FSH and LH, starting a menstrual cycle (Flynn 1991).

Clomiphene is administered on cycle days 5 to 9 after menses, starting in dosages of 50 mg. Intercourse is recommended every other day from about day 12 or 13 until a rise on the basal body temperature chart is seen. If the woman fails to ovulate at the 5-mg dose, this can be increased to 100 mg in the next cycle. Most pregnancies occur at clomiphene dosages of 50 to 100 mg. Clomiphene can be given in amounts up to 250 mg/day before other therapies are considered. Once ovulation has occurred at a specific dose, there is no advantage to increasing the dose. Among women treated with clomiphene, ovulation is achieved in 75 percent of women and conception in 35 percent of women. Multiple gestations, usually twins, occur in approximately 10 percent to 12 percent of pregnancies. Less than 1 percent of deliveries are triplets or more (Flynn 1991).

Side effects of clomiphene include hot flashes, headaches, ovarian enlargement, and multiple gestation. Other infrequent symptoms include nausea and visual disturbances. The estrogenic properties of clomiphene may cause wild but troubling alterations of mood—lability (rapid mood changes), irritability, or depression. If pregnancy has not resulted in 6 to 12 months of therapy, other medications should be considered.

The next step in ovulation induction is direct stimulation of the ovary with use of Metrodin (FSH) or Pergonal (human menopausal gonadotropins), a preparation of FSH and LH in a 1:1 ratio. This therapy is indicated when women receiving clomiphene fail to ovulate. Dosage is carefully monitored daily by serum estrogen levels and ovarian ultrasound scan. Ovulation is triggered by administration of human chorionic gonadotropin (hCG). Since Pergonal administration often results in the development of multiple follicles, hCG may be withheld when there are more than three mature follicles to limit the chance of multiple gestation. While 80 percent of Pergonal births will be singletons, the multiple gestation rate is 20 percent, with less than 5 percent of that being three or more. If the woman becomes pregnant with more than triplets, the issue of selective reduction of one or more fetuses must then be discussed with the couple. The prospect of aborting one or more of the fetuses can be traumatic for couples and for care providers. The other serious side effect of Pergonal therapy is ovarian hyperstimulation. This syndrome presents with pelvic distention and weight gain (Hahn et al. 1994). Early diagnosis and treatment of ovarian hyperstimulation are essential, as death can result if the condition progresses (Flynn 1991).

Coordination of Ovulation Induction

Instructions regarding the basal body temperature graph are straightforward. Couples should be cautioned not to try to interpret the graph themselves. Nursing care of the woman undergoing ovulation induction requires adequate education of the patient regarding mechanism of action, expected results, and potential side effects. The patient's compliance with specified regimens is essential. Ovulation induction can be expensive and requires a time commitment with Pergonal therapy because of the necessity of daily monitoring. Couples must be carefully counseled about the prospect of multiple births, and this counseling must be documented in the chart.

Egg Donation

While donated sperm have been used for more than 100 years in situations of male infertility, it is only recently that egg donation has been technically possible. The advent of in vitro fertilization (IVF) techniques has provided this solution for female infertility.

Egg donation involves the removal of eggs from one woman (donor) for the purpose of placement in another woman (recipient) with the goal of achieving a pregnancy. The eggs are removed from the donor's ovaries and fertilized in the laboratory with sperm from the recipient's male partner. The developing embryo is then placed in the recipient's uterus, where it is hoped that implantation and pregnancy will occur. The recipient does not need to have functioning ovaries, but she must have a uterus that is able to carry a pregnancy.

Newspaper advertisements from fertility and reproductive endocrinology centers appeal to women who have proven fertility and are within the 21- to 34-year-old age range. The copy may read, ". . . donate eggs anonymously to help infertile couples achieve pregnancy. You will receive compassionate, expert medical care and financial compensation."

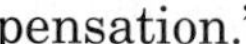

Male Factors

DESCRIPTION

Little information is usually available for nursing practice in the area of male infertility, and yet 40 to 60 percent of fertility is related to a male factor. Careful explanation of the normal physiology of the man (see Chapter 9) and the components of the evaluation of the male partner should be provided at the initial examination. A systematic history of physical development, general health, and sexual habits is necessary to identify potential problems. Because spermatogenesis is an ongoing process, the man is much more susceptible to environmental factors, such as drug, alcohol, and cigarette use and high scrotal temperatures. Questions about drug use, illnesses, past episodes of sexually transmitted disease, and the adequacy of ejaculation are essential to the male history.

Causes of male infertility include pituitary and hypothalamic dysfunction, which can be diagnosed by serum FSH and LH levels. Low FSH and LH levels may indicate hypothalamic dysfunction, while elevated gonadotropins (FSH, LH) indicate testicular failure. Hormonal problems at the level of the testes can be detected by serum testosterone levels. Undescended testes after 2 years of age may result in permanent damage from excessive heat to the testes. Congenital anomalies, such as hypospadias, in which the urethral outlet is on the shaft of the penis rather than at the end, may result in semen being deposited in the vagina rather than at the cervix. This condition is sometimes associated with maternal cocaine use during pregnancy. Mumps, particularly after adolescence, can result in permanent damage to the testes. Recurrent venereal disease may cause scarring and blockage of the reproductive tract. A low-grade prostate infection can also affect sperm count. Any injury, such as testicular torsion, can result in ischemia to the testes, causing permanent damage (Amar 1991).

A varicocele, or varicose vein of the scrotum, is thought to affect sperm motility and form by increasing the heat of the scrotum. Other factors that can adversely affect spermatogenesis are marijuana and tobacco use; alcohol abuse; radiation and chemotherapy; and drugs such as anabolic steroids, antihypertensives such as methyldopa (Aldomet), and anticholinergics such as cimetidine (Tagamet). Men should be counseled about overall health factors that can contribute to their infertility (Amar 1991).

Antisperm antibodies may develop and cause fertility problems. Normally, the male reproductive tract does not come into direct contact with the circulatory system. When there is a breakdown of the reproductive tract that allows sperm into the general circulation, the immune system forms antibodies to sperm. Conditions that can cause antibody formation include recurrent venereal infections and vasectomy. The titer of antibodies, which can either immobilize or agglutinate sperm, is significant in projecting overall chances of pregnancy. Men should be counseled about obtaining a serum antisperm antibody titer before attempting a vasectomy reversal (Amar 1991).

Semen Analysis

Laboratory evaluation of the man starts with semen analysis. Traditionally done with a hemocytometer, semen analysis is changing with the introduction of computerized technology. Normal semen parameters are an ejaculate volume of 1.5 to 5.0 ml, count of at least 20 million motile sperm, morphology (number of normally shaped sperm) greater than 60 percent, and motility (number of sperm swimming progressively forward) greater than 60 percent (see Normal Semen Parameters). No semen analysis will have 100 percent motility or normal forms. The problem with low motility or abnormally developed sperm is that they are not able to navigate the cervix so that fertilization can occur in the fallopian tubes. This is not correlated with birth defects. Degrees of oligospermia (reduced count) or reduced motility and morphologic appearance will have bearing on the types of therapy available to the couple (Amar 1991).

The semen sample is ideally collected by masturbation into a sterile container after no less than 2 days but no more than 7 days of abstinence. The sample should be examined within 2 hours of collection. Sterile, unlubricated condoms can be used for collection when there are religious or cultural objections to masturbation.

Two or more abnormal samples must be obtained before a definitive diagnosis is made. Serum levels of FSH, LH, and testosterone and a physical examination are then appropriate for further diagnosis. Additional testing for sperm-mucus interaction, antisperm antibodies, and sperm penetration may be necessary before a prognosis can be given and treatment recommended.

Normal Semen Parameters

On at least two occasions

- Ejaculate volume: 1.5 to 5.0 ml
- Sperm density: >20 million per milliliter or >50 to 60 × 10^6 total sperm
- Motility: >60%
- Forward progression: >2+ (scale 0 to 4)
- Morphology: >60% normal

And

- No significant sperm agglutination
- No significant pyospermia
- No hyperviscosity or inadequate liquefaction

From Amar, L., *Male Infertility,* 98, in *Principles of Infertility Nursing,* Garner, C., Ed., CRC Press, Boca Raton, FL, ©1991. With permission.

The sperm penetration assay is an evaluation of the functional ability of sperm to penetrate hamster eggs. The sperm penetration assay has been shown to be a reliable predictor of the ability of human sperm to fertilize human eggs (Johnson et al. 1985). This test may be ordered when there is a question about the ability of sperm to fertilize an egg. Sperm, obtained by masturbation, are incubated with hamster eggs. After a period, the hamster eggs are examined for evidence of penetration by the human sperm. There is no fusion of the hamster egg and the human sperm.

MANAGEMENT

Treatment is tailored to the individual problem. Medical therapy for low FSH and LH levels includes clomiphene citrate to stimulate FSH and LH production. Antibiotics are indicated when infection is present. Lifestyle changes may be necessary to correct self-induced fertility factors. Surgical therapy to correct blockages or ligate varicose veins may also be appropriate. Approximately 60 to 70 percent of men will see an improvement in semen quality after varicocelectomy, which is the ligation and excision of the enlarged veins of a scrotal varicocele, but the effect of a varicocelectomy on increasing fertility rates is less certain (Amar 1991). Other therapies, such as artificial insemination and intrauterine insemination of the husband's semen, involve the manipulation of the semen.

Artificial Insemination

Artificial insemination of the husband's sperm involves collecting the semen sample by masturbation and placing it into the cervix by use of a catheter or a cervical cap or into the uterus directly (intrauterine insemination).

Intrauterine insemination allows direct placement of sperm into the uterus, thus bypassing the cervix. This is of benefit when there is a problem with cervical mucus production. Sperm are processed to remove the seminal plasma and to concentrate the motile sperm before placement. This procedure is also performed when there is low motility and low sperm count, although overall pregnancy rates when male factors exist are poor (Dalgish 1991).

Both of these procedures require precise timing with menstrual cycles and may be taxing to the couple emotionally. Artificial insemination can provoke feelings of inadequacy and abnormality, as it often interferes with the normal sexual relationship of the couple. Nursing sensitivity to these issues is important. Male partners should be encouraged to be present during the insemination to support their partners and to feel included in the process.

Therapeutic Donor Insemination

Therapeutic donor insemination with donor semen is indicated in cases with severely low count or no sperm (azoospermia), sex-linked genetic diseases, and severe antisperm antibodies. In a 1987 survey, the Office of Technology Assessment found that approximately 172,000 women underwent artificial insemination. Approximately 65,000 live births (38 percent) resulted from these procedures (OTA 1988). Couples require extensive counseling regarding this option, as there are a number of psychological issues involved. The couple may need to grieve over the inability to achieve a biologic union between both partners as well as discuss any religious objections they may have. Most donor insemination programs in the United States are coordinated by nurses, who counsel couples about the procedure, assist them in selecting a donor from a written description of the donor profile, and then perform the inseminations. Nursing care requires exceptional sensitivity (Prattke and Gass-Sternas 1993). The nurse must be able to detect problems with the couple's acceptance of the procedure and, ultimately, of the child produced. Nurses must be knowledgeable about the ethical, religious, legal, and medical aspects of the procedure.

Sperm are usually obtained from a semen bank that screens donors for sexually transmitted diseases, health risk factors, and congenital defects. Sperm must be quarantined for 6 months and the donor retested for the human immunodeficiency virus (HIV) before release for use, as semen is the primary route of transmission for the HIV. Sperm are frozen in liquid nitrogen in the interim.

Physical characteristics of husband and donor are matched, and insemination is accomplished with thawed donor semen by intracervical or intrauterine insemination. Donor and husband semen are not mixed because of immunologic incompatibility.

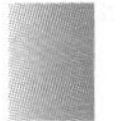

Cervical Factors

DESCRIPTION

The precise role and relative importance of cervical mucus in human fertilization continue to be controversial. The secretions of the cervical canal serve as a filter for the millions of spermatozoa that are deposited into the vagina. Perhaps as few as 100 sperm pass through the cervical canal into the uterine cavity. While there is no absolute proof that cervical mucus is necessary for the fertilization process to occur, abnormalities of quantity and quality of the cervical mucus have been associated with infertility. Although the true incidence of abnormal cervical mucus–sperm interaction is unknown, it is estimated that it is a causal factor in between 5 and 15 percent of infertility.

The postcoital test is an evaluation of cervical mucus–sperm interaction. The test provides information on the receptivity of the cervical mucus to the sperm and the ability of the sperm to reach the mucus and survive (Amar 1991). Couples are asked to have sexual intercourse around the time of ovulation. Cervical mucus is aspirated from the internal os of the woman's cervix and examined under a microscope for the presence of motile sperm. At the time of aspiration, cervical mucus is evaluated for quality and quantity. Because of the influence of estrogen, mucus should be clear and abundant. Scant, viscous mucus with a low basal body temperature may indicate that the test was scheduled too early in the preovulatory period. The use of a urinary LH testing kit, which can be obtained over-the-counter in drugstores, can help to predict ovulation more precisely. Evidence of LH in the urine should indicate periovulatory estrogenic mucus. The couple should be instructed to have intercourse sometime in the next 24 hours and to schedule the postcoital test for 2 to 24 hours after intercourse. Testing immediately after intercourse is not necessary, as sperm will survive in cervical mucus for the length of time that mucus is receptive, sometimes as long as 72 hours.

The results are reported as the number of sperm per high-power field. Greater than five sperm per high-power field is considered to be consistent with proven fertility. Sperm that are immotile or observed to "shake" may be related to antisperm antibodies in the cervical mucus.

The most common cause for a poor postcoital test result is poor timing. There is a window of only 48 to 72 hours when cervical mucus is receptive to sperm. At any other time, cervical mucus serves as a protective barrier to sperm. A careful evaluation of timing in relation to ovulation is important.

Coital difficulties can include premature ejaculation and obesity, which cause sperm to be deposited in the outer two thirds of the vagina. Impotence before or with vaginal penetration may also be a factor. Psychologically, couples may feel that the postcoital test is an evaluation of their sexual performance as well as their reproductive capacity. Many couples are simply unable to complete the act of intercourse on demand. Repeated cancellations of office visits should be investigated to determine whether they are due to psychological difficulties.

Poor cervical mucus can be caused by cervical stenosis; cervical infection; or cervical trauma due to removal of portions of the cervical canal through biopsy, laser therapy, cauterization, or resection. Coital lubricants, such as petroleum jelly, act as spermicides and should be avoided in attempting pregnancy. A poor postcoital test result with normal cervical mucus may be due to cervical mucus antisperm antibodies. These antibodies can be found in both the serum and cervical mucus of women and interfere with normal conception.

MANAGEMENT

Treatment depends on the cause. Infections are treated with antibiotics. Estrogen is occasionally given to enhance mucus production. When cervical problems are severe, sperm are placed directly into the uterus by intrauterine insemination. If repeated intrauterine inseminations are unsuccessful, IVF may be recommended.

Tubal Factors

DESCRIPTION

One of the most common causes of female infertility is damage or blockage of the fallopian tubes. Careful evaluation is needed. Any history of previous pelvic infection should be noted, although tubal damage can occur without symptomatic infection. Tubal infertility is one of the most common causes of infertility and has been on the increase in the last decade owing to an increase in the number of pelvic infections of *Chlamydia trachomatis* and gonorrhea.

The uterine cavity and fallopian tubes are examined by an x-ray study called hysterosalpingography. X-ray films are taken from several different angles after the uterus is filled with either an oil-based or water-based contrast medium introduced into the uterus through a cannula. The contrast fluid fills the uterine cavity and tubes and is absorbed in time. If tubal obstruction is present, the patient may experience moderate to severe discomfort and will be at slightly higher risk for infection immediately after the procedure.

Women report varying degrees of pain and cramping with the procedure, and prophylactic analgesia with antiprostaglandins or nonsteroidal antiinflammatory agents may be indicated. Because serious pelvic infections occur in between 0.3 and 1.3 percent of patients undergoing hysterosalpingography, prophylactic antibiotics are given when there is a history of PID or blocked tubes or when this is found during the test. Side effects of hysterosalpingography include uterine cramping, bleeding, nausea, and dizziness. Vagal stimulation may occur with cervical manipulation, resulting in mild bradycardia, hypotension, and diaphoresis. There is a slight risk of uterine perforation and allergic reaction to the contrast medium. Most women report some cervical bleeding after the procedure.

Nursing care includes careful explanation of the procedure and the possibility of discomfort. Contraindications are pregnancy and an allergy to the contrast medium. The presence of a support person during hysterosalpingography can provide psychological assistance should the procedure be painful or should the results, which are available minutes after the procedure, be poor.

During hysterosalpingography, the woman is in a physically and psychologically vulnerable position. Every effort should be made to ensure privacy and comfort during the procedure. The patient should be allowed to dress before discussing the results in detail with the physician.

Endometrial Development Factors

Adequate development of the endometrium is necessary for normal implantation of the embryo. The endometrial glands and stroma respond to the progesterone secreted by the corpus luteum in the second half of the luteal phase of the menstrual cycle. Inadequate development during the luteal phase may be due to either inadequate progesterone stimulation from the ovarian follicle or an inappropriate response of the endometrial tissue.

DESCRIPTION

An endometrial biopsy is the classic method of diagnosis to determine an inadequate luteal phase. The biopsy is obtained 1 or 2 days before expected menses and is used to evaluate the endometrial response. A sample of endometrium is obtained from the uterine fundus with a biopsy instrument. Patients may experience pelvic discomfort, uterine cramping or spotting. They should remain supine for 3 to 5 minutes after the procedure. They may experience some vaginal bleeding and should be provided with a tampon or pad. The woman should be instructed to call with the date of her menstrual period, as this is essential to the proper interpretation of the biopsy. The endometrial biopsy is occasionally done during the cycle of conception, so patients may wish to use barrier contraception the month of biopsy. A sensitive urine pregnancy test should be performed immediately before the biopsy to rule out pregnancy (May and Garner 1991).

The biopsy specimen is examined microscopically, and an approximate cycle date is assigned to the endometrial pattern. An out-of-phase biopsy should be confirmed by a second biopsy in a subsequent cycle for a diagnosis to be made of luteal phase inadequacy, as all women occasionally experience an out-of-phase cycle.

MANAGEMENT

Treatment of a luteal phase defect depends on the cause. If the defect is present with other conditions such as elevated serum prolactin level or endometriosis, treatment of the underlying disorder may result in correction of the defect.

There is some debate about the treatment of the true luteal phase deficiency. Some argue that since the cause may involve faulty development of the ovarian follicle, the approach should be to enhance the follicular phase with ovulation induction agents. Others argue that a progesterone deficiency is best treated with progesterone. Both approaches are used with success.

Progesterone supplementation is usually accomplished with oral progesterone or with progesterone rectal or vaginal suppositories. The progesterone is begun 3 days after the midcycle rise of basal body temperature and continued until menstruation, which is rarely delayed beyond 2 days by the progesterone. The dosage may be adjusted to achieve an adequate endometrial response.

Should pregnancy occur, the progesterone is continued until ultrasound scan at 6 to 8 weeks documents a viable pregnancy. At this time, the fetal placental unit should be able to sustain itself through its own progesterone production. The corpus luteum normally declines at this time, so supplemental progesterone may be discontinued.

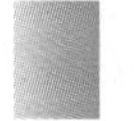

Pelvic Factors

DESCRIPTION

Direct intraabdominal visualization by laparoscopy is usually necessary to establish a diagnosis. Laparoscopy allows direct visualization of the internal organs through a small incision in the umbilicus. A second and occasionally a third incision is necessary to manipulate the pelvic organs for complete evaluation. Six characteristics, the site, shape, surface, color, consistency, and mobility of the uterus, tubes, and ovaries, are noted during diagnostic laparoscopy.

The procedure is commonly done under general anesthesia. Local anesthetic is injected at the incision site when general anesthesia has been accomplished, and a Verres needle is introduced. The abdomen is insufflated with carbon dioxide to distend the abdominal cavity. The laparoscope is introduced through a stabilizing instrument, the trocar. Self-absorbing sutures are usually used to close the incision, which is usually small enough to be covered by two or three adhesive bandages.

Diagnostic laparoscopy is usually performed early in the menstrual cycle. Much operative work can be accomplished through the laparoscope, including lysis of adhesions, vaporization of endometriosis, and surgical excision of ectopic pregnancy. Postoperatively, many patients report some shoulder discomfort due to the insufflation of carbon dioxide. This usually resolves within 24 hours, and discomfort can be relieved by assuming the knee-chest position. A sore throat from the endotracheal intubation is not uncommon. The degree of abdominal discomfort depends on the amount of surgical manipulation and the individual's threshold of pain. Nausea and vomiting may occur as a consequence of anesthesia or manipulation of the bowel during surgery.

Short-acting anesthetic agents are generally used for laparoscopy. The patient should recover and be able to ambulate and tolerate clear liquids within 1 to 2 hours postoperatively. Instructions about sexual intercourse are individualized. If cervical manipulation occurred, some vaginal bleeding may be noted. Some bruising around the incision or secondary puncture sites is occasionally noted. The woman should be told to report signs of infection around the incision, fever, or excessive abdominal pain.

MANAGEMENT

Treatment of intrauterine defects is usually performed by hysteroscopy, a procedure using a telescope-like instrument through the cervix to examine the inside of the uterine cavity. This may be done at the time of laparoscopy or as a separate procedure. Evaluation and removal of a uterine defect, such as adhesions, polyps, or a septum, may be accomplished through the hysteroscope. It is valuable for the lysis of adhesions with Asherman's syndrome, a condition in which there is internal scarring of the uterus. Postoperatively, the patient should expect some vaginal bleeding and needs to refrain from intercourse for a time.

Unexplained Infertility

There is still much to be learned about human reproduction. In the early 1950s, perhaps 40 percent to 50 percent of infertility cases were called unexplained. As the knowledge base has expanded, this diagnosis is applied in less than 5 percent of cases. This is particularly frustrating to couples, as there is nothing to correct or to treat. After prolonged infertility, intrauterine insemination and the assisted reproductive technologies are used to treat the couple, even in the absence of a known disorder.

COMMON INFERTILITY CONDITIONS

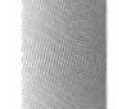

Ectopic Pregnancy

DESCRIPTION

Any condition that alters the function of the fallopian tube can contribute to the occurrence of ectopic pregnancy. Disease processes outside the tube that can lead to tubal problems include appendicitis, endometriosis, ruptured ovarian cyst, and peritubular adhesions from abdominal or pelvic surgery. Implantation of the embryo in the fallopian tube is similar to uterine implantation with the development of a placenta and intervillous space. Tubal rupture is probably secondary to the distention of the growing embryo. Ectopic pregnancy accounts for approximately 12 percent of maternal deaths and is the leading cause of maternal mortality in the first trimester. The number and rate of ectopic pregnancies have increased steadily since 1970. The risk of ectopic pregnancy is greater for nonwhite women and increases with age among women of all ages, with the highest rate occurring among women 25 to 44 years of age. Barrier methods of contraception and oral contraceptive use are associated with a decreased risk of ectopic pregnancy (May and Garner 1991).

Except for those patients presenting with acute rupture with signs and symptoms of hemorrhagic shock, the physical findings are variable. Abdominal pain is the most common presenting symptom and represents 90 to 95 percent of all complaints. It may be either acute or chronic. Abdominal tenderness is generally present with palpation. Patients with ectopic pregnancy frequently experience pain with movement of the cervix during pelvic examination.

Abnormal vaginal bleeding is seen in 70 percent to 80 percent of cases; but the bleeding is seldom heavy, does not resemble normal menses, and frequently occurs later than when menses was expected.

If an ectopic pregnancy is suspected, a sensitive pregnancy test, the beta-hCG, is an important test. Beta-hCG is produced by the developing embryo and is detectable as early as 8 days after fertilization. The beta-hCG level normally doubles approximately every 48 hours until the eighth week of pregnancy. If samples taken every 2 days have an abnormal doubling time, an ectopic pregnancy should be suspected and early ultrasound examination scheduled.

When the level of beta-hCG approaches 6500 mIU/ml, an abdominal ultrasound scan can be used to determine the location of the pregnancy. With the use of vaginal ultrasound, a fetal sac can often be seen at beta-hCG levels of 2500 mIU/ml. Although it has some margin of error, ultrasound scanning can visualize the embryo by the fifth week with an intrauterine pregnancy. If an intrauterine pregnancy is detected, it is unlikely but not impossible that an ectopic pregnancy coexists. An absent gestational sac in the uterus with a positive pregnancy test result at 5 weeks' gestation is compatible with ectopic pregnancy (May and Garner 1991).

MANAGEMENT

Depending on the location of the ectopic pregnancy and the amount of damage, the products of conception may be excised and the tube repaired by microsurgical techniques through the laparoscope. The conceptus can sometimes be milked out of the fallopian tube by gentle manipulation of the tube. More extensive surgical removal through a salpingectomy of part of the tube with reanastomosis of the remaining parts may be necessary to remove the ectopic pregnancy. If the ectopic pregnancy is detected early, a linear salpingostomy is performed. This requires an incision in the involved portion of the tube; the tube is then repaired without removing an entire section (Fig. 12–2). Ectopic pregnancy can also be treated with chemotherapeutic agents such as methotrexate, thus decreasing the need for surgical intervention. When future pregnancies are not desired or the tube is damaged beyond repair, a complete salpingectomy is performed. With the advent of IVF, surgeons now do not remove the ovaries unless it is medically necessary. The risk of recurrence in a repaired tube depends on the extent of tubal disease and damage from the ectopic pregnancy. Careful tissue handling with the use of fine, absorbable, nonreactive suture such as Vicryl and Dexon is important. Recurrence in the other tube also depends on the extent of tubal disease.

Early and aggressive treatment of sexually transmitted diseases may help to reduce the severity of the inflammatory disease process. Any sexually active woman should be educated about the symptoms and risks of sexually transmitted diseases. Prompt reporting of symptoms is essential.

Any woman who has a history of an episode of PID, tubal surgery, ectopic pregnancy, or IUD use should inform her clinician as soon as she suspects pregnancy. Early clinical monitoring will include serial beta-hCG determinations and early pelvic ultrasound examination. Any unusual bleeding, cramping, or pelvic pain should be reported immediately.

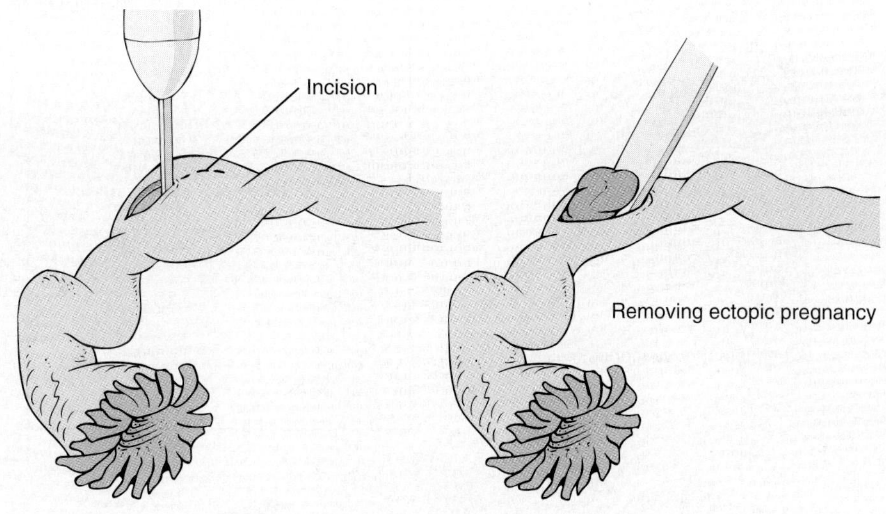

Figure 12–2
Surgical removal of an ecotopic pregnancy with the linear salpingostomy procedure • An incision is made in the fallopian tube over the area of the ectopic pregnancy • Then the pregnancy is shelled out, electrocoagulation is used to stop any bleeding, and the tube is left open and allowed to heal by secondary intention.

Endometriosis

Endometriosis is a condition in which the cells normally lining the uterus grow on organs outside the uterus, usually within the pelvis. The etiology of endometriosis is poorly understood, as is the mechanism by which endometriosis causes infertility.

DESCRIPTION

Endometriosis is observed at laparoscopy and staged according to severity from stage 1 (minimal) to stage 4 (severe) (American Fertility Society 1985). Endometriosis sometimes presents as chronic pelvic pain and can be present in early adolescence. There is no correlation, however, between the extent of the disease and the symptoms. Many women with severe cases have no symptoms at all.

MANAGEMENT

Therapy may involve laser treatment or more conventional surgical removal of the disease. Medical therapies most effective are danazol (Danocrine) 800 mg daily for 6 months and Gn-RH agonists (leuprolide [Lupron], nafarelin [Synarel], and goserelin [Zoladex]). They work by suppressing ovarian production of estrogen and progesterone, both hormones that promote growth of endometrium. Laser vaporization of the disease is also commonly used. No matter what the form of treatment, endometriosis returns in 40 percent of cases. Thus, for many, endometriosis represents a chronic disease and requires nursing management of the manifestation of this condition, whether it is chronic pelvic pain or infertility.

ASSISTED REPRODUCTIVE TECHNOLOGIES

While 20 million motile sperm are required for natural conception, as few as 50,000 to 500,000 sperm are necessary for IVF or gamete intrafallopian transfer (GIFT). The availability of these procedures has led to an increase in couples choosing them because of infertility caused by a male factor.

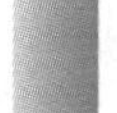

In Vitro Fertilization

In vitro (within an artificial environment) fertilization, which is frequently equated with test-tube babies, evolved as a procedure to assist women with blocked or absent fallopian tubes to achieve pregnancy. Very simply, the ovaries are hyperstimulated with a combination of ovulation induction agents to obtain a number of oocytes. Once the ovary has been sufficiently stimulated, oocytes are

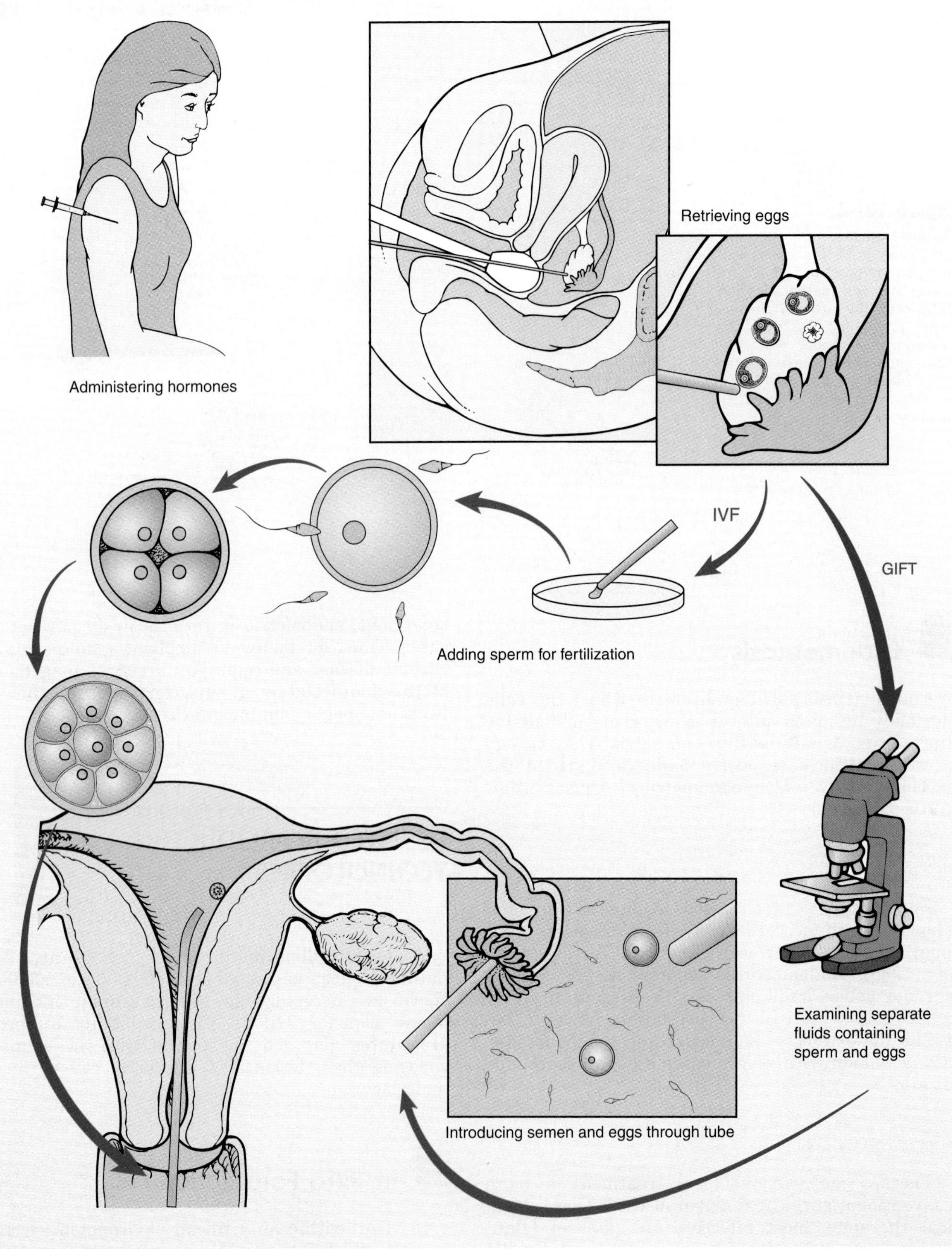

Figure 12–3

Assisted reproductive technology includes in vitro fertilization (IVF) and gamete intrafallopian transfer (GIFT) • In both procedures, drug therapy is used to stimulate egg production, and the mature oocytes are retrieved vaginally • IVF is a procedure in which the egg and sperm are placed together in an artificial environment (Petri dish) to aid fertilization • After fertilization occurs, the four- to eight-cell embryos are transferred by a small catheter directly into the uterus, where they may implant • GIFT is a variation of the IVF procedure in which the sperm and eggs are placed sequentially into the fimbriated ends of the fallopian tubes by means of laparoscopy • This method may be used when the fallopian tubes are patent, and it allows fertilization to take place naturally within the body.

removed by laparoscopy or vaginal ultrasound-guided aspiration and placed into an incubator with sperm. After 48 hours, if fertilization and division of oocytes have occurred, four- to eight-cell emybryos are transferred into the uterus by use of a small catheter (English 1991) (Fig. 12–3). More than 15,000 births have resulted from this technology since its introduction in 1980 (Chartrand 1989). Success rates vary widely depending on the age of the woman, the cause of the infertility condition, and the skill of the professionals at the IVF center.

Gamete Intrafallopian Transfer

GIFT is a variation of IVF; oocytes are removed, identified, and then placed back into the end of a fallopian tube with the sperm (Fig. 12–3). Fertilization is allowed to occur naturally in vivo (within the body). GIFT is an option for women with one normal fallopian tube and unexplained infertility or recurrent endometriosis (Patrizio and Asch 1994). Both IVF and GIFT are performed if the man has a compromised semen analysis.

When transfer of embryos or eggs is accomplished, one of the major concerns is the possibility of multiple births. Many centers are limiting the number of embryos transferred to three to significantly decrease the likelihood of multiple gestation. The question then becomes what to do with excess embryos. Embryos can be frozen (cryopreserved) for indefinite periods, thawed, transferred into the uterus, and progress through pregnancy and birth. Couples who do not become pregnant as a result of the procedure can return in a subsequent menstrual cycle for a transfer of embryos from the freezer to the uterus.

The issue of cryopreservation of human embryos presents numerous ethical and religious dilemmas. Couples must be comfortable with their decisions and the lifetime consequences. What happens, for instance, if the couple dies before the transfer? Nursing roles must focus on education and working through acceptable alternatives with couples. The consent form must encompass possibilities such as death, divorce, or simply that the couple does not want the embryo at a later date.

Cost is a significant factor when couples are deciding about assisted reproductive technologies. The average cycle costs $6000 to $8000, and insurance companies rarely cover this procedure. With success rates averaging 15 to 25 percent for IVF and 25 to 30 percent for GIFT, this is a significant gamble for many couples. Issues that couples must resolve include the religious acceptance of procedures, feelings about cryopreserving human embryos, and family acceptance of their decision and their child's origins.

There are two other assisted reproductive technologies, zygote intrafallopian transfer (ZIFT) and tubal embryo transfer (TET), that as yet have not achieved widespread use or acceptance (Surrey and Kerin 1995). Both are similar to the GIFT procedure. For the ZIFT procedure, oocyte retrieval is done, usually by transvaginal ultrasound aspiration. The oocytes are cultured and inseminated in vitro (IVF). Once normal fertilization has been confirmed, about 18 hours after insemination, the fertilized eggs are transferred via laparoscope into the fimbriated end of the fallopian tube, usually within 24 hours after insemination. Tubal embryo transfer (TET) is the same as ZIFT except that the fertilized eggs are allowed to develop to the four- to eight-cell embryo stage before they are replaced via a laparoscope into the fallopian tube.

Reproductive technologies are expanding rapidly and currently allow donor eggs, donated embryos, and transfer of an embryo into the uterus of a gestational surrogate mother. The ethical and legal implications are significant. Nurses are critical participants in providing expert care to these families with infertility.

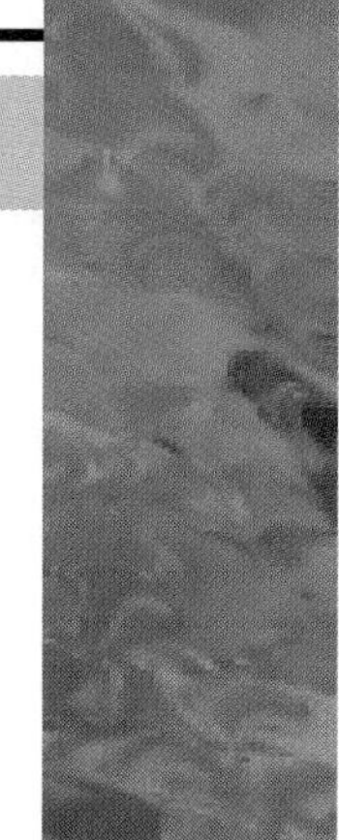

Nursing Practice

Nursing Process

When the medical diagnosis has been established, the physician outlines the various treatment options for the couple. No infertility therapy is mandatory. All couples have the choice to forgo any medical therapy, and they have the options of adoption or child-free living.

▼ Assessment

Assessment includes comprehensive physical and psychological assessment of the infertile couple. The essential components of physical assessment are personal and family medical history; review of systems; and a detailed sexual, menstrual, and reproductive history (see Assessment Tool, p. 282). During psychological assessment, the nurse elicits information about the couple's feelings about their infertility problems, their cultural and personal expectations for parenting, and the adequacy of their coping strategies for dealing with the grief associated with infertility.

▼ Diagnosis

The nursing diagnosis depends on the education level, clinical diagnosis, and treatment decisions as well as the overall goal of the patient and her partner. It is simplistic to assume that the only goal is achievement of pregnancy. For some, it is the answer to the question of why the problem is occurring. For others, it will be the achievement of a pregnancy that results from the *biologic* union. For others still, it will be the process of becoming a parent through pregnancy or adoption. A number of nursing diagnoses are common for individuals with infertility. These potential nursing diagnoses are

- Knowledge deficit: lack of knowledge related to human reproduction, infertility evaluation, treatment options, stress of infertility, or pregnancy and parenting
- Ineffective individual or family coping related to stress of infertility, lack of family support and understanding, ethical or religious conflicts, or poor marital communication
- Self-esteem disturbance related to inability to conceive or cultural expectations of fertility
- Grieving related to anticipated or perceived loss, actual loss of own childbearing potential, or loss of biologic parenting
- Altered sexuality patterns related to infertility testing (situational) or the stress of infertility on the relationship
- Risk for altered parenting related to perceived or real high-risk pregnancy, poor resolution of infertility issues, or overprotection of child

▼ Planning

Treatment for infertility can be prolonged, expensive, and personally frustrating. While specific goals are established according to each individual's needs, the general goals for nursing care for individuals with infertility are

- Educate couples about human reproduction, factors that interfere with normal conception, and the basic infertility evaluation
- Provide couples with complete and accurate information about their infertility diagnosis and

THE CHALLENGE OF HELPING INFERTILE COUPLES

Infertility may be one of the most difficult crises couples face in their lives. Dealing with patients' disappointments, frustrations, sometimes anger, emotional suffering, and ever present grief is a daily challenge for nurses who work in infertility clinics. Nurses are frequently the key individuals who provide the help that enables infertile couples to meet the crisis of infertility and even be strengthened by the experience.

The following are essential guidelines for helping infertile couples:

- Face your own doubts, needs, and fears about yourself and your value and adequacy as a helper.
- Understand and be comfortable with suffering, knowing that somehow it fits into the tapestry of each person's life and that it often brings positive growth.
- Believe that the process of healing takes time and that you cannot make it happen more quickly for others; healing occurs primarily through the efforts of the wounded.
- Acknowledge your own suffering and the way it has enhanced your life; this enables you to relate more authentically to those in pain.
- Recognize and respect the unique pain of the infertile couples with whom you work.
- Listen with your heart and not your critical mind, or, said another way, hear the music and not the words.
- Comfort with the comfort with which you have been comforted.

Adapted from Mahlstedt, P. P., *What Is Essential Is Invisible to the Eye: Dealing with Patient Disappointment,* in *Principles of Infertility Nursing,* Garner, C., Ed., CRC Press, Boca Raton, FL, ©1991. With permission.

the various treatment options open to them, including adoption and child-free living
- Provide support and counseling to the couple during the decision-making process
- Evaluate the need for referral of couples or individual partners to other resources including religious support and psychological counseling
- Assist couples in their pursuit of solutions to infertility
- Support couples pursuing alternative routes of parenting including adoption and donor gametes

▼ Intervention

The role of the nurse is to provide further facts and information about the therapies after the physician has told the couple of the diagnosis and reviewed the treatment options so that they can make an informed decision. The nurse can provide education, facilitate the diagnosis and treatment phases of infertility, assist with the decision-making process, and help with resolution of infertility by either assisting the grief process or facilitating parenting. Providing emotional support for the couple during therapy is essential, particularly when a particular treatment proves unsuccessful.

▼ PROVIDING PSYCHOLOGICAL SUPPORT

The couple with infertility faces many uncertainties and multiple losses. Mahlsteadt (1991) described infertility as (1) a loss of self-esteem, (2) loss of a dream, and (3) loss of balance of a relationship, security, and fantasy. While common behaviors of couples with infertility are observed, Sandelowski (1994) emphasized that these behaviors have different meanings for different couples. Thus, while scientific generalizations are helpful in understanding the infertility experience, nursing care must be individualized on the basis of the couple's perception of their infertility experience.

As with all losses, grief must be worked through. Multiple losses can cripple an individual emotionally. Support groups such as RESOLVE (see Appendix VIII), the national support network for infertile couples, and individual counseling can be important parts of recovery. Recognition of specific aspects of grief and of marital strain is essential during the infertility evaluation and treatment phase. Infertility is not a life-threatening condition and, as such, has sometimes been considered to be less important than illnesses such as cancer that are always perceived of as serious. Yet, the feelings of infertility can be devastating to individuals and to a couple's relationship.

Family and cultural backgrounds sometimes reinforce feelings of inadequacy and of a wrathful God. Parenting means different things to different people. Cultural expectations, family pressure, and a general acceptance of fertility as a matter of choice all influence reactions. Many find infertility problems embarrassing and are at a loss as to what to tell inquisitive friends and relatives.

Nurses help couples understand the physical implications of fertility and infertility, the purpose of testing, and the options available for treatment. The special skills that a nurse has in counseling and education are essential to successful management of the infertile couple.

Assessment of the emotional response of the couple is readily accomplished as the nurse obtains general and specific reproductive information. Observation of nonverbal behavior, such as supportive gestures between the couple or complete absence of such behavior, gives clues as to the marital situation. Lack of eye contact and other signs of discomfort during the interview will give you an indication of the level of comfort the couple has in discussing reproduction. Statements should be informational and supportive. Many feel as though they are the only ones experiencing difficulty with infertility. Sample statements are "One of six couples experience difficulty achieving pregnancy" or "Many of our patients don't have friends or family available to discuss these problems with, so they have formed a group to provide education and support for each other. I have included that information in your initial packet."

At some point, it is important to acknowledge that infertility has both a physical and psychological component and that diagnostic procedures can be stressful. Simple things, such as allowing choices between a morning and afternoon appointment, can help give the couple some degree of control over a schedule that must be determined by menstrual cycle days. Questions about the sociocultural issues are sometimes more difficult. Questions such as "Do you come from a large family?" or "Had you planned a small or large family for yourself?" are good opening remarks. Cultures that place more emphasis on the self-worth of the individual related to ability to procreate can add a great deal of stress.

▼ DIAGNOSTIC PHASE

As the couple presents at the initial visit, the nurse should ascertain their particular goal and then provide the appropriate framework for meeting that goal. For instance, if the couple has been attempting pregnancy for more than a year and wants to achieve pregnancy, the first step is education about normal reproduction and common problems that can prevent conception, such as the use of lubricants with intercourse. Next is an outline of the basic infertility evaluation, with explanations about each test, the purpose, timing, and cost. It is also important to set psychological goals, such as maintaining marital communication; decreasing stress on the sexual relationship; and developing a support system through family, friends, or RESOLVE.

▼ TREATMENT PHASE

Once the medical diagnosis has been established and the treatment plan decided, it is the nursing role to provide further education about these options and to assist the couple with the decision-making process. During this phase, it may be best to provide educational pamphlets, books, or referral to other resources so that the couple can make an informed decision (see Appendix VIII, Society of Assisted Reproductive Technology). It is not uncommon for partners to have difficulty communicating their real feelings at this stage. One partner may feel reluctant about a procedure but will agree because of fear of hurting the spouse's feelings. Providing a time to talk with each partner separately can elicit clues as to background conflicts.

Sandelowski and colleagues (1990), from their extensive qualitative research with infertile couples, described the infertility experience as one of pain, not pleasure; struggle, not ease; separation, not unity; public exposure, not intimacy; and artificial, not natural. "These couples labored, frequently for years to make it happen! Lovemaking had become a coercive chore, almost exclusively a means to an end. Lives were lived in 30-day segments and the generally simple and pleasurable means of conceiving were transformed into a series of painful hurdles to be overcome" (Sandelowski et al. 1990; Sandelowski 1994).

One husband described the couple's attempts to achieve a pregnancy as follows:

> *"We make up a chart with the days of the month. I set the alarm clock for the same hour every morning, wake up and take Suzanne's temperature, and note it on the chart. Every morning on which we discover a low thermometer reading we make love* immediately *after temperature taking. One morning we made love* during *temperature taking. It is, frankly, not the most efficient way to get an accurate reading.*
>
> *We try to make love every morning during fertile periods, even if we are still asleep, even if we aren't in the mood, even if we have a headache, even if we have had a fight the night before and are still smoldering."*
>
> G. Johnston (1994)

Couples need to be encouraged to talk about their feelings and their experiences. Support groups offer a safe environment in the eyes of many couples who fear being dropped from treatment if they express negative feelings to health care providers.

Open communication can decrease stress and circumvent resentment in the relationship. At the initiation of any therapy, the possibility should be raised that the therapy will not work. Infertility therapy may result in a pregnancy and leave the marriage in ruins (Halman et al. 1994). Steps to strengthen the relationship should be developed by the couple. Sharing experiences unrelated to childbearing is important. One couple may schedule a dinner date once in a while to allow time to talk. Others deliberately seek out couples without children. Couples need to explore the possibilities of childlessness and adoption. This process cannot be rushed and must occur as the couple is ready. The nurse, however, must raise this possibility. The treatment phase is described as a roller coaster of emotions, as hopes rise early in the cycle, only to be dashed with the onset of menses. Patients should be encouraged to discuss their feelings and referred for counseling as appropriate.

▼ PREGNANCY AFTER INFERTILITY

Pregnancy may be the overriding goal, but nursing care does not stop when pregnancy occurs. Many couples assume that the achievement of pregnancy will solve all of the emotional problems associated with infertility. Pregnancy does not necessarily dissolve all of the anxiety and concerns that affected the couple before. Many times, the attainment of pregnancy does not bring all of the satisfaction the couple envisioned. Olshansky (1990) described couples experiencing an identity shift after becoming pregnant, straddling the two worlds of infertility and fertility, not feeling completely a part of either world. Couples are at risk for distress if they have unresolved marital issues, conflicts with the medical profession, self-image problems, general or specific anxiety, or unrealistic expectations about pregnancy. Nursing care should include discussion of the significance of the infertility diagnosis and treatment on both the individuals and the couple. Education about normal adaptations of pregnancy can alleviate some of the anxieties if pregnancy occurs. Reading materials, book lists, and emergency telephone numbers can help reassure couples. Frequent appointments early in pregnancy can have a positive influence. Crisis intervention is essential should a spontaneous abortion or ectopic pregnancy occur.

▼ FACILITATING GRIEF

Grief over either unsuccessful individual treatment or the inability to achieve pregnancy requires work. Feelings must be acknowledged to be dealt with openly and honestly. Resolution of infertility takes time. Depression is not uncommon and should be referred for appropriate mental health care. Resolution of infertility is not a finite phenomenon. The identity of oneself as an infertile person does not change even when pregnancy occurs.

Even after adoption, many couples still describe themselves as infertile. The first task for couples pursuing adoption is to recognize and express their feelings about their infertility and how it has affected their lives and work toward the resolution of their infertility (Sherrod 1992). A part of the resolution process is accepting their infertility. Couples must redefine their relationship and fantasies about the future. Couples must learn to be comfortable living out their lives in a fertile world. Some couples cope by becoming proactive. Joining forces through RESOLVE for community education or for legislative efforts to provide insurance coverage for infertility is a healthy way to channel feelings and energies. Positive results that have an impact on others experiencing the same difficulty can be tremendously rewarding (Hahn 1991).

Skills that can help couples move through this process include open communication, positive self-esteem, and mutual support. The nurse's role as educator, counselor, and facilitator can support this process. Feelings about infertility will recur at various points, and couples should be told to expect this. The birth of a baby into the extended family or to a friend or the anniversaries of a pregnancy loss may trigger feelings of sadness, envy, or decreased self-worth.

▼ Evaluation

Evaluation is a continual process in the care of the couple receiving infertility treatment. The couple's needs and the goals for nursing care will change, being based on the outcome of infertility treatment. Thus, evaluation should be conducted on a regular basis to determine the degree to which the goals have been met and their continued appropriateness.

Risk Management

Couples have choices about infertility treatment. Health care professionals have a responsibility to present the risks and benefits of each therapy along with expected outcomes. Unfortunately, some infertility clinics inflate their pregnancy rates to attract clients. The dishonesty of this manipulation of statistics is both unethical and cruel. Nurses need to be careful about presentation of statistics so that they represent a true picture of that couple's chances of pregnancy. Risks such as multiple gestation must be presented before the initiation of pregnancy so that this becomes part of the informed decision-making process. The physical and emotional pain of infertility cannot be separated. Couples sometimes become desperate in their attempts to conceive and do not listen

Guidelines for Clients Considering Assisted Reproductive Technologies

In the absence of federal regulation of fertility clinics and in the wake of ethical, legal, and procedural problems that have been uncovered in some fertility clinics, clients considering assisted reproductive technologies should consider

- Clinic success rates: Find out the clinic's success rates. Standardized statistics on birth rate results are available for participating clinics from the Society of Assisted Reproductive Technology (SART) in Birmingham, Alabama.
- Credentials: Ask about qualifications. Physicians should be board-certified reproductive endocrinologists. The laboratory's director, who oversees the facility and staff, should be an MD or PhD.
- Accreditation: Ask about accreditation. Laboratories should be accredited by the federal Clinical Laboratory Improvement Act (CLIA) and SART in collaboration with the College of American Pathologists (CAP).
- Facility: Ask about the clinic's affiliations and design. A clinic that handles more than 150 cases per year and is affiliated with a university medical center should have good outcomes-based experience, administrative oversight, and the sophisticated on-site equipment and laboratory space necessary for all of the assisted reproductive technologies available.
- Informed consent: Make sure that you have a complete and accurate understanding of the procedure to be performed. Fill out and sign only clear and detailed consent forms. The forms should specify how sperm and retrieved eggs and embryos will be used, stored, donated, or discarded. Do not leave any questions blank on the forms. Date the form and keep a copy.

See Appendix VIII for resource information. Data from Gabriel, T. (1996). High-tech pregnancies test hope's limit. *The New York Times,* January 7, 1, 10–11, and Wexler, K. (1996). Fertile ground for deception: For those seeking help conceiving, news of medical misdeeds can be chilling. *The Washington Post,* January 2, 1, 8.

to or internalize the risks of pregnancy or the true statistics presented. The nursing role is to see that these facts are at least presented in a manner that the couple can understand.

The nursing role in infertility has expanded rapidly into areas of primary care responsibility, such as coordination of donor insemination programs or IVF programs. Much of the responsibility for education, care, and reviewing the informed consent documents has fallen to the nurse. Careful documentation, development of nursing protocols, and careful exploration of the legal status in these areas are essential.

The laws in this area are limited but can be expected to proliferate as more couples take advantage of the options available. The American Fertility Society has issued guidelines on a number of technologies, including the use of donor insemination. Many IVF programs may voluntarily report their results to a national IVF registry. Interest has been raised in the health policy area with the advent of the assisted reproductive technologies, and in 1992, Congress passed Public Law 102-4773, the Fertility Clinic Success Rate and Certification Act. This law directs the Secretary of Health and Human Services to develop a model program for certification of embryo laboratories for distribution to the states. It also requires assisted reproductive technology programs to provide their pregnancy success rates to the Secretary for yearly publication and distribution to the public on request. One of the unique features of this bill is a provision mandating that the Secretary consult with both appropriate professional and consumer groups to assist with this task (Lawrence and Rosenwaks 1993).

Implications for Research

Fertility and infertility are relatively new areas for the nurse specialist. Reproductive endocrine and infertility nursing was first considered a subspecialty area in the early 1980s. The first certification examination for reproductive endocrinology and infertility was offered by the National Certification Corporation in 1989. This evolving specialty offers numerous opportunities and innovative clinical programs for research.

There is a need to examine the coping skills of infertile couples and what can be done to enhance a healthy outcome, from both a health care and a psychosocial standpoint. Assisted reproductive technologies are expanding rapidly, and too little is known about their effect on pregnancy and parenting after infertility. Researchers are just beginning to study the psychosocial effects of reproductive technologies on the families we are helping to create. The following research questions can be asked.

- What are the most effective strategies for increasing an infertile couple's coping ability during the treatment phase?
- What are the most effective interventions for facilitating an infertile couple's resolution of infertility?
- How does past infertility affect a couple's perceptions of pregnancy and parenting?
- What are the responses of the past infertile couple to pregnancy and parenting, particularly as they relate to differences in sexual relationships, parent-infant attachment behaviors, and early parenting behaviors?
- What are the past infertile couple's educational needs during the pregnancy, childbirth, and parenting periods?
- How does the experience of infertility before a pregnancy affect the decision-making process about subsequent pregnancies?

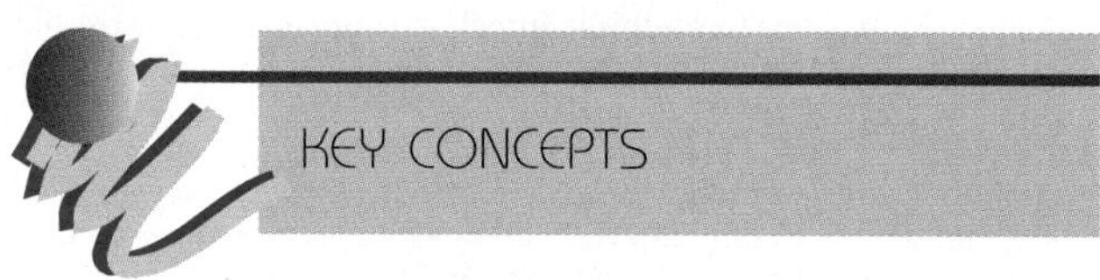

▼ Infertility is a relatively common problem for couples in their childbearing years. Incidence increases for women with age, particularly after 35 years.

▼ Infertility is a couple problem. When diagnosis is finally made, 40 percent will be attributable to a male factor, 40 percent to a female factor, and 20 percent to both partners.

▼ The evaluation should proceed in an orderly, timely fashion, looking at six factors: (1) ovulation, (2) sperm count, (3) sperm–cervical mucus interaction, (4) fallopian tube anatomy, (5) endometrial development, and (6) pelvic disorders.

▼ Disorders of ovulation account for 20 percent to 30 percent of factors affecting women. Diagnosis is complex, and treatment is often prolonged. Ovulation disorder is usually amenable to medical therapy, which may result in multiple births.

▼ Less is known about male infertility, and treatment is generally designed to maximize the sperm through preparation and artificial insemination. New reproductive technologies such as IVF offer hope to men with very low sperm counts.

▼ The male partner is much more susceptible to poor lifestyle habits, such as smoking, absence of cardiovascular exercise, and drug ingestion. Careful education about healthy lifestyle habits can be beneficial for men.

▼ The rising incidence of PID due to gonorrhea and chlamydial infection has contributed to fallopian tube damage. This damage can result in ectopic pregnancy or sterility. Early identification of and intervention for women at risk are critical to reducing the incidence of this problem.

▼ Endometriosis is a disease in which the tissue that normally lines the endometrium grows on pelvic organs, often causing pelvic pain and infertility. It is more common in women who have delayed childbearing beyond the age of 30 years. Even when medical or surgical therapy corrects this condition, it returns in 40 percent of patients.

▼ Assisted reproductive technologies may be appropriate for as many as 15 percent of infertile couples. These technologies require careful education and counseling of couples because of a number of ethical considerations.

▼ A couple faces many uncertainties and multiple losses with infertility. Couples experience many phases of the grief response, including anger, denial, and depression. Support groups such as RESOLVE offer psychological support for couples.

▼ Many people still believe in a number of myths surrounding fertility and conception. The nurse should educate all couples about the facts of reproduction and work to dispel these myths.

▼ Nurses are just beginning to explore the issues surrounding parenting after infertility. Couples have been described as experiencing an identity shift, straddling the infertile and fertile worlds, but not belonging to either one.

▼ Infertility nursing offers exciting opportunities as a new specialty practice evolves in this area.

References

Amar, L. (1991). Male infertility. In C. Garner (Ed.). *Principles of infertility nursing* (pp. 83–110). Boca Raton, FL: CRC Press.

Amar, L. (1994). Caffeine linked to miscarriage . . . and to reduced fertility. *Science News,* Jan 22, 145, 61.

American Fertility Society. (1985). Revised American Fertility Society classification of endometriosis. *Fertility and Sterility,* 43 (3), 351.

Chartrand, S. (1989). Experts assess a decade of in vitro fertilization. *New York Times,* Apr 11, 7.

Clements, D. (1988). Not crazy, after all of these years. *RESOLVE Newsletter,* Apr, 3.

Dalgish, C. S. (1991). Therapeutic donor insemination. In C. Garner (Ed.). *Principles of infertility nursing* (pp. 111–125). Boca Raton, FL: CRC Press.

English, M. E. (1991). Frontiers of reproductive technology: A review of assisted methods of reproduction. In C. Garner (Ed.). *Principles of infertility nursing* (pp. 137–156). Boca Raton, FL: CRC Press.

Flynn, M. T. (1991). Ovulation disorders. In C. Garner (Ed.). *Principles of infertility nursing* (pp. 31–55). Boca Raton, FL: CRC Press.

Fraser, I. S., and Weisberg, E. (1982). Fertility discontinuation of different methods of fertility control. *Contraception,* 26, 389.

Garner, C. (1991). An overview of infertility. In C. Garner (Ed.). *Principles of infertility nursing* (pp. 1–8). Boca Raton, FL: CRC Press.

Hahn, S. (1991). Caring for couples considering alternatives in family-building. In C. Garner (Ed.). *Principles of infertility nursing* (pp. 179–205). Boca Raton, FL: CRC Press.

Hahn, S. J., Butkowski, C. R., Capper, L. L. (1994). Ovarian hyperstimulation syndrome: Protocols for nursing care. *Journal of Obstetric, Gynecologic, and Neonatal Nursing,* 23 (3), 217–226.

Halman, L. J., Andrews, F. M., Abbey, A. (1994). Gender differences and perceptions about childbearing among infertile couples. *Journal of Obstetric, Gynecologic, and Neonatal Nursing,* 23 (7), 593–600.

Johnson, A. R., Lipshultz, L. I., Smith, R. C. (1985). Sperm penetration assay: Relationship between motile sperm per ejaculate and fertilizing potential. *Abstract 34, 41st Annual Meeting, American Fertility Society.* Chicago.

Johnston, G. P. (1994). *The wish, the wait, the wonder: A book of wisdom for expectant parents* (p. 12). New York: Harper Collins.

Kabanitz, A. M., Grimes, D. A., Daunitz, K. K. (1987). A physician's guide to adoption. *Journal of the American Medical Association,* 258, 3537–3541.

Lawrence, L. D., and Rosenwaks, Z. (1993). Implications of the Fertility Clinic Success Rate and Certification Act of 1992. *Fertility and Sterility,* 59 (2), 285–290.

Mahlstedt, P. (1991). Psychological aspects of infertility. In C. Garner (Ed.). *Principles of infertility nursing* (pp. 157–167). Boca Raton, FL: CRC Press.

May, J., and Garner, C. (1991). Uterine, tubal, and pelvic factors. In C. Garner (Ed.). *Principles of infertility nursing* (pp. 57–81). Boca Raton, FL: CRC Press.

Mosher, W. D., and Pratt, W. F. (1990). Fecundity and infertility in the United States, 1965–1988. *Advance Data,* 192. DHHS publication (PHS) 91-1250. Hyattsville, MD: National Center for Health Statistics.

Office of Technology Assessment. (1988). *Infertility: Medical and social choices* (OTABA 358) (p. 25). Washington, DC: Office of Technology Assessment.

Olshansky, E. F. (1990). Psychological implications of pregnancy after infertility. *NAACOG's Clinical Issues in Perinatal and Women's Health Nursing,* 1 (3), 342–347.

Patrizio, P., and Asch, R. H. (1994). Gift procedure. In F. P. Zuspan and E. J. Quilligan (Eds.). *Current therapy in obstetrics and gynecology* (pp. 55–57). Philadelphia: W. B. Saunders.

Pratt, W. F., Mosher, W. D., Bachrach, C., Horn M. (1984). Understanding US fertility: Findings from the National Survey of Family Growth, Cycle III. *Population Bulletin,* 39, 27.

Prattke, T. W., and Gass-Sternas, K. A. (1993). Appraisal, coping and emotional health of infertile couples undergoing donor artificial insemination *Journal of Obstetric, Gynecologic, and Neonatal Nursing,* 22 (6), 516–527.

Sandelowski, M. (1994). On infertility. *Journal of Obstetric, Gynecologic, and Neonatal Nursing,* 23 (9), 749–752.

Sandelowski, M., Harris, B. A., Hoditch-Davis, D. (1990). Pregnant moments: The process of conception in infertile couples. *Research in Nursing and Health,* 13, 273–282.

Sherrod, R. A. (1992). Helping infertile couples explore the option of adoption. *Journal of Obstetric, Gynecologic, and Neonatal Nursing,* 21 (6), 465–470.

Surrey, E. S., and Kerin, J. F. (1995). Extended techniques in assisted reproductive technologies. In W. R. Keye, R. J. Chang, R. W. Rebar, M. R. Soules (Eds.). *Infertility: evaluation and treatment.* Philadelphia: W. B. Saunders.

Wilcox, L. S., and Mosher, W. D. (1993). Use of infertility services in the United States. *Obstetrics and Gynecology,* 82 (1), 122–127.

Chapter 13

Genetics

Mira L. Lessick

Quite suddenly, in the last decade, biologists began to spell out human nature in an entirely new way. At a breathtaking pace, they have proceeded to characterize it in nature's own terms, in the language of molecules we call genes. Their research began with the study of heredity, by observing people within their families. Every family has its stories to tell, and others that it keeps secret. Another kind of story is written in our genes. We can read parts of it by looking at each other, but most of the details are obscure. Usually, the specifics of any family's genetic heritage are blessedly mundane. Sometimes, however, they reveal a story so momentous that it redefines a person's concept of who he is.

LOIS WINGERSON (1991)

HIGHLIGHTS

- ▼ Human Genetics in Perspective
- ▼ Review of Genetic Principles
- ▼ Chromosome Disorders
- ▼ Patterns of Mendelian Inheritance and Alterations
- ▼ Multifactorial Inheritance
- ▼ Genetic Screening, Assessment, and Diagnosis
- ▼ The Genetic Counseling Process
- ▼ Nursing Practice
- ▼ Risk Management
- ▼ Implications for Research

THE GENETIC BASIS OF HUMAN DISEASE

Human genetics deals with human variation: its nature, extent, origin, and maintenance; its distribution in families and populations; its interaction with the environment; and its consequences for normal development. Unprecedented scientific and technologic advances have been made in human genetics during the past decade. Accompanying these advances are rapidly expanding service capabilities: the capacity to undertake mass screenings to identify carriers of deleterious genes, the opportunities for prenatal diagnosis, the technology to sustain the lives of seriously ill and malformed newborns, and the ability to increase the life expectancy of people affected by genetic disorders. Rapid developments in genetics have also resulted in heightened public awareness of and concern for enhanced health and optimal reproduction.

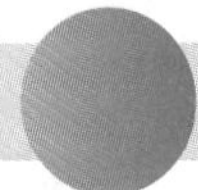

DEFINITIONS

Carrier—An individual who has a copy of a disease-causing gene but does not express the disease. The term is used to denote heterozygotes for a recessive disease gene.

Centromere—The primary constriction of a chromosome that separates the short arms from the long arms of the chromosome. Centromeres are the sites of attachment of spindle fibers during cell division.

Chromosomes—Microscopic structures present in the cell nucleus composed of chromatin. Chromosomes contain genetic information and are constant in number in a species; humans have 46 chromosomes, 22 autosome pairs, and 2 sex chromosomes.

DNA (deoxyribonucleic acid)—A double-helix molecule that consists of a sugar-phosphate backbone and four nitrogenous bases (adenine, cytosine, guanine, and thymine). DNA bases encode messenger RNA (mRNA), which in turn encodes amino acid sequences.

Gamete—A reproductive cell (sperm and ovum) with the haploid chromosome number, or 23 chromosomes.

Genes—The fundamental units of heredity. Genes are segments of DNA that direct the process of protein synthesis.

Haploid—The chromosome number of a normal gamete, with only one member of each chromosome pair. In humans, the haploid number is 23.

Heterozygote (heterozygous)—An individual or genotype with two different alleles at a given locus on a pair of homologous chromosomes.

Homozygote (homozygous)—An individual or genotype with identical alleles at a given locus on a pair of homologous chromosomes.

Karyotype—A photomicrograph of the chromosomes of an individual arranged in a standard classification.

Meiosis—Cell division process in which gametes containing the haploid chromosome number are produced from diploid germ cells.

Mitosis—The process of somatic cell division, resulting in the formation of two cells genetically identical to the parent cell.

Nondisjunction—The failure of two members of a chromosome pair to separate appropriately during cell division, resulting in abnormal chromosome numbers in gametes or cells.

Recessive—A trait expressed when two copies of the gene are present.

RNA (ribonucleic acid)—A single-stranded molecule that consists of a sugar (ribose), phosphate group, and nitrogenous bases (adenine, cytosine, guanine, and uracil).

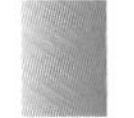

Human Genetics in Perspective

Genetic disorders and congenital malformations have become major causes of morbidity and mortality in infants and children since the reduction or control of many communicable diseases. Genetic and related disorders are also of increasing importance in the case of adults, particularly pregnant women and adults of reproductive age. Genetic disease and congenital malformations occur in 2 to 5 percent of live births and account for 30 percent of pediatric hospital admissions (Weatherall 1991; Connor and Ferguson-Smith 1993). About 40 percent of all congenital abnormalities have a known genetic or environmental etiology. Genetic causes of birth defects include chromosome, single-gene, and multifactorial disorders. Chromosome abnormalities are a significant cause of birth defects and fetal loss, occurring in about 1 in 200 (0.5 percent) newborns, 50 percent of all spontaneous abortions, and 7 percent of stillbirths (Robinson and Linden 1993). Birth defects may also be due to environmental factors such as drugs, infections, alcohol, and radiation. Finally, chronic diseases with a genetic component affect about 10 percent to 20 percent of the adult population (Connor and Ferguson-Smith 1993). The overall costs of genetic and related disorders to individuals, families, and society are incalculable.

Intense emotions are aroused when an actual or potential genetic disorder is identified. Fears of being different or undesirable as a mate may arise. Pregnant women, or their partners, may have fears about the normality of the fetus. Guilt may also occur by the disclosure that a child was affected with a disorder transmitted by one or both parents. As the capabilities to identify individuals and families at risk for genetic disorders continue to increase, so will the demand for genetic services. Maternal-child health nurses can play an active role in the delivery of services to families with real or potential genetic concerns. By applying principles of health promotion, maintenance, and illness prevention coupled with an understanding of cultural differences, family dynamics, growth and development, counseling, and other professional skills, nurses can help meet the biopsychosocial needs of families threatened by a genetic disorder in ways that can ensure an effective outcome.

This chapter provides a review of basic genetic principles; an overview of various types of genetic disorders including chromosome aberrations, single-gene patterns of inheritance, and multifactorial defects; an understanding of genetic screening and counseling services as applied to maternal and newborn care; and an appreciation of the roles of the nurse in genetic assessment and counseling.

Review of Genetic Principles

GENES AND CHROMOSOMES

Genes are the basic units of heredity that determine the unique physical, chemical, and mental characteristics and traits of all individuals. More specifically, genes are defined as segments of DNA (deoxyribonucleic acid) that direct the process of protein synthesis. Genes determine protein and enzyme structure as well as control their regulation and rate of synthesis. Chromosomes are microscopic structures in the nucleus of cells; they carry the genes that convey genetic information. Chromosomes consist of DNA and histone and nonhistone proteins. DNA is a macromolecule composed of a five-carbon sugar (deoxyribose); a phosphate group; and a nitrogenous base, of which there are two types, purines and pyrimidines. In DNA, the purine bases are adenine (A) and guanine (G), and the pyrimidine bases are thymine (T) and cytosine (C). Each unit of purine or pyrimidine base together with the attached sugar and phosphate group is referred to as a nucleotide.

A molecule of DNA is composed of two nucleotide chains that are coiled around one another in a clockwise fashion to form a double helix or spiral structure. The two chains run in opposite directions and are held together by hydrogen bonds between the bases. Adenine (A) in one chain is always bonded to thymine (T) in the other chain, whereas cytosine (C) in one chain is bonded to guanine (G) in the other. This base pairing is specific; that is, a given base on one DNA strand determines the base at the same position on the other strand because they are complementary.

The genetic code is a series of triplet sequences of the A, G, T, and C nitrogenous bases. Each sequence of three bases (called a codon) specifies an amino acid, which is the building block of proteins. Proteins, whether structural components, enzymes, hormones, carrier molecules, or receptors, are all composed of a series of amino acids. There are 20 known amino acids and 64 possible combinations or codons (4^3). The sequence of the amino acids determines the form and function of the resulting protein. Protein synthesis occurs in the cell cytoplasm at intracellular structures known as ribosomes. Messenger RNA (mRNA), or ribonucleic acid, molecules copy the genetic information coded within the DNA and migrate to the cytoplasm, where they then form a template for the formation of proteins as directed by the original DNA.

Genes are arranged in a linear fashion along the length of chromosomes, each gene having a specific location (locus). There are thousands of genes on each chromosome, and a person's total genetic makeup (or genome) is thought to contain between 50,000 and 100,000 genes. The majority of genes consist of alternating protein-coding segments, or exons, and noncoding segments called introns, whose function is unknown. Genes may be categorized into two types: structural genes, which control the production of proteins; and regulatory genes, which control the activity of structural genes.

Genetic mutations may involve alterations in the sequence of DNA nitrogenous bases. These may be due, for example, to a change in one or more bases, the loss of genes from chromosome breakage, or the addition of bases to a gene sequence as a result of chromosome replication or rearrangement. The outcome of such changes is a misreading of the genetic code, which can lead to overproduction, underproduction, or absent production of the product or production of a structurally abnormal product.

CHROMOSOME CLASSIFICATION, MORPHOLOGY, AND ANALYSIS

Chromosomes are present in the nucleus of all body cells. Each species has a characteristic chromosome constitution with respect to number and structure of chromosomes. The normal human chromosome number in somatic cells and in the zygote (fertilized ovum) is 46. These 46 chromosomes exist in pairs; one member of each pair comes from the individual's mother and one from the father. The 46 chromosomes, or 23 pairs, represent the diploid (2N) number. The first 22 pairs of chromosomes are common to both males and females and are called autosomes. The autosome pairs are homologous chromosomes since each pair has a similar size and shape and contains the same linear arrangement of genes. The twenty-third pair of chromosomes are the sex chromosomes. Normal females have two X chromosomes,

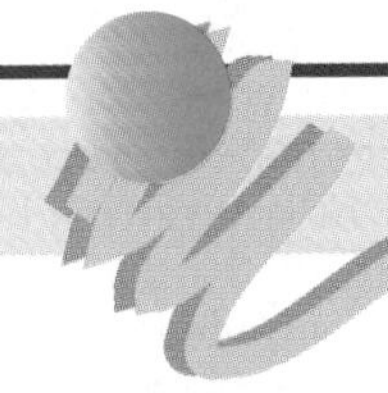

HISTORICAL PERSPECTIVES

GENETICS

1859 Charles Darwin published *On the Origin of the Species*

1865 Gregor Mendel advanced the principles of segregation and independent assortment

1869 Friedrich Miescher discovered DNA

1900 Hugo de Vries, Carl Correns, and Erich von Tschermak rediscovered Mendel's principles

1902 Archibald Garrod noted the first genetic disease
Walter Sutton and Theodor Boveri proposed the chromosome theory

1908 G. H. Hardy and Wilheim Weinberg formulated the Hardy-Weinberg principle

1913 A. H. Sturtevant constructed a genetic map

1915 Thomas Morgan and Calvin Bridges demonstrated that genes are on chromosomes

1927 H. J. Muller induced mutation by x-rays

1931 Harriet Creighton and Barbara McClintock obtained physical evidence for recombination

1941 George Beadle and E. L. Tatum proposed the one gene–one enzyme hypothesis

1944 Oswald Avery, Colin McLeod, and Maclyn McCarty identified DNA as the material genes are made of

1953 James Watson, Francis Crick, Rosalind Franklin, and Maurice Wilkins determined the structure of DNA

1958 Mathew Meselson and Franklin Stahl demonstrated the semiconservative replication of DNA

1961 Sidney Brenner, François Jacob, and Mathew Meselson discovered messenger RNA

1966 Marshall Nirenberg and Har Gobind Khorana finished unraveling the genetic code

1972 Paul Berg made the first recombinant DNA in vitro

1973 Herb Boyer and Stanley Cohen first used a plasmid to clone DNA

1977 Walter Gilbert and Frederick Sanger worked out methods to determine the sequence of bases in DNA
Frederick Sanger determined the base sequence of an entire viral genome (ϕX174)
Phillip Sharp, Richard Roberts, and others discovered interruptions (introns) in genes

1985 Alec Jeffreys discovered DNA fingerprinting

1988 Nancy Wexler, Michael Conneally, and James Gusella located the Huntington disease gene on human chromosome 4

1990 Lap-Chee Tsui, Francis Collins, and John Riordan found the gene that is responsible for cystic fibrosis
James Watson and many others launched the Human Genome Project to map the entire human genome and, ultimately, to determine its base sequence

1991 W. French Anderson and others performed the first successful gene therapy for severe combined immunodeficiency syndrome in two girls

1993 The Huntington Disease Group identified the Huntington disease gene

1994 Donna Shattuck-Eidens, Mark H. Skolnick, and others located the gene *(BRCA1)* responsible for an inherited form of breast cancer

Data from Weaver, R. F., and Hedrick, P. W. (1995). *Basic genetics* (2nd ed.). Dubuque, IA: William C. Brown Publishers; Connor, J. M., and Ferguson-Smith, M. A. (1993). *Essential medical genetics* (4th ed.). Oxford: Blackwell Scientific Publications; Nash, J. M. (1994). Cornering a killer. *Time,* Sept 26, 70.

and normal males have one X and one Y chromosome. While the two X chromosomes in the female are also homologous, the X and Y male chromosomes are nonhomologous since they are different from one another. Gametes (ova and sperm) each have 23 chromosomes, consisting of 22 autosomes and 1 sex chromosome. These 23 chromosomes in gametes are referred to as the haploid (N) number.

Two types of cell division are necessary for transmitting genetic information: mitosis and meiosis. Mitosis is the process of somatic cell division whereby growth of the organism occurs and cells normally repair and replace themselves.

Every individual begins life as a single cell, the zygote, which is formed by the fusion of a 23-chromosome–bearing ovum and sperm. The zygote thus has 46 chromosomes, and each parent has equally contributed to the offspring's genetic makeup. After fertilization, the organism grows by cell division; the genetic information of each cell is passed to two new daughter cells, which are precisely identical to the parent cell in chromosome complement. The process of mitosis therefore maintains the diploid chromosome number of 46 (Fig. 13–1).

Meiosis is the process by which reproductive or germ cells divide to form gametes. During meiosis,

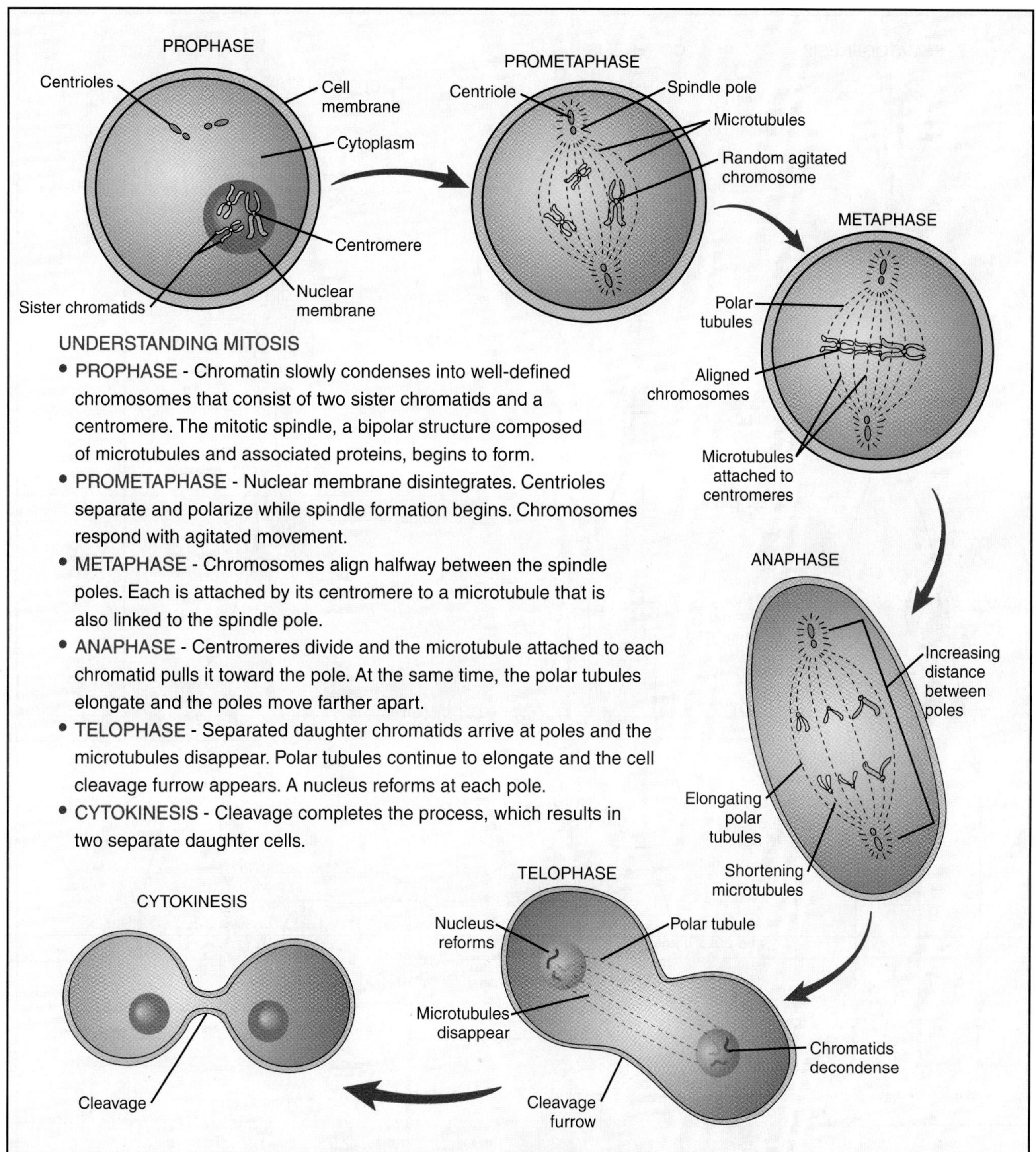

Figure 13–1
The process of mitosis.

the homologous chromosomes join together and may exchange genetic material before each of the 23 paired chromosomes separates and is incorporated into a daughter cell having 23 chromosomes. This exchange of genetic material allows new gene combinations and enhances genetic variability among individuals. A second meiotic division then occurs in which each of the 23 individual chromosomes divides, and this process ends with the formation of mature haploid gametes with 23 chromosomes (Fig. 13–2). The fusion of male and female gametes at fertilization restores the diploid chromosome number of 46 and promotes genetic variability.

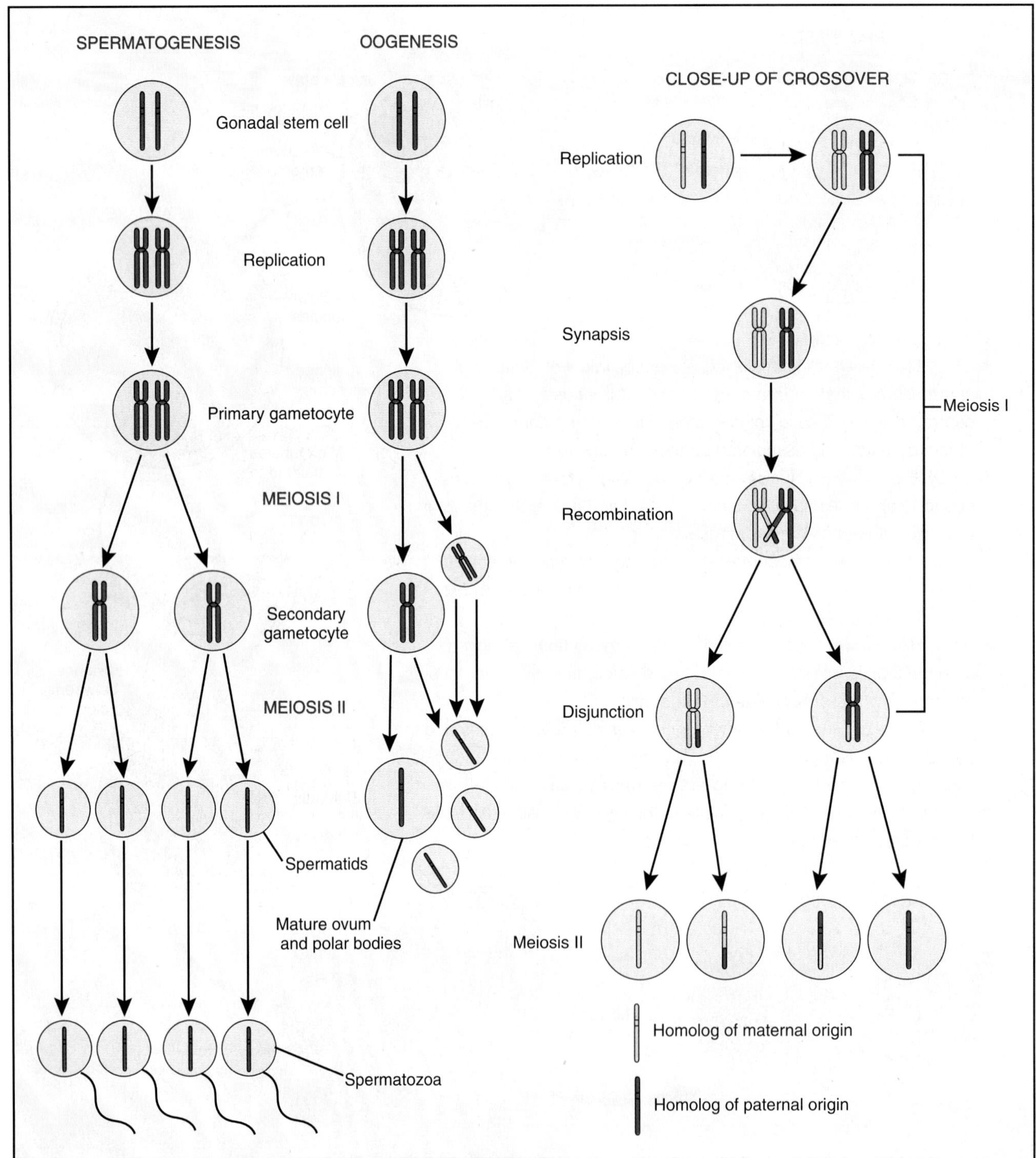

Figure 13–2
The process of meiosis in spermatogenesis and oogenesis.

Chromosomes can best be identified during the metaphase or prophase stage of cell division (see Fig. 13–1). In metaphase, the chromosomes consist of two complementary halves, called sister chromatids. The sister chromatids are joined to each other at the centromere, a primary constriction, that separates the short arms (p) from the long arms (q) of the chromosome and serves as the site of spindle attachment during cell division (Fig. 13–3).

The chromosomal constitution of an individual can be determined by studying many different tissues. The tissues most commonly used are peripheral lymphocytes, skin fibroblasts, and amniotic fluid cells. Other tissues, such as bone marrow cells, gonadal tissue, and fibroblasts from other organ tissues, are also used in specific situations. When prepared for analysis, the chromosomes of a single cell appear under the microscope as a chromosome spread (Fig. 13–4). To analyze a spread, the chromosomes are photographed and arranged in pairs in a standard classification according to their size and centromere position. This process is referred to as karyotyping, and the completed picture is a karyotype (Fig. 13–4). Typically, at least 20 spreads are examined before karyotyping, and the number of chromosomes in each cell is counted. The process of karyotyping is now performed with computers so the amount of time needed for preparing and interpreting the karyotype is significantly reduced. When the karyotype is completed, it is then examined for any abnormalities in number or structure of chromosomes.

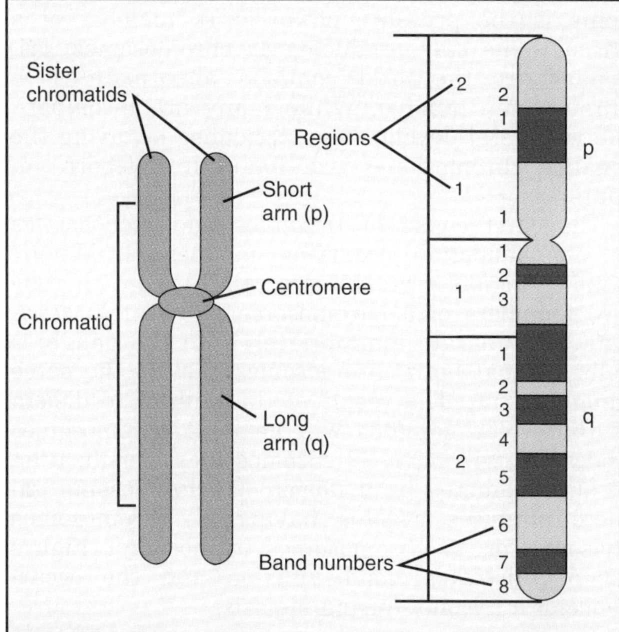

Figure 13–3

Diagrammatic representation of the parts of a chromosome at metaphase, and a single chromatid structure marked with band and region numbers.

Advances in banding techniques have led to the rapid identification of individual chromosomes and enabled more precise identification of aberrations. Banding techniques are methods of manipulating chromosome preparations to elicit banding patterns along the length of each chromosome. Giemsa (G) banding is a widely used method for routine clinical evaluation. Other common types of banding are quinacrine (Q), reverse (R), centromere (C), and prophase banding. Bands are distinct markings that appear along the chromosomes after the preparations have been treated and stained in a specific manner. Alternate light and dark bands give unique patterns for each chromosome (see Fig. 13–3). Each arm is divided into regions and given numbers, and each region is further divided into band numbers that allow precise identification of sites on chromosomes.

Gene mapping involves the assignment of genes to specific locations on specific chromosomes. Mapping is crucial for improving prenatal diagnosis and carrier detection for particular genetic disorders. The mapping of a genetic disorder to a chromosome region may also represent the first step toward cloning the gene and discovering its function (so-called reverse genetics). There are various techniques used to map genes, including family linkage studies, gene dosage methods, in situ hybridization, interspecific somatic cell hybridization, and flow-sorted chromosome dot blot analysis (Connor and Ferguson-Smith 1993).

Mapping of the human genome is a major goal of the federally sponsored Human Genome Project, which began in 1990 (Jordon 1992; Antonarakis 1990). This project will produce extensive new knowledge about the genes involved in inherited disorders, birth defects, and adult-onset disorders with a genetic component—including heart disease, neurologic disorders, mental illness, and many cancers. Risk factors for common disorders will be identified and new treatment modalities developed. These advances raise many social, ethical, and legal issues that will affect the delivery of health care and need to be carefully considered. Among these are the possibility of discrimination related to employment or insurance; social stigma of carrying the genes for a particular disorder; and concerns about informed consent, privacy, confidentiality of information, and individual versus societal rights (Cook-Deegan 1990; Lessick and Forsman 1995).

Genetic disorders can be classified into three major etiologic categories. Disorders in which there is a demonstrable change in the number or structure of a person's chromosomes are termed chromosome disorders. Disorders due to a single-gene mutation and that follow specific patterns of inheritance are called single-gene disorders. Disorders due to the interaction of both genetic and environmental factors are called multifactorial disorders. An understanding of these three categories is

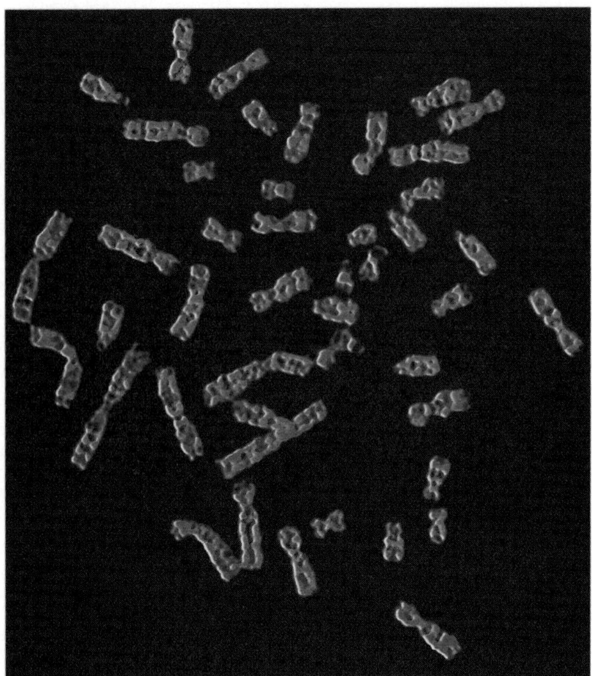

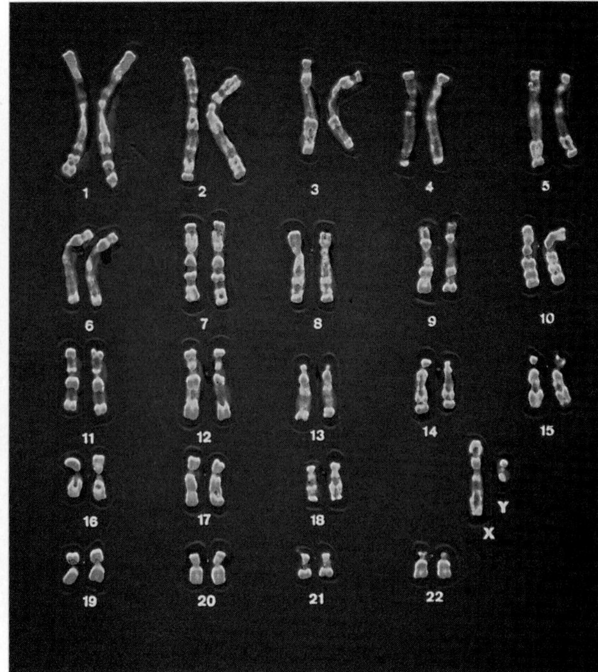

Figure 13–4

The microscopic appearance of metaphase chromosomes from a single cell shown on a false-color light micrograph of normal human chromosomes, obtained by amniocentesis. • A normal trypsin/Leishman–banded male karyotype (46, XY), the full complement of male chromosomes arranged in numbered homologous pairs, shown on a false-color light micrograph. (From CNRI/Science Photo Library/PHOTO Researchers, Inc.)

central to the delivery of effective genetic health care.

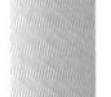

Chromosome Disorders

Chromosome disorders are conditions associated with changes in either chromosome number or structure and may involve one or more autosomes, sex chromosomes, or both simultaneously. In addition, a particular abnormality may be present in all or in only some of the body cells.

CHANGES IN CHROMOSOME NUMBER

Numerical changes in individual chromosomes represent loss or gain of chromosome sets. The term euploidy denotes the correct complete chromosome set, that is, in humans, the diploid (2N = 46) and haploid (N = 23) numbers of chromosomes. Two types of deviations in chromosome number are polyploidy and aneuploidy. Polyploidy refers to an exact multiple of the haploid set. An example is 69 (3N) chromosomes with three copies of each chromosome instead of two. Polyploidy is generally incompatible with life and observed commonly in abortuses. Aneuploidy is a numerical deviation that is not an exact multiple of the haploid set, such as 45 or 47 chromosomes. An aneuploid state in which one member of a chromosome pair is absent, resulting in 45 chromosomes, is called monosomy. Monosomy for the X chromosome (Turner syndrome) is relatively common, but monosomy for an autosome is usually lethal. Trisomy is the presence of an extra member of a chromosome pair, producing 47 chromosomes. Trisomies are the most common abnormalities in chromosome number. While many are incompatible with fetal development, trisomies involving the smaller chromosomes are found in liveborn infants.

The chief cause of trisomies and monosomies is nondisjunction occurring in meiosis. Meiotic nondisjunction is an error in cell division whereby two members of a chromosome pair fail to separate and migrate appropriately into the daughter cells, so that both chromosomes pass to the same daughter cell. The result of this failure to disjoin is that some gametes will have 24 chromosomes and some will have 22 chromosomes. Fertilization of such gametes by a normal 23-chromosome gamete produces zygotes having 47 chromosomes (trisomy) or 45 chromosomes (monosomy). Figure 13–5 illustrates nondisjunction and the occurrence of a trisomy during meiosis.

The occurrence of nondisjunction during mitosis results in another numerical change called mosaicism. An individual who is mosaic has two or more cell lines with different chromosome constitutions (e.g., 46- and 47-chromosome cell lines)

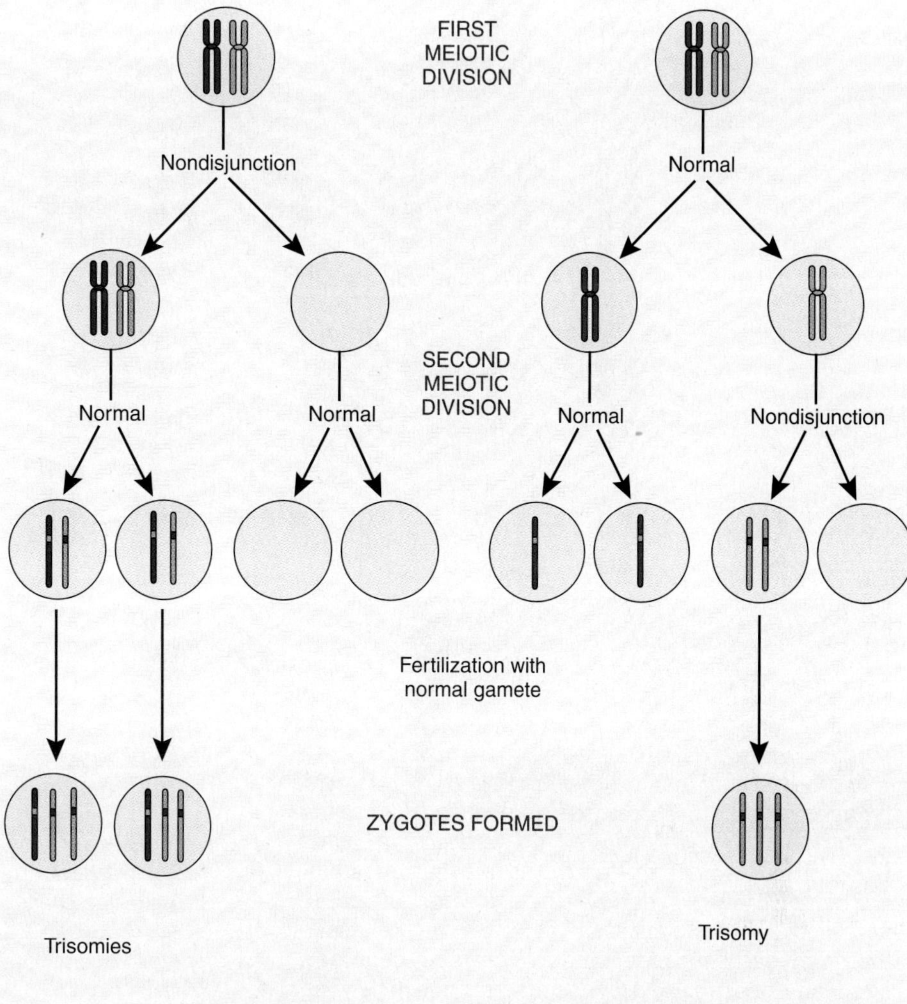

Figure 13–5
The process of nondisjunction and the occurrence of a trisomy during meiosis.

originating from a single zygote. The clinical effects of mosaicism vary, depending on how early the error occurs in the postzygotic cell division and the proportion of abnormal cell lines in different tissues.

Autosomal Chromosome Disorders of Number

There are several well-defined chromosome disorders in which a numerical abnormality of an autosome is present. Three disorders common among liveborn infants are trisomy 21, trisomy 18, and trisomy 13.

▼ **Trisomy 21.** Trisomy 21 (or Down syndrome) is the most common autosomal abnormality and one of the most common causes of mental retardation; its overall incidence is 1 in 700 live births. In approximately 95 percent of cases, the affected child has three copies of chromosome 21 instead of two (Fig. 13–6). This complete (or regular) trisomy 21 arises from meiotic nondisjunction in either parent. The extra chromosome has been found to be of maternal origin in about 85 percent of cases and of paternal origin in 15 percent (Connor and Ferguson-Smith 1993). Advanced maternal age is an important factor in the incidence of Down syndrome.

The diagnosis of Down syndrome can generally be made shortly after birth by clinical findings (Fig. 13–6) and is confirmed by chromosome analysis. Common clinical features are hypotonia, poor Moro reflex, brachycephalic head, flat facial profile, speckling of the outer portion of the iris (Brushfield spots), upslanting palpebral fissures, epicanthal folds, small nose with low nasal bridge, small ears, protruding tongue secondary to a

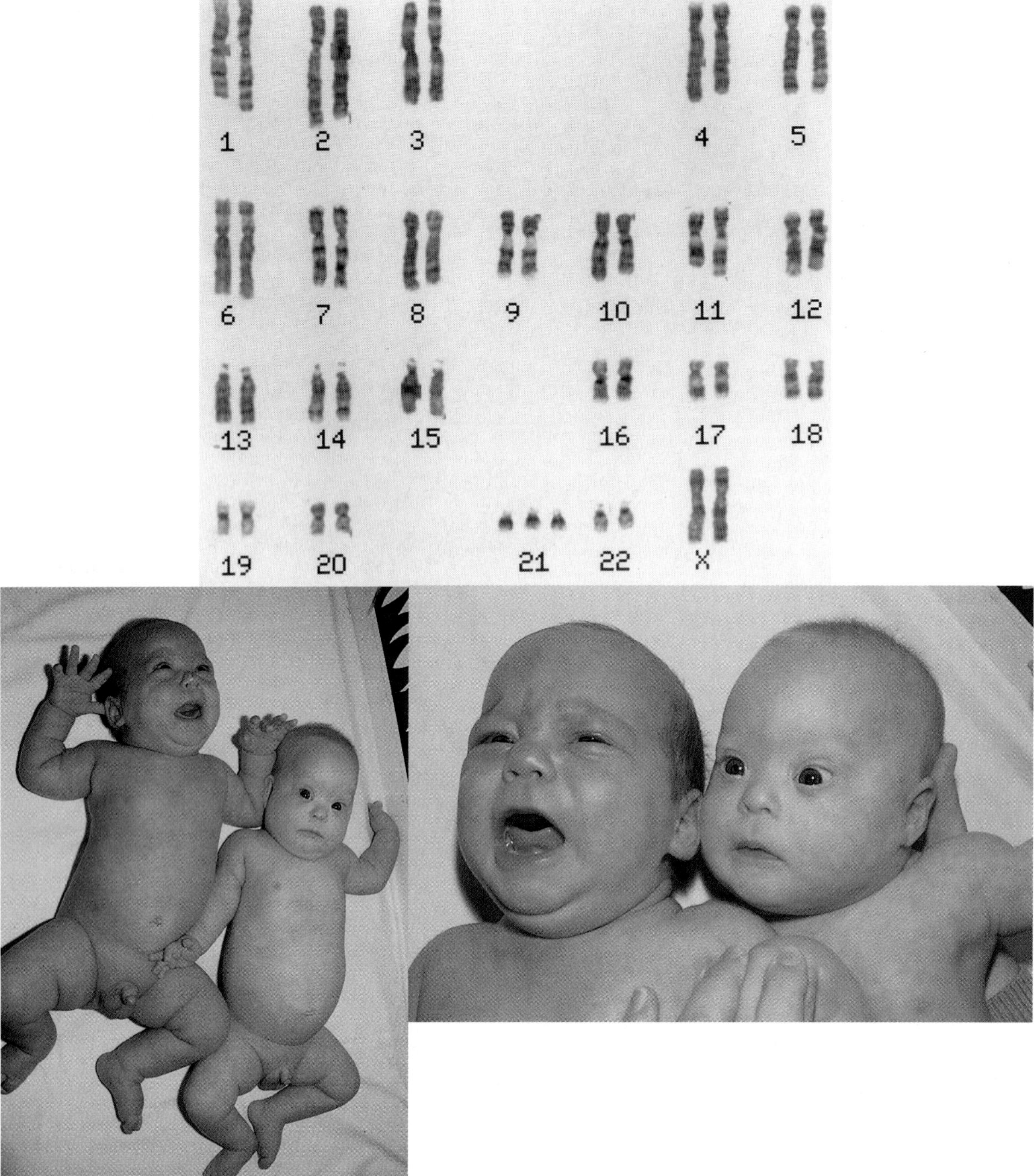

Figure 13–6

Male karyotype of trisomy 21 shows the extra or third copy of the number 21 chromosome. • Dizygotic (fraternal) male twins who are discordant for Down syndrome (trisomy 21); the twin on the right is smaller and hypotonic compared with the unaffected twin. • Close-up shows the characteristic facial features of Down syndrome in the twin on the right (upslanting eyes, flat nose bridge, small ears). (Karyotype courtesy of Rush-Presbyterian-St. Luke's Medical Center, Chicago, IL; photos courtesy of Dr. A. E. Chudley, Professor of Pediatrics and Child Health, Children's Hospital, Winnipeg, Manitoba, Canada.)

small maxilla and narrow palate, short and broad hands with a single palmar crease and incurving of the fifth finger (clinodactyly) (Fig. 13–7), excess skinfolds on the back of the neck, and hyperflexible joints. Mental retardation varies from mild to severe. Congenital heart defects occur in 40 to 60 percent of patients and are a major cause of early mortality. Other complications may include thyroid

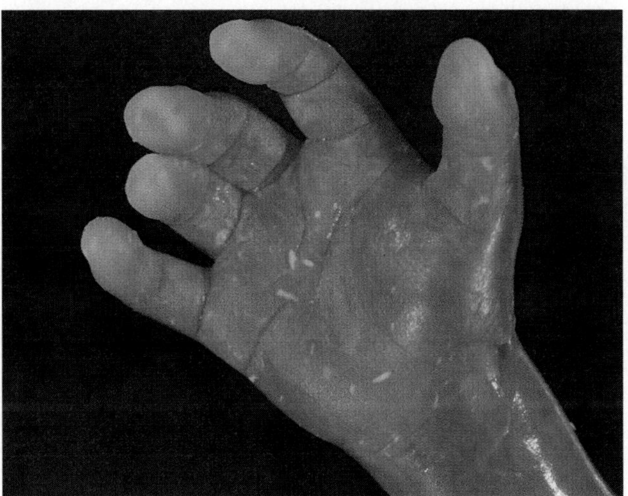

Figure 13–7

A fetal hand shows a single, transverse palmar crease and clinodactyly (incurving) of the fifth finger. (Courtesy of Dr. A. E. Chudley, Professor of Pediatrics and Child Health, Children's Hospital, Winnipeg, Manitoba, Canada.)

problems, gastrointestinal disorders, and an increased incidence (about 1 percent) of leukemia.

Two other forms of Down syndrome exist that account for a small percentage of cases. About 4 percent of cases are due to a translocation in which the third chromosome 21 is attached to another chromosome. In this situation, the child may have received the extra copy of chromosome 21 from one parent who is clinically normal but a carrier of a balanced translocation involving chromosome 21 (see Changes in Chromosome Structure, p. 315). The clinical features of this form are indistinguishable from those of regular trisomy 21. Mosaicism occurs in at least 1 percent of infants with Down syndrome. A child with mosaic Down syndrome has a mixture of normal and abnormal (trisomy 21) chromosome cells and therefore may exhibit milder manifestations.

▼ **Trisomy 18.** Trisomy 18 (Edwards syndrome) is the second most common autosomal trisomy; its incidence is about 1 per 3500 live births. Roughly 95 percent of affected fetuses abort spontaneously. There is a preponderance of female infants at birth, which may reflect a preferential survival. This syndrome is associated with severe defects and poor postnatal survival. Clinical features are low birth weight, failure to thrive, severe mental and growth retardation, congenital heart disease, micrognathia, prominent occiput, low-set malformed ears, short sternum, clenched fists with the second and fifth digits overlapping the third and fourth, and rocker-bottom feet (Fig. 13–8). Anomalies of the kidneys and other organs may also be present. Among affected infants, 30 percent die within the first month, and only 10 percent survive beyond the first year (Jones 1988).

The extra copy of chromosome 18 is usually caused by parental nondisjunction at either the first or second meiotic division. Translocation is rare, but occasionally mosaicism consisting of a normal cell line and a trisomy 18 line is found.

▼ **Trisomy 13.** Trisomy 13 (Patau syndrome) is a severe multiple malformation disorder with an incidence of about 1 per 5000 live births. Clinical features include severe mental and motor retardation, defects of the forebrain, microphthalmos, cleft lip and palate, polydactyly, clenched fists, low-set malformed ears, microcephaly with sloping forehead, congenital heart disease, and urogenital anomalies (Fig. 13–9). About 50 percent of affected infants die within the first month, and only 10 percent survive beyond the first year (Connor and Ferguson-Smith 1993; Jones 1988).

In trisomy 13, three copies of chromosome 13 are present. Most affected infants have a regular trisomy due to meiotic nondisjunction in either parent. However, translocation and mosaicism (a mixture of normal and trisomy 13 cells) can also occur.

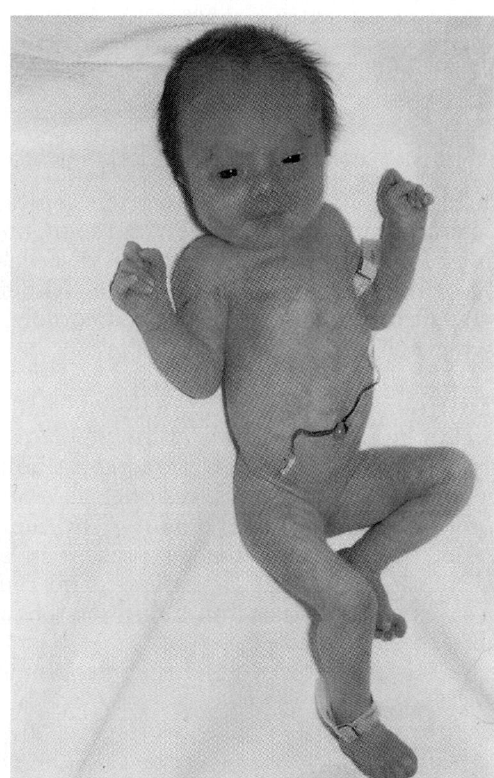

Figure 13–8

A female neonate with trisomy 18 shows the characteristic growth retardation, clenched fists with overlapping second and fifth fingers, short sternum, and narrow pelvis. (Courtesy of Dr. A. E. Chudley, Professor of Pediatrics and Child Health, Children's Hospital, Winnipeg, Manitoba, Canada.)

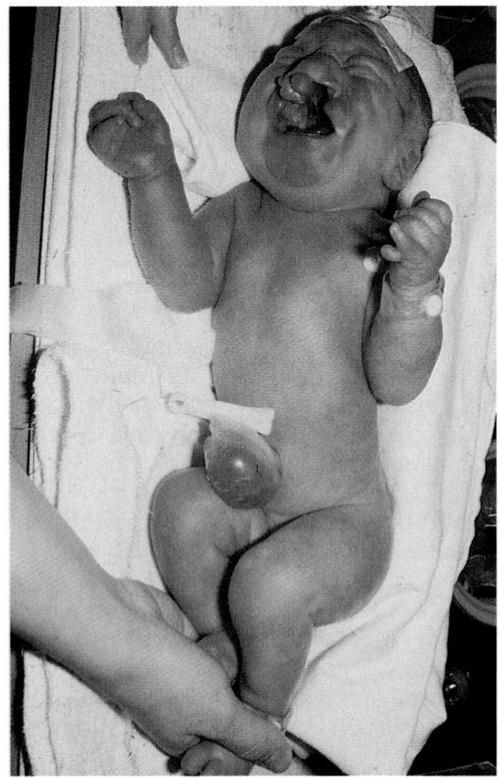

Figure 13–9

Female neonate with trisomy 13. Note the bilateral cleft lip, low-set ears, and polydactyly (extra fingers). (Courtesy of Dr. A. E. Chudley, Professor of Pediatrics and Child Health, Children's Hospital, Winnipeg, Manitoba, Canada.)

Sex Chromosome Disorders of Number

Numerical changes of the sex chromosomes, like those of autosomes, arise chiefly through nondisjunction. Common sex chromosome disorders in newborns are Turner (XO) syndrome, Klinefelter (XXY) syndrome, triple X (XXX) syndrome, and XYY syndrome.

▼ **Turner Syndrome.** Turner syndrome (45, XO) occurs in approximately 1 in 2000 to 2500 live female births and is also a frequent finding in spontaneous abortions. This disorder is the only monosomy compatible with viability. The complete absence of the X chromosome is present in about 50 percent to 60 percent of patients. The remaining cases have a structural alteration of the X chromosome or mosaicism.

Characteristic features of Turner syndrome are short stature, low posterior hairline, webbing of the neck, broad chest with widely spaced nipples, cubitus valgus (increased carrying angle of the arms), hypoplastic nails, multiple pigmented nevi, and failure of secondary sexual development. The ovaries begin to develop normally in early fetal life but then degenerate so that at birth they are represented by streaks, and this results in failure of secondary sexual development. While primary amenorrhea and infertility are usual, about 5 to 10 percent of affected girls may initiate menses, and a small number have borne children (Jorde et al. 1995). Turner syndrome can be detected in newborns by the presence of a webbed neck, lymphedema of the hands and feet, and coarctation of the aorta or another cardiac defect. Intelligence is normal, but deficits in spatial perception and orientation are common in this disorder. Other clinical problems may include an increased risk of thyroid, renal, and gastrointestinal disorders; hearing impairment; diabetes mellitus; and tumors of the reproductive system (Hall 1987). With appropriate guidance and management, girls with Turner syndrome are capable of leading normal and productive lives.

Monosomy X may arise from parental nondisjunction. Since the maternal X chromosome is present in many cases, it has been suggested that the error occurred in spermatogenesis or after fertilization (Connor and Ferguson-Smith 1993). Girls with Turner syndrome may also have mosaicism (XX and XO cell lines) or a structural alteration of the X chromosome, such as an isochromosome or a short arm deletion of one X chromosome.

▼ **Triple X Syndrome.** Triple X syndrome (47, XXX) has a birth frequency of about 1 per 1000 female infants. Affected girls do not demonstrate any consistent physical abnormal features. Clinical characteristics may include a tendency to tallness with increased height velocity between 4 and 8 years of age, menstrual irregularities, delay in speech and language development, mild mental retardation, problems in interpersonal relationships, and an increased risk for premature ovarian failure. Fertility is usually not impaired, and offspring tend to be chromosomally normal. Meiotic nondisjunction in either parent is the cause of 47, XXX.

▼ **Klinefelter Syndrome.** Klinefelter syndrome (47, XXY) is considered the most common single cause of hypogonadism and infertility; it occurs in about 1 in 850 live male births. Behavioral problems or dull mentality, long limbs, and small penis or small testes may provide clinical clues toward diagnosis in childhood. However, it is usually not until after adolescence that the characteristics of Klinefelter syndrome appear. Features include small testes, incomplete development of secondary sex characteristics, inadequate testosterone production, gynecomastia (about 40 percent of cases), tall and slim stature, and infertility with hyalinization and fibrosis of the seminiferous tubules. Infertility may be the first presenting complaint in patients (Garver and Marchese 1986). Affected boys may have normal intelligence or varying degrees of mental retardation.

The extra X chromosome usually arises as a result of meiotic nondisjunction in either parent. Mosaicism (46, XY and 47, XXY cell lines) may also occur in some cases. There are several variants of Klinefelter syndrome, such as XXXY and XXXXY, which cause more severe features, including a greater degree of mental retardation, hypogenitalism, and other physical abnormalities (Jones 1988).

▼ **XYY Syndrome.** XYY syndrome occurs in approximately 1 in 1000 male newborns. The frequency is increased among men in penal and mental institutions (Connor and Ferguson-Smith 1993). Since there are few physical features that characterize this disorder, it often goes undetected during childhood or even in the adult. Clinical findings may include tall stature, large teeth, severe acne at adolescence, behavioral problems with aggression, and dull mentality. Intelligence tends to be about 10 to 15 points less than that of the normal siblings (Jones 1988). XYY men are usually fertile, and there does not appear to be an increase in chromosome abnormalities in offspring. The psychological effects (e.g., antisocial behavior) associated with the XYY karyotype are not yet clear (Nora and Fraser 1989). The origin of 47, XYY is obviously paternal, arising from the production of a YY sperm during meiotic division or postfertilization nondisjunction of the Y.

The buccal smear for Barr bodies is a useful screening test in patients in whom abnormalities of X chromosome number are suspected. This test involves a light scraping of cells from inside the cheek (buccal mucosa); the cells are then spread on a slide, fixed, and stained to reveal the presence or absence of sex chromatin, or the Barr body. This densely staining chromatin mass is located against the inner surface of the nuclear membrane in cells containing two or more X chromosomes. The number of Barr bodies is one less than the number of X chromosomes. Accordingly, a normal XY male and XO female have no Barr bodies, an XXY male and normal XX female have one, an XXX female has two, and so forth.

CHANGES IN CHROMOSOME STRUCTURE

Minor variations in chromosome structure that involve regions of chromosomes having few active genes are known to exist in normal human populations and have little or no effect. However, structural alterations may produce adverse effects with varying degrees of severity if there is loss, duplication, or exchange of genetic material within or between chromosomes.

Structural alterations result from chromosome breakage or errors in the division of chromosomes. The term deletion refers to loss of a portion of a chromosome. It can occur at the ends of a chromosome by a single break or within the body of a chromosome, which involves two breaks and reattachment of the broken pieces. A well-known disorder resulting from a deletion is cri du chat syndrome. This syndrome is due to a deletion of the short arm of chromosome 5. It is characterized by a distinctive catlike cry of the infant, slow growth, microcephaly, hypotonia, round face, poorly formed or low-set ears, hypertelorism, epicanthal folds, and severe mental retardation.

Isochromosomes and translocations are two additional types of structural alterations. Isochromosomes result from abnormal division (transverse rather than longitudinal division) of the centromere of a chromosome so that chromosomes are formed that have long arms but no short arms or short arms with no long arms. The most common kind of isochromosome is one involving the long arms of the X chromosome, which is found in some patients with Turner syndrome. A translocation is the transfer of a segment of one chromosome to another chromosome after breakage has occurred. A balanced translocation is one in which no genetic material is lost or added by the exchange of chromosome pieces. Individuals with a balanced translocation are clinically normal but carriers of the abnormal rearrangement. An unbalanced translocation has loss or gain of genetic material. If genetic material is lost during a translocation with a piece of a chromosome missing, a partial monosomy results. If genetic material is gained with a piece of a chromosome present in triplicate, a partial trisomy results.

Translocations can arise de novo (for the first time), or they can be inherited. The clinical significance of the inherited form is that carriers of a balanced translocation can form unbalanced gametes and therefore have an increased risk for producing abnormal offspring with a chromosome rearrangement. When an infant with anomalies is found to have an unbalanced translocation, chromosome analysis and genetic counseling should be offered to the parents to determine whether one of them is a translocation carrier and to inform them of the possible risks in future pregnancies. In the case of an inherited translocation, chromosome analysis should also be offered to other family members, such as siblings, who may be carriers as well.

CAUSES OF CHROMOSOME ABNORMALITIES

While the mechanisms that produce chromosome abnormalities are generally understood, little is known about the underlying risk factors contributing to their cause. Three classes of environmental agents have been shown to induce chromosome breaks and other damage: ionizing radiation; chemicals such as toxins, alkylating agents, and antibiotics; and viral infections such as measles. A specific cause in individual cases, however, becomes difficult to determine. Pregnant women exposed to these agents should be referred for genetic counseling to ascertain the possible risks to the fetus. Specific genes predisposing individuals in some families to the occurrence of nondisjunction may be another contributing factor in chromosome disorders, but this awaits further confirmation.

Perhaps the most significant factor associated with chromosome abnormalities, particularly Down syndrome, is advanced maternal age. Figure 13–10 illustrates the relationship between the risk for Down syndrome and increased age of the mother. This maternal age effect begins to assume importance at about 35 years. Hence, the matter of genetic counseling and prenatal diagnosis of chromosome abnormality should be raised with any pregnant woman who will be 35 years of age or older at the time of delivery. The reason for the association of advanced maternal age with the nondisjunctional event that results in Down syndrome remains unknown (Gardner and Sutherland 1989). However, it has been hypothesized that the older the oocyte, the greater the chance that the chromosomes will fail to disjoin correctly.

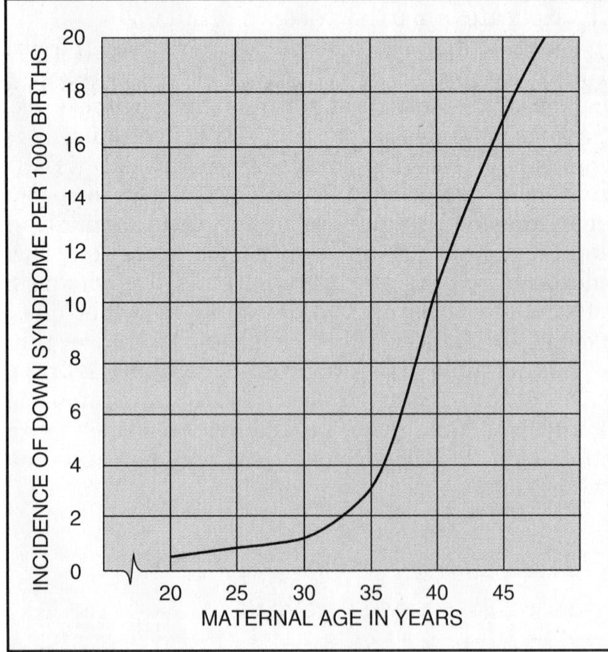

Figure 13–10

Incidence of Down syndrome births compared with maternal age. (From Klug, W. S., and Cummings, M. R. [1994]. *Concepts of genetics* (4th ed.) (p. 180). Upper Saddle River, NJ: Prentice-Hall.)

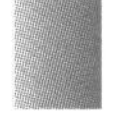

Patterns of Mendelian Inheritance and Alterations

SINGLE-GENE TRANSMISSION AND PRINCIPLES

The transmission of traits or disorders according to specific patterns first described by the Austrian monk Gregor Mendel is known as mendelian inheritance. Mendelian disorders are also called single-gene disorders. In contrast to chromosome abnormalities, which involve an excess or deficiency of whole chromosomes or chromosome segments, single-gene disorders are caused by a mutation of a gene at a single locus (location) on a chromosome. These disorders represent a single major error in the genetic information.

There are four major patterns of mendelian (single-gene) inheritance: autosomal dominant, autosomal recessive, X-linked recessive, and X-linked dominant. Genes located on the autosomes are autosomal, whereas genes on the X chromosome are X-linked. Y-linked inheritance has little clinical significance since few genes are located on the Y chromosome.

Because chromosomes come in pairs (called homologous chromosomes), genes also exist in pairs. Genes at the same locus on a chromosome pair that govern a particular trait may occur in different or alternative forms called alleles. If the two alleles of a gene pair are identical, they are referred to as homozygous. If the two alleles are different, they are called heterozygous.

The term genotype refers to the genetic constitution of an individual, with respect to either a specific gene pair or, less often, the total complement of genes. The total genetic complement of a person may also be called the genome. Letters are often used to symbolize the genotype. For example, a person who is heterozygous for one gene pair may be represented Aa, whereas one who is homozygous might be AA or aa. Phenotype refers to the observable expression of a specific trait or characteristic, either visibly apparent or biochemically detectable. Brown eyes, webbed toes, and hypoglycemia are examples of phenotypic features. Dominant and recessive are terms used to describe the phenotype. A trait expressed when the gene is present in a single dose or copy is dominant. A recessive trait is expressed only when two copies of the gene are present. Codominance occurs when both alleles at a locus are equally expressed, as in the case of the AB blood group antigens.

Most disorders determined by single-gene mutation follow the laws of inheritance described by Mendel. Two main laws were derived from his experiments with garden peas, in which he crossed pure lines differing in one or more characteristics and observed the offspring of the crosses for several generations. These laws include

1. Law of segregation (Mendel's first law). The two members of a single pair of genes (alleles) are never found in the same gamete but instead segregate and pass to different gametes during meiosis.
2. Law of independent assortment (Mendel's second law). Members of different gene pairs, or nonalleles, assort to gametes independently of one another. There is random recombination of the paternal and maternal chromosomes in the gametes. For example, if a parent cell contains genes for brown and red hair color and genes for ability and inability to taste phenylthiocarbamide, a bitter-tasting drug detected by persons with the dominant gene (taster) but undetected by individuals homozygous for the recessive genes (nontaster), the following combinations may occur: brown hair/taster, red hair/taster, brown hair/nontaster, and red hair/nontaster. In regard to two traits, then, a germ cell could produce four possible combinations of traits in the gametes.

The construction of a family tree or pedigree is a first step in assessing the genetic transmission of any disorder. A pedigree is a pictorial representation or diagram of the family history, wherein information is summarized by the use of standardized symbols to indicate individuals, relationships, and significant details associated with them (Fig. 13–11). A pedigree can clarify the pattern of inheritance in a particular family and indicate which members are at risk and need examination or testing. It also helps provide information about the natural history of the disorder and variation in its clinical expression, assists in risk estimates, serves as a quick reference source for other health professionals who work with the family, and allows patients an opportunity to raise issues of concern from their family history that were not previously discussed.

AUTOSOMAL DOMINANT INHERITANCE

Disorders that follow autosomal dominant inheritance are due to mutant genes located on the autosomes. Only one copy or dose of a mutant gene is necessary to produce the disorder, and affected individuals are typically heterozygous. The rare occurrence of an autosomal dominant condition in a homozygous state (two copies of the mutant gene) results in severe effects and is usually lethal. Examples of autosomal dominant disorders include achondroplasia, polydactyly, Huntington disease, Marfan syndrome, and neurofibromatosis.

The following are major characteristics of autosomal dominant inheritance: (1) the trait appears in every generation without skipping and is often described as being vertically transmitted, that is, from grandparent to parent to child; (2) males and females are equally likely to have or to transmit the condition; (3) male-to-male transmission is possible; (4) each offspring of an affected individual has a 50 percent chance of being affected; and (5) normal offspring do not transmit the condition to their own children. The characteristics of autosomal dominant inheritance as shown in a pedigree and the mechanism of transmission of autosomal dominant traits are illustrated in Figure 13–12. When one parent is affected and the other normal, the risk for each child to inherit the mutant gene and thus be affected is 50 percent, regardless of sex. The chance for a normal, unaffected child is also 50 percent. These risks remain the same for each pregnancy and are not influenced by the outcome of previous pregnancies.

Certain features of autosomal dominant inheritance may modify the pedigree and genetic counseling in a given family. An autosomal dominant disorder in a child may have been caused by a new mutation. A careful physical examination of both parents in this situation is crucial since fresh gene mutations are not uncommon in these disorders. If the disorder can confidently be classified as a new mutation, then the risk for the parents to have another similarly affected child is negligible. If one of the parents actually had the disorder, however, the risk for recurrence is 50 percent. Variable expressivity and penetrance are two additional characteristics of autosomal dominant inheritance. Variable expressivity refers to variation in the clinical expression of a trait, ranging from mild to severe. A severely affected parent, for instance, may have a mildly affected child and vice versa. Penetrance refers to whether a mutant gene is clinically expressed. If the gene is expressed, no matter how slightly, it is considered penetrant. If a disorder is not clinically manifested in a person despite the fact that he or she possesses the mutant gene, it is called nonpenetrant. Nonpenetrance accounts for what appear to be skipped generations in some pedigrees. A person whose parent and child are both affected must have the mutant gene, even if that person has no clinical manifestations of the disorder.

▼ **Achondroplasia.** Achondroplasia is an example of an autosomal dominant disorder characterized by short-limbed dwarfism, large head, prominent forehead with a low nasal bridge, midfacial hypoplasia, lumbar lordosis, and caudal narrowing of the spinal canal. This disorder is the most common skeletal dysplasia, affecting approximately 1 in 10,000 to 1 in 12,000 newborns. Approximately 90 percent of cases represent new

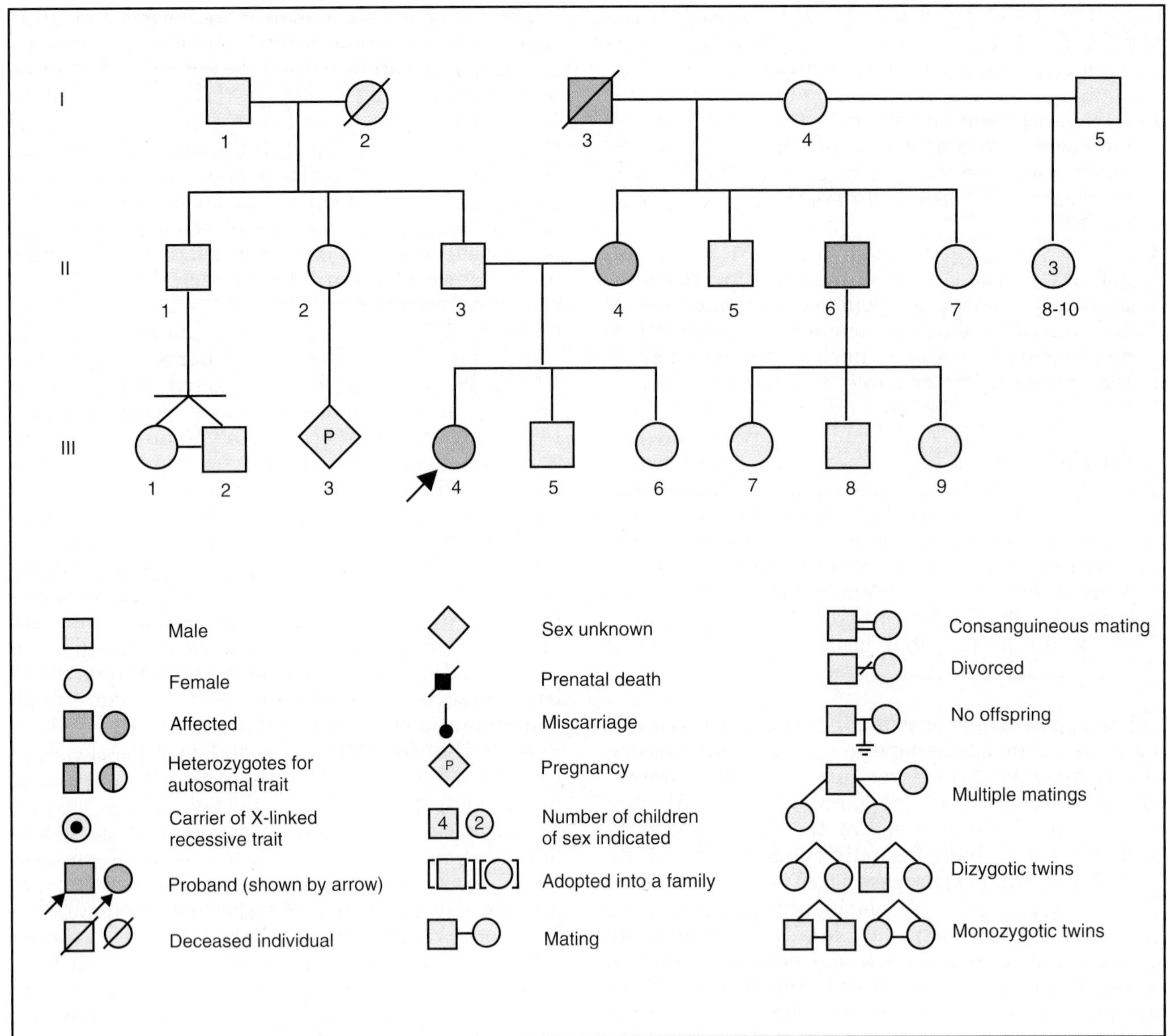

Figure 13–11

Sample pedigree and commonly used pedigree symbols.

mutations, and older paternal age has been implicated as a contributing factor (Jones 1988). Most individuals with achondroplasia have normal intelligence and can lead normal lives within their physical capabilities. True achondroplasia can be distinguished from other forms of dwarfism by clinical and radiographic study (Pauli 1995). The fact that this disorder demonstrates complete penetrance and little variation in expressivity is also helpful in establishing the diagnosis.

It is not unusual that an individual with achondroplasia marries someone with short stature. Since other forms of short stature may also carry a significant recurrence risk, information may need to be modified after marriage, with the couple counseled together. When two affected persons with achondroplasia mate, the risk is 25 percent for having an affected child who is homozygous for the achondroplasia gene; 50 percent for having an affected child who is heterozygous, similar to the parents; and 25 percent for having a normal child. The homozygous achondroplastic offspring are usually severely affected and do not survive.

The social and emotional consequences of short stature are profound. For achondroplasia, there is no effective treatment to increase adult height. An integral part of management in this disorder involves ongoing discussion with parents about potential problems the child is likely to face. People will generally consider the child to be younger than his or her actual age. Other concerns may include difficulty in getting clothes and shoes, teasing by other children, and the possibility of discrimination. Various support groups are available

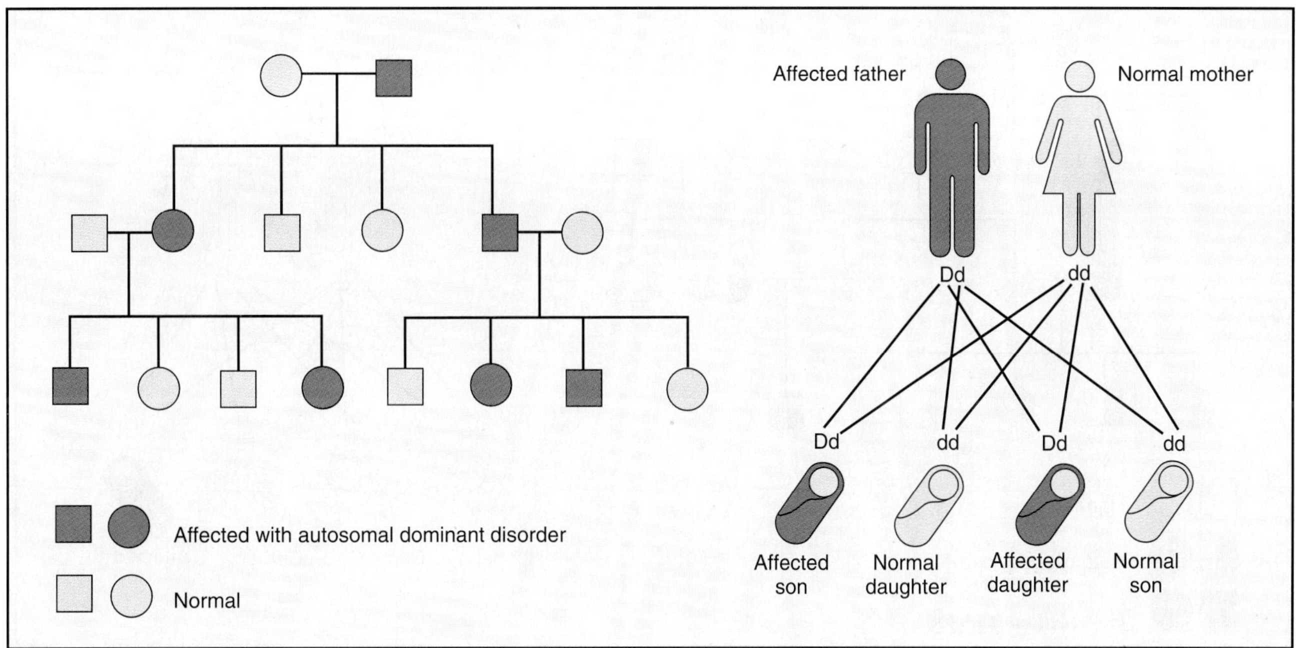

Figure 13–12

Pedigree and the mechanism of transmission found in autosomal dominant inheritance.

that address the special concerns of families of children with achondroplasia and other growth problems (Hall 1985).

AUTOSOMAL RECESSIVE INHERITANCE

Autosomal recessive disorders are expressed only when the mutant gene is on both members of a homologous pair of autosomes. Affected individuals receive one copy of the same mutant gene from each heterozygous (carrier) parent and are therefore homozygous at a given locus, having two copies of the defective gene. Figure 13–13 presents a pedigree of autosomal recessive inheritance and illustrates the transmission of a recessive condition.

In autosomal recessive inheritance, males and females are equally likely to be affected. Heterozygous individuals are usually clinically normal but, depending on the disorder, may demonstrate biochemical differences that form the basis for carrier detection tests. Each child of carrier parents has a 25 percent chance of being affected with the disorder; a 50 percent chance of being a carrier like the parents; and a 25 percent chance of being normal, without receiving the defective recessive gene. These risks remain the same for each pregnancy.

Autosomal recessive disorders tend to show a horizontal pattern of transmission in that they characteristically appear only in siblings, not in the parents or other relatives. If an affected person marries someone who does not carry the same recessive gene, all of their offspring will be normal, but they are carriers. In the unusual situation of a mating between an affected person and a carrier for the same recessive gene, there is a risk for having an affected child. Autosomal recessive disorders commonly involve an enzyme defect or deficiency, and new mutations are rare.

Another important feature of autosomal recessive disorders is that the rarer the disorder, the more likely is consanguinity (mating of blood-related individuals) to be found among carrier parents. Although everyone carries a few harmful recessive genes, most of these are rare, so the likelihood of selecting a partner with the same recessive genes is remote. However, the chances of two parents being heterozygous for the same mutant gene are increased if they are related and have a common ancestor from whom they have inherited the gene.

Several examples of autosomal recessive disorders are phenylketonuria (PKU), sickle cell disease, cystic fibrosis, galactosemia, Tay-Sachs disease, and adrenogenital syndrome.

▼ **Phenylketonuria.** Classic PKU is an inborn error of metabolism of the amino acid phenylalanine caused by a deficiency of phenylalanine hydroxylase, the liver enzyme that normally converts phenylalanine to tyrosine. When this enzyme is deficient, phenylalanine accumulates in the blood and is broken down through alternative pathways to phenylpyruvic acid and other metabolites that may be toxic. The overall incidence of PKU in the general population is approximately 1 in 11,000 live births.

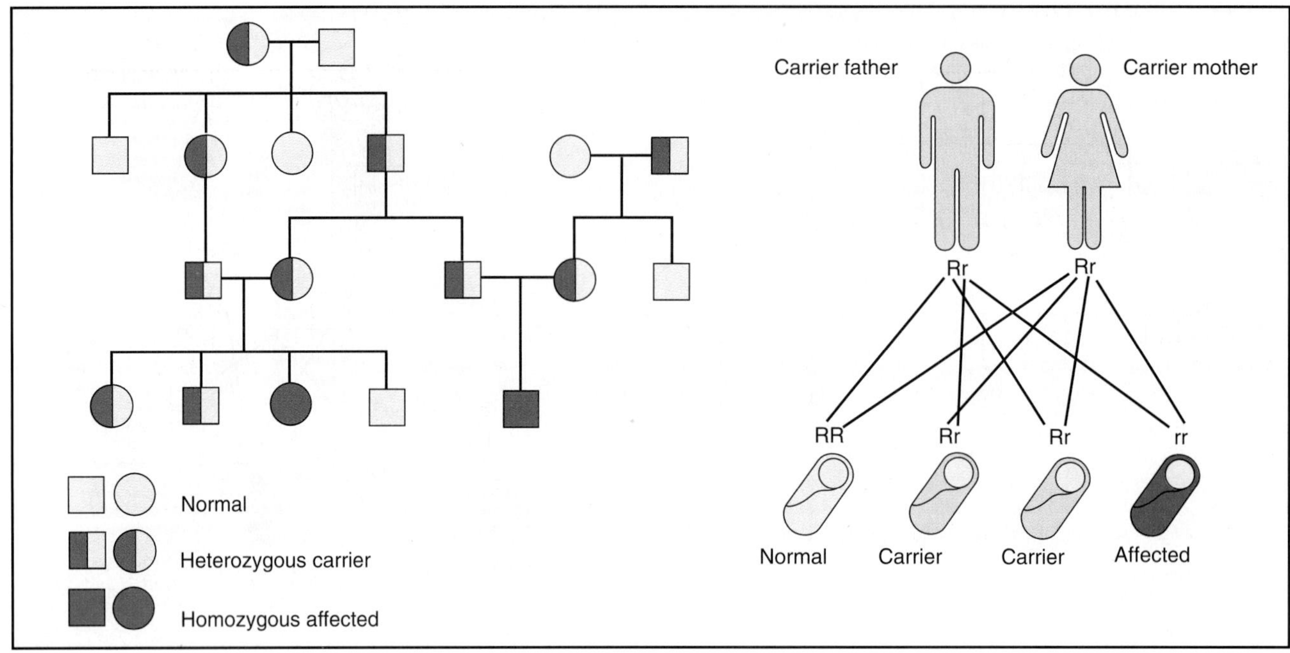

Figure 13–13

Pedigree and the mechanism of transmission found in autosomal recessive inheritance.

The major feature of untreated PKU is severe mental retardation. Affected children appear normal at birth and become retarded if phenylalanine is ingested for some time. Clinical manifestations that can occur are a progressive delay in developmental milestones, seizures, irritability, hyperactivity, increased muscle tone, and agitated behavior. Fair hair and blue eyes are common as a result of decreased melanin production and reduced pigment in the disturbed metabolic pathway.

PKU is the prototype metabolic disorder for which early detection through mass newborn screening is appropriate. The screening test is simple, involving a capillary blood sample that is analyzed for its phenylalanine content by a bacterial inhibition assay (Guthrie test), chromatography, or fluorimetric method (Scriver et al. 1989). The Guthrie test is most widely used. Heel stick blood samples are collected on filter paper slips from newborns before nursery discharge and sent to a central laboratory for assay.

Treatment of PKU consists of a low-phenylalanine diet, which must begin early in life (within 1 month of birth) before brain damage has occurred. The aim of treatment is to restrict dietary phenylalanine enough to prevent its buildup in the blood, allowing the infant to reach normal intellectual potential while providing sufficient nutrients for normal growth and metabolism. As an essential amino acid, some phenylalanine must be added to the diet to prevent breakdown of the body's proteins. Infants are usually started on the low-phenylalanine diet with Lofenalac. Phenylalanine levels must be monitored frequently and a dietary prescription developed by establishing the infant's phenylalanine, protein, and energy needs. Although dietary treatment was in the past discontinued in childhood, evidence that significant neuropsychological deficits can occur after treatment termination (Seashore et al. 1985; Fishler et al. 1987) has prompted centers to recommend continuation of phenylalanine restriction throughout life (Steele 1989; Scott and Cederbaum 1990).

Successful early treatment of affected children has prevented mental retardation and resulted in women with PKU who are having children. Pregnant women who are no longer on the low-phenylalanine diet expose the fetus to a phenylketonuric environment having high maternal plasma phenylalanine levels. The outcomes of infants born to mothers with untreated PKU are well known, including mental retardation, microcephaly, intrauterine growth delay, and congenital heart defects (Acosta and Wright 1992). Avoidance of the effects of maternal PKU can be achieved if treatment is begun before conception and continued throughout the pregnancy (Krywawych et al. 1991). Registers for tracking women with hyperphenylalaninemia have been recommended for purposes of reproductive counseling (Ghavami et al. 1986). The gene for phenylalanine hydroxylase has been identified on chromosome 12. Within affected families, prenatal diagnosis and carrier detection are possible by DNA analysis.

Sickle Cell Disease. Sickle cell disease (or hemoglobin S disease) is a hemolytic disorder characterized by a tendency of the red blood cells to become sickle in shape under conditions of decreased oxygen tension. These sickle cells have a short life span and are capable of occluding vessels throughout the body. The clinical manifestations include chronic hemolytic anemia; susceptibility to infection; and episodes of sickle cell crises marked by intravascular sickling, vascular occlusion, and painful infarcts in various tissues such as the bones, spleen, and lungs. Some patients may have more severe manifestations than others.

Adult hemoglobin is composed of two alpha-globin chains and two beta-globin chains. Individuals with sickle cell disease have a substitution of one amino acid, valine, for the normal glutamic acid in the beta-hemoglobin chain and thus form sickle cell hemoglobin (HbS) instead of the normal adult hemoglobin (HbA). Persons who are carriers for the sickle cell gene are said to have sickle cell trait. Individuals with sickle cell trait are generally asymptomatic, although occasionally they may experience exercise intolerance or splenic infarction under conditions of reduced oxygen pressure, such as at high altitudes.

Because sickle cell disease is autosomal recessive in inheritance, both parents must have sickle cell trait; that is, they have both hemoglobin S (HbS) and hemoglobin A (HbA), the amount of HbS varying from approximately 25 to 45 percent. Carrier detection is available by hemoglobin electrophoresis or laboratory demonstration of the sickling phenomenon of red cells. When both parents have sickle cell trait, there is a 25 percent risk with each pregnancy of having a child affected with sickle cell disease. One study of genetic counseling of sickle trait–carrying couples found that concern for producing a child with sickle cell anemia was often offset by a strong desire to have children regardless of risk (Neal-Cooper and Scott 1988). Many states now include sickle cell disease in their newborn screening programs.

Sickle cell disease is found primarily in the black population. Approximately 1 in 400 to 600 black Americans are born with this disorder, and about 1 in 10 individuals in this ethnic group are carriers (Motulsky 1973). The disorder may also occur among people whose ancestors come from the Mediterranean area, Middle East, and parts of India. There is no successful treatment at present for sickle cell disease, although there has been considerable improvement in symptomatic management and survival of patients (Powars 1989). Prenatal diagnosis is available for carrier couples and can be performed in either the first trimester of pregnancy (by chorionic villus sampling) or the second trimester of pregnancy (by amniocentesis), using DNA analysis (Weatherall et al. 1989; Thompson et al. 1991).

Cystic Fibrosis. Cystic fibrosis is the most common autosomal recessive disorder in white populations; the incidence is estimated to be 1 in 2500 live births. About 1 in 25 whites is a carrier of the cystic fibrosis gene. The disorder is less frequent in American blacks, Indians, Asians, and other groups. Cystic fibrosis is primarily a disorder of exocrine glands of the skin, gastrointestinal tract, pancreas, respiratory tract, and reproductive tract. Symptoms usually occur between birth and early childhood, but individuals with a milder form of the disease may go undetected until adolescence or adulthood. Most of the clinical problems in cystic fibrosis are caused by obstruction of organ ducts and other structures by abnormally thick mucous secretions. Clinical features include neonatal meconium ileus; malabsorption; pancreatic insufficiency with failure to thrive; recurrent and persistent pulmonary infection; chronic obstructive lung disease; infertility in men; and elevated concentrations of sodium, chloride, and potassium in sweat. A suspected diagnosis is confirmed by sweat chloride levels greater than 60 mEq/L.

Management of cystic fibrosis involves a comprehensive approach to provide chest physical therapy, antibiotics, pancreatic enzyme supplementation, proper nutrition, psychosocial support, and teaching and counseling to the patient and the family. Because of improved symptomatic therapy, the life expectancy of patients has increased; 75 percent survive to the late teens, 50 percent survive to the mid-20s, and about 40 percent survive to the fourth decade (Boat et al. 1989). Intense research efforts are under way to develop a variety of drug and gene therapy approaches for the treatment of cystic fibrosis, but the success of these efforts is still being studied (American Society of Human Genetics 1992; Beaudet 1992).

The gene responsible for cystic fibrosis lies on chromosome 7 and results in a protein product called the cystic fibrosis transmembrane conductance regulator (CFTR). The most common mutation causing cystic fibrosis is known as delta F508, a deletion of an amino acid at the 508 position in the gene (Collins 1992; U. S. Congress 1992). It accounts for approximately 70 percent of cystic fibrosis mutations among individuals of European ancestry. Besides delta F508, more than 200 additional mutations in the cystic fibrosis gene also cause cystic fibrosis.

With recognition of the gene for cystic fibrosis, it is now possible to directly analyze DNA from any individual for the presence of cystic fibrosis mutations. Population-based carrier screening is a possibility in the future, and this could provide an important approach to identifying high-risk couples and allowing prenatal diagnosis before the birth of an affected child (Wilfond and Fost 1990). Furthermore, newborn screening, while not routinely performed, can be accomplished with use of dried blood samples for measurement of immunoreactive trypsin (Boat et al. 1989). Its use may also increase if early medical intervention is demonstrated to be of value.

X-LINKED INHERITANCE

Both recessive and dominant X-linked disorders are due to mutant genes located on the X chromosome. A key characteristic of X-linked inheritance is that genes on the X chromosome have no counterpart (or corresponding locus) on the Y chromosome. Since males have only one X chromosome, they are said to be hemizygous, rather than heterozygous or homozygous, with respect to X-linked genes. A mutant gene on the X chromosome will therefore always be expressed in the male. Females have two X chromosomes and are either heterozygous or homozygous for X-linked mutant genes. Since no serious human diseases are known to be associated with the Y chromosome, sex linkage is synonymous with X linkage.

X-Linked Recessive Inheritance

Most X-linked disorders are inherited in the recessive pattern. X-linked recessive disorders appear almost always in males whose mothers are unaffected but are carriers of the mutant gene (Fig. 13–14). Each son of a carrier female has a 50 percent chance of inheriting the mutant gene and thus being affected; each daughter has a 50 percent chance of being a carrier, similar to the mother. As in the other patterns of single-gene inheritance, these risks hold true for each pregnancy. If an affected male mates with a normal noncarrier female, all of their daughters will be carriers and all the sons will be normal. There is no male-to-male transmission of X-linked traits because males never transmit their X chromosome to their sons. An affected male cannot have affected daughters who are homozygous for the mutant gene unless he mates with a carrier female for the same disorder. Several examples of X-linked recessive disorders are color blindness, hemophilia A and B, Duchenne muscular dystrophy, glucose-6-phosphate dehydrogenase (G6PD) deficiency, and fragile X syndrome.

In X-linked recessive disorders, it may be difficult to tell whether an isolated case represents a new mutation or whether the mother is a carrier. Detection of carrier status may be a problem because of overlapping test values between normal and carrier females. This is seen, for example, in hemophilia A and Duchenne muscular dystrophy, for which 20 to 30 percent of known carriers have test results falling within normal limits (Harper 1993). Such situations need careful consideration to avoid inaccurate genetic counseling.

An important genetic principle relevant to X-linked disorders is the Lyon hypothesis. This well-accepted principle asserts that early in the embryonic development of the XX female, one of the two X chromosomes in each somatic cell becomes genetically inactivated, and the same X chromosome remains inactivated in all subsequent generations of that cell. Whether the maternal or paternal X chromosome is inactivated in any given cell is random. The inactive X chromosome can be seen in the interphase nuclei of cells as condensed chromatin (the Barr body).

Because inactivation of one of the X chromosomes is random, the percentage of cells containing the X chromosome with the normal gene turned off (inactive) is occasionally high, leading to a greater preponderance of cells with active X chromosomes bearing the mutant gene. This explains why some female carriers of an X-linked recessive disorder may have mild clinical manifestations of the disorder (called a manifesting heterozygote) and also why carrier detection may be difficult in view of the variation in range of enzyme activity values.

▼ **Color Blindness.** The common forms of color blindness (deutan and protan) demonstrate X-linked recessive inheritance and occur in approximately 8 percent of males. Because of this high frequency, matings of an affected male and carrier female are not uncommon, and each offspring therefore has a 50 percent chance of being affected. About 0.4 percent of females have color blindness (Harper 1993). Red-green color blindness has been mapped to the long arm of the X chromosome, which will enable molecular analysis of color vision defects and provide a useful marker for nearby genes.

▼ **Fragile X Syndrome.** Fragile X syndrome is a common form of X-linked mental retardation and associated with a "marker" X chromosome. The marker, or fragile site, is a secondary constriction near the end of the long arm of the X chromosome and requires special cytogenetic techniques to show it. The combination of a defect caused by a mutant gene but associated with a specific chromosome alteration is unique in human genetics.

Affected males with fragile X syndrome generally have large testes (macroorchidism) after puberty, large or prominent ears, and long narrow faces. The degree of mental retardation ranges from severe to mild. Behavioral problems are often present in childhood, including attention deficit disorder or hyperactivity, poor eye contact, and stereotypic hand movements (Cronister and Hagerman 1989). Even though the fragile X mutation is present in every cell, expression of the fragile site is seen in only a proportion (10 percent to 50 percent) of cultural cells in affected males (Nussbaum and Ledbetter 1989).

While most males who inherit the fragile X gene exhibit at least some clinical abnormalities, an interesting finding in the genetic analysis of fragile X families is that a significant minority of males (about 20 percent) who have the gene appear to be clinically normal (Sherman et al. 1984; Nelson 1993). Such clinically normal males are called "transmitting" males, since they transmit the gene to their daughters and hence to their affected grandsons. This atypical inheritance needs to be considered in counseling family members at risk.

Female carriers of the fragile X gene are usually clinically normal, although approximately one third have mental impairment (Nussbaum and Ledbetter 1989). This may be the result of X chromosome inactivation (Lyon principle) wherein affected females may have a higher frequency of active X chromosomes bearing the fragile X gene. Many intellectually normal carrier females, and up to 10 percent of females who are mentally retarded, may not show the fragile site (Sherman et al. 1984; Nussbaum and Ledbetter 1989). In those who do show it, the frequency is much lower than in affected males.

Fragile X syndrome affects about 1 in 1000 males and 1 in 2000 females, making it the single most common form of inherited mental retardation (Brown 1990). The gene causing fragile X syndrome has been identified and is known as *FMR1*. Prenatal diagnosis is possible in the first trimester with chorionic villus sampling or in the second trimester with amniocentesis, using both chromosome and DNA analysis techniques. Management of fragile X syndrome depends on supportive therapy directed toward alleviating behavioral and neurologic manifestations, extensive family testing, and genetic counseling.

▼ **Hemophilia A.** Hemophilia A (classic hemophilia) is an X-linked recessive disorder in which the blood fails to clot normally because of a deficiency of factor VIII, the antihemophilic factor. This disorder is the most common of all coagulation disorders and occurs in about 1 in 5000 male births (Connor and Ferguson-Smith 1993). It is characterized by recurrent episodes of bleeding that develop spontaneously or follow minor injury. Hemorrhage into the joints and muscles is frequent and may lead to crippling deformities, if untreated. Knees, ankles, hips, and elbows are commonly affected sites. Large bruises or subcutaneous hematomas may be noticed in the early months of infancy, which sometimes causes suspicion of child abuse with needless psychological trauma to parents. Frequent bleeding episodes, especially into the large joints, occur as the infant begins to actively crawl. About 5 percent of carrier females have a low enough factor VIII level to be classified as mild hemophiliacs (Vehar et al. 1989). These females may sometimes experience traumatic bleeding and require precaution if surgery is indicated.

The availability of factor VIII concentrates and the institution of home care programs have simplified management and led to dramatic improvements in the lives of affected individuals with hemophilia. These therapeutic advances have unfortunately been overshadowed by the acquired immunodeficiency syndrome (AIDS) tragedy in these families. The number of new cases of HIV infection resulting from blood products is being reduced with better methods of donor blood screening and focused efforts on improved plasma products and recombinant DNA production systems (Nora and Fraser 1989; Vehar et al. 1989).

The gene for hemophilia A is a large gene located at the distal end of the long arm of the X chromosome where a number of other genes have been confirmed, such as G6PD and color blindness. Prenatal diagnosis is possible by fetal sexing and DNA analysis after first-trimester chorionic villus sampling. Fetal blood sampling in the second trimester to measure factor VIII levels in male pregnancies may be considered in families when DNA analysis is not applicable (Connor and Ferguson-Smith 1993). Carrier detection is also available by DNA analysis and in certain situations may be supplemented with determination of factor VIII activity by immunologic and coagulation assays.

X-Linked Dominant Inheritance

Disorders that follow X-linked dominant inheritance are relatively uncommon. These disorders are due to mutant genes that need be present in only a single copy to be phenotypically manifested and that are located on the X chromosome. In X-linked dominant inheritance, both males and females can be affected (although approximately twice as many females are affected as males), and both can transmit the disorder to their offspring. The pedigree pattern (Fig. 13–14) resembles autosomal dominant disorders except that all the daughters and none of the sons of affected males will be affected. Hence, there is no male-to-male transmission as is often seen in autosomal dominant disorders. Because of the Lyon principle of random X chromosome inactivation, females affected with X-linked dominant disorders tend to be less severely affected than males. These disorders are often lethal in males since males have no normal gene counterpart. With each pregnancy, affected heterozygous females have a 50 percent chance of transmitting the condition to their offspring of either sex. Affected homozygous females (although rare) transmit the condition to all their children.

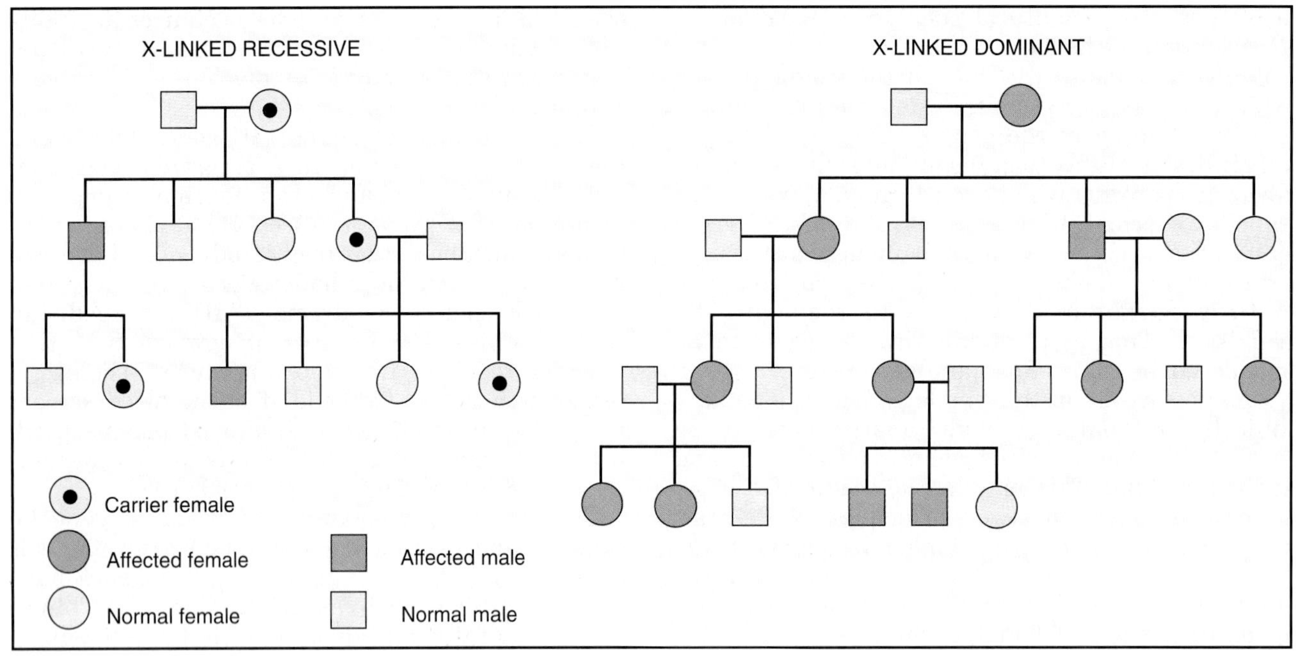

Figure 13–14

Pedigrees for X-linked recessive and X-linked dominant inheritance.

Vitamin D–resistant rickets, also called hypophosphatemic rickets, is an example of an X-linked dominant disorder. This disorder is due to defective membrane transport of phosphate, especially the reabsorption of phosphate in the proximal renal tubule. Clinical manifestations include mild to moderate growth deficiency, hypophosphatemia, hyperphosphaturia, rickets unresponsive to physiologic amounts of vitamin D, bowing of legs with weight bearing, short stature, and slow growth (Chan et al. 1985; Jones 1988). Growth is usually normal in early infancy until about 6 months of age, when the serum phosphorus concentration drops to low levels. The gene for vitamin D–resistant rickets has been located on the distal short arm of the X chromosome (Machler et al. 1986).

Multifactorial Inheritance

A group of disorders exists in which there is a considerable genetic component, but they do not fit a single-gene inheritance pattern and show no identifiable chromosome abnormality. The term multifactorial inheritance is used to designate this group, which includes many common congenital malformations and isolated birth defects. Multifactorial inheritance refers to those traits and disorders that are determined by the interaction of both genetic and environmental factors, with each contributing some effect. The genetic factor comprises a number of genes (polygenic) at different loci, each having a small additive effect. The process of multifactorial causation may be represented by a threshold model whereby the combined effects of genetic and environmental factors exceed a threshold that is required for expression of the trait. A useful analogy for explaining multifactorial inheritance is the water glass analogy wherein the genetic contribution of each parent is shown as water poured from two partially filled glasses. The rim of the glass is the threshold. When the water from the parents' glasses (representing the parents' unfavorable genes) is poured into the third glass (representing the child) that has a rock in it (representing unfavorable environmental factors), the water overflows the threshold and thus the child manifests the defect.

Some common congenital defects with a multifactorial basis are neural tube defects, cleft lip and cleft palate, congenital heart defects, clubfoot, pyloric stenosis, congenital dislocation of the hip, and Hirschsprung disease. Most normal human traits, such as height, intelligence, body build, and blood pressure, are also multifactorial. In addition, examples of common adult diseases that occur secondary to multifactorial causation include diabetes mellitus, schizophrenia, coronary artery disease, hypertension, peptic ulcer disease, and some forms of cancer.

The genetic counseling of families affected by multifactorial disorders may be more difficult than for those with single-gene disorders, since empirical (observed) risk figures are given that are derived from population and family studies. Such risk figures are not universal in their application, as are mendelian ratios with precise probabilities. A number of characteristics are unique to multifactorial inheritance. In contrast to single-gene inheritance, in which the recurrence risk remains the same with each pregnancy, the risk of recurrence in multifactorial inheritance increases with the number of affected family members. For ventricular septal defect, for example, the recurrence risk in subsequent siblings of an affected child is about 3 percent; but if two siblings are affected, this rises to 10 percent (Nora and Nora 1988).

The severity of the defect also influences recurrence risk estimates. That is, the more severe the defect, the higher will be the risk of recurrence. This is observed in Hirschsprung disease, for instance; the risk for siblings of patients with long-segment disease is greater than for those with a short segment affected (Harper 1993).

An important factor in multifactorial inheritance is the number of genes an individual shares in common with the affected person. The closer the relationship, the greater the number of genes shared in common (Table 13–1). Specific to multifactorial disorders, the risk to relatives is sharply lower for second-degree than for first-degree relatives and declines at a lower rate for third-degree and more distant relatives. For example, for cleft lip with or without cleft palate, the empirical risks for first-, second-, and third-degree relatives are 40, 7, and 3 times that of the general population incidence of 1 per 1000 (Thompson et al. 1991).

Table 13–1

MULTIFACTORIAL DISORDERS—RISK TO RELATIVES BASED ON DEGREES OF RELATIONSHIP

RELATIONSHIP	PROPORTION OF GENES IN COMMON
First-degree relatives	½
Parents	
Offspring	
Siblings	
Second-degree relatives	¼
Grandparents, grandchild	
Half-siblings	
Uncles, aunts	
Nephews, nieces	
Third-degree relatives	⅛
First cousins	

Multifactorial disorders tend to occur more frequently in one sex than in the other. Pyloric stenosis, for example, is more common in males than in females. Accordingly, another characteristic of this type of inheritance is that the risk to relatives is greater when the affected individual is a member of the less frequently affected sex (Emery and Mueller 1992). In such cases, the threshold is assumed to be higher for that sex and thus takes more unfavorable factors to exceed it.

It is important to exclude specific identifiable causes of a disorder before assessing risk in genetic counseling for a multifactorial disorder. A common error is the assumption that a major malformation was multifactorially determined when in fact the malformation was the feature of a chromosome disorder or single-gene syndrome. A thorough understanding of the disorder in the affected individual as well as a detailed family history is essential in determining the recurrence risk to be used in genetic counseling.

CLEFT LIP

Cleft lip with or without cleft palate is considered etiologically distinct from cleft palate alone. While most oral clefts are multifactorial, they may also be a feature of single-gene disorders (e.g., orofaciodigital syndrome), chromosome disorders (e.g., trisomy 13), syndromes resulting from teratogenic influences (e.g., fetal hydantoin syndrome), and nonfamilial syndromes.

Cleft lip with or without cleft palate results from a failure of fusion of the frontal prominence with the maxillary process at about day 35 of fetal development. Clefts of the upper lip may be unilateral or bilateral and may extend to include various portions of the maxillary alveolar process posteriorly, the hard or soft palate, or the nose superiorly. More males than females are affected, and the frequency of the disorder varies considerably in different ethnic groups: 1 per 1000 in whites, 1.7 per 1000 in Japanese, and 0.4 per 1000 in American blacks (Thompson et al. 1991). When neither parent is affected, the recurrence risk in subsequent siblings of an affected child is about 4 percent. If two children are affected, the risk increases to approximately 9 percent (Thompson et al. 1991). The recurrence risk is also somewhat higher in the siblings of affected females than of affected males and in the siblings of patients with a severe defect.

CLEFT PALATE

Isolated cleft palate is failure of fusion of the secondary palate. This condition is less common than cleft lip with or without cleft palate, having an average frequency in whites of about 0.45 per 1000 births (Nora and Fraser 1989). More females than males are affected. Incomplete forms of cleft palate include bifid uvula and congenital palatopharyngeal incompetence, a condition in which the individual speaks as though the palate is cleft, but there is no cleft apparent. The recurrence risk of cleft palate in siblings is about 2 percent, although the risk is higher for siblings of affected males than for siblings of affected females.

NEURAL TUBE DEFECTS

Neural tube defects encompass a group of malformations in which there is failure of closure of the neural tube, the embryonic structure that gives rise to the central nervous system during the fourth week of gestation. These defects include anencephaly, encephalocele, and spina bifida. Anencephaly is the absence of skull, skin, overlying membranes, forebrain, and midbrain, which is not compatible with survival. Affected infants with this defect are either stillborn or die shortly after birth. An encephalocele is due to a defect of the skull bones and, depending on the severity, can sometimes be successfully repaired (Garver and Marchese 1986). Spina bifida is a failure of fusion of the bony spinal arch ranging in severity from spina bifida occulta, in which the defect is limited to the bony arch and covered by skin, to spina bifida cystica, in which the spinal cord or its covering, the meninges, protrudes through the opening in the spine (meningocele, myelomeningocele).

The long-term effects of these congenital defects can range from no obvious physical defects to paralysis of the lower extremities with loss of bladder and bowel control; hydrocephalus may also occur. Although the majority of neural tube defects are multifactorial, some are secondary to chromosome abnormalities (e.g., trisomy 13) or single-gene disorders (e.g., Meckel syndrome), and some may be due to teratogenic influences (e.g., valproic acid, maternal diabetes). Neural tube defects show marked geographic and ethnic variation. The frequency tends to be higher in western than eastern Britain and in eastern than western North America; high in the Irish, Welsh, and Sikhs; low in Asians and blacks; and higher in lower socioeconomic groups (Mortimer 1980). The incidence in the United States is approximately 1 to 2 per 1000 liveborn infants. Neural tube defects tend to occur more frequently in females than in males.

Spina bifida and anencephaly are related genetically and in pathogenesis, and they are generally discussed together in counseling situations. After the birth of one child with anencephaly or spina bifida, the risk of recurrence is for either one or the other. The recurrence risk in the United States after one affected child is estimated to be 3 to 4 percent. After two affected siblings, the risk increases to about 10 percent (Nora and Fraser 1989).

Prenatal diagnosis of neural tube defects is possible by a combination of ultrasound scanning and measurement of amniotic fluid concentrations of alpha-fetoprotein and acetylcholinesterase. These methods can detect virtually all subsequent cases of anencephaly and about 90 percent of cases of spina bifida, those undetected being covered or small open defects. In pregnancies with an elevated amniotic fluid level of alpha-fetoprotein and a nondiagnostic ultrasound scan, assay of amniotic fluid acetylcholinesterase activity becomes an especially important test.

Since the majority of infants with neural tube defects are born into families without any previous history, the measurement of maternal serum alpha-fetoprotein levels in pregnant women has become a routine prenatal screening test. Measurement of maternal serum alpha-fetoprotein is less sensitive and specific than amniotic fluid measurement. However, an elevated maternal serum alpha-fetoprotein level can indicate a problem and the need for further evaluation through amniocentesis and real-time ultrasonography to confirm the diagnosis. Some studies indicate that maternal serum alpha-fetoprotein screening is an anxiety-provoking test in and of itself (Fearn et al. 1982; Burton et al. 1985).

A recent approach to the prevention of neural tube defects is the preconception use of folate and multivitamin regimens. A number of studies have demonstrated that multivitamin and folic acid supplementation before conception and during pregnancy reduces the recurrence or occurrence of neural tube defects (Smithells et al. 1983; Milunsky et al. 1989; Jorde et al. 1995). The encouraging results of these studies have prompted the Centers for Disease Control and Prevention to publish two recommendations regarding the use of folate in pregnancy. The recommendations are that all women who have had a child with a neural tube defect should take 4 mg/day of folic acid if they are planning to become pregnant and that all women of reproductive age should take 0.4 mg/day of folic acid throughout their reproductive years (Jorde et al. 1995). Furthermore, advances in medical and surgical management have also led to a reduced risk of life-threatening central nervous system infection and hydrocephalus and to improved functioning in infants and children with spina bifida. The findings from one study, for example, suggest that cesarean delivery before the onset of labor may result in improved motor function, compared with delivery after the onset of labor by either cesarean section or vaginal delivery, without affecting intellectual performance (Luthy et al. 1991).

CLINICAL APPLICATIONS OF GENETICS IN HEALTH CARE

Genetic Screening, Assessment, and Diagnosis

Genetic screening involves the testing of a specific population to identify individuals who are affected with a genetic disorder, those who are carriers of a mutant gene and at risk for having affected offspring with a genetic disorder, and those with certain genotypes who are known to be predisposed to the development of illness. Screening programs are not appropriate for all genetic diseases because certain criteria must be met. Among these criteria are a clearly defined disorder having a significant burden and an appreciable frequency in the population; the availability and efficacy of treatment or preventive measures; and a simple, cost-effective screening test that is accurate with high sensitivity and specificity and that causes little inconvenience or health risk to the individuals being tested (Nora and Fraser 1989). Major types of screening programs relevant to maternal and newborn care are preconception screening, prenatal screening and diagnosis, and neonatal screening.

PRECONCEPTION SCREENING

An important dimension of preconception screening is heterozygote (or carrier) detection. The purpose of carrier screening is to identify clinically normal carriers of a harmful recessive gene who are at risk for having offspring with a genetic disorder. Screening for carrier detection is performed essentially for preventive purposes. The occurrence of genetic disease in the future children of someone who is an identified carrier could be prevented by selecting a mate who is not a carrier for the same disorder or, in the case of a carrier couple, by exercising various reproductive options. Depending on whether the couple chooses to have natural children or not, such options may include, for example, prenatal diagnosis, contraception, artificial insemination by donor, in vitro fertilization, or adoption.

Carrier screening programs are often offered to members of ethnic groups known to have a high frequency of the disorder under investigation. Tay-Sachs disease, beta-thalassemia, and sickle cell anemia represent three autosomal recessive disorders that are relatively common in particular ethnic groups and have carrier screening available. For such disorders, both prospective parents must be carriers to be at risk for having affected offspring. If a high-risk couple is identified by screening, genetic counseling should be offered to make sure that the genetic risk, its implications, and available reproductive options are understood. This knowledge is important in helping the couple make an informed decision about future family plans. The reader should refer to the detailed discussion of sickle cell disease (p. 321).

Tay-Sachs disease is a degenerative neurologic disorder common among Jews of eastern European (Ashkenazi) ancestry. The incidence in the Ashkenazi Jewish population is approximately 1 per 3600 live births, and about 1 in 30 individuals are carriers of the Tay-Sachs gene (Connor and Ferguson-Smith 1993). Affected infants appear normal until about 6 months of age, when the child fails to achieve normal developmental milestones. Subsequently, developmental retardation progresses to dementia, seizures, blindness, paralysis, and death usually between 3 and 4 years of age.

The basic defect underlying this disorder is lack of the enzyme hexosaminidase A, which is needed for metabolizing a body lipid called GM_2 ganglioside. Because of the deficient enzyme, GM_2 ganglioside accumulates in cells of the nervous system, resulting in progressive neurologic damage.

Similar to other autosomal recessive disorders, Tay-Sachs disease often occurs in families with no prior history. There is no cure or treatment for this disorder. Prevention is possible, however, through prenatal diagnosis and screening programs that detect carrier individuals. Carrier screening involves assay of hexosaminidase A activity in the serum. Carriers have a detectable reduction in activity of the enzyme compared with control subjects. Prenatal diagnosis is performed by assay of hexosaminidase A in amniocytes or chorionic villi. The incidence of Tay-Sachs disease has dropped dramatically in North America as a result of voluntary screening followed by prenatal diagnosis (Thompson et al. 1991).

Beta-thalassemia (or Cooley anemia) is a hemoglobin disorder caused by a decreased or absent synthesis of the beta-globin chains. The disorder most often occurs in persons of Mediterranean ancestry, especially from Italy, Greece, and Cyprus. Clinical manifestations of thalassemia present during the first few months of life, with severe anemia, frequent infections, stunting of growth, hepatosplenomegaly, failure to thrive, prominence of skull bones, and maxillary overgrowth. Repeated blood transfusions are necessary and may lead to chronic iron overload with resultant cardiac complications. Iron-chelating agents, such as deferoxamine, have been used to treat the iron burden brought about by transfusion.

Heterozygotes for beta-thalassemia with one

normal and one abnormal beta-globin gene are usually asymptomatic, although they may exhibit mild anemia and splenomegaly. The carrier state is detected by hemoglobin electrophoresis and red blood cell morphology. Prenatal diagnosis can be carried out either in the first trimester of pregnancy by chorionic villus sampling and DNA analysis or in the second trimester by fetal blood sampling or DNA analysis of amniotic fluid cells (Alter 1985).

The taking of a family history is an essential aspect of preconception screening in helping to identify couples who may be at risk for having a child with a birth defect or inherited disorder. The history should cover at least three generations of relatives and include such information as racial and ethnic background; age and cause of death of deceased individuals; the presence of birth defects, retardation, and familial traits; and miscarriages, stillbirths, and severe infant and childhood illnesses. The possibility of parental consanguinity should also be assessed, since this is associated with birth defects and recessively inherited disorders. A physical examination or other testing (e.g., chromosome analysis) of one or both members of the couple may also be necessary if an actual or potential genetic problem is suspected.

PRENATAL SCREENING AND DIAGNOSIS

The development of technologies for diagnosing certain genetic disorders in utero has proved to be one of the most significant advances in human genetics that has altered the outlook for families at risk for having affected children. Prenatal diagnosis involves all aspects of embryonic and fetal diagnosis (Connor and Ferguson-Smith 1993). Examples of techniques for prenatal diagnosis include amniocentesis, chorionic villus sampling, cordocentesis, ultrasonography, and maternal serum screening (Wright 1994). Several new research techniques that hold promise for prenatal diagnosis, such as genetic tests on fetal cells isolated from maternal blood and preimplantation diagnosis, have also emerged (Simpson and Elias 1994).

Information about the genetic health of a fetus through prenatal diagnosis provides a couple with several options to consider. A limited number of conditions may be amenable to in utero medical treatment or surgical intervention. However, in most cases when therapy is not possible, the parents have the choice of terminating the pregnancy if the fetus is found to be affected with a serious abnormality. Parents who decide to continue a pregnancy when a fetal abnormality has been detected can also benefit from this information by preparing emotionally and medically for the birth of an infant who will need special care. In most cases (about 96 percent), the prenatal diagnostic tests will have normal results for the condition in question. The reader is referred to Chapter 15, Fetal Development, for a detailed discussion of prenatal diagnoses.

NEONATAL SCREENING AND ASSESSMENT

The objective of neonatal screening programs is to identify newborns with a genetic disorder so that prompt treatment can be initiated before symptoms and permanent damage occur. The number of disorders for which a newborn is screened varies by state and is usually mandated by state law. Among the major elements required in any newborn screening program are informed parental consent and education about the reasons for and process of screening; follow-up testing; provision for genetic and other counseling; and provision for treatment and ongoing management of the infant and family. The screening sample taken from the newborn may be cord blood, capillary blood, or urine. It is important that the sample taken be appropriate to the disorder in question and that all specimens be properly collected and transported to the designated laboratory within the appropriate time for accurate testing. Specimens are often obtained just before hospital discharge. Examples of genetic and metabolic disorders that may be routinely included in newborn screening programs are PKU, galactosemia, maple syrup urine disease, homocystinuria, tyrosinemia, hemoglobinopathies, congenital hypothyroidism, congenital adrenal hyperplasia, and biotinidase deficiency.

Since screening tests are not diagnostic tests, any positive tests results must be further confirmed by more sensitive methods that can distinguish a true from a transient abnormality or artifact as well as determine the particular cause in an individual case. Many parents are unaware that their infant has been screened unless there is an abnormal finding, thus producing much anxiety. Nurses can help minimize anxiety by explaining to parents before hospital discharge the reasons for screening, what it shows and does not show, and how the communication of results is handled (Wright et al. 1992). It is also important to assess family response to screening, since potential risks associated with routine newborn screening may include interference with parent-child attachment, overprotection of the child, and guilt feelings (Andrews et al. 1994). Genetic counseling is a crucial component of any screening program and should be offered to parents whose infant is found to have a genetic disorder.

Assessment of the newborn for suspected genetic problems also involves the collection of information from histories, physical examination, and laboratory tests. The family, pregnancy, and birth histories can suggest specific areas for physical assessment. Certain clinical findings, in turn, can indicate a possible genetic or related disorder and the need for further evaluation. For example, a newborn girl with lymphedema and neck webbing should have a chromosome analysis because of the possibility of Turner syndrome. In general, the presence of two or more minor anomalies in a newborn should alert the clinician to search carefully for one or more major defects. About 20 percent of infants with multiple minor malformations have an associated major malformation (Connor and Ferguson-Smith 1993). During assessment, particular attention should be paid to the head, face, skin, and limbs since the majority of abnormal development has some reflection in these areas. Other investigations that may be necessary to help identify or confirm a suspected disorder are x-ray studies, skin or muscle biopsy, photographs, biochemical testing, or dermatoglyphics. Dermatoglyphics refers to the dermal ridge configurations on the digits, palms, and soles. Certain syndromes include unusual combinations of dermatoglyphic patterns and may provide important clues to a particular diagnosis. Even when a specific syndrome cannot be identified, abnormal patterns are evidence of prenatal developmental disturbance and thus may have some diagnostic value in cases in which there is a question of perinatal or prenatal cause.

The Nature and Characteristics of Genetic Counseling

Genetic counseling, as defined by the American Society of Human Genetics (1975), is

a communication process which deals with the human problems associated with the occurrence, or the risk of occurrence, of a genetic disorder in a family. This process involves an attempt by one or more appropriately trained persons to help the individual or family (1) comprehend the medical facts, including the diagnosis, the probable course of the disorder and the available management; (2) appreciate the way heredity contributes to the disorder, and the risk of recurrence in specified relatives; (3) understand the options for dealing with the risk of recurrence; (4) choose the course of action which seems appropriate to them in view of their risk and family goals and act in accordance with that decision; and (5) make the best possible adjustment to the disorder in an affected family member and/or to the risk of recurrence of that disorder.

This definition is broad and encompasses the long-term physical, psychological, and sociologic adaptations that accompany the occurrence of a genetic disorder in an individual and the family.

The usefulness of genetic counseling depends partly on the timing of information provided to families. Since many emotions are involved in a genetic disorder, it is not always helpful to provide genetic counseling soon after the birth of an affected child or soon after a serious diagnosis has been made in a family member. During the initial early stages of a genetic diagnosis, information may be directed to explaining the nature of the disorder, describing the short-term prognosis, and providing support services for ongoing counseling. Parents, for example, will often feel that their child's defect is a sign that they themselves are abnormal in some way and may benefit by having these feelings aired. Once the initial crisis is over and the parents become aware of the long-term significance of their baby's defect and wonder about its cause and whether it may happen again, specific genetic counseling may be offered.

Examples of the kinds of families that are likely to be referred for genetic assessment and counseling are couples who have a child with a birth defect or known genetic disorder; those who are known carriers of a specific genetic disorder; those who have a known or suspected inherited condition in the family; those who have experienced reproductive problems, such as multiple miscarriages or stillbirth; those with exposure to environmental agents during pregnancy; those with ethnic backgrounds at high risk for genetic disease; and women 35 years of age or older (see Indications for Genetic Assessment and Referral).

Genetic counseling is best provided in a multidisciplinary team setting that enables individuals and families to receive expert care from a variety of professionals who specialize in the management and counseling of genetic and related disorders. Because of rapid advances in human genetics and the need for clients to have access to the latest methods of genetic diagnosis and treatment, this team approach to the delivery of genetic care is especially crucial. An effective genetics team includes expertise in genetic analysis, diagnosis, and treatment; skills in objective and subjective data collection; experience in information presentation; and family support. Accordingly, the team may be composed of a medical geneticist, cytogeneticist, biochemical geneticist, genetic counselor, pediatrician, obstetrician, nurse, social worker, and psychologist. Other specialists, such as a neurologist or endocrinologist, may be consulted as needed. In one study of prenatal management of fetal anomalies, team counseling was found effective in offering a clear definition of the problem, avoiding unnecessary confusion and anxiety for families, and providing a supportive environment during the crisis (Lorenz and Kuhn 1989).

GENETIC COUNSELING PROCESS

There are five major steps in the process of genetic counseling: obtaining a family history, estab-

Indications for Genetic Assessment and Referral

- Known or suspected congenital abnormalities: congenital malformations of any type; mental retardation (cause unknown); ambiguous genitalia
- Known or suspected chromosome abnormality
- Known or suspected inherited disorder
- Identified carriers of metabolic, biochemical, or chromosome disorders
- Multiple miscarriages, stillbirths
- Infertility
- Consanguinity
- Ethnic background at risk for specific disorder
- Fetal or parental exposure to environmental agents (drugs, certain infections, radiation, maternal factors)
- Delayed or altered rate of development
- Advanced maternal age (35 years or older)
- Parental concern or anxiety about potential offspring

lishing a diagnosis, establishing the recurrence risk, communicating information, and following up. The family history, in association with a physical examination and various confirmatory or supplementary tests, forms the basis on which a particular diagnosis is made. In taking a detailed family history, both members of a couple should be present, if possible, to obtain accurate information about both sides of the family. Information should be recorded about relatives as far back as three generations, including grandparents, siblings, half-siblings, parents, offspring, aunts, uncles, and cousins. Among the kinds of information to be gathered are names, ages, and health status; early infant deaths, stillbirths, or miscarriages; parental consanguinity; ethnic origin; and presence of birth defects, retardation, and familial traits in the various family members. If a child is affected, information about the pregnancy and birth history should be noted with particular attention to maternal infections and fever; metabolic disorders; x-ray, drug, and chemical exposures; labor and delivery details; Apgar scores; and birth weight, head circumference, and other relevant data. Information collected from the history should be assembled in the form of a pedigree or family tree (see Fig. 13–11). Tests that may be necessary to help confirm or establish a diagnosis are, for example, chromosome analysis, x-ray studies, skin or muscle biopsy, electromyography, immunologic studies, and biochemical tests appropriate to the disorder in question. Photographs may also be useful for consulting with experts about a rare or unknown disorder.

Establishing the recurrence risk involves placing the disorder in one of several categories: single-gene, chromosome aberration, multifactorial, or major environmental agents. The risk can then be calculated either from mendelian ratios or by selection of the appropriate empirical estimate. Once the recurrence risk is estimated, the next step is to inform the individual or couple about the condition, its consequences, the risk figures, and therapeutic and reproductive options available for dealing with the problem. The communication of information must take into account the educational level of the couple. Since most people have little knowledge of the medical or genetic aspects of the disorder for which they are receiving counseling, the counselor must take adequate time to explain information in simple terms and repeat content in different ways. Explaining information with the use of pictures and diagrams is useful. A follow-up letter summarizing the information provided is also helpful, as it gives the couple something tangible to refer to when needed.

Follow-up visits may be needed to make sure that individuals understand and remember the information they are given. Many families are seen by a genetics team for a period of years for ongoing treatment, to keep current on new therapies and diagnostic procedures, or when new family members develop the disorder or want information to assist them in reproductive planning. As part of follow-up, parents should be informed about community agencies that can assist in the care of an affected infant, such as infant stimulation programs, physical therapy, and support groups (Mackta and Weiss 1994). Home visits by a nurse are also beneficial to assess coping and family adjustment, identify problems, clarify information, and answer further questions.

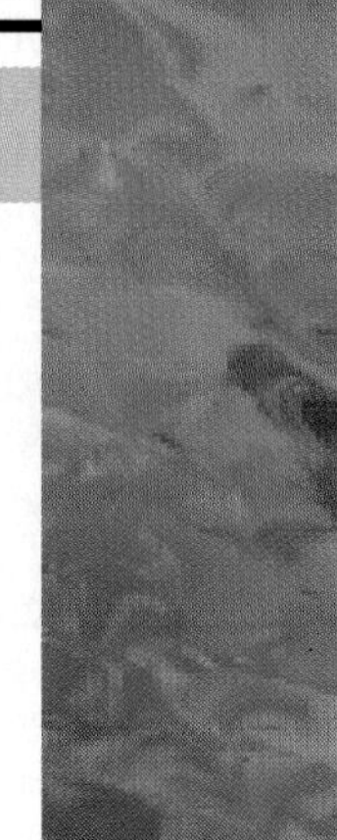

Nursing Practice

Nurses may play a variety of roles in delivery of genetic health care, depending on their educational preparation, understanding of genetics, practice setting, and job description (see Roles of the Nurse in Genetic Health Care). While some nurses may specialize in genetics and provide genetic counseling, most nurses act in a liaison position between the family and specialized genetic resources.

Roles of the Nurse in Genetic Health Care

- Identify and refer families for genetic services
- Record family histories and construct pedigrees
- Educate children and family about the genetic counseling process
- Evaluate the family's understanding of genetic counseling and reinforce information
- Identify meaning of the genetic problem involved for the client and family
- Support the family through the grief process
- Assess coping mechanisms of the client or family and build on strengths
- Assess adjustment of siblings
- Refer the client or family to community resources
- Provide health teaching and anticipatory guidance
- Support and assist families in decision making by clarifying and identifying viable options
- Manage home care and treatment plans
- Plan, implement, or evaluate screening programs
- Become involved with public education about genetic disorders and their prevention
- Increase public awareness of the availability of genetic services

Nursing Process

The application of the nursing process provides direction for the nurse working with children and families affected by or at risk for genetic disorders and related defects (Lea et al. 1994). Implementation of this process requires skills in interviewing, history taking, teaching, and counseling. The first step in the nursing process is assessment, which includes the gathering of physical, emotional, sociocultural, and cognitive data to determine the needs of patients.

▼ Assessment

Identifying individuals and families at risk for genetic problems and initiating referrals for genetic counseling are important nursing responsibilities. The nurse may be the first health professional to suspect a genetic problem in a child and the first to whom parents turn for information about genetic concerns. Risk factors may be identified through the recording of a detailed family history. If a pregnancy resulted in an affected child, information should be gathered that can assist in the determination of the type of defect presented. The taking of a family history from potential parents may also indicate the risks involved in having future offspring with a genetic disorder, problems associated with an affected child, and the value of genetic counseling concerning reproductive options. The nurse should record the family history in pedigree form in preparation for genetic counseling. Medical records are often needed as well to further evaluate the occurrence or possible occurrence of a disorder in a family.

The physical assessment can provide clinical clues that suggest the possibility of a genetic component and the need for further evaluation and testing. For the infant and child, measurements of height, weight, and head circumference are needed. Other measures, such as interpupillary distances, arm span, upper and lower body segment ratios, chest circumference, ear measurements, and various craniofacial measurements, are done when suspicion so dictates. The physical assessment should also include a health, reproductive, pregnancy, birth, and developmental history as well as laboratory tests. The Denver Developmental Screening test and the Brazelton Neonatal Behavioral Assessment Scale are examples of commonly used tools for developmental assessment.

Many factors influence the impact of a birth defect or genetic disorder on the family and the way in which they respond and cope. Some of these are the size and structure of the family unit, religious beliefs and practices, availability of and relationship with extended family members, coping resources, visibility and severity of the disorder, past experiences with previous crises, and lifestyle and plans of the family. Hence, the gathering of emotional, sociocultural, and cognitive data is an essential dimension of nursing assessment.

Interviewing skills are extremely important in obtaining an emotional assessment about family dynamics and coping. The nurse can help the parents cope with the idea that a genetic referral is needed. The realization that a child may have a genetic condition represents a painful loss of their idealized child, which often initiates grieving. Since the possibility of a genetic disorder may also raise concerns about the normality of other children, the nurse should emphasize the child's uniqueness and differences from other siblings. Nurses can also help clarify any misconceptions about genetic counseling and the purpose of referral. Some parents fear that they will be told not to have more children or that they will be blamed for their child's defects. They need reassurance that genetic counseling's purpose is to help them make their own decisions. The family needs opportunities to verbalize their feelings, worries, and fears. For instance, how will the family accept the test results? In the case of an affected fetus, is the possibility of terminating the pregnancy acceptable or not acceptable? What are the present family relationships in terms of their potential for support as well as their vulnerability to strain?

The nurse must also be sensitive to and identify the cultural values, religious beliefs and practices, and socioeconomic considerations of the family. The gathering of sociocultural data is important, since ethnic and religious backgrounds influence attitudes toward a genetic defect, reproductive choices, and responses to the birth of an affected child. In addition, socioeconomic and occupational status will affect the family's capacity to provide care for an affected child, especially in terms of financial resources, health insurance coverage, and access to expert health services.

Recognition of certain cognitive characteristics that indicate whether a parent or potential parent has the capacity to use genetic information effectively or whether special help will be needed is crucial. Any cognitive deficit, such as mental handicap or impaired concentration or memory, may require further evaluation. Also, a precounseling assessment of the parents' genetic knowledge is important, since those having high and low levels of knowledge may have different needs (Seidenfeld and Antley 1981).

▼ Diagnosis

On the basis of data gathered during the initial assessment, nursing diagnoses can be identified. The diagnoses should reflect identified needs in all four dimensions of assessment, that is, physical, emotional, sociocultural, and cognitive. Examples of nursing diagnoses relevant to genetic counseling are

- Situational low self-esteem related to the parents' knowledge of having transmitted a disorder to their child
- Decisional conflict: possible genetic defect related to religious and personal values against termination of pregnancy of an affected fetus
- Altered parenting related to difficulty in accepting a genetic etiology of the child's disorder
- Altered family processes related to blaming the partner's family for having "bad genes"
- Knowledge deficit: genetic aspects, related to difficulty in understanding the disorder

▼ Planning

Once the nursing diagnoses have been identified, a plan of care can be developed. The plan should reflect the needs of the child, parents, other family members such as siblings, or prospective parents, depending on the situation. Measurable objectives should be developed that cover the physical, emotional, sociocultural, and cognitive dimensions and can assist the nurse to implement and evaluate intervention goals. Examples of objectives might include the following. The parents will

- Correctly explain the cause of the disorder, risk of recurrence, and reproductive options available for future family planning
- Discuss attitudes and feelings regarding the birth of the affected child
- Ask questions and voice concerns that will assist in the process of making genetic-related decisions
- Plan a timetable that includes the needs of normal siblings in the family and time alone for the parents; tension-reducing activities
- Plan for what supplies and equipment will be needed for care of the child (e.g., special diet)
- Describe clinical manifestations and physical signs associated with the disorder that indicate the need for prompt treatment (e.g., respiratory infections)

▼ Interventions

Nursing interventions relative to genetic disorders are based on the assessment data and the identified plan of care. Physical interventions depend on the genetic disorder in question but in general might include such actions as demonstrating the use of special care procedures (e.g., feeding the infant with cleft lip and palate), managing home care and therapeutic regimens, nutrition planning, following up on positive newborn screening test results, and monitoring growth and development.

Interventions that relate to the emotional, sociocultural, and cognitive needs of children and families are most often carried out by the nurse through teaching, support, and counseling. Many families who have genetic counseling are reluctant to acknowledge that they do not understand the genetic information provided in counseling. While parents are learning about the diagnosis, they also experience various stages of grief and may have difficulty remembering information they received after diagnosis. Nurses should review, reinforce, and clarify information given by the geneticist to help increase parents' understanding and to correct misconceptions.

Grief, sorrow, depression, guilt, anger, and denial are intense emotions experienced by parents of a newborn with a defect. They are not encouraged by knowing that the situation could have been worse, because this is as bad as things can get for them, even if the defect appears minor to professional staff. Parents need time to sort through their exhausting and discouraging feelings. The nurse can help parents by providing opportunities for them to verbalize their feelings and fears, building on the family's strengths, and reestablishing feelings of self-esteem. Parents may need help in communicating with each other and finding assistance for the daily responsibility and demands created by a child with a genetic disability (Olsen 1994). Siblings may also be anxious about their own health and may be reluctant to ask their parents questions about the disorder. They may also feel guilt and resentment over the unique position that the affected infant now holds in the family. The nurse should help parents to think through possible approaches in discussing the disorder with siblings and to plan time that includes their needs. The nurse may also provide guidance to parents in dealing with the questions and concerns raised by relatives, neighbors, friends, and others.

The nurse as a resource person should be familiar with community resources and help families obtain whatever supplies and equipment may be needed; locate parent and sibling support groups; and identify agencies that can provide financial aid, special educational treatment, daycare, and other supportive services.

Providing support and information for family members at various stages of the life cycle is another important nursing responsibility. The nurse must anticipate and deal with ongoing and exacerbated periods of stress and provide appropriate coping measures and support services at times when they may most be needed. In childhood, success for school, opportunities for independence, and the need to be like one's peers are areas that should be addressed. The nurse may also help parents understand normal growth and development since they may not know which behaviors result from their child's disorder and which are related to their child's developmental level. The major needs of adolescents include the desire to be like one's peers, establishment of identity, self-determination, independence, a need for respect, and opportunities for exploring sexual relationships. Future education, employment, and independent living should be considered. Adolescents will also desire information about their own reproductive risks.

Genetic-related decisions are emotionally painful ones, whether they involve the birth of an affected newborn, termination of a pregnancy, or other reproductive options. Meeting the emotional, sociocultural, and cognitive needs of the couple during the process of decision making is essential. Although the couple should make the ultimate decision for options, the nurse may encourage them to think it over for a while, if time is not a critical factor in their situation. The nurse should support the family in the process of making a decision and after the decision is made. Religious and cultural influences can be explored, social and financial factors can be identified, and genetic information and risks can be clarified or reinforced. The nurse can also help to make arrangements to facilitate decisions. If the family has sought genetic services because of the need to ascertain what the condition is in a family member, then decision making centers around the need to plan for the resources necessary for coping. Long-term help with coping may be provided by the nurse in collaboration with the genetics team, or referral arrangements may be made for ongoing care.

The following cognitive and emotional factors of parents are to be considered as influencing both the perception of genetic information and the decision-making process (Reif and Baitsch 1985):

- Previous knowledge regarding diagnosis, etiology, and prognosis
- Assessment of the problem (diagnosis, etiology, prognosis): degree of burden
- Impairment of self-esteem: that of the partner or of both partners
- Attribution of guilt (to oneself, to the partner)
- Anxiety closely connected with or independent of given risks: desire for security, absolute assurance
- Ethical dilemma: whether and under what condition to have an abortion
- Problems developing or already developed in the partner relationship and in relationships with the family and the environment

▼ Evaluation

Evaluation is an essential step in the nursing process. After genetic counseling, parents need to review and assimilate information; have time to grieve; verbalize feelings, concerns, and fears; know where to find help for practical problems; and know where to turn when new problems arise. Nurses should ensure that appropriate information, support, and guidance are available to families on an ongoing basis and should evaluate the outcomes of care. In particular, the nurse needs to know whether knowledge of the disorder has increased, whether psychological distress was reduced, whether a course of action taken by the family was appropriate, and whether realistic plans for management of the affected child are identified and implemented. Evaluation is usually carried out by scheduling follow-up visits to reassess cognitive understanding of the disorder, adjustment to physical aspects of care, and emotional adaptation. The plan of care and interventions can then be modified, depending on outcomes and the additional expressed needs of family members.

Risk Management

The psychosocial and ethical issues associated with proliferating genetic services are varied and complex. Besides reproductive decisions, individuals and families may need to make major readjustments in their conception of themselves and their relationships to others and perhaps their total lifestyles. If genetic services are to develop as a need-fulfilling human service, nurses involved in the process must become sensitive to these issues and their implications.

Religious beliefs and ethnic background strongly influence attitudes and interpretation of the meaning of a genetic disorder. The condition may be interpreted, for example, as punishment for unacceptable thoughts, wishes, or deeds or as a test or trial of the parents. Such beliefs influence use as well as interpretation of genetic information. They also influence the manner of coping with a child's defect and attitudes concerning reproductive alternatives. Nurses involved in providing genetic health care should assess the cultural and ethnic values of individuals and couples, encouraging them to discuss their expectations about family size and constitution, reproductive attitudes, and views of the disorder.

Nurses also need to examine their own biases to relate in a nonjudgmental way toward parents. A nonjudgmental attitude is particularly important for certain topics about which there is public controversy, such as abortion. The wrong words or attitude can be most destructive to people going through crises. So that personal prejudices do not influence the counseling process, nurses and other health providers need to recognize their own values and strive to separate them from professional responsibilities. A family can be made to feel comfortable with their right to make their own decisions, or uncomfortable or guilty because their feelings and needs meet with disapproval from the experts.

The issues of informed consent and patient rights are relevant at all levels of clinical genetics, from practice to research investigation. They are particularly important in several areas: the right to privacy; the efficacy and consequences of genetic screening programs; the use and limitations of prenatal diagnosis; and the diagnostic and therapeutic measures of an investigative nature that require informed consent.

There are numerous complexities regarding the right to privacy. Since the genetic health care provider's obligation is not only to the individual client but also to other family members at risk either for having affected offspring or for development of the disorder, an ethical dilemma may arise when clients refuse to share information about genetic risks with members of their extended families. There is a fine line between the client's right to privacy and the health professional's responsibility to disclose information to other at-risk family members. Nurses can help parents to appreciate the value of the possible need to share genetic information with other relatives, especially in assembling a family pedigree.

For prenatal diagnosis, informed consent means ensuring that the pregnant woman and her partner fully understand the indications for the procedure, potential positive and negative consequences, limitations, and risks of the procedure involved. The question of informed consent in genetic testing also raises the important issue of individual autonomy. As health care professionals, nurses share the responsibility to ensure that the individual's autonomy is protected when decisions are made regarding genetic testing (Lessick and Williams 1994). The major reason for information acquisition in genetic counseling is its use in decision making. This process is a uniquely personal matter, since clients themselves are the ones who must decide how best to weigh their own situational factors.

It is generally agreed that nondirective genetic counseling is the best approach in informing patients and families. This approach assumes that the responsibility of the counselor is educational and that couples should be free to make their own decisions based on an understanding of the risks and options that they face. Whatever the decision, the counselor must be careful not to impose his or her own judgment, especially if it differs from that of the couple. However, ethical dilemmas may be encountered in nondirective counseling. Adequately counseled intelligent couples generally will make responsible decisions, but occasionally the clients may be mentally retarded, be emotionally unstable, or simply refuse to participate in the counseling process.

The issue of genetic parenthood has medicolegal and ethical importance and can be a problem in genetic counseling. While questionable paternity is the most common reason for determination of genetic parenthood, it may also be done to determine maternity, especially when infants may have been exchanged in the hospital or when a woman claims a kidnapped baby to be her own. DNA fingerprinting, discovered in 1985, has become a central technique in determining genetic parenthood (Connor and Ferguson-Smith 1993). The probes used identify multiple dispersed DNA sequences of variable size, and the pattern produced is characteristic for an individual. A child's fragment pattern is a combination of some of the fragments from each parent, so that paternity can be either excluded or positively identified. DNA fingerprinting has also found applications in twin zygosity determination and forensic medicine.

Implications for Research

As scientific and technologic advances in human genetics continue to evolve and service capabilities increase, the incorporation of genetic knowledge and skills into nursing practice will become crucial to meet the needs of families in health promotion, health maintenance, illness prevention, and health restoration.

Conducting research is an important responsibility of the nurse in genetics. While medical research has primarily focused on diagnostic, therapeutic, and preventive aspects of genetic disorders and services, little is known about the psychological, sociocultural, or cognitive aspects associated with genetic health care. Nursing research could make a significant contribution to providing new and important information in these areas. Research questions that could be addressed by nurses might include the following:

- Are there differences in maternal-fetal attachment between women who undergo prenatal genetic testing and those who do not?
- Is there a relationship between mothers' personal beliefs about the causes of their children's genetic disorders and acceptance of information provided in genetic counseling?
- What teaching and counseling strategies are most effective in regard to understanding of genetic risks?
- Are there differences between counseled and noncounseled couples for a genetic disorder in terms of knowledge of recurrence risks, initiation of subsequent pregnancies, or use of prenatal diagnosis?
- Is there a relationship between sources of social support and parental attitudes about having transmitted a defect to a child?

Research findings will help expand the knowledge base in nursing and improve the quality of care delivered to individuals and families affected by or at risk for genetic disorders and birth defects.

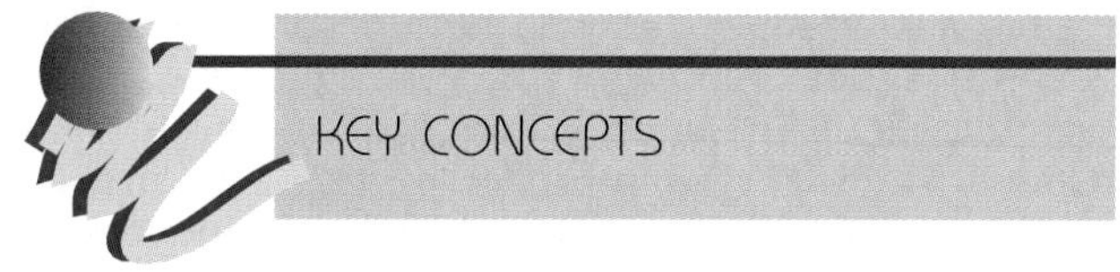

KEY CONCEPTS

- Genes, the basic units of heredity, are contained in chromosomes and consist of DNA (deoxyribonucleic acid). Genes direct the process of protein synthesis and ultimately influence all aspects of body structure and function.
- The DNA molecule has three basic components: a five-carbon sugar (deoxyribose); a phosphate group; and nitrogenous bases, of which there are two types, purines and pyrimidines. The purine bases are adenine (A) and guanine (G), and the pyrimidine bases are thymine (T) and cytosine (C).
- The DNA molecule is composed of two chains of nucleotides arranged in a double-helix structure. The two chains are held together by hydrogen bonds between complementary base pairs: adenine (A) in one chain is always bonded to thymine (T) in the other chain, whereas cytosine (C) in one chain is bonded to guanine (G) in the other.
- Somatic cells are diploid, having 23 pairs of chromosomes (22 pairs of autosomes and 1 pair of sex chromosomes). Gametes (ova and sperm) have the haploid number of chromosomes, 23.
- Two types of cell division are necessary for transmitting genetic information: mitosis and meiosis. Mitosis maintains the diploid chromosome number in successive generations of somatic cells. Meiosis results in the haploid chromosome number during production of gametes.
- Chromosome bands help to identify individual chromosomes and structural abnormalities in chromosomes.
- Chromosome disorders are conditions associated with changes in either chromosome number or structure and may involve one or more autosomes, sex chromosomes, or both simultaneously.
- There are four major patterns of mendelian (single-gene) inheritance: autosomal dominant, autosomal recessive, X-linked recessive, and X-linked dominant.
- Traits that follow autosomal dominant inheritance are manifested in the heterozygous state, are usually transmitted from one generation to the next, and affect both males and females equally. Each offspring of an affected parent has a 50 percent chance of being affected, and normal offspring do not transmit the condition to their own children.
- Traits that follow autosomal recessive inheritance are manifested in the homozygous state, are usually seen only in siblings, and affect both males and females equally. Each child of carrier (heterozygous) parents has a 25 percent chance of being affected with the condition; a 50 percent chance of being a carrier like the parents; and a 25 percent chance of being normal, without receiving the abnormal recessive gene.
- X-linked recessive conditions appear almost always in males, whose mothers are unaffected but carriers of the abnormal gene. Each son of a carrier female has a 50 percent chance of inheriting the gene and thus being affected; each daughter has a 50 percent chance of being a carrier like the mother.
- Traits that follow X-linked dominant inheritance are relatively uncommon. Females tend to be less severely affected than males, and male-to-male transmission is not seen.
- Many traits are determined by the interaction of both genetic and environmental factors, with each contributing some effect. These traits are referred to as multifactorial and include many common congenital malformations and isolated birth defects.
- Risks for multifactorial conditions usually increase if more family members are affected, the condition has more severe expression, and the affected individual is a member of the less commonly affected sex. The risk to relatives is sharply lower for second-degree than for first-degree relatives and declines at a lower rate for third-degree and more distant relatives.
- Genetic screening involves the testing of a specific population to identify individuals who are affected with a genetic disorder, those who are carriers of a mutant gene and at risk for having affected offspring with a genetic disorder, and those with certain genotypes who are known to be predisposed to the development of illness.
- Major types of screening programs relevant to maternal and newborn care are preconception screening, prenatal screening and diagnosis, and neonatal screening.
- Genetic counseling is best provided in a multidisciplinary team setting that enables individuals and families to receive expert care from a variety of professionals who specialize in the management and counseling of genetic and related disorders.
- There are five major steps in the process of genetic counseling: obtaining a family history, establishing a diagnosis, establishing the risk of

occurrence or recurrence, communicating information, and following up.

- ▼ Nurses play a variety of roles in delivery of genetic health care. While some nurses may specialize in genetics and provide genetic counseling, many nurses act in a liaison position between the family and specialized genetic resources.
- ▼ The application of the nursing process provides direction for the nurse working with children and families affected by or at risk for genetic disorders and related defects. Nursing interventions may include teaching, support, counseling, anticipatory guidance, referral to genetic services and community resources, and managing physical and related aspects of care.

References

Acosta, P. B., and Wright, L. (1992). Nurses' role in preventing birth defects in offspring of women with phenylketonuria. *Journal of Obstetric, Gynecologic, and Neonatal Nursing,* 21, 270–276.

Alter, B. P. (1985). Antenatal diagnosis of thalassemia: A review. *Annals of the New York Academy of Sciences,* 445, 393–407.

American Society of Human Genetics. (1975). Genetic counseling. *American Journal of Human Genetics,* 27, 240–242.

American Society of Human Genetics. (1992). Statement of the American Society of Human Genetics on cystic fibrosis carrier screening. *American Journal of Human Genetics,* S1, 1443–1444.

Andrews, L. B., Fullarton, J. E., Holtzman, N. A., Motulsky, A. G. (1994). *Assessing genetic risks: Implications for health and social policy.* Committee on assessing genetic risks, Institute of Medicine. Washington, DC: National Academy Press.

Antonarakis, S. E. (1990). The mapping and sequencing of the human genome. *Southern Medical Journal,* 83 (8), 876–878.

Beaudet, A. (1992). Genetic testing for cystic fibrosis. *Pediatric Clinics of North America,* 39, 213–228.

Boat, T. F., Welsh, M. J., Beaudet, A. L. (1989). Cystic fibrosis. In C. R. Scriver, A. L. Beaudet, W. S. Sly, D. Valle (Eds.). *The metabolic basis of inherited disease* (pp. 2649–2680) (6th ed.). New York: McGraw-Hill Information Services Co.

Brown, W. T. (1990). Invited editorial: The fragile X: Progress toward solving the puzzle. *American Journal of Human Genetics,* 47, 175–180.

Burton, B. K., Dillard, R. G., Clark, E. N. (1985). The psychological impact of false positive elevations of maternal serum alpha-fetoprotein. *American Journal of Obstetrics and Gynecology,* 151, 77–82.

Chan, J. C. M., Alon, U., Hirschman, G. M. (1985). Renal hypophosphatemic rickets. *Journal of Pediatrics,* 106 (4), 533–544.

Collins, F. (1992). Cystic fibrosis: Molecular biology and therapeutic implications. *Science,* 256 (5058), 774–779.

Connor, J. M., and Ferguson-Smith, M. A. (1993). *Essential medical genetics* (4th ed.). Oxford: Blackwell Scientific Publications.

Cook-Deegan, R. M. (1990). Social and ethical implications of advances in human genetics. *Southern Medical Journal,* 83 (8), 879–882.

Cronister, A. E., and Hagerman, R. J. (1989). Fragile X syndrome. *Journal of Pediatric Health Care,* 3, 9–19.

Emery, A. E. H., and Mueller, R. F. (1992). *Elements of medical genetics* (8th ed.). New York: Churchill Livingstone.

Fearn, J., Hibbard, B. M., Laurence, K. M. (1982). Screening for neural tube defects and maternal anxiety. *British Journal of Obstetrics and Gynaecology,* 89, 218–221.

Fishler, K., Azen, C. G., Henderson, R., Friedman, E. G., Koch, R. (1987). Psychoeducational findings among children treated for phenylketonuria. *American Journal of Mental Deficiency,* 92 (1), 65–73.

Gardner, R. J. M., and Sutherland, G. R. (1989). *Chromosome abnormalities and genetic counseling.* New York: Oxford University Press.

Garver, K. L., and Marchese, S. G. (1986). *Genetic counseling for clinicians.* Chicago: Year Book Medical Publishers.

Ghavami, M., Levy, H. L., Erbe, R. W. (1986). Prevention of fetal damage through dietary control of maternal hyperphenylalaninemia. *Clinical Obstetrics and Gynecology,* 29 (3), 580–585.

Hall, J. G. (1985). Support groups for families of children with growth problems. *Growth, Genetics, and Hormones,* 1 (4), 7–8.

Hall, J. G. (1987). Turner syndrome: An update. *Growth, Genetics, and Hormones,* 3 (2), 4–7.

Harper, P. S. (1993). *Practical genetic counseling* (4th ed.). Oxford: Butterworth-Heinemann Ltd.

Jones, K. L. (1988). *Smith's recognizable patterns of human malformation* (4th ed.). Philadelphia: W. B. Saunders.

Jorde, L. B., Carey, J. C., White, R. L. (1995). *Medical genetics.* St. Louis: Mosby-Year Book.

Jordon, E. (1992). Invited editorial: The human genome project: Where did it come from, where is it going? *American Journal of Human Genetics,* 51, 1–6.

Krywawych, S., Haseler, M., Brenton, D. P. (1991). Theoretical and practical aspects of preventing fetal damage in women with phenylketonuria. In J. Schaub, F. Van Hoof, H. L. Vis (Eds.). *Inborn errors of metabolism* (pp. 125–135). New York: Raven Press.

Lea, D. H., Williams, J. K., Tinley, S. T. (1994). Nursing and genetic health care. *Journal of Genetic Counseling,* 3, 113–124.

Lessick, M., and Forsman, I. (1995). Advances in genetic health care: New challenges for pediatric nursing. *Capsules and Comments in Pediatric Nursing,* 1, 3–12.

Lessick, M., and Williams, J. (1994). The human genome project: Implications for nursing. *MEDSURG Nursing,* 3, 49–58.

Lorenz, R. P., and Kuhn, M. H. (1989). Multidisciplinary team counseling for fetal anomalies. *American Journal of Obstetrics and Gynecology,* 161 (2), 263–266.

Luthy, D. A., Wardinsky, T., Shurtleff, D. B., Hollenbach, K. A., Hickok, D. E., Nyberg, D. A., Benedetti, T. J. (1991). Cesarean section before the onset of labor and subsequent motor function in infants with meningomyelocele diagnosed antenatally. *New England Journal of Medicine,* 324 (10), 662–666.

Machler, M., Frey, D., Gal, A., Orth, U., Wienker, T. F., Fanconi, A., Schmid, W. (1986). X-linked dominant hypophosphatemia is closely linked to DNA markers DXS 41 and DXS 43 at Xp 22. *Human Genetics,* 73, 271–275.

Mackta, J., and Weiss, J. O. (1994). The role of genetic support groups. *Journal of Obstetric, Gynecologic, and Neonatal Nursing,* 23, 519–523.

Milunsky, A., Jick, H., Jick, S. S., Bruell, C. L., MacLaughlin, D. S., Rothman, K. J., Willett, W. (1989). Multivitamin/folic acid supplementation in early pregnancy reduces the prevalence of neural tube defects. *Journal of the American Medical Association,* 262 (20), 2847–2852.

Mortimer, E. A. (1980). The puzzling epidemiology of neural tube defects. *Pediatrics,* 65 (3), 636–637.

Motulsky, A. G. (1973). Frequency of sickling disorders in U.S. blacks. *New England Journal of Medicine,* 288 (1), 31–33.

Neal-Cooper, F., and Scott, R. B. (1988). Genetic counseling in sickle cell anemia: Experiences with couples at risk. *Public Health Reports,* 103 (2), 174–178.

Nelson, D. L. (1993). Fragile X syndrome: Review and current status. *Growth, Genetics, and Hormones,* 9, 1–4.

Nora, J. J., and Fraser, F. C. (1989). *Medical genetics: Principles and practice* (3rd ed.) Philadelphia: Lea & Febiger.

Nora, J. J., and Nora, A. H. (1988). Update on counseling the family with a first-degree relative with a congenital heart defect. *American Journal of Medical Genetics,* 29, 137–142.

Nussbaum, R. L., and Ledbetter, D. H. (1989). The fragile X syndrome. In C. R. Scriver, A. L. Beaudet, W. S. Sly, D. Valle (Eds.). *The metabolic basis of inherited disease* (pp. 327–341) (6th ed.). New York: McGraw-Hill Information Services Co.

Olsen, D. G. (1994). Parental adjustment to a child with genetic disease: One parent's reflections. *Journal of Obstetric, Gynecologic, and Neonatal Nursing,* 23, 516–518.

Pauli, R. M. (1995). Osteochondrodysplasias with mild clinical manifestations: A guide for endocrinologists and others. *Growth, Genetics, and Hormones,* 11, 1–5.

Powars, D. (1989). Diagnosis at birth improves survival of children with sickle cell anemia. *Pediatrics,* 83, 830–833.

Reif, M., and Baitsch, H. (1985). Psychological issues in genetic counseling. *Human Genetics,* 70, 193–199.

Robinson, A., and Linden, M. G. (1993). *Clinical genetics handbook* (2nd ed.). Boston: Blackwell Scientific Publications.

Scott, C. R., and Cederbaum, S. D. (1990). Disorders of amino acid metabolism. In A. E. H. Emery and D. L. Rimoin (Eds.). *Principles and practice of medical genetics* (Vol. 22, pp. 1639–1673) (2nd ed.). New York: Churchill Livingstone.

Scriver, C. R., Kaufman, S., Woo, S. L. C. (1989). The hyperphenylalaninemias. In C. R. Scriver, A. L. Beaudet, W. S. Sly, D. Valle (Eds.). *The metabolic basis of inherited disease* (pp. 495–544) (6th ed.). New York: McGraw-Hill Information Services Co.

Seashore, M. R., Friedman, E., Novelly, R. A., Bapat, V. (1985). Loss of intellectual function in children with phenylketonuria after relaxation of dietary phenylalanine restriction. *Pediatrics,* 75 (2), 226–232.

Seidenfeld, M. J., and Antley, R. M. (1981). Genetic counseling: A comparison of counselee's genetic knowledge before and after. *American Journal of Medical Genetics,* 10, 107–112.

Sherman, S. L., Morton, N. E., Jacobs, P. A., Turner, G. (1984). The marker (X) syndrome: A cytogenetic and genetic analysis. *Annals of Human Genetics,* 48, 21–37.

Simpson, J. L., and Elias, S. (1994). Fetal cells in maternal blood: Overview and historical perspective. *Annals of the New York Academy of Sciences,* 731, 1–8.

Smithells, R. W., Nevin, N. C., Seller, M. J., Sheppard, S., Harris, R., Read, A. P., Fielding, D. W., Walker, S., Schorah, C. J., Wild, J. (1983). Further experience of vitamin supplementation for prevention of neural tube defect recurrences. *Lancet,* 1, 1027–1031.

Steele, S. (1989). Phenylketonuria: Counseling and teaching functions of the nurse on an interdisciplinary team. *Issues in Comprehensive Pediatric Nursing,* 12, 395–409.

Thompson, M. W., McInnes, R. R., Willard, H. F. (1991). *Thompson and Thompson genetics in medicine* (5th ed.). Philadelphia: W. B. Saunders.

U. S. Congress, Office of Technology Assessment. (1992). *Genetic counseling and cystic fibrosis carrier screening: Results of a survey-background paper,* OTA-BP-BA-97. Washington, DC: U. S. Government Printing Office.

Vehar, G. A., Lawn, R. M., Tuddenham, E. G. D., Wood, W. I. (1989). Factor VIII and factor V: Biochemistry and pathophysiology. In C. R. Scriver, A. L. Beaudet, W. S. Sly, D. Valle (Eds.). *The metabolic basis of inherited disease* (pp. 2155–2170) (6th ed.). New York: McGraw-Hill Information Services Co.

Weatherall, D. J. (1991). *The new genetics and clinical practice* (3rd ed.). New York: Oxford University Press.

Weatherall, D. J., Clegg, J. B., Higgs, D. R., Wood, W. G. (1989). The hemoglobinopathies. In C. R. Scriver, A. L. Beaudet, W. S. Sly, D. Valle (Eds.). *The metabolic basis of inherited disease* (pp. 2281–2339) (6th ed.). New York: McGraw-Hill Information Services Co.

Wilfond, B. S., and Fost, N. (1990). The cystic fibrosis gene: Medical and social implications for heterozygote detection. *Journal of the American Medical Association,* 263 (20), 2777–2783.

Wingerson, L. (1991). *Mapping our genes: The genome project and the future of medicine.* New York: Penguin Books.

Wright, L. (1994). Prenatal diagnosis in the 1990s. *Journal of Obstetric, Gynecologic, and Neonatal Nursing,* 23, 506–515.

Wright, L., Brown, A., Davidson-Mundt, A. (1992). Newborn screening: The miracle and the challenge. *Journal of Pediatric Nursing,* 7, 26–42.

Chapter 14

Termination of Pregnancy

Bobbie S. Frye

> . . . Even among groups committed to confirming a woman's right to legal abortion there was consensus that any abortion represented a failure in some part of society's support system—individual, family, church, public health, economic, or social.
>
> C. Everett Koop, MD (1989)

HIGHLIGHTS

- ▼ Epidemiology of Induced Legal Abortion
- ▼ Abortion Providers and Services
- ▼ Abortion and Health Care Policy
- ▼ Abortion: Two Opposing Views
- ▼ Reasons Women Choose Abortion
- ▼ The Decision-Making Process
- ▼ Physical and Psychological Effects of Abortion
- ▼ Types of Abortion Procedures
- ▼ Complications of Abortion
- ▼ Nursing Practice
- ▼ Impact of Providing Nursing Care
- ▼ Implications for Research

Termination of pregnancy is a social, public health, and women's health issue that generates intense moral and ethical debate. Elective termination of pregnancy is one of the most frequently performed gynecologic procedures in the United States today (Wallach and Zacur 1995).

Induced abortion is not a new phenomenon. Instruments used and descriptions of techniques for uterine evacuation are found as early as the era of ancient Rome and Greece (Dueveraux 1960). Abortion is found among all cultural groups and today is thought to be the most frequent "fertility control" method used worldwide (DeCherney and Pernoll 1994).

Ethical issues related to induced abortion are examined in Chapter 8, and a comprehensive discussion of spontaneous abortion is found in Chapter 21. Aspects of induced legal abortion covered in this chapter include statistics on legal abortion and abortion services, the characteristics of women seeking legal abortions, health care policy related to abortion, the controversy surrounding abortion, decision making related to choosing abortion, the psychological and physical effects of abortion, types of abortion procedures, and nursing practice.

DEFINITIONS

Abortion Rate—The number of legal abortions per 1000 women aged 15 to 44 years.

Abortion Ratio—The number of legal abortions per 1000 live births.

Abortion-Related Death—A death that results from a direct complication of an abortion, from an indirect complication caused by the chain of events initiated by an abortion, or from the aggravation of a preexisting condition by the physiologic or psychological effects of an abortion.

Curettage—Suction or sharp scraping procedure performed at 12 weeks or less of gestation to remove contents of uterus.

Dilatation and Curettage (D & C)—When used in referring to abortion, D & C is the termination of pregnancy during the first trimester by either suction (the most commonly used) or sharp (the oldest method) curettage.

Dilatation and Evacuation (D & E)—The termination of pregnancy during the second trimester by presurgical dilatation of the cervix followed by suction curettage.

Fertility Rate—The number of live births per 1000 women aged 15 to 44 years.

Intra-Amniotic Instillation—The instillation of a hyperosmotic fluid into the amniotic sac that causes fetal death and induces labor.

Legal Abortion—An abortion performed by a licensed physician or by someone acting under the supervision of a licensed physician. Also referred to as induced or elective abortion.

Medical Abortion—An abortion induced through the means of a drug such as RU 486 (mifepristone).

Multifetal Pregnancy Reduction (MFPR)—A procedure in which the number of fetuses in a multifetal pregnancy is decreased during the first trimester to improve the outcome of pregnancy.

Surgical Abortion—An abortion induced by surgical means of curettage, D & E, intra-amniotic instillation, hysterotomy, or hysterectomy.

EPIDEMIOLOGY OF INDUCED LEGAL ABORTION

Abortion Rate, Abortion Ratio, and Fertility Rate

The number of legal abortions increased from a low of 193,491 in 1970 to a high of 1,429,577 in 1990 (CDC 1993). Beginning in 1991, the number of legal abortions has decreased each year. In 1992, a total of 1,359,145 legal abortions were reported to the Centers for Disease Control and Prevention (CDC), a 2.1 percent decrease from the number of abortions reported in 1991 (CDC 1994).

The fertility rate (the number of live births per 1000 women aged 15 to 44 years) was 68.9 in 1992, a decrease of 1.1 percent from 1991. As a result, the national abortion ratio (number of legal abortions per 1000 live births) decreased from 339 in 1991 to 335 in 1992. From 1972 to 1980, the national abortion rate (number of legal abortions per 1000 women aged 15 to 44 years) increased each year, from 13 in 1972 and peaking at 25 in 1980. Since 1980, this rate has fluctuated relatively little, remaining between 23 and 24. In 1992, the national abortion rate was 23 (CDC 1994) (Fig. 14–1).

Characteristics of Women Who Have Legal Abortions

In 1992, women who obtained legal abortions in the United States were predominantly 24 years or younger (54.7 percent), white (62.9 percent), unmarried (79.3 percent), and with no previous liveborn children (46.3 percent).

Although most women who obtain abortions are white, the abortion rate for black women is three times higher than that for white women (CDC 1994). The younger the woman, the more likely she is to obtain an abortion later in pregnancy (16 gestational weeks or more). The older the woman, the more likely she is to obtain an abortion early in pregnancy (8 gestational weeks or fewer). Since 1980, the abortion ratio has declined for almost all age groups, especially for the youngest women (teenagers) and oldest women (35 years and above), indicating that women in these

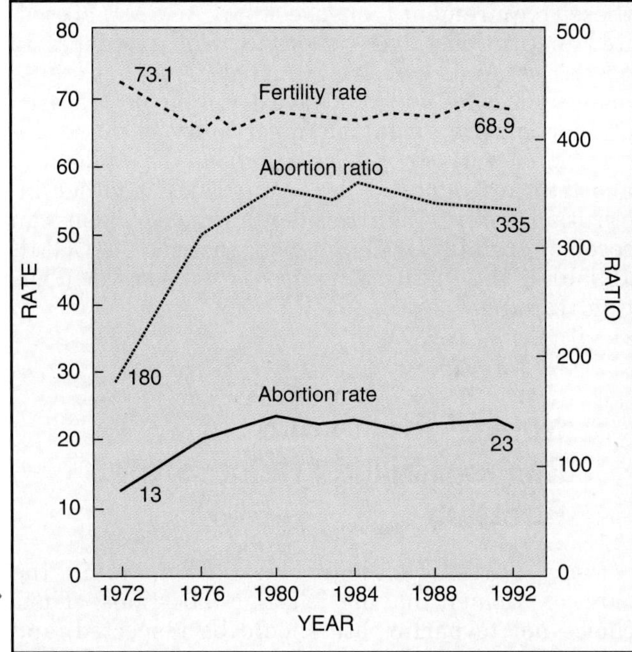

Figure 14–1

Fertility rate, abortion ratio, and abortion rate by year, United States, 1972–1992. (From Centers for Disease Control and Prevention. [1994]. CDC Surveillance Summaries. *MMWR,* 43 (50), 931.)

age groups are having fewer abortions (CDC 1993).

Abortion Mortality

Maternal deaths related to abortion are reported to the CDC from a variety of sources: state health departments, health care providers, medical examiner reports from death certificates, private citizens, the media, and maternal mortality committees. The medical definition of abortion-related deaths is "deaths that result from a direct complication of an abortion, from an indirect complication caused by the chain of events initiated by an abortion, or from the aggravation of a preexisting condition by the physiologic or psychological effects of an abortion (Lawson et al. 1994, p. 1366).

Abortion ranked as a leading cause of maternal mortality in the years before the 1973 Supreme Court decision on abortion, Roe v. Wade. The annual number of deaths from legal abortions decreased by 75 percent between 1972 and 1987, from 24 deaths in 1972 to 6 deaths in 1987. The mortality rate for induced legal abortion fell sharply (more than 90 percent) from 4.1 per 100,000 abortions in 1972 to 0.4 per 100,000 abortions in 1987. During this 16-year period, white women had the lowest mortality rate, while the mortality rate was 2.5 times higher for black and other minority women (Fig. 14–2). In 1987, black and other minority women were still significantly more at risk after an abortion and were twice as likely to have an abortion-related death (Lawson et al. 1994).

The risk from an abortion increases with age. Women under 20 years of age have the lowest risk of mortality (1 per 100,000 abortions), while the risk of an abortion-related death is three times as high for women 40 years and older (3 per 100,000). Increasing parity increases the risk of an abortion-related death. Women who have given birth three or more times have a statistically significant increased risk of an abortion-related death. The risk of death increases markedly with increasing gestational age. Women who have a legal abortion during the first 8 weeks of gestation have the lowest risk of an abortion-related death (0.4 per 100,000 abortions). Women who have an abortion beyond 8 weeks of gestation have a 31 times higher risk of an abortion-related mortality than if the procedure had been performed during the first 8 weeks of pregnancy (Lawson et al. 1994).

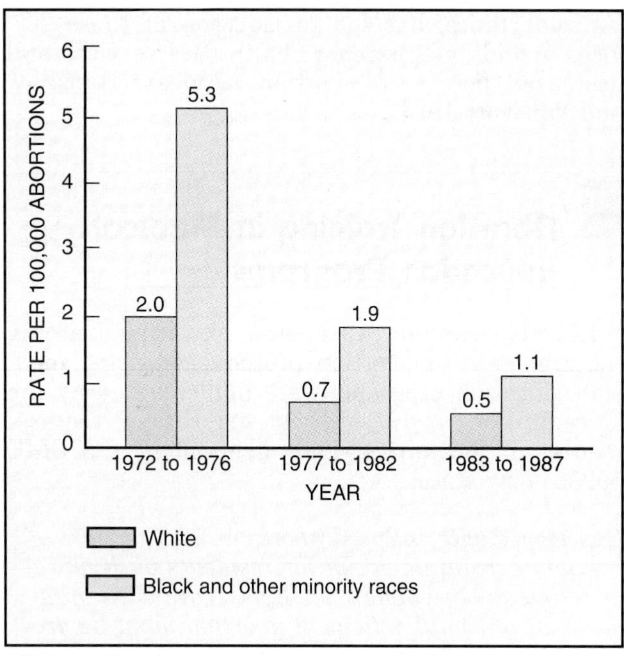

Figure 14–2

Mortality trends for legal abortion by race, United States, 1972–1976, 1977–1982, and 1983–1987. (From Lawson, H. W., Frye, A., Atrash, H. K., Smith, J. C., Shulman, H. B., Ramick, M. [1994]. Abortion mortality, United States, 1972 through 1987. *American Journal of Obstetrics and Gynecology,* 171 (5), 1369.)

ABORTION PROVIDERS AND SERVICES

In 1992, there were 2380 abortion providers in the United States. The number of hospitals, clinics, and physician's offices that provide abortion services has been gradually, but steadily, decreasing since 1988. The biggest decline has been in the number of hospitals that provide abortion services. In 1992, 69 percent of all abortions were performed in abortion clinics, about 7 percent were performed in hospitals, and less than 25 percent were performed in doctor's offices or other sites. Less than 1 percent of women undergoing an abortion have an inpatient hospital stay (Henshaw and Van Vort 1994).

This decrease in providers has led to a decrease in the availability of abortion services. Most abortions are performed in metropolitan areas. However, 33 percent of all metropolitan areas either do not have an abortion provider or have none that serve at least 50 women per year. Most U. S. counties do not have an abortion provider, and in nonmetropolitan areas 94 percent of counties do not have an abortion provider. These changes, along with the concentration of abortion services in specialized clinics, has led to isolation of these services outside mainstream health care services and decreased access to abortion services (Henshaw and Van Vort 1994).

Abortion Training in Medical Education Programs

Effective January 1996, new physician training requirements in abortion procedures during medical education programs were implemented by the accreditation body. Medical education requirements in obstetrics and gynecology (ACGME 1995a) now state:

Experience with induced abortion must be part of residency training, except for residents with moral or religious objections . . . Experience with management of complications of abortion must be provided to all residents . . .

The Accreditation Council for Graduate Medical Education (ACGME) emphasizes that these new program requirements do not force any individual or institution with a moral or religious objection to abortion into performing abortions. Rather, these requirements ensure that ACGME-accredited institutions that choose to train residents in obstetrics and gynecology must see that those physicians who wish to have training in the area of abortion are given the opportunity to do so. Institutions with moral or religious objections to abortion are required to contract with another institution where their residents who so wish can receive training in induced abortion (ACGME 1995b), if the institution chooses not to offer abortion training.

Nurses' Rights and Responsibilities Related to Abortion

Many nurses choose not to participate in the care of women having elective abortions. Their choice not to participate should be respected, and this right should be included as written policy in health care facilities that provide elective abortion services. The 1993 Association of Women's Health, Obstetric and Neonatal Nurses (AWHONN) position statement on reproductive health services expresses a view that supports both the right of individuals to make informed decisions regarding their reproductive health care choices and the right of health care providers to decide not to participate in procedures that are in conflict with their own beliefs. Some agencies maintain the position that staffing patterns often do not allow for absolute patient care choices, and that any nurse employed in the facility may at some time be called on to participate in an abortion procedure. Nurses already employed at an agency that issues such a policy may find that their only choice is to leave that facility and seek employment elsewhere.

Nurses have the responsibility to provide care to all clients who need emergency care. They also have the responsibility to inform their potential employer before employment about their attitudes and beliefs regarding abortion and caring for clients who have abortions.

ABORTION AND HEALTH CARE POLICY

In the United States, the first law specific to the performance of abortions was passed by Connecticut in 1821 (David 1990). This law and most other early laws prohibited abortion after "quickening"

AWHONN Position Statement: Reproductive Health Services

AWHONN believes that any reproductive health care decision is best made by the informed woman in consultation with her health care provider.

AWHONN believes these personal and private decisions are best made within health care systems whose providers respect the woman's right to confidentiality and the values and ethics of each individual woman and health care provider.

Therefore, AWHONN supports and promotes a woman's right to accurate and complete information and access to reproductive health care services.

AWHONN recognizes that abortion is a controversial issue. AWHONN respects the values and ethics of each of our members, as well as of the women in our care.

AWHONN respects the right of all individuals to make informed choices, including the right of health care providers to choose not to participate in interventions that conflict with their own system of values and ethics.

Position statements are reviewed every two years and are either reaffirmed or withdrawn. Reaffirmed by the Executive Board, March 1995.

except to preserve the life of the mother. By 1900, abortion was illegal in all American jurisdictions. Interruption of pregnancy at any point was considered a crime, and this doctrine remained in force for the next 70 years. Because of the high mortality rates of all surgical procedures at the turn of the century, early laws were developed on the premise that they were needed to protect women from the high risks of abortion procedures. However, most early legislative arguments probably reflected moral and religious beliefs.

During the 1960s, state laws slowly began to change, but it was not until 1973 that the major change regarding abortion occurred. The U. S. Supreme Court ruled that termination of an unwanted pregnancy in the first trimester was to be resolved solely by the pregnant woman and her physician (Roe v. Wade, 1973). This court decision was based on a constitutional right to privacy, and

AWHONN Position Statement: Nurses' Rights and Responsibilities Related to Abortion and Sterilization

AWHONN is aware of the nurse's role in meeting the health care needs of a woman seeking an abortion or sterilization. There may be concern, however, regarding nursing participation in this particular area of health care. Therefore, AWHONN supports the protection of the individual nurse's rights through written policies.

AWHONN supports the following principles:

1. Nurses have the responsibility to provide nursing care to all patients needing emergency care.
2. Nurses have the responsibility to provide nursing care to all patients either directly or through appropriate and timely referral.
3. Nurses have the right to refuse to assist in the performance of abortion and/or sterilization procedures, in keeping with their personal, moral, ethical, or religious beliefs. This refusal should not jeopardize the nurses' employment, nor should nurses be subjected to harassment or embarrassment because of their refusal.
4. Nurses should not impose their personal beliefs on patients or other personnel.
5. Nurses have an obligation to inform their employers, at the time of employment, of their attitudes and beliefs regarding abortion and sterilization.
6. Nurses have the right to expect their employers to maintain policies that ensure safe practice regarding abortion and sterilization.

Position statements are reviewed every two years and are either reaffirmed or withdrawn. Revised and reaffirmed, November 1993, 1995.

the justices in the majority opinion report offered three reasons for reversal of early laws. First, the existing laws were based on moralistic grounds meant to discourage extramarital sex. Second, the laws were developed to protect women from highly dangerous procedures. Third, the majority rejected the state's supposed interest in protecting the un-

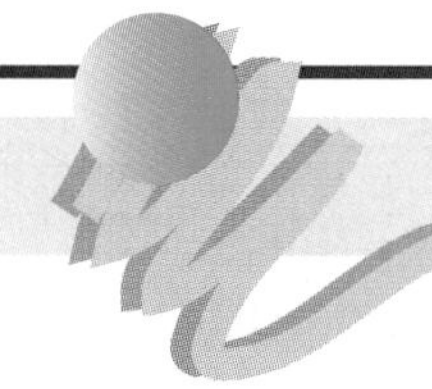

HISTORICAL PERSPECTIVES

SUPREME COURT DECISIONS ON ABORTION LAW

1965 The Supreme Court ruled in Griswold v. Connecticut that married persons have the right to use birth control under the constitutionally protected right to privacy. The decision laid the groundwork for Roe v. Wade.

1973 On January 22, abortion was legalized nationally. In the landmark case Roe v. Wade, the Supreme Court, citing the right to privacy in reproductive matters established in Griswold v. Connecticut, overturned a Texas law that made abortion a crime except to save a pregnant woman's life; the Court ruled that the constitutional right to privacy encompassed a woman's decision to terminate a pregnancy. Over the next few years, safe and legal abortion services became available. States where there was strong sentiment against abortion immediately began to pass laws restricting abortions. Also on January 22, in Roe v. Bolton, the Court struck down restrictions on places that could be used to perform abortions. The decision gave rise to the abortion clinic.

1976 The first post-Roe abortion challenge reached the Supreme Court. On July 1 in Planned Parenthood v. Danforth, the Supreme Court struck down a Missouri law requiring a married woman to obtain her husband's consent for an abortion. The Court also said that parents of minor unwed girls could not be given an absolute veto over abortions.

1977 On June 20 in Maher v. Roe, the Supreme Court held that a state is not constitutionally required to pay for abortion for poor women. States were allowed to cut off their Medicaid funding for abortions.

1979 On January 29, in Colautti v. Franklin, the Supreme Court ruled unconstitutional a Pennsylvania law that required a doctor performing an abortion to choose the abortion method most likely to save the life of a fetus that might be old enough to survive outside the womb. On July 2, in Bellotti v. Baird, the Court ruled that a state may not require teenagers to have their parents' consent for an abortion unless the law also provides, as an alternative procedure, that teenagers can obtain permission from a judge.

1980 On June 30, in Harris v. McRae, the Supreme Court upheld the Hyde Amendment, Federal law banning the use of Federal Medicaid money for abortions for poor women.

1981 On March 23, in H. L. v. Matheson, the Supreme Court ruled that a state may require a doctor to inform a teenaged girl's parents before performing an abortion or face criminal penalties, at least when the girl is still living at home and dependent on her parents.

1982 The Reagan Justice Department urged the Supreme Court to overturn Roe v. Wade. In an Associated Press NBC News poll, 75 percent of Americans said they opposed a proposed constitutional amendment to ban abortion.

1983 Over 26,000 people marched on Washington, D.C. to protest abortion on the tenth anniversary of Roe v. Wade. On June 15, in three decisions, led by City of Akron v. Akron Center for Reproductive Health, the Supreme Court struck down a law requiring women seeking abortions to wait at least 24 hours after receiving counseling that included the statement that "the unborn child is a human life from the moment of conception."

1986 On June 11, in Thornburgh v. American College of Obstetricians and Gynecologists, the Supreme Court struck down the 1982 version of Pennsylvania's Abortion Control Act, requiring that women be given specific "informed consent" information intended to discourage abortions. Later, in the 1992 Casey decision, the court reversed itself, upholding this same counseling law.

1987 President Reagan nominated ultraconservative Robert Bork to the Supreme Court. A pro-choice coalition helped defeat the nomination. Anthony Kennedy, a moderate conservative whose views on abortion were unclear, was confirmed as Supreme Court Justice.

Continued on facing page

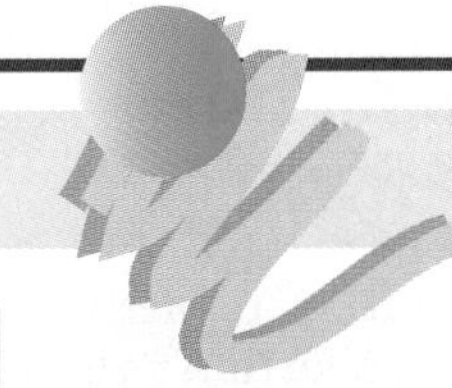

HISTORICAL PERSPECTIVES Continued

1989 On July 3, in Webster v. Reproductive Health Services, the Court upheld a Missouri law that barred the use of public hospitals or clinics for abortions, with an analysis that for the first time indicated that a majority of the Court no longer considered abortion to be a "fundamental" constitutional right. Webster v. Reproductive Health Services mobilized pro-choice forces. National Organization for Women (NOW) membership increased by more than 40,000. Students Organizing Students and other groups dedicated to protecting reproductive rights were formed all over the United States. Money poured in to support pro-choice candidates at the state and federal levels. An estimated 300,000 to 500,000 abortion rights advocates marched on the Capitol. Polls showed that abortion became a pivotal issue for voters. In the first statewide elections following the decision, abortion played a decisive role in electing pro-choice governors in New Jersey and Virginia.

1990 On June 25, in Hodgson v. Minnesota and Ohio v. Akron Center for Reproductive Health, the Supreme Court again addressed the question of parental notification. In the Minnesota case, the Justices said that a state may require a teenaged girl to notify both parents before obtaining an abortion, as long as the law provides the alternative of a judicial hearing. In the Ohio case, the Court upheld the state's law requiring notification of only one parent while also allowing the judicial alternative.

1991 The Supreme Court decision Rust v. Sullivan sanctioned gag rules that prohibited federally funded family planning programs from providing abortion counseling or referrals.

1992 On June 29, in Planned Parenthood of Southeastern Pennsylvania v. Casey, the Supreme Court reaffirmed what it called the "essence" of the constitutional right to abortion while at the same time permitting some new state restrictions. This decision effectively stopped legislation in Louisiana, Utah, and Guam that would have outlawed abortion completely. However, the Supreme Court allowed some significant state restrictions and upheld Pennsylvania's mandatory waiting period and requirements for counseling that discourage women from having abortions.

1993 On January 13, in Bray v. Alexandria Women's Health Clinic, the Supreme Court ruled that a Reconstruction-era civil rights law enacted to protect blacks from the Ku Klux Klan did not give Federal judges jurisdiction to bar antiabortion protesters from blockading abortion clinics. Also in January, in NOW v. Scheidler, the Supreme Court allowed antiabortionists to be charged under federal Racketeer Influenced and Corrupt Organizations (RICO) law, which could help prosecute antiabortion activists who conspired to close abortion clinics through organized criminal activity.

1994 On June 30, in Madsen et al. v. Women's Health Center, the Supreme Court upheld an injunction that barred antiabortion protesters from picketing within 36 feet of a Florida abortion clinic.

Data from Butler, J. D., and Walbert, D. F. (1992). *Abortion, medicine, and the law* (4th ed.). New York: Facts on File, Inc.

born life by refusing to accept the fetus as a person because of substantial disagreement on the concept of personhood (Bandman and Bandman 1990). In the years since the 1973 decision on Roe v. Wade, the Supreme Court has in subsequent rulings limited its effects (see Historical Perspectives).

Abortion is a moral and religious issue that cuts to the very core of individual beliefs about human life. As such, the legal battle over the right to abortion will most likely continue for years to come. In reality, the issue is whether abortion will be legal. The outcome of the controversy can be expected to have little influence on whether abortion will continue to exist in the future. History shows that many women throughout the years have sought and had abortions regardless of the law (O'Dowd and Philipp 1994).

ABORTION: TWO OPPOSING VIEWS

The issues surrounding legalization of abortion are grounded in the question of moral permissibility. Beliefs about the status of the products of conception guide opinions about abortion. The two viewpoints that are diametrically opposed are: (1) abortion should never be allowed under any circumstances at any time and (2) abortion is completely a private choice of the woman.

The issue of abortion is even more complex, however, because there are many differing individual beliefs between these views. Neither the groups that support nor those that oppose abortions reflect totally unified beliefs related to abortion. For example, some individuals opposed to abortion equate contraception with abortion. However, other individuals opposed to abortion, while also dedicated to preserving the life of the fetus, do not consider contraception wrong either morally or religiously. Within the pro-choice group, some individuals personally oppose abortion but support a woman's right to choose abortion. Also, within the pro-choice group, individuals have differing beliefs about the rights of the fetus versus the rights of the mother (Koop 1992). Other differences in belief arise about timing of abortion, the rights of the spouse, the rights of biological unmarried fathers, and the rights of parents of minors.

The Belief That Abortion Should Never Be Allowed

The antiabortion view is that the fetus is human from the moment of conception and should be protected from abortion, which ends life. The belief holds that the fetus' right to life outweighs the woman's right to decide what happens in and to her body. This group, often called the "pro-life" group, believes that abortion is killing and immoral under all circumstances even when the mother's life is endangered (Bandman and Bandman 1990). Ethical and Religious Directives Regarding Reproductive Care, which is the position of the Catholic Church on abortion, states one expression of total opposition to abortion. Other churches or religious groups that also oppose abortion may agree with all or only some parts of this position.

The Belief That Women Have the Right to Choose Abortion

Beginning in the 1960s, a coalition of activists from the women's movement, abortion rights movement, and population control movement carried out political actions based on the view that women have the sole right to make decisions about what happens to them and thus have the right to choose abortion (Staggenborg 1991). This view holds that since the previable fetus is dependent on the host environment of the woman, it has no rights as an independent person. Individuals may call their position "pro-choice" and point out that pro-choice does not mean pro-abortion, but rather the right to choose. Many individuals who believe that women have the right to choose abortion also believe that abortion should be used as a last resort, with contraception, adoption, or giving birth and raising the child as alternatives.

The Controversy

Both groups have intense moral and religious beliefs inspired by concern for an individual's rights, with such beliefs resulting in exactly opposite conclusions. Both sides argue eloquently and emotionally for the person's right to life, the difference being the individual who has the right, the fetus or the woman. Leaders in philosophy, theology, and health care have been unable to reach a consensus on the issues surrounding abortion, and resolution of the issues appears unlikely.

REASONS WOMEN CHOOSE ABORTION

There have always been multiple reasons why women choose abortion. However, an unintended or unwanted pregnancy that may have occurred because of the lack of the use of contraceptive measures or despite the use of contraception has been linked to induced abortion (CDC 1993) and is one of the primary reasons women choose abortion. Most women who choose abortion believe they are ill prepared for how a baby would change their lives in terms of work, school, or other responsibilities. Many women who have an abortion believe they cannot afford a child. Approximately 20 percent of women who choose abortion have a

Ethical and Religious Directives for Catholic Health Care Services Regarding Reproductive Care

The church's commitment to human dignity inspires an abiding concern for the sanctity of human life from its very beginning, and with the dignity of marriage and of the marriage act by which human life is transmitted. The church cannot approve medical practices that undermine the biological, psychological and moral bonds on which the strength of marriage and the family depends.

Catholic health care ministry witnesses to the sanctity of life "from the moment of conception until death." The church's defense of life encompasses the unborn, and the care of women and their children during and after pregnancy . . .

With the advance of the biological and medical sciences, society has at its disposal new technologies for responding to the problem of infertility. While we rejoice in the potential for good inherent in many of these technologies, we cannot assume that what is technically possible is always morally right.

DIRECTIVES

- When the marital act of sexual intercourse is not able to attain its procreative purpose, assistance that does not separate the unitive and procreative ends of the act, and does not substitute for the marital act itself, may be used to help married couples conceive.
- Those techniques of assisted conception that respect the unitive and procreative meanings of sexual intercourse, and do not involve the destruction of human embryos or their deliberate generation in such numbers that it is clearly envisaged that all cannot implant and some are simply being used to maximize the chances of others implanting, may be used as therapies for infertility.
- Heterologous fertilization (that is, any technique used to achieve conception by the use of gametes coming from at least one donor other than the spouses) is prohibited because it is contrary to the covenant of marriage, the unity of the spouses and the dignity proper to parents and the child.
- Homologous artificial fertilization (that is, any technique used to achieve conception using the gametes of the two spouses joined in marriage) is prohibited when it separates procreation from the marital act in its unitive significance, e.g., any technique used to achieve extracorporeal conception.
- Because of the dignity of the child and of marriage, and because of the uniqueness of the mother-child relationship, participation in contracts or arrangements for surrogate motherhood is not permitted. Moreover, the commercialization of such surrogacy denigrates the dignity of women, especially the poor.
- A Catholic health care institution that provides treatment for infertility should offer not only technical assistance to infertile couples but also should help couples pursue other solutions, e.g., counseling, adoption.
- A Catholic health care institution should provide prenatal, obstetric and postnatal services for mothers and their children in a manner consonant with its mission.
- Abortion, that is, the directly intended termination of pregnancy before viability or the directly intended destruction of a viable fetus, is never permitted. Every procedure whose sole immediate effect is the termination of pregnancy before viability is an abortion, which, in its moral context, includes the interval between conception and implantation of the embryo. Catholic health care institutions are not to provide abortion services even based upon the principle of material cooperation. In this context, Catholic health care institutions need to be concerned about the danger of scandal in any association with abortion providers.
- Catholic health care providers should be ready to offer compassionate physical, psychological, moral and spiritual care to those persons who have suffered from the trauma of abortion.
- Operations, treatments, and medications that have as their direct purpose the cure of a proportionately serious pathological condition

Continued on following page

Ethical and Religious Directives for Catholic Health Care Services Regarding Reproductive Care Continued

of a pregnant woman are permitted when they cannot be safely postponed until the unborn child is viable, even if they will result in the death of the unborn child.

- In case of extrauterine pregnancy, no intervention is morally licit which constitutes a direct abortion.
- For a proportionate reason, labor may be induced after the fetus is viable.
- Prenatal diagnosis is permitted when the procedure does not threaten the life or physical integrity of the unborn child or the mother and does not subject them to disproportionate risks, when the diagnosis can provide information to guide preventative care for the mother or pre- or postnatal care for the child, and when the parents, or at least the mother, give free and informed consent. Prenatal diagnosis is not permitted when undertaken with the intention of aborting an unborn child with a serious defect.
- Nontherapeutic experiments on a living embryo or fetus are not permitted, even with the consent of the parents. Therapeutic experiments are permitted for a proportionate reason with the free and informed consent of the parents or, if the father cannot be contacted, at least of the mother. Medical research that will not harm the life or physical integrity of an unborn child is permitted with parental consent.
- Catholic health institutions may not promote or condone contraceptive practices, but should provide, for married couples and the medical staff who counsel them, instruction both about the church's teaching on responsible parenthood and in methods of natural family planning.
- Direct sterilization of either men or women, whether permanent or temporary, is not permitted in a Catholic health care institution when its sole immediate effect is to prevent conception. Procedures that induce sterility are permitted when their direct effect is the cure or alleviation of a present pathology and a simpler treatment is not available.
- Genetic counseling may be provided in order to promote responsible parenthood and to prepare for the proper treatment and care of children with genetic defects, in accordance with Catholic moral teaching and the intrinsic rights and obligations of married couples regarding the transmission of life.

Excerpted from U. S. Bishops' Meeting. (December 15, 1994). Ethical and religious directives for Catholic health care services. *Origins,* 24 (27), 456–458.

wanted pregnancy but choose to terminate the pregnancy because of fetal defects or maternal health (Gold 1990).

Multifetal Pregnancy Reduction

The widespread use of assisted reproduction techniques has resulted in a dramatic increase in the number of multifetal pregnancies and an increasing use of multifetal pregnancy reduction (MFPR) procedures in which the number of fetuses is decreased during the first trimester to improve the outcome of pregnancy (Evans et al. 1993). The most widely used MFPR technique is the transabdominal injection of potassium chloride (which causes cardiac standstill) into the intrathoracic cavity of a fetus by means of ultrasound guidance (Evans et al. 1993; Tabsh 1993). The major risk of the MFPR procedure is loss of the pregnancy, the incidence of which has been cited as approximately 16 percent. Data on the number of women who have MFPR procedures are not included in published statistics on abortion and are limited to published research studies.

Maternal and fetal morbidity are directly related to the number of fetuses (Tabsh 1993). The risk of fetal and maternal complications is significantly decreased when the number of fetuses is reduced to triplets (Evans et al. 1993). The effectiveness of further reduction of fetuses to twins or a singleton in an attempt to further improve outcome is unclear. MFPR raises serious ethical questions. Evans and colleagues assert that better assisted reproduction techniques are needed that would eliminate the necessity for MFPR (Evans et al. 1993).

THE DECISION-MAKING PROCESS

The decision to terminate an unwanted pregnancy is complex and influenced by personal beliefs and values, past experiences, support from significant others, and the amount of fear associated with each option. The decision to abort is often arrived at as the result of an extended, circuitous process. In general, each woman makes the choice for or against abortion based on the impact she believes it will have on her life. Women with unintended and unwanted pregnancies often view abortion as the only solution available to them.

On the other hand, for women with wanted pregnancies complicated by maternal disease or fetal anomaly, the decision to abort usually follows an extended period of testing and is generally accompanied by a pattern of bereavement, beginning at diagnosis of the fetal or maternal condition (Rayburn and LaFerla 1986). Women who conceive multiple fetuses as a result of infertility treatment find the decision to reduce the number of fetuses by abortion (MFPR) extremely difficult and require extensive counseling about potential risks (Berkowitz et al. 1988). The issues that women generally consider when seeking an abortion are the overall experience of the abortion, time limits on the efficacy of the method, the individual who is in control of the process or procedure, the time it takes to complete the abortion, the abortion setting, the number of clinic visits required, the individual who can use the method, expected physical effects, and possible adverse effects (Berer 1992).

On the basis of a review of the literature, David (1990) described a seven-phase decision-making process that women who consider abortion are likely to undergo:

1. Acknowledgment of pregnancy
2. Formulation of alternative forms of pregnancy resolution
3. Extensive consideration of the merit of each option
4. Commitment to one option
5. Adherence to the chosen option
6. Delay of choice
7. Failure to follow through

Acknowledgment of Pregnancy

Denial, particularly prevalent in teenagers, may preclude recognition of symptoms and acknowledgment of pregnancy. For some women, the actual discovery of an unwanted pregnancy may be more stressful than any subsequent decision.

Formulation of Alternatives

Formulation of alternatives is seldom necessary for women who want to carry a pregnancy to term, and they rarely consider abortion or adoption. Unintended conception and unwanted pregnancy make decision making more complex, leading to a review of available options and the ramifications of each.

Consideration of Options

In this phase, the woman undertakes extensive consideration of abortion, adoption, and motherhood as perceived within her present life circumstances. Alone, or with significant others, each woman must weigh cultural, religious, socioeconomic, and environmental factors within the context of her current and future life. For a time, there may be considerable indecision and ambivalence, dependent in part on the woman's perception of support for her decision and her susceptibility to potentially conflicting pressures from others. Good evidence exists that, in some cultures, adoption is not an option, so that the only choice remaining is between abortion and motherhood (Zabin et al. 1989).

Commitment to One Option

Commitment to one option over another signals the woman's entry into phase four. An attitude is developed in favor of her choice and reinforced by informational materials that support the choice. New information about other options is rejected. If the woman chooses pregnancy termination, she may seek a facility before telling others. A small proportion of women continue to be ambivalent, postponing a decision until the second trimester or until it is too late for a safe and legal abortion. In this instance, the decision to carry the pregnancy to term is made by default.

Adherence to the Chosen Option

Phase five is when the woman actually keeps her appointment with an abortion provider. At this point, most women continue with pregnancy termination. Those women with considerable ambivalence or pressure from others need to be referred for counseling. Most women have reached this stage of decision making when they enter the health care system.

Delay of Choice

Women in the last two phases of the abortion decision-making process include those who delay decision making past the first trimester and those who fail to keep appointments. Delay is particularly relevant, because increased mortality and complication risks are associated with increasing gestational age, procedures are more expensive and require greater skill, and abortion is more difficult to obtain. Women who delay decision making are more likely to be unmarried, primigravid teens with lower levels of completed education and socioeconomic status. Economically disadvantaged and rural black women are disproportionately represented in women having second-trimester abortions (Gold 1990). Delays are often caused by lack of information on the availability and location of services, financial difficulties, bureaucracy, or parental notification regulations. In addition, younger women may fear telling significant others or may fail to recognize or deny pregnancy until it becomes obvious. Such delays reflect an inability to carry through because of ambivalence about the decision.

Failure to Follow Through

Women who fail to keep appointments after making initial contact regarding an abortion represent the final phase. In a study of women who decided against termination of pregnancy, three reasons were dominant (David 1990): public controversy concerning the morality of abortion, the partner's desire for a baby, and fear of the procedure and possible complications.

PHYSICAL AND PSYCHOLOGICAL EFFECTS OF ABORTION

Probably the most comprehensive review of the scientific literature on the physical and psychological effects of abortion was conducted by Dr. C. Everett Koop, former Surgeon General, U. S. Public Health Service, in response to President Reagan's request in July 1987 (Koop 1989, 1992). The findings of this review were as follows:

- In 1987, the available scientific evidence did not support that abortion *does* or *does not* cause or contribute to psychological problems.
- The scientific data do not provide conclusive evidence about the physical health effects of abortion.
- The incidence of physical injury is greater when abortions are performed or attempted by individuals unqualified to do them or when abortions are conducted in unsterile conditions.

Koop (1992) pointed out that anecdotal reports on the effects of abortions abound, that the scientific studies reviewed had major methodologic flaws, and that both antiabortion and pro-choice groups had preconceived beliefs about the effects of abortion that lacked scientific support.

Researchers who conducted studies in the 1990s on the psychological effects of abortion concluded that the development of psychiatric problems after abortion was almost always found to have developed in the context of other significant risk factors such as previous psychiatric disturbances or poverty (Zolese and Blacker 1992; Stotland 1991).

Grief Response After Abortion

Most women who have an abortion experience feelings of guilt, sadness, or regret that disappear when successful crisis resolution occurs (David 1990). Women who have an elective abortion for an unplanned or unwanted pregnancy usually have a milder intensity of grief response than do women with wanted pregnancies.

The grief responses of women who terminate wanted pregnancies because of fetal anomaly have been shown to be similar to those of women who experience spontaneous perinatal loss. Women who terminate wanted pregnancies may experience profound maternal grief, may require counseling and follow-up (Zeanah et al. 1993), and benefit from approaches similar to those used for spontaneous perinatal loss (see Chapter 38). Grieving after an abortion includes the typical feelings of shock and disbelief, anger, guilt and anxiety, despair and depression, and finally acceptance.

TYPES OF ABORTION PROCEDURES

The types of surgical abortion procedures currently used are categorized in consistency with the classification used in abortion surveillance activities by the CDC for statistical reporting purposes. These are curettage (sharp and suction), intra-amniotic instillation, hysterotomy, and hysterectomy. Medical abortion using RU 486 (mifepristone) is discussed, but the use of this drug in the United States is still under investigation by the Food and Drug Administration (FDA).

In clinical practice, the terms *dilatation and curettage (D & C)* and *dilatation and evacuation (D & E)* are often used when referring to abortion procedures. D & C is a minor gynecologic surgical procedure that may be indicated for diagnostic or therapeutic reasons. When used for the termination of pregnancy during the first trimester, it can be done by suction (most commonly used) or sharp (the oldest method) curettage. D & E is the termination of pregnancy during the second trimester by presurgical dilatation of the cervix followed by suction curettage.

Curettage

Curettage is a procedure in which either a sharp curet (a sharp, metal, spoon-shaped instrument) or a hollow curet through which suction is applied is used to remove the uterine contents from the wall and cavity of the uterus (Stubblefield 1993). Sharp curettage is the oldest method of abortion and can be done up to 12 weeks of gestation. It is used infrequently today because suction curettage is considered safer.

Curettage (suction and sharp) is the primary abortion method used in the United States, accounting for 98.9 percent of all such procedures. Approximately 89 percent of all abortions are performed during the first 12 weeks of pregnancy, with 52.6 percent of these performed during the first 8 weeks of gestation (CDC 1994). These statistics have remained similar since 1969 when data on abortions were first collected by the CDC in an attempt to reduce preventable causes of

Table 14–1

TYPES OF ABORTION PROCEDURES BY TRIMESTER

FIRST TRIMESTER	SECOND TRIMESTER
Suction curettage	Suction curettage
Sharp curettage	Intra-amniotic instillation
RU 486 (mifepristone)*	Induction of labor
	Hysterotomy and hysterectomy

* Had not received final approval by the FDA as of September 1996.

morbidity and mortality associated with abortion (CDC 1993).

Suction curettage is classified as D & C when used during the first trimester and D & E when used in the middle trimester. The cervix is dilated to enable the insertion of an aspiration cannula. The uterine contents are then aspirated. The procedure usually requires less than 5 minutes. With the use of *Laminaria* or synthetic osmotic dilators to dilate the cervix, suction curettage can be performed up to 20 weeks of gestation. Both sharp and suction curettage can be performed in a physician's office, clinic, or hospital.

Intra-amniotic Instillation

Intra-amniotic instillation procedures are used during the second trimester. A solution of hypertonic saline, prostaglandin $F_{2\alpha}$, or hypertonic urea is injected into the amniotic sac after removal of some of the amniotic fluid. Fetal death occurs and uterine contractions usually begin within 8 to 48 hours. Oxytocin may be given if labor contractions do not start within the expected time. Prostaglandins, PGE_2 and PGF_2, are also used to induce labor but have numerous side effects such as fever, nausea, and diarrhea (Brown and Crombleholme 1993). There is an increased risk of complications with instillation abortions.

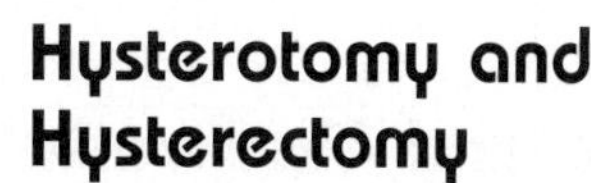

Hysterotomy and Hysterectomy

Hysterotomy is accomplished via an abdominal incision, and the uterine contents are removed. It is usually done during the second trimester, after uterine instillation has been unsuccessful. Hysterectomy should be used only when there is preexisting gynecologic pathology. Both procedures have increased risks and carry a higher incidence of complications, and are rarely used as a method of abortion today (Wallach and Zacur 1995). Potential complications and nursing care are similar to those in cesarean delivery.

RU 486

RU 486 (mifepristone) is a progesterone antagonist that is used to induce abortion in European countries. It has not yet been approved by the FDA for use in the United States, but clinical trials are now in progress and its future use now appears certain. The effectiveness rate for RU 486 is 65 to 95 percent when used alone. When prostaglandin is given 36 to 48 hours after a one-time 600-mg dose of RU 486, the effectiveness rate exceeds 95 percent (Donaldson et al. 1994).

RU 486 is used for very early abortion and is most effective when given within fewer than 48 days of amenorrhea (Cottrell 1995). If given after that time, the woman may have an incomplete abortion. By 63 days of amenorrhea, placental production of progesterone has increased to the point that RU 486 is usually ineffective in blocking progesterone and inducing abortion. The effectiveness of RU 486 has been documented only after implantation. Also, for reasons that are not understood, the drug consistently fails to induce abortion in women who have an ectopic pregnancy (Donaldson et al. 1994).

RU 486 is contraindicated for women with high blood pressure, high cholesterol levels, heart conditions, bronchial asthma, kidney disorders, and fibroid tumors; for women who smoke; and for women over 35. The safety of RU 486 is controversial. In European countries the drug is promoted as safe and a less expensive alternative to surgical abortion. However, opponents in the United States claim that its safety has not been documented and that the cost is equal to that of a first-trimester surgical abortion (Cottrell 1995).

In July 1996, after an 8-hour meeting, the FDA Advisory Committee on Reproductive Health Drugs determined that RU 486 was safe and effective. This was an important step in the FDA approval process. RU 486 was expected to become available in the United States in 1997 (The Feminist Majority Foundation 1996).

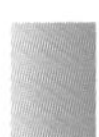

Methotrexate and Misoprostol

Both methotrexate and misoprostol have long been approved by the FDA for purposes other than abortion. However, in recent years a number of physicians have used methotrexate in combination with misoprostol to induce abortion early in pregnancy. Using a drug for other than approved purposes is termed "off-label" use of the drug. In September 1996, Planned Parenthood Federation of America received FDA clearance to conduct a nationwide study of early medical abortion using methotrexate and misoprostol. The study is to include data from 3000 women who were given methotrexate and misoprostol to induce abortion early in pregnancy. If the study demonstrates that methotrexate and misoprostol are safe and effective for early medical abortion, Planned Parenthood Federation of America will request that the FDA recommend a change in labeling for these drugs (Planned Parenthood Federation of America 1996).

COMPLICATIONS

Gestational age and the method of abortion are the two most important determinants of complica-

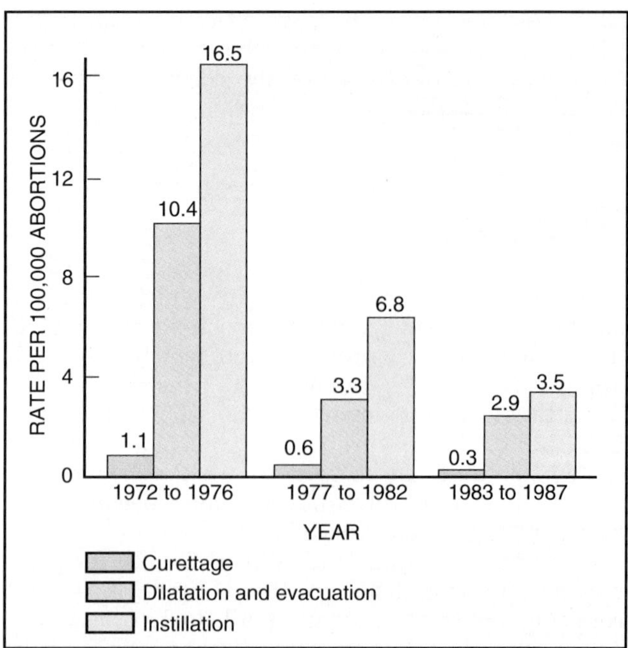

Figure 14–3

Mortality trends for legal abortion by method, United States, 1972–1976, 1977–1982, and 1983–1987. (From Lawson, H. W., Frye, A., Atrash, H. K., Smith, J. C., Shulman, H. B., Ramick, M. [1994]. Abortion mortality, United States, 1972 through 1987. *American Journal of Obstetrics and Gynecology,* 171 (5), 1370.)

tions (Wallach and Zacur 1995). The relative risk of death to the woman from an abortion doubles for every 2 weeks of delay after 8 weeks of gestation (Gant and Cunningham 1993).

Infection is the most common complication, but the routine use of antibiotics has decreased this risk. Other possible complications are hemorrhage, cervical lacerations, uterine perforation and rupture, bowel and bladder injury, embolism, disseminated intravascular coagulopathy, postabortion pain syndrome, and failed abortion (Wallach and Zacur 1995; Brenner and Ballard 1994; Stubblefield 1993). The rate of complications increases with increasing gestational age. Complications from second-trimester abortions are three to four times higher than from first-trimester abortions (Chez and Mishell 1994).

From 1974 to 1976, mortality from abortion varied significantly according to the procedure used. D & C—sharp or suction curettage before 12 weeks—had the least risk, followed by D & E—suction aspiration between 12 to 20 weeks. Instillation carried a higher risk (Fig. 14–3). Between 1977 and 1982, mortality rates from abortion fell for all types of procedures, and by 1983 to 1987, although differences in mortality rates between the type of procedure used still existed, with curettage having the least risk, these differences were not statistically significant (Lawson et al. 1994).

Infection, embolism, hemorrhage, and anesthesia together accounted for 82 percent of abortion-related deaths between 1972 and 1987, each accounting for approximately 20 percent of the deaths during this 16-year period. A review of abortion-related deaths by time periods during the years from 1972 to 1987 provides additional information about abortion-related deaths. In the early period from 1972 to 1976, infection and embolism accounted equally for the greatest number of deaths. However, during the most recent period in this review, 1983 to 1987, anesthesia emerged as the most frequent cause of abortion-related deaths and continues to be the most frequent cause of abortion-related mortality (Lawson et al. 1994).

Nursing Practice

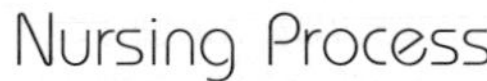

Nursing Process

Nursing roles and responsibilities vary with setting, type of procedure, and patient needs. In some facilities the nurse and physician may be the only health care providers, while other environments include social workers, counselors, and a variety of other support services. In either setting, the nursing role is essential to optimal patient care outcomes. An examination of one's values and beliefs related to abortion is essential before assuming responsibility for the care of women who choose to have an abortion (see Improving Your Practice).

▼ Assessment

▼ HEALTH HISTORY

A comprehensive health history is essential for identifying risk factors, determining patient needs,

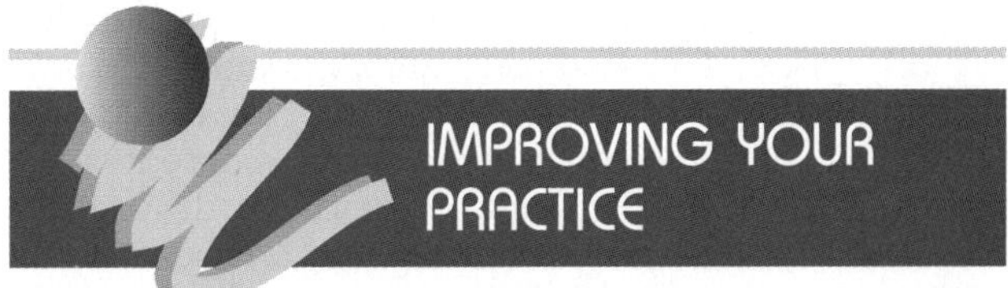

PROVIDING OPTIMAL CARE FOR WOMEN SEEKING TERMINATION OF PREGNANCY

The nurse is key to optimal patient care for women who seek termination of pregnancy. The following steps will help the nurse provide the most effective nursing care possible:

- IDENTIFY YOUR ATTITUDES ABOUT PREGNANCY TERMINATION. Honestly evaluate your own feelings about abortion and the woman's right to choose. Recognize the impact and influence your religion, culture, and social group have on your beliefs.
- UPDATE YOUR KNOWLEDGE BASE. Obtain current accurate information about abortion procedures, their indications and contraindications, and the risks of each. Read the lay literature on abortion so that you are knowledgeable about general sources of information.
- INVESTIGATE THE STATUS OF HEALTH POLICY AND SOCIAL CONTROVERSY CONCERNING PREGNANCY TERMINATION. Examine how social, political, and religious controversy over pregnancy termination affects access to health care services.
- REVIEW THE PROFESSIONAL LITERATURE AND STANDARDS OF PRACTICE RELATED TO PREGNANCY TERMINATION. Evaluate clinical practice in your setting using current research findings.
- PARTICIPATE IN CONTINUING EDUCATION ACTIVITIES RELATED TO ABORTION. Discuss with colleagues ways to provide better care. Continue to upgrade your knowledge and skills.
- AVOID VALUE JUDGMENTS. If you have strong beliefs against abortion, don't work in areas where women seek pregnancy termination. Choose another clinical area that is compatible with your own personal beliefs.

and formulating a plan of care. Regardless of the alternative chosen, gestational age must be determined through history taking, physical examination, and/or ultrasound examination.

Menstrual History. Determine the age of onset and usual frequency and duration of menstrual periods. Also, ask about the type of flow and symptoms related to menses. Irregular or erratic menstrual periods make determining gestational age more difficult.

Obstetric History. Any complications of pregnancy, birth, or the postpartum period should be determined, as well as the number of previous pregnancies, the outcome of each, and the number of living children.

Current Obstetric History. Determine the last menstrual period and whether it was normal or abnormal. Has the woman used contraception, and if so which method? Ascertain whether the woman has pregnancy-related symptoms such as fatigue, nausea, vomiting, and breast tenderness. Also, determine whether the woman is sexually active, so that proper follow-up related to pregnancy prevention and safer sex practices can be conducted.

Gynecologic History. Gather information related to surgery, infertility, or trauma to the reproductive system. Current symptoms of pelvic inflammatory disease or sexually transmitted diseases usually indicate the need for additional laboratory testing and possible procedure(s) before abortion.

Medical History. This should include serious illnesses, surgeries, accidents, or hospitalizations and their sequelae. Determine whether there are any drug, food, or other allergies; the Rh type; and information about which medications are taken regularly or sporadically.

Family History. Family history should include chronic diseases such as diabetes, hypertension, cardiac disease, cancer, and genetic disorders, because of hereditary risks.

Health Habits. Knowledge of the usual health behavior of the client will assist the nurse in developing a teaching plan. The information should include last health visit, Papanicolaou smear, mammogram, breast self-examination, bowel and bladder habits, sleep patterns, and nutrition. Ascertain whether the woman uses alcohol, nicotine, or street drugs and whether there are any other potentially destructive social habits.

▼ PHYSICAL ASSESSMENT

Physical assessment of the woman presenting for termination of an unwanted pregnancy does not differ significantly from that of other women. Basic physical assessment includes vital signs, blood pressure, height, weight, and complete systems assessment (general appearance, skin, neurologic, respiratory, cardiovascular, gastrointestinal, and genitourinary).

▼ PSYCHOLOGICAL ASSESSMENT

Psychological assessment for a woman considering pregnancy termination is made to determine her available support and needed resources. One must first determine at what point the woman is in the decision-making process, her ability to make decisions, and her feelings about her pregnancy. Conflicting emotions may occur with any pregnancy, and ambivalence is common. However, most women appear to resolve these conflicts once they make a decision.

The woman's ability to cope with her pregnancy and decision making may be affected by the quality or quantity of her support systems. If opinions of significant others are in direct conflict with the woman's beliefs and actions, she may be isolated from her usual support.

Other questions are: Is the woman in a stable relationship? Does her partner know about the pregnancy? Who lives in the home? Is she employed or in school? Who knows about the pregnancy and are they supportive? Is the pregnancy a result of rape or incest?

▼ EDUCATIONAL AND COUNSELING NEEDS ASSESSMENT

The woman's current knowledge about pregnancy and options for unwanted pregnancy, communication skills, and level of anxiety will affect her ability to learn and should be determined first. Once the woman makes a decision, her educational needs will be specific to her choice of an option and her feelings about family planning and future sexual activity.

▼ LABORATORY ASSESSMENT AND DIAGNOSTIC TESTS

Hemoglobin, hematocrit, urinalysis, blood group and RH, and pregnancy test are the essential laboratory tests needed. An ultrasound examination to determine gestational age is necessary when there is a discrepancy between clinical examination and menstrual history. Additional laboratory tests may be needed, depending on each woman's unique situation, medical history, and stage of pregnancy.

▼ Diagnosis

Nursing diagnoses develop from the initial assessment and form the basis of the care plan. The complexity of the plan varies greatly with the type of procedure, whether it occurs in an ambulatory or inpatient facility, and the psychosocial status of the woman. Applicable diagnoses are

- Anxiety and/or fear related to the procedure
- Knowledge deficit: abortion, related to specific unknown aspects of the procedures, expectations, and postabortion care
- Risk for injury to mother related to potential complications from procedure
- Pain related to the procedure
- Anticipatory grieving related to having an abortion, loss of a pregnancy, or feelings of guilt

▼ Intervention

Although most women have already made the decision to terminate the pregnancy before arrival at the facility, the health care provider must offer supportive interventions. To some extent, all women will require the following:

- An environment conducive to determining the best alternative at this point in their lives
- Data necessary to make an informed choice, considering all alternatives
- Assistance with exploring the potential impact of factors affecting the decision to continue or terminate the pregnancy
- Assistance with identification and mobilization of resources
- Freedom to make their own decisions, and support once the choice is made

The nurse may become the primary contact and support person for women during this process of decision making.

A primary problem for all women who are undergoing a pregnancy termination procedure is anxiety and/or fear related to the procedure itself. The nurse and other health care providers need to be supportive and reassuring. A closely related problem is knowledge deficit related to specific unknown aspects of the procedure. One explanation is seldom sufficient, and some women require several repetitions in order to fully comprehend the details. This difficulty with understanding is almost always associated with fear and anxiety about the procedure.

After the abortion is completed, patient teaching should always include the expected physiologic changes and symptoms that may precede complications. Increase in body temperature, excessive or continued vaginal bleeding, malodorous vaginal discharge, and abdominal pain are unusual circumstances and should be reported to health care providers immediately. In addition, postprocedure instructions should include delay in sexual intercourse for 1 to 2 weeks, contraception counseling, and follow-up care.

Because of the potential for immediate complications related to uterine perforation and uterine atony, observation for associated symptoms is crucial. Vital signs, particularly blood pressure, pulse, and respiration, are taken frequently the first 1 to 2 postabortion hours to identify early symptoms of hypovolemic shock. Hematocrit testing is usually done before discharge.

Since the risk of sensitization is always present for Rh-negative women, care should be taken to decrease the risk. Blood typing in all women will identify the ones at risk. Rh-negative women should receive immune globulin D (RhoGAM) before discharge, since approximately 5 percent of RH D-negative women who have an abortion become sensitized (Gant and Cunningham 1993).

Women who have pregnancy terminations because of maternal disease or fetal anomaly present other nursing management problems. In addition to already discussed problems, these women and their families will require support and resources to assist with their grief and adjustment to the loss of an infant. Most want to see the aborted fetus, and for later gestations, many women want to hold the fetus. Women and their families should be supported in their grief and encouraged to express feelings. They should be provided with mementos, pictures, footprints, and so forth, as appropriate (see Chapter 38).

Since women having medically indicated abortions are frequently cared for by the same health care providers as those having elective abortions, it is important for the nurse to recognize the difference. Women who have medically indicated abortions have different needs and require highly individualized care. Ideally, the nurse should not be asked to care for both types of women within the abortion patient population. The role dichotomy that arises from the continual necessity to switch approaches in caring for "elective" or "medically indicated" abortion clients is very stressful for most nurses.

Women having pregnancy termination procedures are a challenge for nursing, whether the abortion is elective or medically indicated. Although almost all terminations are performed in ambulatory settings, some women continue to require hospitalization and more complex procedures.

Most women have already made the decision to terminate their pregnancies by the time of initial contact with health care providers. Their major needs from providers are information and support. Usually women choose abortion because they believe it is the only solution for them at that time in their lives.

The decision of whether or not to terminate a wanted pregnancy complicated by maternal disease or fetal anomaly is extremely difficult for the individuals involved. In the case of maternal illness, the option to abort a pregnancy is weighed against a real threat to the woman's life. The decision to abort a fetus with a genetic abnormality will vary in difficulty, particularly if the defect is not universally lethal or catastrophic. In situations in which the pregnancy was wanted but a decision for abortion was made because of maternal disease or fetal abnormality, the psychosocial approach for providing care is different in some aspects from that for women having an elective abortion for an unwanted pregnancy. Women should be encouraged to seek out friends, family, and clergy during their period of grief.

▼ Evaluation

Established criteria to determine outcomes are essential, and patient status should be evaluated against these criteria. The following are essential client outcomes:

- Physiologic integrity is maintained as evidenced by vital signs and laboratory tests within normal limits.
- The woman displays signs of coping with grief as evidenced by the ability to express concerns, fears, and feelings.
- The woman verbalizes knowledge about conception and family planning as evidenced by statements about future plans.

IMPACT OF PROVIDING NURSING CARE

Providing care for abortion clients in general can be stressful, but nurses have the greatest difficulty in caring for women having second-trimester abortion procedures. Several factors that contribute to this difficulty are exacerbated by the environment and level of care needed. Women undergoing elective second-trimester abortion procedures are frequently part of a busy patient care assignment on an inpatient gynecology unit. Women undergoing indicated abortions for maternal or fetal reasons are usually placed in the labor and delivery unit, and the nurse assumes primary responsibility for their care throughout the procedure. After completion of the abortion, disposition of the fetus is usually the nurse's responsibility.

Labor nurses often suffer increased stress associated with providing intense care in cases involving a known negative outcome and an already grieving family. A nurse on a busy gynecology unit may feel abandoned by other health care team members as she provides care for women having a second-trimester abortion.

Implications for Research

To determine the health effects of abortion on women, Koop (1992) stated there is a need for a prospective study on a cohort of women of child-bearing age that provides a complete examination of the variables of mating. This should include the following:

- What are the psychological effects of failure to conceive?
- What are the physical and psychological effects of pregnancy—planned and unplanned, wanted and unwanted—whether carried to delivery, miscarried, or terminated by abortion?
- The discrepancy between the number of abortions on record and the number of women who admit having an abortion on surveys points out a problem of "denial." How can this problem be addressed and resolved before further research investigations are undertaken?

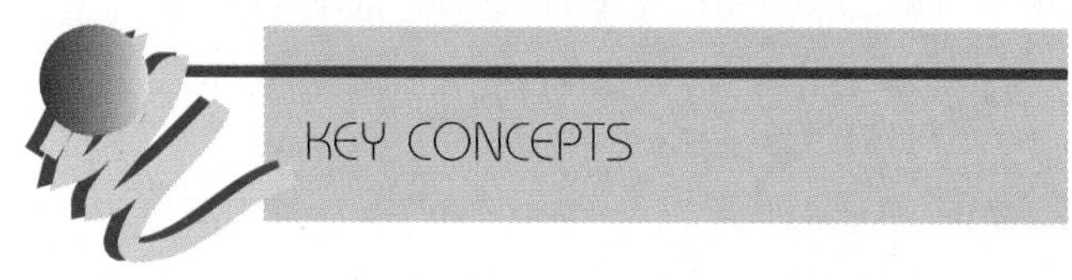

- ▼ Elective termination of pregnancy is one of the most frequently performed gynecologic procedures in the United States today.
- ▼ The number of legal abortions increased from a low of 193,491 in 1970 to a high of 1,429,577 in 1990. Since 1991, the number of legal abortions has decreased each year.
- ▼ In 1992, most women who obtained legal abortions were 24 years or younger (54.7 percent), white (62.9 percent), unmarried (79.3 percent), and with no previous liveborn children (46.3 percent).
- ▼ Approximately 89 percent of all abortions are performed during the first 12 weeks of pregnancy. The primary abortion method used is curettage (suction and sharp).
- ▼ The abortion rate for black women is three times higher than that for white women. The mortality rate is 2.5 times higher for black and other minority women than for white women.
- ▼ The risk from an abortion increases with age. Teenagers have the lowest risk of mortality, while the risk of an abortion-related death is three times as high for women 40 years and older.
- ▼ Abortion ranked as a leading cause of maternal mortality in the years before the 1973 Supreme Court decision on abortion, Roe v. Wade. After abortion was legalized, mortality decreased significantly.
- ▼ Subsequent Supreme Court rulings have limited the effects of Roe v. Wade.
- ▼ Controversy surrounds abortion in the United States. There are also differences in individual beliefs within each of the major ideologies.
- ▼ Unintended or unwanted pregnancy, which may have occurred because of the lack of contraceptive measures or despite the use of contraception, has been linked to legal abortion as one of the primary reasons women choose abortion.
- ▼ Approximately 20 percent of women who have abortions choose abortion to terminate a wanted pregnancy because of fetal defects or maternal health.
- ▼ Women who consider abortion typically follow a decision-making process, which may include acknowledgment of pregnancy, formulation of alternative forms of pregnancy resolution, extensive consideration of the merit of each option, commitment to one option, adherence to the chosen option, delay of choice, and failure to follow through.
- ▼ The types of surgical abortion procedures currently used in the United States are curettage (sharp and suction), intra-amniotic instillation, hysterotomy, and hysterectomy.
- ▼ Gestational age and the method of abortion are the two most important determinants of complications; the relative risk of death from an abortion doubles every 2 weeks of delay after 8 weeks of gestation.
- ▼ Suction curettage at 8 weeks of gestation or less is the safest method of abortion.
- ▼ Anesthesia continues to be the most frequent cause of abortion-related death. Other primary causes include infection, embolism, or hemorrhage.
- ▼ Women seeking an abortion may need an environment conducive to determining the best alternative at this point in their lives; data necessary to make an informed choice, considering all alternatives; assistance with exploring the potential impact of factors affecting the decision to continue or terminate the pregnancy; assistance with identification and mobilization of resources; and freedom to make their own decisions, and support once the choice is made.

References

Accreditation Council for Graduate Medical Education (ACGME). (1995a). Program requirements for residency education in obstetrics and gynecology. Chicago, IL: Author.

Accreditation Council for Graduate Medical Education

(ACGME). (1995b). Program requirements for residency education in obstetrics and gynecology. Press release.

Bandman, E. L., and Bandman, B. (1990). *Nursing ethics through the life span* (2nd ed.). Norwalk, CT: Appleton & Lange.

Berer, M. (1992). Inducing a miscarriage: Women-centered perspectives on RU 486/prostaglandin as an early abortion method. *Law, Medicine, & Health Care,* 20 (3), 199–200.

Berkowitz, R. L., Lynch, L., Wilkins, I. A., Mehalek, K. E., Alvarez, E. (1988). Selective reduction of multifetal pregnancies in the first trimester. *The New England Journal of Medicine,* 318 (6), 1043–1047.

Brenner, P. F., and Ballard, C. A. (1994). Management of complications of first-trimester pregnancy termination. In D. Mishell, and P. Brenner (Eds.). *Management of common problems in obstetrics and gynecology* (3rd ed.) (pp. 858–863). Boston: Blackwell Scientific Publications.

Brown, J. S., and Crombleholme, W. R. (1993). *Handbook of gynecology and obstetrics.* Norwalk, CT: Appleton & Lange.

Butler, J. D., and Walbert, D. F. (1992). *Abortion, medicine, and the law* (4th ed.). New York: Facts on File, Inc.

Centers for Disease Control and Prevention. (1993). CDC Surveillance Summaries. *MMWR,* 42 (SS-6), 29–57.

Centers for Disease Control and Prevention. (1994). CDC Surveillance Summaries. *MMWR,* 43 (50), 930–939.

Chez, R., and Mishell, D. (1994). Control of human reproduction: Contraception, sterilization, and pregnancy termination. In J. R. Scott, P. J. Disaia, C. B. Hammond, W. N. Spellacy (Eds.). *Danforth's obstetrics and gynecology* (7th ed.). Philadelphia: J. B. Lippincott.

Cottrell, B. H. (1995). RU 486 (letter to the Editor). *Journal of Obstetric, Gynecologic, and Neonatal Nursing,* 24 (5), 389–390.

David, H. P. (1990). Induced abortion: Psychosocial aspects. In J. J. Sciarra (Ed.). *Gynecology and obstetrics,* Vol. 6. Philadelphia: J. B. Lippincott.

DeCherney, A. H., and Pernoll, M. L. (1994). *Current obstetric & gynecologic diagnosis & treatment.* Norwalk, CT: Appleton & Lange.

Donaldson, K., Briggs, J., McMaster, D. (1994). RU 486: An alternative to surgical abortion. *Journal of Obstetric, Gynecologic, and Neonatal Nursing,* 23 (7), 555–559.

Dueveraux, G. (1960). *A study of abortion in primitive societies.* London: Thomas Yaseloff.

Evans, M., Dommergues, M., Wapner, R., Lynch, L., Dumez, Y., Goldberg, J., Zador, I., Nicolaides, K., Johnson, M., Golbus, M., Boulot, P., Berkowitz, R. (1993). Efficacy of transabdominal multifetal pregnancy reduction: Collaborative experience among the world's largest centers. *Obstetrics and Gynecology,* 82 (1), 61–66.

The Feminist Majority Foundation. (1996). The fight to make RU 486 available to U.S. women. The Feminist Majority Foundation and New Media Publishing, Inc. (Available through the Internet.)

Gant, N. F., and Cunningham, F. G. (1993). *Basic gynecology and obstetrics.* Norwalk, CT: Appleton & Lange.

Gold, R. B. (1990). *Abortion and women's health: A turning point for America?* New York: Guttmacher Institute.

Henshaw, S. K., and Van Vort, J. (1994). Abortion services in the United States, 1991 and 1992. *Family Planning Perspectives,* 26 (3), 100–112.

Koop, C. E. (1989). Letter to President Reagan, January 9, 1989. Washington, D.C.: White House Press Office.

Koop, C. E. (1992). The U. S. Surgeon General's Report on Health Effects of Abortion (Appendix I). In J. D. Butler, and D. F. Walbert (Eds.). *Abortion, medicine, and the law* (4th ed.). New York: Facts on File, Inc.

Lawson, H. W., Frye, A., Atrash, H. K., Smith, J. C., Shulman, H. B., Ramick, M. (1994). Abortion mortality, United States, 1972 through 1987. *American Journal of Obstetrics and Gynecology,* 171 (5), 1365–1372.

O'Dowd, M. J., and Philipp, E. E. (1994). *The history of obstetrics and gynecology.* New York: Parthenon Publishing Group.

Planned Parenthood Federation of America. (September 11, 1996). Planned Parenthood gets FDA clearance for new medical abortion study; could lead to "on-label" status for early abortion using methotrexate. (Press release.)

Rayburn, W. F., and LaFerla, J. J. (1986). Mid-gestational abortion for medical or genetic indications. *Clinics in Obstetrics and Gynecology,* 13 (1), 71–82.

Roe v. Wade. (1973). Supreme Court of the U. S., 410 U. S. 113.

Staggenborg, S. (1991). *The pro-choice movement.* New York: Oxford University Press.

Stotland, N. (1991). *Psychiatric aspects of abortion.* Washington, D.C.: American Psychiatric Press.

Stubblefield, P. G. (1993). First and second trimester abortion. In D. H. Nichols (Ed.). *Gynecologic and obstetric surgery.* St. Louis: Mosby-Year Book.

Tabsh, K. M. (1993). A report of 131 cases of multifetal pregnancy reduction. *Obstetrics and Gynecology,* 82 (1), 57–60.

U. S. Bishops' Meeting. (December 15, 1994). Ethical and religious directives for Catholic health care services. *Origins,* 24 (27), 456–458.

Wallach, E. E., and Zacur, H. A. (1995). *Reproductive medicine and surgery.* St. Louis: Mosby-Year Book.

Zabin, L. S., Hirsch, M. B., Emerson, M. R. (1989). When urban adolescents choose abortion: Effects on education, psychological status and subsequent pregnancy. *Family Planning Perspectives,* 21, 248–255.

Zeanah, C. H., Dailey, J. V., Rosenblatt, M. J., Saller, D. N., Jr. (1993). Do women grieve after terminating pregnancies because of fetal anomalies? A controlled investigation. *Obstetrics and Gynecology,* 82 (2), 270–275.

Zolese, G., and Blacker, C. V. (1992). Psychological complications of therapeutic abortions (review). *British Journal of Psychiatry,* 160, 742–749.

Unit 3

Nursing Care During Pregnancy

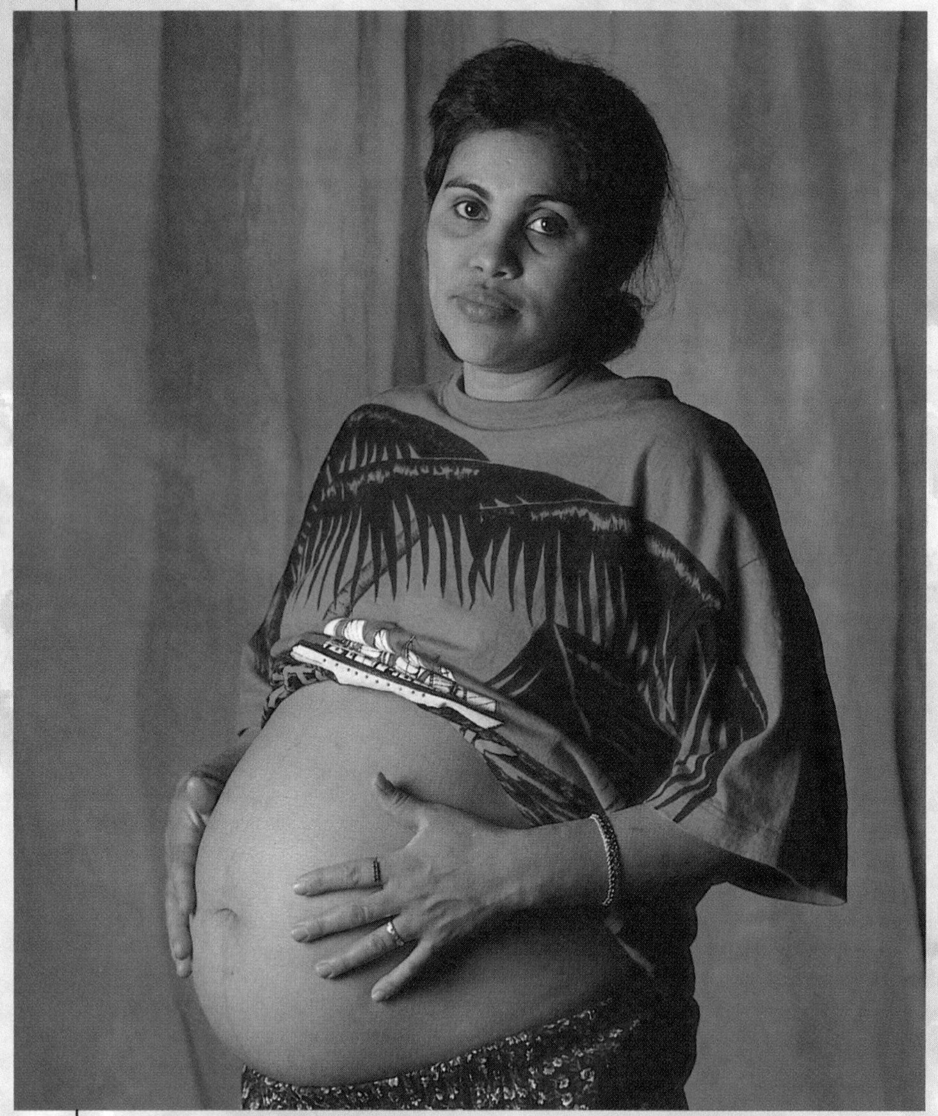

Pregnancy is an emotional experience that can trigger major psychological responses. It is a time of conflicting emotions—excitement, delight, awe, and joy—and, as is apparent in this woman's face, contemplation, a search for meaning as an individual and as a mother, often evidenced by ambivalence, emotional lability, and mood swings.

Trends in Research

PSYCHOLOGICAL RESPONSES TO PREGNANCY

Contrasting views of pregnancy range from the *fulfillment* of a woman's deepest and most powerful wish to a maturational or developmental life *crisis.*

Pregnancy has been viewed in different ways: a developmental milestone, a psychosocial crisis, a time in which earlier emotionally charged conflicts emerge, a stage during which the woman must develop a nurturing relationship with her child, and an opportunity for personal growth and enhancement of self.[1] These contrasting views of pregnancy range from the fulfillment of a woman's deepest and most powerful wish to a maturational or developmental life crisis.

CONCLUSIONS FROM RESEARCH

Major research findings richly portray the psychological nature of the behavioral manifestations that occur.

- Deutsch and Benedek described pregnancy as a developmental task of great maturational importance that enables the woman to prepare for parenthood and establish a more secure and independent adult identity by resolving earlier childhood conflicts.[1]
- Bibring and colleagues viewed pregnancy as a crisis during which earlier conflicts could emerge to provide an opportunity for constructive resolution. It also allows the new organization of the personality and personal growth.[1]
- According to Mercer,[2] pregnancy represents a transition between two lifestyles—from being a couple to being parents with the full-time responsibility for a child. Parenthood alters the balance of established marital and gender roles, leading to new conflicts and different patterns of interactions.
- Colman and Colman[3] reported that pregnancy alters the state of a woman's consciousness and a new inner experience develops, unique to the state of pregnancy. The woman's entire attention is focused on her pregnancy and the events that are occurring.
- Rubin[4] and Lederman[5] characterized pregnancy as a developmental turning point that presents a series of necessary tasks and requires adaptations to prepare the woman and her partner for the birth of the baby and the role of parenting.
- The degree of crisis experienced during pregnancy depends on the nature of the pregnancy (normal or high risk), the status of the woman's and family's existing resources, and their perception of the pregnancy.[6]
- Emotional lability increases, especially in early pregnancy, and is manifested in frequency and intensity of emotional highs and lows.[4,5]
- Ambivalence is a common emotional response during pregnancy and is usually limited to the first and second trimesters.[2,3]
- Pregnant women may experience vivid dreams and fantasies about their unborn baby, which often begin during the second trimester.[3–5]
- Pregnant women usually experience changes in body image, which may be either positive or negative, as their bodies enlarge and change in shape.[3–5]
- Most women experience a mixture of anticipation and dread about the impending childbirth experience.[3–6]
- A woman initially perceives her developing baby as a part of her self rather than a separate person. As pregnancy progresses, the baby is increasingly viewed as a separate, distinct individual. This emotional investment in her unborn child forms the foundation for the critical element of attachment.[1]

IMPLICATIONS FOR PRACTICE

Common emotional responses to pregnancy exist; however, each woman's response to pregnancy is unique, depending on her situation. The nurse's understanding of the typical emotional dimensions of pregnancy is essential to design appropriate interventions. A thorough assessment of the meaning of this pregnancy to each woman and her support system is required for development of an individualized plan of care.

---

[1] Leon I. G. (1992). The psychoanalytic conceptualization of perinatal loss: A multidimensional model. *American Journal of Psychiatry,* 149 (11), 1464–1472.

[2] Mercer, R. (1986). *First-time motherhood: Experiences from teens to forties.* New York: Springer.

[3] Colman, L., and Colman, A. (1991). *Pregnancy: The psychological experience.* New York: The Noonday Press.

[4] Rubin, R. (1984). *Maternal identity and the maternal experience.* New York: Springer.

[5] Lederman, R. (1984). *Psychosocial adaptation in pregnancy.* Englewood Cliffs, NJ: Prentice-Hall.

[6] Arizmendi, T., and Affonso, D. (1987). Stressful events related to pregnancy and postpartum. *Journal of Psychosomatic Research,* 31 (6), 743–756.

–FRANCINE H. NICHOLS

15 Chapter

Every day during the first few weeks after conception, new developments occur which are crucial to future growth. Fertilization, the safe journey through the fallopian tube, implantation in the uterus, the first signals to the ovaries and the brain, early cell division and the emergence of a nurturing placenta: each event is as vital as the last. When one considers all the possible hazards and disturbances that could interrupt this process, the development and birth of a new human being seems all the more miraculous.

LARS HAMBERGER (NILSSON AND HAMBERGER 1990)

Fetal Development

Mary C. Brucker

HIGHLIGHTS

- Ovulation and Conception
- Preembryonic Development
- Implantation
- Embryonic and Fetal Development
- Teratology
- Placental Development
- Embryonic and Fetal Assessment Techniques
- Future Methods for Fetal Surveillance
- Implications for Research

During a woman's lifetime, she usually ovulates no more than 400 times. However, it is during one of these episodes that fertilization may occur and pregnancy ensue. Historically, this period was treated as a miraculous event. Even today, as more is understood about the physiologic mechanisms involved, the processes of conception, implantation, and fetal development serve as reminders of the sophistication of the human body.

OVULATION AND CONCEPTION

A major purpose of the ovary is the production of female eggs or ova. At birth, it is estimated that a woman has a million primary ovarian follicles. Unlike in the male reproductive system, no new germ cells are ever created. The majority of the follicles are eventually lost to atresia and degeneration. Only a few hundred primary follicles fully mature to ova.

DEFINITIONS

Antrum—Fluid-filled space in the follicle that marks the maturation of the ovum.

Blastocyst—Stage of growth and development that follows a morula; at this point, approximately 100 cells exist.

Blastomere—Stage of growth and development that follows the zygote; at this point, approximately two to eight cells exist.

Blocking polyspermy—Normal physiologic changes that make more than one sperm unable to fertilize the same ovum.

Cephalocaudal—Growth from the head down the body.

Chorionic villus—Tissue is formed into projections; part of the placenta.

Decidua—Endometrium during pregnancy; subdivided into basal, capsular, and parietal sections.

Embryo—Stage of growth and development from implantation to the end of the seventh postconceptional week.

Fertilization—Uniting of mature ovum and sperm.

Fetus—Stage of growth and development after the embryo until birth.

Human chorionic gonadotropin (hCG)—Hormone produced by cells of the cytotrophoblast layer; the measurement of hCG levels is the basis of pregnancy tests.

Implantation—Nidation or the embedding of the fertilized ovum, usually in the uterine decidua.

Placenta—Organ of exchange between the pregnant woman and her fetus.

Teratology—Study of congenital malformations or of agents producing such malformations.

Zygote—Fertilized ovum.

Gametogenesis

The process of gametogenesis, by which maturation of the sex cells occurs, is related to the hormonal milieu (Speroff et al. 1994; Blackburn and Loper 1992; Moore and Persaud 1993). For women, gametogenesis can also be referred to as oogenesis. For men, gametogenesis is termed spermatogenesis. Although the woman has all the ova she will ever produce present in her ovary at the time of her birth, these ova are not mature (Moore and Persaud 1993; Sadler 1995). Oogonial cells exist in the ovary from which eventually ova will emerge. Meiosis first occurs during the intrauterine period. The oogonial cells give rise to oocytes. However, meiosis is arrested before the first division. This state remains until puberty. During puberty, a primary oocyte (46, XX) continues through meiotic division; disproportionately sized cells are produced, one called the secondary oocyte and the other the polar body (see Fig. 13–2). The secondary oocyte contains 23 chromosomes (23, X), including 22 autosomes and 1 sex chromosome. An arrest again occurs, this time in the stage of metaphase, and the oocyte remains until the time of ovulation, when a second meiotic division begins immediately and division continues as the oocyte travels through the fallopian tube. This secondary oocyte completes the second meiotic division and becomes a mature ovum at the time of fertilization. Two second polar bodies, which are smaller in size than the ovum, are also produced. All three of the small polar bodies produced during gametogenesis disintegrate eventually (Moore and Persaud 1993; Sadler 1995). The similar process of spermatogenesis can also be seen in Figure 13–2; a detailed discussion of meiosis is found in Chapter 13.

Ovulation

Simultaneously with the genetic changes that are occurring, the ovary is also undergoing a number of structural variations. As a follicle develops, there is a characteristic increase in the size of the ovum and surrounding granulosa cells. The ovum eventually becomes separated from the granulosa cells by a thick membrane, the zona pellucida. In spite of the zona pellucida, the ovum remains associated with the granulosa cells through cytoplasmic processes traversing the zona pellucida and forming gap junctions with the ovum. New cell layers form as the follicle continues to grow. Therefore, in addition to the ovum and surrounding layers of granulosa cells, the follicle develops outer layers of cells termed the theca. The granulosa cells secrete fluid, and eventually a fluid-filled space is formed in their midst, known as the antrum. When the antrum has formed, the ovum reaches full growth. However, the follicle continues to grow, largely because of an increase in the size of the antrum. Eventually, the ovum, which is surrounded by the zona pellucida and several layers of granulosa cells (also known as the cumulus), becomes a peninsula surrounded by the fluid of the antrum. The antrum is so large (approximately 1.5 cm) that a completely mature follicle can visibly protrude from the surface of the ovary (Vander et al., 1989; Cunningham et al. 1993).

As discussed in Chapter 9, after approximately 2 weeks of increasing levels of estrogen, sensitivity of the anterior pituitary is raised to the degree that a surge in luteinizing hormone occurs. The increased amount of luteinizing hormone causes ovulation to follow by causing the ovarian membrane to dissolve at the bulge of the mature follicle. The ovum, covered with the zona pellucida and cumulus, is carried out of the ovary by the antral fluid. Some women complain of an ovulatory pain, also known as mittelschmerz, which has traditionally been attributed to intra-abdominal irritation at the time of ovulation. Physiologists have questioned the timing of the events, and although the phenomenon is clear, the scientific reasons for it remain more elusive (Vander et al. 1989; Boston Women's Book Collective 1991).

When the ovum erupts from the ovary (Fig. 15–1, step 1), it must first gain entry into the fallopian tube, or oviduct. To facilitate this mission, the fallopian tubes have long projections called fimbriae, which are lined with ciliated epithelium. The smooth muscles of the fimbriae pass over the ovary around the time of ovulation, and the ovum is swept into the cilia; ciliary action and regular peristaltic actions of the muscle layer within the tube transport the ovum toward the uterine cavity (Moore and Persaud 1993; Moore et al. 1994) (Fig. 15–1, step 2). It is the combination of ciliary activity and peristalsis of the smooth muscle of the tube that provides motion for the ovum. Without such intervention, the ovum is motionless. Although the peristalsis occurs rapidly immediately after ovulation, the contractions ultimately diminish within a few minutes. Tubal transport eventually slows, so that it takes several days for the ovum to traverse the fallopian tube into the uterine cavity. It is during this time that fertilization must transpire for pregnancy to occur. If fertilization does not occur, the ovum slowly disintegrates and is phagocytosed by the lining of the uterus.

Fertilization

Mature sperm must be present to unite with the mature ovum as a prerequisite for fertilization. The timing of intercourse is important for fertilization to occur. It is estimated that sperm live for approximately 24 to 72 hours. The ovum itself is fertile for approximately 10 to 24 hours after ovulation. Therefore, for pregnancy to ensue, intercourse should occur no longer than 48 hours before or 15 hours after ovulation, on the basis of these averages. These times are averages, since wide variations in the survival times of both the sperm and ova have been found. For example, ova from a more mature woman are older and may not be fertile for as long a period.

When intercourse does occur, approximately 300 million sperm are deposited into the vagina. Although millions of sperm are deposited, most die before they reach the fallopian tube in which the ovum is being transported. Those that remain in the vagina die relatively rapidly because of the acidic vaginal environment. However, those sperm that reach the ovulatory cervical mucus find a favorable alkaline environment. The elastic mucus (termed spinnbarkeit) that accompanies the hormonal changes surrounding ovulation, together with the mobility of sperm itself and fluid pressure of the ejaculate, facilitates the movement of the sperm through the cervix and uterus. Muscle contractions have also been identified within the uterus and oviducts as another method to promote sperm transportation. During orgasm, the cervix tips down into the seminal fluid, thus providing another method of facilitating sperm transportation. Sperm have been identified at the site of fertilization within 30 minutes of ejaculation.

Not only does the female reproductive system positively influence the transportation of the sperm to the ovum, but it also enables the sperm to fully mature. Although the sperm have matured to a great degree in the epididymis, it is during the transportation time that the sperm are allowed to reach maturity and undergo capacitation, or penetration of the zona pellucida that surrounds the ovum. Capacitation is the enzymatic process that enables penetration of the ovum to occur. The manner by which sperm maturity is facilitated is not well understood. However, maturity allows the sperm to release acrosomal enzymes on contact with the zona pellucida, which helps to dissolve the membranes of the ovary so penetration by one sperm may occur (Fig. 15–1, step 3).

Penetration (capacitation) usually occurs when the ovum has been transported to the ampulla of the fallopian tube. The acrosomal cap enzymes break down cell connections and intermolecular bonds. After entering the ovum, the sperm fuses with the ovum's plasma membrane and passes into the cytoplasm. By this time, the sperm has commonly lost its tail. The ovum completes its last division, and the second polar body (the daughter cell with little, if any, cytoplasm) is extruded. Then the nuclei of the sperm and ovum unite. At this time, the cell has its complete complement of 46 chromosomes, and fertilization is completed.

Future viability of the fertilized ovum is contingent on many factors, the most immediate being the ability to block polyspermy, or the entry of additional sperm. Several mechanisms appear to be involved in the blocking actions. Enzymes are released during the breakdown of secretory vesicles when the sperm fuses with the plasma membrane of the ovum. The enzymes break down binding sites for the zona pellucida. In addition, calcium appears to be a major agent in this reac-

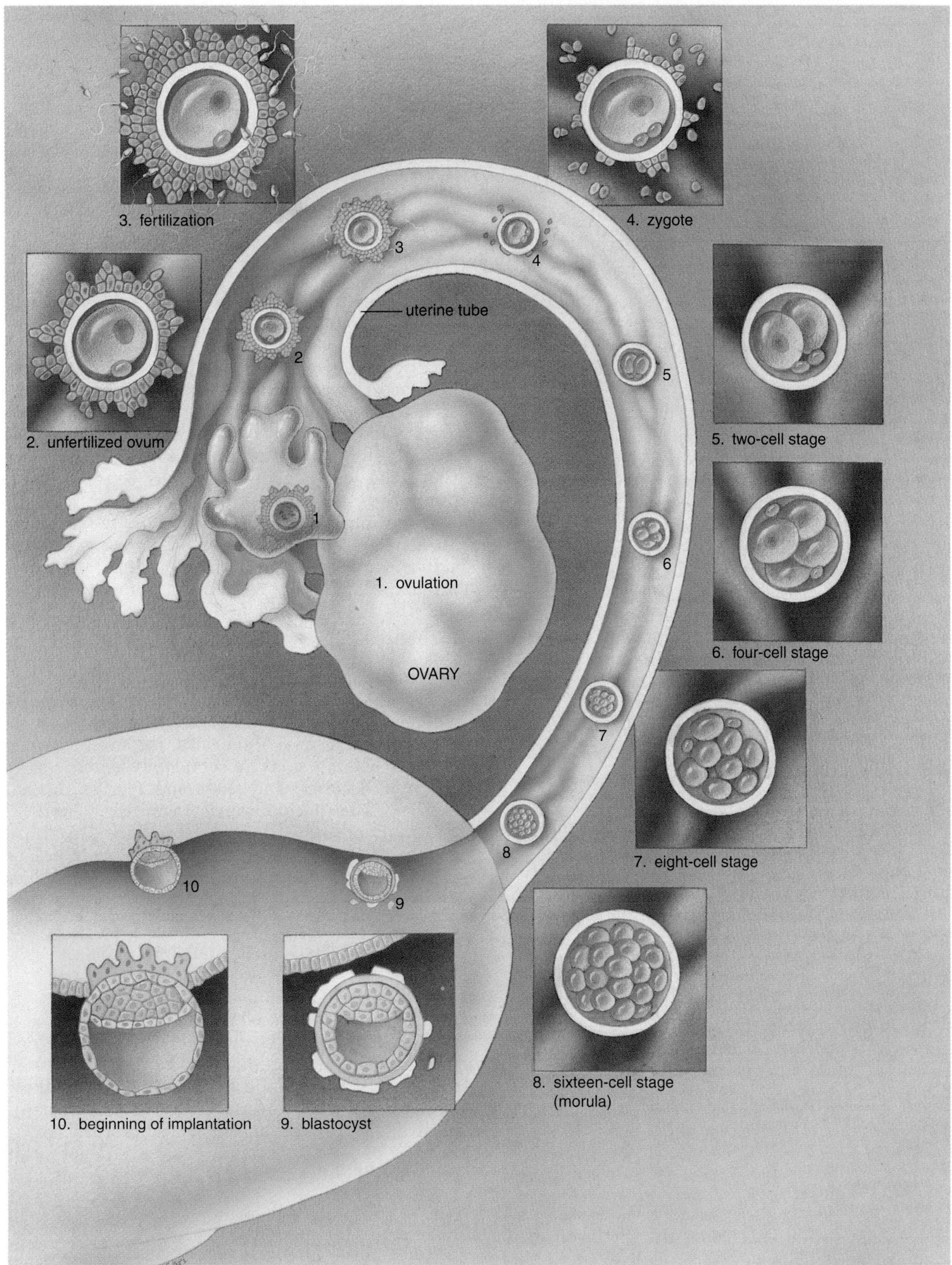
3. fertilization
4. zygote
3
4
uterine tube
2
5
2. unfertilized ovum
5. two-cell stage
1
6
1. ovulation
6. four-cell stage
OVARY
7
8
7. eight-cell stage
10
9
8. sixteen-cell stage
(morula)
10. beginning of implantation
9. blastocyst

Figure 15–1

The ten beginning steps of development during the first week of life proceed from ovulation through fertilization and cleavage of the zygote to implantation of the blastocyst in the endometrium of the uterus. (From Moore, K. L., Persaud, T. V. N., Shiota, K. [1994]. *Color atlas of clinical embryology* [p. 3]. Philadelphia: W. B. Saunders.)

tion, since it is released with membrane fusion and is also theorized to be required for activation of enzymes in the ovum needed for cell divisions and embryogenesis (Moore and Persaud 1993; Sadler 1995).

PREEMBRYONIC DEVELOPMENT

Zygote

After fertilization, the organism is termed a zygote. The zygote continues its passage through the fallopian tube (Fig. 15–1, step 4). This is usually a 3- to 4-day passage. On rare occasions, the ovum is not transported at the usual rate of speed and remains within the tube (Cherry and Merkatz 1991; Cunningham et al. 1993; Creasy and Resnik 1994). Such a tubal, or ectopic, pregnancy cannot continue indefinitely within the confined space of the fallopian tube. Ectopic pregnancies can be life threatening and are discussed in more detail in Chapter 21.

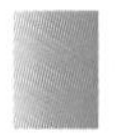

Blastomere to Morula

Approximately 12 hours after the zygote has formed, it divides into two daughter cells, termed blastomeres. Divisions then continue at a rate of approximately every 12 to 15 hours. This cell division process is termed cleavage. While cleavage occurs, the fertilized egg continues to move through the fallopian tube (Fig. 15–1, steps 5 to 8). When 16 cells exist, the fertilized egg is called a morula, a Latin term derived from the word for the fruit of the mulberry tree. The morula passes into the uterine cavity, where it continues to float for several days while undergoing additional cell division.

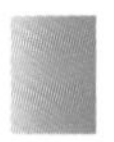

Blastocyst

Seven days after ovulation, the fertilized ovum is known as a blastocyst, or a ball of more than 100 cells surrounding a recently formed central fluid-filled cavity. At this time, the blastocyst loses the zona pellucida in preparation for embedding into the endometrium (Fig. 15–1, step 9).

IMPLANTATION

Development of the Decidua

The process of implantation, or nidation, is enhanced by the status of the endometrium since the endometrial lining has changed dramatically in the postovulatory phase. During this phase, the endometrium becomes extremely vascular and rich in glycogen. By the time of ovulation, the zona compacta, or compact zone, which is the endometrial surface, develops a large number of coiled or spiral arteries that break into capillaries and reach progressively closer to the surface. At this time, the endometrial layer is between 5 and 6 mm deep.

When implantation takes place, (Fig. 15–1, step 10), the endometrium becomes known as the decidua. The progesterone produced by the corpus luteum allows the decidua to continue its soft, vascular state that is necessary for successful implantation and early development. The areas of the decidua are often defined by their proximity to the implanting blastocyst. The decidua immediately underneath the blastocyst is the basal decidua, and it will eventually unite with the chorion and form the placenta; the area surrounding the blastocyst as it completely embeds is the capsular decidua; and the remainder is the parietal or true decidua (see Figs. 15–4 and Fig. 15–5). Eventually, as the intrauterine conceptus grows, the capsular and true decidua meet and blend together (Cunningham et al. 1993).

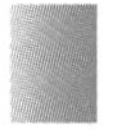

Process of Implantation

After the zona pellucida has disappeared, a specialized area of cells of the blastocyst becomes apparent. These are the trophoblasts, which provide the nutrient membranes for the fetus. They form the outer lining of the blastocyst and rapidly enlarge and make contact with the endometrium, most likely through an enzymatic process. Implantation appears to stimulate an even more rapid growth of the trophoblasts.

Development of Separate Types of Cells

As the trophoblastic cells implant, they differentiate into separate types. Those closest to the endometrium fuse to form the syncytiotrophoblast; the next proximate cells form the cytotrophoblast. Next to the inner cytotrophoblast is a layer of mesoderm or primitive mesenchyme. An inner cell mass lies proximate to the mesoderm.

SYNCYTIOTROPHOBLAST

The syncytiotrophoblast is composed of nucleated protoplasm. This protoplasm breaks down tissue during implantation and erodes the walls of blood vessels of the decidua to make nutrients in the maternal blood available to the developing organism.

CYTOTROPHOBLAST

The cytotrophoblast is a single layer of cells that produce human chorionic gonadotropin (hCG). It is this hormone on which modern pregnancy tests are based. As the hCG level rises, the corpus luteum is maintained and continues to produce estrogen and progesterone and inhibit menstruation.

MESODERM AND INNER CELL MASS

The mesoderm is loose connective tissue that is similar to the inner cell mass. Both the mesoderm and inner cell mass are contiguous at the point at which they join in the body stalk. While the trophoblast will form the placenta, the inner cell mass of the trophoblast eventually forms the fetus itself. The cells of the inner cell mass include those that ultimately form the ectoderm, the mesoderm, the endoderm, the amniotic cavity, and the yolk sac.

After implantation and until 8 weeks conceptional age (10 weeks menstrual age), the intrauterine organism is called an embryo. It is during the embryonic period that the major cell differentiation and rudimentary organ development are accomplished. After this period, the embryo is referred to as a fetus.

EMBRYONIC AND FETAL DEVELOPMENT

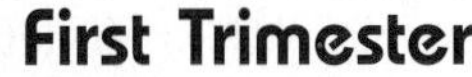

First Trimester

The first trimester traditionally includes the first 12 weeks of gestational age. This period includes the entire zygotic and embryonic periods as well as 2 weeks of fetal age. One of the greatest areas of confusion centers on the use of different language to describe age. Most clinicians who care for pregnant women use the term gestational age and begin calculation of pregnancy at the time of the last normal menstrual period. However, embryologists and some neonatologists may prefer to discuss the "actual" age of the conceptus, beginning their calculations at the time of fertilization.

To help avoid confusion caused by the different terminology, health professionals should be aware of the common terms for describing pregnancy dating and use them appropriately. Menstrual age and gestational age both refer to the number of weeks starting with the first day of the last normal menses; full-term pregnancy is commonly calculated as 280 days or 40 weeks. For the normal woman, this includes 2 weeks before ovulation, thus 2 weeks before she could possibly be pregnant. Maternity health care providers often use this measure since the last menstrual period is usually known and provides a clear reference point.

Lunar months also use the woman's last menstrual period as the beginning reference point. However, rather than discussing age in days or weeks, the calculation is based on a 28-day or 4-week month. Therefore, there would be 10 lunar months in a pregnancy.

Embryologists commonly use the terms ovulation age, fertilization age, and conceptional age for their reference points. These measurements do not reflect the first 2 weeks of the menstrual cycle before pregnancy was possible.

Varying terminology is used in different contexts, so to avoid misunderstandings, it is important that health professionals be cognizant of which measures are being discussed. In addition, the calculation used should be clearly marked on charts and records to diminish the possibility of a 2-week discrepancy. The nurse should also acknowledge the confusion that can be caused by the different calculations in discussing and teaching an expectant couple about fetal development. Many couples want to follow the development of their baby through available books and pamphlets but are unsure "how pregnant" they are because of the varying nomenclature.

TIME OF IMPLANTATION

At the time of implantation, the embryo is referred to as a bilaminar embryo since the inner cell mass consists of two layers of cells: the embryonic ectoderm and the embryonic endoderm. The embryonic endoderm is the origin of the three germ layers from which all tissue, organs, and structures arise. These germ layers are also the site of origin of the fetal membranes and umbilical cord. As discussed later, the endoderm is also partially responsible for the development of the placenta.

THREE WEEKS AFTER CONCEPTION

By 3 weeks after conception, a primitive streak has developed from the embryonic disk (Fig. 15–2). This is the growth center for the embryo for approximately 2 weeks more, after which time it begins to disintegrate. Simultaneously with the development of the primitive streak, a third germ layer, the embryonic mesoderm, appears between the other two layers. Thus, the embryo is referred to as a trilaminar embryo. By the end of the week, somite development begins. Eventually, 42 to 44 pairs of somites will appear. These somites are responsible for most of the skeleton of the head and trunk, accompanying musculature, and general skin dermis. It is also during this week that the neural tube, notochord (rudiment of the vertebrae), coelomic spaces (rudiment of body cavities), a primitive cardiovascular system, and primitive blood cells develop. During this time, the yolk sac assists in nourishment of the embryo. In addition, red blood cells develop on the walls of the yolk sac and continue to form here for approximately 3 more weeks, when hematopoietic activity begins in the liver.

FOUR WEEKS AFTER CONCEPTION

By 4 weeks after conception, a woman may first seriously suspect pregnancy, since her menses should have started approximately 2 weeks before. Inside the uterus, not only does the conceptus have a cardiac system at this time, but the heart has begun to beat. The fourth conceptional week is characterized by rapid growth that causes both transverse and longitudinal folding of the embryonic disk. Transverse folding transpires with right and left transverse areas enfolding to the midline. This process transforms the organism from a flat form to a cylindric form. The longitudinal folding that occurs includes a head fold and a tail fold, changing the embryo from a straight organism to one with a curved form (Cunningham et al. 1993; Moore and Persaud 1993; Sadler 1995). By the end of this week, the embryo demonstrates rudimentary ears (otic pits), arms (arm buds), legs (leg buds), and the first four branchial arches for the face and neck. During the fourth week, the dorsal part of the yolk sac is incorporated into the embryo and becomes the primitive gut. This process is called gastrulation, and the embryo may be called a gastrula at this time. The yolk sac detaches by the end of the following week and begins to shrink.

FIVE WEEKS AFTER CONCEPTION

It is during the fifth postconceptional week that there is rapid brain growth. During this week, the brain becomes grossly larger than the rest of the body. Development is said to occur in a cephalocaudal pattern, with growth moving from the head down the body. For example, the arms develop almost a week before the legs. It is during this period that the lens, vesicles, optic cups, and nasal pits form, and the developing eye becomes apparent.

SIX WEEKS AFTER CONCEPTION

The facial development continues during the sixth postfertilization week. The nose, mouth, and palate begin to form. The extremities begin to evidence well-differentiated areas such as wrists, elbows, fingers, and toes. During this week, a woman misses her second menses.

SEVEN WEEKS AFTER CONCEPTION AND BEYOND

By the end of the seventh postconceptional week, urogenital development is beginning. The external ears are manifested, although they are not fully functional, and the tip of the nose is distinct. During the eighth postfertilization week, fingers are distinct; the upper limbs are longer, and the elbows are manifested. The end of this week completes the embryonic period. All essential internal and external structures are present, even though the conceptus will continue to grow and mature for 30 more weeks in the intrauterine environment (Fig. 15–2; Table 15–1).

Teratology

DEFINITION

As illustrated in the preceding discussion, the embryonic period is a critical time for development. Therefore, the first 8 weeks after conception constitute the most vulnerable time frame for malformations to occur. It has been estimated that 3 percent to 7 percent of all infants have some birth defect or structural abnormality, although the majority are minor (Cunningham et al. 1993). Teratology is the study of "monsters." In modern usage, it means the study of congenital anomalies or of agents producing such malformations. A teratogen is an agent that increases chances of an infant's being born with a structural or functional abnormality. It has been estimated that 65 percent of major birth defects are caused by a multifactorial influence, that is, a combination of genetics and environmental factors. Genetics and chromo-

Table 15–1

PREEMBRYONIC AND EMBRYONIC DEVELOPMENTAL MILESTONES

DAY	DEVELOPMENTAL MILESTONE
1	Fertilization
2	Blastomere
3	Morula
4	Early blastocyst
5	Late blastocyst
7	Implantation
8	Bilaminar germ disk
9	Trophoblast with lacunae
13	Uteroplacental circulation begins
14	Primitive streak apparent
15	Approximate beginning of embryonic period (usual time of missed menses for women)
16	Trilaminar germ disk
17	Notochordal process apparent
19	Formation of central nervous system
20	Appearance of somites
24–25	Villus formation
28	Ear placodes, eye anlagen, and arm buds apparent
29	Umbilical cord apparent
31	Tail bud apparent
34	Developing limb buds apparent
38	Finger rays and foot rays apparent
41	Chorionic villi, amnion, and yolk sac apparent
46	Placenta apparent
47	Fingers
48	Toes

some transmissions alone have been implicated in an additional 25 percent of birth defects or teratisms, and 10 percent have been found to be related to the environment. Of the environmental influences, radiation has been linked to less than 1 percent; maternal infection, 2 percent to 3 percent; maternal disorders (e.g., diabetes), 1 percent to 2 percent; and drugs or chemicals, less than 5 percent (Niebyl 1988; Cunningham et al. 1993). Thus, when an infant is born with a birth defect, it is the exception rather than the rule that an outside agent can be identified as the causative factor in the development of the malformation. Women should be informed that for most birth defects, some underlying genetic or chromosome activity is involved.

However, of all of the possible causes of teratologic malformations, the agents most investigated by scientists appear to be in the area of drugs and chemicals. These may be the most investigated for several reasons. Modern society appears to be predisposed to use drugs and chemicals relatively freely, even during pregnancy. It has been estimated that more than 90 percent of women take prescribed drugs and 65 percent take over-the-counter medications during pregnancy (Cunningham et al. 1993). A woman may be using some agent in early pregnancy, during a critical developmental period, yet she may not even suspect that she is pregnant. Researchers desire to intervene appropriately to decrease the risks of teratogenicity. Although scientists may be at the forefront of genetic manipulation, there is much more to be accomplished before such interventions are commonplace. However, identification of teratogenic drugs and chemicals can culminate in rapid changes through the dissemination of information and suggestions for avoidance of harmful substances.

BASIC PRINCIPLES OF TERATOLOGY

Teratology is based on several principles of embryonic development. These include the following:

- Manifestations of teratogenesis may include no observable effect or malformation, a malformation, growth retardation, functional disorders, or death. In other words, a dose-effect curve may exist that ranges from no effect to lethality for the conceptus, depending on such factors as host susceptibility and amount or duration of exposure.
- The susceptibility of the organism depends on the developmental stage at exposure, or the "critical moment." For example, between conception and implantation, exposure to a teratogen usually results in an all-or-nothing phenomenon. The conceptus either is aborted spontaneously or emerges unharmed since the exposure happens before cell differentiation.
- Even the most potent teratogenic agent may have little or no effect on the mother while causing severe damage to the embryo or fetus.
- Teratogenic agents act on specific cells in specific ways. That is, characteristic malformations exist with a teratogenic agent. When a drug is implicated in a wide variety of malformations, it is most likely expressing a multifactorial effect and not a specific teratogenic effect.
- Susceptibility to teratogenesis is contingent on both the agent and the conceptus. Thus, not every conceptus will be affected or affected to the same degree since biologic variability is in operation.
- Essentially any drug or chemical to which the mother is exposed will pass to the conceptus. The concept of "placental barrier" is a myth. Although agents that are nonionized, soluble, not bound to protein, and of low molecular weight

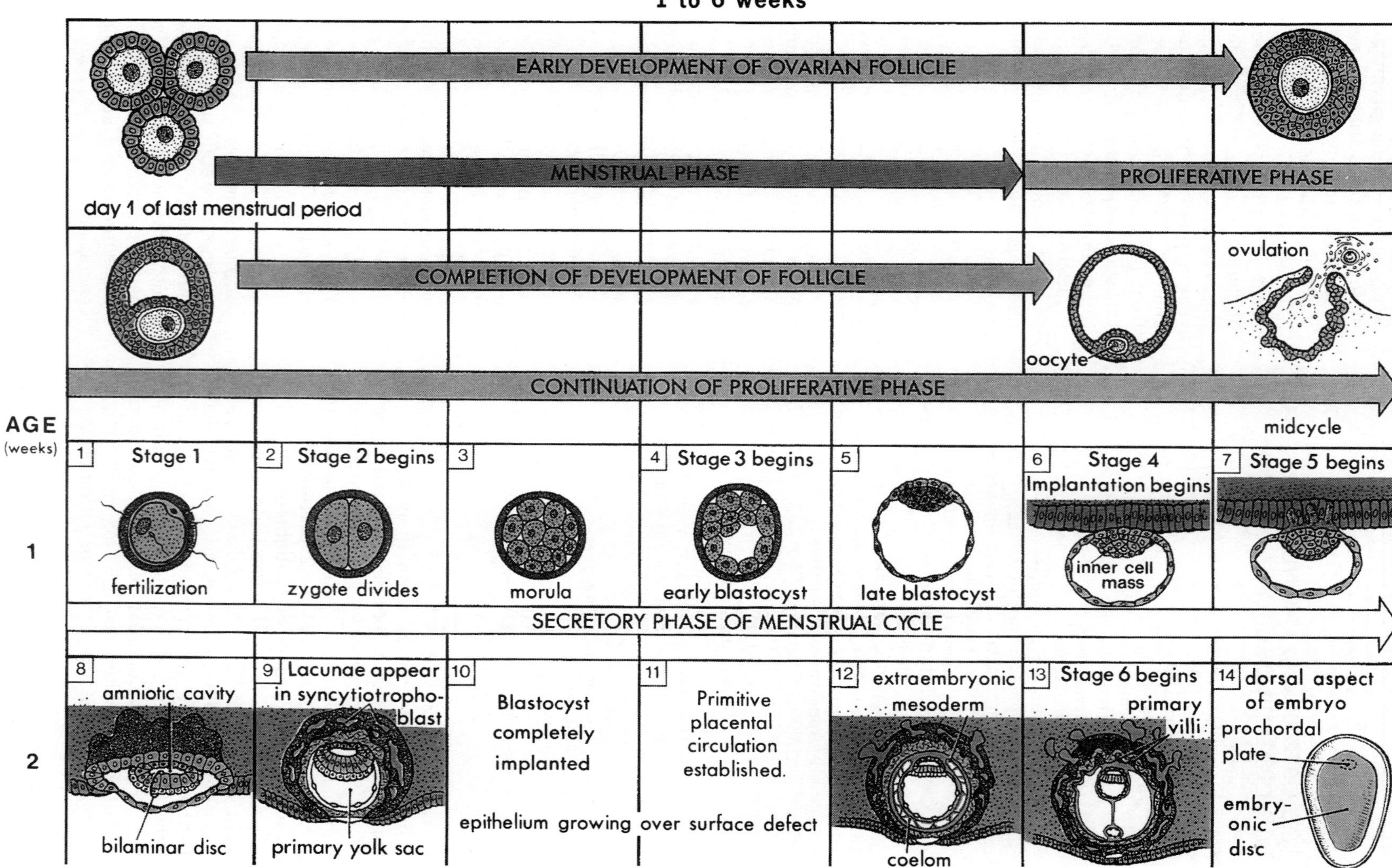

TIMETABLE OF HUMAN PRENATAL DEVELOPMENT
1 to 6 weeks
AGE
(weeks)
1
2
EARLY DEVELOPMENT OF OVARIAN FOLLICLE
MENSTRUAL PHASE
PROLIFERATIVE PHASE
day 1 of last menstrual period
COMPLETION OF DEVELOPMENT OF FOLLICLE
oocyte
ovulation
CONTINUATION OF PROLIFERATIVE PHASE
midcycle
1 Stage 1
fertilization
2 Stage 2 begins
zygote divides
3
morula
4 Stage 3 begins
early blastocyst
5
late blastocyst
6 Stage 4
Implantation begins
inner cell mass
7 Stage 5 begins
SECRETORY PHASE OF MENSTRUAL CYCLE
8
amniotic cavity
bilaminar disc
9 Lacunae appear in syncytiotrophoblast
primary yolk sac
10
Blastocyst completely implanted
11
Primitive placental circulation established.
epithelium growing over surface defect
12 extraembryonic mesoderm
coelom
13 Stage 6 begins
primary villi
14 dorsal aspect of embryo
prochordal plate
embryonic disc

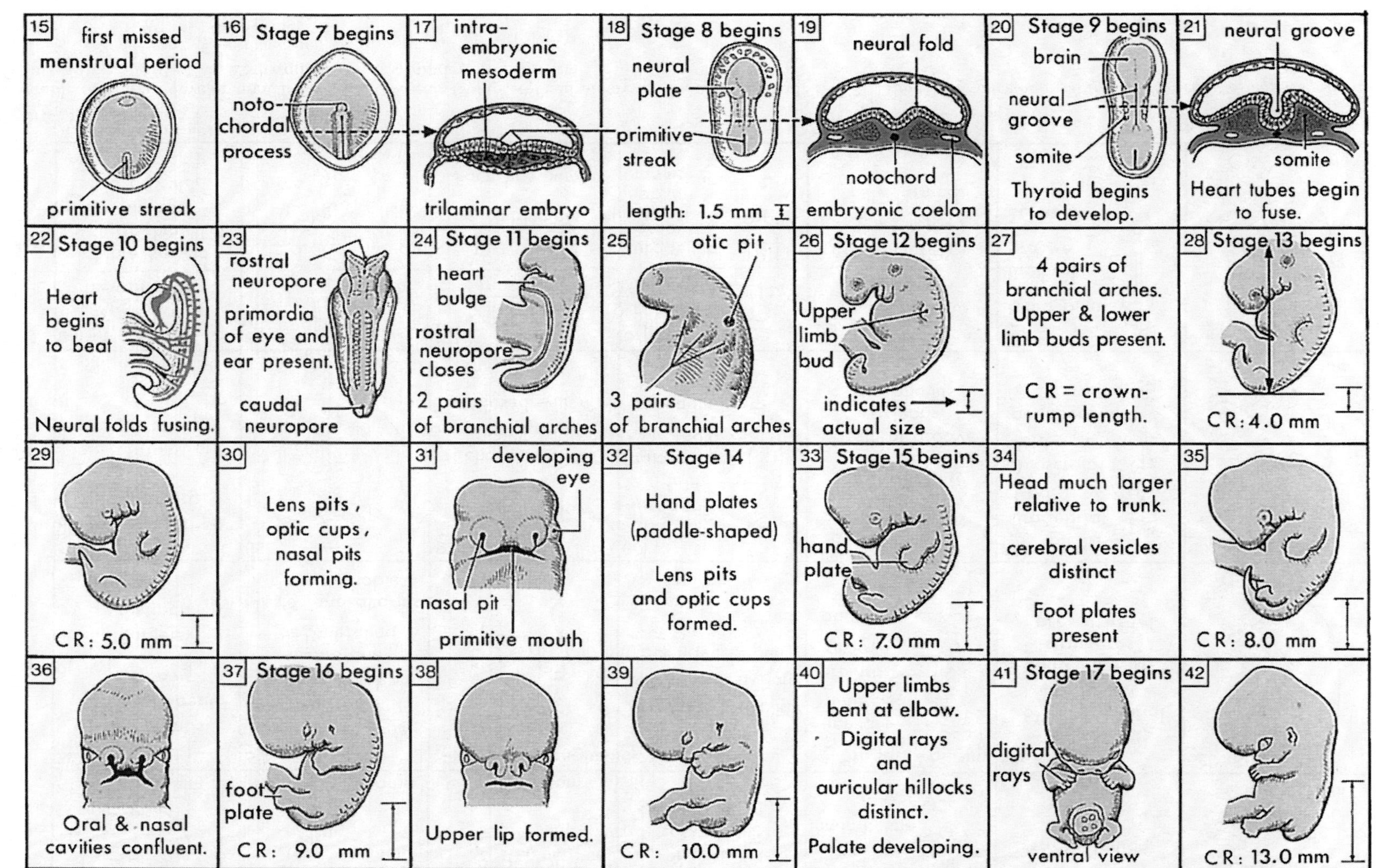

Figure 15–2

Continued on following page

TIMETABLE OF HUMAN DEVELOPMENT
7 to 10 weeks

AGE (weeks)							
7	43 CR: 16.0 mm	44 Stage 18 begins. Eyelids beginning	45 Tip of nose distinct. Digital rays appear in foot plates. CR: 17.0 mm	46 Loss of villi. Smooth chorion forms.	47 genital tubercle; urogenital membrane; anal membrane; ♀ or ♂	48 Stage 19 begins. Trunk elongating and straightening.	49 CR: 18 mm
8	50 Upper limbs longer & bent at elbows. Fingers distinct.	51 Anal membrane perforated. Urogenital membrane degenerating. Testes and ovaries distinguishable.	52 Stage 21 begins	53 Stage 21. External genitalia still in sexless state but have begun to differentiate.	54 Stage 22 begins. genital tubercle; urethral groove; anus; ♀ or ♂	55 Beginnings of all essential external & and internal structures are present.	56 Stage 23. CR: 30 mm
9	57 Beginning of fetal period.	58	59 Genitalia show some ♀ characteristics but still easily confused with ♂.	60 phallus; urogenital fold; labioscrotal fold; perineum; ♀	61 Genitalia show fusion of urethral folds. Urethral groove extends into phallus.	62 phallus; urogenital fold; labioscrotal fold; perineum; ♂	63 CR: 50 mm
10	64 Face has human profile. Note growth of chin compared to day 44.	65	66 Face has human appearance.	67 clitoris; labium minus; urogenital groove; labium majus; ♀	68 Genitalia have ♀ or ♂ characteristics but still not fully formed.	69 glans penis; urethral groove; scrotum; ♂	70 CR: 61 mm

Figure 15–2

Timetable of human development from 1 to 10 weeks. (Adapted from Moore, K. L., and Persaud, T. V. N. [1993]. *The developing human: Clinically oriented embryology* [5th ed.] [pp. 470–472]. Philadelphia: W. B. Saunders.)

pass more easily than their counterparts, it should never be assumed that an agent cannot pass into fetal circulation.

Just as there are several principles of teratology, so are there several proposed mechanisms that make an agent teratogenic. An agent does not become a teratogen in only one way. The mechanism by which an agent causes a teratogenic effect can be one of many. Among the common mechanisms are mutations; chromosome nondisjunctions and breaks; mitotic interference, which can cause mosaicism (or chromosomes of nonequal status) and is most likely a result of radiation; altered nucleic acid integrity of function (common with antineoplastic drugs); lack of precursors and substrates needed for biosynthesis; altered energy sources (e.g., a possible link has been proposed between lack of adenosine triphosphate [ATP] in the fetus and intrauterine hypoxia); enzyme inhibitions; osmolar imbalances (abnormal fluid accumulations and malformations are associated, but which is the cause and which is the effect is not clear); and altered membrane characteristics (a theoretical mechanism, but one needing more research to clarify). Additional information on genetics can be found in Chapter 13.

LIMITATIONS OF CURRENT STUDIES

The major difficulty in the scientific investigation of teratogenesis is the problem in predicting the effects of drugs and chemicals on humans. Much of the scientific knowledge about teratogenesis emanates from animal studies. Yet extrapolating findings, about mechanism of action or ultimate effect, is a problem from an animal model (Niebyl 1988). Animal models provided the basis for the concepts of multifactorial causes, specificity, and even teratogenicity of drugs with the discovery in 1951 of cleft palates among mice receiving corticosteroids. Since the gestational period for most animals is less than that of humans, studies can be conducted in a shorter period. The disadvantages of the animal research include the fact that teratogenicity in one species does not always predict teratogenicity in another. For example, although a potent teratogen for humans, thalidomide was rarely teratogenic in other species and never manifested the classic phocomelia, or flipper-like limb malformation, in species other than humans. In addition, it has been estimated that half of all the drugs on the market can cause teratogenic effects in small animals, and such animals are more likely to evidence major abnormalities from environmental effects such as malnutrition. Moreover, in some animals, the relative embryonic period is much longer than in humans and can last half the period of gestation. The ethics of animal research have been called into question, especially with the appreciation of the problem of application of the findings to humans.

Another method of investigation of teratogens is personal history from women with affected offspring. Much of the time, this is a retrospective investigation based on recall of the woman. Not only can this cause a woman to assume a great deal of guilt (especially since the most common mechanism of a malformation is multifactorial and will never be known), but recall data may result in an overreporting of a drug. For example, two women may use the identical over-the-counter preparation, but the woman giving birth to a normal infant may never remember it. On the other hand, a woman who is scrupulously trying to recall all drugs she used in pregnancy because her child has a malformation may remember the drug and report it. Thus, it can appear that only the women who have taken this drug have abnormal babies, suggesting a strong link of teratogenicity based on recall data.

In spite of the problems with animals and recall data about drug ingestion or chemical exposure, it is likely that they will remain as major investigational methods. Other methods of human research are not possible, for it is unreasonable to assume a woman would knowingly subject her embryo or fetus to the effects of an "unknown" agent simply in the quest of scientific knowledge in general.

KNOWN OR STRONGLY SUSPECTED TERATOGENS

It is surprising that the list of known teratogens is so short. Table 15–2 includes the agents generally accepted as teratogenic. Probably the first teratogenic agent was a nonpharmaceutical one, rubella. It was identified as teratogenic in the 1940s. More teratogenic agents may be discovered in the future, for the entire marketplace for pharmaceutical agents is enlarging. The teratogenic agents on the list include nonmedications such as alcohol and radiation as well as such pharmaceutical agents as thalidomide. It is a list of consensus, not an absolute list. There are several drugs whose teratogenicity remains unproven, but they are best avoided in pregnancy because of potential harm. These include oral contraceptives and live virus vaccines.

FOOD AND DRUG ADMINISTRATION DRUG CLASSIFICATIONS

In the United States, the Food and Drug Administration (FDA) is responsible for ensuring the safety of pharmaceutical agents for human use (see Historical Perspectives). In 1979, the FDA established five categories for drugs and medications

Table 15–2

KNOWN OR STRONGLY SUSPECTED TERATOGENS

CHEMICALS AND DRUGS	
Alcohol	Goitrogens (antithyroids)
Aminopterin	Isotretinoin
Androgenic hormones	Lithium
Angiotensin-converting enzyme (ACE) inhibitors	Methimazole
Busulfan	Methotrexate
Carbamazepine	Organic mercury
Chlorbiphenyls	Penicillamine
Coumarins	Phenytoin
Cyclophosphamide	Tetracycline
Danazol	Thalidomide
Diethylstilbestrol (DES)	Trimethadione
Etretinate	Valproic acid
INFECTIONS	
Cytomegalovirus	Toxoplasmosis
Rubella virus	Venezuelan equine virus
Syphilis	
MATERNAL DISORDERS	
Alcoholism	Endemic cretinism
Connective tissue diseases	Hyperthermia
Diabetes	Virilizing tumors
RADIATION	
Atomic weapons	Radiotherapy
Radioactive iodine	

Adapted with permission from Cunningham, F. G., MacDonald, P. C., Gant, N. F., Leveno, K. J., Gilstrap, L. C. III. (1993). *Williams obstetrics* (19th ed.)(p. 960). Norwalk, CT: Appleton & Lange.

in regard to possible adverse fetal effects (see FDA Pregnancy Risk Categories). Although the classification list is not without flaw, it provides one of the few standardized methods of categorizing drugs for both patients and providers. Few drugs fall into the category A classification. For example, class A may include vitamins, but not the megavitamins that are potentially teratogenic. Class B drugs are suggested to be "safe" but have not had controlled studies undertaken. An example of a class B drug is penicillin, which has been used for years in pregnancy. Class C drugs may have demonstrated teratogenicity with the animal model but not for humans, or (most likely of all) they have not had any study undertaken as to their effects on pregnancy. This is the most difficult of all the classifications for clinical practice. Most drugs fall into this category. Some agents, like the corticosteroids, are class C because of the first half of the definition (animal teratogenicity only), whereas most drugs, especially new ones, lack any scientific information on safety in pregnancy. Class D drugs encompass those for which the risks and benefits must be carefully weighed. Anticonvulsants are an excellent example of a drug placed in this problem category. Uncontrolled seizures threaten a fetus because of trauma and potential hypoxia; however, phenytoin has potential teratogenic effects. Each situation must be individualized and the woman informed as to the known risks involved. Class X drugs are pharmaceuticals that are known teratogens and offer no lifesaving effect. For example, other teratogenic hypnotics and sedatives exist besides thalidomide. Isotretinoin (Accutane), a drug used to treat acne, is a known teratogen, and no maternal mortality has resulted from acne during pregnancy.

One of the major difficulties with the FDA classification listing is that almost 2 decades after its introduction, not all drugs are categorized. It was initially proposed that the manufacturer would categorize a drug when it was manufactured. Today, many of the classifications have been given on the basis of information in the general domain by researchers in obstetrics and gynecology. Briggs and colleagues (1994) have written a text on drugs in pregnancy and breastfeeding and used the FDA classifications. In most cases, they awarded the classification on the basis of available research, the minority of cases being provided by the manufacturer.

INFORMATION SOURCES FOR DRUGS IN PREGNANCY

In clinical practice, there are few more perplexing situations than having a woman question the safety of a drug she has taken or wishes to take. Obviously, the best solution is for all women to abstain from drugs and chemicals during pregnancy. However, this is not always pragmatic advice. Common references on drugs include the *Physicians' Desk Reference* (PDR). This book is a compendium of manufacturers' information as provided to the FDA. It rarely includes useful information about advisability of use in pregnancy. An alternative reference is often termed the USPDI, the *United States Pharmacopeia Dispensing Information* (USPDI 1997). This text is updated annually, like the PDR. However, the information is not strictly from manufacturers but includes extrapolations from other published studies of both prescribed and nonprescribed drugs. FDA classifications are listed, and the known information about use in pregnancy and lactation is summarized. A companion volume, *Advice for the Patient,* is composed of material that can be photocopied to give to women using particular pharmaceuticals (USPDI 1997).

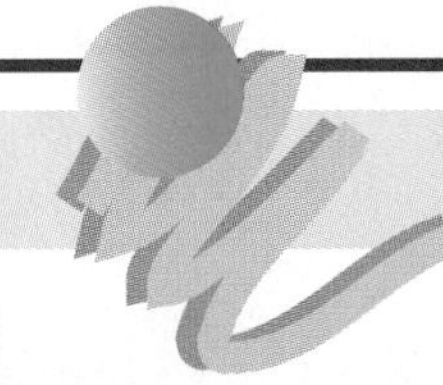

HISTORICAL PERSPECTIVES

HIGHLIGHTS OF U. S. FOOD AND DRUG REGULATIONS RELATING TO SAFETY

Regulation of food in the United States dates from early colonial times. Federal controls over the drug supply began with inspection of imported drugs in 1848.

1785 MASSACHUSETTS enacted the first general food adulteration law in the United States.

1820 Eleven physicians met in the Capitol at Washington to establish the U. S. PHARMACOPEIA, the first compendium of standard drugs for the United States.

1848 DRUG IMPORTATION ACT passed by Congress required U. S. customs inspection to stop entry of adulterated drugs from overseas.

1862 PRESIDENT LINCOLN appointed a chemist, Charles M. Wetherill, to serve in the new Department of Agriculture—the beginning of the Bureau of Chemistry, now the Food and Drug Administration in the Department of Health and Human Services.

1879 PETER COLLIER, chief chemist, U. S. Department of Agriculture, began investigation of food adulteration. The following year, he recommended a national food and drug law. In the next 25 years, more than 100 food and drug bills were introduced in Congress.

1902 BIOLOGICS CONTROL ACT was passed to ensure purity and safety of serums, vaccines, and similar products used to prevent or treat diseases in humans.

Congress appropriated funds to establish FOOD STANDARDS and to study the effects of chemicals on digestion and health.

1906 The original FOOD AND DRUGS ACT was passed by Congress and signed by President Theodore Roosevelt. It prohibited interstate commerce in misbranded and adulterated foods, drinks, and drugs.

1911 Congress enacted the SHERLEY AMENDMENT to prohibit labeling medicines with false therapeutic claims intended to defraud the purchaser.

1927 A separate law enforcement agency was formed, first known as the Food, Drug, and Insecticide Administration and then, in 1930, as the Food and Drug Administration (FDA).

CAUSTIC POISON ACT required warning labels and antidotes to protect children from being injured by lye and other dangerous chemicals.

1937 An ELIXIR OF SULFANILAMIDE containing a poisonous solvent killed 107 persons, mostly children, dramatizing the need to establish drug safety before marketing and to enact the pending food and drug law.

1938 The Federal FOOD, DRUG, AND COSMETIC ACT was passed by Congress after a 5-year legislative battle, containing new provisions:

- Extending control to cosmetics and therapeutic devices
- Requiring new drugs to be shown safe before marketing—starting a new system of drug regulation
- Eliminating the Sherley Amendment requirement to prove intent to defraud in drug misbranding cases
- Providing that safe tolerances be set for unavoidable poisonous substances
- Authorizing standards of identity, quality, and fill-of-container for foods.
- Authorizing factory inspections
- Adding the remedy of court injunctions to the previous penalties of seizures and prosecutions.

1945 PENICILLIN AMENDMENT required FDA testing and certification of safety and effectiveness of all penicillin products.

1951 DELANEY COMMITTEE started congressional investigation of the safety of chemicals in foods and cosmetics, laying the foundation for effective controls over pesticides, food additives, and colors.

DURHAM-HUMPHREY AMENDMENT defined the kinds of drugs that cannot be safely used without medical supervision and restricted their sale to prescription by licensed practitioners.

1954 PESTICIDES AMENDMENT spelled out procedures for setting safety limits for pesticide residues on raw agricultural commodities.

Continued on following page

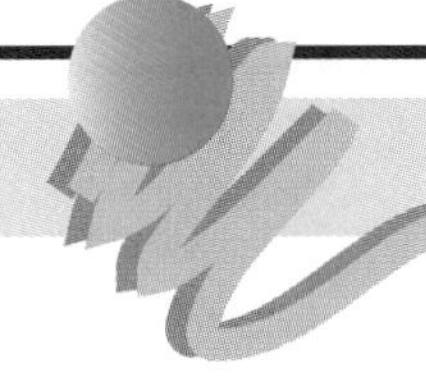

HISTORICAL PERSPECTIVES Continued

1962 THALIDOMIDE, a new sleeping pill, was found to have caused birth defects in thousands of babies born in Western Europe. News reports on the role of Dr. Frances Kelsey, FDA medical officer, in keeping the drug off the U. S. market aroused public support for stronger drug regulations.

KEFAUVER-HARRIS DRUG AMENDMENTS were passed to ensure greater drug safety. For the first time, drug manufacturers were required to prove the effectiveness of their products to the FDA before marketing them.

CONSUMER BILL OF RIGHTS was proclaimed by President John F. Kennedy in a message to Congress. It included the right *to safety*, the right *to be informed*, the right *to choose*, and the right *to be heard*.

1966 FDA contracted with the National Academy of Science/National Research Council to evaluate the effectiveness of 4000 drugs approved on the basis of safety alone between 1938 and 1962.

CHILD PROTECTION ACT enlarged the scope of the Federal Hazardous Substances Labeling Act to ban toys and other articles so hazardous that adequate label warnings could not be written.

1970 ENVIRONMENTAL PROTECTION AGENCY was established; it took over the FDA program for setting pesticide tolerances.

1971 BUREAU OF RADIOLOGICAL HEALTH was transferred to the FDA. Its mission: protection against unnecessary human exposure to radiation from electronic products in the home, industry, and the healing arts.

1976 VITAMINS AND MINERALS AMENDMENTS stopped the FDA from establishing standards limiting potency of vitamins and minerals in food supplements or regulating them as drugs solely on the basis of potency.

1977 SACCHARIN STUDY AND LABELING ACT was passed by Congress to stop the FDA from banning the chemical sweetener but requiring a label warning that it has been found to cause cancer in laboratory animals.

1985 HIV ANTIBODY TEST FOR SERUM was approved by the FDA, developed, and first used to screen donated blood for HIV in order to protect transfusion recipients.

1993 REGULATIONS ON DATA MONITORING OF CLINICAL TRIALS were issued by the FDA; all data submitted to the FDA were now to be audited.

Adapted from Food and Drug Administration. (1991). *FDA background: Current and useful information from the Food and Drug Administration.* Washington, DC: Author.

LITIGATION RISKS RELATED TO TERATOGENS

The last several decades have demonstrated that a litigation crisis exists in the United States. In the last decade, a popular antihistamine and vitamin combination (Bendectin) that had been widely used to treat morning sickness was withdrawn from the market by its manufacturer after it had been implicated as a teratogen in a large lawsuit. The court system had declared it a teratogen in spite of the lack of clear evidence. Rather than assuming risks and costs for additional legal battles, the manufacturer withdrew the drug to minimize legal exposure and risk. Other suits have suggested that spermicidal jellies may also be teratogens, even though no data appear to support the contention. The advent of "legal teratogens" has given rise to a new term, a litogen. A litogen is an agent that is not associated with teratogenic malformations but is associated with litigation risk.

FETAL TERATOLOGY

As mentioned previously, the critical period for teratogenesis is the embryonic period. However, it is now proposed that teratogenicity can occur later in pregnancy as well. In the second and third trimesters, such agents as nicotine (smoking) and maternal malnutrition can affect the conceptus. For example, in the broad use of the term teratogenesis, decreased uterine blood flow or oxygenation may result in functional malformations as a result of exposure to smoking. Thus, even after the structures have been formed during the first trimester, the conceptus remains vulnerable to insult (Fig. 15–3).

FDA Pregnancy Risk Categories

CATEGORY A

Controlled studies in women fail to demonstrate a risk to the fetus in the first trimester (and there is no evidence of a risk in later trimesters), and the possibility of fetal harm appears remote.

CATEGORY B

Animal reproduction studies have not demonstrated a fetal risk but there are no controlled studies in pregnant women; animal reproduction studies have shown an adverse effect (other than a decrease in fertility) that was not confirmed in controlled studies in women in the first trimester (and there is not evidence of a risk in later trimesters).

CATEGORY C

Studies in animals have revealed adverse effects on the fetus (teratogenic or embryocidal or other) and there are no controlled studies in women and animals are not available. Drugs should be given only if the potential benefit justifies the potential risk to the fetus.

CATEGORY D

There is positive evidence of human fetal risk, but the benefits from use in pregnant women may be acceptable despite the risk (e.g., if the drug is needed in a life-threatening situation or for a serious disease for which safer drugs cannot be used or are ineffective).

CATEGORY X

Studies in animals or human beings have demonstrated fetal abnormalities or there is evidence of fetal risk based on human experiences or both, and the risk of the use of the drug in pregnant women clearly outweighs any possible benefit. The drug is contraindicated in women who are or may become pregnant.

From Food and Drug Administration. (1980). Pregnancy risk categories. *Federal Register,* 44, 37434–37467.

Second Trimester

The second trimester is said to include weeks 13 through 27 after the last menstrual period (weeks 11 to 25 after conception), and the third trimester includes weeks 28 through 40 after the last menstrual period (weeks 26 through 38 after conception). It is during these trimesters that the conceptus grows and matures. The nurse can help the parents-to-be visually clarify the developmental timeline with a gestational wheel (see Improving Your Practice).

FETAL GROWTH

At the beginning of the second trimester, the fetus weighs less than 1 ounce. The eyelids are fused at this time, and the growth of the head that was so prominent a few weeks ago begins to slow. The fetus still has a disproportionately large head. Taste buds are present. Growth continues cephalocaudally, and therefore it is not surprising that fingernails are apparent before toenails.

DEVELOPMENT OF FETAL HEMOGLOBIN

Blood cells are being formed in the bone marrow during the second trimester. Although the fetus has a genetic predisposition to a particular blood type that is based on inheritance patterns, the major blood type at this time is HbF, or fetal hemoglobin, which has a greater affinity for oxygen. Bile is now being secreted in the pancreas, and the intestines manifest their characteristic formation. The kidney is now able to secrete urine.

QUICKENING

During gestation weeks 13 to 16, the fetus becomes increasingly more active, with head rotation, facial movements, and even breathing mo-

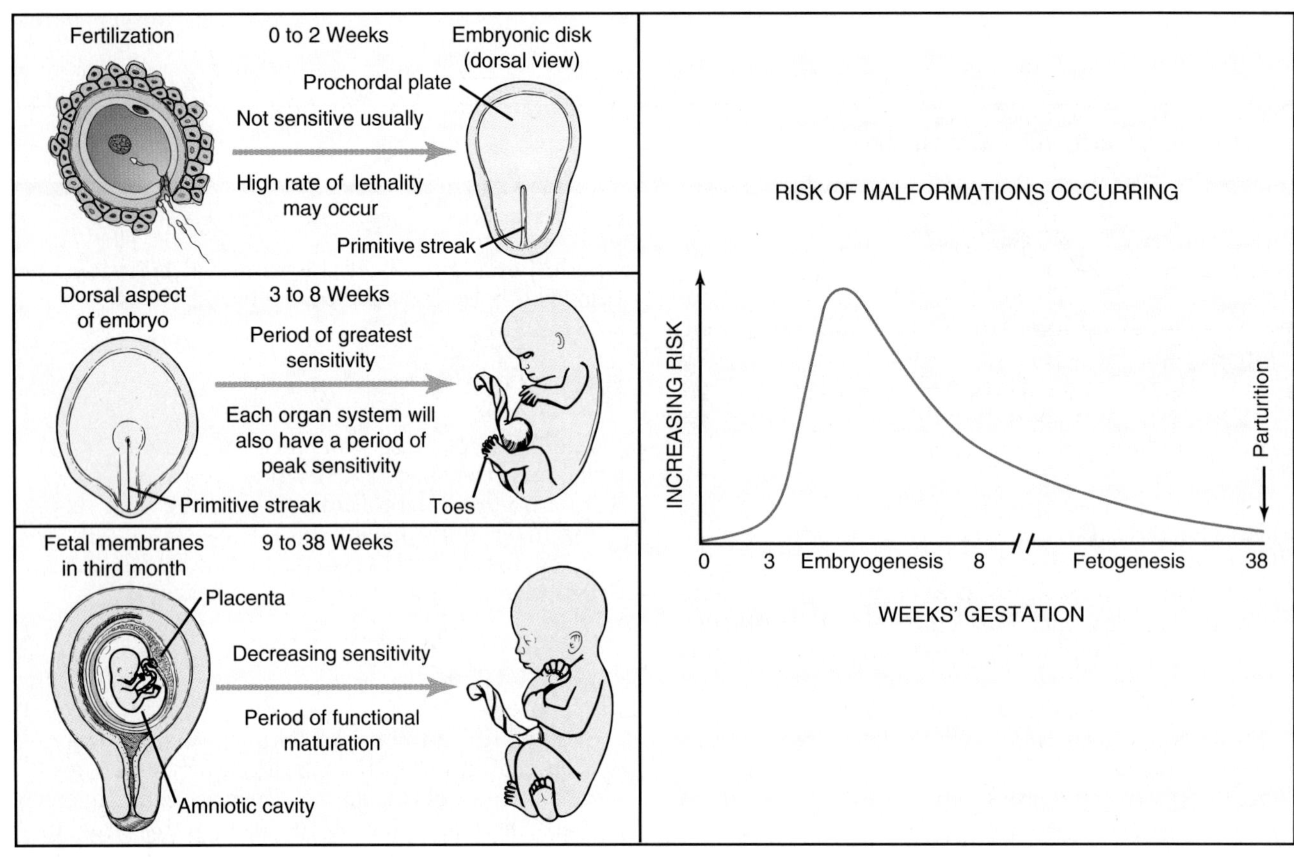

Figure 15–3

Developmental periods of susceptibility to teratogenesis. (Adapted from Sadler, T. [1995]. *Langman's medical embryology* [7th ed.] Baltimore: Williams & Wilkins.)

tions occurring. The fetus is too small for most women to be able to identify these movements, although by week 16 some women, especially those who are multigravid, may correctly identify the sensation as quickening. Quickening is the first time a woman identifies fetal movement during a pregnancy.

The sex is clearly identifiable by gestational weeks 14 to 16. Ossification has occurred to such a degree that bones would be apparent on x-ray examination (a process not indicated in pregnancy because of teratogenic risk). The fetus is able to react to sound at this time, and the external ear begins to be visible. By gestational week 16, the fetus has a crown-rump length of 4.5 inches and weighs between 3.5 and 4.0 ounces. The byproduct of bile and fetal waste, meconium, is now being produced in the bowel, and the bronchioles appear in the lung.

By gestational weeks 18 to 20, the fetus is large enough that most women, including primigravida women, have noticed quickening. Eyelashes, eyebrows, and head hair are visible, and lanugo, a fine downy hair, covers most of the external epidermis. The purpose of lanugo is still not clear. It is shed by the last few weeks of intrauterine development. However, it has been hypothesized that the fine hair may retain the secretion that is formed from the sebaceous glands around the hair follicles. This secretion, vernix caseosa, tends to be a protective agent for the baby's skin both intrauterinely and immediately extrauterinely.

The hands can form fists, and the fetus may spend some of the time suckling a hand or fist. By the end of gestational week 25, the fetus has formed brown fat. Brown fat is a major source of energy, heat production, and heat regulation for the newborn. However, subcutaneous fat is lacking, making the skin look thin and transparent. During this time, the eyelids remain fused, but some vision has been hypothesized because a fetus will recoil from a bright, focused light. The fetus remains aware of sounds and becomes more discriminatory, appearing to be stimulated by some sounds and irritated by others. At this time, the fetus is just more than 8 inches for the crown-rump measurement and weighs slightly more than a pound.

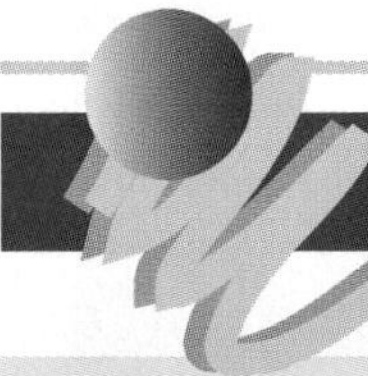

IMPROVING YOUR PRACTICE

FOLLOWING FETAL GROWTH AND DEVELOPMENT

During the second trimester, most women voice a desire to learn about and understand the process of fetal growth and development. This is an ideal time to discuss the stages of the baby's growth with the parents.

- USE A GESTATIONAL WHEEL OR ELECTRONIC GESTATIONAL BIRTH CALCULATOR TO EXPLAIN HOW THE ESTIMATED DATE OF THE BABY'S BIRTH IS ESTABLISHED.

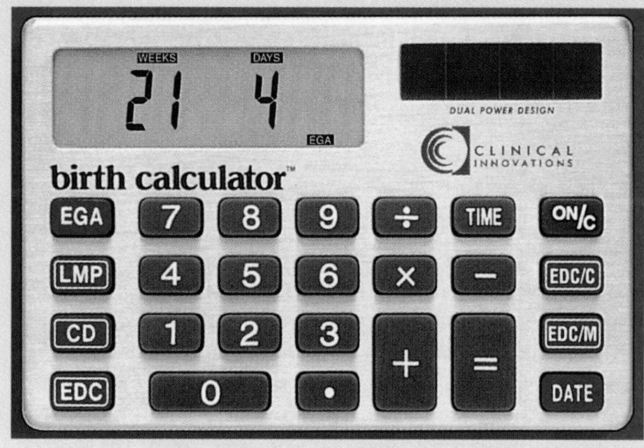

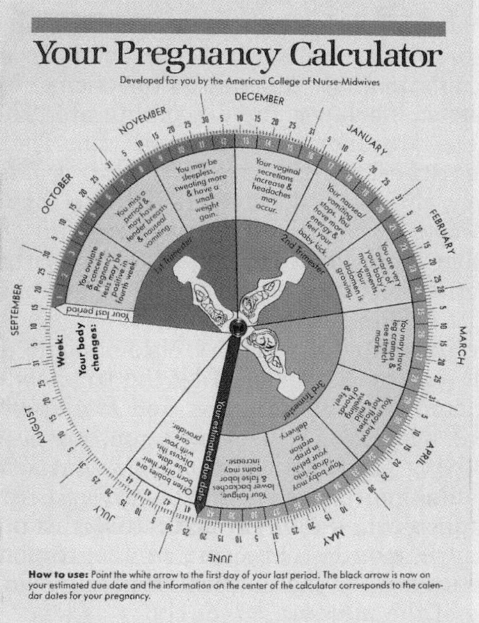

- USE BOOKS, PAMPHLETS, AND VIDEOS TO HELP EXPECTANT PARENTS UNDERSTAND FETAL DEVELOPMENT. Many are available from a variety of sources; some address weekly or monthly changes that take place during pregnancy and are easy to understand. Pamphlets are particularly good teaching tools since they may be taken home for further reference.
- LOOK FOR SPECIAL TOOLS TO SHARE WITH CLIENTS. *A Child Is Born* by Nilsson and Hamberger (1990) is an excellent lay publication that shows each step of fetal development with color photographs and accompanying text. It will help the expectant couple appreciate the many changes that the fetus undergoes.

Gestational wheel courtesy of the American College of Nurse-Midwives, Washington, D.C. Electronic gestational calculator courtesy of Clinical Innovations, Murray, UT.

Third Trimester

FETAL GROWTH AND ACTIVITY

Gestational weeks 26 to 32 tend to be weeks of steady growth. During weeks 26 to 27, some lecithin begins to appear in the amniotic fluid, and the alveolar ducts and sacs are present in the lungs. Overall subcutaneous fat begins to form slowly, causing the rounding of contours and smoothing of some of the wrinkles previously evidenced. The fetus is now covered with thick vernix caseosa, and lanugo remains except on the face, where it has been shed. The fetus manifests regular breathing motions and evidences a sleep-wake cycle. The eyelids are no longer fused, and they open and close regularly. The fetus may demonstrate a period of hiccups, occasionally to the dismay of the pregnant woman because of the rhythmic movements she feels. Surfactant, the substance needed to facilitate neonatal breathing, begins to be produced by approximately week 28. By the end of gestational week 32, the fetus is almost 4 pounds in weight and 11 inches in length.

During the ninth lunar month (gestational weeks 33 to 36), the fetus continues to deposit subcutaneous fat. If the fetus is male, the testes have descended into the scrotum. Plantar creases are visible on the feet of the fetus. Lanugo has essentially disappeared, and the baby weighs approximately 5.5 pounds with a crown-rump length of slightly more than 12.5 inches by week 36. By this time, the fetus is still producing some fetal hemoglobin but is also producing the blood type he or she will have throughout life.

GESTATIONAL AGE

▼ **Preterm.** By the last 4 weeks of pregnancy, the fetus begins to gain approximately half a pound weekly. A fetus born after 20 weeks of gestation, but before completion of 37 weeks, is a preterm or premature infant. Because the intrauterine development has not been completed, the infant is susceptible to a variety of potentially life-threatening conditions. The preterm infant is discussed in Chapter 36.

▼ **Term.** During the last weeks of pregnancy, the pregnant woman, especially the primigravida, may notice the fetus nestle into the pelvis so that the presenting part drops to the level of the ischial spines. When the presenting part is at the level of the ischial spines, it is termed engagement. The process of the baby's dropping or engaging is called lightening. Primigravidas tend to notice engagement approximately 2 weeks before delivery. Women may also notice an associated increased pelvic pressure and decreased pressure on the diaphragm.

The term or full-term fetus has firm bones, including a firm skull that is malleable because of elasticity afforded by suture lines and fontanelles. The head remains slightly disproportionately large. The chest is prominent, with protruding nipples for both male and female infants. The crown-rump length is approximately 14 inches. At this point, approximately 280 days after the last menstrual period, the fetus is ready to begin the journey from an intrauterine environment to an extrauterine environment and from fetal life to neonatal life. It is at birth that the fetal circulation ends and neonatal circulation begins.

▼ **Postterm.** A fetus who is born after 42 gestational weeks, or 294 days after the last menstrual period, is often called postterm or postmature. By this time, placental changes have included increased fibrin deposits, which impair the actions of the villi and thus compromise fetal oxygenation. Not only does the postmature infant not have lanugo, it does not have the vernix caseosa apparent with the term infant. The postmature baby is susceptible to a variety of clinical problems discussed in Chapter 36.

PLACENTAL DEVELOPMENT

Origin

The placenta, an organ of exchange between mother and fetus, consists of two parts: (1) the maternal portion, which includes the basal decidua and its circulation; and (2) the fetal portion, which contains the chorionic villi and their circulation. The placenta is formed by union of chorionic villi and the basal decidua. Although the organ is not completed until 10 to 12 weeks of gestational age, the placenta begins to emerge at the time of initial implantation. As the trophoblast burrows into the decidua, nutrients are provided through the maternal bloodstream to the syncytiotrophoblast. However, this is adequate only for the first few weeks while the embryo's demands for nutrition are small. Projections from the trophoblastic layer rapidly proliferate. These projections are known as chorionic villi. The villi become richest in the area of most profuse blood supply, the basal decidua. It is there that the trophoblasts expand and break down an increased number of decidual capillaries. This process allows maternal blood to ooze into the spaces surrounding it, forming lakes or sinuses. Clotting appears to be prevented by the presence of some anticoagulant substance produced by the trophoblasts. The chorionic villi differentiate, and two trophoblastic layers appear: (1) the syncytium, an outer layer consisting of syncytiotrophoblasts that secrete the placental hormones of pregnancy; and (2) the cytotrophoblast, an inner layer that disappears by the fifth month. This part of the trophoblast is then known as the chorion frondosum and is the basis of the placenta.

A few villi become deeply attached to the decidua and are called anchors; others begin the foundation for maternal-embryonic and maternal-fetal exchange, which is possible because of simultaneous changes occurring with the embryo. While the villi are burrowing into the decidua, the developing embryo has begun to project the major blood vessels through the umbilical cord or funis.

The system uses a variety of transport mechanisms (Fig. 15–4). For example, oxygen and carbon dioxide are carried by simple passive diffusion, while other substances may be carried by active transport. Even as the placenta grows and matures, the maternal and the embryonic and fetal bloodstreams never blend. Each chorionic villus has a branching structure that arises from a single stem. The center consists of mesoderm and

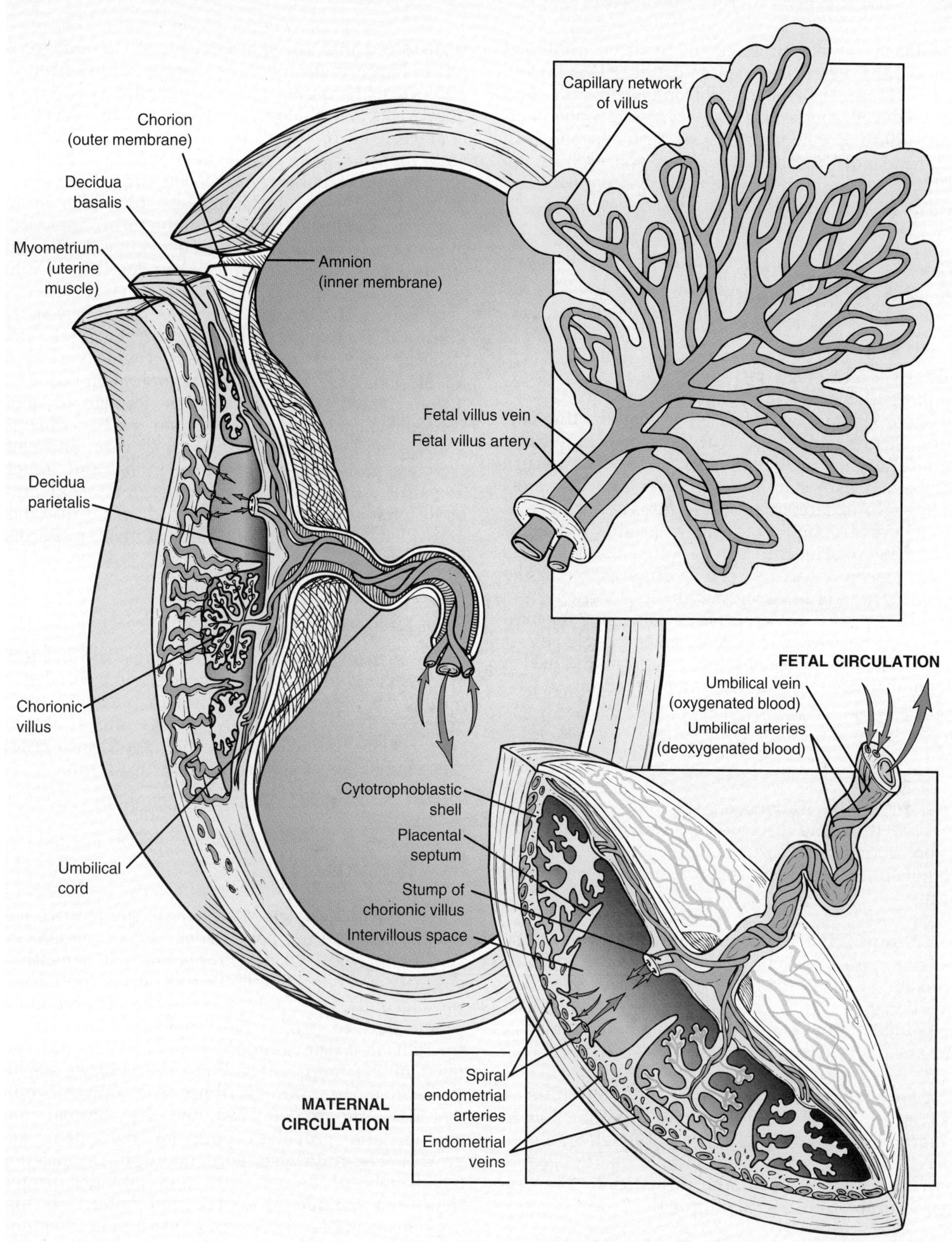

Figure 15–4

Maternal-fetal circulation is accomplished through the placenta • Arrows indicate the direction of blood flow from the expectant mother and placenta through the endometrial arteries and veins as well as between the fetus and placenta through the umbilical arteries and vein • This blood flow allows the placenta to function as a metabolic, transfer, and endocrine organ • Top inset shows the fetal capillary network within a chorionic villus, which is located on the fetal side of the placenta; bottom inset details how blood flows between the maternal and fetal sides.

fetal blood vessels, branches of the true umbilical arteries and veins. The center of the villus is covered by a single layer of cytotrophoblast cells, and the external layer by the syncytiotrophoblast. Thus, there are four layers of tissue separating maternal blood in the intervillous spaces from fetal blood in the villi, and any interchange between the two is not possible in the intact system.

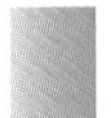

Placental Functions

METABOLISM

By 10 weeks after fertilization, the placenta is completely formed and functioning (Fig. 15–4). Between 12 and 24 weeks of gestation, the placenta weighs more than the fetus. At this time, the fetal organs are insufficient to perform mature metabolism. However, as fetal liver and other organs begin to function, the cytotrophoblast and the syncytiotrophoblast begin to gradually degenerate. The relationship of the fetus in the uterus to the placenta can be seen in Figure 15–5. The placenta functions as a metabolic, transfer, and endocrine organ. In terms of metabolism, the placenta synthesizes glycogen in early pregnancy. It also synthesizes cholesterol and fatty acids needed for energy used in transfer and endocrine activities.

TRANSFER

As an organ of transfer, the placenta uses at least six different mechanisms, which include diffusion, active transport, and pinocytosis, to transfer substances to and from the intrauterine conceptus.

▼ **Simple Diffusion.** Simple diffusion is the transfer across a concentration gradient. Simple diffusion is most likely the mechanism used for transfer of oxygen, carbon dioxide, water, most electrolytes, and many drugs, including analgesic and anesthetic drugs.

▼ **Facilitated Diffusion.** Facilitated diffusion also occurs across a concentration gradient, but in a more rapid manner. Glucose, although found in fairly low maternal concentrations, is thought to be transferred by facilitated diffusion to the embryo to promote more rapid growth.

▼ **Active Transport.** Active transport uses energy to transport against the usual physiologic principles. Iron and ascorbic acid are theorized to be transferred by active transport.

▼ **Pinocytosis.** Pinocytosis allows a substance to be invaginated by the chorionic villus and transferred into the bloodstream of the embryo or fetus. Large molecules are usually transported by pinocytosis. Immune gamma globulin G is an example. Two pathologic methods of transport include breaks in the cells, by which maternal and embryonic or fetal bloods may intermix with potential catastrophic results for an Rh-negative woman, and placental infections, by which protozoal and bacterial (and possibly viral) infections may reach the intrauterine environment. Rh sensitization is discussed in more detail in Chapter 21.

Although at one time scientists thought that the placenta was a barrier against harmful substances, today it is known that a wide variety of agents can pass into the embryonic or fetal circulation. Among the substances known to pass through the placenta are oxygen, carbon dioxide, and water; lactic acid, vitamins, glucose, and electrolytes; amino acids, proteins, lipids, and minerals; urea and bilirubin hormones; maternal antibodies for some diseases; most drugs (prescribed and illicit); and a large number of viral, protozoal, and bacterial infections.

ENDOCRINE ORGAN

The placenta functions as an endocrine organ by synthesizing, producing, and secreting a number of hormones, including hCG, human placental lactogen (HPL), estrogen, and progesterone. It is also theorized that the placenta may synthesize chorionic thyrotropin and chorionic corticotropin.

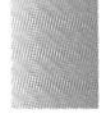

Amniotic Fluid

Two membranes exist as part of the mature placenta. The chorion is a thick, tough membrane that is derived from the trophoblast. It is continuous with the chorionic plate that forms the base of the placenta. The amnion is the thin, friable membrane derived from the inner cell mass. It is thought that the amnion is involved in development of the fluid surrounding the embryo and fetus, called the amniotic fluid. The amniotic fluid distends the sac formed by the amnion and chorion and provides space for movement and growth. The fluid also helps maintain a consistent environmental temperature and provides protection from outside pressures and impact. It also provides some protection from ascending infections from the vagina and cushions the umbilical cord to prevent compression and problems with oxygenation. In labor, not only does the intact amniotic fluid continue to cushion the fetus and cord, but it promotes effacement (or thinning) of the cervix and even dilatation when the presenting part is not applied well to the cervix.

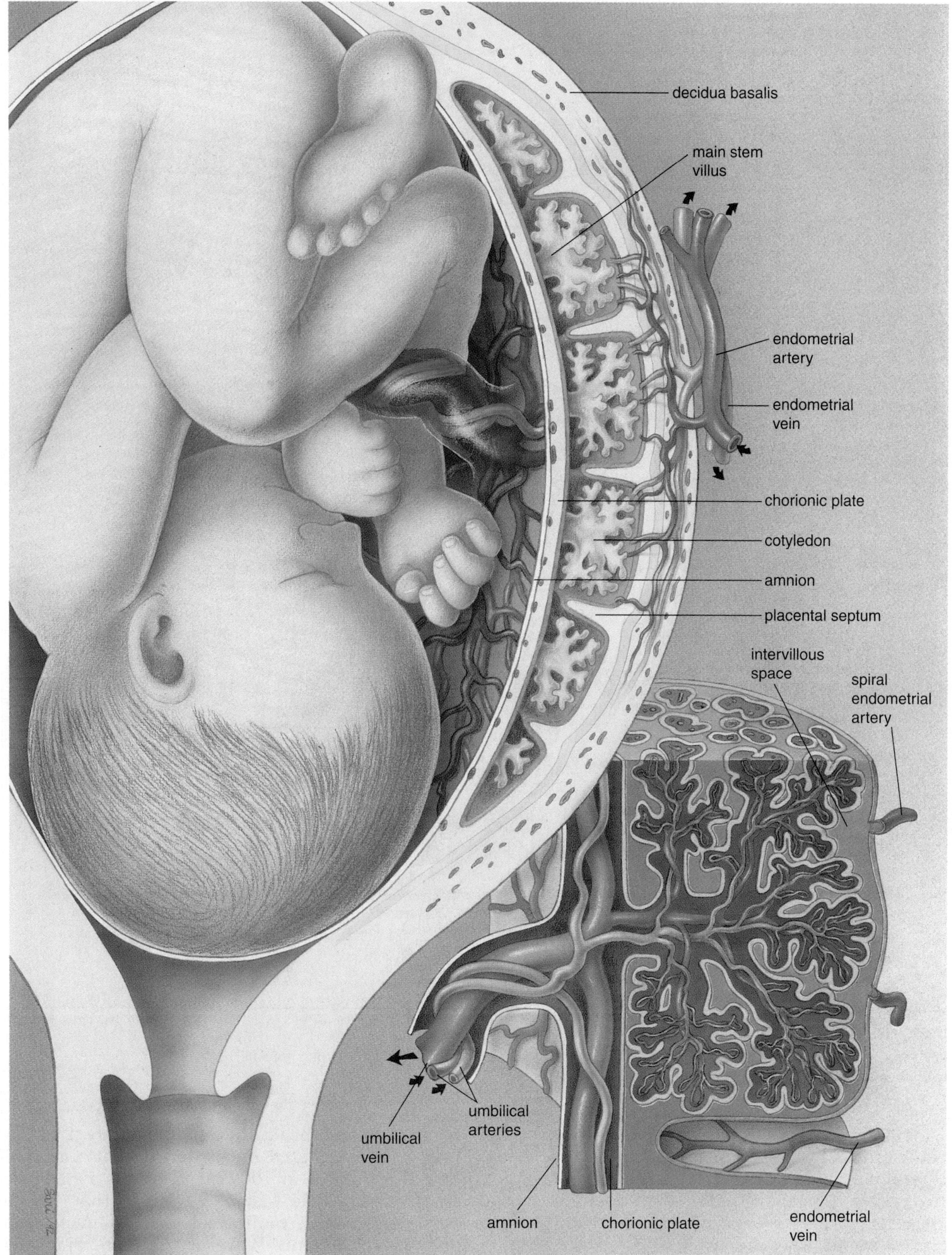

Figure 15–5

The near-term fetus in the uterus is surrounded by amniotic and chorionic sacs with little room for movement. (From Moore, K. L., Persaud, T. V. N., Shiota, K. [1994]. *Color atlas of clinical embryology* [p. 85]. Philadelphia: W. B. Saunders.)

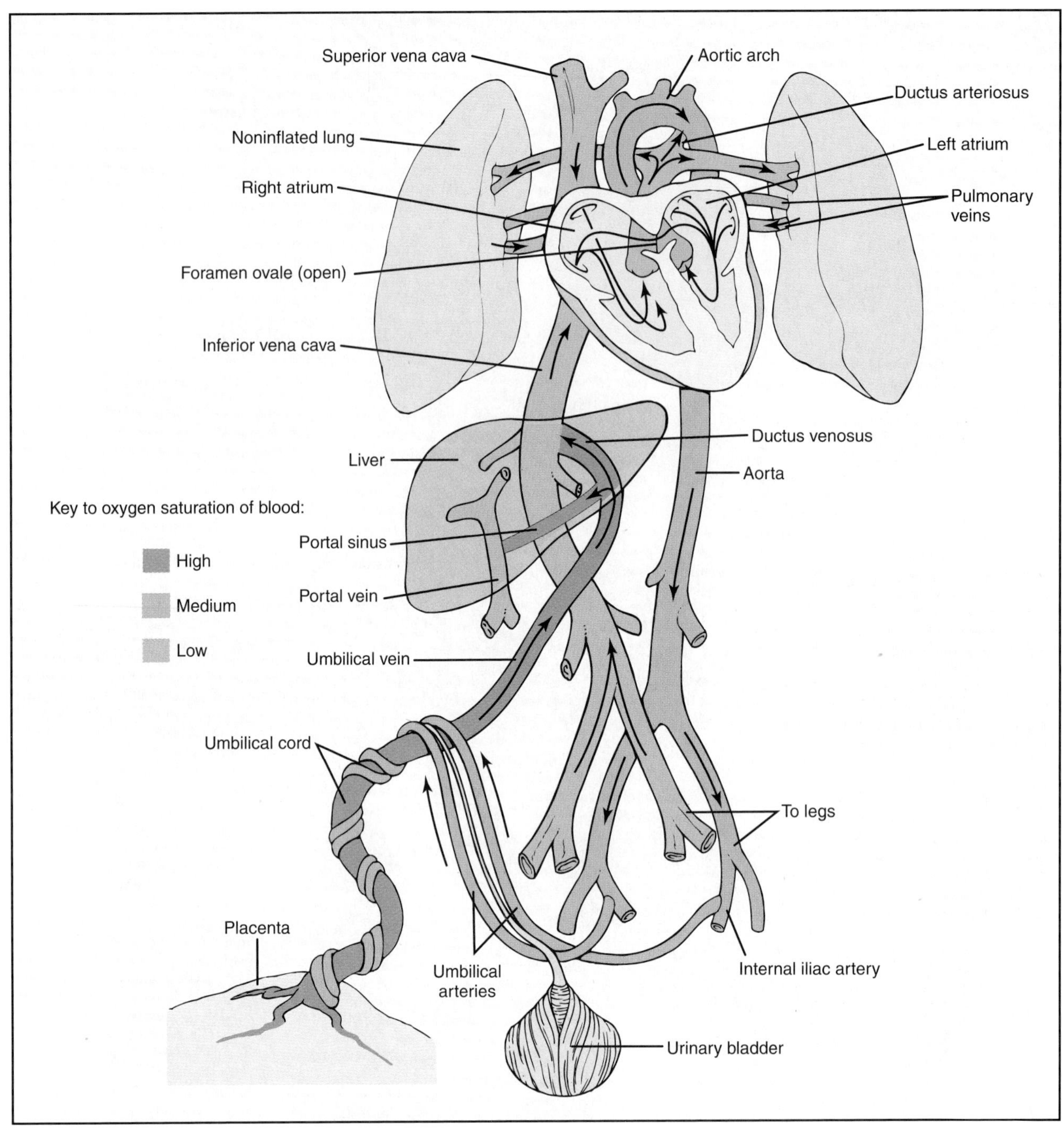

Figure 15–6

Fetal circulation • Three shunts that permit fetal blood to bypass the liver and lungs can be seen in this schematic drawing: ductus venosus, foramen ovale, and ductus arteriosus.

Amniotic fluid is composed primarily of water. It is secreted by the amnion, maternal vessels in the decidua, and fetal vessels in the placenta. Approximately 1 percent of the fluid contains fetal skin cells, vernix caseosa, lanugo, and the results of fetal waste (predominantly fetal urine). Aspiration of the amniotic fluid is one method of fetal assessment and is discussed further in this chapter.

The volume of amniotic fluid increases during pregnancy and peaks at approximately 2 weeks before the estimated due date. At that time, volume is estimated at 1000 mL. There is a slight decrease during the last 2 weeks so that by the estimated date of confinement, the volume is approximately 800 mL. However, there are wide variations in the amount. Less than 300 mL at term is called oligohydramnios; more than 1500 mL is termed polyhydramnios or hydramnios. These conditions may indicate fetal jeopardy. Amniotic fluid volume is assessed during abdominal assessments, including fundal height measurements, as well as by ultrasonic techniques.

Fetal Circulation

Blood, pumped by the embryo's heart, leaves the embryo through two umbilical arteries and is transported along their branches to the capillaries of the chorionic villi. Once oxygenated through the villi, the blood is then returned by one umbilical vein. These three umbilical vessels are protected within an umbilical cord, which is about 2 feet long at birth and surrounded by a gelatinous substance called Wharton's jelly. Wharton's jelly prevents cord kinking, which could interfere with umbilical circulation. Maternal blood is transported to the placental bed by spiral arteries in the decidua, and the blood flows into the blood spaces surrounding the villi. There are no pain receptors in the umbilical cord.

During fetal life, the conceptus manifests a unique circulatory system (Fig. 15–6). The fetal circulation has several unusual elements. Prominent among them are the number of temporary structures that are integral components as well as the fact that, unlike in the adult, the oxygenated blood is carried by the umbilical vein and the deoxygenated blood by the umbilical arteries. Among the temporary structures are the following:

- The ductus venosus connects the umbilical vein to the inferior vena cava. When connected, the blood mixes with deoxygenated blood that is returning from the lower parts of the body. Thus, the blood throughout the body is, at best, partially oxygenated.
- The foramen ovale is a temporary opening between the right and left atria that allows the majority of blood that enters from the inferior vena cava to pass across into the left atrium. Thus, little flow goes into the lungs since they are not a major organ of importance for the fetus. The ductus arteriosus arises from a bifurcation of the pulmonary artery to the descending aorta.
- The hypogastric arteries branch off from the internal iliac arterioles and become the umbilical arteries when they enter the umbilical cord. These arteries carry the blood back to the placenta to remove waste and oxygenate.

By term, fetal blood takes approximately 30 seconds to circulate in the conceptus. It follows this path:

- Oxygenated blood is transported from the placenta by the umbilical vein through the abdominal wall to the undersurface of the liver.
- The ductus venosus carries blood to the inferior vena cava, where it intermixes with blood from the lower body.
- The blood then passes into the right atrium, where most of it is transported across the foramen ovale into the left atrium.
- The blood then follows the usual adult course through the left ventricle and passes into the aorta. (The heart and brain are well supplied through early branching of the aorta into the coronary and carotid arteries. Cephalocaudal development may also be enhanced by the rich supply of the subclavian arteries to the arms and the greater amount of oxygen in the upper region of the body.)
- Blood collected from the upper parts of the body returns to the right atrium in the superior vena cava and passes into the right ventricle. Partial oxygenation is obtained for this blood from some sharing of blood passing from the inferior vena cava to the right ventricle. Only a small amount of blood enters the pulmonary artery and continues into the lungs. Most of the remaining blood continues along the aorta.
- The internal iliac arteries lead to the hypogastric arteries. They in turn return blood to the placenta through the umbilical arteries.
- Physiologic changes that occur at birth include a major metamorphosis as the fetal circulation becomes a neonatal circulation. Newborn adaptation to extrauterine life is discussed in Chapter 30.

EMBRYONIC AND FETAL ASSESSMENT TECHNIQUES

Today several different strategies exist to facilitate assessment of the intrauterine environment. Prominent among them are ultrasound scanning, Doppler flow studies, amniocentesis, chorionic villus sampling (CVS), and percutaneous umbilical blood sampling (PUBS). Some are assessments of the embryo, some of the fetus, and others of both. Additional fetal assessment tests that are not discussed in this chapter, including the nonstress test, vibroacoustic stimulation, the contraction stress test, and the biophysical profile, are covered in Chapter 26. The field of assessment of the intrauterine environment is a rapidly growing area. As new technology becomes available, it is often quickly adopted into use. In some cases, long-term data are lacking regarding effects, and efficacy with a low-risk population has never been demonstrated. However, these assessment techniques have proved to be invaluable for certain high-risk populations.

Psychological Implications of Antepartum Testing

One area that is frequently overlooked in the application of the newer assessment techniques is the psychological impact of such technology. Rothman explored the effects that prenatal testing can have for the modern woman. She noted that attachment to the intrauterine conceptus often appears to be delayed until the woman is assured of the normalcy of the fetus. Only then can the woman truly accept the pregnancy and proceed with normal psychological adaptation. Until then, the pregnancy is psychologically viewed in tentative terms. Thus, not only is it important that the childbearing couple receive clear information about the risks and benefits of all prenatal testing, but the practitioner must recognize that such testing may influence the couple's acceptance of the pregnancy and of the baby (Rothman 1987; Heidrich and Cranley 1989).

Ultrasound Scanning

DESCRIPTION OF PROCEDURE

The technique of ultrasonic scanning, or sonography, has revolutionized assessment of the intrauterine world (Thornton 1992). Unlike x-ray study, ultrasound examination uses a high-frequency sound source (3.5 to 7.0 MHz) instead of radiation. These sound waves are intermittent and at a frequency that is above the highest range of hearing. With this method, an image is created in shades of gray, depending on the intensity of echoes derived from spaces in the tissues (Catanzarite and Maida 1992; Callen 1994). Real-time ultrasound scanning allows the ultrasonographer to observe fetal motion, including breathing, cardiac action, and vessel pulsations. There are two levels of ultrasound examination. A level I (basic) ultrasound scan is performed by a technician and can assess the number of fetuses, presentation, lie, viability (cardiac motion is usually visible by 7 weeks of gestational age), placental site, and amniotic fluid volume. A level II (targeted) ultrasound scan is more detailed. It is performed when fetal anomaly is likely. A level II scan includes the aforementioned aspects found in a level I scan, but it adds a detailed study of fetal anatomy.

The ultrasound procedure is done on an outpatient basis. The woman is asked to come for the testing with a full bladder so that the uterus will be elevated out of the pelvis, facilitating better visualization on the ultrasound scan. The full bladder also serves as a landmark in reading the ultrasound image, but it may provide a measure of discomfort for the woman throughout the procedure.

The woman should be made as comfortable as possible on the examination table. A pillow under her head and knees helps to alleviate back or abdominal discomfort. A conductive gel is spread on the abdominal wall to diminish the loss of ultrasound waves at the surface of the skin and to reduce friction as the transducer is moved across the skin. A vaginal probe transducer may also be used during the first trimester to obtain a clearer image of the fetus and placenta. The image of the fetus appears on the monitor screen of the machine as the transducer is passed back and forth over the abdomen (Fig. 15–7).

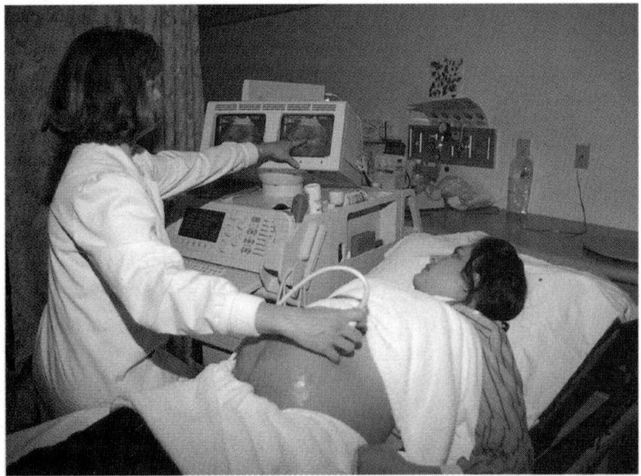

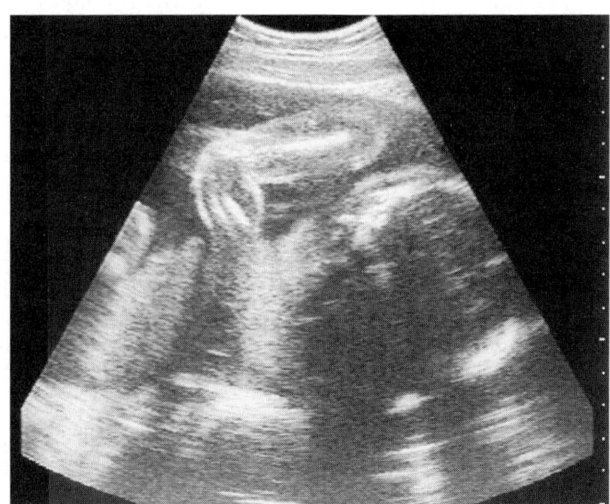

Figure 15–7

Ultrasonography uses high-frequency sound waves to create an image of the fetus and intrauterine environment on a monitor screen • Ultrasound scan for fetal assessment outlines the hand, arm, and head of the fetus. (Scan courtesy of Melissa and Mark Schroeder.)

BENEFITS AND RISKS

The benefits of ultrasonography relate to its use in monitoring the pregnancy and detecting abnormalities. These aspects are discussed in detail in the next section. Currently, few data exist to disprove the safety of ultrasonography (Cunningham et al. 1993). The technique became widely adopted only in the middle to late 1960s; therefore, long-term or multigenerational data are only now becoming available. Ultrasonography was initially used only when fetal problems were suspected. Today, however, ultrasound scanning is used routinely with many pregnancies. The cost effectiveness of routine scans has not been demonstrated, nor has the general usefulness of routine ultrasound scans in a population of women not at medical risk been proved. A large multicity study revealed no significant perinatal outcome differences between two groups of women, one with routine ultrasound scans during pregnancy and the other without (Ewigman et al. 1993).

Although there seems to be little benefit to routine screening, routine ultrasound examinations are still administered in many practice settings. Some practitioners suggest that it is the woman's right to choose this technology since no major risks have been established. Others question the allocation of health care dollars for "baby pictures." Yet other clinicians advocate continuing routine scans in an effort to protect themselves from unnecessary litigation by confirming normalcy of the fetus as much as is feasible (Berkowitz 1993). Additional problems related to ultrasonography that have been discussed in the literature include professional roles, interpretation of ultrasound findings, and initiation of unnecessary interventions as a result of testing (Fresquez and Collins 1992; Gegor 1992; Merritt 1992; Seeds 1992; Wilson and Foster 1992). Ultrasound findings must be interpreted by a health professional; however, errors may occur in interpretation. In some areas, ultrasound scans are offered without cost at health fairs or shopping malls to interest prospective parents in receiving care at some specific birth site. In such situations, interpretation is not ideal. Minor, or perhaps major, congenital anomalies may be overlooked. Ultrasound examination is a procedure assumed by departments of obstetrics and radiology. Marked differences of opinion on the qualifications of the interpreter of an ultrasound scan exist, especially among representatives from both groups.

Variations in fetal size may sometimes be constitutional in origin, and confirmation by an ultrasound examination of a large or small infant may initiate a chain of interventions that ultimately prove to be unnecessary. Although ultrasound scanning has enabled early diagnoses to be made and interventions to be started that in some cases have made major positive contributions, questions arise as to the role of ultrasound examination in selective termination of pregnancy and advanced reproductive technologies.

REASONS FOR USE

Dating of the pregnancy (and determination of gestational age) is a common reason to employ ultrasound examination (Gegor et al. 1991; Catanzarite and Maida 1992; Gegor and Paine 1992; Thornton 1992). The single best parameter for establishing the estimated date of delivery is a known date of the last normal menstrual period for a woman who usually has regular, predictable cycles. However, there are times when a reliable last menstrual period date is unavailable. Examples include the breastfeeding woman who becomes pregnant, the woman who has discontinued oral contraceptives and conceives before menses, or the woman who has unusual or unpredictable cycles. In cases of uncertain last menstrual periods, an ultrasound scan may be used to establish or confirm the estimated date of delivery. The earlier in pregnancy an ultrasound scan is performed, the more accurate it is. For example, for some infertility patients, ovulation may be demonstrated on ultrasound imaging. In the embryonic period, ultrasound scans measure crown-rump lengths; later in the fetal period, biparietal diameters, femur lengths, head circumferences, and estimated fetal weights can be approximated. These are less accurate than crown-rump lengths since the fetus evidences more variation than the embryo at the same gestational period. However, later ultrasound examinations can provide additional information, such as fetal growth assessments.

Ultrasound examination is often employed to identify a variety of congenital structural anomalies that may be diagnosed prenatally (Carlson and Platt 1992). Another major use of ultrasound scanning is to identify the number of fetuses and rule out multifetal pregnancy. By 7 weeks of gestation, the cardiac motion can be seen for more than one embryo. Even earlier, double sacs may be visible, but the appearance of a double sac may be secondary to another factor, such as subchorionic hemorrhage. Twin pregnancy is discussed in Chapter 21.

Ultrasound examination is employed to assess fetal growth, especially serial ultrasound scans to assess fetal growth retardation. Asymmetric fetal growth retardation is the most common type found on ultrasound examination. It is associated with placental insufficiency, although Doppler fetal cerebral blood studies have demonstrated that shunting occurs that allows adequate circulation to the brain. This phenomenon, in turn, encourages adequate head growth, which is disproportionate to the rest of the body, making it asymmetric. Symmetric growth retardation is associated with an idiopathic reduction in growth

Congenital Structural Anomalies Potentially Identifiable by Ultrasonography

Cardiac anomalies

Central nervous system anomalies

- Anencephaly
- Spina bifida
- Encephalocele
- Dandy-Walker syndrome

Fetal tumors

- Teratoma
- Cystic hygroma
- Intracranial tumors

Gastrointestinal anomalies

- Gastroschisis
- Pyloric atresia
- Duodenal atresia
- Colonic obstruction

Genitourinary tract anomalies

- Obstructive uropathy
- Renal agenesis
- Polycystic kidney disease
- Ovarian cysts

Pulmonary system anomalies

- Diaphragmatic hernia
- Pleural effusion

Skeletal anomalies

- Short-limb dysplasia
- Achondrogenesis
- Osteogenesis imperfecta
- Phocomelia

Other

- Fetal hydrops
- Facial anomalies

potential that is so severe (e.g., severe malnutrition, congenital anomalies) that brain sparing is not operational. The ratio of head circumference to abdominal circumference provides one technique to differentiate between symmetric and asymmetric fetal growth retardation. The outcome for infants born with fetal growth retardation is discussed in Chapter 36. Ultrasound scanning has also been used as a technique to assess macrosomatia. Macrosomatia occurs when a fetus is at or above the 90th percentile for normal weight. It is a condition usually associated with infants of diabetic mothers. Diabetes in pregnancy is discussed in Chapter 21.

Not only may the fetus be assessed for size, but other fetal well-being patterns can also be observed with ultrasound examination. These include amount of amniotic fluid, placental grading (to rule out calcifications associated with an aging placenta), and fetal activity (Catanzarite and Maida 1992). The fetal activity is often observed as spontaneous actions (such as fetal breathing movements) or in response to stimulation, such as vibroacoustic stimulation or nipple stimulation (Willson 1991; Curtis et al. 1989; Inglis et al. 1993). These fetal assessments under ultrasound visualization are frequently performed with a nonstress electronic fetal monitoring assessment and are commonly termed a biophysical fetal profile (Gegor et al. 1991; Gegor and Paine 1992; Sabey and Clark 1992; Gebauer and Lowe 1993). Fetal monitoring is discussed in Chapter 26. In summary, ultrasound scanning has taken an important role in the delivery of prenatal care, especially for the woman at medical risk. Some questions remain regarding appropriate routine use of the technology.

Doppler Flow Studies

DESCRIPTION OF PROCEDURE

Doppler flow ultrasonic studies are another method of prenatal fetal assessment (Cundiff 1990; Lunell and Nylund 1992). They allow the study of blood flow in deep-lying vessels and can be useful in the management of pregnancies complicated by hypertension, diabetes, multifetal gestation, intrauterine growth retardation, or preterm labor. The ultrasound study enables the moving column of red blood cells to be visualized. The frequency of movement is proportionate to the velocity. The returning signal allows the display of flow-velocity waveforms (*Lancet* staff 1992).

REASONS FOR USE

Most Doppler flow studies have been performed in experimental research projects. The modality is not yet a common fetal assessment tool. However, the method holds promise for screening of early placental insufficiency that could be distinguished by a diminished umbilical flow or perhaps flow through the circle of Willis. It is likely that future studies in this area may find wide clinical applications for Doppler flow studies, even as an adjunct to, or perhaps instead of, electronic fetal monitoring in the intrapartum period.

Maternal Alpha-Fetoprotein Screening

DESCRIPTION OF PROCEDURE

The maternal serum alpha-fetoprotein (MSAFP) test is designed to screen, not diagnose, open neural tube defects (American Academy of Pediatrics 1991). It requires a tube of maternal blood. Alpha-fetoprotein is a glucoprotein produced by the fetal yolk sac, gastrointestinal tract, and liver. It passes through the placenta to the maternal circulation and is then excreted through fetal urine into the amniotic fluid. By the seventh week of pregnancy, alpha-fetoprotein is usually detectable in maternal serum. It then shows a progressive rise throughout pregnancy until it peaks in the third trimester. Normal ranges exist for each week of pregnancy. The optimal time for MSAFP screening is between 16 and 18 weeks' gestation.

BENEFITS AND RISKS

Early studies of MSAFP demonstrated that there were marked variations of serum levels among different laboratories. To better standardize the findings, data are now commonly reported in multiples of the individual laboratory's own median level in unaffected pregnancies, categorized by gestational weeks. An elevated multiple of the median suggests an open neural tube defect; a low level may suggest Down syndrome. Since the test is a screening test only and has high sensitivity but low specificity, the MSAFP is usually repeated if indicated. An ultrasound scan may be done to rule out structural anomalies. An amniocentesis is the diagnostic method for detection of a neural tube defect or Down syndrome. It measures alpha-fetoprotein in the amniotic fluid and provides the cells needed for chromosomal analysis. An informed consent should be obtained using terms the patient understands and in her native language. Information must be provided about the potential of the test and procedures that will be followed if the test result is positive. This is important because the MSAFP test is a screening procedure and may produce a false-positive result, especially since there is a wide variation of normal levels even among healthy women and fetuses. Some parents may elect to not be tested to avoid being confronted with the dilemmas posed by an abnormal test result. Counseling should be made available to help parents with their decision. If the decision is made to not have the MSAFP screening, this should be recorded in the patient's chart along with her written signature (American Academy of Pediatrics 1991; Evans et al. 1992a).

REASONS FOR USE

Several factors can cause the MSAFP level to be either elevated or low. The MSAFP test has currently been proposed by the American Academy of Pediatrics (1991) to be offered to all pregnant women for prenatal screening since neural tube defects frequently occur without prediction. The most common neural tube defects are anencephaly and spina bifida, both of which are termed open lesions since the meninges or neural elements are either directly exposed or covered with a thin membrane. The cause of neural tube defects is unknown, although two prominent theories are genetic predisposition and vitamin deficiency. The vitamin deficiency theory has been supported by findings suggesting a decrease in neural tube defects for women who have taken folic acid preconceptionally.

Studies have shown that the MSAFP test may also be useful in screening for Down syndrome. Low alpha-fetoprotein values can be used in conjunction with maternal age and other serum markers (unconjugated estriol and chorionic gonadotropin) to predict risks for Down syndrome. If these markers indicate a high risk for Down syndrome, the blood tests should be followed by amniocentesis (Cunningham et al. 1993).

Amniocentesis

DESCRIPTION OF PROCEDURE

Among the contents of the amniotic fluid are fetal cells. Amniocentesis is a procedure designed to harvest the fetal cells and allow them to be karyotyped for analysis of genetic makeup. Although the classic timing for an amniocentesis is approximately 16 to 20 weeks of gestation, some practitioners are now performing it at approximately 12 weeks of gestation. The procedure is performed under ultrasonic visualization so that the largest pocket of fluid may be identified. An empty bladder helps to eliminate confusion. Positioning the woman supine for 15 to 20 minutes before the procedure may facilitate the rising of fetal cells in the fluid, and thus obtaining them with the procedure is more likely. A needle is inserted transab-

Factors Linked to Abnormal Maternal Serum Alpha-Fetoprotein Concentrations

ELEVATED LEVELS

- Open neural tube defect
- Underestimated gestational age
- Multiple gestation
- Intrauterine death (transient rise)
- Low birth weight
- Pilonidal cysts
- Esophageal or intestinal obstruction
- Oligohydramnios
- Decreased maternal weight
- Urinary obstruction
- Liver necrosis
- Abdominal wall defects
- Renal anomalies
- Congenital nephrosis
- Congenital skin defects
- Cloacal exstrophy

LOW LEVELS

- Overestimated gestational age
- Chromosomal trisomies
- Overdilution of serum (e.g., secondary to maternal obesity)
- Gestational trophoblastic disease
- Fetal death

Adapted with permission from Cunningham, F. G., MacDonald, P. C., Gant, N. F., Leveno, K. J., Gilstrap, L. C. III. (1993). *Williams obstetrics* (19th ed.) (p. 941). Norwalk, CT: Appleton & Lange.

dominally or suprapubically and placed into the pocket of fluid, from which 15 to 20 mL of amniotic fluid is obtained. Physical discomfort tends to be mild for a woman, but psychologically most women are concerned and possibly frightened about the interventive nature of the procedure (Fig. 15–8).

BENEFITS AND RISKS

Risks with an amniocentesis are not common (less than 1%), but the procedure is not necessarily innocuous. Thus, a woman should receive an informed consent about the advantages and disadvantages to her and her fetus. The risks include inadvertent rupture of membranes, preterm labor, fetal trauma, infection, and isoimmunization for an Rh-negative woman. Because of Rh isoimmunization risk, anti-D serum is usually administered after the procedure.

REASONS FOR USE

Like CVS, amniocentesis allows fetal genetic profiles to be obtained (Wapner et al. 1993). Genetic diseases, including sex-linked diseases, can be diagnosed during this intrauterine period. Unlike CVS, amniocentesis is the method of choice for diagnosing a suspected neural tube defect. Since an amniocentesis uses fetal cells instead of the fetal tissue used by CVS, it may take longer to grow the cells and extricate the needed genetic material. It is not uncommon for results to take 2 to 3 weeks to become available. During this period of waiting, the expectant couple needs realistic support and counseling. An amniocentesis is occasionally performed late in pregnancy to ascertain maturity of the fetus. Lung maturity can be assessed by the presence of phosphatidylglycerol and phosphatidylcholine and a mature lecithin/sphingomyelin ratio.

Chorionic Villus Sampling

DESCRIPTION OF PROCEDURE AND REASONS FOR USE

CVS is a method employed to obtain genetic fetal tissue (Evans et al. 1989; Stringer et al. 1991; Evans et al. 1992b). Since the chorionic villi are rapidly growing during the embryonic stage, CVS is performed at approximately 9 to 12 weeks of gestation. The technique may be transabdominal or transvaginal. Under ultrasound visualization, chorionic villi are obtained (Fig. 15–9). Karyotyping can be performed on this tissue or other tissue obtained from cell growth to establish a genetic profile.

BENEFITS AND RISKS

The advantage of CVS compared with an amniocentesis, another procedure designed to obtain fetal genotyping, is the early stage of pregnancy during which it is performed. Should a woman choose to terminate the pregnancy, it can be done during the first trimester when such surgery has less physical risks, although psychological issues are similar regardless of week of pregnancy. The disadvantages of CVS include the inability to screen for neural tube defects and the possible increased risk for spontaneous abortion, which is under study since the data are confounded by the

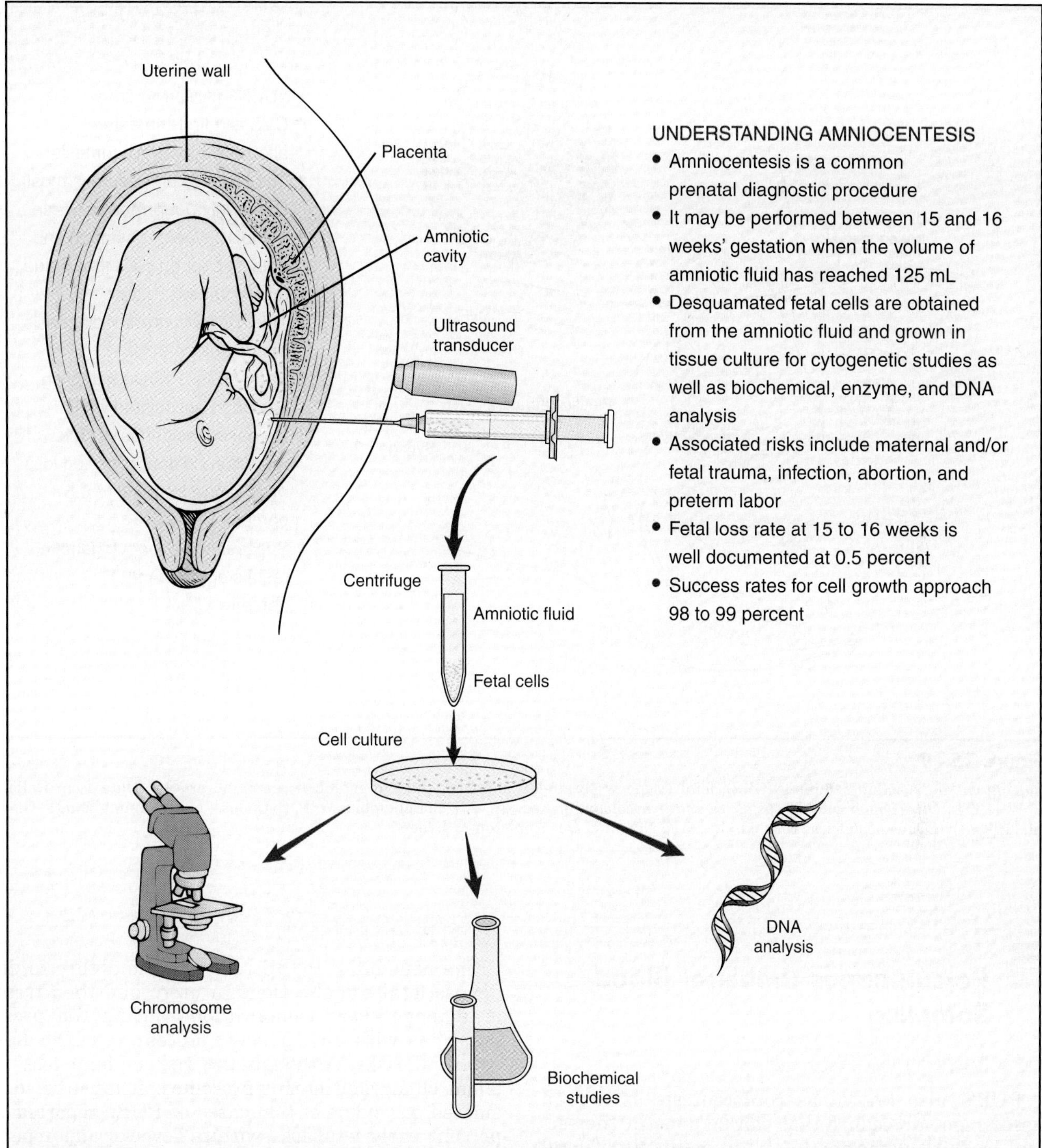

Figure 15–8

During amniocentesis, a sample of amniotic fluid containing fetal cells is removed from the amniotic cavity. (Data from Callan, P. W. [1994]. *Ultrasonography in obstetrics and gynecology* [3rd ed.] [p. 17]. Philadelphia: W. B. Saunders; and Cunningham, F. G., et al. [1993]. *Williams obstetrics* [19th ed.] [p. 946]. Norwalk, CT: Appleton & Lange.)

fact that spontaneous abortions are normally more common in the first trimester than in the second trimester when an amniocentesis is performed. A study showed that women who had experienced CVS gave birth to a disproportionately high number of infants with limb defects (Burton et al. 1992; Cunningham et al. 1993). Subsequent studies have questioned the association of the two factors; however, in some areas, practitioners have been increasingly hesitant about performing CVS because of potential malpractice risk in the event of an infant's being born with a birth defect. Instead, some clinicians have been advocating early amniocentesis (Henry and Miller 1992).

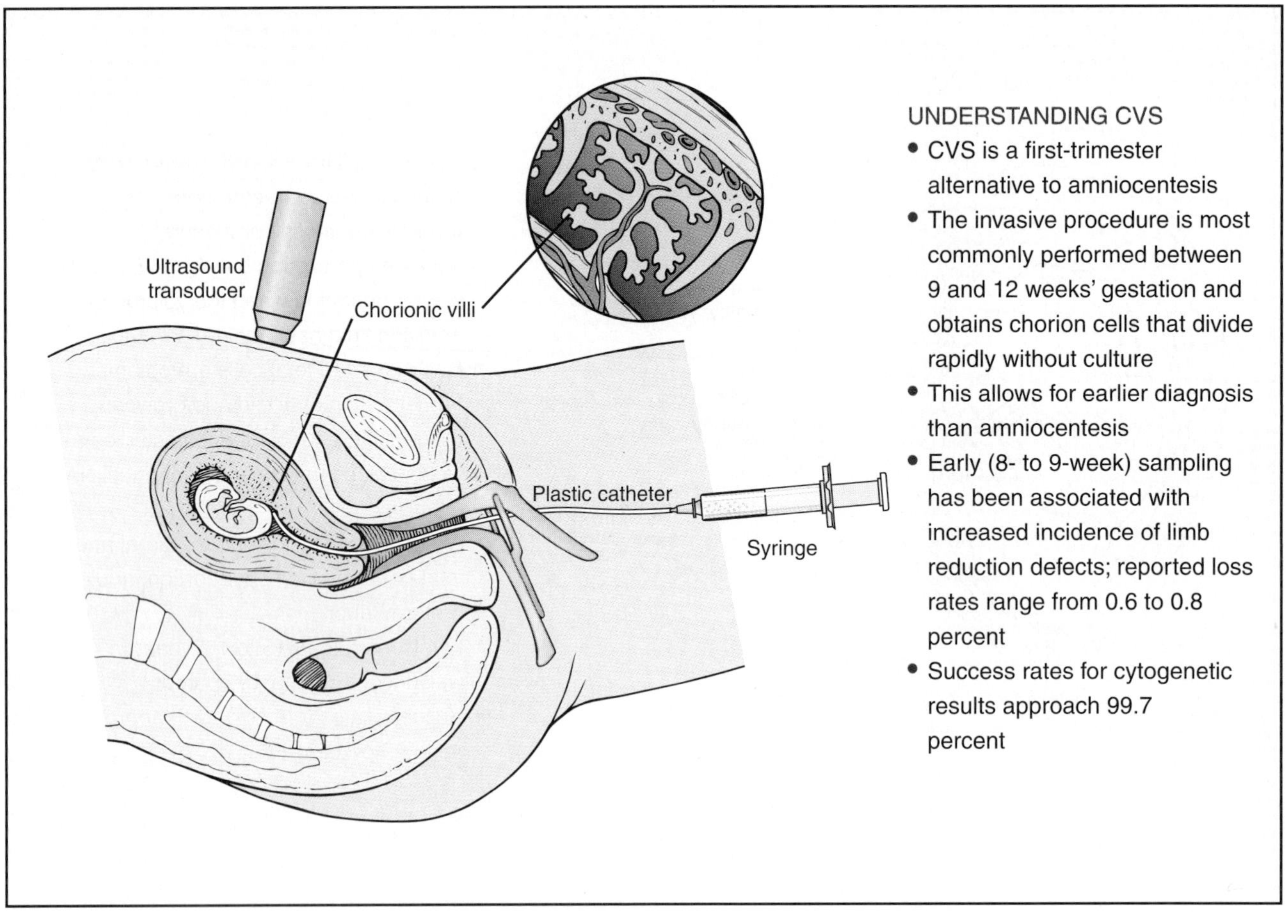

Ultrasound transducer

Chorionic villi

Plastic catheter

Syringe

UNDERSTANDING CVS

- CVS is a first-trimester alternative to amniocentesis
- The invasive procedure is most commonly performed between 9 and 12 weeks' gestation and obtains chorion cells that divide rapidly without culture
- This allows for earlier diagnosis than amniocentesis
- Early (8- to 9-week) sampling has been associated with increased incidence of limb reduction defects; reported loss rates range from 0.6 to 0.8 percent
- Success rates for cytogenetic results approach 99.7 percent

Figure 15–9

During chorionic villus sampling (CVS), fetal tissue is obtained for karyotyping to establish a genetic profile. (Data from Callen, P. W. [1994]. *Ultrasonography in obstetrics and gynecology* [3rd ed.] [p. 20]. Philadelphia: W. B. Saunders; and Cunningham, F. G., et al. [1993]. *Williams obstetrics* [19th ed.] [p. 951]. Norwalk, CT: Appleton & Lange.)

Percutaneous Umbilical Blood Sampling

DESCRIPTION OF PROCEDURE

PUBS, also known as cordocentesis, is a fetal assessment procedure that can be done in the second or third trimester to obtain a sample of fetal blood from the umbilical cord for prenatal testing. The umbilical cord is first located through the use of high-resolution ultrasound scanning. A needle is then inserted through the abdominal and uterine walls and then directly into a fetal umbilical vessel, and a blood sample of 1 to 4 mL is aspirated. A site 1 to 2 cm from the insertion of the cord into the placenta is desirable, for the cord is well anchored and less likely to move, and the risk of obtaining maternal blood from the placenta is slight (Fig. 15–10). After the sample is obtained, it is tested by the Kleihauer-Betke procedure to ensure that it is fetal blood (Cunningham et al. 1993).

BENEFITS AND RISKS

The benefits of PUBS relate to the ability to diagnose fetal complications in utero and then treat or manage these complications during the pregnancy. As with any invasive procedure, PUBS has potential risks. Although the risk of fetal loss is slight as a result of this procedure, it must be considered. A review of 928 cases of PUBs reported 1 percent early fetal loss within 2 weeks and 1 percent fetal deaths within 4 to 20 weeks (Cunningham et al. 1993, p. 953). Other complications that might result include leakage of blood from the umbilical puncture site, fetal bradycardia, and chorioamnionitis. Research is ongoing to determine the safety of this procedure.

REASONS FOR USE

PUBS might be done during pregnancy to diagnose isoimmunization and platelet disorders, congenital infections, chromosome abnormalities, abnormal blood-clotting factors, or metabolic disor-

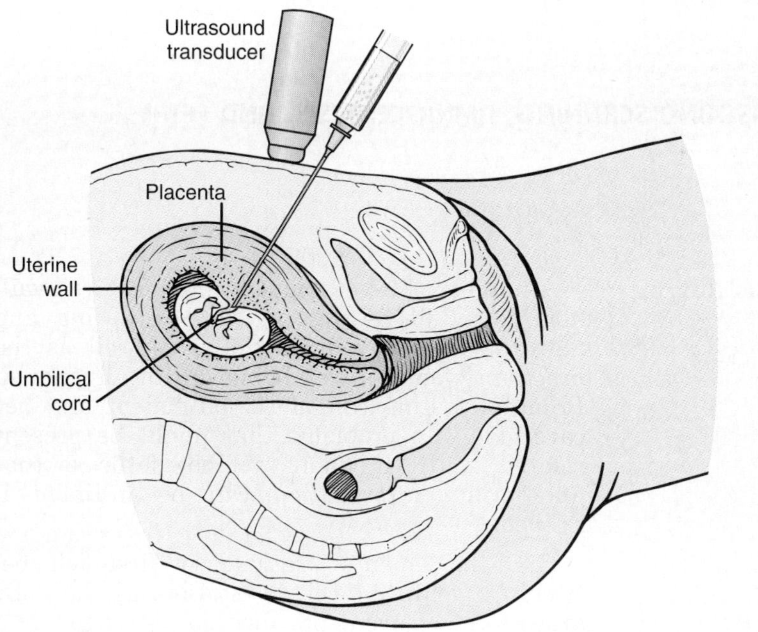

Ultrasound transducer

Placenta

Uterine wall

Umbilical cord

UNDERSTANDING PUBS

- PUBS can be used to confirm abnormal findings resulting from amniocentesis and/or chorionic villus sampling
- Rapid analysis of fetal blood (48 to 72 hours) is possible compared with 2 to 3 weeks for amniocentesis
- PUBS is revolutionizing the fields of fetal physiology, diagnosis, and therapy
- Indications for use include: prenatal diagnosis for blood disorders, isoimmunization, metabolic disorders, and fetal infections; fetal karyotyping; evaluation of fetal hypoxia; and fetal therapy
- Associated risks are the same as for amniocentesis
- Fetal loss rates have been documented at 1 percent

Figure 15–10

During percutaneous umbilical blood sampling (PUBS), a sample of fetal blood is obtained by insertion of a needle through the expectant mother's abdomen and into the umbilical vein. (Data from Callen, P. W. [1994]. *Ultrasonography in obstetrics and gynecology* [3rd ed.] [p. 21]. Philadelphia: W. B. Saunders; and Cunningham, F. G., et al. [1993]. *Williams obstetrics* [19th ed.] [p. 953]. Norwalk, CT: Appleton & Lange.)

ders; to evaluate fetal hypoxia; or to determine the acid-base balance of a fetus suspected of having intrauterine growth retardation. PUBS can also be used for intrauterine transfusion or fetal drug therapy. During labor, PUBS might be used to assess fetal distress when fetal scalp sampling is not possible (Cunningham et al. 1993).

Fetal Activity Counting

DESCRIPTION OF PROCEDURE

The counting of fetal movements is an age-old assessment technique that has been shared throughout generations by women with childbirth wisdom. Many women discuss how each of their children differs in utero in terms of activity pattern. Although fetal activity (quickening) may be present as early as 16 weeks of gestation, the activity increases as the fetus grows and becomes more neurologically competent. The greatest normal fetal activity is usually reported between 29 and 30 weeks. After 40 weeks, movements tend to decrease slightly.

Several studies within the last two decades have attempted to quantify fetal activity and use it to predict perinatal outcome. Some practitioners call fetal movement studies "kick counts." Some studies have suggested that universal implementation of fetal activity charts kept by pregnant women can decrease unexpected stillbirth, whereas other studies have not been able to replicate any statistically significant difference (Coleman 1981; Davis 1987). Other researchers have strongly advocated either the Sandovsky approach (count four movements three times a day after meals) or the Cardiff method (count the first ten movements each morning). The major difference has seemed to center on which method a woman is most likely to perform on a regular basis. Freda and associates (1993) discovered that there was no difference in compliance between the two methods. The woman needs to be given clear instructions (see Teaching Guide) about the type of fetal activity counting desired.

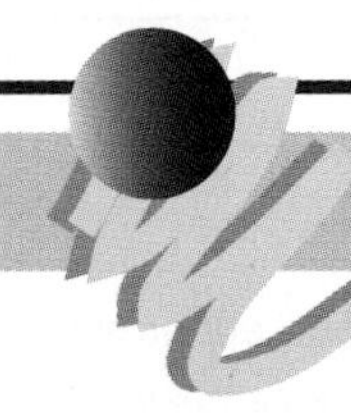

TEACHING GUIDE

ASSESSMENT OF FETAL STATUS: ULTRASOUND SCANNING, AMNIOCENTESIS, AND FETAL ACTIVITY COUNTING

TOPIC	*MAJOR CONCEPTS*
Reasons for assessment of the fetus during pregnancy • Mother's well-being • Baby's well-being	A number of assessment techniques are available today for evaluating the well-being and maturity of a developing fetus as well as the pregnant woman's well-being during pregnancy. Prenatal testing can alert your client and her care givers to problems that might be present related to the pregnancy or the fetus so that appropriate intervention can be initiated if needed.
Fetal movement counts	Fetal movements are usually first felt between 18 and 20 weeks' gestation; as the baby grows, the movements become stronger and more regular. Most babies move at least ten times in a 12-hour period. The amount of movement your client feels may vary and be influenced by the time of day (babies have sleep and awake periods in the uterus) and the level of the woman's activity. A change in fetal activity (increase or decrease) should be reported to her health care provider. Your client may be asked to keep a record of her baby's activity for continuing evaluation. This assessment of the well-being of the baby can easily be done in the client's home. Sometimes the woman is asked to keep a time record of either four fetal movements three times a day after meals (the Sandovsky method) or the first ten movements felt each morning (the Cardiff method). Instruct your client to lie on her side and place her fingers over her abdomen to feel the baby's movements; noting the time she begins, counting the number of movements requested, and noting the time that number is reached. It may take only 15 to 20 minutes or a couple of hours to feel the number of movements requested. The results should then be reported to her health care provider.

Continued on facing page

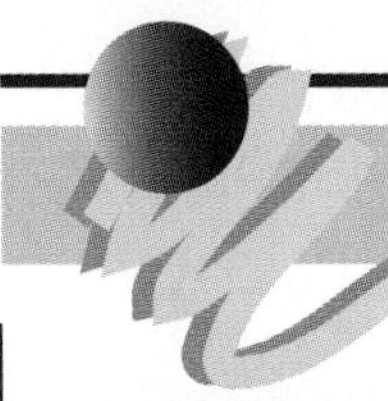

TEACHING GUIDE Continued

ASSESSMENT OF FETAL STATUS: ULTRASOUND SCANNING, AMNIOCENTESIS, AND FETAL ACTIVITY COUNTING

TOPICS	*MAJOR CONCEPTS*
Ultrasound scanning • Can usually reassure that baby is developing normally • Confirms due date	Ultrasound examination uses high-frequency sound waves to create an image of the developing fetus and placenta in the uterus. This is a safe technique that is used to determine whether the baby is developing normally and growing as it should, to identify whether a multiple gestation is present (twins, triplets), or to help confirm the gestational age of the baby and your client's due date. An ultrasound scan can be done at any time during pregnancy.
• Bladder needs to be full	Before the test, instruct your client to allow her bladder to become full, as it serves as a landmark on the scan and raises the uterus out of the pelvis for better viewing. She will need to drink at least 1 quart of water (4 glasses) in the 2 hours before the examination.
• Procedure is painless • Scanner moves on outside of abdomen • Image will be on monitor screen	The ultrasound procedure is painless, but sometimes it is uncomfortable because of the full bladder. Instruct your client to lie on her back on the examining room table; a gel is spread over the abdomen to allow the ultrasound scanner to move easily over the skin. As the scanner is moved across her abdomen, the image of the baby will be seen on the monitor of the ultrasound machine.
Amniocentesis • Sample of fluid is taken to examine fetal cells	An amniocentesis is a procedure in which a sample of amniotic fluid is removed from the sac surrounding the fetus in the uterus. It is done between 16 and 20 weeks' gestation to examine fetal cells in the fluid to identify the presence of genetic diseases or abnormalities of the fetus. Later in pregnancy, amniocentesis is performed to assess the maturity of the fetal lungs. It is possible to determine the sex of the baby from an amniocentesis; however, that alone is not the reason to do one.

Continued on following page

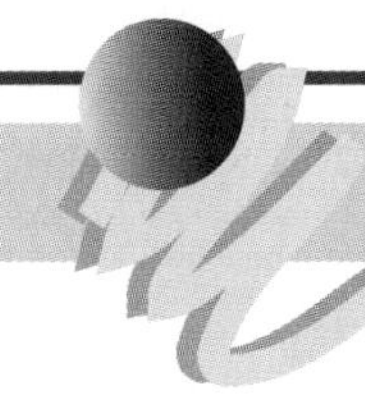

TEACHING GUIDE Continued

ASSESSMENT OF FETAL STATUS: ULTRASOUND SCANNING, AMNIOCENTESIS, AND FETAL ACTIVITY COUNTING

TOPIC	*MAJOR CONCEPTS*
Amniocentesis *(Cont'd)*	Ask your client to empty the bladder and get comfortable. An ultrasound scan is first used to locate the baby, the placenta, and a pocket of amniotic fluid. The patient's skin is cleansed with an antiseptic solution. A local anesthetic may be used to numb the skin. A needle is inserted through the abdominal wall into the uterus and amniotic sac. A small amount of amniotic fluid is withdrawn into a syringe. Sometimes slight pressure is felt at this time. The fluid is placed in a test tube and sent to a laboratory for testing. After the procedure, the woman may feel some soreness or cramping; however, instruct your client to notify her care provider immediately if she notices any bleeding, leaking of amniotic fluid, signs of infection, persistent uterine contractions, or decreased fetal movement. There are advantages and disadvantages of this procedure. The advantages include the information gained from the test; the disadvantages include risks of rupture of the membranes, hemorrhage, preterm labor, fetal trauma, infection, and isoimmunization for an Rh-negative woman. These complications are less than 1 percent, however.

Teaching Aids

1. Chart for fetal movement counting
2. Posters or illustrations showing technique for ultrasound scan and amniocentesis

Increasing Your Teaching Effectiveness

Your success in teaching a woman about prenatal fetal assessment tests will be enhanced by using the following approaches:

1. Establish a comfortable rapport with the woman and identify her knowledge of the reason that she may need to have fetal testing done.
2. Give her the information she needs in a clear, concise, and honest manner; use visual aids whenever possible to increase the clarity of the information you give.
3. Ask her if she has questions; ask her to repeat her understanding of the information you have presented.
4. Identify her feelings and concerns about the need for prenatal fetal testing; allow her to express her emotions; offer reassurance and support.

BENEFITS AND RISKS

The major advantage of fetal activity monitoring is that it is a low-technology intervention that is performed by the pregnant woman and even helps her become more aware of the uniqueness of her intrauterine fetus. The disadvantages are the lack of clear association with perinatal outcome and the need to perform such monitoring regularly before fetal jeopardy is suspected so that a healthy baseline of activity can be established. Fetal movement counting is also discussed in Chapter 26.

REASONS FOR USE

Throughout pregnancy, a woman begins to recognize a normal pattern of movement or activity for her baby. These movements will deviate from this established pattern when the fetus is in distress, which often serves as the first indicator that something is wrong. Counting and recording fetal movement enables the woman to identify a normal activity pattern for her fetus that can serve as a baseline and to identify deviations from the normal pattern should they be suspected. The woman should contact her health care provider if she notices no fetal movement for 8 hours, feels less than ten movements in 12 hours, or experiences a sudden increase in violent movements followed by decreased activity.

Future Methods for Fetal Surveillance

As mentioned earlier, high-technology interventions such as amniocentesis or CVS often lead to high levels of anxiety and apprehension for the childbearing couple. In some areas of the country, special hospital units exist solely to perform fetal assessment procedures (Curtis et al. 1989; Willson 1991; Sabey and Clark 1992; Gebauer and Lowe 1993; Inglis et al. 1993).

A couple may occasionally ask why it is not possible to simply take a blood sample from the mother and assess the fetus indirectly. In the future, this may be possible. Sophisticated biochemical screening is being explored so that, like the MSAFP test, fetal assessment testing could be performed with less intervention but, it is hoped, with reasonable sensitivity and specificity (Drugan et al. 1992; Holzgreve et al. 1992). Even today, there is evidence that some fetal cells may be extricated from maternal serum. It can be expected that as knowledge increases about the intrauterine environment, changes will become apparent in the clinical assessment of the intrauterine conceptus.

Implications for Research

The following questions are examples of those that could serve as the basis for inquiry for nursing research related to human intrauterine development.

- What is the level of knowledge of pregnant women and their partners regarding fetal development in each of the three trimesters?
- What do expectant parents know about the environmental teratogens that could influence the healthy development of the fetus?
- What health behaviors are altered by pregnant women to facilitate the healthy development of the fetus?
- Does the use of ultrasound imaging enhance parents' understanding of fetal development and encourage the implementation of health behaviors during pregnancy?

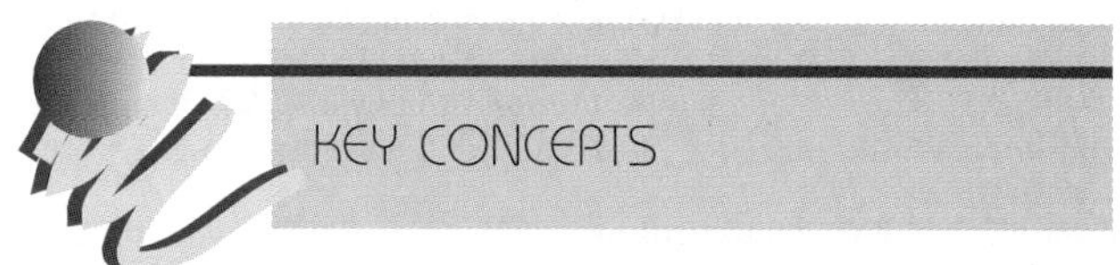

KEY CONCEPTS

- ▼ The process of conception is dependent on several sophisticated physiologic events of the body, including gametogenesis, fertilization, and implantation.
- ▼ The normal growth and development of the intrauterine conceptus includes an orderly progression through the stages of zygote, blastomere, morula, blastocyst, embryo, and fetus.
- ▼ The period of oogenesis is the most vulnerable period for threats from teratogenic agents.
- ▼ Most birth defects are multifactorial in etiology, not the result of exposure to drugs or chemicals.
- ▼ Although drugs and chemicals account for less than 5 percent of causative agents for congenital malformations, much research is focused on them since they are potentially avoidable.
- ▼ The fetus during the second and third trimesters remains at risk from external insults, including nicotine, alcohol, illicit drugs, and malnutrition.
- ▼ No perfect fetal assessment modality exists. All current techniques have both advantages and disadvantages. Yet, appropriately used, these modalities can add insight into fetal well-being and facilitate interventions when necessary.

References

American Academy of Pediatrics, Committee on Genetics. (1991). Maternal serum alpha-fetoprotein screening. *Pediatrics,* 88 (6), 1282–1283.

Berkowitz, R. (1993). Should every pregnant woman undergo ultrasonography? *The New England Journal of Medicine,* 329 (12), 874–875.

Blackburn, S., and Loper, D. (1992). *Maternal, fetal, and neonatal physiology.* Philadelphia: W. B. Saunders.

Boston Women's Book Collective. (1991). *Our bodies, ourselves.* New York: Simon & Schuster.

Briggs, G., Freeman, R., Yaffe, S. (1994). *Drugs in pregnancy and lactation* (4th ed.). Baltimore: Williams & Wilkins.

Burton, B. K., Schulz, C. J., Burd, L. I. (1992). Limb anomalies associated with CVS. *Obstetrics and Gynecology,* 79 (5), 726–730.

Callen, P. W. (1994). *Ultrasonography in obstetrics and gynecology* (3rd ed.). Philadelphia: W. B. Saunders.

Carlson, D., and Platt, L. (1992). Ultrasound detection of genetic anomalies. *Journal of Reproductive Medicine,* 37 (5), 419–426.

Catanzarite, V., and Maida, C. (1992). Practical sonography. *Contemporary Obstetrics and Gynecology,* 37 (9), 44–68.

Cherry, S. H., and Merkatz, I. R. (1991). *Complications of pregnancy: Medical, surgical, gynecologic, psychosocial, and perinatal* (4th ed.). Baltimore: Williams & Wilkins.

Coleman, C. (1981). Fetal movement counts: An assessment tool. *Journal of Nuclear Medicine,* 26 (1), 15–23.

Creasy, R., and Resnik, R. (1994). *Maternal-fetal medicine: Principles and practice* (3rd ed.). Philadelphia: W. B. Saunders.

Cundiff, J. (1990). Umbilical artery Doppler flow studies during pregnancy. *Journal of Obstetric, Gynecologic, and Neonatal Nursing,* 19 (6), 475–481.

Cunningham, F. G., MacDonald, P. C., Gant, N. F., Leveno, K. J., Gilstrap, L. C. III. (1993). *Williams obstetrics* (19th ed.). Norwalk, CT: Appleton & Lange.

Curtis, P., Evens, S., Resnick, J., Thompson, C. J., Rimer, R., Hisley, J. (1989). Patterns of uterine contractions and prolonged uterine activity using three methods of breast stimulation for CST. *Obstetrics and Gynecology,* 73 (4), 631–638.

Davis, L. (1987). Daily fetal movement counting. *Journal of Nuclear Medicine,* 32 (1), 11–19.

Drugan, A., O'Brien, J. E., Gambino, R. S., Evans, M. I. (1992). Prenatal biochemical screening. *Journal of Reproductive Medicine,* 37 (5), 403–409.

Evans, M. I., Drugan, A., Koppitch, F. C. III, Zador, I. E., Sacks, A. S., Sokol, R. J. (1989). Genetic diagnosis in the first trimester: The norm for the 1990s. *American Journal of Obstetrics and Gynecology,* 160 (6), 1332–1338.

Evans, M. I., Dvorin, E., O'Brien, J. E., Moody, J. L., Drugan, A. (1992a). Alpha-fetoprotein and biochemical screening. In M. I. Evans (Ed.). *Reproductive risks and prenatal diagnosis.* Norwalk, CT: Appleton & Lange.

Evans, M., Johnson, M., Holgrene, W. (1992b). Chorionic villus sampling. *Journal of Reproductive Medicine,* 37 (5), 389–394.

Ewigman, B. G., Crane, J. P., Frigloetto, S. D., LeFevre, M. L., Bain, R. P., McNellis, D. (1993). Effect of prenatal ultrasound screening on perinatal outcome. *The New England Journal of Medicine,* 329 (12), 821–826.

Food and Drug Administration. (1980). Pregnancy risk categories. *Federal Register,* 44, 37434–37467.

Food and Drug Administration. (1991). *FDA background: Current and useful information from the Food and Drug Administration.* Washington, D.C.: Author.

Freda, M., Mikhail, M., Mazloom, E., Polizzotto, R., Damus, K., Merkatz, I. (1993). Fetal movement counting: Which method? *Maternal-Child Nursing,* 18 (6), 314–321.

Fresquez, M., and Collins, D. (1992). Advancement of the nursing role in antepartum fetal evaluation. *Journal of Perinatal Neonatal Nursing,* 5 (4), 16–22.

Gebauer, C., and Lowe, N. (1993). The biophysical profile: Antepartal assessment of fetal well-being. *Journal of Obstetric, Gynecologic, and Neonatal Nursing,* 22 (2), 115–124.

Gegor, C. (1992). Obstetric ultrasound: Who should perform sonograms? *Birth,* 19 (2), 92–99.

Gegor, C., and Paine, L. (1992). Antepartum fetal assessment techniques. *Journal of Perinatal Neonatal Nursing,* 5 (4), 1–15.

Gegor, C. L., Paine, L. L., Johnson, T. R. (1991). Antepartum fetal assessment. *Journal of Nurse-Midwifery,* 36 (3), 153–167.

Heidrich, S., and Cranley, M. (1989). Effects of fetal movement ultrasound scans and amniocentesis on maternal fetal attachment. *Nursing Research,* 38 (2), 81–84.

Henry, G., and Miller, W. (1992). Early amniocentesis. *Journal of Reproductive Medicine,* 37 (5), 396–402.

Holzgreve, W., Garritsen, H., and Ganshirt-Ahlert, D. (1992). Fetal cells in the maternal circulation. *Journal of Reproductive Medicine,* 37 (5), 410–418.

Inglis, S. R., Druzin, M. L., Wagner, W. E., Kogut, E. (1993). The use of vibroacoustic stimulation during the abnormal or equivocal biophysical profile. *Obstetrics and Gynecology,* 82 (3), 371–374.

Lunell, N. O., and Nylund, L. (1992). Uteroplacental blood flow. *Clinical Obstetrics and Gynecology,* 35 (1), 108–118.

Merritt, C. (1992). Obstetric ultrasound. *Birth,* 19 (2), 100–101.

Moore, K. L., and Persaud, T. V. N. (1993). *The developing human* (5th ed.). Philadelphia: W. B. Saunders.

Moore, K. L., Persaud, T. V. N., Shiota, K. (1994). *Color atlas of clinical embryology.* Philadelphia: W. B. Saunders.

Niebyl, J. (1988). *Drugs in pregnancy.* Philadelphia: Lea & Febiger.

Nilsson, L., and Hamberger, L. (1990). *A child is born* (p. 75). New York: Delacorte Press/Seymour Lawrence.

Rothman, B. (1987). *Tentative pregnancy.* New York: Doubleday.

Sabey, P., and Clark, S. (1992). Establishing an antepartum testing unit. *Journal of Perinatal Neonatal Nursing* 5 (4), 23–32.

Sadler, T. (1995). *Langman's medical embryology* (7th ed.). Baltimore: Williams & Wilkins.

Seeds, J. (1992). Who should perform sonograms? *Birth,* 19 (2), 101–102.

Speroff, L., Glass, R., Kase, N. (1994). *Clinical endocrinology and infertility.* (5th ed.). Baltimore: Williams & Wilkins.

Staff. (1992). Doppler ultrasound in obstetrics. *Lancet,* 339, 1083–1084.

Stringer, M., Librizzi, R., Weiner, S. (1991). Establishing a prenatal genetic diagnosis. *Maternal-Child Nursing,* 16 (3), 152–156.

Thornton, K. (1992). Principles of ultrasound. *Journal of Reproductive Medicine,* 37 (1), 27–32.

USPDI. (1997). *Drug information for the health care provider* (14th ed.). Maryland: U. S. Pharmacopeia Convention.

Vander, A., Sherman, J., Luciano, D. (1989). *Human physiology: The mechanisms of body function.* New York: McGraw-Hill.

Wapner, R. J., Johnson, A., Davis, G., Uban, A., Morgan, P., Jackson, L. (1993). Prenatal diagnosis in twin gestations: A comparison between second-trimester amniocentesis and first-trimester chorionic villus sampling. *Obstetrics and Gynecology,* 82 (1), 49–56.

Wilson, J., and Foster, D. (1992). *Textbook of endocrinology.* Philadelphia: W. B. Saunders.

Willson, N. (1991). A legal/ethical issue in prenatal diagnosis. *TexGene,* 2 (2), 8.

Chapter 16

Physiologic Changes of Pregnancy

Elaine Zwelling

> The output of hormones is colossal. For instance, at any time during an average menstrual cycle, the maximum daily output of one key hormone, progesterone, would be a few milligrams a day; towards the end of pregnancy this rises to as much as 250 mg a day. While progesterone output increases 50–60 times, that of another key hormone, estrogen, increases 20–30 times. . . . No organ escapes the effects of these biochemical alterations.
>
> DR. MIRIAM STOPPARD (JOHNSTON 1994)

HIGHLIGHTS

- ▼ Diagnosis of Pregnancy
- ▼ Presumptive Signs of Pregnancy
- ▼ Probable Signs of Pregnancy
- ▼ Positive Signs of Pregnancy
- ▼ Physiology of Pregnancy
- ▼ Nursing Practice
- ▼ Procedure 16–1: Leopold Maneuvers
- ▼ Procedure 16–2: Assisting with Pelvic Examination
- ▼ Procedure 16–3: Testing Urine with Urinary Dipstick
- ▼ Risk Management
- ▼ Implications for Research

Pregnancy has been a source of fascination and wonder for centuries. This fascination may be seen in paintings and sculptures of pregnant women, in films or television, and in the glances of people passing a pregnant woman on the street. Yet there is an interesting contrast between the portrayals of pregnancy in any medium and the reality of the experience. The true experience of pregnancy is a series of slowly unfolding physical changes accompanied by many highs and many lows. Pregnancy is not always the dramatic or humorous experience portrayed in the movies, but it can be a joyous growth experience. It is an all-encompassing life event identified variously as a developmental crisis, a normal transitional event, and a maturational challenge.

The physiologic changes of pregnancy result from a response of the woman's body to normal hormonal changes, fetal growth, and maternal adaptation to both of these. All organs of a woman's body change in some way during pregnancy to adapt to the needs of the developing fetus. These physical changes and the resultant symptoms would be warnings of illness or abnormal pathology in any state other than pregnancy. Pregnancy is not

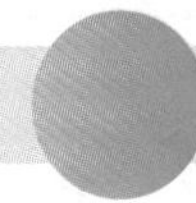

DEFINITIONS

Ballottement—A maneuver done with palpation to test for a floating object in the body; in pregnancy done during vaginal or abdominal examination to detect the rebound movement of the fetus; light tapping or pushing of the fingers causes the fetus to move away and then return to touch the examiner's fingers.

Braxton Hicks contractions—Mild, painless, irregular uterine contractions that occur normally throughout pregnancy in response to uterine growth and stretching; may occur more frequently as pregnancy progresses, but do not progress or dilate the cervix like true labor contractions.

Chadwick's sign—Bluish coloration of the vaginal mucosa caused by increased vascularity of pregnancy; observed at about 4 weeks' gestation.

Fetal age—The age of the fetus as calculated in weeks from the time of conception.

Fundus—The upper portion of the uterus.

Gestation—The period of fetal development from the time of fertilization of the ovum to birth.

Goodell's sign—The softening of the cervix and vagina that occurs around the second month of pregnancy.

Gravida—A woman who is pregnant.

Hegar's sign—The softening of the lower uterine segment that occurs around the second month of pregnancy.

Leopold maneuvers—A series of abdominal palpation maneuvers that give information regarding fetal presentation, position, presenting part, attitude, and descent.

LMP—The date of the first day of the last menstrual period.

McDonald's sign—The ease with which the body of the uterus can be flexed against the cervix; a physical change that can be diagnostic of pregnancy.

Parity—The number of pregnancies that have been carried to viability.

Quickening—The first maternal perception of fetal movement, usually between the 16th and 20th weeks of pregnancy.

Viability—The period of gestation at which the fetus is capable of sustaining life outside the uterus; now considered to be between 20 and 24 weeks' gestation.

an illness but a state of wellness. In pregnancy, the changes are a result of normal physiology.

The length of pregnancy is important to the woman and her family as a factor that guides their adaptation and planning. It is even more important to the woman's health care providers, who use the length of pregnancy as a guide for assessing normal progress and fetal development and for planning care. A full-term pregnancy lasts 280 days or 40 weeks. This represents nine calendar or ten lunar months. The period of pregnancy is divided into three equal trimesters; the first trimester includes the first through third months of pregnancy, the second trimester includes months 4 through 6, and the third trimester includes the seventh through ninth months. Each of these trimesters is characterized by predictable physical and emotional maternal changes and predictable patterns of fetal development.

DIAGNOSIS OF PREGNANCY

Presumptive Signs of Pregnancy

The woman is the first to suspect the diagnosis of pregnancy from the symptoms she experiences. Although these initial symptoms are indicative of pregnancy, they could be caused by other physical conditions and therefore are not positive. Presumptive or subjective symptoms need to be confirmed by further assessment (see Diagnosis of Pregnancy).

▼ **Amenorrhea.** The first sign of pregnancy experienced by the woman is likely to be a missed menstrual period. Although amenorrhea can indicate pregnancy in a healthy woman whose cycles are regular, it can be caused by other factors such as stress, nutritional status, excessive exercise, or gynecologic problems.

▼ **Nausea and Vomiting.** Nausea and vomiting are symptoms noticed early in the pregnancy by about half of all pregnant women. These symptoms are caused by elevated levels of human chorionic gonadotropin (hCG) and altered carbohydrate metabolism and usually subside by 12 weeks of pregnancy.

▼ **Breast Sensitivity.** Many women notice increased breast sensitivity, often accompanied by a tingling sensation in the nipples. This symptom may be the first to appear, even before the first

Diagnosis of Pregnancy

PRESUMPTIVE OR SUBJECTIVE SIGNS

- Amenorrhea
- Nausea and vomiting
- Breast sensitivity
- Urinary frequency
- Fatigue
- Weight gain
- Quickening

PROBABLE OR OBJECTIVE SIGNS

- Hegar's sign
- Goodell's sign
- McDonald's sign
- Chadwick's sign
- Fetal outline
- Ballottement
- Positive pregnancy test
- Abdominal changes
- Braxton Hicks contractions

POSITIVE OR DIAGNOSTIC SIGNS

- Fetal heart tones
- Uterine souffle
- Funic souffle
- Observed fetal movement
- Observation of fetus on ultrasound

missed menstrual period, and is caused by hormone-induced growth of the secretory ductal system in the breasts.

▼ **Urinary Symptoms.** Urinary symptoms, particularly frequency, occur in the first trimester and are caused by the pressure of the enlarging uterus on the bladder.

▼ **Fatigue.** Some women experience fatigue very early after conception and complain of not being able to get enough sleep. The fatigue is caused by the many hormonal changes of early pregnancy.

▼ **Weight Gain.** Weight gain may be a presumptive sign of pregnancy; however, the amount of weight gained in the first trimester is usually small and weight gain can be attributed to many factors other than pregnancy.

▼ **Quickening.** Quickening, the subjective perception of fetal movement or feeling of life, can be felt by most women between 16 and 20 weeks of gestation. It is perceived as a fluttering sensation that becomes stronger over time and at first may be confused with gastrointestinal peristalsis. A woman's ability to feel fetal movement is thought to be dependent on the size of the fetus in relation to the amount of amniotic fluid, the number and strength of fetal movements, and the extent to which the uterus is in contact with the anterior abdominal wall.

Probable Signs of Pregnancy

Probable or objective signs of pregnancy are those that can be observed by the health care provider. Although these signs are more indicative of pregnancy than presumptive symptoms, they still do not confirm pregnancy. Pelvic changes are usually the first observable signs that indicate pregnancy and can be observed on pelvic examination. They occur as a result of hormonal changes and increased vascular congestion.

CHANGES IN PELVIC STRUCTURES

Hegar's sign is the softening of the isthmus of the uterus in the lower uterine segment (Fig. 16–1), Goodell's sign is the softening of the cervix and vagina, and McDonald's sign is the easy flexion of the fundus of the uterus toward the cervix. These changes in consistency of the tissue can be palpated on pelvic examination.

Chadwick's sign is the purplish or bluish coloration of the cervix, vagina, and vulva caused by vasocongestion. The size and shape of the uterus begin to change early in pregnancy, as it progresses from a pear-shaped organ to a more globular shape. As the pregnancy progresses, the uterus enlarges and moves out of the bony pelvis.

FETAL OUTLINE AND BALLOTTEMENT

The fetal outline can be palpated easily by an examiner after 24 weeks' gestation. Although feeling fetal parts by doing Leopold maneuvers is strongly indicative of pregnancy, it is not positive confirmation.

Ballottement of the fetus can be felt on pelvic examination as an upward movement followed by a rebounding of the fetus elicited by tapping the cervix with two fingers (see Fig. 16–1).

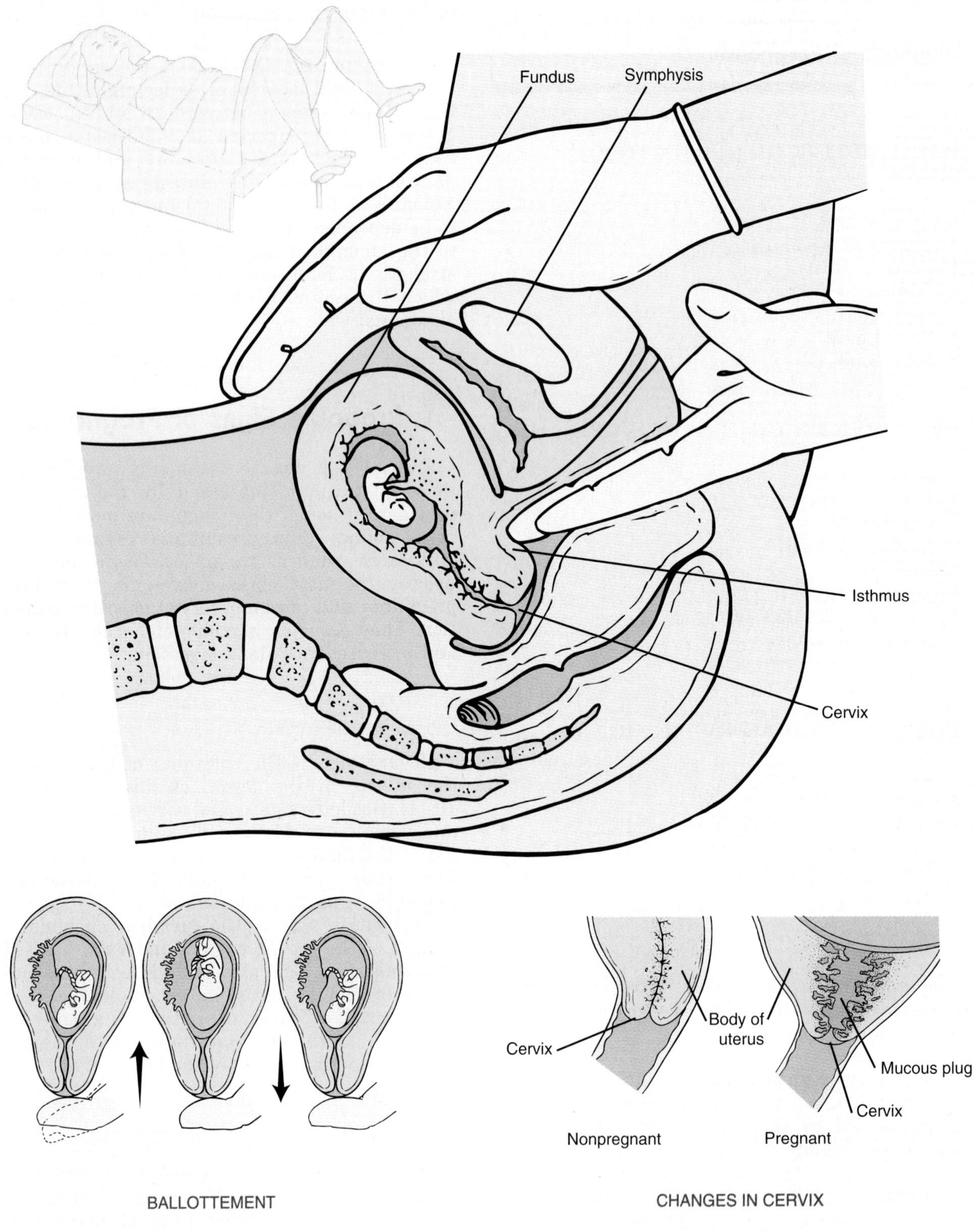

Figure 16–1
Bimanual examination is performed with the client in the lithotomy position, allowing the examiner to assess the cervix and palpate Hegar's sign. Ballottement, the upward rebounding of the fetus against the uterus, may also be tested.

PREGNANCY TESTS

Positive pregnancy tests are only a probable sign of pregnancy because although they suggest pregnancy, they are not considered absolute indicators. The similarity of hCG, secreted by the trophoblast, and luteinizing hormone (LH), secreted by the pituitary, may occasionally result in cross-reactions. It is also possible that other medical conditions could cause elevated hCG levels. There has been a significant increase in the number and variety of pregnancy tests that are available to the woman and her health care provider. Pregnancy testing can be done by the physician or nurse-midwife in a health care setting or by the woman in her home.

All pregnancy tests are based on the ability to detect hCG in maternal blood or urine, but today most tests are performed on the first urine specimen voided in the morning. hCG is secreted by the trophoblastic cells of the fertilized ovum shortly after conception, and it continues to rise after that time. A rapid increase in serum hCG values can be observed in the pregnant woman approximately 1 week after conception. A peak is reached 6 weeks after conception. Pregnancy tests can be used to detect normal or ectopic pregnancy, to predict threatened abortion, or to follow up spontaneous abortion. Unlike the pregnancy tests of previous years, today's tests can detect pregnancy long before the first missed menstrual period.

There are far too many pregnancy tests on the market today to discuss each one in this textbook. Pregnancy tests are either immunoassay tests based on the antigenic property of hCG or radioreceptor assay tests based on the use of radioiodine. All pregnancy tests fall into one of seven categories (Cunningham et al. 1993).

Latex agglutination inhibition (LAI) tests. Available as slide or tube tests; agglutination of latex particles is inhibited in the presence of urine containing hCG; positive pregnancy is indicated by a clear milky solution; accurate from 4 to 10 days after the first missed menstrual period (examples: Pregnosticon slide, Gravindex slide, Placentex tube test).

Hemagglutination inhibition (HAI) tests. Tube tests in which agglutination of red blood cells is inhibited in the presence of urine containing hCG; positive pregnancy is indicated by a ring at the bottom of the test tube formed by red cells settling to the bottom; most tests are accurate 4 days after the first missed menstrual period (the Neocept test gives accurate results at or before the missed period).

Radioreceptor assay (RRA) tests. Radioiodine-labeled hCG attaches to receptor cell membranes; a positive test indicated by the amount of free radiolabeled hCG measured in a cell membrane preparation; accurate at the time of the first missed menstrual period (example: Biocept G).

Beta subunit radioimmunoassay (RIA) tests. Radioiodinated hCG is added to urine or serum as an antigen to specific antibodies; a positive test is indicated by free radioiodinated hCG in the test solution; this is the most reliable test as it can identify the beta subunit of hCG; accurate as early as 6 days before the first missed menstrual period (examples: Beta Tec, Chorio Quant).

Direct agglutination tests. Two different monoclonal antibodies are introduced into urine; a positive test results if agglutination or ring formation occurs in response to the presence of hCG; accurate results are possible at or before the first menstrual period.

Enzyme-linked immunosorbent assay (ELISA) tests. Complex monoclonal anti-hCG with enzymes is used to bind with hCG in urine; a positive test is indicated by a visible color change; accurate results are possible about 4 days before the first missed menstrual period (examples: Pregnospia, Tandem ICON, Confidot).

Home pregnancy tests. The many tests now available over the counter for home use are based on either hemagglutination inhibition tube tests or enzyme immunoassay tests and are performed on a first-voided urine sample; the latest kits can be used within a few days of a missed period and give results in less than 30 minutes (examples: e.p.t., Confidot, Fact, Clearblue Easy, Daisy-2). Accuracy is equal to that of the less sensitive hemagglutination tests. A false-positive rate of 5 percent and a false-negative rate of approximately 20 percent have been reported. Almost one third of pregnant women have used a home pregnancy test kit at least once during their pregnancy (Fig. 16–2). Women use home pregnancy tests because they are fast, convenient, and confidential. Whether home pregnancy testing encourages or discourages early prenatal care is controversial. The woman should be encouraged to seek care, despite having identified a pregnancy herself with a home test.

Knowledge regarding the type of pregnancy test used, how it detects hCG levels, the sensitivity of the test, when after conception it accurately yields positive results, and the woman's medical and gynecologic history is essential in interpreting the results of a given pregnancy test. The nurse must either read the package insert for the test used or call the laboratory at which the test was done to obtain information about the test. Data about the woman's menstrual cycle and previous pregnancy history are needed when interpreting a pregnancy test. Information about factors that could influence the results of the pregnancy test is also im-

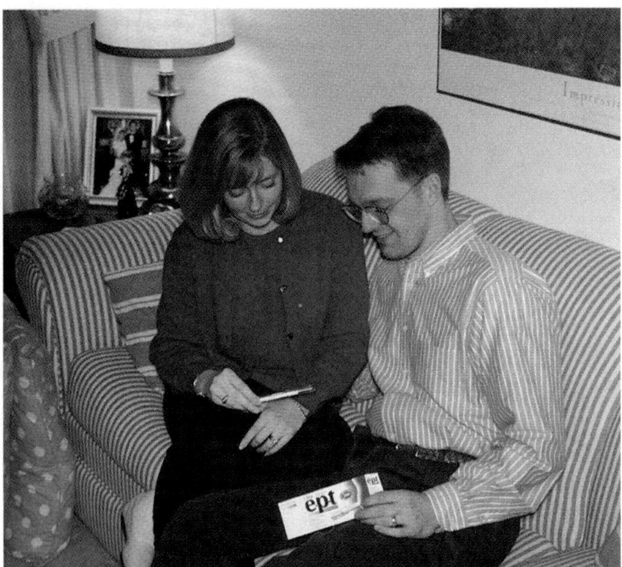

Figure 16–2

Home pregnancy tests enable a woman to determine whether she is pregnant very soon after missing a menstrual period • However, to decrease the chance of a false-negative result, she should wait 6 to 9 days after the missed period to use the test • Benefits of home pregnancy tests include the convenience of doing the test at home and sharing the news with her partner.

portant, such as how the specimen was collected or whether the woman was using any medications or drugs that might alter the test results. If there is a question about the results of a pregnancy test, it should be repeated.

ABDOMINAL CHANGES

Abdominal changes occur gradually in the first trimester as the growing uterus begins to move out of the pelvis. Abdominal enlargement may be earlier and more pronounced in the multigravida than in the primigravida. Although abdominal changes are a good indicator of pregnancy, particularly when accompanied by continuing amenorrhea, they could be a result of pathology, which needs to be ruled out.

Uterine contractions, called Braxton Hicks contractions, can be palpated through the abdominal wall during the second trimester. These painless contractions occur throughout pregnancy and may not be perceived by the woman until the end of the third trimester. These contractions facilitate muscle tone and uterine blood flow but do not cause cervical dilatation.

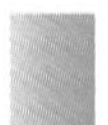

Positive Signs of Pregnancy

Only three signs are considered to be positive or diagnostic indicators of pregnancy.

FETAL HEART TONES

The auscultation of fetal heart tones by the examiner gives positive confirmation of pregnancy. Fetal heart tones usually cannot be heard with a fetoscope until 16 to 20 weeks' gestation. It may be possible to pick up the fetal heartbeat earlier by using an electronic Doppler fetoscope or fetal monitor.

UTERINE SOUNDS

Additional uterine sounds may be heard as well. The uterine souffle is a sound made by the rushing of maternal blood going to the placenta. The rate of this sound is the same as that of the woman's pulse. The funic souffle is caused by fetal blood moving through the umbilical cord. This sound is heard at the same rate as the fetal heart tones, between 120 and 160 beats per minute.

FETAL MOVEMENT

Fetal movement observed or palpated through the abdominal wall by an examiner is the second sign that gives positive confirmation of pregnancy, even though the woman has probably been feeling fetal movement before this time. This objective evaluation of fetal movement can usually be made around 16 to 20 weeks' gestation. Observation of the fetus by ultrasonography is also positive confirmation of the pregnancy. The gestational sac can be visualized with ultrasound around 6 weeks' gestation (4 weeks after conception); fetal breathing movements (FBMs) can be observed around 11 weeks' gestation; the fetal heart can be seen beating between 8 and 12 weeks; and the skeletal form of the fetus and fetal movement can be viewed around 12 to 14 weeks (see Fig. 15–7).

Calculating the Delivery Date

EXPECTED DATE OF CONFINEMENT

Once the pregnancy has been confirmed, the woman and her health care provider are both interested in knowing the expected date of confinement (EDC) or due date. In some health care settings the term expected date of delivery (EDD) is preferred. This date is important to the woman and her family in guiding their expectations and preparations for the baby. It is essential information for the physician or nurse-midwife to use as a parameter for assessing the progression of fetal development and physical changes manifested by the woman throughout the pregnancy. The average length of pregnancy is 280 days, 9 calendar months, or 10 lunar months. The expected delivery date can be calculated in several ways.

NÄGELE'S RULE

The first method, called Nägele's rule, is based on the woman's menstrual cycle. The first day of the last menstrual period (LMP) is identified, 3 months are subtracted, and then 7 days are added to that date. For example:

First day of LMP → January 14, 1997

Subtract 3 months → October 14, 1997

Add 7 days → October 21, 1997

If the pregnancy spans more than one given year, a year must be added to the date. Also, changing the months to numbers may make calculation easier for some people. For example:

First day of LMP → 8-26-1997

Subtract 3 months; add 1 year → 5-26-1998

Add 7 days → 6-02-1998

Accurate use of Nägele's rule requires that the woman have a regular 28-day menstrual cycle. A cycle that is irregular or deviates from 28 days probably indicates that she is not ovulating 14 days before the start of menstruation and makes the date identified by Nägele's rule inaccurate. If this is the case, it may be desirable to use additional methods for calculating the EDC.

GESTATIONAL WHEEL OR CALCULATOR

A gestational wheel is used as a quick and easy method for identifying the EDC (see Improving Your Practice in Chapter 15). The wheel is turned so that the arrow labeled "last menses began" points to the first day of the woman's LMP. The term arrow found at 40 weeks' gestation on the wheel then points to the expected date of delivery. This wheel can also be used postpartally to determine the woman's actual length of gestation or the infant's gestational age. Information from ultrasound readings and fundal height measurements can also help in determining the date of delivery. A new gestational calculator is also now available to determine the EDC.

PHYSIOLOGY OF PREGNANCY

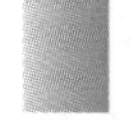

Endocrine System

The endocrine system plays a critical role in the early initiation and later maintenance of the pregnancy. In addition to the endocrine organs (the thyroid, pituitary, adrenals, and pancreas), the corpus luteum and placenta have major functions in the hormonal control of the pregnancy, development of the fetus, and return to the nonpregnant state during the postpartal period (Cunningham et al. 1993; Guyton and Hall 1996).

CORPUS LUTEUM AND MATERNAL-FETAL-PLACENTAL UNIT

The corpus luteum and maternal-fetal-placental unit serve as the primary regulators of endocrine function during pregnancy. After conception, the pituitary inhibits the formation of new ovarian follicles, which maintain the existing corpus luteum. This change in the usual hypothalamic-pituitary-ovarian cycle takes place immediately after conception. Human chorionic gonadotropin, a glycoprotein that is similar to LH, also functions to prevent the normal involution of the corpus luteum at the end of the female sexual cycle. Secreted by the syncytial trophoblast cells of the blastocyst, hCG reaches its peak concentration at 8 to 10 weeks of gestation and then begins to decline as placental function takes over. In the first 8 to 10 weeks of pregnancy, hCG causes the corpus luteum to secrete even larger quantities of its usual sex hormones, progesterone and estrogens (Fig. 16–3). These hormones cause the endometrium to continue to develop and store large

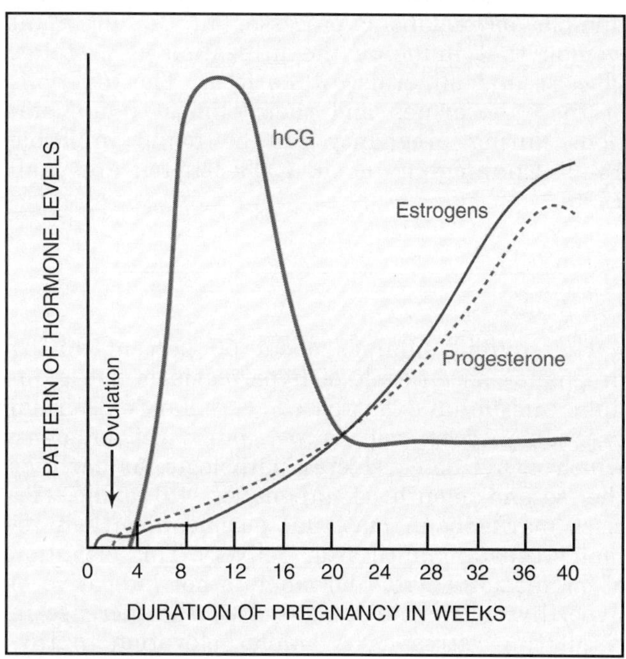

Figure 16–3

Hormone levels change dramatically during different stages of pregnancy. (Adapted from Guyton, A. C., and Hall, J. E. (1996). *Textbook of Medical Physiology* (9th ed.) (p. 1037). Philadelphia: W. B. Saunders.)

amounts of nutrients in preparation for the implantation of the blastocyst. Estrogens and progesterone promote development of the embryo and maintain the pregnancy until the placenta begins to function as the primary organ of pregnancy. The corpus luteum also secretes relaxin, which is responsible for softening and increased mobility of the joints.

After the first 8 to 10 weeks, the maternal-fetal-placental unit begins to function and takes over the secretion of estrogen, progesterone, hCG, human placental lactogen (hPL), also known as human chorionic somatomammotropin, and prostaglandin. The production of estrogen increases to a level about 30 times normal by the end of pregnancy. This hyperestrogenic state of the pregnant woman terminates abruptly after delivery of the fetus and placenta. Estrogens cause proliferation, resulting in the enlargement of the uterus, breasts, and external genitalia; relaxation of pelvic ligaments and joints; and increase in vascularity, causing vasodilation. The secretion of progesterone increases about tenfold as the pregnancy progresses, reaching a level of 250 mg/day. Progesterone is essential in maintaining the pregnancy, decreasing the contractility of the uterus, and helping to prepare the breasts for lactation. In addition to its other functions, hCG is thought to have a role in the sexual differentiation of the male embryo, for it stimulates the testes to synthesize testosterone throughout pregnancy until the time of birth. The amount of hPL secreted by the placenta also increases throughout the pregnancy. It promotes fetal growth by stimulating a number of metabolic processes in the pregnant woman that influence the utilization of proteins, glucose, and minerals by the fetus. The functions of these hormones and their clinical manifestations during pregnancy can be found in Table 16–1 (Cunningham et al. 1993; Guyton and Hall 1996).

THYROID

The thyroid enlarges about 50 percent during pregnancy as a result of hyperplasia of the glandular tissue and increased vascularity. Normal pregnancy does not cause goiter development, which would be considered pathologic. As early as the second month of pregnancy, thyroxine (T_4) rises markedly in maternal plasma and then remains constant until after delivery. This elevation of circulating thyroid hormone is not indicative of hyperthyroidism but is caused by the increase in circulating estrogens. A similar elevation in thyroid hormone levels has been observed in nonpregnant women who take oral contraceptives. The basal metabolic rate (BMR) increases progressively up to as much as 25 percent during pregnancy. Most of the increase in oxygen consumption is a result of the metabolic activity of the fetal-placental unit. Although blood studies and the elevated BMR would normally indicate hyperthyroidism, clinical symptoms do not appear (see Table 16–1) (Cunningham et al. 1993; Guyton and Hall 1996).

PARATHYROID

The parathyroid glands also enlarge during pregnancy, especially if the woman has a calcium-deficient diet. Enlargement of these glands causes calcium absorption from the woman's bones, which maintains the normal calcium ion concentration in maternal extracellular fluids as the fetus removes calcium for its own bones. Parathyroid hormone concentrations in maternal plasma decrease during the first trimester and then increase progressively through the remainder of pregnancy. This increase represents a physiologic hyperparathyroidism of pregnancy that results in an increased supply of calcium and vitamin D for the fetus (Cunningham et al. 1993; Guyton and Hall 1996).

PITUITARY

The pituitary gland enlarges during pregnancy, with the greatest enlargement occurring during the last month. The anterior lobe increases up to 50 percent in size; the posterior lobe does not show a marked increase. The hormones of both the anterior and posterior lobes play a number of important roles throughout the pregnancy (see Table 16–1). The most significant changes in anterior lobe hormone production related to pregnancy include suppression of follicle-stimulating hormone (FSH) and LH and an increase in prolactin. The posterior lobe secretes oxytocin during labor and lactation (Cunningham et al. 1993; Guyton and Hall 1996).

PANCREAS

During the first trimester of pregnancy, the production of insulin decreases in response to a drop in maternal glucose stores caused by early fetal development. In the second and third trimesters, insulin production rises at a steady rate until term. This increasing demand for insulin is triggered by the hormones secreted by the maternal-fetal-placental unit as well as increased cortisol production by the adrenals. Estrogen, progesterone, hCG, hPL, and cortisol all decrease the ability of the pregnant woman to utilize insulin. The placenta also produces insulinase, an enzyme that counteracts maternal insulin. The resultant diabetogenic effect of pregnancy ensures an adequate supply of glucose to the maternal-fetal-placental unit. The islets of Langerhans in the pancreas are usually able to meet the increased demand for insulin during pregnancy and maintain an acceptable balance between glucose and insulin. If increased insulin production does not occur, the woman may develop gestational diabetes (see Chapter 21) (Cunningham et al. 1993).

ADRENAL GLANDS

In normal pregnancy little structural change occurs in the maternal adrenal glands. An increase in the circulating levels of cortisol is thought to result from lowered renal excretion and estrogen stimulation. In early pregnancy the levels of circulating adrenocorticotropic hormone (ACTH) are reduced, followed by a rise as pregnancy progresses. The cause of this shift is not completely understood. Increased levels of aldosterone are also noted during pregnancy. Aldosterone levels are even higher if the woman is given a sodium-restricted diet. This increase is thought to be the body's protective response to the increased sodium excretion associated with progesterone (Cunningham et al. 1993).

Reproductive System

The reproductive system is most directly affected during pregnancy. All organs change in some way in both structure and function and then return to prepregnancy functioning after the pregnancy is over.

UTERUS

▼ **Size.** The size of the uterus increases dramatically throughout the pregnancy. It is transformed from an organ the size of a small pear into a thin-walled muscular organ that is large enough to accommodate the fetus, placenta, and amniotic fluid. In its nonpregnant state, the uterus measures 2 inches (4 cm) by 4 inches (6.5 cm), weighs approximately 2 ounces (60 to 70 g), and has the capacity to hold about 10 mL of fluid; by term the uterus measures 10 inches (24 cm) by 12 inches (32 cm), weighs approximately 2.2 pounds (1200 g), and has a total volume of about 5000 mL, although it can accommodate 20 L or more. These changes account for a 500- to 1000-fold greater capacity than in the nonpregnant state. This significant change in size is the result of stretching and marked hypertrophy of existing muscle cells, as well as the development of some new muscle cells (hyperplasia). An accumulation of fibrous tissue, particularly in the external muscle layer, as well as a considerable increase in elastic tissue also takes place and adds to the strength of the uterine wall. There is also a great increase in the size and number of blood vessels and lymphatics to accommodate the circulatory requirements of pregnancy. By the end of pregnancy, one sixth of the total maternal blood volume is contained within the uterine vascular system. During the first few months of the pregnancy the uterine changes related to size result from the influence of estrogen and progesterone. After the first trimester uterine enlargement is primarily the result of mechanical pressure from the growing fetus. The enlargement of the uterus is not symmetric but occurs most in the area of the fundus (Cunningham et al. 1993; Guyton and Hall 1996).

▼ **Shape.** The uterus changes from its nonpregnant pear shape to a more globular shape and then, as the baby grows, to an ovoid shape. The position of the uterus changes as pregnancy progresses. As the uterus grows out of the pelvic area it can be palpated above the symphysis pubis between 12 and 14 weeks' gestation. It turns slightly to the right (dextrorotated) because of pressure from the rectosigmoid colon on the left side of the pelvis. The uterus reaches the level of the umbilicus at about 22 to 24 weeks and almost reaches the xiphoid process at term (Fig. 16–4). When the baby engages into the pelvis (lightening) between 38 and 40 weeks of gestation, the fundal height drops slightly. As the uterus enlarges it comes in contact with the abdominal wall and displaces the intestines both laterally (sideways) and superiorly (upward). The abdominal wall supports the uterus anteriorly and maintains its position in relation to the bony pelvis. When the woman is supine the uterus rests upon the vertebral column, the inferior vena cava, and the aorta. As a result, the woman may experience supine hypotensive syndrome (inferior vena cava syndrome) caused by compression of these vessels, with resultant decreased blood flow to the brain and uterus. This is discussed further in relation to the cardiovascular system.

▼ **Consistency.** During the first trimester, the consistency of the uterus changes as the walls of the uterus become considerably thicker than in the nonpregnant state. As gestation progresses, the uterine walls become very thin. The softening of the lower uterine segment, known as Hegar's sign, can be felt on pelvic examination (see Fig. 16–1). By 40 weeks' gestation the walls of the corpus of the uterus are 1.5 cm or less in thickness. Early in pregnancy the uterus loses its characteristic firmness and the walls become soft and readily indentable. This can be observed when palpating the fetus through the abdominal wall or observing fetal movement. Because of its softness, the uterus often becomes anteflexed in the early

Table 16–1

HORMONAL INFLUENCES DURING PREGNANCY

ENDOCRINE ORGAN AND HORMONES	INFLUENCE IN PREGNANCY	CLINICAL MANIFESTATIONS
Corpus Luteum and Maternal-Fetal-Placental Unit; Ovary; Adrenal Cortex		
Estrogen Principal source is placenta; also ovary and adrenal cortex; increases 1000-fold	Level of circulating estriol rises in pregnancy and can be measured in urine and amniotic fluid; in late pregnancy may stimulate prostaglandin production	Measurement of estriol in urine is index of fetal well-being: • Decrease indicates fetal anomaly or demise; maternal illness or drug use • Increase indicates multiple gestation or erythroblastosis Increased uterine vascularity and responsiveness to oxytocin stimulation in late pregnancy triggers rhythmic contractions
	Controls growth and function of uterus: • Hypertrophy and hyperplasia of muscle cells • Proliferation of endometrium • Increased blood supply to maternal-fetal-placental unit	Changes in uterus noted on pelvic examination; probable signs of pregnancy
	Stimulates breast development: • Growth of glandular tissue, ducts, alveoli, and nipples	Increased size of breasts and tenderness
	Increased pliability of connective tissue; relaxation of pelvic joints and ligaments	Cervical dilatation Lordosis, backache Tenderness of symphysis pubis or coccyx
	Enlargement of external genitalia	
	Decreased gastric secretion of hydrochloric acid and pepsin	Decreased absorption of fat; heartburn, nausea, indigestion
	Increased deposition of fat	Nourishment of developing fetus; preparation for breastfeeding
	Increased pigmentation of skin: • Stimulates increased production of melanin-stimulating hormone	Chloasma, linea nigra, darkened areolae and external genitalia
	Sodium and water retention by kidneys	Increased plasma volume and resultant physiologic anemia; increased interstitial fluid volume and resultant edema
	Hematologic changes: • 50% increase in clotting potential of blood fibrinogen (factor I)	Increased sedimentation rate; increased tendency to develop thrombosis
	Vascular changes: • Decreased peripheral vascular resistance	Vascular spiders; palmar erythema
	Psychological alterations	Mood swings; emotional lability; possible changes in sexual libido
Progesterone Source is corpus luteum for 7 wks; then maternal-fetal-placental unit; increases tenfold in pregnancy	Maintenance of pregnancy: • Stimulates development of decidual cells in endometrium • Suppresses maternal immunologic response to fetus • Decreases uterine contractility	Prepares for implantation; prevents sloughing of endometrium as menses; glycogen needs of embryo provided; prevents uterine contractions and spontaneous abortion

Table 16–1

HORMONAL INFLUENCES DURING PREGNANCY Continued

ENDOCRINE ORGAN AND HORMONES	INFLUENCE IN PREGNANCY	CLINICAL MANIFESTATIONS
Corpus Luteum and Maternal-Fetal-Placental Unit; Ovary; Adrenal Cortex		
Progesterone (cont'd)		
	Relaxation of smooth muscle: • Gastric and colonic motility decreases • Tone of bladder and ureters decreases • Decreased vascular tone	Nausea, heartburn, indigestion, constipation; urinary stasis, urinary tract infections, loss of urinary control; decreased diastolic blood pressure; dependent edema; varicosities
	Breast development: • Development of secretory capabilities of lobular-alveolar system	Preparation for lactation; breast tenderness
	Resetting of hypothalamic centers: • Stimulates respiratory center causing decreased maternal P_{CO_2}, which facilitates transfer of CO_2 from fetal to maternal blood	Physiologic hyperventilation; decreased maternal alveolar and arterial P_{CO_2}
	• Increases basal body temperature by 0.5°F	Feelings of increased warmth; increased perspiration
	• Increases storage of maternal fat	Protection of mother and fetus in times of starvation or physical exertion; 7–8 lb of weight gain attributed to fat storage
	Stimulation of sodium secreted in urine: • Aldosterone secreted to maintain water and electrolyte balance	Hyponatremia could develop
Human Chorionic Gonadotropin (hCG) Produced by syncytiotrophoblasts of placenta; present as early as 8 days post conception, peaks at 60–90 days, then falls steadily	Maintenance of corpus luteum in early pregnancy: • Stimulates production of estrogen and progesterone until placenta fully developed • Prevents menstruation	Contributes to nausea and vomiting of early pregnancy
	May regulate steroid production in fetus • Testosterone levels of male fetus rise	Basis of pregnancy testing before 16–20 wk; increased levels in multiple gestation; decreased levels with threatened abortion; persistent levels indicative of hydatidiform mole or choriocarcinoma
Human Placental Lactogen (hPL) Produced by syncytiotrophoblasts of placenta; present by 5–6 wk gestation and rises steadily throughout pregnancy; amount secreted related to fetal and placental weight	Exerts action similar to that of pituitary growth hormone	Blood levels related to placental function and provide basis for screening for complications
	Alters glucose metabolism: • Anti-insulin effect • Spares maternal glucose by increasing lipolysis • Increases glycogen storage	Provides adequate glucose to fetus throughout pregnancy; increased protein synthesis diabetogenic effect in mother (increased insulin production); can lead to gestational diabetes
	Alters protein metabolism: • Increases protein synthesis • Decreases protein breakdown and use of protein for energy • Increases circulating fatty acids	Protein available for maternal and fetal growth; possible maternal ketosis

Continued on following page

Table 16–1

HORMONAL INFLUENCES DURING PREGNANCY Continued

ENDOCRINE ORGAN AND HORMONES	INFLUENCE IN PREGNANCY	CLINICAL MANIFESTATIONS
	Corpus Luteum and Maternal-Fetal-Placental Unit; Ovary; Adrenal Cortex	
Human Placental Lactogen (hPL) (cont'd)	Contributes to breast development • Development of alveoli • Casein synthesis • Milk production	Preparation for lactation
Prostaglandins Found in amniotic fluid, decidua, and maternal venous blood before labor; also widely distributed throughout human body	Thought to contribute to the following in pregnancy: • Formation of corpus luteum • Uterine motility • Milk ejection	May be contributing factor in initiation of labor; prostaglandin E used to induce second-trimester abortions or labor at term
	Production inhibited by anti-inflammatory drugs such as aspirin or indomethacin	Indomethacin used to stop preterm labor
Relaxin Produced by ovary, corpus luteum, and placenta	Inhibits uterine activity	Helps to prevent preterm labor
	Softens cervix	Facilitates cervical ripening
	Softens and increases mobility of sacroiliac, sacrococcygeal, and pubic joints of bony pelvis	May make woman more prone to injury with exercise during pregnancy if jerky movements are not avoided; contributes to low backache of pregnancy; facilitates passage of fetal head through pelvis during labor
	Thyroid Gland	
Thyroxine T_3 decreases until end of first trimester, then stabilizes; T_4 increases during pregnancy	Basal metabolic rate increases 25% by late pregnancy	Cardiac palpitations and tachycardia; emotional lability; heat intolerance; fatigue; increased perspiration
	Increased protein-bound iodine	
	Pituitary Gland	
Follicle-Stimulating Hormone (FSH) Produced by anterior pituitary	Decreases markedly during pregnancy and in immediate postpartum period; increases to follicular phase levels about third week postpartum	Ovulation ceases
Prolactin Produced by anterior pituitary	Facilitates lactation: • Stimulates production of fat, lactose, and casein by glandular cells of breasts after delivery of placenta • Milk production inhibited during pregnancy by inhibitory effect of estrogen	Preparation for breastfeeding
Oxytocin Produced by posterior pituitary	Stimulates uterine contractions: • Counteracted by progesterone until near term • Triggered by Ferguson reflex during second stage of labor	Role in onset of labor not clear; augments intensity of uterine contractions during labor
	Stimulates letdown and ejection of milk: • Released by stimulation from baby sucking on nipple	Facilitates lactation

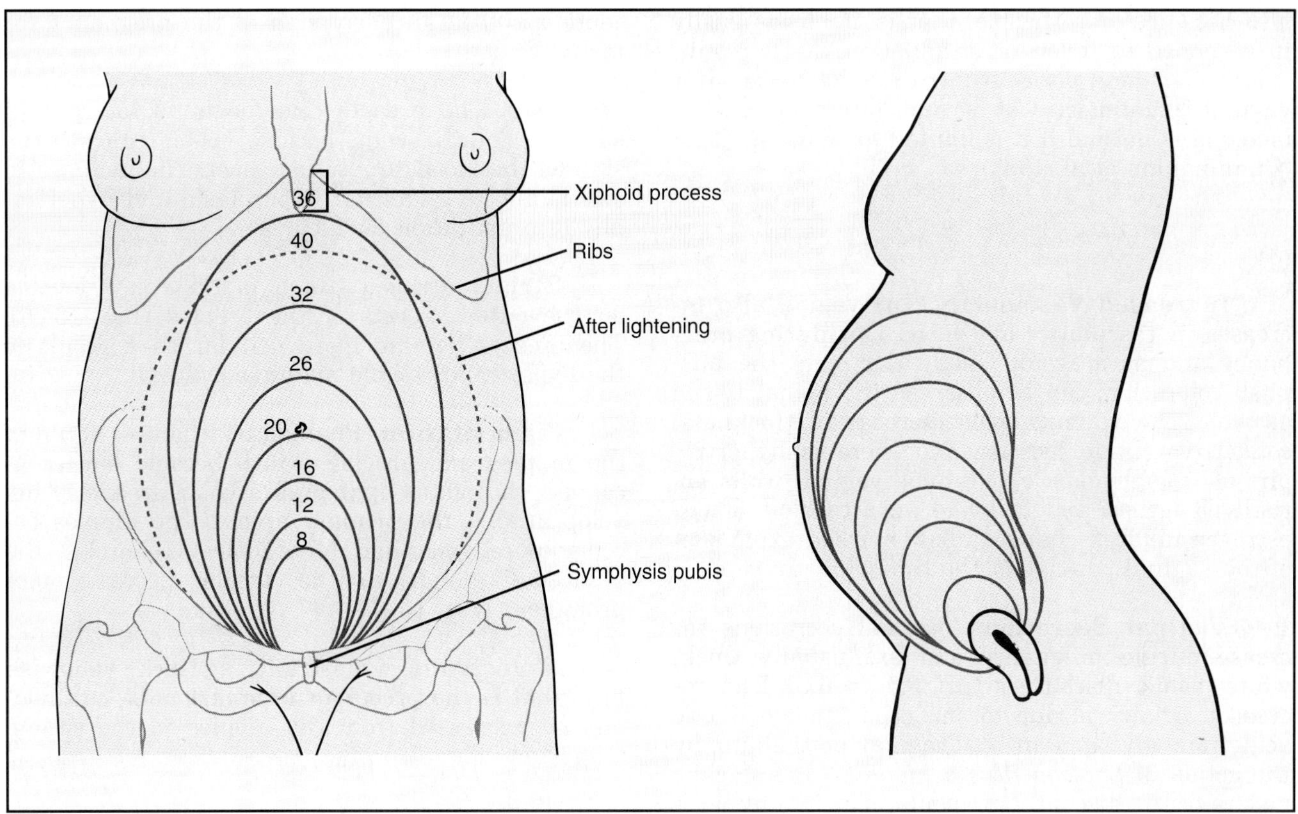

Figure 16–4

Changes in uterine size during pregnancy show the height of the uterine fundus at progressing weeks of gestation and where the enlarging uterus may be palpated at the fundus.

weeks of pregnancy but then straightens as it becomes larger.

▼ **Contractions.** The uterus contracts from the first trimester until delivery. These contractions are irregular and painless and are not usually perceived by the woman until some time in the third trimester. These normal contractions, called Braxton Hicks contractions, can be palpated by an examiner on bimanual examination or by abdominal palpation. The uterus, which is typically soft and indentable, becomes tight or hard for a brief period and then returns to its relaxed state. Uterine contractions occur in response to the stretching of the myometrium as it grows, and they serve to keep the muscle in good tone. Braxton Hicks contractions become more frequent, regular, and noticeable as the woman nears term. If they become strong and regular for a period of time, the woman may mistake them for labor. If no cervical changes occur as a result of these contractions (i.e., ripening, effacement, or dilatation), they are often called false labor. It is important to assess for cervical changes or other accompanying physical symptoms if a woman complains of frequent Braxton Hicks contractions to rule out preterm labor (see Chapter 21, Teaching Guide: Identification and Prevention of Preterm Labor).

CERVIX

▼ **Goodell's Sign and Chadwick's Sign.** The earliest signs of pregnancy can often be noted in the cervix. A pronounced softening occurs (Goodell's sign), along with a bluish coloration (Chadwick's sign). These changes can be palpated and observed on pelvic examination. The changes in consistency and color of the cervix are caused by estrogen, which stimulates increased vascularity, edema, and blood flow in the entire cervix, along with hypertrophy and hyperplasia of the cervical glands. The cervix becomes edematous and thickens. The glands of the cervical mucosa undergo such marked proliferation that by the end of pregnancy they occupy approximately half of the entire mass of the cervix, rather than the small portion occupied in the prepregnant cervix.

▼ **Mucus and Bloody Show.** The glands secrete a thick mucus that blocks bacterial invasion of the cervical os and protects the fetus from infection (see Fig. 16–1). When labor begins this mucous plug is gradually released as the cervix begins to efface and dilate. The mucus is often tinged with blood from ruptured capillaries as the cervix dilates, and this "bloody show" is observed by the woman as an early sign of labor. The cervix also becomes more friable; that is, it bleeds easily in response to touch or stimulation. As a result, the woman may notice a few drops of blood after vaginal examination or sexual intercourse. This bleeding is normal if it is limited to slight spotting (Cunningham et al. 1993).

VAGINA

▼ **Increased Vascularity.** The vagina also increases in vascularity and blood flow during pregnancy and as a result Chadwick's sign, the purplish coloration, can be observed in vaginal tissue as well. The vaginal walls increase in thickness, connective tissue loosens, and there is hypertrophy of smooth muscle cells. The vaginal walls actually lengthen and fold like an accordion. These estrogen-induced changes allow marked expansion of the vaginal passage at the time of birth.

▼ **Vaginal Secretions.** Vaginal secretions increase during pregnancy and are usually thick, white, acidic discharges (pH 3.5 to 6.0). The increased acidity is due to the production of lactic acid from glycogen in the vaginal epithelium by the action of *Lactobacillus acidophilus.* The acidic nature of the discharge prevents invasion by pathogenic organisms, but favors moniliasis (yeast infections). An increase in leukocytes in the vaginal discharge results in a characteristic leukorrhea (Cunningham et al. 1993).

OVARIES

The maturation of new follicles is blocked and the ovaries cease their production of ova during pregnancy. The theca cells that line the immature ovarian follicles become active in the production of hormones in pregnancy and are therefore called the interstitial glands of pregnancy. The corpus luteum functions by producing estrogen and progesterone during the first 6 to 7 weeks of pregnancy, until the placenta is developed enough to assume this function. The corpus luteum then degenerates. The increase in estrogen and progesterone is responsible for the cessation of menses during pregnancy.

BREASTS

A number of changes occur in the breasts during pregnancy as a result of estrogen and progesterone influence.

▼ **Sensitivity.** Initially, the woman experiences increased sensitivity, noted as tingling, tenderness, or heaviness of the breasts. This sensitivity may be particularly pronounced during sexual intercourse. This can occur within a few weeks of conception and is an early sign of the pregnancy for many women.

▼ **Size.** The breasts then begin to increase in size and delicate veins become visible beneath the skin as the blood supply increases. The increase in size is due to glandular hyperplasia and hypertrophy in preparation for lactation.

▼ **Striae.** Striae (stretch marks) may develop on the outer aspects of the breasts (Fig. 16–5). The breasts become more nodular as a result of the hypertrophy of the mammary alveoli.

▼ **Pigmentation.** Pigmentary changes occur in the nipples and areolae, which become darker in color. A secondary light pink areolar area may develop around the primary areola. The nipples become more erect and Montgomery tubercles, the sebaceous glands in the areola, become more prominent (Fig. 16–5).

▼ **Colostrum.** Colostrum, a thick yellowish fluid that is the precursor of breast milk, can usually be expressed from the nipples in the second trimester.

Cardiovascular System

The changes that take place in the cardiovascular system are essential to the well-being of the mother and her baby throughout the pregnancy. Next to the reproductive system, the cardiovascular system shows the most dramatic adaptations.

HEART

Pregnancy causes several anatomic or mechanical changes of the heart.

▼ **Position.** The position of the heart shifts slightly in the chest. As the uterus grows upward in the abdominal cavity, the diaphragm is elevated and the heart is displaced upward, forward, and to the left; the apex of the heart is moved laterally from its nonpregnant position (Fig. 16–6).

▼ **Volume.** The cardiac volume increases by about 10 percent or 75 mL between early and late pregnancy. As a result of these changes in position and volume, the heart appears to be slightly increased in size when viewed on radiographs. This slight enlargement may also be a result of increased blood volume and cardiac workload.

▼ **Heart Sounds.** Auscultatory changes occur as a result of the changes in position and size of the heart. Ninety percent of pregnant women have

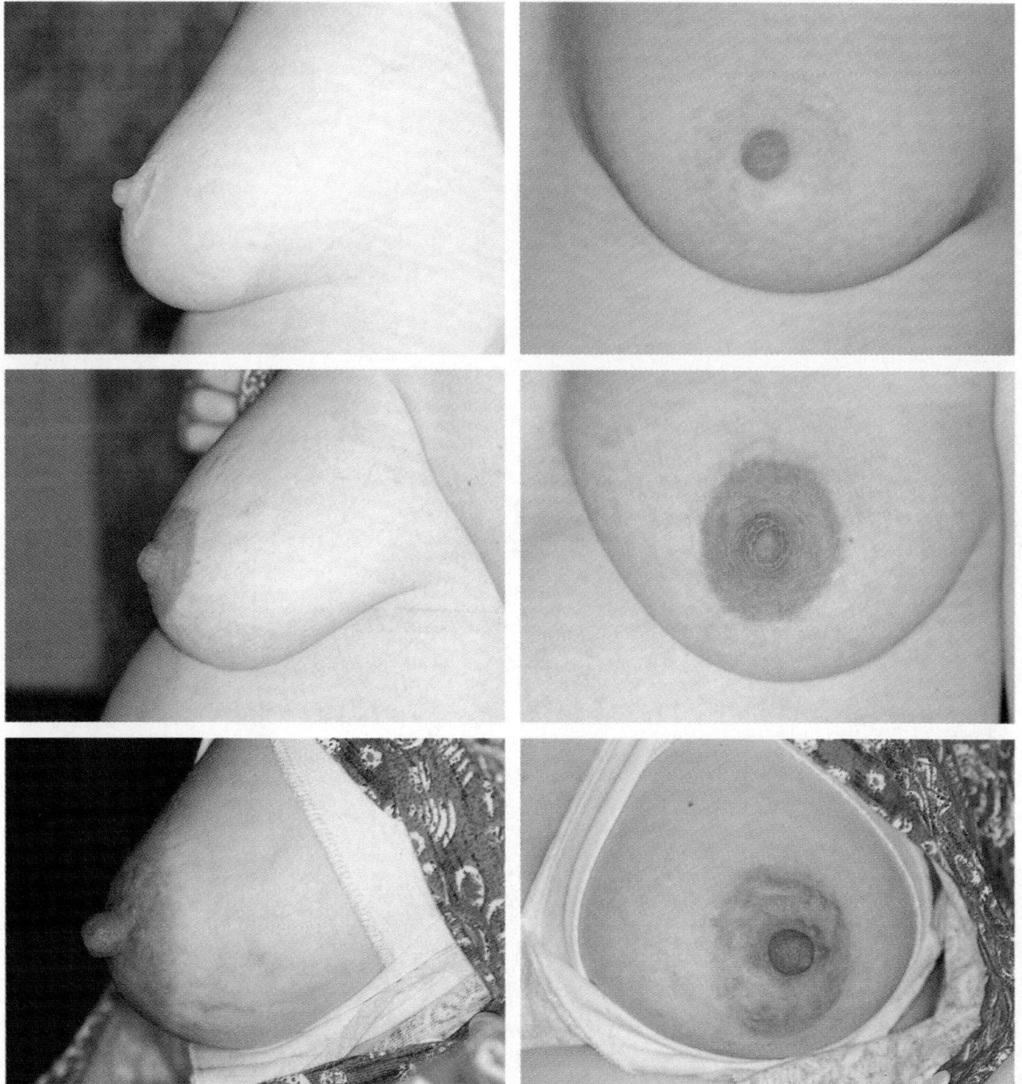

Figure 16–5

This series of photographs shows how the breasts change from before pregnancy *(top row, left and right),* through pregnancy *(middle row, left and right),* to lactation *(bottom row, left and right)* • During pregnancy, the breasts increase in size and sensitivity; pigmentary changes and striae may be observed.

a systolic murmur, which is physiologic and disappears shortly after delivery; 19 percent of women have a soft transient diastolic murmur; and 10 percent of women have continuous murmurs arising from the breast vasculature. These physiologic murmurs, which are normal during pregnancy, should be differentiated from those that are organic. Organic murmurs can be heard in any position, during both inspiration and expiration, and are louder with increased heart rate. This is not usually true of the physiologic murmurs of pregnancy. Normal pregnancy induces no characteristic changes in the electrocardiogram (Cunningham et al. 1993).

▼ **Cardiac Output.** Cardiac output increases 30 to 50 percent by the end of the second trimester and remains elevated during the third trimester (Fig. 16–7). The increase in cardiac output during pregnancy is influenced by decreased arterial blood pressure and vascular resistance and by increases in circulating estrogen, blood volume, stroke volume, tissue demands for oxygen, maternal weight, and BMR. In late pregnancy cardiac output is 22 percent higher when the woman is in the lateral recumbent position than when she is supine, because the uterus occludes venous return to the heart when the woman is lying on her back (Fig. 16–8). As a result, cardiac output is decreased and the blood pressure drops rapidly (supine hypotensive syndrome). Symptoms of dizziness, nausea, or diaphoresis when lying on the back indicate that the pregnant woman should turn to her side immediately to relieve the com-

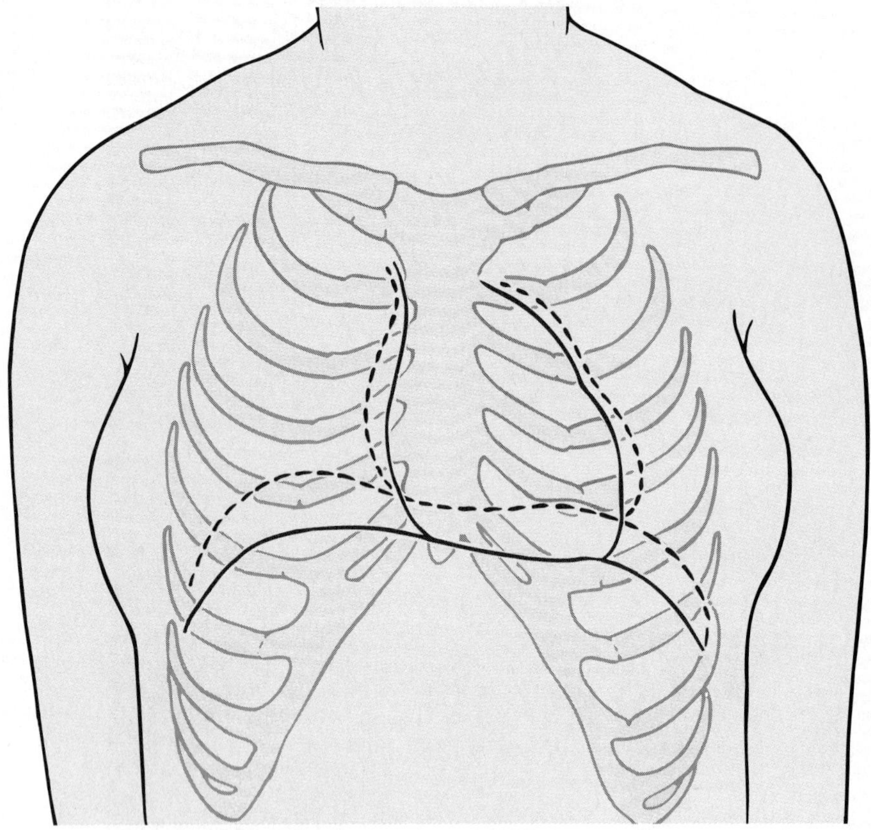

Figure 16–6

The elevation of the diaphragm caused by uterine growth during pregnancy displaces the heart upward, forward, and to the left *(blue dotted line);* the rib cage also expands.

pression and restore adequate circulation. Cardiac output is also increased during pregnancy in response to physical exercise and the process of labor and birth.

The distribution of cardiac output favors the organs that have an increased workload during pregnancy. The uterus and maternal-fetal-placental unit receive 10 percent of the total cardiac output (500–1000 mL/min by term). This represents a 1000 percent increase in blood flow to the uterus. Uterine blood flow can be compromised during pregnancy as a result of contractions, alterations in blood pressure, smoking, prolonged strenuous exercise, or complications such as pregnancy-induced hypertension (PIH) or placenta previa. Bed rest in the left lateral position is often prescribed to facilitate blood flow to the uterus. The kidneys also receive an increase in blood flow during pregnancy as a result of the increased cardiac output. These increases are necessary to provide oxygen and nutrients to the developing fetus and to remove metabolic wastes.

CIRCULATORY CHANGES

▼ **Peripheral Changes.** Peripheral circulatory changes are due to decreased blood vessel tone and peripheral vascular resistance. Stagnation of blood in the lower extremities is common and is due to a rise in femoral venous pressure caused by pressure from the enlarged uterus. As a result, women may experience dependent edema and varicose vein formation in the legs, vulva, and rectum. The woman may experience postural hypotension and feel dizzy upon rising from a prone position. Vasodilatation allows increased blood flow to the skin, resulting in palmar erythema, nosebleeds, or feelings of warmth.

▼ **Blood Volume.** By the end of the second trimester, a 30 to 50 percent (1200–1700 mL) increase in plasma volume occurs as estrogen stimulates the adrenals to release aldosterone, resulting in sodium and water retention. This additional fluid volume increases blood volume and helps to

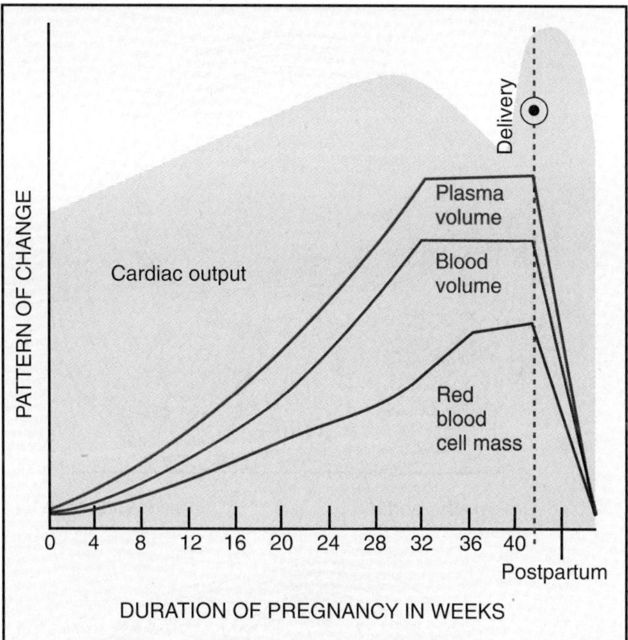

Figure 16–7

Over the duration of pregnancy, increases are seen in cardiac output, blood volume, plasma volume, and red blood cell production.

meet the increased circulatory demands of the maternal-fetal-placental unit during pregnancy, birth, and the postpartum period. By 40 weeks' gestation the woman has approximately 1 to 2 liters of additional blood in her circulatory system, which serves as a reserve against fluid loss that might occur during childbirth (Fig. 16–7). At the same time, erythrocyte production increases; however, the increase in red blood cell volume is only about 25 to 30 percent. Because the increase in red blood cells is less than the increase in plasma volume, the pregnant woman experiences a physiologic anemia. The clinical manifestation of these blood volume changes is a 10 to 15 percent decrease in hemoglobin and hematocrit. The hemoglobin may drop from the normal range of 12 to 16 g/dL to about 10 to 14 g/dL. The hematocrit may drop from the normal 36 to 48 percent level to about 32 to 46 percent (Table 16–2). An increase in iron intake is necessary to meet the expanded need resulting from fetal growth and increased red blood cell production. Part of this iron should come from dietary sources (see Chapter 19); however, dietary sources of iron may not be enough to meet the need during pregnancy, so an iron supplement is often prescribed.

Production of white blood cells (WBCs) begins to increase during the second trimester and peaks in the third trimester. This increase is equal to or slightly greater than the increase in blood volume. The WBC count increases from the nonpregnant range of 4500 to 11,000/mm^3 to 15,000 to 18,000/mm^3 during pregnancy. During labor and the early postpartum period the WBC count may rise even higher in response to physiologic stress. By term, the fibrin level in the blood increases by up to 40 percent and the plasma fibrinogen by as much as 50 percent. This accounts for a physiologic rise in sedimentation rate that is seen clinically. Because of increases in various clotting factors, there is a tendency for coagulation during pregnancy. Fibrinolytic activity (dissolution of blood clots) is depressed during pregnancy and the early postpartum period. As a result, the woman is more prone to develop venous thrombosis.

VITAL SIGNS

▼ **Heart Rate.** The heart rate increases by up to 10 to 15 beats per minute during pregnancy to facilitate oxygen transport and kidney filtration. Palpitations may occur as a result of the increase in BMR caused by increased thyroxine.

▼ **Blood Pressure.** The blood pressure remains relatively stable because of the balance established between estrogen and progesterone (which relax blood vessels and lower blood pressure) and vasopressin (which constricts blood vessels and raises blood pressure). The lowest diastolic pressures (5–10 mm Hg below prepregnant readings) are seen in the first and second trimesters as a result of high progesterone levels and vasodilatation. Systolic pressure may also decrease by 2 to 3 mm Hg. The highest blood pressure levels are likely to be seen in the last week of pregnancy (see Table 16–2). The blood pressure also varies with the woman's position. It is usually highest when she is sitting, intermediate when supine, and lowest when in the left lateral position. The woman is diagnosed as having mild preeclampsia if she has a rise from her early pregnancy baseline value of 30 mm Hg in systolic pressure or 15 mm Hg in diastolic pressure on two occasions 6 hours apart. Hypertensive disorders in pregnancy can be a serious alteration of pregnancy and require additional assessment and intervention (see Chapter 21) (Cunningham et al. 1993; Guyton and Hall 1996).

Respiratory System

Along with changes in the cardiovascular system, the changes in the respiratory system are also essential to maternal-fetal well-being. Both anatomic and functional changes in the respiratory system take place during pregnancy.

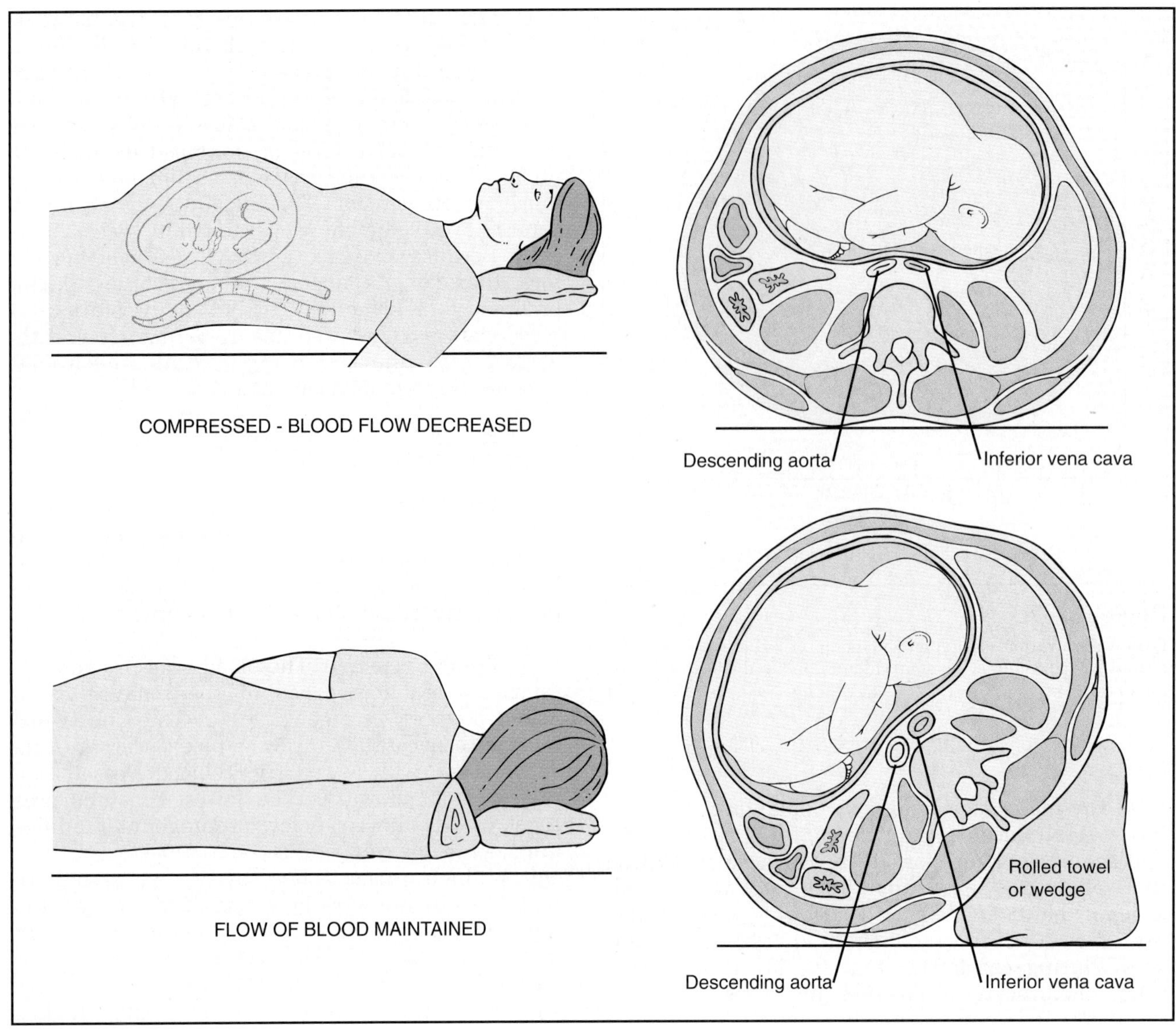

Figure 16–8

The supine position in pregnancy causes the uterus to compress the inferior vena cava, decreasing blood flow return to the heart and causing maternal hypertension, which may lead to supine hypotensive syndrome.

ANATOMIC CHANGES

▼ **Chest.** As the uterus becomes larger, the diaphragm rises about 4 cm and the substernal angle of the rib cage increases. This causes the rib cage to flare, resulting in a decrease in the vertical diameter and an increase in the anterior-posterior and transverse diameters (see Fig. 16–6). The circumference of the chest may increase by as much as 6 cm. These changes in the diameters of the chest compensate for the elevation of the diaphragm, so there is no significant loss of intrathoracic volume. The chest may not return to its prepregnant size when the pregnancy is over.

▼ **Respiration.** The respiratory rate remains stable and respiration becomes thoracic rather than abdominal. The depth of respiration may increase slightly to maintain adequate ventilation. Increased vascularization resulting from estrogen stimulation may cause nasal stuffiness or epistaxis (nosebleed).

FUNCTIONAL CHANGES

▼ **Hyperventilation.** Functional changes in the respiratory system include a slight degree of hyperventilation related to the increased tidal volume throughout pregnancy. The tidal volume of 500 mL in the nonpregnant state increases to 700 mL in pregnancy.

▼ **Oxygenation.** Oxygen consumption rises 15 to 20 percent in the second and third trimesters as a result of the increased basal metabolic rate,

Table 16–2

NORMAL LABORATORY VALUES: NONPREGNANT AND PREGNANT WOMEN

	NONPREGNANT	PREGNANT
Endocrine		
Total thyroxine concentration	4.5–12.5 μg/dL thyroxine	↑ 2–4 μg/dL
Aldosterone		1 mg/24 hr by third trimester
Cardiovascular		
Pulse	60–100 bpm	↑ 10–20 bpm
Blood pressure	120/80 mm Hg	↓ in second trimester; return to baseline by third trimester
Cardiac output	3–5 L/min	5–7 L/min
Hemoglobin	12–16 g/dL	11–13 g/dL
Hematocrit	36%–48%	33%–39%
Red cell volume	1600 mL	1900 mL
Plasma volume	2400 mL	3700 mL
Red blood cell count	4.2–5.4 million/mm^3	3.8–4.4 million/mm^3
White blood cell count (total)	4000–11,000/mm^3	5000–15,000/mm^3
Prothrombin time	12–14 sec	Slight ↓
Bleeding time	3–8 min	No change
Coagulation time	5–15 min	No change
Platelets	150,000–350,000/mm^3	150,000–450,000 mm^3 (see ↑ 3–5 days post partum)
Fibrinogen	200–400 mg/dL	450 mg/dL
Blood sugar		
Fasting	70–80 mg/dL	65 mg/dL
2 hr postprandial	60–110 mg/dL	Below 140 mg/dL
Respiratory		
Respiratory rate	15/min	16/min
Tidal volume	485 mL	680 mL
Minute ventilation	7270 mL	10,340 mL
Vital capacity	3260 mL	3310 mL
Inspiratory capacity	2625 mL	2745 mL
Residual volume	965 mL	770 mL
Renal		
Bladder capacity	500–1000 mL	1000–1500 mL
Glomerular filtration rate (GFR)	80–100 mL/min	120–150 mL/min
Blood urea nitrogen (BUN)	10–16 mg/dL	7–10 mg/dL
Creatinine	15–25 mg/kg/24 hr	May ↑ or ↓
Glucose	Negative	Present
Gastrointestinal		
Cholesterol	140–310 mg/dL	↑ 40%–60%
Alkaline phosphatase	20–90 U/L	Doubled
Serum albumin	4.3 g/dL	3.5 g/dL

From Black, J., and Matassarin-Jacobs, E. (1993). *Medical-Surgical Nursing.* Philadelphia: W.B. Saunders Co.; Blackburn, S. and Loper, D. (1992). *Maternal, Fetal, and Neonatal Physiology.* Philadelphia: W.B. Saunders Co.; Cunningham, F., MacDonald, P., Gand, N., Leveno, K., Gilstrap, L. (1993). *Williams Obstetrics* (19th ed). Norwalk, Conn: Appleton and Lange; Harvey, M. (1992). Critical care for the maternity patient. *MCN: The American Journal of Maternal Child Nursing.* 17 (6): 296–309.

the woman's increased size, and the demands of the maternal-fetal-placental unit. This, along with the influence of progesterone, which increases the sensitivity of the respiratory center to carbon dioxide, causes the minute ventilation to increase 30 to 50 percent. The vital capacity also increases slightly; however, lung compliance and pulmonary diffusion remain at the prepregnancy levels (see Table 16–2).

Airway Resistance. Progesterone causes decreased airway resistance and relaxation of smooth muscle. Estrogen increases the pliability of connective tissue, which results in decreased pulmonary resistance. These changes allow increases in oxygen consumption, CO_2 production, and respiratory functional reserve. The pregnant woman may experience dyspnea because of the increase in uterine pressure and the decrease in CO_2 levels (Cunningham et al. 1993; Guyton and Hall 1996).

Urinary System

Pregnancy also leads to anatomic and functional changes in the urinary system. These changes often produce annoying symptoms for the woman during pregnancy.

ANATOMIC CHANGES

Bladder. The uterus compresses the bladder against the pelvis as it enlarges, which decreases the bladder capacity and results in urinary frequency. This bladder compression is most evident in the first trimester before the uterus rises out of the pelvis and again near term, when the presenting part of the baby engages into the pelvis. The bladder mucosa becomes congested with blood, and estrogen stimulates hypertrophy of the bladder walls as pregnancy progresses. This results in edema of the bladder tissue and causes it to be more susceptible to trauma and infection during labor and birth.

Ureters. The ureters are also compressed as they pass over the pelvic brim. This compression is especially evident on the right side, because the sigmoid colon cushions the left side. The compression of the ureters, along with the smooth muscle relaxant effects of progesterone, may result in dilatation of both ureters above the point of compression and the renal pelves.

Kidneys. The kidneys increase slightly in size during pregnancy as a result of increased blood volume and enlargement of their interstitial spaces. The clinical consequences of these anatomic changes are stasis of urine and an increased susceptibility to urinary tract infections (UTIs) throughout pregnancy. The ureters may dilate enough to contain as much as 200 mL of urine.

FUNCTIONAL CHANGES

Urine Formation. Functional changes are also evident in the urinary system. The rate of urine formation is slightly increased because of an increased load of excretory products. Reabsorption of sodium, chloride, and water by the renal tubules is increased by as much as 50 percent as a result of increased production of steroid hormones by the placenta and adrenal cortex. The renal plasma flow (RPF) increases early in pregnancy but only by a moderate amount. The glomerular filtration rate (GFR) increases by as much as 50 percent by the second trimester and the increased rate persists until term (see Table 16–2). The increased GFR tends to increase the rate of water and electrolyte loss in the urine; however, this loss is balanced by the increased reabsorption, so that the woman accumulates only about 6 pounds of extra water and sodium throughout the pregnancy.

Physiologic Edema. Physiologic edema may occur as a result of the water retention. Estrogen, progesterone, and aldosterone work together to allow the appropriate amounts of sodium retention and excretion during pregnancy. Sodium intake should not be severely limited by diet or use of diuretics during pregnancy, because decreased kidney function and urine volume may result. A decreased BUN is observed because of the increased renal function. Therefore, a better test of renal function during pregnancy is a measurement of serum creatinine clearance. Renal function is most efficient when the woman lies in the left lateral recumbent position and least efficient when she assumes a supine position.

Glycosuria. Because of the increased GFR and decreased tubule glucose reabsorption, physiologic glycosuria occurs in one sixth of pregnant women. This glycosuria is a reflection of the kidneys' inability to reabsorb all of the glucose being filtered by the glomeruli. It is important to evaluate whether any observed glycosuria is a normal response to these functional changes or a sign of gestational diabetes resulting from the diabetogenic effects of pregnancy (Cunningham et al. 1993; Guyton and Hall 1996).

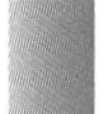

Gastrointestinal System

The changes that occur in the gastrointestinal system are often those that are most noticeable to the pregnant woman, for most of the changes are accompanied by uncomfortable symptoms. However, the changes that occur benefit the developing fetus by providing greater absorption of nutrients and enhancing their utilization.

STOMACH AND INTESTINES

Heartburn, Constipation, and Hemorrhoids. The enlarging uterus places pressure on the stomach and intestines. This mechanical change, as well as relaxation of the cardiac sphincter related to the effects of progesterone, contributes to heartburn or pyrosis (reflux of acidic secretions from the stomach into the lower esophagus) and constipation. A number of physical changes resulting from increased hormone levels also contribute to gastrointestinal symptoms during pregnancy. Heartburn and indigestion are caused not only by mechanical pressure but also by an estrogen-stimulated decrease in gastric secretion of hydrochloric acid and pepsin. The effects of progesterone on smooth muscle relaxation cause decreased gastric emptying time (peristalsis) and intestinal motility, which also contribute to constipation. The increase in electrolyte and water absorption during pregnancy adds to the problem of constipation as well. If constipation is a problem during pregnancy, it may increase the likelihood of the development of hemorrhoids.

Nausea, Vomiting, and Alterations in Taste or Smell. Nausea and vomiting of early pregnancy, which may be aggravated by the decreased tone and mobility of the smooth muscles of the gastrointestinal tract, is thought to be caused by both hCG and progesterone. A change in carbohydrate metabolism also contributes to nausea and vomiting. Many women describe alterations in taste and smell during pregnancy, and these changes can contribute to the nausea. Nausea has also been found to be related to fatigue during early pregnancy (Van Lier et al. 1993).

Epulis. Swollen spongy gums (epulis) that are hyperemic and softened may bleed easily with brushing. This condition is thought to result from the effect of estrogen on fibers in collagenous tissue. Pregnancy does not affect the teeth, and the old wives' tale "for every child a tooth" is unfounded. If the woman maintains a good diet, dental caries should not occur more frequently in pregnancy than at any other time.

Alteration in Appetite. Several symptoms related to the gastrointestinal system are of unknown origin. Some women experience a sensation of ptyalism, an increase in the production of saliva, although studies have shown that saliva production does not increase during pregnancy. This sensation can be annoying and may be related to nausea. Pica, a craving to eat substances that are not food, may be caused by physiologic or sociocultural factors. Examples of such substances are clay, laundry starch, soap, and plaster. Many pregnant women report more normal cravings for foods that are sweet or salty. These cravings are thought to occur because the sense of taste is often dulled during pregnancy. The woman's appetite fluctuates during pregnancy. It may diminish initially if nausea and vomiting occur but then increase in the late first trimester and early second trimester. Toward the end of the pregnancy the appetite may diminish again (Van Dinter 1991; Cunningham et al. 1993).

LIVER AND GALLBLADDER

Only minor changes in liver function are thought to occur during pregnancy. Liver volume remains the same, despite increased circulation and metabolic activity. Metabolic changes result in increased levels of cholesterol, lipoproteins, and triglycerides (see Table 16–2). The spider nevi and palmar erythema seen during pregnancy are caused not by liver disease but by estrogen and disappear in the early postpartum period. The gallbladder empties more slowly during pregnancy as a result of the smooth muscle relaxation caused by progesterone. Incomplete emptying could cause the formation of cholesterol crystals and increase the incidence of gallstones. However, this occurs infrequently during pregnancy (Cunningham et al. 1993).

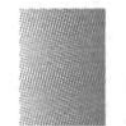

Musculoskeletal and Neurologic Systems

POSTURE

The enlarging uterus causes several mechanical changes in the musculoskeletal system, and hormonal influences contribute to changes as well. The pregnant woman experiences an altered center of gravity as the uterus increases in size and weight. The increased weight of the uterus causes a forward pull of the bony pelvis. This leads to lordosis, an accentuation of the lumbodorsal spinal curve. The change in the woman's posture, which allows a redistribution of the center of gravity over the extremities, often results in low backache. These alterations in posture may also cause aching, numbness, or weakness in the upper extremities related to flexion of the neck and slumping of the shoulders. The resulting stress and traction on peripheral nerves can cause pain. Carpal tunnel syndrome can be caused by compressing the ulnar and median nerves, leading to paresthesia, weakness, or tenderness in the wrist and thumb. Numbness and tingling of the hands (acroesthesia) may be experienced as a result of traction on segments of the brachial plexus caused by a stoop-shouldered posture.

UTERINE LIGAMENTS AND ABDOMINAL MUSCLES

Round ligament pain may be experienced as the uterus enlarges and pulls on the ligaments that anchor it in the abdominal cavity. It may be experienced as an aching sensation or shooting pain.

The abdominal muscles are greatly stretched as the pregnancy advances, often leading to a diastasis or separation of the two halves of the rectus abdominis muscle. This diastasis can be palpated when the woman lies supine and contracts the abdominal muscles by raising her chin to her chest. The muscle separation should resolve after the pregnancy.

LOWER EXTREMITIES

Leg cramps or sensory changes in the legs are caused by both uterine pressure on nerves and altered calcium and phosphorus levels. The increases in estrogen and relaxin during pregnancy cause relaxation of the sacroiliac, sacrococcygeal, and pubic joints. The increased flexibility in these joints contributes to the waddling gait seen in pregnancy and facilitates movement of the baby through the pelvis during birth. Because all joints are more flexible during pregnancy, the woman should use more caution when exercising (see Chapter 19).

SYNCOPE

Some women may experience light-headedness or syncope in early pregnancy. Factors that could cause faintness include postural hypotension, vasomotor instability, and hypoglycemia (Cunningham et al. 1993).

Integumentary System

A number of changes are seen in the skin during pregnancy as a result of mechanical stretching or hormonal influence. The breasts show increased pigmentation in the nipples and areola and the genitalia become darker in color. All of the pigmentary changes of the skin usually disappear when the pregnancy is over.

Sweat and sebaceous gland activity increases during pregnancy as a result of increased blood flow and basal metabolic rate. As a result, the woman may perspire more readily and may develop oily skin and acne. Hair and nail growth may also increase noticeably as a result of the effects of estrogen. An increase in fine hair growth on the body may be observed (hirsutism), and the nails may become thinner and softer. Cutaneous allergic responses may be enhanced (Gagnon 1992; Cunningham et al. 1993).

▼ **Striae and Linea Nigra.** The stretching of the abdomen by the enlarging uterus and separation within underlying connective tissue causes striae, or "stretch marks." The development of striae may also be related to hormonal changes. Striae appear as reddish or purplish depressed streaks and can occur on the breasts, buttocks, and thighs as well as the abdomen. After the pregnancy the striae fade to a silver color that is not as noticeable. Some women develop more striae than others, which may be a function of familial tendency as well as the amount of stretching. The striae may be accompanied by a sensation of itching (Gagnon 1992). The linea nigra is a

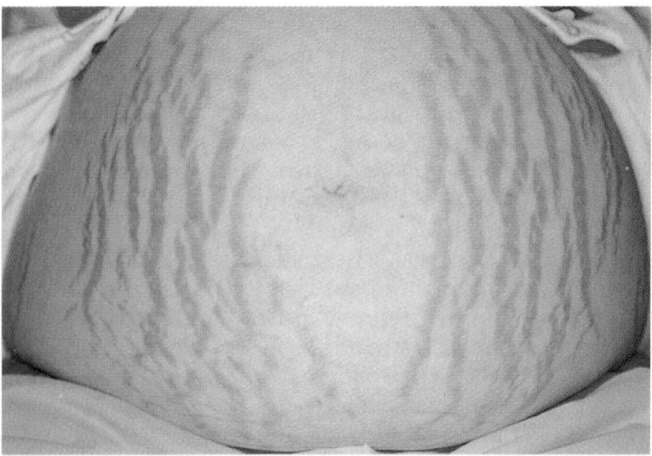

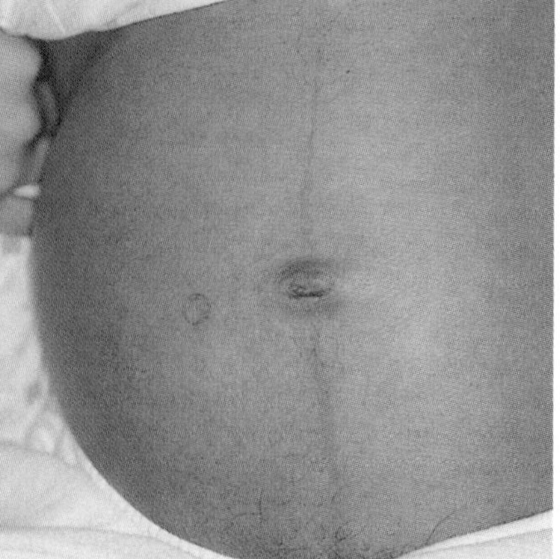

Figure 16–9

Two changes of the integumentary system are often seen on the pregnant abdomen: striae and linea nigra.

pigmented line that extends in the midline of the abdomen from above the umbilicus to the pubis (Fig. 16–9).

Vascular Spiders and Palmar Erythema. Vascular spiders, also called spider angiomas, spider nevi, or vascular telangiectases, often appear on the woman's face, neck, chest, arms, or legs. These are spider-shaped clusters of thin-walled dilated capillaries caused by increased subcutaneous blood flow in response to estrogen. The spiders have a bluish color and do not blanch with pressure (Gagnon 1992). Redness of the palms of the hands, called palmar erythema, may also be observed. Neither of these conditions has any clinical significance, and both disappear after the pregnancy.

Chloasma. A number of pigmentary changes in the integumentary system result from an estrogen- and progesterone-stimulated increase in the anterior pituitary hormone melanotropin. Chloasma, or the "mask of pregnancy," may be seen on the woman's face. This pigmentation is a blotchy brownish coloration over the cheeks, nose, and forehead and is accentuated by sun exposure. It is more common in dark-complected women but is seen in approximately 70% of women during pregnancy (Gagnon 1992).

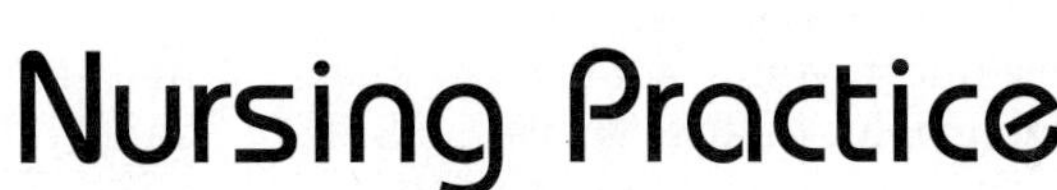

Nursing Practice

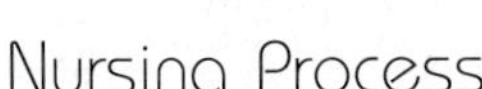

Nursing Process

The purpose of prenatal care is to decrease maternal mortality and morbidity, fetal loss, and unnecessary intervention in pregnancy. Prenatal care is the primary factor that has decreased maternal and fetal mortality and morbidity in the past 50 years. The management of the woman's health during pregnancy is a responsibility shared by the woman and the team of health care providers who work with her. Thus it is important to establish a positive, supportive relationship with the pregnant woman and her family at the initial prenatal visit and at all succeeding visits. The nature of this relationship and the tone that is set in the health care setting are major influences on the woman's motivation and willingness to continue regular prenatal care.

The objective of prenatal care is to ensure that every pregnancy results in the delivery of a healthy baby without impairing the health of the mother (Cunningham et al. 1993). Ideally, prenatal care is merely an extension of the regular health care received by the woman throughout her life. In reality, however, the first prenatal visit may be the first contact the woman has had with the health care system in many years. Prenatal care should begin as soon as the pregnancy is confirmed and continue until delivery. Unfortunately, far too many women in the United States delay prenatal care or do not receive sufficient prenatal care.

Universal access to prenatal care does not yet exist in the United States. This is of major concern, for prenatal care is the first step in preventing low birth weights of infants. The Surgeon General's goals for 1990 to reduce the number of low-birth-weight infants and to ensure that at least 90 percent of all pregnant women receive prenatal care in the first trimester of pregnancy were not met (U.S. Department of Health and Human Services 1988). Women who are most likely to receive inadequate prenatal care are adolescent, unmarried, high parity, minority status, non–English speaking, poor, or rural, or have less than 12 years of education (Mattson and Lew 1992; Mc-

Clanahan 1992). Reasons women cite for delaying prenatal care are denial or delayed acceptance of the pregnancy, lack of understanding or motivation regarding the importance of prenatal care, financial issues, or conflicting family responsibilities (Young et al. 1989). The most frequent complaints women have about the prenatal care offered in our health care system are poor accessibility, lack of transportation, no third-party payment, crowded or inadequately staffed clinic services, lack of continuity of care, and failure to provide care for small children during the visit (McClanahan 1992).

Health care professionals need to identify and implement creative alternatives for the provision of prenatal care to make it more attractive and accessible to hard-to-reach groups of women. Examples of successful programs that target minority cultural groups and adolescents or involve community public and private support have been reported in the literature (Helton 1990; Aaronson 1991; Mattson and Lew 1992). Alternatives that might make prenatal care more desirable to women are suggested by Mahan and McKay (1984) in Table 16–3. A primary goal of any nurse involved in the provision of prenatal care should be to work to improve the accessibility of services for all women and to make each prenatal visit comfortable and individualized so that the woman is motivated to return.

Controversy has arisen regarding the number and frequency of prenatal visits that have been the standard of practice for many years (i.e., 13 total prenatal visits: one visit per month until 28 weeks, one visit every 2 weeks from 28 to 36 weeks, and a weekly visit from 36 weeks until delivery). As a result of the publication of the 1989 report of the U.S. Public Health Service's Expert Panel on the Content of Prenatal Care, this routine schedule for all women has been challenged. It is proposed that good prenatal care may be provided in fewer visits for women showing no signs of risk, that laboratory tests that have become routine may not need to be done as often, and that more must be done for women who experience a high-risk pregnancy (Mahan and McKay 1984; Public Health Service 1989; Young 1990).

The nursing process provides an excellent framework in which to ensure the best quality of care for the woman and her baby, for it can be applied to the physical, emotional, and sociocultural aspects of care and can include the expectant woman as a partner in her care.

▼ Assessment

As in any situation, assessment is a critical component of the provision of health care throughout pregnancy. Because pregnancy is a normal physiologic process, the primary purpose of prenatal care is to consistently make assessments that the pregnancy is proceeding normally and that no alterations have occurred. Assessment begins at the first prenatal visit and is repeated at each contact throughout the pregnancy. At each of these contacts it must include the following components: an initial comprehensive health history or history update since the last visit, a physical examination, laboratory tests, screening for high-risk alterations, and counseling and education on healthful behavior. The initial prenatal visit should be scheduled for at least 1 hour. If this is not possible, two 30-minute visits should be scheduled 1 week apart (Public Health Service 1989; Cunningham et al. 1993).

▼ INTERVIEW

The initial interview with the woman who is pregnant is critical, for it is the time to begin establishing a therapeutic relationship and to collect essential information about her health history. A warm, friendly approach that conveys sincere interest and concern about the woman is important. The environment selected for the initial interview is also important. It should be as private and quiet as possible. These factors facilitate the woman's trust and encourage open communication. It is important to identify the woman's desires and expectations regarding her prenatal care at this time. The partner or other family members can be included in the interview if the woman desires. This helps the nurse to evaluate the family relationships and identify the nature of the woman's support system. Family members can often add important information about the health history that the woman may not remember. Some of the assessment data can be collected by a self-administered questionnaire; however, this method should not be the only one used to obtain information. If a questionnaire is used, it should be followed by an interview to validate and clarify the information collected and to establish rapport with the woman and her family.

It is important to collect both subjective and objective data. Subjective data include the nurse's observations of the woman's appearance, affect, behavior, attitudes, and response to being pregnant. Objective data consist of demographic data, a medical and gynecologic history, family health history, history of past pregnancies, and history of the current pregnancy. This information serves as a basic screen to identify any factors that may adversely affect the course of the pregnancy. At each subsequent visit throughout the pregnancy a shorter update of the initial history is completed to identify recent events, the woman's current health status, and symptoms since the last visit (see Components of Prenatal Health History). All data collected must be carefully documented on

Table 16–3

CURRENT ROUTINES AND SUGGESTED ALTERNATIVES*

CURRENT	SUGGESTED
Patients' records are "owned" by the health facility	Make each woman responsible for her own obstetric folder. If her first language is not English, make provisions to record pregnancy information so she can read it.
Pregnant women are impersonally scheduled for their initial antepartal visit, usually by phone	View the initial phone contact as an important communication opportunity. Have the person making phone contact convey interest, as well as information about self-care practices. Obtain preliminary assessment of risk status using a brief checklist. Give women a specific person's name as a phone contact for pregnancy-related questions. Send a follow-up welcoming letter.
Time between initial booking and the first prenatal visit is 3–6 wk	Have the pregnant woman seen within a week, either in a group orientation session, individually by a health team member, or, if her risk status warrants it, by a physician.
In many settings, women still meet the health care provider at the first visit when they are partially or completely undressed and lying on an examination table	At the first visit, the woman should be seen first fully clothed and upright, before the physical examination. She should have the opportunity to discuss the pregnancy, health history, and social or psychological issues with the health care provider in this manner.
The woman's family member or other support person is not welcomed to accompany her throughout the examination if she desires	Invite and encourage family members and friends to come for antepartal visits. Allow them to enter the examination room and participate in all aspects of care to the extent desired by the pregnant woman.
In some settings, blood pressure, weight, and urine checks are done in a waiting room or other public area, in view of other pregnant women and their families	Provide privacy for all assessments. Teach pregnant women and their family members to take responsibility for doing and recording some of the basic prenatal assessments (e.g., weight, urine checks).
Office or clinic visits are scheduled only during weekdays in many settings	Make evening and weekend hours available for prenatal care.
In many clinics or large private group practices, the woman may see a different nurse, midwife, or physician on each visit	Try to provide continuity of care and allow some choice among care providers. Assign a primary care nurse to the family for the duration of pregnancy to coordinate plan of care.
Women are addressed by their first or last names, according to established local custom; health care providers often neglect to introduce themselves and inform women of their names	Ask women how they would like to be addressed and record this information on their records; be sure that women know your name.
Waiting time is unpredictable and in some settings may be an hour or more	Minimize waiting time by better use of care team members and careful scheduling. Plan antepartal care educational activities for waiting periods, including programs for those with special needs, such as high-risk or non–English-speaking women.
Decisions about prenatal and intrapartal care may still be made by health care providers, without informing pregnant women of their options or asking them about their preferences	Educate pregnant women about care options and encourage them to participate in decision making. Develop preference profiles with each woman and her family and include them in the prenatal records sent to the birth facility.

*Since the original publication of this table, progress has been made in improving many maternity care practices. However, the changes suggested here are still not available to pregnant women and their families in all areas of the country, particularly those without private health care.

From Mahan, C., and McKay, S. (1984). Let's reform our antenatal care methods. *Contemporary Obstetrics and Gynecology,* 23 (May), 147.

PHYSIOLOGIC CHANGES OF PREGNANCY

Assessment is an integral component of antepartal care. In many settings, the role of the professional nurse has changed to include responsibility for in-depth nursing assessments. For these reasons, it is important that nurses develop and refine their assessment skills. The following steps can help the nurse to accomplish this goal.

- TAKE A HEALTH ASSESSMENT COURSE. This is particularly important if advanced health assessment skills were not part of the nurse's basic nursing education. Completion of a health assessment course should prepare the nurse to obtain a health history and perform a physical examination.
- PRACTICE SKILLS REGULARLY. Skill in physical assessment is lost if not used regularly. Seek opportunities to use assessment skills frequently in the clinical setting.
- SEEK GUIDANCE AND REAFFIRMATION AS NEEDED. Use another nurse, a nurse-midwife, or a physician as a preceptor when first learning new assessment skills. If uncertain of techniques or findings, do not hesitate to ask for help.
- USE A PHYSICAL ASSESSMENT TEXTBOOK FOR REFERENCE. Purchase a textbook that provides an excellent description of the skills you will be using. Periodically review the information to improve your theoretic understanding and techniques.
- ATTEND INSERVICE EDUCATION CLASSES. Many health care settings or hospitals regularly offer inservice education to enable staff to maintain skills or to become informed about new techniques or equipment. These classes are an important component of continuing professional education.
- BECOME INVOLVED IN SETTING POLICY. Most health care settings have developed written policies regarding the role of the nurse in health assessment. Become involved in the writing of these policies so that the interest of the nurse is represented and the nurse's full potential can be utilized in the provision of health care.

the woman's prenatal record (Assessment Tool: Prenatal Laboratory Data).

The interview provides an excellent opportunity to begin teaching the woman about the importance of prenatal care. Explanations should be given about the importance of the data being collected and how the information is related to pregnancy. The nurse should use terminology that is understood by the woman or explain the meanings of terms that the woman will hear throughout her pregnancy. Some prenatal caregivers have found it helpful to involve the woman in the responsibility for her prenatal care by making her record accessible to her so that she can confirm the data recorded and follow her progress or by establishing a contract with the woman that outlines her responsibilities and those of the health care providers in her care during pregnancy.

▼ PHYSICAL EXAMINATION

After data about the woman's health history have been collected, the physical examination is performed. The initial examination provides baseline data for each of the body systems that serve as a basis of comparison regarding changes that occur throughout the pregnancy. The nurse can help the woman relax before the examination by having her empty her bladder (and provide a clean catch specimen if one has not previously been collected), ensuring her comfort and privacy in the examination room, and explaining what will be done. In conducting the physical examination, an organized sequence of some type should be followed so that nothing is omitted. Most health care providers prefer to follow either a systems approach (collecting data about each body system) or a cephalocaudal approach (collecting data by moving from head to toe). As the examination proceeds, the examiner should describe what is being assessed and explain why each observation is important in pregnancy so that the woman understands why regular assessments are necessary. The components of the initial physical examination are seen in Components of Prenatal Examination.

Vital Signs, Height, and Weight. The vital signs are taken and height and weight are measured. Blood pressure is a critical measurement throughout pregnancy. Any change from the initial baseline reading should be noted in the chart. A blood pressure of 140/90 is indicative of PIH, as is any rise of 30 mm Hg in the systolic or 15 mm Hg in the diastolic component. The blood pressure should be measured with the woman in the same position at each visit in order to eliminate variations that might occur with positional changes. The pulse, respirations, and temperature should also be recorded for baseline data. Measurements of height and weight are also helpful as baseline

Components of Prenatal Health History

Demographic Data

1. Age
2. Race or ethnic group (necessary to identify need for genetic testing)
3. Religion (necessary to identify beliefs that might influence health care)
4. Occupation (necessary to identify potential fetal and maternal risks)
5. Address and telephone

Medical and Gynecologic History

1. Childhood illnesses
2. Immunizations
3. Disease conditions (hypertension, cardiovascular disease, diabetes, renal disorders, bleeding disorders, hepatitis)
4. Injuries or handicapping conditions
5. Surgery or hospitalizations
6. Previous blood transfusions
7. Blood type and Rh factor
8. Use of alcohol, illicit drugs, or cigarettes
9. Prescription or over-the-counter medications taken
10. Drug allergies
11. Exposure to teratogenic factors (x-rays, employment risks, cat in the home—toxoplasmosis, viral infections)
12. Weight
13. Menstrual history (age at menarche; regularity, frequency, and duration of flow; dysmenorrhea)
14. Sexual history
15. Contraceptive history
16. Infections (vaginal, cervical, tubal, sexually transmitted)

Family and Partner Health History

1. Hypertension, cardiovascular disease, diabetes, hematologic disorders, allergies, pregnancy-induced hypertension
2. Drug or alcohol use
3. Blood type and Rh factor
4. Congenital diseases or deformities
5. Multiple births
6. Cesarean births

History of Past Pregnancies

1. Gravity and parity (number of pregnancies, number of spontaneous or elective abortions, stillbirths, number of living children)
2. Medical problems (pregnancy-induced hypertension, gestational diabetes, infections, preterm labor)
3. Labors and deliveries (length of labor, type of delivery, complications, interventions needed)
4. Neonatal (weeks' gestation at birth; birth weights; Apgar scores; respiratory, infectious, or hematologic health problems; feeding method)

History of Current Pregnancy

1. First day of last menstrual period
2. Estimated dates of conception and delivery
3. Cramping, spotting, or bleeding since last period
4. Results of pregnancy test
5. Discomforts (e.g. nausea, vomiting, headache, pain, urinary frequency, fatigue)
6. Exposure to teratogens or contagious illnesses
7. Drugs, alcohol, or cigarettes
8. Childbirth education

Components of a Psychological History—See Chapter 17

Components of a Sociocultural History—See Chapter 18

REVISIT

Questions, Complaints, or Concerns Since Last Visit

1. Changes noted in body since last visit
2. Minor discomforts of pregnancy
3. Appetite, nutritional practices, typical 24-hr diet
4. Maintenance or interference with daily activities, work, or exercise
5. Sexual concerns

Continued on following page

Components of Prenatal Health History Continued

Presence of Danger Signs

1. Vaginal bleeding
2. Edema of face or fingers
3. Severe or continuous headache
4. Blurred vision
5. Abdominal pain
6. Persistent vomiting
7. Escape of fluid from the vagina
8. Frequent or regular uterine contractions
9. Pelvic pressure
10. Dysuria
11. Chills or fever
12. Excessive weight gain

Exposure to Potential Teratogens

1. Use of medications and reasons
2. Alcohol, drug, or cigarette use

Emotional Responses to Pregnancy

1. Feelings about pregnancy
2. Father's adjustment, siblings' adjustment
3. Anxieties about birth or new parenting role

Sociocultural Adaptation to Pregnancy

1. Family adjustments
2. Work adjustments and plans
3. Financial management
4. Preparation for baby
5. Plans for infant feeding

Education About Pregnancy, Birth, Parenting

1. Reading
2. Childbirth classes
3. Teaching posters
4. Films seen
5. Practicing breathing and relaxation for birth

Data from Block, G., and Nolan, J. (1986). *Health assessment for professional nursing: A developmental approach.* Norwalk, CT: Appleton-Century-Crofts, and Public Health Service, Expert Panel on the Content of Prenatal Care. (1989). *Caring for our future: The content of prenatal care.* Washington, DC: U.S. Department of Health and Human Services.

data and are used to guide counseling regarding diet and nutrition. Weight gain should occur gradually during pregnancy, averaging 2 to 4 total pounds in the first trimester, 1 pound per week in the second trimester, and a little less than a pound per week in the third trimester. The total weight gain should average 24 to 28 pounds; a range of 20 to 30 pounds is within accepted limits. The recommended weight gain is influenced by the woman's prepregnancy weight and her body mass index (BMI) (see Chapter 19). The vital signs and weight should also be recorded at each revisit. It is helpful if they are recorded in such a way that patterns of change can easily be seen, as on a graph.

General Well-Being. An initial examination for general well-being should include an assessment of the integumentary system, cardiovascular system, respiratory system, and musculoskeletal system. Observation of skin color and the condition of the hair and nails gives an indication of general health and nutritional status. The presence of lesions, moles, scars, striae, linea nigra, and chloasma should be noted. The mouth and gums should be pink and moist. Hypertrophy and redness of gum tissue may be noted and is due to the influence of estrogen. The thyroid is palpated for enlargement and irregularities. It should remain small with smooth lateral lobes palpable on each side of the trachea.

Examination of the chest and lungs should reveal no retraction or bulging of intercostal spaces during inspiration or expiration. On auscultation the upper lobes should reveal equal bronchovesicular sounds on inspiration and expiration above the sternum and scapulas. In the remainder of the chest, vesicular breath sounds should be heard without rales, rhonchi, or wheezes. Heart rate and rhythm should remain normal with no abnormal heart sounds or murmurs. Any murmurs or extra sounds should be noted. The woman's posture and range of motion should be noted. Reflexes should be normal and symmetric. The extremities should be observed for color, pulses, and edema. Examination of the legs should include inspection for varicose veins and dorsiflexion of the foot with the legs extended to check for Homans' sign and thrombophlebitis.

Assessment Tool:

HOLLISTER maternal/newborn RECORD SYSTEM

Prenatal Laboratory Data

Patient's Name ______
ID. No. ______

Initial Screening

Date	Test	Result
	Blood Type/Rh (Mother)	☐ O ☐ A ☐ B ☐ AB +/−
	Blood Type/Rh (Father)	☐ O ☐ A ☐ B ☐ AB +/−
	Rh Antibody Screen	☐ Neg ☐ Pos Titer____:____
	Hgb/Hct	______gms/dL____%
	CBC	☐ Normal ☐ Abnormal
	RPR	☐ Non-Reactive ☐ Reactive
	FTA-ABS	☐ Non-Reactive ☐ Reactive
	Rubella Antibody Titer	☐ Immune ☐ Non-Immune
	Hepatitis Screen	☐ Neg ☐ Pos (type______)
	HTLV-3 or HIV	☐ Neg ☐ Pos
	CMV Screen	☐ Neg ☐ Pos
	PPD/Chest X-Ray	☐ Neg ☐ Pos / ☐ Neg ☐ Pos
	Serology for Toxoplasma gondii	☐ Neg ☐ Pos
	______	______
	Hgb Electrophoresis (Mother)	☐ Neg ☐ Pos HgS______% HgA_2____% HgF______%
	Hgb Electrophoresis (Father)	☐ Neg ☐ Pos HgS______% HgA_2____% HgF______%
	Tay-Sachs Screen (Mother)	☐ Neg ☐ Pos ______
	Tay-Sachs Screen (Father)	☐ Neg ☐ Pos ______
	______	______
	Urinalysis (Macro)	☐ Normal ☐ Abnormal
	Urine (Micro)	______
	Urine Culture	☐ No Growth ☐ Growth ____Organism/ml
	Toxicology Screen	☐ Neg ☐ Pos ______
	______	______
	PAP	☐ Normal ☐ Abnormal
	Gonorrhea	☐ Neg ☐ Pos
	Chlamydia Culture	☐ Neg ☐ Pos
	Herpes Culture	☐ Neg ☐ Pos
	Beta Streptococcus	☐ Neg ☐ Pos

Follow-Up, Repeat Labs

Date	Test	Result
	Diabetes Screen (24-28 Wks)	☐ Neg ☐ Pos ______
	GTT	____FBS ____1 Hr ____2 Hr ____3 Hr
	______	______
	______	______

Follow-Up, Repeat Labs (Cont'd.)

Date	Test	Result
	Hgb/Hct	______gms/dL____%
	Hgb/Hct	______gms/dL____%
	Rh Antibody Screen (28 Wks)	☐ Neg ☐ Pos Titer____:____
	______	______
	Cervical or Vaginal Culture	☐ Neg ☐ Pos ______
	______	______
	Urine Culture	☐ No Growth ☐ Growth ____Organism/ml

Tests of Fetal Well-Being

Date	Test	Result
	Serum AFP (15-18 Wks)	☐ Normal ☐ High ☐ Low
	Repeat Serum AFP	☐ Normal ☐ High ☐ Low
	Ultrasound	Findings
	Ultrasound	Findings
	Ultrasound	Findings
	Fetal Movement Count	☐ Normal ☐ Abnormal
	Biophysical Profile	☐ Normal ☐ Equivocal ☐ Abnormal
	NST	☐ Reactive ☐ Unsatisfactory ☐ Non-React.
	NST	☐ Reactive ☐ Unsatisfactory ☐ Non-React.
	NST	☐ Reactive ☐ Unsatisfactory ☐ Non-React.
	NST	☐ Reactive ☐ Unsatisfactory ☐ Non-React.
	NST	☐ Reactive ☐ Unsatisfactory ☐ Non-React.
	NST	☐ Reactive ☐ Unsatisfactory ☐ Non-React.
	CST	☐ Negative ☐ Suspicious ☐ Positive
	CST	☐ Negative ☐ Suspicious ☐ Positive
	CST	☐ Negative ☐ Suspicious ☐ Positive

Hollister
HOLLISTER INCORPORATED, 2000 HOLLISTER DR, LIBERTYVILLE, IL 60048

PRENATAL LABORATORY DATA FORM #5705
691

MATERNAL RECORD COPY

Components of Prenatal Examination

Vital Signs

1. Blood pressure
2. Pulse
3. Respiration

Height and Weight

General Well-being

1. Skin, hair, nails
2. Mouth, gums
3. Thyroid
4. Chest and lungs
5. Heart
6. Posture and range of motion
7. Extremities

Breast Examination

1. Symmetry and pigmentation
2. Firmness and consistency
3. Nipples
4. Colostrum
5. Axillary nodes

Abdominal Examination

1. Size and conformation
2. Pigmentation
3. Fundal height (as soon as possible)
4. Leopold maneuvers (as soon as possible)
5. Diastasis rectus
6. Fetal heart tones (as soon as audible)
7. Maternal and fetal souffle (as soon as audible)

Pelvic Examination

1. Vaginal color and discharge
2. Cervical color and appearance
3. Uterine size, position, shape
4. Ovaries
5. Pelvic measurements

Laboratory Tests

1. Hemoglobin or hematocrit
2. Rh antibody screen
3. Syphilis test
4. Random blood glucose level
5. Gonococcal culture
6. *Chlamydia* culture
7. Hepatitis B
8. HIV screen (encourage)
9. Urine culture
10. Urine dipstick
    Protein
    Glucose
11. Pap smear
12. Tuberculosis
13. Rubella titer

REVISIT

Vital Signs

1. Blood pressure (each visit)

Weight (each visit)

Abdominal Examination

1. Fundal height and growth (16 wk and after)
2. Leopold maneuvers (24 wk and after)
3. Fetal heart tones (20 wk and after)

Pelvic Examination (after 36 wk)

1. Cervical assessment
2. Reassessment of bony pelvis

Laboratory Tests

1. Repeat hemoglobin or hematocrit (after 24 wk)
2. Repeat Rh antibody screen (26–28 wk)
3. Diabetic screen (26–28 wk)
4. Repeat syphilis test if needed (third trimester)
5. Repeat gonococcal culture if needed (36 wk)
6. Repeat HIV screen if needed (36 wk)
7. Maternal serum alpha-fetoprotein (14–16 wk)
8. Obstetric ultrasound examination if indicated

Data from Public Health Service, Expert Panel on the Content of Prenatal Care. (1989). *Caring for our future: The content of prenatal care.* Washington, DC: U.S. Department of Health and Human Services.

Breast Examination. The breast examination is important not only for assessing breast changes that have taken place as a result of the pregnancy but also for teaching the woman about doing routine breast self-examination. The breasts should be symmetric in size and contour. Pigmentary changes in the nipples and areolar areas may be noted, as well as the development of striae and superficial venous patterns. If the woman is planning to breastfeed, the nipples should be assessed for erectility. The axillary nodes should be either unpalpable or the size of small pellets. Breast tissue may become more nodular as the ductal system grows, and colostrum may be present after the first trimester. Although the nodular changes in the consistency of the breast tissue may make it more difficult for the woman to examine her own breasts, she should be strongly encouraged to do so (see Teaching Guide). The changes that occur in pregnancy are gradual and can be monitored monthly. Changes related to breast cancer would be inconsistent and might include masses or lumps that are hard or fixed, breast pain, nipple retraction, or skin changes such as redness, dimpling, edema, ulceration, or rashes. If any of these changes are noted, the woman should be referred immediately for further evaluation.

Abdominal Examination. The abdominal examination is an important component of the physical examination and should take place at every prenatal visit. It consists of visual inspection, palpation and measurement, and auscultation and is important because abdominal changes serve as a rough guideline to fetal growth. Before doing the abdominal examination, the nurse should help the woman get into a comfortable position on the examination table. The woman should lie on her back with her knees flexed and a small pillow under her head. The abdomen should be exposed, but her chest and pelvic area can remain covered. If the woman becomes dizzy while lying flat on her back (because of the supine hypotensive syndrome), she should be helped immediately to her side to move the weight of the uterus off the inferior vena cava. Symptoms then subside quickly.

Initial visual inspection includes notation of normal skin changes such as striae and linea nigra, rashes or lesions, status of the umbilicus (whether inverted or protruding), presence of previous scars, and size and configuration of the abdomen. The size of the abdomen should be related to the estimated gestational age, and the configuration of the abdomen may give initial clues to fetal position. For example, an abdomen that appears distended in width may suggest a transverse lie of the fetus. These initial observations are verified by palpation and measurement.

Abdominal palpation enables the nurse to assess both uterine size and fetal position. As the uterus enlarges throughout pregnancy, the height of the fundus serves as a guide to the estimation of gestation. The symphysis pubis and umbilicus are used as landmarks for various points during gestation. For example, by the 12th week of pregnancy, the fundus is palpable just above the symphysis. At 16 weeks, the fundus is approximately halfway between the symphysis and the umbilicus. By 20 weeks' gestation, the fundus usually reaches the lower border of the umbilicus (see Fig. 16–4). After the 20th week, the uterus increases in height approximately 1 cm per week until weeks 34 to 36, when the fundus almost reaches the xiphoid process. During this time the measurement in centimeters should equal the gestational age. After 36 weeks the fundal measurement either remains the same or begins to decrease as the fetal head drops into the pelvis (lightening).

When measuring fundal height, the top of the uterus is located by moving the ulnar side of the hand downward from above the uterus in small progressive steps until the examiner can differentiate between the softness of the abdomen and the firm, round surface of the fundus (see Fig. 16–4). A tape measure is used to measure the height of the fundus in centimeters. When the fundal edge is located, its distance from the symphysis is measured by placing the zero point of the tape at the top rim of the symphysis. The tape is then held in place at the symphysis with the right hand while the left hand pulls the tape up over the abdominal curve to the fundus.

Two methods can be used to obtain the measurement. The first method avoids measuring the fundal curve and adipose tissue and therefore is considered more accurate. The left hand presses down slightly to identify the fundus, but the tape is held straight over the abdomen and is not brought up over the curve of the fundus. The second method keeps the tape in contact with the skin and brings the tape up over the curve of the fundus. This method is sometimes called McDonald's measurement (Fig. 16–10). The examiner should choose one of these methods for measuring fundal height and use it consistently. If the same examiner is not seeing the woman at each revisit, the method used should be noted in the chart along with the measurement.

McDonald's rule can be used to add precision to the fundal height measurement. The formula for McDonald's rule is:

$$\text{Height of fundus in cm} \times 2/7 = \text{duration of pregnancy in lunar months}$$

$$\text{Height of fundus in cm} \times 8/7 = \text{duration of pregnancy in weeks}$$

Other methods that have been used in the past for measuring fundal height are not advised today. These include (1) reporting the position of the uterus in finger breadths (FBs) above or below a

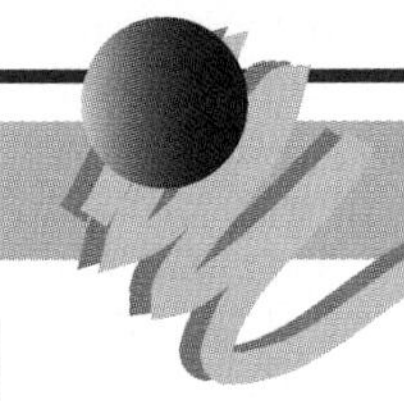

TEACHING GUIDE

BREAST SELF-EXAMINATION

TOPIC	*MAJOR CONCEPTS*
Importance of regular breast examination	Early detection of breast cancer is very important for its treatment and cure. Clients should be taught the three methods of breast cancer detection. The first, mammography, is an x-ray examination of the breast that should be done every 1–2 yrs after age 40; annually after age 50. The second is a clinical breast examination done by a doctor or nurse every 3 yrs between the ages of 20 and 40 and every year thereafter. The third is breast self-examination.
Breast self-examination	Women can monitor their own breasts every month, in the privacy of their home and at no cost. The optimum time for premenopausal women is a week after the menstrual period. Pregnant and postmenopausal women should pick a date that is easy to remember and mark it on their calendars.
Step 1: Look for Changes	Your client should begin the procedure by standing in front of a mirror.

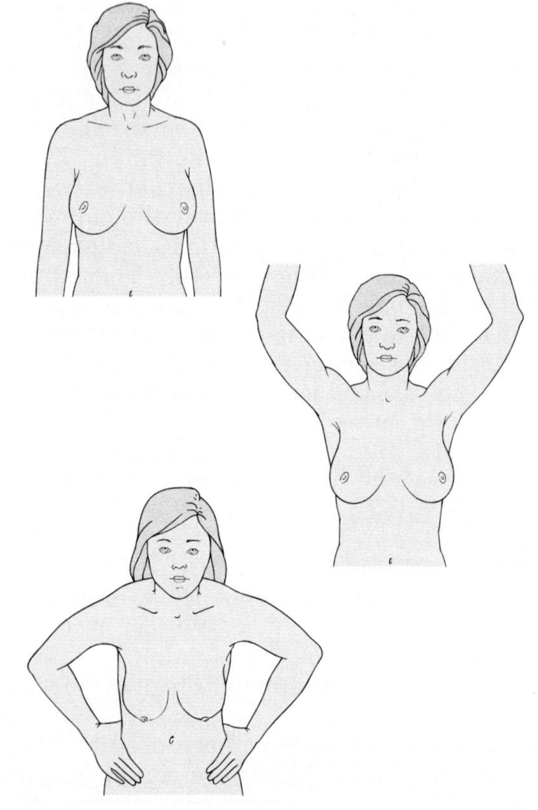

1. Keeping her hands at her sides, she should look for changes in shape and color of the breasts. Next she should check for puckering, dimpling, skin changes, or nipple discharge.
2. Raising her hands over her head, she should check for symmetry, puckering, or dimpling, both from the front and from the side.
3. Placing her hands on her hips, she should press down and bend forward. She should check the symmetry, nipple direction, and general appearance of her breasts, noting anything that looks unusual.

Continued on facing page

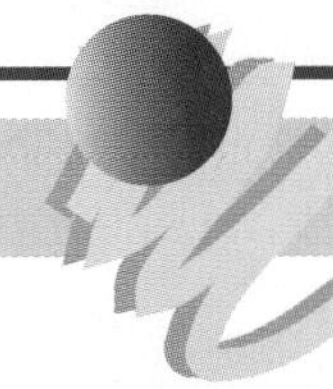

TEACHING GUIDE Continued

Step 2: Feel for Changes

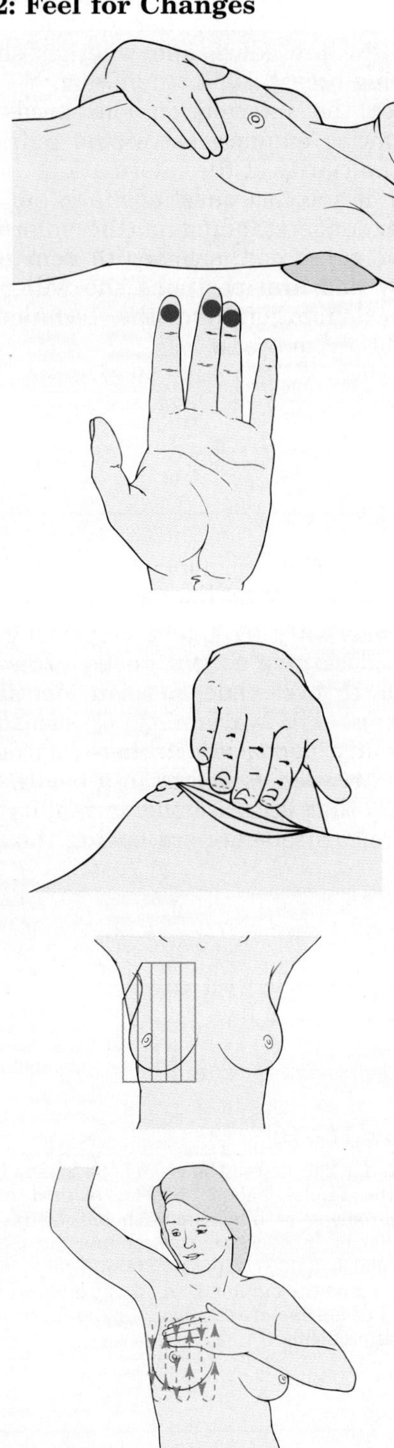

She should continue the procedure by lying down with a towel under her right shoulder and raising her right arm over her head.

1. Using the pads of the three middle fingers of her left hand (triple touch), she should examine her right breast; her hand should be in a bowed position and the fingers moved in dime-size circles.

2. Using light, medium, and firm pressure, she should examine her breast in four segments.

    - From the underarm down one side of the breast to the lower bra line
    - Across the breast to the breast bone
    - Up the other side of the breast to the collar bone
    - Back across the upper half of the breast to the armpit

3. She should examine the entire breast area using a vertical strip pattern.

Now, she should repeat this procedure using her right hand to examine her left breast. She should notify her health care provider immediately if she notices any lumps, knots, or changes in the breast tissue.

Data from *American Cancer Society guidelines for early detection*. (1994). New York: Author.

Continued on following page

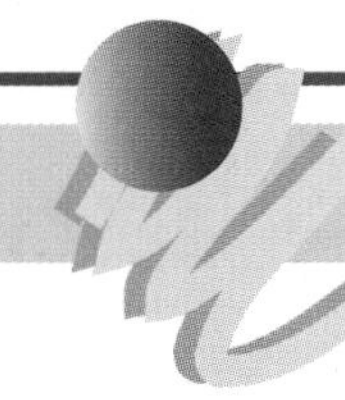

TEACHING GUIDE Continued

Teaching Aids

1. Posters or illustrations showing the technique for breast self-examination.
2. Breast models for identification of lumps or other alterations and to use when practicing correct palpation techniques.
3. Your own body to illustrate positioning and technique for the procedure.
4. Pamphlets illustrating the procedure that can be given to the woman to take home.

Increasing Your Teaching Effectiveness

Your success in teaching a woman about breast self-examination is enhanced by using the following approaches:

1. Establish a comfortable rapport with the woman and determine her current knowledge of the procedure and whether she has been doing breast self-examination.
2. Give her the information she needs in a clear, concise manner; use visual aids to increase the clarity of the information.
3. Ask her if she has questions; ask her to repeat her understanding of the information you have presented; ask her to demonstrate the body and arm positions she will use for breast examination and the technique for palpation of the breast.

selected landmark such as the symphysis, umbilicus, or xiphoid (example: the uterus is 2 FBs above the umbilicus); (2) estimating uterine position between two landmarks in fractions (example: the uterus is one half the distance between the symphysis and umbilicus); and (3) comparing the uterus with the sizes of selected fruits such as pears, oranges, grapefruits, or melons (Engstrom 1988).

The measurement of fundal height is approximate and may vary by 1 to 2 cm among examiners, but it does give a continuous assessment of uterine growth over time and can identify potential problems. The variability of measurements can be greatly decreased if there is consistency within and between clinicians in a health care setting. Factors that decrease the variability between sequential measurements are having the same ex-

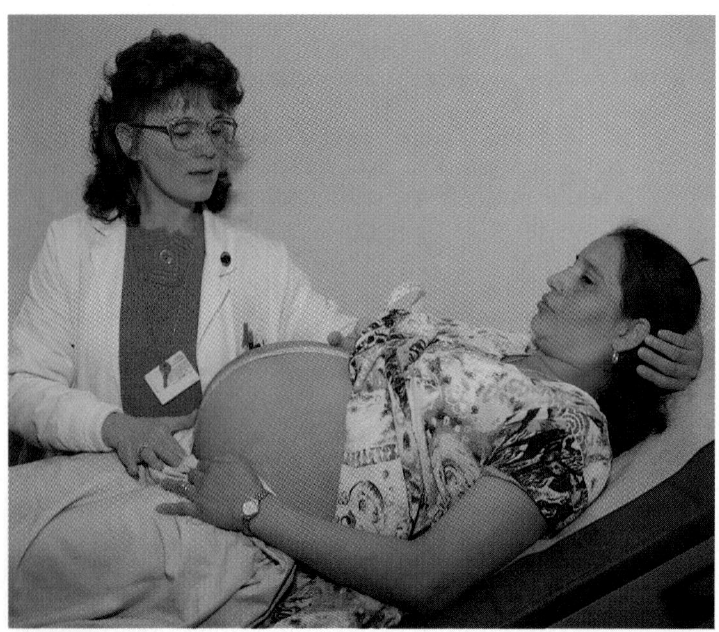

Figure 16–10

The nurse can assess the size of the uterus by measuring the fundal height • The method (McDonald's measurement is illustrated) should be recorded and used for each assessment • While the measurement of fundal height is approximate and may vary by 1 or 2 cm among examiners, it does give a continuous record of uterine growth over time and can identify potential problems.

aminer measure the uterus at each revisit, obtaining the measurement within 30 minutes of when the woman last voided, and obtaining the measurement with the woman in the same position.

If the fundal height measurements are not consistent with gestational age, further assessment with ultrasonography may be indicated. Inadequate uterine size is associated with complications such as intrauterine growth retardation (IUGR), fetal demise, oligohydramnios, and inaccurate estimation of the gestational interval. Excessive uterine size is associated with complications such as fetal macrosomia, hydramnios, multiple gestation, hydatidiform mole, and inaccurate estimation of the gestational interval (Engstrom 1988; Cunningham et al. 1993).

In addition to the measurement of fundal height, the abdomen is palpated to determine fetal position if the pregnancy is in the latter part of the second trimester or the third trimester, when the fetus has become large enough for the outline to be felt through the abdominal wall. This is done by using a method called Leopold maneuvers (Procedure 16–1). These maneuvers are a series of abdominal palpations that give information about fetal presentation, position, presenting part, attitude, and descent. It is helpful to do the Leopold maneuvers to find the baby's back before listening to the fetal heart tones (FHTs), as the FHTs are best heard through the back. Assessment of fetal size and single versus multiple gestation can also be accomplished by doing Leopold maneuvers.

When doing Leopold maneuvers, the examiner may also feel fetal movement. This is considered a positive sign that the baby is doing well and can add information about the position of the baby. When fetal movement is first felt by the woman, between 16 and 20 weeks' gestation, it may be perceived as a faint flutter. By the time the nurse is able to feel the baby moving, the movements are usually brisk kicks. This movement can often be observed by watching the abdomen, as well as felt by the hands. The date of the first perceived fetal movement (quickening) may be used as an indicator of gestational age. However, because of the wide variation in the time when fetal movement is felt and the subjective nature of this assessment, the use of quickening as the only method of assessing the gestational interval of the pregnancy is not valid (Cunningham et al. 1993).

The final abdominal palpation is done to evaluate the rectus abdominis musculature for a diastasis. This is done to determine the amount of separation that has occurred in the rectus muscle as a result of the pregnancy. The woman is instructed to lie on her back, take a deep breath, and gently exhale. This forces the diaphragm downward and decreases the size of the abdominal cavity. A separation in the rectus muscle may be palpated during exhalation or observed as a ridge between the muscles when the intra-abdominal pressure is increased by raising the head and shoulders. A separation does not pose a threat to the function of abdominal organs and usually corrects itself during the postpartum period. Identification of a diastasis is important in guiding teaching about posture and exercise during pregnancy (see Chapter 19).

Abdominal auscultation follows the palpation of the abdomen and is the last component of the abdominal examination. The abdomen is auscultated during pregnancy for the primary purpose of listening to the FHTs. FHTs are much easier to locate after the Leopold maneuvers have been done, because identification of the position of the baby suggests where the heart tones can best be heard. The location of the fetal back suggests the side of the abdomen on which to listen for heart tones. If the baby is in a cephalic presentation, the FHTs are more likely to be heard in the lower half of the abdomen, below the umbilicus. If the baby is in a breech presentation, the FHTs are more likely to be heard above the umbilicus. Knowing both the side of the abdomen where the baby's back is located and the presentation of the baby allows the nurse to select a quadrant of the abdomen where the heart tones are most likely to be heard.

Fetal heart tones can be heard with a Doppler ultrasound stethoscope as early as 8 to 11 weeks' gestation and with a fetoscope by 18 to 20 weeks' gestation (Fig. 16–11). The Doppler stethoscope magnifies the sound, and the fetoscope uses bone conduction from the nurse's head to enhance auscultation. A regular stethoscope can be used but may not be as effective. Auscultation of the abdomen should be part of the assessment at every revisit during pregnancy.

The normal fetal heart rate is 120 to 160 beats per minute. The sound heard may be soft and muffled or loud and bounding, depending on the baby's position. Because the rate is rapid, it is sometimes helpful to use the index finger to tap the beat as it is heard to assist in counting it. The FHTs should be counted for a full minute to identify any irregularities. Hearing the FHTs can add confirming information regarding gestational age, but this assessment alone is not a valid method for determining gestational age. Hearing the FHTs helps to assure that the fetus is viable and provides confirmation and reassurance to the mother about the reality of the pregnancy and the status of her baby. At each revisit during pregnancy, the parents should always be given the opportunity to listen to the FHTs; usually this provides a sense of excitement and can contribute to prenatal attachment. Further discussion of assessment of the FHTs can be found in Chapter 26.

In addition to the FHTs, other sounds may be heard in the abdomen. A uterine souffle (maternal souffle) or funic souffle (fetal souffle) may be heard as a swishing sound. The uterine souffle results from the blood rushing through the placenta

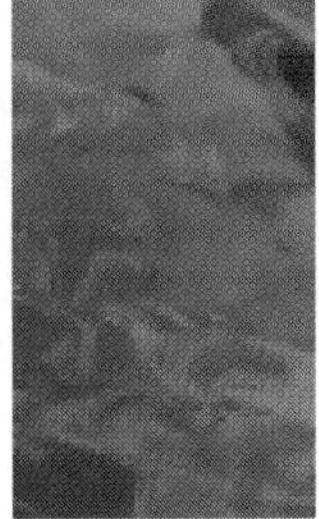

Leopold Maneuvers

▼ PURPOSE

To provide information about fetal presentation, position, presenting part, lie, attitude, and descent. Can aid in location of fetal heart tones, assessment of fetal size, and determination of single versus multiple gestation. Performed in latter part of second trimester or third trimester, after fetus has become large enough for outline to be felt through abdominal wall.

▼ EQUIPMENT

- Flat examination bed

1 Instruct the woman to empty her bladder and to lie on her back on the examination bed with her knees bent. **An empty bladder contributes to the woman's comfort during the examination. The bent-knee position relaxes the abdominal muscles, facilitating palpation of the fetal parts.**

2 Provide a wedge under the woman's right or left hip to maintain a slight lateral tilt. **A wedge under the woman's hip displaces the uterus sufficiently to prevent compression of the maternal blood vessels and subsequent supine hypotension.**

3 With warm hands, perform each maneuver systematically using gentle but firm motions. Stand by the woman's side, facing her head for the first three maneuvers. **Warm hands help prevent tightening of the abdominal muscles and promote the woman's comfort. Position facilitates the ease and accuracy of performing the procedure.**

First Maneuver

4 Palpate the uterine fundus with both hands to identify the fetal part (either the breech or the head) and the fetal lie. **Determines whether the fetal presentation is cephalic (breech in fundus) or breech (head in fundus). The breech is softer, broader, less uniform, and less movable than the head. Also determines whether the fetal lie is longitudinal, transverse, or oblique.**

Second Maneuver

5 Move your hands to the sides of the abdomen to locate the fetal back. With one hand in place to steady the uterus, use the other hand to palpate the opposite side of the uterus with firm, circular motions to identify either a smooth fetal back or knobby small parts, such as knees or feet. Repeat the maneuver, but palpate the opposite side of the uterus to confirm your findings. **Determines the position of the fetus in relation to the uterus.**

Third Maneuver

6 With the thumb and fingers of one hand, gently grasp the lower portion of the abdomen just above the symphysis pubis to hold the presenting part (the part nearest the cervix). Attempt to move the presenting part side to side between your thumb and fingers to determine whether the part is the head (hard and smooth) or the breech (soft and irregular) and whether it is floating above the pelvis, dipping into the pelvis, or engaged (immobile) in the pelvis. **Confirms data on presentation of fetus from first maneuver. Provides information about the level of descent of the presenting part in the pelvis.**

Fourth Maneuver

7 To do the fourth maneuver, turn and face the woman's feet. Place the palmar surface of your hands on each side of the abdomen. Move your hands down the sides of the abdomen toward the symphysis pubis, palpat-

Continued on facing page

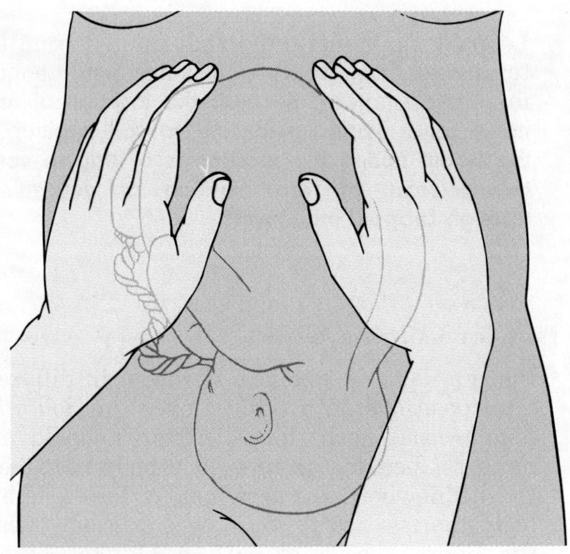
First maneuver

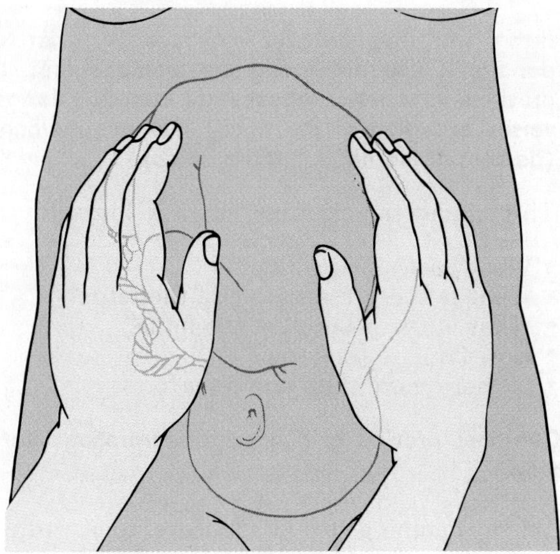
Second maneuver

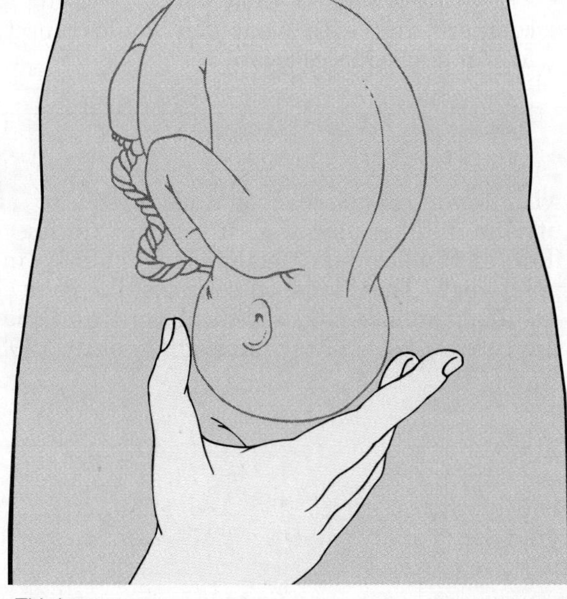
Third maneuver

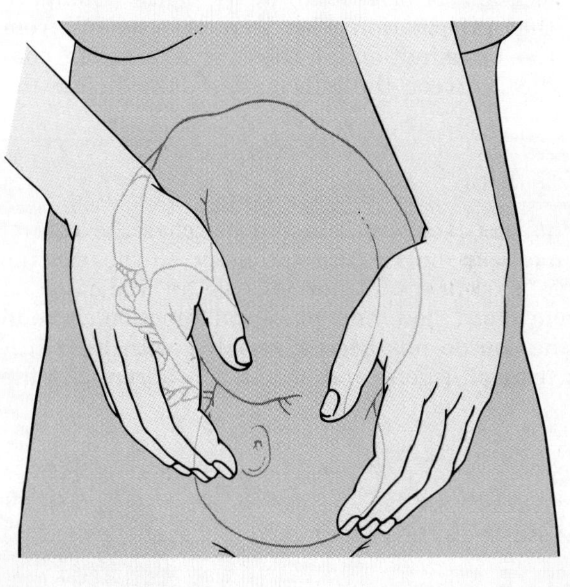
Fourth maneuver

ing with your fingertips for resistance on either side, to locate the cephalic prominence. One of your hands will continue, unimpeded, toward the symphysis pubis. Your other hand will feel resistance because it has come upon the cephalic prominence. If you first feel resistance on the side opposite the fetal back, the cephalic prominence is the fetal brow (forehead); this indicates that the fetal head is well flexed. If you first feel resistance on the same side as the fetal back, the cephalic prominence is the occiput; this indicates that the fetal head is not well flexed. Note whether the head is free and floating or

Continued on following page

PROCEDURE 16–1 Continued

flexed and engaged. **The maneuver is easier to perform if you are facing the woman's feet. It provides information about fetal attitude (flexion versus extension of the head) and engagement (descent of the head into the pelvis).**

8 Throughout the examination, ask yourself:

- What part am I feeling?
- What is the presentation of the fetus?
- What is the position of the fetus?
- How large is the fetus?
- Is there more than one fetus?

Questions provide guidance for interpreting information.

9 When listening to fetal heart tones after completing the Leopold maneuvers, note the location of the fetal heart tones. Compare that information with your assessment from the examination. If there is a possible conflict between the information gained from the Leopold maneuvers and that gained from listening to fetal heart tones, perform Leopold maneuvers again. **Because the location of fetal heart tones varies according to the position of the baby, noting the location is a way to verify the accuracy of fetal position as determined through Leopold maneuvers.**

Tips for Gaining Skill

- Place a doll the size of a newborn in different fetal positions on a table. Cover the doll with a pillowcase each time. Perform Leopold maneuvers, focusing on how each body part feels.
- In the newborn nursery, gently feel a baby's body parts—with your eyes closed—while the baby is covered with a blanket in the crib.
- Practice visualizing what you are feeling and compare that with what you would expect to feel in a specific position.

and uterine blood vessels and matches the rate of the mother's pulse. The intensity of the uterine souffle has been interpreted as an indicator of uterine blood flow and placental function. A loud uterine souffle has been associated with high urinary estriol levels and a soft or absent souffle with lower estriol levels. Thus, a soft or absent uterine souffle may indicate poor uterine blood flow and placental function, particularly in late pregnancy. The funic souffle results from blood rushing through the umbilical cord and matches the rate of the FHTs (Cunningham et al. 1993).

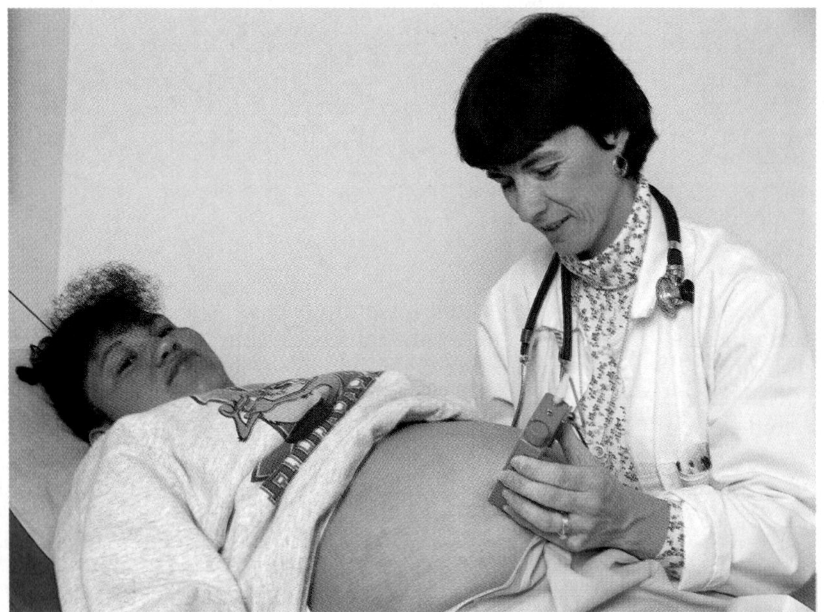

Figure 16–11

The nurse uses a Doppler ultrasound stethoscope to locate and count the fetal heart tones (FHTs) • Women are usually very curious about their baby's heartbeat • After the nurse has completed the assessment, she or he should teach the client about the normal range of fetal heart rate (FHR) and discuss the baby's heart rate • The mother should then be offered the opportunity to listen to her baby's heart tones.

Pelvic Examination. The pelvic examination is done at the initial prenatal visit to provide information about the presumptive and probable signs of pregnancy and to note any pelvic abnormalities that might influence the pregnancy, labor, or birth (Procedure 16–2). It also provides an opportunity to obtain cytologic specimens for laboratory evaluation and to assess the bony pelvis. After the initial prenatal visit, pelvic examinations are not usually repeated until the last month of pregnancy.

The pregnant woman may be uneasy about having a pelvic examination, particularly if she is a teenager or if this is the first pelvic examination she has experienced. Even the most experienced woman may be nervous or embarrassed about this part of the physical assessment, and the nurse can do a great deal to put the woman at ease and provide support throughout the examination. The woman should be prepared for the pelvic examination by explaining what will be done, what she will feel, and what information will be obtained. It is helpful to have charts or other visual aids to illustrate the pelvic organs. Her bladder should be empty, for a full bladder not only makes the examination more uncomfortable but also makes accurate assessment of uterine size more difficult. The woman should be positioned in the lithotomy position (see Fig. 16–1). Although it has been traditional to drape the woman for a pelvic examination, Willard and colleagues (1986) found that a large percentage of women preferred to see the examiner's face during the examination and disliked the air of mystery created by having the examiner hidden behind a drape.

During the examination the nurse can help the woman relax by remaining at her side, encouraging her to relax her pelvic floor muscles, and showing her how to do a slow, relaxed breathing technique. Teaching about what is being assessed should continue throughout the examination. Allowing the woman to examine a speculum before the examination may relieve her anxiety, although it may heighten anxiety. The needs of each woman must be assessed individually. Some women may appreciate having a mirror available to visualize the cervix and other anatomic structures being evaluated. This allows the woman to become an active participant in the examination, learn about her body, voice concerns, and share in decisions regarding her care. The study by Willard and colleagues (1986) showed that the majority of women in the sample preferred the educational format of a pelvic examination created with use of a mirror.

The pelvic examination has several components. The first step is visual inspection of the external genitalia. This is done to identify any abnormalities or infections that can be treated before labor and birth. The speculum examination is done to visualize changes in the introitus, vagina, and cervix. Changes in the color of the cervix and vagina (Chadwick's sign) are noted, and cervical specimens are taken for the Papanicolaou test and gonococcal screen. The amount and character of the vaginal discharge are noted. The speculum component of the pelvic examination is not usually repeated during pregnancy unless a problem arises. A bimanual examination is the third component of the pelvic assessment. In the first trimester, uterine enlargement, shape, position, and location can be noted. Changes in the consistency of the cervix (Goodell's sign) and lower uterine segment (Hegar's sign) can be palpated. The effacement (thinning) and dilation (opening) of the cervix can also be assessed. The final component of the pelvic examination is an assessment of the bony pelvis (see Chapter 22). This is done to determine the adequacy of the pelvic diameters for delivery. If the pelvis is not large enough, the baby will not be able to pass through during labor and birth. Bimanual examinations are not usually repeated after the initial prenatal visit until 36 weeks' gestation. They are done at that time to assess cervical changes that indicate readiness for labor and the descent of the baby into the pelvis. The bimanual pelvic examination may be repeated at each weekly revisit in the last month of pregnancy (Cunningham et al. 1993).

Laboratory Tests. Laboratory evaluation of urine and blood specimens is an important part of prenatal physical assessment, for laboratory tests provide data that support information obtained during the interview or physical examination. Most laboratory tests are done on the initial prenatal visit and not repeated again until the second or third trimester. Evaluations of prenatal care for women who are not at high risk suggested that laboratory tests that have become routine may not need to be done as often (Public Health Service 1989; Young 1990).

A urine sample for testing is obtained at every prenatal visit by having the woman bring her first voided specimen with her or obtaining a midstream clean catch specimen from the woman when she arrives for her appointment. At the initial visit and all return visits, a dipstick reading is taken to assess glucose, protein, and ketones (Procedure 16–3). During pregnancy, glucose may occasionally appear in the urine in small amounts. This is usually a reflection of the increased glomerular filtration rate and decreased tubular reabsorption during pregnancy. However, if large amounts of glucose are noted on more than one occasion, further screening should be done for gestational diabetes (see Chapter 21). Traces of protein may also be found in the urine as a result of vaginal secretions or blood, but large amounts of protein can be indicative of preeclampsia (see Chapter 21). A dipstick reading of zero, trace, or one plus is considered to be within normal limits; two plus or greater is a finding that warrants further investigation. Ketones in the urine during

PROCEDURE 16-2

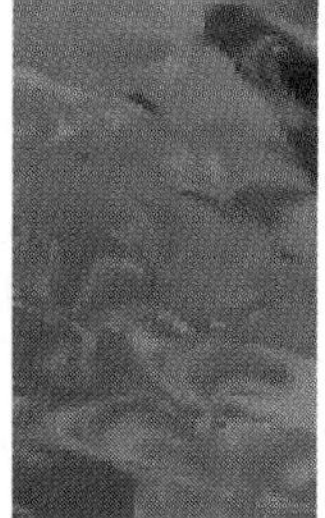

Assisting with Pelvic Examination

▼ PURPOSE

To help the woman feel at ease throughout the examination and to assist the woman's health care provider as needed. The woman's health care provider performs the examination at the first prenatal visit and again toward the end of pregnancy unless otherwise indicated. The first examination is performed to detect any pelvic abnormalities that would influence pregnancy, labor, or birth; to assess uterine size and pelvic size and shape; and to collect cytologic specimens. The later examination is done to assess cervical readiness for labor, as well as fetal descent into the pelvic cavity, and to obtain cultures if necessary.

▼ EQUIPMENT

- Sterile gloves
- Vaginal speculum
- Water-soluble lubricant
- Materials for Pap smear and cultures, including biohazard bag and labels for cultures
- Other culture media for additional specimens
- Mirror
- Light
- Sheet
- Examination table with stirrups

1 Greet the woman warmly and make her feel at ease. Instruct her to empty her bladder and to undress from the waist down. Give her a sheet to place around her and ask her to sit on the end of the table. **Feeling that the nurse is interested and concerned about her decreases the woman's apprehension and anxiety. An empty bladder promotes comfort during the examination and helps assure accurate assessment of the uterus during the bimanual examination. A sheet helps decrease the woman's self-consciousness by providing privacy.**

2 Explain the purpose of the pelvic examination. Describe the procedure and what the woman will feel. Show her the equipment that will be used. **Knowledge of the procedure decreases apprehension and fear.**

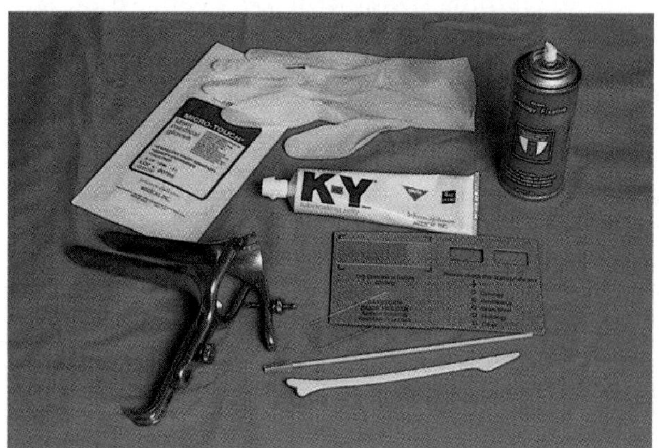

3 Assist the woman into the lithotomy position for the examination, making her as comfortable as possible. If the fetus is large enough to compress maternal blood vessels, place a wedge under the woman's right or left hip to maintain a slight lateral tilt. Elevate her head and shoulders slightly. Her arms should rest either at her side or on her chest. Position her buttocks at the bottom of the table. Place her feet in the stirrups, with her legs wide apart. Drape the sheet over her from the waist down. **Correct positioning enhances the health care provider's ability to perform the examination and increases the woman's ability to relax during the examination. Placing a wedge under the woman's hip displaces the uterus sufficiently to prevent compression of maternal blood vessels and subsequent supine hypotension. The sheet provides privacy and helps decrease the woman's self-consciousness.**

Continued on facing page

PROCEDURE 16–2 Continued

4 When the examination begins, encourage the woman to remain relaxed. Show her how to do slow-paced breathing. Involve her in the procedure as much as she wishes. For example, offer her a mirror if she would like to observe the procedure. Inform the woman about what to expect at each point of the examination (inspection of external genitalia, speculum examination, bimanual examination, and assessment of the bony pelvis). Instruct her to bear down as the speculum is being inserted. **Relaxation and slow-paced breathing enable the woman to minimize discomfort. Involvement in the procedure promotes learning. A mirror enables her to learn about her own anatomy during the examination. Bearing down helps relax pelvic floor muscles, open the vaginal orifice, and decrease intravaginal pressure.**

5 Assist the woman's health care provider with the examination as needed. Before handling specimens, wash hands and put on gloves. Prepare specimens for transfer to the laboratory. **Washing hands, wearing gloves, and correct handling of specimens help prevent cross-contamination and infection.**

6 Assist the woman to a sitting position, assuring that she remains covered with the sheet. Offer her a towel to wipe lubricant from the perineal area. Provide privacy as she dresses. Ask whether she has any questions before she leaves. **Assistance in moving to a sitting position is sometimes needed because lying supine may cause postural hypotension. Wiping off lubricant and vaginal secretions makes the woman feel more comfortable. Providing privacy whenever possible helps decrease self-consciousness. Giving the woman an opportunity to ask more questions after the examination helps promote learning and decrease anxiety.**

pregnancy can be detrimental to the developing fetus and may result from inadequate food intake or strenuous exercise. Nitrites in the urine can indicate a UTI. At the initial prenatal visit a urine culture and sensitivity (C & S) test is also done to identify bacteria, blood, or white blood cells in the urine. Any of these are indicative of a UTI, which should be treated immediately with antibiotics. Urinary tract infections are associated with increased risk for the mother and fetus, especially for premature labor and low birth weight. If the results of the C & S test are negative, this test is not repeated unless indicated.

A number of blood tests are done at the initial prenatal visit and some may be repeated later in the pregnancy, depending on assessed need (see Table 16–2). Hemoglobin and hematocrit (H/H) testing is done to identify anemia during pregnancy. Although the H/H values are lower during pregnancy because of the normal physiologic anemia discussed earlier in this chapter, diet counseling and iron supplementation may be needed if the H/H values are too low. The blood type and Rh factor are identified early in pregnancy. It is important to identify an Rh incompatibility between mother and baby as soon as possible (see Chapter 21).

Tests for sexually transmitted diseases (STDs) should also be done. Syphilis is identified by the Venereal Disease Research Laboratory (VDRL) serology test and can cause prematurity, intrauterine death, or congenital syphilis in the infant; if this test is positive, treatment should begin early in pregnancy (Holland and O'Mahony 1989; Cunningham et al. 1993). Hepatitis B antigen screening is recommended for all women because of the prevalence of the disease in the general population. This virus can be extremely detrimental to the developing fetus. Even if the woman has no symptoms, infants born to mothers who have the virus have a 70 to 90 percent chance of contracting the virus during delivery and are at high risk for developing liver disease or cancer as young adults. For women at high risk (those who have a past history of liver disease; have exposure to blood or blood products; use illegal intravenous drugs; are of Asian, Eskimo, Haitian, or African descent; have multiple sexual partners; or have a sexual partner who is at risk), nonimmunity for the hepatitis B antigen raises consideration of the need for vaccination.

Infections with the human immunodeficiency virus (HIV) are becoming increasingly common among women of reproductive age. The effects of these infections on maternal and child health are substantial. Evidence has shown that testing only women who are recognized by themselves or their caregivers as being at risk fails to identify considerable numbers of infected patients. The US Public Health Service now recommends that *all* pregnant women *routinely* be counseled about the HIV virus and educated about the benefits of knowing

PROCEDURE 16–3

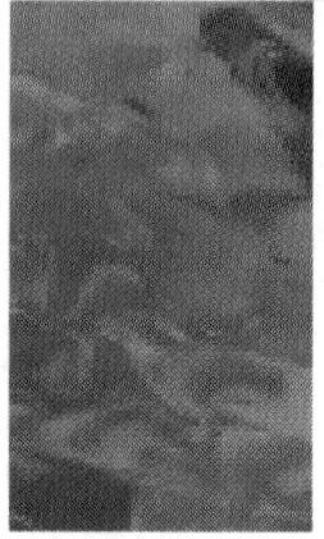

Testing Urine with Urinary Dipstick

▼ PURPOSE

To detect the presence of substances in the urine that indicate a potential problem requiring further investigation. To identify trends by comparing current specimen results with those collected previously. Performed at each prenatal visit throughout pregnancy.

▼ EQUIPMENT

- Fresh urine specimen
- Dipsticks
- Gloves

1 Ask woman to collect urine midstream in a clean specimen cup. **The chance of contamination or inaccurate test results is reduced by obtaining a fresh midstream urine specimen in a clean cup.**

2 With gloved hands, pull a dipstick from the bottle and check the date on the bottle that indicates when it was opened. **The shelf life of an open bottle of urinary dipsticks is 30 days.**

3 Dip the stick into the urine specimen until all the colored tabs are wet. **An accurate result is obtained only if all the colored tabs are immersed in the specimen.**

4 Wait sufficient time (according to directions on the bottle) for the colors on the stick to change. **Waiting a sufficient amount of time is essential for obtaining an accurate result.**

5 Compare the colors on the stick to the color chart on the bottle. **The color chart on the bottle indicates how to interpret the colors on the stick. The presence of glucose, protein, ketones, or nitrites in the urine could indicate a potential problem (see text).**

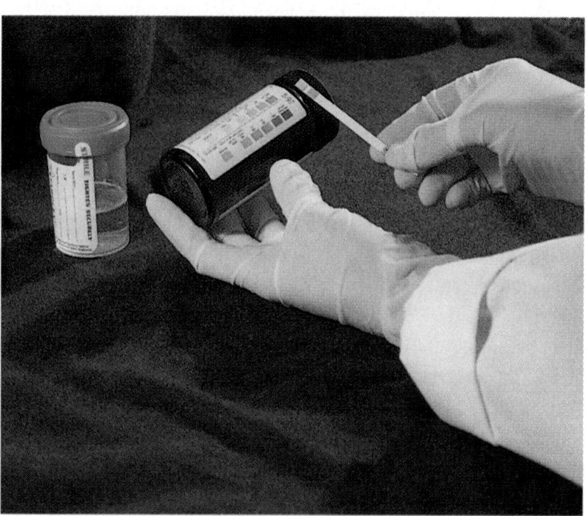

6 Remove gloves, wash hands, and record your findings. **Removing gloves and washing hands prevent cross-contamination. Recording findings enables the nurse to compare results from previous appointments and look for trends.**

their status and the options for reducing transmission to their fetus, were they to be infected. It is recommended that testing for HIV be voluntary because mandatory testing or testing without informed consent, counseling, and education has the potential to impair the provider-patient relationship and may cause some women to avoid prenatal care altogether (MMWR 1995) (see Chapter 40 for a full discussion of HIV/AIDS). Toxicology screening for drugs should also be recommended to women at risk (Public Health Service 1989; Cunningham et al. 1993).

Screening for gestational diabetes should be done for all women between 26 and 28 weeks' gestation. Gestational diabetes can result in the development of a macrosomic infant who is at risk for developing hypoglycemia, respiratory distress, or jaundice after birth (see Chapters 21 and 36). Screening is done with a glucose challenge test (GCT). If the results are abnormal, the more sensitive glucose tolerance test (GTT) is done (Cunningham et al. 1993). An alpha-fetoprotein (AFP) test on a blood sample from the woman is suggested between 14 and 16 weeks' gestation to detect open neural tube defects. AFP is normally made by the fetus in amounts that increase with gestational age. It is normally secreted into the amniotic fluid and crosses the placenta into the mother's circulation. Fetuses with open neural tube defects secrete increased amounts of AFP into the amniotic fluid. The amount absorbed into the maternal blood also tends to be greater. An elevated level of AFP can lead to the identification of 90 percent of neural tube defects.

Rubella screening should be done to determine whether the woman has had German measles. If she has not, it is possible for the rubella virus to cross the placenta and infect the fetus with varying degrees of harm, including deafness, cataracts, mental retardation, and heart defects. If she is not immune, she should be counseled to avoid contact with any suspected cases of rubella and to receive the rubella vaccine as soon as the pregnancy is over. The suspected exposure of a nonimmune woman to someone with probable rubella calls for monitoring the woman's antibody level to see if it rises. A rising level indicates infection in the mother and possibly in the fetus. Infection in the mother raises the question of aborting the pregnancy, because at present there is no treatment for rubella in either the mother or the fetus.

Screening for infections such as toxoplasmosis and cytomegalovirus (CMV) is more effective when done before conception. Toxoplasmosis is a parasitic infection that can be transmitted by cat feces, undercooked meat, and other sources. Although this disease normally causes only mild, flulike symptoms in the mother, it can damage or cause the death of an unborn baby whose mother contracts the infection. Women who are immune to the infection cannot transmit it to the baby. A woman who is not immune should not clean cat litter boxes or eat undercooked meat (see Chapter 40). All black and Asian women should be routinely screened for the inherited disease sickle cell anemia, which is most often seen in these populations. Screening for tuberculosis is restricted to women at risk.

Ultrasound testing is currently recommended only if the duration of gestation is uncertain or if problems for the fetus are anticipated. Research in this area continues to be given high priority, for long-term effects of frequent or multiple ultrasonographic examinations on the fetus are unknown (see Chapter 15) (Public Health Service 1989). Parents often enjoy seeing an ultrasound image of their baby, and studies have suggested that this may promote attachment (Grace 1984) and decrease anxiety (Brown 1988). However, these reasons are not sufficient for doing routine ultrasound examinations.

High-Risk Screening. Because pregnancy is a normal physiologic process, the focus of prenatal health assessment is on screening women routinely for medical, psychosocial, or environmental high-risk factors that may develop and be indicative of further problems. All of the components of the prenatal examination already discussed are part of risk assessment, including the history, the monitoring of weight and blood pressure; the abdominal, breast, and pelvic examinations; and laboratory tests. Throughout the initial prenatal assessment and subsequent visits, all caregivers who are involved with the pregnant woman must be alert for the development of risk factors that might signal potential problems or lead to complications in the pregnancy (see Identifying Risk Factors in Pregnancy).

Many health care settings now use a special risk assessment form as part of the prenatal record to assist in the identification of high-risk factors. Not all risk factors are of equal severity, and these forms provide a means of assigning a score for each problem identified. The total score gives an indication of the woman's high-risk status and alerts all health care providers to be particularly observant. The risk scoring form can be changed and updated as the pregnancy progresses. It is important, however, that caregivers not become lulled by a risk score. Continual observation and assessment are still necessary. If risk factors are identified during the pregnancy, it is essential that the woman be informed. Additional time must be spent in educating her about the potential problem and ways in which she can assist in its management. A complete discussion of high-risk pregnancy may be found in Chapter 21.

▼ Diagnosis

The extensive assessment that is done at the initial prenatal visit, followed by continued assessments at each revisit, enables the nurse to identify and revise nursing diagnoses throughout the pregnancy. Nursing diagnoses may be related to emotional or sociocultural factors identified during the interview or to physical factors identified during the physical examination. For the normal childbearing woman who has no problems and is progressing well through pregnancy and childbirth, nursing diagnoses focus on patterns of wellness, healthy responses, client strengths, or teaching needs. For high-risk maternity clients, nursing

Identifying Risk Factors in Pregnancy

MATERNAL CHARACTERISTICS

- Age (under 16 or over 35)
- Unmarried, especially adolescent
- Race (nonwhite)
- Poverty
- Height (less than 5 ft)
- Weight (20% overweight or underweight before pregnancy)
- Inadequate diet
- Emotional conflict regarding pregnancy
- Lack of social support; family disorganization
- Drug or regular alcohol use
- Smoking during pregnancy

HISTORY OF PROBLEMS IN PREVIOUS PREGNANCIES

- History of infertility
- Para V or more
- Pregnancy-induced hypertension
- Premature labor or delivery, prolonged labor, cesarean section
- Difficult midforceps delivery
- Uterine or cervical anomaly
- Myomas
- Ovarian masses
- Ectopic pregnancy or spontaneous abortion
- Stillbirth or neonatal death
- Infant less than 2500 g
- Infant over 4000 g
- Infant of ABO incompatibility
- Infant with neurologic deficit, birth injury

MEDICAL HISTORY

- Heart disease
- Pulmonary disease
- Metabolic disease—particularly diabetes mellitus, thyroid disease
- Chronic renal disease, repeated urinary tract infections, repeated bacteriuria
- Gastrointestinal disease or endocrine disorders (pituitary, adrenal)
- Chronic hypertension
- Hemoglobinopathies
- Seizure disorder
- Viral, bacterial, or protozoal infectious disease
- Malignancy or surgery during pregnancy
- Major congenital anomalies of the reproductive tract
- Mental retardation, major emotional disorders

PRESENT PREGNANCY STATUS

- Late or no prenatal care
- Rh sensitization
- Fetus inappropriately large or small for gestation
- Premature labor
- Pregnancy-induced hypertension
- Multiple gestation
- Polyhydramnios
- Premature rupture of the membranes
- Antepartum bleeding
  - Placenta previa
  - Abruptio placentae
- Abnormal presentation
- Postdatism
- Abnormality in test for fetal well-being
- Maternal anemia

From Aumann, G. M.-E., and Baird, M. M. (1993). Risk assessment for pregnant women. In Knuppel, R. A., Drukker, J. E. (Eds.), *High-risk pregnancy: A team approach* (pp. 8–35). Philadelphia: W. B. Saunders.

diagnoses focus on both areas of strength and areas of risk. The following nursing diagnoses are examples of those that might be stated for the woman during pregnancy after her initial prenatal examination. The diagnoses that are identified at one prenatal visit may change by the following visit. Therefore, it is important to reevaluate and update the nursing diagnoses throughout pregnancy:

- Knowledge deficit: lack of information related to expected physical changes and symptoms during the first trimester of pregnancy
- Anxiety related to fear of pelvic examination
- Pain and discomfort related to muscle tension during pelvic examination
- Risk for altered health maintenance related to psychosocial problems and inaccessibility of health care services

▼ Planning

The nursing diagnoses that are developed as a result of the assessment at each prenatal visit serve as the basis for developing a plan of expected outcomes for the interventions that are needed at that time in the pregnancy. As the identified nursing diagnoses change, the plan and objectives for intervention also change as the pregnancy progresses. The plan for the woman at any point during pregnancy should address both physical and psychological needs and should represent the goals of the woman as well as those of the health care providers. Because contact with a woman is often limited during a prenatal visit, it may be necessary to establish priorities regarding the identified plan. If the plan is recorded in the woman's prenatal record, objectives that cannot be met at one prenatal visit can be met at succeeding visits. The following measurable objectives and expected outcomes are examples of those that might be written in response to the foregoing nursing diagnoses. The pregnant woman should:

- Verbally describe the physical changes that will occur in the first trimester and discuss the physical symptoms she experiences
- Demonstrate decreased fear of the pelvic examination through a relaxed body, decreased facial tension, and verbal confirmation
- Relax pelvic floor muscles, perform slow paced breathing, and express a decrease in discomfort during the pelvic examination
- Return for prenatal visits regularly according to identified needs

▼ Intervention

The nursing or medical interventions that are necessary throughout pregnancy are identified from the nursing diagnoses and planned objectives for care. Interventions are planned on the basis of priorities that are evident. All aspects of care for the pregnant woman and her family should be addressed, including physical, emotional, cognitive, and sociocultural factors, and the woman and her family should be consulted in the planning of interventions. What seems to be a high-priority concern to the nurse may not be viewed as such by the woman or her family. Obviously, if a particular intervention is essential to the well-being of the woman or her baby, safety must take priority over concerns of the family. If the woman is experiencing a healthy pregnancy, medical interventions are limited. The primary focus of the interventions needed throughout the pregnancy is health promotion.

Counseling about healthful behavior should take place at every prenatal visit. Teaching is a continuous process and should include information about nutrition, exercise, stress reduction, and relief of discomforts of pregnancy and helping the woman identify and avoid tobacco, alcohol, illicit and teratogenic drugs, and environmental toxins (see Chapter 19). Women also need to expand their knowledge about pregnancy, birth, and parenting. Both maternal and fetal changes should be explained at every visit. The warning signs to report to the health care provider during pregnancy should be reinforced repeatedly (see Warning Signs to Report in Chapter 19) and the woman should be informed of the signs of preterm labor (see Chapter 21). The emotional and sociocultural aspects of pregnancy should also be addressed, and help with problems related to these dimensions should be made available (see Chapters 17 and 18). In the third trimester, women begin to focus on the impending birth and are receptive to information about the signs of labor, the process and management of labor and birth, hospital procedures, and pain management strategies. Pregnant women and their partners should be encouraged to attend childbirth classes; however, participation in these classes does not relieve the nurse of the responsibility for reinforcing information at every prenatal visit. Questions are often stimulated in childbirth classes that can be answered at a prenatal visit. Information about the woman's proposed care and treatment should not be overlooked. If the woman is to become an active participant in her health care, she must be informed of her health status at all times. The results of her physical examination or laboratory tests should be explained in terms she can understand. If a rationale is given for suggested interventions, the woman is more likely to comply. For example, the woman is more willing to follow a recommendation if she knows how an increased calcium intake will benefit her baby or why a particular exercise will make her more comfortable. A complete list of suggested health promotion activities throughout pregnancy is given in Assessment Tool: Prenatal Education and Counseling.

▼ Evaluation

Both short-term and long-term evaluations of the outcomes of prenatal care are important. Short-term evaluation of outcomes takes place at every prenatal visit as the nurse assesses changes that have taken place since the last visit related to the woman's health status and health behaviors. Short-term evaluation is likely to be based on the measurable objectives identified in the woman's plan for care. Long-term evaluation of outcomes is based on the perinatal outcome of the pregnancy and birth. Factors such as maternal and fetal mortality and morbidity, incidence of complications, and infant birth weight are easy to

Assessment Tool:

HOLLISTER maternal/newborn RECORD SYSTEM

Prenatal Education and Counseling

Patient's Name__________

ID. No.__________

	Date	Init	Date and Initial When Topic is Addressed / Patient Needs/Comments
Plan of Care During Pregnancy			
1. Visit Schedule and Content			
2. Screening and Diagnostic Tests			
3. Prescribed Medications			
4. Early Prenatal Classes			
5. Prepared Childbirth Classes			
6. Self Care Needs			
7.			
Changes of Pregnancy			
8. Fetal Growth and Development			
9. Maternal Physical Changes			
10. Maternal Emotional Changes			
11. Management of Common Discomforts			
12. Signs and Symptoms of Labor			
13. Attachment			
14. Family Adjustment			
15.			
Prevention of Complications			
16. Danger Signs to Report			
17. Use of Alcohol, Tobacco, Drugs			
18. Exposure to Teratogens			
19. Signs and Symptoms of Preterm Labor			
20. Stress Management			
21. Seat Belts			
22.			
23.			
Promotion of Health			
24. Nutrition			
25. Activity, Exercise			
26. Rest, Sleep			
27. Hygiene, Clothing			
28. Employment, Travel			
29. Sexuality			
30.			
Birth Plan (32-38 Wks)			
31. Participation of Support Person			
32. Other Family Members in L & D			
33. Method of Delivery ☐ Vaginal ☐ VBAC ☐ Cesarean			
34. Episiotomy			
35. Site of Delivery ☐ LDR ☐ LDRP ☐ DR ☐ Birthing Room ☐ OR			
36. Position For Delivery			
37. Analgesia/Anesthesia			
38. Technology (IVs, Monitor)			
39. Early Interaction with Infant			
40.			
Discharge Plan (32-38 Wks)			
41. Infant Care Giver			
42. Method of Feeding ☐ Breast ☐ Formula			
43. Rooming-in			
44. Tubal Ligation Candidate ☐ No ☐ Yes; Authorization Signed ☐ No ☐ Yes			
45. Circumcision ☐ Yes ☐ No			
46. Length of Stay			Initials / Signature
47. Follow-up Home Visit by RN			
48. Infant Car Seat			Initials / Signature
49. Family Planning Preference			
50. Social Service Referral			Initials / Signature
51.			

Hollister
HOLLISTER INCORPORATED, 2000 HOLLISTER DR, LIBERTYVILLE, IL 60048

PRENATAL EDUCATION AND COUNSELING FORM #5706
691

MATERNAL RECORD COPY

measure. Factors that are not as easy to quantify but are also important evaluation measures are the woman's satisfaction with her health care, her feelings about pregnancy and birth, and her self-esteem related to parenting roles. The findings of the nurse's evaluation lead to reassessment and alteration of the identified goals and expected outcomes and plan of care.

Collaborative Process

Many health care providers work together to provide care for the pregnant woman and her baby. The nurse's role throughout pregnancy is one of the most important, for the nurse can help to organize the implementation of care, oversee all components of service, influence the approach and tone of the professional relationship with the woman and her family, and provide continuity of care. Nursing roles have expanded in relation to prenatal care and may include those of the certified nurse-midwife, the nurse-practitioner, and the childbirth educator. The nurse's approach to pregnancy is based on the view of pregnancy as a normal physiologic process rather than a disease and a holistic experience that includes emotional and sociocultural aspects as well as physical components. This view guides the manner in which the nursing process is implemented. However, the nurse cannot meet all of the woman's needs throughout pregnancy. It is important that she work closely and collaboratively with the physician, nutritionist, physical therapist, social worker, or other health care team member in making the pregnancy and birth a healthy, positive experience for the woman and her family.

Risk Management

Regular antepartal care and risk management might be viewed as synonymous terms. Antepartal care provides a system whereby a normal physiologic process can be monitored, any deviation can be immediately identified and treated, and risk can thus be decreased or avoided. Even though pregnancy is a normal process, it does have the potential for risk and requires frequent and regular assessment. Because the pregnant woman is essentially healthy and pregnancy is normal, antepartal care could begin to seem routine or unnecessary. It is possible that either the pregnant woman or her health care providers might begin to feel lax about maintaining a regular schedule of antepartal care. It is critical that this attitude does not develop. All components of health assessment during pregnancy that are discussed in this chapter contribute to the management of maternal or fetal risk. For example, by identifying early in the pregnancy that the woman's blood pressure is higher than normal, the risks of PIH can be avoided through early treatment. By identifying during an interview with the pregnant woman that her family system is experiencing stress, intervention can be used to avert problems such as abuse, financial crisis, or cessation of health care.

Risk management during antepartal care involves inclusion of the family, as well as the woman, in all aspects of the care. A woman who is involved in her health care is more likely to feel that she is a part of the process, be more compliant, and be more satisfied with the treatment she receives. Constant teaching and explanation must take place so that the expectant family understands what is happening and why. Families must also be given some control over their environment. It is important during the antepartal period to acquaint the woman and her family with all of the services and personnel they will encounter during the pregnancy. A tour of the hospital where the woman will deliver should also be arranged so that the family can see the environment where birth will take place and learn about the options that are available to them.

Another component of risk management is careful documentation throughout the pregnancy. At each prenatal visit it is important that every member of the health care team who interacts with the pregnant woman record all information in the prenatal record. This information should be accurate, concise, and objective. Accurate record keeping also prevents duplication of services, promotes collaboration among health care team members, and saves time in the long run. If all of these components of care during the antepartal period are included, the goal of decreasing maternal and fetal mortality and morbidity can be achieved through successful risk management.

Implications for Research

Research has repeatedly demonstrated the physical benefits of prenatal care to both the woman and her baby. Outcomes such as the incidence of various maternal complications or infant birth weight have been measured and shown to improve with prenatal care. However, little research has been done to date on the woman's perception of prenatal care, factors that might improve the quality of care, or factors that contribute to the woman's compliance with prenatal care. There is also little research related to the nurse's role during the antepartal period. The following research questions might provide findings that would improve the care provided during the antepartal period:

- How do pregnant women view the care they receive during pregnancy?
- Is there a relationship between the amount of time spent in individual teaching and counseling activities and patients' compliance during the prenatal period?
- What factors influence regular attendance at prenatal appointments?
- How can prenatal care services be organized to allow more patient involvement and education of the patient during the antepartal period?

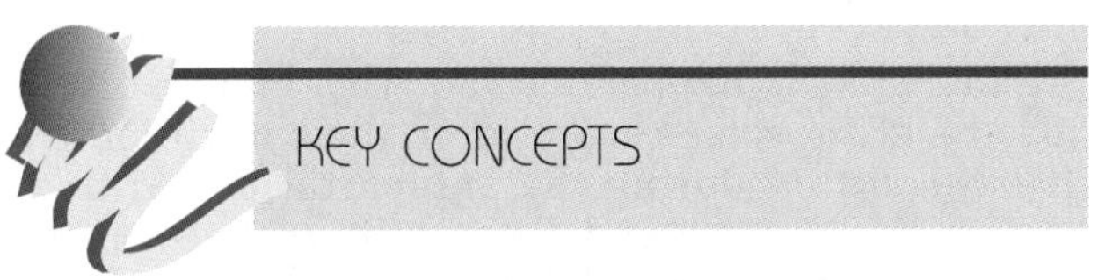

KEY CONCEPTS

▼ All organs of a woman's body change in some way during pregnancy to adapt to the needs of the developing fetus; these changes are a result of normal physiology; pregnancy is not an illness but a state of wellness.

▼ A full-term pregnancy lasts 280 days, 40 weeks, 9 calendar months, or 10 lunar months; the first trimester consists of months 1 to 3, the second months 4 to 6, and the third months 7 to 9.

▼ Presumptive (subjective) signs of pregnancy include amenorrhea, nausea, and vomiting, breast sensitivity, urinary symptoms, fatigue, weight gain, and quickening.

▼ Probable (objective) signs of pregnancy include changes in the consistency of pelvic structures (Hegar's sign, Goodell's sign, and McDonald's sign), changes in the color of pelvic structures (Chadwick's sign), changes in the size and shape of pelvic structures, abdominal palpation of the fetal outline, ballottement of the fetus, and positive pregnancy testing, abdominal enlargement, and Braxton Hicks contractions.

▼ Positive (diagnostic) signs of pregnancy include fetal heart tones, uterine sounds (souffles), and fetal movement.

▼ To calculate the expected day of confinement (EDC) using Nägele's rule, identify the first day of the last menstrual period (LMP), subtract 3 months, and add 7 days.

▼ The corpus luteum and maternal-fetal-placental unit are primary regulators of endocrine function during pregnancy; the corpus luteum secretes estrogen and progesterone and the maternal-fetal-placental unit secretes estrogen, progesterone, human chorionic gonadotropin (hCG), and human placental lactogen (hPL).

▼ The thyroid enlarges about 50 percent during pregnancy; maternal plasma thyroxine (T_4) rises markedly; the basal metabolic rate (BMR) increases up to 25 percent. The parathyroid glands also enlarge and help to maintain an adequate calcium level for mother and fetus.

▼ The pituitary gland enlarges; the changes in anterior lobe hormone production include suppression of follicle-stimulating hormone (FSH) and luteinizing hormone (LH) and an increase in prolactin; the posterior lobe secretes oxytocin during labor and lactation.

▼ Insulin production decreases in the first trimester and then rises until term; the hormones of pregnancy decrease utilization of insulin, resulting in a diabetogenic effect of pregnancy that ensures adequate glucose for the maternal-fetal-placental unit.

▼ The reproductive system is most directly affected during pregnancy; the uterus changes in size, shape, and consistency and may contract with Braxton Hicks contractions; the cervix softens (Goodell's sign), becomes bluish (Chadwick's sign), and forms a mucous plug that is discharged as "bloody show" in early labor; the vagina increases in vascularity, secretions, and acidity; ovulation ceases; and the breasts increase in size and sensitivity, develop pigmentary changes and striae, and can express colostrum.

▼ Changes occur in the position and volume of the heart, resulting in a physiologic systolic murmur; cardiac output increases 30 to 50 percent with the distribution favoring the organs that have an increased workload during pregnancy; blood volume increases 30 to 50 percent, resulting in a physiologic anemia caused by hemodilution; heart rate increases by up to 10 to 15 beats per minute; and blood pressure remains stable.

▼ The respiratory rate remains stable, although the depth may increase; slight hyperventilation occurs because of an increased tidal volume; the vital capacity also increases slightly; airway resistance is decreased by progesterone.

▼ A decrease in bladder capacity caused by pressure by the enlarging uterus results in urinary frequency; stasis of urine can result from compression of the ureters and relaxation of smooth muscle by progesterone, resulting in an increased susceptibility to urinary tract infections (UTIs); the glomerular filtration rate (GFR) increases up to 50 percent; a physiologic edema may occur as a result of water retention; a physiologic glycosuria may occur because of the inability of the kidneys to reabsorb all of the glucose being filtered by the glomeruli.

- Pressure by the enlarging uterus on the gastrointestinal system results in heartburn, constipation, and hemorrhoids; nausea and vomiting may occur in early pregnancy as a result of hCG, progesterone, and altered carbohydrate metabolism; alterations in taste and smell may occur; appetite fluctuates and some women experience food cravings or pica.
- Changes in the musculoskeletal system include alterations in posture that can lead to spinal lordosis and low backache; pain may be experienced as the uterus enlarges and pulls on the round ligaments that anchor it; an abdominal muscle diastasis may occur because of stretching of the muscles; leg cramps result from uterine pressure on nerves or alteration in calcium and phosphorus levels; an increase in joint flexibility and alteration in center of gravity result in a wide, waddling gait.
- The integumentary changes that occur in pregnancy include abdominal or breast striae; vascular spiders on the face, neck, chest, arms, or legs; palmar erythema or redness; chloasma, or the "mask of pregnancy," increased pigmentation in the nipples and areolae of the breasts and in the genitalia; and increased sweat gland activity and hair growth.
- Early and regular prenatal care has been shown to decrease maternal mortality and morbidity, fetal loss, and unnecessary intervention in pregnancy. However, universal access to prenatal care does not yet exist in the United States.
- Assessment of the woman during pregnancy should include the following: (1) an interview to collect both subjective and objective data; (2) a physical examination, including observation of vital signs, height, and weight; a review of all systems; a breast examination; and an abdominal examination, including visual inspection, palpation, measurement of fundal height, Leopold maneuvers, assessment of fetal movement, and auscultation for fetal heart tones and uterine souffles; (3) a pelvic examination, including visual inspection, a speculum examination, a bimanual examination, and assessment of the bony pelvis; (4) laboratory tests, including urine testing, blood tests, and screening for infections; (5) ultrasound testing, and (6) screening for high-risk factors.
- Risk management during pregnancy includes the initiation of early and regular prenatal care, involvement of the pregnant woman and her family in the plan of care, and careful documentation of care.

References

Aaronson, R. (1991). Grassroots strategies for promoting maternal and infant health. *Birth,* 18 (2), 93–97.

Block, G., and Nolan, J. (1986). *Health assessment for professional nursing: A developmental approach.* Norwalk, CT: Appleton-Century-Crofts.

Brown, G. (1988). Short-term impact of fetal imaging on paternal stress and anxiety. *Pre- and Perinatal Psychology Journal,* 3 (1), 25–40.

Cunningham, F. G., MacDonald, P. C., Gant, N. F., Leveno, K. J., Gilstrap, L. C. (1993). *Williams obstetrics* (19th ed.). Norwalk, CT: Appleton & Lange.

Engstrom, J. (1988). Measurement of fundal height. *Journal of Obstetric, Gynecologic, and Neonatal Nursing,* 17 (3), 172–178.

Gagnon, L. (1992). Healthy skin care for mother and baby. *Journal of Perinatal Education,* 1 (3), 21–45.

Grace, J. (1984). Does a mother's knowledge of fetal gender affect attachment? *MCN,* 9 (1), 42–45.

Guyton, A. C., and Hall, J. E. (1996). *Textbook of medical physiology* (9th ed.). Philadelphia: W. B. Saunders.

Helton, A. (1990). A buddy system to improve prenatal care. *MCN,* 15 (4), 234–237.

Holland, E., and O'Mahony, C. (1989). Is it time to review antenatal screening for syphilis? *British Journal of Obstetrics and Gynecology,* 96 (8), 1005–1006.

Johnston, G. P. (1994). *The wish, the wait, the wonder: A book of wisdom for expectant parents.* New York: HarperCollins Publishers.

Mahan, C., and McKay, S. (1984). Let's reform our antenatal care methods. *Contemporary Obstetrics and Gynecology,* 23, 147.

Malasanos, L., Barkauskas, V., Stoltenberg-Allen, K. (1986). *Health assessment.* St. Louis: C. V. Mosby.

Mattson, S., and Lew, L. (1992). Culturally sensitive prenatal care for Southeast Asians. *Journal of Obstetric, Gynecologic, and Neonatal Nursing,* 21 (1), 48–54.

McClanahan, P. (1992). Improving access to and use of prenatal care. *Journal of Obstetric, Gynecologic, and Neonatal Nursing,* 21 (4), 280–284.

Public Health Service, Expert Panel on the Content of Prenatal Care. (1989). *Caring for our future: The content of prenatal care.* Washington, D.C.: U.S. Department of Health and Human Services.

U.S. Department of Health and Human Services. (1988). Progress toward achieving the 1990 objectives for pregnancy and infant health. *Morbidity and Mortality Weekly Report,* 37 (26), 405–408, 413.

Van Dinter, M. (1991). Ptyalism in pregnant women. *Journal of Obstetric, Gynecologic, and Neonatal Nursing,* 20 (3), 206–211.

Van Lier, D., Manteuffel, B., Dilorio, C., Stalcup, M. (1993). Nausea and fatigue during early pregnancy. *Birth,* 20 (4), 193–197.

Willard, M., Heaberrg, G., Pack, J. (1986). The educational pelvic examination: Women's responses to a new approach. *Journal of Obstetric, Gynecologic, and Neonatal Nursing,* 15 (2), 135–140.

Young, C., McMahon, J., Bowman, V., Thompson, D. (1989). Maternal reasons for delayed prenatal care. *Nursing Research,* 38 (4), 242–243.

Young, D. (1990). How can we enrich prenatal care? *Birth,* 17 (1), 12–13.

17 Chapter

Pregnancy is clearly one of the most profound psychological events in a human life. It is the ultimate psychosomatic experience.

DONALD SLOAN, M.D.
(JOHNSTON 1994)

Psychological Responses to Pregnancy

Elaine Zwelling

HIGHLIGHTS

- ▼ Psychological Fulfillment and Maturational Crisis
- ▼ Maternal Psychological Adaptation
- ▼ Developmental Tasks
- ▼ Maternal Tasks
- ▼ Prenatal Attachment
- ▼ Paternal Psychological Adaptation
- ▼ Developmental Tasks and Styles of Involvement
- ▼ Psychological Adaptation of Siblings and Grandparents
- ▼ Factors Altering Psychological Adaptation
- ▼ Nursing Practice
- ▼ Risk Management
- ▼ Implications for Research

Pregnancy is most often viewed from a physiologic perspective because of the dramatic physical changes that occur from conception, through the pregnancy and birth, and during the immediate postpartal period. The primary focus of the pregnancy experience, as viewed by the health care providers, friends, and family of the expectant parents, is centered on the woman's physical changes and health status. Perhaps one reason this occurs is that the physical changes are those we can most readily see. The primary focus for the woman and her partner, however, may or may not be the physiologic aspects of the pregnancy. Pregnancy is a very emotional experience. The changes that a pregnancy and the birth of a baby initiate for expectant parents often trigger major psychological responses. These emotional responses may be as much, or more of, a focus for the parents as the physical changes that occur.

Because emotional well-being is known to influence physical well-being, any plan for the woman's care during pregnancy must include an assess-

DEFINITIONS

Ambivalence—Mixed feelings regarding pregnancy; feeling happy and excited at one moment and then unhappy or depressed the next.

Binding-in—The commitment that the pregnant woman forms to her baby by the end of pregnancy; similar to prenatal attachment.

Body image—The subjective mental picture of her body that the woman develops in her mind during pregnancy.

Crisis—A critical life event that results in the disruption of one's normal equilibrium and requires some form of coping effort; caused by normal maturational experiences in the life cycle (developmental crises) or by unexpected life situations (situational crises).

Developmental tasks of pregnancy—Necessary adaptations that need to be accomplished to prepare the woman and her partner for the birth of the baby and the role of parenting.

Emotional lability—Frequency and/or extremes in emotional changes experienced by a woman during pregnancy.

Fetal embodiment—Recognition of the developing fetus as part of the woman's body image.

Maladaptation—Failure to adapt to the normal developmental or psychological tasks of pregnancy, resulting in potential alterations in parenting.

Nesting behavior—The psychological need experienced by some pregnant women at the end of pregnancy to make preparations for the baby.

Prenatal attachment—The beginning development of affiliation, love, or bonding to the fetus that begins during pregnancy.

ment of her psychological responses. Attention to this component of the woman's health status is also crucial because her psychological adaptation during pregnancy will most certainly be directly related to her adaptation to the mothering role after birth. An assessment of the father's emotional responses to the pregnancy, as well as those of other family members, is also an important component of family-centered care. A holistic plan of care must include interventions as needed to assist the emotional adaptation of both parents.

PREGNANCY: PSYCHOLOGICAL FULFILLMENT AND MATURATIONAL CRISIS

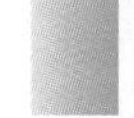

Fulfillment

In her classic developmental text on the psychology of women, Deutsch (1945) described pregnancy as being the fulfillment of the deepest and most powerful wish of a woman, an expression of creation and self-realization. It has been said that pregnancy confirms the woman's sexuality, her ability to reproduce, her femininity, and her self-esteem. It is a natural manifestation of the life process. The childbearing year (i.e., the 9 months of the pregnancy and the first 3 months of adjustment to the mothering role) can be thought of as the most important year of the woman's lifetime, for it alters and influences all aspects of her life. More contemporary thought, while viewing reproduction as an important component of feminine identity, does not emphasize the necessity of having a baby in order to feel whole. Although pregnancy and motherhood continue to be of primary importance to many women, other satisfying roles are also available to women today (Robinson and Stewart 1989).

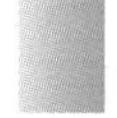

Crisis

In contrast to the view that pregnancy represents a woman's greatest fulfillment, it has also been described as a maturational or developmental life crisis (Lederman 1984; Tilden 1980). A maturational crisis is a critical period in which a normal situation in the life cycle alters one's equilibrium, resulting in the initiation of coping mechanisms to adapt. If these coping mechanisms do not work, a sense of crisis occurs. If coping mechanisms are effective, growth or change is often the result. The life situations that most likely precipitate a crisis are those that represent a major change. Classic theorists have proposed that psychological conflicts from previous developmental phases are often revived during this time, and psychological growth can occur as a result of resolution of those conflicts. Therefore, a crisis is neither a negative nor a positive entity, but it provides for potential positive outcomes (Bibring 1959; Caplan 1957).

Even though pregnancy is normal and in most situations is a happy event, it is an event that creates major change in the lives of the woman and her family. Pregnancy represents a major transition between two lifestyles, from being an individual or part of a couple with responsibilities only to oneself or to each other, to having full-time responsibility for a child. The multiple roles that parents must balance along with marriage and job responsibilities contribute to the feelings of being overwhelmed. These changes can easily threaten to disrupt the usual balance in the woman's life.

The Resiliency Model of Family Stress, Adjustment, and Adaptation (McCubbin and McCubbin 1993) discussed in Chapter 4 is a useful framework for considering the maturational crisis of pregnancy. As shown in the diagram of the adjustment phase of the model (see Fig. 4–7), family adjustment in response to a stressor (A factor) varies along a continuum from bonadjustment, or a positive outcome, to maladjustment, which may lead to a crisis situation (X factor). Whether a family experiences bonadjustment or maladjustment and crisis depends on the interplay of a number of components that include family vulnerability, family type and established patterns of functioning, family resistance resources, family appraisal of the stressor, and problem-solving and coping strategies.

Figure 17–1 depicts the event of pregnancy as the stressor in this model. Whether a family experiences bonadjustment or maladjustment and crisis in response to pregnancy depends on (1) the nature of the pregnancy (A factor—normal vs. high risk; planned vs. unplanned); (2) family vulnerability (V factor—status of family relationships such as single mother without support systems vs. a married dyad); (3) family type and established patterns of functioning (T factor—communication regarding the pregnancy); (4) family resistance resources (B factor—family capabilities and strengths, including support, financial stability, housing); (5) family appraisal of the pregnancy (C factor—whether the family is pleased or unhappy about the pregnancy); (6) problem-solving and coping skills (PSC factor—adjustments the family is able to make to accommodate the pregnancy).

Some families experience the stressor event of pregnancy with relative ease. In these families the coping mechanisms initiated to adjust to the pregnancy are effective, and bonadjustment is the result. In families in which the coping mechanisms initiated to adjust to the stressor are not effective,

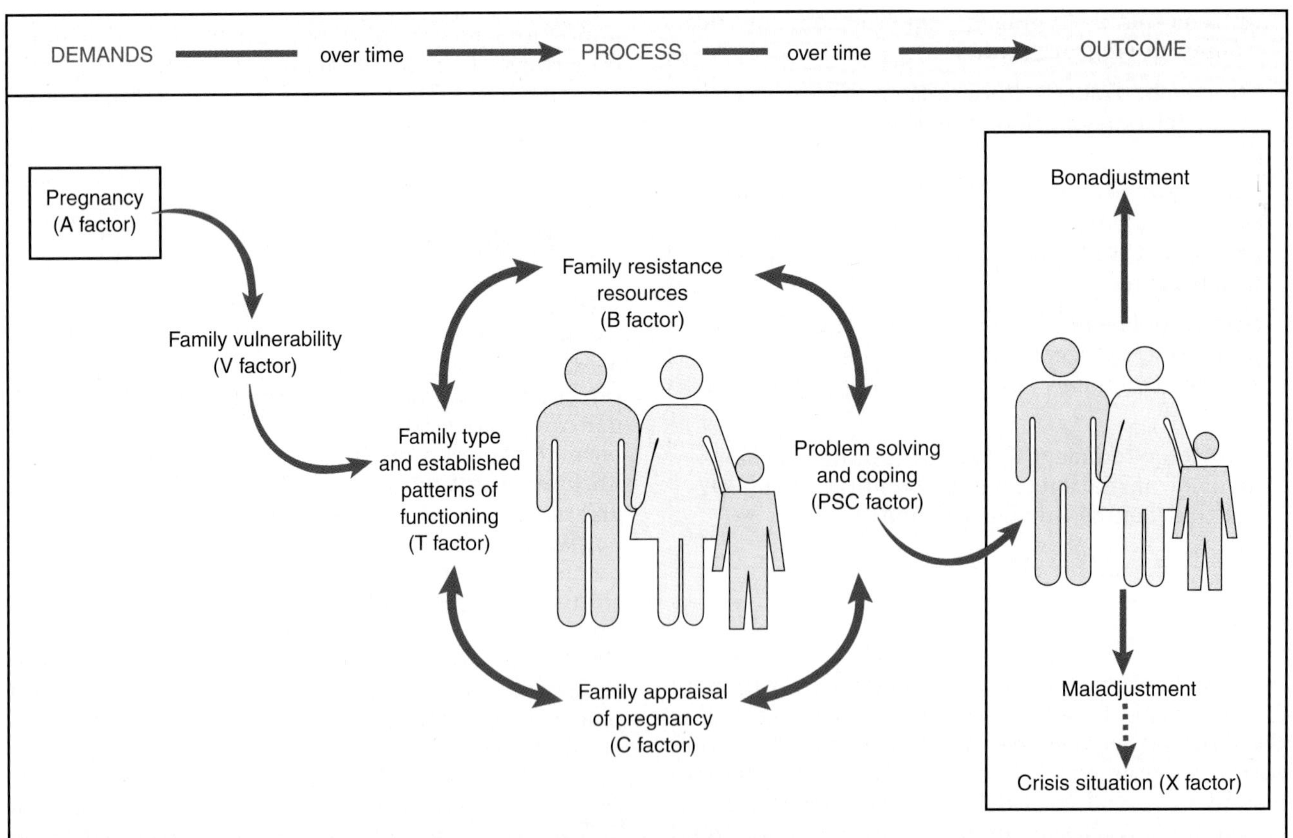

Figure 17–1

Whether a family experiences bonadjustment or maladjustment and crisis in response to pregnancy depends on the interplay of a number of components, such as the nature of the pregnancy, the family's resources, and the family's appraisal of the pregnancy event. (Adapted from Danielson, C. B., Hamel-Bissell, B., Winstead-Fry, P. [1993]. *Families, health, & illness: Perspectives on coping and intervention [p. 101]. St. Louis: C. V. Mosby.)*

the outcome is maladjustment, which can result in a crisis situation. Although the pregnancy as a stressful life event may not change, the existing resources and the appraisal of the pregnancy can be altered through education, counseling, and interventions aimed at resolving the crisis (Arizmendi and Affonso 1987). The nurse may also help the individual and family focus their coping strategies to restore the balance between demands and resources.

MATERNAL PSYCHOLOGICAL ADAPTATION IN PREGNANCY

Although every pregnancy is unique, a fairly predictable sequence of emotional responses occurs. These emotional changes may vary from one pregnancy to another or even from moment to moment within the same pregnancy. There is a certain quality of inner experience that seems to be distinctive of the pregnant state and sets it apart from life at any other time. This has been described as an altered state of consciousness. The woman's whole psyche becomes focused on her pregnant state, and life becomes a new experience centered around the major changes that are occurring (Colman and Colman 1991). It has long been hypothesized that a woman may even have a different way of thinking about her world or conceptualizing things during pregnancy (Rubin 1970, 1984). A study conducted to test earlier concepts proposed by Rubin suggests a cognitive process during pregnancy that involves a search for meaning, a sense of mastery, and self-enhancement. These cognitive processes help the woman understand and adapt to the pregnancy and its effects on her life (Affonso and Sheptak 1991). Research to date does not support claims that pregnant women become cognitively impaired. In fact, in one study, performance in cognitive tests improved during pregnancy (Schneider 1989).

Developmental Tasks

Developmental theory tells us that as individuals move from one stage to another throughout the life span, developmental tasks arise that must be accomplished. A similar theoretic model exists regarding pregnancy. Pregnancy poses a series of necessary tasks and adaptations that prepare the woman and her partner for the birth of the baby and the role of parenting (Colman and Colman 1991; Lederman 1984; Rubin 1984; Tanner 1969). It is hypothesized that the inability of a woman to complete these tasks successfully during pregnancy may affect her subsequent adaptation to the mothering role.

Table 17–1 outlines two classic perspectives on the psychological tasks of maternal adaptation in pregnancy: Tanner's developmental tasks and Rubin's maternal tasks. A number of emotional reactions and psychological changes (Table 17–2) accompany these tasks during the course of pregnancy. Rubin's maternal tasks are discussed later in this chapter. Tanner identified three developmental tasks that parallel the three trimesters of pregnancy: (1) accepting the fetus, (2) perceiving the fetus as a separate being, and (3) establishing a caretaking relationship.

ACCEPTING THE FETUS

The first task the woman must accomplish is to incorporate and integrate the fetus as part of her body. This is achieved as the marked physiologic changes of the first trimester cause her to focus on herself and on the pregnancy (Tanner 1969). This acceptance is easier for women who had planned or hoped for a pregnancy. Women may feel a sense of excitement, delight, awe, joy, or spirituality upon discovering that they are pregnant. However, acceptance does not occur auto-

Table 17–1

MATERNAL PSYCHOLOGICAL ADAPTATION IN PREGNANCY: TWO PERSPECTIVES

TANNER'S DEVELOPMENTAL TASKS	RUBIN'S MATERNAL TASKS
Accepting and integrating the fetus as a part of her body ("I am pregnant")	Ensuring safe passage
Perceiving the fetus as a separate being, not as an extension or integral part of oneself ("I am going to have a baby")	Seeking acceptance of the child by others
Preparing for giving up the fetus and establishing a caretaking relationship with the infant ("I am going to be a mother")	Binding-in (emotional attachment) to the child
	Learning to give of oneself on behalf of one's child

Data from Rubin, R. (1984). *Maternal identity and the maternal experience.* New York: Springer; and Tanner, L. (1969). Developmental tasks of pregnancy. In B. S. Bergersen, et al. (Eds.). *Current concepts in clinical nursing* (Vol. II, pp. 292–297). St. Louis: C. V. Mosby.

Table 17–2

PSYCHOLOGICAL CHANGES IN PREGNANCY

FIRST TRIMESTER	SECOND TRIMESTER	THIRD TRIMESTER
Maternal Changes		
Acceptance vs. denial Shock and disbelief Ambivalence Emotional lability Self-focus	Latent period—introverted Increased dependence Altered body image Dreams and fantasies Alteration in sexual responsiveness Increased awareness of fetus Prenatal attachment ("binding-in") Seeking acceptance of fetus by others Beginning to give of self to fetus	Increased anxiety Self-absorption Anticipation vs. dread Concerns re safety Giving of self to fetus Nesting
Paternal Changes		
Joy/excitement vs. anger/disappointment Pride Ambivalance	Emotional distancing Introspection Detachment vs. involvement Jealousy	Acceptance of reality Protectiveness Active involvement Increased anxiety Altered sexual desire Prenatal attachment

matically: it may take time, and other emotional reactions may occur before full acceptance is reached (Colman and Colman 1991).

Denial as Initial Coping Mechanism. For women who had not planned or wanted a pregnancy, acceptance may be more difficult, and feelings of despair, fear, or anger may accompany the news. Denial may be a coping mechanism used initially by women who are not pleased about being pregnant.

Shock and Disbelief. Most women react with shock and disbelief upon learning they are pregnant, even if the pregnancy had been planned. Rubin (1970, 1984) describes this reaction as "Someday, not now," indicating that although pregnancy had been hoped for, this hope always related to some time in the future. The readiness for the experience right now may be uncertain. The initial response may be "Wait! I had wanted first to . . . ." (e.g., finish school, pay off debts, get a new job, move to a bigger apartment, and so forth).

Emotional Lability. Another psychological characteristic of early pregnancy is increased emotional lability (Colman and Colman 1991; Joffe 1989; Lederman 1984). This lability is manifested as frequency in the change of emotional states or extremes in emotional highs or lows. The woman may initially be unaware of these changes until her family or friends point them out to her. She may cry more easily, become angry more readily, laugh uncontrollably, or experience euphoria about life events that are routine to others. This emotional lability varies from one woman to another, depending on personality structure, the amount of stress, and the quality of support received from family or friends. Hormonal changes may also influence emotional lability. Progesterone, estrogen, corticosteroids, and other hormones involved in the changes of pregnancy are thought to have some effect in mediating emotions, particularly depression and elation. Pregnant women often view their emotional lability as abnormal and think they are "going crazy" when they burst into tears without warning or become fearful in situations that normally would cause no distress. Significant others, especially fathers, also have concerns about the woman's mood swings and don't know how to respond. Women may worry that their mood swings will influence the baby. Reassurance is needed that the emotional lability is normal and is unlikely to affect the baby. Fathers should be encouraged to remain calm, be patient and loving, and understand that the emotional lability will pass.

Factors Influencing Acceptance. Factors that may be related to acceptance of the pregnancy are the woman's readiness for the experience and her identification with the motherhood role. For example, a pregnancy may be more readily accepted when the woman is in her 20s or 30s than when she is in her teens or 40s. The woman's identity or perception of herself also influences acceptance. Fear of helplessness, pain, loss of control, or loss of self-esteem during labor is another factor that may influence acceptance. Cultural or religious background may be an influence in how the woman accepts the pregnancy. Finally, the relationship the woman had with her own mother may be an influencing factor. Total acceptance at all times during pregnancy may be rare (Lederman 1984; Mercer 1986).

Evaluating Acceptance of the Pregnancy. Lederman (1984) identifies five ways that the degree of acceptance of the pregnancy can be evaluated:

1. Whether the woman consciously planned and wanted the pregnancy. Although this is one factor that may influence acceptance, it is important to note that a planned pregnancy is not necessarily associated with wanting to be a mother. The pregnancy could be motivated by family or community pressure. An unplanned pregnancy does not necessarily indicate that the baby will not be loved and wanted.
2. Whether the woman is happy or depressed during the pregnancy. Usually there is congruence between feeling happy during pregnancy and acceptance of the pregnancy. Some women may not be happy about being pregnant but are looking forward to the baby. Women who are happy usually feel gratified by their biologic fulfillment. They enjoy fetal movement; experience few minor discomforts or tolerate them well; and demonstrate self-confidence about outcomes for themselves, the baby, or their career. All women may experience depression for short intervals at some time during the pregnancy, but if it occurs consistently throughout the pregnancy it may be caused by fears about labor and birth, anxiety about motherhood, concern regarding finances, concern about bodily changes, worry about the status of the baby, or career interruption.
3. The amount of discomfort the woman experiences during the pregnancy. The prevalence of physical symptoms may be related to the desire for the pregnancy, the amount of anxiety during pregnancy, and the general emotional well-being of the woman. When the pregnancy is accepted and the baby is wanted, the discomforts of pregnancy tend to be perceived as a minor imposition, and measures to relieve them usually have some success.
4. Whether the woman accepts or rejects changes in her body. Although pregnant women may not like the change in body size, particularly with today's societal pressure for being thin, women who accept the pregnancy are not greatly troubled by the changes and accept them as a part of the pregnancy experience. Women who accept the pregnancy believe that the bodily changes are reversible and have self-confidence that the previous body size will return after the birth.
5. Whether ambivalence or conflict about the pregnancy is experienced in the third trimester. Ambivalence is common for most women during pregnancy but is usually limited to the first or second trimesters (Brown 1984; Caplan 1957; Colman and Colman 1991). Women may occasionally express a wish not to be pregnant or voice doubts about the impending responsibilities of motherhood. Concerns about financial security and changed lifestyle are the primary contributors to ambivalence. However, if ambivalence about pregnancy and motherhood is still prevalent in the third trimester, acceptance is probably being blocked by unresolved conflicts.

PERCEIVING THE FETUS AS A SEPARATE BEING

The second developmental task the woman must accomplish is to perceive the fetus as a separate being, not just an extension or integral part of the self (Tanner 1969). This represents the next necessary step that must follow the acceptance of being pregnant. It is accomplished as the woman gradually sees the infant's needs as separate from her own. She must first recognize the developing fetus as a part of her body image and then eventually come to recognize the fetus as a separate, unique person.

Focus on the Developing Fetus. This developmental task usually takes place during the second trimester. During this time, women begin to move from focusing on their own physical and emotional symptoms to focusing on the development of the fetus. Increased interest regarding fetal growth and development is shown by women at this time as they read everything they can find about fetal development, ask questions of health care providers regarding their baby, or express a desire to see an ultrasound picture of the fetus. The occurrence of quickening around 20 weeks of gestation adds to the increasing focus on the baby as a separate human being. It is during this time that prenatal attachment to the baby begins. This is discussed further later in the chapter.

Latent Period. This period of the pregnancy is often experienced as a quiet, latent period emotionally. Anxieties that may have been present in the first trimester seem to decrease. The woman may begin to feel an increased sense of accomplishment and physical well-being. On one hand, the woman may become more introverted as she begins to focus on her developing baby, evaluate her life, and think about her future plans. This introspectiveness helps the woman to prepare for her role as a mother. On the other hand, the woman may at times feel more open in her interactions with others. As the development of the baby becomes evident with the woman's increased body size, she may begin to feel pride in her pregnant state and be eager to talk with others about being pregnant. She may also begin to feel a sense of increased dependence on others in her life (Campbell and Field 1988; Joffe 1989; Robinson and Stewart 1989).

▼ **Dreams and Fantasies.** Although dreams and fantasies about the baby or the birth can occur at any time during the pregnancy, they often begin during the second trimester (Colman and Colman 1991; Lederman 1984; Rubin 1984). Most pregnant women experience vivid dreams and need to be reassured that they are normal. The fantasies may take the form of daydreams while the woman is awake. She may find herself drifting off into space, imagining what the baby will be like or how she will act in her role as a mother. Dreams that occur during sleep may be positive and happy in nature or may be frightening. Dreams with positive themes reflect ecstatic anticipation, joy about the fullness of life, the love of a man, or unity with a world alive with growing things (Colman and Colman 1991). Dreams often mirror the actual concerns the woman may be feeling about her pregnancy. Lederman (1984) in her study of pregnant women found that five categories of dreams commonly occurred: reliving childhood, school dreams, motherhood-career conflict, confidence in maternal skills, and food dreams that reflect infant intactness. Sherwen's 1981 survey of women in the third trimester of pregnancy identified dreams relating to having an abnormal infant, being attacked, being enclosed or drowning, forgetting or losing things, being unprepared, or sexual encounters.

The fact that the frightening dreams often revolve around themes of being trapped or in grave danger may reflect the woman's feelings about pregnancy being unchangeable and the approaching birth being somewhat threatening. The dreams that reflect bizarre thoughts or fears about losing the baby may be an expression of the fact that the woman will lose the baby from her body when she gives birth. It is not unusual for a woman to dream that her baby is born with a deformity or is stillborn. Women need to be reassured that a dream of this nature is not in any way predictive of future events. These fantasies and dreams provide some of the most dramatic evidence of the woman's psychological changes during the pregnancy (Blake and Reimann 1993).

▼ **Body Image.** As the woman's body begins to change in the second trimester, she may begin to experience alterations in body image. Body image is defined as the subjective picture or mental image of oneself that is formed in the mind. This image incorporates physiologic, psychological, and social factors and is closely related to self-esteem. Formation of the body image is a dynamic process shaped by experiences in life and by cognitive development. The changes in the woman's perception of her image during pregnancy occur gradually and may be either positive or negative. Some women may view their changing shape as beautiful, representative of their fertility and femininity.

Unfortunately, many women express a more negative body image during pregnancy, reflecting their view of themselves in relation to the ideal thin body image prevalent in the United States. Research has shown that the body image declines as pregnancy progresses (Hofmeyr et al. 1990; Strang and Sullivan 1985). By the media's standards in our society, the pregnant woman is overweight, has curves in many of the wrong places, and can't fit into the latest fashions. Pregnant women may describe themselves with such adjectives as fat, blimp, watermelon, ugly, elephant, or barn. These negative perceptions are unfortunate in view of the unique experience and function that pregnancy represents.

The physical changes and symptoms that the woman experiences during pregnancy contribute to her body image. For example, she becomes warmer faster and may have a tendency to feel faint or weak; she needs more physical space because of her increased size, making her feel fat; it is more difficult to move or bend, making her feel awkward; she becomes tired more easily and may experience backache or other bodily aches, making her feel old. All these physical changes contribute to an altered view of herself.

The woman's partner, family members, or friends also influence her perception of her body image. The woman values highly her partner's feelings toward the appearance of her body. If he finds her physically attractive during pregnancy and communicates this to her, her body image will be influenced positively. If, on the other hand, he conveys feelings of disgust or sexual disinterest, or even teases her about her size, her body image will be negatively influenced. If friends and family members give her positive rather than negative feedback about her changing appearance, she will feel better about herself. Women need to be reassured that their bodily changes are normal and attractive, and that their body will return to its prepregnant state after the birth of the baby.

Alteration in Sexual Responsiveness. Women may also experience an alteration in sexual responsiveness during pregnancy. The physical changes in the woman and the psychological demands on both woman and partner have an influence on their sexual relationship. The changing roles that the woman and her partner experience as a result of pregnancy and impending parenthood also have an effect. Some women find pregnancy a time of increased sexual enjoyment, while others may find their sexual interest decline. Many factors already discussed, such as acceptance of the pregnancy, emotional lability, body image, and reaction of the partner, influence the woman's sexual responsiveness during pregnancy. Unfortunately, sexuality in pregnancy is often given little attention by health care providers, and information given is scant, inconsistent, or based on tradition rather than on scientific study (Masters et al. 1995) (See Chapter 10 for a complete discussion of sexuality in pregnancy.)

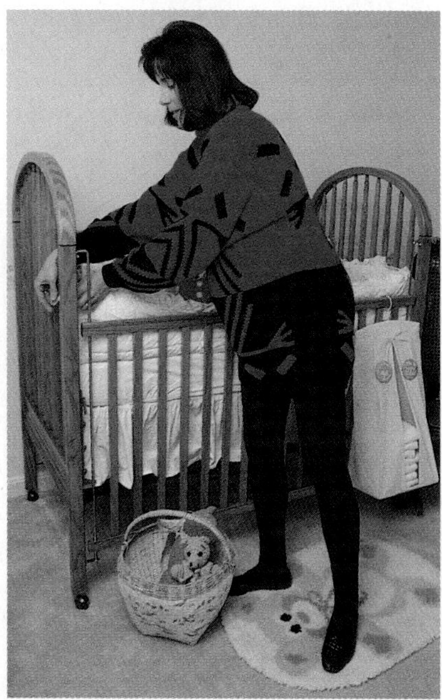

Figure 17–2
Making preparations for the baby. Women often exhibit nesting behavior as they make preparations for the baby's arrival.

ESTABLISHING A CARETAKING RELATIONSHIP

The final developmental task is to prepare for giving up the fetus, giving birth, and establishing a caretaking relationship with the infant (Tanner 1969). The woman begins to work on this task toward the end of pregnancy as she approaches delivery. After accomplishing the second task of recognizing the baby as a separate human being, she must then prepare emotionally to give birth and begin the task of parenting. As she works through this developmental task, she begins to view herself not just as a pregnant woman, but as the mother who will be responsible for nurturing the baby. Even though she is eager to have the pregnancy end and see her baby, she may have some feelings of sadness at the thought of letting her baby go from her body and ending the special relationship that has existed.

Nesting. At this time the woman begins to show an increase in activities to prepare for this reality. She becomes more interested in coping with the birth and attends childbirth classes. Preparations for the baby take place in earnest as the prospective parents obtain supplies, attend baby showers, and get the nursery ready (Fig. 17–2). The increase in such physical symptoms as fatigue, backache, urinary frequency, clumsiness, and Braxton Hicks contractions toward the end of pregnancy helps to increase the woman's emotional readiness for birth, and she becomes very impatient to have the pregnancy come to a conclusion.

Anxiety. By the third trimester, women have resolved most of the ambivalence about pregnancy and motherhood that existed in the earlier part of pregnancy. They have come to accept the reality of the pregnancy, the baby, and all the life changes that result. However, an increase in anxiety and self-absorption may be observed as women focus on concerns about life, death, separation, and attachment. Many women begin to think more about the health and safety of the baby. They worry about their behavior and ability to cope in labor. Of particular concern is the fear that they will lose control of themselves and act foolishly. There is a mixture of anticipation and dread about the impending birth (Colman and Colman 1991; Lederman 1984; Rubin 1984).

Maternal Tasks

In addition to the developmental tasks of pregnancy, another way to conceptualize the emotional changes that a woman experiences is seen in Rubin's classic theory of maternal tasks of pregnancy (1984) (see Table 17–1). Although this framework provides a basis for the consideration of emotional processes during pregnancy, it must be remembered that it is a theory proposed several decades ago. It may not be as relevant today in light of modern technology and increased parental awareness (Gay et al. 1988). The advent of ultrasonography as a means of prenatal testing enables women to visualize and identify with their babies very early in pregnancy. Prenatal education also increases the parents' focus on their unborn child.

Rubin discussed four emotional tasks that the woman must accomplish during pregnancy: (1) ensuring safe passage, (2) seeking acceptance of the child by others, (3) binding-in to the child, (4) learning to give of oneself on behalf of one's child.

ENSURING SAFE PASSAGE

From the moment she realizes that she is pregnant, the woman consciously and unconsciously begins to carry out activities that will contribute to the safety of herself and her baby. Initially, in the first trimester, these activities are focused on her own well-being, for she is not yet physically aware of the fetus. Choosing a competent physician or nurse midwife and obtaining prenatal care are examples of early activities to ensure safety. By the second trimester the woman is more aware of her baby because of size and movement, and the focus of concern shifts to the baby. She begins to engage in data gathering, seeking information about every aspect of pregnancy and childbirth, so that she can do all that she can to protect her infant. Activities that she undertakes include trying to eat well, exercise, and obtain sufficient rest. The focus shifts again in the third trimester and the woman now becomes concerned with the safety of both herself and the baby. Her protectiveness can be seen in her cautious behavior related to everyday environmental hazards such as crossing streets, walking in crowds, or moving through revolving doors. She begins to become involved in reading, discussions with other mothers, or childbirth classes to identify information and coping mechanisms that will ensure safe passage through childbirth.

SEEKING ACCEPTANCE OF THE CHILD BY OTHERS

As discussed in Chapter 18, pregnancy and childbirth change the relationships that exist within a family system or within the woman's other social systems. From an emotional perspective, it is important to the pregnant woman that those around her, and particularly her partner, accept the pregnancy and the changes that will result after the birth of the baby. Acceptance of the coming of a child requires an awareness on the part of all family members, particularly the partner, siblings, and grandparents, that personal sacrifices may be necessary. It may be necessary to let go of some ego-satisfying pleasures, such as activities or possessions, to accommodate the new baby. Also, the time available for interaction between any two family members will be altered by a new baby, and this is often the most difficult change to accept. The family must be willing to make these changes, and the woman watches carefully during her pregnancy to assess the acceptance of others.

Acceptance of the pregnancy by others is usually the greatest in the second trimester. In the first trimester, others' awareness may be limited; in the third trimester, there is mounting social pressure for the pregnancy to end as people become impatient with the pregnant state. Statements such as "Are you still pregnant?" or "You haven't delivered yet?" may be heard. The increasing impatience of others only adds to the woman's own impatience, and it takes a strongly formed maternal identity to cope with the pressures from others regarding continuing the pregnancy.

BINDING-IN TO THE CHILD

Fetal movement begins the process of transforming the baby in the woman's mind from a theoretic fantasy to a real, living being. It begins the natural discovery process of commitment that the woman forms to her child and to the successful completion of the pregnancy. Rubin calls this commitment "binding-in," a process of seeking commitment and acceptance of oneself as a mother. This process is thought to result from the intimacy of sensory experience, the exclusive communication between mother and baby, and the hidden nature of the unborn child. Today, "binding-in" is more likely to be called prenatal attachment. This is discussed further in the next section.

LEARNING TO GIVE OF ONESELF ON BEHALF OF ONE'S CHILD

Giving of oneself is probably the greatest and most complex task of pregnancy, childbirth, and early parenting. The progressive, all-consuming demands and challenges of pregnancy and parenting cannot be passively endured without purpose. The woman is able to balance the physical, emotional, and social changes resulting from the pregnancy only because of her growing awareness of and commitment to her baby. The baby gives her a cause for all the changes she must make. The act of giving for the sake of the baby is continual. It may be the first time in the woman's life that such unconditional giving has been required, and it may require a great deal of emotional work. As a result of this experience, there may be qualitative changes in the personality of a woman in the course of pregnancy and childbearing resulting from her mastery of self-deprivation and giving of herself.

Prenatal Attachment

RESEARCH FINDINGS

For many years, the concept of the woman attaching emotionally to her baby was considered

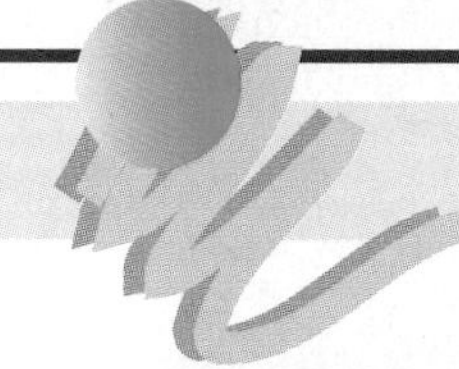

HISTORICAL PERSPECTIVES

THE PSYCHOLOGY OF PREGNANCY: A MODERN-DAY LUXURY?

It is difficult to determine with absolute certainty the nature of the emotional experience of pregnancy for women from centuries past, or the views of early midwives and physicians about the psychology of pregnancy, because little was documented in the literature about the psychological adaptation to pregnancy, birth, or early parenting. However, on the basis of what is known about the pregnancy and birth experience in the eighteenth and nineteenth centuries, it is easy to speculate that the primary emotions of concern were those of worry, fear, and grief.

An important part of women's experiences during pregnancy and childbirth in past centuries was their anticipation of dying, of being permanently injured during the event, or of losing the baby. Concerns about completion of the developmental and psychological tasks of pregnancy or prenatal attachment did not exist when the physical aspects of pregnancy and childbirth were associated with such danger and risk. Attention to the emotional aspects of pregnancy therefore held little priority. If women's emotional responses were mentioned, they were often described as "hysterias" that resulted from their delicate condition or female gender. The fact that many "advice manuals" were written for pregnant women to inform them how "nature" decreed they should conduct themselves when pregnant indicates that anxiety was a common emotion. Unfortunately, the table of contents of an advice manual in 1834 included only one topic ("Despondency") that related to the emotional aspects of pregnancy. The primary emotional support given to women in days past was from their mothers, sisters, or female friends.

Anxiety during labor and birth was of concern to early midwives and physicians because it was believed to have the potential to affect the viability of the fetus or to impair the physiologic progression of labor, not because of concern for the woman's holistic well-being. In 1727, Dr. James Blondel proposed the theory of "maternal impressions," which stated that the condition and viability of the fetus was profoundly influenced by the mother's mental and emotional state. In 1806, another physician wrote, "Much will depend upon the skill of the practitioner in regulating the passions of the mind . . . so that their undue influence may not interfere with the regular process of parturition" (Oakley 1986, p. 264). It is unclear from early writings how the passions of the mind were regulated. Most likely the use of drugs or anesthesia was the only means at that time of dealing with women's emotions.

As the twentieth century evolved, a number of factors allowed for our continuing increased interest in and attention to the emotional experience of pregnancy and childbirth. The fact that the physiologic events of pregnancy and birth are now relatively safe, owing to comprehensive prenatal care and medical technology, is no doubt the primary reason that attention can be focused on all aspects of the pregnancy experience. The influence of childbirth education since the 1960s, the women's movement in the 1970s, and the emphasis on holistic health since the 1980s have all increased our awareness of the psychological experience of pregnancy and childbirth.

Data from Leavitt, J. (1986). *Brought to bed: Childbearing in America: 1750–1950.* New York: Oxford University Press; and Oakley, A. (1986). *The captured womb: A history of the medical care of pregnant women.* Oxford: Basil Blackwell.

only in relation to the early postpartal period. However, close observation of pregnant women and studies conducted in the 1980s by researchers such as Cranley (1981) and Gaffney (1988), as well as those done in the 1990s (Lumley 1990; Muller 1990, 1992), have revealed that the attachment process begins long before birth. A number of factors may be related to the development of prenatal attachment: (1) the physical symptoms of pregnancy, particularly quickening (Lerum and

LoBiondo-Wood 1989), (2) the mother's perception of her infant (Cranley 1981), (3) maternal state anxiety (Gaffney 1986), and (4) social support (Cranley 1981). However, other variables such as maternal age, race, educational level, socioeconomic status, number of previous pregnancies, desire for the pregnancy, self-esteem, and pregnancy risk status have not been found to relate significantly to prenatal attachment (Cranley 1981; Gaffney 1988; Kemp and Page 1987). Although a number of studies of prenatal attachment have been performed, small sample sizes, instruments that have not shown good validity and reliability, and lack of consistent findings make generalization of these study findings risky (Muller 1992).

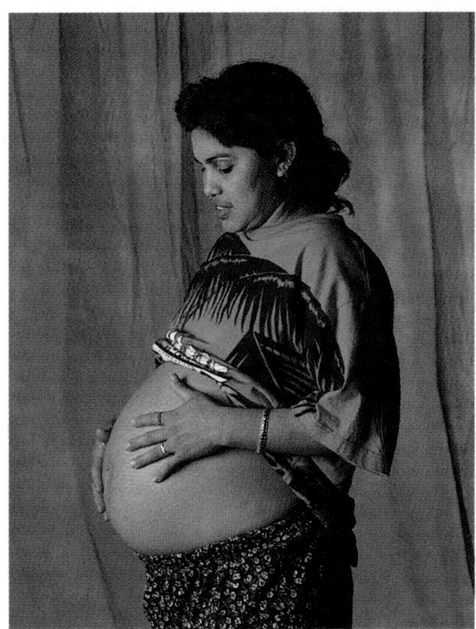

Figure 17–3

Prenatal attachment to the baby begins long before the birth. Mothers begin to interact with the baby during the pregnancy, often talking to and calling him or her by a name.

PRENATAL ATTACHMENT BEHAVIORS

A pregnant woman demonstrates many behaviors that illustrate her growing affiliation and interaction with her developing infant. In the first trimester, although the baby may still seem somewhat unreal, the woman begins her attachment process by fantasizing and daydreaming about the baby. In the second trimester, attachment may be enhanced when fetal movement is felt, the fetal heart rate is heard, or an ultrasound picture is seen. By the third trimester, obvious attachment behaviors may be observed. For example, the woman pats or rubs her tummy as she talks lovingly to her baby (Fig. 17–3), she assigns pet names to the baby, or she eats particular foods that she tells the baby are for him or her (Rubin 1984). Fathers also interact with their unborn infant during pregnancy. Both parents can describe individual characteristics of their baby in relation to appearance, gender, temperament, and sleep-wake cycle. From the expectant parent's point of view, the baby is an individual that responds in unique and predictable ways (Stainton 1990).

FACILITATING PRENATAL ATTACHMENT

On the basis of the premise that prenatal experience influences postnatal maternal attachment, a number of research studies have been conducted to establish factors that might enhance prenatal attachment (Muller 1992). Researchers have been interested in the effects that modern obstetric technology such as ultrasound examination and amniocentesis might have on the process of prenatal attachment (Grace 1984; Heidrich and Cranley 1989; Kohn et al. 1980; Milne and Rich 1981). In addition, nurses have been encouraged to routinely plan prenatal interventions that promote attachment. Suggested interventions include teaching the pregnant woman to feel for the parts of the baby to determine fetal position; encouraging the woman to become aware of fetal activity and factors that influence that activity; and encouraging the woman to rub, stroke, and massage her abdomen (Carter-Jessop 1981; Davis and Akridge 1987). The findings of these research studies have been inconclusive: some demonstrate a relationship between prenatal intervention and postnatal attachment and others show no relationship (Carson and Virden 1984). The wisdom of actively intervening in the prenatal attachment process through the use of technology and interventions, in contrast with allowing the process to unfold naturally, has been challenged (Muller 1990). Although interventions or technology that heighten the woman's awareness of her infant are unlikely to cause harm, the process of prenatal attachment seems to proceed predictably with or without these interventions.

PATERNAL PSYCHOLOGICAL ADAPTATION IN PREGNANCY

Historically, the emotional adaptation to pregnancy experienced by the father has been given far less attention than that of the mother. This is probably understandable since there is no obvious physical change in the father during pregnancy, and it is uncommon for men to seek assistance or support for the emotional stresses that a pregnancy may cause. Expectant fathers must struggle for recognition as a parent from their partner, family, friends, and society. They must work hard at carving out their role when often there are no available role models in their social network. Men are often recognized not as expectant parents but as helpmates or breadwinners, which can interfere with validation of the reality of the pregnancy or developing baby (Jordan 1990). However, it is important to recognize that pregnancy, childbirth, and parenting are emotional experiences for men. The emotional needs of fathers also need to be met. In the past 25 years, such social changes as increased involvement and participation of the father in the childbirth process, childbirth education, and egalitarian maternal and paternal parenting roles have made families, health care professionals, and researchers more aware that pregnancy is an emotional experience for fathers. Like expectant mothers, expectant fathers face developmental tasks that contribute to the adjustments and role changes necessary during the childbearing phase of life (Fawcett 1989).

Developmental Tasks

May (1982b) suggests that first-time fathers experience a characteristic pattern of developmental change and emotional involvement during pregnancy. The data from her research with 20 expectant fathers suggest a pattern consisting of three phases (Table 17–3). A number of emotional reactions and psychological changes (see Table 17–2) accompany these phases during the course of pregnancy.

ANNOUNCEMENT PHASE

The first phase is called the announcement phase. It occurs during the time in which the pregnancy is first suspected and confirmed, and lasts a few hours to several weeks. The task of fathers during this phase is to accept the pregnancy. The process of acceptance may come more slowly for fathers than for mothers because fathers do not experience physical symptoms or changes that require frequent attention to the pregnant state, although some men do experience physical manifestations in response to the pregnancy as part of the couvade syndrome (Fawcett and York 1986; Ferketich and Mercer 1989; Strickland 1987). These phenomena are discussed in more detail in Chapter 18. Fathers may experience either great joy and excitement if the pregnancy was desired, or shock, anger, and disappointment if it was not. Some men may feel a sense of pride at the news of their partner's pregnancy, resulting from a belief that the pregnancy is proof of their masculinity. Ambivalence is common for both men and women in this early phase of pregnancy. The pregnancy may seem exciting and desirable at some times and then overwhelming and undesirable at other times.

MORATORIUM PHASE

The second phase of adaptation for expectant fathers is the moratorium phase. This period usually occurs while there is still not much visual evidence of the pregnancy, so that conscious thought about the pregnancy can be put aside for a time; it ends when the pregnancy becomes visible. The moratorium may last for several days after the announcement to several months. The tasks of fathers during this phase are to accept the fetus, adjust to reality, and come to terms with the pregnancy. The moratorium phase may be characterized by the emotional distance of the father. He may become introspective and not talk about the pregnancy unless encouraged to do so by his partner. The pregnancy does not seem real at this point, there is no concrete evidence of its existence, and physical changes are not the major focus of attention for fathers. As a result, the father is more able than the mother to concentrate on other life concerns. This discrepancy in the experience between mothers and fathers at this time may result in marital tension and disrupted communication; the expectant mother may feel hurt that the father is not as focused on the pregnancy or emotionally involved as she is.

FOCUSING PHASE

The final period of developmental change for fathers is the focusing phase. The task in this phase is to accept the birth of the baby and the future

Table 17–3

PATERNAL PSYCHOLOGICAL ADAPTATION IN PREGNANCY: THREE PHASES

PHASE	DEVELOPMENTAL TASK	POSSIBLE RESPONSE
Announcement	Accepting pregnancy	Ambivalence
Moratorium	Accepting fetus	Introspection, emotional distancing
Focusing	Accepting birth of baby and future parenting role	Active preparation

Data from May, K. (1982b). Three phases of father involvement in pregnancy. *Nursing Research,* 31(6), 337–342.

parenting role. During this phase the man begins to feel that the pregnancy is real and he focuses on its importance in his life. He redefines himself as a father and feels more in tune with his wife in regard to the pregnancy. Fathers continue to feel pride as the pregnancy progresses, and become more tender and protective of their partners. They may start to show more active involvement with the pregnancy and fetus and demonstrate evidence of prenatal attachment (Fig. 17–4). The strength of the feelings of prenatal attachment experienced by fathers may be related to their investment in the pregnancy and the strength of the marital relationship (Weaver and Cranley 1983). Prenatal attachment in men has not been shown to be related to the couvade syndrome or to the degree of maternal prenatal attachment (Schodt 1989).

Expectant fathers can experience varying emotional reactions to the changing physical appearance of their partners. Some men may be "turned off" by their partner's changing body; others may respond positively and view her as being more feminine and beautiful than ever. These feelings, along with fear that lovemaking may harm the baby, can alter the expectant father's sexual desire during pregnancy. As the time of birth nears, fathers may begin to become increasingly anxious about the labor, the birth, the well-being of his partner and baby, finances, or increased responsibilities. It is helpful if the man negotiates with his partner in advance the roles he will assume during the birth and parenting. Attendance at childbirth classes often facilitates these discussions. The focusing phase usually begins around the twenty-fifth to thirtieth weeks of gestation and ends with the onset of labor (Colman and Colman 1991; Joffe 1989; May 1982b).

Styles of Involvement

May (1980) interviewed expectant fathers and found that their responses to pregnancy fell along a continuum from detachment to involvement. Three distinct styles of detachment/involvement were identified: (1) observer, (2) instrumental, and (3) expressive.

OBSERVER STYLE

The observer style is one in which the father feels an emotional distance from the pregnancy and sees himself as a bystander. Fathers with this style of involvement may not feel comfortable accompanying the woman to prenatal appointments or attending childbirth classes. Cultural or religious background often influences this paternal style. Pregnancy and childbirth may be viewed as "woman's work."

INSTRUMENTAL STYLE

The instrumental style is one in which the father is somewhat involved but sees himself as the caretaker or manager of the pregnancy, and is concerned primarily with the concrete tasks that need to be accomplished. For example, the father may not be as comfortable in discussing the woman's diet or hearing about her fears regarding childbirth as he is in painting the nursery, building a cradle, or expanding his life insurance coverage.

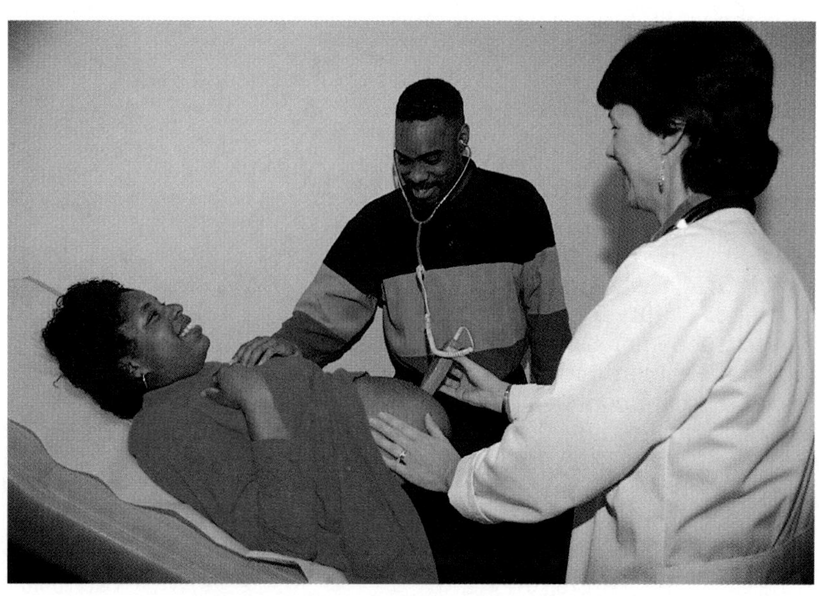

Figure 17–4

Paternal prenatal attachment. Fathers also form an attachment to the baby during the pregnancy. Expectant parents shown here together at a prenatal visit listen to the fetal heartbeat through a transducer.

EXPRESSIVE STYLE

The expressive style is one in which the father becomes highly involved emotionally, sees himself as a full partner, and plays an active role throughout the pregnancy. This father is likely to be eager to attend childbirth classes, encourage the woman to do her daily exercises, or talk to the health care provider about options for the labor and birth experience. According to May, the father who exhibits the expressive style is likely to be most in tune with the expectant mother and experience the pregnancy in much the same manner as she does.

Identification of these styles of emotional response in expectant fathers provides a helpful framework, but one that should be used with caution. It is quite possible for a discrepancy to exist between observable behavior and actual feelings or emotional involvement.

Dreams and Fantasies/Jealousy

During the pregnancy the father may experience dreams or fantasies just as the mother does. These fantasies may differ in frequency or description from the mother's and are probably influenced by the father's sex role orientation and involvement in the pregnancy (Sherwen 1981). If they do occur, however, they probably help the father adapt emotionally to the pregnancy and visualize his role as a parent. Expectant fathers may begin to experience some jealousy at some point in the pregnancy as they see the amount of attention being given to the pregnancy and developing fetus by their partners and other family members.

Factors Influencing Paternal Response

Factors that influence the father's response to and acceptance of pregnancy include his age and developmental status, the power balance in the partner's role relationship, whether or not he had intended to be a father at some point in his life, his sense of financial security, the stability in the couple's relationship, his preparation for the event (Taubenheim and Silbernagel 1988), and a feeling of closure to the childless period of the relationship with his partner (May 1980, 1982a). The father's perception of his role during pregnancy and parenting is probably influenced by his memories of the fathering he received from his own father, his cultural background, his self-esteem, and his readiness for the fathering experience.

PSYCHOLOGICAL ADAPTATION OF OTHER FAMILY MEMBERS

Siblings

EMOTIONAL REACTIONS

A pregnancy and the subsequent addition of another child to a family cause a wide range of emotional reactions in the other children. These feelings may include excitement, jealousy, interest, anger, or embarrassment, depending on the age of the sibling and the family circumstances. The psychological adaptation of the siblings may also vary from the onset of the pregnancy to the actual introduction of the baby into the family. For example, a child under 2 years of age will be affected very little during the pregnancy but may show extreme jealousy when the baby is brought home. A school-age child may be excited and eager to learn about pregnancy and birth but react with anger when the reality of the baby's influence on family life becomes apparent. Adolescents may be embarrassed about their mother being pregnant but become nurturing and helpful when the baby is brought home.

MATERNAL CONCERNS

The pregnant woman is usually very concerned about the reactions of her children to her pregnancy. The development of a new life within her often increases her awareness and precipitates an examination of her relationship with her other children. She may worry about the increased demands on her life that the addition of another child will make. The effects of the pregnancy on her other children represent an area of concern that most pregnant women need to discuss with a health care professional. The woman may need only to verbalize her concerns and thoughts or she may need specific guidance about how to manage the adjustment of her other children. The possible behavioral responses of the children, depending on their developmental level, should be discussed so that she can anticipate these responses and plan for ways to deal with them. The behavioral response of most concern is usually that of jealousy and sibling rivalry. Some jealousy is no doubt inevitable, but it can be lessened if the parents continue to show love and attention and include the sibling in the care of the baby.

HELPING SIBLINGS ADJUST

It is important for parents to inform siblings about the pregnancy at a time appropriate for them (e.g., a 2-year-old need not be told until later in the pregnancy, whereas an adolescent should be informed in the first trimester). Explanations about pregnancy and birth should be given at a level appropriate for the age of the child. The preschool child can begin to understand concepts about fetal development and may enjoy reading books with the mother or listening to the baby's heartbeat (Fig. 17–5); the school-age child may show a great deal of interest in the process of pregnancy and birth and ask many questions; adolescents may be somewhat uncomfortable in discussing the pregnancy as it confirms the sexuality of the parents or promotes a realization of their own sexuality.

Whenever possible, siblings should be included in the family planning and preparations for the baby. For example, if an adjustment in sleeping arrangements of the children will need to be made to accommodate the new baby, this will be more readily accepted if children are included in a family problem-solving meeting in which they have input into the decision. Involving the children in the health care of the mother may help them to adjust. Accompanying mother to prenatal appointments, feeling the baby kick or hearing the heartbeat, and participating in the preparation of a healthy diet all make children feel involved. Taking children to the sibling classes now offered at many hospitals as part of a complete childbirth education program will help them to learn about the birth and care of their new baby brother or sister. (See Chapter 20 for a further discussion of sibling classes.) It is important that parents do all they can to provide consistency in the lives of their other children, both during the pregnancy and after the baby comes home. If a number of things in life that seem normal and familiar continue to occur in the lives of the siblings, their adaptation to a new baby will be easier.

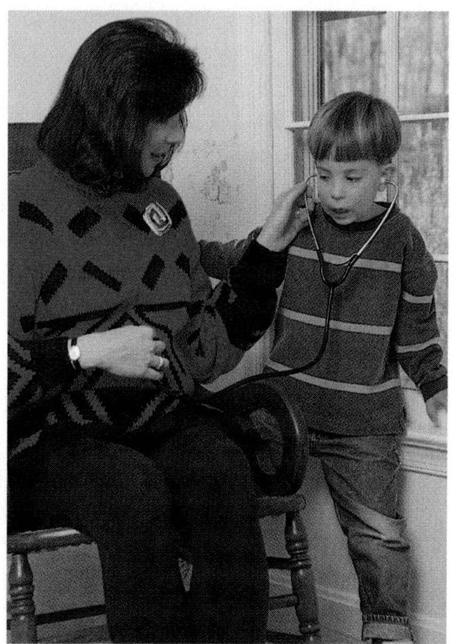

Figure 17–5

Sibling involvement. Expectant parents can help siblings adjust to the idea of a new baby by giving them age-appropriate information, showing them love and attention, and including them in the family preparations for the baby.

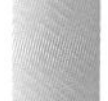

Grandparents

EMOTIONAL REACTIONS

The announcement of a pregnancy will trigger a wide range of emotions for the parents of the expectant couple. The realization that one is about to become a grandparent is most likely to cause feelings of great joy and excitement. On the other hand, some grandparents may feel nostalgic with the realization that the pregnancy marks the beginning of a new generation, is a reminder of one's own aging, and marks changes in expected roles. Impending grandparenting often triggers memories that had been forgotten, and grandparents often enjoy reviewing the events of their own pregnancies, births, and parenting experiences. The expectant parents may examine their relationship with the grandparents and seek to foster closer ties (Kornhaber 1986).

MATERNAL-GRANDMOTHER RELATIONSHIP

The reactions of the pregnant woman's own mother (i.e., the baby's grandmother) are particularly important to the woman's emotional adaptation to the pregnancy. Lederman (1984) discusses four components of the woman's relationship with her mother that were found to be important: (1) the availability of the grandmother to the pregnant woman, both in the past and during this pregnancy; (2) the grandmother's reactions to the pregnancy, especially her acceptance of the grandchild and her acknowledgment of the daughter as a mother; (3) the grandmother's respect for her daughter's autonomy, as demonstrated by relating to the woman as a mature adult rather than as a child; and (4) the grandmother's willingness to reminisce with her daughter about her own childbearing and childrearing experiences. If the relationship between mother (grandmother) and daughter (pregnant woman) is not a good one, the pregnant woman may try to reconcile differences during the pregnancy. Lederman suggests that a poor mother-daughter relationship may be related to a persistent negative attitude toward pregnancy, difficulty with labor and birth, and difficulty in adjusting to parenthood. A study by Zachariah (1994) found that the mother-daughter relationship was a significant predictor of the psychological well-being of the woman during pregnancy.

STYLES OF GRANDPARENTING

Grandparents may differ in their style of grandparenting. Some choose to become highly involved with grandchildren, offering to care for them regularly, visit them often, or contribute to their financial needs. Others may be less involved and see their grandchildren only on occasion. Many factors influence the degree of involvement, including age and health status, geographical location, financial status, and work status. It is helpful if grandparents and expectant parents discuss the desired degree of grandparent-grandchildren involvement before the birth, so that the needs of both can be met. During pregnancy and the early parenting period, expectant parents often express an increased awareness of the importance of their parents and a greater understanding of the issues their parents faced in raising them.

EDUCATIONAL PROGRAMS

Educational programs that include grandparents have been developed as part of the total childbirth education curriculum offered by many health care providers. Grandparents delight in learning information they did not have available to them during their pregnancies. Classes for grandparents serve to involve them in the birth experience of their children and help them to support the choices made by the expectant couple regarding birth, infant feeding, or childrearing. (See Chapter 20 for further discussion of grandparenting classes.)

FACTORS ALTERING PSYCHOLOGICAL ADAPTATION

A number of variables can influence the psychological adaptation of parents to the pregnancy. It is important that these potential factors be identified during pregnancy, for an alteration in psychological adaptation to pregnancy can be of as much concern as an alteration in physical adaptation to pregnancy.

High-Risk Pregnancy

The woman experiencing a high-risk pregnancy is dealing with two simultaneous crises: (1) the normal developmental crisis of pregnancy and (2) the situational crisis of a high-risk pregnancy that may not progress in line with expected patterns to end with a healthy mother-infant dyad. (See Chapter 21 for a discussion of the physiologic aspects of high-risk pregnancy.) This additional stress may result in interference with the usual emotional reactions to pregnancy and may alter the developmental tasks of pregnancy (Gilbert and Harmon 1993; Kemp and Page 1986). In fact, the woman experiencing a high-risk pregnancy has additional developmental tasks to complete. Not only must she accept that she is pregnant, but she must also accept that she is a high-risk pregnant woman and that her pregnancy is high risk; not only must she accept the developing fetus, she may question whether her pregnancy and fetus will remain viable and must accept the reality of an uncertain outcome; not only must she prepare to give up the fetus by giving birth, she must adapt to the possibility of a less than perfect outcome.

EMOTIONAL REACTIONS

The pregnancy and its successful completion take on special value when it is complicated by maternal or fetal illness. Any risk factor that endangers the outcome of the pregnancy is viewed as a threat and usually leads to many emotional reactions that may be experienced by the woman, her partner, or other family members.

▼ **Anxiety and Stress.** Anxiety and stress are common during a high-risk pregnancy and can be manifested in such behaviors as helplessness, apathy, restlessness, irritability, depression, or anger (Avant 1988; Mercer et al. 1986, 1988). Anxiety is often caused by worry about the woman's health or the status of the baby. It can be increased if cognitive or emotional needs are not addressed. The treatment regimens during a high-risk pregnancy, such as complete bedrest, prenatal testing, or hospitalization, can also contribute to anxiety.

▼ **Denial.** Some women or their partners may demonstrate denial during a high-risk pregnancy. Denial may be expressed as failure to seek care, to acknowledge the risk factor, or to be compliant with medical treatment. It may be easy for parents to deny a problem if they have had previous normal pregnancies or if the woman is not feeling ill. Denial may be an effective coping mechanism to decrease stress, but it is maladaptive if the health status of the mother or infant is in danger.

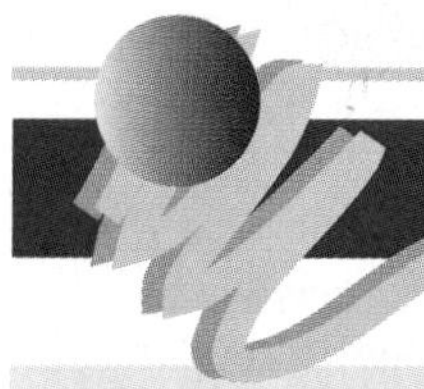

IMPROVING YOUR PRACTICE

MAINTAINING AWARENESS OF PSYCHOLOGICAL ADAPTATION TO PREGNANCY

It is important in all situations for the nurse to remember that the psychological adaptation of the pregnant woman and her partner is as important as the woman's physical status. Prenatal care is not complete unless the emotional reactions to the pregnancy and birth experience are recognized and given attention. Unfortunately, the psychological experience of pregnancy is not as easy to observe or measure and thus is often neglected when the realities of providing maternity care in our health care system are experienced. The following suggestions will help the nurse to include the emotional components of the pregnancy experience in her holistic care:

- IDENTIFY YOUR PERSONAL FEELINGS RELATED TO PREGNANCY AND CHILDBEARING. By giving thought to how you have felt or think you would feel about being pregnant and giving birth, you will become more sensitive to the importance of the emotional experience of the childbearing year.
- BECOME KNOWLEDGEABLE REGARDING CURRENT PSYCHOLOGICAL THEORIES OF PREGNANCY. Read professional journals and attend continuing education offerings to remain up-to-date regarding current research and theory about the emotional aspects of the pregnancy, birth, and early parenting experience.
- MAKE TIME. Vow to find creative ways to allow time in every prenatal visit to talk with the pregnant woman and her partner about how they feel emotionally. Be an actor if necessary! No matter how stressed or hurried you are, learn to hide your own frustrations in order to appear willing to listen and show sincere interest in what the woman or her partner has to say. Sit down with them, if only for a few minutes, establish eye-to-eye contact, and use good listening skills.
- ACCEPT AND ACKNOWLEDGE FEELINGS. Feelings are not right or wrong, they just are! The feelings a woman or partner expresses may not be those you might have in the same situation and may even be startling or negative. However, the feelings exist and have been shaped by a number of factors. Feelings should not be judged, but instead dealt with in light of the expectant parents' life circumstances. If you show judgmental disapproval, they are not likely to confide in you further. A better strategy is to say, "I am concerned about what you are telling me. I'd like to talk further with you to help you work through these feelings."
- PROVIDE CONTINUITY AND FOLLOW-THROUGH. Document your assessment of the woman's or partner's emotional status and interventions so that at the next prenatal visit you, or another member of the health care team, can follow up with what was discussed. One conversation about emotions and feelings during pregnancy is not enough; psychological adaptation is an ongoing process throughout pregnancy.

▼ **Ambivalence.** As discussed earlier in this chapter, ambivalence is common for parents in early pregnancy. However, it may be seen in even greater frequency and for longer periods during a high-risk pregnancy. Parents often feel confused about whether they want the high-risk pregnancy to continue or whether it might be better for the woman or the baby for it to end.

▼ **Blame and Guilt.** Another emotional response of parents experiencing a high-risk pregnancy can be blame and guilt. Parents may worry that something they did caused the health problem. Blame can be self-directed, directed at the partner, or directed at a health care provider. If the blame is directed at the partner, that, along with all the other heightened emotional responses, can place a tremendous strain on the marital relationship. If the blame is directed at health care providers, the woman's compliance with her treatment can be threatened. If the blame is self-directed, guilt is experienced. Feelings of failure may also be expressed. The expectant mother or father may feel a loss of self-esteem because they cannot produce or carry out a "normal" pregnancy.

▼ **Anticipatory Grief.** High-risk parents also experience anticipatory grieving during the pregnancy, as they face the possibility of loss of the baby or a health alteration for the baby. As a re-

Maternal Psychological Adaptation in High-Risk Pregnancy: Additional Developmental Tasks

- Accepting self as high-risk mother

  (Seeing pregnancy as high risk)

- Accepting uncertain outcome

  (Questioning whether pregnancy will remain viable)

- Adapting to possibility of less than perfect outcome

  (Accepting pregnancy as it is)

sult, parents may not allow themselves to attach to their developing baby for fear the emotional pain would be too difficult to bear. If the normal prenatal attachment is interrupted, parents may have difficulty attaching to the baby after birth, and the early parent-child relationship may be impaired. Chapter 38 presents a complete discussion of perinatal loss and grief.

Demographic Characteristics

AGE/DEVELOPMENTAL LEVEL

Several demographic characteristics of the woman may affect her psychological adaptation during pregnancy. Her age and developmental level may influence her emotional responses to pregnancy. Mercer (1986), in her study of three age groups of women during pregnancy, found that older women were more likely than teenage expectant mothers to view their pregnancy as positive and rate their feelings about pregnancy as good or very good. The older women felt proud rather than ashamed, were less worried, and thought that the pregnancy was as welcome as planned and had occurred at a good time. In contrast, however, teenagers were less likely to describe emotional symptoms during pregnancy, while the older women more often reported feeling depressed, happy, serene, or having mood swings. Winslow's 1987 study of pregnant women over 35 revealed that older mothers may approach pregnancy in a more deliberate and thoughtful way than do younger mothers, often employing coping strategies that they had used successfully in the past. Several of the women in this study actually described their pregnancies as projects. These findings no doubt reflect the developmental readiness that women have for the pregnancy and birth experience. Gottesman (1992) found that later ages of childbearing (30 and over) were related to motivation for motherhood, maternal-fetal relationship, and maternal role conceptualization. Further discussion of age as an influence in adolescent pregnancy can be found in Chapter 39.

PARITY

Although, in common belief, increased parity is viewed as influencing pregnancy in a positive manner, resulting in easier pregnancies for multiparous women, this has not been demonstrated in relation to the emotional experience of pregnancy in either empirical observations or clinical research (Norr et al. 1980). Each pregnancy is a new experience for a woman and her family, and although some issues may be easier or even resolved in subsequent pregnancies, others may evolve for the first time as each child is added to the family. The developmental tasks of pregnancy always exist and emotional responses are always part of the holistic experience of pregnancy, no matter how many times a woman has been pregnant.

CULTURE/RELIGION

The cultural background or the religion of the woman and her partner can also have an impact on the emotional responses to pregnancy. The way that procreation, pregnancy, women's roles, men's roles, childbirth, and parenting are viewed by a particular culture or religion brings influence to bear on the woman's emotional responses. For example, if cultural lore or religious doctrine states that pregnancy is a blessed gift from God, emotional adaptation to the event is likely to be influenced. Research is needed in this area to identify the relationship between specific cultural differences or religious beliefs and emotional adaptation during pregnancy.

MARITAL STATUS

The marital status or marital relationship is another demographic factor that can influence psychological adaptation to pregnancy. Single parenthood or an unhappy marital relationship can add additional stressors and negatively influence the emotional responses to pregnancy, making completion of the developmental tasks of pregnancy more difficult. One study reported that a poor relationship between partners during pregnancy was significantly associated with depression during pregnancy and also predictive of depression after childbirth

(Dimitrovsky et al. 1987). On the other hand, a positive relationship between the expectant couple can greatly enhance the emotional changes that occur in pregnancy (Saunders and Robins 1987).

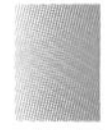

Social Support

The social support available to expectant parents from family, friends, or community services most certainly influences the emotional adaptation to pregnancy. If the pregnancy is accepted by the social network of the expectant couple, their emotional responses will be positively influenced and their completion of developmental tasks enhanced. The socioeconomic status and financial status of the parents may also influence psychological adaptation. If financing the cost of the pregnancy and new baby is a major consideration, worry about money will influence all the other emotional responses taking place.

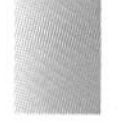

Previous Experience

If the expectant woman has had previous negative experiences related to pregnancy or birth, her emotional responses are likely to be more negative and her completion of developmental tasks altered. Stressful events in the life of the woman, whether they relate to family, job, or community situations, may alter her feelings about the pregnancy. The expectant couple's educational preparation for childbearing also influences emotional adaptation. The more factual information parents have and the more coping skills they acquire, the more positive their psychological adaptation to the pregnancy and birth is likely to be.

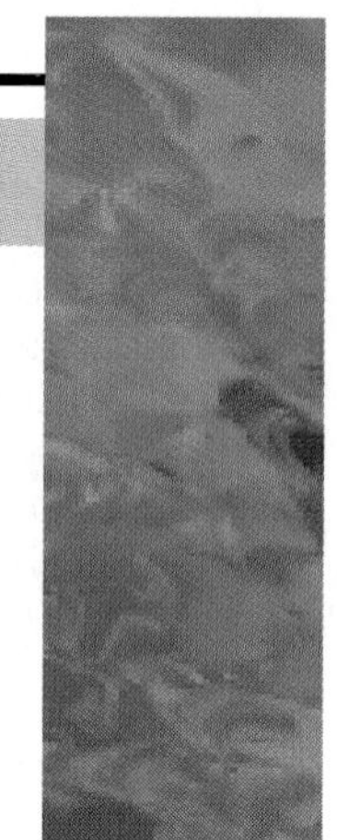

Nursing Practice

Nursing Process

Because the psychological changes and adaptations discussed in this chapter are normal during pregnancy, medical intervention is not usually necessary. Nursing management of these emotional changes becomes a part of each prenatal visit and is as important as the management of the woman's physical care.

▼ Assessment

The psychological history should be included as part of the complete health history during pregnancy (see Components of a Psychological History). Assessment of psychological adaptation in pregnancy can be made through casual conversation, direct interview, and careful observation of the pregnant woman and her significant others. Although the emotional state of the woman and her partner can often be detected by conversational cues, tone of voice, body language, and facial expressions, the couple should also be questioned directly about what they are feeling and experiencing emotionally each month of the pregnancy. By having direct attention paid to their feelings at each prenatal visit, the expectant couple are shown that the emotional responses of pregnancy are indeed important and of interest to their health care providers.

Components of a Psychological History

Developmental tasks of pregnancy

- Acceptance vs. denial of pregnant status
- Feelings about being pregnant
- Emotional affect, behavior, facial expression
- Pregnancy planned/unplanned
- Effects of pregnancy on life situation/plans
- Acceptance of body discomforts and changes

Relationships

- Relationship with father of baby
- Acceptance of pregnancy by father; father's feelings
- Effects of pregnancy on father's life situation/plans
- Relationship with other family members
- Reactions of other family members to pregnancy

Prenatal attachment

- Has mother experienced quickening? Is she aware of daily fetal movement?
- Have mother and father heard fetal heart tones?
- Have mother and father viewed ultrasound image?
- Have mother and father palpated fetal parts?
- Do mother and father talk to baby?
- Have names been selected for baby?
- Is mother able to describe what she thinks her baby is like?

Knowledge and fears

- Understanding of pregnancy, birth, and postpartal period
- Fears/anxiety re pregnancy, birth, or early parenting
- Dreams/fantasies experienced
- Opportunity for group support
- Plans for childbirth/parenting education

Choices

- Wishes/desires for care during pregnancy
- Wishes/desires for care during labor and birth (i.e., a birth plan)
- Desires for early postpartal period

In assessing emotional status, it is important to gather information about factors that could alter emotional responses during pregnancy. For example, an assessment of the developmental level of the woman and her partner will help the nurse focus on the emotional needs likely to be most relevant for the couple. Information about the nature of the relationship between the expectant parents is important, as well as the relationship between the couple and other family members and support systems. Identifying whether the pregnancy was planned or unplanned will guide the nurse in helping the parents work through the developmental tasks of pregnancy and the accompanying emotional changes. It is important to assess the level of knowledge and understanding of pregnancy, birth, and parenting so that referral for education and/or counseling can be made. An assessment of the status of prenatal attachment should be made several times during the pregnancy. Identifying the woman's desires and choices for her pregnancy and birth experience is helpful in meeting her emotional needs (Morcos et al. 1989). By gathering and recording all of this information, health care providers can be alerted to any alterations in emotional status that might occur in relation to these variables and can identify expectant parents who may be at risk for psychological adaptation.

▼ Diagnosis

The nursing diagnoses related to psychological adaptation in pregnancy are based on the information gathered from the assessment of the woman and her family. Because developmental tasks and emotional responses change as the pregnancy progresses, these diagnoses also change. The nursing diagnoses related to psychosocial adaptation are more likely to be potential diagnoses rather than actual diagnoses, but if an alteration in emotional adaptation is identified, the diagnosis will be specific to that alteration. Examples of diagnoses related to psychosocial adaptation are as follows:

- Anxiety related to unexpected pregnancy and disruption of life plans
- Risk for self-esteem disturbance related to altered body image
- Knowledge deficit: childbirth, related to first experience with childbirth
- Risk for altered parent/infant attachment related to high-risk pregnancy
- Altered role performance related to father and sibling adjustment to new baby

▼ Planning

The nursing diagnoses identified will guide the plan of care to meet the woman's and the father's emotional needs during pregnancy. Although the emotional changes and needs of most parents during pregnancy are similar, the plan should be developed in relation to the specific needs of each individual couple and their unique situation. The plan is written in terms of objectives that can be measured and evaluated. The pregnant woman or her partner will

- Verbally express decreased anxiety by the second trimester after adjusting to being pregnant and identifying alternative life plans
- Verbally express comfort and demonstrate through her appearance a positive self-concept and body image
- Verbally express decreased fear about childbirth after attending a series of prepared childbirth classes
- Demonstrate such prenatal attachment behaviors as talking to the fetus, calling the fetus by a name, stroking the fetus through the abdominal wall or feeling body parts, and expressing love and concern for the fetus
- Discuss plans for helping father and siblings adjust to the addition of a new baby

▼ Intervention

The role of the nurse during the prenatal period in relation to psychological adaptation is that of counselor, teacher, role model, and resource. Because of the extended relationship possible during the perinatal period, nurses are in a position to evaluate the expectant couple's mastery of developmental tasks and emotional adaptation.

▼ ANTICIPATORY GUIDANCE

Anticipatory guidance regarding the expected emotional changes of pregnancy should be a part of the teaching plan throughout the pregnancy. Through knowing in advance about the emotional changes that many women and men experience, the expectant couple's concerns about what they are feeling emotionally will be put to rest. Offering factual information about what is commonly experienced during each trimester of pregnancy is a helpful strategy for making the pregnant woman and her partner comfortable about sharing what they are currently experiencing emotionally. For example, stating, "During pregnancy, many women occasionally have dreams about the pregnancy, the birth, or the baby. Have you had any dreams? Can you tell me about them?" will encourage the woman to discuss her emotional status. Saying to the father, "Sometimes men feel jealous of the woman or of the baby during pregnancy. Have you ever felt this way?" will make him feel accepted and comfortable in sharing his feelings. This intervention requires that the nurse establish a comfortable, consistent relationship with the woman and her partner; demonstrate a sincere interest in their feelings about the pregnancy; and allow a little time in each visit for such discussions. In reality, this can be a challenge in a busy clinic or physician's office, but it is an important part of holistic prenatal care. If the expectant parents are made to feel that their health care providers are always changing, hassled, or hurried, they are not likely to reveal any psychological problems that might exist.

▼ COUNSELING AND TEACHING

If alterations from the expected developmental and emotional adaptation are identified, interventions then include counseling and teaching. If the nurse discovers that the woman is not moving through the developmental tasks of pregnancy as expected, or that the father is not coping well with an emotional response to pregnancy, it is essential that this information be recorded on the woman's chart so that all her health care providers be made aware of her need for additional support. Additional time should be scheduled with the woman or her partner to talk about their emotional concerns, just as additional time would be scheduled if a medical problem were identified. The goal of these counseling sessions is to help the expectant couple verbalize concerns, identify reasons for the concerns, and make suggestions for coping with the situation. For example, if the woman is having difficulty in completing the first development task of pregnancy (i.e., accepting the pregnancy), the nurse might help her to identify and verbalize the conflicts she faces in her life, the reasons the pregnancy is not welcomed at this time, the impact that a baby will have on her life, and how she is feeling physically. Suggestions can then be made to help her deal with these problems. If the expectant parents are having difficulty accepting the changes that having a baby will bring to their life, marital or family counseling might be advised.

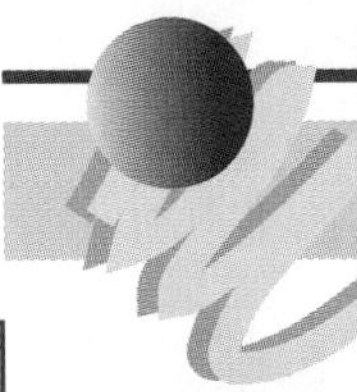

TEACHING GUIDE

PRENATAL ATTACHMENT

TOPIC	*MAJOR CONCEPTS*
Introduction of concept	Attachment to the baby begins during pregnancy as the woman accepts being pregnant, recognizes the reality of a developing fetus, and prepares to give birth to the baby. By the time the baby is born, the parents feel very "attached" to him or her.
Landmarks of fetal development	The fetus has capabilities and is responsive to parents early in development: • 6 weeks: heart begins beating. • 8 weeks: brain activity begins; moves in response to touch; 1 inch long. • 16 weeks: baby begins sucking response; 3½ inches long. • 20 weeks: baby's hearing begins to develop; can respond to external sounds in environment; 10 inches long. • 28 weeks: baby can perceive light; baby is "thinking" and "perceiving"; all senses are functional; sleep-wake periods; 16 inches long; viable.
Identification of woman's awareness of her baby in utero	Has the woman experienced quickening? Is the woman aware of daily fetal movement? Has the woman heard the fetal heartbeat? Has the woman seen an ultrasound image? Has the woman palpated fetal parts?

Continued on next page

Teaching interventions can have a positive impact on the couple's emotional adaptation to pregnancy. For example, if the woman is having difficulty accepting her changing body image, the use of pictures to show her the development of the baby and the internal maternal anatomic changes that result from this growth can help her understand and accept the external changes she sees. The nurse can reinforce the normalcy and beauty of the physical changes during pregnancy and discuss clothing, grooming, and personal care that would help the woman feel better about herself. If the woman is not demonstrating signs of prenatal attachment to her fetus, the nurse can intervene by teaching her to feel for fetal parts and position, asking her to keep a record of fetal movement, and demonstrating how to rub or massage her baby in utero (see Teaching Guide: Prenatal Attachment). If the father seems irritated by the woman's emotional mood swings, the nurse might intervene by teaching him about the normal emotional changes of pregnancy and suggesting strategies he might try to help his partner when she is upset.

▼ REFERRAL

If these interventions do not meet the desired goals, if the nurse does not feel qualified to deal with an identified emotional problem, or if assis-

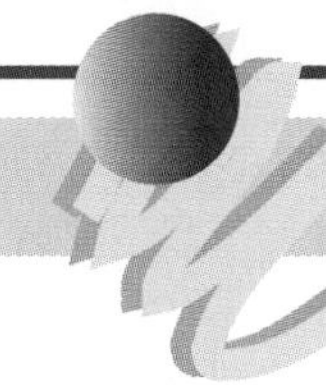

TEACHING GUIDE Continued

PRENATAL ATTACHMENT

TOPIC	*MAJOR CONCEPTS*
Strategies for interacting with baby in utero	The woman can stimulate her baby and interact with him or her in the following ways: • Talk to baby; play music • Call baby by a name • Stroke/pat/massage the baby through the abdominal wall

Teaching Aids

1. Birth Atlas or Nilsson photographs showing fetal development
2. Plastic models of developing embryo showing size
3. Fetascope to hear fetal heart tones
4. Sonogram picture of woman's developing baby

Increasing Your Teaching Effectiveness

Your teaching about prenatal attachment will be more effective by using the following approaches:

1. Determine the weeks of gestation to take into consideration the size and development of the fetus and the woman's probable emotional adaptation to the pregnancy.
2. Ask the woman questions that will allow you to determine her awareness of her developing fetus; identify what attachment behaviors she may already be demonstrating.
3. Use visual aids as you explain the level of development and capabilities of the fetus.
4. Perform Leopold maneuvers to show the woman the position of her baby and to locate body parts; encourage the woman to feel her baby with her own hands.
5. Explain ways that the woman can begin to interact with her baby in utero; demonstrate the use of massage on the woman's abdomen; ask for a return demonstration.

tance from other members of the health care team is needed, referral for additional psychological help is important. For example, if the expectant woman or the father has still not accepted the pregnancy by the third trimester and shows no signs of prenatal attachment to the fetus, additional intervention from a mental health professional or social worker is indicated. If social problems such as food, housing, finances, or social support are influencing their emotional adaptation, social services can help by guiding them toward resources that will help them meet these needs. Referral to childbirth or parenting classes is essential, for classes can help women gain knowledge that will assist them in their emotional adaptation to pregnancy and give them the opportunity to discuss feelings with other pregnant women.

▼ Evaluation

Evaluation of the objectives selected for the plan of care is based on ongoing assessment of the woman's and father's emotional status and their attainment of the developmental tasks of pregnancy. This evaluation includes observation of the woman's behavior, information gathered from discussions with the woman and her partner, her compliance with the health care plan, and her expressed interest in her developing baby.

Risk Management

The risk of concern related to psychological adaptation to pregnancy is that the infant will be neglected or even abused because of the woman's or her partner's failure to complete the developmental tasks of pregnancy or to adapt emotionally to pregnancy and early parenting. An understanding of the psychological developmental tasks of pregnancy and the expected normal emotional responses of pregnant women and the fathers is essential for all health care providers, including maternity nurses, nurse midwives, and obstetricians. This understanding is the first line of defense against psychological maladaptation in the pregnant woman and her partner. Risk management is then accomplished by ensuring that the emotional status of every pregnant woman and every father is evaluated throughout pregnancy, that the woman's and her partner's emotional status are documented in the medical record, and that interventions are planned and executed if alterations are identified.

Implications for Research

Although existing theories serve to explain the psychological adaptation that is necessary for women and men during pregnancy, many theories are not based on a large body of research. Nurses have conducted studies related to the emotional aspects of pregnancy, as well as to prenatal attachment, but the findings of these studies are often based on small, nonrandom sample groups and have not been replicated. Psychological adaptation is always more difficult to study than physiologic adaptation, so that existing instruments must be further tested and new measures developed. Qualitative research may lend itself more easily than quantitative designs to the study of maternal and paternal emotions. Examples of research questions that might be studied are as follows:

- Do culture and religion influence the expectant parents' acceptance of the pregnancy? the woman's body image? prenatal attachment to the baby?
- Are emotional responses to pregnancy related to the positive or negative outcomes of the pregnancy and birth?
- What nursing strategies are effective in helping the woman and her partner deal with the emotional adaptation to pregnancy?

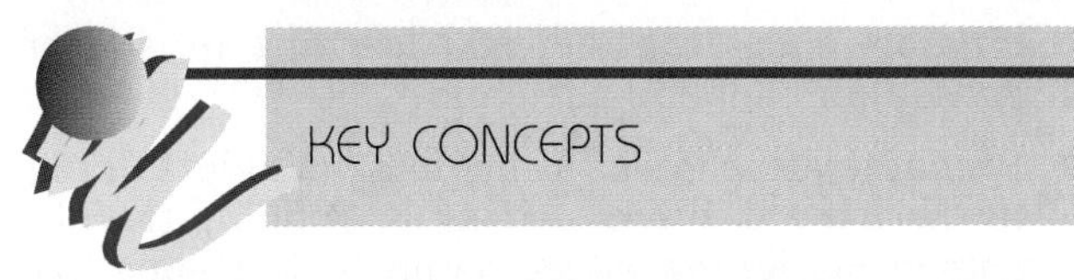

KEY CONCEPTS

- ▼ Pregnancy is often viewed as a maturational or developmental crisis, the nature of which is influenced by the characteristics of the pregnancy, the family's resources, and the family's appraisal of the pregnancy event.
- ▼ Pregnancy poses a series of developmental tasks and adaptations that prepare the woman and her partner for birth and parenting.
- ▼ The first developmental task for the woman is to accept the fetus as part of her body. In the process of acceptance, some women may experience shock and disbelief or denial in regard to the pregnancy, particularly in the first trimester.
- ▼ The woman's acceptance of the fetus can be assessed by whether the pregnancy was planned or unplanned, whether she seems happy or depressed, the amount of discomfort she experiences, whether she accepts or rejects changes in her body, and whether ambivalence about the pregnancy remains unresolved by the third trimester.
- ▼ The second developmental task of pregnancy is to perceive the fetus as a separate being. This often occurs in response to feeling quickening in the second trimester, and it facilitates prenatal attachment.
- ▼ Many mothers and fathers experience dreams or fantasies about the baby or the birth. These dreams may be positive or negative, may mirror the concerns the parents are feeling, and reflect the normal ongoing process of psychological adaptation.
- ▼ The woman's body image is often altered during pregnancy. She and her partner may view her changing body shape as being a positive, beautiful change that represents fertility and femininity or may see the changes as being negative in contrast to the American ideal of being thin.
- ▼ The third task of pregnancy is to prepare to give up the fetus, give birth, and establish a caretaking relationship with the infant. Completion of this task does not usually take place until sometime during the third trimester, and women are often observed to engage in nesting behavior as they prepare for the baby.
- ▼ Rubin's maternal tasks of pregnancy include ensuring safe passage for the woman and her baby, seeking acceptance of the child by others,

binding-in to the child, and learning to give of oneself on behalf of the child.

- ▼ Prenatal attachment behaviors include talking to the baby in utero, patting or rubbing the abdomen, assigning a pet name to the baby, responding to fetal movement or kicking, and eating particular foods for the baby.
- ▼ May proposed three developmental phases for fathers during pregnancy: the announcement phase, in which fathers deal with acceptance of the pregnancy; the moratorium phase, in which they may become introspective and emotionally distance themselves; and the focusing phase, in which active preparation for the birth and parenting role takes place.
- ▼ May also identified three styles of paternal involvement during pregnancy: the observer style, in which the father maintains an emotional distance; the instrumental style, in which he sees himself as caretaker or manager of the pregnancy; and the expressive style, in which he becomes highly involved and sees himself as a full partner in the pregnancy.
- ▼ Siblings and grandparents also experience emotional changes and a need to adapt throughout the pregnancy. They can be helped by being included in the preparations for the baby, through discussions about the pregnancy and birth, by recognition and acceptance of their feelings, and by attending sibling or grandparenting classes.
- ▼ Factors that may alter the parents' psychological adaptation to the pregnancy include a high-risk pregnancy; demographic characteristics such as age, developmental readiness, parity, marital status, and culture; social support; and previous experiences.
- ▼ Application of the nursing process to psychological adaptation to pregnancy is just as important as the physical aspects of care. Nursing interventions include anticipatory guidance, teaching and counseling, and referral to other members of the health care team as necessary.

References

Affonso, D., and Sheptak, S. (1991). Maternal themes during pregnancy. *Maternal-Child Nursing Journal,* 18, 147–166.

Arizmendi, T., and Affonso, D. (1987). Stressful events related to pregnancy and postpartum. *Journal of Psychosomatic Research,* 31 (6), 743–756.

Avant, K. (1988). Stressors on the childbearing family. *Journal of Obstetric, Gynecologic, and Neonatal Nursing,* 17(3), 179–186.

Bibring, G. (1959). Some considerations of the psychological process in pregnancy. *Psychoanalytic Study of the Child,* 14, 113–121.

Blake, R. L., and Reimann, J. (1993). The pregnancy-related dreams of pregnant women. *Journal of the American Board of Family Practice,* 6 (2), 117–122.

Brown, S. (1984). Late-pregnancy ambivalence. *Childbirth Education,* Summer, 37–40.

Campbell, I., and Field, P. (1989). Common psychological concerns experienced by parents during pregnancy. *Canada's Mental Health,* 37 (1), 2–5.

Caplan, G. (1957). Psychological aspects of maternity care. *American Journal of Public Health,* 47, 25–31.

Carson, K., and Virden, S. (1984). Can prenatal teaching promote maternal attachment? Practicing nurses test Carter-Jessop's prenatal attachment intervention. *Health Care for Women International,* 5, 355–369.

Carter-Jessop, L. (1981). Promoting maternal attachment through prenatal intervention. *MCN,* 6, 107–112.

Colman, L., and Colman, A. (1991). *Pregnancy: The psychological experience.* New York: Noonday Press.

Cranley, M. (1981). Development of a tool for the measurement of maternal attachment during pregnancy. *Nursing Research,* 30, 281–284.

Davis, M., and Akridge, K. (1987). The effect of promoting intrauterine attachment in primiparas on postdelivery attachment. *Journal of Obstetric, Gynecologic, and Neonatal Nursing,* 16 (6), 430–437.

Deutsch, H. (1945). *The psychology of women: Motherhood* (Vol. 2). New York: Grune & Stratton.

Dimitrovsky, L., Perez-Hirshberg, M., Itskowitz, R. (1987). Depression during and following pregnancy: quality of family relationships. *Journal of Psychology,* 121 (3), 213–218.

Fawcett, J. (1989). Spouses' experiences during pregnancy and the postpartum: a program of research and theory development. *Image: Journal of Nursing Scholarship,* 21 (3), 149–152.

Fawcett, J., and York, R. (1986). Spouses' physical and psychological symptoms during pregnancy and the postpartum. *Nursing Research,* 35 (3), 144–148.

Ferketich, S., and Mercer, R. (1989). Men's health status during pregnancy and early fatherhood. *Research in Nursing and Health,* 12 (3), 137–148.

Gaffney, K. (1986). Maternal-fetal attachment in relation to self-concept and anxiety. *Maternal-Child Nursing Journal,* 15 (2), 91–101.

Gaffney, K. (1988). Prenatal maternal attachment. *Image: Journal of Nursing Scholarship,* 20 (2), 106–109.

Gay, J., Edgil, A., Douglas, A. (1988). Reva Rubin revisited. *Journal of Obstetric, Gynecologic, and Neonatal Nursing,* 17, 394–398.

Gilbert, E., and Harmon, J. (1993). *Manual of high risk pregnancy and delivery.* St. Louis: C. V. Mosby.

Gottesman, M. M. (1992). Maternal adaptation during pregnancy among adult early, middle, and late childbearers: similarities and differences. *Maternal-Child Nursing Journal,* 20 (2), 93–110.

Grace, J. (1984). Does a mother's knowledge of fetal gender affect attachment? *Maternal-Child Nursing Journal,* 9, 42–45.

Heidrich, S., and Cranley, M. (1989). Effect of fetal movement, ultrasound scans, and amniocentesis on maternal-fetal attachment. *Nursing Research,* 38 (2), 81–84.

Hofmeyr, G., Marcos, E., Butchart, A. (1990). Pregnant women's perceptions of themselves: A survey. *Birth,* December, 17, 205–206.

Joffe, H. (1989). Emotional factors in pregnancy. *Australian Family Physician,* 18 (5), 493, 496–497.

Johnston, G. P. (1994). *The wish, the wait, the wonder: A book of wisdom for expectant parents* (p. 49). New York: Harper Collins.

Jordan, P. (1990). Laboring for relevance: expectant and new fatherhood. *Nursing Research,* 39 (1), 11–16.

Kemp, V., and Page, C. (1986). The psychosocial impact of a high-risk pregnancy on the family. *Journal of Obstetric, Gynecologic, and Neonatal Nursing* 15 (3), 232–235.

Kemp, V., and Page, C. (1987). Maternal prenatal attachment

in normal and high-risk pregnancies. *Journal of Obstetric, Gynecologic, and Neonatal Nursing,* 16 (3), 179–184.

Kohn, C., Nelson, A., Weiner, S. (1980). Gravidas' responses to realtime ultrasound fetal image. *Journal of Obstetric, Gynecologic, and Neonatal Nursing,* 9, 77–80.

Kornhaber, A. (1986). The grandparent-grandchild bond. *Childbirth Educator,* 6 (1), 40–44.

Leavitt, J. (1986). *Brought to bed: Childbearing in America: 1750–1950.* New York: Oxford University Press.

Lederman, R. (1984). *Psychosocial adaptation in pregnancy.* Englewood Cliffs, NJ: Prentice-Hall.

Lerum, C., and LoBiondo-Wood, G. (1989). The relationship of maternal age, quickening, and physical symptoms of pregnancy to the development of maternal-fetal attachment. *Birth,* 16 (1), 13–17.

Lumley, J. (1990). Through a glass darkly: ultrasound and prenatal bonding. *Birth,* 17 (4), 214–217.

Masters, W., Johnson, V., Kolodny, R. (1995). *Human sexuality* (5th ed.). New York: HarperCollins.

May, K. (1980). A typology of detachment/involvement styles adopted during pregnancy by first-time expectant fathers. *Western Journal of Nursing Research,* 2 (2), 445–461.

May, K. (1982a). Factors contributing to first-time fathers' readiness for fatherhood: an exploratory study. *Family Relations,* 31, 353–361.

May, K. (1982b). Three phases of father involvement in pregnancy. *Nursing Research,* 31 (6), 337–342.

McCubbin, M., and McCubbin, H. (1993). Families coping with illness. In C. B. Danielson, B. Hamel-Bissell, P. Winstead-Fry (Eds.). *Families, health, and illness: Perspectives on coping and intervention.* St. Louis: C. V. Mosby.

Mercer, R. (1986). *First-time motherhood: experiences from teens to forties.* New York: Springer.

Mercer, R., Ferketich, S., DeJoseph, J., May, K., Sollid, D. (1988). Effect of stress on family functioning during pregnancy. *Nursing Research,* 37 (5), 268–275.

Mercer, R., May, K., Ferketich, S., DeJoseph, J. (1986). Theoretical models for studying the effect of antepartum stress on the family. *Nursing Research,* 35 (6), 339–346.

Milne, L., and Rich, O. (1981). Cognitive and affective aspects of the responses of pregnant women to sonography. *Maternal-Child Nursing Journal,* 10, 15–39.

Morcos, F., Snart, F., Harley, D. (1989). Choices, expectations, and the experience of childbirth. *Canada's Mental Health,* 37 (1), 6–8.

Muller, M. (1990). Binding in: still a relevant concept? *NAACOG's Clinical Issues in Perinatal and Women's Health Nursing,* 1, 297–302.

Muller, M. (1992). A critical review of prenatal attachment research. *Scholarly Inquiry for Nursing Practice,* 6 (1), 5–26.

Norr, K., Blodk, C., Charles, A., Meyering, S. (1980). The second time around: parity and birth experience. *Journal of Obstetric, Gynecologic, and Neonatal Nursing,* 9 (1), 30–36.

Oakley, A. (1986). *The captured womb: A history of the medical care of pregnant women.* Oxford: Basil Blackwell.

Robinson, G., and Stewart, D. (1989). Motivation for motherhood and the experience of pregnancy. *Canadian Journal of Psychiatry,* 34 (9), 861–865.

Rubin, R. (1970). Cognitive style in pregnancy. *American Journal of Nursing,* 70 (3), 502–508.

Rubin, R. (1984). *Maternal identity and the maternal experience.* New York: Springer.

Saunders, R., and Robins, E. (1987). Changes in the marital relationship during the first pregnancy. *Health Care Women International,* 8 (5–6), 361–377.

Schneider, Z. (1989). Cognitive performance in pregnancy. *Australian Journal of Advanced Nursing,* 6 (3), 40–47.

Schodt, C. (1989). Parental-fetal attachment and couvade: a study of patterns of human-environmental integrality. *Nursing Science Quarterly,* 2 (2), 88–97.

Sherwen, L. (1981). Fantasies during the third trimester of pregnancy. *MCN,* 15 (3), 398–401.

Stainton, C. (1990). Parents' awareness of their unborn infant in the third trimester. *Birth: Issues in Perinatal Care and Education,* 17 (2), 92–96.

Strang, V., and Sullivan, P. (1985). Body image attitudes during pregnancy and the postpartum period. *Journal of Obstetric, Gynecologic, and Neonatal Nursing,* 14, 332–337.

Strickland, O. (1987). The occurrence of symptoms in expectant fathers. *Nursing Research,* 36 (3), 184–189.

Tanner, L. (1969). Developmental tasks of pregnancy. In B. S. Bergersen, et al. (Eds.). *Current concepts in clinical nursing* (Vol. II, pp. 292–297). St. Louis: C. V. Mosby.

Taubenheim, A., and Silbernagel, T. (1988). Meeting the needs of expectant fathers. *MCN,* 13 (2), 110–113.

Tilden, V. (1980). A developmental conceptual framework for the maturational crisis of pregnancy. *Western Journal of Nursing Research,* 2 (4), 667–679.

Weaver, R., and Cranley, M. (1983). An exploration of paternal-fetal attachment behavior. *Nursing Research,* 32 (2), 68–72.

Winslow, W. (1987). First pregnancy after 35: what is the experience? *Maternal Child Nursing,* 12, 92–96.

Zachariah, R. (1994). Mother-daughter and husband-wife attachment as predictors of psychological well-being during pregnancy. *Clinical Nursing Research,* 3 (4), 371–392.

18 Chapter

A society's way of conceptualizing birth constitutes the single most powerful indicator of the general shape of its birthing system. In all settings, the definition of the event is of fundamental importance in that it informs participants regarding the proper who, where and how of birth.

BRIGITTE JORDAN
(JORDAN 1993)

Sociocultural Aspects of Pregnancy

Elaine Zwelling

HIGHLIGHTS

- Family and Pregnancy
- Culture and Pregnancy
- Religion and Pregnancy
- Development of Maternal Role
- Social Adaptation of Fathers
- Couvade
- Social Support During Pregnancy
- Risk Management
- Implications for Research

The experience of pregnancy does not occur in isolation. Although the woman is the one who experiences the pregnancy from a physical perspective, those around her are also influenced by it. Relationships with family members, friends, and others who interact with the pregnant woman change in subtle to significant ways. New roles must be learned as the woman and her family prepare for the addition of a baby to the family system. The pregnant state is difficult to ignore. At the least it evokes acknowledgment or comment from others, while at most it stimulates major changes between people. These changes can be positive, contributing to growth, or negative, resulting in the disintegration of relationships.

Just as the pregnancy experience affects those in the woman's social network, the social environment also influences the course of the pregnancy. The woman's physical status, behaviors, and responses are influenced by the social context in which they occur. Factors that shape the pregnancy are family, culture, religion, and the social, political, economic, and intellectual climate. Each generation of childbearing women perceives pregnancy and birth differently. The meaning of these events at any given time reflects the society's shifting attitudes toward women, babies, families, and family life, as well as the changing capabilities of preserving and protecting life and manipulating the reproductive process (Simkin 1989). It is important that

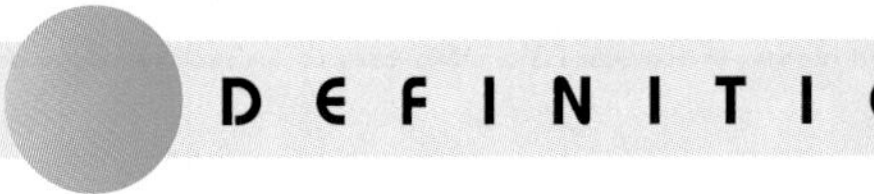

DEFINITIONS

Couvade—Physical symptoms of pregnancy or birth experienced by some expectant fathers during their partner's pregnancy.

Culture—The ideas, customs, skills, and arts of a given people in a given period of history.

Emotional support—A type of social support in which communication of empathy, caring, love, and trust are given to an individual.

Ethnicity—Affiliation with a homogeneous population as distinguished by customs, characteristics, language, or common history.

Family developmental tasks—Skills or competencies acquired by a family at a particular stage of development.

Fantasy—A stage in the process of maternal role development in which the woman engages in a form of daydreaming about how she will behave as a mother.

Health behavior—Behavior directed at maintenance of health or prevention of illness.

Identity—The final stage in the process of maternal role development in which the woman comfortably takes on the behaviors associated with the maternal role.

Maternal role—Behaviors learned by a woman either indirectly or directly for the nurturing of a child.

Mimicry—A stage in the process of maternal role development in which the woman copies behaviors that manifest the mothering role.

Race—A population of people that differs from others according to genetic traits, geographical location, ancestry, lineage, habits, and ideas.

Role—Pattern of socially accepted behaviors that guide the functions of an individual in a given social situation.

Role conflict—Stress resulting from two or more competing roles assumed by an individual at the same time.

Role play—A stage in the process of maternal role development in which behaviors are acted out or tried on for size.

Social support—Feelings of being cared for, loved, esteemed, valued, and part of a network of communication and mutual obligation.

nurses recognize the relationships between pregnancy and sociocultural factors, assess these aspects of the pregnancy experience, and plan interventions accordingly.

SOCIOCULTURAL FACTORS AND THE PREGNANCY EXPERIENCE

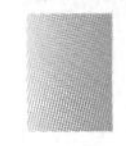

Family

The woman's family experiences the pregnancy most intimately. The course of the pregnancy influences family functioning. On the other hand, the home environment, living conditions, and financial status of the family affect the woman's physical and emotional adaptation during pregnancy. All pregnant families experience some stress and change. If the pregnancy deviates from the normal course and complications occur, there is further stress on family functioning. Studies of pregnancy within a family system have shown that there are relationships between a number of interacting variables, including psychosocial factors, health status, self-esteem, social support, anxiety, depression, family functioning, life events, family structure, and the outcome of pregnancy. Any number of these variables can influence the pregnancy experience of the woman (Keeping et al. 1989; Mercer et al. 1988; Mercer and Ferketich 1990).

Family relationships can have a positive or negative influence on health and pregnancy. If family members are not supportive of the pregnancy or are angry, disappointed, or resentful about its occurrence, the woman's attitudes and responses are affected. If the home environment is less than adequate, the woman's physical health may suffer. The financial status of the family also has an influence on the adaptation to pregnancy. If adequate resources are not available, nutritious food and proper health care are not seen as priorities during the woman's pregnancy. These situational factors compound the normal maturational crisis of pregnancy. (See Chapter 17 for a further discussion of pregnancy as a maturational crisis.) Identification of these possible variables is a critical component of the pregnant woman's prenatal care.

Pregnancy can be viewed as an individual developmental task, as discussed in Chapter 17, and as a developmental task for the family. Because pregnancy is a period of change, all family members must begin to adapt and prepare for the changes that a new baby will bring. This is particularly true for the pregnant woman and her partner, but

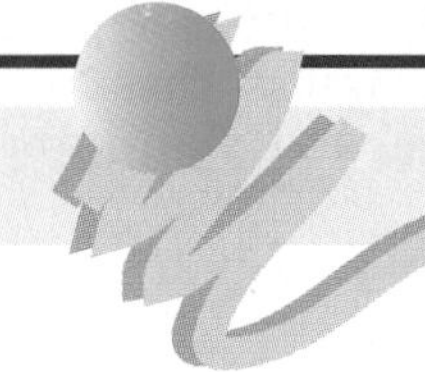

HISTORICAL PERSPECTIVES

PREGNANCY AND CHILDBEARING

In the prehospital era of the late eighteenth and nineteenth centuries, the pregnancy and childbearing experiences of American women were definitely influenced by cultural group, socioeconomic level, rural or urban location and time period. In her book, *Brought to Bed,* Judith Walzer Leavitt categorizes childbearing experiences of that time into four groups.

The "institutionals" were the poorest urban women who were usually unmarried and had no financial or social options available to them during their pregnancies and confinements. They turned to charity and public institutions for their care as their last resort. Medical aid was often received in exchange for the clinical experience they provided for medical students. In the nineteenth century, the hospitals to which these poor women went for their births varied greatly in quality of care. In some training centers, there was adequate staff to serve the needs of the women; in others, extreme neglect characterized their treatment. For example, at Bellevue Hospital in 1860, a reporter observed that one woman gave birth entirely unattended, after which rats attacked her baby before anyone noticed!

The second group of women, the "traditionalists," were a diverse group of some urban but increasingly rural women, working class, lower-middle and some middle class, immigrant and native-born, who had limited choices available during their pregnancies and deliveries. They remained within the traditional female-centered network for their births, until childbirth moved to the hospital in the twentieth century. Many of the immigrant women in this group chose midwives because they did not approve of the American custom of male birth attendants or because medical care was not available in their community. Their pregnancies and births incorporated varied practices according to their cultural group. For example, Polish women had a tradition of "scrubbing," perhaps for exercise during pregnancy; Jewish women insisted on placing a pan of water under the birthing bed to draw away poisons; and Italian women feared bathing during pregnancy. The traditionalist group of women shared the common expectations that birth rarely needed outside consultation with the medical profession, and that

Continued on following page

siblings, grandparents, and other family members must also adapt. Duvall (1985), a family theorist, proposed that childbearing families face a number of developmental tasks that must be accomplished during the pregnancy (see Developmental Tasks of the Childbearing Family). If these tasks are not accomplished, Duvall proposed that the adjustments to new parenthood will be more difficult, family coping may be inadequate, and a crisis situation can develop within the family system.

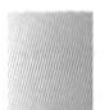

Culture

Pregnancy and birth are described as biosocial events, meaning that the universal biologic experience of pregnancy is shaped by the social or cultural context in which it occurs (Jordan 1993). The woman's cultural and ethnic background influences her attitudes about and adaptation to pregnancy. Cultural beliefs and traditions are present in all families during pregnancy and can shape the woman's view of her fetus, her attitudes about health care, the clothing she wears, her activity and rest patterns, her diet, and her beliefs about sexual activity during pregnancy (Judkins and Judkins 1992). Cultural beliefs have usually been handed down from generation to generation and are sometimes referred to as "old wives' tales." These beliefs are evident not only in primitive cultures, but also frequently in contemporary culture in the United States. Cultural beliefs are usually related to one of three categories: (1) practices that might influence the fetus (e.g., viewing ugly or violent things during pregnancy could damage the fetus); (2) activities that would ensure a healthy baby and safe delivery (e.g., avoiding exercise or coitus to prevent miscarriage, or eating only in moderate amounts so that the baby will

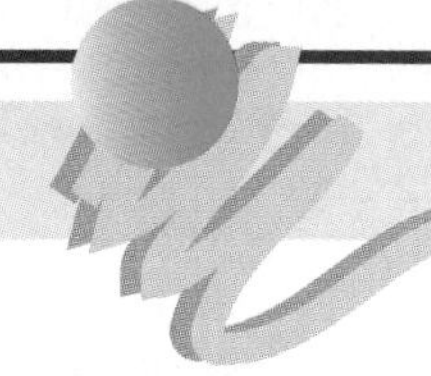

HISTORICAL PERSPECTIVES Continued

birth took place within a comfortable environment with the family and close friends of the birthing woman in attendance.

The third group, "integrationists," were largely urban middle-class women who had financial options and social networks that allowed them wide-ranging options during their pregnancies and deliveries, and who included physicians in their birthing plans. These women were able to integrate medical practices into the traditional practices to create their ideal birth experience. They believed that medicine could offer increased safety, and they were willing to spend the extra money necessary to get the benefits of that promise. After anesthesia became available in the middle of the nineteenth century, these women wanted the relief it provided and called upon physicians specifically for this purpose. Many of these women continued to ask midwives to help out as well, and birthing women asked friends and relatives to be with them to provide the needed domestic help and emotional support.

The final group were the "privileged," wealthy upper-middle-class and upper-class women living in major urban centers who had access to medical services of the highest repute. Because finances were not a consideration, these women could make choices limited only by their own knowledge of the available options. Because they lived in the major urban centers, they chose not just medical care, but medical care from the physicians with the best reputations in their community, usually professors at medical schools. Midwives were not a part of their care. This group of privileged women were quickest to incorporate the newest techniques as they became available. By the end of the nineteenth century, these women had made the transition from using general practitioners to using specialists in obstetrics for their medical birth attendants, and in the twentieth century they moved into luxurious private maternity hospitals or private suites in general hospitals where they could receive their obstetricians' full attention.

Excerpted from *Brought to Bed: Childbearing in America, 1750–1950* by J. W. Leavitt. Copyright © 1986. Reprinted by permission of Oxford University Press, Inc.

remain small for an easier delivery); or (3) practices related to gender determination of the fetus (e.g., a male infant is carried "low" while a female infant is carried "high").

CULTURAL PRACTICES

Examples of cultural beliefs relating to pregnancy and birth can be seen in Table 18–1. A review of the literature also provides a rich source of information regarding cultural practices during pregnancy.

Hispanic Practices

In the Hispanic culture, some people believe in the phenomenon of the "evil eye," which can harm the mother or baby and can be caused if someone stares at them during the pregnancy. For this reason, a female relative, usually an older experienced woman, may accompany the pregnant woman to prenatal visits to protect her against the "evil eye." The relative is very watchful and often places herself between a stranger and the pregnant woman. Red ribbons, red clothing, or charms may also be used to prevent the "evil eye." All family members may come to the hospital with the woman during labor and take turns attending her. A female relative often remains with a new mother and her baby for up to 40 days after childbirth, going everywhere with her in public to protect her from the "evil eye."

Strict rules about food (avoidance of chili and other spices, cold foods, fish, pork, or citrus fruits), exercise and activities (no coitus, bathing, or washing of hair) may be followed during pregnancy. It is believed that failure to follow such restrictions may have serious consequences, including illness, infertility, infection, or even death. Tradition does encourage eating tortillas and chicken soup and binding the abdomen during the postpartum period. Despite the fact that many Hispanic women are attached to the values of the

Developmental Tasks of the Childbearing Family

- Acquiring knowledge and plans for the specific needs of pregnancy, childbirth, and early parenthood
- Preparing to provide for the physical care of the expected baby
- Adapting financial patterns to meet increasing needs
- Defining evolving role patterns
- Adjusting patterns of sexual expression to accommodate pregnancy
- Expanding communication to meet present and future emotional needs
- Reorienting relationships with relatives
- Adapting relationships with friends and community to take account of the realities of pregnancy and the anticipated child
- Maintaining a healthy morale and philosophy of life

Data from Duvall, E. (1985). *Marriage and family development.* Philadelphia: J.B. Lippincott.

old country and are the keepers of traditions, they are open to change during pregnancy because they believe it is for the benefit of their families. However, the value of routine prenatal visits to a health care provider must be repeatedly emphasized, otherwise some Hispanic women may stop the visits because they are feeling well and are used to crisis intervention health care (Khazoyan and Anderson 1994).

Haitian Practices

In the Haitian culture, a strong contrast emerges between the attitudes of women toward the antepartum and postpartum periods. Pregnancy, labor, and birth are seen as inevitable courses. Once the woman conceives, it is believed that the baby grows, labor begins, and the birth happens regardless of what the woman does. The woman is passive, allowing the midwife or physician to assume the active role. During pregnancy the woman eats whatever she can tolerate, depending on the "desires of the baby." There are few prescriptions or proscriptions for pregnancy or labor, other than the need to protect the baby against "werewolves." It is believed that werewolves can consume babies before they are born and harm small children as well. As a result of the belief that pregnancy follows a normal inevitable course, Haitian women may not seek health care until the time for delivery.

Haitian custom may dictate that men not involve themselves in childbirth. The Haitian father often drops the woman off at the hospital door and picks her up when it is time to go home. The Haitian woman may chant and call on the saints during her labor to cleanse the spirit and heal the body. This chanting appears to produce a state of euphoria. It is believed that the sex of the baby determines the kind of labor pain. During the postpartum period the woman takes a much more active role, as do the women who care for her. There are clear ideas of what should happen to a woman and her baby after birth. Special vapor baths, drinking special teas, and dressing warmly are seen as good ways to become healthy and clean again after a birth (Harris 1987).

Indian Practices

Becoming pregnant is very important for a woman in India. It is a tragedy for her if she is unable to conceive, for motherhood is considered the woman's chief role and fulfillment. An Indian woman lives a submissive role within the family that remains unaltered until she has borne a child. If the first baby is a boy, the young woman's position within the family does not alter, but her status is improved considerably. To be without a son is a terrible stroke of fate, for it is the son who inherits, who will provide for the parents in their old age, and who participates in the ritual of death and mourning that guarantees the passage of the parents into Heaven. As a result, Indian women may experience emotional despair if only girls are born, and may have successive pregnancies in order to give birth to at least one son. This profound belief may even affect physical adaptation to the pregnancy, causing complaints of backache, headache, abdominal pain, or fatigue (Ahmed and Watt 1986).

Hmong Practices

The Hmong tribe in Laos does not have a tradition of seeking assistance for birth and as a result are reluctant to use hospitals or medical doctors for delivery. Hmong women prefer to rely on their own strength to deal with pregnancy and birth. As residents in the United States, they tend to enter the health care system at 5 months' gestation, the point at which they define pregnancy. A squatting position is used for birth. It is usually the husband or a relative of the husband who delivers the baby, and it is tradition that the husband cut the umbilical cord. Because arranged marriages for very young women are a common practice, there is a potential for the health risks of early adolescent

Table 18–1

OVERVIEW OF CULTURAL BELIEFS RELATED TO PREGNANCY AND CHILDBIRTH

CULTURAL GROUP	GENERAL ATTITUDE AND BELIEFS ABOUT PREGNANCY AND CHILDBIRTH	ROLE EXPECTATIONS OF WIFE, HUSBAND, FAMILY AND SIGNIFICANT OTHERS	OTHER CULTURAL FACTORS RELATED TO CHILDBIRTH
African-American (Crib Sheet 1991; Spector 1991)	Approach childbirth with a mixture of feelings of happiness, worry, fear, ambivalence. Many believe that pregnancy is a state of wellness and prenatal care is not necessary; others regard pregnancy as a delicate physical condition, like an illness, and the woman is discouraged from engaging in certain activities. Childbearing is a natural process and should not be interfered with by employing birth control methods or abortion. To many people, birth control is considered a form of "black genocide" and a way of limiting the growth of the community.	Flexible in family roles (Crib Sheet 1991). Women are socialized to be strong because they more than likely will have to use their resourcefulness. Stoic during labor and delivery to hide weakness. Males are socialized to be strong, aggressive, and independent. Strong kinship network and extended family are an effective mechanism in providing extra emotional and economic support.	Self-care and folk medicine prevalent. Emphasis on health prevention through use of tried traditions. Inactivity during pregnancy to prevent nuchal cord. Use of pica (eating nonedible substances, e.g., clay, Argo corn starch, refrigerator frost) (Crib Sheet 1991). Orthodox Muslims oppose use of narcotic drugs.
Arab-American (Meleis and Sorrell 1981; Meleis et al. 1992)	Pregnancy increases status and self-esteem of women. Sex of child more of a concern than health and growth and development of baby. Birth of a son more welcomed than birth of a daughter.	Women are expected to manage household and observe modesty in dress and words; they do not discuss sex and related matters with men and strangers. Pain tolerance is low and expressed verbally. Do not readily accept breathing and relaxation techniques yet seldom request anesthesia. Overuse of pain pill in postpartum period. Males are involved in all aspects of health care; may be construed as excessive control. Intense eye-to-eye interaction and repetition in speech pattern. Children are expected to be part of all events that affect the family. Grandparents participate in child care.	Planning ahead has potential for defying God's will and will bring "evil eye." Time does not dictate needs, it is need that dictates time—"Allah willing"; believe pregnancy does not occur during postpartum period and breastfeeding. Respect of verbal agreements and mistrust of written words; problem with written consent.

Continued on following page

Table 18–1

OVERVIEW OF CULTURAL BELIEFS RELATED TO PREGNANCY AND CHILDBIRTH Continued

CULTURAL GROUP	GENERAL ATTITUDE AND BELIEFS ABOUT PREGNANCY AND CHILDBIRTH	ROLE EXPECTATIONS OF WIFE, HUSBAND, FAMILY AND SIGNIFICANT OTHERS	OTHER CULTURAL FACTORS RELATED TO CHILDBIRTH
Asian-American	Childbearing is strictly a family-centered event; most significant event in family. Considered a natural process but also a time to seek special assistance and counsel. Harmony and moderation as means of maintaining health.	Strong mother-daughter relationship during pregnancy and childbirth; doctrines of childbearing behavior take precedence over health provider's prenatal instructions. Family support shows in extra consideration by freeing woman from home responsibilities. Chinese: husband's presence preferred during childbirth but wife's mother expected to be present too (Pillsbury 1982). Japanese: generally an indulgent attitude toward expectant mothers in contemporary Japan. No husband is present during childbirth.	Chinese: use of acupuncture analgesia is increasing; yin and yang theory (Spector 1991). Japanese: pragmatic interest in health education. Mothering is a major source of social status for Japanese women and is almost synonymous with selfless devotion to the child (Bernstein and Kidd 1982).
Jewish-American Orthodox (Feldman 1992; Waterhouse 1994)	During pregnancy, no planning for baby in advance; no baby showers or naming the baby. Because of modesty, seek care from nurse-midwife. Refrain from use of contraception. "State of separation" during menstruation to 7 days after and from onset of "show" to 7 days after disappearance of lochia.	Husband has to choose to participate in labor and delivery, either (1) actively by preparing to communicate verbally, as he will not touch wife during labor; or (2) spiritually only by sitting in the corner and reciting from the book of Psalms. Childbirth preparation classes taught by their own women, and men are asked to leave during exercise practice because they are not allowed to view another's wife doing exercise. Husbands are not allowed to view the genital area during labor and delivery and may view the baby only after it is lifted from the perineum.	Children and others are not permitted to view birth; no home births. Childbirth classes are held with couples sitting around the table, not sitting on the floor, as it is a sign of mourning. Circumcision and naming of boys on 8th day. Girls named and presented first Saturday after birth.
Mexican-American	Childbearing is a privilege and an obligation of a married woman. Pregnancy is a delicate and perilous time for the fetus. Maintain a state of equilibrium and harmony between the natural and supernatural forces of the world.	Women solve everyday problems, manipulating a dominant man to get what they need. The man is the unquestioned head of the family and wage earner. Gives strength, honor, and protection to the female (machismo); he is a disciplinarian but has few other responsibilities for childrearing. The elderly are well respected, care for the children, and help in their rearing.	Mild sickness is treated at home by the mother or grandmother. Severe illness is referred to curandera (uses prayers, artifacts) or yerbero (herbalist). There is belief in folk healing, use of prayers, diet, rituals, and herbs (Spector 1991). Pregnancy cravings (autojos) need to be satisfied, otherwise the baby will be born with a birthmark (Crib Sheet 1990).

Table 18–1

OVERVIEW OF CULTURAL BELIEFS RELATED TO PREGNANCY AND CHILDBIRTH Continued

CULTURAL GROUP	GENERAL ATTITUDE AND BELIEFS ABOUT PREGNANCY AND CHILDBIRTH	ROLE EXPECTATIONS OF WIFE, HUSBAND, FAMILY AND SIGNIFICANT OTHERS	OTHER CULTURAL FACTORS RELATED TO CHILDBIRTH
Mexican-American *(Cont'd)*		Most social relationships are still determined by kinship. The family is nuclear, but the extended family concept is still retained–includes such relatives as grandparents, aunts, uncles, cousins, and the "compadre" system (friends or relatives are given special privileges of being allowed to become members of the extended family by baptism, confirmation, or marriage) (Enriquez 1982).	Milk avoided and activity decreased to decrease baby weight. The woman sleeps flat on her back to protect the fetus.
Mormon (Stark 1982)	Importance of marriage and parenthood in individual and spiritual life. Importance of regular and good prenatal care is acknowledged. Birthing is considered a normal body function without negative connotations. Breastfeeding is encouraged. Health is the only valid reason to limit family size.	The wife considers it a duty to have as many children as possible; expected be expert provider for children, husband, and church. During labor and delivery, the woman should remember that she is of strong pioneer stock and should behave as a strong woman would. During the postpartum period, there is help from family members: mother-in-law, unmarried aunts, or other family members. Man as the holder of priesthood is the spiritual and actual head of household.	Prenatal education is not discouraged by the church. Most accept physicians as major caregivers during pregnancy and delivery but prefer a woman doctor, ideally a church member. Boy babies are usually circumcised because this is the accepted medical procedure, rather than a religious requirement. The baby receives a name and a special religious blessing for health, strength, and good life on the first Sunday of the month after birth. Wearing of a "garment" (received during the first visit to the temple, somewhat like long underwear, which provides its wearer with special protection and comfort) while in the hospital is controversial; some believe it is all right not to wear it, others feel more comfortable keeping it on.
Neo-Oriental American (Hubbell 1982) (group of people found in ashrams: members of 3HO Foundation (Happy, Health, Holy) and members of the religious sect Sikh Darhma).	Concept of family is a most important aspect. Size of family is determined mainly by family income.	The woman is thought to be the grace of God. She does not tell anyone in the household about the pregnancy until the 120th day. The soul enters the fetus on this day and calls for celebration. No restrictions in activity until 120th day, then specific exercises to strengthen and stretch all the muscles in the groin area. Posture is emphasized.	3HO Foundation offers classes in nutrition, prenatal yoga, and meditation. Chanting is encouraged, and there is customary reading from the scriptures during labor and after birth.

Continued on following page

Table 18–1

OVERVIEW OF CULTURAL BELIEFS RELATED TO PREGNANCY AND CHILDBIRTH Continued

CULTURAL GROUP	GENERAL ATTITUDE AND BELIEFS ABOUT PREGNANCY AND CHILDBIRTH	ROLE EXPECTATIONS OF WIFE, HUSBAND, FAMILY AND SIGNIFICANT OTHERS	OTHER CULTURAL FACTORS RELATED TO CHILDBIRTH
Neo-Oriental American *(Cont'd)*	Contraception is individualized; methods used are abstinence and rhythm; diaphragm is acceptable; pill not used because it is not natural. Pregnancy is a glorious event. The woman is very open during pregnancy and receives vibrations from the environment. Natural childbirth at home is the preferred method.	Rules for the husband: (1) Be strong and stable, protect the wife from the openness, and defend her from all negativity. (2) Refrain from lovemaking while the wife is pregnant to spare the child from over-powering sexual vibration of the love act. (3) Chant with her, study the growth and development of the child and the birth process; for a truly spiritual birth experience, suggest the wife have the birth at home. The husband or midwife massages the perineum during crowning. Birth itself is without medications, and no episiotomy is performed.	Women have a 40-day postpartum period in seclusion with the infant and helped by the husband and Sevadar (the mother's helper trained to serve the mother in her daily needs). Mothers who breastfeed often chant and pray during actual breastfeeding.

Contributed by Irene dela Torre, CNM, MSN, Los Angeles, CA.

pregnancy. Hmong families also seem to lack concern for the immediate postpartum needs of women and expect them to return to work prematurely (Faller 1992; Judkins and Judkins 1992; Lee 1986).

Cambodian Practices

Childbearing for Cambodian women begins early and ends late in the reproductive years. The fertility rate is considerably higher than in the United States. Many women from Southeast Asia believe that both the woman's and the man's body must be "cool" in order for the woman to become pregnant. A Cambodian medicine can be given to make the body cool. It is thought that infants born in odd months (e.g., the seventh or ninth month) are viable, whereas infants born in even months (e.g., the eighth month) will die. Cold foods (e.g., poultry, fish, fruits, and vegetables) are thought to be essential for a healthy infant, and hot foods (e.g., red peppers, spicy soups, red meat, onion, coffee, and sweets) are to be avoided entirely or eaten only in small amounts, as they could lead to excess fetal movement, abortion, or preterm labor.

Southeast Asians may not seek prenatal care in the United States until their third trimester because of cost, fear, or lack of perceived need. It is believed that an unhealthy or undesirable infant can result for three reasons. First, bathing or showering at night could cause an infant to become so large that it would be difficult to deliver, for water might pass through the woman's body and into the fetus. Second, sexual intercourse is considered dangerous after 7 months of pregnancy because it could cause the amniotic fluid to thicken, leading to respiratory distress in the fetus and resulting in a long labor. Third, falling, reaching high, jumping, or drinking hot substances could cause an unhealthy infant (D'Avanzo 1992; Kulig 1990; Mattson and Lew 1992).

HEALTH VERSUS ILLNESS BEHAVIOR

Some cultures view pregnancy as a normal healthy state, while others believe that the woman is ill during pregnancy. The way pregnancy is viewed determines whether women respond with health or illness behavior. Health behavior occurs in the absence of illness and includes behavior directed at maintenance of health or prevention of illness. In American culture, during pregnancy, health behaviors include seeing a nurse-midwife or physician at regular intervals for assessment, following a nutritious well-balanced diet, exercising regularly, and getting sufficient rest. Unfortunately, in some cultures, health behavior is not given the same sanctions or attention as illness behavior. In 1969, Baric proposed that health behavior does not offer any rights but only imposes duties, has no formal recognition or reinforcement from the medical profession or from society, has no time limit for its duration, is based on abstract qualities rather than symptom realities, and requires the individual to be responsible for the actions that will promote health. In the United States, the concept of health behavior during the prenatal period is valued, but in reality women are often not given positive reinforcement for assuming health behavior. Access to health care is difficult in many areas, and many insurance providers do not reimburse women for preventive health care.

In some cultures or social groups, illness behavior may be seen during pregnancy. Illness behavior includes the adoption of the sick role and may include such privileges as exemption from normal role responsibilities, not being responsible for being ill, and dependence. If the woman demonstrates no actual physiologic alterations during pregnancy, adoption of a sick role might imply that she, or her cultural group, identifies the symptoms she experiences as being more than normal manifestations of pregnancy. She may be unwilling to integrate her discomforts with her usual social involvements, and may focus increased attention on her body and its functions. The woman exhibiting illness behavior during pregnancy may initiate frequent consultations with her nurse midwife or physician and demonstrate increased dependent behaviors.

Over the past 30 years there has been criticism of the "cultural warping" of childbirth in the United States, where pregnancy is often treated as illness and birth as an operative procedure (Haire 1976; Jordan 1993). Other variables that influence behavioral responses during pregnancy include the age of the woman, her educational preparation for the event, the attitudes of her family and friends, the attitudes of her health care providers, and the philosophy of the maternity care system where she receives care.

GENETIC CONSIDERATIONS

A final consideration relating to culture during pregnancy is the increased risk of genetic disease in some racial or ethnic groups. Because of these known risks, screening should be initiated when a woman from an identified high-risk group receives antepartal care (see Chapter 13). For example, thalassemia, a genetic disorder affecting the hemoglobin, is most commonly found in people of Mediterranean origin, especially Italians, Greeks, Africans, and Indians; sickle cell anemia, a disorder in which red blood cells are produced with a sickle shape, is a disease seen in those of African-American and Mediterranean ancestry; cystic fibrosis and phenylketonuria are almost always found in whites; and Tay-Sachs disease, a disorder that causes brain destruction, blindness, and eventually death, is found almost exclusively in the Ashkenazic Jewish population. Thus, information about the pregnant woman's racial and ethnic background is important for many reasons in order to provide comprehensive prenatal care.

Religion

The association between religion and health is a topic of interest, but there are few studies on the relationship between religious involvement and pregnancy outcomes. The results of a study from Australia suggest that higher levels of religious commitment are associated with more favorable pregnancy outcomes (e.g., in terms of length of gestation and birth weight), and women who profess minority Christian sect affiliations have the best pregnancy outcomes (Najman et al. 1988). These differences can be attributed to the healthy lifestyle and large, supportive social networks of the groups studied, and represent a major influence of religious affiliation. In this study the women in the religious groups ingested less alcohol and did not smoke during pregnancy; these behaviors were more likely to be seen in people who were not as involved in a religious group.

Religious practices have influenced the conduct of pregnancy and birth for centuries, and even today religious customs may be followed during pregnancy. For example, throughout the centuries, many cultures have accepted the belief of a hot-cold opposition in the spiritual and material universe. Evil spirits are associated with destructive heat, while prayer is a cooling opposing force. Health results from a balance of these opposing elements in the body.

Islamic Malays believe in the concept of destructive spiritual heat and perform rituals during the reproductive process in an attempt to balance the fire and air of the spirit world by adding cooling earthy and watery elements to the prospective mother's body. Such spiritual practices are most important during a woman's first pregnancy, since she has not yet become adept at her womanly task. The woman is bathed in cold water into which humorally cold lime juice has been squeezed. A rice paste is added to the water and painted on the foreheads of both the midwife and her patient. This is believed to neutralize the spirits' fire and air because it is made from rice and water from the cooling earth. Spiritual heat is further balanced by the midwife's breath, cooled by the power of her incantations and blown toward her patient. The fetus is protected from heat by cooling herbs strung around the mother's waist. All these measures are expected to help a prospective mother deliver her baby safely, yet the measures may not achieve their goal if she is not in harmony with the midwife she has chosen (Laderman 1987, 1988; Lantican 1987).

SOCIOCULTURAL INFLUENCES ON MATERNAL ROLE DEVELOPMENT

Pregnancy and parenthood stimulate modifications in almost all aspects of family life. These changes take place whether it is the first, second, or succeeding baby being added to the family, for each new addition requires modifications in family structure. The addition of a baby to a family system changes the interrelationships of all the members of the family. New roles must be learned, because mothering, fathering, and grandparenting are not necessarily innate. Several theorists have studied how the maternal role is attained and which factors influence its development.

Role Theory

Every member of a family assumes a role within that family, since roles are the basic unit of socialization in any social system. A role provides a pattern of behavior that guides us in social situations. Most people have more than one role in their daily lives. The behaviors that accompany a particular role are learned from childhood through either intentional instruction or incidental learning. These role behaviors are culturally determined. For example, in one culture the accepted behavior of a mother may be very different from accepted maternal behavior in another culture. Roles within a family system do not exist in isolation, for there is always a role partner and reciprocal interaction with others. Therefore, role relationships occur within a family system. The roles of mother and father are an example of reciprocal roles. Role conflict can occur when two or more roles that an individual assumes are in opposition to one another in relation to time or behavioral demands. Many women today find that the multiple roles of wife, mother, and career woman conflict as a result of multiple demands.

Development of Maternal Role

Development of the maternal role was first described by Rubin in 1967. It is defined as the process by which a woman achieves competence in the role of a mother and is able to integrate culturally determined mothering behaviors into her established behavior patterns. This process takes place over the woman's lifetime. Work on maternal role development by Rubin and by other researchers, such as Mercer, continued in the 1970s and 1980s and is still accepted today as basic theory. The maternal role is learned in two ways. It is learned indirectly as the woman experiences mothering from her own mother and as she observes other mother-child relationships (Fig. 18–1). The maternal role can also be learned directly after the birth of the baby as the woman begins to "experiment" with maternal role behaviors. This direct learning is shaped by the expectations of others in the woman's social context and by her own unique style (see Chapter 34).

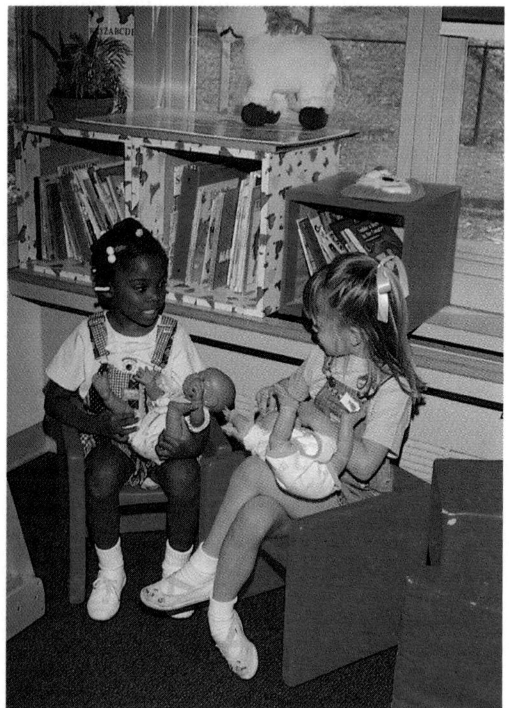

Figure 18–1
Playing with dolls allows little girls to learn the maternal role indirectly.

TAKING-ON

Rubin (1967a) identified three processes involved in maternal role development (see Steps in Maternal Role Development). Each of these processes consists of characteristic behaviors that help the woman to achieve the maternal role. The first process is called taking-on. In this phase the expectant woman begins her work of incorporating a new role by practicing in two ways, mimicry and role play.

▼ **Mimicry.** Mimicry is the adoption of simple behavioral manifestations such as dress, speech affects, or gestures that are recognizable symbols of the mothering role. An example is seen in the woman who is eager to wear maternity clothes to announce her pregnant state, long before they are needed.

▼ **Role Play.** Role play behaviors move a step beyond mimicry, in that behaviors related to the mothering role are actually acted out or "tried on for size." For example, role play might take place as the pregnant woman baby-sits for her friend's baby.

TAKING-IN

The next three behavioral manifestations occur as the woman "takes-in" or internalizes the maternal role. Rubin views this process as a higher level of role development than taking-on.

▼ **Fantasy.** Fantasy is a form of daydreaming, an internalized "trying on for size," in which the woman thinks about how she will act as she mothers her baby. She imagines situations she may encounter as a mother and ways in which she will cope. She fantasizes about the baby's appearance and behavior. Fantasy incorporates her wishes, fears, and ideals.

▼ **Introjection-Projection-Rejection.** This is another behavior that is part of the process of internalizing the maternal role. It is similar to mimicry but includes actual evaluation of the maternal behavior the woman has observed in relation to how that behavior would actually fit for her. If the fit seems good, the behavior will be remembered; if not, it will be rejected. This process is the major substance of "woman talk" and is the basis for many of the decisions that must be made about mothering (e.g., childbirth classes? breast- or bottlefeeding? diaper service? return to a career?).

▼ **Identity.** Identity occurs when the woman has comfortably taken in the maternal role and integrated it into her own behavioral patterns. It is the end point of the process of incorporating a new role. At this stage, the woman actually feels comfortable with the image of herself as a mother and is eager to carry it out.

Steps in Maternal Role Development

Taking-on

- Mimicry
- Role play

Taking-in

- Fantasy
- Introjection—projection—rejection
- Identity

Letting-go

- Grieving for previous identity

Data from Rubin, R. (1967a). Attainment of the maternal role: Part I. Processes. *Nursing Research,* 16 (3), 237–245.

LETTING-GO

▼ **Grief Work.** The final process of maternal role development is letting-go, and this incorporates the task of grief work. The woman's former identities and behaviors that are now incompatible with the assumption of the new role of mother must be abandoned. This is not done easily and may be accompanied with some grieving for her previous identity that will never be again.

VARIABLES INFLUENCING THE DECISION TO PARENT

▼ **Cultural Pressure.** Considerable pressure still exists for young women to become pregnant and take on a maternal role at some point in their lives. Maternity and parenthood are still viewed in many families as necessary steps to female fulfillment and to female status as an adult. This cultural pressure can result in negative feelings toward the role, or the assumption of the role, before the woman is emotionally and socially ready.

▼ **Nature of the Decision.** A second factor related to the parental role is that its occurrence is not always the result of a voluntary decision. If the pregnancy is unplanned and its termination is not socially sanctioned, the adjustment to the resultant parenting role may be very difficult.

▼ **Irrevocable Role.** A third characteristic of parenthood is that it is irrevocable. Once a baby is born, there is little socially accepted possibility of undoing the commitment to that child. As Rossi (1968) states in her classic work on the transition to parenthood, "We can have ex-spouses and ex-jobs but not ex-children."

▼ **Preparation for the Role.** A final factor related to parenthood is the degree of preparation for the role. In the United States, for the most part, women approach motherhood with no previous child care experience beyond sporadic babysitting, a course in child psychology, or occasional care of younger siblings. Most women do not attend a parenting course during pregnancy, either because courses are not available or because attendance is not viewed as necessary. The transition to the maternal role is very abrupt; from the moment of birth, the new mother has immediate 24-hour responsibility for her role. There is no gradual initiation period in which the role can be learned as an apprentice (Rossi 1968).

VARIABLES INFLUENCING MATERNAL ROLE DEVELOPMENT

Many variables can influence the woman's ease in taking on the maternal role and its accompanying behaviors. In a number of research studies conducted within the past 30 years by Lederman (1984), Majewski (1986), Mercer (1985, 1986a, 1986b), Mercer and Ferketich (1994), and Rubin (1967a, 1967b, 1984), the following variables have been identified from interviews with new mothers:

- Acceptance of the pregnancy
- Commitment to and motivation for the pregnancy
- Perception of the birth experience
- Preparation and competence for the maternal role
- Value given to the maternal role
- Perceived conflicts with the maternal role
- Attitudes about childrearing
- Maternal age, ethnic background, marital status, and socioeconomic status
- Maternal health status
- Pregnancy risk status
- Maternal personality traits
- Maternal self-concept
- Role models
- Social resources and support
- Social stress
- Early contact with the infant
- Temperament of the infant
- Health status of the infant

The relationship of these variables is complex: they may influence the process of role development for some women but not for others, and the variables have an ever-changing interrelationship with one another. It is important to identify which of these variables are present in a pregnant woman's social context so that anticipatory guidance and support can be given to help her adapt to the maternal role.

EVALUATION OF MATERNAL ROLE ATTAINMENT

Once the woman assumes her maternal role, she evaluates her success in regard to the feedback she receives from the baby (her role partner) and from her other significant family members. If the baby responds positively to her maternal behaviors (e.g., stops crying, smiles, cuddles), the woman feels rewarded, her self-esteem is maintained, and her behaviors are reinforced. The same response takes place if family members praise her for the good job she is doing or support her in her maternal role. On the other hand, if the baby responds negatively to her or family members are critical, she evaluates her behaviors negatively and the maternal role is not reinforced. Unfortunately, no written job description exists to guide the new mother and help her evaluate her mothering. Because of this, the mothering role lacks clarity, specificity, and consensus, all of which make transition to the role more difficult. The initial incorporation of the maternal role into the woman's identity may take up to 3 months after the birth of the baby. An even longer period may be necessary for teenagers, many of whom report that they did not feel like mothers until the baby was 6 to 10 months of age (Mercer 1986b).

Social Adaptation of Fathers

Fathers also experience the sociocultural aspects of the pregnancy, childbirth, and parenting experience. For many years, society did not fully acknowledge the role that fathers played in the parenting experience. Pregnancy, childbirth, and parenting were seen as women's domain. Today, many in our society expect fathers to play a large part during the pregnancy and birth experience, but often little social support is offered for men to assume these roles. For example, men are seldom given parental leave benefits from their jobs to care for a pregnant wife or newborn infant. Because today's expectations are a shift from those of previous generations, new fathers may have had no role models as examples of involved fathering and may find it difficult to feel comfortable with their role expectations (Conner and Denson 1990; Ferketich and Mercer 1994).

The response of family members and peers to the man's impending fatherhood will influence his perception of the fathering role and adoption of it. His behavior as a father will be shaped by cultural expectations of the father's role in regard to parenting. In some family and cultural groups the father is expected to be intimately involved in all aspects of childrearing (Fig. 18–2), while in other social groups the father is viewed as an authoritative figure who does not give direct child care. Fathers do not usually experience the same degree of role conflict that women do in Western culture. Despite the current egalitarian view of parental roles in the family, men are still not viewed as the parent having the primary responsibility for childrearing, and are expected to uphold their work and career as the primary roles in their lives.

COUVADE

Some expectant fathers in the United States may experience a sociocultural phenomenon known as the couvade syndrome. They may have physical discomforts during their partner's pregnancy that mimic her symptoms. In studies on the couvade syndrome conducted since the early 1980s, men have reported a variety of physical symptoms throughout the period of the pregnancy. For example, men reported more colds, unintentional weight gain, appetite changes, food cravings, nausea and vomiting, constipation, abdominal pain and bloating, nervousness, inability to concentrate, headaches, backache, fatigue, and insomnia. The reasons for these physical symptoms in men during pregnancy are not clear but may be related to the man's involvement in the pregnancy and his identification with his pregnant partner. The couvade syndrome is influenced by demographic factors such as education, ethnic group, income, and age or by factors such as relationships with others, affective responses to the pregnancy, and previous health status (Brown 1988; Clinton 1986; Conner and Denson 1990; Fawcett 1989; Ferketich and Mercer 1989).

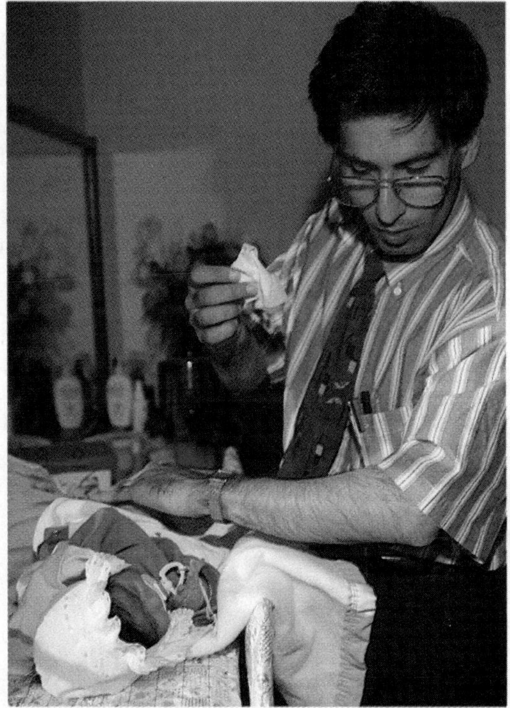

Figure 18–2

Each cultural group has its own beliefs about the role of the father. In the United States, fathers are encouraged to be intimately involved in childrearing.

SOCIAL SUPPORT DURING PREGNANCY

There is a growing recognition that supportive relationships in people's lives play an important role in promoting health, preventing health problems, buffering against the effects of stress, and strengthening coping efforts. The same is true for women who are pregnant. The support received from significant others in the social network has a positive impact on the woman's pregnancy experience, while lack of support can negatively influence the experience.

Concept of Social Support

TYPES OF SOCIAL SUPPORT

The social network of an individual, and the feelings of being cared for, loved, esteemed, valued, and part of a network of communication and mutual obligation, are important to health and emotional well-being. In classic work done by Caplan (1974), social support was defined as being either objective (support observed by others) or subjective (support perceived by an individual), psychological (emotional support) or tangible (help with finances, workload, baby-sitting, and so forth), and potential (resources available) or actual (support being given). House (1981) identified four types of social support: (1) emotional support: communication of empathy, caring, love, and trust; (2) instrumental support: direct aid such as gifts of money or help with work; (3) informational support: sharing of information people can use in coping with problems; and (4) appraisal support: sharing information to help people evaluate themselves or the situation. Social support is believed to buffer stress, enhance coping, and facilitate positive health practices and thus prevent or modify illness. The effects of social support are influenced by many variables, such as the characteristics of the individual, the life context in which the support takes place, and the type of social support.

EFFECTS OF SOCIAL SUPPORT ON HEALTH STATUS

Studies of pregnant women have demonstrated that social support can buffer the effects of life stress and anxiety during pregnancy (Brown 1987; Cronenwett 1985; Mercer and Ferketich 1988; Norbeck and Anderson 1989a, 1989b). Cronenwett (1985) examined the role of social support in enhancing the individual's sense of well-being during pregnancy. She found that the average social network for women in her sample was 8.5 members, most of whom were relatives. Emotional support was the type of support most frequently received by both mothers and fathers and was a predictor of their satisfaction with the parenting role and infant care. Norbeck and Tilden (1983) found that women with high stress before pregnancy and low social support had the highest rate of gestational and infant complications, and women with low stress but also low levels of social support had higher rates of labor and delivery complications. It is interesting to note that a woman experiencing a normal pregnancy may receive more support from her social network than a woman with a high-risk pregnancy, because her pregnancy makes fewer demands on others and follows the course expected by society (Richardson 1987; Snyder 1979). Studies in the 1980s found that the amount of perceived social support may also increase adaptation and promote healthy relationships and practices (Aaronson 1989; Brown 1986a, 1986b). Thus, positive social support can influence help-seeking behavior, decrease pregnancy complications, and enhance adherence to health practices that are beneficial to fetal growth and development, as well as the health of the pregnant woman (Aaronson 1989).

EFFECTS OF SOCIAL SUPPORT ON PARENTING

Social support is a strong predictor of satisfaction with the parent role and infant care, a sense of parental competence, feelings of well-being, and positive marital interaction (Cronenwett 1989). It is also a useful predictor of both the mother's and the father's health (Brown 1986c). Mothers and fathers may find different types of social support helpful to them. For example, one study showed that mothers preferred emotional support received from the marital relationship and the social network, while fathers responded more positively to support from a parenting group (Wandersman and Wandersman 1980). Other studies found that mothers valued assurance about being attractive, and fathers needed acceptance of their work schedule (Brown 1986b, 1987).

CHARACTERISTICS OF A SOCIAL NETWORK

▼ **Size.** The characteristics of the social network determine its effectiveness. For example, the size of the network is related to its degree of effectiveness in providing support (Cronenwett 1985). If a network is too large, support can become conflicting; if it is too small, support may be insufficient.

▼ **Composition.** The composition of the social network (family, friends, or professionals) influences its effectiveness for each person. Some expectant parents respond more positively to family members, while others may prefer friends or professionals (Cronenwett 1985).

▼ **Degree of Involvement.** The degree of involvement of the social network is either a positive or negative influence. For example, the family that is too involved (enmeshed) may cause expectant parents to feel a lack of privacy, autonomy, or psychological space.

▼ **Demographic Characteristics.** The age of the pregnant woman and her socioeconomic status are also influencing factors. The older the woman and the higher her socioeconomic status, the fewer social network conflicts she is likely to experience. Sex differences may exist. Expectant mothers and expectant fathers may prefer different types of support (Cronenwett 1985).

▼ **Type of Support.** The type of support offered (emotional, instrumental, informational, or appraisal) can influence its effectiveness. One study found that although most advice given to a pregnant woman by her social network was sound, some advice conflicted with recommendations by health care providers (St. Clair and Anderson 1989).

CHANGES IN SOCIAL NETWORK

In studies by Richardson (1981, 1983), pregnant women described more changing than stable relationships throughout their pregnancies. In the early weeks, the women described relationships with their husbands and children as changing more than their relationships with parental figures and peers. By the middle weeks of pregnancy, all important relationships were described as changing more than they had been in early weeks. During the late weeks, the women reported fewer changing relationships with husbands and parental figures than in earlier weeks, reflecting a trend toward increasing stability. In contrast, relationships with children were experienced as increasingly changing and less satisfactory in the late weeks. Although the women described their relationships during pregnancy as more satisfactory than unsatisfactory overall, the changes experienced reflect the complexity of reorganizing lives to accommodate the addition of an expected baby to a family system.

▼ **Family.** The woman's family members become particularly important to her, and she views them differently and depends on them in different ways, because of her pregnancy and anticipated motherhood. Rubin (1984) found that the woman's mother is of particular importance as a role model for maternal behavior. Lederman (1984) found that the effectiveness of the support offered by the woman's mother is shaped by her availability, her reactions to the pregnancy, her respect for her daughter's autonomy, and her willingness to reminisce about her own experiences.

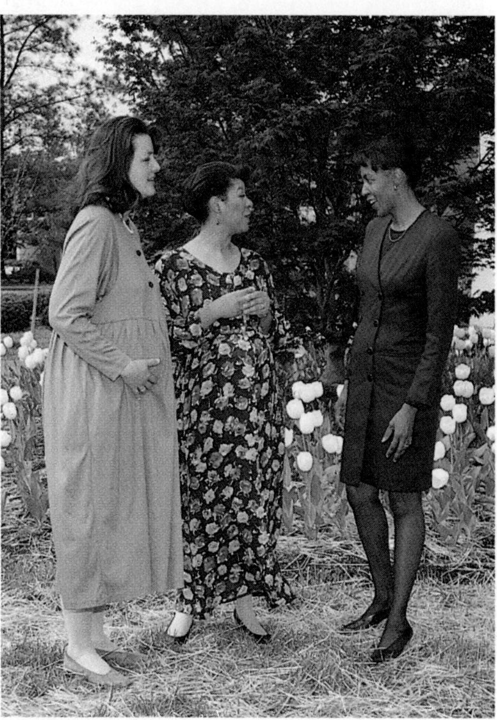

Figure 18–3

The subculture of pregnancy. Pregnant women begin to make changes in their peer group as they are drawn to social relationships with other pregnant women and new mothers.

▼ **Friends.** The responses the woman receives from those in her social network give her information regarding the ease or difficulty with which she will make the important transition to motherhood. With the exception of the father of the baby, relationships shared with women seem to be of greater importance during pregnancy, labor, birth, and the early postpartum period. Pregnant women are likely to identify more closely with other pregnant women or new mothers. The woman's peer group is likely to change as she withdraws from her usual contacts and develops social relationships that are more supportive of the pregnancy (Fig. 18–3).

▼ **Father of the Baby.** Probably the most important relationship for the woman during pregnancy is the one with her partner or father of the baby. This relationship is the one most likely to be affected by a pregnancy, whether in a positive or negative way (Saunders and Robins 1987). The woman who perceives that she is loved and supported by her partner will feel that her baby will also be nurtured and loved. On the other hand, if her partner is not accepting of the expected child, she may feel rejection, and her pregnancy may become an unwanted burden. In contemporary U.S. society, fathers are expected to be active participants in the pregnancy and birth process. If the father is not comfortable doing this, the woman may feel very isolated if she has no other support system (Richardson 1982).

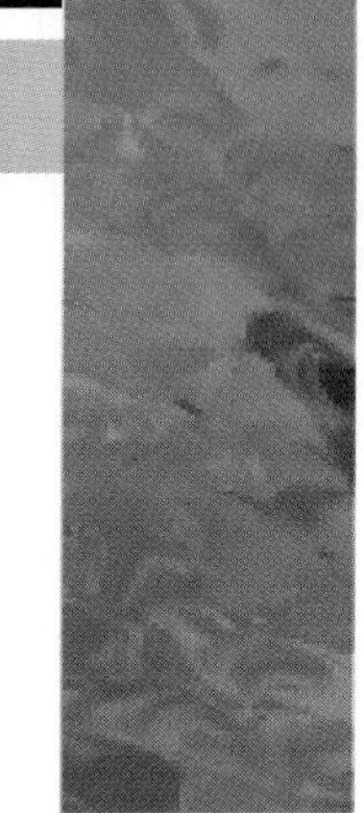

Nursing Practice

Nursing Process

Comprehensive care of the pregnant woman and her partner includes attention to the sociocultural components of their life that might influence the course of pregnancy, birth, and adaptation to parenthood. The nursing process should be applied to determine the influence that family, culture, religion, and other social factors might have on the pregnancy experience, as well as the support the expectant parents are receiving from their social network. Interventions to identify and support the sociocultural aspects of the pregnancy experience can be planned and implemented along with other aspects of care.

▼ Assessment

Assessment of the sociocultural components influencing the expectant parents' pregnancy experience should be a part of the initial prenatal interview. Identification of the sociocultural factors that will influence the course of the pregnancy will alert the health care team to any interventions that might be needed. Components of a sociocultural history can be seen in the box on page 491. A general profile of the family structure and other support systems is important in order to identify whether additional social support might be helpful during the pregnancy. Identification of family living conditions and financial resources alerts the nurse to potential problems that could affect the woman's health status or ability to obtain health care. Knowledge of the woman's and father's (or partner's) religious beliefs and cultural backgrounds allows the health care team to understand the influences that might be responsible for behavior or attitudes during the pregnancy and to plan care so that it will be as congruent as possible with their beliefs.

By knowing the woman's occupational history, the nurse can provide appropriate suggestions for comfort and safety during pregnancy in accordance with the woman's educational level. Identification of the social habits and lifestyle patterns of the woman's family will alert the nurse to potential risk behaviors and the need for the provision of information about healthy practices during pregnancy. Knowledge of family stresses is important so that interventions can be planned to decrease stresses that may be a potential threat to the well-being of the woman or her baby. Family coping patterns can be either reinforced or altered through counseling and education. Family members can be encouraged to explore the implications of the role changes they will experience as a result of the birth of the baby.

▼ Diagnosis

The nursing diagnoses identified from the sociocultural assessment may be based on actual problems identified or may be areas identified as potential high-risk situations. If problems are identified within the family system, diagnoses will be specific and will guide the planning of actual interventions. On the other hand, if no immediate sociocultural concerns are identified, diagnoses will be related to potential alterations. The sociocultural diagnoses should be periodically reevaluated throughout the pregnancy to identify changes in the family or other social influences. Examples of diagnoses that relate to the sociocultural domain are as follows:

Components of a Sociocultural History

Family living conditions

- Economic level: person responsible for family income; adequacy of income
- Housing: adequacy of housing arrangements
- Support system: people living in household; relationships of household members; responsibilities for housework, food selection and preparation; significant others not in household

Religious/cultural history

- Religious preference
- Beliefs/practices that could influence health care (dietary restrictions; opposition to blood products; beliefs about childbirth, circumcision)
- Beliefs about baptism

Educational/occupational history

- Educational level achieved
- Occupation (typical work responsibilities that might affect pregnancy, exposure to harmful substances, opportunity for breaks, provision for maternity leave)
- Plans for continued employment during pregnancy and early postpartum period

Social habits

- Exercise, stress reduction
- Use of drugs such as alcohol, cigarettes, or crack cocaine
- Use of health care system

- Altered family processes related to stress resulting from financial problems caused by pregnancy
- Anxiety related to identified deficits in the social support system
- Knowledge deficit: lack of understanding regarding changes in family roles and relationships resulting from birth of the baby

▼ Planning

A plan of care related to sociocultural influences on the pregnancy can be made along with the other areas of the health care plan. It is particularly important that this plan be developed in conjunction with the woman and her family, for unless they also see the need for interventions or change related to sociocultural aspects of their life, the development of a plan will be futile. The following objectives are examples that might be developed in conjunction with the nursing diagnoses identified. The pregnant woman and her partner will

- Meet with a referred social services worker to discuss resources available to assist with financial problems
- Apply for a Women, Infants, and Children (WIC) nutritional program
- Attend an expectant parents' support group to develop an additional network of social support
- Participate in discussions with the nurse at prenatal appointments and with members of the parents' group to identify ways to plan for changes in family roles and relationships

▼ Intervention

The interventions related to sociocultural aspects of the woman's pregnancy are guided by the diagnoses and planned goals. Interventions in this area most likely relate to either anticipatory guidance by the nurse or other members of the health care team, or referral to supporting health care professionals. By talking with the woman and her partner at each prenatal visit, the nurse can give information and guidance about areas of social or family change that might be encountered during the pregnancy. Discussions can center on expected family role changes, the importance of family and social network support, occupational or financial issues, and family health habits. If the woman or her partner is from a cultural or religious background that has particular beliefs about pregnancy and birth, the nurse can develop a plan with them for how their specific needs might be met within the health care system. If the nurse identifies family or social problems that are beyond his or her scope of assistance, referral should be made to the appropriate resource. Additional services that should be arranged may include assistance with housing, finances, family therapy, legal intervention, or use of community resources (Dawson et al. 1989). Helping the woman and her partner enroll in expectant parent classes, classes

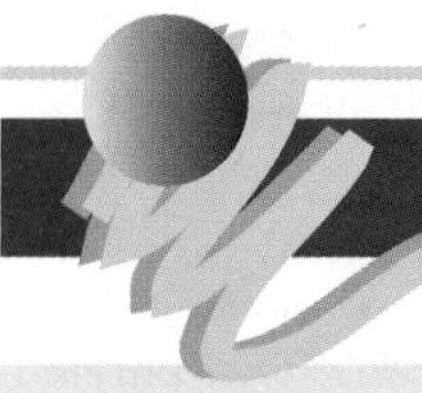

IMPROVING YOUR PRACTICE

HOW TO HELP EXPECTANT CLIENTS FROM VARIOUS CULTURAL GROUPS

Provision of comprehensive care to the pregnant woman and her family includes understanding and acceptance of their social, cultural, and religious background. It requires the willingness of nurses to interact with a family in a nonjudgmental way, no matter how the behaviors, attitudes, or values of the family differ from their own. It requires that nurses put aside any preconceptions or prejudices they may have and approach the woman and her family with an open mind. To achieve this goal, it may help nurses to first evaluate their own beliefs, values, and biases about people from other cultural groups.

- IDENTIFY YOUR PERSONAL CULTURAL, RELIGIOUS, AND SOCIAL INFLUENCES. Think about the factors in your own background that shape who you are and what you value. What is your own cultural or ethnic heritage? What is your religious background? What is your socioeconomic status? Do these factors influence your view of yourself? Do they influence how you interact with others?
- IDENTIFY THE BELIEFS YOU MAY HOLD ABOUT OTHER CULTURAL GROUPS. Honestly admit to yourself what you may hold to be true about others. Try to determine how these beliefs originated and whether they are based on actual experience and information or on hearsay. Evaluate how these feelings could affect your care of women during pregnancy and birth.
- DISCUSS YOUR BELIEFS WITH OTHERS. Contrast and evaluate the views of others with your own. Identify ways that you might overcome biases that you hold and provide nonjudgmental nursing care to all clients.
- BECOME CULTURALLY SENSITIVE TO OTHERS. Take every opportunity that you can to learn about the viewpoints of people from other cultural groups. Take the time to talk with women or their family members about their beliefs and values; read books or articles about other cultural groups; or attend films that give insight into ethnic, cultural, or religious experiences different from your own.

for new parents, or a discussion group for fathers gives additional support.

▼ Evaluation

Evaluation of the plan of care is made on the basis of verbal feedback from the pregnant woman or her family; discussion with representatives from referral agencies; or direct observations regarding the woman's behavior, attitudes, or social situation. If the planned goals are written in specific, measurable outcomes, evaluation will be easier. Evaluation should take place at each prenatal visit, so that the degree of progress can be identified and revision of diagnoses or plans made if needed. Data regarding the sociocultural aspects of the woman's pregnancy are important and should be carefully recorded in her health record, along with the other assessment data.

Risk Management

Management of risk in relation to the sociocultural aspects of childbirth requires members of the health care team to identify cultural or religious beliefs that might interfere with care. This information should be identified during the initial prenatal assessment. For example, the beliefs of some groups oppose the administration of all blood products. For the pregnant woman, this presents a serious risk if a blood transfusion or RhoGAM administration is needed. Dietary restrictions during pregnancy or the postpartum period are common cultural practices for some groups and may pose a threat to fetal development or postpartum healing. In situations such as these, it is essential to document in the woman's medical record that she and her family were informed of the need for a particular health practice or medical intervention but refused it.

Implications for Research

A number of studies have been conducted regarding the sociocultural aspects of the pregnancy, birth, and parenting experience. Nurses have contributed to this body of research, particularly in the areas of maternal role development and social support. Additional research in these areas, as well as descriptive research regarding cultural practices during pregnancy and childbirth, would add to our body of knowledge. The following research questions could provide additional information to help in the planning of comprehensive nursing care during the prenatal period.

- What practices from other cultures can be safely integrated with health care practices in the United States to provide a more meaningful pregnancy and birth experience for women from other ethnic or cultural backgrounds?
- What effects do religious beliefs have on the pregnancy and birth experience?
- What interventions demonstrate effectiveness in helping parents in the transition to their maternal and paternal roles?
- What intervention strategies are useful to strengthen the expectant couple's existing social support network during pregnancy?

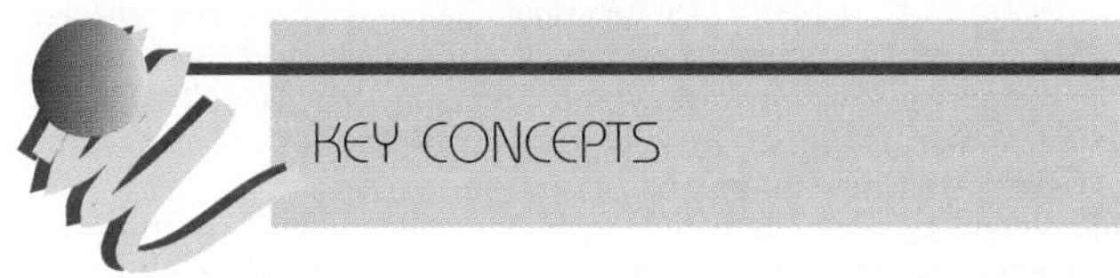

KEY CONCEPTS

- ▼ Pregnancy and birth are biosocial events; i.e., these universal biologic experiences are shaped by the social and cultural context in which they occur.
- ▼ The pregnancy experience affects everyone in the woman's social network, and the social environment influences the course of the pregnancy.
- ▼ Sociocultural factors that influence pregnancy include the family, culture, and religion.
- ▼ Cultural beliefs are handed down from generation to generation and are usually related to one of three categories: (1) practices that might influence the fetus, (2) activities that would ensure a healthy baby and safe delivery, and (3) practices related to gender determination of the fetus.
- ▼ Some cultures view pregnancy as a normal healthy state, while others believe the woman is ill during pregnancy. The way pregnancy is viewed determines whether the woman responds with health or illness behavior during pregnancy.
- ▼ An increased risk of genetic disease exists in some racial groups. For example, thalassemia is most commonly seen in people of Mediterranean origin; sickle cell anemia is seen most often in people of African-American or Mediterranean ancestry; cystic fibrosis and phenylketonuria are found most often in white people; and Tay-Sachs disease is found almost exclusively in the Ashkenazic Jewish population.
- ▼ Rubin's maternal role theory identifies three processes involved in the development of the maternal role from childhood through pregnancy: (1) taking-on, which includes the behaviors of mimicry and role play; (2) taking-in, which includes the behaviors of fantasy, introjection-projection-rejection, and identity; and (3) letting-go, which involves grieving for her previous identity as she prepares to take on a new role.
- ▼ Variables that influence the decision to parent include cultural pressure, whether the decision is voluntary or involuntary, the irrevocable nature of the role, and the degree of preparation for the role.
- ▼ Society influences the role that fathers play in pregnancy, childbirth, and parenting. Some fathers may experience the couvade syndrome—the manifestation of physical discomforts during the partner's pregnancy that mimic her symptoms.
- ▼ The social support that parents receive during pregnancy and early parenting can greatly influence their adaptation to the experience. Social support can be emotional (empathy, caring, love), instrumental (direct aid such as gifts), informational (sharing of information), or appraisal (help with evaluation of a situation).
- ▼ The characteristics of the expectant couple's social network (e.g., the size, composition, degree of involvement, demographic characteristics of the people involved, and type of support given) influence the usefulness of the support network.
- ▼ Expectant parents often notice a change in their social network. Family members may become more important and there is increased dependency on family. Pregnant women and new mothers tend to withdraw from their usual

contacts and draw more closely to other women experiencing the same life events.

- ▼ A sociocultural assessment should be part of the initial prenatal interview and include information about family living conditions, religious and cultural practices, educational and occupational background, and social habits.
- ▼ Nursing interventions related to the sociocultural aspects of pregnancy include anticipatory guidance regarding social and family changes that might be encountered, and referral to other members of the health care team to assist with identified social needs.

References

Aaronson, L. (1989). Perceived and received support: Effects on health behavior during pregnancy. *Nursing Research,* 38 (1), 4–9.

Ahmed, G., and Watt, S. (1986). Understanding Asian women in pregnancy and confinement. *Midwives Chronicle,* 99 (1180), 98–101.

Baric, L. (1969). Recognition of the "at-risk" role: A means to influence health behavior. *International Journal of Health Education,* 12, 24–32.

Bernstein, G. L., and Kidd, Y. A. (1982). Childbearing in Japan. In M. A. Kay (Ed.). *Anthropology of human birth* (pp. 101–117). Philadelphia: F. A. Davis.

Brown, M. (1986a). Social support during pregnancy: A unidimensional or multidimensional construct? *Nursing Research,* 35 (1), 4–9.

Brown, M. (1986b). Marital support during pregnancy. *Journal of Obstetric, Gynecologic, and Neonatal Nursing,* 15 (6), 475–483.

Brown, M. (1986c). Social support, stress, and health: A comparison of expectant mothers and fathers. *Nursing Research,* 35 (2), 72–76.

Brown, M. (1987). How fathers and mothers perceive prenatal support. *MCN,* 12, 414–418.

Brown, M. (1988). A comparison of health responses in expectant mothers and fathers. *Western Journal of Nursing Research,* 10 (5), 527–549.

Caplan, G. (1974). *Support systems and community mental health.* New York: Behavioral Publications.

Clinton, J. (1986). Expectant fathers at risk for couvade. *Nursing Research,* 35 (5), 290–295.

Conner, G., and Denson, V. (1990). Expectant fathers' response to pregnancy: Review of literature and implications for research in high-risk pregnancy. *Journal of Perinatal and Neonatal Nursing,* 4 (2), 33–42.

Crib Sheet, Vol. 4, No. 1. (Autumn 1990). Cross-cultural perinatal care I: The Latina patient. Available from USCD Medical Center Regional Perinatal Center, 225 Dickinson St. H-410, San Diego, CA 92103.

Crib Sheet, Vol. 5, No. 1. (Spring, 1991). Cross-cultural perinatal care II: The African American patient. Available from USCD Medical Center Regional Perinatal Center, 225 Dickinson St. H-410, San Diego, CA 92103.

Cronenwett, L. (1985). Network structure, social support, and psychological outcomes of pregnancy. *Nursing Research,* 34 (2), 93–99.

Cronenwett, L. (1989). Parental network structure and perceived support after birth of first child. *Nursing Research,* 34 (6), 347–352.

D'Avanzo, C. (1992). Bridging the cultural gap with Southeast Asians. *MCN,* 17 (4), 204–208.

Dawson, P., VanDoorninck, W., Robinson, J. (1989). Effects of home-based, informal social support on child health. *Developmental and Behavioral Pediatrics,* 10 (2), 63–67.

Duvall, E. (1985). *Marriage and family development.* Philadelphia: J. B. Lippincott.

Enriquez, M. S. (1982). Studying maternal infant attachment: A Mexican-American example. In M. A. Kay (Ed.). *Anthropology of human birth* (pp. 61–79). Philadelphia: F. A. Davis.

Faller, H. (1992). Hmong women: Characteristics and birth outcomes, 1990. *Birth,* 19 (3), 144–148.

Fawcett, J. (1989). Spouses' experiences during pregnancy and the postpartum: A program of research and theory development. *Image: Journal of Nursing Scholarship,* 21 (3), 149–152.

Feldman, P. (1992). Sexuality, birth control and childbirth in orthodox Jewish tradition. *Canadian Medical Association Journal,* 146 (1), 29–33.

Ferketich, S., and Mercer, R. (1989). Men's health status during pregnancy and early fatherhood. *Research in Nursing and Health,* 12, 137–148.

Ferketich, S., and Mercer, R. (1994). Predictors of paternal role competence by risk status. *Nursing Research,* 43 (2), 80–85.

Haire, D. (1976). Maternity practices around the world: How do we measure up? In D. Stewart and L. Stewart (Eds.). *Safe alternatives in childbirth.* Chapel Hill, North Carolina: NAPSAC.

Harris, K. (1987). Beliefs and practices among Haitian American women in relation to childbearing. *Journal of Nurse Midwifery,* 32 (3), 149–155.

House, J. (1981). *Work, stress, and social support.* Reading, MA: Addison-Wesley.

Hubbell, K. M. (1982). The neo-oriental American: Childbearing in the Ashram. In M. A. Kay (Ed.). *Anthropology of human birth* (pp. 305–320). Philadelphia: F. A. Davis.

Jordan, B. (1993). *Birth in four cultures* (4th ed.). Prospect Heights, IL: Waveland Press.

Judkins, R., and Judkins, A. (1992). Commentary: Cultural dimensions of Hmong birth. *Birth,* 19 (3), 148–150.

Keeping, J., Najman, J., Morrison, J., Western, J., Andersen, M., Williams, G. (1989). A prospective longitudinal study of social, psychological and obstetric factors in pregnancy: Response rates and demographic characteristics of the 8556 respondents. *British Journal of Obstetrics and Gynaecology,* 96 (3), 289–297.

Khazoyan, C., and Anderson, N. (1994). Latina's expectations for their partners during childbirth. *MCN,* 19 (4), 226–229.

Kulig, J. (1990). Childbearing beliefs among Cambodian refugee women. *Western Journal of Nursing Research,* 12 (1), 108–118.

Laderman, C. (1987). Destructive heat and cooling prayer: Malay humoralism in pregnancy, childbirth, and the postpartum period. *Social Science and Medicine,* 25 (4), 357–365.

Laderman, C. (1988). Cross-cultural perspectives on birth practices. *Birth,* 15 (2), 86–87.

Lantican, L. (1987). Social support among Filipino pregnant women in an atmosphere of socioeconomic political uncertainty. *Health Care of Women International,* 8 (4), 261–276.

Lederman, R. (1984). *Psychosocial adaptation in pregnancy.* Englewood Cliffs, NJ: Prentice Hall.

Lee, P. (1986). Health beliefs of pregnant and postpartum Hmong women. *Western Journal of Nursing Research,* 8 (1), 83–93.

Majewski, J. (1986). Conflicts, satisfactions, and attitudes during transition to the maternal role. *Nursing Research,* 35 (1), 10–14.

Mattson, S., and Lew, L. (1992). Culturally sensitive prenatal care for Southeast Asians. *Journal of Obstetric, Gynecologic, and Neonatal Nursing,* 21 (1), 48–54.

Meleis, A. I., Lipson, J. G., Paul, S. M. (1992). Ethnicity and health among five Middle Eastern immigrant groups. *Nursing Research,* 41 (2), 98–103.

Meleis, A. I., and Sorrell, L. (1981). Arab American women and their birth experience. *MCN,* 3 (3), 171–176.

Mercer, R. (1985). The process of maternal role attainment over the first year. *Nursing Research,* 34 (4), 198–204.

Mercer, R. (1986a). The relationship of developmental variables to maternal behavior. *Research in Nursing & Health,* 9, 25–33.

Mercer, R. (1986b). *First-time motherhood: Experiences from teens to forties.* New York: Springer.

Mercer, R., and Ferketich, S. (1988). Stress and social support as predictors of anxiety and depression during pregnancy. *Advances in Nursing Science,* 10 (2), 26–39.

Mercer, R., and Ferketich, S. (1990). Predictors of family functioning eight months following birth. *Nursing Research,* 39 (2), 76–82.

Mercer, R., and Ferketich, S. (1994). Predictors of maternal role competence by risk status. *Nursing Research,* 43 (1), 38–43.

Mercer, R., Ferketich, S., DeJoseph, J., May, K., Sollid, D. (1988). Effect of stress on family functioning during pregnancy. *Nursing Research,* 37 (5), 268–275.

Najman, M., Williams, G., Keeping, J., Morrison, J., Anderson, M. (1988). Religious values, practices and pregnancy outcomes: A comparison of the impact of sect and mainstream Christian affiliation. *Social Science and Medicine,* 26 (4), 401–407.

Norbeck, J., and Anderson, N. J. (1989a). Life stress, social support, and anxiety in mid and late pregnancy among low income women. *Research in Nursing and Health,* 12 (5), 281–287.

Norbeck, J., and Anderson, N. J. (1989b). Psychosocial predictors of pregnancy outcomes in low-income black, Hispanic, and white women. *Nursing Research,* 38 (4), 204–209.

Norbeck, J., and Tilden, V. (1983). Life stress, social support, and emotional disequilibrium in complications of pregnancy: A prospective, multivariate study. *Journal of Health and Social Behavior,* 24, 30–46.

Pillsbury, B. L. K. (1982). Doing the month: Confinement and convalescence of Chinese women after childbirth. In M. A. Kay (Ed.). *Anthropology of human birth* (pp. 119–146). Philadelphia: F. A. Davis.

Richardson, P. (1981). Women's perceptions of their important dyadic relationships during pregnancy. *Maternal-Child Nursing Journal,* 10 (1), 159–174.

Richardson, P. (1982). Significant relationships and their impact on childbearing: A review. *Maternal Child Nursing Journal,* 11 (1), 17–40.

Richardson, P. (1983). Women's perceptions of change in relationships shared with children during pregnancy. *Maternal Child Nursing Journal,* 12 (1), 75–88.

Richardson, P. (1987). Women's important relationships during pregnancy and the preterm labor event. *Western Journal of Nursing Research,* 9 (2), 203–222.

Rossi, A. (1968). Transition to parenthood. *Journal of Marriage and Family,* 30, 26–39.

Rubin, R. (1967a). Attainment of the maternal role: Part I. Processes. *Nursing Research,* 16 (3), 237–245.

Rubin, R. (1967b). Attainment of the maternal role: Part II. Models and referrants. *Nursing Research,* 16 (4), 342–346.

Rubin, R. (1984). *Maternal identity and the maternal experience.* New York: Springer.

Saunders, R., and Robins, E. (1987). Changes in the marital relationship during the first pregnancy. *Health Care for Women International,* 8, 361–367.

Simkin, P. (1989). Childbearing in social context. *Women and Health,* 15 (3), 5–21.

Snyder, D. (1979). The high-risk mother viewed in relation to a holistic model of the childbearing experience. *Journal of Obstetric, Gynecologic, and Neonatal Nursing,* 8 (3), 164–170.

Spector, R. (1991). *Cultural diversity in health and illness* (8th ed.). East Norwalk, CT: Appleton & Lange.

Stark, S. (1982). Mormon childbearing. In M. A. Kay (Ed.). *Anthropology of human birth* (pp. 341–360). Philadelphia: F. A. Davis.

St. Clair, P., and Anderson, N. (1989). Social network advance during pregnancy: Myths, misinformation, and sound counsel. *Birth,* 16 (3) 103–108.

Wandersman, L., and Wandersman, A. (1980). Social support in the transition to parenthood. *Journal of Community Psychology,* 10, 332–342.

Waterhouse, C. (1994). Midwifery care for orthodox Jewish women. *Modern Midwife,* 4 (9), 11–14.

19 Chapter

Pregnancy itself is a healthy, normal occurrence—humans, unfortunately, are the only species with the ability to worry about it.

FRITZI KALLOP
(JOHNSTON 1994)

Promoting a Healthy Pregnancy

Elaine Zwelling

HIGHLIGHTS

- ▼ Discomforts of Pregnancy and Relief Measures
- ▼ Warning Signs in Pregnancy
- ▼ Nutrition in Pregnancy
- ▼ Variables Influencing Good Nutrition
- ▼ Nutritional Requirements
- ▼ Weight Gain in Pregnancy
- ▼ Nutritional Risk Factors in Pregnancy
- ▼ Exercise in Pregnancy
- ▼ Recommendations for a Safe Exercise Program in Pregnancy
- ▼ Stress Management in Pregnancy
- ▼ Common Concerns During Pregnancy
- ▼ Nursing Practice
- ▼ Nursing Care Planning Guide: Healthy Pregnancy
- ▼ Assessment Tools: Health History Summary, Initial Lifestyle Profile, Initial Pregnancy Profile
- ▼ Collaborative Process
- ▼ Risk Management
- ▼ Implications for Research

Attention to health and physical well-being is important throughout our lives; however, it is critical during pregnancy. Good health practices during pregnancy are known to have positive effects on the mother and on her developing baby. Despite the fact that the normal discomforts of pregnancy may at times make the woman feel as though she is ill, pregnancy remains a normal physiologic process. This process can best be supported by a

DEFINITIONS

Anthropometric measurements—Measurements of size, weight, and proportions of the human body.

Body mechanics—Safe movements of the body when rising from a lying position, bending, or lifting to protect abdominal and low back muscles during pregnancy.

Braxton Hicks contractions—The normal painless contractions of the uterus that occur throughout pregnancy; caused by increased estrogen and uterine distention.

Fetal alcohol syndrome—A group of physical and mental alterations in the newborn caused by the ingestion of alcohol during pregnancy.

Flush-back effect—Rapid return of blood flow to the uterus and placenta after a period of exercise during pregnancy.

Health promotion—Education and counseling to maintain and enhance health, support healthful behaviors, and facilitate decision making regarding health care.

Intrauterine growth retardation (IUGR)—Fetal growth retardation; can be caused by many factors, including malnutrition during pregnancy.

Kegel exercises—Alternate contraction and release of the pubococcygeal muscle to strengthen the pelvic floor muscles; done during pregnancy to promote elasticity for birth; done throughout life to maintain tone for support of abdominal organs and to enhance sexuality.

Lactose intolerance—Sensitivity to milk products containing lactose, resulting in gastrointestinal disturbances.

Pelvic rock—An exercise done during pregnancy to prevent or relieve low backache and tone abdominal muscles.

Pica—The practice of ingesting substances that have no nutritive value.

Recommended dietary allowances (RDAs)—Guidelines for daily intake of essential food nutrients.

Risk assessment—The identification of the presence or absence of medical, obstetric, or psychosocial risks throughout pregnancy through history taking, physical examination, or laboratory tests.

Teratogens—Environmental substances that can cause alterations in fetal growth and development during pregnancy.

Warning signs—Symptoms in pregnancy that are not normal discomforts but may signal the development of a complication.

lifestyle that incorporates balance and homeostasis through good nutrition, frequent exercise, stress reduction, and attention to safety. All of these components of good health shape the course of pregnancy and influence maternal and fetal health during the pregnancy and in the postpartum period. Women who maintain a healthy lifestyle during pregnancy can decrease the discomforts they experience and can help prevent pregnancy complications (Thompson 1989; Thompson and Culpepper 1989; Vogt 1987).

Pregnancy is a time in the life of a woman and her family when many "teachable moments" occur. Families are open to change and are interested in improving their health. During the past decade, the American public has shown a dramatic increase in its interest in health promotion and illness prevention. All forms of the media have proclaimed the message that nutrition, exercise, stress reduction, and safety are important components of good health. This increased national focus on healthy lifestyles, along with openness to change during pregnancy, makes the childbearing year a time when people are receptive to health teaching and positive lifestyle changes can be made (Abrums 1986; Lewallen 1989; Lowenstein 1989).

The nurse is one member of the health care team who provides a great deal of information to expectant families about positive health practices during pregnancy. Along with the nutritionist, the physical therapist, and the childbirth educator, nurses have a wonderful opportunity in a variety of settings to provide counseling about the woman's diet, her activity, the stresses in her life, and ways to ensure safety during the pregnancy. This health teaching can take place in physicians' or nurse-midwives' offices, clinics, childbirth classes, homes, or hospital inpatient antepartum units. Teaching and counseling women about healthy lifestyle practices during pregnancy is as important a component of antepartum care as are the physical assessment components of care (Public Health Service 1989). This chapter presents information about the common discomforts of pregnancy; nutrition, exercise, stress reduction, and safety during pregnancy; and the nursing process related to the promotion of a healthy pregnancy.

DISCOMFORTS OF PREGNANCY AND RELIEF MEASURES

The discomforts that women experience throughout pregnancy are often called minor discomforts of pregnancy. This phrase is no doubt used because most discomforts are a result of normal physiologic changes due to hormonal changes and the influence of the developing pregnancy on supporting organs. However, at the time the woman is experiencing these symptoms, she may not feel that they are "minor," for they can be bothersome and interfere with daily living. In this chapter, the most frequent discomforts of pregnancy are identified and discussed for each trimester of pregnancy. Table 19–1 provides a summary of these discomforts and their causes and relief measures. A universal and critical factor in dealing with each discomfort is the woman's knowledge and understanding of the normal physiologic reasons for the symptoms she experiences. Education must be a primary component of intervention in helping the pregnant woman deal with the discomforts of pregnancy.

First Trimester

NAUSEA AND VOMITING

▼ **Description.** Nausea and vomiting are often the first symptoms that a woman experiences in early pregnancy. Seventy percent of pregnant women experience these symptoms (Jimenez 1992; Petitti 1986). They usually begin soon after the first missed menstrual period and are normally limited to the first trimester. They are commonly called morning sickness because of the time of day that they usually occur; however, they can occur at any time throughout the day. Although some degree of nausea occurs for most women at some point in the first trimester, the majority of women do not experience vomiting.

The exact cause of nausea and vomiting in pregnancy is unknown, but several theories are accepted today. The increase of the hormones human chorionic gonadotropin (hCG) and progesterone early in pregnancy is thought to be the primary cause of nausea. Levels of hCG rise soon after the first missed menstrual period and remain elevated until about the fourth missed period. Progesterone causes increased gastric emptying time as a result of smooth muscle relaxation. Alterations in carbohydrate metabolism resulting in a decreased blood glucose level are also thought to contribute to nausea in pregnancy. Other causes of nausea may be decreased gastric secretion of hydrochloric acid and pepsin, hunger, an empty stomach, dehydration, ptyalism, maternal hypotension, emotional factors, and fatigue.

▼ **Management.** A number of remedies for nausea and vomiting have been suggested by professionals and by pregnant women (Alley 1984; Bennett 1984; Jimenez 1992). If nausea occurs early in the morning, it is often helpful to eat a dry carbohydrate food before arising. Having crackers at the bedside is a common practice for many women. Drinking a glass of milk or taking two calcium tablets may help to neutralize stomach acid. Eating frequent, small high-protein or complex carbohydrate meals throughout the day is advisable. Fluids should be consumed between meals rather than with a meal, and unsweetened carbonated beverages are particularly helpful. Some women find that sucking or chewing ice relieves nausea; others may find that chamomile tea gives relief. Preparation of meals may bother the pregnant woman in the first trimester. Avoiding bothersome food odors or greasy, highly seasoned foods will help, as will making certain that the kitchen is well ventilated. Vitamin B_6 supplements taken after meals or at bedtime have been found to decrease nausea (Herold 1981; Jimenez 1992). Other over-the-counter antinausea medications should be avoided without consultation from the physician or midwife (see Chapter 15). Getting adequate rest and rising slowly to avoid maternal hypotension may help to decrease nausea.

If nausea and vomiting become persistent, cause dehydration, or do not cease by the fourth month of pregnancy, they should not be considered a "normal" symptom of pregnancy. The health care provider should be informed and additional assessment implemented. Other problems, such as intestinal flu, hyperemesis gravidarum, gastric ulcers, cholecystitis, pancreatitis, hepatitis, gastroenteritis, or appendicitis, should be ruled out.

BREAST TENDERNESS

▼ **Description.** Breast discomfort during pregnancy can be experienced as tenderness, fullness, tingling, or nipple sensitivity. One or more of these sensations are often early signs of pregnancy and may continue throughout the pregnancy. These symptoms result from hypertrophy of mammary glandular tissue and increased vascularization caused by elevations in levels of estrogen and progesterone.

▼ **Management.** Breast discomfort can be decreased by wearing a supportive bra with wide adjustable straps. Sleep positions may need to be changed to decrease pressure on the breasts. As pregnancy progresses, the woman should avoid us-

Table 19–1

DISCOMFORTS OF PREGNANCY AND RELIEF MEASURES

DISCOMFORT	CAUSE	RELIEF
First Trimester		
Nausea and vomiting (morning sickness)	hCG Progesterone Altered carbohydrate metabolism Emotional factors Decreased gastric motility	Frequent, small meals Dry carbohydrate food before arising; protein or complex carbohydrate snack before bedtime Fluids between meals Avoid cooking odors Vitamin B_6 Adequate rest
Urinary frequency	Pressure from uterus or fetal presenting part Progesterone	Empty bladder frequently Maintain daytime fluid intake Decrease fluids before bedtime Avoid caffeinated and carbonated beverages Wear panty liners Kegel exercises
Fatigue and drowsiness	Increasing hormone levels Increased basal metabolic rate	Get 7–8 hours sleep per night Naps or relaxation breaks during the day Exercise Social activity Decrease workload
Breast tenderness	Elevated estrogen and progesterone	Wear supportive bra Change sleep position Avoid soap on nipple Cleanse colostrum with water Alter lovemaking techniques
Increased vaginal discharge	Increased estrogen Increased pelvic pressure	Good hygiene Mild bath powder or cornstarch Cotton underwear Avoid tight clothing or pantyhose Panty liners Avoid douching
Nasal stuffiness or epistaxis	Increased estrogen	Normal saline nose drops Cool-air vaporizers Avoid oral decongestants
Ptyalism	Increased estrogen Nausea	Good oral hygiene Astringent mouthwash Hard candy or gum Good nutrition
Syncope	Hormonally triggered vasomotor lability Increased blood volume Anemia Hypoglycemia Sudden position changes Fatigue	Recognize symptoms Sit or lie down with head lowered Avoid sudden position changes Use side-lying recumbent position Avoid warm, crowded areas Moderate exercise Iron and vitamin supplements
Second Trimester		
Constipation	Increased progesterone Increased pelvic pressure	Increase fluids High-fiber diet

Continued on following page

Table 19–1

DISCOMFORTS OF PREGNANCY AND RELIEF MEASURES Continued

DISCOMFORT	CAUSE	RELIEF
	Second Trimester (Cont'd)	
Constipation *(Cont'd)*	Iron supplements	Warm beverages Regular bowel habits Exercise Mild laxative, stool softener, or suppository
Hemorrhoids	Increased blood volume Increased pelvic pressure Constipation	Ice packs Warm or cool sitz baths Gentle cleansing Topical ointments Kegel exercises Gentle reinsertion
Braxton Hicks contractions	Increased estrogen Uterine distention	Evaluate Rest in left lateral position Mild exercise Practice relaxation and breathing techniques
Round ligament pain	Uterine growth and stretching	Use good body mechanics Avoid strenuous exercise Knees to chest Rest, relaxation Heat Massage
Varicosities	Hormone-triggered relaxation of venous walls Increased blood volume Stasis and pooling of blood Increased pelvic pressure (large baby; multiple gestation) Heredity Age Obesity	Elevate legs Frequent position changes Avoid lengthy standing Exercise Support hose Avoid crossing legs Avoid garters or knee-high hose
	Third Trimester	
Dyspnea	Decreased thoracic space Decreased vital capacity Vena cava syndrome	Use good posture Tailor reach exercise Avoid overexertion Sleep in semi-Fowler with extra pillows or in left lateral position Eat small meals Stop smoking
Backache	Compensatory lordosis Poor posture Lax abdominal muscles Estrogen and relaxin Fatigue High-heeled shoes	Use good posture Use good body mechanics Pelvic rock exercise Flat, supportive shoes Maternity girdle Avoid overexertion Sleep in lateral position on firm mattress Massage
Leg cramps	Uterine pressure on nerves or blood vessels in legs Calcium/phosphorus imbalance in diet	Dorsiflexion of foot Stand on cold surface Warm baths Elevate legs

Continued on facing page

Table 19–1

DISCOMFORTS OF PREGNANCY AND RELIEF MEASURES Continued

DISCOMFORT	CAUSE	RELIEF
Third Trimester (Cont'd)		
Leg cramps *(Cont'd)*	Pointing the toes Fatigue	Massage Exercise Evaluate calcium intake—increase or decrease Calcium supplement Decrease soft drinks
Epulis	Increased estrogen	Oral hygiene Warm saline or astringent mouthwash Well-balanced diet Dental checkups
Insomnia	Difficulty with comfortable positioning Fetal activity Urinary frequency Indigestion, heartburn Leg cramps Dyspnea Emotional stress	Use extra pillows for positioning Open window for fresh air Back massage Relaxation techniques Warm milk before bedtime Warm shower Avoid caffeinated beverages late in day Regular exercise Avoid sleeping medications
Heartburn	Increased progesterone causing decreased gastrointestinal motility Displacement of stomach and duodenum by uterus	Small, frequent meals Avoid fatty, fried foods Avoid coffee and cigarettes Gum Frequent sips of milk, hot tea, or water Mild antacids (avoid those containing aspirin or sodium)
Edema	Hormonal influence on sodium and water retention Increased blood volume Varicose veins Prolonged sitting or standing Hot weather High-sodium or low-protein diet	Rest in left lateral position Drink 6–8 glasses fluid Elevate legs Support hose Ankle rotations Regular exercise Avoid garters or knee-high hose Increase protein in diet Avoid diuretic drugs

ing soap on the nipple and areola area to prevent drying of the tissues. If there is leakage of colostrum, it should be gently massaged into the nipple area, as it serves as an excellent moisturizer to prepare the nipples for breastfeeding. The woman should be instructed to wear soft-textured clothing to decrease nipple tenderness and to use breast pads inside the bra if leakage of colostrum is a problem. If breast discomfort is annoying during lovemaking, the woman should inform her partner so that alternative types of foreplay or positions for intercourse can be explored (Jimenez 1992).

PTYALISM

▼ **Description.** Ptyalism is the production of excessive, sometimes bitter saliva during pregnancy. It is characterized by its sudden onset at 2 to 3 weeks' gestation and the production of saliva in excess of 1900 mL/day (Van Dinter 1991).

Ptyalism may decrease after the first trimester or can continue throughout the entire pregnancy. The excess saliva is often difficult to swallow and may require frequent expectoration or contribute to nausea and vomiting. The woman may experience a dry tongue, swollen salivary glands, irritated perioral skin, and speech difficulties.

Although causative factors are uncertain, ptyalism is thought to most likely result either from increased estrogen levels or from the woman's reluctance to swallow because of nausea. Other theories include the possibility of salivary gland stimulation by starch intake, increased acidity of saliva leading to gland production of excess saliva, or unusual food cravings or pica.

▼ **Management.** There are few remedies for ptyalism; however, good oral hygiene and the use of an astringent mouthwash are helpful. Small, frequent meals and sucking on hard candy or chewing gum may also help. It may be advisable to limit starch intake and maintain good nutrition (Van Dinter 1991). If excess saliva becomes a major problem, differential diagnosis should be made for oral infections or lesions; tonsillitis; or a gastric, pancreatic, or hepatic disorder.

URINARY FREQUENCY

▼ **Description.** Urinary frequency, often accompanied by urgency, occurs at two points in the pregnancy. In the first trimester, frequency occurs as the growing uterus exerts pressure on the bladder. By the second trimester when the uterus is large enough that it moves out of the pelvis, the pressure is temporarily relieved and frequency may subside, despite the fact that the glomerular filtration rate increases. Frequency again becomes a problem in the third trimester as the large uterus and the presenting part of the baby press against the bladder. The muscle relaxant effects of progesterone may decrease the tone of the bladder and urethra, so that leakage of urine is common.

▼ **Management.** Urinary frequency during pregnancy can be relieved in several ways. The bladder should be emptied frequently as soon as the urge to void is perceived to avoid bladder distention and urinary stasis. The bladder should be emptied completely as well. Fluids should not be decreased during the day. However, as evening approaches, the woman may decrease fluids to prevent nocturia and interrupted sleep. Caffeinated beverages such as tea, coffee, or cola should be avoided. Kegel exercises should be done daily to improve pelvic floor muscle tone (see Teaching Guide: Kegel Exercises later in this chapter). If urinary leakage is a problem, panty liners can be worn (Jimenez 1992).

If no other symptoms of a urinary tract infection are present, the symptoms of frequency, urgency, and leakage are considered to be normal in pregnancy. However, if pain, burning, or hematuria occurs, the physician should be notified immediately.

FATIGUE AND DROWSINESS

▼ **Description.** Many women experience profound fatigue or drowsiness in early pregnancy. The exact cause of fatigue is unknown, but it is thought to be due to increasing levels of estrogen, progesterone, hCG, or relaxin. The normal 25 percent elevation in the basal metabolic rate during pregnancy may also contribute to fatigue as well as to shortness of breath, energy depletion resulting from the physiologic and psychological changes occurring during the first trimester, anemia, and increased weight (Bennett 1984; Poole 1986; Jimenez 1992).

▼ **Management.** The best way for the pregnant woman to counter fatigue is to sleep at least 7 to 8 hours each night. If her schedule permits, afternoon naps are also helpful. If she is working, brief rest periods and use of relaxation techniques during coffee breaks are advisable. A well-balanced diet should be maintained with the addition of an iron supplement. Regular exercise and social activity are stimulating and can decrease the feeling of fatigue; however, overexertion should be avoided. The woman should also avoid medications advertised for increasing energy and excessive caffeine intake (Jimenez 1992). If fatigue is profound or constant, additional contributing factors should be explored, such as inadequate nutrition, anemia, excessive weight gain, infection, lack of exercise, excessive activity, or emotional responses to pregnancy.

INCREASED VAGINAL DISCHARGE

▼ **Description.** Many women notice an increased thin, colorless or yellow vaginal discharge throughout pregnancy. The increase in the amount of discharge may be bothersome, but it is usually a normal alteration.

Increased vaginal discharge is caused by the increase in estrogen levels, which stimulates increased production of mucus by the endocervical glands and hyperplasia of the vaginal mucosa. Increased pelvic pressure also contributes to the increase in vaginal discharge. The discharge is often profuse, thin, and usually light yellow or white in color (leukorrhea).

▼ **Management.** Good hygiene is important in dealing with this increased discharge. Keeping the perineal area clean and dry prevents irritation and infection from occurring. It is advisable to wear cotton underwear, which is cooler and allows air to circulate. Tight clothing and pantyhose should be avoided for the same reason. If the vaginal discharge is profuse, panty liners may be desirable, but the woman should not wear tampons as they may increase the likelihood for development of an infection or toxic shock syndrome. The panty liners should be changed frequently. Douching should not be used as a method of cleansing during pregnancy as it can force bacteria upward in the reproductive tract or inject air that could result in an air embolus. Feminine hygiene sprays and powders should be avoided (Jimenez 1992).

If the vaginal discharge has a foul odor or changes in character or color or if the woman has pruritus, she should contact her caregiver. If the amount of discharge is too much for a panty liner, she should see her caregiver to rule out rupture of membranes. Because vaginal secretions become less acidic during pregnancy, organisms are able to grow more easily. Differential diagnosis should be made to rule out *Candida albicans* or sexually transmitted infections. The woman's partner should also be evaluated if signs of a vaginal infection persist.

NASAL STUFFINESS OR EPISTAXIS

▼ **Description.** Some women experience nasal congestion or stuffiness during pregnancy, feeling as though they have an allergy or cold. Other women may have occasional nosebleeds.

Elevated estrogen levels may cause edema of the nasal mucosa. Increased nasal dryness, discharge, obstruction, or nosebleeds (epistaxis) may result.

▼ **Management.** Normal saline nose drops or spray may be safely used in pregnancy to counteract nasal stuffiness. Cool-air vaporizers or humidifiers may also help. The woman should avoid the use of oral decongestants and antihistamines as they may have an effect on fetal development (see Chapter 15) or raise maternal blood pressure. If a nosebleed occurs, the woman should pinch the nostrils shut for about 10 minutes; an ice pack applied to the bridge of the nose is also helpful. If the bleeding continues, the nose can be packed with cotton or gauze (Jimenez 1992). If epistaxis becomes frequent or profuse and does not respond to the preceding treatment, the woman should consult her physician to rule out more serious respiratory tract problems or hypertension.

SYNCOPE OR HYPOTENSION

▼ **Description.** In the first trimester of pregnancy, the woman may experience dizziness or faintness from vasomotor lability or postural hypotension caused by hormonal changes. Increased blood volume, anemia, hypoglycemia, peripheral venous pooling, sudden changes in position, and fatigue may also be contributing factors. Later in pregnancy, the woman may experience supine hypotension (also known as the inferior vena cava syndrome) and dizziness caused by the pressure of the uterus on the ascending vena cava when she is supine.

▼ **Management.** The first step in dealing with syncope or hypotension is to recognize the symptoms. Lightheadedness, dizziness, or a narrowing of the field of vision is commonly described. The woman should then be instructed to sit or lie down immediately and lower her head. Applying pressure with the thumbnail or fingernail to the skin just above the center of the upper lip for 60 seconds may prevent the fainting spell. The woman should avoid prolonged standing or sitting in one position for this allows pooling of the blood and leads to syncope. Sudden changes in position should be avoided, and the woman should move slowly and deliberately. When recumbent, she should lie on either side rather than on her back. Warm, crowded areas should be avoided, and fresh air should always be plentiful. Moderate exercise and deep breathing may be helpful. Eating frequent small meals throughout the day will prevent hypoglycemia. Sufficient rest and iron and vitamin supplements are important (Jimenez 1992). If symptoms persist or become more serious, the physician should be consulted to rule out more serious circulatory or neurologic problems.

Second Trimester

HEMORRHOIDS

▼ **Description.** Hemorrhoids are enlarged veins, similar to the varicose veins that develop in some women's legs. They may be internal or protrude externally through the anus, feeling like a soft lump or bulge. Hemorrhoids can cause bleeding, itching, or pain.

Hemorrhoids during pregnancy are caused by several factors. Increased blood volume places additional pressure on venous circulation in the rectum and anus, and increased pressure from the enlarging uterus restricts venous return from blood vessels in the perineal area. Constipation from relaxation of the smooth muscle of the bowel and the resultant straining at stool contribute to hemorrhoid development. Symptoms of hemorrhoids usually include itching, swelling, pain, or bleeding with defecation. If hemorrhoids are not a problem for the woman in pregnancy, they may become evident in the early postpartum period as a result of pushing in the second stage of labor. Hemorrhoids may be internal, located above the anal sphincter, or external, located outside the anal sphincter. By the end of the puerperium, hemorrhoids usually become asymptomatic and may disappear.

▼ **Management.** Remedies for the symptoms of hemorrhoids include ice packs, warm or cool sitz baths, gentle cleansing, or topical ointments and anesthetic agents. Kegel exercises help strengthen the perineum and control hemorrhoids (see Teaching Guide: Kegel Exercises later in this chapter). Prevention of constipation, achieved by the methods suggested later in this chapter, is important. If the hemorrhoids are external, relief of discomfort may be achieved by gently reinserting the hemorrhoid. This can be done by the woman as she lies on her side or places pillows under her hips. The woman should first place pressure against the rectal sphincter for a few minutes to relax it. A lubricant is then used on the finger to press the hemorrhoids inside, holding them in place for a couple of minutes. Once the finger is withdrawn, the anal sphincter should then hold the hemorrhoids inside the rectum (Jimenez 1992). If bleeding or pain becomes excessive, the woman should consult her caregiver to assess whether thrombosis of the hemorrhoids has occurred.

BRAXTON HICKS CONTRACTIONS

▼ **Description.** Braxton Hicks contractions are the normal irregular, painless contractions of the uterus that occur throughout the pregnancy. The woman will feel her uterus harden for a number of seconds and then soften again. Some women even notice the uterus rising in the abdomen. Braxton Hicks contractions may be triggered by activity or exercise, or they may occur for no reason at all. They may also be noticed after sexual intercourse, especially if the woman has experienced an orgasm.

Braxton Hicks contractions are caused by increased estrogen levels and distention of the uterus. They probably begin in the first trimester but are not felt by the woman or palpated by her physician until about the fourth month. Multiparous women usually perceive these contractions earlier and experience more of them than do primiparous women. Braxton Hicks contractions help to promote uteroplacental circulation and enhance good uterine muscle tone in preparation for labor.

▼ **Management.** Braxton Hicks contractions are usually not bothersome enough to interrupt the woman's daily routine or to warrant comfort measures. However, if they are bothersome, the woman should evaluate their character (frequency, interval, duration) to assess whether they seem to be progressing to an early labor pattern (see Chapter 23 for a contrast of true and false labor). She can rest in the left lateral position or try a mild exercise such as walking. Massage of the abdomen may decrease any discomfort experienced. Braxton Hicks contractions provide an excellent time to practice relaxation and breathing techniques (Horan 1984; Jimenez 1992).

If more than four contractions per hour are experienced, the woman should begin to keep a written log of the contractions. If the contractions do not stop or if they progress to a regular pattern, the woman should call her caregiver immediately and be evaluated for preterm or true labor.

ROUND LIGAMENT PAIN

▼ **Description.** The round ligaments are like guidewires that suspend the uterus in the abdominal cavity (see Figs. 9–8 and 9–9). The stretching of these ligaments as the uterus becomes larger may cause occasional sensations of tenderness or sharp pain.

▼ **Management.** The woman can decrease discomfort from round ligament stretching by using good body mechanics when bending or lifting to avoid overstretching or sudden twisting or jerking movements. Bending at the waist toward the area of discomfort lets the ligament relax and relieves the pain. Strenuous exercise should be avoided. Bringing the knees to the chest, either when lying prone or by squatting, may help. Rest, relaxation techniques, heat, and effleurage of the area of discomfort may also relieve painful sensation (Horan 1984; Jimenez 1992). If round ligament pain becomes constant (lasting longer than 2 minutes) or severe, differential diagnosis should be made for preterm labor, ovarian cyst, ectopic pregnancy, constipation, appendicitis, urinary tract infection, or inguinal hernia.

CONSTIPATION

▼ **Description.** Minor alterations in the gastrointestinal system caused by the hormonal changes of pregnancy result in a number of gastrointestinal symptoms for the pregnant woman. She may experience bloating, abdominal tenderness, or fatigue as a result.

The increased levels of progesterone that cause smooth muscle relaxation and increased water reabsorption result in bowel sluggishness. In addition to the hormonal influence, the pressure of the enlarging uterus on the colon and rectum also contributes to constipation. Other factors that can contribute to constipation during pregnancy include iron supplements, diet, insufficient fluids, and lack of exercise.

▼ **Management.** Constipation can be treated with increased fluids (six to eight glasses per day) and a diet high in fiber and roughage. Juices or warm beverages in the morning are helpful. Even though many women have hectic, busy lives, attention should be paid to establishing a regular schedule for bowel habits. Increasing exercise is an excellent way to improve gastric motility. If none of these natural remedies works, mild laxatives, stool softeners, or suppositories recommended by the physician or midwife may be used. Mineral oil should never be used as a stool softener since it inhibits the absorption of fat-soluble vitamins. Caution should be taken not to become dependent on laxatives for regular bowel function. If constipation becomes a serious problem, the woman should be assessed to rule out fecal impaction, irritable colon, or atonic colon.

VARICOSITIES

▼ **Description.** Varicose veins are enlarged, distended, tortuous superficial veins. They are most commonly located in the legs and rectum. They may cause aching or a sensation of heaviness in the affected area. Varicose veins seem to be familial.

During pregnancy, varicose veins are caused either by relaxation in the walls of veins due to hormonal influences and increased blood volume or by poor valve functioning resulting in stasis and pooling in the veins of the lower extremities. The weight of the pregnant uterus in the pelvis also contributes to the development of varicosities in the pelvic area and lower extremities by preventing good venous return. Not all pregnant women have varicosities. Other influencing factors, such as heredity, age, weight gain, a large baby, or multiple gestation, play a part in their development. Women who have varicosities experience a tired, aching, or throbbing feeling in the legs. The veins of the legs may become discolored and prominent. Vulvar or perineal varicosities may also develop as a result of increased pelvic pressure.

▼ **Management.** Preventive measures or treatments for varicose veins include measures to promote venous return, such as frequently elevating the legs above the level of the body (Fig. 19–1), changing positions often and not standing for long periods, exercising regularly, and wearing supportive hose. Supportive hose should be placed on the legs before arising while the legs are elevated. Measures to prevent constriction of veins include avoidance of garters, knee-high hosiery with constrictive bands, or crossing the legs at the knees. Relief of vulvar varicosities can be achieved by wearing a perineal pad for support. If varicosities become severe, the woman should be evaluated for the development of phlebothrombosis and thrombophlebitis (Jimenez 1992).

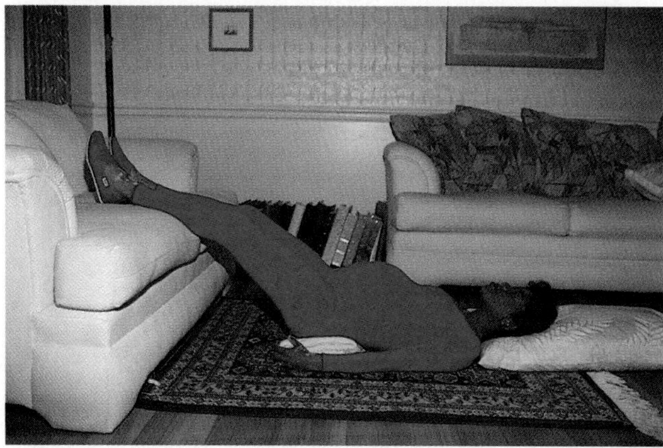

Figure 19–1
Elevating the legs above the level of the body helps increase venous return and promotes comfort. After the fourth month of pregnancy, a pillow or wedge should be placed under the hip to help prevent supine hypotension.

Third Trimester

BACKACHE

▼ **Description.** One of the most common complaints of pregnant women is backache. Although it is usually perceived in the low back, some women have pain in the upper back too. This discomfort may be noticed in relation to activity or prolonged periods of standing, or it may occur for no reason at all.

Backache in pregnancy is caused by the increased weight of the growing baby and uterus pulling forward on the low back muscles. The changing center of gravity that results and poor support from lax abdominal muscles cause a compensatory lordosis (increased curvature of the lumbosacral vertebrae) and muscle strain. The influence of estrogen and relaxin on pelvic ligaments also contributes to backache. Other contributing factors might include excessive weight gain, fatigue, high-heeled shoes, and poor posture.

▼ **Management.** Backache can be prevented or relieved in several ways. The pelvic rock exercise, which can be done in a standing position or on the hands and knees, is an excellent technique for relieving backache (see Fig. 19–8). Good posture to correct the lordosis and good body mechanics to prevent muscle strain are probably the most important measures for preventing backache.

Good posture in pregnancy involves standing up straight so that the head, upper trunk, pelvis, and lower extremities are in alignment. The knees should be slightly bent and buttocks tucked under (Fig. 19–2).

Good body mechanics include rising properly from a recumbent position and bending and lifting so that back muscles are not strained. When rising from a recumbent position, the woman should not do a "sit-up." This places too much strain on low back and abdominal muscles. Instead, she should roll over to her side and use her arms to walk her body to a sitting position. When bending or lifting, the woman should not lean forward

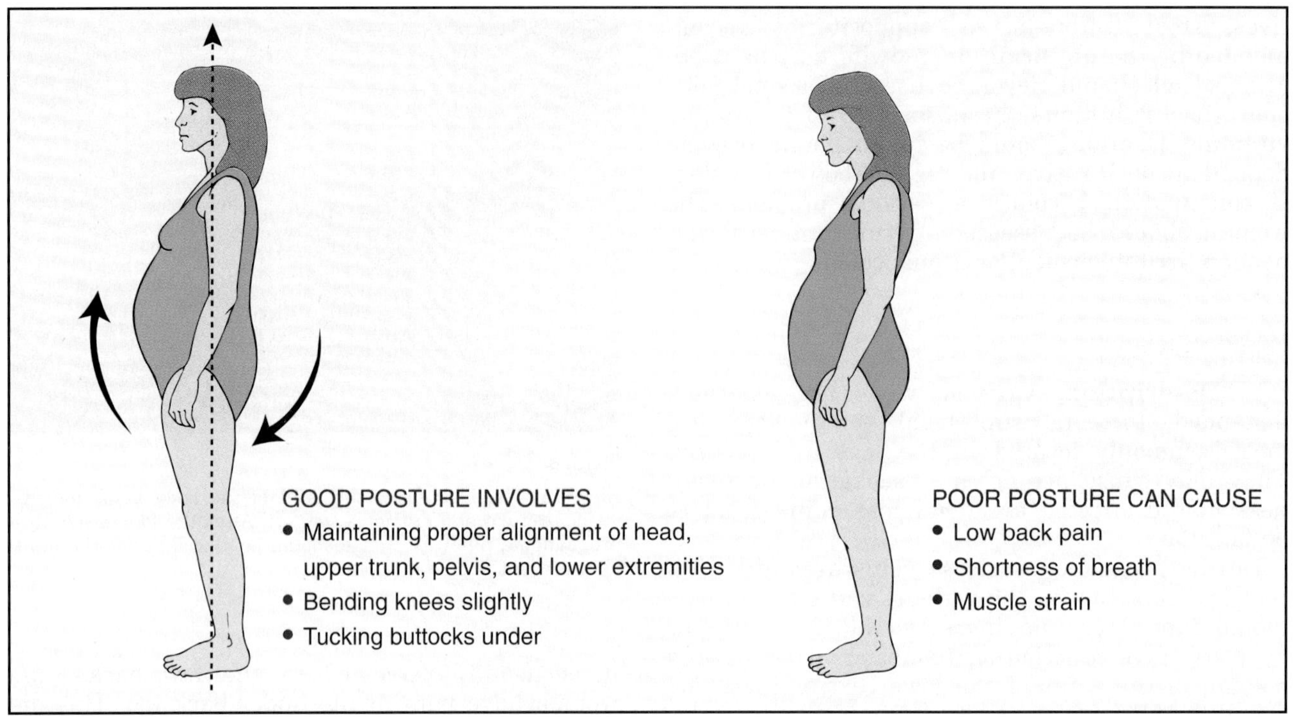

Figure 19–2
Maintaining good posture during pregnancy helps prevent backache by countering lordosis (increased curvature of the lumbosacral vertebrae).

from the waist. This places too much strain on low back muscles. Instead, she should use a squatting position with legs wide apart. If lifting an object, the woman should hold it close to the body. The thigh muscles should be used to straighten the body to a standing position (Fig. 19–3).

Wearing flat, supportive shoes during pregnancy also helps relieve backache. The woman may want to try a supportive maternity girdle. Avoiding overexertion, resting frequently in the side-lying position, sleeping on a firm mattress, using relaxation techniques, and applying heat to the area of discomfort are also helpful. Use of a small pillow to support the abdomen while in the side-lying position has been found to prevent or alleviate backache (Thomas et al. 1989). A good back massage from the partner or a friend usually feels wonderful and promotes muscle relaxation (Horan 1984; Jimenez 1992).

If backache becomes severe, the woman should notify her caregiver so that other problems can be ruled out, such as acute back muscle strain, anatomic musculoskeletal defects, or preterm labor.

LEG CRAMPS

▼ **Description.** Leg cramps, or "charley horses," in the third trimester of pregnancy are spasms of the gastrocnemius muscles. They are experienced as a sudden stabbing pain that grabs the calf. Leg cramps often occur at night during sleep or in the morning on stretching.

Leg cramps are caused by compression of the uterus on the nerves supplying the lower extremities or by blood vessel occlusion in the legs. These cramps may also be aggravated by a disturbance in the calcium/phosphorus ratio (too little calcium; too much phosphorus), poor peripheral circulation, pointing the toes on stretching, or muscle strain and fatigue. They most often occur at night but may occur at any time of day.

▼ **Management.** Leg cramps can be relieved by stretching the affected muscle. Methods for stretching the affected muscle include dorsiflexing the foot with the knee extended (Fig. 19–4), using heat over the affected muscle, or standing on a cold surface. Warm baths, elevating legs on a pillow, loosening the covers while sleeping, and regular exercise help to decrease leg cramps. The woman should avoid pointing her toes to avoid contracting muscles that may begin to cramp. The woman should evaluate her calcium intake and maintain it at four servings of dairy products a day. If calcium intake is insufficient, oral supplementation with calcium carbonate or calcium lactate tablets may be helpful. The amount of phosphorus in the diet can be decreased by lowering soft drink intake or by taking antacids containing aluminum hydroxide to bind the phosphorus (Ho-

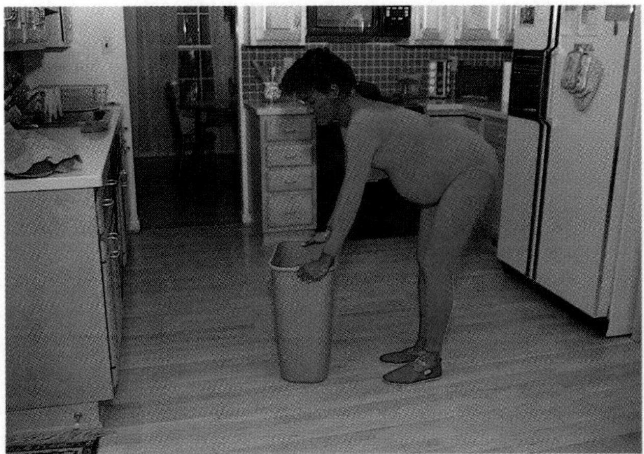

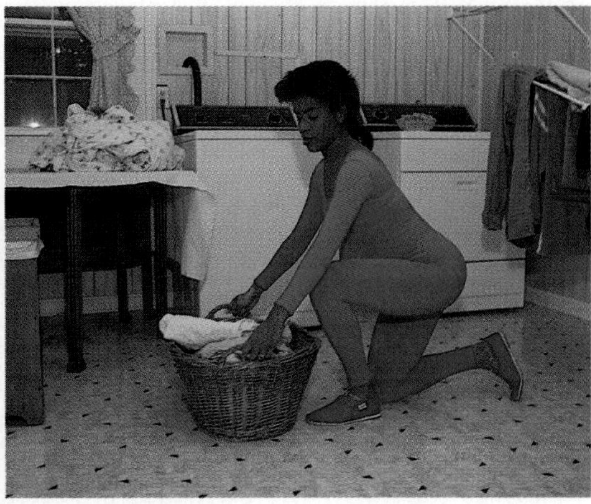

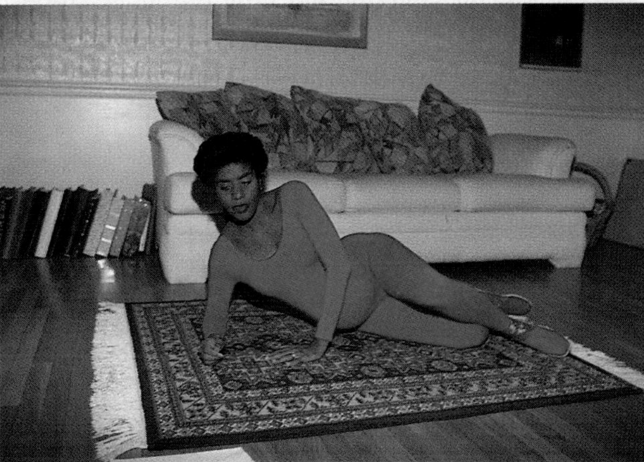

Figure 19–3

Using good body mechanics during pregnancy helps prevent muscle strain and backache. • When lifting objects, avoid bending at the waist because it strains low back muscles. • When bending and lifting, squat down close to the object to be lifted and hold the object close to the body while using the thigh muscles (not back muscles) to straighten the body to a standing position. • When rising from a recumbent position, roll to your side and use your arms to push your body up to a sitting position.

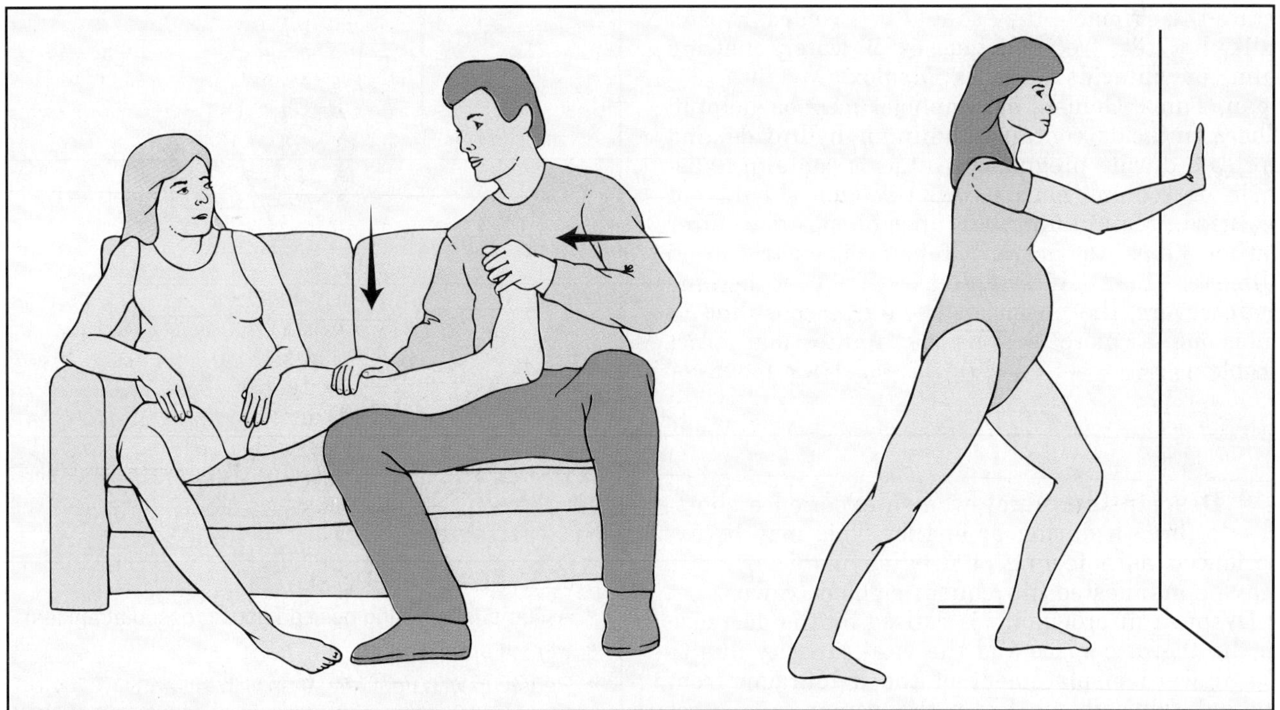

Figure 19–4

Leg cramps can be relieved by stretching the affected muscle. Two methods for stretching the affected muscle are (1) dorsiflexing the foot with the knee extended and (2) standing on the leg and leaning the body weight forward.

ran 1984; Jimenez 1992). If leg cramps become persistent or severe, the woman should be evaluated for phlebitis or thrombophlebitis by checking for the Homans sign, the occurrence of pain when the leg is extended and the foot dorsiflexed.

HEARTBURN

Description. Heartburn, also known as acid indigestion during pregnancy, is experienced as a burning or painful sensation in the stomach or esophagus. Some women experience a sudden sensation of burning acid in the throat, particularly when they are lying in a prone position.

Heartburn is caused by the increased production of progesterone, which causes decreased gastrointestinal motility and increases relaxation of the cardiac sphincter. Relaxation of tone in the gastrointestinal tract, along with displacement of the stomach and duodenum by the enlarging uterus, causes delayed emptying of the stomach and regurgitation of acidic gastric contents into the esophagus. Reflux causes a burning sensation in the esophagus that may even radiate upward, causing burping and leaving an unpleasant taste in the mouth.

Management. Remedies for heartburn consist of eating small and more frequent meals and avoiding fatty, fried, spicy, or gas-producing foods. It may also help to eliminate drinking liquids with meals. The woman should avoid eating just before going to bed. Since coffee and cigarettes irritate the stomach, they should be avoided. Sips of milk, hot tea, frequent glasses of water, chewing gum, or antacids such as Maalox, Mylanta, Riopan, Tums, Gelusil, or Amphojel may be helpful. These antacids contain aluminum hydroxide and are safe during pregnancy. Antacids containing aspirin or sodium, such as Alka-Seltzer, should not be used. Maintaining an upright position after eating helps to prevent reflux of gastric fluid (Jimenez 1992). If symptoms persist or become more severe, the physician should be consulted to rule out a more serious gastrointestinal tract problem.

DYSPNEA

Description. Many women experience shortness of breath during pregnancy. This may be experienced as a feeling of needing more air, or it may be manifested in frequent sighs or yawns.

Dyspnea in pregnancy is caused by the decrease in the thoracic space and the vital capacity due to the upward displacement of the diaphragm from the enlarging uterus. When the woman is in a recumbent position, dyspnea is further aggravated by uterine compression of the vena cava, causing decreased venous return to the heart and arterial hypotension. The woman will experience some relief of shortness of breath when the baby drops, lightening occurs, and thoracic space is increased.

Management. Dyspnea can be relieved by using good posture (see Fig. 19–2). The tailor reach exercise (Fig. 19–5) is helpful because it expands the thoracic space. Overexertion should be avoided, and the woman should rest after exercising. If the woman experiences shortness of breath at night, she should sleep in the semi-Fowler position with extra pillows or in the left lateral position. These positions help by allowing better lung expansion. Eating small meals will promote comfort. If the woman smokes, she should stop immediately, for smoking not only influences fetal development (see Chapter 15) but also contributes to shortness of breath (Jimenez 1992). If symptoms become severe, the woman should be evaluated for anemia, thoracic deformities, emphysema, asthma, or other pulmonary disease.

INSOMNIA

Description. Insomnia during the third trimester of pregnancy is a common occurrence for many women and can be caused by a number of

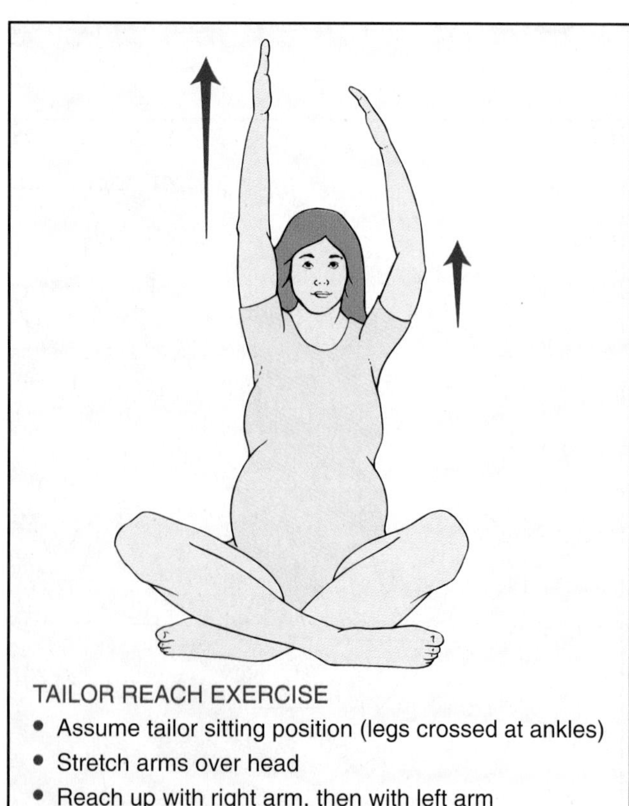
TAILOR REACH EXERCISE
• Assume tailor sitting position (legs crossed at ankles)
• Stretch arms over head
• Reach up with right arm, then with left arm

Figure 19–5

The tailor reach exercise helps relieve symptoms of dyspnea or heartburn during pregnancy by expanding the thoracic space.

factors. Difficulty finding a comfortable position for sleeping due to the large uterus is often a primary cause. Fetal activity may make it difficult for the woman to sleep as well. Urinary frequency may awaken the woman, and then she may find it difficult to go back to sleep. Other factors that interrupt sleep may be indigestion, heartburn, leg cramps, dyspnea, and anxiety.

▼ **Management.** Measures to assist with comfortable positioning may be helpful in promoting sleep. Extra pillows to elevate the head and chest to counteract dyspnea or heartburn or to place under the legs for support in the lateral recumbent position can be used. It may help to sleep with a window open for fresh air. A back massage and use of conscious relaxation techniques should be employed. Avoiding caffeinated beverages and decreasing fluid intake before bedtime help with nocturia and sleeplessness. Warm milk and a warm shower just before bedtime may promote sleep. Milk contains a natural element called tryptophan that helps induce relaxation. A cup of chamomile or lemon tea with honey before bedtime may also help. Daily exercise may help to relieve tension or anxiety and promote fatigue. If insomnia becomes regular, the woman should consult her physician. She should not use sleeping medications without consultation because of the potential effects on fetal development (Jimenez 1992) (see Chapter 15).

EPULIS

▼ **Description.** The increased vascularity and proliferation of connective tissue caused by increased estrogen in pregnancy may cause gingivitis and epulis (hyperemia, hypertrophy, bleeding, or tenderness) of the gums. The gums may bleed when touched or with brushing of the teeth.

▼ **Management.** Epulis can be treated with good oral hygiene to prevent infection. This includes gentle brushing with a soft brush, flossing, and use of a warm saline or astringent mouthwash. A well-balanced diet high in protein, vitamin C, fruits, and vegetables is helpful. Regular visits to the dentist for routine cleaning are important. The dentist or physician should be consulted if gums become infected or if more serious symptoms appear.

EDEMA

▼ **Description.** Most women experience some edema during pregnancy, and it becomes most pronounced in the third trimester. Normal edema in pregnancy is usually limited to the lower extremities (pedal edema), but it may also occur in the hands. The woman may notice that her rings or her shoes are tighter than usual.

Edema is caused by the influence of hormonal changes on sodium and water retention and capillary permeability. Increased aldosterone leads to increased sodium retention, resulting in increased water retention. Factors that also contribute to edema are increased venous pressure due to increased blood volume, decreased venous return from dependent body parts, varicose veins, prolonged standing or sitting, hot weather, increased intake of sodium, and protein deficiency in the diet.

▼ **Management.** Edema can be prevented or relieved by incorporating regular rest periods in the left lateral position to facilitate circulation. Wearing support hose and elevating the legs when sitting also help. Frequent rotation of the ankles and dorsiflexion of the feet when sitting are helpful. Regular exercise enhances circulation. Tight garters or knee-high hosiery should be avoided. Dietary alterations should be made to decrease sodium, fat, and carbohydrate intake and increase protein. The woman should drink six to eight glasses of fluid a day to aid in diuresis. Diuretic drugs should not be taken (Jimenez 1992). If edema becomes generalized, is present on arising, or is accompanied by other symptoms of preeclampsia, the woman should notify her caregiver to be evaluated further. (See Chapter 21 for a discussion of hypertensive disorders of pregnancy.)

Warning Signs in Pregnancy

Although the majority of physical symptoms experienced during pregnancy are a result of normal physiologic processes, symptoms may occur that signal alterations from the normal. It is essential that the pregnant woman be informed about the symptoms that are warning signs of potential complications of pregnancy and that she be instructed to report these symptoms at once should they occur. A printed list of these symptoms should be given to the woman for reference at home (see Warning Signs to Report).

▼ **Vaginal Bleeding.** Any vaginal bleeding other than a light pink mucous spotting or brownish spotting at term may indicate the occurrence of a threatened abortion, ectopic pregnancy, placenta previa, or abruptio placentae. The woman should be instructed to call her caregiver immediately and to go to the hospital emergency department.

▼ **Premature Rupture of Membranes.** Premature rupture of membranes, experienced as a

Warning Signs to Report

- Vaginal bleeding
- Premature rupture of membranes
- Preterm uterine contractions
- Change in or absence of fetal activity
- Severe headaches
- Visual disturbances
- Rapid weight gain
- Epigastric pain
- Generalized or facial edema
- Persistent vomiting
- Abdominal pain
- Signs of infection

sudden gush or trickling or steady leak of clear fluid from the vagina before the estimated date of confinement, needs to be reported immediately.

▼ **Preterm Labor Contractions.** Preterm labor contractions, experienced as a regular, progressive pattern of uterine contractions accompanied by menstrual-like cramps, low backache, or pelvic pressure, should be reported at once so that infection can be prevented and preterm labor can be ruled out (see Chapter 21).

▼ **Change in Fetal Activity.** Any change in fetal activity for a period of 24 hours should be reported. This might include an increase, a decrease, or a cessation of fetal movement and could indicate fetal distress or fetal demise.

▼ **Symptoms of Preeclampsia.** Symptoms such as severe headaches, visual disturbances, jitteriness, rapid weight gain, epigastric pain, and generalized or facial edema may indicate preeclampsia and should be brought to the attention of the physician as soon as possible (see Chapter 21).

▼ **Vomiting or Abdominal Discomfort.** Persistent vomiting and abdominal pain are not normal pregnancy discomforts and may be indicative of complications such as hyperemesis gravidarum, appendicitis, or abruptio placentae.

▼ **Signs of Infection.** Any signs of infection, such as fever, chills, burning with urination, or diarrhea, should have medical attention.

NUTRITION IN PREGNANCY

Many factors, such as age, inherited characteristics, sociocultural influences, trauma, stress, illness, exposure to harmful chemicals, smoking, or alcohol, interact to determine the woman's health status and the progress and outcome of a pregnancy. Nurses who maintain healthy lifestyles themselves are more effective in teaching their clients sound health habits that promote healthy pregnancies (see Improving Your Practice: How to Help Pregnant Clients Maintain a Healthy Lifestyle). Probably the most important influence on the health of the pregnant woman is her nutritional status, both before and during the pregnancy. Poor nutrition has been found to result in low-birth-weight babies; an increased risk of fetal anomalies; increased risks during pregnancy, labor, and birth; and an increased susceptibility of the newborn to illness in the first year of life. Poor nutrition during pregnancy can also negatively influence brain development in the fetus and newborn (Winick 1970, 1986; Worthington-Roberts and Williams 1993).

One commonly held theory regarding the effects of poor nutrition on the baby relates to the potential effects of malnutrition on placental efficiency. During pregnancy, the woman and her fetus have a synergistic relationship, that is, they interact and function together through the placenta. The efficiency of the placenta throughout pregnancy is influenced by its size, and the size of the placenta is influenced by the woman's nutritional status. If the placenta is small because of maternal malnutrition, there will be decreased placental blood flow to and from the fetus. Maternal malnutrition can also result in reduced maternal blood volume expansion and an adequate increase in cardiac output. The potential result of these alterations is decreased nutrient, oxygen, and metabolic end-product transport leading to fetal growth retardation. Despite the common acceptance of this theory, it is difficult to obtain substantial proof from human research that placental insufficiency alone limits the supply of nutrients to the baby when the circulation on both sides is intact. Other, yet unproven, factors in the maternal organism may also influence malnutrition (Committee on Maternal Nutrition, Food and Nutrition Board 1970; Lechtig et al. 1975; Winick 1970, 1986).

Pregnant women are often bombarded with information and advice about their diet by health professionals, childbirth classes, books, news reports, or radio and television commercials. Unfor-

IMPROVING YOUR PRACTICE

HOW TO HELP PREGNANT CLIENTS MAINTAIN A HEALTHY LIFESTYLE

Nurses can more effectively promote healthy pregnancies for their clients if they live healthy lifestyles themselves. A nurse cannot be effective in teaching health promotion if the nurse's own health habits are not sound. The following steps assist nurses to improve their own health status.

- COMPLETE A PERSONAL HEALTH ASSESSMENT. Evaluate your own nutrition, exercise, health habits, and stress levels. Be honest. Make plans to improve the behaviors that are not contributing to your own good health.
- KEEP A FOOD DIARY FOR A WEEK. Record all foods that you eat and your pattern of eating. Evaluate whether your diet includes the appropriate food groups and nutrients. Assess the influence that fatigue, stress, or socialization has on your eating patterns. Make an attempt to decrease "junk foods."
- INCREASE YOUR EXERCISE. Plan your daily schedule so that you can incorporate some type of regular exercise into your routine, even if only for 15 to 20 minutes each day.
- STOP SMOKING, STOP RECREATIONAL DRUGS, OR DECREASE YOUR ALCOHOL INTAKE. If you engage in any of these habits, make a plan to alter them in some way. Enlist the support of a friend or colleague.
- TRY A STRESS REDUCTION TECHNIQUE. The next time you experience a stressful situation, respond by trying a new relaxation strategy. Practice the relaxation you teach to pregnant women in your own life.
- ATTEND A WELLNESS SEMINAR OR READ A BOOK ON HEALTH PROMOTION. These learning experiences not only will enhance your personal life but can also be beneficial continuing professional education that will enable you to promote healthy behavior with your clients more effectively.

tunately, these sources may be conflicting, and the information they communicate may change from time to time. Much of the nutritional counseling given to pregnant women has been based on beliefs gained through life experiences, informal observations, or old wives' tales rather than on a scientific basis resulting from controlled research studies. Knowledge about the effects of nutrition on health and on pregnancy is still developing. It is difficult to design studies with humans that can show a direct relationship between what a woman eats during the 9 months of gestation and the course and outcome of the pregnancy. However, it is important that nurses base their nutritional counseling on current research that is available and current dietary recommendations. Pregnancy is a time when women are often highly motivated to make positive changes in their nutritional habits. These changes can become part of their lifestyle even after the pregnancy is over and can contribute to better nutritional health for the entire family (Wilkerson 1988).

Variables Influencing Good Nutrition

LIFESTYLE

Many factors influence the woman's ability to maintain a good diet during pregnancy. The complexities of our American lifestyles can make it difficult to eat well. For example, busy schedules interrupt regular mealtimes and decrease the time necessary for good meal preparation. As a result, families either prepare convenience foods or eat out, often at fast-food restaurants. Sixty percent of the American diet is now composed of convenience foods, and 30 percent of the meals Americans consume are eaten outside the home. These foods are often high in calories, sodium, and fat and low in essential nutrients. The hectic American lifestyle may lead to increased stress, which may also negatively influence eating habits.

MYTHS

Myths and old wives' tales about foods that should or should not be eaten in pregnancy can influence good nutrition. For example, in the late nineteenth century, women were encouraged to eat a diet consisting only of fruit. This was thought to decrease pain in childbirth by producing a baby with small flexible bones. Women have been advised to avoid salty or sour foods so that the infant would not have a "sour" disposition (Worthington-Roberts and Williams 1993).

PHYSICAL HEALTH

The woman's physical health status, including how well she feels and the minor discomforts of pregnancy that she experiences, also influences her appetite and her desire to eat well. Emotional, sociocultural, and cognitive factors affect good nutrition as well and are discussed in more detail later in this chapter.

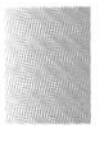

Physical Aspects of Nutrition in Pregnancy

NUTRITIONAL REQUIREMENTS

During pregnancy, there should be an increase in all nutrients to meet the physiologic demands of maternal changes and fetal growth. The food guide pyramid (Fig. 19–6) and Table 19–2 provide guidelines for a healthy diet. Table 19–3 (p. 514) gives all recommended dietary allowances (RDAs) for pregnancy and lactation. The amount of increase in essential nutrients for each woman depends on a number of factors. The general nutritional status before pregnancy, current health status, age and parity, amount of time between pregnancies, height and bone structure, weight, and activity level all influence prenatal diet. If the woman's health status is poor, her illness places additional demands on her body that may increase nutritional requirements. Adolescents who are pregnant before the cessation of their own growth do not have the physiologic maturity to withstand the additional stresses of pregnancy and have greater nutritional requirements than do adults. Adolescent pregnancies have been associated with low birth weight, short gestational periods, and perinatal mortality (see Chapter 39). High parity or conceptions that occur more often than 12 months apart deplete the woman's nutritional reserves. Low pre-pregnancy weight and insufficient weight gain during pregnancy may result in low-birth-weight infants and other pregnancy complications. All these factors should be considered in planning a diet for a pregnant woman.

KEY
○ Fat (naturally occurring and added)
▽ Sugars (added)
These symbols show fats, oils, and added sugars in foods
USE SPARINGLY
Fats, oils, and sweets
2–3 SERVINGS
Milk, yogurt, and cheese group
2–3 SERVINGS
Meat, poultry, fish, dry beans,eggs, and nuts group
3–5 SERVINGS
Vegetable group
2–4 SERVINGS
Fruit group
6–11 SERVINGS
Bread, cereal, rice, and pasta group

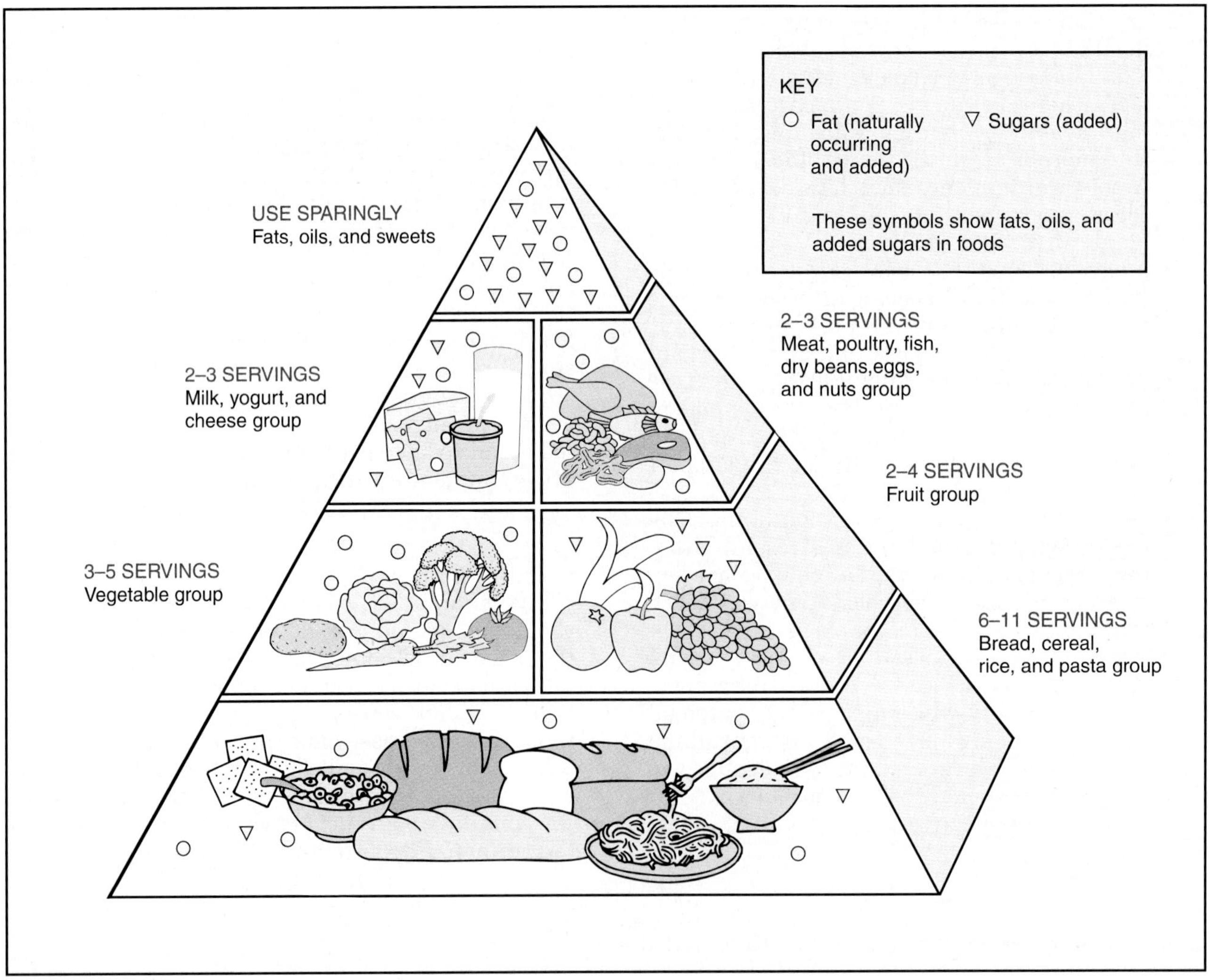

Figure 19–6

The food guide pyramid is an excellent teaching tool to help pregnant women learn about the foods they need to eat during pregnancy. (From U. S. Department of Agriculture/U. S. Department of Health and Human Services, Washington, D.C.)

Table 19–2

USE OF THE DAILY FOOD GUIDE

What Counts as One Serving?

Breads, Cereals, Rice, and Pasta
1 slice of bread
½ cup of cooked rice or pasta
½ cup of cooked cereal
1 ounce of ready-to-eat cereal

Vegetables
½ cup of chopped raw or cooked vegetables
1 cup of leafy raw vegetables

Fruits
1 piece of fruit or melon wedge
¾ cup of juice
½ cup of canned fruit
¼ cup of dried fruit

Milk, Yogurt, and Cheese
1 cup of milk or yogurt
1½ to 2 ounces of cheese

Meat, Poultry, Fish, Dry Beans, Eggs, and Nuts
2½ to 3 ounces of cooked lean meat, poultry, or fish

Count ½ cup of cooked beans, or 1 egg, or 2 tablespoons of peanut butter as 1 ounce of lean meat (about ⅓ serving)

Fats, Oils, and Sweets
Limit calories from these, especially if you need to lose weight.

Note: The amount you eat may be more than one serving. For example, a dinner portion of spaghetti would count as two or three servings of pasta.

How Many Servings Do You Need Each Day?

	Women and Some Older Adults	Children, Teen Girls, Active Women, Most Men	Teen Boys and Active Men
Calorie level*	About 1600	About 2200	About 2800
Bread group	6	9	11
Vegetable group	3	4	5
Fruit group	2	3	4
Milk group	2–3†	2–3†	2–3†
Meat group	2, for a total of 5 ounces	2, for a total of 6 ounces	3, for a total of 7 ounces

*These are the calorie levels if you choose low-fat, lean foods from the five major food groups and use foods from the fats, oils, and sweets group sparingly. The calorie level of pregnant women should be about 2500, and that of women who are breastfeeding should be about 2700.

†Women who are pregnant or breastfeeding, teenagers, and young adults to age 24 years need three servings.

A Closer Look at Fat and Added Sugars

The small tip of the pyramid (see Fig. 19–6) shows fats, oils, and sweets. These are foods such as salad dressings, cream, butter, margarine, sugar, soft drinks, candies, and sweet desserts. Alcoholic beverages are also part of this group. These foods provide calories but few vitamins and minerals. Most people should go easy on foods from this group.

Some fat or sugar symbols are shown in the other food groups. That is to remind you that some foods in these groups can also be high in fat and added sugars, such as cheese or ice cream from the milk group or French fries from the vegetable group. When choosing foods for a healthful diet, consider the fat and added sugars in your choices from all the food groups, not just fats, oils, and sweets from the pyramid tip.

From U.S. Department of Agriculture/U.S. Department of Health and Human Services, Washington, D.C.

Calorie Increase

Calorie requirements must be increased between 10 and 15 percent during pregnancy to meet the increased energy demands created by the physiologic changes of the woman's body and the development of the fetus. The total energy cost during pregnancy is approximately 80,000 calories. Therefore, an increase of about 300 calories (kcal) per day is needed during pregnancy (National Research Council 1989). This increase may be insufficient for many active or nutritionally deficient women. This is not a large increase compared with the needs for extra protein, vitamins, and minerals. Carbohydrates and proteins provide 4 calories per gram, and fats provide 9 calories

Table 19–3

NUTRITIONAL REQUIREMENTS DURING PREGNANCY AND LACTATION

NUTRIENT	RECOMMENDED DIETARY ALLOWANCE (RDA) For Nonpregnant Female (15–18 yr/19–24 yr/25–50 yr)	During Pregnancy	During Lactation (first 6 mo/second 6 mo)	FOOD SOURCE
Calories	2200/2200/2200	2500	2700	50% carbohydrates 30% fats 20% protein
Protein (g)	44/46/50	60	65/62	Milk, cheese, eggs, meat, fish, poultry, grains, legumes, and nuts
		Fat-soluble Vitamins		
Vitamin A (μg RE)*	800/800/800 (4000 IU/4000 IU/4000/IU)	800 (4000 IU)	1300/1200 (6500 IU/6000 IU)	Organ meats, egg yolks, butter and fortified margarine, fruits, and green and yellow vegetables
Vitamin D (μg)[†]	10/10/5 (400 IU/400 IU/200 IU)	10 (400 IU)	10/10 (400 IU/400 IU)	Fortified milk and margarine, egg yolks, liver, canned sardines, salmon, and fresh fruits and vegetables
Vitamin E (mg α-TE)[‡]	8/8/8 (11 IU/11 IU/11 IU)	10 (13 IU)	12/11 (16 IU/14 IU)	Vegetable fats and oils, whole grains, greens, and eggs
Vitamin K (μg)	55/60/65	65	65/65	Green leafy vegetables fruit, cereals, dairy products, and meat
		Water-soluble Vitamins		
Vitamin B_1 (mg) (Thiamine)	1.1/1.1/1.1	1.5	1.6	Pork, liver, milk, potatoes, enriched breads, and cereals
Vitamin B_2 (mg) (Riboflavin)	1.3/1.3/1.3	1.6	1.8/1.7	Milk, liver, eggs, enriched breads, and cereals
Vitamin B_6 (mg) (Pyridoxine)	1.5/1.6/1.6	2.2	2.1/2.1	Fish, liver, pork, potatoes, lentils, wheat germ, and yeast
Vitamin B_{12} (μg) (Cobalamin)	2.0/2.0/2.0	2.2	2.6/2.6	Milk, meat, liver, eggs, and cheese
Niacin (mg NE)[§]	15/15/15	17	20/20	Meat, poultry, fish, liver, whole grains, enriched breads, cereals, and nuts
Folic acid (μg) (Folate)	180/180/180	400	280/260	Fresh green leafy vegetables, oranges, bananas, organ meats, yeasts, dried beans peanuts, broccoli, and asparagus

Continued on facing page

Table 19–3

NUTRITIONAL REQUIREMENTS DURING PREGNANCY AND LACTATION Continued

NUTRIENT	RECOMMENDED DIETARY ALLOWANCE (RDA) For Nonpregnant Female (15–18 yr/19–24 yr/25–50 yr)	During Pregnancy	During Lactation (first 6 mo/second 6 mo)	FOOD SOURCE
		Water-soluble Vitamins (Cont'd)		
Vitamin C (mg) (Ascorbic acid)	60/60/60	70	95/90	Citrus fruits, green leafy vegetables, cantaloupe, strawberries, tomatoes, potatoes, and broccoli
		Minerals		
Iron (mg)	15/15/15	30	15/15	Lean meats, liver, shellfish, eggs, dark green leafy vegetables, legumes, whole-grain and enriched breads and cereals, and molasses
Zinc (mg)	12/12/12	15	19/16	Liver, shellfish, wheat bran, milk, oysters, eggs, and meat
Copper (mg)	3/3/3	Exact RDA unknown	Exact RDA unknown	Oysters, nuts, liver, corn oil margarine, dried legumes, and drinking water
Calcium (mg)	1200/1200/800	1200	1200/1200	Milk, yogurt, egg yolk, cheese, leafy vegetables, and whole-grain cereals and breads
Phosphorus (mg)	1200/1200/800	1200	1200/1200	Meat, chicken, eggs, milk, and cheese
Sodium (g)	2–3	Exact RDA unknown	Exact RDA unknown	Most natural foods
Magnesium (mg)	300/280/280	320	355/340	Milk, whole grains, beet greens, legumes, nuts, and tea

*Retinol equivalents; 1 RE = 1 μg retinol or 6 μg beta-carotene.

†As cholecalciferol; 10 μg cholecalciferol = 400 IU of vitamin D.

‡Alpha-tocopherol equivalents; 1 mg *d*-alpha-tocopherol = 1 alpha-TE.

§Niacin equivalents; 1 NE = 1 mg of niacin or 60 mg of dietary tryptophan.

Reprinted with permission from RECOMMENDED DIETARY ALLOWANCES: 10TH EDITION. Copyright 1989 by the National Academy of Sciences. Courtesy of the National Academy Press, Washington, D.C. "Food source" data from Whitney, E., Cataldo, C., Rolfes, S. (1994). *Understanding normal and clinical nutrition* (4th ed.). Minneapolis/St. Paul: West Publishing Company; and Worthington-Roberts, B., and Williams, S. (1993). *Nutrition in pregnancy and lactation* (5th ed.). St. Louis: C. V. Mosby.

per gram. On the average, a well-balanced diet consisting of about 2500 calories a day should meet the nutritional demands of pregnancy (Table 19–4). Calorie needs are greater in the last two trimesters than in the first. The increased calorie requirements may be partially offset by a tendency to decrease physical activity in late pregnancy. Since women differ in body size, individual needs can be calculated by allowing approximately 18 calories per pound of body weight. The simplest methods of evaluating calorie intake in pregnancy are to assess the woman's appetite and pattern of weight gain (Heslin 1993; Wilkerson 1988; Worthington-Roberts 1985).

Protein

Protein should be increased from 44 to 50 g/day in the nonpregnant woman to 60 g/day for the pregnant woman (National Research Council 1989). This increase is a general guideline, however. An individualized protein level may be calculated by allowing 1.3 g of protein per kilogram of nonpregnant desirable body weight. For adolescents, the level should be 1.5 g per kilogram of body weight. There has been some controversy among researchers regarding the desired amount of increase in protein during pregnancy, for study findings have been conflicting. For example, toxemia of pregnancy (pregnancy-induced hypertension) has been linked with both low- and high-protein diets. It is currently suggested that protein be limited to 20 percent of the total calories in the diet. An adequate protein intake without adequate calories is undesirable, for the protein is then used for maternal energy needs rather than for building tissue (Heslin 1993; Wilkerson 1988).

Protein is needed to provide additional amino acids to support rapid fetal and placental growth, enlargement of the breasts and uterus, and expansion of maternal blood volume. The demands of labor, birth, and lactation also require additional protein reserves. Protein should be of the highest quality. Recommended food sources for complete proteins include milk, cheese, eggs, meat, fish, poultry, grains, legumes, and nuts. Women who are vegetarians or who have allergies to milk (lactose intolerance) can try canned soy milk in cooking, and goat's milk or cheese, or tofu. Plant foods can also be a source of protein; however, these are incomplete proteins that lack some of the essential amino acids. Vegetable proteins can be combined with complete proteins, or two vegetable proteins that complement each other's amino acid deficiencies can be eaten together to make a complete protein. Examples might be milk and cereal, tuna and rice, rice with beans, cheese and noodles, peanut butter with whole-wheat bread, or eggs and toast.

Table 19–4

DAILY FOOD PATTERN AND SUGGESTED MENU FOR A PREGNANT WOMAN

Daily Food Pattern

Food	*Amount*
Milk, nonfat or low fat; yogurt; cheese	3 to 4 cups
Meat (lean), poultry, fish, egg	2 servings (total of 4–6 oz)
Vegetables, cooked or raw dark green or deep yellow; starchy, including potatoes, dried peas, and beans; all others	3–5 servings, all types often
Fruits, fresh or canned; dark orange including apricots, peaches, cantaloupe	2–4 servings, all types often
Whole-grain and enriched breads and cereals	7 or more servings
Fats and sweets	In moderate amounts

Suggested Menu*

Breakfast
Orange juice, ½ cup
Oatmeal, ½ cup
Whole-grain or enriched toast, 1 slice
Peanut butter, 2 tsp
Decaffeinated coffee or tea

Midmorning
Apple
High-bran cereal, ¼ cup
Nonfat yogurt, ½ cup

Lunch
Turkey (2 oz) sandwich on rye or whole-grain bread with lettuce and tomato and 1 tsp mayonnaise
Green salad
Salad dressing, 2 tsp
Fresh peach
Nonfat or low-fat milk, 1 cup

Midafternoon
Nonfat or low-fat milk, 1 cup
Graham crackers, 4 squares

Dinner
Baked chicken breast, 3 oz
Baked potato with 2 tbsp sour half-and-half
Peas and carrots, ½ cup
Green salad
Salad dressing, 2 tsp
Fresh pear

Evening
Nonfat frozen yogurt, 1 cup
Fresh strawberries

*Quantities of food should be adjusted to meet individual energy needs to promote appropriate weight gain. The pregnant adolescent, very active woman, or underweight woman will require more.

Adapted from Mahan, L. K., and Escott-Stump, S. (1996). *Krause's food, nutrition and diet therapy* (9th ed., p. 194). Philadelphia: W. B. Saunders.

Carbohydrates and Fats

The roles of carbohydrates and fats during pregnancy are to contribute to the total calorie intake required for maternal and fetal growth and thus spare protein from being used as an energy source. Carbohydrates provide protective substances and bulk, while fats are stored in the mother and baby for energy. Fats are more completely absorbed during pregnancy. Thus, the pregnant woman may have elevated serum lipid, lipoprotein, and cholesterol levels while she is pregnant. Sources of carbohydrate goods include fruits, vegetables, whole-grain cereal and bread, and milk. Fats are found in butter, cream cheese, cream, whipped cream, mayonnaise, oil, and nuts.

Vitamins

Vitamin intake should be maintained or increased during pregnancy and lactation. The RDAs for pregnant women can be found in Table 19–3. This intake should be obtained through a well-balanced diet as well as the commonly prescribed prenatal vitamin tablet. The role of vitamins in the diet is to maintain the normal cell structure and function and to support the growth of new tissues. The fat-soluble vitamins, A, D, E, and K, are stored in the liver in moderate amounts. They are absorbed along with the dietary fats eaten. The major complication with these vitamins is not deficiency but a toxic effect due to overdose. Water-soluble vitamins, B complex, folic acid, and C, are not able to be stored in the body; any excesses are excreted in the urine. Therefore, a daily supply of the water-soluble vitamins is needed. Health care providers do not agree on the use of vitamin and mineral supplements in pregnancy. If the woman has a well-balanced diet, supplementation other than iron and folic acid is usually unnecessary. However, accepted practice in antepartum care today is the routine prescription of prenatal vitamins. The pregnant woman should be reminded that taking a prenatal vitamin tablet each day does not preclude the importance of eating a well-balanced diet, for vitamins in their natural form are often better used than those that are synthesized. It is also important to counsel the woman about the inadvisability of taking "megadoses" of vitamins during pregnancy, for some vitamins in large doses can be toxic.

▼ **Vitamin A.** During pregnancy, a daily intake of 800 μg retinol equivalents of vitamin A is recommended (National Research Council 1989). Vitamin A is essential for cell development, tooth formation, and bone growth. It plays a role in the metabolism of carbohydrates and fats and affects night vision. Food sources are usually adequate to provide the needed amounts of vitamin A and include organ meats, egg yolks, butter and fortified margarine, fruits, and green and yellow vegetables. Excessive amounts of vitamin A are toxic and during pregnancy could be teratogenic, causing congenital fetal malformations. For that reason, pregnant women should be questioned about their use of vitamin A supplements.

▼ **Vitamin D.** The intake of vitamin D should be maintained for women ages 15 to 24 years and doubled for women age 25 years or older (National Research Council 1989). Vitamin D is needed to enhance the absorption and use of the increased amounts of calcium and phosphorus needed during pregnancy. Calcium and phosphorus are needed for fetal skeletal and tooth bud formation. Vitamin D can be found in fortified milk and margarine, liver, egg yolks, canned sardines, salmon, and several fresh fruits and vegetables. Sun exposure can cause vitamin D synthesis in the skin; however, this is an unreliable source. A deficiency in vitamin D can cause rickets, a disease characterized by improper calcification of the bones. Megadoses of vitamin D can cause calcium to be deposited in soft tissue, resulting in irreversible kidney damage. During pregnancy, excessive vitamin D could contribute to the production of severe maternal and neonatal hypercalcemia.

▼ **Vitamin E.** The primary function of vitamin E is as an antioxidant. It takes on oxygen so that another substance will not undergo chemical change. For example, vitamin E helps spare vitamin A by preventing its oxidation in the intestinal tract and the tissues. It is also involved in enzymatic and metabolic reactions. Its role during pregnancy is not known, but the recommended intake increases from 8 to 10 mg alpha-tocopherol equivalents for pregnant women (National Research Council 1989). Vitamin E is found in many foods, especially vegetable fats and oils, whole grains, greens, and eggs. Deficiency symptoms of vitamin E are related to long-term inability to absorb fats. In excessive amounts, it can interfere with vitamin K metabolism and blood coagulation. Depression and fatigue may occur after ingestion of more than 900 mg/day.

▼ **Vitamin K.** Vitamin K is essential for the synthesis of prothrombin and the prevention of hemorrhage in the newborn; it is synthesized by bacteria in the bowel. However, because the normal newborn has a sterile bowel, vitamin K manufacture is limited. Common practice is to supplement the newborn immediately after birth with an injectable form of synthetic vitamin K rather than administer vitamin K to the woman before birth. The RDA for pregnant women is 65 μg/day (National Research Council 1989). Intake of vitamin K is usually adequate in a well-balanced diet; it can be found in green leafy vegetables, fruit, cereals, dairy products, and meat.

▼ **Vitamin B.** The entire B complex of vitamins, B_1 (thiamine), B_2 (riboflavin), B_6 (pyridoxine), B_{12} (cobalamin), niacin, and folic acid, have the important function of being coenzymes in metabolic functions, such as cell respiration, glucose oxidation, and energy metabolism. Therefore, the quantities needed during pregnancy increase as calorie intake increases to meet metabolic and growth needs. Vitamin B_1 requirements increase from 1.1 mg/day to 1.5 mg/day (National Research Council 1989). Food sources include pork, liver, milk, potatoes, enriched breads, and cereals.

Vitamin B_2 requirements increase to 1.6 mg/day (National Research Council 1989). Sources include milk, liver, eggs, enriched breads, and cereals. Vitamin B_6 is associated with amino acid metabolism, so that if the protein intake is higher than average, vitamin B_6 intake should be higher. Vitamin B_6 plays a part in the development of the baby's central nervous system, including the brain cells. The requirements increase in pregnancy to 2.2 mg/day (National Research Council 1989). Dietary sources that can supply this needed increase include fish, liver, pork, potatoes, lentils, wheat germ, and yeast. Vitamin B_6 deficiencies have been related to oral contraceptive use.

Vitamin B_{12} is the cobalt-containing vitamin and is found only in animal sources. Unless the woman is a vegetarian, it is unusual to find a deficiency of this vitamin. It is found in milk, meats, liver, eggs, and cheese. Vitamin B_{12} is thought to be involved in the formation of red blood cells in the mother and fetus during the fourth month of pregnancy. The RDA during pregnancy is 2.2 μg/day (National Research Council 1989). Low maternal levels of vitamin B_{12} are associated with anemia and prematurity and occur more often in smokers than in nonsmokers.

Although few research data on the niacin requirements of pregnant women are available, 17 mg niacin equivalents per day of niacin is recommended (National Research Council 1989). Sources of niacin include meat, poultry, fish, liver, whole grains, enriched breads, cereals, and nuts. Folic acid (folate) is important for the promotion of adequate fetal growth and prevents macrocytic, megaloblastic anemia of pregnancy. Deficiency of folic acid has been related to spontaneous abortion, fetal malformations such as neural tube defects, preeclampsia, abruptio placentae, and other bleeding complications of pregnancy. The RDA for folic acid increases during pregnancy from 180 to 400 μg/day (National Research Council 1989). Good dietary sources of folic acid are limited but include fresh green leafy vegetables; oranges and bananas; kidney, liver, and other organ meats; food yeasts; and dried beans and peanuts. Folic acid is sensitive to high heat, and as much as 80 percent may be lost in cooking. Research has shown that 50 to 75 percent of fetal neural tube defects, such as spina bifida and anencephaly, can be prevented by maternal ingestion of a minimum of 0.4 mg (400 μg) of folic acid daily. Therefore, supplementation of folic acid is recommended and is part of the prenatal vitamin (Heslin 1993).

▼ **Vitamin C.** Vitamin C (ascorbic acid) requirements increase in pregnancy from 60 to 70 mg/day (National Research Council 1989). During pregnancy, vitamin C aids in the formation and development of connective tissue, collagen, skin, tendons, and the vascular system. It also enhances the absorption of iron from the gastrointestinal tract and is essential for the transfer of iron to the liver for storage. A deficiency in vitamin C causes scurvy. A well-balanced diet provides the required amounts of vitamin C. Foods rich in this vitamin include citrus fruit, cantaloupe, strawberries, tomatoes, potatoes, broccoli, and green leafy vegetables. Even though vitamin C is water soluble, toxic effects can occur. Megadoses can cause nausea, abdominal cramps, and diarrhea. In pregnant women, high doses can cause neonatal bleeding (Heslin 1993).

Minerals

Minerals such as iron, zinc, copper, calcium, phosphorus, sodium, and magnesium also have important roles during pregnancy.

▼ **Iron.** Iron is essential in the synthesis of hemoglobin in maternal and fetal red blood cells. Unfortunately, many women enter pregnancy with low iron stores. The development of increased maternal blood volume and physiologic anemia of pregnancy (see Chapter 16), increased fetal demands for iron, and blood loss associated with childbirth must be offset by an increased iron intake during pregnancy. Inadequate iron stores and intake can result in the development of iron deficiency anemia during pregnancy; low hemoglobin level has been associated with complications of pregnancy such as spontaneous abortion, stillbirth, perinatal death, low birth weight, and premature birth. If dietary iron is not sufficient to meet maternal and fetal needs, fetal iron reserves will not be impaired but maternal iron stores will be depleted. Women who are at greatest risk for iron deficiency are adolescents, women with pregnancies occurring less than 12 months apart, women with a multiple gestation, and women with poor diets (Green and Harry 1987; Worthington-Roberts 1985). The recommended amount of iron in the daily diet from natural food sources plus an iron supplement is 30 mg for pregnant women (National Research Council 1989). Dietary sources of iron include lean meats, liver, shellfish, eggs, dark green leafy vegetables, legumes, whole-grain and enriched breads and cereals, and molasses. Because absorption of iron is generally higher from animal products than from vegetable products, the absorption of vegetable sources can be enhanced by combining them with a meat or a vitamin C source. For example, eating meat with potatoes, tomato and lettuce on a cheeseburger, or orange juice with an enriched cereal promotes iron absorption. Although iron can be obtained easily from food sources, the amount that is needed in pregnancy is difficult to obtain from the diet, and only about 25 percent of the available iron in food is absorbed by pregnant women. A well-balanced diet with good iron-rich foods will provide only about 15 to 18 mg/day of iron. Therefore, a supplement of iron, such as ferrous gluconate, ferrous fumarate, or ferrous sulfate, is needed (Heslin 1993).

▼ **Zinc.** Zinc requirements increase during pregnancy because zinc is essential for normal fetal growth and development, antibacterial activity of amniotic fluid, and uterine contractility for the initiation of labor. Research has shown that low levels of zinc have been associated with infection, pregnancy-induced hypertension, fetal distress or malformations, low birth weight, labor dystocia, intrapartum hemorrhage, and tissue fragility leading to vaginal lacerations during birth. Daily zinc supplementation in pregnant women with relatively low concentrations of the mineral is associated with increased infant birth weight and head circumference. The RDA for zinc during pregnancy is 15 mg/day (National Research Council 1989). Since zinc is found in most high-protein foods, such as liver, shellfish, wheat bran, and milk, a protein-sufficient diet most likely provides the necessary requirements (Green and Harry 1987; Wilkerson 1988).

▼ **Copper.** The exact requirements for copper during pregnancy are not known, nor is the effect of copper deficiency in humans during pregnancy. Trace amounts of copper are normally found in all tissues in the body but especially in the eye, liver, heart, and brain. Copper aids in the absorption, storage, and release of iron. A few studies of copper deficiency have shown teratogenic effects on the fetus, such as neural tube defects. The RDA for copper in the nonpregnant woman is 3 mg/day. It has been suggested that adequate copper in maternal serum is not possible without the use of a supplement. Food sources of copper are liver, meat, oysters, nuts, corn oil margarine, dried legumes, and drinking water (Wilkerson 1988; Worthington-Roberts 1985).

▼ **Calcium.** Calcium is essential in pregnancy for the mineralization of fetal skeletal tissue, tooth formation, and regulation of nerve and muscle activity. Although calcium is not used for fetal development until the last trimester, the mineral is probably stored in the woman's body in anticipation of the increased requirements in late pregnancy. By the third trimester, the fetus accumulates calcium at an average rate of 300 mg/day. If calcium intake is inadequate, fetal needs will be met by demineralization of the maternal skeleton. Adequate calcium intake in pregnancy has also been linked to prevention of pregnancy-induced hypertension, although research findings are conflicting. The balance of calcium to phosphorus in relation to leg cramps has been studied for a number of years. The prevailing opinion today is that the amount of milk in the diet should not be limited to prevent leg cramps, but foods high in phosphorus should be limited (Wilkerson 1988). The RDA for calcium during pregnancy is 1200 mg/day (National Research Council 1989). The RDA for pregnant teenagers is 1600 mg/day. Inadequate prenatal calcium intake has been associated with an increase in the incidence of neonatal hypocalcemia. Milk and milk products are the primary source of calcium. Additional sources are leafy green vegetables and whole-grain and enriched cereals and breads (Heslin 1993).

▼ **Phosphorus.** Phosphorus is necessary for the rapid division and growth of new fetal cells, and it also contributes to the early formation of the baby's skeleton and tooth buds. The RDA for phosphorus during pregnancy is the same as that for calcium, 1200 mg/day (National Research Council 1989). Phosphorus is widely available in foods such as meat, chicken, eggs, milk, and cheese, so a deficiency is rare. In fact, the intake of phosphorus may easily exceed that of calcium, particularly if the woman includes high quantities of snack foods, processed meats, or carbonated soft drinks in her diet. This imbalance between phosphorus and calcium is often the cause of the leg cramps experienced in pregnancy, so snack foods should be limited.

▼ **Sodium.** There is a slight increase in the need for sodium in pregnancy to maintain fluid levels for expanded maternal blood volume. The accepted medical practice for many years was to restrict sodium intake in an effort to prevent edema and pregnancy-induced hypertension. This practice is now viewed as being unphysiologic and unfounded, and it may actually place the woman and fetus at unnecessary risk. During pregnancy, the glomerular filtration rate is increased by approximately 50 percent. The increased fluid normally retained during pregnancy actually increases the body's need for sodium. Aldosterone increases in pregnancy and conserves sodium, a protective response to the increase in sodium excretion related to progesterone. The practice of restricting sodium causes the woman to undergo a series of hormonal and biochemical changes in an effort to conserve sodium (Worthington-Roberts

1985). The RDA for sodium in the nonpregnant woman is 2 to 3 g/day obtained from natural dietary sources. The exact RDA for sodium during pregnancy is unknown; however, the sodium content of a pregnant woman's daily diet should not fall below 2 to 3 g (Worthington-Roberts 1992). Sources of excess sodium, such as canned and processed foods, junk foods, bouillon cubes, table salt, and medications such as bicarbonate of soda, are discouraged.

Magnesium. Magnesium is also important during pregnancy and can be found in milk, whole grains, beet greens, legumes, nuts, and tea. It is necessary for cellular metabolism and structural growth. The RDA for pregnancy is 320 mg/day.

Water and Fluids

Fluid intake during pregnancy is an important component of a well-balanced diet to support the physiologic changes taking place. The woman's body retains about 6.5 additional liters of water during pregnancy. This represents 3.5 liters from the water content of the fetus, placenta, and amniotic fluid as well as 3.0 liters more that accumulates as a result of the increases in maternal blood volume and the size of the uterus and breasts. An adequate fluid intake also helps by assisting with digestion and in the management of constipation. Eight to 12 glasses of liquids (1500 to 2000 mL), in addition to the daily milk requirement, are recommended every day. This fluid should be water or fruit and vegetable juices rather than carbonated soft drinks.

WEIGHT GAIN IN PREGNANCY

Weight gain during pregnancy is a topic of interest to all pregnant women and an important indicator of maternal-fetal well-being. Although weight gain can be an indicator that the woman's calorie intake and nutritional status are adequate, that maternal physiologic processes are taking place to support gestation, and that the baby's growth is proceeding normally, weight gain alone should not be assumed to be a valid measure of actual nutritional status. It may also be associated with the woman's body mass index before pregnancy and with the amount of edema she experiences (Aaronson 1989b; Institute of Medicine 1990). The accepted standards for the amount of weight gain have changed considerably during the past several decades. For many years, women were rigidly restricted in their amount of weight gain, with 20 pounds usually set as the limit. This strict management was observed because of the belief that weight gain was a contributing factor in the development of preeclampsia.

Further empirical evidence and research have convinced caregivers today that strict weight gain limitation is more detrimental than beneficial in pregnancy (Dohrmann and Lederman 1986; Taffel 1986; Institute of Medicine 1990). Women who gain within the current recommended range of weight have the fewest risks and complications associated with the pregnancy and healthier babies. The amount of weight a woman should gain varies, depending on her pre-pregnancy weight and her health status. In fact, the body mass index is a better indicator of maternal nutritional status than is weight alone. Body mass index is defined as pre-pregnancy weight/height^2, where weight is measured in kilograms and height is measured in meters. Table 19–5 shows the body mass index weight-for-height categories and recommendations for total weight gain during pregnancy according to those categories.

The pattern of weight gain is actually more important than the total amount of weight and should be gradual during the course of pregnancy. The pregnant woman's weight should be recorded at each prenatal appointment so that the pattern of weight gain can be monitored. Although specific grids for recording weight gain have substantial limitations, most are useful in the clinical setting because they permit visual tracking of weight gain by week of gestation. They provide the nurse with a visual impression of the progress of weight gain and simplify detection of an abnormal change in weight over time (Fig. 19–7). A smooth, progres-

Table 19–5

WEIGHT GAIN RECOMMENDATIONS BY PRE-PREGNANCY BODY MASS INDEX (BMI)

WEIGHT-FOR-HEIGHT CATEGORY*	RECOMMENDED TOTAL GAIN†	
	Kilograms	Pounds
Low (BMI < 19.8)	12.5–18	28–40
Normal (BMI 19.8–26.0)	11.5–16	25–35
High (BMI > 26.0–29.0)‡	7.0–11.5	15–25

*BMI is calculated by use of metric units.

†Young adolescents and black women should strive for gains at the upper end of the recommended range; short women (<157 cm, or 62 in) should strive for gains at the lower end of the range.

‡The recommended target weight gain for obese women (BMI > 29.0) is at least 6.8 kg (15 lb).

Reprinted with permission from NUTRITION DURING PREGNANCY. Copyright 1990 by the National Academy of Sciences. Courtesy of the National Academy Press, Washington, D.C.

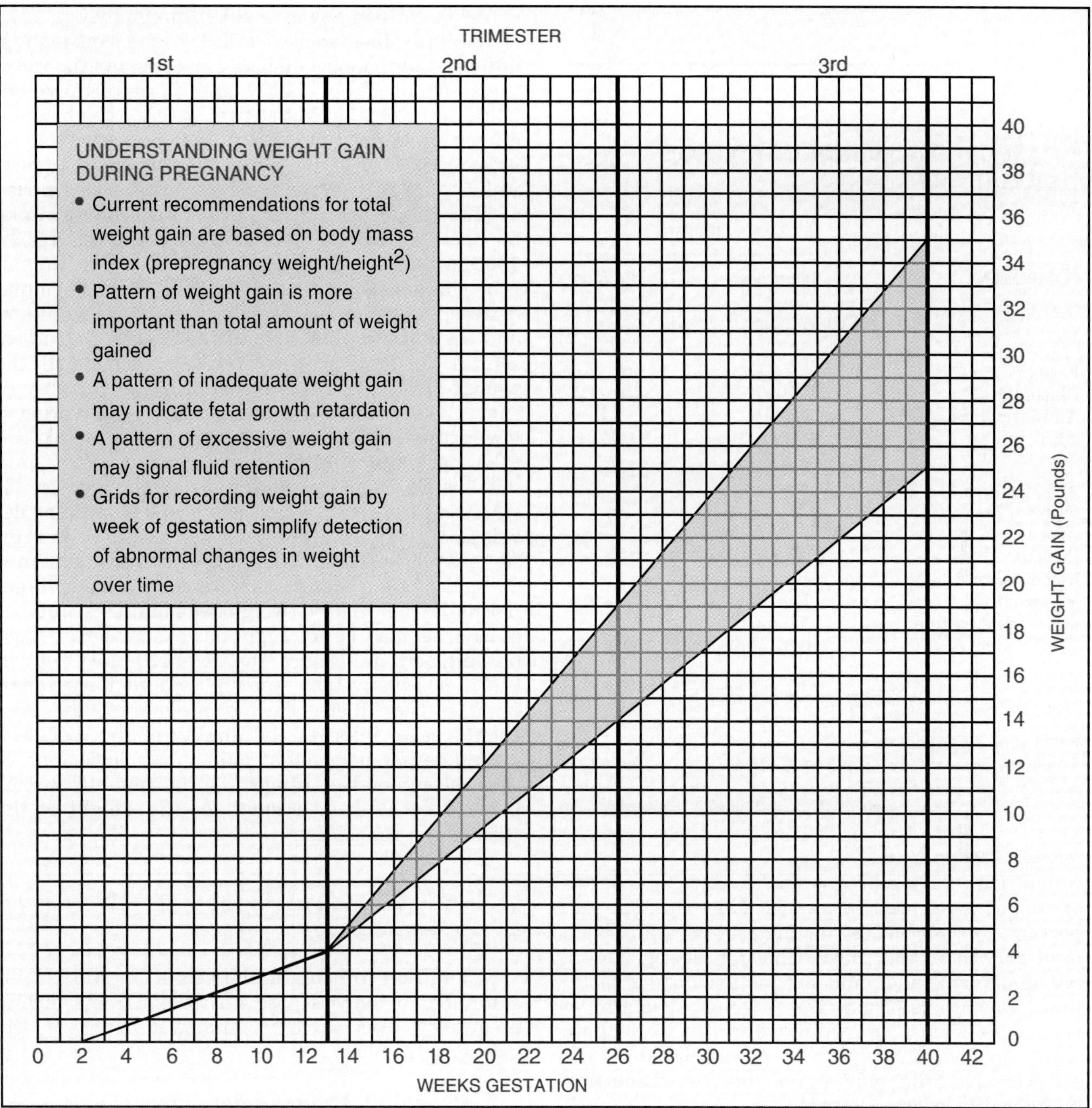

Figure 19–7

Weight gain should be assessed regularly, because the pattern of weight gain is one indication of whether the fetus is growing normally. Weight gain should progress gradually during pregnancy, with a total average gain of 2 to 4 pounds in the first trimester and approximately 1 pound per week during the second and third trimesters. This grid illustrates an average range for weight gain (25 to 35 pounds) over a period of full-term gestation.

sive weight gain generally represents a gain of lean and fat tissue, whereas erratic or high weight gain is likely to represent excessive fluid retention (Institute of Medicine 1990).

During the first trimester, the average amount of expected weight gain is 2 to 4 pounds total. This is due to beginning changes in maternal tissue and increased blood volume. The weight gain in the second trimester is more rapid and averages about 1 pound per week. Most of this gain reflects an increase in blood volume, an enlargement of the breasts and uterus, and the deposition of maternal fat. In the third trimester, the rate of weight gain may slow slightly but still approximates 1 pound per week. The weight gain in late pregnancy represents placental development, amniotic fluid, and fetal growth. Table 19–6 shows the maternal and fetal distribution of average

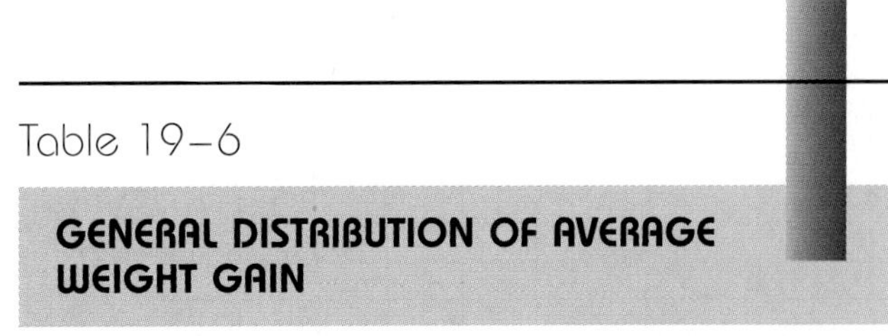

Table 19–6

GENERAL DISTRIBUTION OF AVERAGE WEIGHT GAIN

COMPONENT	WEIGHT Kilograms	WEIGHT Pounds
Fetal Components		
Fetus	3.2–3.4	7.0–7.5
Placenta	0.5–0.7	1.0–1.5
Amniotic fluid	0.9	2.0
Total weight	4.6–5.0	10.0–11.0
Maternal Components		
Uterus	1.1	2.5
Breasts	0.7–1.4	1.5–3.0
Blood volume	1.6–1.8	3.5–4.0
Maternal fat stores	1.8–4.3	4.0–9.5
Extracellular fluid	1.6–2.3	3.5–5.0
Total weight	6.8–10.9	15.0–24.0
Total Average Weight Gain		
Fetal plus maternal components	11.4–15.9	25.0–35.0

weight gain during pregnancy. The 4 to 9.5 pounds of weight attributed to maternal fat stores is important, for it provides the energy to sustain rapid fetal growth in the third trimester, energy for labor and birth, and milk production during lactation. Deviations from the average pattern of weight gain must be evaluated, for an inadequate gain may indicate fetal growth retardation, while an excessive gain may signal fluid retention and be indicative of preeclampsia.

Alterations in the average recommended amount of weight gain should be calculated for the underweight or overweight woman (see Table 19–5). Being underweight during pregnancy is associated with maternal anemia, cardiopulmonary problems, premature rupture of membranes, intrauterine growth retardation, small-for-gestational-age babies, preterm delivery, and low Apgar scores. The underweight woman should increase her calorie intake to 500 calories per day above the nonpregnant RDA, and her protein intake should be increased to 20 g/day. At least 10 pounds should be gained by week 20 of the pregnancy, and her total weight gain should range between 28 and 40 pounds (Abrams et al. 1989; Dohrmann and Lederman 1986).

Although being overweight in pregnancy is associated with an increased risk for hypertensive disorders of pregnancy, diabetes, pyelonephritis, infections, dystocias of labor, and large-birth-weight babies, the major risk with excess weight gain during pregnancy is obesity after delivery. Women who are overweight should not attempt to lose weight during the pregnancy, for this poses a risk of inadequate nutrient, calorie, and protein intake for fetal development (Dohrmann and Lederman 1986). Counseling the overweight pregnant woman is a challenge, because a balance must be found between keeping her weight gain to a minimum and encouraging her to gain the weight that is essential for fetal growth and development. If the woman's weight gain is not sufficient, even though she is overweight, she is at risk for delivering a low-birth-weight infant. An inadequate dietary intake, particularly a diet that is insufficient in protein, will result in maternal catabolism of fat stores and ketosis, which can jeopardize fetal development. Optimal protein use requires energy. At least 30 kcal per kilogram of body weight in a 24-hour period is necessary to metabolize protein normally. For the overweight woman, this number of calories may be too high; however, calories must be sufficient to ensure the required nutrients in the diet. Overweight women tend to have nutritionally poor diets. During pregnancy, the goal should be to improve the quality of the diet. She should target her weight gain to the lower end of the recommended range (i.e., about 15 to 25 pounds) to at least account for the weight of the products of conception.

NUTRITIONAL RISK FACTORS IN PREGNANCY

In addition to being underweight or overweight, a number of factors pose nutritional risks during pregnancy and threaten the well-being of the mother and infant.

▼ **Frequent Pregnancies.** Frequent pregnancies, those that occur more often than 12 months apart, make it difficult for the woman to replenish her nutritional reserves.

▼ **High-Risk Health History.** A history of medical or obstetric problems requires additional nutritional assessment and counseling, for many health problems can be positively or negatively influenced by the quality of the diet.

▼ **Fad Diets.** Fad diets are dangerous in pregnancy, for most fad diets are focused on eating only one type of food or an unusual combination of foods. This type of diet is likely to be lacking in all the essential nutrients needed for fetal development.

Eating Disorders. Eating disorders such as anorexia or bulimia pose challenging problems in the maintenance of good nutritional balance for the woman and her baby (Mogul 1989; Ramchandani and Whedon 1988). Society's pressures for a woman to be thin are not necessarily altered during pregnancy; as a result, women may have to deal with psychological conflicts that influence good eating habits (McBride 1982).

Vegetarian Diets. Vegetarian diets present the challenge of providing the necessary amount of protein and vitamin B_{12} for fetal growth and development and maternal physiologic adaptation. The type of vegetarian diet determines the degree of difficulty in meeting essential nutrients during pregnancy (Table 19–7). The strict vegetarian (vegan) presents the greatest challenge, for no foods of animal origin are included in the diet. This eliminates meat, poultry, fish, eggs, cheese, and milk. Foods that are eaten include fruits, vegetables, legumes, grains, and nuts. The lactovegetarian eats no meat, poultry, or fish but adds dairy products (lacto) to the diet; the ovolactovegetarian also adds eggs (ovo) to the diet. The fruitarian eats only fruits, nuts, honey, and olive oil.

Protein requirements can be met with a vegetarian diet; however, knowledge, planning, and commitment on the part of the pregnant woman are required. Because plant foods do not contain the eight essential amino acids for complete protein, a strict vegan vegetarian needs to be more aware of the quality of foods chosen. Although it is not essential, the pregnant woman may wish to improve the quality of her diet by using "mutual supplementation," the practice of combining plant foods with complementary amino acid composition to obtain a complete protein (see Table 19–7).

Table 19–7

GUIDELINES FOR THE PREGNANT VEGETARIAN

PROTEIN COMBINATIONS			EXAMPLES
The following combinations of foods provide "complete" proteins with all the essential amino acids.			
For the Vegan Vegetarian			
Cereal grains	+	*Legumes*	
Barley	+	Dried beans	Bean taco
Oats	+	Dried peas	Lentils and rice
Rice	+	Peanuts	Peanut butter sandwich
Whole-grain breads	+	Soy products	Tofu with rice
Pasta			
Cornmeal			
Legumes	+	*Seeds and Nuts*	
Dried beans	+	Sesame seeds	Hummus (chickpea and sesame paste)
Dried lentils	+	Sunflower seeds	Split-pea soup and sesame crackers
Dried peas	+	Walnuts	
Peanuts	+	Cashews	
Soy products	+	Nut butters	
For the Ovolactovegetarian			
Eggs or Milk Products	+	*Vegetable-Protein Foods*	
Eggs	+	Legumes	Macaroni and cheese
Milk	+	Nuts	Vegetable omelet
Yogurt	+	Seeds	Eggplant Parmesan
Cheese	+	Whole grains	Broccoli with cheese sauce
Cottage cheese	+	Vegetables	French toast
			Cereal with milk

Data from Whitney, E., Cataldo, C., Rolfes, S. (1994). *Understanding normal and clinical nutrition* (4th ed.). Minneapolis/St. Paul: West Publishing Company; and Worthington-Roberts, B., and Williams, S. (1993). *Nutrition in pregnancy and lactation* (5th ed.). St. Louis: C. V. Mosby.

Knowing which foods can be combined to make these essential proteins requires time and effort. The woman who follows a vegetarian diet during pregnancy should have the consultation of a professional nutritionist or registered dietitian. As for any pregnant woman, the diet of the vegetarian woman should be supplemented with iron and folic acid (Mutch 1988; Whitney et al. 1994).

▼ **Adolescence.** Adolescence presents another nutritional risk factor during pregnancy. Because the adolescent's own growth and development are not complete, the added developmental needs of the fetus result in significant nutritional requirements during pregnancy. Unfortunately, these added requirements are imposed on a young woman in an age group that typically follows a poor diet. It is common for the diet of an adolescent to consist primarily of junk foods and few foods of nutritional value. High activity levels and erratic eating schedules influence the adolescent's diet as well. Because body image is of great concern to the adolescent, many teens follow calorie-restricted diets to remain "thin." The developmental need to achieve independence from parents may cause the adolescent to reject what may have been taught in the home about eating a well-balanced diet. Attitude and acceptance of the pregnancy will influence the adolescent's motivation to eat well. Her living situation, food resources, relationship with the father of the baby, and peer relationships are additional influencing factors (see Chapter 39).

During pregnancy, therefore, the diet of an adolescent must actually exceed the nutritional requirements for the adult pregnant woman. The RDAs for pregnant teenagers are calculated by adding the RDAs for nonpregnant teenagers to the RDAs for pregnant women. Special attention should be paid to ensure that protein, iron, calcium, and folic acid are higher in the diet of the pregnant adolescent. Adolescents gain more weight during pregnancy because of their own growth as well as the pregnancy. It is advised that adolescents gain the amount of weight equal to that usually gained per year in their stage of physical development in addition to the recommended amount of weight for pregnancy. For example, in one study of pregnant teens, the mean weight gain was 37 pounds. Special attention must be given to assessment, teaching, and evaluation to prevent the adolescent from developing maternal or fetal complications that could be prevented with good nutrition. This nutritional counseling is often challenging, for the psychological and sociocultural factors that may be associated with teen pregnancy often interfere with the ability of the adolescent to focus on eating well (Dohrmann and Lederman 1986; Worthington-Roberts 1985).

▼ **Substance Abuse.** Finally, substance abuse presents a nutritional risk factor as well as the risks related to fetal development (see Chapter 15 for a discussion regarding substance abuse in pregnancy). Smoking, alcohol, drugs, and caffeine can all influence the woman's nutritional status during pregnancy because use of any one of these substances can result in decreased appetite and decreased essential nutrient intake (Heslin 1989; Public Health Service 1989; Vogt 1987; Wilkerson 1988). It has been estimated that 25 percent of women continue to smoke throughout pregnancy (Floyd et al. 1991). Smoking has been related to spontaneous abortion, ectopic pregnancy, preterm labor, abruptio placentae, placenta previa, low birth weight due to intrauterine growth retardation, and small-for-gestational-age infants (Aaronson and Macnee 1989; Floyd et al. 1991; Handler et al. 1989; Public Health Service 1989). In general, women who smoke during pregnancy may not eat as well and may have lower intakes of most nutrients than do nonsmokers. Smoking increases the metabolism of some nutrients, such as vitamin C, leading to potential nutritional deficiencies (Brooten et al. 1987; Haste et al. 1990). During the postpartum period, maternal smoking can result in the passage of nicotine to breast milk and a higher incidence of respiratory problems in the first year of life from exposure of the infant to passive smoke. Sudden infant death syndrome is also associated with maternal smoking during pregnancy and the postpartum period (Alexander 1987; Costa 1989; Floyd et al. 1991; Mayer et al. 1990; Schoendorf and Kiely 1992).

Alcohol and drug abuse can be teratogenic during fetal development (see Chapter 15). Moderate alcohol ingestion can result in the birth of a baby with subtle defects; heavy alcohol ingestion can result in the birth of a baby with fetal alcohol syndrome and may also result in the birth of a stillborn or a low-birth-weight baby (Aaronson and Macnee 1989). Both the timing and the amount of alcohol ingestion in pregnancy can influence fetal outcomes. No safe levels of alcohol ingestion have been established to date, and there is concern that even minimal to moderate alcohol intake harms the fetus. An indirect effect of alcohol or drug abuse during pregnancy is the poor nutritional status of the addicted woman (Public Health Service 1989; Vogt 1987; Walpole et al. 1989).

The research findings regarding the effects of caffeine on pregnancy outcome are the least consistent and least conclusive. Most of the research on the effects of caffeine in pregnancy has been done with laboratory animals; however, because abnormalities have been found in fetal development in animals exposed to caffeine, it is advised that use in pregnancy be limited. There is little evidence of caffeine-induced birth defects or spontaneous abortion. The strongest reproductive caffeine hazard is thought to be decreased fetal growth and low birth weight. Studies have also found that caffeine use before pregnancy may inhibit male fertility. Pregnant women should be advised to become aware of common sources of caffeine, such as coffee, tea, chocolate, soft drinks, and some over-the-counter drugs, and to avoid the use of these caffeine sources as much as possible (Aaronson and Macnee 1989; Mille et al. 1993).

Emotional Aspects of Nutrition in Pregnancy

During pregnancy, as throughout our lives, emotions can influence appetite, choice of food, and resultant nutritional status. Food can hold many meanings and symbols for people. For example, most significant events in our lives are associated with some type of food. Eating certain foods may promote feelings of comfort, nurturance, warmth, or reward. Some foods may trigger childhood memories and give a sense of comfort or security.

During pregnancy, food may hold particular meaning for a woman as she thinks about being loved by her mother or dreams about nurturing her own baby. Eating habits established before the pregnancy may offer emotional security. These habits are derived from one's total life experience and as a result may be difficult to change. The food selections that are made as a result of emotional influence may or may not be wise nutritional choices. If a woman is depressed during pregnancy or does not want the pregnancy, her depression may result in reduced calorie and nutrient intake, leading to poor weight gain, a low-birth-weight infant, and even perinatal mortality.

Sociocultural Aspects of Nutrition in Pregnancy

Social practices, culture, or religion can influence eating habits and food selections during pregnancy. The sharing of food on social occasions is a major form of social interaction or a source of pride and identity in most cultures. Eating usually denotes happiness, good times, or celebration. Some foods may have symbolic significance and be related to major life experiences. Throughout history, special attention has been given to the diets of pregnant women. In many cultures, foods were either restricted or prohibited. Some foods were regarded as necessary to ward off catastrophe for the pregnant woman or her infant. Such food prohibitions still exist today. For example, some black Americans believe that craving a particular food during pregnancy will cause the baby to be "marked" in the shape of that food; Chinese women may eat only "hot" or "cold" foods to maintain balance, for different stages of pregnancy are considered to be "cold" or "hot" periods. In many cultures, there are myths or old wives' tales related to diet in pregnancy. For example, common beliefs such as "eating for two," "a lost tooth for every pregnancy," or "prunes will cause the baby to be wrinkled" may strongly influence the woman's eating habits.

A practice called pica has cultural roots and can greatly influence nutrition in pregnancy. Pica is the practice of ingesting nonfood substances that have no nutritive value. Although pica may be observed in any socioeconomic group, it is most often seen in poverty areas where nutritious diets are lacking. It may be rooted in the tradition of families or communities. Substances most commonly eaten are laundry starch, clay, or dirt; however, ingestion of many other types of substances has been reported. Women who practice pica may actually crave these nonfood substances. In addition to contributing to poor nutritional status, the practice of pica can also cause such health complications as iron deficiency anemia, intestinal fecal impaction, or excessive weight gain. Because women who practice pica may be embarrassed about their strange cravings, they may be reluctant to share information about the practice with health care providers. It is therefore important that a nonjudgmental approach be used when asking about food cravings during the nutritional assessment.

Lactose intolerance is common in some ethnic groups, particularly among blacks, Native Americans, Mexican Americans, Asians, and Ashkenazi Jews. Lactose is a sugar found in milk and dairy products. For some people, symptoms such as abdominal distention, cramping and diarrhea, or nausea and vomiting occur after the consumption of milk. These symptoms occur because intolerant individuals have an inadequate amount of the enzyme lactase, which is necessary to break down lactose into digestible substances. For lactose-intolerant individuals, protein and calcium intake must be obtained through sources other than milk. Tofu (soybean cake) is a good source of calcium and contains no lactose. Dairy products that are fermented, such as cheese and yogurt, may be tolerated, and Swiss cheese contains little lactose. Milk may be tolerated in cooked form, such as in custards or other dishes. The enzyme lactase is available in tablet or liquid form and may be used before drinking milk to alleviate the problem.

The living situation of the pregnant woman will influence eating habits. Her housing, the facilities for cooking, cooking practices, the number of people living in the household, and her employment all influence her nutrition. If housing conditions are crowded or there are not adequate facilities for cooking, it is likely that junk foods requiring no preparation will be eaten in place of nutritious foods. Some cooking practices diminish the nutritional value of food by depleting vitamin content, adding unnecessary fat, or breaking down protein. If the woman is employed, traditional food preparation patterns may give way to the use of "convenience foods" because of fatigue or lack of time. Ethnic or language differences may cause nutritional problems for a pregnant woman. Even while attempting to follow a specific cultural food pattern in a new location, the woman may be unable to obtain foods that are familiar to her. As a result, these foods may be replaced by less nutritious items found in local markets. For example, guava juice may be replaced by carbonated beverages. If English is not a familiar language, the woman may not be able to read or understand information about foods eaten in this country. In many cases, ethnic or language differences have been associated with anemia and inadequate or sporadic weight gain during pregnancy.

The socioeconomic status and financial situation of the pregnant woman and her family also directly influence nutrition. Low income has been related to an inadequate nutrient intake. Pregnant women with limited food budgets may be unable to purchase enough of the quality foods necessary to meet their nutritional requirements. As a result, low-birth-weight babies are more prevalent in low socioeconomic groups. Food assistance programs are available for women who do not have the resources necessary to purchase nutritious foods. It is important that women receive counseling regarding their current diet, the foods needed in pregnancy, and the assistance programs available to help with the purchase of nutritious foods. Assistance may be offered through local church or community groups or through state or federal programs. The woman may qualify for food stamps or for the WIC (Women, Infants, and Children) nutritional supplement program.

Cognitive Aspects of Nutrition in Pregnancy

The pregnant woman's cognitive understanding of the importance of nutrition during pregnancy, and the direct influence that her diet can have on the development of her baby, will greatly influence her willingness to eat well. If she has no understanding of various nutrients and their food sources, her motivation to ensure a well-balanced diet throughout her pregnancy will be lacking. Because learning often means change, obtaining information alone may not be adequate for altering lifetime eating patterns that may be culturally rooted. Therefore, in addition to receiving cognitive information about good nutrition, the woman must also receive continual support and encouragement to eat a diet consisting of all the essential nutrients for pregnancy (Worthington-Roberts and Williams 1993).

EXERCISE IN PREGNANCY

Historically, a great deal of confusion has existed about the benefits or risks of exercise during pregnancy (see Historical Perspectives: Exercise During Pregnancy). During the eighteenth and nineteenth centuries, beginning recognition of the positive influences of exercise on maternal and fetal outcome was countered with numerous restrictions on activity during pregnancy. For example, many prescriptions for exercise permitted housework while prohibiting any type of social or sports activity, despite the fact that housework could be more exhausting than sports (Artal et al. 1991). Today, there is a great deal of interest in exercise and fitness for all individuals. This interest has influenced the emphasis on exercise for pregnant women as well, and now there is a growing realization that pregnant women can safely participate in a number of physical activities and that exercise during pregnancy offers many benefits (see Benefits of Exercise During Pregnancy).

Physical Aspects of Exercise in Pregnancy

The increased interest in exercise for pregnant women has triggered concern about its safety during pregnancy. Both animal and human research studies have been conducted, and the findings are now being used to give guidance to pregnant women.

Although some research on exercise in pregnancy has been done with pregnant women, most has been conducted with animals, primarily ewes and goats. Three primary concerns about exercise during pregnancy have emerged from the animal studies:

1. The effects of prolonged increased maternal core body temperature on the developing fetus. The possibility of fetal hyperthermia resulting from strenuous and prolonged exercise has been suggested. The fetus's ability to dissipate heat through the placenta may be compromised by a decrease in uterine blood flow and an elevation of maternal temperature during exercise.

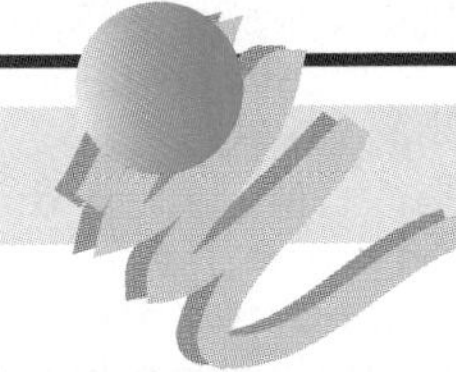

HISTORICAL PERSPECTIVES

EXERCISE DURING PREGNANCY

Throughout history, the amount of exercise undertaken by pregnant women was influenced by the observations of birth outcomes made by a cultural group at a particular time. Even in biblical times, people recognized that the Hebrew slave women had easier labors than their Egyptian masters. It is written in the Bible that "the Hebrew women are not as the Egyptian women; for they are lively, and are delivered ere the midwife come unto them" (Exodus 1:19). Of course, other factors may have influenced the ease of birth at that time. It is possible that in addition to being physically active, the Hebrew slave women delivered small or preterm infants while the sedentary Egyptian women delivered large babies.

Aristotle also attributed difficult childbirth to a sedentary maternal lifestyle in the third century BC. By the eighteenth century, the prevailing philosophy seemed to encourage exercise during pregnancy, although many limitations were advised. In 1781, Alexander Hamilton published his *Treatise of Midwifery* and wrote in the chapter "Rules and Cautions for the Conduct of Pregnant Women" that pregnant women should exercise only in moderation. He stated that women should avoid "agitation of the body from violent or improper exercise, as jolting in a carriage, riding on horseback, dancing and whatever disturbs the body or mind." In 1788, James Lucas, a surgeon at the Leeds General Infirmary in England, presented a paper to the Medical Society of London in which he strongly advocated maternal exercise. He suggested that maternal exercise could decrease the size of the baby and allow easier passage through the maternal pelvis.

The concept of moderation prevailed throughout the nineteenth century and was reinforced by both unscientific moral admonitions and beginning research on the relationship between physical activity and birth outcomes. By the twentieth century, there was concern in many countries about the effects of strenuous physical labor on pregnant women. Legislation in a number of European countries prohibited the employment of pregnant women in factories during the 2 weeks preceding childbirth and the 4 to 6 weeks after birth. A number of books published for pregnant women in the first half of the twentieth century advised moderation in exercise and the need for fresh air. Women who did their own housework were thought to obtain sufficient physical exercise. Walking was considered to be the best exercise, and outdoor sports were not encouraged.

After the 1930s, a number of prenatal exercise programs were initiated that included specific exercises to promote comfort in pregnancy and prepare for childbirth. Kathleen Vaughan and Grantly Dick Read in England, the psychoprophylactic method in Russia, and Fernand Lamaze in France all taught exercises to provide the pregnant woman a sense of control and active participation in pregnancy and birth. Squatting, tailor sitting, pelvic floor, and breathing exercises were introduced. Many books and exercise programs have followed, and today pregnant women are encouraged to lead active lives throughout pregnancy.

From Artal, R., Wiswell, R. A., Drinkwater, B. L. (Eds.). (1991). *Exercise in pregnancy* (2nd ed., pp. 1–7). Baltimore: Williams and Wilkins.

The fetus is unable to reduce temperature through respiration or perspiration. An increase in maternal temperature exceeding 1.5°C during embryogenesis has been observed to affect the developing fetal brain. Such findings have suggested that there is a possible maternal threshold for human teratogenesis of 39.2°C, also explaining the observed increases in congenital anomalies seen with hot tub use in early pregnancy (Artal et al. 1991).

2. The effects of decreased uterine blood flow on the fetus. During exercise, blood flow to the uterus can decrease by as much as 59 to 70 percent as blood is shifted to priority organs and skeletal muscles. Maternal exercise increases circulating catecholamines, which can

Benefits of Exercise During Pregnancy

- Strengthens and tones muscles
- Increases joint flexion and mobility
- Increases maternal-fetal circulation
- Decreases discomforts of pregnancy
- Positively affects bowel function
- Assists in weight management
- Improves energy level and endurance
- Increases psychological well-being and self-esteem

cause visceral vasoconstriction. This could lead to fetal hypoxia and bradycardia (Fishbein and Phillips 1990; Vogt 1987).

3. The effects of activation of the sympathetic nervous system. A predominant rise in both epinephrine and serum norepinephrine occurs during exercise. Although epinephrine inhibits uterine activity, norepinephrine can act as a stimulant to the uterus and increase the frequency and amplitude of uterine contractions. These changes do not necessarily negate one another, and increased norepinephrine levels may precipitate preterm labor in women at risk for this complication (Artal et al. 1991; Fishbein and Phillips 1990).

The applicability of these animal studies to human pregnant subjects is not entirely clear. The findings have limited generalization to humans because of the anatomic and physiologic differences in animals and humans. Also, the physiologic effects observed when animals are forced to exercise may be more a function of the resultant stress than of the effects of the exercise. It is a challenge to conduct safe research and control for the many variables of both exercise and pregnancy with human pregnant subjects. The following preliminary conclusions can be drawn from the animal and human research studies done to date:

- No correlation has been found between fetal heart rate responses and gestational age, exercise intensity, and maternal circulating catecholamines (Fishbein and Phillips 1990; Vogt 1987).
- A "flush-back" effect occurs after exercise is completed. The decreased blood flow that occurs during exercise is rapidly reversed. This compensatory increase of blood flow beyond normal levels seems to protect the fetus during maternal exercise if the exercise is not prolonged (Fishbein and Phillips 1990; Vogt 1987).
- When exercise is performed for a moderate duration at a submaximal heart rate level, the healthy pregnant woman and her fetus are not compromised and exercise may have some beneficial effects (Mogul 1989; Thomas et al. 1989).
- If the pregnant woman is not healthy or is experiencing high-risk factors, exercise may accentuate those risk factors and thus should be individually evaluated and prescribed (Mogul 1989; Thomas et al. 1989).

CHANGES IN PREGNANCY INFLUENCING EXERCISE

The normal physiologic changes that occur during pregnancy influence the need for adaptation of exercise (see Chapter 16 for a complete discussion of physiologic changes of pregnancy). The most important maternal changes that need to be considered are the changes occurring in the respiratory, cardiovascular, and musculoskeletal systems. Metabolic changes also influence exercise tolerance.

Respiratory System

During pregnancy, respiratory vital capacity increases as a result of enlargement of the rib cage, due in part to relaxation of the ligamentous attachments. Increased oxygen consumption occurs, even when at rest, as a result of increased inspiratory capacity, decreased expiratory reserve volume, and decreased functional residual capacity. The development of a physiologic pulmonary hyperventilation early in pregnancy also contributes to increased oxygen consumption, as do additional body weight and tissue mass, increased red cell mass, and elevated blood volume. Increased oxygen consumption during exercise may also be caused in part by the increased work of the respiratory and cardiac muscles in hypeventilation. The added demands of pregnancy on the woman's body require more work, and thus more oxygen is consumed. The effect of exercise on oxygen consumption is not clear, although most studies seem to indicate that exercise further increases oxygen consumption over and above physiologic demands (Fishbein and Phillips 1990; Ketter and Shelton 1984; Nakahata 1988; Woodward 1988).

Cardiovascular System

The cardiovascular changes that influence exercise during pregnancy include increased blood volume, increased heart rate, increased stroke volume, increased cardiac output, and decreased cardiac reserve. When the pregnant woman exercises, there is further increase in heart rate, depending on the physical strain of the exercise. No change occurs in diastolic pressure, but systolic pressure increases. This is a normal response for any individual during exercise. Increased blood volume has no apparent effect on the circulatory system's response to exercise. The hemodilution that results from increased blood volume may cause a physiologic anemia during pregnancy. As discussed previously, blood is shunted from some internal visceral organs to the working skeletal musculature and priority organs during exercise (Fishbein and Phillips 1990; Ketter and Shelton 1984; Nakahata 1988; Woodward 1988).

Musculoskeletal System

Changes in the musculoskeletal system during pregnancy may alter the safety of activities that were possible before pregnancy. The increased laxity of joints, ligaments, and connective tissue fibers caused by hormonal changes and the shift in the center of gravity may predispose the woman to discomfort or injury from exercise that is not designed for her special needs. All joints and muscle attachments are more vulnerable to injury, particularly with sudden, forced movements. The amount of joint laxity varies with individuals and with parity. Postural changes resulting from generalized weight gain and the enlarging uterus shift the center of gravity forward and upward. These changes require ongoing adjustments, particularly in standing activities. Balance may also be altered by the increase in weight and the spinal lordosis (Ketter and Shelton 1984; Nakahata 1988).

Basal Metabolic Rate

Metabolic changes also influence the effects of exercise. The basal metabolic rate is higher, and increased metabolism is accompanied by a rise in heat production. Epinephrine and norepinephrine levels increase during exercise. During mild to moderate exercise, the changes are minimal and transient, returning to normal levels within 15 to 30 minutes (Artal et al. 1991; Fishbein and Phillips 1990).

RECOMMENDATIONS FOR A SAFE EXERCISE PROGRAM IN PREGNANCY

In light of the physiologic changes of pregnancy and the documented beneficial effects of exercise on the mother and fetus, a number of recommendations can be made to promote safe exercise during pregnancy (see Recommendations for Safe Exercise During Pregnancy). Ideally, women should begin an exercise program before they become pregnant. Women who exercise during pregnancy should be encouraged to do so regularly. Intermittent exercise is more likely to predispose the woman to injury. Women who have not been exercising before pregnancy should begin gradually

Recommendations for Safe Exercise During Pregnancy

1. Exercise regularly at least three times per week.
2. Always include a warm-up and cool-down period of exercise.
3. Avoid forced passive stretches; avoid deep flexion or extension of joints.
4. Avoid movements that hurt, jerking or bouncing movements, and sudden changes in position; exercise only on wood or tightly carpeted surfaces.
5. Limit aerobic activity to low impact only; stop if fatigue occurs; limit aerobic activity to 15 to 20 minutes if you have not exercised before pregnancy or to 30 minutes if you have previously exercised.
6. Do not overstrain abdominal muscles.
7. Avoid positions that exaggerate a lordotic curve or place the head lower than the stomach.
8. Maintain a pelvic tilt in standing or in the supine position.
9. Avoid use of the supine position after the first trimester; rise slowly from the floor; continue some form of activity involving the legs for a brief period after rising.
10. Measure heart rate at times of peak activity; do not exceed 140 beats per minute, and not for longer than 15 minutes.
11. Avoid overheating; drink plenty of water; do not exercise in hot, humid weather or when febrile.
12. Use controlled breathing; avoid the Valsalva maneuver.
13. Avoid competitive or high-risk sports.
14. Discontinue exercise if any unusual symptoms occur (see pp. 534–535).

Data from American College of Obstetricians and Gynecologists. (1994). *Exercise during pregnancy and the postpartum period* (ACOG Technical Bulletin, Number 189). Washington, DC: Author; Artal, R., Wiswell, R. A., Drinkwater, B. L. (Eds.). (1991). *Exercise in pregnancy* (2nd ed.). Baltimore: Williams & Wilkins; and Noble, E. (1988). *Essential exercises for the childbearing year.* Boston: Houghton Mifflin.

and increase exercise periods slowly. Warm-up and cool-down periods before and after exercise also prevent injury by gently stretching muscles. Because of the relaxation of joints and connective tissue due to relaxin and progesterone, activities that could cause injury should be avoided. This includes forced passive stretches; deep flexion or extension of joints; sudden changes in position; or jumping, jerking, and bouncing movements. Aerobic activity should be low impact only. Heart rate should be monitored before exercise and at times of peak activity and should not exceed 140 beats per minute. To avoid prolonged periods of shunting of uterine circulation and a prolonged rise in core body temperature, aerobic exercise should continue no longer than 15 to 20 minutes if the woman has not been exercising before pregnancy or 30 minutes if she was more active before the pregnancy. Exercise should take place for short periods, in the cool portion of the day, in an environment where the temperature and humidity are such that maternal mechanisms for heat dissipation are not compromised. Hydration should be maintained by drinking fluids frequently before, during, and after exercise.

Because abdominal muscles are already stretched, abdominal exercises should be monitored carefully. The rectus abdominis muscles may split if traditional abdominal exercises are done during pregnancy. Therefore, full sit-ups or double leg lifts should not be used. To protect the low back muscles, decrease the incidence of low backache, and promote good posture (see Fig. 19–2), a pelvic tilt should always be maintained in standing or in the supine position. This helps to counter the spinal lordosis that occurs during pregnancy. Use of the supine position should be limited, if used at all, to prevent orthostatic hypotension. After doing floor exercises, women should be cautioned to rise slowly from the floor and to use proper body mechanics when rising from a recumbent position or when bending or lifting (see Fig. 19–3). Exercising the legs should be continued for a brief period after floor activity to enhance venous return. The woman should never hold her breath while exercising but should maintain controlled breathing (American College of Obstetricians and Gynecologists 1994; Clapp 1989; Noble 1988).

EXERCISES TO INCLUDE

A number of exercises are recommended for women during pregnancy to promote comfort, to maintain good muscle tone, to promote a positive body image and to prepare for birth. Making the woman aware of good posture and body mechanics during pregnancy is a starting point and will promote comfort and decrease backache.

Traditional advice to pregnant women has been to continue those exercises that they have been doing on a regular basis but not to initiate new forms of exercise. Women who are conditioned to regular aerobic exercises before pregnancy can probably feel safe in continuing such activities as mild calisthenics or other aerobic programs. This type of exercise is beneficial for improving general cardiorespiratory status and physical fitness. Women who have not been participating regularly in an aerobic exercise program before pregnancy could begin such a program, but only if it is done slowly and under the supervision of an instructor who is knowledgeable about exercise in pregnancy.

Non–Weight-Bearing Exercises

Non–weight-bearing exercise (e.g., bicycling, swimming, or rowing) is preferable to weight-bearing exercise (e.g., jogging, cross-country skiing, and tennis), as it will decrease the risk of injury and facilitate the continuation of exercise throughout the pregnancy. Weight-bearing exercise can be performed if the appropriate safety guidelines are followed (see Recommendations for Safe Exercise During Pregnancy). However, it has been found that most women experience a decline in weight-bearing exercise performance during the course of the pregnancy. Non–weight-bearing exercises not only eliminate the bouncing caused by weight-bearing exercises but also decrease the workload and energy cost, and they may be better tolerated physically by the pregnant woman. Competitive or high-risk sports, such as scuba diving, water skiing, downhill skiing, horseback riding, basketball, volleyball, and gymnastics, should be avoided. Long-endurance exercises are not recommended since they delay the flush-back effect of returning blood supply to the uterus. Any exercise that can cause an air embolism to enter the uterine blood vessels should be discouraged. Because of the proximity of the uterine sinuses to the expansive vagina, the introduction of air into the circulation is possible. Examples of exercises to avoid are shoulder-standing and bicycling with the legs in the air. Use of the knee-chest position should also be avoided (American College of Obstetricians and Gynecologists 1994; Artal et al. 1991; Fishbein and Phillips 1990; Skinner 1993).

Pelvic Floor Exercises

The pelvic floor muscles support the uterus and other pelvic organs. Strengthening the pelvic floor muscles through pelvic floor and Kegel exercises helps the woman learn to relax the muscles in preparation for birth and helps promote healing and tone in the postpartum period (Sampselle et al. 1989) (see Teaching Guide: Kegel Exercises). After learning the location of the pelvic floor muscles, the woman learns to contract the muscles as though she were trying to prevent the flow of

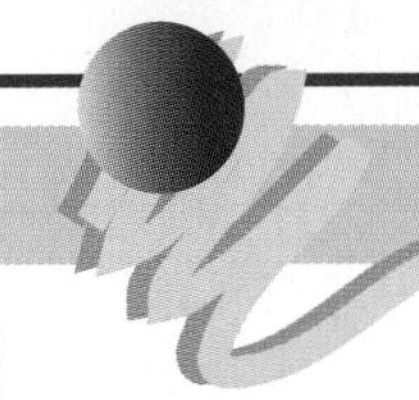

TEACHING GUIDE

KEGEL EXERCISES

TOPIC	*MAJOR CONCEPTS*
Description of the Kegel muscle	The Kegel muscle, also known as the pubococcygeal muscle, serves as the major muscle of support for the pelvic floor. The Kegel muscle is like a hammock that attaches in the front at the symphysis pubis and in the back at the coccyx.
Purpose of the Kegel muscle	The Kegel muscle provides support for the uterus, bladder, rectum, and vagina. Proper position and good tone of the Kegel muscle prevent prolapse of these pelvic organs and also prevent stress incontinence. At the time of birth, the Kegel muscle stretches to allow the baby to be born.

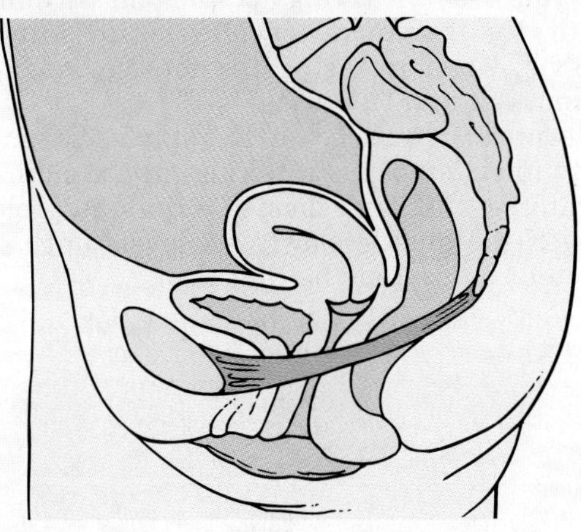

Proper position and good tone of the pubococcygeal muscle provide support for the pelvic organs

Rationale for exercising the Kegel muscle	If not exercised regularly, the Kegel muscle can lose tone and begin to sag, allowing the pelvic organs to prolapse or contributing to stress incontinence. At the time of birth, the Kegel muscle is more elastic and stretches more readily if it has been exercised. When the Kegel muscle is in good tone, it provides support to the vaginal walls, contributing to increased sexual enjoyment during coitus.

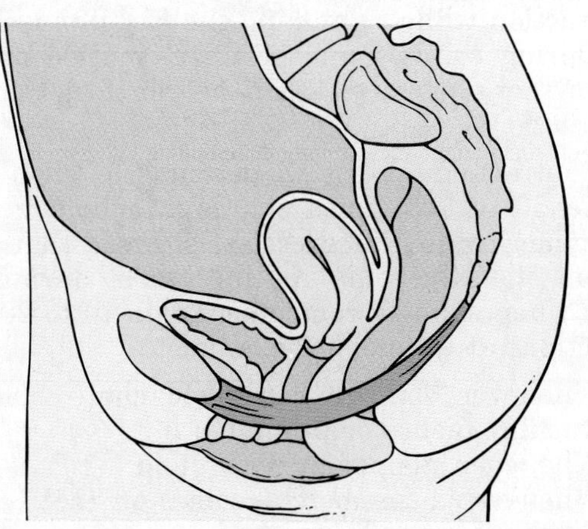

Incorrect position and poor tone of the pubococcygeal muscle can result in prolapse of the pelvic organs

Continued on following page

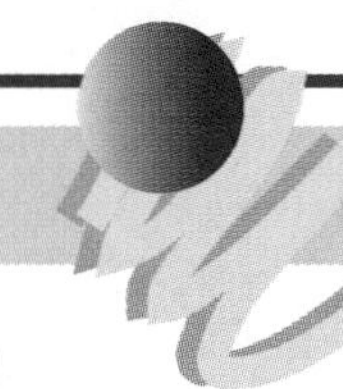

TEACHING GUIDE Continued

KEGEL EXERCISES

TOPIC	*MAJOR CONCEPTS*
Description of Kegel exercises	The Kegel muscle is exercised by contracting and releasing it; two forms of the exercise can be done: 1. Contract-release: When contracting the muscle, tighten around the urethra, vagina, and rectum—as if trying to prevent urination. Pull the hammock of muscle up into the pelvis; when releasing the muscle, relax the hammock and feel it sag. 2. Elevator: Contract the Kegel muscle gradually in six steps, as if taking an ascending elevator to the sixth floor of a building; release the Kegel muscle slowly six levels until completely relaxed at the first floor.

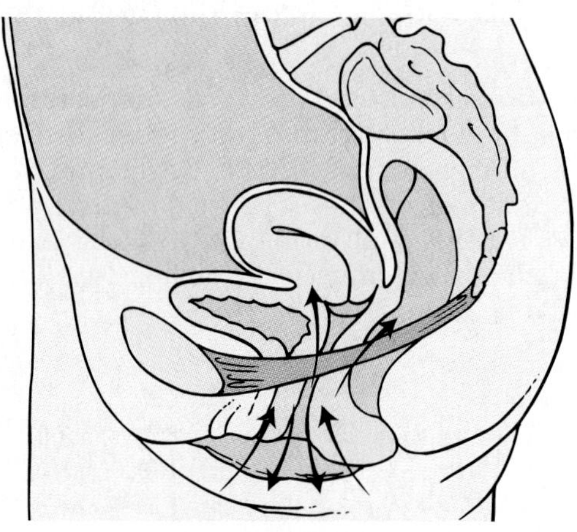

Contraction and release of the pubococcygeal muscle (Kegel exercises) can improve muscle tone, thereby providing better support for the pelvic organs

TOPIC	*MAJOR CONCEPTS*
Ways to check correct use of the Kegel muscle during exercise	The following checks can be made to ensure correct performance of the exercise. • When voiding, begin flow of urine, then contract the Kegel muscle to stop flow of urine midstream. • Insert one finger into vagina and feel for contraction while tightening the Kegel muscle. • During coitus, contract Kegel muscle around partner's penis to see if he can feel the contraction.
Instructions for practice	Contraction of the Kegel muscle should be done 50 to 100 times per day; to help her remember to do the exercise, suggest that your client identify some routine times during the day when she will remember to do 10 to 20 contractions at a time. For example: • Whenever doing a household chore, such as washing dishes or ironing • Whenever stopped at a red light • Whenever a commercial comes on TV • Whenever standing in a line, such as at the bank or grocery store

Continued on facing page

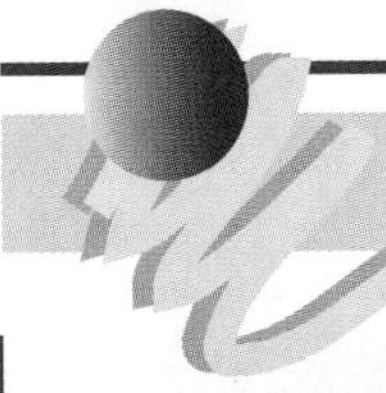

TEACHING GUIDE Continued

KEGEL EXERCISES

Teaching Aids

1. Posters or illustrations showing (1) pelvic floor muscles, (2) contrast of position of muscles and pelvic organs in good and poor tone, and (3) baby moving through pelvic floor muscles at delivery.
2. Use of hands to illustrate Kegel muscle attaching at pubis and coccyx; the hand can also illustrate how the Kegel muscle is pulled up as it is contracted and released as it is relaxed.
3. Empty coffee can with both ends removed; latex glove; rubber band. Place rim of cuff on glove around one end of can and secure with strong rubber band; fingers of glove are inside can. Latex across opening of can illustrates the pelvic floor muscles. Using your hand inside can, gently and slowly pull fingers of glove upward, showing how the Kegel muscle is tightened and released.

Increasing Your Teaching Effectiveness

Your success in teaching the Kegel exercises will be enhanced by using the following approaches:

1. Establish a comfortable rapport with the woman before teaching the exercises; the somewhat intimate nature of the exercises could embarrass her if she does not feel comfortable with you.
2. Use visual aids and teaching materials to demonstrate the exercises.
3. Emphasize the importance of the Kegel exercises by providing the rationale for their use.
4. Ask for feedback or questions throughout your teaching presentation.
5. Follow up your teaching during your next contact with the woman to identify whether she had problems or questions and to encourage her to practice.

urine. Once she is able to isolate the pubococcygeal muscle, which serves as the major muscle of support for the pelvic floor, she should imagine contracting around the urethra, vagina, and rectum. Women should do 100 of these contractions each day. During pregnancy, these should be done in groups of 10 at a time, and each contraction should be held for a count of five. An "elevator" form of the exercise can also be done in which the woman contracts and releases the pubococcygeal muscle in steps. The pelvic floor exercises can be done in any position and incorporated easily into the woman's day.

Pelvic Rock Exercise

The pelvic rock/pelvic tilt exercise is important in pregnancy to prevent or relieve low backache. It is also useful in helping the woman to maintain good posture and to strengthen abdominal muscles. The pelvic tilt can be taught in many positions, including standing, sitting, lateral recumbent, and on hands and knees. When doing the exercise on hands and knees in the third trimester, the woman should be cautioned to always maintain a flat position of the back and not allow the back to sag, as this could increase back discomfort. To do the exercise, the woman first tilts or rocks the pelvis toward the face by tucking the buttocks under her pelvis, tightening her abdominal muscles, and arching her back slightly. The second step of the exercise reverses this process. The pelvis is tilted away from the face, abdominal muscles are relaxed, and the back is flat. These two steps are repeated in a slow rocking movement (Fig. 19–8).

Abdominal Exercise

Abdominal strengthening exercises help to maintain tone in the abdominal muscles to provide support to the spine during pregnancy, to prepare for expulsion in the second stage of labor, and to promote return of muscle tone in the postpartum period. Several forms of abdominal exercises can be taught. Partial or "mini" sit-ups can be taught safely in pregnancy. The woman begins in a supine position with knees bent and feet on the floor. A pillow or wedge should be placed under one hip so that she is not flat on her back. As she exhales, the woman tightens abdominal muscles and raises her head and shoulders off the floor while reaching for her knees with her arms. She then inhales as she returns to the starting

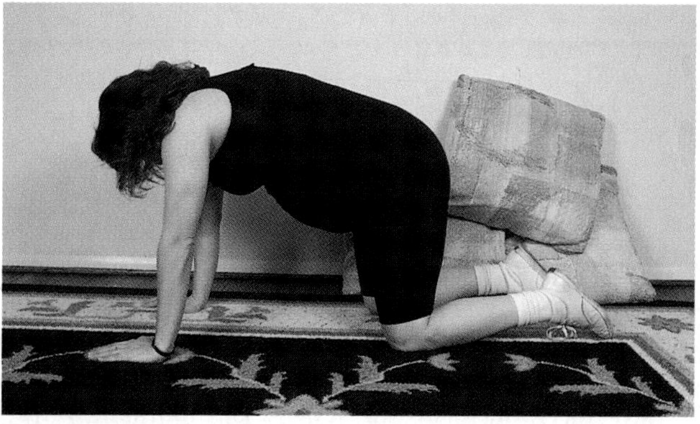
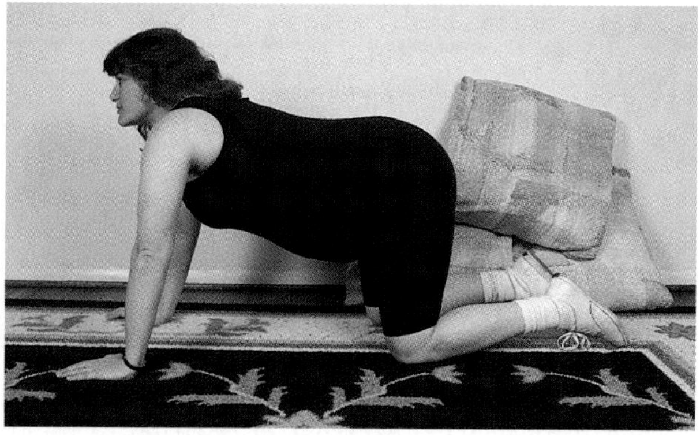

Figure 19–8

Pelvic rock exercise • helps prevent or relieve low backache • strengthens abdominal muscles • helps pregnant women maintain good posture • can be done in standing, sitting, lateral recumbent, or hands and knees position. Pelvic rock exercise in the hands and knees position involves two steps, which are repeated in a slow rocking movement. *Left,* The woman tilts or rocks her pelvis toward her face by tucking her buttocks under her pelvis, tightening her abdominal muscles, and arching her back slightly. *Right,* The woman reverses the process by gently tilting or rocking her pelvis away from her face, relaxing her abdominal muscles, and flattening her back.

position (Fig. 19–9, *left*). An alternative way of doing an abdominal exercise is known as a let-back. With this exercise, the woman begins in a sitting position with knees bent and feet on the floor. With arms stretched out toward her knees, she leans back slightly toward the floor as she tightens abdominal muscles and exhales. She then inhales as she returns to the starting position. These exercises should be done slowly in repetitions of ten (Fig. 19–9, *right*).

CONTRAINDICATIONS TO EXERCISE IN PREGNANCY

There are a number of contraindications to exercise during pregnancy. Any factors that could compromise physiologic adaptation to exercise should be evaluated by the physician or midwife before an exercise program is begun. Contraindications include risk for preterm labor, multiple gestation, hypertension, diabetes, cardiovascular disease, pregnancy-induced hypertension, vaginal or uterine bleeding, premature rupture of membranes, incompetent cervix/cerclage, malnutrition or poor weight gain, anemia, intrauterine growth retardation, fetal distress, kidney disease, endocrine disorders, and neurologic or psychiatric disorders. If the woman experiences any unusual symptoms while exercising, she should discontinue exercise immediately and report her symptoms to her health care provider. Such symptoms include chest, back, pubic, or hip pain; headache; uterine contractions at intervals of 20 minutes or less;

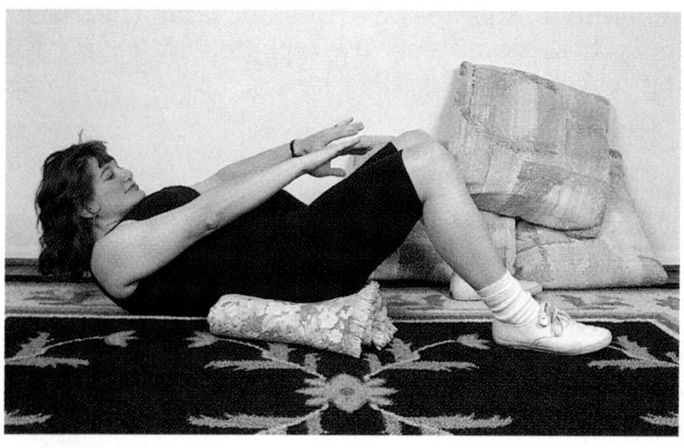
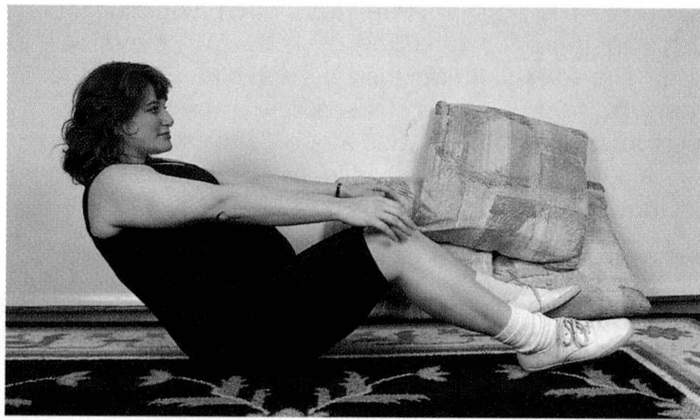

Figure 19–9

Abdominal strengthening exercises help maintain abdominal muscle tone during pregnancy. Strong abdominal muscles provide support to the spine during pregnancy • support expulsion in the second stage of labor • promote return of muscle tone in the postpartum period. *Left,* In the mini sit-up, the woman begins the exercise in a supine position with knees bent and feet on the floor. She exhales, tightens her abdominal muscles, and raises her head and shoulders off the floor while reaching for her knees with her hands. She then inhales and returns to the starting position. During this exercise, a towel roll or wedge should be placed under the woman's hip so that she is not flat on her back. *Right,* In the let-back exercise, the woman begins in a sitting position with knees bent and feet flat on the floor. She stretches her arms forward toward her knees and leans back slightly toward the floor as she tightens her abdominal muscles and exhales. She then inhales as she returns to the starting position.

dizziness, faintness, shortness of breath, palpitations, or tachycardia; persistent nausea and vomiting; difficulty walking; generalized edema; and decreased fetal activity (American College of Obstetricians and Gynecologists 1994; Artal et al. 1991).

Emotional Aspects of Exercise in Pregnancy

In nonpregnant individuals, many studies have shown that the psychological benefits of exercise include increased self-esteem, confidence, and happiness. Exercise seems to be related to a decrease in depression, anxiety, and minor medical complaints. Few studies have examined the psychological effects of exercise on pregnant women. The few studies that have been done have reported an increased sense of well-being, fewer physical complaints, improved appetite, better sleep patterns, and improved self-image and self-esteem. Because pregnancy is a time when many women express feelings of a negative body image, the positive emotional aspects of exercise are significant. Exercise may help decrease the pregnant woman's anxiety about the birth process by giving her a sense of control over her body. These findings should be viewed with caution, however, for most studies compare self-selected exercising and nonexercising groups, rather than using random assignment. It is possible that women who choose to exercise may already have a higher self-concept or a more positive body image. It is safe to assume, however, that a program of regular exercise in pregnancy can provide positive emotional benefits. Exercise is usually an enjoyable activity and can be a source of fun during pregnancy, particularly if it is integrated into the woman's daily routine (Reich 1987; Wallace et al. 1986; Wallace and Engstrom 1987).

Sociocultural Aspects of Exercise in Pregnancy

Exercise can provide an important social activity for women during pregnancy. A group exercise class for pregnant women can provide a chance to meet with other pregnant women, give the needed motivation to continue exercise regularly, and be a source of enjoyment. As with exercise at any stage of the life span, it is more difficult to maintain discipline when exercising alone.

The woman's sociocultural background may influence her willingness to participate in an exercise program during pregnancy. If her culture or religion views exercise as taboo or if cultural beliefs or old wives' tales suggest negative outcomes from exercise, the woman is not likely to participate in an exercise program. It is important to assess the influence of culture and religion before prescribing exercises. If such influences are identified, it is possible that cognitive information could counteract sociocultural aspects, but continual support and encouragement would be needed.

Cognitive Aspects of Exercise in Pregnancy

Without a cognitive understanding of the benefits and safety precautions of exercise during pregnancy, the woman may not become involved in a regular exercise program or may become involved in exercise that is not safe. It is important, therefore, that information be given to pregnant women about the value of exercise and exercises that are helpful. This can be done through the use of printed information, in one-to-one teaching during antepartum appointments, or in group childbirth classes.

STRESS MANAGEMENT IN PREGNANCY

Stress is an unavoidable component of life in modern society. All individuals experience some level of stress each day and learn to adapt in ways that are effective for them. Stress is not always negative and can be a motivating or protective factor in life. Selye (1976) defined stress as the nonspecific response of the body to any demand or stimulus. A nonspecific response is one that affects all or most parts of the body without selectivity and occurs as a result of either a positive or negative stimulus. Thus, the stress response is the body's physical, mental, and chemical reactions to frightening, unknown, exciting, joyful, confusing, endangering, or irritating situations.

The situations that trigger the stress response are called stressors. Stressors may be of a beneficial or a harmful nature, depending on the individual, the situation, or the intensity of the stressor. As a result, stress can be either "eustress," a pleasant stress, or "distress," an unpleasant or unhealthy stress (Selye 1976). Stress can be caused by such factors as family life, physical exertion or injury, trauma, job or career, urban or national problems, role overload, or social situations. Pregnancy is a stressor for many women. Women may experience additional stress during pregnancy as a result of the necessary physical and emotional adaptations that are required.

Physical Aspects of Stress

Stress responses may include physiologic and psychological symptoms that can lead to illness. In the 1950s, Selye described a physiologic response to stress called the general adaptation syndrome. This theory proposes that a universal pattern of physiologic reactions occurs in three progressive stages (i.e., an alarm reaction, the stage of resistance, and the stage of exhaustion) as a result of stress. In time, if the stress is severe and prolonged, the body undergoes neurophysical and hormonal changes that can result in adaptation problems and illness.

It is unhealthy for the body to remain in a heightened state of arousal. The body's immune system is suppressed in response to stress through the effects of cortisol. Cortisol has been shown in the laboratory to increase the level of cholesterol and other lipids in the blood and to increase the development of atherosclerosis. Symptoms of stress include lack of energy, muscle tension, headaches, loss of appetite, diarrhea, gastrointestinal ulcers, backaches, and insomnia (Queenan 1986).

Whenever people encounter stress, they attempt to adapt to it. If adaptation is successful, the individual's balance will not be disturbed or will be restored. Physical adaptation to stress is accomplished by the brain, the central and autonomic nervous systems, and the pituitary and adrenal glands. The pituitary and adrenals release hormones that specifically combat stress and inhibit or stimulate the body's defense mechanisms. Selye calls the hormones produced by the pituitary and adrenal glands adaptive hormones. Antiinflammatory corticoids or glucocorticoids (e.g., cortisone) inhibit excessively defensive activities on the part of the body. Proinflammatory corticoids or mineralocorticoids (e.g., aldosterone) stimulate the body's defenses. The stress response can be influenced by such conditioning factors as age, diet, climate, heredity, marital status, education, social support, past exposure to stress, and typical coping patterns. These factors are responsible for the varying individual ways in which different persons react to the same degree of stress.

During pregnancy, stress can affect both maternal and fetal adaptation. One study found that stress may trigger a drop in salivary immunoglobulin A during pregnancy and parturition (Annie and Groër 1991). A number of studies have been done that relate stress during pregnancy with poor perinatal outcomes. Although both animal and human studies have shown conflicting findings, stress during pregnancy has been associated with maternal obstetric complications, fetal and neonatal abnormalities, and low birth weight (Ascher 1978). During labor, high anxiety scores and epinephrine levels were associated with longer labors, poorer quality uterine contractions, and neonates who experienced more health problems (Lederman et al. 1978, 1981). The stress of having a high-risk pregnancy has been associated with less optimal family functioning (Mercer et al. 1988).

Emotional Aspects of Stress

There is increasing recognition that emotion and cognition are closely linked in the stress response. After the cognitive evaluation of a stressor, a person determines the degree of threat and the resources available to meet the demand. Almost simultaneously, a fluctuation in general anxiety takes place, followed by a refinement of the energy into one or more specific emotions. The stimulation of the sympathetic nervous system also contributes to emotional responses. Emotions such as fear, sadness, anticipation, anger, and surprise are common responses to stress. The resultant response of these emotions is then a subsequent translation of the emotion into a coping behavior. With activation of the parasympathetic nervous system after the stressor has passed, the feelings perceived are comfortable, pleasurable, and relaxing (Scott et al. 1980).

Emotional adaptation to stress often occurs as a result of coping strategies. Coping strategies are categorized as affective (emotional), cognitive (informational), and instrumental (tangible). They can be either a direct action to resolve the problem or palliative measures to reduce the anxiety. Palliative responses include symptom-directed strategies such as relaxation techniques and exercise or defense mechanisms such as denial and projection (Lazarus 1976). Coping can be employed consciously or unconsciously. Coping strategies can be beneficial in reducing stress and related anxiety, or they may be ineffective and actually increase stress and anxiety. Many people gain confidence in themselves, achieve goals, and develop new potentials as a result of successfully adapting to a stressful situation. If adaptation is consistently faulty, illness may result.

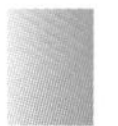

Sociocultural Aspects of Stress

Sociocultural factors can influence the individual's physical stress response, the cognitive perception of a stressor, and the emotional response. The environment or context in which the stressor occurs, the presence or absence of a social support system, and demographic characteristics such as age, educational level, marital status, or occupation all play a part in shaping a stressful situation. For example, the degree of fatigue and stress of a pregnant woman's job has been shown to relate to early uterine activity (Public Health Service 1989). Coping responses may be influenced by culture or religion. The behavior seen in a stressful situation is often influenced by the beliefs or taboos of a sociocultural group.

Cognitive Aspects of Stress

The cognitive branch of stress research is based on Piaget's developmental psychology. Using this framework, cognitive psychologists suggest that a mental operation underlies and affects the physiologic level of the stress response. The individual continuously scans the environment for stimuli and then operates on the stimulus through a careful and continual evaluation of the threat to system survival. One of three possible appraisals of the stressor occurs: (1) irrelevent; (2) benign, resulting in positively toned emotions; or (3) stressful, resulting in negatively toned emotions. If the stimuli are appraised as stressful, further differentiation occurs and includes (1) harm—loss, injury, or damage has already been done; (2) threat—anticipated trauma has not yet occurred in a perceived hostile and dangerous environment, with the self lacking in the resources to master it; or (3) challenge—opportunity for growth, mastery, or gain in view of demands that are difficult but not impossible with existing or acquirable skills.

The essential point of the cognitive approach is that in the progression of events occurring after the introduction of a stressor, cognitive functioning encompasses all neurological levels of system control, autonomic regulation, elicitation of feeling states, sensory selection processes, memory, and mental operation. In coping with stress, it is the cognitive appraisal of the situation that occurs first. Emotional and physiologic responses to stress occur only after cognitive appraisal. The cognitive phase of the primary appraisal of the stressor determines the intensity and the quality of the emotional response (Scott et al. 1980).

Stress Management Techniques

Because stress is part of our lives and cannot be avoided, it is essential to develop adaptive responses to it. Holistic approaches to stress management include attention to diet, exercise, and relaxation strategies. Diet and exercise have already been discussed in this chapter. Both scientific research and empirical observations have shown the benefits of various relaxation techniques in decreasing stress. During the childbearing year, women can be taught these techniques to decrease stress during pregnancy, to cope with the pain and stress of labor and birth, and to deal with the stress of new parenthood in the postpartum period. Relaxation skills can be taught individually to a woman during an antepartum visit or in prepared childbirth classes.

Relaxation techniques are useful in reducing the damaging psychophysiologic effects of stress and promoting a sense of physical and mental well-being. They can result in an altered state of consciousness and produce a decrease in sympathetic nervous system activity. All relaxation strategies require four basic elements for them to be maximally effective: (1) a calm, quiet environment with minimal distractions; (2) a mental focus; (3) a passive attitude so that distracting thoughts are pushed aside; and (4) a comfortable position that reduces the need for muscle effort. A number of different relaxation strategies can be used to decrease stress. These are also discussed in Chapter 20.

▼ **Progressive Relaxation.** Progressive relaxation consists of the systematic tensing and releasing of muscles to develop body awareness and identify the difference between tension and release of a muscle group.

▼ **Neuromuscular Dissociation.** Neuromuscular dissociation, also called selective relaxation, teaches women to tense some muscles and relax others simultaneously in preparation for maintaining a relaxed body during uterine contractions in labor.

▼ **Touch and Massage.** Touch relaxation and massage are a means for the partner to help the woman relax muscle groups, to promote comfort, and to facilitate communication (Fig. 19–10).

▼ **Visual Imagery and Music.** Visual imagery and music can be used along with any of these relaxation techniques to enhance a relaxed state and alter the stress response.

▼ **Biofeedback.** Biofeedback, a strategy for helping people develop an awareness of body processes, can also be taught to pregnant women to facilitate stress reduction and relaxation (see Chapter 24).

▼ **Controlled Breathing.** Controlled breathing techniques are taught not only to alter pain perception in labor but also to facilitate relaxation.

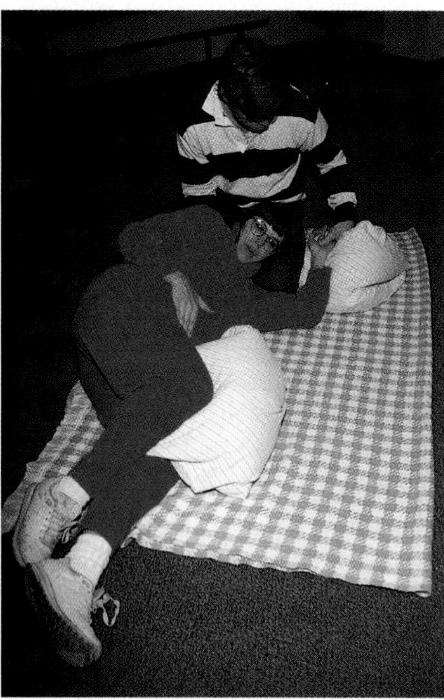

Figure 19–10

During the childbearing year, women can learn techniques such as touch relaxation for decreasing stress during pregnancy. Practicing touch relaxation with her partner can promote the woman's physical comfort, reduce stress, and facilitate communication.

Other activities during pregnancy are also useful as a means of stress management. Social or volunteer activities allow the pregnant woman to remain involved in her community and focus on issues other than her pregnancy. Hobbies such as painting, crafts, or photography allow her to remain mentally active and provide relaxation. Exercise, as discussed earlier, is helpful in decreasing discomforts, providing a social outlet, and decreasing stress. Support groups consisting of other pregnant women may also be a helpful way to manage stress by providing a forum for sharing and discussion of concerns.

COMMON CONCERNS DURING PREGNANCY

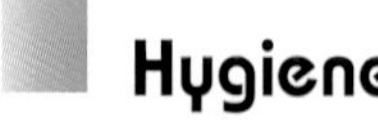

Hygiene

Daily hygiene becomes even more important to the woman during pregnancy because of the increase in perspiration and vaginal discharge caused by hormonal changes. Both showers and tub baths are safe during pregnancy, although tub baths should not be advised if the woman is bleeding or if she suspects that her membranes have ruptured, because of the risk that bacteria might be introduced into the vaginal tract. The woman should also be aware of safety as she gets into and out of the tub so that she does not fall. Prolonged submersion in hot tubs is not advised during pregnancy because of the potential harmful effects of elevated core body temperature on the fetus. Dental hygiene and care are also important components of health care during pregnancy and should not be neglected (Blau 1987; Chenger and Kovacik 1987).

Comfortable clothing should be worn during pregnancy to allow comfort and prevent restriction of venous circulation. Attractive clothing during pregnancy also contributes to the woman's self-esteem. Clothing can be fashionable as well as comfortable and might include larger sizes of regular fashions or maternity fashions. Although girdles are seldom worn by women today, if the woman has a large pendulous abdomen during pregnancy, a supportive girdle will promote good posture and help to prevent backache. A good supportive bra should be worn to accommodate the increasing size of the breasts. Shoes should be either flat or with a small heel. High-heeled shoes not only add to back discomfort, they may be unsafe as the woman begins to experience alterations in balance as her center of gravity changes.

Adequate Rest and Sleep

Because of the physical demands that pregnancy places on the pregnant woman, many women express fatigue throughout pregnancy. This fatigue may be greatest in the first trimester when drowsiness is a common symptom and again in the third trimester as the baby and uterus reach full size. Adequate rest and sleep are an important component of daily health care to counteract these symptoms. The pregnant woman should plan her schedule so that she can get 7 to 8 hours of sleep each night. Regular periods of rest during the day are also essential. Ideally, one or two of these rest periods should be spent lying down, either in the side-lying position to promote placental perfusion or with legs elevated to relieve edema in the lower extremities. Establishing a good pattern of sleep and rest periods may be a challenge for the woman with small children or the woman who is employed; however, making an effort to do so will enable the woman to deal with the stressors of pregnancy and prepare her for the stresses of the postpartum period.

Safety

TRAVEL

Most forms of travel are safe during pregnancy; however, women should make provisions for frequent rest periods, consider diet and exercise options while away from home, and make plans for access to maternity care if needed. Some pregnant women express a sense of uneasiness regarding travel during pregnancy as they become more aware of the risks in relation to the safety of their unborn baby. Several precautions for travel during pregnancy are important to consider.

Travel by automobile may be tiring and uncomfortable, particularly for long distances. The woman should stop every 2 hours to walk about. The use of seat belts is essential in traveling by car. Many people, including pregnant women, continue to be ambivalent about seat belt use, despite the fact that seat belts have been proved effective in reducing deaths and serious injuries. One study showed that less than 50 percent of a sample of pregnant women used seat belts regularly during pregnancy, and for those who did, use was often incorrect (Arneson et al. 1986; Hammond et al. 1990). Some controversy has existed regarding the safety of lap-type seat belts alone for pregnant women; however, any risk to the fetus from the lap portion of the seat belt at the time of the impact is far less than the risk from the mother's being ejected from the automobile. The pregnant woman should use both a lap belt and a shoulder harness to decrease the force of an impact and prevent the woman's body from flexing forward over the lap belt. The lap belt should be worn snugly and as low as possible across the abdomen and hips, so that it is under the fetus. The shoulder restraint should be over the shoulder and across the chest and upper abdomen (Fig. 19–11) (Chang et al. 1987; Hammond et al. 1990; Krozy and McColgan 1986).

Travel by other means also requires additional precautions during pregnancy. Air or train travel is safe and often recommended for long-distance travel as pregnancy progresses, although many airlines will not allow pregnant women to fly in the last month of pregnancy. Airplane travel should be in a pressurized cabin only. Provisions should be made for regular movement and ambulation. An aisle seat on a airplane or train is most desirable for this purpose. The woman should get up and move about frequently; pelvic rocking, foot circles, and relaxation exercises can be done while sitting in the seat (Reukema 1985).

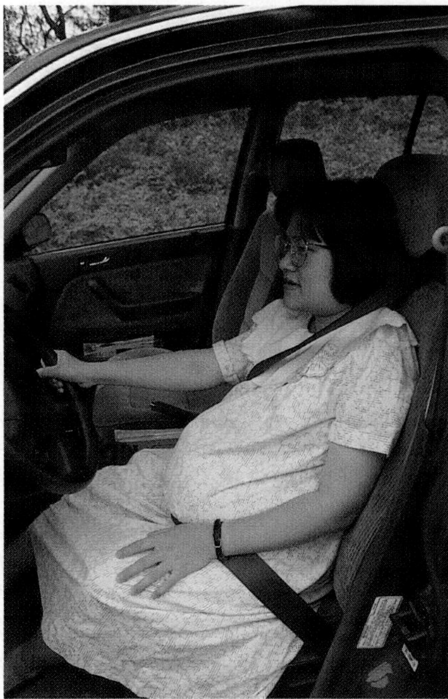

Figure 19–11

The pregnant woman should always use both a lap belt and a shoulder restraint during automobile travel. The lap belt should be worn as low as possible across the abdomen and hips, so that it is under the fetus. The shoulder restraint should be across the chest and upper abdomen.

MEDICATIONS

Most medications taken by the woman during pregnancy pass through the placenta and thus have the potential of affecting the fetus in some way (Ericson 1987). The teratogenic effects of some medications are not yet known. It is important that the pregnant woman consult with her caregiver regarding any over-the-counter drug that she plans to take, and she should keep a record of medications taken during pregnancy (Brackbill 1987). Even substances that are not commonly thought to be detrimental can be teratogenic during pregnancy. For example, megadoses of some vitamins can cause problems with fetal development. Isotretinoin (Accutane), a synthetic derivative of vitamin A, has been linked with a variety of birth defects (Thompson and Cordero 1989). In the past few years, a number of medications that were previously available only by prescription have now become available over-the-counter. The woman should always read package inserts and consult with her physician before taking antacids or using medicated vaginal creams that might not be safe during pregnancy. The greatest risk of teratogenic effects from medications is during the first trimester when early fetal development is occurring (see Chapter 15).

EMPLOYMENT

Since one of every two women in the childbearing years is employed, concerns regarding the safety of work during pregnancy have increased.

Many pregnant women today work until the time they go into labor. The decision to work may not be an option for some pregnant women because of financial need, while others may work because of a strong investment or commitment to a career. Pregnant women often express concern regarding the safety of their job, how long they can work during pregnancy, and when it is advisable to return to work after the baby is born. Concern has also been expressed regarding the psychological effects of working during pregnancy (Homer et al. 1990). Many women today experience role strain or role overload as they attempt to balance employment, management of the home, and marital and parental roles. However, many women find work to be a positive psychosocial diversion and a social stimulus.

Potential workplace and environmental hazards during pregnancy include physical hazards (gravity, radiation, temperature, noise, vibration, and humidity) and chemical hazards (metals, anesthetic gases, vinyl chloride, solvents, pesticides, antineoplastic agents, and sterilants) (Ericson 1987; Hein 1989; Moore 1989). Some occupations pose a greater work-related risk than others. Operating room personnel, x-ray technicians, dental assistants, and some laboratory or pharmacy workers may be exposed to chemicals, drugs, gases, and radiation that could be harmful to the fetus unless precautions are taken. Industrial settings vary so widely that it is difficult to make generalizations about possible harmful exposures. Home industries, such as arts and crafts, where chemicals such as solvents may be used, are of concern because individuals often lack the knowledge, resources, and regulatory supervision that can help to minimize similar exposures in large-scale industrial settings. Jobs that require physical stamina or balance may become unsafe as the pregnancy progresses. Sedentary jobs may require regular short breaks for the purpose of ambulation, stretching, and leg exercise. It is advisable that the woman spend some time lying down in the left lateral position during her midday lunch break. Fatigue is the factor that often determines how long the woman is able to continue her full job schedule as she nears term (Bernhardt 1990; Bryant 1985; Holt 1984).

One particular concern regarding job safety is the effect of video display terminals (VDTs) during pregnancy. Measurements have confirmed that the low-voltage cathode ray tube and thick glass of the VDT produce no x-rays outside the terminal. Scientists do not know what, if any, biologic damage the electrical field can cause, but the electrical field or radiation is well below currently acceptable levels of exposure. There is no convincing evidence to date that VDTs affect the outcome of pregnancy. Although a few studies have related VDT use with miscarriage, on evaluation, other factors such as socioeconomic status or chance seem to be more likely to be influencing pregnancy outcome. Even though VDTs do emit several types of electromagnetic radiation, studies from the National Institute for Occupational Safety and Health indicate that the machines do not emit enough radiation to pose any health threat to either the woman or the fetus. Further studies are being planned to evaluate this potential risk (Mayo Clinic 1989).

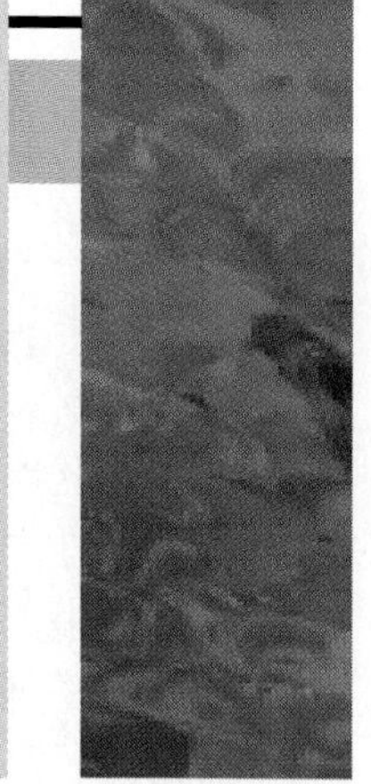

Nursing Practice

Nursing Process

To promote a healthy pregnancy, the management of the pregnant woman's health care should include both risk assessment and health promotion. This health promotion should actually begin before the pregnancy occurs. Once pregnant, the woman should be encouraged to seek health care early in the pregnancy and to continue it regularly (Thompson 1989; Thompson and Culpepper 1989; Vogt 1987; Young et al. 1989). Using the nursing process in establishing a care plan helps the nurse ensure comprehensive management of the woman's care. Beginning at the end of this chapter on page 554, Nursing Care Planning Guide: Healthy Pregnancy shows how the nursing process is applied in creating a plan of care designed to meet an individual's needs.

▼ Assessment

Early and continuing assessments should be made with special attention to the pregnant woman's discomforts, nutritional status, exercise, stress levels, and safety. Attention to all of these factors provides the nurse with a holistic basis for planning care. Assessment tools, such as the Health History Summary (pp. 556–557), the Initial Lifestyle Profile (p. 558), and the Initial Pregnancy Profile (p. 559), enable the nurse to gather the data pertinent to the planning and implementation of prenatal care. By obtaining this information early and throughout the pregnancy, the nurse will be able to determine the woman's need for information or intervention and can influence the woman's health status during the pregnancy.

▼ DISCOMFORTS OF PREGNANCY

The assessment of pregnancy discomforts can be done verbally by the nurse, through a written checklist given to the woman during her antepartum visit, or by asking her to keep a diary of her symptoms. It is essential that this assessment be repeated at regular intervals, however, for discomforts will change as the pregnancy progresses. Obtaining the data is of no value unless the information is then followed with teaching and counseling interventions that will help the woman manage the discomforts she is experiencing. This assessment also allows the nurse to differentiate between symptoms that represent normal discomforts of pregnancy and symptoms that may signal the onset of more serious complications (Moore et al. 1985).

▼ NUTRITIONAL STATUS

A nutritional assessment is a critical component of the health assessment and should include physical, emotional, cognitive, and sociocultural data regarding the woman's nutritional status. The physical nutritional data should include weight-height analysis, laboratory data, physical inspection, and dietary history.

Weight-Height Analysis. The weight-height analysis includes information about the woman's prepregnant weight, her weight gain during pregnancy, and the rate of her gain. Skinfold measurements may also be done to assess body fat stores. Key elements for assessing weight gain during pregnancy are provided in Assessment of Maternal Weight During Pregnancy.

Laboratory Data. Routine laboratory data should include measurement of hemoglobin and hematocrit to identify anemia; urine testing for glucose and ketone bodies to screen for gestational dia-

Assessment of Maternal Weight During Pregnancy

- Before conception, use consistent and reliable procedures to accurately measure and record the woman's weight and height without shoes.
- Determine the woman's pre-pregnancy body mass index (weight/height^2, calculated in metric units of kilograms and meters). The result is then compared with the classifications seen in Table 19–5.
- Measure height and weight at the first prenatal visit by using careful procedures that have been rigorously standardized at the site of prenatal care; compare this weight with the pre-pregnancy weight, which provides the baseline for monitoring weight change during the course of pregnancy.
- Use consistent, reliable procedures to measure weight at each subsequent visit.
- Estimate the woman's gestational age from the onset of her last menstruation; supplement with estimates based on the clinical examination and early ultrasound examination.
- Record weight in a table and plot it on a chart included in the prenatal record; week of gestation should be shown on the horizontal axis and weight on the vertical axis.
- Set a weight gain goal together with the pregnant woman at her first prenatal appointment, and explain why weight gain is important.
- Base the recommended range of total weight gain and pattern of gain mainly on pre-pregnancy weight for height (for a woman of normal pre-pregnancy weight for height carrying a single fetus, this will be 25 to 35 pounds).
- Monitor the prenatal course to identify any abnormal pattern of gain that may indicate a need to intervene. Assess the pattern of gain at each visit relative to the established weight gain goal and the course leading to that goal.
- When abnormal gain appears to be real, rather than a result of an error in measurement or recording, try to determine the cause and then develop and implement corrective actions jointly with the woman.

betes; and urine testing for protein to screen for hypertensive disorders of pregnancy (see discussion of laboratory tests, p. 437, in Chapter 16 for further information). Tests of serum protein and other vitamin and mineral levels may also be performed; however, these are not usually routine.

Physical Inspection. Physical inspection includes an impression of general appearance and examination of the skin, mucous membranes, lips, gums and teeth, tongue, eyes, nails, and hair (Table 19–8).

Dietary History. A dietary history can be obtained through a nutrition interview conducted by the nurse or nutritionist (see Assessment Tool: Dietary History Interview), a 24-hour food recall completed by the pregnant woman during her antepartum visit, or a food record that the woman keeps for a week at home (see Assessment Tool: Food Record). The choice of method used depends on the amount of time available during the antepartum visit, the skills of the nurse, and the reliability of the client.

Tools such as the Dietary History Interview and the Food Record help the nurse focus on the client's dietary habits and nutrient intake. Completing such tools gives both nurse and client an opportunity to discuss nutrition practices appropriate for the prenatal period. They also help the nurse identify and promote dietary changes the client should make to meet the physiologic demands of pregnancy and lactation. From the Dietary History Interview and the Food Record, the nurse can also obtain data concerning the emotional, cognitive, and sociocultural influences on a client's diet.

Emotional Influences. To assess emotional influences, the nurse should determine the woman's feelings regarding food, how her emotional state influences eating patterns, and her eating behaviors.

Cognitive Influences. Cognitive influences include the woman's knowledge regarding food groups and their nutrients and her understanding of the nutritional needs of her growing baby.

Table 19–8

PHYSICAL SIGNS OF NUTRITIONAL STATUS

BODY AREA	SIGNS OF GOOD NUTRITION	SIGNS OF POOR NUTRITION
General appearance	Alert, responsive	Listless, apathetic, cachectic
Weight	Normal for height, age, body build	Overweight or underweight
Posture	Erect, arms and legs straight	Sagging shoulders, sunken chest, humped back
Muscles	Well developed, firm, good tone	Flaccid, poor tone, underdeveloped, tender, "wasted" appearance
General vitality	Endurance, energetic, sleeps well, vigorous	Easily fatigued, no energy, falls asleep easily, looks tired, apathetic
Hair	Shiny, lustrous, firm, not easily plucked, healthy scalp	Stringy, dull, brittle, dry, thin and sparse, depigmented, can be easily plucked
Skin	Smooth, slightly moist, good color	Rough, dry, scaly, pale, pigmented, irritated, bruises, petechiae
Face and neck	Skin color uniform, smooth, healthy appearance, not swollen	Greasy, discolored, scaly, swollen, skin dark under eyes, lumpiness or flakiness of skin around nose and mouth
Lips	Smooth, good color, moist, not chapped or swollen	Dry, scaly, swollen, redness and swelling, or angular lesions at corners of the mouth or fissures or scars
Mouth, oral membranes	Reddish pink mucous membranes in oral cavity	Swollen, boggy oral mucous membranes
Gums	Good pink color, healthy, red, no swelling or bleeding	Spongy, bleed easily, marginal redness, inflamed, gums receding
Tongue	Good pink color or deep reddish in appearance, not swollen or smooth, surface papillae present, no lesion	Swelling, scarlet and raw, magenta color, beefy, hyperemic and hypertrophic papillae, atrophic papillae
Teeth	No cavities, no pain, bright, straight, no crowding, well-shaped jaw, clean, no discoloration	Unfilled caries, absent teeth, worn surfaces, mottled color, malpositioned
Eyes	Bright, clear, shiny, no sores at corner of eyelids, membranes moist and healthy pink color, no prominent blood vessels on sclera, no fatigue circles beneath	Eye membranes pale, redness of membrane, dryness, signs of infection, redness and fissuring of eyelid corners, dryness of eye membrane, dull appearance of cornea
Nails	Firm, pink	Spoon shape, brittle, ridged
Legs, feet	No tenderness or weakness, good color	Tender calf, tingling, weakness

From Worthington-Roberts, B., and Williams, S. (1993). *Nutrition in pregnancy and lactation* (5th ed.). St. Louis: C. V. Mosby.

Sociocultural Influences. The sociocultural influences on diet include family eating patterns, cultural or religious practices that influence diet, favored ethnic foods, cooking habits, food allergies or intolerances, and medications or supplements. An assessment of habits that may influence nutritional status, such as smoking, drug abuse, and alcohol use, should also be made (Public Health Service 1989).

▼ EXERCISE

A physical, emotional, cognitive, and sociocultural assessment of the woman's exercise habits gives helpful medical information and allows early intervention.

Physical Influences. The physical dimension of these data should consist of the identification of the woman's current exercise pattern, including

Assessment Tool: Dietary History Interview

Date:________________

Name:______________________________
ID#:______________________________
Birthdate:______________________________

				Comments
1. Have you ever talked to anyone about what you have been eating?		Yes	No	
If yes, when?________________				
What were you told?________________				
2. Have you ever had any problems with your weight?		Yes	No	
If yes, what were they?________________				
3. Have you ever been on a special diet? (low-salt, diabetic, weight reduction, low-fat, other)		Yes	No	
If yes, what kind of diet?________________				
4. In the past month, have you had:	Heartburn	Yes	No	
	Constipation	Yes	No	
	Diarrhea	Yes	No	
	Nausea	Yes	No	
	Vomiting	Yes	No	
	Weight loss	Yes	No	
	Weight gain	Yes	No	
5. Are you taking any of the following:	Vitamins/minerals	Yes	No	
	Laxatives	Yes	No	
	Antacids	Yes	No	
	Diet pills	Yes	No	
	Birth control pills	Yes	No	
6. How many times a week do you generally eat out or away from home?___				
Where do you generally go for these meals?________________				
7. Do you buy and prepare most of your own food?		Yes	No	
If yes, how often do you shop?________________				
How much money do you spend?________________				
How many people do you cook for?________________				
If no, who does most of the cooking for you?________________				
8. Have there been any changes in your appetite in the past few months?		Yes	No	
If yes, explain.________________				
9. Do you have a working:	Refrigerator	Yes	No	
	Stove	Yes	No	
	Sink	Yes	No	
10. Do you receive:	Food stamps	Yes	No	
	AFDC	Yes	No	
	Medicaid	Yes	No	
	Medicare	Yes	No	
	Meals on Wheels	Yes	No	
	WIC	Yes	No	
11. Do you have any trouble chewing your food?		Yes	No	

12. How much exercise do you get every day? (please check)

❐ A little (desk work, cooking, watching TV)   ❐ Moderate (walking, light housework)   ❐ A lot (running, farm work, heavy housework)

PREGNANT WOMEN ONLY	POSTPARTUM WOMEN ONLY
1. When is your baby due?________________	1. When was your baby born?________________
2. If you have been pregnant before, how many pounds did you gain during your last pregnancy?_________lb	2. How many pounds did you gain during your pregnancy? _________lb
3. Do you plan to breastfeed or bottle feed? ❐ Breastfeed ❐ Bottlefeed ❐ Both	3. Are you breastfeeding? ❐ Yes ❐ No

Data from Human Resource Service, Florida Women, Infants, and Children (WIC) Program.

Assessment Tool: Food Record

Food Frequency

Circle any of the following you have had in the last 2 days.

Milk (whole, low-fat, or skim)	Crackers	Oranges	Broccoli	Coffee (reg. or decaf.)
Cheese	Bread	Grapefruits	Carrots	Tea (reg. or decaf.)
Ice cream	Rolls	Orange juice	Greens	
Yogurt	Biscuits	Grapefruit juice	Spinach	Coke/soda
Pudding	Cornbread	Other fruit or juice What kind?	Sweet potatoes	Diet soda
	Cereals		Tomatoes	Gatorade
Meat	Grits	________	Pumpkin	Koolaid
Chicken/turkey	Rice	________	Other vegetables What kind?	Water
Fish	Spaghetti	________		Beer
Eggs	Noodles	________	________	Wine/wine cooler
Dried peas	Macaroni	________	________	Liquor
Dried beans	Corn	________	________	Tobacco
Peanut butter	White potatoes			Street drugs
	Clay/plaster			
	Starch			

24-Hour Recall

Please write down everything you have had to eat or drink (including water) in the last 24 hours.

Time	Food or Beverage	Amount

Is this the way you usually eat? ❐ Yes ❐ No

Comments:____

____

____

Reviewed by:______________________________ Date:____________

Name, Title

Data from Human Resource Service, Florida Women, Infants, and Children (WIC) Program.

type and frequency of exercise. Physical symptoms or discomforts arising from exercise should also be identified.

Emotional Influences. To assess emotional influences, the woman can be questioned regarding her feelings and attitudes about exercise and how those feelings have influenced her exercise patterns in the past. For example, if she fears that exercise will harm her baby, she is not likely to be active during the pregnancy.

Cognitive Influences. Cognitive influences on exercise include the woman's knowledge regarding the benefits and detriments of exercise, current recommendations for exercise in pregnancy, and potential effects of exercise on the baby.

Sociocultural Influences. Assessment of the sociocultural influences on exercise includes typical family exercise and activity patterns and cultural beliefs regarding exercise during pregnancy.

▼ STRESS

Many prenatal assessments do not include psychosocial data regarding the pregnant woman's stress levels. By identifying the woman's common life stressors and stress responses, the nurse can offer anticipatory guidance and counseling regarding stress management during the pregnancy.

Physical Influences. Physical indicators of stress should be identified by questioning the woman about symptoms that she has previously experienced or may currently be experiencing that could be stress related. These data then need to be explored further in relation to the other dimensions of stress, for physical symptoms of stress may parallel some symptoms or discomforts of pregnancy.

Emotional Influences. The emotional dimension of stress can be explored by assessing the woman's usual responses and coping patterns in stressful situations.

Cognitive Influences. Determining how the woman identifies stress in her life and whether she is aware of the symptoms and effects of stress gives information about her cognitive understanding of stress.

Sociocultural Influences. Sociocultural data provide information about the woman's current life stressors. This might include information about her home and family life, her employment, or her financial concerns.

▼ SAFETY

A risk assessment regarding factors that could potentially cause problems during the pregnancy should be part of the prenatal interview. Many opportunities for counseling are offered and important data are yielded from information about the woman's plans for travel; her medication/drug, smoking, and alcohol use; and her employment.

▼ Diagnosis

On completion of the assessment, nursing diagnoses may be identified that relate to pregnancy discomforts, nutritional status, exercise, or stress. These diagnoses are based on the data gathered during the assessment process from an interview, client questionnaires or diaries, laboratory data, or physical examination. Examples of these nursing diagnoses might be

- Risk for altered comfort:* nausea and vomiting, related to elevated hormonal levels, altered carbohydrate metabolism, or decreased gastric motility
- Altered nutrition: more than body requirements, related to excessive dietary intake
- Altered nutrition: less than body requirements, related to endocrine disorder
- Knowledge deficit: pregnancy, related to lack of information about exercise in pregnancy
- Ineffective individual coping: stress, related to lack of support system during pregnancy
- Risk for injury: fatigue and stress, related to employment during pregnancy

▼ Planning

The plan for nursing interventions is based on the formulated nursing diagnoses. This plan should reflect the holistic components of the assessment and might include both the woman and her family. By developing measurable objectives as part of the planning process, the nurse will be able to direct and evaluate her interventions more effectively. The following objectives are examples of those that might be written to promote a healthy pregnancy. The pregnant woman will

- Report a relief of nausea and vomiting as a result of eating small frequent meals, avoiding cooking odors, and getting adequate rest
- Gain 2 pounds during the month between prenatal visits and report an improvement in eating habits
- Walk 2 miles three times a week during the month between prenatal visits
- Identify the stressors in her life and state one coping strategy that she will implement
- Report two coping strategies she has implemented to decrease fatigue and stress during her workday

*Although "risk for altered comfort" is not a current NANDA-approved nursing diagnosis, it is used advisedly here to describe a condition that creates "discomfort" rather than "pain."

Intervention

The interventions necessary for the promotion of a healthy pregnancy are based on the assessment, the nursing diagnoses, and the plan and focus primarily on the health promotion activities of teaching and counseling. The physical, emotional, cognitive, and sociocultural dimensions of care need to be considered at all times.

PHYSICAL

The physical dimension of health promotion consists of continual assessment to identify changes that may have occurred since the initial evaluation. Medication to relieve persistent discomforts of pregnancy or vitamins to supplement dietary intake may be prescribed. Referral to other members of the health care team, such as the nutritionist or physical therapist, may be helpful.

EMOTIONAL

The woman's emotional needs can be met by providing regular opportunities for her to discuss aspects of her pregnancy and prenatal care; by using a caring, supportive approach; and by offering praise and reinforcement. The nurse should discuss the emotional changes of pregnancy, family alterations, and changes in marital relationships that may occur. Sexuality during pregnancy should also be included (see Chapter 10).

COGNITIVE

The cognitive aspect of health promotion should consist of three parts: (1) counseling to promote and support healthful behavior, (2) general knowledge about pregnancy and parenting, and (3) specific information concerning proposed care and treatment (Public Health Service 1989). Information that should be given to women regarding healthy behavior during pregnancy includes the following:

- Nonpharmacologic self-help measures to counter the discomforts of pregnancy (see Table 19–1)
- List of warning signs in pregnancy (see Warning Signs to Report, p. 510), including signs of preterm labor (see Chapter 21)
- Nutrition counseling and dietary planning (see Fig. 19–6 and Tables 19–2, 19–3, 19–4, 19–5, and 19–7)
- Encouragement and guidelines for safe exercise (see Recommendations for Safe Exercise During Pregnancy, p. 529)
- Methods of stress reduction (see preceding discussion, p. 535)
- Avoidance of teratogens (see Chapter 15)
- Smoking cessation (see preceding discussion, p. 524)
- Drug and alcohol avoidance (see Table 15–2)
- Maternal seat belt use (see Fig. 19–11)
- Work counseling (see preceding discussion, p. 539)
- General health and hygiene habits (see preceding discussion, p. 538)
- Information on proposed antepartum care (see Chapter 16)

By ensuring that the pregnant woman is informed about all these aspects of her health during pregnancy, the nurse in many ways is also serving in an advocacy role. It is helpful to incorporate a health teaching checklist, such as the Prenatal Education and Counseling form in Chapter 16, with suggested timelines as part of the woman's antepartum record to ensure that all essential components of information are taught. Additional guidelines for providing pregnant women with information about pregnancy and parenting and about the proposed antepartum care and treatment can be found in Chapters 16 and 20.

SOCIOCULTURAL

Interventions that reflect the sociocultural aspects of the pregnant woman's care might include the provision of information to dispel cultural myths or old wives' tales and referral to team members or agencies to meet financial or social needs. For example, a social worker may be able to help the woman and her family find housing or employment. The WIC nutritionist may be able to help the woman improve her diet with nutritional supplements. Enlisting the help and involvement of family members may also provide support to the woman in making health behavior changes (Aaronson 1989a; Jennings 1989).

Evaluation

The evaluation of these health promotion measures is based on the initial assessment, diagnoses, and objectives. Just as all other components of the nursing process are ongoing throughout pregnancy, evaluation should occur at each prenatal visit to determine the success of previous interventions and the need for further assessment or revision of goals. Evaluation may be based on direct observation and assessment or verbal feedback from the woman. Direct observations might include the woman's general appearance, weight gain, laboratory values, physical examination findings, and emotional affect and attitude. Verbal feedback might include reports about physical signs and symptoms, discomforts, feelings, and stress levels.

Collaborative Process

Although the nurse plays a primary role in the activities that are involved in the promotion of a healthy pregnancy, other health care professionals have important contributions to make as well. Team members might include a nutritionist, a physical therapist, a childbirth educator, a social worker, and the physician or midwife. As with other aspects of prenatal care, verbal and written communication between these team members must take place on a regular basis to prevent duplication or omission of risk assessment and health promotion activities. A health promotion teaching checklist in the woman's prenatal record helps to provide continuity of teaching efforts. Reinforcement regarding various aspects of health during pregnancy can be given by a number of members of the team to increase the likelihood that positive lifestyle changes are made.

Risk Management

The information given to women to help them have a healthy pregnancy is not only beneficial in promoting comfort and improving general health status but essential in managing potential risks through the prevention of complications. It is essential, therefore, that a comprehensive risk assessment be completed at the first prenatal visit and updated at each succeeding visit. The risks to health during pregnancy have been discussed earlier in this chapter and in Chapters 13, 15, and 21. For example, the risks of maternal malnutrition during pregnancy might include fetal growth retardation, poor brain development, fetal anomalies, or low birth weight. The risks of inappropriate exercise might include fetal hypoxia or bradycardia. The risks of substance abuse could include fetal alcohol syndrome, fetal anomalies, or fetal growth retardation and prematurity. Thus, health assessment and promotion become essential in the risk management of women during pregnancy. Pregnant women should be given direct teaching, either individually or in groups, about all aspects of health during pregnancy. In addition to direct teaching, written materials relating to the promotion of a healthy pregnancy should be provided. Teaching should not be done once and then forgotten, but reinforced at each prenatal contact.

Implications for Research

Research relating to all aspects of health during pregnancy is ongoing. The majority of the research done to date relates to the effects of a particular variable on maternal or fetal outcome. Many of the studies that have been done are retrospective or descriptive in design because of the ethical impossibility of conducting experimental research with humans during pregnancy. For example, research studies have documented the effects of poor nutrition or environmental teratogens in populations of women experiencing an adverse fetal or maternal outcome. The experimental research relating to exercise in pregnancy has been conducted primarily with animals. Research that documents the relationship of a health variable to pregnancy outcome must continue to be done in carefully designed studies that are both safe and ethical.

Perhaps the area of research that has received the least attention is the study of ways that health care professionals can conduct more thorough risk assessments and provide health promotion education and counseling. These areas of research could easily be carried out by nurses in their clinical settings. Research questions might include

- What teaching methods are most effective in stimulating a change in dietary habits and intake during pregnancy?
- Is there a relationship between exercises taught to pregnant women and physical discomforts during pregnancy?
- Which relaxation strategies are most effective in helping expectant parents reduce their perception of the stress in their lives?
- What do pregnant women know about the effects of drugs, alcohol, smoking, and other environmental teratogens on the development of their babies during pregnancy?

Research in the area of health promotion during pregnancy will become even more important as insurance costs rise and subsidized health care funding decreases. Knowledge regarding ways to improve maternal and fetal outcomes through cost-effective health practices will be critical in future years.

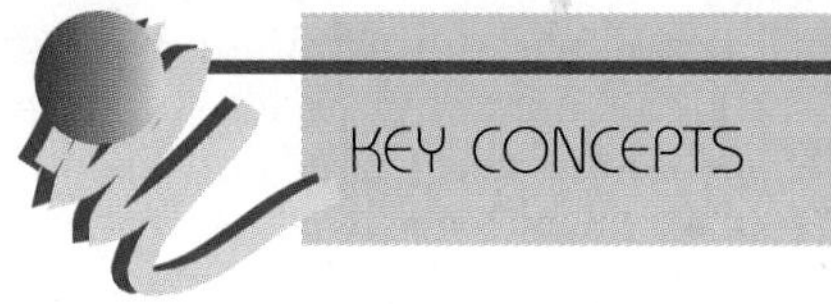

KEY CONCEPTS

- Nausea and vomiting in pregnancy, called morning sickness, often occur in the first trimester. They are thought to be caused by the effects of hCG and progesterone on the gastrointestinal tract. Comfort measures include frequent small protein or carbohydrate meals, crackers at the bedside before arising in the morning, and vitamin B_6 supplements.
- Urinary frequency may occur in the first trimester and again in the third trimester as the growing uterus places pressure on the bladder. It can be relieved by voiding regularly, decreasing fluids before bedtime, and avoiding caffeinated or carbonated beverages.
- Fatigue or drowsiness in early pregnancy is caused by increased levels of estrogen, progesterone, and hCG and the increased basal metabolic rate. Women can counter fatigue by getting 7 to 8 hours of sleep each night, taking brief rest periods during the day, eating a well-balanced diet, and exercising regularly.
- Breast tenderness in early pregnancy is caused by hypertrophy of mammary glandular tissue and increased vascularization caused by elevations of estrogen and progesterone. Wearing a supportive bra, altering sleep positions, and avoiding soap on the nipple and areola area may provide relief.
- Increased vaginal discharge is caused by the increase in estrogen, which stimulates increased production of mucus by the endocervical glands and hyperplasia of the vaginal mucosa. Increased pelvic pressure also contributes. Good hygiene, cotton underwear, loose comfortable clothing, and panty liners promote comfort.
- Edema of the nasal mucosa, increased nasal discharge, or nosebleeds (epistaxis) can result from elevated estrogen levels. Normal saline nose drops and cool-air vaporizers can be used to relieve discomfort.
- The excessive production of saliva (ptyalism) is experienced by some pregnant women and is thought to be caused by increased estrogen levels or nausea. Good oral hygiene, astringent mouthwash, hard candy, or gum may relieve this discomfort.
- Dizziness or faintness caused by vasomotor lability or postural hypotension may result from hormonal changes in pregnancy. Supine hypotension in late pregnancy can be caused by pressure from the uterus on the ascending vena cava when the woman is supine. The woman should avoid sudden changes in position and move slowly and deliberately. She should lie on either side rather than on her back.
- Increased progesterone causes smooth muscle relaxation and increased water reabsorption in the gastrointestinal tract, resulting in constipation. The pressure of the enlarging uterus on the colon and rectum also contributes. Constipation can be treated by increasing fluid intake, eating a diet high in fiber and roughage, and increasing exercise.
- Hemorrhoids during pregnancy are caused by increased blood volume, pressure from the enlarging uterus on blood vessels in the perineal area, and constipation. Remedies include ice packs, sitz baths, topical ointments, and anesthetic agents.
- Braxton Hicks contractions of the uterus occur normally throughout pregnancy and are caused by increased estrogen and distention of the uterus. If they are bothersome, the woman should rest in the left lateral position, try mild exercise, or practice relaxation and breathing techniques.
- The stretching of the round uterine ligaments as the uterus grows may cause tenderness or pain. It can be relieved by bringing the knees to the chest, rest, heat, or massage.
- Varicose veins in pregnancy are caused by relaxation in the walls of veins due to hormonal influences and increased blood volume or by poor valve functioning resulting in stasis and pooling in the veins of the lower extremities. Elevation of the legs, changing position frequently, avoiding long periods of standing, regular exercise, and supportive hose can help provide relief.
- Dyspnea during pregnancy is caused by the decrease in thoracic space and vital capacity due to upward displacement of the diaphragm from the growing uterus. It can be relieved by use of good posture, the tailor reach exercise, rest after exercise, sleeping in the semi-Fowler or left lateral position, and eating small meals.
- The increased weight of the growing baby and uterus pulling forward on low back muscles, the influence of estrogen and relaxin on pelvic ligaments, excessive weight gain, and poor posture can all contribute to backache in pregnancy. Backache can be relieved by use of good posture and body mechanics, the pelvic rock exercise, wearing a maternity girdle or flat supportive shoes, sleeping in a lateral position, and massage.
- Leg cramps in the third trimester of pregnancy

are caused by compression of the uterus on the nerves supplying the lower extremities, by blood vessel occlusion in the legs, or by an alteration in the calcium/phosphorus ratio in the diet. They can be relieved by stretching the affected muscle by dorsi-flexing the foot with the knee extended, using heat, standing on a cold surface, taking warm baths, or elevating the legs.

- ▼ Gingivitis and epulis (hyperemia, hypertrophy, bleeding, or tenderness) of the gums is caused by the increased vascularity and proliferation of connective tissue caused by estrogen. It can be treated with good oral hygiene, gentle brushing, flossing, and use of a warm saline or astringent mouthwash.
- ▼ Insomnia often occurs in the third trimester because of difficulty finding a comfortable position for sleeping, fetal activity, urinary frequency, heartburn, leg cramps, dyspnea, or anxiety. Measures to relieve insomnia include extra pillows for comfort, an open window for fresh air, a back massage, use of relaxation techniques, warm milk, or a warm shower.
- ▼ Heartburn (pyrosis) is caused by the increased production of progesterone, which causes decreased gastrointestinal motility and increases relaxation of the cardiac sphincter, resulting in delayed emptying of the stomach and regurgitation of gastric contents into the esophagus. Remedies consist of eating small meals and avoiding fatty, fried, or gas-producing foods.
- ▼ Edema of the lower extremities is common in the third trimester because of the influence of hormonal changes in sodium and water retention and capillary permeability. It can be relieved by regular rest in the left lateral position, elevation of the legs, support hose, ankle rotation, and exercise.
- ▼ Warning signs in pregnancy include vaginal bleeding, premature rupture of membranes, preterm labor contractions, a change in fetal activity, severe headaches, visual disturbances, rapid weight gain, epigastric pain, generalized or facial edema, persistent vomiting, abdominal pain, and signs of infection.
- ▼ Calorie requirements during pregnancy increase 300 calories per day to 2500 calories.
- ▼ Protein should be increased from 44 to 50 g/day to 60 g/day. Protein is needed to provide additional amino acids to support rapid fetal and placental growth, enlargement of the breasts and uterus, and expansion of maternal blood volume. Food sources include milk, cheese, eggs, meat, fish, poultry, grains, legumes, and nuts.
- ▼ Carbohydrates and fats contribute to the total calorie intake required for maternal and fetal growth. Sources of carbohydrate foods include fruits, vegetables, whole-grain cereal and bread, and milk. Fats are found in butter, cream cheese, cream, mayonnaise, oil, and nuts.
- ▼ All vitamin intake should be either maintained or increased during pregnancy. Vitamin A is essential for cell development, tooth formation, and bone growth. It plays a role in the metabolism of carbohydrates and fats and affects night vision. Vitamin D is needed to enhance the absorption and use of the increased amounts of calcium and phosphorus needed during pregnancy. Vitamin E is an antioxidant, taking on oxygen so that another substance will not undergo chemical change. Vitamin K is essential for the synthesis of prothrombin and the prevention of hemorrhage in the newborn. The B complex vitamins have the function of being coenzymes in metabolic functions, such as cell respiration, glucose oxidation, and energy metabolism. Vitamin C aids in the formation and development of connective tissue, collagen, skin, tendons, and the vascular system. A well-balanced diet during pregnancy provides all the essential vitamins, but prenatal vitamin supplements are often prescribed.
- ▼ Minerals have an important role in pregnancy. Iron is essential in the synthesis of hemoglobin in maternal and fetal red blood cells. Zinc is needed for normal fetal growth and development, antibacterial activity of amniotic fluid, and uterine contractility for the initiation of labor. Copper aids in the absorption, storage, and release of iron. Calcium is essential for the mineralization of fetal skeletal tissue, tooth formation, and regulation of nerve and muscle activity. Phosphorus is necessary for the rapid division and growth of new fetal cells, and it also contributes to the early formation of the baby's skeleton and tooth buds. Sodium is needed in pregnancy to maintain fluid levels for expanded maternal blood volume.
- ▼ The amount of weight a woman should gain varies, depending on her pre-pregnancy weight and health status. The body mass index (BMI) is used to determine her recommended total weight gain during pregnancy. For women with a normal BMI (weight/height^2) before pregnancy, a total gain of 25 to 35 pounds is suggested. The pattern of weight gain is important and should be gradual during the course of pregnancy, with a total gain of 2 to 4 pounds in the first trimester and 1 pound per week in the second and third trimesters.
- ▼ Nutritional risk factors in pregnancy include frequent pregnancies, a history of medical or obstetric problems, fad diets, eating disorders, vegetarian diets, adolescence, and substance abuse.

- Three potential concerns about exercise in pregnancy relate to the effects of prolonged raised body temperature on the developing fetus, the effects of decreased uterine blood flow on the fetus, and the effects of activation of the sympathetic nervous system. The consensus of the research to date is that when exercise is performed for a moderate duration at a submaximal heart rate level, the healthy pregnant woman and her fetus are not compromised and exercise may have some beneficial effects.
- Safe exercises for pregnancy include non–weight-bearing exercise (e.g., bicycling, swimming, or rowing); brisk walking; and pregnancy exercises such as the pelvic floor/Kegel exercise, the pelvic rock/pelvic tilt exercise, and partial or mini sit-ups.
- Stress during pregnancy has been associated with maternal obstetric complications, fetal and neonatal abnormalities, and low birth weight. Stress during labor is associated with longer labors, poorer quality uterine contractions, and neonates who experience more health problems. Stress management techniques useful in pregnancy include progressive relaxation, neuromuscular dissociation, touch relaxation, visual imagery, music, biofeedback, and controlled breathing techniques.
- A prenatal assessment should include information about the woman's discomforts of pregnancy, her nutritional status, her exercise, and her stress levels.
- Nursing interventions aimed at promoting a healthy pregnancy include providing comfort measures for discomforts; teaching about causes of and remedies for the discomforts of pregnancy, nutritional needs and diet for pregnancy, exercises, and stress reduction strategies; counseling to meet emotional or sociocultural needs; and making referrals to other members of the health care team as needed.

References

Aaronson, L. (1989a). Perceived and received support: Effects on health behavior during pregnancy. *Nursing Research,* 38 (1), 4–9.

Aaronson, L. (1989b). The relationship between weight gain and nutrition in pregnancy. *Nursing Research,* 38 (4), 223–227.

Aaronson, L., and Macnee, C. (1989). Tobacco, alcohol, and caffeine use during pregnancy. *Journal of Obstetric, Gynecologic, and Neonatal Nursing,* 18 (4), 279–287.

Abrams, B., Newman, V., Key, T., Parker, J. (1989). Maternal weight gain and preterm delivery. *Obstetrics and Gynecology,* 74 (4), 577–583.

Abrums, M. (1986). Health care for women. *Journal of Obstetric, Gynecologic, and Neonatal Nursing,* 15 (3), 250–255.

Alexander, L. (1987). The pregnant smoker: Nursing implications. *Journal of Obstetric, Gynecologic, and Neonatal Nursing,* 16 (3), 167–173.

Alley, N. (1984). Morning sickness: The client's perspective. *Journal of Obstetric, Gynecologic, and Neonatal Nursing,* 13 (3), 185–189.

American College of Obstetricians and Gynecologists. (1994). *Exercise during pregnancy and the postpartum period* (ACOG Technical Bulletin, Number 189). Washington, D.C.: Author.

Annie, C. L., and Groër, M. (1991). Childbirth stress: An immunologic study. *Journal of Obstetric, Gynecologic, and Neonatal Nursing,* 20 (5), 391–397.

Arneson, S., Beltz, E., Hahnemann, B., Smith, R., Triplett, J., Witt, V. (1986). Automobile seat belt practices of pregnant women. *Journal of Obstetric, Gynecologic, and Neonatal Nursing,* 15 (4), 339–344.

Artal, R., Wiswell, R. A., Drinkwater, B. L. (Eds.). (1991). *Exercise in pregnancy* (2nd ed.). Baltimore: Williams & Wilkins.

Ascher, B. (1978). Maternal anxiety in pregnancy and fetal homeostasis. *Journal of Obstetric, Gynecologic, and Neonatal Nursing,* 7 (3), 18–21.

Bennett, E. (1984). The first trimester. *Journal of Obstetric, Gynecologic, and Neonatal Nursing,* 13 (2), 93s–96s.

Bernhardt, J. H. (1990). Potential workplace hazards to reproductive health: Information for primary prevention. *Journal of Obstetric, Gynecologic, and Neonatal Nursing,* 19 (11), 53–63.

Blau, B. (1987). Dental care during pregnancy. *Childbirth Educator,* 6 (4), 41–45.

Brackbill, Y. (1987). Medication in maternity. *Childbirth Educator,* 6 (2), 28–35.

Brooten, D., Peters, M., Glatts, M., Gaffney, S., Knapp, M., Cohen, S., Jordan, C. (1987). A survey of nutrition, caffeine, cigarette and alcohol intake in early pregnancy in an urban clinic population. *Journal of Nurse-Midwifery,* 32 (2), 85–90.

Bryant, H. (1985). Antenatal counseling for women working outside the home. *Birth,* 12 (4), 227–232.

Chang, A., Magwene, K., Frand, E. (1987). Increased safety belt use following education in childbirth classes. *Birth,* 14 (3), 148–152.

Chenger, P., and Kovacik, A. (1987). Dental hygiene during pregnancy: A review. *MCN: American Journal of Maternal–Child Nursing,* 12 (5), 342–343.

Clapp, J. (1989). The effects of maternal exercise on early pregnancy outcome. *American Journal of Obstetrics and Gynecology,* 161, 1453–1457.

Committee on Maternal Nutrition, Food and Nutrition Board, National Research Council. (1970). *Maternal nutrition and the course of pregnancy: Summary report.* Washington, D.C.: National Academy of Sciences.

Costa, A. (1989). Smoking cessation. *Ohio Medicine,* December, 982–983.

Dohrmann, K., and Lederman, S. (1986). Weight gain in pregnancy. *Journal of Obstetric, Gynecologic, and Neonatal Nursing,* 15 (6), 446–453.

Ericson, A. (1987). What is a teratogen? *Childbirth Educator,* 6 (2), 44–49.

Fishbein, E. G., and Phillips, M. (1990). How safe is exercise during pregnancy? *Journal of Obstetric, Gynecologic, and Neonatal Nursing,* 19 (1), 45–52.

Floyd, R., Zahniser, C., Gunter, E., Kendrick, J. (1991). Smoking during pregnancy: Prevalence, effects, and intervention strategies. *Birth,* 18 (1), 48–53.

Green, M., and Harry, J. (1987). *Nutrition in contemporary nursing practice* (2nd ed.). New York: John Wiley & Sons.

Hammond, T., Mickens-Powers, B., Strickland, K., Hankins, G. (1990). The use of automobile safety restraint systems during pregnancy. *Journal of Obstetric, Gynecologic, and Neonatal Nursing,* 19 (4), 339–343.

Handler, A., David, F., Ferre, C., Yeko, T. (1989). The relationship of smoking and ectopic pregnancy. *American Journal of Public Health,* 79 (9), 1239–1242.

Haste, F., Brooke, O., Anderson, H., Bland, J., Shaw, A., Griffin, J., Peacock, J. (1990). Nutrient intakes during pregnancy: Ob-

servations on the influence of smoking and social class. *American Journal of Clinical Nutrition,* 51, 29–36.
Hein, D. (1989). What makes a pregnant woman special: Medical, obstetric, and genetic risks. *Childbirth Educator,* 8 (4), 37–39.
Herold, V. (Ed.). (1981). *Natural remedies for pregnancy discomforts.* (Over-the-Counter Drug Committee of the Coalition for the Medical Rights of Women, 82936-206 10-81 50M CS OSP). Sacramento, CA: Department of Consumer Affairs.
Heslin, J. (1989). Guide to caffeine consumption. *Childbirth Educator,* 90, 11–12.
Heslin, J. (1993). Nutrition during pregnancy. *Childbirth Instructor,* 3 (2), 14–19.
Holt, L. (1984). Expecting and employed. *Childbirth Educator,* Spring, 50–56.
Homer, C., Sherman, J., Siegel, E. (1990). Work-related psychosocial stress and risk of preterm, low birthweight delivery. *American Journal of Public Health,* 80 (2), 173–177.
Horan, M. (1984). Discomfort and pain during pregnancy. *MCN: American Journal of Maternal-Child Nursing,* 9 (4), 267.
Institute of Medicine, National Academy of Sciences, Food and Nutrition Board. (1990). *Nutrition during pregnancy.* Washington, D.C.: National Academy Press.
Jennings, R. (1989). The other half: Evaluating one's partner for health. *Childbirth Educator,* 8 (4), 26–36.
Jimenez, S. (1992). *The pregnant woman's comfort guide.* Garden City Park, NY: Avery Publishing Group.
Johnston, G. P. (1994). *The wish, the wait, the wonder: A book of wisdom for expectant parents* (p. 42). New York: Harper Collins Publishers.
Ketter, D., and Shelton, B. (1984). Pregnant and physically fit, too. *MCN: American Journal of Maternal-Child Nursing,* 9, 120–122.
Krozy, R., and McColgan, J. (1986). Auto safety: Pregnancy and the newborn. *Journal of Obstetric, Gynecologic, and Neonatal Nursing,* 14 (1), 11–21.
Lazarus, R. (1976). *Patterns of adjustment.* New York: McGraw-Hill.
Lechtig, A., et al. (1975). Effect of moderate maternal malnutrition on the placenta. *American Journal of Obstetrics and Gynecology,* 123, 191.
Lederman, R., Lederman, E., Work, B., McCann, D. (1978). The relationship of maternal anxiety, plasma catecholamines, and plasma cortisol to progress in labor. *American Journal of Obstetrics and Gynecology,* 132, 495–500.
Lederman, E., Lederman, R., Work, B., McCann, D. (1981). Maternal psychological and physiologic correlates of fetal-newborn health status. *American Journal of Obstetrics and Gynecology,* 139, 956–958.
Lewallen, L. (1989). Health beliefs and health practices of pregnant women. *Journal of Obstetric, Gynecologic, and Neonatal Nursing,* 18 (3), 245–246.
Lowenstein, V. (1989). Who's in control: Personal behaviors and pregnancy. *Childbirth Educator,* 8 (4): 20–25.
Mayer, J., Hawkins, M., Todd, R. (1990). A randomized evaluation of smoking cessation interventions for pregnant women at a WIC clinic. *American Journal of Public Health,* 80 (1), 76–78.
Mayo Clinic. (1989). Video display terminals (VDTs). *Mayo Clinic Health Letter,* September, 5–6.
McBride, A. (1982). Obesity of women during the childbearing years. *Nursing Clinics of North America,* 17 (2), 217–225.
Mercer, R., Ferketich, S., DeJoseph, J., May, K., Sollid, D. (1988). Effect of stress on family functioning during pregnancy. *Nursing Research,* 37 (5), 268–275.
Mille, J., Holmes, L., Aarons, J., et al. (1993). Moderate caffeine use and the risk of spontaneous abortion and intrauterine growth retardation. *Journal of the American Medical Association,* 269 (5), 593–597.
Mogul, S. (1989). Sexuality, pregnancy, and parenting in anorexia nervosa. *Journal of the American Academy of Psychoanalysis,* 17 (1), 65–88.
Moore, L., Burns, A., Thomas, L., Skaria, M. (1985). Self-assessment: A personalized approach to nursing during pregnancy. *Journal of Obstetric, Gynecologic, and Neonatal Nursing,* 15 (4), 311–318.
Moore, R. (1989). Environmental risks and pregnancy. *American Baby,* March, 22 and 28.
Mutch, P. (1988). Food guide for the vegetarian. *American Journal of Clinical Nutrition,* Supplement 48 (3), 913.
Nakahata, A. (1988). Exercise. In F. Nichols and S. Humenick (Eds.). *Childbirth education: Practice, research, and theory.* Philadelphia: W. B. Saunders.
National Research Council, National Academy of Sciences, Food and Nutrition Board. (1989). *Recommended dietary allowances* (10th ed.). Washington, D.C.: National Academy Press.
Noble, E. (1988). *Essential exercises for the childbearing year.* Boston: Houghton Mifflin.
Petitti, D. (1986). Nausea and pregnancy outcome. *Birth,* 13 (4), 223–226.
Poole, C. (1986). Fatigue during the first trimester of pregnancy. *Journal of Obstetric, Gynecologic, and Neonatal Nursing,* 15 (5), 375–379.
Public Health Service, Expert Panel on the Content of Prenatal Care. (1989). *Caring for our future: The content of prenatal care.* Washington, D.C.: U. S. Department of Health and Human Services.
Queenan, L. (1986). Stress: One of life's certainties. Part II: The physiology of stress. *National Women's Health Report,* 6 (2), 1 and 3.
Ramchandani, D., and Whedon, B. (1988). The effect of pregnancy on bulimia. *International Journal of Eating Disorders,* 7 (6), 845–848.
Reich, C. (1987). Exercise in pregnancy: A review for nurse practitioners. *Health Care for Women International,* 8, 349–360.
Reukema, B. (1985). Air travel during pregnancy. *Childbirth Educator,* 4 (4), 48–49.
Rubin, R. (1967a). Attainment of the maternal role: Part I. Processes. *Nursing Research,* 16 (3), 237–245.
Rubin, R. (1967b). Attainment of the maternal role: Part II. Models and referrants. *Nursing Research,* 16, 342–346.
Sampselle, C., Brink, C., Wells, T. (1989). Digital measurement of pelvic muscle strength in childbearing women. *Nursing Research,* 38 (3), 134–138.
Schoendorf, K., and Kiely, J. (1992). Relationship of sudden infant death syndrome to maternal smoking during and after pregnancy. *Pediatrics,* 90 (6), 905–908.
Scott, D., Oberst, M., Dropkin, M. (1980). A stress-coping model. *Annals of Nursing Science,* 3 (1), 9–24.
Selye, H. (1976). *The stress of life* (2nd ed.). New York: McGraw-Hill.
Skinner, J. (Ed.). (1993). *Exercise testing and exercise prescription for special cases* (2nd ed.). Philadelphia: Lea & Febiger.
Taffel, S. (1986). Association between maternal weight gain and outcome of pregnancy. *Journal of Nurse-Midwifery,* 31 (2), 78–81.
Thomas, I., Nicklin, J., Pollock, H., Faulkner, K. (1989). Evaluation of a maternity cushion (Ozzlo pillow) for backache and insomnia in late pregnancy. *Australian and New Zealand Journal of Obstetrics and Gynaecology,* 29, 133–138.
Thompson, E., and Cordero, J. (1989). The new teratogens: Accutane and other vitamin-A analogs. *MCN: American Journal of Maternal-Child Nursing,* 14 (4), 244–248.
Thompson, J. (1989). Pregnant: To be or not to be. *Childbirth Educator,* 8 (4), 42–45.
Thompson, J., and Culpepper, L. (1989). Prenatal care: It begins before pregnancy. *Childbirth Educator,* 8 (4), 18–19.
Van Dinter, M. (1991). Ptyalism in pregnant women. *Journal of Obstetric, Gynecologic, and Neonatal Nursing,* 20 (3), 206–211.
Vogt, B. (1987). Pregnancy healthlines. *Childbirth Educator,* 6 (2), 50–55.
Walker, L. O. (1995). Rethinking weight gain during pregnancy. *Journal of Perinatal Education,* 4(4), 49–54.
Wallace, A., and Engstrom, J. (1987). The effects of aerobic ex-

ercise on the pregnant woman, fetus, and pregnancy outcome: A review. *Journal of Nurse-Midwifery,* 32 (5), 277–290.

Wallace, A., Boyer, D., Dan, A., Holm, K. (1986). Aerobic exercise, maternal self-esteem, and physical discomforts during pregnancy. *Journal of Nurse-Midwifery,* 31 (6), 255–262.

Walpole, I., Zubrick, S., Pontre, J. (1989). Confounding variables in studying the effects of maternal alcohol consumption before and during pregnancy. *Journal of Epidemiology and Community Health,* 43, 153–161.

Whitney, E., Cataldo, C., Rolfes, S. (1994). *Understanding normal and clinical nutrition* (4th ed.). Minneapolis/St. Paul: West Publishing.

Wilkerson, N. (1988). Nutrition. In F. Nichols and S. Humenick (Eds.). *Childbirth education: Practice, research, and theory.* Philadelphia: W. B. Saunders.

Winick, M. (1970). Fetal malnutrition. *Clinical Obstetrics and Gynecology,* 13, 526.

Winick, M. (1986). Maternal nutrition and fetal growth. *Perinatal Neonatology,* 10 (5), 28.

Woodward, S. (1988). How does strenuous maternal exercise affect the fetus? A review. *Birth and the Family Journal,* Spring (1), 17–24.

Worthington-Roberts, B. (1985). The role of nutrition in pregnancy course and outcome. *Journal of Environmental Pathology, Toxicology, and Oncology,* 5 (6), 1–80.

Worthington-Roberts, B. (1992). Nutrition during pregnancy and lactation. In L. K. Mahan and M. T. Arlin (Eds.). *Krause's food, nutrition and diet therapy.* Philadelphia: W. B. Saunders.

Worthington-Roberts, B., and Williams, S. (1993). *Nutrition in pregnancy and lactation* (5th ed.). St. Louis: C. V. Mosby.

Young, C., McMahon, J., Bowman, V., Thompson, D. (1989). Maternal reasons for delayed prenatal care. *Nursing Research,* 38 (4), 242–243.

NURSING CARE PLANNING GUIDE

Healthy Pregnancy

This Nursing Care Planning Guide was developed to be used as a planning tool. You will need to modify and adapt it to individual clients as appropriate.

Performing a *complete and thorough assessment* is the first step in providing effective nursing care for a client. Major nursing diagnoses used in care that promotes a healthy pregnancy include

1 Altered nutrition: less than, or more than, body requirements

2 Altered maternal and fetal tissue perfusion

3 Risk for urinary tract infection

4 Risk for altered comfort:* nausea and/or vomiting

5 Risk for low back pain

6 Risk for hemorrhoid pain

7 Risk for altered comfort:* heartburn

8 Risk for leg cramp pain

9 Risk for constipation

10 Risk for ineffective breathing pattern

11 Risk for sleep pattern disturbance

12 Risk for altered sexuality patterns

13 Risk for injury with exercise

14 Knowledge deficit: pregnancy

15 Risk for fetal injury

16 Risk for body image disturbance

17 Risk for altered growth and development: parenting

18 Altered role performance: anticipating the maternal role

---

*Although "risk for altered comfort" is not a current NANDA-approved nursing diagnosis, it is used advisedly here to describe a condition that creates "discomfort" rather than "pain."

Continued on facing page

NURSING CARE PLANNING GUIDE Continued

ASSESSMENT

Assessment of the client during the prenatal period plays a critical role in enhancing maternal and fetal health and in promoting healthy lifestyle practices. To collect data, use the following Assessment Tools: Health History Summary (pp. 556–557), Initial Lifestyle Profile (p. 558), and Initial Pregnancy Profile (p. 559). In the data collected, identify defining characteristics to use as a basis for formulating nursing diagnoses that are appropriate for your client. Areas requiring special attention in care that promotes a healthy pregnancy include nutrition, maternal and fetal tissue perfusion, fetal well-being, and maternal role performance.

NURSING CARE PLANNING GUIDE Continued

HOLLISTER maternal/newborn RECORD SYSTEM

Health History Summary

Date___/___/___ Page 1 of 2

Patient's Name________________

ID. No.________________

Demographic Data

Date of Birth________ Age______ Religion____________ Race/Ethnicity________

Marital Status S M SEP D W Father of Baby's Name____________

	Education	Occupation	Full	Part	Self	Unemp	Work Tel No	Home Tel No
Patient			☐	☐	☐	☐		
Father of Baby			☐	☐	☐	☐		

Referring Physician Primary Physician

Contraceptive History ☐ None

Type	Dates Used

Menstrual History

Menarche	Interval	Length	Abnormalities
yrs	days	days	

Positive Pregnancy Test___/___/___ ☐ Blood ☐ Urine

LMP___/___/___ Certain ☐ Yes ☐ No Normal ☐ Yes ☐ No EDD By Dates___/___/___ By Ultrasound___/___/___

Pregnancy History

Gravida	Full Term	Premature	Spontaneous Ab	Induced Ab	Ectopic	Multiple Births	Live

No	Month/ Year	Infant Sex	Weight At Birth	Wks Gest	Hours In Labor	Type of Delivery	Anesthesia	Comments/Complications
1								
2								
3								
4								
5								
6								
7								

Medical History

Check and detail positive findings below. Use reference numbers.

Obstetric (Patient / Family)

1. Anemia ☐
2. Fetal/Neonatal Death or Anomaly ☐ ☐
3. Gestational Diabetes ☐
4. Hemorrhage ☐
5. Hyperemesis ☐
6. Incompetent Cervix ☐
7. Intrauterine Growth Retardation ☐
8. Isoimmunization ☐
9. Polyhydramnios ☐
10. Postpartum Depression ☐
11. Pregnancy Induced Hypertension ☐
12. Preterm Labor or Birth ☐
13. PROM-Chorioamnionitis ☐
14. Rhogam Given ☐
15. RH Neg ☐

Gynecologic

16. Abnormal PAP ☐
17. GYN Surgery ☐

Gynecologic (Cont'd.) (Patient / Family)

18. Infertility ☐
19. In Utero Exposure to DES ☐
20. Uterine Anomaly ☐

Sexually Transmitted Diseases

21. Chlamydia ☐
22. Gonorrhea ☐
23. Herpes (HSV) ☐
24. Syphilis ☐

Vaginal/Genital Infections

25. Trichomonas ☐
26. Condylomata ☐

Other Infections

27. Toxoplasmosis ☐
28. Group B Streptococcus ☐
29. Rubella ☐
30. Chicken Pox ☐
31. Cytomegalovirus (CMV) ☐
32. AIDS (HIV) ☐
33. Hepatitis (type____) ☐

Hollister. HOLLISTER INCORPORATED, 2000 HOLLISTER DR, LIBERTYVILLE, IL 60048

HEALTH HISTORY SUMMARY FORM #5700 (Page 1 of 2) 691

MATERNAL RECORD COPY

NURSING CARE PLANNING GUIDE Continued

HOLLISTER maternal/newborn RECORD SYSTEM

Health History Summary

Page 2 of 2

Patient's Name__________

ID. No.__________

Check and detail positive findings below. Use reference numbers.

Cardiovascular	Patient	Family
34. Heart Disease	☐	☐
35. Rheumatic Fever	☐	
36. Mitral Valve Prolapse	☐	
37. Chronic Hypertension	☐	☐
38. Varicosities Thrombophlebitis	☐	☐
39. Previous Pulmonary Embolism	☐	
40. Blood Disorders	☐	☐
41. Anemia/ Hemoglobinopathy	☐	☐
42. Blood Transfusions	☐	
Pulmonary		
43. Asthma	☐	
44. Tuberculosis	☐	
45. Chronic Obstructive Pulmonary Disease	☐	☐
Endocrine		
46. Diabetes	☐	☐
47. Thyroid Dysfunction	☐	☐
48. Maternal PKU	☐	
49. Endocrinopathy	☐	☐
50. Gastrointestinal	☐	
51. Liver Disease	☐	

Renal Disease	Patient	Family
52. Cystitis	☐	
53. Pyelonephritis	☐	
54. Asymptomatic Bacteriuria	☐	
55. Chronic Renal Disease	☐	☐
56. Neurologic/ Seizure Disorder	☐	☐
57. Autoimmune Disease	☐	☐
58. Cancer	☐	☐
59. Other______	☐	
Other		
60. Psychiatric Disease	☐	☐
61. Abuse or Neglect	☐	☐
62. Addiction (Drug, Alcohol, Nicotine)	☐	☐
63. Major Accidents	☐	
64. Surgery	☐	
65. Anesthetic Complications	☐	
66. Non-Surgical Hospitalization	☐	
67. Medication Allergy/ Sensitivities (identify______)	☐	
68. Other______	☐	
69. No Known Disease/Problems	☐	

Genetic History

	Patient	Father of Baby	Family
70. Age ≥ 35 (♀) ≥ 50 (♂)	☐	☐	☐
71. Cerebral Palsy	☐	☐	☐
72. Congenital Anomalies	☐	☐	☐
73. Cystic Fibrosis	☐	☐	☐
74. Down's Syndrome	☐	☐	☐
75. Hemophilia	☐	☐	☐
76. Huntington's Chorea	☐	☐	☐
77. Mental Retardation	☐	☐	☐
78. Muscular Dystrophy	☐	☐	☐
79. Neural Tube Defect	☐	☐	☐
80. Sickle Cell Disease or Trait	☐	☐	☐
81. Tay-Sachs Disease	☐	☐	☐
82. Test for Fragile X	☐	☐	☐
83. Thalassemia A or B	☐	☐	☐
84. Other______	☐	☐	☐
85. Other______	☐	☐	☐

Historical Risk Status ☐ No Risk Factors Noted

☐ At Risk (Identify)

Signature__________

Hollister. HOLLISTER INCORPORATED, 2000 HOLLISTER DR, LIBERTYVILLE, IL 60048

HEALTH HISTORY SUMMARY FORM #5700
(Page 2 of 2) 691

MATERNAL RECORD COPY

NURSING CARE PLANNING GUIDE Continued

HOLLISTER maternal/newborn RECORD SYSTEM

Patient's Name________

ID. No.________

Initial Lifestyle Profile

Nutritional Assessment

24 Hour Diet History

Usual Pattern ☐ No ☐ Yes

Eating Disorder ☐ None ☐ Anorexia ☐ Bulimia ☐ Pica

Breakfast	Lunch	Dinner	Snacks
Fluids:	Fluids:	Fluids:	Fluids:

	No	Yes	
Special Diet	☐	☐	
Food Intolerance	☐	☐	
Vitamin/Mineral Supplement	☐	☐	
Other____	☐	☐	

Nutritional Habits	No	Yes	Frequency/Amount
Artificial Sweeteners	☐	☐	
Caffeine	☐	☐	
Excessive Vitamin Intake	☐	☐	
Raw Meat/Fish	☐	☐	

Activity Assessment

	No	Yes
1. Job Outside Home	☐	☐
2. Work At Home	☐	☐
3. Travel/Commuting	☐	☐
4. Exercise	☐	☐
5. Leisure Activities	☐	☐
6. Other____	☐	☐

Comments

Sexuality Assessment

7. Partners ☐ None ☐ One ☐ Many
8. Physical Changes ☐ None (identify)____
9. Psychological Changes ☐ None (identify)____

Psychosocial Assessment

Emotional Status ☐ Happy ☐ Ambivalent ☐ Anxious ☐ Depressed ☐ Angry

Basic Needs Met	Yes	No
10. Housing	☐	☐
11. Clothing	☐	☐
12. Food	☐	☐
13. Finances	☐	☐
14. Transportation	☐	☐
15. Ability to Read/ Communicate	☐	☐
16. Other____	☐	☐
Life Stress		
17. Free From Apparent Abuse (physical, emotional)	☐	☐
18. Major Change	☐	☐
19. Serious Illness or Death	☐	☐

Life Stress (Cont'd.)	Yes	No
20. Other____	☐	☐
Social Support		
21. Biological Father Involved	☐	☐
22. Others Available	☐	☐
Adaptation to Pregnancy		
23. Planned Pregnancy	☐	☐
24. Self Care Needs	☐	☐
25. Other____	☐	☐
Other		
26.____	☐	☐
27.____	☐	☐

Initial Lifestyle Risk Status

☐ No Risk Factors Noted

☐ At Risk (Identify)

Signature

Date___ /___ /___

Hollister

HOLLISTER INCORPORATED, 2000 HOLLISTER DR, LIBERTYVILLE, IL 60048

INITIAL LIFESTYLE PROFILE FORM #5702
691

MATERNAL RECORD COPY

NURSING CARE PLANNING GUIDE Continued

HOLLISTER maternal/newborn RECORD SYSTEM

Patient's Name____

ID. No.____

Initial Pregnancy Profile

History Since LMP

Pregnancy Complications (✔)

1. Vaginal Bleeding ☐
2. Abdominal or Epigastric Pain ☐
3. Headache/Dizziness ☐
4. Change in Vision ☐
5. Hyperemesis ☐
6. Urinary Complaint ☐
7. Febrile Episode ☐
8. Rash with Viral Illness ☐
9. Physical Trauma or Surgery ☐
10. Other____ ☐

Exposure To

11. HIV ☐
12. Rubella ☐
13. Heavy Metal, Organic Solvent, Radiation ☐
14. Toxoplasmosis ☐
15. Tuberculosis ☐
16. Other____ ☐

Check and detail positive findings below. Use reference numbers.

Substance Use

17. Alcohol ☐ type____ amt/day____
18. Tobacco ☐ type____ amt/day____
19. Non-Prescribed Drugs ☐ type____ amt/day____
20. Prescribed Drugs ☐ type____ amt/day____ type____ amt/day____ type____ amt/day____
21. Street Drugs ☐ type____ amt/day____ type____ amt/day____

Physical Assessment

Height	Weight	Pregravid Weight	B.P.	Pulse

System	Normal	Abnormal
22. Skin	☐	☐
23. HEENT/Fundi	☐	☐
24. Mouth/Teeth	☐	☐
25. Neck/Thyroid	☐	☐
26. Breasts/Nipples	☐	☐
27. Heart	☐	☐
28. Lungs	☐	☐
29. Abdomen	☐	☐
30. Extremities	☐	☐
31. Neurologic	☐	☐
32. Other____	☐	☐
Pelvic Examination		
33. Vulva	☐	☐
34. Vagina	☐	☐
35. Cervix	☐	☐
36. Uterus Size____Wks	☐	☐
37. Adnexa	☐	☐
38. Rectum	☐	☐

Check and detail abnormal findings below. Use reference numbers.

39. Pelvic Type ☐ Gynecoid ☐ Anthropoid ☐ Android ☐ Platypelloid
40. Measurements ☐ Adequate ☐ Inadequate ☐ Borderline
41. Diagonal Conjugate Reached ☐ Yes ☐ No ____ cms
42. Ischial Spines ☐ Average ☐ Prominent ☐ Blunt
43. Intertuberous Diameter ____ cms
44. Sacrum ☐ Concave ☐ Anterior ☐ Straight
45. Coccyx ☐ Moveable ☐ Malpositioned ☐ Fixed
46. Pubic Arch ☐ Normal ☐ Narrow ☐ Wide

Examined by____

Date____/____/____

Hollister. HOLLISTER INCORPORATED, 2000 HOLLISTER DR, LIBERTYVILLE, IL 60048

INITIAL PREGNANCY PROFILE FORM #5701
691

MATERNAL RECORD COPY

NURSING CARE PLANNING GUIDE Continued

1

Analysis: ▼ NURSING DIAGNOSIS

Altered nutrition: less than, or more than, body requirements, related to

Less than Body Requirements

- Endocrine disorder
- Inadequate income
- Nausea, vomiting
- Heartburn
- Stress
- Inadequate dietary intake for pregnancy
- Lack of transportation
- Lack of knowledge
- Substance abuse
- Eating disorder

More than Body Requirements

- Dysfunctional eating patterns, excessive dietary intake
- Using food for rewards
- Eating in response to cues other than hunger
- Low self-esteem
- Obesity in one or both parents
- Depression
- Diabetes/gestational diabetes

Defining Characteristics

SUBJECTIVE

Less than Body Requirements

States occurrence of nausea

States unable to eat

States heartburn occurs

Unable to relay knowledge of the food pyramid and necessary number of servings required in each group to meet pregnancy requirements

OBJECTIVE

Less than Body Requirements

Fundal height less than expected for gestational age

Nutritional intake less than the following recommended daily requirements for pregnancy:

6–11 servings bread/cereal group

3–5 servings vegetable group

2–4 servings fruit group

3 servings dairy group

2–3 servings meat group

Intake of adequate amount of calories

Dehydration

Lack of interest in food

Continued on facing page

NURSING CARE PLANNING GUIDE Continued

More than Body Requirements	More than Body Requirements
States always hungry	Excessive dietary intake Frequent interest in food Excessive weight gain

Client Goal / ▼ EVALUATION CRITERIA

Client will demonstrate nutritional intake adequate for body requirements. / ▼ **Client will evidence absence of dehydration symptoms, verbalization of minimal nausea and vomiting, adequate intake of calories, adequate intake of nutrients, normal pattern of weight gain during pregnancy, normal increases in fundal height.**

▼ NURSING INTERVENTIONS	Rationale
Less than Body Requirements and More than Body Requirements	
• Obtain 24-hour diet recall.	• Baseline data are necessary to assess adequacy of dietary intake.
• Assess whether dietary intake meets nutritional requirements for pregnancy. Determine nutritional adequacy of calories, proteins, calcium, iron, and vitamins.	• There should be an increase of 300 calories per day (unless calorie intake is already excessive) to provide for the increased metabolic rate and growth of the fetus. Protein is necessary for increased production of red blood cells (RBCs) and growth of fetal and maternal tissue. Calcium is necessary for bone and tooth development of the fetus. Iron is necessary for production of RBCs and for the fetal store of iron that will be used after birth to produce RBCs. Vitamins and minerals are needed for metabolic processes. Typical nutritional requirements include 6 to 11 servings from the bread/cereal group, 3 to 5 servings from the vegetable group, 2 to 4 servings from the fruit group, 3 servings from the dairy group, and 2 to 3 servings from the meat group. At least 30 calories per kilogram is needed every 24 hours so that catabolism does not produce ketones that could affect fetal development.
• Obtain information about dietary preferences, including cultural preferences.	• Dietary intake is influenced by preferences, including cultural practices in relation to food. The client is more likely to eat dietary requirements if they can be provided in preferred foods. Clients may be more motivated to "eat right" if instruction is geared to preferences.
• Obtain information about daily routine, schedule, who prepares meals.	• Daily schedules and meal preparation influence dietary practices.
• Refer to Women, Infants, and Children (WIC) food program if applicable.	• The WIC program helps supplement available food so that the client is more likely to meet nutritional requirements.
• Assess knowledge level of nutritional needs.	• Pregnant women may not have knowledge about nutritional requirements of pregnancy.

Continued on following page

NURSING CARE PLANNING GUIDE Continued

- Weigh client at each visit.

- Gaining weight according to the normal pattern is one indicator of adequate calorie intake. A typical weight gain pattern is a gain of 2 to 4 pounds in the first trimester and then approximately 1 pound per week.

  Inadequate weight gain is less than 2.2 pounds per month in the second and third trimesters. Pregnant women should not diet because the resultant catabolism produces ketones that could affect fetal development.

  Outcomes of pregnancies in women who are underweight include greater probability of hypertensive disorders of pregnancy, low-birth-weight neonate, and intrauterine growth retardation. There is a greater probability of a longer labor, cesarean delivery, and preeclampsia/eclampsia in overweight women. With inadequate intake of nutrients (not merely calories), there is greater likelihood of low birth weight or intrauterine growth restriction.

<u>Less than Body Requirements</u>

- Assess frequency and severity of nausea and vomiting

- Nausea and vomiting are thought to be caused by hCG and progesterone. They are enhanced by decreased tone and mobility of smooth muscles of the gastrointestinal tract. Alterations in taste and smell may influence nausea. Dietary intake is influenced by nausea and vomiting.

- Assess hemoglobin level in first and third trimesters, or more often if necessary.

- Hemoglobin is assessed to determine presence of anemia. Normally, the hemoglobin level drops during pregnancy because of hemodilution. A level of 10 g/dL or less is considered abnormal. Counseling about which foods are high in iron and iron supplementation are necessary.

- Assess for presence and severity of heartburn.

- Relaxation of the cardiac sphincter and pressure of the enlarging uterus contribute to reflux of acidic secretions of the stomach to the lower esophagus. Heartburn may influence appetite.

- Assess for cravings and alteration in appetite.

- Many report food cravings during pregnancy, which is thought to occur because of dulling of taste. Appetite varies with nausea and vomiting as well as with alterations in metabolism.

<u>More than Body Requirements</u>

- Test urine for acetone, albumin, and glucose at each prenatal visit.

- Excessive urinary glucose on several occasions may be suggestive of gestational diabetes. Presence of albumin may indicate urinary tract infection or preeclampsia. Ketones in the urine may be related to inadequate food intake or strenuous exercise.

- Plan physical activity schedule.

- Exercise increases weight loss through loss of fat rather than muscle and improves muscle tone, cardiopulmonary status, and mental attitude.

- Use behavior modification strategies.

- Analyzing eating patterns and planning rewards help the client to modify dietary intake.

Continued on facing page

NURSING CARE PLANNING GUIDE Continued

2

Analysis: ▼ **NURSING DIAGNOSIS**

Altered maternal and fetal tissue perfusion, related to

- Increased blood plasma and RBCs with resultant hemodilution
- Increased cardiac output
- Relaxed blood vessel walls
- Increased oxygen needs of maternal and fetal tissues
- Decreased hemoglobin and hematocrit
- Inadequate intake of iron
- Interrupted arterial flow
- Interrupted venous flow

Defining Characteristics

SUBJECTIVE

Complains of dizziness, nausea on arising rapidly

Complains of dizziness when lying on back in second and third trimesters

Complains of edema

Complains of leg varicosities with dull, aching pain in legs after standing

OBJECTIVE

Blood pressure increases above normal baseline level

Blood pressure decreases below normal baseline level

Systolic murmur

Pulse or heart rate increases >15 heartbeats per minute

Supine hypotension; dizziness, nausea, diaphoresis

Decreased hemoglobin <10 g/dL

Decreased hematocrit <32%

Postural hypotension; dizziness, nausea

Varicose veins

Pathologic edema

Elevated hematocrit (dehydration)

Protein in urine

Inadequate intake of iron foods

Client Goal / ▼ **EVALUATION CRITERIA**

Client will demonstrate adequate tissue perfusion. / ▼ **Client will evidence normal maternal blood pressure; normal maternal pulse; maternal urine without protein; physiologic, not pathologic, edema; absence of organic murmur; normal hemoglobin and hematocrit for pregnancy.**

Continued on following page

NURSING CARE PLANNING GUIDE Continued

▼ NURSING INTERVENTIONS	Rationale
• Check blood pressure at each prenatal visit. Systolic blood pressure should not increase more than 30 mm Hg and diastolic blood pressure not more than 15 mm Hg from baseline levels.	• Cardiac function results in ejection of blood, causing it to circulate throughout the body to subsequently perfuse tissues. Blood pressure is the pressure exerted by the ejection and circulation of the blood. If it is lowered, circulation and tissue perfusion are reduced. If it is increased as the result of increased peripheral resistance, circulation and tissue perfusion are also altered. With increased blood volume, cardiac output increases by 30%–50% in the second trimester. Blood pressure remains relatively stable, however, because of the balance between vasodilatation and vasoconstriction. Preeclampsia occurs when systolic pressure increases 30 mm Hg or when diastolic pressure increases 15 mm Hg from baseline level on two occasions 6 hours apart.
• Obtain heart rate if indicated.	• Cardiac function results in ejection of blood. Heart rate measures the frequency with which the heart contracts and ejects blood. When it is altered, circulation and tissue perfusion are also altered. With increased blood volume and cardiac workload, the heart rate increases slightly. If the pulse increases more than 15 beats per minute, there may be cardiac stress.
• Auscultate heart sounds, differentiating systolic from organic murmur.	• As a result of the enlarging uterus, the position of the heart changes; it is displaced upward, forward, and to the left. With increased blood volume and workload, physiologic systolic murmurs may occur. They must be differentiated from organic murmurs, which are heard in any position. Organic murmurs alter cardiac function and circulation, which consequently alters tissue perfusion.
• Obtain information about supine or postural hypotension. Recommend side-lying position later in pregnancy. Recommend rising slowly.	• When postural or supine hypotension occurs, there is reduced cardiac output with resultant redirection of circulation to maternal and fetal tissues. Later in pregnancy, the weight of the uterus occludes venous return to the heart when the mother-to-be lies on her back, and supine hypotension may occur. Symptoms include drowsiness, nausea, and diaphoresis. Blood may have pooled in the legs when a woman lies down, reducing venous return. With reduced venous return, cardiac output is diminished, and blood pressure falls. The reduced cardiac output decreases blood supply to the fetus as well as to maternal tissues.
• Assess edema; distinguish between physiologic and pathologic edema. Assess edema in tibial area, feet, abdominal wall, fingers, back of hands, and face. Ask if edema is present in morning on arising.	• Edema is associated with reduced circulation and tissue perfusion. Physiologic, dependent edema may occur in the legs because of decreased blood vessel tone and peripheral vascular resistance. Stagnation of blood occurs in the lower extremities because there is pressure on blood vessels from the enlarging uterus. There is an increased plasma volume and release of aldosterone that results in

Continued on facing page

NURSING CARE PLANNING GUIDE Continued

	sodium and water retention, contributing to edema. Edema present on arising, on the back of the hands, in the face, or on the abdominal wall indicates pathologic edema.
• Assess hemoglobin and hematocrit in first and third trimesters and more often if indicated.	• Anemia is associated with reduced oxygen-carrying capacity. With reduced oxygen-carrying capacity, there is less oxygen available to perfused tissues. Plasma volume and number of RBCs increase. The increase in RBCs is less than the increase in plasma volume and hemodilution, or physiologic anemia occurs. Laboratory values show a 10%–15% decrease in hemoglobin and hematocrit. Thus, hemoglobin may decrease to 10–14 g/dL from 12–16 g/dL, and the hematocrit may drop from 36%–58% to 32%–46%.
• Instruct client to increase intake of foods high in iron and to take iron supplements starting in second trimester. The best dietary source of iron is meat. Give instructions about self-administration of iron supplements.	• Iron is necessary to form RBCs, which carry oxygen to tissues. When RBCs are diminished, the amount of oxygen available to tissues is altered. An increase in iron is necessary for fetal production of RBCs, for increased production of maternal RBCs, and to provide a fetal store of iron. Part should come from dietary sources and part from iron supplementation. Iron supplementation typically begins in the second trimester. Iron should not be taken with milk or antacids since absorption is decreased. Taking iron with vitamin C sources, such as orange juice, increases absorption. Iron supplementation contributes to constipation and makes the stools a black, tarry color. Iron can be toxic to children, and therefore it should be kept away from children. If there is inadequate iron, the mother-to-be will first use her iron store, then increase total iron-binding capacity. Next there will be a reduced number of RBCs, followed by hypochromic RBCs (RBCs with less hemoglobin) and then microchromic RBCs (RBCs that are a smaller size). These changes result in less oxygenation of fetal and maternal tissues.
• Assess legs and vulva for varicosities.	• Varicosities are distended vein walls that result in altered circulation to tissues. Increased circulating volume and hormonal relaxation of blood vessel walls predispose to vascular wall distention and venous stasis or varicosities. Symptoms include dull, aching pain in legs and visible distention of leg veins. In the vulva, varicosities cause aching, heaviness, and pain.
• Instruct client in ways to improve circulation. These include elevating legs, walking rather than standing in one place, abstaining from crossing legs, omitting restrictive knee-high stockings or socks, and dorsiflexing the foot periodically.	• Adequate circulation is necessary to adequately perfuse tissues. Walking increases circulation, thereby decreasing venous stasis. Crossing the legs restricts circulation. Dorsiflexion constricts the calf muscle, enhancing venous return. Knee-high stockings restrict circulation.
• Support stockings may be recommended.	• Support stockings should be applied in bed before arising, before leg veins have the opportunity to become distended; these stockings provide support to distended vascular walls.

Continued on following page

NURSING CARE PLANNING GUIDE Continued

- Try to elicit the Homans sign; if present, report to physician.
- Homans sign may indicate venous thrombosis. Clotting results in reduced circulation and tissue perfusion. Fibrinolytic activity decreases because of the increases in various clotting factors. There is, therefore, a tendency to coagulation.
- Counsel in relation to smoking. Work with client to reduce amount of smoking or to quit. Refer to smoking cessation programs.
- Smoking causes vasoconstriction and resultant restriction of circulation to fetal and maternal tissues. In addition, it produces byproducts that take the place of oxygen on hemoglobin, thereby reducing oxygen-carrying capacity to the fetus. Research indicates that smoking reduces oxygen to the fetus regardless of diet; the amount of reduction is related to the number of cigarettes smoked per day. Smoking results in higher risk for intrauterine growth restriction, low birth weight, and prematurity.

3

Analysis: ▼ NURSING DIAGNOSIS

Risk for urinary tract infection, related to

- Pressure on bladder from enlarging uterus, which reduces bladder capacity
- Increased glomerular filtration rate
- Increased renal tubular reabsorption
- Edema of bladder tissue, which renders it more susceptible to infection
- Compression of ureters as they pass over pelvic brim
- Dilatation of ureters due to compression and muscle relaxation from progesterone

Defining Characteristics

SUBJECTIVE	*OBJECTIVE*
States voids frequently	Frequency
States has urge and must void immediately	Urgency
States has discomfort or burning with voiding	Stress incontinence (with stress, like cough or sneeze)

Continued on facing page

NURSING CARE PLANNING GUIDE Continued

Client Goal / ▼ EVALUATION CRITERIA

Client will not have urinary tract infection. / ▼ **Client will evidence absence of urinary tract infection symptoms.**

▼ NURSING INTERVENTIONS	Rationale
• Assess for symptoms of cystitis. These include frequency, urgency, and dysuria.	• Reduced bladder capacity results in urinary frequency. Bladder mucosal congestion and hypertrophy of wall with estrogen stimulation lead to edema and greater susceptibility to infection. Presence of lactose in urine may predispose to infection.
• Assess for symptoms of pyelonephritis. These include costovertebral tenderness, fever or chills, and symptoms of cystitis.	• Glomerular filtration increases in pregnancy, which increases water and electrolyte loss in urine. Reabsorption of sodium, chloride, and water in renal tubules increases. These changes as well as the changes in the bladder contribute to susceptibility to infection. If cystitis is not treated, pyelonephritis may result.
• Assess knowledge of urinary tract infection symptoms to report.	• Client may be unaware of symptoms that need to be reported. A low-grade infection may go unnoticed.
• Teach hygiene with perineal measures as needed. These include wiping vulva from front to back after voiding, voiding after intercourse, and wearing underwear with cotton crotch.	• Cleansing from front to back minimizes introduction of microorganisms from vagina or rectum into urinary tract. Voiding after intercourse fosters washing away of microorganisms with urinary stream. Cotton underwear minimizes moisture, which fosters growth of microorganisms.
• Instruct client to drink 8+ glasses of liquid daily. Encourage to drink cranberry juice.	• Drinking liquids increases urinary output, which reduces stasis of urine. Cranberry juice acidifies urine, which is thought to alter the environment in the urinary tract, making it less favorable for growth of microorganisms.
• Obtain clean voided urine specimen. Instruct client to wash hands, separate the labia and hold, cleanse perineum from front to back, void and collect specimen. Routinely assess urine in first and third trimesters. Assess urine at other times if symptoms occur.	• Analysis of urine specimen determines whether an infection is present. The urine specimen should not contain blood or white blood cells. A colony count >100,000/mL indicates an infection. Approximately 2%–10% of pregnant women have asymptomatic bacteriuria or a colony count >100,000/mL without symptoms of infection. Therefore, routine analysis of urine is advised. A urinary tract infection predisposes to preterm labor.
• Teach Kegel exercises.	• Kegel exercises that tighten perineal muscles aid in support of urinary tract organs. When urinary tract organs are properly supported, cystocele is avoided.
• Instruct client about proper self-administration of oral antibiotics. This includes instructions to take all the medication and to take it at appropriate intervals.	• The appropriate oral antibiotic will treat the infection. Ampicillin or erythromycin is typically ordered. The entire course of the antibiotic must be taken, and the medication must be taken at proper intervals to maintain a blood level of the medication that will eradicate the microorganism.

Continued on following page

NURSING CARE PLANNING GUIDE Continued

4

Analysis: ▼ NURSING DIAGNOSIS

Risk for altered comfort:* nausea and/or vomiting, related to

- Elevated hCG
- Elevated progesterone

Defining Characteristics

SUBJECTIVE	*OBJECTIVE*
States presence of nausea	Vomiting
States frequency of vomiting	Decreased intake, intolerance of food

Client Goal / ▼ EVALUATION CRITERIA

Client will demonstrate comfort in relation to nausea and vomiting. / ▼ **Client will evidence adequate intake, absence of nausea and vomiting.**

▼ NURSING INTERVENTIONS	Rationale
• Obtain data about nausea and vomiting: frequency and severity, factors that aggravate it, measures taken to relieve it, and effectiveness of those measures.	• Baseline data are necessary to assess severity of nausea and vomiting. These data serve as the basis for nursing interventions.
• Assess knowledge of the cause of nausea and vomiting.	• The nurse can supplement and clarify information as necessary.
• Suggest self-care activities as appropriate. These include 1. crackers or carbohydrate food 2. carbonated beverages 3. elimination of fatty foods 4. small, frequent high-carbohydrate meals 5. someone else's preparing meals	• High-carbohydrate foods often decrease nausea. Fatty foods have been known to aggravate nausea. At times, particular food odors may trigger nausea. Small, frequent meals allow continuing digestion and avoidance of an empty stomach. Many state that carbonated beverages relieve nausea.
• Caution against taking antiemetic medications.	• There is no approved medication for nausea during pregnancy.

*Although "risk for altered comfort" is not a current NANDA-approved nursing diagnosis, it is used advisedly here to describe a condition that creates "discomfort" rather than "pain."

Continued on facing page

NURSING CARE PLANNING GUIDE Continued

• Assess nutritional intake by obtaining dietary recall.	• Nausea and vomiting may result in inadequate nutritional intake.
• Assess weight gain.	• Nausea and vomiting, coupled with inadequate intake, may result in minimal weight gain or even weight loss.
• Assess for dehydration.	• Symptoms of dehydration include reduced skin turgor, dry mucous membranes, elevated urine specific gravity, and elevated temperature.

5

Analysis: ▼ NURSING DIAGNOSIS

Risk for low back pain, related to

- Altered center of gravity
- Lordosis

Defining Characteristics

SUBJECTIVE	*OBJECTIVE*
Complains of low back pain	Waddling gait Lordosis

Client Goal / ▼ EVALUATION CRITERIA

Client will demonstrate minimal back pain. / ▼ **Client will evidence statements of comfort, minimal lordosis.**

▼ NURSING INTERVENTIONS	Rationale
• Recommend pelvic tilt exercises.	• Pelvic tilt exercises decrease the curvature of the spine, which strains muscles and contributes to low back pain.
• Instruct client about proper posture and body mechanics.	• Proper posture that reduces curvature of the spine and proper bending and lifting reduce strain and subsequent low back pain.
• Recommend wearing low-heeled shoes.	• Low-heeled shoes reduce the curvature of the spine.

Continued on following page

NURSING CARE PLANNING GUIDE Continued

- Recommend tailor sitting.
- Recommend side-lying position in bed with proper supports.

- This position reduces curvature of the spine.
- The side-lying position with proper pillow support reduces strain on back muscles.

6

Analysis: ▼ NURSING DIAGNOSIS

Risk for hemorrhoid pain, related to

- Pressure of enlarging uterus on veins in rectal area
- Restricted circulation in rectal area
- Reduced gastrointestinal mobility

Defining Characteristics

SUBJECTIVE	*OBJECTIVE*
States presence of itching in anal area	Swelling in anal area
States presence of rectal bleeding	Blood with stools

Client Goal / ▼ EVALUATION CRITERIA

Client will demonstrate comfort in relation to hemorrhoids. / ▼ **Client will evidence minimal anal itching and swelling, absence of bleeding with stools.**

▼ NURSING INTERVENTIONS	Rationale
• Assess for symptoms of hemorrhoids. These include itching, swelling, and discomfort in anal area or rectal bleeding.	• Hemorrhoids are anal varicosities, or distended, dilated vein walls. Internal hemorrhoids occur above the anal sphincter; the predominant symptom is rectal bleeding. External hemorrhoids may be visible and often cause itching and discomfort. Reduced gastrointestinal motility, pressure on the bowel, and pressure on the vasculature created by the enlarging uterus lead to distended vein walls.
• Suggest self-care activities. These include 1. high-fiber diet 2. topical ointments, suppositories 3. sitz bath	• A high-fiber diet minimizes the potential for constipation; constipation further restricts circulation and accentuates hemorrhoids. Topical ointments and suppositories reduce swelling, soothe, and may

Continued on facing page

NURSING CARE PLANNING GUIDE Continued

provide a local anesthetic that reduces hemorrhoidal discomfort. Examples are Americaine spray (local anesthetic), Wyanoids suppositories (zinc oxide and a local anesthetic), and Anusol suppositories (zinc oxide and hydrocortisone). A sitz bath is warm, increases circulation, and soothes the area.

7

Analysis: ▼ NURSING DIAGNOSIS

Risk for altered comfort:* heartburn, related to

- Stomach acid reflux to esophagus
- Pressure of enlarging uterus on stomach
- Relaxation of cardiac sphincter due to progesterone
- Decreased motility of gastrointestinal tract
- Anxiety, which increases stomach acidity

Defining Characteristics

SUBJECTIVE

States presence of heartburn

OBJECTIVE

Nonverbal facial expression indicating discomfort

Decreased appetite

Decreased dietary intake

Sternal or substernal pain or discomfort occurring at intervals

Client Goal / ▼ EVALUATION CRITERIA

Client will be comfortable in relation to heartburn. / ▼ **Client will evidence absence of sternal or substernal pain, adequate appetite and intake.**

▼ NURSING INTERVENTIONS	Rationale
• Obtain data about heartburn: frequency of occurrence, length of discomfort, measures taken to relieve it, effectiveness of those measures, factors that aggravate it.	• Baseline data are necessary to assess existence and severity of heartburn. This information serves as the basis for nursing interventions.

*Although "risk for altered comfort" is not a current NANDA-approved nursing diagnosis, it is used advisedly here to describe a condition that creates "discomfort" rather than "pain."

Continued on following page

NURSING CARE PLANNING GUIDE Continued

- Assess knowledge of the cause of heartburn.
  - The nurse can supplement and clarify information as necessary.
- Suggest self-care activities to lessen symptoms. These include
  1. small, frequent meals
  2. minimal intake of high-fat foods, coffee, tea, spicy foods
  3. oral antacids
  - Small, frequent meals are believed to minimize production of acid. Coffee, tea, fat, and spicy foods stimulate stomach acid production. Oral antacids minimize the effect of stomach acid, neutralizing it.

8

Analysis: ▼ NURSING DIAGNOSIS

Risk for leg cramp pain, related to

- Calcium/phosphorus imbalance
- Pressure on nerves

Defining Characteristics

SUBJECTIVE	*OBJECTIVE*
States presence of leg cramps	Nonverbal facial expression indicating discomfort
	Grasping, holding leg
	Tension in calf muscle

Client Goal / ▼ EVALUATION CRITERIA

Client will demonstrate comfort in relation to leg cramps. / ▼ **Client will evidence minimal leg cramps, ability to relieve leg cramps when they occur.**

▼ NURSING INTERVENTIONS	Rationale
• Obtain data about leg cramps: frequency, severity, measures taken to relieve leg cramps, effectiveness of those measures.	• Baseline data are necessary to assess severity. These data serve as the basis for nursing interventions.
• Suggest self-care activities as appropriate. These include 1. reduction in amount of dairy products	• Excessive intake of dairy products increases level of phosphorus in relation to calcium, which creates a phosphorus/calcium imbalance that results in leg cramps.

Continued on facing page

NURSING CARE PLANNING GUIDE Continued

2. dorsiflexion of foot with leg extended when cramp occurs	Dorsiflexion of foot with leg extended increases blood supply to the muscle, which stops the muscle spasm.
3. intake of calcium supplements daily when dietary calcium is reduced.	Calcium supplements help restore the phosphorus/calcium balance.

9

Analysis: ▼ NURSING DIAGNOSIS

Risk for constipation, related to

- Relaxation of smooth muscles in gastrointestinal tract due to progesterone
- Reduced peristalsis in gastrointestinal tract
- Increased reabsorption of water from stool
- Taking iron supplements
- Decreased activity
- Diet with minimal fiber and liquids

Defining Characteristics

SUBJECTIVE	*OBJECTIVE*
States stools are hard and difficult to pass	Infrequent bowel elimination Hard stools Straining with stool

Client Goal / ▼ EVALUATION CRITERIA

Client will demonstrate normal bowel elimination. / ▼ **Client will evidence normal pattern of elimination, soft stools.**

▼ NURSING INTERVENTIONS	Rationale
• Assess bowel elimination; assess frequency, consistency, difficulty with passage.	• The physiologic changes in the bowel during pregnancy predispose to constipation. In addition, activity is often decreased; activity increases peristalsis. Iron supplementation predisposes to constipation. A diet low in fiber and with minimal fluid also predisposes to constipation (fiber increases peristalsis; with increased peristalsis, less water is absorbed from the stool).

Continued on following page

NURSING CARE PLANNING GUIDE Continued

- Obtain information regarding knowledge about influences of diet and activity on bowel elimination and clarify as needed.
- Client may lack knowledge about factors influencing bowel elimination.
- Provide information about the role of fiber and liquids in preventing constipation. Teach which foods are high in fiber, if needed, and number of servings recommended per day.
- Fiber stimulates peristalsis in the gastrointestinal tract. With peristalsis, stool is eliminated before an excess amount of water is absorbed from the stool. Liquid in the diet helps provide a proper consistency to the stool; many advise 8 to 10 glasses a day. Foods with fiber are fresh fruits and vegetables (not cooked), whole grains, and cereals. Many recommend at least two servings of high-fiber foods per day.
- Obtain information about daily activities, exercise. Devise an individualized exercise regimen with the client.
- Exercise increases peristalsis. Knowledge of the daily schedule as well as of preferences for particular exercise allows the nurse to assist in planning a schedule to which the client is most likely to adhere.
- Instruct client about proper self-administration of medication, if ordered.
- Various stool softeners may be prescribed. These often contain wetting agents that lower the surface tension so the stool is more easily penetrated by water (an example is Colace). Others contain a combination of a wetting agent and a chemical that stimulates peristalsis (Peri-Colace). Still others provide bulk, or fiber (Metamucil).

10

Analysis: ▼ NURSING DIAGNOSIS

Risk for ineffective breathing pattern, related to

- Increased vital capacity
- Diaphragm rises when uterus enlarges
- Increased circumference of chest
- Thoracic rather than abdominal respirations that occur during pregnancy

Defining Characteristics

SUBJECTIVE	*OBJECTIVE*
Complains of shortness of breath	Shortness of breath, dyspnea
	Hyperventilation
	Smokes
	Increased respiratory rate

Continued on facing page

NURSING CARE PLANNING GUIDE Continued

Client Goal / ▼ EVALUATION CRITERIA

Client will demonstrate effective breathing pattern. / ▼ **Client will evidence normal respiratory rate, absence of hyperventilation, and absence of shortness of breath.**

▼ NURSING INTERVENTIONS	Rationale
• Assess for shortness of breath.	• Shortness of breath may occur as a result of a rising diaphragm and an enlarged uterus.
• Assess for hyperventilation. Teach ways to stop hyperventilation (breathe into paper bag).	• Increased tidal volume and functional changes result in tendency for hyperventilation. Breathing into a paper bag increases inspired carbon dioxide.
• Assess rate and depth of respirations.	• Respiratory rate remains the same in pregnancy, but the depth of respirations may increase to meet increased demands for oxygen created by increased metabolic rate, tissue growth, and demands of the fetus. Progesterone decreases airway resistance, and estrogen decreases pulmonary tissue resistance.
• Assess preexisting respiratory conditions, such as allergic rhinitis, asthma, or a sinus condition. Caution client about taking medications during pregnancy.	• These conditions may alter breathing patterns further. Medications may harm the fetus.
• Recommend self-care activities to ease breathing. These include	
1. reducing or eliminating smoking	• Smoking decreases oxygen availability.
2. good posture 3. semi-Fowler position for sleeping if necessary 4. intercostal breathing	• Good posture, upright positioning, and intercostal breathing increase lung expansion.

11

Analysis: ▼ NURSING DIAGNOSIS

Risk for sleep pattern disturbance, related to

- Increased basal metabolic rate resulting in fatigue
- Conflict or anxiety about pregnancy
- Fetal movement, activity
- Muscle-skeletal strains
- Insomnia

Continued on following page

NURSING CARE PLANNING GUIDE Continued

Defining Characteristics

SUBJECTIVE	*OBJECTIVE*
States feelings of fatigue	Difficulty concentrating
States difficulty in falling asleep	Appears fatigued
States is waking up at night	Sleeps less than 8 hours per night
Describes anxiety about being pregnant	Unable to take a nap daily

Client Goal / ▼ EVALUATION CRITERIA

Client will demonstrate adequate sleep pattern. / ▼ **Client will evidence absence of fatigue and absence of insomnia; client will evidence signs of feeling refreshed; and client will fall asleep readily, sleep 8 hours per night, and nap if necessary.**

▼ NURSING INTERVENTIONS	Rationale
• Obtain information about usual sleep pattern and typical schedule.	• The nurse can assist in adjusting the daily schedule to "fit in" a nap or rest period. Suggestions to aid relaxation just before sleep can be provided (such as quiet time with minimal noise and activity, meditation, soft music, use of relaxation techniques).
• Recommend a nap or rest period each day.	• Sleep is needed to feel refreshed, restored.
• Recommend positions for sleep that provide adequate support.	• Proper support with pillows for side-lying position promotes relaxation and aids sleep.

12

Analysis: ▼ NURSING DIAGNOSIS

Risk for altered sexuality patterns, related to

- Nausea and vomiting
- Breast tenderness
- Decreased desire by both partners associated with body changes of pregnancy
- Pelvic vasocongestion
- Uterine enlargement
- Shortness of breath
- Fatigue
- Decreased mobility
- Fear of fetal injury
- Fear of initiating labor

Continued on facing page

NURSING CARE PLANNING GUIDE Continued

Defining Characteristics

SUBJECTIVE	*OBJECTIVE*
Discusses sexual concerns	Unable to engage in intimate physical activities other than intercourse
Shares feelings about alteration in sexual desire	Unable to alter position for intercourse as necessary
Discusses how body changes of pregnancy affect sexual activity	Unable to engage in sexual activity at desired frequency
Verbalizes fear associated with sexual activity	

Client Goal / ▼ EVALUATION CRITERIA

Client will demonstrate adjusted sexuality patterns. / ▼ **Client will evidence sharing feelings about alteration in desire, discussing concerns, verbalizing mutual satisfaction.**

▼ NURSING INTERVENTIONS	Rationale
• Obtain information about usual pattern of sexual activity and desire.	• Information about usual patterns provides a baseline for comparison. Sexual desire may decrease with feelings of nausea and with changing energy levels and body changes.
• Obtain information about body changes of pregnancy and the impact of these on sexual activity.	• Perceptions about the influence of body changes on sexual activity influence the client's behaviors. Once there is awareness of effect of changes, acceptance of or alteration in behavior can occur.
• Provide information about physiologic changes of pregnancy.	• Knowledge of normalcy of changes helps the client to accept those changes.
• Obtain data about feelings associated with changes in sexual activity.	• Verbalizing feelings helps with self-recognition as well as with acceptance by the partner. Communication is essential to resolve concerns. The client may feel unattractive with body changes. The male partner may feel increased desire, may feel repulsed, or may fear injury to the fetus.
• Assess feelings about changes in body shape.	• The body image is related to one's identity as a female. Changes in body shape associated with pregnancy may conflict with usual body image. One's body image and the other's conception of it are associated with feelings of attractiveness and attraction to the other.
• Discuss ways to enhance intimacy through physical contact other than intercourse (hugging, stroking, kissing).	• Physical contact provides emotional support, meets needs for affection and attention.
• Suggest alternative positions for intercourse if this is necessary.	• The nurse provides information that is the basis for selecting behaviors from alternatives. The enlarging uterus may require a change in position.

Continued on following page

NURSING CARE PLANNING GUIDE Continued

- Advise not to let partner blow air into the vagina.
  - Air embolism with resultant mortality has occurred when air is blown into the vagina.
- Encourage client to verbalize fears related to sexual activity. Clarify misconceptions.
  - Many fear miscarriage, fetal injury, infection, or premature labor. Most studies indicate that intercourse has not been the cause of premature rupture of membranes, onset of labor, infection, or fetal injury.
- Refer for counseling if necessary.
  - Counselors can assist in resolving sexual concerns.
- Be alert for occurrence of inappropriate sexual behaviors.
  - The literature indicates that the frequency of rape, incest, violence, and extramarital affairs is higher during pregnancy.

13

Analysis: ▼ NURSING DIAGNOSIS

Risk for injury with exercise, related to

- Altered center of gravity
- Lordosis
- Increased elasticity of tissues
- Softening of connective tissue
- Relaxation of joints

Defining Characteristics

SUBJECTIVE

Symptoms of round ligament pain

Complains of aching numbness or weakness in upper extremities

Complains of paresthesia, weakness, or tenderness in wrist and thumb

OBJECTIVE

Waddling gait

Lordosis

Injuries from fall

Client Goal / ▼ EVALUATION CRITERIA

Client will demonstrate absence of injury with exercise. / ▼ **Client will evidence absence of pain, abrasions, bruises.**

Continued on facing page

NURSING CARE PLANNING GUIDE Continued

▼ NURSING INTERVENTIONS	Rationale
• Recommend exercise that will not injure muscles or joints.	• Exercises that require jogging, bouncing, or ballistic movements can lead to sprain and injury.
• Recommend warm-up, stretching, and cool-down.	• These allow stretching that minimizes injury.
• Advise avoidance of stretching to point of maximal resistance.	• Stretching to maximal resistance may increase potential for injury.
• Recommend adequate hydration; drink liquids before and after exercise.	• During exercise, fluid is lost in perspiration and with respiration.
• Recommend avoiding exercises that require balance.	• The center of gravity is altered during pregnancy and the curvature of the spine is accentuated. These changes result in greater difficulty in maintaining balance.

14

Analysis: ▼ NURSING DIAGNOSIS

Knowledge deficit: pregnancy, related to

- First experience with pregnancy
- Lack of understanding of physiologic and psychological changes of pregnancy
- Lack of knowledge of warning signs in pregnancy
- Lack of knowledge of self-care activities that promote health in pregnancy
- Lack of knowledge of newborn caretaking skills

Defining Characteristics

SUBJECTIVE	*OBJECTIVE*
Unable to explain physiologic or psychological changes of pregnancy	Lack of attendance at childbirth education classes
Unable to demonstrate self-care activities promoting health	
Unable to state warning signs to report	
Unable to explain fetal growth and development	
Unable to state signs of labor	
Unable to decide type of anesthesia desired	
Unable to decide whether will breastfeed or bottle feed	

Continued on following page

NURSING CARE PLANNING GUIDE Continued

Client Goal / ▼ EVALUATION CRITERIA

Client will demonstrate adequate knowledge about pregnancy. / ▼ **Client will evidence adequate ability to explain normal physiologic and psychological changes of pregnancy, demonstrate self-care behaviors that promote health, identify warning signs to report.**

▼ NURSING INTERVENTIONS	Rationale
• Assess knowledge level of normal physiologic and psychological changes of pregnancy, fetal growth and development, and changes in sexual patterns.	• Knowledge allows the client to anticipate changes and reduces anxiety that may occur with those changes.
• Assess knowledge of warning signs in pregnancy.	• Knowledge of warning signs to report allows early recognition and reporting so treatment can be instituted promptly.
• Assess knowledge of self-care activities that promote health, including self-help strategies for discomforts, proper exercise, appropriate hygiene measures, aids for rest and sleep, information about proper nutrition, how to avoid teratogens, and work environment counseling.	• Information related to self-care activities that promote health allows the client the opportunity to perform those activities.
• Assess knowledge about labor and delivery.	• Mothers-to-be are often fearful of the labor and birth experience. Information aids decision making and decreases anxiety coming from the unknown.
• Assess knowledge of newborn caretaking skills, including breastfeeding and infant safety.	• Mothers-to-be begin to conceptualize the maternal role during pregnancy.
• Assess knowledge of family role adjustment.	• Addition of a new family member necessitates role adjustments. Mothers-to-be progress through stages in transition to the maternal role.
• Clarify any misconceptions.	• Information allows the client to operate on a sound basis.
• Supply additional information as needed. Answer questions.	• The nurse provides information useful in making choices and carrying out self-care activities that promote health.
• Encourage enrollment in childbirth education classes.	• Information reduces anxiety associated with the unknown.
• Provide written information as necessary.	• Supplemental information reinforces learning and provides a reference at home, which enhances learning.

Continued on facing page

NURSING CARE PLANNING GUIDE Continued

15

Analysis: ▼ NURSING DIAGNOSIS

Risk for fetal injury, related to

- Exercise program that elevates core temperature
- Maternal dehydration with exercise that contributes to elevated core temperature
- Hemoconcentration and reduced cardiac reserve with maternal exercise
- Back-lying exercise later in pregnancy
- Back-lying position later in pregnancy
- Maternal anemia
- Maternal smoking
- Hypertensive disorders of pregnancy
- Gestational diabetes

Defining Characteristics

SUBJECTIVE	*OBJECTIVE*
Continued maternal smoking	Low-birth-weight infant
	Premature birth
	Birth defect
	Fundal height lower than expected for gestational age
	Ultrasound examination indicating intrauterine growth retardation
	Abnormal fetal heart rate
	Late decelerations during labor
	Fetal demise

Client Goal / ▼ EVALUATION CRITERIA

Client will demonstrate absence of fetal injury. / ▼ **Client will evidence normal maternal hemoglobin level; minimal or no maternal smoking; exercise so maternal heart rate does not exceed 140 beats per minute; absence of maternal hypertensive disorders of pregnancy; diabetes, or infection symptoms; normal fundal height; normal fetal heart tones; normal term infant.**

Continued on following page

NURSING CARE PLANNING GUIDE Continued

▼ NURSING INTERVENTIONS	Rationale
• Recommend exercise program with 1. warm-up, stretching, cool-down 2. maternal heart rate not exceeding 140 beats per minute at peak activity 3. no back-lying exercises later in pregnancy 4. adequate increase in calories and fluid to compensate for exercise	• With exercise, there is hemoconcentration, which contributes to reduced cardiac reserve and oxygen-carrying capacity. The back-lying position causes the weight of the uterus to restrict venous return to the heart and, with exercise, can lead to abruptio placentae. The respiratory reserve is lowered during pregnancy; with moderate to strenuous exercise, lactic acidosis can occur. With exercise, the core temperature increases; renal tube defects have occurred in baby animals exposed to elevated core temperature of the mother during pregnancy.
• Assess fetal heart rate at each visit. A normal fetal heart rate ranges from 120 to 160 beats per minute.	• A normal heart rate indicates a developing fetus that is adequately oxygenated.
• Assess fetal movement. Ask mother about fetal movement pattern.	• Fetal movement indicates a live, active fetus that is growing appropriately.
• Assess fundal height at each visit. Compare with previous visit and number of weeks' gestation.	• Fundal height increases according to a typical pattern; the increase indicates appropriate growth of the fetus and absence of intrauterine growth restriction.
• Assess for hypertensive disorders of pregnancy. Assess maternal blood pressure, edema, and urine for protein.	• In hypertensive disorders of pregnancy, vasoconstriction with subsequent reduced oxygenation of the fetus occurs. Maternal convulsions result in reduced oxygenation and possible placental separation.
• Assess for maternal anemia.	• Maternal anemia results in reduced RBCs and oxygenation of the fetus.
• Recommend and assist mother in reducing or quitting smoking.	• Smoking causes vasoconstriction and also reduces oxygenation of the fetus because oxygen is replaced on hemoglobin by cigarette byproducts.
• Assess maternal alcohol and drug intake.	• Excessive, chronic intake of alcohol during pregnancy can result in fetal alcohol syndrome. Over-the-counter medication may harm the fetus. Use of illegal drugs may harm the fetus.
• Assess for gestational diabetes. Check urine for glucose at each visit; if elevated, check blood sugar. Do glucose tolerance screening test at 24 to 28 weeks' gestation.	• Altered metabolic states accompanying maternal diabetes during pregnancy may cause fetal defects, demise, or hypoglycemia after birth. Macrosomatia and dystocia problems can also occur.
• Assess for maternal infection, including gonorrhea, chlamydia, syphilis, herpes, condyloma, and vaginitis (due to *Candida, Trichomonas,* or *Gardnerella*). Obtain appropriate blood tests or cultures. Treat as appropriate.	• Infections can be transmitted to the fetus transplacentally or at the time of birth, causing various infections, defects, or conditions. Treatment of infection can be instituted to minimize detrimental effects.
• Advise against changing cat litter box. Advise wearing gloves for gardening.	• *Toxoplasma gondii* infection is transmitted by cat feces.
• Obtain maternal serum for alpha-fetoprotein (AFP) assessment. Screen for elevated AFP levels in high-risk populations (previous child with chromosome abnormalities, gravidas older than 35 years).	• AFP is a protein produced by the yolk sac and fetal liver. When there is an open neural tube defect, it appears in maternal serum at a much elevated level at 8 to 15 weeks' gestation, and then it decreases.

Continued on facing page

NURSING CARE PLANNING GUIDE Continued

• Assess for high-risk factors for genetic disorders; discuss options.	• Clients at higher risk for genetic disorders may desire counseling.
• Provide information about potential teratogens, such as x-rays, medications, alcohol, viral infections, and rubella. Assess rubella titer.	• Information provides the opportunity to avoid exposure. Rubella exposure and infection can lead to fetal defects; if the client is not immune, she should avoid exposure and obtain immunization after delivery. A rubella titer of 1:10 is necessary to be considered immune.
• Refer for substance abuse treatment if necessary.	• Treatment is necessary for resolution.

16

Analysis: ▼ NURSING DIAGNOSIS

Risk for body image disturbance, related to

- Changing body shape
- Other body changes, such as chloasma and striae
- Fear or anxiety about safe birth
- Fear or anxiety about normality of baby

Defining Characteristics

SUBJECTIVE	*OBJECTIVE*
Negative statements about changing body image	Inappropriate maternity clothing
	Wearing high-heeled shoes
	Not well groomed

Client Goal / ▼ EVALUATION CRITERIA

Client will demonstrate positive body image as pregnancy progresses. / ▼ **Client will wear appropriate maternity clothing, make positive statements about body changes, appear well groomed.**

▼ NURSING INTERVENTIONS	Rationale
• Assess reaction to pregnancy, to changing body image. Obtain information about reactions of significant others.	• Feelings influence adjustment to the pregnancy and ability to accept it as a positive life event. Significant others influence how the mother-to-be views herself and her degree of acceptance of body changes.

Continued on following page

NURSING CARE PLANNING GUIDE Continued

- Review physiologic and body changes.
- Obtain information about conceptualizations of body image, how the mother-to-be views herself, and how body changes of pregnancy will affect this.
- Provide information about normalcy of mood swings, fears, and anxiety.
- Assess social network for ability to provide emotional and appraisal support.
- Suggest available sources of maternity clothing.

- Anxiety is lessened if changes can be anticipated.
- In developing the "self," feedback from others and one's own perception influence the image of the physical self.
- Reaction to physiologic changes and anticipated changes as well as processes involved in maternal role attainment contributes to anxiety, fear, and mood swings. Lack of information may also contribute to anxiety.
- The social network can provide positive feedback that increases self-esteem.
- Clothing to enhance appearance during pregnancy enhances self-esteem.

17

Analysis: ▼ NURSING DIAGNOSIS

Risk for altered growth and development: parenting, related to

- Pregnancy is a period of change
- Individual developmental task for a pregnant woman, becoming a mother
- Individual developmental task for the husband or significant other, becoming a father
- Family developmental tasks (siblings, grandparents)

Defining Characteristics

SUBJECTIVE

States feelings about pregnancy

Discusses relationship with own mother

OBJECTIVE

Does not plan for physical needs of the baby; does not obtain furniture, car seat, clothing, or supplies

Does not adjust financial patterns

Takes over-the-counter medications

Nutritional intake inadequate for pregnancy

Does not adjust work schedule, activities to adjust for pregnancy

Continued on facing page

NURSING CARE PLANNING GUIDE Continued

Client Goal / ▼ EVALUATION CRITERIA

Client will demonstrate adequate adjustment to pregnancy and birth. / ▼ **Client will evidence successful accomplishment of developmental tasks, adequate individual coping (mother and father), adequate family coping.**

▼ NURSING INTERVENTIONS	Rationale
• Provide information about normal physiologic and psychological changes of pregnancy and self-care. This includes physiologic changes, warning signs to report, growth and development of the fetus, psychological changes, and self-care to minimize discomforts. It includes warning signs, like bleeding, as well as identifying agents harmful to the fetus, like drugs, smoking, and alcohol.	• Parents may not be aware of the pattern of fetal growth and development or of self-care activities to promote such growth. Parents may not be aware of psychological adjustments to the natural process of pregnancy.
• Provide information and resources related to physical care of the baby. This involves housing, furniture, clothing, supplies, and car seat.	• The newborn will need to have a safe place to sleep, clothing and diapers, feeding equipment, and an approved car seat. Parents may not be aware of regulations regarding car seats or type of clothing and supplies available. Either finances may need to be adjusted to provide for purchase of these items, or other resources may be used to provide for them.
• Discuss work patterns and activities and help plan alterations that promote health. This may involve breaks, finding a place to relax at lunch or midafternoon, altering activities to avoid long periods of standing, providing a way to elevate legs, and learning good posture. In addition, hazards in the environment need to be identified and avoided (such as chemicals, x-rays).	• Activities may need to be adjusted to promote circulation, minimize backache, and lessen edema. Hazards need to be avoided to prevent injury to the fetus.
• Discuss alterations in sexual expression, providing recommendations as needed (see nursing diagnosis of altered sexual patterns).	• As the uterus enlarges, adjustment in position for sexual activity may be required. There may be fears or anxieties associated with sexual expression during pregnancy.
• Encourage parents to discuss feelings about the pregnancy and feelings related to adjustments necessary to accommodate the new family member.	• There are many psychological reactions to pregnancy. First, the mother-to-be realizes she is pregnant and focuses on the meaning of pregnancy to herself and her lifestyle; she incorporates the fetus into her self. Next, the mother-to-be focuses on the developing baby and examines her relationship with her own mother to begin developing her own maternal role conceptions. This brings emotional responses. Finally, the mother pictures the baby and the mothering role while she prepares for birth.
• Identify support persons; include them in prenatal care and planning for birth. This may involve grandmother, aunt, sister, or support person in childbirth classes.	• Emotional, instrumental informational, and appraisal support from significant persons helps the mother adjust to pregnancy and to develop role conceptions. The woman's cultural background influences attitudes about, and adjustment to, pregnancy. Social support buffers stress, enhances coping, facilitates positive health practices, and helps prevent complications.

Continued on following page

NURSING CARE PLANNING GUIDE Continued

• Suggest childbirth education classes.	• These classes provide additional information about pregnancy, labor and birth, and preparing for care of the new baby.
• Identify complications and intervene promptly.	• Complications influence not only physiologic but psychological and sociocultural aspects of pregnancy as well. Minimizing complications promotes health.

18

Analysis: ▼ NURSING DIAGNOSIS

Altered role performance: anticipating the maternal role, related to

- Learning the maternal role
- Learning the grandparent role
- Adjustments in family roles
- Adjustments in the occupational role
- Resources available to assist transition to mothering role
- Support persons available

Defining Characteristics

SUBJECTIVE	*OBJECTIVE*
Does not describe imagined maternal role	Does not purchase supplies and equipment for baby
Negative verbal feedback from father	Does not attend childbirth education classes
States others do not praise her for maternal behaviors (family members and others)	Does not observe mothering behavior of others
Negative verbalizations about baby	

Client Goal / ▼ EVALUATION CRITERIA

Client will demonstrate effective transition to maternal role. / ▼ **Client will evidence positive feedback from father, family members, others, and baby; appropriate caretaking tasks.**

▼ NURSING INTERVENTIONS	Rationale
• Assess response to pregnancy.	• If the mother-to-be achieves developmental tasks, she will progress through a series of emotional responses to pregnancy, essentially accepting the pregnancy and having positive feelings about it.

Continued on facing page

NURSING CARE PLANNING GUIDE Continued

- Assess economic situation and financial resources.
- Prenatal care requires financial or insurance resources. Preparation for the baby also involves expenditures. Proper nutrition is necessary and also requires financial resources.

- Discuss necessary alterations in family roles. Recommend strategies to aid adjustment.
- Roles are patterns of behavior that are learned and that provide guides for behavior. The behaviors are learned predominantly within the family, and therefore there are cultural beliefs and values involved. Role behaviors accompany positions within the family structure (mother and father, husband and wife are positions).

  Formal roles in the family typically include roles like breadwinner, child socializer, physical caretaker of children, meeting emotional needs, and housekeeper. These may be shared and will need to be altered to accommodate care of the new baby.

- Encourage talk about her relationship with her own mother.
- The mother-to-be often uses her own mother as a role model for parenting. During pregnancy, the mother-to-be reviews this relationship and begins to conceptualize her own behaviors as a mother.

- Provide suggestions about reading material regarding adjustment to parental role.
- Information increases awareness and helps to reappraise family roles.

- Assist mother-to-be with the taking-on process. Observe maternity clothing. Obtain data about practice of role behaviors.
- According to Rubin (1967a and b), taking-on is the first of three processes involved in the maternal role development. Part of this process is practicing "mimicry" or adopting simple behaviors of mothers, like dress, speech affects, and gestures. An example might be wearing maternity clothes before they are necessary. Role play is also involved, when maternal behaviors are actually tried out. An example might be baby-sitting.

- Assist mother-to-be with taking-in process. Obtain data about maternal "daydreams" and conceptualizations of what she will do as a mother.
- According to Rubin (1967a and b), taking-in is the second of three processes in maternal role attainment. In this process, the maternal role is internalized. This involves "fantasy" or daydreaming about the role, imagining herself playing the maternal role. It also involves "introjection, projection, rejection," which is evaluating maternal behavior she has observed, then remembering or rejecting it. Finally, it involves maternal "identity"; the mother-to-be has conceptualized the role and feels comfortable with it, and the conceptualization is integrated into her self.

- Assist mother-to-be with letting-go process. Encourage mother to express feelings associated with letting-go.
- According to Rubin (1967a and b), letting-go is the third and last process in attaining the maternal role. This involves abandoning former identities and behaviors so the new maternal identity can be integrated. Grief accompanies the letting-go.

- Identify factors hindering maternal role development and work toward overcoming these barriers. Some of these factors are degree of commitment to pregnancy, perceptions of birth experience, preparation for the maternal role, value of the maternal role, perceived conflicts with the maternal role, maternal health status, available role models, available social support and resources, and maternal age.
- Many factors influence the transition to the maternal role. Identification of factors hindering a positive adjustment allows interventions to overcome these barriers.

Continued on following page

NURSING CARE PLANNING GUIDE Continued

• Obtain information about strategies that were effective in adjusting to other new roles.	• One tends to use coping strategies that were effective in the past. Effective strategies can be reinforced by the nurse.
• Suggest additional coping strategies as necessary.	• The nurse can suggest additional strategies that will enhance maternal role development.
• Assist fathers in the transition to paternal role. Encourage discussion of paternal role behaviors. Identify paternal role models. Obtain information about cultural beliefs regarding fathering.	• Fathers must also develop conceptualization of fathering behaviors.

Chapter 20

Perinatal Education

Francine H. Nichols
Elaine Zwelling

> A student once said to me, It never occurred to me not to learn how to give birth. After all, everything I have ever done in my life, from learning to walk, talk, read and write, to preparing myself for a career, I had to learn. It did not come by itself. It seems obvious to me that I had better learn to give birth to my child in order to do it well and as efficiently as possible.
>
> ELISABETH BING (JOHNSTON 1994)

HIGHLIGHTS

- What Is Perinatal Education?
- Prepared Childbirth: A Psychoeducational Intervention
- Components of Prepared Childbirth Classes: Information, Coping Skills, Support
- Paced Breathing Strategies
- Breathing for Birth
- Role of the Perinatal Educator and Types of Practice
- Professional Preparation and Certification
- Nursing Practice
- Risk Management
- Implications for Research

Today, perinatal education is an integral part of maternal-newborn nursing practice, having grown from a one-to-one approach in the early years to a comprehensive program. This recognized specialty area has a firmly established scientific basis, and maternal-newborn nurses who wish to teach perinatal education classes should have formal specialized preparation for the role as perinatal educators (Association of Women's Health, Obstetric and Neonatal Nurses [AWHONN] 1993).

DEFINITIONS

Bradley Husband-Coached Childbirth—A method of prepared childbirth developed by Robert Bradley and published in 1965 in *Husband-Coached Childbirth.* This method advocates deep relaxation techniques and slow abdominal breathing to promote comfort. The woman's spouse is viewed as the most effective support person for her during labor.

Consumer advocacy—Informing, supporting, and encouraging clients to participate in making decisions that affect their well-being and that of their unborn child.

Change agent—An individual or a group who initiates change or assists others to initiate change within a system.

Dick-Read Prepared Childbirth—A method of prepared childbirth developed by Dr. Grantly Dick-Read and published in 1933 in *Natural Childbirth.* Information, muscular relaxation techniques, and slow abdominal breathing strategies were advocated to interrupt the fear-tension-pain cycle.

Labor support—Activities that include both affective and psychomotor behaviors that enhance the woman's participation in childbirth and that foster activity enabling her to cope more effectively. Support can be given by the woman's partner, a family member, a nurse, or a doula (a woman with special training to give labor support).

Lamaze Prepared Childbirth—A method of prepared childbirth that includes information about pregnancy and childbirth, the use of relaxation and paced breathing strategies, other noninvasive pain management techniques, and labor support techniques for childbirth. This method was adapted from the Russian psychoprophylaxis model by French obstetrician Fernand Lamaze.

Paced breathing strategies—Controlled types of breathing strategies that can be used to decrease stress and anxiety, and relieve pain.

Perinatal education—Health education for the family unit during pregnancy, childbirth, and the early parenting period.

Psychoeducational intervention—An intervention that uses educational and psychological strategies to decrease pain, enhance recovery, promote psychological well-being, and increase satisfaction with health care. Psychoeducational interventions include three areas of content: information about events, procedures, sensations, or self-care activities; skills to reduce discomfort and complications; and psychological support to reduce anxieties and enhance coping.

Psychoprophylaxis—A method of childbirth preparation known in North America as the Lamaze method.

WHAT IS PERINATAL EDUCATION?

Perinatal education is health education for the family unit during pregnancy, childbirth, and the early parenting period. As the childbearing family expands, the roles of family members change and the interactions between family members increase in number and complexity (Fig. 20–1) (Peterson and Peterson 1993). Thus, perinatal education is composed of a variety of different types of classes that address the needs of all family members as the family moves from one developmental life cycle stage to another during the childbearing years. Perinatal education uses both the psychoeducational model, which focuses on information, skills, and social support; and the health education model, which focuses on prevention, informed choice, and healthy lifestyle practices as a framework for classes (Nichols 1988b). These models are based on the research literature from developmental psychology, maternal-newborn nursing, childbirth education, and multidisciplinary studies on stress and on the family.

The overall goal of perinatal education is to provide information, coping skills for pain management, and support for family members based on individual needs related to childbearing and parenting. Specific goals vary according to the type of class and the audience. For example, prenatal classes stress information about pregnancy and childbirth rather than development of psychomotor coping skills and support systems. In contrast, prepared childbirth classes give equal emphasis to all three areas: providing information, developing coping skills for childbirth, and using support systems.

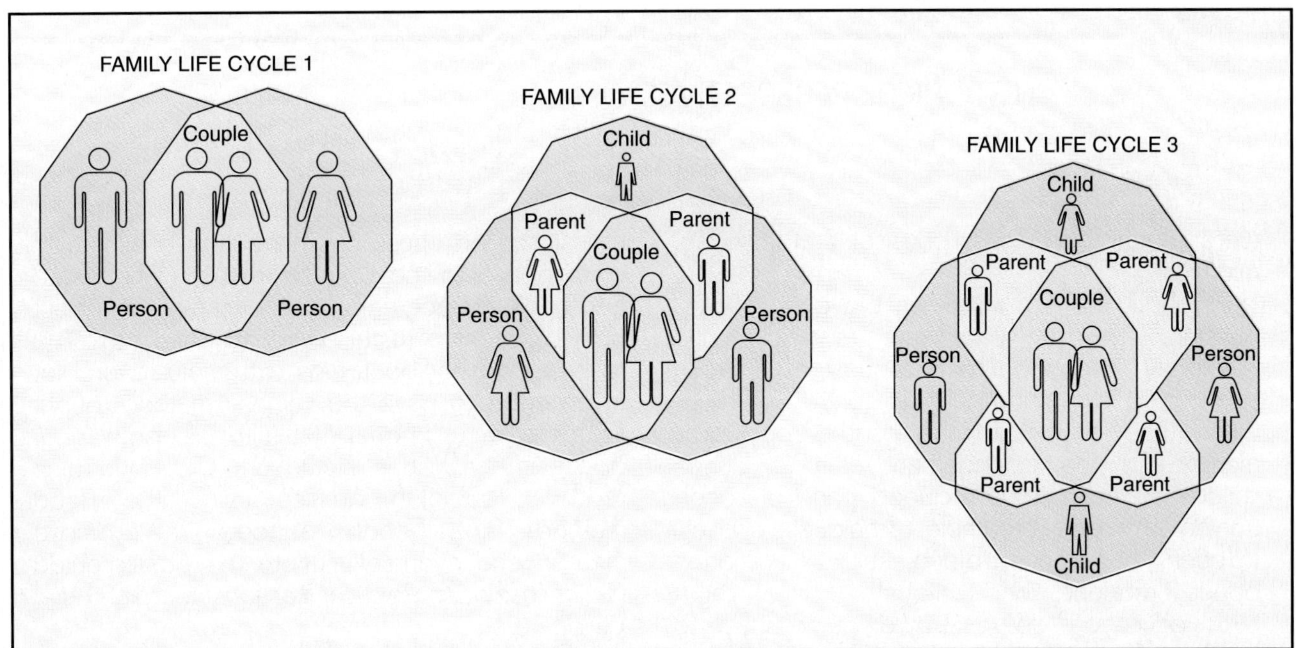

Figure 20–1

Stages of the family life cycle. Relationships, communications, and individual roles become increasingly complex as a family changes from a couple to a family that also includes one child and then additional children. (From Peterson, K. J., and Peterson, P. L. [1993]. Family-centered perinatal education. In F. H. Nichols [Ed.]. *Perinatal education. AWHONN's clinical issues in perinatal and women's health nursing* [pp. 1–4]. Philadelphia: J. B. Lippincott.)

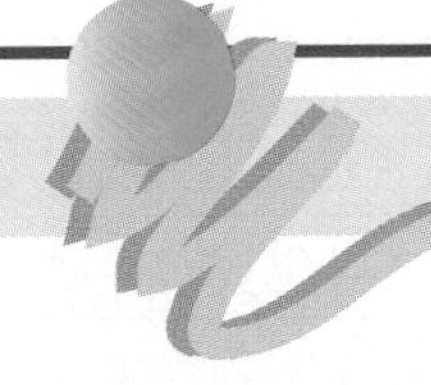

HISTORICAL PERSPECTIVES

THE DEVELOPMENT OF PERINATAL EDUCATION

For centuries, the only education for childbirth that existed took place within the family system. Information about pregnancy and birthing was passed down from one generation of women to another. Often the information was incorrect and based on "old wives' tales." While no formal mechanism for education existed, some information was no doubt given to women by midwives as well.

In the early 1900s, formal childbirth education emerged as a result of two separate forces with distinctly different missions. To meet public health needs and improve the health of women and children, the American Red Cross started childbirth classes in 1908 and the Maternity Center Association in New York City started childbirth classes in 1919.

Later, other childbirth education classes developed to prepare women for childbirth and to meet their pain management needs. It is difficult to trace when the first formal childbirth education class was started to teach pain management techniques, as these classes were developing at the same time in both England and Russia. In England in 1933, a physician, Grantly Dick-Read, published his book, *Natural Childbirth.* The book was based on years of observations of his patients giving birth and his resultant belief that most of the pain women experienced was caused by fear due to a lack of knowledge. Dick-Read's intent was that his book would be used by obstetricians to instruct women about birth. The concept of formal childbirth education classes apparently did not occur to him at first. However, when obstetricians did not use Dick-Read's book as he had anticipated, he established childbirth classes that

Continued on following page

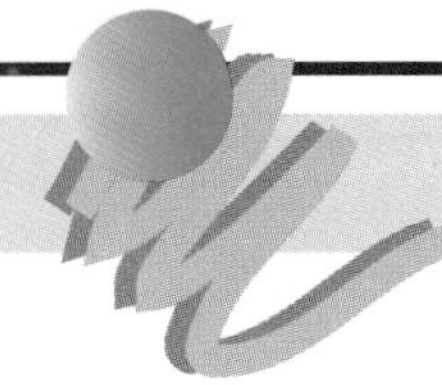

HISTORICAL PERSPECTIVES Continued

were taught by nurses, physical therapists, or midwives.

At about the same time in the early 1930s, Russian scientists Velvovsky, Platonov, and Nikolayev responded to a request from Stalin to develop a method of pain control for childbirth. They developed the psychoprophylactic method for the management of pain during childbirth. The method included physical conditioning exercises, breathing techniques, and relaxation techniques along with information about pregnancy and childbirth. Formal childbirth education classes were established to teach women the psychoprophylactic method of childbirth.

In January 1951, the Academy of Medical Sciences and the Ministry of Health in Russia organized a conference on the psychoprophylactic method. Nikolayev called for its nation-wide adoption as the standard method of childbirth in all obstetric institutions in Russia. Obstetricians from many countries were then invited to Russia to view their childbirth education classes and women using the psychoprophylactic method during labor and birth.

One of the physicians who went to Russia was Fernand Lamaze, the Chief of Obstetrics at the Metalworkers Hospital in Paris. Lamaze was very impressed with the Russian psychoprophylactic method of childbirth. He made a few changes, adapting the method to the European culture, and began to teach the psychoprophylactic method to his patients in Paris. As it spread throughout Europe, it became known as the Lamaze method.

An American woman named Marjorie Karmel introduced the method in the United States in 1959 with the publication of her book, *Thank You, Dr. Lamaze.* Karmel and her husband lived in Paris at the time of the birth of their first baby. Dr. Lamaze was her obstetrician and she used the psychoprophylactic method for childbirth. When Karmel and her husband returned to the United States and she was about to give birth to their second child, Karmel discovered that American physicians were not familiar with or receptive to the Lamaze method. She wrote her book at that time to inform women about her experiences with prepared childbirth. The response to her book was extremely favorable. In an effort to have the Lamaze method taught in this country, Karmel met with Elisabeth Bing, a physiotherapist in New York City, who was teaching childbirth classes using the Read method. Bing began to teach the Lamaze method and eventually wrote the classic guide for its use, *Six Practical Lessons for an Easier Childbirth.*

In 1974, a physician named Robert Bradley also played a major role in the development of childbirth education. In his book *Husband-Coached Childbirth,* he encouraged expectant fathers to take an active role as labor coach during childbirth. He also developed the Bradley method of childbirth preparation.

Early prepared childbirth education classes focused on the use of "specific methods" proposed by their proponents Dick-Read, Lamaze, and Bradley. Today, the "specific methods" approach has evolved to one that is scientifically based. Often, proponents of a specific method attempt to point out the unique differences of their method, but the main difference between the various methods of childbirth preparation today is primarily a philosophical one. All methods include information related to childbearing, relaxation and breathing techniques, and labor support training. A blurring of distinct lines between the traditional methods of prepared childbirth education will continue as educators base their practice on research findings. Perinatal education as we know it today, which includes many types of classes encompassing the needs of all family members, evolved from the practice of childbirth education.

In 1960, two formal organizations committed to influencing and changing maternity care services developed: the American Society for Psychoprophylaxis in Obstetrics (ASPO/Lamaze) and the International Childbirth Education Asso-

Continued on facing page

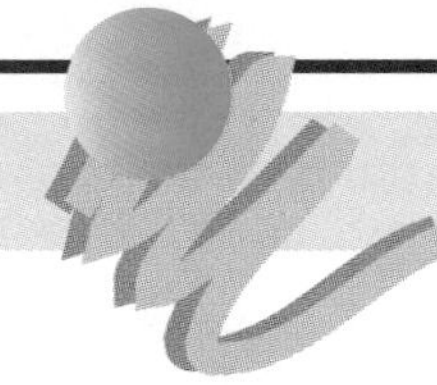

HISTORICAL PERSPECTIVES Continued

ciation (ICEA). In addition to promoting perinatal education, through the efforts of these two organizations, many significant improvements have been made in maternity care services through the years, such as allowing fathers to be present during birth, sibling visiting, a family-centered approach to childbirth, and changes in obstetric practices. Both of these organizations have had a tremendous influence in the areas of childbirth education and family-centered maternity care for over 35 years.

Prepared childbirth education is accepted as a standard of good prenatal care today because of the influence of many individuals throughout this century and the influence of consumer demands for preparation for childbirth. It is available in most areas of North America but is still unknown in many countries and just developing in others.

Data from Bing, E. (1969). *Six practical lessons for an easier childbirth.* New York: Bantam Books; Bradley, R. (1974). *Husband-coached childbirth.* New York: Harper & Row; Dick-Read, G. (1933). *Natural childbirth.* London: Heinemann; Karmel, M. (1959). *Thank you, Dr. Lamaze.* New York: J. B. Lippincott; Nichols, F. H., and Humenick, S. S. (1988). *Childbirth education: Practice, research, and theory.* Philadelphia: W. B. Saunders; Public Health Service, Department of Health and Human Services. (1989). Caring for our future: The content of prenatal care. *A report of the public health service expert panel on the content of prenatal care.* Washington, DC: Author; Velvovsky, I., Platonov, K., Ploticher, U., Shungom, E. (1960). *Painless childbirth through psychoprophylaxis.* Moscow: Foreign Languages Publishing House; and Velvovsky, I. (1972). Psychoprophylaxis in obstetrics: A Soviet method. In J. Llowells (Ed.). *Modern perspectives in psycho-obstetrics.* New York: Brunner/Mazel.

PERINATAL EDUCATION CLASSES

Since the introduction of childbirth preparation classes in the early 1900s, a significant increase in the variety of course offerings has taken place. Childbirth education has grown from a basic course to prepare women for pregnancy and birth to a comprehensive program that teaches about all aspects of the childbearing years and includes the entire family.

Preconceptional Counseling Classes

Public health nurses, family planning nurses, and nurse midwives have delivered elements of preconceptional care for decades. Studies have shown that the condition of the woman before pregnancy affects the pregnancy outcome, and a healthy pregnancy begins well in advance of conception (Frede and Strohbach 1992). Pregnancy can be viewed as a 12-month experience that begins 3 months before conception takes place. A Healthy People 2000 objective is to increase to at least 60 percent the proportion of primary care providers who provide age-appropriate preconception care and counseling (DHHS 1995). Many childbirth educators have already developed and teach preconceptional counseling classes. These classes offer potential parents information about healthy lifestyle activities that are beneficial to maternal and fetal health and behaviors that are detrimental to maternal and fetal health. A preconceptional health assessment is an important aspect of preconceptional care because it provides the foundation on which to plan care (see Preconceptional Health Assessment). Preconceptional counseling can be offered in a traditional classroom format through individual counseling or community education programs, or in junior high and high schools.

Prenatal Classes

A wide array of prenatal classes are now available to expectant parents. Prenatal classes are primarily informational in their focus, although they may introduce some muscle-toning exercises and relaxation and breathing skills. There is less em-

Preconceptional Health Assessment

The following preconceptional health assessment form is derived from the screening questions recommended in the text of this book. This assessment tool can be used in various ways: (1) it can be mailed to patients in advance of their appointment with instructions to complete it and bring it to their counseling session; (2) it can be completed by the patient in the waiting room just before the session; or (3) it can be completed by the health care professional during the initial interview. The first approach has advantages in that it encourages the patient to organize potentially important information before the counseling session, such as the amounts of vitamin supplementation or the types of chemical exposures, and to review pertinent questions with her partner if he is unable to attend the actual session. If the population being served has limited reading skills, the form or its use should be modified to accommodate their abilities.

PRECONCEPTIONAL HEALTH ASSESSMENT

What is your main interest in seeking preconceptional counseling?

____

____

____

____

So that we can address your specific interests and concerns, we ask that you complete the following questionnaire. You may use the reverse sides of the form to provide additional information when necessary.

Place an X next to any item that applies to you.

SOCIAL HISTORY

Do you:

_____ Drink beer, wine, or hard liquor

_____ Smoke cigarettes or use any other tobacco products

_____ Use marijuana, cocaine, or any recreational drugs

_____ Use lead or chemicals at home or at work. If yes, list the specific chemicals if you know what they are:

____

____

_____ Work with radiation

_____ Participate in an exercise program

Are you:

_____ 34 years of age or older

NUTRITION HISTORY

On the back of this sheet, list by meal everything you ate and drank yesterday, including the approximate amount; indicate snacks separately.

Do you:

_____ Practice vegetarianism

_____ Eat unusual substances, such as laundry starch or clay

_____ Have a history of bulimia or anorexia

_____ Follow a special diet. If yes, describe

____

____

_____ Supplement your diet with vitamins. If yes, list vitamins and dosages:

____

____

_____ Take a folic acid supplement. If yes, give dosage:

____

____

_____ Take medications, including oral contraceptives

_____ Have an intolerance for milk

MEDICAL HISTORY

Do you now have, or have you ever had:

_____ diabetes

_____ thyroid disease

_____ phenylketonuria (PKU)

_____ asthma

_____ heart disease

Continued on facing page

Preconceptional Health Assessment Continued

_____ high blood pressure
_____ deep venous thrombosis (blood clots)
_____ kidney disease
_____ systemic lupus erythematosus (SLE)
_____ epilepsy
_____ sickle cell disease
_____ cancer
_____ other health problems that require medical or surgical care. If yes, describe:______________________________
____

INFECTIOUS DISEASE HISTORY

Do you or your partner have a history of:
_____ recurrent genital infections
_____ herpes simplex
_____ *Chlamydia* infection
_____ human papillomavirus (genital warts)
_____ gonorrhea
_____ syphilis
_____ viral hepatitis or high-risk behavior, including use of intravenous street drugs, intimate bisexual/homosexual contact, or multiple sexual partners
_____ acquired immunodeficiency syndrome (AIDS) or high-risk behavior, including use of intravenous street drugs, intimate bisexual/homosexual contact, or multiple sexual partners
_____ occupational exposure to the blood or bodily secretions of others
_____ blood transfusions

Do you:
_____ own or work with cats
_____ have documented immunity to rubella

Do you:
_____ Routinely or occasionally take prescribed medications. If yes, list names and dosages:
____
____
_____ Routinely or occasionally take over-the-counter medications. If yes, list names and dosages:
____
____

REPRODUCTIVE HISTORY

Do you have a history of:
_____ uterine or cervical abnormalities
_____ two or more pregnancies that ended in first-trimester miscarriages
_____ one or more pregnancies that ended between 14 and 28 weeks of gestation
_____ one or more fetal deaths
_____ one or more infants who weighed less than 5½ pounds at birth
_____ one or more infants who were admitted to a neonatal intensive care unit
_____ one or more infants with a birth defect

FAMILY HISTORY

Do you, your partner, or members of either of your families, including offspring, have:
_____ hemophilia
_____ thalassemia
_____ Tay-Sachs disease
_____ sickle cell disease or trait
_____ phenylketonuria (PKU)
_____ cystic fibrosis
_____ a birth defect
_____ mental retardation

Are you and your partner related outside of marriage (such as cousins)?

Do you and your partner have the same ethnic or racial background, such as Ashkenazic Jew, Mediterranean, or black?

Modified from Cefalo, R. C., and Moos, M. K. (1995). *Preconceptual health care: A practical guide* (2nd ed.). St. Louis: C. V. Mosby.

phasis on the psychomotor coping skills of relaxation, breathing strategies, and positioning in preparing for birth than in prepared childbirth classes.

Early Pregnancy Classes

These classes are usually offered during the first trimester of the pregnancy and deal with topics of most concern at that time. Information included in these classes usually includes human sexuality, signs and symptoms of pregnancy, minor discomforts of pregnancy and comfort measures, fetal growth and development, emotional responses and changes of pregnancy, nutrition and health promotion during pregnancy, and danger signs. Muscle-toning exercises and relaxation are often introduced in these early classes. Early pregnancy classes also provide a forum for group sharing and support, allowing expectant parents to deal with their personal needs and feelings related to pregnancy, childbirth, and parenting.

Middle and Late Pregnancy Classes

The learning needs of expectant parents change as pregnancy advances (Table 20–1). Midpregnancy classes are designed to be offered during the second trimester of pregnancy, and late preg-

Table 20–1

LEARNING NEEDS OF EXPECTANT PARENTS: PREGNANCY, CHILDBIRTH, AND PARENTING

Note: Strong research support exists for some of the learning needs during pregnancy, childbirth, and parenting. Others are based on health care professionals' beliefs about what expectant parents and new parents need to know. The most appropriate time for the introduction of these topics in perinatal education classes is as yet undetermined from a scientific perspective. Systematic documentation of the learning needs of expectant parents and new parents, and the extent to which these topics should be included in childbirth education classes, is needed.

FIRST TRIMESTER	SECOND TRIMESTER	THIRD TRIMESTER	PARENTING
• Physical changes of pregnancy • Emotional changes of pregnancy • Sexuality Changing relationships Sexual concerns • Minor discomforts of pregnancy Frequent urination Nausea Cramps Vaginal discharge Fatigue • Danger signs Vaginal bleeding Persistent vomiting • Nutrition • General hygiene Rest and sleep Exercise • Use of drugs Smoking Alcohol OTC drugs Prescription drugs Illegal drugs	• Physical changes of second trimester • Emotional changes of second trimester • Sexuality Changing needs Sexual concerns • Minor discomforts of pregnancy Backache Varicose veins Braxton Hicks contractions Leg cramps Vaginal discharge Constipation Round ligament pain • Danger signs Vaginal bleeding Abdominal pain Edema of face, hands, feet Severe headache Visual disturbances Rupture of membranes • Nutrition • General hygiene	• Physical changes of third trimester and postpartum period • Emotional changes of third trimester and postpartum period • Sexuality Changing needs Sexual expression (different methods) Sexual concerns Problem solving • Minor discomforts of pregnancy Frequent urination Backache Dyspnea Varicose veins Braxton Hicks contractions Leg cramps Vaginal discharge Constipation Round ligament pain Fatigue • Danger signs Vaginal bleeding Abdominal pain	• Parent-infant interaction and attachment • Infant behavior • Infant growth and development • Infant caretaking skills • Infant feeding • Infant needs • Infant health • Infant safety • Circumcision • Role changes • Parenting caretaking roles • Resources for new parents

Continued on facing page

Table 20–1

LEARNING NEEDS OF EXPECTANT PARENTS: PREGNANCY, CHILDBIRTH, AND PARENTING Continued

FIRST TRIMESTER	SECOND TRIMESTER	THIRD TRIMESTER	PARENTING
• Fetal development • Financial considerations • How to use the health care system • Resources for pregnancy and childbirth • Myths about pregnancy and childbirth	Rest and sleep Exercise • Use of drugs Smoking Alcohol OTC drugs Prescription drugs Illegal drugs • Fetal growth • Preparation for newborn Feeding methods Physical arrangements Selection of pediatrician Infant care	Edema of face, hands, feet Severe headache Visual disturbances Rupture of membranes (prior to 38 weeks) • Nutrition • General hygiene Rest and sleep Exercise • Use of drugs Smoking Alcohol OTC drugs Prescription drugs Illegal drugs • Fetal growth • Preparation for breast-feeding • Support systems • Preparation for childbirth Common fears and anxieties Father involvement in childbirth The issue of choice Anatomy and physiology of childbirth Comfort measures Pain management strategies Variations in childbirth Hospital routines Obstetric interventions Special needs of multiparas • Parenting Lifestyle changes Role changes Role conflict Balancing family demands Maternal role acquisition Maternal development tasks • Preparation for newborn • Family planning	

Adapted from Roberts, J. (1976). Prenatal teaching guide. *Journal of Obstetric, Gynecologic, and Neonatal Nursing,* 5, 18; and Nichols, F. H. (1988b). The content. In F. H. Nichols and S. S. Humenick (Eds.). *Childbirth education: Practice, research, and theory* (pp. 456–457). Philadelphia: W. B. Saunders.

nancy classes are offered during the third trimester. Information is presented as a continuum of that begun in early pregnancy classes and specifically deals with second- or third-trimester issues. It is designed to stimulate expectant parents to plan for labor and birth, infant care, and infant feeding.

Pregnancy Fitness Classes

With the interest in physical fitness seen in the last decade, there has been an increased awareness of the importance of exercise during pregnancy. As a result, many childbirth educators have developed pregnancy fitness classes, the purpose of which is to increase general well-being, flexibility, and fitness during pregnancy and in preparation for labor and early parenting. The classes include stretching, toning, and some aerobic exercises that are safe during pregnancy.

Breastfeeding Classes

Although information about infant feeding is included in early, middle, and late pregnancy classes, separate breastfeeding classes are offered in some areas to prepare women and their partners for the breastfeeding experience. This course usually consists of one or two classes that include information about the anatomy and physiology of the breasts, the benefits of breastfeeding, the process of milk production, prenatal preparation for breastfeeding, maternal nutrition, and tips for initiating and maintaining lactation. Breastfeeding is covered in depth in Chapter 33.

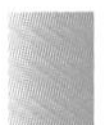

Other Prenatal Classes

Some of the changes seen in maternity care over recent years have precipitated other types of prenatal classes. Because many parents are waiting to begin their families until a later age, classes for mature gravidas have been started by some childbirth educators. These classes enable parents, who may be older than the average expectant couple in a childbirth class, to meet with other couples of similar age to share their unique situations and concerns. Information can be tailored to meet the needs of these older parents.

With the increase in the rate of multiple gestation due to the use of fertility drugs, some childbirth educators have started preparation for multiple birth classes. The physical, emotional, and medical aspects of a multiple gestation pregnancy and birth are unique, and when classes can be formed for a group of parents experiencing a multiple gestation, their needs can be met in a more meaningful way. The information presented includes prevention of preterm labor and tips for caring for more than one baby.

Classes for adoptive parents are also offered by some childbirth educators to meet the needs of parents who plan to adopt a baby. These classes include information on parenthood, lifestyle changes, infant characteristics, infant illness, and family coping strategies.

Prepared Childbirth Classes

Prepared childbirth classes focus on readying expectant parents for childbirth and the immediate postpartum period. Cognitive information about the labor and birth experience is offered as well as in-depth emphasis on developing the psychomotor skills of relaxation and controlled breathing and on establishing support systems. Parents are prepared physically and emotionally as well as intellectually for the birth experience (see Objectives for a Prepared Childbirth Education Course).

The basic information and skills taught in all types of prepared childbirth classes are similar, whether they be Lamaze (see below), Bradley, or generic programs. All emphasize relaxation, controlled breathing, comfort measures, and use of support systems. Since all information and skills taught in classes should be based on the scientific literature, this similarity is not surprising. Proponents of the various methods are often quick to point out what they consider unique differences between methods. However, the primary difference is a philosophical one related to differing views on working with the obstetric health care system and the emphasis on *not* using medical intervention during childbirth. For example, while all childbirth preparation methods oppose the routine use of medication and medical intervention during childbirth, some methods emphasize that "you should not take any medication during childbirth" while others clearly point out that "there is no safe medication during pregnancy and childbirth; you should use medication only if you absolutely need it, and if you need medication, use the least amount possible" (Nichols 1990).

Some childbirth education advocates prefer to work outside the obstetric health care system to bring the need for changes in obstetric care to the public's attention. This is often the approach chosen by the International Childbirth Education Association (ICEA). Other childbirth education advocates choose to work directly with the obstetric health care system, promoting needed changes in obstetric care from within the system. Since its in-

Objectives for a Prepared Childbirth Education Course

COGNITIVE DOMAIN

By the end of the course class, members will be able to

- Describe the common biological, psychological, and social responses to pregnancy, childbirth, and postpartum processes as well as associated comfort measures
- Define vocabulary terms useful in facilitating communication with health care providers or in reading literature on childbearing
- Use objective information to develop a plan that can serve as a basis for active participation in health care decisions, including commonly encountered interventions
- Plan assertive strategies for negotiating support from family members and from health care providers

AFFECTIVE DOMAIN

By the end of the course, class members will be able to

- View pregnancy and birth as a normal maturational process that includes stressors but also the potential for growth
- View themselves as central figures in their own health care and become actively involved in decisions concerning their care
- Use values clarification strategies to facilitate making realistic but flexible plans and choices

PSYCHOMOTOR DOMAIN

By the end of the course, class members will be able to

- Demonstrate physical exercises designed to promote comfort in pregnancy, prepare the body for birth, and promote postpartum recovery
- Demonstrate relaxation techniques designed to minimize tension and to promote the body's ability to function at maximal efficiency
- Demonstrate techniques using breathing and attention focusing for increasing relaxation
- Demonstrate activities that enhance relaxation and comfort in labor, such as positioning, mobility, massages, application of heat or cold, and water therapy
- Demonstrate expulsion techniques that support the physiologic process of second-stage labor

Adapted from Nichols, F. H. (1988b). The content. In F. H. Nichols and S. S. Humenick (Eds.). *Childbirth education: Practice, research, and theory* (p. 461). Philadelphia: W. B. Saunders.

ception in 1960, the American Society for Psychoprophylaxis in Obstetrics (ASPO)/Lamaze has usually followed the inside approach. Neither approach is wrong and both strategies are necessary to create long-lasting changes in the obstetric health care system.

LAMAZE CLASSES

The best known prepared childbirth program is Lamaze, originally called the psychoprophylaxis method. Adapted from the Russian model by French obstetrician Fernand Lamaze, this method was introduced to America in 1959 by Marjorie Karmel in her book, *Thank You, Dr. Lamaze.* These classes prepare expectant parents for the childbirth experience by presenting information about the physical and emotional aspects of pregnancy and childbirth, hospital procedures, possible medical interventions, and cesarean prevention techniques. Muscle-toning, relaxation, and breathing skills are taught for use during labor and birth and as future life skills. Consumer advocacy and informed decision making are also emphasized.

A Lamaze course is usually 6 to 8 weeks long and is ideally taken in the last trimester of pregnancy so that it ends about 2 weeks before the expected delivery date (Fig. 20–2). A complete Lamaze course should have a minimum of 12 hours of direct classroom content (ASPO/Lamaze 1993), typically taught over a period of multiple weeks to allow feedback from the instructor to the pregnant couple during the development of psychomotor skills.

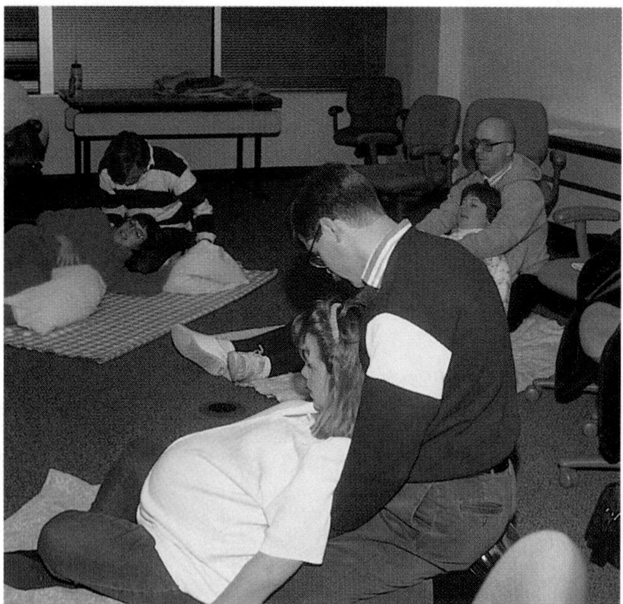

Figure 20–2

Practice in developing the psychomotor skills of relaxation and breathing strategies during class and at home is important to the woman's ability to learn to cope effectively during childbirth.

▼ **Weekend Lamaze Classes.** Weekend Lamaze classes in which expectant parents completed an entire Lamaze course in one weekend were established in response to consumer demands stemming from work obligations, conflicting time constraints, and family responsibilities (Bowden and Rose 1994). To be most effective, these classes require highly motivated expectant parents who assume responsibility for reading in preparation for the class, and practicing the childbirth skills of relaxation and controlled breathing after completion of the class until childbirth (Andreoli and Moran 1994). A negative aspect of weekend Lamaze classes is the lack of time needed to acquire the psychomotor skills of breathing and relaxation and the decreased opportunity for instructor feedback.

The primary objective guiding the development of weekend Lamaze classes was to offer an educationally sound alternative to a traditional childbirth education program during a restful weekend at a reasonable rate. Bowden and Rose (1994), in an analysis of the data from 126 expectant couples over a 2-year period, found that those who attended weekend Lamaze classes learned and retained the class content, and that the close group contact fostered intimate sharing and group bonding. Participants indicated satisfaction with the course content, method of instruction, and class environment. The data were obtained by questionnaire, but a direct measurement of psychomotor skill acquisition was not made.

▼ **Refresher Lamaze Classes.** Refresher classes for Lamaze are offered by many childbirth educators for parents who have taken a Lamaze course with a previous pregnancy. These classes are popular with parents who have other children at home and find it difficult or do not want to attend a complete Lamaze course. Such classes prepare parents both physically and emotionally for their next delivery, and provide an opportunity to share their residual fears or regrets from their first birth experience while planning for the upcoming birth. Refresher classes are composed of all experienced parents who can benefit from mutual sharing. Since refresher courses are short, lasting 3 to 4 weeks, some childbirth educators ask that couples meet certain requirements, such as having attended a previous Lamaze course within the last 3 years.

▼ **Vaginal Birth After Cesarean Classes.** A new type of prepared childbirth class has grown out of the recent increase in vaginal birth after a previous cesarean birth (VBAC). These classes are designed for parents who will be experiencing their first vaginal birth. Parents planning a VBAC need more preparation than a simple refresher course. Classes include discussion and sharing about the circumstances and the emotional responses of the parents' previous birth experience, and confidence building for parents who may feel that they "failed" with their first birth. Anxieties and unresolved feelings about a previous birthing experience are discussed. Parents are encouraged to have realistic expectations and open communication with their physician. Heavy emphasis is placed on cesarean prevention and pain management techniques for labor and birth. Flamm and colleagues (1994) have stated that while VBAC classes may not affect the mode of this birth (vaginal versus cesarean), they may "profoundly affect patient satisfaction."

Cesarean Birth Classes

Both research (Fawcett and Henklein 1987) and clinical observation have shown that parents' responses to cesarean birth, particularly if it is unanticipated, have indicated the need for detailed information about the events surrounding a cesarean delivery. Although some information about cesarean birth is usually offered in a late pregnancy course or a Lamaze course, many childbirth educators have developed separate cesarean birth classes for parents who anticipate a cesarean delivery. The course includes information about the surgery and related procedures, choices available to the parents, and postpartum physical recovery. Lamaze relaxation and breathing skills are taught for use before and after the birth.

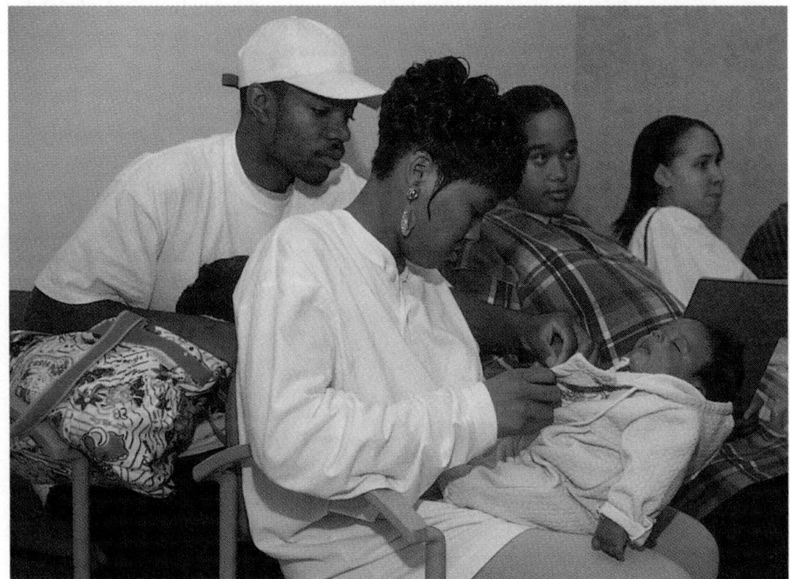

Figure 20–3

Parenting classes can assist parents in understanding their baby's physical, emotional, and developmental needs. Parents are also helped to develop coping skills for parenting as well as being given a realistic picture of being a parent.

Cesarean birth prevention information may be taught in prepared childbirth classes to help parents learn what they can do to try to avoid a cesarean delivery if safely possible. Information about the physiologic approach to birth includes positioning, ambulation, upright expulsion, minimal use of drugs, and avoidance of routine interventions.

Postpartum Classes

Preparation for the birth experience does not end with delivery of the baby, and a number of classes have been developed to meet the needs of parents during the postpartum period.

▼ **Parenting Classes.** Parenting classes include information about the physical and emotional adjustments to the postpartal period, role changes, coping skills, infant growth and development, and newborn care, along with consumer information on the selection of baby furniture and safe toys. The opportunity for group discussion and sharing is particularly helpful to new parents during this transitional time in their lives (Starn 1993). With the increase in mothers working outside the home, classes for working parents have become an important addition to parenting courses. These classes offer information about balancing the multiple role demands of parenthood, family, and career. Daycare options for the infant are also explored (Shapiro 1993).

▼ **Postpartum Exercise Classes.** Postpartum exercise classes focus on physical fitness for the new mother and a return to her prepregnancy physical state. The exercise program is designed to include stretching, muscle strengthening, and aerobic exercises that are safe during the postpartum period.

▼ **Infant Care Classes.** Infant care classes are offered during both the antepartum and postpartum periods. There is no consistent evidence de-fining the best time to teach infant care skills (Bliss-Holtz 1988). Infant care classes usually cover the normal characteristics of the newborn, bathing and hygiene, infant feeding, first aid and safety, signs of illness, and when to call the doctor. These classes may also include demonstrations with an actual newborn, video tapes, and cardiopulmonary resuscitation (CPR). Infant care classes vary in length from one session to a program several weeks in length (Fig. 20–3).

Outreach Classes

Many perinatal educators have become concerned because the courses offered are not accessible to or affordable by all parents. Classes are generally attended by middle to upper middle class parents in their 20s or 30s who are married or in a committed relationship. Thus, a large segment of the pregnant population is not being served by the traditional perinatal course offerings. As a result, childbirth educators have begun to develop perinatal classes for hard-to-reach groups (see Chapter 39).

▼ **Teen Pregnancy Classes.** Teen pregnancy classes include the same pregnancy and childbirth course material from a developmental perspective but approach the information in a format that is more appropriate for and meaningful to teens. Teenagers are encouraged and reinforced to adopt healthy lifestyle changes during pregnancy when they are with their peers, and can feel more comfortable in sharing their feelings and asking questions. School-based teen pregnancy and parenting classes can be effective in providing teenagers with the immediate information they need related to pregnancy and parenting as well as encouraging them to remain in school and graduate (Podgurski 1993).

▼ **Homeless Shelter Classes.** Women in homeless shelters present unique challenges to the perinatal educator. Many of the women are transient, are at different stages of pregnancy, may have difficulties such as substance abuse and nutritional problems, and lack the skills required to be a good parent. Teaching childbirth classes in shelters requires a motivated, resourceful, and flexible perinatal educator because of constantly changing populations and limited resources. However, childbirth education classes can have a powerful and positive effect on improving the health of women in shelters and their childbirth experiences (O'Connell 1993), which may lead to improved infant outcomes and parenting skills.

▼ **Other Outreach Classes.** Classes for handicapped individuals are being developed in some areas to meet the unique needs of physically or mentally handicapped women and their partners during the childbearing year (Rogers 1993). Additional outreach efforts provide perinatal education classes for minority populations, low-income populations, low-literacy populations, refugees, and women experiencing a high-risk pregnancy. These outreach classes contain the basic pregnancy and childbirth information essential in other prepared childbirth classes but are designed to meet the needs of a unique audience (Pitzer and Toussant 1995). Childbirth education for low-income populations has been effective in improving pregnancy outcomes (Jeffers 1993).

Classes for Other Family Members

At the same time that the variety of perinatal course offerings has increased for the pregnant woman and her partner, courses for other family members involved in the pregnancy and birth experience have also developed. This wide variety of classes helps meet the learning needs of all family members involved in a birth and parenting experience.

▼ **Sibling Preparation Classes.** Sibling preparation classes are offered by many hospitals or birthing centers for the brothers and sisters of the expected baby to prepare them for the events of pregnancy, birth, and life with a newborn. Class activities are fast-paced, participatory, and appropriate for the age group. Spero (1993) found that sibling preparation classes eased the transition of children becoming big brothers or sisters.

▼ **Expectant Fathers Classes.** Classes for expectant fathers are offered by some childbirth educators to meet their special needs during the childbearing year. Sometimes the class is taught by an experienced father along with the childbirth educator. These classes provide group support, allow for sharing of feelings and concerns, give fathers an opportunity to practice infant care skills, and offer strategies for coping with lifestyle changes that occur with the birth of the baby.

▼ **Grandparent Classes.** Classes for grandparents are also available in some areas and help grandparents-to-be update their knowledge about childbirth, maternity care, and infant care. These classes often help to improve communication between the expectant parents and their own parents during the childbearing year (Biasella 1993).

PREPARED CHILDBIRTH: A PSYCHOEDUCATIONAL INTERVENTION

A psychoeducational intervention uses educational and psychological strategies to decrease pain, enhance recovery, promote psychological well-being, and increase satisfaction with health care. According to the model, psychoeducational interventions are divided into three content areas: information about events, procedures, sensations, or self-care activities; skills to reduce discomfort and complications; and psychological support to reduce anxieties and enhance coping (Devine and Cook 1986). The psychoeducational model is very helpful in structuring prepared childbirth classes (Fig. 20–4). It provides an effective guide for selecting essential class content from large amounts of information that is available on childbirth. It is impossible to include everything that the educator

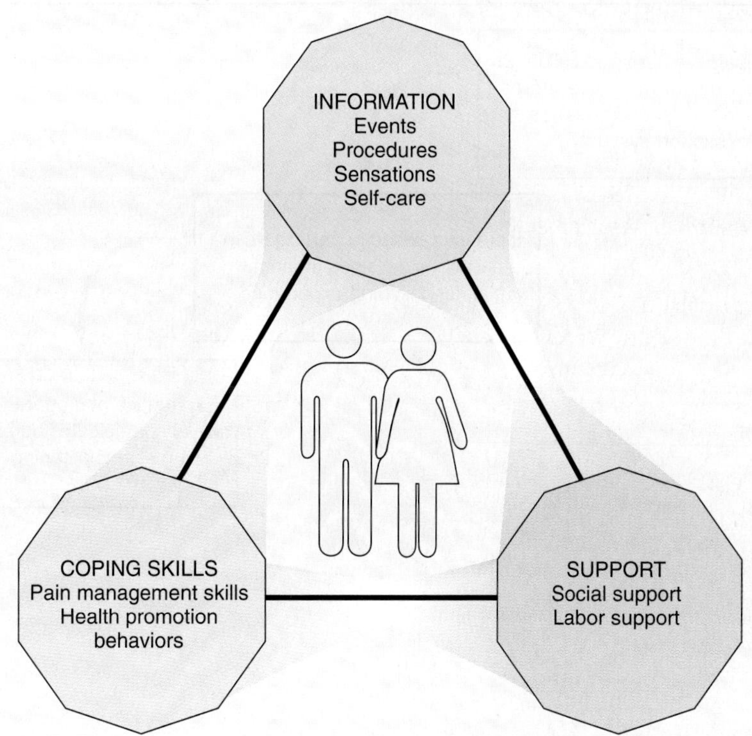

Figure 20–4

The psychoeducational model of prepared childbirth education. Psychoeducational interventions that can be used to decrease pain, enhance recovery, and promote psychological well-being and satisfaction with health care are in three content areas: information about the event, skills to reduce discomfort and complications, and psychological support that reduces anxieties and promotes the individual's ability to cope. (Adapted from Koehn, M. L. [1993]. The psychoeducational model of prepared childbirth. In F. H. Nichols [Ed.]. *Perinatal education. AWHONN's clinical issues in perinatal and women's health nursing* [pp. 66–71]. Philadelphia: J. B. Lippincott.)

would like to teach expectant parents in classes. Using the psychoeducational model, the childbirth educator can prioritize information and skills that should be taught in classes and then organize classes according to essential content. In planning classes, the educator structures classes according to three dimensions: information, skills, and support.

The fundamental belief of prepared childbirth is that childbirth is a normal physiologic process that benefits from support and observation but generally does not require medical intervention. Childbirth should be accomplished in a manner that promotes biological safety and enhances the emotional and spiritual aspects inherent in birth. Pregnancy, childbirth, and early parenting are significant events in the lives of those who experience them (see Philosophy of Prepared Childbirth). The meaning of childbirth and the goals for the childbirth experience are different for the pregnant woman and her family.

The overall goals of prepared childbirth classes are to increase coping ability for childbirth, decrease complications, and increase childbirth satisfaction. The scientifically documented positive effects of prepared childbirth are primarily psychological in nature: increased satisfaction with

Philosophy of Prepared Childbirth

- Birth is normal, natural, and healthy
- The experience of birth profoundly affects women and their families
- Women's confidence and ability to give birth is either enhanced or diminished by the care provider and place of birth
- Women have the right to give birth free from routine medical intervention
- Birth can safely take place in birth centers and homes
- Childbirth education empowers women to make informed choices in health care, to assume responsibility for their health, and to trust their inner wisdom

From American Society for Psychoprophylaxis in Obstetrics, Inc. (ASPO/Lamaze). (1994). *Philosophy of birth.* Washington, DC: Author.

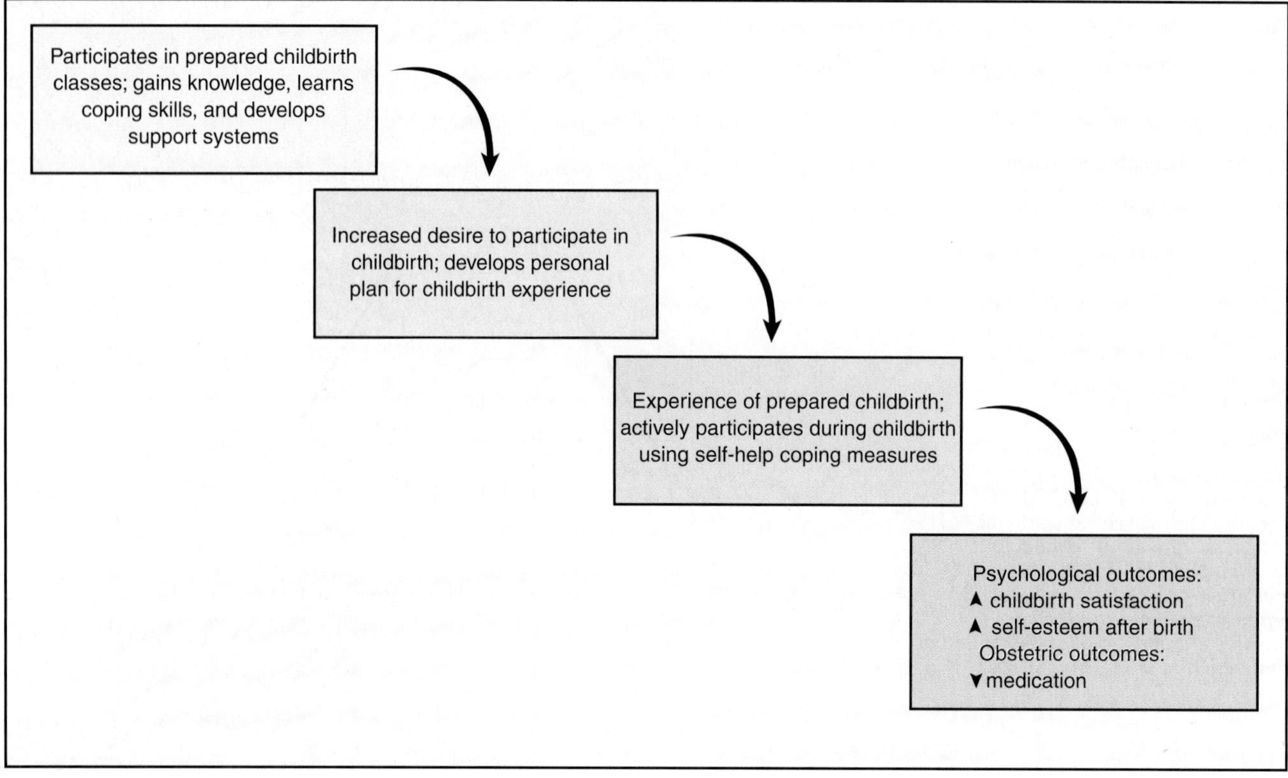

Figure 20–5

The effects of prepared childbirth. (Adapted from Nichols, F. H. [1992b]. The psychological effects of prepared childbirth on single adolescent mothers. *Journal of Perinatal Education,* 1 [1], 41–49.)

the childbirth experience and increased self-esteem after birth. The one consistently documented obstetric effect of prepared childbirth is decreased use of medication (Nichols 1992b) (Fig. 20–5). Although not documented for childbirth education, the health education and lifestyle change information have the potential to decrease the number of obstetric complications.

COMPONENTS OF PREPARED CHILDBIRTH CLASSES

There are three components of Lamaze prepared childbirth classes: information, coping skills, and support.

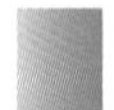

Information

Parents want to know what will happen to them during their childbirth experience. Some topics are of common interest to both expectant parents, but women and men are often interested in different topics, so an individualized approach is important (Moore and Billings 1993). Parents ask "What should I expect?," "How will I feel?," and "What should I do?" (Koehn 1992).

The curriculum should be balanced and ideally should cover cognitive and affective information as well as fears and feelings relating to the birth process. Consumer advocacy, values clarification, and informed decision making should also be included. The content has been established by ASPO/Lamaze (see Content for Prepared Childbirth Classes).

Coping Skills

The second component of prepared childbirth classes is the teaching of skills that the pregnant woman can use to cope more effectively during childbirth. These include relaxation techniques such as progressive relaxation, imagery, and other strategies that enhance relaxation (e.g., massage and music); breathing strategies; positioning; and physical conditioning exercises. The use of nonpharmaceutical pain management techniques during childbirth is also discussed in Chapter 24.

RELAXATION TECHNIQUES

Relaxation is the foundation for all pain management techniques in Lamaze prepared childbirth. A variety of relaxation techniques are taught, including progressive relaxation, neuromuscular dissociation, autogenic training, biofeedback, therapeutic touch, massage and acupressure, imagery, music, water therapy, and controlled breathing using paced breathing strategies.

Relaxation is a learned skill, and practice is essential to successful skill development. The nurse should emphasize to the pregnant woman the importance of practice sessions and the importance of evaluation and feedback from the instructor or partner (Fig. 20–6).

BREATHING STRATEGIES

Early childbirth theorists advocated various breathing patterns, either the slow abdominal breathing of the Dick-Read and Bradley methods or the more rapid and structured breathing patterns advocated by Lamaze in the early years. There was little agreement about which breathing strategies were the best, and information regarding the effectiveness of various strategies was sup-

Content for Prepared Childbirth Classes

Theory of the Lamaze method

Anatomy and physiology as they relate to

- Pregnancy
- Labor and birth
- The postpartum period (the mother)
- The newborn

Emotional responses of expectant parents to

- Pregnancy experience
- Childbirth experience
- Early parenting experience (include role changes)

Physical conditioning for childbirth

- Prenatal exercises
- Posture/body mechanics
- Guidelines for exercises

Stages and phases of labor

- Overview
- First stage
    - Latent phase
    - Active phase
    - Transition phase
- Second stage
- Third stage
- Woman's physical responses
- Woman's emotional responses
- Coach's role

Nonpharmacologic analgesia

- Progressive relaxation
- Touch relaxation
- Imagery
- Focusing techniques
- Effleurage
- Massage
- Comfort measures (back rub, positioning, and the like)
- Support (role of the coach, birthing agency staff, and physician or midwife)

Pharmacologic analgesia and anesthesia

- Types used (describe and explain)
- How and when administered
- Effects on expectant mother and baby

Breathing techniques

- Respiratory theory and principles
- Respiratory techniques
    - Slow paced
    - Modified paced
    - Patterned paced
- Second stage expulsion
    - Physiologic technique
    - Modified valsalval technique

Birthing process

- Vaginal birth

Continued on following page

Content for Prepared Childbirth Classes Continued

Birthing process (Cont'd)

- Cesarean birth
    - Indications
    - Procedures
    - Use of prepared childbirth techniques
    - Coach's role
- Precipitous birth

Variations in labor and birth

- Back labor
- Amniotomy
- Fetal monitoring
    - External
    - Internal
- Induction and augmentation
- Forceps and vacuum extraction
- Episiotomy (use of perineal massage)

Birthing agency procedures

- Admission
- Labor and birth
- Postpartum care (mother and baby)
- Parent-infant interaction

Provision for other content

- Nutrition
- Infant feeding (breast or bottle)
- Signs of premature labor (prevention of prematurity)
- Grieving and loss in unexpected outcomes
- Postpartum "blues"
- Family planning (contraception)

Consumer advocacy (integrated throughout classes)

- A balanced viewpoint (positive and negative aspects) of procedures is presented.
    - Regarding pregnancy
    - Regarding childbirth
    - Regarding parenting
- Family-centered options are presented.
- Alternatives to "standard" or "routine" practices that are inconsistent with the philosophy of family-centered maternity care and a physiologic approach to childbirth are explored.
- The development of effective communication skills is promoted between
    - Pregnant woman and her labor partner
    - Pregnant woman and her obstetric care provider
- Realistic expectations and birth plans are promoted.
- Information and guidelines are provided so that expectant parents can make informed decisions.

From Guidelines for Developing a Teaching Plan. (1987). *ASPO/Lamaze teacher certification program for childbirth educators.* Washington, DC: American Society for Psychoprophylaxis in Obstetrics.

ported by clinical experience rather than scientific data.

Paced Breathing Strategies

In 1983, ASPO/Lamaze held a symposium of leading experts in the field of childbirth education in which the scientific data on respiratory effects on pain control were reviewed and analyzed. The terminology for prepared childbirth breathing strategies was revised so that it was consistent with the scientific literature; *paced breathing* was chosen as the term most appropriate for all childbirth breathing strategies. Paced breathing describes the type of breathing used in studies on response to stress, attempts to relieve pain, and the role of respiration and responses of the autonomic nervous system (Rose and Hilbers 1988). There are four components to paced breathing.

▼ **Cleansing Breath.** The cleansing breath is an effortless, relaxed breath to a comfortable depth, similar to a sigh. During labor, a cleansing breath should be taken at the beginning and end of each contraction. During the second stage, two or more cleansing breaths are taken at the beginning of a contraction and one at the end of every contraction. The cleansing breath serves to ventilate the woman's lungs, enhancing oxygenation and serving as a signal for relaxation. Taking two or more cleansing breaths at the beginning of a contraction ensures that the woman uses her en-

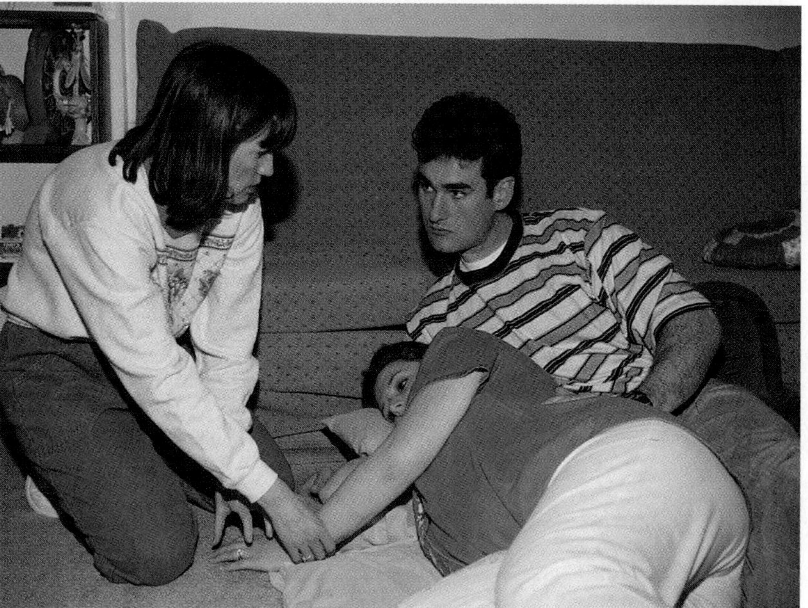

Figure 20–6
A childbirth educator works with a couple during relaxation practice in Lamaze class. Relaxation is the foundation of all childbirth preparation skills. The expectant woman needs feedback on her state of relaxation as well as on how to achieve an even higher degree of relaxation. Here, her partner is assisted in checking her state of relaxation.

ergy most efficiently with the contraction and that pushing is most effective.

▼ **Slow-Paced Breathing.** This is a slow, rhythmic, repetitive breathing pattern. The slowest rate should be no less than one half the woman's normal respiratory rate. The woman's comfort is more important than the style of breathing. She can breathe in nose/out mouth, in mouth/out mouth, or in mouth/out nose. The goal is relaxation, so lips and face should be relaxed (see Paced Breathing Strategies).

▼ **Modified-Paced Breathing.** Modified-paced breathing is done at a slightly faster rate than slow-paced breathing. The rate should be no greater than twice the woman's normal respiratory rate. She can breathe in nose/out mouth, in mouth/out mouth, or in mouth/out nose. Modified-paced breathing should be used when slow-paced breathing is not enough to help the woman relax during a contraction.

▼ **Patterned-Paced Breathing.** Pattern-paced breathing is a variation of modified-paced breathing. Soft blows are interspersed between breaths to create a pattern. Patterned-paced breathing can be done in any manner that is comfortable for the woman, but most women find that in mouth/out mouth is the easiest. Patterned-paced breathing is used during transition or a period of intense discomfort to maintain control.

Purpose of Paced Breathing Strategies

The purpose of paced breathing strategies during childbirth is to increase physical and mental relaxation, provide a means of attention focusing and concentration to decrease the perception of pain, and decrease ineffective responses to pain and stress. Paced breathing strategies should be carried out using the following principles:

- A slow rate of breathing should be used for all patterns
- The slowest breathing pattern should be one half the woman's normal rate of respirations
- The fastest breathing pattern should be no more than twice the woman's normal rate of breathing
- The woman should always use the slowest breathing pattern that supports relaxation and decreases pain during labor
- The woman should breathe in a manner, through either the nose or mouth, that is most comfortable for her

Breathing for Birth

Two types of breathing patterns are taught for birth: the modified Valsalva maneuver and controlled exhalation pushing. The woman should learn both patterns and then choose the one she can do most effectively.

▼ **Modified Valsalva Maneuver.** Using the modified Valsalva maneuver or short breath-holding breathing for second-stage pushing, the woman takes two or more cleansing breaths, then takes a breath and holds it for a maximum of 5 to 6 seconds. She should then blow her breath out, catch another breath while maintaining pressure in the lower abdominal muscles, and continue to push for another 5 to 6 seconds, repeating the pro-

Paced Breathing Strategies

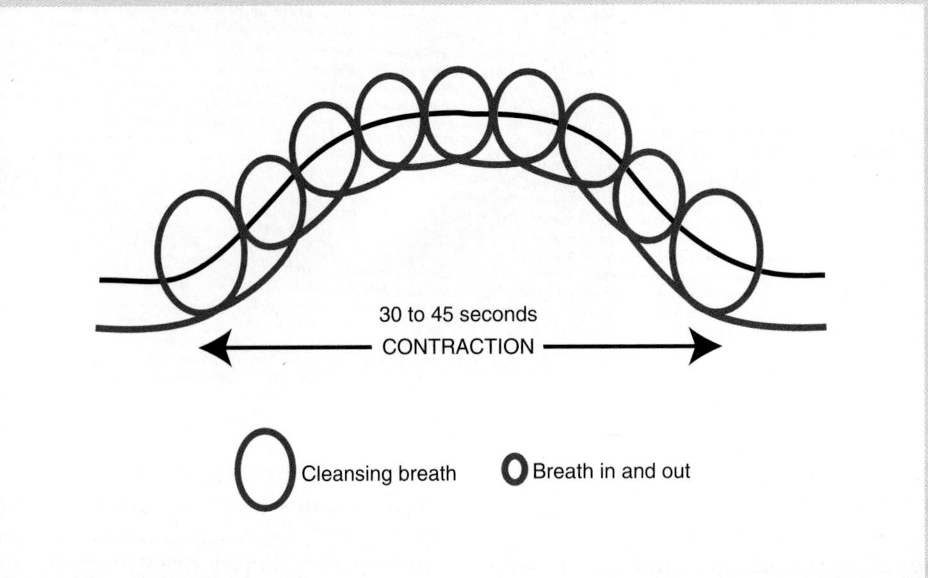

SLOW-PACED BREATHING

Slow-paced breathing has a relaxing and calming effect and conserves energy. This technique should be started when relaxation and diversion are no longer effective in keeping the woman comfortable. The technique can be used throughout labor as long as it is effective in helping the woman cope with pain.

Instruct the woman to

- Assume a comfortable, relaxed position when contraction begins
- Take a cleansing breath (1) and focus on relaxing the body
- Concentrate on a focal point (either visual or internal)
- Breathe in and out in a slow, comfortable, relaxed, rhythmic manner
- Breathe at a rate of **one half normal respiratory rate** (approximately 6 to 9 breaths per minute) (2)
- Use the breathing style that is most comfortable for her (breathing through nose or mouth)
- Take a cleansing breath and concentrate on totally relaxing the body when the contraction ends

1. A cleansing breath is a comfortable, full, relaxed breath—in through the nose and out through the mouth. It is a signal for the individual to relax.
2. Count the woman's normal respiratory rate for 1 full minute during a period when she is relaxed and divide by two.

Continued on facing page

cedure for the length of the contraction. She should take a cleansing breath at the end of each contraction. It is important that the length of time a woman holds her breath while she pushes be limited to 5 to 6 seconds because of the detrimental effects that prolonged breath holding can have on the fetus (see Breathing Strategies for Birth).

▼ **Controlled Exhalation Pushing.** The woman takes two or more cleansing breaths as she begins controlled exhalation pushing, also called gentle open glottis or physiologic pushing. She then takes a deep, comfortable breath and pushes as she lets the air escape slowly. Next she catches another breath, maintaining pressure with

Paced Breathing Strategies Continued

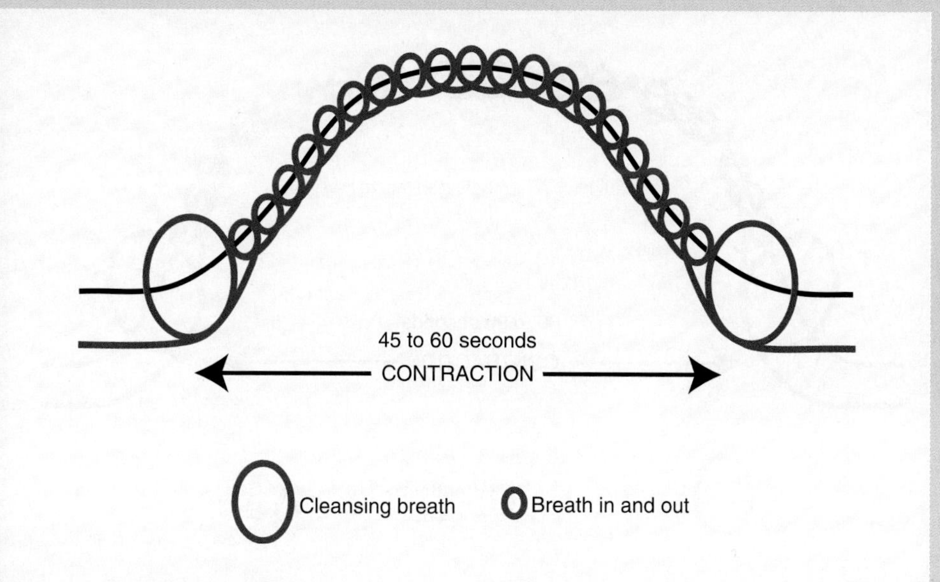

MODIFIED-PACED BREATHING

Modified-paced breathing has an increased rate of breathing. It requires more concentration, thus decreasing the perception of pain from a contraction. Modified-paced breathing should be used when slow breathing is no longer effective. The woman should return to slow-paced breathing when she no longer needs modified-paced breathing.

Instruct the woman to

- Assume a comfortable, relaxed position when contraction begins
- Take a cleansing breath (1) and focus on relaxing the body
- Concentrate on a focal point (visual or internal)
- Breathe in and out in a light, comfortable, relaxed, rhythmic manner
- Use the breathing style that is most comfortable for her (breathing through nose or mouth)
- Increase the breathing rate slowly until she finds a comfortable rate that helps decrease the pain experienced from a contraction
- Breathe at a rate **no more than twice normal respiratory rate** (approximately 24 to 32 breaths per minute) (2)
- Take a cleansing breath and concentrate on totally relaxing the body when the contraction ends

Continued on following page

her abdominal muscles, and repeats the sequence for the length of the contraction. Several studies have found no significant difference in the length of second stage whether open glottis or modified Valsalva maneuver pushing is used (Nelsson-Ryan 1988). These methods of breathing/pushing provide better use of the abdominal muscles and increased pelvic floor relaxation, and prevent the negative effects of the Valsalva maneuver (Fig. 20–7).

PHYSICAL CONDITIONING

Another coping skill taught in prepared childbirth classes is physical conditioning. Physical conditioning exercises help the pregnant woman

Paced Breathing Strategies Continued

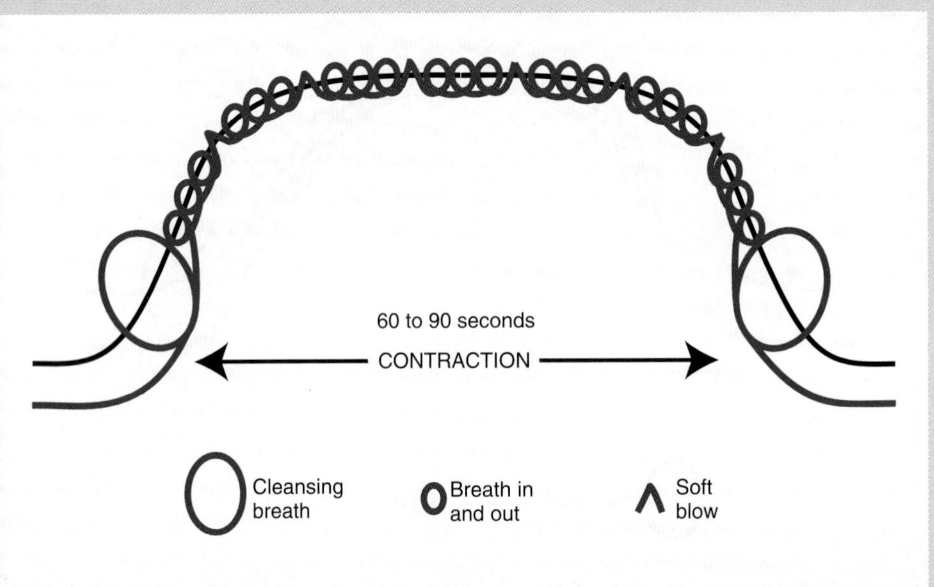

PATTERNED-PACED BREATHING

Patterned-paced breathing is an adaptation of modified-paced breathing. It is done in the same basic manner with the addition of a "soft blow" at regular intervals. A variety of rhythmic patterns can be used to increase concentration and decrease pain during the more difficult periods of labor. The woman should return to a slower breathing pattern when patterned-paced breathing is no longer needed.

Instruct the woman to

- Assume a comfortable, relaxed position when contraction begins
- Take a cleansing breath (1) and focus on relaxing the body
- Concentrate on a focal point (visual or internal)
- Breathe in and out in a light, comfortable, relaxed, rhythmic manner
- Use the breathing style that is most comfortable for her (breathing through nose or mouth)
- Increase the breathing rate slowly until she finds a comfortable rate that helps decrease the pain experienced from a contraction
- Breathe at a rate **no more than twice normal respiratory rate** (approximately 24 to 32 breaths per minute) (2)
- Use a pattern such as three breaths: one soft blow at regular intervals. The rate and volume of air exchange of the breaths and soft blows are the same. There are many other common patterns such as 4:1, 5:1, 6:1
- Use continuous light "blows" to control a premature urge to push
- Keep the face and lips relaxed during the contraction
- Take a cleansing breath and concentrate on totally relaxing the body when the contraction ends

deal with the discomforts of pregnancy and contribute to her overall health and well-being. Although some form of physical conditioning has always been taught in perinatal education, today's rising national interest in fitness motivates pregnant women to seek out exercise programs. Physical conditioning exercise is included in most pregnancy and prepared childbirth classes and may also be offered as a specialty course. When it is offered as a separate course, a great deal of time

Breathing Strategies for Birth

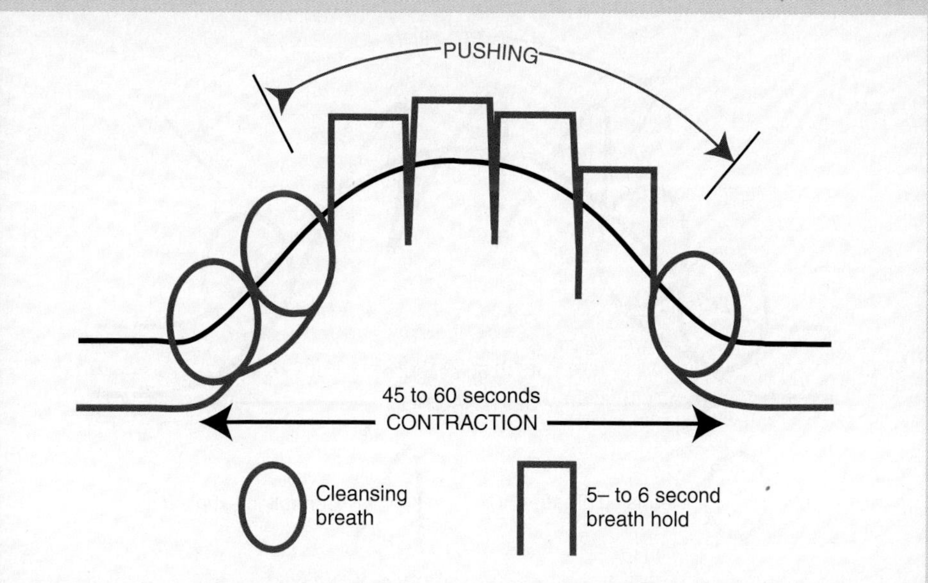

TRADITIONAL PUSHING

(also called "modified Valsalva maneuver," "breath holding," or "closed glottis" pushing)

Instruct the woman to

- Assume an upright, comfortable, relaxed position and maintain pelvic tilt when contraction begins
- Take two cleansing breaths
- Focus on keeping the perineum relaxed and concentrate on directing pushing out the vagina
- Take a comfortable, full breath; hold it, tighten the abdominal muscles, and bear down for no longer than 5 to 6 seconds, keeping the face and perineum relaxed
- When more air is needed, keep the abdominal muscles tightened while breathing out and taking another breath, and then bear down again for 5 to 6 seconds
- Repeat this process until the contraction is over
- Take one cleansing breath and relax when the contraction ends

Continued on following page

can be spent with warm-up and cool-down stretching, moderate aerobic activity, and attention to the nine areas of exercise that are important in pregnancy: pelvic floor contractions; posture reeducation; pelvic tilt; abdominal strengthening; low back and hamstring stretches; neck, shoulder, and upper torso exercises; foot rotation; squatting; and adductor stretches. When exercise is taught as a component of a childbirth course, it is important to include at least the following: pelvic tilt, pelvic floor contractions, posture reeducation, abdominal strengthening, and squatting (see Chapter 19 for additional discussion and guidelines on exercise during pregnancy).

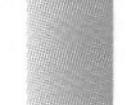

Support

The third dimension of prepared childbirth classes is support. Support has been an integral component of childbirth education since the proponents of prepared childbirth first published works describing their beliefs. The benefits of support are well documented in the literature. Studies have shown that women with a support person require less medication, have shorter labors, and experience a more positive childbirth experience (Klaus et al. 1993). Women should be encouraged to have

Breathing Strategies for Birth Continued

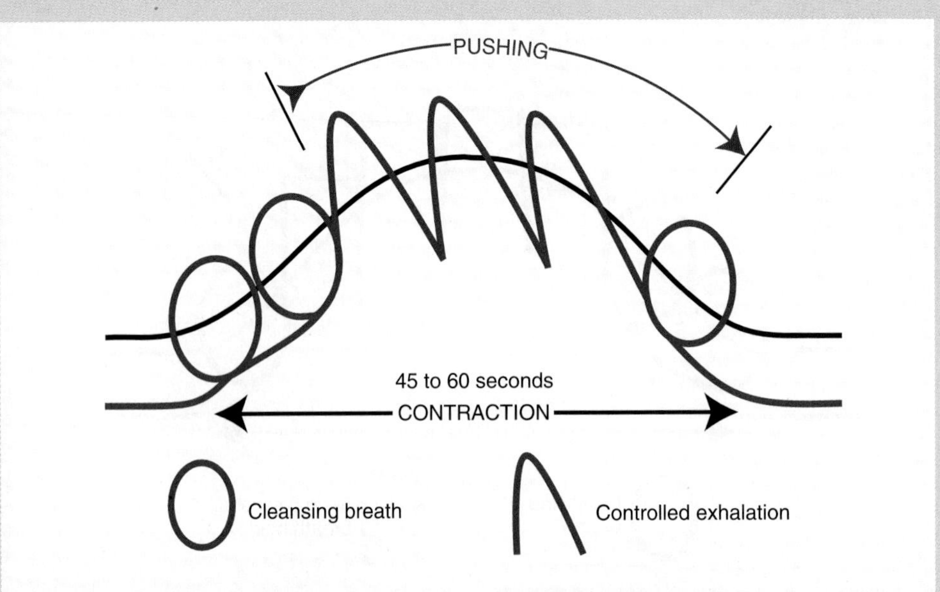

CONTROLLED EXHALATION PUSHING

(also called "physiologic," "open glottis," or "gentle" pushing)

Instruct the woman to

- Assume an upright, comfortable, relaxed position and maintain pelvic tilt when contraction begins
- Take cleansing breaths until she feels the urge to push
- Focus on keeping the perineum relaxed and concentrate on directing pushing out the vagina
- Take a deep breath, tighten the abdominal muscles, and bear down, releasing the breath slowly while continuing to push, keeping the face and perineum relaxed
- When more air is needed, keep the abdominal muscles tightened while taking another breath, and then repeat bearing down while slowly releasing the breath again
- Repeat this process until the contraction is over
- Take as many cleansing breaths as needed and relax when the contraction ends

their support person attend childbirth classes with them as well as being with them during childbirth. However, for support to be most effective, it requires a supportive birth environment and care providers who provide support during the experience.

SOCIAL SUPPORT

Social support is defined as information leading to the belief that one is cared for, loved, esteemed, valued, and part of a network of communication and mutual obligation (Cobb 1976). Supportive relationships during pregnancy have been shown to influence the number of pregnancy complications that occur, the decision to breastfeed, adjustment to parenthood, and parent-infant interaction (Fig. 20–8). By participating in a childbirth class, parents are exposed to a social network of other pregnant people. Involvement in this "subculture of pregnancy" allows expectant parents to compare their experiences with those of others in the same situation. This social reinforcement increases satisfaction with the pregnancy experience (Jones 1988).

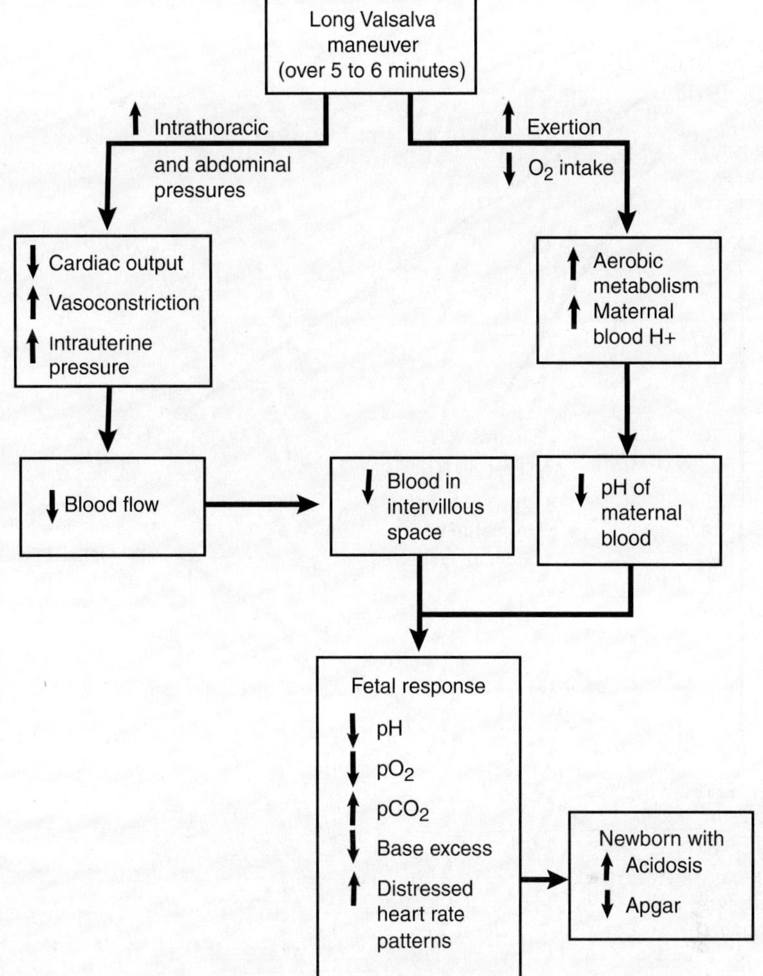

Figure 20–7

Consequences of the Valsalva maneuver. This maneuver causes a high intrathoracic pressure, decreasing venous return to the woman's heart. This in turn causes maternal hypotension, decreased cardiac output, and decreased blood flow to the uterus, which results in fetal hypoxia.

Not only do perinatal classes provide a forum for group social networking and support, they can also teach parents how to anticipate and obtain the support they need during pregnancy, labor, and early parenting and how to strengthen the existing support systems. Fathers and mothers often have different perceptions of what behaviors are supportive during pregnancy and the postpartum period, and these perceptions can be identified and discussed in a prenatal or childbirth class. Encouragement to evaluate the existing support network and to seek other sources of support can balance the woman-partner team emphasis that is usually promoted in perinatal classes (Jones 1988).

LABOR SUPPORT

The supportive role of labor companion is also taught in childbirth classes. This supportive role goes beyond the usual definition of support, including both affective and psychomotor coaching behaviors. The goal of support during labor is to enhance the woman's participation in childbirth and foster activity that enables her to cope more effectively. The labor coach is a caring partner, giving feedback to the woman by visual, verbal, and tactile means; and offering encouragement, reassurance, praise, and reinforcement. Labor partners are taught strategies for helping the laboring woman relax, encouraging her to use the pain management skills she has learned, giving supportive verbal feedback and instruction, and assisting with physical comfort measures.

Another part of the supportive role of the labor companion is assuming the role of her advocate during labor and birth. This role complements the dependency role that the woman may assume during labor. The components of the supportive coaching role are discussed and practiced in childbirth preparation classes. Role playing may be used so

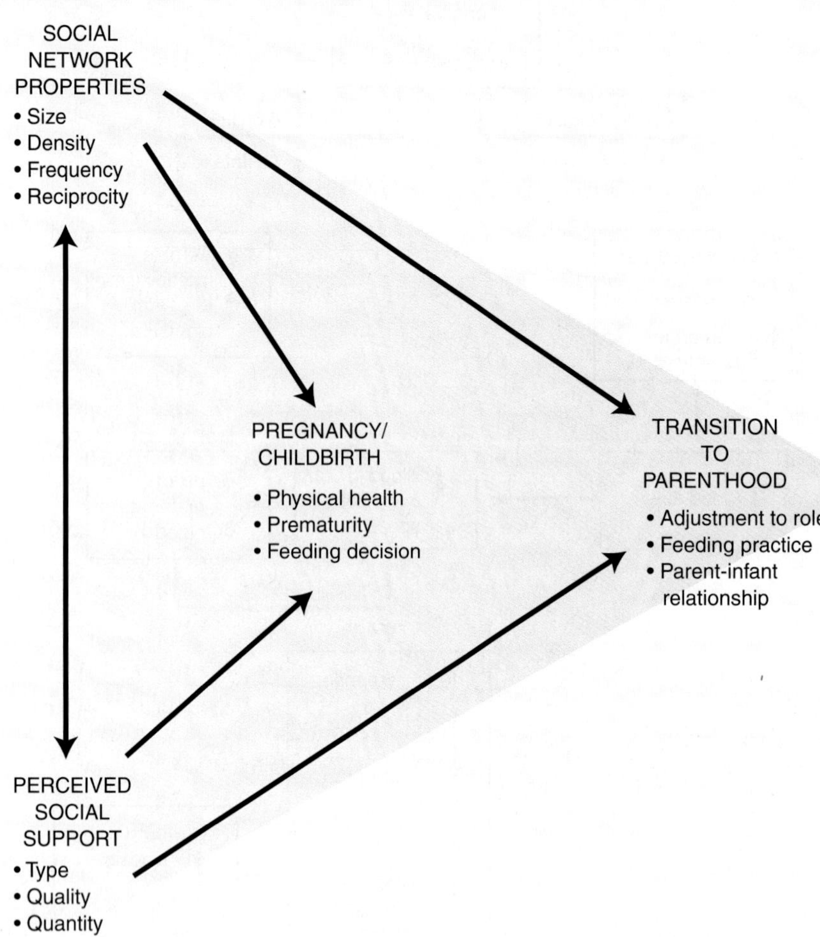

Figure 20–8

Social network and social support variables can influence pregnancy, childbirth, and the transition to parenthood. Supportive relationships from family, friends, and health care providers buffer the effects of stress, increase individual coping ability, and promote increased positive health outcomes. (Adapted from Jones, L. C. [1988]. Support systems. In F. H. Nichols and S. S. Humenick [Eds.]. *Childbirth education: Practice, research, and theory* [pp. 362–373]. Philadelphia: W. B. Saunders.)

that labor coaches can try out their newly learned skills (Butler et al. 1988). Some expectant parents enlist the services of a doula, a woman with special training in labor support, to assist them during labor and birth.

DIMENSIONS AND ISSUES IN PREPARED CHILDBIRTH CLASSES

Five critical dimensions of perinatal education have been identified by ASPO/Lamaze (1992): presenting information, enhancing coping skills, fostering support systems, promoting informed decision making, and incorporating client advocacy. Each one of these major themes must be addressed by the perinatal educator when teaching perinatal education classes. Lothian (1993), in a review of the five critical dimensions, points out:

- Basic knowledge and understanding about pregnancy, birth, infants, and parenting is essential for families, but basic information is often overshadowed by an emphasis on medical tests and interventions and the complications of childbirth.
- Families should be helped to identify their own particular ways of coping, to enhance those skills, and to add to each individual family member's repertoire of coping skills.
- All families should be helped to identify their current support system and what type of support is most valuable to them, and helped to strengthen their support networks of family, friends, and community.

- Perinatal education should help each family to see choices and alternatives and to make informed decisions based on their personal desires and goals; the role of the perinatal educator is to provide an environment that encourages and supports individuals' right to make informed decisions, to facilitate their ability to analyze alternatives, and to help them make appropriate decisions.
- The perinatal educator should inform and support families so that they can make the best possible decision for themselves, and should work within the health care system to ensure that families have alternatives and are able to have the decisions they make become reality.

The three major issues in perinatal education are the new expectations of prospective parents today, the dilemma of consumer advocacy, and the high-risk obstetric climate (Nichols 1993).

Today's Expectant Parents

Most expectant parents who attend perinatal education classes today are different from their counterparts in the 1960s and 1970s. Then, expectant parents attended classes because they wanted a special type of birth experience with a minimum of intervention and medication. They were crusaders and rebels who walked to the beat of a different drum, often in total opposition to the health care establishment. It is in large measure because of the personal investment, commitment, and energies of these expectant parents that perinatal education has achieved its current recognition.

Today, many expectant parents attend childbirth classes because it is the expected thing to do. They often value medication, technology, and instant relief from pain (Nichols 1992a). Also, many of these pregnant women are employed and plan to manage their pregnancy and childbirth in the same way as they would projects at the office. Therefore, today's expectant parents require a different approach in the classroom from that offered to their predecessors. Information must be presented in a manner that motivates them to prepare for childbirth and parenting.

Consumer Advocacy

Promoting consumer advocacy in childbirth classes while also being responsive to the demands of the health care agency sponsoring those classes sometimes creates a dilemma or source of conflict for the perinatal educator. Health care agencies may try to control the curriculum and teaching methods used. Perinatal educators may be asked to present information that conflicts with the promotion of informed decision making in perinatal education classes. They must balance the role of consumer advocate for families against the expectations of the employer, negotiating areas of disagreement.

High-Risk Obstetric Climate

Technology has changed the character of modern obstetrics and childbirth in the hospital setting. The benefits of technology cannot and should not be denied; it has improved the prognosis of high-risk pregnancies and childbirth, making excellent outcomes possible for women who could not have given birth safely in the past. However, the routine use of technology for all women has become the norm in obstetric care today (Wagner 1994) and has influenced what is taught in perinatal education classes. Before high-risk information is taught in classes, the rationale for its inclusion should be identified and considered carefully. A fundamental premise of perinatal education classes is that women should be prepared for a normal, healthy childbirth, and the focus in classes should be on preventive and health promotion strategies rather than high-risk technology.

ROLE OF THE PERINATAL EDUCATOR

The activities of a perinatal educator involve many roles and functions. While the primary role is that of teacher, a perinatal educator is also a counselor, motivator, change agent, and liaison between the lay and professional communities (Nichols 1988a). The multiplicity of roles provide an exciting, challenging, and rewarding vocation.

▼ **Teacher and Counselor.** As a teacher, the perinatal educator takes the responsibility of bringing current, factual information to the expectant parents in her classes. Her or his approach is not that of a stern authoritarian but of a caring facilitator or resource person. As a counselor, the perinatal educator works to establish a therapeutic rapport with each member in the class; creates a warm, supportive atmosphere; identifies problems or concerns that parents may have; and either helps the parents to problem-solve independently or refers them for additional help.

Motivator. Perinatal educators may find themselves being a motivator for expectant parents during the childbearing year. They may use their expertise to stimulate parents to incorporate healthy lifestyle behaviors, such as eating nutritious diets or incorporating exercise into their daily life. They may motivate parents to consider using the least medication possible for birth or to breastfeed the baby. A cautionary fine line must be drawn between this role of motivator and the inappropriate practice of forcing the educator's own biases or beliefs on parents, or making parents feel guilty if their desires differ from the educator's personal beliefs.

Change Agent and Liaison. Perinatal educators are also change agents as they work within the maternity care system to generate new ideas, introduce innovations, develop a climate that will overcome resistance, and implement change. Their goal in these roles is to improve maternity health care services for the expectant woman and her family. As a liaison between expectant parents, who are the consumers, and members of the health care system, who are the providers, the perinatal educator serves as a link between the two, facilitating communication and problem solving.

PROFESSIONAL PREPARATION AND CERTIFICATION

The perinatal educator is responsible for gaining adequate professional preparation and maintaining current knowledge in the area of perinatal education. Health care agencies and consumers increasingly seek well-prepared childbirth educators.

Academic Preparation. A professional education in nursing or an allied health profession serves as the requisite basic preparation. However, additional preparation is also important to teach parents about pregnancy, childbirth, and parenting, and for the educator to learn creative teaching and group process skills. Although this preparation can be accomplished independently through reading or clinical observation, a more effective way to achieve such specialized preparation is to complete a nationally recognized educational program for perinatal educators. Many educational programs may prepare childbirth educators, but the only academic university programs available are accredited by ASPO/Lamaze. Attendance at such a recognized program ensures the quality of the preparation received and provides the opportunity to take the national certification examination for childbirth educators offered by ASPO/Lamaze.

Certification. Certification as a childbirth educator indicates to consumers and health care agencies that the individual has demonstrated competency in that area. Thus, certification can be beneficial to both the childbirth educator and the health care agency. An increasing number of health care agencies are requiring perinatal educators to be certified by a national organization, and such certification is usually required for the educator to receive third-party reimbursement for teaching perinatal education classes (Nichols 1993). ASPO/Lamaze oversees the oldest and largest childbirth educator certification programs. To be eligible to take the ASPO/Lamaze Certification Examination, you must complete an ASPO/Lamaze accredited program or be an experienced childbirth educator with specific academic credentials. To become certified by other organizations such as ICEA, Bradley, or the National Association of the Council of Childbirth Education Specialists (NACES), the appropriate organization's educational program must be completed.

Continuing Education. In addition to formal educational preparation, the professional perinatal educator must maintain current knowledge in the area by seeking out continuing education. Rapid developments in the field of maternal-newborn care and childbirth education make it necessary for a perinatal educator to update knowledge and skills on a regular basis in order to maintain competency. Attendance at conferences, seminars, and continuing education programs keeps skills current. Membership in professional organizations is also helpful to the perinatal educator. Specialty organizations relating to maternal-newborn care or perinatal education provide support and networking and are a source of continued professional growth.

TYPES OF PRACTICE

In past years, most childbirth educators taught independently in their homes or with a community group before prepared childbirth classes became accepted by the medical community. Today the options for practice are numerous and varied; three primary practice patterns have been identified and each has advantages and disadvantages.

Agency Practice. A perinatal educator may be hired by a hospital, health maintenance organization, or other health care agency to teach the classes offered by that agency. This option is advantageous to the perinatal educator who does not want to spend the time to build a private practice. The agency assumes the responsibility for many of the management details of the classes, such as recruitment of expectant couples, registration, purchase of equipment and teaching aids, and bookkeeping.

The disadvantages of this option are those of any salaried position. Disagreement may arise regarding salary, teaching load, hours, or class size. The major disadvantage, however, may be interference from agency or medical staff in the objectives or curriculum for the classes. Sometimes the perinatal educator is told what may or may not be taught and what teaching methods are appropriate. It may also be difficult for the perinatal educator to provide true consumer-oriented advocacy.

However, it is wrong to assume that, because a health care agency sets standards for perinatal education classes, this is a negative aspect. Many perinatal education programs are established and managed by competent certified childbirth educators who have increased the quality of the perinatal education provided by the agency, gaining its approval of standards of content for classes and qualifications for the childbirth educators hired to teach the classes.

Private Practice. Private practice is a second practice pattern and may consist of an individual or partnership. The advantages of this option are the professional independence it affords, the potential for a good income if the practice is successful, and the potential for offering other related perinatal services. Disadvantages include the risk that the practice will not be successful, the required management responsibilities, and the energy and finances necessary to promote the practice in a competitive market.

Contractual Practice. Contracted services have emerged as an alternative for perinatal educators to private or agency practice. The perinatal educator is an independent contractor who may contract services to hospitals, health departments, health maintenance organizations, or physician practice groups that do not have their own established childbirth education program. Educators retain more autonomy than agency employees and at the same time can promote their own philosophy. Independent contractors must maintain records and meet Internal Revenue Service guidelines, and they are responsible for any financial and managerial aspects of their practices.

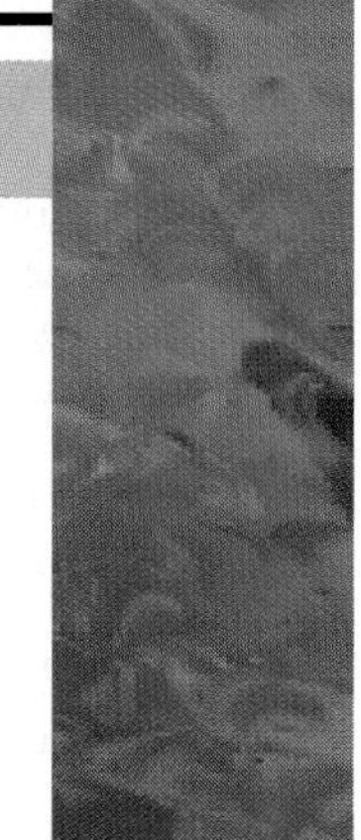

Nursing Practice

Nursing Process

This section describes the use of prepared childbirth techniques during labor and birth.

▼ Assessment

On admission to the labor-delivery unit, in addition to assessing the pregnant woman for the physical, obstetric, and psychological factors related to labor and birth (see Chapter 19), it is of utmost importance that the nurse assess both the woman and her partner's educational preparation for childbirth. This assessment should include evaluation of three areas: the woman's level of preparation for this childbirth, her response to labor contractions and effective use of coping techniques, and her confidence in her own ability to cope with childbirth. Assessment should also determine the knowledge of the labor support role of the woman's labor support companion as well as how that person wishes to be involved during this childbirth.

The following questions should be asked:

- Did the woman attend formal childbirth education classes in preparation for this birth? Did her partner or a labor support person attend classes with her?
- If she attended an educational program for this birth, what type of childbirth education classes were they? How many classes did she attend? Did her labor support companion attend classes too? How many classes? What type of coping techniques does the woman plan to use during labor? How confident does she feel in her ability to use the prepared childbirth techniques she learned in class? What are her plans and goals for this birth? Does she or her partner have any special requests?
- If she did not attend an educational program in preparation for this birth, has she ever attended any type of childbirth classes? Has she read any books about labor and birth? Does she know how to do any of the relaxation and breathing techniques for childbirth? What does her labor support companion, if she has one, know about coping techniques for childbirth? What are the woman's plans and goals for this birth? Does she or her partner have any special requests?

▼ Diagnosis

Nursing diagnoses are based on the data the nurse has gathered and may change as the woman progresses through labor and birth. Potential nursing diagnoses for the laboring woman include

- Knowledge deficit: lack of information related to childbirth and coping techniques for childbirth
- Anxiety related to process of labor and delivery
- Fear related to process of labor and delivery
- Pain related to uterine contractions
- Ineffective individual coping related to lack of knowledge about coping techniques or failure to use coping techniques

Potential nursing diagnoses for the woman's labor support companion include

- Knowledge deficit: lack of information related to childbirth and coping techniques for childbirth
- Anxiety related to ability to support woman during labor

Intervention

Noninvasive prepared childbirth techniques are an integral part of nursing care during labor and birth. The use of these techniques during childbirth is discussed in Chapter 24. Interventions are selected on the basis of the nursing diagnoses for each individual. In general, interventions during childbirth can be categorized in three areas: promoting support and guidance and assisting women to use noninvasive prepared childbirth pain management techniques to cope with labor contractions; providing knowledge about coping techniques as needed; and promoting normal labor through the use of ambulation and positioning.

Support, Guidance, and Assistance. Support, guidance, and assistance in the use of noninvasive pain management techniques to cope with labor contractions and childbirth pain are critical. Noninvasive pain management techniques, relaxation, and paced breathing techniques are the first line of defense in helping the woman cope effectively with the labor contractions and childbirth pain. The prepared woman needs to be reinforced in using the techniques she has learned, and guided to change positions or use other types of breathing strategies or relaxation techniques. Her labor partner will also benefit from the nurse's support and encouragement throughout the process of labor.

The unprepared woman needs to be taught breathing strategies and given concrete feedback by the nurse on how to relax during labor. Her labor partner needs instruction in how he or she can best help the woman cope with contractions, for example, with back rubs or counterpressure.

Information on Childbirth Coping Techniques. Knowledge about childbirth coping techniques should be provided according to individual needs. Accurate assessment of the woman and her labor partner's knowledge is the first step. The nurse can then provide information, demonstrate how to perform certain techniques, give feedback to the expectant woman and her partner, and help the laboring woman make changes as needed.

Promotion of Normal Labor. The use of proper positioning and ambulation is key to promoting a normal labor (see Chapters 23 and 24). Many expectant parents, especially those who are unprepared, do not realize the importance of positioning and ambulation during labor. Even prepared individuals, who know and understand the importance of these two strategies, often agree to stay quietly in bed if they believe this is what is expected of them. Thus, the nurse needs to make sure that the laboring woman uses ambulation and position effectively.

Evaluation

Care can be evaluated in two ways. An immediate evaluation consists of objective information related to a woman's increased ability to cope using prepared childbirth techniques, and her decreased anxiety and fear about childbirth. The effectiveness of care can also be evaluated by ascertaining how satisfied the woman is about her birth experience after childbirth. The nurse plays a pivotal role in determining whether the woman's childbirth experience is positive or negative through astute assessment of individual needs, accurate diagnosis of the nursing problems, and implementation of interventions to resolve these problems. Thus, the nurse's knowledge of prepared childbirth coping techniques, and her ability to apply them effectively with both prepared and unprepared women during childbirth, is essential.

Risk Management

Perinatal educators, just like any professionals, are accountable and liable for their practice. Since their primary function is the provision of information to expectant parents and their families, they should ensure that the information provided is correct and complete and presented in a professional manner. This will be possible if they are well prepared through a strong educational preparation for childbirth educators and have maintained a current knowledge base through continuing education. It is possible that a childbirth educator could be held liable for giving incorrect or incomplete information. When controversial issues are discussed in the classroom, it is wise to present all facets of the issue so that expectant parents can make an informed decision. The use of personal opinions without scientific evidence to support them is inappropriate in the classroom setting.

Confidentiality is also important to risk management. The supportive role of the childbirth educator often encourages the client to share confidential information that might not be known to the health care providers. It is important that educators safeguard the client's right to privacy and protect information of a confidential nature. If they feel that any information they have obtained affects the health care of the woman or her baby, that information should be shared with other health care providers only with the woman's permission.

Implications for Research

Implications for research in the area of perinatal education impinge on three areas: the effectiveness of perinatal education, the learning needs of family members, and the teaching of perinatal education classes. Some specific questions that can be asked include

- What are the obstetric, psychological, and neonatal effects of prepared childbirth classes?
- What are the learning needs of family members related to pregnancy, childbirth, parenting, and role changes within the family?
- What are the most effective teaching strategies for content taught in the different types of perinatal education classes?

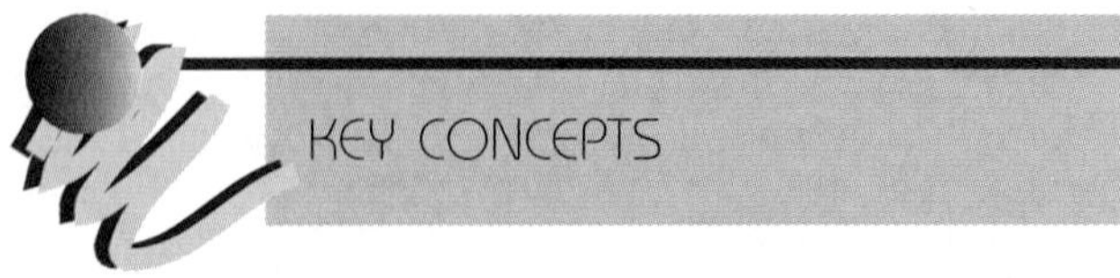

KEY CONCEPTS

- ▼ Perinatal education has grown from a primarily one-to-one approach in the early years to the comprehensive programs of today. Perinatal education is an integral part of maternal-newborn nursing practice and a recognized specialty area with a firmly established scientific basis.
- ▼ In the early 1900s, formal childbirth education emerged as a result of two separate forces with different missions. To meet public health needs and improve the health of women and children, the American Red Cross started childbirth classes in 1908, and the Maternity Center Association in New York City started childbirth classes in 1919. Later, beginning in the 1930s with Dick-Read in England and Velvosky, Platonov, and Nikolayev in Russia, and followed by Lamaze and Bradley, other childbirth education classes developed to prepare women for childbirth and to meet pain management needs.
- ▼ The overall goal of perinatal education is to provide information, coping skills, and support for family members based on individual needs related to childbearing and parenting. Specific goals of perinatal education vary according to the type of perinatal education class and the audience.
- ▼ Perinatal classes can be classified as prenatal classes, prepared childbirth classes, cesarean birth classes, postpartum classes, outreach classes, or classes for other family members.
- ▼ Prenatal classes are primarily informational in their focus, although they may introduce some psychomotor skills such as muscle-toning exercises, relaxation techniques, and breathing strategies.
- ▼ Prepared childbirth classes, in contrast to general prenatal classes, focus on preparing expectant parents for childbirth and the immediate postpartum period. Prepared childbirth classes not only offer cognitive information about the labor and birth experience, but also emphasize the development of the psychomotor skills of relaxation and controlled breathing and the establishment of support systems.
- ▼ For perinatal education programs to be most effective, they should be developed in a planned and systematic manner.
- ▼ The primary role of the perinatal educator is that of teacher, but a perinatal educator is also a counselor, motivator, change agent, and liaison between lay and professional communities.
- ▼ The fundamental belief of prepared childbirth is that childbirth is a normal physiologic process that benefits from support and watchful observation but generally does not require medical intervention.
- ▼ The major goals of prepared childbirth classes are to increase coping ability for childbirth, decrease complications, and increase childbirth satisfaction.
- ▼ The scientifically documented positive effects of prepared childbirth are primarily psychological in nature: increased satisfaction with the childbirth experience and increased self-esteem. The only consistently documented obstetric effect of prepared childbirth is decreased use of medication.
- ▼ The purpose of paced breathing strategies during childbirth is to increase physical and mental relaxation, provide a means of attention focusing and concentration to decrease the perception of pain, and decrease ineffective responses to pain and stress.
- ▼ There are five dimensions of perinatal education identified by ASPO/Lamaze: presenting information, enhancing coping skills, fostering support systems, promoting informed decision making, and incorporating client advocacy.

References

American Society for Psychoprophylaxis in Obstetrics, Inc. (ASPO/Lamaze). (1987). *ASPO/Lamaze teacher certificate program for childbirth educators.* Washington, DC: Author.

American Society for Psychoprophylaxis in Obstetrics, Inc. (ASPO/Lamaze). (1992). *Position paper on perinatal education.* Washington, DC: Author.

American Society for Psychoprophylaxis in Obstetrics, Inc. (ASPO/Lamaze). (1993). *Standards for prepared childbirth classes* (position paper). Washington, DC: Author.

American Society for Psychoprophylaxis in Obstetrics, Inc. (ASPO/Lamaze). (1994). *Philosophy of birth.* Washington, DC: Author.

Andreoli, E., and Moran, B. A. (1994). Lamaze getaway weekend classes. *Journal of Perinatal Education,* 3 (3), 1–6.

AWHONN. (1993). *Competencies and program guidelines for nurse providers of perinatal education.* Washington, DC: Author.

Biasella, S. (1993). A comprehensive perinatal education program. In F. H. Nichols (Ed.). *Perinatal education: AWHONN's clinical issues in perinatal and women's health nursing* (pp. 5–19). Philadelphia: J. B. Lippincott.

Bliss-Holtz, V. J. (1988). Primiparas' prenatal concern for learning infant care. *Nursing Research,* 37, 20–24.

Bowden, J., and Rose, A. T. (1994). Weekend lamaze classes: From hospital to hotel. *Journal of Perinatal Education,* 3 (4), 27–33.

Butler, M., Luther, D., and Frederick, A. (1988). Coaching: The labor companion. In F. H. Nichols and S. S. Humenick (Eds.). *Childbirth education: Practice, research, and theory* (pp. 275–290). Philadelphia: W. B. Saunders.

Cefalo, R. C., and Moos, M. K. (1995). *Preconceptional health promotion: A practical guide* (2nd ed.). St. Louis: C. V. Mosby.

Cobb, S. (1976). Social support as a moderator of life stress. *Psychosomatic Medicine,* 38 (5), 300–314.

Department of Health and Human Services. (1995). Healthy People 2000 midcourse review and 1995 revisions. Washington, DC: Author.

Devine, E., and Cook, T. (1986). Clinical and cost-savings effects of psychoeducational interventions with surgical patients: A meta-analysis. *Research in Nursing and Health,* 9, 89–105.

Enkin, M., Keirse, M. J. N. C., Renfrew, M., Neilson, J. (1995). A guide to effective care in pregnancy and childbirth (2nd ed.). Oxford: Oxford University Press.

Fawcett, J., and Henklein, J. C. (1987). Antenatal education for cesarean birth: Extension of a field test. *Journal of Obstetric, Gynecologic, and Neonatal Nursing,* 16, 61–65.

Flamm, B. L., Goings, J. R., Creed, S., Ancheta, R., Newman, J. (1994). Vaginal birth after cesarean (VBAC) education classes at ten California hospitals. *Journal of Perinatal Education,* 3 (4), 35–38.

Frede, D. J., and Strohbach, M. E. (1992). The state of preconceptional health education. *Journal of Perinatal Education,* 1 (2), 19–26.

Jeffers, D. F. (1993). Outreach childbirth education classes for low-income families: A strategy for program development. In F. H. Nichols (Ed.). *Perinatal education. AWHONN's Clinical Issues in Perinatal and Women's Health Nursing* (pp. 95–101). Philadelphia: J. B. Lippincott.

Johnston, G. P. (1994). *The wish, the wait, the wonder: A book of wisdom for expectant parents.* New York: HarperCollins.

Jones, L. C. (1988). Support systems. In F. H. Nichols and S. S. Humenick (Eds.). *Childbirth education: Practice, research, and theory* (pp. 362–375). Philadelphia: W. B. Saunders.

Klaus, M. H., Kennell, J. H., Klaus, P. H. (1993). *Mothering the mother.* New York: Addison-Wesley.

Koehn, M. L. (1992). Effectiveness of prepared childbirth and childbirth satisfaction. *Journal of Perinatal Education,* 1 (2), 33–43.

Koehn, M. L. (1993). The psychoeducational model of prepared childbirth. In F. H. Nichols (Ed.). *Perinatal education. AWHONN's clinical issues in perinatal and women's health nursing* (pp. 66–71). Philadelphia: J. B. Lippincott.

Lothian, J. A. (1993). Critical dimensions in perinatal education. In F. H. Nichols (Ed.). *Perinatal education. AWHONN's clinical issues in perinatal and women's health nursing* (pp. 20–28). Philadelphia: J. B. Lippincott.

Moore, M. L., and Billings, S. (1993). Learning interests of men and women attending childbirth classes. *Journal of Perinatal Education,* 2 (2), 37–41.

Nelsson-Ryan, S. (1988). Positioning: Second stage labor. In F. H. Nichols and S. S. Humenick (Eds.). *Childbirth education: Practice, research, and theory* (pp. 256–274). Philadelphia: W. B. Saunders.

Nichols, F. H. (1988a). Roles. In F. H. Nichols and S. S. Humenick (Eds.). *Childbirth education: Practice, research, and theory* (pp. 18–33). Philadelphia: W. B. Saunders.

Nichols, F. H. (1988b). The content. In F. H. Nichols and S. S. Humenick (Eds.). *Childbirth education: Practice, research, and theory* (pp. 452–470). Philadelphia: W. B. Saunders.

Nichols, F. H. (1992a). The "give me drugs" generation (editorial). *Journal of Perinatal Education,* 1 (2), iii–iv.

Nichols, F. H. (1992b). The psychological effects of prepared childbirth on single adolescent mothers. *Journal of Perinatal Education,* 1 (1), 41–49.

Nichols, F. H. (1993). Issues in perinatal education. In F. H. Nichols (Ed.). *Perinatal education. AWHONN's clinical issues in perinatal and women's health nursing* (pp. 55–59). Philadelphia: J. B. Lippincott.

Nichols, F. (1990). Pain relief during childbirth. *Lamaze Parents' Magazine,* 60–61.

O'Connell, M. L. (1993). Childbirth education classes in homeless shelters. In F. H. Nichols (Ed.). *Perinatal education. AWHONN's clinical issues in perinatal and women's health nursing* (pp. 102–112). Philadelphia: J. B. Lippincott.

Peterson, K. J., and Peterson, P. L. (1993). Family-centered perinatal education. In F. H. Nichols (Ed.). *Perinatal education. AWHONN's clinical issues in perinatal and women's health nursing* (pp. 1–4). Philadelphia: J. B. Lippincott.

Pitzer, M., and Toussant, K. (1995). Bench clinics: A creative way to present childbirth education. *Journal of Perinatal Education,* 4 (3), 9–16.

Podgurski, M. J. (1993). School-based adolescent pregnancy classes. In F. H. Nichols (Ed.). *Perinatal education. AWHONN's clinical issues in perinatal and women's health nursing* (pp. 80–94). Philadelphia: J. B. Lippincott.

Rogers, J. G. (1993). Perinatal education for women with physical disabilities. In F. H. Nichols (Ed.). *Perinatal education. AWHONN's clinical issues in perinatal and women's health nursing* (pp. 141–146). Philadelphia: J. B. Lippincott.

Rose, A. T., and Hilbers, S. M. (1988). Relaxation: Paced breathing techniques. In F. H. Nichols and S. S. Humenick (Eds.). *Childbirth education: Practice, research, and theory* (pp. 216–233). Philadelphia: W. B. Saunders.

Shapiro, H. R. (1993). Prenatal education in the work place. In F. H. Nichols (Ed.). *Perinatal education. AWHONN's clinical issues in perinatal and women's health nursing* (pp. 113–121). Philadelphia: J. B. Lippincott.

Spero, D. (1993). Sibling preparation classes. In F. H. Nichols (Ed.). *Perinatal education. AWHONN's clinical issues in perinatal and women's health nursing* (pp. 122–132). Philadelphia: J. B. Lippincott.

Starn, J. (1993). Strengthening family systems. In F. H. Nichols (Ed.). *Perinatal education. AWHONN's clinical issues in perinatal and women's health nursing* (pp. 35–43). Philadelphia: J. B. Lippincott.

Wagner, M. (1994). *Pursuing the birth machine: The search for appropriate birth technology.* Camperdown, Australia: ACE Graphics.

21 Chapter

. . . although specialized, intensive perinatal care has been shown to result in improved fetal and neonatal outcomes, it is equally clear that there must be attention to the psychologic as well as physical aspects of care for mothers who are particularly at risk for poor pregnancy outcomes.

JANE M. MURPHY AND DEBORAH ROBBINS (1993)

High-Risk Pregnancy

Mary K. Barger
Elizabeth Fein

HIGHLIGHTS

- What Is Normal and What Is High Risk?
- Conditions Resulting from the Pregnancy Related to Spontaneous Abortion, Incompetent Cervix, Ectopic Pregnancy, Gestational Trophoblastic Diseases, Fetal Death
- Conditions Occurring During the Pregnancy Related to Hyperemesis Gravidarum, Multiple Gestation, Hypertensive Disorders of Pregnancy, Rh Isoimmunization and ABO Incompatibility, Preterm Labor, Trauma, or Surgery
- Procedure 21–1: Assessing Pitting Edema, Deep Tendon Reflexes, and Clonus
- Procedure 21–2: Administration of Rh_0(D) Immune Globulin (RhoGAM or Mic-RhoGAM) and Other Blood Products
- Systemic Diseases Coincident with the Pregnancy Related to Diabetes in Pregnancy, Anemia, Heart Disease, Asthma, Acquired Immunodeficiency Snydrome (AIDS), Perinatal Infections
- Psychosocial Situations Related to Eating Disorders, Battering During Pregnancy, Substance Abuse
- Risk Management
- Implications for Research

When is a pregnancy normal and when is it high risk? The current view of pregnancy and childbirth as a natural process (meaning medically uncomplicated and low risk) is in a sense distinctly different from that which most women have experienced across the continuum of time and place. While pregnancy and birth were natural, the process was not without risks by today's standards. In fact, within living memory, maternal mortality rates (not to mention perinatal mortality rates) were considerably higher than they are now. Today 7.8 women die per 100,000 live births, but in 1935

DEFINITIONS

Disseminated intravascular coagulation (DIC)—A hypocoagulation syndrome resulting from inappropriate activation of the clotting process; the underlying disease process causes intravascular consumption of plasma clotting factors and platelets such that hemorrhage occurs.

Ectopic pregnancy—Implantation of the blastocyst outside the uterine cavity.

Gestational diabetes—Carbohydrate intolerance that is diagnosed during pregnancy and disappears after delivery; can be insulin-dependent (IDDM) or diet-controlled (NIDDM).

Gestational trophoblastic disease—The spectrum of diseases resulting from abnormal proliferation of the placental trophoblast; it includes hydatidiform mole and both metastatic and nonmetastatic trophoblastic neoplasias.

HELLP syndrome—A unique syndrome that appears in some women with preeclampsia; includes intravascular hemolysis, elevated liver enzymes, and low platelets.

Hydatidiform mole—Abnormal development of the placenta in which the fetal part of the pregnancy fails to develop; the chorionic villi of the placenta become a mass of cystlike clear vesicles that hang in clusters, resembling a bunch of grapes.

Hyperemesis gravidarum—Intractable, excessive vomiting during pregnancy.

Hypertensive disorders of pregnancy—Disorders characterized by hypertension and classified as preeclampsia-eclampsia, chronic hypertension, and transient hypertension. Preeclampsia is characterized by hypertension with edema and/or proteinuria; preeclampsia becomes eclampsia in the presence of maternal convulsions; transient hypertension is elevated blood pressure without edema or proteinuria.

Incomplete abortion—Incomplete expulsion of the products of conception; usually occurs after 10 weeks' gestation, when the placenta may be retained after the fetus has been expelled.

Inevitable abortion—The presence of cervical dilatation and/or spontaneous rupture of membranes in addition to vaginal bleeding.

Megaloblastic anemia—A folic acid deficiency that causes a low hematocrit and low hemoglobin; in rare cases, it is due to vitamin B_{12} deficiency.

Peripartum cardiomyopathy—Congestive heart failure with myocardial disease that occurs either late in pregnancy or in the first 5 months postpartum.

Physiologic anemia of pregnancy—A normal decrease in hematocrit, which peaks at 28 to 32 weeks' gestation; caused by a larger proportional increase in blood plasma than in red blood cell mass.

Preterm labor—Labor that begins before 37 completed weeks of gestation.

Spontaneous abortion—The naturally occurring termination of a pregnancy before viability, which is usually defined as either before 20 weeks' gestation or weight less than 500 g.

the rate was 582 per 100,000 live births (Cunningham et al. 1993). In previous centuries the prospects of maternal death, and associated feelings about pregnancy, were quite grim: "Seventeenth century [American] women approached birth not with joy but with dread; some found pregnancy the proper occasion for meditation upon their impending death" (Wertz and Wertz 1977).

Improvements in general health care have enabled large numbers of women who in previous generations might have been too sick, or who might not even have survived long enough, to become pregnant and give birth. This has been true most notably for women with heart disease and diabetes. Medical advances such as improved anesthesia, the availability of blood products, and antibiotics have made giving birth much safer for high-risk women. The advent of new technologies such as ultrasonography and sampling of amniotic fluid and fetal blood has improved fetal surveillance and enabled maternal-newborn health care providers to treat the fetus as well as the mother. With these advances have come new ethical dilemmas, among them how to balance the needs of the mother against the needs of the fetus.

These advances have radically changed basic prenatal management. Women have more options for pregnancy continuation and fetal treatment with improved fetal outcomes. However, there are some costs as well. The challenge for the maternal-newborn nurse is to help women with high-risk pregnancies maintain a human perspective while, at the same time, comprehending the value of the technologic innovations that increase options and improve outcomes.

In high-risk pregnancy there is a high probability of a poor maternal or perinatal outcome because of social, demographic, medical, or obstetric risk factors in the mother (Selwyn 1990; Gabbe et al. 1991). The purpose of classifying pregnancies into low- and high-risk categories is to provide an appropriate level of care for each group and to better allocate health care resources. It also enables better assignment of women to appropriate birth settings, such as out-of-hospital birth centers or regionalized tertiary care centers.

The risk probability is estimated by using a risk assessment tool to attempt to distinguish women who will develop problems from those who will not. Screening tools are variably accurate in predicting which women are at risk. A tool that could correctly classify every women who will develop a significant problem could also falsely label many normal pregnancies as high risk (false positive). Such a tool would not be helpful in allocating health care resources. Most screening tools try to balance the number of false positives with the number of high-risk women incorrectly labeled as low risk (false negatives). Most existing obstetric risk scoring systems do only a moderately good job in predicting which pregnancies are at high risk for poor outcomes (Selwyn 1990). Risk assessment tools may do a better job in assessing multiparas versus nulliparas, particularly for preterm delivery, since nulliparas have no previous pregnancy history on which to score obstetric risk factors.

HIGH-RISK CONDITIONS RESULTING FROM THE PREGNANCY

Spontaneous Abortion

Spontaneous abortion or miscarriage is defined as a naturally occurring termination of the pregnancy before the fetus is viable (capable of extrauterine life)(Moore et al. 1992). Traditionally, viability has been defined as 20 weeks of gestation or 500 g. As technology has become increasingly successful in saving lower weight fetuses, some weighing slightly under 500 g, the line between viable and nonviable has become less certain. Clinical and ethical dilemmas for parents and health care providers are the result.

The incidence of spontaneous abortion is about 15 percent of all recognized pregnancies; however, another 30 percent of women abort very early, unaware that they were pregnant (Moore et al. 1992). Thus, an overall early spontaneous abortion rate is thought to reach 45 percent (Rubin and Farber 1988). There are two basic causes of spontaneous abortion: (1) abnormal development of the fetus with subsequent maternal rejection and (2) poor implantation of the blastocyst with subsequent failure of the trophoblast to support the growing embryo. First-trimester losses are usually a result of abnormal chromosomes in the sperm or the egg. Second-trimester losses can be attributed to either maternal or fetal causes (Mueller 1991) (see Etiology of Spontaneous Abortion). There are four types of spontaneous abortion: threatened, inevitable, missed, and habitual (Fig. 21–1). The management of each type can be quite different.

THREATENED ABORTION

Threatened abortion is the occurrence of any vaginal bleeding or spotting before 20 weeks' gestation. The bleeding is characteristically slight and may vary in color from dark brown to bright red.

Etiology of Spontaneous Abortion

CAUSES OF FIRST-TRIMESTER LOSSES

Chromosomal abnormalities (50–60%)

- Autosomal trisomy
- Polyploidy
- Autosomal monosomy
- Monosomal x

Structural abnormalities

- Translocation
- Structural defects

CAUSES OF SECOND-TRIMESTER LOSSES

- Cervical incompetence (from DES exposure)
- Uterine abnormalities
- Systemic maternal diseases—infections
- Chromosomes (30%)
- Placental abruption
- Exposure to teratogens

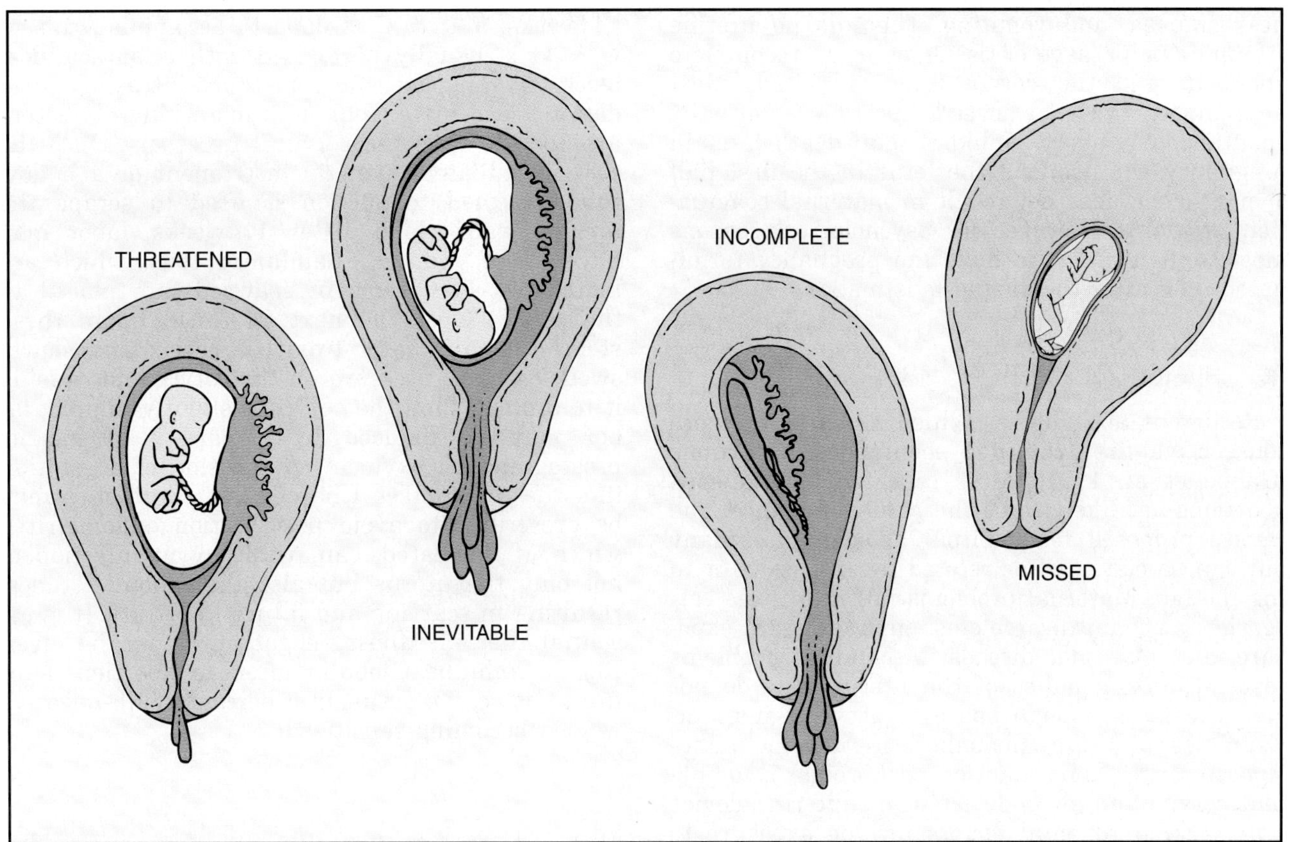

Figure 21–1
Maternal-newborn nurses need to be aware of four types of spontaneous abortion: threatened, inevitable, incomplete, and missed.

The bleeding can occur over days or weeks and may or may not be accompanied by cramping pain or low backache. There is no passage of tissue and the cervical os remains closed. Since 20 to 25 percent of women experience some kind of spotting in the first half of pregnancy, threatened abortion is a common diagnosis. Only one half of these women actually abort the pregnancy. If fetal life has been documented by ultrasonography during the first trimester, 90 percent of these pregnancies continue. Another common type of spotting early in pregnancy is implantation spotting, which occurs at about the time of the first missed period when the blastocyst attaches to the endometrium.

INEVITABLE ABORTION

Inevitable abortion occurs with the gross rupture of membranes and the presence of cervical dilatation. Bleeding and uterine cramping are moderate. These events usually result in uterine contractions and expulsion of the products of conception or the development of uterine infection. The expulsion of the products of conception is further defined as a complete or incomplete abortion.

COMPLETE ABORTION

Complete abortion is defined as the cessation of pain and bleeding after the entire conceptus has been passed. Before 10 weeks' gestation, the fetus and placenta are expelled together, usually resulting in complete emptying of the uterus. After 10 weeks' gestation, the placenta may be partially or completely retained. If it is retained, further bleeding may occur at some point, indicating an incomplete abortion. Action such as dilatation and curettage (D & C) must be taken to evacuate the uterus completely, since either profuse bleeding or uterine infection can result from retained placental fragments.

MISSED ABORTION

A missed abortion occurs when the conceptus dies but is not aborted before 20 weeks' gestation. There is no clear understanding of why some pregnancies with nonviable fetuses continue. Typically, there is no increase in fundal height and fetal heart tones are absent. The woman continues to be amenorrheic but notes a regression of symptoms of pregnancy, such as loss of breast tenderness, nausea, and vomiting. There is no uterine cramping or passage of tissue, as in an incomplete abortion, and the cervix remains closed. Most pregnancies with a missed abortion eventually spontaneously abort. Unlike a fetal death later in pregnancy, the death of the fetus in the first half of pregnancy does not result in maternal coagulation problems. However, for psychological reasons most women prefer to have the pregnancy terminated soon after the diagnosis is made.

RECURRENT OR HABITUAL ABORTION

Recurrent abortion is defined as three or more consecutive first-trimester spontaneous abortions (Gabbe et al. 1991). Most repeated spontaneous abortions are likely to be the result of chance. The causes proposed for habitual abortion are many but can be classified as related to the zygote or to the mother. Maternal problems fall into three categories: mechanical problems, environmental exposure, and maternal disease. Mechanical problems result from anomalies of the uterus that do not give the fetus enough space to grow or implant. Examples of these anomalies are uterine adhesions, uterine abnormalities or fibroids, incompetent cervix, and an undetected intrauterine device (IUD). Environmental factors include exposure to infectious agents such as Listeria or Ureaplasma, which cause chronic uterine infection, or chemicals such as anesthetic gases, lead, arsenic, benzene, and formaldehyde. Tobacco and alcohol use can also contribute to abortion. The most commonly diagnosed maternal endocrine problem is a menstrual luteal phase defect with a progesterone deficiency. In this case, the corpus luteum is not maintained until the placenta is able to take over the role of progesterone production, resulting in a pregnancy loss. Other endocrine problems affecting successful pregnancy outcomes are thyroid disorders and diabetes. Maternal autoimmune diseases, the presence of lupus anticoagulant, and anticardiolipin antibodies are also associated with pregnancy loss. Among women who suffer spontaneous abortions, 40 to 50 percent of those who have had no previous live birth eventually have a successful pregnancy, as do 70 percent of women who have previously delivered one live infant.

MANAGEMENT

A woman experiencing symptoms of a threatened abortion should be placed on bed rest and given sedation if necessary. When a complete abortion takes place, usually no further intervention is necessary if the uterine contractions are strong enough to prevent hemorrhage and no signs of infection are present. A woman with an inevitable or incomplete abortion needs to have all products of conception removed to avoid infection. Before 14 weeks, a D & C is done to accomplish this. A D & C is usually performed with a paracervical block for analgesia and sometimes intravenous sedation. Firm metal rods with increasing diameters are used to open the cervix if necessary. Once the cervix is dilated, a metal instrument or a hollow tube attached to suction is used to scrape the uterine walls clean. After 14 weeks, labor may have to be induced. Laminaria rods, which are matchstick-size stems of seaweed, are placed in the cervix. Over the next 24 to 48 hours these stems take up water from the cervix and slowly swell, exerting pressure on the cervix and causing it to dilate. When the cervix is slightly dilated, labor may be induced by a variety of means: prostaglandins, oxytocin, or infusion of a solution into the uterus (see Chapter 25). Antibiotics may be prescribed to avoid postabortion endometritis, which, if untreated, can result in an infection of not only the uterus but also the fallopian tubes, resulting in scarring and future infertility. It is essential that all Rhesus-negative women be given Rh_0(D) Immune Globulin after an abortion. Failure to do so can result in 5 percent of Rh-negative women becoming sensitized.

Nursing Process

▼ Assessment

A nurse's initial assessment of a woman with a spontaneous abortion is likely to be by telephone. Crucial to nursing assessment is accurate estimation of gestational age. If the woman is unable to provide a known last menstrual period (LMP), the nurse may have to ask other questions to determine gestational age (see Chapter 16). The nurse must inquire about the amount, duration, timing, and character of the bleeding. She should determine whether any products of conception have been expelled and instruct the woman to save any tissue if she does expel it. Other signs that must be assessed are the presence of pain or cramping and infection. The presence of significant pain or signs of hypovolemia such as syncope or confusion requires immediate referral to rule out ectopic pregnancy. Any pregnant woman complaining of bleeding or spotting should be scheduled for an appointment within 24 hours.

When the woman is seen in an ambulatory health care setting, the nurse needs to obtain the above history as well as vital signs. Orthostatic vital signs should be obtained if significant bleeding is suspected from the elicited history. Frequently, the hematocrit is obtained to determine the severity of the woman's bleeding. A urine pregnancy test may be done to identify changes in results.

The woman's emotional status should also be assessed, for she may be grieving at the potential loss of her pregnancy.

Diagnosis

On the basis of an assessment that includes the client's history, physical examination, and laboratory findings, the following diagnoses are suggested:

- Risk for injury related to bleeding or infection
- Pain related to uterine contractions
- Knowledge deficit: lack of information related to the cause of pregnancy loss and the effect of the loss on future childbearing
- Anticipatory grieving related to pregnancy loss

Planning

The plan of care that is chosen for the woman with a spontaneous abortion might include the following outcome goals:

- The woman will demonstrate no signs of infection as evidenced by a normal temperature
- The woman will verbalize decreased pain and increased comfort
- The woman will explain the possible causes of her abortion and its likely effect on her future childbearing
- The woman will verbalize her feelings related to the pregnancy loss

Intervention

All pregnant women in their first trimester should be instructed to call their health care provider if they have any spotting, bleeding, or increased temperature. Any woman who complains of bleeding should be scheduled for an appointment within 24 hours to assess the situation. If threatened abortion is the likely diagnosis, information about activity restriction and signs and symptoms of infection should be given. In addition, the woman should be told to save any expelled tissue and report any worsening of symptoms.

A pregnancy loss, even this early in gestation, can precipitate a grieving process. This response is normal and healthy. The role of the nurse is threefold: to support, facilitate, and educate (Hutti 1988). It is helpful for the nurse to facilitate the grieving process by acknowledging the emotions the client is currently expressing and giving guidelines on what to expect during the grieving process (see p. 636 and Chapter 38 for more extensive discussion). A woman may complete her grieving but have a second episode of grief at the time of the expected delivery of the lost baby. It is important that all office or ambulatory staff be aware of the abortion so that inappropriate remarks about the pregnancy such as "Is the baby moving yet?" can be minimized. One way to accomplish this is to maintain a perinatal loss checklist in the woman's chart so that staff is aware of the loss, the interventions the woman has received, and the ones she still needs.

The nurse's role during a medical procedure to remove the products of conception is twofold: providing support to the mother and assisting the physician with the procedure. The nurse must first ensure that the woman understands the procedure and why she is having it done. The nurse needs to ask the woman to empty her bladder and then provide her with a drape to cover herself after she removes her underwear. A prophylactic antibiotic, usually doxycycline, may be administered at this time, along with a nonsteroidal anti-inflammatory agent to lessen uterine cramping after the procedure. Assistance to the physician requires obtaining the necessary equipment: a speculum; cleansing solution, either iodine or benzalkonium chloride solution; and sterile gloves. A sterile field should be set up with cervical dilators and suction along with a paracervical kit with lidocaine, a syringe, and a long needle with a trumpet.

Once everything is ready, the nurse can assist the woman into the lithotomy position and verbally give her instructions on how to relax. During the procedure the nurse monitors the woman for symptoms of a vasovagal reaction such as diaphoresis, dizziness, visual disturbance, lightheadedness, or syncope. The woman's pulse may be weak and thready and her blood pressure may drop. If the woman experiences a vasovagal reaction, the nurse should be prepared to lower her head and offer her spirits of ammonia. If circulatory or respiratory depression continues, 0.4 to 0.5 mg of atropine sulfate should be given intramuscularly. The use of paracervical block can decrease the incidence of vasovagal reactions. However, the woman should report any symptoms of nausea, dizziness, or tingling of the lips after the onset of the block. These symptoms may be normal but indicate that the nurse should monitor the woman's vital signs to rule out lidocaine toxicity (Lichtman and Papera 1990). Another common response to be prepared for is vomiting, either during or after the procedure. After the procedure the nurse should give the woman adequate time to recover. Her pulse and blood pressure should be monitored if she has any symptoms or if any complications, such as a uterine perforation, were encountered during the procedure. Before the woman is discharged, she should be made aware of signs of possible infection or excessive bleeding, instructed to avoid anything in her vagina for 2 weeks or until her bleeding has stopped, and advised when her follow-up appointment is scheduled.

▼ Evaluation

Evaluation of the nursing care for a woman experiencing a spontaneous abortion is based on the planned goals and outcomes. Her plan of care is successful if she develops no signs of infection, remains comfortable, can verbalize her understanding of the abortion, and is able to express her feelings about her loss.

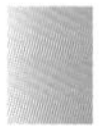

Incompetent Cervix

DESCRIPTION

Incompetent cervix, although somewhat negative in its connotation, is the term used to describe a cervix that begins to dilate in the second or third trimester without uterine contractions. The result of this early dilatation, which occurs in about 0.1 to 1 percent of all pregnancies, is usually a spontaneous abortion. An incompetent cervix may result from trauma, such as a forceful D & C, a previous cone biopsy procedure, cervical cauterization, or a difficult birth, or from anatomic abnormalities, such as a short cervix, abnormal uterus, or decreased collagen in the cervix. It may also be caused by the drug diethylstilbestrol (DES) taken by the woman's own mother during pregnancy. An incompetent cervix is usually suspected when a woman experiences habitual second-trimester abortions. Pelvic examinations show progressive cervical effacement and dilatation along with bulging of the membranes, which present a characteristic hourglass shape. Serial ultrasonography can provide information on the dilatation of the internal cervical os even before dilatation of the external os is apparent.

MANAGEMENT

Management of an incompetent cervix usually begins with bed rest (sometimes in a Trendelenburg position), fluid replacement, no sexual activity (vaginal rest), and tocolysis (inhibition) of uterine contractions. If this management approach is not successful in preventing further dilatation, a cervical cerclage procedure may be performed. This procedure uses either a McDonald cerclage, nonabsorbable ribbon (Mersilene), or a band of homologous fascia to constrict the internal os and prevent dilatation (Fig. 21–2). These cerclages are left in place until term and then removed to allow labor to begin. Because the cerclage is removed, these procedures would be repeated in succeeding pregnancies. Another type of cerclage, the Shirodkar-Barter, is a permanent suture that allows the cervix to remain closed for all pregnancies but requires birth to take place by cesarean delivery. Cerclage is done only if the cervix is not more than 3 cm dilated and the membranes are intact. The procedure is successful in 80 to 90 percent of women and allows them to carry the pregnancy to viability or beyond. Any cerclage procedure should be followed by bed rest and vaginal rest. Because of a risk of cervical infection, the woman should be instructed to watch for signs of infection. Weekly examinations should be done to assess the cervical status.

Nursing Process

▼ Assessment

A thorough history is important in identifying a woman who may be experiencing repeated spontaneous abortions as a result of an incompetent cervix. It is important to assess the woman's emotional status as it is related to repeated pregnancy losses, her understanding of an incompetent cervix, and the nature of her support system.

▼ Diagnosis

The following diagnoses are examples of those that might be appropriate for the woman with an incompetent cervix:

- Anticipatory grieving related to the potential loss of the pregnancy
- Knowledge deficit: lack of understanding related to incompetent cervix and its treatment
- Situational low self-esteem related to inability to carry pregnancy to term

▼ Planning

The goals that are developed in collaboration with the woman might include the following:

- The woman will express her feelings about the potential loss of her pregnancy

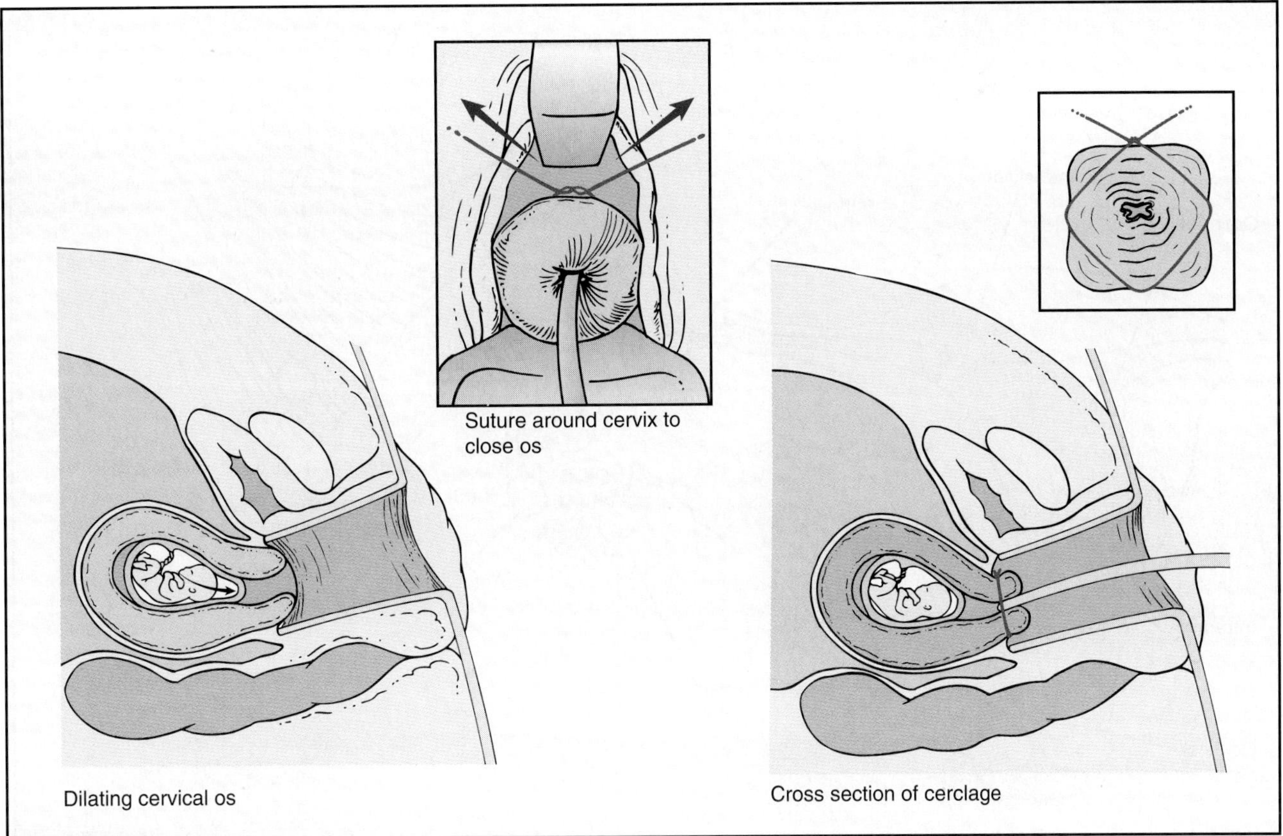

Figure 21–2

Cervical cerclage is a procedure used to prevent dilatation when the cervix is incompetent. (Adapted with permission from Cunningham, F. G., MacDonald, P. C., Gant, N. F., Leveno, K. J., Gilstrap, L. C. III. (1993). *Williams obstetrics* (19th ed.) (p. 674). Norwalk, CT: Appleton & Lange.)

- The woman will verbally explain the diagnosis of incompetent cervix and its expected treatment
- The woman will verbally express her understanding that she is not at fault for a pregnancy loss related to an incompetent cervix

▼ Intervention

Education is an important intervention for the woman experiencing the risk of a pregnancy loss associated with an incompetent cervix. She should be taught about the physiology of the problem, its treatment, and her role in self-care. If she receives a cerclage procedure and is discharged, the woman should be taught the signs and symptoms of infection, rupture of membranes, and preterm labor. Emotional support is also important, for the woman may be experiencing a great deal of anxiety about the potential loss of the pregnancy or grief if she is unable to carry the pregnancy to term.

▼ Evaluation

The plan of care for the woman with an incompetent cervix is evaluated on the basis of her ability to express her feelings, verbalize that she is not responsible, and verbalize her understanding of her medical situation.

Ectopic Pregnancy

DESCRIPTION

An ectopic pregnancy is one in which the blastocyst does not implant within the uterine cavity. The most common site of implantation is the fallopian tube; however, the zygote can implant in numerous places including the abdomen (Fig. 21–3). Ectopic pregnancies occur primarily in only one tube, although cases have been reported of bilateral ectopic pregnancies. Occasionally an ectopic pregnancy can occur with a coexistent intrauterine pregnancy.

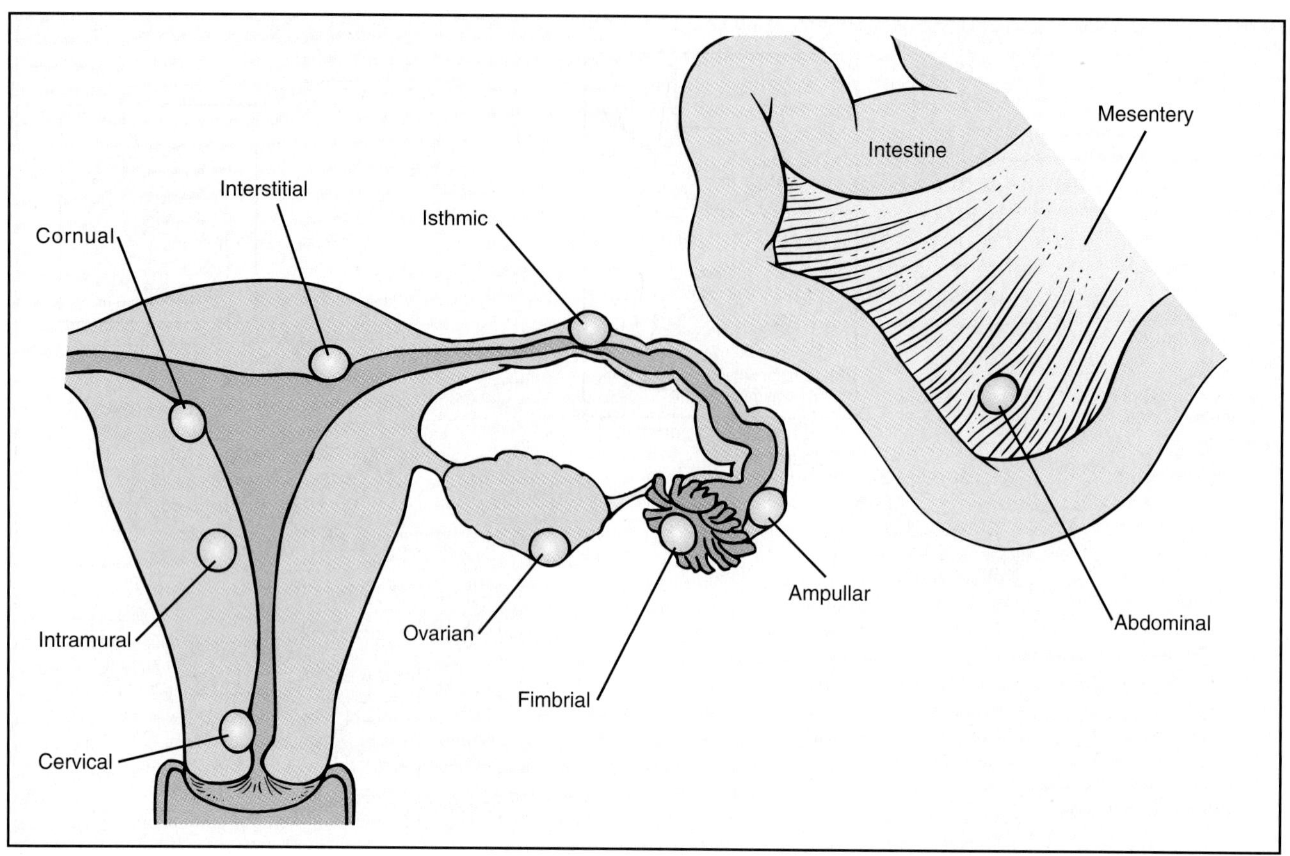

Figure 21–3

An ectopic pregnancy can implant anywhere along the fallopian tube, in the cervix, on the ovary, or in the abdomen.

Ectopic pregnancies have dramatically increased over the last two decades, mirroring the epidemic of sexually transmitted diseases, primarily gonorrhea and chlamydial infection. Currently in the United States, 2 percent of all pregnancies are ectopic. Improved tests for human chorionic gonadotropin (hCG) and surgical techniques have decreased the maternal mortality rate from 3.5 to 0.5 per 1000 ectopic pregnancies. However, ectopic pregnancy is the second leading cause of maternal mortality in the United States, and minority women die as a result of ectopic pregnancies at three times the rate of white women (Moore et al. 1992).

Delayed ovum transport is the primary cause of an ectopic pregnancy. The delay may be due to a tubal abnormality, scarring, or the presence of hormones such as progesterone that slow down transport. The strongest contributing factor to ectopic pregnancy is pelvic inflammatory disease (PID). PID damages the normal ciliary action of the tube and causes scarring, resulting in partial occlusion of the tube. PID can result from a gonorrheal or chlamydial infection, abdominal surgery, or postpartum salpingitis. Another contributing factor is the presence of an IUD. Although there is some evidence that progesterone IUDs have increased the rate of ectopic pregnancies, the apparent increase is due to the fact that IUDs are more effective at preventing intrauterine than extrauterine pregnancies. The use of progestin-only oral contraceptives also increases the risk of an ectopic pregnancy although the risk is still less than for women using no contraceptive method. Combined oral contraceptives exert a protective effect against ectopic pregnancy. Another risk factor for ectopic pregnancy is a history of tubal sterilization. Twelve percent of pregnancies after failure of nonlaparoscopic sterilization and 25 percent after laparoscopic sterilization are ectopic. However, failed sterilization procedures account for less than 2 percent of ectopic pregnancies (Moore et al. 1992). The last important risk factor is the treatment of infertility with medications that induce ovulation or assisted reproductive technologies.

MANAGEMENT

Management of an ectopic pregnancy is dependent on the signs and symptoms, gestational age of the pregnancy, and whether the implantation site remains intact or is ruptured. Early diagnosis improves the prognosis for an ectopic pregnancy. Diagnosis is based on the history, physical examination, pregnancy test, and ultrasonography.

The signs and symptoms of an ectopic pregnancy can vary widely from no symptoms to signs of hemorrhagic shock. Pain is a primary symptom and may vary from sudden and intense to persistent cramping in the lower abdomen, usually unilaterally. The abdominal pain can be so variable that the differential diagnosis includes not only spontaneous abortion, PID, and a uterine pregnancy with a concomitant abdominal problem but also a corpus luteum cyst, appendicitis, and degenerating fibroid. The pain may radiate to the shoulder in the presence of a ruptured ectopic pregnancy. Abdominal tenderness, which is usually unilateral, is also frequently present. Irregular vaginal bleeding after a delayed menses or an abnormally light period is also present in 75 percent of ectopic pregnancies and may be the only sign. Subjective symptoms of pregnancy such as breast tenderness, nausea, urinary frequency, and fatigue may be noted in these cases. Symptoms of syncope and urinary or rectal pressure can be present in the presence of internal bleeding.

Classic physical examination findings in an ectopic pregnancy are a uterus smaller than expected for gestational age with a unilateral, enlarged adnexal mass or cervical motion. Women who have a ruptured ectopic pregnancy have signs of hypovolemia demonstrated by tachycardia and postural hypotension. A rigid abdomen is indicative of peritoneal bleeding. The presence of intraperitoneal bleeding is assessed by performing a culdocentesis. Since the cul-de-sac behind the cervix is the lowest intra-abdominal space, any blood in the abdomen settles there. An 18-gauge needle is introduced through an open speculum and inserted through the posterior vaginal wall, and any fluid present is aspirated into a syringe. The presence of blood can signal a ruptured ectopic pregnancy and the need for rapid treatment.

Laboratory tests now make the diagnosis of ectopic pregnancy much easier and possible earlier in gestation. A serum quantitative pregnancy test and monitoring of beta-hCG levels over 48 hours can confirm the examination findings. In an intrauterine pregnancy, the hCG levels are expected to double over 48 to 72 hours. In an ectopic pregnancy, hCG levels rise more slowly. Adjunct use of ultrasonography, which can reveal the presence of a gestational sac in the uterus as early as 6 to 7 weeks after the LMP, can be helpful in the diagnosis.

The management of an ectopic pregnancy is dependent on signs and symptoms. A primary goal is to preserve the ovary and fallopian tube and maintain future fertility. Early diagnosis permits conservative treatment and preservation of the woman's future fertility. In fact, one study found spontaneous abortion and resorption of the pregnancy in 83 percent of all documented ectopic pregnancies (Carson and Butler 1993). Therefore, early ectopic pregnancies with declining hCG levels may just be observed. Some centers are using methotrexate, a toxic chemotherapeutic agent, on unruptured masses smaller than 4 cm to resorb the trophoblastic tissue of an early ectopic pregnancy (Carson and Butler 1993). This drug causes a medically induced abortion and thereby successfully preserves the fallopian tube. For ectopic pregnancies that are larger, removal of the fetus by laparoscopy or pelviscopy is desirable. If the ectopic pregnancy is tubal or ovarian, excision and repair of the tube or ovary is preferable to removal of the tube or ovary. Abdominal surgery is necessary in the case of a ruptured ectopic pregnancy, an ectopic pregnancy outside the ampulla, or an unstable patient. In the case of an ectopic pregnancy implanted in the cervix, hysterectomy is usually necessary to avoid severe blood loss. Complications of surgery for an ectopic pregnancy include uncontrolled bleeding with subsequent severe blood loss and residual trophoblastic tissue that causes infection or adhesions.

Management of an ectopic pregnancy that has implanted in the abdomen and developed to a significant gestation, an abdominal pregnancy, is different from that of an earlier ectopic pregnancy. An abdominal pregnancy is a rare event (1 in 25,000 births), with almost all cases resulting from a tubal pregnancy that has ruptured into the abdomen (Cunningham et al. 1993). Generally, the placenta remains attached to the oviduct. Perinatal loss in such pregnancies is extremely high, 91 percent, and maternal mortality is around 6 percent (Cunningham et al. 1993). If the pregnancy continues, women are likely to complain of nausea, vomiting, diarrhea, constipation, and abdominal pain. Usually symptoms are not severe enough to warrant extensive investigation. Fetal movements in late pregnancy can cause pain. Abdominal palpation detects a fetus with a transverse or oblique lie. The fetal parts may be easily palpated, but this is not diagnostic of an abdominal pregnancy. A definitive diagnosis can be made by ultrasound examination or abdominal radiography. Delivery is by abdominal surgery. This surgery involves a high risk of massive hemorrhage and all preparations for blood transfusion must be anticipated. There is controversy about the management of the placenta after delivery. Some experts state that it is better to leave the placenta undisturbed and allow it to degenerate spontaneously rather than risk hemorrhage associated with partial removal of a placenta that is implanted over many different organs (Cunningham et al. 1993).

Nursing Process

▼ Assessment

The nurse's accurate assessment of complaints of bleeding and pain in early pregnancy is essential to the successful management of an ectopic pregnancy, especially since it is the nurse who screens the calls of these women. A comprehensive history should be obtained. A history of risk factors such as a previous ectopic pregnancy, PID, infertility or infertility surgery, tubal sterilization, or presence of an IUD should raise the nurse's suspicions of an ectopic pregnancy. Abdominal pain in early pregnancy should be carefully evaluated with directive questioning. The suspicion of an ectopic pregnancy requires immediate referral, unlike that of a threatened abortion, which is less urgent. When a woman of childbearing age presents with a history of abdominal pain and a time since the LMP greater than 4 weeks, vital signs, including orthostatic blood pressure, are important.

▼ Diagnosis

On the basis of an assessment that includes the client's history, physical examination, and laboratory findings, the following diagnoses are suggested:

- Pain related to pregnancy outside the uterus
- Risk for injury related to rupture of ectopic pregnancy and hemorrhage related to placental adherence to tissues or organs
- Knowledge deficit: lack of information related to the causes and treatment of ectopic pregnancy
- Anticipatory grieving related to pregnancy loss and fear for future fertility

▼ Planning

On the basis of the nursing diagnoses formulated from the initial assessment, the nurse might develop the following outcome goals:

- The woman will verbalize decreased pain and demonstrate increased comfort as evidenced by facial expressions and body positioning
- The ectopic pregnancy will be resolved with no resulting injury or hemorrhage
- The woman will explain the causes and treatment of ectopic pregnancy
- The woman will express her feelings about the ectopic pregnancy and her concern for future fertility

▼ Intervention

The primary role of the nurse in dealing with ectopic pregnancy is one of prevention. The nurse is in a position to be the primary educator of women about prevention of sexually transmitted diseases (STDs) and the use of condoms and to encourage women and men with symptoms of an STD to receive prompt treatment. A woman with an early ectopic pregnancy and falling hCG levels who is being treated conservatively must be educated about possible danger signs and the importance of returning for serial hCG tests to ensure that the ectopic pregnancy has totally regressed.

The woman who has an unruptured ectopic pregnancy that requires surgery needs preparation similar to that of a woman undergoing an abortion. However, women undergoing pelviscopy or laparotomy usually have these procedures done under somewhat emergent conditions. The nurse plays an important role in keeping the patient informed about what to anticipate and reinforces any information provided by the physician, since the woman is not likely to recall everything if events are occurring quickly. Preoperative care requires the initiation of an intravenous line usually with at least an 18-gauge angiocatheter in case blood products are needed. Postoperatively, the nurse must be alert to signs of infection and intra-abdominal bleeding. Follow-up beta-hCG levels are essential to confirm that all trophoblastic material was removed.

Women who receive methotrexate therapy must be able to comply with the necessary follow-up evaluations and be knowledgeable about treatment side effects. The nurse can discuss with the woman the fact that she has a 20 percent risk of drug side effects that include mouth ulceration, nausea, abdominal discomfort, and altered liver enzyme values. Three to four days after the start of methotrexate therapy many women have transient pelvic pain for 4 to 12 hours, which signals successful tubal abortion (Carson and Butler 1993). However, women should be informed that it is important to report all abdominal pain, especially if accompanied by dizziness, postural hypotension, or tachycardia, since it may signal a rupturing ectopic pregnancy.

▼ Evaluation

The evaluation of the nursing care of the woman with an ectopic pregnancy is based on the goals and desired outcomes. For example, if the woman has no pain, has experienced no injury or hemorrhage, has demonstrated her knowledge about her medical status, and is able to express her feelings, her plan of care has been successful.

Gestational Trophoblastic Disease

DESCRIPTION

Gestational trophoblastic disease (GTD) is a spectrum of diseases resulting from abnormal proliferation of placental trophoblast. These diseases are hydatidiform moles and gestational trophoblastic neoplasia, which can be nonmetastatic or metastatic. Choriocarcinoma is one of the malignancies, and it commonly metastasizes to the lungs. These diseases can follow a normal pregnancy, a spontaneous abortion, an ectopic pregnancy, or a molar pregnancy. A hydatidiform mole is a pregnancy in which the placenta or trophoblast is abnormally developed. Specifically, the chorionic villi degenerate into a mass of clear vesicles, giving the placenta a characteristic appearance of a bunch of grapes (Fig. 21–4). Molar pregnancies have been further defined as complete or incomplete moles. Complete molar pregnancies are diploid, contain only paternal chromosomes, and have no fetus present. Incomplete moles have triploid chromosomes from either the mother or father and the presence of a fetus, cord, or amniotic sac and some normal villi (Herbst et al. 1992). It is rare for the fetus of a molar pregnancy to survive to delivery.

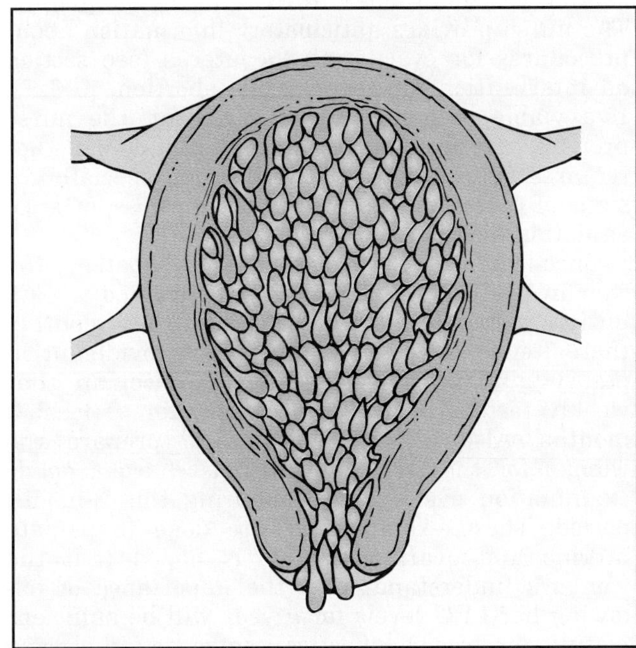

Figure 21–4

Degeneration of the chorionic villi in a hydatidiform mole pregnancy results in a mass of clear vesicles that are visually grapelike.

A molar pregnancy occurs in the presence of an abnormal chromosomal makeup of the zygote. The incidence of this disorder is rare, 1 in 1500 to 2000 pregnancies in the United States (Gabbe et al. 1991). However, marked geographic differences have been noted. Molar pregnancies are five to ten times more frequent in Southeast Asia and the Far East. Nutrition may account for some of the differences. Another important risk factor for a molar pregnancy is maternal age over 40, after which risk increases progressively with age (Herbst et al. 1992). Gestational trophoblastic neoplasia develops after 15 to 20 percent of complete molar pregnancies versus a much smaller percentage (4 percent) for incomplete moles. The sequelae of choriocarcinoma occur after 3 to 4 percent of all moles but are much more common following a complete mole. When a woman has had a molar pregnancy, her risk of a subsequent molar pregnancy is 20 to 40 times higher than that of the general population (Herbst et al. 1992).

MANAGEMENT

Traditionally, a molar pregnancy is suspected when a woman experiences hyperemesis related to elevated serum hCG levels, has signs of preeclampsia in the first 24 weeks of pregnancy, has a uterine size larger than expected for the number of weeks of gestation because of proliferating trophoblastic tissue and clotted blood, and has no fetal heart tones present at the expected time. Women often present with vaginal bleeding, which is either a characteristic brownish color or bright red. If spontaneous abortion occurs, the edematous (hydropic) trophoblastic vesicles are noted at that time. In truth, the clinical signs of a molar pregnancy are variable. The preceding classic signs occur in only about a third of molar pregnancies. When a fetus or amniotic sac is present, the woman may have few signs that differ from those of a normal pregnancy.

Management of a molar pregnancy is based on three principles: diagnosis of the mole, evacuation of the uterus, and monitoring of hCG levels. Diagnosis is made by documenting abnormally elevated hCG levels and by ultrasound visualization of the abnormal placenta. A chest radiograph is obtained to rule out spread of malignant GTD to the lungs. Evacuation of the uterus can be accomplished by suction D & C. Hysterectomy is an alternative for women who have completed childbearing and desire sterilization. This choice significantly decreases the risk of malignant sequelae.

Follow-up of serum beta-hCG levels is essential in diagnosing the presence of a resultant malignancy. Women typically have a spontaneous regression of hCG levels by 15 weeks after evacuation. When hCG levels are normal, the woman's level is monitored monthly for another 12 months to confirm that no malignancy has developed. Women should not become pregnant during this time, since a pregnancy would mask any increase in hCG related to malignancy. Pelvic examinations are also performed to assess uterine and ovarian size every 2 weeks and then every 3 months when hCG levels are negative.

Women whose hCG levels remain the same or increase, who have evidence of metastases, or in whom choriocarcinoma is diagnosed on the tissue from the pregnancy are given chemotherapy. It should be noted that GTD is 100 percent curable in women without metastasis or those with metastasis whose initial hCG levels are less than 40,000 mIU/mL, who have had the disease for less than 4 months, and who have not had previous chemotherapy.

Nursing Process

▼ Assessment

The nurse can be alert to factors associated with a GTD pregnancy such as signs and symptoms of preeclampsia before 24 weeks, hyperemesis, or persistent vaginal bleeding. When a hydatidiform mole is identified the nurse should assess the woman's understanding of her condition and her emotional status on experiencing the loss of a potential pregnancy, as well as her potential risk of developing a malignancy.

The nurse's role as an educator is essential. The nurse provides anticipatory information about probable procedures and informs the woman about the need for follow-up of hCG levels. During this follow-up, the nurse should assess the woman's method of contraception and discuss the fact that a pregnancy at this time might mask the ability to detect a trophoblastic tumor. The woman should be told that after her hCG levels have been normal for a sufficient length of time, there is no restriction on future pregnancies except to inform her provider of her history. The provider may want to document normal placental development early in the pregnancy.

▼ Diagnosis

On the basis of an assessment that includes the client's history, physical examination, and laboratory findings, the following diagnoses are suggested:

- Risk of injury related to hyperemesis, preeclampsia, bleeding, and possible choriocarcinoma
- Anticipatory grieving related to pregnancy loss
- Knowledge deficit: regarding follow-up care related to the effects on future fertility

▼ Planning

The plan of care that is chosen for the woman with GTD might include the following outcome goals:

- The woman's molar pregnancy will be resolved without maternal injury resulting from hyperemesis, preeclampsia, bleeding, or choriocarcinoma
- The woman will express her feelings related to the loss of her pregnancy
- The woman will correctly explain the components of her follow-up care and the effects of the molar pregnancy on her future fertility

▼ Intervention

The nurse's role as the patient's educator is essential for the woman with a molar pregnancy. The nurse provides anticipatory information about procedures for evacuating the uterus (see section on intervention for spontaneous abortion, p. 627). If a viable pregnancy is also present, the nurse prepares the woman for an antenatal course that requires more intensive surveillance, especially for signs of preeclampsia, respiratory distress, or a coagulation disorder.

Once the uterus has been evacuated, the woman's hCG levels should be determined weekly until they become undetectable and then monthly thereafter for 1 year. The nurse can provide anticipatory guidance by informing the woman that weekly tests are usually necessary for at least 3 months. Also, it is important to prepare the woman for the fact that she must have a pelvic examination every 2 weeks during this 3-month period. These examinations are done to palpate uterine and ovarian size. It is hoped that the woman's understanding of the importance of following her hCG levels for a year will be sufficient motivation to use effective contraception during this time. The nurse may help a woman sort out her contraceptive choices and reinforce appropriate teaching to maximize the effectiveness of the method chosen.

In addition to education, the nurse must focus

on the psychosocial aspects of the molar pregnancy. The nurse should elicit how the woman is feeling and assist her in working through her grief. The woman may have a fear of developing cancer and the nurse can support her in expressing and dealing with this fear, as well as giving her realistic reassurance about the excellent prognosis if she does develop a malignancy.

▼ Evaluation

According to the examples given of potential nursing diagnoses and the goals for measuring outcomes, the plan of care for a woman with a hydatidiform mole would be evaluated on the basis of the occurrence of maternal injury, the woman's expression of her feelings related to the loss of the pregnancy, and her ability to demonstrate her understanding of the follow-up care and the effects of the molar pregnancy on her future fertility.

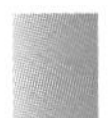

Fetal Death

DESCRIPTION

Fetal death or stillbirth is defined as any birth in which there is no sign of life (Moore et al. 1992). Fetal death rates are calculated as the number of fetal deaths after 20 weeks of gestation per 1000 total births (live births and stillbirths). Fetal deaths before 20 weeks of gestation are considered to be spontaneous abortions and were discussed earlier in this chapter. Fetal death rates have decreased by half over the last 40 years, and the rate was 7.5 per 1000 births in 1989 (Cunningham et al. 1993). Intrapartum fetal deaths are rare events. The causes of these deaths can be divided into four general categories: chronic asphyxia of diverse origin (50 percent); congenital anomalies (20 percent); superimposed complications of pregnancy, including fetal infection, placental accidents, and isoimmunization (5 percent); and unexplained stillbirth (25 percent)(Institute of Medicine 1990).

MANAGEMENT

The primary management of an intrauterine fetal death (IUFD) is to identify normal, viable fetuses who are at risk for fetal demise because of maternal risk factors and follow these pregnancies more closely throughout the antepartal period. Correction or treatment of the underlying maternal disease combined with antepartum fetal monitoring with daily fetal movement counts, nonstress tests, contraction stress tests, and ultrasound examination can significantly decrease intrauterine fetal deaths.

The medical management of an IUFD can be either expectant or active. In 75 percent of pregnancies, spontaneous labor and delivery occur within 2 weeks after the fetal death, and by 3 weeks 90 percent of women have delivered. The expectant approach of waiting for spontaneous labor can avoid potential problems such as a failed induction, infection, and hemorrhage. The risks of continuing a pregnancy with an IUFD include the psychological stress to the mother. There is also a small possibility of developing a hypocoagulation disorder known as disseminated intravascular coagulation (DIC) (see Chapter 35 for additional discussion of DIC). Active management of an IUFD is accomplished by induction of labor and delivery of the baby. In the third trimester, induction can be accomplished with oxytocin or rupture of membranes if the cervix is soft and dilated. If the cervix is unripe, prostaglandin gel may be inserted intravaginally before oxytocin administration.

Nursing Process

▼ Assessment

An initial nursing assessment may elicit the perception of decreased fetal movement by the mother. Early in pregnancy a woman may note loss of symptoms of pregnancy, such as decreases in the size and tenderness of her breasts. This assessment should be followed by careful assessment of the fundal height, looking for a lack of growth or decrease in height. Thorough auscultation for fetal heart tones should also be done. In early pregnancy, when detecting a heart rate is not reliable, a negative pregnancy test after a previous positive one can confirm the diagnosis of IUFD. The absence of fetal heart tones should always be confirmed by ultrasound findings of no fetal heart activity before informing a couple that they have experienced a fetal demise.

▼ Diagnosis

On the basis of an assessment that includes the client's history, physical examination, and laboratory findings, the following diagnoses are suggested:

- Risk for injury related to fetal death
- Knowledge deficit: lack of information related to the causes of IUFD and the proposed management plan

- Anticipatory grieving related to the loss of the anticipated child

Planning

The plan of care that is chosen for the woman experiencing fetal death might include the following outcome goals:

- The pregnancy will be terminated without adverse physiologic effects
- The woman will verbalize her understanding of the causes of the IUFD and her proposed management plan
- The woman will express her feelings regarding the loss of her baby

Intervention

The goal of the nursing intervention for an IUFD is to assist parents in confirming their loss and to provide emotional support through the grieving process. A perinatal loss checklist that is maintained in the woman's prenatal chart is a helpful way to keep all health care staff informed that a loss has occurred and to record the interventions parents have received (Ryan et al. 1991; Ewton 1993).

Parents need confirmation of who and what has been lost (Ewton 1993). This confirmation can be accomplished by sharing sonograms and laboratory slips confirming the pregnancy if it is an early pregnancy loss. Later losses resulting in a stillbirth can be validated by enabling parents to spend time holding their infant after the birth, taking photographs, and giving parents mementos such as footprints, bracelets, or a blanket. Parents need honest, factual information about the condition of their baby and the cause of death, which may be unknown until an autopsy is performed. The nurse can explore the parents' feelings about having an autopsy done so that they can later feel that their decision was the right one for them.

Parents need validation of their feelings of loss and emotional support. Openly discussing the loss and suggesting to the parents that they name their baby are ways of letting parents know that a significant event has happened to them. Parents need privacy to grieve, but not isolation. They need to feel free to express their emotions and know someone will listen to them. Although by instinct we want to alleviate the pain of grieving with tranquilizing drugs, this artificial dulling of grief can actually prolong the process and inhibit thoughtful decision making (Ewton 1993). Options for funeral and burial also need to be explored as appropriate and in accordance with state law. Encouraging the parents to think about a public grieving ceremony is one way to help them validate their feelings of loss. An assessment of social support systems and a discussion of coping methods usually employed under stress can help the nurse evaluate the kind of referrals the couple may need to cope with this loss. Educational material on perinatal loss as well as referral to a perinatal loss support group may be helpful.

The nurse can educate parents about the stages of the grieving process and let them know the process can take 6 months to 2 years (Ewton 1993). Symptoms of grief are similar to those of depression: nightmares, loss of appetite, weight loss, nervousness, and increased or decreased sleep. Normal grief reactions include sadness, anger, guilt, anxiety, loneliness, numbness, confusion, absent-mindedness, social withdrawal, and yearning for the deceased. Couples should know that men and women may experience grief differently, with women needing to talk about their loss and men more commonly busying themselves so they do not have to think about the loss. Open communication with each other, other children, and other family members is essential for successful coping. The nurse can encourage parents to emphasize in their discussion with their children that no one is to blame for the loss and no one else is going to die because of the loss. The nurse can help parents anticipate possible reactivation of grief during upcoming holidays or on the estimated delivery date.

Follow-up care should occur 1 week after the loss by telephone or a visit if it is indicated and then at subsequent visits. The nurse needs to assess whether the couple is undergoing a normal grieving process. Signs that are not normal are the use of drugs and alcohol, inability to carry out activities of daily living, complaints of recurring somatic symptoms, thoughts of worthlessness, suicide or sudden change in lifestyle excluding family and friends, and a wooden manner (Ewton 1993). The woman or her partner should be referred to a mental health provider if she or he exhibits any of these symptoms. Encouraging healthy preventive behaviors such as rest, exercise, good eating habits, and minimal life changes can help parents through this period of stress. Contraceptive counseling is an important component of follow-up to enable the parents to plan the next pregnancy when they are ready. Another pregnancy soon after the loss of this child may interrupt the grieving process, which may then continue after the birth of the next child.

HIGH-RISK CONDITIONS OCCURRING DURING THE PREGNANCY

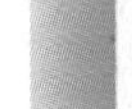

Hyperemesis Gravidarum

DESCRIPTION

Hyperemesis gravidarum is intractable vomiting during pregnancy that results in dehydration and electrolyte imbalance. It occurs in 1 to 4 per 1000 pregnancies (Newman et al. 1993). It is seen more often in primiparous women, young women, and women of increased body weight. The presence of hyperemesis puts a pregnancy at high risk because of lack of maternal weight gain. Many women with this condition lose weight, and loss of more than 5 percent of the prepregnancy weight can result in intrauterine growth restriction (IUGR) and possible fetal anomalies or central nervous system (CNS) malformations. If it is uncontrolled, fetal death can occur. In addition, the risk of preterm delivery is increased four times over that in a normal pregnancy. Hyperemesis differs from common morning sickness in several aspects (Table 21–1). The cause of hyperemesis remains a mystery, just as an explanation for morning sickness is uncertain. The theories fall into the categories of endocrine, psychological, and allergic; however, none of the theories has definitive supporting evidence.

MANAGEMENT

Hyperemesis gravidarum is a diagnosis of exclusion. Other causes that must first be considered are hyperthyroidism; hepatitis; drug-induced nausea, which can also cause jaundice; typical medications (antibiotics, sulfasalazine, digoxin); and pancreatitis. Management of hyperemesis is symptomatic. Women are rehydrated with intravenous fluids combined with vitamins. Frequently this therapy given intermittently makes the symptoms abate enough for adequate nutrition. However, some women may require hyperalimentation during the pregnancy for adequate nutrition. If the vomiting remains intractable, hospitalization may be required. Generally, women need this therapy for only 2 to 4 weeks, although there are documented cases in which therapy was necessary for most of the pregnancy.

Nursing Process

▼ Assessment

The nurse must assess the degree of morning sickness a woman is having and determine whether she has developed hyperemesis. A 2-day diet history assists in determining the degree of vomiting and nutritional intake the woman is experiencing. The nurse must also assess the woman for symptoms of dehydration such as dizziness and thirst. Symptoms of dizziness and fainting should be further evaluated with orthostatic vital signs. Other signs of dehydration include concentrated urine and low urine output. The nurse should also be alert for signs of electrolyte imbalance: ketonuria, irregular heart rate, and signs of thyroid dysfunction, which may result from protein-energy malnutrition. The woman's psychological status may also be indicative of hyperemesis,

Table 21–1

CHARACTERISTICS OF MORNING SICKNESS AND HYPEREMESIS GRAVIDARUM

CHARACTERISTIC	MORNING SICKNESS	HYPEREMESIS GRAVIDARUM
Onset	4–8 wk	Early pregnancy
Resolution	14–16 wk	Persists throughout pregnancy
Weight	Maintained or increased	Loss
Ketosis	Absent	Present
Electrolytes	Normal	Abnormal
Skin turgor	Hydrated	Dehydrated
Liver	Normal	Jaundice possible
Thyroid laboratory values	Normal	Abnormal

since B vitamin deficiency can cause anxiety and depression. An accurate weight is essential to making a differential diagnosis between morning sickness and hyperemesis. Any weight loss greater than 5 percent of body weight is highly indicative of hyperemesis and needs to be brought to the attention of the woman's health care provider (Newman et al. 1993).

▼ Diagnosis

On the basis of an assessment that includes the client's history, physical examination, and laboratory findings, the following diagnoses are suggested:

- Altered nutrition: less than body requirements related to persistent vomiting
- Fluid volume deficit related to decreased fluid intake and persistent vomiting
- Risk for maternal and fetal injury related to malnutrition and dehydration
- Knowledge deficit: lack of understanding related to medical condition, treatment, and possible effects on herself and fetus

▼ Planning

The plan of care that is chosen for the woman experiencing hyperemesis gravidarum might include the following outcome goals:

- The woman will maintain a diet that provides adequate nutritional components for pregnancy
- The woman will maintain an adequate fluid intake
- The woman experiences no further episodes of nausea or vomiting
- The woman verbally states her understanding of hyperemesis, her medical treatment, and the effects on her and her fetus

▼ Intervention

Relief of the nausea and vomiting and resumption of normal appetite and food intake are the goals of nursing intervention. The nurse plays an important role in recognizing the severity of the nausea and vomiting and appropriately referring the client for treatment. The nurse may suggest that the woman try the various measures listed in Strategies to Reduce Nausea and Vomiting. Magnesium- and potassium-rich foods should be encouraged since these elements are depleted with prolonged vomiting. Magnesium can be replaced by chewing on a milk of magnesia tablet two or three times a day. Taking 25 mg of vitamin B_6 every 8 hours for at least 3 days may also be helpful in alleviating vomiting (Newman et al. 1993). Other therapies include the use of antiemetics or acupressure (Beal 1992). Acupressure can be applied easily by wearing a wrist band that has a tiny button on one side to be placed against the inside of the wrist against an acupressure point (see Fig. 24–6). These bands are available commercially. Recumbent rest has also been shown to be effective in alleviating symptoms of nausea and

Strategies to Reduce Nausea and Vomiting in Pregnancy

- Eat small amounts of food every 2 to 3 hours
- Eat foods that appeal to you, even if they are junk food; favorites may be salty, tart, bitter, sour, bland, crunchy, sweet, earthy
- Drink liquids between meals instead of with meals
- Avoid greasy or fried foods unless craved because they are harder to digest
- Avoid food aromas that cause nausea by cooking outside, not being in the kitchen during meal preparation, or using a fan to ventilate odors
- Stay upright for 1 to 2 hours after eating to avoid gastric reflux
- Continue eating until bedtime to avoid low blood sugar in the morning unless vomiting occurs in the evening
- Avoid brushing teeth immediately after eating
- Sleep in a well-ventilated room to avoid stale room smell in the morning
- Eat some bread or crackers before getting out of bed in the morning
- Get out of bed slowly
- Drink herbal teas; flavors such as ginger root, spearmint, raspberry leaf, peppermint, and chamomile may be helpful

Data from Erick, M. (1993). *No more morning sickness: A survival guide for pregnant women.* New York: Plume Books, and Newman, V., Fullerton, J. T., Anderson, P. O. (1993). Clinical advances in the management of severe nausea and vomiting during pregnancy. *Journal of Obstetric, Gynecologic, and Neonatal Nursing,* 22 (6), 483.

vomiting. The nurse should assist a woman in making any changes necessary in her life to allow her to lie down, especially during the part of the day when she experiences her worst symptoms.

Women with hyperemesis may need intravenous therapy with multivitamins and minerals to alleviate symptoms of nausea and vomiting and to correct their electrolyte imbalance. This therapy may be given in hospital or twice weekly on an ambulatory basis. Typically women are able to tolerate clear liquids with gradual progression to small meals after their first intravenous therapy (Newman et al. 1993). Therapy is continued for at least 2 weeks until weight gain is documented and symptoms have subsided.

Some women may need enteral feeding through a nasogastric tube or parenteral nutrition. The solutions used supply up to 2000 calories per day and contain amino acids, fatty acid, vitamins, and minerals. Usually women are hospitalized for this therapy. Each feeding method has its risks. Enteral feeding is successful only when severe vomiting has subsided, but a woman is at risk for aspiration pneumonia if she does vomit. Parenteral nutrition requires peripheral or central venous access. Generally the latter is preferred because of the high rate of infiltration of peripheral veins that cannot tolerate the high osmolality of parenteral nutrition solution. If a woman is hospitalized for hydration or nutrition therapy, the nurse can provide psychological support to the woman. The nurse's psychological assessment of the woman can be valuable input to the physician for appropriate psychological counseling or referral.

▼ Evaluation

The nurse evaluates the plan of care for the woman with hyperemesis gravidarum on the basis of the identified nursing diagnoses and outcome goals. Further plans for intervention depend on the woman's ability to maintain a nutritious diet, maintain an adequate fluid intake, decrease her nausea and vomiting, and maintain her weight. Her understanding of her illness and its management is an important component for evaluation in order to elicit her compliance.

Multiple Gestation

DESCRIPTION

In the United States, approximately 12 in 1000 births result in multiple neonates (twins, triplets, or higher order) (Gabbe et al. 1991). One third of all twins are identical or monozygotic, and this figure is consistent around the world. Monozygosity occurs when a single egg is fertilized and divides into two separate but identical embryos. Depending on when the ovum divides, the resulting embryos may have their own amnion and chorion or may share one or both (Fig. 21–5). Most commonly, each conceptus has its own amnion but they share a chorion. If separation occurs later than 14 to 15 days after conception, the twins may be conjoined within the same amniotic sac.

The other two thirds of twins are dizygotic or fraternal. They arise from two or more separate ova and do not share the same genetic material; thus they are no more alike than any other siblings. The multiple ova may occur spontaneously or as a result of infertility treatments such as ovulation-inducing drugs, in vitro fertilization (IVF), or gamete intrafallopian tube transfer (GIFT). The rate of spontaneous dizygotic twinning is variable around the world, generally being lowest in Asians, intermediate in whites, and highest in blacks. Increased maternal age, increased parity, race, heredity, and malnutrition are factors for dizygotic twins (Gabbe et al. 1991). Higher order gestations may arise from either or both of the foregoing processes. For example, triplets (1 in 9000 births) may arise from one, two, or three ova.

MANAGEMENT

Although multiple gestations account for less than 1 percent of pregnancies, they represent 10 to 11 percent of overall perinatal mortality as well as increased neonatal morbidity because of prematurity, low birth weight, abnormal growth pattern, or congenital anomalies. The mother with a multiple-gestation pregnancy is at three to five times increased risk for preeclampsia than if she had a singleton pregnancy (Moore et al. 1992). The best means of preventing complications is early detection of the multiple gestation, usually confirmed by early ultrasonography.

A multiple-gestation pregnancy is managed by close surveillance of mother and babies. Prenatal visits are usually scheduled every 2 weeks and increased to weekly sometime between 24 and 28 weeks' gestation. Maternal well-being is monitored for signs and symptoms of preeclampsia and preterm labor. Cervical examinations may be performed at each visit, since a woman with a multiple gestation is less likely to perceive premature contractions and therefore "silently" dilate her cervix (Dyson et al. 1991). Many providers may prescribe bed rest either at the first sign of any cervical change or at 24 to 28 weeks, whichever comes first. Bed rest has the benefit of improving uterine blood flow and thereby increasing birth weight by 10 percent and of decreasing uterine activity and preventing preterm labor (Moore et al. 1992).

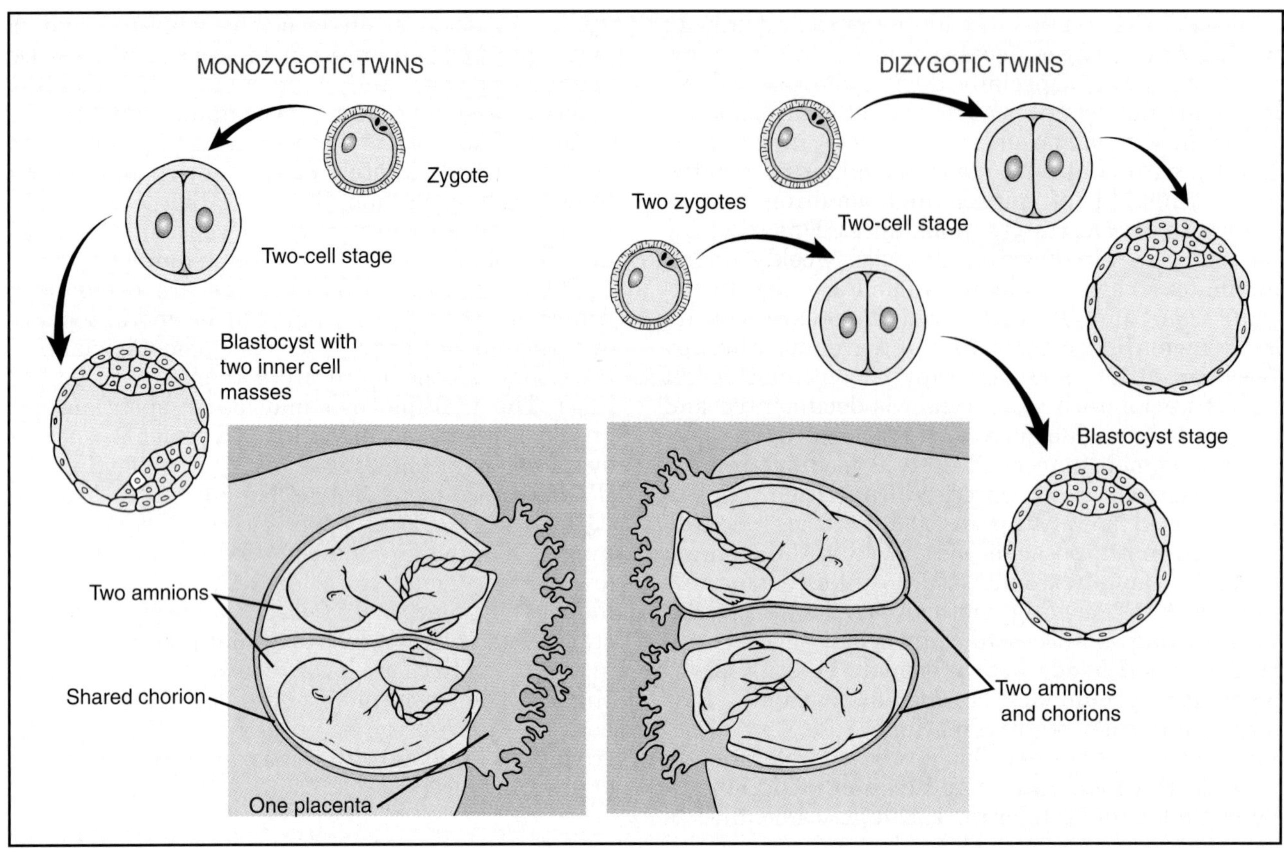

Figure 21–5

Placentation in twin pregnancies differs, depending on when the ovum divides • Fetuses in a monozygotic multiple pregnancy may have their own amnion and chorion or may share both • Dizygotic twins have two separate placentas.

Fetal well-being during a multiple gestation is monitored by ultrasonography and auscultation tests. The initial ultrasound examination attempts to document a membrane between the twins since the management of monoamniotic twins, who experience a much higher mortality rate, differs from that for other types of twins. Serial ultrasound examinations (approximately monthly) can be used to assess fetal growth, rule out discordant growth between twins, or document intrauterine growth restriction (IUGR). Doppler flow studies, which examine the flow of blood through the umbilical artery and vein, may be done in the case of discordant growth. Nonstress tests and biophysical profiles beginning at 28 to 32 weeks can be used to assess fetal well-being (Eganhouse 1992). Careful technique must be used to ensure that each fetus is individually assessed. If antenatal testing reveals that one fetus is in jeopardy, a careful assessment is done to minimize the risk of delivering the healthy fetus prematurely while not increasing the likelihood of morbidity and mortality of the less healthy twin by delaying delivery. In this situation, the lung maturity of each fetus is assessed by obtaining fluid from each sac by means of amniocentesis. The amniotic fluid is examined for the presence of surfactant, which is necessary to reduce the collapsibility of lung alveoli. The lung maturity test is reported as a ratio of lecithin to sphingomyelin (L/S ratio). An L/S ratio greater than or equal to 2 in a nondiabetic pregnancy is indicative of mature fetal lungs (Moore et al. 1992).

The method of delivery in a multiple gestation depends on gestational age, fetal weight, and presentation. Vertex-vertex twins at term may be delivered vaginally. If the presenting twin is breech or transverse, the twins are most likely to be delivered by cesarean section. The delivery method for vertex-breech twins is controversial and varies according to the obstetrician's experience and the gestational age of the fetuses; it is recommended that a nonvertex baby weighing less than 1500 g should be delivered abdominally (Moore et al. 1992). Further discussion of the management of a multiple gestation during the intrapartal period can be found in Chapter 25.

Overdistention of the uterus with multiple gestations can cause postpartum hemorrhage related to uterine atony. Uterine massage and intramuscular or intravenous oxytocics may be used to control bleeding. Immediate postpartum observation is essential to identify the development of abnormal bleeding early.

Specific problems that may be identified in twins include the following:

1. Monoamniotic twins share a common amniotic sac. Since there is no physical separation of the twins, they are at high risk for cord entanglements resulting in cord occlusion and death of one twin. The fetal mortality rate for these twins is 40 to 60 percent (Moore et al. 1992).
2. Twin-to-twin transfusion occurs in monozygotic twins when a single placenta forms an arteriovenous fistula with blood flowing in one direction. The "donor" twin becomes anemic and growth retarded, and the sac contains less than the normal amount of fluid (oligohydramnios). The "recipient" has an elevated hemoglobin level, possibly hydrops, and is in danger of developing congestive heart failure with polyhydramnios being evident.
3. Discordant growth between twins can occur. Commonly each child born from a multiple gestation is smaller than a singleton of the same gestational age, although these babies typically experience "catch-up" growth and by 1 year weigh the same as their singleton peers. Sometimes one baby is much smaller than the other. If the weight difference is more than 25 percent (i.e., discordant growth), the smaller twin has a six times increased risk of fetal death.
4. IUGR can also occur in twins. This growth pattern is usually a result of poor placental implantation causing poor placental perfusion and decreased overall supply of nutrients to the babies. Other causes include chromosomal or major anatomic anomalies, poor cord insertion (velamentous insertion), and hydrops (Moore et al. 1992).
5. Intrauterine demise of a single twin can result in a difficult management dilemma. The incidence of demise of a single twin in the first trimester may be as high as 21 percent on the basis of early ultrasonography. The exact incidence is difficult to ascertain since the gestational sacs visualized on early ultrasound examinations may represent a true viable fetus or a blighted ovum. This "vanished" twin does not pose any hazards to the other viable gestations. However, a demise later in pregnancy can precipitate the onset of labor or clotting abnormalities in the mother. However, induction of labor early in gestation can cause long-term problems of prematurity for the viable twin.
6. Structural anomalies occur twice as often in monozygotic twins as in dizygotic twins. Cardiac anomalies, which may include absence of a heart, also appear to be more prevalent. Conjoined twins develop once in every 1500 twin pregnancies. The degree of conjoining is determined by the timing of the separation during gametogenesis.

Nursing Process

▼ Assessment

The nurse needs to take a careful family history, since a woman's risk of having dizygotic twins is increased if her female relatives have had dizygotic twins. Pregnancy achieved after the use of infertility drugs (7 percent twinning with clomiphene citrate and 20 percent with menotropins [Pergonal]) (Moore et al. 1992) or other assisted technologies should alert the nurse to the strong possibility of twins. A woman whose uterine size is more than 3 cm larger than expected for gestational age may have a multiple gestation. However, it is important to keep in mind that the most common reason for size greater than dates is an incorrect LMP. If a woman's uterine size is larger than dates, the nurse may attempt to auscultate two different heart rates or palpate three fetal poles as a method of detecting more than one fetus in utero. If a woman is sent for an ultrasound examination to diagnose twins, the nurse can begin to explore the woman's initial feelings about the possibility of twins.

The nurse must carefully assess the woman diagnosed with a multiple gestation for signs and symptoms of preeclampsia and preterm labor. It is also important to discuss in detail the common discomforts of pregnancy, since these symptoms are often magnified for women who have a multiple gestation. A nutritional assessment is also important, because the nutritional needs in multiple gestation are greater than those of a singleton pregnancy.

▼ Diagnosis

On the basis of an assessment that includes the client's history, physical examination, and laboratory findings, the following diagnoses are suggested:

- Risk for discomfort related to enlarged uterus
- Risk for injury related to medical complications of pregnancy
- Risk for altered growth and development related to preterm labor or IUGR
- Altered nutrition: less than body requirements related to multiple gestation

- Risk for ineffective family coping: compromised, related to high-risk pregnancy and increased stress

▼ Planning

The plan of care that is chosen for the woman experiencing multiple gestation might include the following outcome goals:

- The woman will verbalize increased comfort
- The pregnancy will proceed without maternal or fetal complications
- The woman will maintain a diet adequate for the development of multiple fetuses
- The woman will verbalize positive stress management and adequate family coping

▼ Intervention

The goal of nursing management is the safe delivery of healthy babies of adequate size with as little morbidity to the mother as possible. The nurse needs to recognize that the large volume of the uterus accentuates most of the common discomforts of pregnancy and at an earlier time in gestation. Abdominal and back pains are common complaints, but it is important to differentiate these symptoms from those of preterm labor. Teaching good body mechanics, use of low-heeled shoes, and use of pillows while lying down may relieve some of the discomfort. As the uterus enlarges upward, pressing on the diaphragm, dyspnea can become a problem. A woman may find that increasing the number of pillows she uses at night is helpful in relieving the dyspnea. Fluid retention and preeclampsia are seen more often with multiple-gestation pregnancies than with singletons. The most helpful measure is to encourage the woman to maintain hydration and improve circulation to the lower extremities and kidneys by lying on her side for several hours at a time. The woman with a multiple gestation must be familiar with the signs and symptoms of preeclampsia and should be encouraged to get in touch with her health care provider if she has any of these symptoms.

The difficulty in meeting the nutritional needs of the pregnancy may result in anemia and increased fatigue. Once diagnosed as having a multiple gestation, a woman should be encouraged to increase her diet by 300 kcal per day per baby as well as receive additional supplementation of folic acid and iron (above regular prenatal vitamins) (Brown and Schloesser 1990; Worthington-Roberts and Williams 1993). Weight gains in multiple-gestation pregnancies associated with the lowest perinatal mortality and lowest proportion of low-birth-weight infants average 40.9 to 44.2 pounds (18.6 to 20.1 kg) (Brown and Schloesser 1990; Institute of Medicine 1990). Because of the greater increase of blood volume (up to 75 percent versus 50 percent in a singleton pregnancy), the woman's hemoglobin status may be checked every trimester to diagnose and treat anemia as early as possible. Adequate hemoglobin is essential not only for the well-being of the fetuses but also because these women are at risk for larger postpartum blood loss.

The initial emotional reaction to a multiple pregnancy may range from disbelief to anger to elation. As the pregnancy progresses, the discomforts and the need for reduced activity may be added stressors to the mother and the family unit. Concern about the health and survival of multiple fetuses may interfere with the normal processes of adaptation to the new family and prenatal attachment. The birth of two or more children can cause a significant strain on family resources. The nurse can support the mother, her partner, and other family members through these difficult times by eliciting their feelings, acknowledging the validity of their concerns, and making appropriate referrals. The nurse can act as a patient's advocate to help the family negotiate the health care system.

As a woman approaches term, which is generally considered 36 to 37 weeks in a multiple gestation pregnancy, the nurse should determine whether she understands the anticipated management plan of her labor and delivery. Once the babies are delivered, the family will need support in coping with the needs of two or more possibly premature infants. Referral to a mothers of twins group for emotional and practical support and to a lactation consultant for assistance with breastfeeding may be appropriate. Return to prepregnancy weight and body status may be prolonged after a multiple pregnancy. Abdominal tone may be poor after delivery when a large diastasis recti is present. The woman should be carefully instructed in exercises that gradually restore abdominal tone without permanently damaging the rectus muscles. A reasonable period for weight loss should be discussed with the woman in the early postpartum period. Accelerated weight loss during the postpartum period may meet a woman's body image needs, but if she is lactating it may decrease her milk supply.

▼ Evaluation

The evaluation of the woman with a multiple gestation is ongoing throughout the entire pregnancy. The initial nursing diagnoses and outcome goals may be altered as events change. The plan of care is successful if the woman and her babies are delivered safely. Evaluation is based on the level of the woman's comfort; the prevention of medical complications, fetal compromise, and IUGR; the woman's ability to maintain an adequate diet; and the ability of the woman and her family to maintain coping and decrease stress.

Hypertensive Disorders of Pregnancy

DESCRIPTION

Hypertensive disorders of pregnancy include preeclampsia-eclampsia, chronic hypertension, preeclampsia superimposed upon chronic hypertension, and transient hypertension (Lenfant et al. 1990). Chronic hypertension is defined as hypertension that is present and observable before pregnancy or is diagnosed before the twentieth week of gestation. Preeclampsia is determined by increased blood pressure after 20 weeks of gestation accompanied by proteinuria, edema, or both (Cunningham et al. 1993; Roberts 1994). Preeclampsia is classified as mild or severe. A woman with the classic symptomatology may be diagnosed as mild preeclampsia if the following criteria are met:

- Increase of 30 systolic or 15 diastolic over the blood pressure before 20 weeks of gestation, or blood pressure >140/90 if there was no evidence of hypertension before pregnancy
- Increase in MAP of 20 mm of MAP ≥120 *and* proteinuria of +1 or 0.3 g/L in 24 hours, or
- Edema, by appearance of generalized edema or rapid weight gain

Severe preeclampsia is diagnosed when the following criteria are present:

- Blood pressure ≥160/110 recorded on at least two occasions at least 6 hours apart
- Proteinuria of +3 or +4, or 5 g/L or more in 24 hours
- Oliguria less than or equal to 500 mL in 24 hours
- Cerebral or visual changes
- Epigastric pain
- Pulmonary edema or cyanosis

Eclampsia denotes the occurrence of convulsions not caused by neurologic disease in a woman who has signs and symptoms of preeclampsia. Transient hypertension is defined as elevated blood pressure during pregnancy or in the first 24 hours post partum without other signs of preeclampsia or preexisting hypertension (Lenfant et al. 1990; Cunningham et al. 1993).

Diagnostic nomenclature for hypertension that occurs before or during pregnancy is a concern for clinicians and researchers. The most recent ACOG Technical Bulletin on hypertension in pregnancy (1996) recommends the use of two terms, chronic hypertension and pregnancy-induced hypertension (PIH), as clinically useful. Such terminology that labels subsets of disorder is discouraged, given the limitations of the current understanding of the disorder. Treatment modalities are generally different for chronic hypertension and PIH, delivery being the only definitive treatment for PIH. Many researchers have noted the difficulty in interpreting studies of hypertensive disorders in pregnancy owing to an inconsistency of terminology. In 1988 a Working Group on High Blood Pressure in Pregnancy, convened by the National High Blood Pressure Education Program of the National Heart, Lung, and Blood Institute, National Institute of Health, endorsed the classification system proposed by ACOG in 1972 (Lenfant et al. 1990) that is presented in this chapter. From the perspective of the researcher, the classification system of the NIH Working Group distinguishes hypertensive disorders that include proteinuria and hyperuricemia from those that do not. This distinction is important to a thorough exploration and understanding of all possible pathophysiologic pathways of this disease process.

Pathophysiology

The primary pathophysiology of preeclampsia is characterized by vasospasm and coagulation abnormalities. It is unknown why these conditions occur. There are several alternative theories regarding the development of preeclampsia. Genetic, immunologic, environmental, and vascular-mediated factors are all hypothesized to play an important role in the development of the disease (Stone et al. 1994). There is substantial evidence that endothelial injury is a pathophysiologic component of preeclampsia (Roberts 1994). The endothelium has many important functions, among them prevention of coagulation and modulation of vascular tone. The vasoconstriction of hypoperfusion in preeclampsia may be due to an increased sensitivity to pressor hormones as can occur in endothelial dysfunction (Cunningham et al. 1993; Roberts 1994). This sensitivity has been documented as early as 11 to 14 weeks of pregnancy in women who later develop preeclampsia.

- Vasospasm in the uterine arterioles leads to degenerative aging of the placenta and decreased placental perfusion, with the potential for IUGR, decreased fetal movement, and fetal hypoxia.
- Decreased renal perfusion results in a decreased glomerular filtration rate (GFR), and increases in creatinine, blood urea nitrogen (BUN), and uric acid. Proteinuria and oliguria occur. In-

creased sodium and water retention causes generalized edema and cerebral edema. Intravascular volume is decreased because of the movement of fluid out of the intravascular compartment, resulting in hemoconcentration and increased blood viscosity (hematocrit).

- Decreased hepatic perfusion results in elevated liver enzymes and possible liver distention, causing epigastric pain.
- Decreased blood to the retina causes visual symptoms such as blind spots (scotomata) and blurring.
- Vasospasm leads to cerebral edema, hemorrhage, thrombosis, and increased central nervous system (CNS) irritability.

The suggestion that immunologic factors play a part in the pathophysiology of preeclampsia is supported by the fact that preeclampsia is ten times more common in first pregnancies than in subsequent ones, and multiparas who have a new partner experience preeclampsia at the same rate as nulliparas. However, a specific immune factor has yet to be identified. Other theories of the cause of preeclampsia include excessive placental mass, since preeclampsia is more common in molar and multiple gestation pregnancies; genetic factors due to familial inheritance patterns of the disease; and dietary deficiencies, particularly calcium.

Much interest has focused on the observation of an abnormality in prostaglandin synthesis in pregnancies complicated with preeclampsia. It is not known whether this imbalance is due to endothelial damage to the vasculature or another reason. Two important prostaglandins, prostacyclin and thromboxane A_2, regulate vascular tone, platelet aggregation, uterine activity, and uterine blood flow. Normally, these two are produced in equal amounts. Women with preeclampsia produce twice as much thromboxane A_2 as prostacyclin. This imbalance, along with endothelial damage, can result in many of the signs and symptoms of preeclampsia. It is possible that the alteration in these prostaglandins may be responsible for the vasoconstriction and increased sensitivity to angiotensin II and the classic symptoms that result. It has been shown that low-dose aspirin, 60 to 80 mg, can selectively inhibit thromboxane A_2 and not affect prostacyclin. In normal therapeutic doses, aspirin inhibits both prostaglandins equally. Studies of the use of low-dose aspirin by women with risk factors for preeclampsia have shown some success in preventing preeclampsia (Imperiale and Stollenwerk 1991; Hines and Jones 1994). Unfortunately, a prospective, double-blind study in which low-dose aspirin was given to a group of healthy, nulliparous women did not show any decrease in preeclampsia or perinatal morbidity but did show an increase in abruptio placentae (Sibai et al. 1993).

Etiology

Preeclampsia occurs in 5 to 6 percent of otherwise normal pregnancies and in as many as 20 to 40 percent of pregnancies complicated by chronic renal or vascular disease. Therefore, about 100,000 births a year in the United States are to mothers with preeclampsia. Data indicate that the rate of severe preeclampsia has increased since the mid-1980s with a concomitant decrease of eclampsia (Saftlas et al. 1990). Despite the relatively low incidence of this disease, it accounts for 20 percent of all maternal mortality (Cunningham et al. 1993). Maternal morbidity and mortality are usually consequences of eclampsia that can result in maternal asphyxia, coma, intracerebral hemorrhage, and aspiration resulting from DIC. Perinatal morbidity and mortality can be due to chronic vasospasm, which can cause growth retardation and abruptio placentae, or to a maternal condition that can lead to asphyxia in the fetus or premature delivery to improve the mother's condition.

There are five risk factors for preeclampsia in normal, healthy women: (1) nulliparity, (2) young age, (3) age greater than 35, (4) African-American race, and (5) history of preeclampsia. As mentioned previously, preeclampsia occurs more frequently in women who have chronic renal or vascular diseases such as diabetes, collagen vascular disease, or chronic hypertension. Preeclampsia also develops more often in molar pregnancies and multiple gestations. A history of preeclampsia in a mother or sister increases a woman's risk of preeclampsia to 25 percent. Preeclampsia is a multisystem disease that causes highly variable signs and symptoms. It can affect one system and not another or may affect several systems at once. Onset may be rapid, and occurrence is more likely with increasing gestational age.

Signs and Symptoms

The signs and symptoms of preeclampsia can be classified by system (see Clinical Manifestations of Preeclampsia). The three classic signs of preeclampsia are hypertension (an increase in systolic pressure of 30 mm Hg or an increase in diastolic pressure of 15 mm Hg above the nonpregnant levels or BP of 140/90), edema (observable swelling of the feet, hands, or face or a sudden rapid weight gain of more than 2 pounds a week), and proteinuria (+1 dipstick analysis or 0.3 g/L in 24 hours). The characteristic appearance of a woman with preeclampsia who has facial edema is seen in Procedure 21–1. Warning symptoms of developing eclampsia are severe headache, visual disturbances, vomiting, epigastric or upper right quadrant pain, increased hyperreflexia, and development of clonus. Assessment of pitting edema, deep tendon reflexes, and clonus is described in Procedure 21–1.

Clinical Manifestations of Preeclampsia

CARDIOVASCULAR

- Hypertension
- Edema (generalized, hand, face)
- Retinal changes (narrowing of arterioles; detachment)

HEMATOLOGIC

- Coagulopathy
- Hemoconcentration

PULMONARY

- Pulmonary edema
- Dyspnea

HEPATIC

- Upper quadrant pain, epigastric pain
- Periportal hemorrhage
- Hepatic enlargement

CNS

- Headache
- Tinnitus
- Blurred vision, scotoma
- Hyperreflexia
- Clonus
- Changes in affect
- Altered mentation
- Grand mal seizure
- Cerebrovascular accident

RENAL

- Proteinuria
- Oliguria
- Hematuria

GASTROINTESTINAL

- Nausea and vomiting
- Hematemesis

PROCEDURE 21 – 1

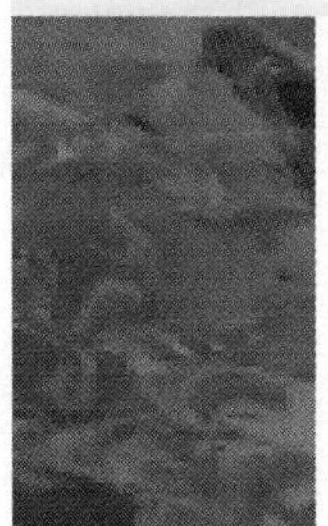

Assessing Pitting Edema, Deep Tendon Reflexes, and Clonus

▼ PURPOSE

An increasing degree of edema or hyperreflexia can indicate preeclampsia or, in a known case of preeclampsia, a worsening of the condition. Edema is assessed routinely at each prenatal visit after 20 weeks' gestation. For women with increasing edema or risk factors for preeclampsia, the evaluation of deep tendon reflexes (DTRs) and clonus is added to this routine assessment

Continued on following page

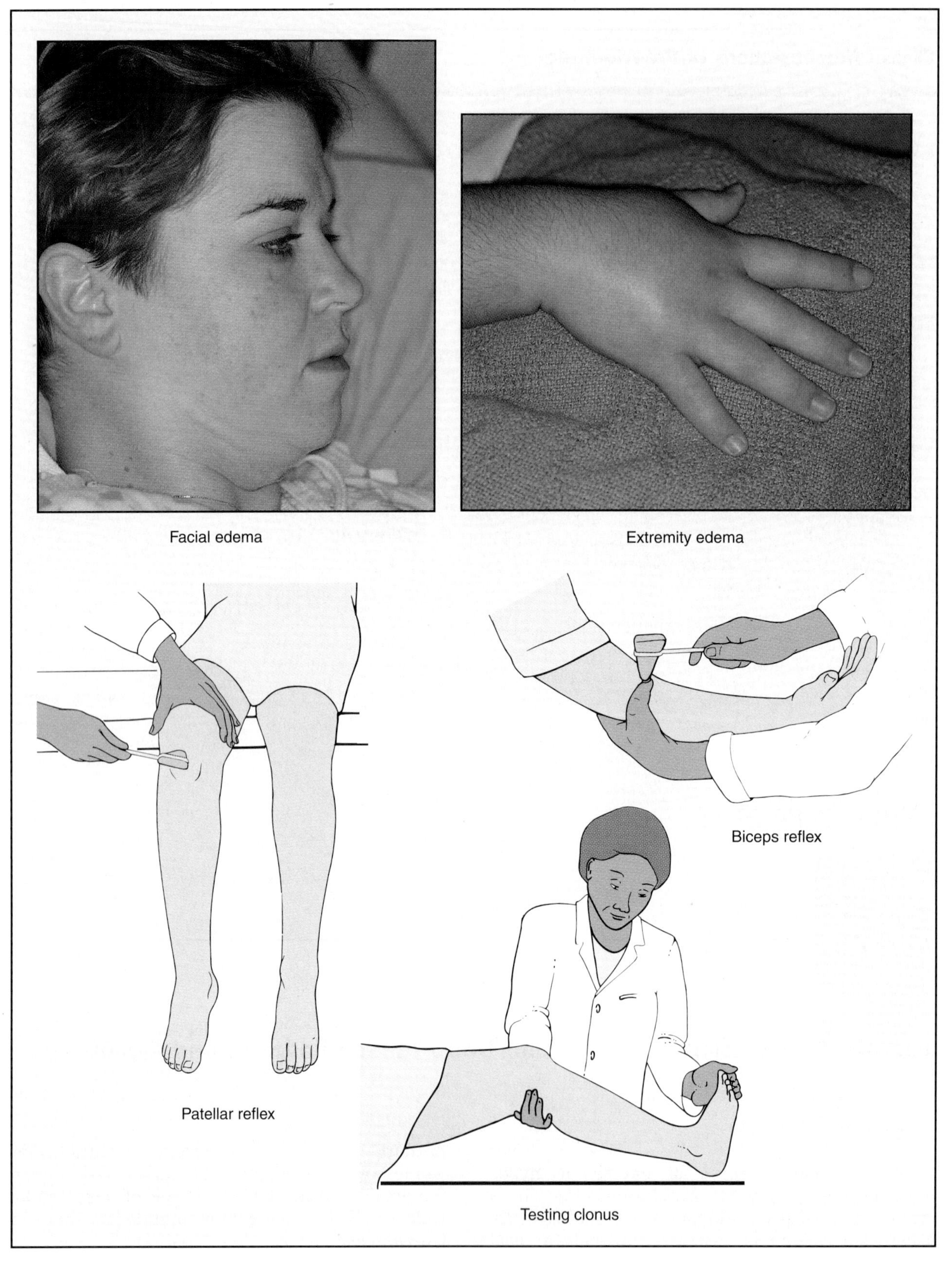

Continued on facing page

PROCEDURE 21–1 Continued

▼ EQUIPMENT

- Reflex hammer or a reasonable substitute, such as the edge of a stethoscope bell, the fingertips, or the sides of the fingers.

Assessing Pitting Edema

1 Ask the woman and/or family members if the woman's face or hands appear swollen. **Nonpitting edema may be found in the patient's fingers, face, and eyelids. It may be best recognized by the woman or family members who are familiar with her normal appearance.**

2 Inspect the woman's face, extremities, and sacral area for signs of pitting edema. **A thorough physical assessment of the woman for edema is important for differentiating dependent edema, which occurs in normal pregnancy, from generalized pitting edema, which may be associated with preeclampsia.**

3 Press each area firmly with the thumb or index finger for several seconds and release. Evaluate the extensiveness of the edema, the depth of the depression, and the length of time it takes to clear. **This technique helps the nurse determine the presence and degree of pitting edema. Pitting edema leaves a depression after finger pressure has been applied to an affected area.**

4 Grade the pitting edema according to the following scale:
1+ = Minimal edema of the lower extremities
2+ = Marked edema of the lower extremities
3+ = Edema of the lower extremities, face, and hands
4+ = Generalized, massive edema
An increasing degree of edema may indicate a worsening condition. The use of a standardized scale lends objectivity and consistency to assessments among health care providers.

5 Record your findings. Compare your findings with those previously recorded. **By recording and comparing findings, trends demonstrating a worsening of or an improvement in the condition can be seen.**

Assessing Deep Tendon Reflexes and Clonus

1 Explain the procedure for assessing DTRs to the woman. Position her so that her arms and legs are flexed or semiflexed and her muscles are relaxed. **Understanding her role in the procedure increases the woman's ability to keep her muscles relaxed. Relaxation of muscles is required in order to elicit the DTR response successfully.**

2 Locate the tendon and the corresponding muscle of the reflex to be tested. For example, prior to assessing the patellar reflex (knee jerk), locate the ligamentum patellae tendon at the base of the patella. Before eliciting the biceps reflex, flex the woman's elbow and place your thumb across the tendon in the antecubital space. **Identifying the correct tendon is essential to eliciting a reflex response.**

3 Tap the tendon directly using the reflex hammer or, in the case of the biceps reflex, firmly tap your thumb, which is pressing on the tendon. **The reflex response occurs when the tendon is briskly tapped. The tendon stimulates the corresponding muscle to contract and the body part to move or jerk (normal response).**

4 Rate the reflex response according to the following scale:
0 = Absent
1+ = Diminished
2+ = Normal
3+ = Brisk
4+ = Hyperactive
Rating helps the nurse evaluate the status of the woman's reflex responses. The use of a standardized scale lends objectivity and consistency to assessments among health care providers. Absent or diminished reflexes are an abnormal finding and may be seen with magnesium toxicity. Brisk or hyperactive reflexes may indicate central nervous system irritability (as in preeclampsia) and require physician follow-up.

5 Repeat the procedure if you are unable to elicit the reflex or to confirm the response as absent or diminished. To confirm absent

Continued on following page

PROCEDURE 21–1 Continued

or diminished reflexes, instruct the woman to contract a group of muscles different from those being evaluated. For example, while testing reflexes in the lower extremities, ask the woman to interlock her fingers and pull her arms outward, contracting the muscles in her arms. **Confirmation of absent or diminished reflexes is essential for an accurate assessment. By having the woman concentrate on muscles other than those being evaluated, a more accurate result may be elicited.**

6 Assess each reflex symmetrically, comparing the reflex response on one side with the reflex response on the other side. **The reflex response for a tendon should be the same on both the right and left sides.**

7 When checking for clonus, explain the procedure to the woman first. Position the woman so that her knee is semiflexed. Support her leg by placing one hand or your arm under her knee. **Understanding the procedure improves cooperation. Relaxation of muscles is required to assess for the presence of clonus.**

8 Using your other hand, sharply dorsiflex the woman's foot, maintaining slight pressure on her foot after dorsiflexion. Release her foot and observe its movement. **Clonus (foot jerks rapidly) is an abnormal neurologic finding that may be elicited when a muscle is sharply stretched and the stretch is maintained in either flexion or extension. The absence of clonus (foot simply returns to its normal position) is a normal finding.**

9 Count the beats of clonus present as you observe for rhythmic contraction and relaxation of the gastrocnemius and soleus muscles. **Clonus is evaluated by counting the number of times the muscle contracts and relaxes after it has been sharply stretched (e.g., "three beats").**

10 Record your findings. Compare your findings with those recorded previously. **By recording and comparing findings, you can see a trend in a worsening or an improving condition.**

HELLP Syndrome

Some women with preeclampsia develop an unusual manifestation of their disease that has been described as the HELLP syndrome (H for intravascular hemolysis; EL for elevated aspartate aminotransferase (AST) and alanine aminotransferase (ALT) liver enzymes; and LP for low platelets (less than 100,000) (Creasy and Resnick 1994). HELLP most often occurs early in the third trimester and is thought to result from a circulating immunologic component. It is classified as class I, less than 50,000 platelets, or class II, 50,000 to 100,000 platelets (Martin et al. 1990). Women with HELLP are managed in the same way as those with severe preeclampsia. Women who develop HELLP may also develop DIC and need intensive medical and nursing care. There is some indication that women with class II HELLP take longer to recover their platelet function (Martin et al. 1990).

MANAGEMENT

Management of preeclampsia begins with early detection, one of the essential reasons for early prenatal care. Once preeclampsia has developed, the only known cure is delivery. The medical management of preeclampsia is based on whether it is mild or severe. As previously noted, the mild versus severe classification is based on signs and symptoms. The laboratory changes noted for mild and severe disease are shown in Table 21–2. Mild preeclampsia is followed conservatively with bed rest to improve uterine perfusion and lower blood pressure. Usually a woman is seen at least twice weekly to monitor her blood pressure, urine, and weight, as well as to assess for more severe symptoms. Blood testing may be done once a week to monitor for changes in liver enzymes or clotting factors as well as to follow kidney function. The fetus is monitored with twice weekly nonstress tests. Delivery of the woman with mild preeclampsia is recommended once the fetus is mature and a safe induction is possible. Severe preeclampsia requires delivery regardless of gestational age. For the fetus younger than 34 weeks, the use of antihypertensives may control symptoms long enough for the mother to receive two doses of betamethasone, which accelerates fetal lung maturation (Cunningham et al. 1993).

Table 21–2

LABORATORY CHANGES ASSOCIATED WITH PREECLAMPSIA

TEST	MILD	SEVERE
Blood pressure	130–140 / 86–95 or ↑ 30 systolic / ↑ 15 diastolic	≥160/110
BUN	10 mg	>20 mg
Creatinine	1 mg	>1.6 mg
Uric acid	4.5	>6
Protein, urine	0.3 g/L in 24 hr	5 g/L or more in 24 hr
Platelets	Normal	<100,000
Clotting factors	Unchanged	Normal or decreased
SGOT and SGPT*	Unchanged	Normal or increased
Bilirubin	Unchanged	Normal or increased

*SGOT, serum glutamic-oxaloacetic transaminase; SGPT, serum glutamic-pyruvic transaminase.

Nursing Process

▼ Assessment

The nurse makes an initial assessment of a woman's risk of developing preeclampsia and is then alert to subsequent symptoms of the disease. The standard prenatal visit schedule with more frequent visits near term has evolved precisely to improve early diagnosis of preeclampsia. Symptoms related to preeclampsia, such as headache, epigastric pain, and visual changes, can be confused with normal symptoms of pregnancy. The nurse can assess a complaint of headache by asking whether it is relieved with rest or an over-the-counter medication, in which case it is not likely to be due to CNS dysfunction. Epigastric pain in normal pregnancy can occur for many reasons: heartburn, pressure on the diaphragm of a fetal part, or rib separation. Epigastric pain in preeclampsia is due to an enlarged liver pressing on the liver capsule. This symptom is a late one in the development of preeclampsia, and once the pain develops it is typically constant and unrelieved by activity or food intake. A nurse who needs to assess the size of the liver must do so cautiously, since palpation may cause the liver capsule to rupture. Visual changes are often difficult for a pregnant woman to characterize. Frequently, asking the woman, "Have you had any blurred vision or spots in front of your eyes?" elicits a positive response. Normal, healthy women frequently report spots before their eyes, but on closer questioning this is related to rapid position changes that cause momentary postural hypotension and hence some visual disturbance. However, these visual changes are of short duration, unlike those associated with preeclampsia, which are caused by increasing central nervous dysfunction.

Another nursing assessment for signs of preeclampsia is difficulty in distinguishing physiologic from pathologic edema. Late in pregnancy, almost all women develop dependent ankle edema. However, pathologic edema of preeclampsia usually does not resolve after lying down as does physiologic edema. In addition, edema associated with preeclampsia occurs in nondependent areas such as the abdomen and particularly the face. A more objective measure of abnormal edema is rapid weight gain. A woman who gains more than 2 pounds in a week should be questioned about her recent nutritional intake. In the absence of increased intake, a careful assessment of other signs and symptoms of preeclampsia should be undertaken.

Since the diagnosis of preeclampsia and classification of its severity are based on blood pressure, it is important that measurements are standardized and accurate. The size of the cuff should be appropriate for the woman's arm. A small cuff on a large woman gives a falsely elevated reading. In the ambulatory setting, it is generally recommended that women have their blood pressures taken in the sitting position with the right arm roughly horizontal at the level of the heart. This measurement is practical as well as accurate in that it gives the blood pressure the woman would experience during the day in her normal daily activities. The diastolic pressure should be taken with both Korotkoff phase IV (muffling sound) and phase V (disappearance of sound) recorded. Diagnosis of preeclampsia should be based on the phase IV sound, since there is a large deviation of the phase V sound in pregnancy related to the blood volume changes (Surratt 1993).

The assessment of proteinuria can also be affected by several factors. If there is some question of the presence of proteinuria, a woman may be instructed to obtain a first-voided morning specimen for testing, since this concentration is most likely to pick up proteinuria. Strips used to test for the presence of protein in the urine can give a false-positive result if the urine contains blood or vaginal secretions (especially those associated with a vaginal infection) or in the presence of a urinary tract infection. If proteinuria is detected in a routine urine specimen, the test should be repeated with a very good clean catch midstream specimen. A urinalysis should be performed to rule out causes of the proteinuria other than kidney dysfunction. The nurse may have to instruct some women with proteinuria in collecting a 24-hour specimen that may be ordered to quantitate the amount of protein they are spilling in 24 hours.

Since preeclampsia causes vasospasm and therefore can affect uteroplacental perfusion, assessment of fetal growth and well-being is crucial for a woman with preeclampsia or chronic hypertension. The nurse's role in this assessment may lie in recording uterine fundal heights.

▼ Diagnosis

On the basis of an assessment that includes the client's history, physical examination, and laboratory findings, the following diagnoses are suggested:

- Risk for maternal injury related to decreased circulating volume, altered renal perfusion, and risk of eclamptic seizure in the presence of elevated blood pressure and vasoconstriction
- Risk for fetal injury related to altered uteroplacental perfusion and increased risk of placental abruption
- Knowledge deficit: lack of information related to preeclampsia and its treatment
- Fear related to maternal and fetal risks and the potential for injury
- Ineffective individual or family coping related to the presence of high-risk pregnancy

▼ Planning

The plan of care that is chosen for the woman experiencing preeclampsia might include the following outcome goals:

- The woman will not develop eclampsia and will give birth with no complications or adverse outcome
- The fetus will not experience distress and will be delivered with no adverse outcome
- The woman will verbally explain preeclampsia and the essential components of her treatment
- The woman will express her fears related to the risks of preeclampsia
- The woman and her family will demonstrate effective coping related to the high-risk pregnancy

▼ Intervention

▼ CARE OF WOMEN WITH MILD PREECLAMPSIA

Unfortunately, there is no primary prevention of preeclampsia, since the cause is unknown. Therefore, the nursing goals are early detection and successful delivery of a healthy mother and infant. Diet may play an important role in preeclampsia, although studies of zinc and magnesium deficiencies have cast doubt on the role these two minerals play (Newman and Fullerton 1990; Repke 1991). Several randomized studies have shown that increased calcium intake (1500 mg per day) may prevent preeclampsia and decrease the incidence of premature delivery and low birth weight (Belizan et al. 1991; Repke 1991). A nurse can obtain an accurate diet history and suggest dietary changes to women who have low calcium intakes. This intervention may be particularly necessary for teenagers who are at increased risk for preeclampsia and who also have increased calcium requirements (Newman et al. 1993). Women with preeclampsia should maintain a moderate salt intake (not greater than 6 g per day). Excessively salty foods should be avoided. In addition, increased water intake is important to maintain blood volume and uterine and kidney perfusion. Since the capillaries are leaking, causing fluid to move from the intravascular to the extravascular space, there is a decrease in blood volume evidenced by an increasing hematocrit as a result of this hemoconcentration. High-protein diets have been recommended in the past, although no randomized studies of their usefulness have been done. In fact, high-protein diets may be detrimental, since the increased osmolality could worsen capillary damage in the kidneys.

All women nearing the end of their second trimester should be educated about the signs and symptoms of preeclampsia and encouraged to call their health care provider if they experience any of the symptoms. Women who develop blood pressure elevations or mild preeclampsia may be advised to be on bed rest to prevent worsening of their disease. The nurse needs to educate women with preeclampsia about the disease in terms of its multiorgan manifestations and its potential consequences for mother and baby. A clear understanding of potential consequences and the plan of management, which is usually for delivery when the fetus is mature and a safe induction is possible, aids the woman in complying with the bed rest regimen. The nurse can prepare the woman for an amniocentesis if preeclampsia occurs before 37 weeks.

Since the vasospasm resulting from preeclampsia can affect uteroplacental perfusion and fetal oxygenation, monitoring fetal well-being is essential. One method for monitoring fetal well-being is fetal movement counting (FMC). FMC provides the mother with a simple, daily method for monitoring her fetus's well-being and includes her as an essential partner in the management of her condition. The nurse can also encourage compliance with other fetal monitoring such as nonstress or contraction stress tests, biophysical profiles, and serial ultrasound examinations for fetal growth.

Women with preeclampsia and their families need to be supported as they deal with the loss of the ideal healthy pregnancy. Bed rest is potentially disruptive to family routines and can contribute to a loss of income for women who had not planned to stop working as early as their bed rest regimen dictates. The woman and her partner may have to alter their birth plans, especially if such plans included delivery at an out-of-hospital birth site. A hospital birth is required, since women with preeclampsia need to have intravenous access, magnesium sulfate, and continuous fetal monitoring. Magnesium sulfate is given to prevent seizures.

▼ CARE OF WOMEN HOSPITALIZED WITH PREECLAMPSIA

Women with severe preeclampsia need to be hospitalized, for the nursing care can be intensive (Keening 1992; Surratt 1993). Women with severe preeclampsia are maintained on strict bed rest in the lateral position but may have bathroom privileges. Generally, the room is kept semidark and other environmental stimuli such as visitors and a ringing phone are kept at a minimum to avoid stimulating the CNS and causing an eclamptic seizure. Seizure precautions must be taken. These precautions include side rails that are kept up and padded if needed, easy access to an airway protector, and a padded tongue blade. Frequently, diazepam (Valium) is kept at the bedside in case of a seizure. Oxygen therapy may be used if maternal respiratory status is compromised or an abnormal fetal heart rate tracing is noted.

A woman with severe preeclampsia requires frequent monitoring of her vital signs. Blood pressure, pulse, and respirations are monitored every 2 to 4 hours. Temperature is usually recorded every 4 to 8 hours unless it is elevated. The nurse should monitor for signs of worsening disease by auscultating the woman's lungs, assessing edema, checking reflexes for clonus, and asking about headache, visual changes, and epigastric pain when she checks the blood pressure. Edema is assessed by taking daily weights and palpating over bony areas of the face, arms, hands, legs, and feet for pitting edema. Assessment of biceps and patellar deep tendon reflexes (DTRs) should be made regularly. Clonus, a hyperactive rhythmic jerking response, is assessed at the ankle joint. Refer to Procedure 21–1, which describes the assessment of pitting edema, deep tendon reflexes, and clonus.

The fetal heart rate is assessed every 4 hours by either auscultation or electronic monitor. If an abnormal pattern is suspected, a continuous monitor strip should be obtained. During labor, all women with preeclampsia need continuous fetal monitoring. Kidney function is monitored by intake and output on every shift. If there is a question of adequate kidney function, an indwelling Foley catheter is used. Output should be greater than 30 mL per hour or 700 mL every 24 hours. Proteinuria should be checked at every void or every 1 to 2 hours if a Foley catheter is in place. Specific gravity should be measured at the same time; readings greater than 1.040 are indicative of proteinuria or oliguria.

Women with preeclampsia who are to be delivered are given magnesium sulfate ($MgSO_4$). Generally, $MgSO_4$ is given intravenously as a 4- to 6-g bolus over 15 minutes and then as a 1- to 3-g continuous infusion that is maintained until 24 hours postpartum. Possible side effects of the $MgSO_4$ are flushing, nausea, drowsiness, and feeling "thick." Respirations are monitored closely, since magnesium levels above 8 to 10 mEq/L can cause respiratory depression. Typically, DTRs are lost at magnesium levels of 4 to 6 mEq/L. Another medication commonly administered is hydralazine to control blood pressures higher than 160/110. Blood pressure must be monitored after administration of hydralazine since a rapid drop could result in decreased uteroplacental perfusion and fetal distress.

Women with severe preeclampsia may need to have invasive hemodynamic monitoring of either central venous pressure (CVP) or pulmonary wedge pressure using a Swan-Ganz catheter. Those who develop pulmonary edema require supplemental oxygen and frequent blood gas determinations.

During labor, special consideration must be given to the analgesia and anesthesia options. A woman with severe preeclampsia that includes clotting abnormalities may not be a candidate for conduction anesthesia. However, pain and increased catecholamines may adversely affect the woman's condition. Pain management must include input from the nurse, the anesthesiologist, and the physician managing the labor.

A woman who has an eclamptic seizure is in grave danger, as is her baby. During the seizure, the nurse can make sure the environment is as safe as possible and, if possible, insert an airway protector. After the seizure, maintaining a patent airway and giving oxygen resuscitate the mother and fetus. The left lateral position further aids fetal recovery. Fetal status should be followed with continuous electronic monitoring. Postseizure prophylactic magnesium sulfate is administered if it is not already being infused; other anticonvulsants are given if $MgSO_4$ was already being infused. Postseizure assessments include careful monitoring for pulmonary edema and circulatory and kidney failure, and neurologic checks for signs of cerebral hemorrhage. In addition, frequent checks should be made for vaginal bleeding from an abrupted placenta. When the woman is stable, a delivery plan is made. The best overall results are obtained if the baby is delivered vaginally (Moore et al. 1992). If a cesarean delivery is necessary, clotting abnormalities should be corrected before surgery with adequate crossmatched blood.

▼ Evaluation

Evaluation of the plan of care for the woman with preeclampsia is critical and continuous. It is based on the measurable outcome goals that were identified and may continually be revised. Evaluation criteria might include such factors as the adverse effects experienced by the woman, the status of the fetus and condition of the newborn, the woman's understanding of her illness and its treatment and her verbalization of her fears, and the family's effective coping with the stress of the high-risk pregnancy.

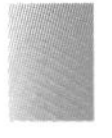

Rh Isoimmunization and ABO Incompatibility

DESCRIPTION

Rh isoimmunization (sensitization) can occur when an Rh-negative mother becomes pregnant with a fetus who is Rh positive. This occurrence is common since 85 to 99 percent of the male population is Rh positive. The classification Rh negative indicates the absence of the Rh_0(D) antigen on the red blood cells; Rh positive indicates the presence of the Rh_0(D) antigen on the red blood cells. During the pregnancy or at delivery, some of the baby's Rh-positive blood can enter the maternal circulation (fetal-maternal hemorrhage). The Rh-negative mother's immune system responds by producing antibodies, since she lacks a means of identifying the Rh_0(D) antigen. The primary response to exposure takes place over several weeks or months with the development of gamma M immunoglobulin (IgM) and the mother becomes isoimmunized. Once this has occurred, the response to a second exposure to the Rh_0(D) antigen, as might occur in a subsequent pregnancy, is the production of anti-Rh_0(D) antibodies. This secondary response is stronger and more rapid, taking place over only a few days. The anti-Rh_0(D) antibodies cross the placenta and enter the fetal circulation. If the fetus has the Rh_0(D) antigen (i.e., is Rh positive), the antibodies attack the fetus's red blood cells, causing hemolysis. The degree of hemolysis varies depending on the amount of the original Rh-positive infusion into the mother, her antibody response, and the gestational age of the fetus in this pregnancy (Fig. 21–6). The hemolysis leads to fetal anemia. If it is not treated, the fetus can develop marked edema (hydrops fetalis), hyperbilirubinemia (icterus gravis), congestive heart failure, and neurologic damage (kernicterus).

A less common way for an Rh-negative mother to develop antibodies is described by the "grandmother" theory. That is, when the Rh-negative mother was herself a fetus, she may have received enough Rh-positive cells from her mother in utero or at delivery to develop anti-Rh_0(D) antibodies (Creasy and Resnik 1994). A third means of sensitization is through blood transfusion. If an Rh-negative woman receives Rh-positive blood, she may develop anti-Rh_0(D) antibodies.

Any time an Rh-negative woman becomes pregnant by an Rh-positive partner she is at risk of carrying an Rh-positive baby and thereby at risk of becoming sensitized. Delivery is the principal event that results in an exchange of blood. Antenatal sensitization occurs in only 1 to 2 percent of all pregnancies (American College of Obstetricians and Gynecologists [ACOG] 1990). A majority of these sensitizations occur during the third trimester but they can occur as early as the first trimester. Obstetric risk factors associated with sensitization include first- or second-trimester abortion, ectopic pregnancy, chorionic villus sampling, amniocentesis, breech version, placenta previa or abruptio placentae, vaginal delivery, cesarean section, and manual removal of placenta.

It should be noted that many other blood antigens can trigger the development of antibodies. As the incidence of Rh isoimmunization decreases with the use of Rh_0(D) Immune Globulin (RhIG), these antibodies are increasing as major causes of isoimmunization. Immunoglobulin G (IgG) is one of the humoral antibodies that crosses the placenta and can cause hemolytic disease of the newborn (HDN) with varying degrees of severity. The most common antigens that can cause an immune response leading to HDN besides the D antigen [Rh_0(D)] are A, B, C, E, Kell, Kidd, and Duffy.

Another type of isoimmunization is called ABO incompatibility. This is much more common than Rh incompatibility and does not pose the same degree of threat to the fetus. Usually ABO incompatibility is seen most often with women who have type O blood who are carrying a fetus with type A or B blood. An incompatibility can occur if the woman has developed anti-A or anti-B antibodies that trigger an interaction with the antigen sites on the fetal red blood cells. It is not unusual for a woman to have developed these antibodies, for they are present in food or arise on exposure to infection by gram-negative bacteria. Hemolysis of the fetal red blood cells can occur when the ma-

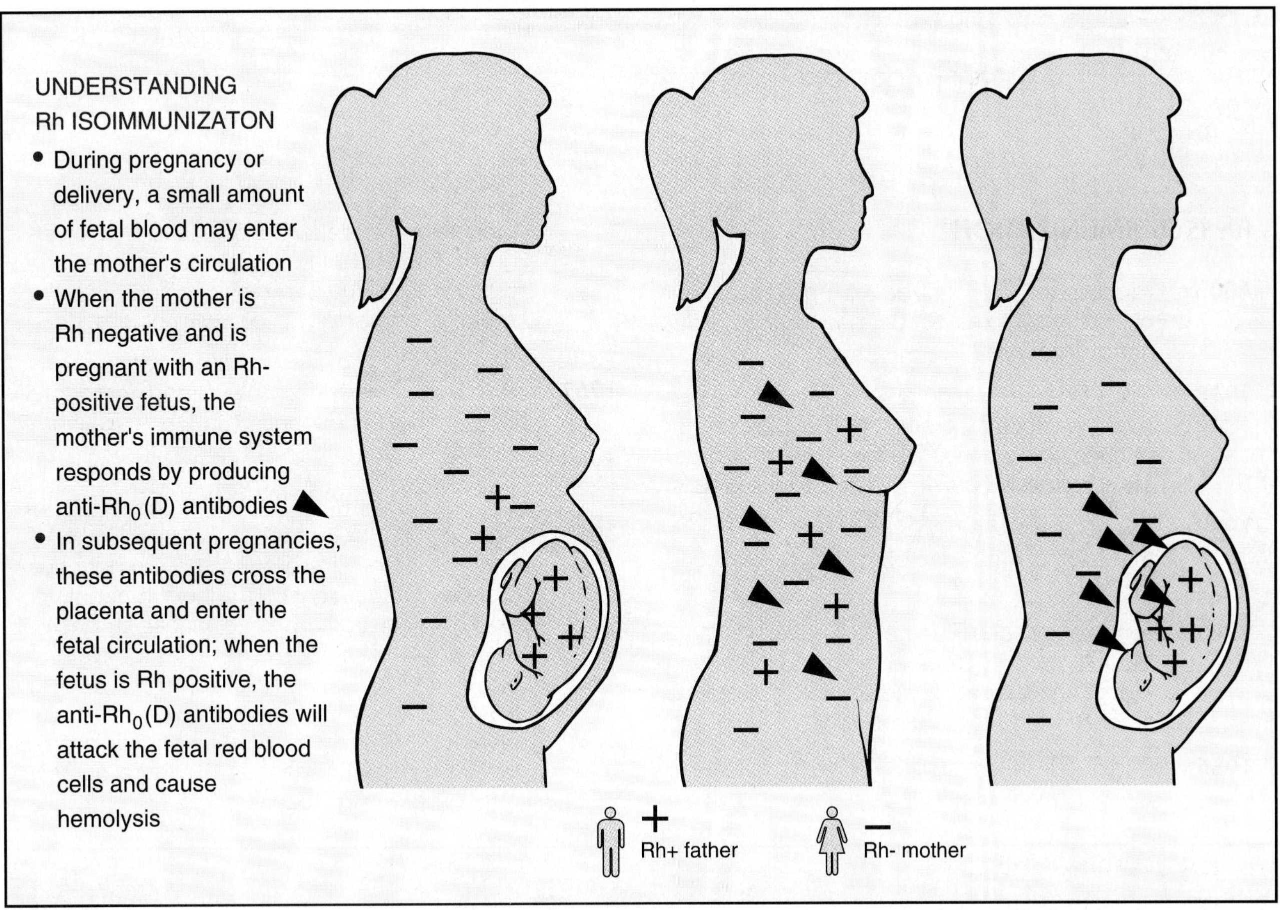

Figure 21–6

If a primiparous Rh-negative woman has an Rh-positive partner, it is likely that her fetus will be Rh positive; during the pregnancy or birth, the expectant mother may become sensitized through exposure to a small amount of fetal blood.

ternal antibodies cross the placenta. Unlike Rh incompatibility, ABO incompatibility affects the first infant; however, treatment is not necessary in the antepartal period. Caregivers should be alert to the possibility of ABO incompatibility at the time of labor and birth, so that the newborn can be watched carefully for the development of hyperbilirubinemia.

MANAGEMENT

Management of Rh isoimmunization begins in the antepartal period. The potential for sensitization is identified by testing the Rh-negative woman's blood type, Rh factor, and antibody titer (indirect Coombs test) at the first prenatal visit. If the woman is not sensitized initially, she should be retested at 28 weeks of gestation (ACOG 1990). If the woman shows evidence of maternal sensitization, her pregnancy is high risk and close fetal monitoring is begun at once. The presence of the anti-Rh_0(D) antibody in maternal serum indicates that sensitization has occurred. After identification, a titer level is obtained and followed at regular intervals (every 2 to 4 weeks in the second trimester and biweekly in the third trimester). If the titer remains at 1:8 or less, the fetus is at low risk of developing hemolytic disease in utero and management is similar to that in a normal pregnancy. If the titer is above 1:8, ultrasonography, amniocentesis, and percutaneous umbilical cord blood sampling (PUBS) are used to monitor the fetal status. Amniotic fluid obtained by amniocentesis is examined for the presence and amount of bilirubin, which is a by-product of hemolysis. This assessment examines the optical density at 450 nm (ΔOD_{450}) of the fluid, which is plotted on a graph called a Liley curve. This curve classifies the hemolysis into three zones. Zone I indicates mild disease, and these fetuses are followed with monthly amniocenteses. Zone II is indicative of moderate disease, and management is dependent on the fetus's gestational age. Zone III indicates severe disease, which requires treatment immediately. Testing also includes serial ultrasound evaluations (to monitor fetal growth and rule out anomalies), assessment of fetal activity (fetal

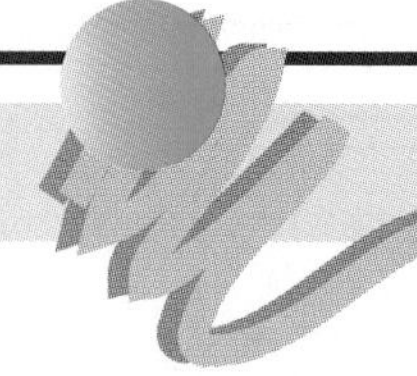

HISTORICAL PERSPECTIVES

Rh ISOIMMUNIZATION

400 BC Hippocrates recognized a disease that caused newborns to be anemic and edematous and die.

1938 Edith Darrow, a mother of several isoimmunized newborns, proposed the theory that antihemoglobin was passed from mother to fetus, causing hemolysis of red blood cells.

1939 Levine and Stetson identified hemolytic disease of the newborn as an immune problem.

1940 Landsteiner and Weiner identified a new blood factor capable of agglutinating blood; they called it rhesus factor after the monkey blood they had examined.

1956 Beginning with Bevis (1956), Walker (1957), and Liley (1961), it was discovered that the delta optical density analysis of the fluid (ΔOD at 450 nm) quantified the amount of bilirubin in amniotic fluid with the severity of hemolytic disease of the newborn (HDN).

1967 Freda, Gorman, and Pollack produced Rh_0(D) Immune Globulin (RhIG).

1968 Rh_0(D) Immune Globulin (RhIG) was licensed under the name RhoGAM.

1995 Injection of RhIG was an accepted component of high-risk care of the Rh-negative woman; it was given to the Rh-negative, unsensitized woman at 28 weeks of gestation and within 72 hours after delivery if her baby was Rh positive; it was also given after an abortion, ectopic pregnancy, amniocentesis, chorionic villus sampling procedure, or any incident of exposure risk occurring before 28 weeks of gestation.

movement counts), heart rate monitoring to assess fetal well-being, and a repeated amniocentesis or PUBS.

Treatment for severe hemolytic disease (zone III) consists of delivery at the earliest possible time or fetal transfusion in utero, since severe fetal anemia can initiate cardiac output failure and fetal hydrops (Knuppel and Drukker 1993; Vomund and Witter 1994). Fetal transfusion is accomplished with ultrasound guidance. A needle is inserted either intravascularly into the umbilical cord through PUBS or into the fetal peritoneal cavity. A fetal hematocrit is obtained and then an appropriate amount of irradiated Rh-negative packed red blood cells (PRBCs) is infused. This procedure involves certain risks for the fetus: fetal distress, infection, fetal-maternal hemorrhage, trauma to internal organs, and death. If hydrops is present, cardiac medications may also be administered in utero if the chance of extrauterine survival is poor. Delivery is undertaken when the risk of fetal demise is greater in utero than if the baby were delivered. Factors in this decision include general fetal well-being and fetal lung maturity. Neonatal treatment of an infant with HDN is dependent on the severity of the hemolysis but may include exchange transfusions, ultraviolet therapy, and circulatory support.

Rh_0(D) Immune Globulin

The primary goal of management of Rh isoimmunization at the time of birth is to prevent any initial sensitization through the use of RhIG. There are several trade names for RhIG, including RhoGAM, Gamulin Rh, HypRho-D, WinRho SD, and Rhesonate. RhIG provides passive immunity by coating any fetal Rh-positive cells as they enter the maternal circulation. This coating prevents the maternal immune system from identifying the cells as foreign, thereby preventing antibody formation. The correct dosage of RhIG is determined by the Kleihauer-Betke laboratory test, which quantifies the amount of fetal-maternal hemorrhage (FMH). One unit of RhIG (300 μg) neutralizes 30 mL of fetal whole blood or 15 mL of fetal red blood cells. For most vaginal deliveries, this amount is more than sufficient. If the amount of fetal blood entering the maternal circulation exceeds this, more RhIG is necessary to prevent an antibody response. Only one half of all spontaneous deliveries result in FMH. Less than 0.5 percent of vaginal deliveries have an FMH greater than 30 mL. Other obstetric events associated with greater FMHs requiring more than one unit of RhIG are cesarean birth, manual removal of the placenta, breech extraction, stillbirth, and pla-

PROCEDURE 21-2

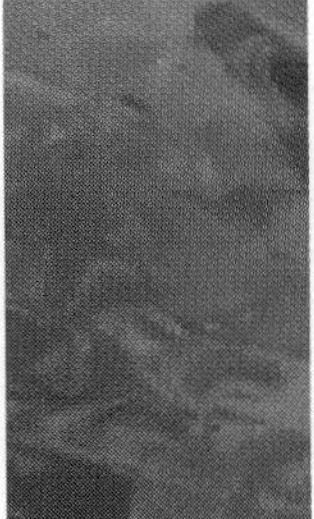

Administration of Rh_0(D) Immune Globulin (RhoGAM or Mic-RhoGAM) and Other Blood Products

▼ PURPOSE

Administration of Rh_0(D) Immune Globulin (RhIG) is indicated to prevent an Rh-negative mother from developing antibodies to the red blood cells of an Rh-positive fetus. Administration of blood products replaces fluid and blood lost after a maternal hemorrhage.

▼ EQUIPMENT

- Requisition slip for blood
- Blood product
- Blood administration set with filter
- Intravenous (IV) bag of normal saline
- Patent IV site with a large-gauge catheter
- Blood documentation form
- Gloves
- Patient's chart
- Thermometer and sphygmomanometer
- Pressure bag
- Vial of RhIG
- Diluent
- Syringe with needle
- Alcohol pad

Rh_0(D) Immune Globulin Administration

1 Review mother's and baby's charts to identify whether RhIG should be administered. **Administration of RhIG (currently available as RhoGAM, 300 μg dose, and as Mic-RhoGAM, 50 μg dose) is indicated when it is known or suspected that fetal red blood cells have entered the circulation of an Rh-negative, unsensitized mother. This can occur during pregnancy or delivery, during amniocentesis or chorionic villus sampling procedures, during an abortion, during fetal surgery, or after an incident of abdominal trauma such as a fall or motor vehicle accident. The Rh-negative, unsensitized mother should receive an RhIG injection under any of the following circumstances:**

- **After an incident of exposure risk that occurs before 28 weeks' gestation**
- **At 28 weeks' gestation (prophylactic administration)**
- **Within 72 hours of delivery if her baby is Rh positive**

A negative indirect Coombs test provides evidence that sensitization of the mother has not already occurred.

2 Provide the woman with a complete explanation of the procedure, its purpose, and its effect on future pregnancies and blood transfusions. Determine that the woman has had no previous adverse reactions to preparations of immune globulin. If required by hospital protocol, have the woman sign a consent form. **Understanding the reason for the procedure helps ease the patient's anxiety. Understanding the importance of taking immune globulin with each pregnancy can affect the type of care the woman seeks in future pregnancies. Identifying previous reactions enables the nurse to inform the physician of adverse reactions to an immune globulin preparation. A signed consent form indicates that the woman acknowledges she has been informed of the risk.**

3 Obtain correct preparation and dosage of RhIG, which is usually stored in the blood bank or pharmacy. Confirm lot number, crossmatch, and patient's identity before administration. **Verifying that the blood product is correct for the patient before its administration is essential to decreasing the occurrence of adverse reactions.**

Continued on following page

PROCEDURE 21–2 Continued

4 Administer injection intramuscularly within 72 hours of exposure risk. If administering a minidose (usually 50 μg), use the deltoid muscle; if administering a full dose (usually 300 μg), use the gluteus maximus muscle or other deep muscle site. **The maximum amount of time from exposure to successful immunization that has been established is 72 hours.**

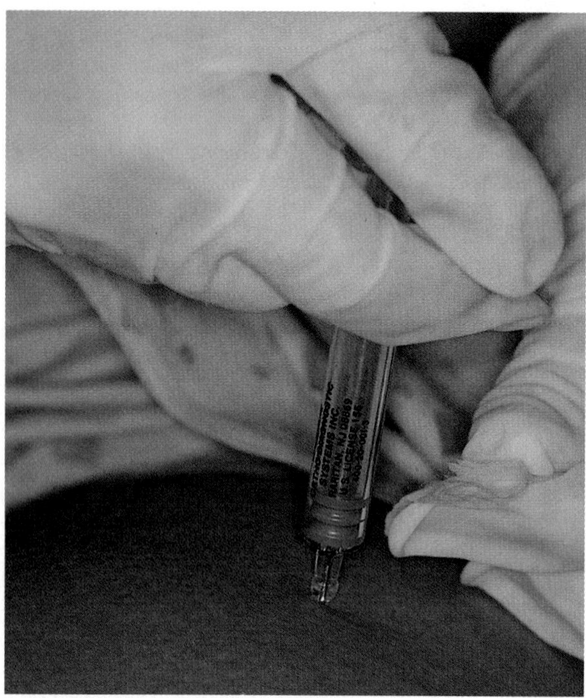

5 Record procedure according to hospital protocol. **Recording procedure provides written documentation in a permanent, legal record that RhIG was given.**

Blood Product Administration

1 Obtain patient's transfusion history and explain procedure. Instruct patient regarding the symptoms of an adverse reaction and the importance of reporting these symptoms. Have patient sign a consent form if required before the transfusion. **An explanation of the procedure and expected sensations helps ease the patient's anxiety. Inform the physician if patient has a history of an adverse reaction to a blood transfusion. A signed consent form indicates that the patient acknowledges having been informed of the risk.**

2 Select or start an IV infusion with a large-gauge catheter, such as an 18-gauge catheter for an adult. **A catheter smaller than 18 gauge can hemolyze RBCs.**

3 Obtain blood product from the blood bank just before use by following hospital protocol. **Strict guidelines regarding this step vary among institutions. Unopened blood products kept at room temperature for more than 30 minutes usually may not be returned to the blood bank because they are potentially unsafe.**

4 Identify the blood product and the patient with another registered nurse. To do this:

- Compare the name and identification number on the patient's wristband with the name and number on the blood bag and order slip.
- Double-check the patient's blood group and Rh type, the donor's blood group and Rh type, unit serial number, the bag's expiration date, and the type and number of blood components ordered.
- Inspect the bag for air bubbles, leaks, and discoloration.

Adverse reactions to blood transfusions often result from failure to identify the blood product or the patient properly.

5 Take baseline vital signs. **A deviation from the baseline assessment can indicate a transfusion reaction.**

6 Prime the Y-type filtered blood administration tubing with normal saline solution. Never add medications to the blood or blood tubing. Wearing gloves, insert the spike of the administration set straight into the port of the blood bag. **Dextrose solutions cause hemolysis of the RBCs, and lactated Ringer solution, which has calcium, could cause clotting. Keeping the blood and blood tubing free of medications helps prevent confusion over the cause of any transfusion reactions that might occur. Inserting the spike straight into the port allows the blood to flow freely from the bag.**

Continued on facing page

PROCEDURE 21–2 Continued

7 Start the transfusion slowly (approximately 2 mL/min). Fill the filter with blood, and monitor the patient closely for the first 15 minutes of the transfusion. Observe for chills, flushing, low back pain, itching, dyspnea, rash, hives, and other signs of a transfusion reaction. **If the patient has an adverse reaction, only a small amount of the blood product will have infused. If a reaction occurs, stop the infusion, keep the vein open with normal saline, and call the physician and blood bank. Follow hospital protocol.**

8 If the patient has no adverse reaction within the first 15 minutes, increase the rate to what the physician ordered. Ideally, the blood should be transfused in 2 hours. Continue to monitor the patient and take vital signs at least every 30 minutes. **Red blood cells begin to deteriorate after 2 hours at room temperature. A pressure bag around the blood bag may help maintain the prescribed rate. Monitoring the patient throughout the transfusion is necessary because adverse reactions can be slow and subtle.**

9 When the transfusion is complete, flush the IV line with normal saline. If another unit is ordered, follow the same procedure, omitting steps 1 and 2. **Using a new blood administration set with each unit of blood ordered helps prevent confusion over the cause of any transfusion reactions that might occur. A new blood administration set also allows blood products to transfuse more quickly because of the new filter in the tubing.**

10 Complete the following required paperwork:
- Signatures of the two persons who identified the blood product and the patient
- The blood product administered
- Patient's baseline vital signs
- Time the transfusion was started and time it was completed
- Total volume of fluid transfused
- Patient's response to the transfusion
- Any nursing action taken in response to an adverse reaction

Written documentation of the procedure becomes part of the patient's permanent record and can be referred to in case of questions.

centa previa or abruptio placentae (Knuppel and Drukker 1993).

Ideally, RhIG should be given to the mother as soon after delivery as possible once the blood type of the baby is known (Procedure 21–2). The maximum amount of time from exposure to successful immunization that has been tested is 72 hours. However, some experts believe that later administration may be effective and RhIG should be given upon identification of a potential sensitization even beyond the 72-hour limit (Knuppel and Drukker 1993). This strategy of immediate postpartum immunization has decreased the incidence of HDN in future pregnancies by 70 percent. However, some women may still become sensitized.

Sensitization occurs because women do not receive RhIG after delivery, the amount they receive is insufficient, or they become sensitized antenatally. Surveys have shown postpartum administration to be nearly 100 percent. Utilization after spontaneous abortions is 81 percent and after induced abortions ranges from 51 to 96 percent. Administration is poorest after ectopic pregnancy (36 percent) and transfusion with Rh-positive blood (52 percent) (Creasy and Resnik 1994). The amount administered is not adequate to provide protection 10 to 15 percent of the time. After administration, maternal blood can be tested for the presence of Rh-positive cells, and more RhIG can be given if these cells are present. It is recommended that this testing be done after procedures involving a high risk of FMH as listed earlier. Since most antenatal sensitization occurs in the third trimester and RhIG is effective up to 12 weeks after injection, prophylactic administration at 28 weeks of gestation is recommended. The recommended doses for obstetric events warranting treatment include (ACOG 1990):

- Rh_0(D) Immune Globulin, 50 μg minidose for first-trimester abortion, ectopic pregnancy, chorionic villus sampling
- Rh_0(D) Immune Globulin, 300 μg full dose for amniocentesis, second-trimester abortion, 28-week prophylaxis, version, trauma, fetomaternal hemorrhage, postpartum

Nursing Process

▼ Assessment

The nurse has an important role in the prevention of Rh isoimmunization. It is the nurse who can alert the primary care provider that the woman being treated is Rh negative. This is particularly true in emergency situations such as a ruptured ectopic pregnancy or severe hemorrhage caused by trauma when type-specific blood is unavailable. When the immediate focus of care is on lifesaving measures, quality-of-life issues may assume lesser importance. However, once the woman in her childbearing years is stabilized, it is important to discover her blood type and administer RhIG if appropriate.

The nurse should determine a woman's blood Rh and type at the initial prenatal visit. If she is Rh negative, the nurse can inquire whether the woman knows the blood Rh and type of the baby's father. If she does not know his blood Rh and type, she may choose to have him tested. If the father is Rh negative, their baby will also be Rh negative and is not at risk for Rh isoimmunization. If he is Rh positive, the woman's chart should be prominently marked with her Rh status. The nurse should also elicit any history of blood transfusions. A positive history puts even Rh-positive women at risk for having antibodies that can cause HDN.

▼ Diagnosis

On the basis of an assessment that includes the client's history, physical examination, and laboratory findings, the following diagnoses are suggested:

- Risk for maternal or fetal injury related to Rh isoimmunization causing maternal antibody production and fetal compromise
- Knowledge deficit: lack of information related to blood type incompatibility and the potential for isoimmunization
- Risk of altered parent-infant-child attachment related to fear of fetal loss

▼ Planning

The plan of care that is chosen for the woman experiencing Rh isoimmunization might include the following outcome goals:

- The fetus will be safely delivered with no complications related to Rh isoimmunization
- The woman will verbalize her understanding of the Rh isoimmunization and its potential effects on her fetus
- The woman will demonstrate appropriate interaction and caregiving with her newborn

▼ Intervention

Education is an essential component of the nursing care for the woman with Rh isoimmunization. It is important for the Rh-negative woman to understand how she can make antibodies and how these antibodies can affect her fetus. Such an understanding heightens her awareness of the necessity for prophylactic administration of RhIG.

The nurse is responsible for ensuring that an Rh-negative woman receives a prophylactic injection of RhIG after procedures such as amniocentesis and breech version (see recommended doses, p. 657). Before RhIG administration at 28 weeks, an antibody screen should be obtained to rule out occurrence of isoimmunization since the initial screen. If her antibody screen is positive for anti-Rh_0(D) antibodies, the woman should not receive RhIG, since it will not modulate her antibody response and will interfere with accurate interpretation of her antibody titers.

In the high-risk isoimmunized pregnancy, the nurse must be familiar with the procedures for fetal surveillance and interventions. These procedures include serial ultrasound examinations to assess the fetal heart and check for fetal ascites, amniocentesis to obtain fluid for ΔOD_{450}, PUBS to assess fetal hemoglobin levels and to transfuse RBCs, and possible intraperitoneal fetal transfusion (Creasy and Resnik 1994). The nursing role entails not only carrying out certain management orders but being able to educate the woman and her family about what to expect during each procedure and provide any postprocedure instructions. After all these procedures except ultrasonography, the woman is at risk for infection and fetal or placental bleeding resulting in a fetal demise. The woman should be instructed to report any elevated temperature, abdominal pain, or change in fetal movements immediately. Women should start daily fetal movement counts at 28 weeks in order to become familiar with their fetus's daily activity pattern.

Nurses must anticipate delayed initiation and development of maternal-infant interactions as in other high-risk pregnancies, especially if a woman has experienced previous perinatal losses as a result of her condition. The nurse can provide emotional support and acceptance of ambivalent feelings. In addition, positive reinforcement of cooperation with invasive, time-consuming procedures may enable a woman to continue to comply with a difficult medical regimen.

Intrapartum management may include induction of labor for fetal indications. If an induction is being attempted without a ripe cervix, the woman may experience a long labor and need a great deal of supportive nursing. Fetal status requires continuous fetal heart rate monitoring. If the fetus's health is in jeopardy, the woman may require a cesarean delivery, which she may have to deal with psychologically.

It is likely that parents will be separated from their infant after delivery, since these infants require intensive care support. The nurse can facilitate communication with parents about the baby's condition and arrange visits to the intensive care unit as early as possible. Also, encouraging the initiation of the lactation process with the use of a breast pump is a positive step a mother can take to contribute to her infant's well-being.

▼ Evaluation

The evaluation of the plan of care for the woman with Rh isoimmunization is based on the measurable goals that were identified. Her care is successful if the infant is delivered without adverse consequences, the woman understands her medical complication and its risks, and she demonstrates appropriate interaction and caregiving with her infant after birth.

Preterm Labor

DESCRIPTION

Preterm births are the major cause of neonatal morbidity and mortality and cause untold anguish for parents and siblings. Approximately 6 to 13 percent of births in the United States are preterm, and the rate varies widely with age and ethnicity, with African-Americans having a rate as high as 13 percent and whites a rate of 5.6 percent (Arnold 1992). The sequelae of preterm labor and birth are responsible for 75 to 90 percent of total neonatal deaths, excluding those caused by lethal congenital malformations. Preterm birth also results in a large proportion of short- and long-term neonatal morbidity. Preterm infants generate $2.5 billion per year in immediate neonatal intensive care costs and another $400,000 in long-term costs per handicapped survivor. If one third of these preterm births could be prevented, prenatal care for 1.3 million women ($600 per woman) could be provided. Ability to prevent or at least stop preterm labor (PTL) would result in greatly improved neonatal health measures (Creasy and Resnik 1994).

The causes of preterm delivery (PTD), which is defined as birth before 36 to 37 completed weeks of gestation, fall into three categories: (1) spontaneous preterm labor with intact membranes, (2) preterm premature rupture of the membranes (PPROM), and (3) elective preterm delivery for indicated maternal or fetal reasons. Generally, each category accounts for one third of the preterm delivery rate, although this proportion may vary by population.

Reasons for spontaneous preterm labor include maternal infection, trauma, and disease. Infections outside the uterus (most commonly urinary tract infections) are thought to cause preterm labor by a mechanism involving the production of interleukins and tumor necrosis factor by maternal macrophages, which trigger the reduction of prostaglandin by the amnion. A large multicenter study that included 10,397 pregnant women found that bacterial vaginosis was associated with the preterm delivery of low-birth-weight infants independently of other recognized risk factors (Hillier et al. 1995). Preterm labor has been associated with maternal disease (e.g., cardiovascular, diabetes, hypertensive disorders), abdominal surgery or trauma during pregnancy, uterine anomalies, exposure to DES, placental abnormalities (e.g., placenta previa or abruptio placentae), fetal pathology or infection, and uterine overdistention (e.g., in multiple pregnancy or polyhydramnios). There is also thought to be a strong correlation between preterm labor and low socioeconomic status (income, education, occupation). Iatrogenic factors (e.g., elective induction or repeated cesarean delivery) can also be a contributing cause.

PPROM often leads to preterm labor and preterm delivery. It has been shown that black populations tend to have a higher proportion of preterm delivery resulting from PPROM than a white population, which has more idiopathic preterm labor (Savitz et al. 1991). The exact causes of PPROM are unknown; however, the role of subclinical chorioamnionitis is becoming increasingly apparent, with possibly one out of four or five preterm deliveries occurring in women with an intra-amniotic infection (Cunningham et al. 1993). Three common pathogens that have been implicated in causing this kind of infection are *Mycoplasma, Fusobacterium,* and *Ureaplasma;* four less common pathogens are *Neisseria gonorrhoeae, Chlamydia,* the pathogen of bacterial vaginosis, and group B *Streptococcus,* especially if it is in the urine. For reasons not well understood, it is theorized that when chorioamnionitis occurs, the barrier between the uterine cavity and the vagina allows the entrance of bacteria into the uterus. The bacteria replicate in the decidua and eventually reach a critical number that can invade the amniotic fluid, the umbilical cord, and other fetal tissues. Often symptoms of intra-amniotic infection such as fever, leukocytosis, uterine tenderness, and fetal tachycardia are not present and preterm labor may be the only sign indicating an active infectious process.

Maternal reasons for preterm deliveries include hypertensive disorders of pregnancy or preeclampsia, kidney disease, worsening diabetes or heart disease, and placental accidents such as placenta previa or abruptio placentae. Fetal indications for preterm deliveries include worsening isoimmunization or hydrops, diaphragmatic hernia, or severe IUGR.

Preterm labor with intact membranes can occur in the presence of fever, such as with pyelonephritis; after maternal abdominal surgery; in the presence of a uterine anomaly; or in the presence of excessive uterine distention as in the case of multiple gestation or polyhydramnios. However, 50 percent of the time the cause of this kind of preterm labor is unknown. The components and symptoms that define preterm labor are shown in Table 21–3.

In light of this information only 30 to 40 percent of preterm births would be amenable to some sort of prevention program. A number of studies of preterm birth prevention programs have been conducted (McLean et al. 1993; Murphy 1993). Preterm labor prevention programs are focused on early detection of preterm labor with the aim of earlier initiation of tocolysis and increased success in stopping labor. These programs determine women at high risk for preterm labor, focus educational efforts on early signs of preterm labor, and offer home monitoring and management by health care providers if necessary. The largest of these studies was carried out in France by Papiernik over a 9-year period and involved 4000 women. Historical studies such as his that compared preterm delivery rates before and after the preterm labor prevention program showed important decreases in the number of premature infants born. However, the studies that have used randomized trials have been unable to show any significant differences related to the preterm labor prevention programs. Although the overall rate of preterm delivery was not decreased, these programs may have resulted in an important decrease in the incidence of very-low-birth-weight infants, or those under 33 weeks. If this is the case, the programs would be cost effective in preventing significant neonatal mortality and morbidity.

Table 21–3

CRITERIA FOR PRETERM LABOR

SIGNS AND SYMPTOMS

• Gestation 20 to 36 weeks	• Uterine contractions (with or without pain)
• Documented uterine contractions (four in 20 min)	• Menstruation-like cramps
• Documented cervical change or cervical dilatation of 2 cm or cervical effacement of 80%	• Pelvic pressure
	• Low dull backache (unrelieved by rest)
	• Intestinal cramping and/or diarrhea
	• Increased vaginal discharge, watery fluid, or blood from vagina

MANAGEMENT

The management of the woman in preterm labor has as its objective prevention of birth until the fetus has less extrauterine than intrauterine risk of complications. It is the goal of management to deliver as close to term as possible. A new immunoassay diagnostic measure for preterm labor was approved by the U.S. Food and Drug Administration in 1995. This biochemical marker, called fetal fibronectin (fFN), is an extracellular protein that is secreted by the anchoring trophoblasts and functions as an adhesive substance in pregnancy to help attach the fertilized egg to the implantation site in the uterus. Fetal fibronectin is found in amniotic fluid and fetal membranes and can normally be detected in vaginal secretions in large quantities from early pregnancy to 22 weeks of gestation. After 22 weeks, it is no longer detected until close to 40 weeks' gestation. If an infection or other process that leads to fetal membrane compromise occurs between 22 and 40 weeks' gestation, fFN is expressed in cervicovaginal secretions. The detection of this protein, normally not present at this time, signifies an abnormal event and identifies the woman as being at increased risk for preterm delivery. A positive fFN test enhances the ability of the clinician to predict preterm delivery in a population with often vague presenting symptoms and allows for better management decisions (Nageotte et al. 1994). Medical management for preterm labor falls into two categories: care for women felt to be at risk and care for those who have had a preterm labor episode. For women in the at-risk group, prenatal care is usually scheduled at more frequent intervals with more frequent cervical examinations done. Women with cervical changes may be asked to limit activities or have a modified bed rest regimen. Frequently, women at risk are told to abstain from vaginal intercourse or orgasm, since these activities can cause the uterus to contract, and women at risk for preterm labor may contract more readily (Main et al. 1993).

When a woman has a documented episode of preterm labor, she may be placed on bed rest at home, hydrated, and started on a tocolytic drug. Bed rest decreases uterine activity by increasing uteroplacental blood flow, decreasing the pressure of the presenting part on the cervix and decreasing the woman's level of activity. An important component of bed rest is the woman's periodic recording throughout the day of uterine and fetal activity (Fig. 21–7) and close surveillance by the nurse. At first the nurse makes a home visit at least once a day augmented by phone calls throughout the day. As the woman stabilizes and learns to manage her own care, the number of home visits is decreased and the nurse telephones the patient daily at the same time each morning and night to determine her status until the physician determines that treatment to forestall labor is no longer necessary.

Hydration is thought to suppress preterm labor by inhibiting the antidiuretic hormone. Often, fluid replacement alone accompanied by rest results in uterine quiescence. If bed rest and hydration alone do not stop uterine activity, drugs known as tocolytics are used. These work in one of several ways: by causing smooth muscle relaxation, stimulating beta-adrenergic receptors in the uterus, inhibiting prostaglandin production, or working as calcium antagonists. They are most effective if the cervix has not effaced more than 50 percent or has not dilated more than 3 cm. The most common ambulatory tocolytics are oral or subcutaneous terbutaline or oral nifedipine (see Chapter 25 for a full description of these drugs). Most women have a circadian rhythm of contractions and frequently note increased uterine activity in the evening. Subcutaneous terbutaline, which is delivered via a constant infusion pump, permits constant low-dose infusion with boluses of the drug given during episodes of increased contractions. This method of administration results in fewer maternal side effects and a lower overall dose of terbutaline per 24 hours, which means a longer period before drug resistance occurs. It also allows the woman to have uninterrupted sleep at night, as she does not have to get up to take medication.

An area of treatment for preterm labor that has advanced rapidly in the past ten years is home monitoring for preterm labor. This is one of the components of preterm labor prevention programs that have been the focus of a number of research studies, as discussed earlier in this section. Both uterine contractions and fetal heart rate can be monitored in the woman's home with a portable electronic fetal monitoring system and then transmitted through a telephone modem to a central location, where they are evaluated several times a day by a staff of specially trained nurses (see Unit 1, Trends in Research, p. 3). One of these nurses may also make regular visits to the woman's home to assess her status. Home monitoring can detect symptoms of preterm labor early and enable the woman to receive further intervention to stop labor if necessary (United States Public Health Service 1993).

If home management of preterm labor is unsuccessful, the woman is hospitalized. In addition to the tocolytic drugs, antibiotics may be administered if the cause of the preterm labor is suspected to be an infection such as pyelonephritis. If delivery seems imminent and it is suspected that the fetal lungs are not mature, a corticosteroid drug called betamethasone is administered. The need for this drug is confirmed by a lecithin/sphin-

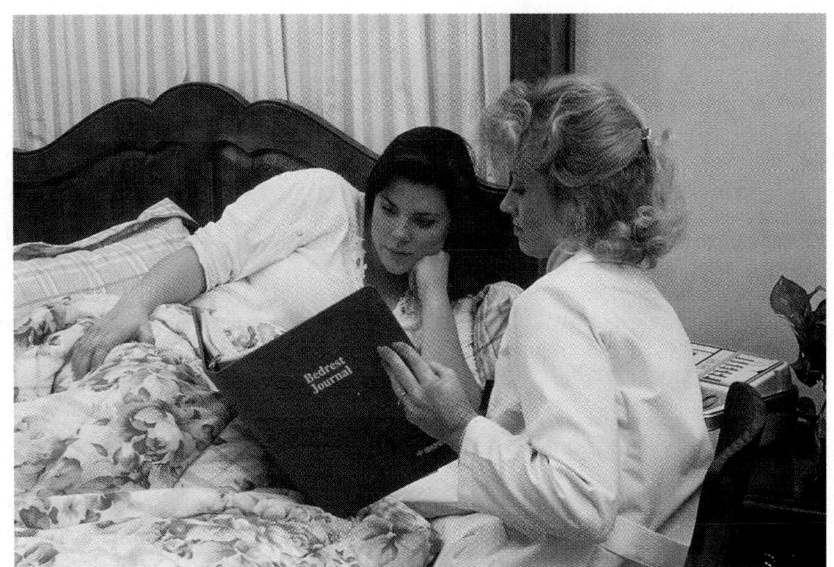

Figure 21–7

Women who experience an episode of preterm labor may be restricted to bedrest to forestall preterm delivery • The patient monitors herself for the presence of uterine contractions, other signs and symptoms of preterm labor, and fetal activity periodically throughout each day and records the results in a bedrest journal. • The home visiting nurse can then review and discuss this record with her at least once daily or more often, depending on the status of the patient • Photo copyright MATRIA, Inc., Marietta, GA.

gomyelin (L/S) ratio less than 2.0 or a negative phosphatidylglycerol test. Betamethasone stimulates the process of fetal lung maturity and thus reduces the risk of respiratory distress syndrome (RDS) if the baby is born preterm. For betamethasone to be effective, the fetus must be between 28 and 34 weeks' gestation and delivery must be delayed for 24 to 48 hours.

Nursing Process

▼ Assessment

The nurse's role at the woman's initial antepartal visit may be to perform the preterm labor risk assessment. Table 21–4 lists factors associated with preterm delivery by Holbrook and associates in 1989. Most preterm labor prevention programs use tools containing similar information, but each has shortcomings that the nurse should keep in mind. By far the most important risk factor for preterm labor is a history of a previous preterm labor or preterm delivery. In fact, a woman with this history has a 2.2 to 5 times increased risk of having another preterm delivery (Moore et al. 1992). If the woman is a primigravida, she has no obstetric history and therefore the risk scoring tool would naturally be less sensitive in predicting her risk of preterm delivery. This issue is a problem, since 50 percent of preterm deliveries are to primigravid women (McLean et al. 1993). Most major risk factors are for causes that are relatively rare and are not subject to any intervention. Among the risk factors, only smoking could be influenced during the course of the pregnancy, with the prevention of pyelonephritis perhaps also included. Another criticism is that this particular risk assessment tool does not include three factors that are known to be associated with preterm labor and could possibly be altered prenatally: (1) poor weight gain, (2) cocaine use, and (3) an adverse working environment that requires repetitive routine work or a stressful environment (Colie 1993). Using this tool or any similar one results in 60 to 80 percent of women who deliver at term being labeled "high risk for PTD"; this label may make these women subject to more interventions such as cervical cerclage and tocolysis (Murphy 1993). In addition, the tool fails to identify 50 percent of preterm deliveries that involve no risk factors.

The nurse should ask about signs of preterm labor on an ongoing basis at prenatal visits and be alert to these signs in telephone conversations with a prenatal client. As certain risk factors for preterm labor arise, such as an episode of pyelonephritis or abdominal surgery, the nurse should reassess the woman's preterm labor risk.

▼ Diagnosis

On the basis of an assessment that includes the client's history, physical examination, and laboratory findings, the following diagnoses are suggested:

Table 21–4

THE HOLBROOK PRETERM LABOR RISK-SCREENING SYSTEM

MAJOR FACTORS	MINOR FACTORS
(Presence of one or more = high risk)	(Presence of two or more = high risk)
Multiple gestation	Febrile illness during pregnancy
Previous preterm labor, term delivery	Bleeding after 12 weeks
Previous preterm labor, preterm delivery	History of pyelonephritis
DES exposure	Cigarette smoking (≥ 10 cigarettes per day)
Hydramnios	One second-trimester abortion
Uterine anomaly	More than two first-trimester abortions
History of cone biopsy	
Uterine irritability (admission to rule out PTL)	
More than one second-trimester abortion	
Cervical dilatation (≥ 1 cm at 32 weeks)	
Cervical effacement (≤ 1 cm at 32 weeks)	

From Holbrook, R. H., Jr., Laros, R. K. Jr., Creasy, R. K. (1989). Evaluation of a risk-screening system for prediction of preterm labor. *American Journal of Perinatology*, 6 (1), 62–68.

- Risk for fetal injury related to preterm delivery
- Risk for maternal injury related to altered nutrition, bowel function, musculoskeletal status, or pain related to prolonged bed rest
- Knowledge deficit: lack of information related to preterm labor risk factors and treatment
- Altered family process related to prevention and/or treatment of preterm labor
- Anxiety related to high-risk pregnancy status

▼ Planning

The plan of care that is chosen for the woman experiencing preterm labor might include the following outcome goals:

- The woman will give birth to a healthy, viable infant
- The woman will remain compliant with her treatment regime and will experience no adverse effects of prolonged bed rest
- The woman will verbalize her understanding of her risks for preterm labor and the plan for her treatment
- The woman and her family will demonstrate adaptation and coping in relation to the imposed restrictions of a high-risk pregnancy
- The woman will express her anxieties related to the high-risk pregnancy

▼ Intervention

The goal of the plan of care for the woman at risk for preterm labor is to deliver a healthy, full-term infant. Education and stress reduction are two of the areas that the nurse can influence during the antepartal period. In an effort to achieve this plan, the nurse can either focus educational efforts on women at risk for preterm labor or, if there is adequate time, educate all women either individually or in groups about altering behaviors that may contribute to a risk of preterm labor. For women who are receiving a tocolytic drug to suppress preterm labor contractions, additional nursing interventions are necessary. These are discussed in Chapter 25.

Education should begin by teaching women about the early and sometimes subtle signs of preterm labor (see Teaching Guide: Identification and Prevention of Preterm Labor). Studies that have examined the sensitivity of these signs show that 5 to 20 percent of women with preterm labor may have none of them. Studies have shown that women may perceive as few as 10 percent of uterine contractions that are detectable by electronic monitor (McLean et al. 1993). However, it is unclear whether these electronically detected contractions cause cervical change. The woman with symptoms of preterm labor should be shown how to palpate and time contractions. She needs to be encouraged to take the time twice a day to "listen to her body." The woman experiencing preterm labor symptoms needs to lie down, drink several glasses of liquid, and monitor for contractions. She should lie on her left side to promote uterine-placental circulation. If, after lying down and resting for an hour, she experiences five or more contractions in an hour or continues to have other symptoms of preterm labor, she should be encouraged to call her health care provider immediately. The woman should feel free to make this contact as often as necessary, since an episode of frequent, mild contractions often precedes a true preterm labor event by 48 to 72 hours.

The nurse can encourage other preventive measures as well. The woman should drink an 8-ounce glass of water or juice every hour while she is awake and empty her bladder frequently. This intervention maintains adequate hydration, which decreases the release of antidiuretic hormone and oxytocin from the posterior pituitary gland. These hormones increase uterine blood flow with the result that arachidonic acid is not freed to be converted into prostaglandins. Adequate hydration can also decrease the risk of urinary infection. If a woman smokes, providing her with an organized, step-by-step method for smoking cessation is another preventive step (Windsor et al. 1993). A discussion of the effect of sexual stimulation and uterine contractions may assist the woman in deciding whether to have vaginal intercourse or whether other types of nonorgasmic intimacy will suffice. Nipple stimulation is contraindicated, however, because of the potential release of oxytocin. If a woman decides that vaginal intercourse is important, the use of a condom may have two purposes: it prevents exposure to semen, which is rich in prostaglandins, a potential initiator of labor; and it decreases exposure to infectious agents, which may increase the risk of infection and premature rupture of the membranes (Brustman et al. 1989).

For women who must continue bed rest, either at home or in the hospital, an important role of the nurse is in assessing the impact of this activity restriction on the woman's family, both economically and psychologically (Maloni 1993; Maloni et al. 1993). Common issues related to bed rest include worries about care for other children, meal preparation, household management, and social isolation (Monahan and DeJoseph 1991).

Some researchers believe that although our knowledge of the physiology of labor is limited and does not permit us to understand fully the causes of preterm labor and delivery, primary preterm labor prevention should include stress reduction and altering an adverse working environ-

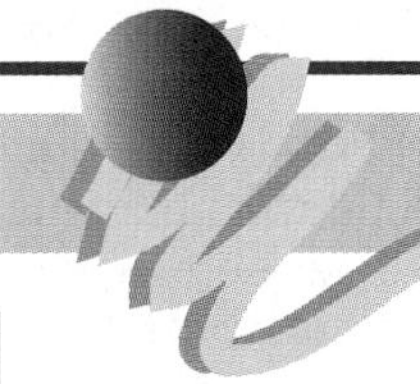

TEACHING GUIDE

IDENTIFICATION AND PREVENTION OF PRETERM LABOR

TOPIC	*MAJOR CONCEPTS*
Definition of Preterm Labor and Birth	When labor begins after 20 weeks of gestation, but before 37 weeks, it is called preterm labor; if the labor cannot be stopped and the baby is born, the birth is called preterm.
Problems Resulting from Preterm Birth	When the baby is born before it is fully mature, it may be very small and typically has a number of problems. Teach your client about the difficulty the neonate may encounter with breathing, eating, keeping its body temperature at a normal level, and development of body organs. Explain that if the baby is too small, it might die.
Risk Factors for Preterm Labor	Factors that might contribute to preterm labor include multiple gestation, a history of previous preterm labor or birth, abnormalities of the uterus or cervix, maternal illnesses such as high blood pressure or diabetes, abdominal surgery or trauma, smoking cigarettes, urinary tract infections, or early rupture of the membranes.
Signs of Preterm Labor	It is sometimes hard to assess preterm labor because the uterus undergoes "practice" or Braxton Hicks contractions on occasion, particularly during the last trimester of pregnancy. These contractions usually stop after an hour or so. Preterm labor contractions do not stop, and your client may notice other symptoms, such as menstrual-like cramps above the pubic bone, pelvic pressure, low dull backache, intestinal cramping or diarrhea, increased vaginal discharge, or watery fluid or blood coming from the vagina.
What To Do if You Suspect Preterm Labor	Instruct your client to call her doctor, midwife, or clinic at once, if she thinks she may be experiencing any symptoms of preterm labor. Explain that she may be asked to come in to be checked. If she is having an episode of preterm labor, she may be sent home to stay in bed on her left side and drink a great deal of fluids. She may also be asked to time and record her contractions. Teach your client to place her hand lightly on her abdomen and feel with her fingertips when the uterus tightens and relaxes. She may also be given medication to stop the contractions.

Continued on facing page

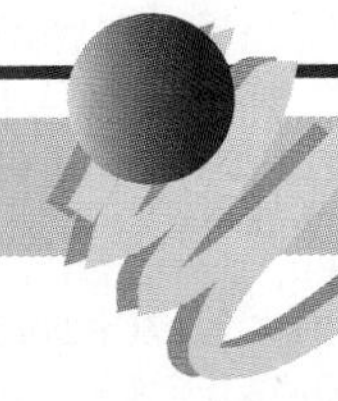

TEACHING GUIDE Continued

IDENTIFICATION AND PREVENTION OF PRETERM LABOR

TOPIC	*MAJOR CONCEPTS*
	If these interventions do not stop the preterm labor, she may have to be admitted to the hospital, where she can be monitored more closely and given stronger medication intravenously.
Ways To Prevent Preterm Labor	Teach your client to • Be aware of uterine activity • Drink plenty of fluids each day • Keep bladder empty • Always wipe from front to back after urinating or having a bowel movement • Wear cotton undergarments • Stop smoking and do not use drugs • Use condoms when having vaginal intercourse • Avoid having sex with multiple partners • Stop physical activity and rest if experiencing contractions that do not stop in a short time
Teaching Aids 1. Pamphlets, booklets, or handouts that include an explanation of preterm labor, its risk factors, prevention measures, and instructions to follow if preterm labor is suspected. 2. Videos explaining preterm labor and birth. 3. Bed rest record or journal for recording contractions. **Increasing Your Teaching Effectiveness** Your success in teaching your client about preterm labor and birth is enhanced by using the following approaches.	1. Identify what your client knows about signs of normal labor, contrast this knowledge with information on Braxton Hicks contractions and the signs of preterm labor. 2. Ask for frequent feedback and clarification of your client's understanding of these differences. Allow ample time for her questions. 3. Use visual aids and teaching materials. 4. Go through the pamphlets and brochures with your client, rather than just handing them to her to take home and read. 5. Show your client how to palpate the fundus of her uterus to feel tightening and relaxation during and after contractions. 6. Show your client how to time and record contractions, including frequency and duration.

ment. The role of stress and preterm labor has been documented in several studies (Alexander et al. 1991; Belizan et al. 1991; Villar et al. 1992). The role of work and preterm labor is less clear, for some studies show an increased relative risk (RR 1.28 to 2.84), whereas other studies show no effect (Colie 1993). Klebanoff and associates (1990), using female residents as subjects, failed to show an increase in preterm delivery except with working more than 100 hours per week. The issue may be related to doing work that the woman enjoys and finds fulfilling, versus work that she finds stressful or boring; international studies have shown that women who do housework have an increased incidence of preterm labor, compared with women who have jobs outside the home (Murphy 1993).

The nurse may not be able to alter a stressful

job but can teach problem-solving and stress reduction techniques. In addition, the nurse may need to advocate for a woman whose job requires prolonged standing or heavy lifting in order to have her duties reduced or at least to have increased rest periods provided. As noted, some studies have found standing longer than 3 to 8 hours to be associated with increased preterm labor (Colie 1993).

It is not uncommon for women experiencing preterm labor to feel anxious about their own well-being, as well as that of their family and their unborn child. The nurse has an opportunity to decrease that anxiety by developing a care plan that promotes control by such means as daily telephone contact, home uterine activity monitoring, participation in telephone support groups, and self-medication. A well-informed woman is the best defense against preterm delivery.

▼ Evaluation

Evaluation is a critical component of the plan of care in working with a woman at risk for preterm labor, because identifying the need for alterations in the plan of care can serve to prevent a preterm delivery. The evaluation is based on the nursing diagnoses and outcome goals. For example, the plan of care can be evaluated as successful if the woman understands and remains compliant with her treatment plan; if the birth can be delayed until the fetus is viable, has achieved lung maturity, and suffers no adverse effects of preterm delivery; if the woman is able to express her anxieties; and if the family is able to cope with the high-risk pregnancy.

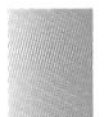

Trauma or Surgery

DESCRIPTION

The occurrence of trauma or surgery during pregnancy can pose a risk to either the woman or her fetus. Probably the most common trauma in pregnancy is falling, for the pregnant woman is often unsteady or awkward as a result of softening of the joints and an altered center of gravity, particularly in the third trimester. In early pregnancy, the fetus is well protected by the bony pelvis, which still surrounds the uterus. In later pregnancy, the fetus is still protected by the amniotic fluid, uterine muscle, and abdominal wall, so that in the case of a fall the force of impact is distributed in all directions and usually causes no serious problems. More serious injuries, such as blunt trauma to the abdomen in an automobile accident or the penetrating trauma of knife or gunshot wounds, can be of much greater concern. The maternal and fetal risks of trauma during pregnancy are related to hemorrhage resulting from uterine rupture or abruptio placentae, preterm labor, maternal head injuries or fractures, and shock (Johnson and Oakley 1991).

Although surgery does impose risks during pregnancy, essential procedures can be safely carried out. The risks include an increased incidence of spontaneous abortion in the first trimester and an increased risk of fetal mortality, intrauterine growth restriction, low birth weight, and preterm labor in the second or third trimester.

MANAGEMENT

The goal of the medical management of trauma is to maintain the stability of the pregnancy and the status of both the woman and the fetus. Management of a traumatic injury must always begin with diagnosis of the location and extent of the injury. Radiology, real-time ultrasonography, and computed tomographic scans are used for this purpose in pregnancy. The physician must always weigh the risk to the fetus of using a diagnostic procedure against the risk to the woman of not obtaining an accurate diagnosis. In the same way, medical interventions must be selected with the effect they will have for both the woman and fetus in mind. The woman or her family may need to help in decision making as treatment is being planned. If the injury is serious, the woman must be hospitalized, often in a regular or an obstetric intensive care unit until she is stable. Mechanical ventilation, hemodynamic monitoring, control of hemorrhage, and fetal monitoring are possible in such specialized units. The support of normal physiology and the treatment of injuries are the same for the pregnant woman as for any other patient, although occasional adaptations may have to be made. A cesarean delivery may be required if allowing the pregnancy to continue poses a serious threat to either the maternal or fetal status.

The management of the preoperative and postoperative care for the woman who requires surgery during pregnancy is the same as for any patient; however, additional considerations are necessary. Fetal heart tones must be monitored continuously with an electronic fetal monitor before, during, and after surgery. The fetus should be shielded if radiographs are needed. To facilitate uterine-placental circulation during surgery, it may be necessary to position the woman so that the uterus is displaced to one side, off the inferior vena cava. Additional respiratory support may be needed for the pregnant woman, who often experiences engorgement of the nasal mucous membranes. A nasogastric tube should be inserted before surgery because of the increased risk of vomiting during anesthesia resulting from the decreased gastrointestinal motility during pregnancy. An indwelling urinary catheter should be inserted before surgery to decrease the risk of injury to the bladder. The type of anesthesia must be selected carefully with consideration of the effects on the fetus. As with trauma, blood loss during surgery should be carefully monitored and fluid or blood replacement given as needed.

Nursing Process

▼ Assessment

Assessment after a trauma or surgical procedure must focus on both the woman and the fetus. In the case of trauma, the first area of concern must be the woman's respiratory status. The nurse must ensure that the woman has an open airway and is breathing freely. When this is established, the second area for assessment is the uterus. It must be determined that the uterus is not ruptured and that there is no uterine activity. Assessment should be made for hemorrhage resulting from a rupture or abruptio placentae. Hemorrhage can be masked by the hypervolemic state of pregnancy, so observation for signs of bleeding is important. Frequent measurement of blood pressure and vital signs is essential. The nurse should be alert for the development of DIC, which can occur as a result of trauma and hemorrhage. Laboratory tests are ordered to assess for hemorrhage and infection. The woman should be typed and crossmatched for blood replacement if needed. The third critical area for assessment is the fetus. Fetal heart rate and fetal activity should be monitored continuously with an electronic fetal monitor. Additional assessments might include those for intake and output, neurologic status, and psychosocial factors. In completing a review of systems to assess for injury, it is important that normal symptoms of pregnancy not be confused with signs of trauma. The assessments necessary for the woman having surgery are the same as for any preoperative or postoperative patient, with the addition of assessment of fetal status (Johnson and Oakley 1991).

▼ Diagnosis

On the basis of an assessment that includes the client's history, physical examination, and laboratory findings, the following diagnoses are suggested:

- Altered tissue perfusion: cardiopulmonary related to decreased oxygenation secondary to trauma, hemorrhage, or general anesthesia
- Pain related to traumatic injury or elective surgery
- Fear related to uncertain outcome of pregnancy and status of the fetus
- Knowledge deficit: lack of information related to the management of the injury or surgery

▼ Planning

The plan of care that is chosen for the woman experiencing trauma or surgery might include the following outcome goals:

- The woman and her fetus will have no adverse outcomes related to the trauma or surgery
- The woman will verbalize that her pain is decreased and demonstrate evidence of increased comfort by facial expression and body positioning
- The woman will explain the plan of care for the management of her injury or surgical procedure

▼ Intervention

An important role of the nurse related to trauma during pregnancy is that of education. In individual counseling sessions with pregnant women or in pregnancy and childbirth classes, the nurse can inform the woman of the importance of safety and caution during pregnancy to prevent accidents. Alterations in the woman's job may be necessary to avoid injury. Simple precautions such as wearing low-heeled shoes, altering physical activities, and wearing car seat belts are important and are discussed further in Chapter 19. Education is also important if the pregnant woman must have surgery. The need for the surgery should be reviewed and the procedure explained to her and her family. Ample time should be given to allow them to ask questions or express concerns. When the woman is ready to go home after recovering from her injury or surgery, discharge teaching is particularly important so that the woman knows what level of activity she can resume, how to care for herself, and what warning signs should be reported to her health care provider.

In addition to the essential assessments already outlined, a number of important nursing interventions are related to the care of the woman who has experienced trauma. The woman should be positioned on her side to facilitate fetal-placental circulation and prevent supine hypotensive syndrome. This can be done by placing a pillow at her back or a wedge under her hip to displace the uterus off the vena cava. Intravenous fluids (usually Ringer's lactate) should be started to provide fluid and electrolyte replacement. If the woman is Rh negative, she should be given Rh_0(D) Immune Globulin. An indwelling urinary catheter should be inserted for drainage and assessment of urine. A nasogastric tube to decrease the risk of vomiting and aspiration should be inserted. Comfort measures, such as oral hygiene, should be provided. The nurse is often the member of the health care team who can best provide the emotional support needed by the pregnant woman and her family.

Care for the pregnant woman who has had surgery requires some adaptations in the usual postoperative plan. As already discussed, it is advisable for the woman to maintain a side-lying position. Support stockings should be used and leg exercises and ambulation encouraged, to prevent the development of thrombophlebitis. The usual routine of coughing and deep breathing to promote oxygenation is essential. The potential effects of medications should be considered before their administration. Maintenance of fluids and nutrition should be monitored closely. And, of course, the fetus should be monitored regularly.

▼ Evaluation

Evaluation of a traumatic injury or surgical recovery is based on the specific measurable outcome goals that were identified. The nurse can be confident that the nursing care has been effective if the woman and her fetus sustain no adverse effects from the trauma or surgery, if the woman is comfortable and free of pain, if the woman is able to verbalize her fears, and if the woman is able to explain correctly the plan of care for her treatment.

SYSTEMIC DISEASES COINCIDENT WITH PREGNANCY

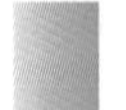

Diabetes in Pregnancy

DESCRIPTION

Pregnancy can complicate diabetes in women with either insulin-dependent diabetes mellitus (IDDM) or diet-controlled non–insulin-dependent diabetes mellitus (NIDDM) because the diabetogenic state of pregnancy helps the fetus grow rapidly. This diabetogenic state can also cause hyperglycemia in a woman who had no signs of abnormal glucose metabolism before the pregnancy; this condition is known as gestational diabetes mellitus (GDM). One to 3 percent of pregnant women develop GDM. Native Americans and Hispanics show an increased incidence, up to 10%, and African-Americans are also more prone to GDM than whites (Cunningham et al. 1993).

An understanding of normal carbohydrate metabolism is essential to an understanding of the signs, symptoms, and consequences of diabetes and the added effect the physiologic changes of pregnancy have on this disease. Carbohydrate metabolism is accomplished by adequate production of insulin by the beta cells of the islets of Langerhans in the pancreas. Insulin is needed to transport glucose from the bloodstream into the muscle cells for use as energy or into the cells in the liver, where it is stored as glycogen for future energy use. Insulin is produced in response to the amount of carbohydrates ingested. The ability of beta cells to respond to varying carbohydrate loads during the day maintains the homeostasis between serum glucose levels and glucose requirements of the body's cells.

During normal pregnancy, dramatic changes in maternal metabolism are brought about by endogenous and placental hormones. These changes permit steady transport of glucose to the fetus for growth and development but frequently, especially in early pregnancy, can result in a fasting hypoglycemic state. In addition, there is progressive insulin resistance as the pregnancy progresses. This resistance is due to rising placental hormones and factors, particularly human placental lactogen (hPL), which results in increased blood sugar levels after meals. Insulin resistance peaks at 24 to 28 weeks of pregnancy. The pregnant woman who has limited pancreatic reserves and is unable to boost her insulin production to offset this insulin resistance becomes a gestational diabetic. For the pregestationally diabetic woman, these changes in pregnancy make it a challenge to balance food intake, exercise, and insulin doses, since requirements are likely to change from month to month during the pregnancy (Cunningham et al. 1993).

Pathophysiology

In diabetes mellitus, the pancreas either cannot produce any insulin or is unable to produce sufficient insulin to meet the demand of carbohydrate intake. If the body does not have sufficient glucose to function, because of either lack of carbohydrate intake or lack of insulin to permit transport into the cells, protein and fat are broken down for energy use, a process called anaerobic metabolism. The result is ketosis resulting from fat metabolism, negative nitrogen balance, an increase of lactic acid from protein metabolism, and ultimately a wasting of muscle cells. This anaerobic metabolism results in the cardinal symptoms of diabetes: (1) polyuria, frequent urination as greater glucose concentration increases osmotic pressure, resulting in inability of the renal tubules to reabsorb fluid; (2) polydipsia, excessive thirst resulting from dehydration caused by polyuria; (3) polyphagia, excessive hunger caused by the lack of glucose in tissues; and (4) weight loss caused by the wasting of muscle as fat and protein are utilized for energy. In addition, the increased blood glucose levels exceed the renal tubules' ability to reabsorb glucose, resulting in glycosuria. The diagnosis of diabetes is based on clinical presentation and laboratory evidence of elevated glucose levels.

Diabetes can have severe effects on fetal health. Diabetic women who become pregnant while in poor control of their glucose levels are at increased risk of spontaneous abortion (as high as 25 to 45 percent) and of having infants with congenital anomalies (7.5 to 13 percent compared with a normal 2 percent rate). However, studies have shown that women in good glucose control at the time of conception can decrease their risk of these problems to a level close to that of healthy women (Cousins 1991). Infants of pregestational diabetics have twice the neonatal mortality of normal women, and perinatal mortality is also increased 4 percent (Moore et al. 1992). The relative risk of perinatal mortality for poorly controlled or undiagnosed gestational diabetics is about four times the normal rate (Coustan 1991). Macrosomia is one of the major consequences of diabetes in pregnancy, occurring in about 25 percent of all diabetic pregnancies. Macrosomia can cause birth injury, severe respiratory distress, and metabolic problems in the neonate. However, one study has shown that strict euglycemic control in gestational diabetics can reduce the risk of macrosomia to nearly zero (Jovanovic-Peterson and Peterson 1990). Other fetal complications resulting from diabetes are small size for gestational age, prematurity, and a predisposition to diabetes.

Maternal consequences for the insulin-dependent diabetic include diabetic ketoacidosis, which can result in fetal mortality and hypoglycemia (Mandeville 1992). All women with diabetes are at increased risk for polyhydramnios, preterm labor, and preeclampsia. The risk of preeclampsia increases with increased vascular involvement, such as occurs in women with nephropathy or chronic hypertension.

Classification

Two systems are used to classify pregnant women with diabetes: the White classification, which is based on duration and complications of the disease (Table 21–5), and the National Diabetes Data Group (NDDG) classification, which is based on pathophysiology (Table 21–6). According to the White classification, gestational diabetic women in class A-1 have demonstrated carbohydrate intolerance in a 100-g, 3-hour glucose tolerance test but have fasting blood sugar levels less than 105 mg/dL and 2-hour postprandial sugar levels less than 120 mg/dL (Gabbe et al. 1991).

Table 21–5

MODIFIED WHITE CLASSIFICATION OF PREGNANT DIABETIC WOMEN

CLASS	DIABETES ONSET AGE (YEARS)		DURATION (YEARS)	VASCULAR DISEASE	INSULIN NEED
		Gestational Diabetes			
A_1	Any		Any	0	0
A_2	Any		Any	0	+
		Pregestational Diabetes			
B	>20		<10	0	+
C	10–19	or	10–19	0	+
D	<10	or	>20	+	+
F	Any		Any	+	+
R	Any		Any	+	+
T	Any		Any	+	+
H	Any		Any	+	+

From Gabbe, S. G., Niebyl, J. R., Simpson, J. L. (1991). *Obstetrics: Normal and problem pregnancies* (2nd ed.) (p. 1104). New York: Churchill Livingstone.

Table 21–6

NATIONAL DIABETIC DATA GROUP PHYSIOLOGIC CLASSIFICATION OF DIABETES IN PREGNANCY

CLASSIFICATION	OTHER TERMS	CLINICAL PRESENTATION
Type I: Insulin-dependent diabetes mellitus (IDDM)	Juvenile-onset diabetes	Ketosis prone, insulin deficient
Type II: Non–insulin-dependent diabetes (NIDDM)	Adult-onset diabetes	Ketosis resistant, insulin resistant; obesity, family history, and age common risk factors
Type III: Gestational diabetes (GDM)	Gestational diabetes	Occurs only during pregnancy; established by glucose tolerance testing; obesity and age common risk factors

From Moore, T. R., Reiter, R. C., Rebar, R. W., Baker, W. W. (1992). *Gynecology and obstetrics: A longitudinal approach* (p. 353). New York: Churchill Livingstone.

Women in class A-2 have fasting and postprandial blood sugar levels above these values and therefore require insulin to maintain normal blood sugar levels. According to the physiologic classification of diabetes in pregnancy, IDDM is known as type I and usually has an onset before age 30. It is characterized by an absolute insulin deficiency state and requires the use of insulin injections. NIDDM is known as type II and is usually seen in adults, although it can occur at any age. It is most often seen in overweight individuals. Rather than causing a total deficiency in insulin, type II is associated with a lack of insulin availability or effectiveness. GDM is known as type III and is characterized by glucose intolerance during pregnancy.

MANAGEMENT

Women who are pregestational diabetics are usually cared for during pregnancy by a team of health care providers; such a team is likely to include a perinatologist, an endocrinologist, a diabetic-nurse educator, a nutritionist, and possibly a social worker and a visiting nurse. The benefits of a multidisciplinary team are that assessments and interventions are better coordinated and women receive the necessary education from the appropriate expert. Insulin requirements can change frequently because of the physiologic changes described previously, and good communication between providers and patients is necessary.

Diagnosis of gestational diabetes is important so that fetal consequences can be prevented. Since insulin resistance peaks at 24 to 28 weeks, it is recommended that all pregnant women be screened with a 50-g, 1-hour glucose challenge test during this time (Cunningham et al. 1993). A value of 140 mg/dL or greater is diagnostic for GDM. If a value greater than 140 mg/dL is obtained, a 3-hour, 100-g glucose tolerance test is needed to make the diagnosis. Table 21–7 shows a comparison of two sets of diagnostic values. The diagnosis of gestational diabetes is made if any two values are elevated or if the fasting value exceeds 130 mg/dL. A study has shown that Carpenter and Coustan's lower values may have better sensitivity in diagnosing GDM but the NDDG values continue to be more universally used and are those recommended by the American College of Obstetrics and Gynecology (Sacks et al. 1989; Coustan 1991; Magee et al. 1993).

Table 21–7

DIAGNOSTIC VALUES FOR GESTATIONAL DIABETES

	PLASMA GLUCOSE (MG/DL)	
Time of Glucose Measurement	NDDG	Carpenter and Coustan
Fasting	105	95
1 h	190	180
2 h	165	155
3 h	145	140

Women with the following risk factors are at increased risk of GDM and should be screened early in pregnancy and then again at 28 weeks (Moore et al. 1992): (1) age >30; (2) family history of NIDDM or GDM; (3) previous macrosomic infant (>4000 g); (4) previous unexplained stillbirth; (5) previous pregnancy with GDM; and (6) obesity (>90 kg).

Antenatal Management

Management of diabetic women in the antepartal period is dependent on the severity of their disease, typically based on the complications they have in the White classification. Generally antenatal visits are scheduled every 2 weeks until 28 weeks and then weekly thereafter. The following sections outline various management aspects of this disease in pregnancy.

▼ **Diet Therapy.** Diet therapy is the mainstay of the management of diabetes, especially for the woman with GDM, who typically can be managed with diet therapy alone. Dietary requirements increase in pregnancy and it is generally recommended that the woman consume 30 to 35 kcal per kilogram of body weight (Hare 1991). Obese women may safely consume a smaller number of calories. This formula permits gradual caloric increase with increasing expected weight gain. The weight gain requirements for the pregnant diabetic woman are the same as for nondiabetic pregnant women. Obese women should have their caloric intake calculated on the basis of their ideal body weight instead of their actual weight.

Meal plans are based on three regular meals with one to three snacks. An evening snack prevents morning ketonuria and, if the woman is taking insulin, prevents hypoglycemia. Calories are divided into 40 to 50 percent carbohydrates, 20 to 25 percent protein, and 30 to 35 percent fat (Department of Health Services [DHS] 1992). Emphasis should be on complex carbohydrates, especially soluble dietary fiber, which appears to lower carbohydrate absorption and improve insulin sensitivity. Concentrated sugars should be eliminated and fruit and juice limited. Saturated fats should be kept at less than 10 percent of intake.

Exercise is considered an adjunct to dietary therapy since exercise increases the effectiveness of insulin, helps prevent excessive weight gain, and improves lipid profiles. Women are advised to exercise after a meal, and walking is recommended as the ideal exercise. Women who are in poor glucose control, with blood sugar levels above 200 mg/dL, should not exercise, since increased glucose, ketones, and anti-insulin hormones produced by exercise worsen their glucose regulation (DHS 1992).

▼ **Glucose Monitoring.** The goals for blood glucose levels are the following: (1) fasting, 60 to 90 mg/dL; (2) preprandial, bedtime, 60 to 110 mg/dL; (3) 1-hour postprandial, below 130 to 140 mg/dL; and (4) 2-hour postprandial, below 120 mg/dL. Generally, women who take insulin need to test their glucose levels four times a day: fasting, before and after meals, and at bedtime. Women may also need to monitor their glucose level if they are experiencing hypoglycemic symptoms. Women with gestational diabetes may test their glucose levels only once a day at home, varying between fasting and postprandial readings, or may have their glucose monitored weekly or biweekly during antenatal visits. Home glucose monitoring can be accomplished by measuring capillary glucose levels on a plastic strip impregnated with glucose oxidase, which either changes color and is read visually to estimate the range of glucose or is inserted into a meter that gives a numerical readout.

Gestational diabetics do not usually need daily monitoring of blood sugar. The American College of Obstetricians and Gynecologists (ACOG) recommendations are to check a fasting and a 2-hour postprandial blood sugar level every 2 weeks. However, many health care providers check blood sugar weekly to ensure euglycemic levels and to be able to initiate insulin sooner if needed (Coustan 1991). Since normal pregnancy induces a ketonemia after a 12- to 16-hour fast, it is generally recommended that morning urine be checked for ketones (Hare 1991). If significant ketones are present and serum levels are normal or modestly elevated, the woman may need additional carbohydrates at the evening meal or bedtime snack.

Women with pregestational diabetes may have testing to assess their glucose control over the previous 1 to 2 months. This laboratory assessment is based on the fact that glucose binds irreversibly with hemoglobin A. The glycosylated hemoglobin test (HbA_{1c}) measures the percentage of hemoglobin attached to a glucose molecule, and these levels correlate with average blood sugar levels over the previous 4 to 8 weeks. Normal levels range from 4 to 8 percent. Levels more than 1 percent above the normal range are associated with increased congenital anomalies (Cousins 1991). The test is also used as a means of assessing blood sugar control, especially if results of home glucose monitoring are questionable.

▼ **Insulin Therapy.** Women diagnosed with gestational diabetes generally need only diet therapy to control their blood sugar levels. However, if their fasting blood sugar levels exceed 105 mg/dL and their postprandial blood sugar levels are greater than 120 mg/dL, they may need insulin. Women who have NIDDM before pregnancy and who take oral hypoglycemic agents must be switched to insulin, preferably before conception, because of the potential teratogenicity of these agents. The number of women who fall into this category is small, since these diabetics are typically diagnosed after age 40 (Hare 1991).

All pregnant women should take human insulin, since it decreases immunoglobulin G (IgG) antibodies that cross the placenta. Women who have been taking bovine or porcine insulin may find they need a smaller dose when they switch to human insulin. It should be stressed that there are no basic patterns of insulin dosage and that a dosage schedule must be individualized for each woman. Nurses should be familiar with the three different types of commonly used insulin and the peak and duration of each (Table 21–8). Insulin may be administered via single injections or with a continuous-infusion insulin pump.

▼ **Fetal Well-being.** Since diabetic women have an increased risk of fetal and neonatal morbidity and mortality, there is more intensive monitoring of fetal well-being during a diabetic pregnancy than with other pregnancies. Alpha-fetoprotein testing is strongly recommended because of the increased risk of neural tube defects. If gestational age is uncertain, an ultrasound examination for dating is important. Many health care providers recommend another ultrasound examination at 20 to 24 weeks to examine fetal anatomy, especially the heart. If there is any question of a cardiac anomaly, a fetal echocardiogram is needed. More frequent visits permit health care providers to monitor for either excessive or lagging fetal growth and the presence of hydramnios. If either of these is evident, it may be further assessed with ultrasonography. At 28 to 32 weeks, weekly nonstress tests are usually initiated for women with IDDM. Nonreactive tests are followed by a contraction stress test and biophysical profiles. Women are instructed to make daily fetal movement counts beginning at 28 weeks. Fetal testing for women with GDM who have normal blood sugar levels is usually not started until 40 weeks of gestation (Gabbe et al. 1991; Landon and Gabbe 1991).

Table 21–8

TYPES OF COMMONLY USED HUMAN INSULIN

TYPE	ACTION	PEAK (H)	DURATION (H)
Regular	Short-acting	2–4	6–8
NPH/Lente	Intermediate	4–10	18–22
Ultralente	Long-acting	8–16	24–26

Before delivery, amniocentesis may be performed for women with poorly regulated IDDM to assess fetal lung maturity. Hyperglycemia during pregnancy delays fetal lung maturity. An L/S ratio greater than 3.5 versus the normal of greater than 2 and a 3 percent phosphatidylglycerol (PG) test are needed to predict that sufficient surfactant is present to prevent infant respiratory distress syndrome (RDS) (Moore et al. 1992).

Intrapartum Management

The timing of delivery in the diabetic pregnancy is dependent on maternal factors (vascular disease complications, diabetes control, ripeness of the cervix, and previous obstetric history) and on fetal factors (estimated fetal weight and suspicion of fetal distress) (Gabbe et al. 1991; Landon and Gabbe 1991). Women who appear to have a large baby may be induced at 37 to 38 weeks' gestation to avoid the risks of birth trauma and prevent the sudden fetal asphyxia and stillbirth associated late in pregnancy with ketoacidosis and blood glucose levels greater than 180 mg/dL. Obviously, induction must be approached only if the risks of RDS outweigh the risks of a term delivery.

During labor, gestational diabetics who have been controlled with diet may need no special intravenous therapy. Insulin-dependent diabetics need continuous intravenous insulin infusion during active labor. Such an infusion permits easy regulation of blood glucose on the basis of hourly capillary tests. Normoglycemic control is essential for the prevention of fetal asphyxia during labor. Oxytocin augmentation for protracted labor and assisted vaginal deliveries are used with caution, since the risk of shoulder dystocia in a macrosomic infant is high. In many studies, the rate of cesarean deliveries for diabetic women remains quite high, ranging from 45 to 81 percent (Cunningham et al. 1993).

Nursing Process

▼ Assessment

The assessment of every pregnant woman for gestational diabetes includes screening for historical risk factors, looking for the presence of physical signs and symptoms, and assisting with diagnostic studies. The history should include reports of excessive weight gain, increased thirst or hunger, frequent urination, frequent urinary tract or vaginal infections (particularly *Monilia* vaginitis), and glucosuria greater than 1+. Since many symptoms of diabetes overlap findings in normal pregnancy, it is essential that screening begin with the first prenatal visit. If historical risk factors are detected, a 50-g, 1-h glucose challenge test should be performed early in pregnancy. Every woman should be screened at 24 to 28 weeks' gestation with a 1-hour screen, including women screened earlier in the pregnancy, since this is the peak time for insulin resistance. Ongoing nursing assessments during the prenatal period include a review of symptoms of exaggerated glucose levels; signs of fetal well-being; and attention to the presence of signs or symptoms of preterm labor, preeclampsia (especially in the woman with nephropathy or chronic hypertension), and infection (especially pyelonephritis).

▼ Diagnosis

On the basis of an assessment that includes the client's history, physical examination, and laboratory findings, the following diagnoses are suggested:

- Risk for altered nutrition related to hypo- or hyperglycemia
- Risk for maternal injury related to vascular changes, ketoacidosis, infection, macrosomia, preterm labor, and preeclampsia
- Risk for fetal injury related to congenital malformations, macrosomia, decreased surfactant production, and decreased uteroplacental perfusion
- Knowledge deficit: lack of information related to gestational diabetes and its management or management if insulin dependent in pregnancy
- Fear related to a high-risk pregnancy

▼ Planning

The plan of care that is chosen for the woman with diabetes might include the following outcome goals:

- The woman will maintain glycemic control and adequate nutrition
- The woman will deliver without complications related to her diabetes
- The infant will experience no complications and will have a normal adaptation to extrauterine life
- The woman will verbalize her understanding of her diabetic condition and its management
- The woman will verbalize her fears regarding her high-risk pregnancy

▼ Intervention

The goal of nursing intervention for the pregnant diabetic woman is to assist her to understand the diabetes in relation to her own health and that of her baby and to assist her in having a healthy outcome. The nurse can play an important part in the prevention of complications of diabetic pregnancies through preconceptional counseling. All diabetic women of childbearing years should be informed of the increased risks of congenital anomalies (7.5 to 13 percent) and miscarriages (30 to 44 percent) when a pregnancy occurs without good glycemic control (Kitzmiller et al. 1991). However, diabetic women can decrease their risk of these conditions to levels approaching those of nondiabetic women if they conceive while in euglycemic control. Diabetic women should be given birth control counseling to avoid unplanned pregnancies (Diamond 1991). Women who are planning pregnancy should have a comprehensive plan of diet control, exercise, and insulin therapy. Women with NIDDM who are taking oral hypoglycemics need to change to insulin therapy. All diabetic women should begin to take 4 mg/day of folic acid to prevent neural tube defects.

Women newly diagnosed with gestational diabetes require extensive education about all aspects of the disease. A structured teaching plan should include understanding of GDM, meal planning, exercise guidelines, signs and symptoms of abnormal blood sugar levels, and routines for glucose monitoring (Keohane and Lacey 1991). Education about glucose monitoring is a frequent role of the diabetic-nurse educator in the high-risk team. Cooperation of the woman and her family is crucial to successful management of her disease. Specific instructions that are reinforced with written information are helpful. Instructions on how to obtain capillary blood should include (1) washing the hands before the puncture, (2) pricking the finger on the side instead of the tip to decrease pain, and (3) warming the hand to increase blood flow to the fingers. Women can be supplied with a spring-loaded device that lances the finger quickly with minimal discomfort. The blood droplet should cover the entire test strip to avoid a falsely low reading. With the visual method, the test strip changes color and is compared with a range on a chart. With the blood glucose meter, the test strip is inserted into the meter and the level is digitally displayed. Although these meters can be very accurate, they must be calibrated according to the manufacturer's instructions. Urine tests to assess for the presence of ketones using another kind of test strip may be ordered. Frequently, women are asked to test their urine in the morning before eating. Women who are sick are at increased risk for ketosis and should check their urine frequently for ketones. The nurse can encourage a woman to keep a diary of her glucose and urine results, as well as a record of any unusual symptoms she may experience.

Women who are started on insulin therapy need to be instructed about (1) careful filling of syringes with the exact dose, (2) the correct method for subcutaneous injection, and (3) rotation of injection sites. Women who must mix two different kinds of insulin should draw up regular or "clear" insulin into the syringe first to avoid accidentally introducing a longer-acting insulin into the short-acting regular insulin. The nurse-educator should teach the woman and her family about possible signs and symptoms of elevated blood sugar and the consequences of these conditions (Hare 1991; Reece et al. 1991) (Table 21–9). They should know how to respond appropriately to each condition. Newly diagnosed women who require insulin should wear a Medic Alert bracelet and carry an identification card.

Hypoglycemic symptoms, also known as insulin reactions, usually occur at times of peak insulin action, when a woman has eaten insufficient food or exercised too much. In pregnancy, hypoglycemia can occur rapidly without the usual warning signs. If possible, the blood sugar level should be checked. If blood glucose is low (50 to 70 mg/dL), it is best treated with the ingestion of a protein-carbohydrate such as 8 ounces of milk or crackers and cheese (DHS 1992). More severe reactions should be treated immediately with a fast-acting carbohydrate in the form of three or four hard candies, 4 ounces of orange juice or regular soda, and a piece of bread. If the woman is unable to ingest anything, especially in early pregnancy when she is experiencing nausea and vomiting, she and her family should be instructed to have injectable glucagon available. After 20 minutes, the blood glucose level should be determined to ensure that it is rising. Women should be prepared for a hypo-

Table 21–9

ABNORMAL GLUCOSE LEVELS AND THEIR EFFECT ON PREGNANCY

HYPOGLYCEMIA	HYPERGLYCEMIA	KETOACIDOSIS
	Symptoms	
Shakiness Dizziness Sweating Clumsy or jerky movements Hunger Headache Sudden moodiness Behavior change Pale skin color Confusion or inability to concentrate Tingling sensation around the mouth	Urinary frequency Increased thirst Headaches Fatigue or tiredness Drowsiness	Dry mouth Thirst Nausea Excessive urination Dry skin Fruity breath Abdominal pain Vomiting Unconsciousness if advanced
	Signs	
Low blood sugar Tachycardia	High blood sugar Glucosuria	High blood sugar Ketonuria
	Maternal Effects	
Somnolence Stupor Coma	Dehydration Hypotension Shock Sodium or potassium depletion	Decreased pH Decreased bicarbonate Rapid deep breathing
	Fetal Effects	
Possible IUGR	Macrosomia Delayed lung maturity	Fetal distress Perinatal mortality

glycemic reaction by carrying a readily available source of carbohydrate and having nonfat milk available at home and at work. If travel in a car for more than 2 hours is anticipated, women should eat some form of carbohydrate.

Hyperglycemia occurs when there is insufficient insulin, too much food has been eaten, or there has been less exercise than planned. It also occurs in the presence of physical stress, such as an illness or a cold, or emotional stress. Progressive insulin resistance increases the risk of this state in pregnancy. Maternal effects of hyperglycemia are dehydration, hypovolemia leading to hypotension, impaired renal function, decreased mental status, and shock, as well as depletion of body sodium and potassium. Most of the fetal complications of diabetes are due to hyperglycemia. These complications are due to diminished availability of amino acids, fetal hyperinsulinemia, and decreased uteroplacental blood flow. Women with hyperglycemia should decrease food intake, increase exercise, or increase insulin to decrease their glucose levels.

Diabetic ketoacidosis (DKA) is a state of hyperglycemia and accelerated ketogenesis, which is a life-threatening condition. DKA may occur in pregnancy at lower glucose levels than in nonpregnant individuals and is most commonly precipitated by emesis, use of betamimetics and/or corticosteroids, and noncompliance (Hagay 1994). Maternal effects of ketosis are decreases in pH and sodium bicarbonate, increased respiratory rate and depth, nausea and vomiting, and abnormal mental state. DKA is associated with a 50 to 90 percent fetal mortality rate related to hypoxia and the effect of ketones on the CNS of the fetus. Nonreassuring fetal heart rate tracings are frequently noted with DKA. Treatment of DKA usually improves the tracing. Principles of management of DKA include volume replacement, continuous intravenous insulin, electrolyte replacement, and identification of precipitating factors. In the nursing assessment of a woman with DKA the nurse evaluates her level of consciousness, auscultates lungs and checks for Kussmaul respirations, and monitors vital signs. An elevated temperature may be indicative of hyperthermia instead of infection, and tachycardia and tachypnea are commonly present. The development of hypotension is an ominous sign.

The nurse can prepare a diabetic woman for anticipated tests or procedures. The woman's compliance with appointments for ultrasonography, antenatal fetal testing, and daily fetal movement counts increases if she thoroughly understands the risks of her diabetes to her infant. During the antepartal period, the nurse can begin to discuss the reasonable expectations for labor and delivery. The woman should be prepared for the high possibility of a cesarean birth. Referral to a support group may help the woman deal with the stresses of a high-risk pregnancy that not only has a profound effect on her own health but also may seriously jeopardize the infant's health.

Intrapartum nursing management includes making hourly blood sugar measurements and communicating with the woman's physician to regulate her intravenous insulin drip accordingly. The nurse should be alert to the possibility of fetal distress and help position the woman in labor to avoid maternal supine hypotension. Frequent position changes, including sitting in a chair while being monitored, may improve the ability of the baby to negotiate the birth canal and avoid a cesarean delivery.

Postpartum insulin requirements decrease dramatically, since the source of insulin resistance, the placenta, has been removed. The nurse must be alert to signs and symptoms of hypoglycemia and be prepared to treat them appropriately. Generally, the woman with GDM does not have to continue her diet or be monitored for blood sugar levels in the postpartum period. However, the woman with GDM should have a 75-g, 2-hour glucose test at 8 to 12 weeks post partum to ensure that she no longer has a problem with carbohydrate metabolism. She should understand that she is at risk of developing gestational diabetes in a subsequent pregnancy and that, if she is overweight, there is a 50 to 60 percent risk of developing type II diabetes (Moore et al. 1992). The diabetic woman should be encouraged to breastfeed. Fluctuating blood sugar levels are reflected in her breast milk, but these do not have significant effects on the baby.

▼ Evaluation

The plan of care for the diabetic pregnant woman is evaluated according to the identified outcome goals. Her care has been successful if she was able to maintain a normal glycemic state throughout the pregnancy, if she and her infant experienced no adverse complications resulting from the diabetes, if she was able to demonstrate an understanding of her diabetes and its treatment, and if she was able to express her fears about having a high-risk pregnancy.

Anemia

DESCRIPTION

Anemia is one of the most common medical problems encountered in pregnancy. Adequate iron is essential for maternal well-being and fetal growth (see Chapter 19). Severe anemia, with a hemoglobin value less than 6 to 7 g/dL, places the pregnant woman at risk for high-output cardiac failure related to decreased oxygen-carrying capacity of the blood. This complication would place both mother and fetus at risk (Williams and Wheby 1992). Hemoglobin values less than 10 g/dL are associated with increased rates of preterm delivery, low birth weight, and perinatal mortality. However, it is not clear whether this association is due to the anemia itself or whether the anemia is a marker for another causative factor, such as nutrition or socioeconomic status. It should be noted that high hemoglobin levels are also associated with poor infant outcomes such as growth restriction, preterm delivery, and perinatal death (Lu et al. 1991). In the postpartum period, anemia increases the risk of hemorrhage, infection, and poor wound healing.

The definition of anemia in pregnancy is dependent on three factors: gestational age, altitude of residence, and smoking. Physiologic changes in pregnancy that cause a larger proportional increase in blood plasma than in red blood cell mass result in physiologic anemia of pregnancy. This anemia results in an expected 3 to 5 percent drop in the hematocrit, which peaks at 28 to 32 weeks' gestation, demonstrating the importance of obtaining an accurate gestational age (Williams and Wheby 1992). Hematocrit levels for nonpregnant women range from 38 to 45 percent. The normal hemodilution of pregnancy results in hematocrit values of 34 to 37 percent. Women who reside at higher elevations have increased hemoglobin levels that compensate for the decreased oxygen concentrations at those elevations. Smoking causes a falsely increased elevated hemoglobin level, and therefore smoking history should be considered. Anemia in pregnancy may be due to nutritional factors, bone marrow suppression, or hemolysis or may be secondary to blood loss. By far the most common types of anemia in pregnancy are iron deficiency, megaloblastic (folic acid deficiency), and hereditary hemolytic types associated with sickle cell or beta-thalassemia.

▼ **Iron Deficiency Anemia.** Iron deficiency anemia accounts for 90 percent of all anemias in pregnancy. It is common in pregnancy, because diet alone cannot replace the normal gestational iron losses. Therefore, even a woman who follows an excellent nutritional diet requires oral iron supplementation (ferrous sulfate). The iron requirement in pregnancy is 4 mg per day, with a slight increase in the latter part of gestation to 6 to 8 mg/day. During pregnancy, the ability to absorb ingested iron is increased, but the amount of iron absorbed is dependent on body iron stores, rate of erythropoiesis, and use of iron supplements. Unfortunately, as many as two thirds of women of reproductive age in the United States have signs of iron deficiency, and 5 percent of them are anemic because of a decreased ability to absorb dietary iron. Iron is needed during pregnancy for fetal development, manufacture of the increased maternal RBC mass in the increased circulating blood volume, and placental development. The woman who has iron deficiency anemia during pregnancy may be asymptomatic; however, she is at increased risk of developing PIH, infections, fatigue, and postpartum hemorrhage. Her fetus has an increased risk of prematurity, low birth weight, stillbirth, or neonatal death.

▼ **Folic Acid Deficiency Anemia.** A deficiency in folic acid can cause megaloblastic anemia during pregnancy. Folate, an essential coenzyme for DNA, RNA, and protein synthesis, is used extremely rapidly by the developing fetus. If folate is deficient, immature maternal RBCs can fail to divide, are decreased in number, and are enlarged (megaloblastic). Evidence has shown that women must have adequate folate levels before conception for normal neural tube development in the fetus. In 1992 the Public Health Service recommended supplementation of 0.4 mg of folate for all women of reproductive age. Folate requirements during pregnancy increase from 100 to 150 to 200 to 250 μg per day. Requirements for multiple gestations are higher. In women receiving routine prenatal supplements, folate deficiency anemia is relatively rare. However, in Western countries with supplementation it can be prevalent in 25 percent of women, and in developing countries is as high as 60 percent (Williams and Wheby 1992). It can be due to poor diet, home canning of vegetables, or preparation of food in large amounts of water.

▼ **Sickle Cell Anemia.** The inherited hemolytic anemias are sickle cell hemoglobinopathy and thalassemia. Sickle cell anemia is an autosomal recessive, hereditary anemia seen most often in women of African-American or Mediterranean ancestry. It results from the presence of an abnormal sickle-shaped hemoglobin cell (hemoglobin A) in the blood. If a woman is heterozygous for the disease, she is a carrier for sickle cell anemia and is said to have sickle cell trait. In this condition, she has sickling of the RBCs, but the RBCs have a normal life span. Sickle cell trait does not usually cause maternal anemia or problems for the baby. However, a woman who is homozygous for the sickle cell gene manifests symptoms. Because of capillary occlusion by the abnormal sickle-shaped cells, sickle cell anemia can cause recurrent attacks of fever and pain in the abdomen and extremities. During pregnancy it can result in neonatal death, prematurity, or low birth weight. The woman with sickle cell anemia is at risk for thromboembolic events such as pulmonary embolus or stroke, heart problems, preeclampsia, and increased infections. Sickle cell anemia is usually further complicated by iron and folic acid deficiencies (Cunningham et al. 1993).

▼ **Beta-thalassemia.** Beta-thalassemia (also

known as Cooley anemia) is also a hereditary condition and is seen more frequently in African-Americans, Southeast Asians, and those of Mediterranean descent. It is caused by abnormal synthesis of the alpha or beta chains of hemoglobin; however, beta-thalassemia is seen most often in the United States. The abnormal hemoglobin production results in premature death of RBSs, causing anemia. Two forms of the disease exist, depending on the pattern of inheritance. The homozygous form of the disease is known as thalassemia major; the heterozygous form is thalassemia minor. Thalassemia major is associated with an increased risk for the development of preeclampsia, IUGR, fetal distress, and low-birth-weight infants. Thalassemia minor does not cause any particular problem in pregnancy except that it may be misdiagnosed as iron deficiency anemia and treated with iron. Iron supplementation is potentially dangerous in the presence of thalassemia since the condition causes increased iron absorption, which might result in iron overload.

MANAGEMENT

Medical management of anemia is dependent on identifying the cause of the anemia and correcting it if possible. Diagnosis is based largely on laboratory tests. The complete blood count (CBC) provides the initial screen not only for the amount of hemoglobin and the hematocrit but also for the mean cell volume (MCV) and color (mean corpuscular hemoglobin concentration, MCHC). The CBC with a peripheral smear is usually all that is needed to make the diagnosis. Iron deficiency anemia is characterized by small, pale red blood cells (microcytic, hypochromic anemia) with decreased hemoglobin. Folic acid deficiency is characterized by the presence of macrocytic, hyperchromic cells with hypersegmented neutrophils. Normal physiologic changes in pregnancy in combination with iron deficiency may make cells appear normal, confusing the diagnosis of folic acid deficiency. The CBC can also indicate possible beta-thalassemia if the hematocrit is below 30 percent and the MCV is less than 80 femtoliters (fL). Definitive diagnosis of a congenital hemoglobinopathy requires a hemoglobin electrophoresis (Cunningham et al. 1993).

Other laboratory tests can be expensive and are usually required only if there is no response after 4 weeks of iron supplementation. These tests include serum ferritin, which is diagnostic for iron deficiency anemia. Ferritin levels less than 35 μg/L indicate iron depletion, and 10 to 12 μg/L is diagnostic for iron deficiency in the bone marrow (Bushnell 1992). Total iron-binding capacity (TIBC) and transferrin saturation may also be measured. Additional tests for folate may be misleading in pregnancy since serum folate decreases with plasma volume expansion. However, a normal serum folate value can rule out folate deficiency. The red cell folate level may be more reliable but usually shows a decrease more slowly.

Nursing Process

▼ Assessment

The nurse must take a complete nutritional history to assess the adequacy of iron and folate intake for the pregnant woman. Vegetarians may be at risk of iron deficiency, although frequently they are better versed in nutrition and know they need to make up for the iron they miss by not eating red meat. In addition, the presence of the nutritional disorder called pica (eating clay, starch, or ice) must be assessed since it is common in iron deficiency and interferes with iron absorption.

Other risk factors for iron deficiency anemia that the nurse should look for include a second pregnancy within a year, a history of chronic aspirin use, donation of blood more than three times a year, and possibly adolescence (Worthington-Roberts and Williams 1993). Factors that may put a woman at risk for folate deficiency include multiple gestation, urinary tract infection, or the use of drugs that interfere with folate metabolism (e.g., phenytoin, barbiturates, nitrofurantoin, and ethanol). In the physical assessment, the nurse should be alert for signs and symptoms that may be indicative of anemia. Symptoms include fatigue, orthopnea, dyspnea on exertion, palpitations, headache, irritability, and lightheadedness or vertigo bulimia. Other signs include skin or conjunctival pallor, glossitis or stomatitis, heart murmur, tachycardia, cardiac hypertrophy, and edema.

▼ Diagnosis

On the basis of an assessment that includes the client's history, physical examination, and laboratory findings, the following diagnoses are suggested:

- Risk for injury related to increased risk of hemorrhage, infection, poor tissue turgor
- Altered nutrition: less than body requirements related to iron or folate deficiency
- Risk for fetal injury related to diminished utero-placental perfusion
- Risk for noncompliance: recommended diet related to prescribed treatment

▼ Planning

The plan of care chosen for the woman with anemia might include the following outcome goals:

- The woman will complete her pregnancy and deliver safely without developing complications related to anemia
- The woman's hemoglobin or folate levels will return to normal
- The fetus will develop normally and be delivered without complication
- The woman will comply with her prescribed treatment

▼ Intervention

Since prevention is the primary goal in the management of anemia, good nutritional counseling is essential. The woman should be informed about a varied diet that includes adequate iron intake as well as dark green leafy vegetables rich in folate. Women experiencing pica should be encouraged to choose alternative activities when they have the pica urge, such as taking a walk or chewing sugarless gum. Women who have ice pica may try freezing fruit juice instead of water. In addition, women should be encouraged to take their prenatal vitamins daily to avoid iron deficiency.

If supplemental iron is prescribed for the woman, the maximum should be 60 to 120 mg of elemental iron a day (including the 60 mg of iron contained in the prenatal vitamin) (Freund et al. 1993). Iron should be taken at separate times during the day to improve the amount absorbed—for example, a prenatal vitamin in the morning, an iron tablet in the afternoon, and another at bedtime. Iron supplements should be taken between meals or at bedtime with fluids other than milk, tea, or coffee (Institute of Medicine 1990). Women who have difficulty swallowing tablets can obtain iron supplements in liquid or chewable forms. Liquid iron may be ingested with a straw to avoid staining the teeth. Compliance is a common problem with iron supplementation because of the prevalence of side effects, which increase with increasing doses. Women should be aware of the potential side effects: nausea, heartburn, epigastric pain, abdominal cramps, diarrhea, constipation, and blackened stools (Bushnell 1992). The best way to improve compliance is to give the smallest therapeutic dose, start with one tablet a day with meals, and then gradually switch to taking the tablet without meals. It may be better to start taking iron at bedtime, when symptoms may not be as noticeable. If constipation is a problem, the nurse should discuss increasing fluid and fiber intake. Occasionally, women late in pregnancy with severe anemia may need to receive parenteral iron, which must be given using the z-track technique to avoid leakage into subcutaneous tissue and potential local abscess. Compliance can also be improved if the nurse ensures that the woman understands the benefits of having adequate iron stores for herself and her baby. The postpartum risks of hemorrhage and poor healing and the prospect of being less fatigued are usually potent motivators for pregnant women, as is improving the chance of having a healthy baby.

▼ Evaluation

The evaluation of the outcome of the plan of care for the woman with anemia is based on the identified measurable goals. For example, the treatment has been successful if she and her fetus develop no complications related to the anemia, if she is able to maintain a normal hemoglobin or folate blood level, and if she is compliant with the treatment.

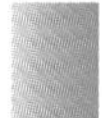

Heart Disease

DESCRIPTION

The combination of maternal heart disease and pregnancy can result in severe disability or death of the mother. Heart disease occurs in 1 percent of pregnancies and is the fourth leading cause of maternal mortality (Gabbe et al. 1991). The hemodynamic changes of pregnancy can worsen cardiac symptoms, resulting in an overload of the cardiac and/or pulmonary system. Maternal mortality can be as high as 50 percent with some types of cardiac disease (Table 21–10). Because of improved management and surgical techniques, the incidence of pregnant women with cardiac disease is increasing. In fact, 27 successful pregnancies have been documented in heart transplant recipients (Scott et al. 1993). However, this fact does not alter the potential for dire outcomes. Maternal cardiac disease also has consequences for the fetus, since normal fetal growth and development depend on a steady supply of well-oxygenated blood. Also, the fetus is at increased risk of being born with a congenital heart defect if either parent has congenital heart disease, and this risk is increased if the parent is the mother.

A brief review of the physiologic changes that occur during pregnancy that can affect heart disease may be helpful. Cardiac output is increased by 40 percent, reaching its peak at 28 to 32 weeks. Some types of heart disease may benefit

Table 21–10

RISKS FOR MATERNAL MORTALITY RELATED TO HEART DISEASE

CARDIAC DISORDER	MORTALITY (%)
Group 1	**0–1**
Atrial septal defect	
Ventricular septal defect	
Patent ductus arteriosus	
Pulmonic or tricuspid disease	
Fallot tetralogy, corrected	
Bioprosthetic valve	
Mitral stenosis, NYHA class I and II	
Group 2	**5–15**
2A: Mitral Stenosis, NYHA Class III and IV*	
Aortic stenosis	
Aortic coarctation without valvular involvement	
Fallot tetralogy, uncorrected	
Previous myocardial infarction	
Marfan syndrome, normal aorta	
2B: Mitral Stenosis with Atrial Fibrillation	
Artificial valve	
Group 3	**25–50**
Pulmonary hypertension	
Aortic coarctation with valvular involvement	
Marfan syndrome with aortic involvement	

*NYHA, New York Heart Association.

From American College of Obstetricians and Gynecologists: Cardiac Disease in Pregnancy. Technical Bulletin No. 168. Washington, DC, ACOG, © 1992.

from the increased output, but women with fixed cardiac lesions may not be able to handle the increased load. Therefore, careful monitoring for pulmonary edema is important at the beginning of the third trimester. In addition, the increase in heart rate during pregnancy may result in poorer diastolic filling of the heart. There is also a decrease in peripheral vascular resistance, which, if not compensated by the heart, results in a fall in blood pressure. This hypotension can result in syncopal episodes in the mother, and the decreased uterine blood flow can compromise the baby. Supine hypotension in later pregnancy is a common phenomenon and must be avoided in women with heart disease.

The intrapartum and immediate postpartum periods are also times of significant cardiovascular changes. During a uterine contraction, venous return to the heart is increased and central venous pressure (CVP) and arterial pressure are elevated. Supine positioning and conduction anesthesia, commonly used for pain relief during labor, can also cause hypotension and a decrease of venous return. Pushing during the second stage can result in dramatic changes in cardiac output and blood pressure if prolonged Valsalva maneuvers are utilized. These procedures may not be well tolerated by healthy women. Therefore, they should be avoided and in specific instances may be contraindicated for women with cardiac disease. With the delivery of the placenta and the subsequent decreased size of the uterus, the blood going to the myometrium is returned to the general circulation, resulting in a further increase in blood volume. Thus, the immediate postpartum period is a high-risk period for women with borderline cardiac function.

MANAGEMENT

All women with heart disease should have the consequences of pregnancy discussed with them preconceptionally. In the case of a woman or partner with a congenital heart defect, genetic counseling regarding the risk to the offspring must be included. A woman and her partner can then make an informed decision about the risks and benefits of having a child. A woman may also have an option for cardiac surgery before pregnancy to correct the heart problem, which would dramatically lower her risk of mortality or morbidity during the pregnancy. Women with heart disease may be taking several drugs to control symptoms, and some of these are potentially teratogenic (e.g., coumarin and spironolactone). In addition, immunization status should be assessed, since infection during pregnancy may be an added stressor that can precipitate cardiovascular failure. The issue of antibiotic prophylaxis to prevent subbacterial endocarditis (SBE) during procedures involving risk such as dental work, surgery, and delivery should be discussed before pregnancy.

Although the primary goal of medical management is to maintain the well-being of the mother during pregnancy, the well-being of the fetus is also important when deciding among different drug regimens that could affect the fetus's growth and development. Diagnosis of worsening cardiac disease is difficult during pregnancy, since many signs and symptoms such as edema and shortness of breath are common complaints. Prevention of infection is a primary goal of medical management. This is accomplished not only with SBE prophylaxis but also with adequate treatment of asymptomatic bacteriuria and respiratory infections, as well as prevention of anemia.

Generally, conservative management of cardiac symptoms in pregnancy is attempted first; this plan may include changes in activity and diet. If these measures fail, cardiac glycoside, antiarrhythmics, antihypertensives, and antianginals as well as diuretics may be used. Diuretics must be used cautiously since they have the potential to decrease uteroplacental perfusion. Women with artificial heart valves and those with arrhythmias are given heparin to prevent emboli. The management of specific heart conditions may vary according to the cardiac problem (Cunningham et al. 1993).

▼ **Mitral Stenosis.** Rheumatic fever is the most common cause of heart disease in pregnancy (Institute of Medicine 1990). There is also evidence for an increased incidence of rheumatic fever during pregnancy. Mitral stenosis is almost exclusively the sequela of rheumatic fever. The stenosis of the mitral valve reduces cardiac output, resulting in the symptom of fatigue. Increased severity of the stenosis causes elevated pressures in the left atrium and the pulmonary vessels, ultimately causing pulmonary congestion. The increased cardiac output of pregnancy as well as fluid retention and tachycardia can result in dyspnea by 20 weeks' gestation, which stabilizes by 32 weeks. Delivery is the next period in which a significant increase of symptoms is expected. Women with significant disease may require invasive hemodynamic monitoring intrapartally.

Mild stenosis is managed by prophylactic treatment with antibiotics against rheumatic fever during pregnancy and delivery. More symptomatic disease requires activity restriction, a low-sodium diet, and cautious use of diuretics. Surgical intervention to perform a commissurotomy or valve replacement is considered if these medical interventions are unsuccessful. Patients with concomitant atrial fibrillation are at increased risk of mortality and require digitalization and possibly cardioconversion. A primary presentation of mitral stenosis may be an embolic event, and these patients require heparin anticoagulation.

▼ **Mitral Regurgitation.** Mitral regurgitation allows blood back into the left atrium because of a prolapse of the mitral valve during diastole. Although it can be caused by rheumatic fever, its occurrence in 10 percent of young adults suggests a different etiology in the United States. Most women are asymptomatic and tolerate pregnancy well. Prophylaxis at delivery is warranted if rheumatic fever is the known cause.

▼ **Mitral Valve Prolapse.** Generally, women with mitral valve prolapse (MVP) are asymptomatic. The defect can occur in 12 to 17 percent of the childbearing population. Most women with MVP tolerate pregnancy well and require prophylaxis only at delivery. In fact, the hemodynamic changes of pregnancy may improve signs and symptoms in some women. However, complications of cardiac arrhythmias, infective endocarditis, and cerebral ischemic events have been reported.

▼ **Congenital Defects: Left-to-Right Shunts.** These defects include atrial septal defect (ASD), ventricular septal defect (VSD), and patent ductus arteriosus (PDA). Generally, if women are asymptomatic these defects do not cause a problem in pregnancy. Women who have pulmonary hypertension are at high risk of developing problems and may be counseled to terminate the pregnancy. Most women tolerate labor well, but care should be taken to maintain venous return and immediately correct any hypovolemia with a blood transfusion if necessary.

▼ **Tetralogy of Fallot.** Tetralogy of Fallot is the most common right-to-left shunt defect. Frequently the defects are surgically corrected in childhood. For women with totally corrected defects, pregnancy poses no increased risk. However, women with uncorrected defects should be counseled against pregnancy since there is a high mortality rate for both mother and baby. Decrease of peripheral vascular resistance during pregnancy can worsen the right-to-left shunt. Also, maintenance of venous return is essential. The most vulnerable time for loss of venous return is during late pregnancy, because of supine hypotension associated with the large uterus, and the early postpartum period. All measures to maintain venous return and blood pressure are appropriate, as is SBE prophylaxis.

▼ **Marfan Syndrome.** Marfan syndrome is an autosomal dominant connective tissue disorder characterized by joint deformities, ocular lens dislocation, and cardiovascular abnormalities. There is a wide variability of clinical expression, which makes cardiovascular assessment before pregnancy essential for accurate counseling. Genetic counseling on risk of inheritance is an important component of preconception discussions. Many authors feel that pregnancy is contraindicated for women with this diagnosis. During pregnancy, aortic dissection and rupture is a significant risk. Its symptoms are excruciating chest pain radiating posteriorly, hypertension, and tachycardia. After a large dissection, hypotension is present. Propranolol is used to decrease pulsatile pressures and avoid such a disaster. SBE prophylaxis is warranted at delivery. If a cesarean is necessary, retention sutures may be needed because of generalized connective tissue weakness.

▼ **Peripartum Cardiomyopathy.** Peripartum cardiomyopathy is defined as the presence of congestive heart failure with cardiomyopathy during late pregnancy or in the first 5 postpartum months in a woman with no history of heart disease or exposure to agents that cause cardiomyopathy. The cause of this illness is unknown, although the functional and structural cardiac changes of pregnancy have been implicated.

The signs and symptoms include fatigue, dyspnea, chest pain, hemoptysis, pulmonary rales, third heart sound, and pedal edema. Management includes bed rest, sodium restriction, digitalis, and diuretic use. Thromboembolic episodes are not uncommon, and anticoagulation therapy may be needed. The long-term prognosis is dependent on the size of the heart several months after diagnosis. Persistent cardiomyopathy carries a significant 5-year mortality risk.

▼ **Valvular Prostheses.** Women who have had heart valves replaced are at high risk during pregnancy, just as are other women with valve disease. Preconception cardiac status needs to be assessed before pregnancy is undertaken. Risks during pregnancy can be due to heart failure, a thromboembolic event, or endocarditis. Women with mechanical valves require long-term anticoagulation therapy. Even with anticoagulation, these women are at high risk for emboli and hemorrhage during the pregnancy. Women with porcine valves do not require long-term anticoagulation unless they have had an embolus. Some studies indicate better outcomes for mother and baby with this type of valve. For this reason, it is advocated that this type of valve be used for women of childbearing age even though it requires replacement in 5 to 10 years. The mortality rate from prosthetic valve endocarditis exceeds 40 percent. Therefore, SBE prophylaxis is mandatory for any dental or surgical procedures and at delivery. If the infection cannot be controlled with antibiotics, the valve may need to be replaced.

New York Heart Association Heart Disease Classification

CLASS I
Uncompromised

- No limitation of physical activity
- No symptoms of cardiac insufficiency
- No angina

CLASS II
Slightly Compromised

- Slight limitation of physical activity
- Ordinary physical activity can result in excessive fatigue, palpitation, dyspnea, or anginal pain

CLASS III
Markedly Compromised

- Marked limitation of physical activity
- Less than ordinary activity can precipitate the symptoms noted in class II

CLASS IV
Severely Compromised

- Inability to perform *any* physical activity without discomfort

Nursing Process

▼ Assessment

The nurse who has contact before conception with women who have heart disease should assess their knowledge of their disease and its potential effect on maternal and fetal well-being during pregnancy. Women who are pregnant should have their functional status assessed using the New York Heart Association classification system (see New York Heart Association Heart Disease Classification). Generally, women with class I and II disease do well in pregnancy, whereas women with class III and IV disease have a 4 to 7 percent risk of maternal mortality (Cunningham et al. 1993).

The usual prenatal care assessment activities provide good indicators of the woman's cardiac health status during pregnancy, along with the other data that are not routinely collected. A review of respiratory symptoms and the symptoms experienced with activity should be done at each prenatal visit. Many of the symptoms of heart disease can be confused with normal changes of pregnancy: fatigue, dyspnea, orthopnea, dizziness, syncope, cardiomegaly, systolic murmurs, dependent edema, cardiomegaly, rales, tachycardia, and electrocardiographic changes. However, the following symptoms are not commonly found in pregnancy and should be further investigated: severe dyspnea, paroxysmal nocturnal dyspnea, syncope with exertion, chest pain on exertion, and hemoptysis. Signs of heart disease that are not typically related to pregnancy are harsh murmurs (especially diastolic), cyanosis, clubbing, and cardiac arrhythmias.

▼ Diagnosis

On the basis of an assessment that includes the client's history, physical examination, and laboratory findings, the following diagnoses are suggested.

- Decreased cardiac output related to the normal increase in circulating volume (50 percent) and cardiac output (40 percent) during pregnancy
- Risk for fetal injury related to decreased placental perfusion in the presence of cardiac or vascular disease
- Knowledge deficit: lack of information related to the effects of pregnancy on heart disease and the consequent need to alter self-care activities
- Anxiety related to high-risk pregnancy with concern for self and fetus

▼ Planning

The plan of care that is chosen for the woman with heart disease might include the following outcome goals.

- The woman will experience no alteration in cardiac output
- The fetus will not be compromised during pregnancy and will be delivered without complications
- The woman will verbalize her understanding of her heart disease, its effects on her pregnancy, and her necessary self-care activities
- The woman will express her feelings about her high-risk pregnancy

▼ Intervention

The goal of nursing care is to maintain a pregnant woman's prepregnancy functional cardiac status and safely deliver a healthy infant. Diet is an important aspect of the management plan for women with heart disease. Although these women have the same nutritional needs as other pregnant women, some women may need to limit their weight gain to the lower end of the acceptable range or even less (15 to 20 pounds), because excessive weight places a further demand on the heart (Creasy and Resnik 1994). The nurse can review a woman's diet and help her eliminate calories that do not provide high nutritional value. In addition, a "no salt added" diet (2 g of sodium per day) is appropriate and women with congestive heart failure may need sodium restriction. It should be noted that most of sodium intake in the United States does not come from using a salt shaker but from eating processed foods. A woman may need to be taught how to interpret food labels to assess the salt content of foods. Prevention of anemia with iron supplementation is also essential to avoid further compromise of oxygen-carrying capacity and to prevent infections.

The nurse can assist in the prevention of infection by reinforcing the need for antibiotics if the woman experiences a dental or surgical procedure. Also, if a woman has a history of previous urinary tract infections (UTIs), the nurse can teach her UTI prevention measures, such as wiping from front to back after a bowel movement, maintaining adequate hydration, and urinating after vaginal intercourse. Women should be encouraged to avoid people with any infectious diseases if possible. Women who develop a respiratory infection should report any signs of a superimposed bacterial infection so that they can receive appropriate antibiotics.

Activity limits should be assessed and discussed with the woman and her family. The gradual increase of cardiac output may mean that activity limits change from week to week. Women should know potential symptoms of worsening disease and limit their activities accordingly. Activity during pregnancy is tolerated poorly with certain cardiac diseases such as cardiomyopathy and mitral stenosis. These women may need strict bed rest during the pregnancy. Women with infants at risk for or those experiencing IUGR may have modified bed rest in the left lateral position to increase uteroplacental perfusion and promote fetal growth.

The nurse may have to instruct a woman about the medications she may need to take during pregnancy. Women who take oral warfarin must be switched to heparin, since warfarin crosses the placenta and can cause multiple congenital malformations in the first trimester; in later trimesters it has been associated with ophthalmic abnormalities and mental retardation (Cunningham et al. 1993). Women may have fear and anxiety about switching to heparin, which must be given subcutaneously. The nurse should instruct the woman or a member of her family in safe, clean injection technique and how to rotate injection sites. A potential adverse effect of long-term heparin in pregnancy is bone loss. Mild weight-bearing exercise may moderate this loss and should be encouraged. Other common medications for the management of heart disease are propranolol (Inderal), digitalis, and nitroglycerin.

Anxiety and feelings of ambivalence about this high-risk pregnancy and the well-being of the fetus are normal responses. Nurses should validate these feelings with the woman and her family. The normal psychosocial adjustments to pregnancy may be prolonged or delayed when a woman has heart disease. A nurse should not attempt to accelerate the process but observe that a progression in family adjustment is occurring. Stress, coping abilities, and support systems should be assessed continually and appropriate referrals made to other members of the health care team when necessary.

▼ Evaluation

Evaluation of the plan of care for the woman with heart disease in pregnancy is based on the specific outcome goals that were developed on the basis of her medical situation and the nursing diagnosis. Her plan of care has been successful if she is able to maintain her pregnancy without alterations in cardiac output, the fetus is not compromised and is delivered without complications, she demonstrates her understanding of her heart disease and is compliant with its necessary treatment, and she can express her concerns about her pregnancy and the status of her baby.

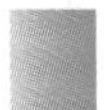

Asthma

DESCRIPTION

Asthma is a chronic lung disease characterized by airway hyperresponsiveness with acute exacerbations of exaggerated bronchoconstriction in response to many physical, chemical, or pharmacologic agents. It is associated with three primary characteristics: (1) airway obstruction that is partially or completely reversible either spontaneously or with treatment, (2) airway inflammation, and (3) airway responsiveness to a variety of stimuli (National Institute of Health [NIH] 1993). Although studies show that about 4 percent of pregnancies are complicated by bronchial asthma, the true prevalence may be much higher. Asthma may occur for the first time during pregnancy or, if diagnosed before the pregnancy, may be worsened by the pregnancy. About one third of pregnant women with asthma are adversely affected, one third remain the same, and one third improve. Women with asthma usually have a return to their prepregnancy level of disease severity by 3 months postpartum. Characteristic symptoms of asthma include cough, wheezing, dyspnea, and chest tightness. These symptoms may be intermittent or more apparent at night, seasonally, or after exposure to allergens, environmental irritants, viral respiratory infections, cold air, or exercise.

If bronchial asthma is uncontrolled during pregnancy, it can produce serious maternal and fetal complications. Maternal complications include preeclampsia, gestational hypertension, hyperemesis gravidarum, vaginal hemorrhage, and complications of labor. Fetal complications include increased risk of perinatal mortality, IUGR, preterm birth, low birth weight, and neonatal hypoxia. However, if asthma is controlled, the woman can maintain a normal pregnancy with little or no increased risk to herself or her baby (NIH 1993).

MANAGEMENT

It is recommended that asthma be treated as aggressively in pregnant women as it is in nonpregnant women (NIH 1993). There are four components of management: (1) objective measures for assessment and monitoring of maternal lung function and fetal well-being; (2) avoidance or control of asthma triggers (factors that induce inflammation or precipitate acute obstruction) in the woman's environment; (3) pharmacologic therapy (anti-inflammatory drugs, bronchodilators, antihistamines, decongestants, cough medications, and antibiotics); and (4) education of the patient. Although no drugs are viewed as absolutely safe in pregnancy, usual medications for the treatment of asthma can be continued. Doses of oral medications may have to be adjusted to maintain therapeutic blood levels because of the increase of blood volume in pregnancy. As with any chronic illness, compliance with long-term medication can be a problem. Acute asthmatic episodes require hospital evaluation with arterial blood gases, supplemental oxygen, and possible intravenous administration of bronchodilators. Mechanical nebulizers may also be used to deliver inhaled bronchodilators.

Nursing Process

▼ Assessment

Assessment of asthma is based on the woman's medical history, a physical examination, and review of the objective measures of maternal lung function and fetal well-being. Maternal vital signs and fetal heart rate should be assessed at each antepartal visit and at regular intervals if the woman is hospitalized. Laboratory values (blood gases, CBC with differential, theophylline levels, electrolytes, sputum with Gram stain and culture, chest radiography, and steroids) should be reviewed as needed. The nurse can play an important role in helping the woman review environmental or dietary factors and over-the-counter medications that induce her bronchospasm. Assessment of the woman's level of knowledge regarding the use of medications is essential (Knuppel and Drukker 1993).

▼ Diagnosis

The following nursing diagnoses should be considered for the client experiencing asthma:

- Impaired gas exchange related to airway obstruction or inflammation
- Risk of fetal injury related to decreased maternal oxygenation
- Knowledge deficit: lack of information related to the effects of asthma on pregnancy and the necessary treatment

▼ Planning

The plan of care that is chosen for the woman experiencing asthma might include the following outcome goals:

- The woman will maintain adequate air exchange without obstruction or inflammation
- The fetus will not be compromised and will be delivered without complications
- The woman will verbalize her understanding of asthma and the treatment plan

▼ Intervention

The nurse's role in caring for the pregnant woman with asthma is to carry out treatment plans and keep the woman informed about the tests and treatments that she will receive. The nurse can educate the woman about the importance of taking medications as prescribed and the implications for herself and her baby if she experiences a worsening of her condition. The woman should be alert to any signs and symptoms of a respiratory infection and be seen promptly for treatment if they occur. Respiratory infections can worsen bronchospasm and also progress more rapidly to pneumonia during pregnancy. All women with asthma should be encouraged to breastfeed, since human milk has anti-infective properties that confer some protection against respiratory tract allergies in the newborn. Women with significant allergies may also want to adhere to a diet free of common allergens during lactation to prevent sensitization of their infant. Most medications in the doses used for control of asthma are safe during lactation.

▼ Evaluation

Evaluation of the care of the pregnant woman with asthma is based on whether the goals and desired outcomes are achieved. The medical and nursing intervention is successful if the pregnancy progresses without complications, the woman's respiratory status remains normal, and the status of the fetus is not compromised.

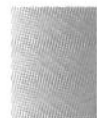

Acquired Immunodeficiency Syndrome (AIDS)

DESCRIPTION

Since its initial recognition in the United States in 1981, the human immunodeficiency virus (HIV), and its end-stage disease acquired immunodeficiency syndrome (AIDS), has evolved to have increasing impact on women and children. In fact, women comprise the fastest growing subgroup of the HIV epidemic worldwide, which is thought to be aggravated by physical, cultural, economic, and political factors (Tinkle et al. 1992). The effectiveness of male-to-female transmission is aided by the large mucosal surface area of the vagina. Additionally, the subordinate role of women in many societies results in their inability to insist on condom use to protect themselves from HIV infection (Smeltzer and Whipple 1991; Persson 1994).

Most women with HIV infection are of reproductive age, which has resulted in an increase in perinatal-acquired HIV infection (vertical transmission) in their infants. In fact, women are often first identified as being HIV antibody positive during pregnancy or upon identification that the newborn is positive. HIV infection is a progressive, severe weakening of the immune system that makes an individual highly susceptible to other infections and types of cancer. It primarily attacks the T4 lymphocytes of the immune system. Because pregnancy is considered a mildly immunosuppressive state, it is thought that HIV among pregnant women may show an enhanced progression (see Chapter 40 for a complete discussion of AIDS/HIV).

MANAGEMENT

Maternal HIV infection during the pre-, intra-, and postnatal period rarely presents in the acute manner associated with events of toxemia, diabetes, or placental abnormalities. The basic nursing and medical care of a woman with HIV during pregnancy and delivery is the same as that of any other patient. However, a woman and her family affected by HIV often require longer visits, more anticipatory guidance, and education, as well as psychological and social services. Also, a woman with HIV is possibly suffering from or dealing with one or more other conditions that complicate her health and pregnancy, such as poverty, substance abuse or recovery, homelessness, and dysfunctional family relationships.

Nurses should play a central role in the care of the woman with HIV, beginning with the education and counseling necessary before HIV antibody screening through providing the support needed by the family as they wait for the diagnosis of the newborn. Components of nursing care include

- Routine HIV counseling and education on the testing recommendations and treatment possibilities for all prenatal patients
- Counseling and factual information for the woman with HIV who becomes pregnant that allow her to make an informed decision about whether or not to terminate the pregnancy
- Nurses being part of the team that communicates positive HIV antibody test results to a patient and assesses the patient's immediate and long-term risks

Nursing Process

▼ Assessment

A detailed health history, physical assessment, psychological assessment, and laboratory data assessment are essential for pregnant women with HIV. A medical and obstetric history provide a baseline of information that help in planning prenatal care and monitoring the progression of the virus. The medical history should include a sexual history, an estimate of when the woman was exposed to HIV, the date and type of HIV testing, and a review of the symptoms the woman has experienced that may be related to HIV (Acosta et al. 1992). The nurse should also assess the woman's support network, risk for violence or legal discrimination, risk for suicide or psychological decompensation, and risk of substance abuse relapse as a result of a new HIV diagnosis.

The physical assessment done at the first prenatal visit, as well as all subsequent visits, should include careful monitoring for early signs of HIV-related symptoms. This is important since progression from early symptoms to more serious disease can be prevented with early diagnosis and treatment. The nurse should be alert to changes in the patient's weight and temperature; shortness of breath; persistent headache or diarrhea; unusual bleeding; localized weakness, paralysis, or change in balance or sensation; seizure or loss of consciousness; visual changes; and changes in mental status. For instance, an elevated temperature (greater than 103°F at any time or 101°F for three consecutive days) can indicate an underlying infection or neoplasm, or weight loss greater than 10 percent in the second or third trimester may indicate HIV wasting syndrome (Hecht and Soloway 1991).

The fetus of an HIV antibody–positive woman should also be monitored closely throughout the high-risk pregnancy. Serial ultrasound screenings are done to identify intrauterine growth restriction. Weekly nonstress testing after 32 weeks of gestation and biophysical profiles may also be indicated (Acosta et al. 1992). The patient's capacity to care for her infant after birth relative to her own health status should also be assessed.

▼ Diagnosis

On the basis of an assessment that includes the client's history, physical examination, psychological assessment, and laboratory findings, the following diagnoses are suggested:

- Ineffective individual coping related to the HIV/AIDS infection process and changes in lifestyle
- Altered nutrition: less than body requirements related to anorexia, diarrhea, and medications secondary to HIV infection
- Risk for infection related to altered immune system secondary to HIV infection

▼ Planning

The plan of care chosen for the woman with HIV/AIDS might include the following outcome goals:

- The woman will express her feelings and demonstrate problem-solving and decision-making skills to deal with lifestyle changes
- The woman will eat a well-balanced diet and gain weight appropriately throughout the pregnancy
- The woman will remain free of HIV-related infections throughout the pregnancy

Intervention

Teaching, counseling, and emotional support are important components of the nurse's role in caring for the woman with HIV/AIDS. These interventions should be given in a private setting and with a nonjudgmental approach. The woman needs to understand the status of her disease, estimated perinatal transmission rates, and prognosis.

The nurse may assist the patient in disclosing her HIV status to significant others. The nurse will also need to educate the patient and her significant others about the meaning of being HIV antibody positive and support the patient through the further testing necessary to stage her infection. It is important that the woman understand that repeated exposure to HIV, through unsafe sex practices or intravenous drug use, can increase the risk of transmission to the fetus. Culturally relevant information should be provided orally and in written form so that the patient will have it to review. This material should cover information on basic HIV transmission, the prevention of secondary infections, and medications, including how to take the medication, the side effects that may be experienced from the medications, ways to prevent those side effects, and the risks and benefits of the medications.

The nurse should assist the patient in obtaining substance abuse treatment when necessary and refer the patient to the multidisciplinary team members who will be part of her care: social services, nutrition, HIV specialist, pediatrics.

During labor, care of an asymptomatic HIV-infected woman will not usually differ from routine care. Strict adherence to Standard Precautions is always important during labor, and especially so with the HIV-infected patient to prevent horizontal transmission (Acosta et al. 1992).

The nurse will also provide appropriate newborn care, assessment, and family education as well as assist the woman with postpartum decisions about birth control. The nurse needs to ensure that the patient has the supports she needs to follow through on medical care for herself and her infant.

Evaluation

Evaluation of the care of the woman who is HIV antibody positive during pregnancy will be based on whether the status of the HIV infection remains stable. Such evaluation should also include the woman's coping responses to her high-risk pregnancy as well as her efforts to maintain a healthy lifestyle.

Perinatal Infections

It is now commonly recognized that infections acquired during pregnancy can affect either mother or baby. However, this knowledge is relatively recent. It was not until Gregg, an Australian ophthalmologist, discovered in 1948 that mothers of infants with congenital cataracts in his caseload all had German measles during pregnancy that it was even considered that maternal infections could affect babies. Since then, much study has been done of the effects of many infections on the pregnant woman and her infant. The acronym TORCH (T for toxoplasmosis, O for other infections such as syphilis, R for rubella, C for cytomegalovirus, and H for herpes) is used in discussing common perinatal infections known to affect infants.

Three common alterations of pregnancy may make the mother and/or fetus more susceptible to infections (Adimora et al. 1994). First, the vaginal walls become engorged and hypertrophied, which exposes a larger area of the columnar epithelium to microorganisms. Second, the vaginal epithelium produces more glycogen, which increases the vaginal pH and alters the flora of the vagina. This alteration in normal flora increases the incidence of acquisition of some infections such as bacterial vaginosis. Third, the mother's immune system is depressed, as evidenced by suppressed lymphocyte function and decreased counts of CD4+ T lymphocytes. The formation of the thick cervical mucous plug may limit ascent of microorganisms into the uterus, but the effectiveness of this protection has not been well studied.

Acquisition of congenital or neonatal infections can occur in three time periods: during pregnancy, intrapartally, or neonatally. Infection during pregnancy can occur by two routes: by transfer of the infecting agent across the placenta or by an ascending infection of bacteria from the vagina, which usually causes an infection of the fetal membranes, chorioamnionitis, resulting in either premature rupture of the membranes or preterm labor with intact membranes. Transplacental infection is limited to infections that involve a causative organism that can cross the placenta such as *Treponema pallidum,* or infections against which the mother does not develop IgG antibodies, which can cross the placenta and protect the baby. Intrapartal infection results from either chorioamnionitis exposure during delivery to an infected cervix or vagina, or exposure to maternal blood.

Infections in pregnancy are relatively common complications, occurring in 5 to 15 percent of pregnancies (ACOG 1993). Generally, infections earlier in pregnancy have more severe consequences, disrupting normal organogenesis. However, later infections can affect the neurologic system, which develops throughout pregnancy. Perinatal infections include those that are transmitted sexually and other viral infections. Perinatal infections are discussed in detail in Chapter 40.

PSYCHOSOCIAL SITUATIONS THAT CAN AFFECT PREGNANCY

Eating Disorders

DESCRIPTION

Five to 10 percent of adolescent and young women experience eating disorders (Burke and Vangellow 1990). Since these women are in their prime childbearing years, one can expect to encounter women with an eating disorder who are pregnant. The most common forms of eating disorders are anorexia nervosa and bulimia. Although these are separate entities, a client may have both anorexia and bulimia.

▼ **Anorexia.** Women with anorexia gain control of their life or their anxiety through strict control of their weight. This can be done by restricting their diet and/or increasing their exercise or through episodes of binges and purges. The profile of anorexia is that of a woman from a white, upper-middle-class background who is a perfectionist, has poor self-esteem, and experiences performance-related stress (Burke and Vangellow 1990). She is generally hyperactive, experiences anxiety if not energetic, and suffers from insomnia. Her body weight tends to be at least 15 percent below normal for age and height. Her body image is distorted so that even in an emaciated state she sees herself as fat. Primary or secondary amenorrhea may also be noted. Paradoxical satiety is a major component of anorexia (Giannini et al. 1990). While starving, the woman feels full, but when she eats, each bite increases her hunger. The onset of anorexia occurs at two ages; the first is just before the onset of menses, and the second is at the time of separation from her family at age 17 to 18 (Burke and Vangellow 1990). Women with late-onset anorexia have a poorer prognosis for recovery.

Anorexia can be a fatal disease; mortality rates range from 4 to 20 percent (Burke and Vangellow 1990). The physical characteristics of anorexia are a thin, cachectic appearance with increased lanugo over the body, alopecia of the scalp and pubic hair, and suppressed menses and secondary sexual characteristics resulting in breast and vaginal introital atrophy. Complaints of constipation, multiple respiratory infections, and cold sensitivity with cyanosis of the extremities are common. Anorexia affects the functioning of many body systems, causing bradycardia, orthostatic hypotension, cardiac arrhythmia, decreased thyroid function, renal changes, and ketonuria. Decreased serum levels of calcium, potassium, sodium, and albumin are also noted (Giannini et al. 1990). It is important that nurses be familiar with these systemic changes, since pregnancy can exaggerate some of the symptoms of anorexia. The laboratory values used as measures of assessment during pregnancy may not be valid in diagnosing certain conditions such as preeclampsia when a woman has an eating disorder.

▼ **Bulimia.** Bulimics use eating and purging as a way to deal with anxiety. Persons with bulimia ingest large amounts of food with a plan to purge themselves to prevent weight gain. Purging is performed by the use of cathartics, diuretics, emetics, self-induced vomiting, or excessive exercise (Burke and Vangellow 1990). Pure bulimics are not underweight but may be undernourished because they undergo large weight fluctuations of 10 or more pounds. They average two eating binges a week and show persistent overconcern with body shape and weight. Bulimia occurs mostly in women, but men can also experience this disease. Generally, women with bulimia are white and come from a high socioeconomic background. They are outgoing, sexually active, and impulsive, with increased risk for chemical dependence, and feel out of control during eating binges. Their family history is positive for depression in either sex, and one or both parents are obese. The onset of bulimia is later than that of anorexia, ranging from 18 to 35 years (Burke and Vangellow 1990).

The most notable physical characteristic of bulimia is the "chipmunk-like" appearance caused by swelling of the parotid gland. The swelling is related to frequent contact with acidic gastric contents, which also causes tooth decay. Other commonly noted signs and symptoms are dizziness, fatigue, abdominal distention, constipation, anal tears or fissures, and hematemesis. Bulimic women report abuse of diuretics, laxatives, and high-fiber foods. The systemic changes associated with bulimia are cardiac arrhythmias secondary to hypokalemia and renal and liver changes similar to those in anorexia. About 20 percent of bulimics are amenorrheic, and this figure increases with decreased body weight. Generally, mortality is rare in a person with pure bulimia and is usually caused by aspiration of vomitus. Unlike those with anorexia, persons with bulimia acknowledge they have a problem and seek help.

Nursing Process

▼ Assessment

Nursing assessment of an eating disorder starts with the recognition that eating disorders are a major women's health issue. Nurses should take the opportunity during general health visits to inquire about a woman's eating habits, desired weight and shape, and use of over-the-counter diuretics and laxatives. A study has shown that the following two questions are highly sensitive in identifying women with bulimia and may also detect anorexia (Freund et al. 1993): (1) Are you satisfied with your eating patterns? (2) Do you ever eat in secret? Responses of "no" and "yes," respectively, to these questions identifies most women with bulimia.

Antenatally, women with eating disorders are at high risk of having growth-retarded babies. Therefore, serial ultrasound examinations may be performed to document adequate growth. If IUGR is suspected, antenatal testing is initiated. As mentioned earlier, laboratory values may already be elevated and normal baseline blood pressure may be low. Therefore, the criterion of an increase of 30 mm Hg systolic and 15 mm Hg diastolic above baseline must be used to assess for preeclampsia. Laboratory values must be compared with baseline data obtained at the beginning of pregnancy to determine whether preeclampsia is present.

Women identified as having eating disorders should receive preconceptional counseling, since studies show that women in remission have much better pregnancy outcomes than women with active disease (Burke and Vangellow 1990). Nurses who see patients for infertility should be alert to the association between eating disorders and infertility. Use of the previous assessment questions may obviate a further medical work-up and expensive treatment for infertility. Rather, a more appropriate referral for treatment of the woman's eating disorder can be made.

▼ Diagnosis

On the basis of an assessment that includes the client's history, physical examination, and laboratory findings, the following diagnoses are suggested:

- Altered nutrition: less than body requirements related to food intake
- Body image disturbance related to self-concept, self-esteem, or personal identity as well as body changes associated with pregnancy
- Ineffective individual coping related to control of life and anxiety
- Risk for fetal injury related to intrauterine growth restriction

▼ Planning

The plan of care that is chosen for the woman experiencing eating disorders might include the following outcome goals:

- The woman will increase and maintain her nutritional intake to meet body requirements
- The woman will make positive verbal statements and demonstrate positive behaviors related to her self-concept and personal identity
- The woman will demonstrate effective coping responses to her personal stress and her disease
- The fetus will not show evidence of compromise related to the woman's eating disorder

▼ Intervention

Normal issues in pregnancy such as weight gain, body image, sexuality, and autonomy versus independence are accentuated for women with eating disorders. Anorectics do not gain weight because it may imply loss of control. They may handle their guilt about not gaining weight and harming the fetus by not seeking health care during the pregnancy. The fears of bulimics may be easier to allay, as their fear of harming the baby can overcome their fear of gaining weight.

The nurse has a difficult role in encouraging appropriate weight gain but not to the degree of removing all the woman's coping mechanisms and alienating her from the health care system. The use of contracts for weight gain and weekly food diaries may be helpful. Comparison of intake reported in the diary with the nutritional needs of pregnancy is an objective method for reassuring a woman that she is not overeating. Contracts may be necessary so that the woman understands that not meeting her obligation will result in hospitalization for feeding. Women may need weekly visits with the nurse, since psychological support is needed frequently. A strategy for decreasing anxiety about weight is to weigh women with their back to the scale or, if appropriate, omit obtaining a weight altogether. A dipstick of urine should include the assessment of ketones. The presence of ketones indicates the body's use of protein for energy.

Hospitalization may be required during the pregnancy, especially for anorectics. These women should be admitted to a high-risk antenatal center or psychiatric unit. Nutrition can be delivered intravenously via feeding tube, or by central hyperalimentation. One author noted that in her experience the only feeding method that anorectic women have not discontinued themselves is central hyperalimentation (Burke and Vangellow 1990).

There are two intrapartal and postpartum concerns for the pregnant woman with an eating disorder. First, electrolyte abnormalities must be corrected intravenously during labor. Potassium is of particular concern, since hypokalemia can result in cardiac arrhythmias. During the postpartum period, the parents may need to deal with the problems of a small-for-gestational-age (SGA) infant who may require prolonged hospitalization. Although lactation should be encouraged, anorectic women must be closely followed since they are at high risk for breastfeeding failure related to insufficient milk supply and vitamin-mineral depletion, which are likely to affect the quality of their breast milk (Bowles and Williamson 1990; Weekly 1992; Riordan and Auerbach 1993). These women should be encouraged to eat 1800 kcal a day and to take a multivitamin supplement. Sources are in conflict as to whether the course of women's eating disorders in the first postpartum year is likely to be the same as during pregnancy or whether relapses are more likely (Burke and Vangellow 1990; Weekly 1992).

Nurses must be prepared for the frustration that can arise when working with women who have eating disorders. These women require much time and emotional energy in efforts that may not always be deemed successful from the nurse's viewpoint. Nurses must be realistic about what they can do to assist pregnant women with eating disorders, and not view the need for hospitalization or poor pregnancy outcome as a personal failure.

▼ Evaluation

The outcome for the pregnant woman with an eating disorder is evaluated on the basis of her ability to maintain adequate nutritional requirements, improve her body image, and cope effectively with stress and on the delivery of a healthy infant who has not been compromised by the woman's disease.

Battering During Pregnancy

DESCRIPTION

The physical and emotional abuse of women by their intimate partners has reached epidemic proportions in the United States. Every 12 seconds a woman is beaten by someone she knows, and each year 1000 women are killed by their partners. One third of these women seek medical treatment for their injuries and one half of all injuries seen in emergency rooms are a result of abuse (McFarlane 1993). However, too frequently health providers fail to identify these women as having been abused; only 5 to 10 percent of battered women are identified on emergency room records (Worcester 1992).

The cycle of violence (Fig. 21–8) is a pattern experienced by most battered women. Partners use isolation to remove women from their social and emotional supports and make the women dependent on their partners for information about their own value (Worcester 1992). Statements such as "No one else will ever love you" or "You deserve to be beaten" become powerful tools in the absence of other validation. The pattern of violence is usually one of increasing tension, climaxing in the battering event, which may be a welcome release from the tension. This battering incident is followed by the honeymoon stage, when the batterer frequently asks for forgiveness and promises never to beat again. Unless there is intervention, the cycle of violence inevitably escalates, with abusive events increasing in frequency and severity.

Our society has many myths about the physical abuse of women, and these myths play a role in perpetuating the belief that the abused woman is responsible for her victimization. The prevalence of abuse in a current pregnancy ranges from 4 to 8 percent, although one study found it to be as high as 17 percent; this represents one out of six pregnant women (McFarlane 1993). There is some controversy about whether battering increases in pregnancy, since studies that showed this association did not adjust for the age of the women. However, 40 to 60 percent of women with a history of being battered are battered during the pregnancy, and some women experience battering for the first time in pregnancy (Campbell et al. 1993). There is evidence that pregnant teenagers experience abuse at a much higher rate (about 22 percent), and most of this abuse starts after the onset of pregnancy (Parker 1993). One study identified four reasons for battering during pregnancy: (1) jealousy of the infant, (2) the pregnancy interfering with the woman's performance of her expected roles, (3) anger toward the infant (a type of prenatal child abuse), and (4) business as usual (Campbell et al. 1993). There was evidence in this study that the severity and frequency of violence increased during pregnancy. Pregnancy is a risk factor for homicide (Campbell 1986). During pregnancy, battered women tend to experience blows not only to the head but also to the abdomen, breasts, and genital area, along with being sexually assaulted. About 8 percent of abused women experience miscarriages, stillbirths, and preterm deliveries attributable to their abuse.

Nursing Process

▼ Assessment

An assessment for abuse should be included as part of routine antepartal assessment. It must occur at the first prenatal visit and at all subse-

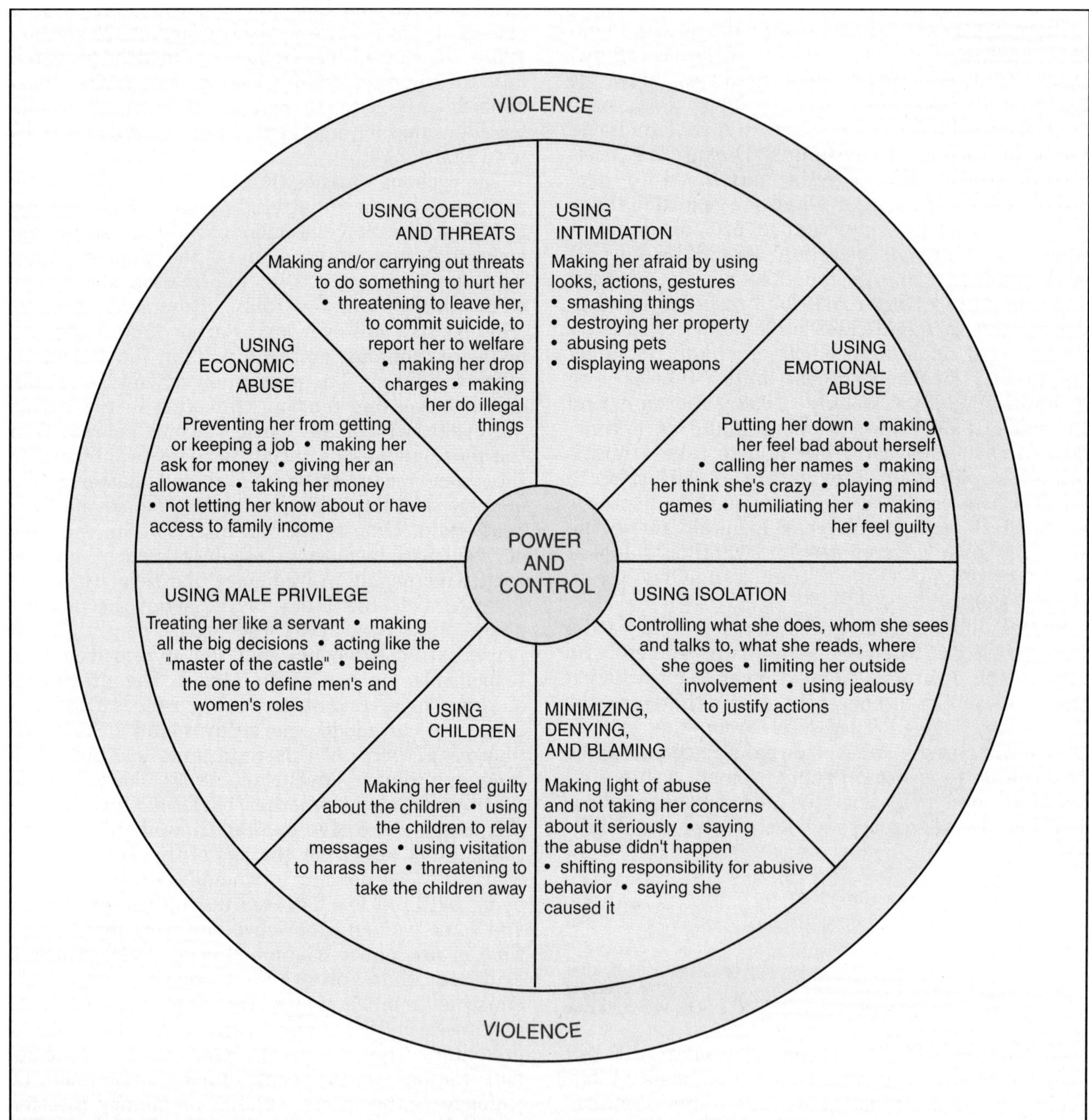

Figure 21–8

Battered women often experience a pattern of physical and sexual behaviors from their abuser when he attempts to demonstrate power and control.

quent visits, since the onset of abuse can occur during the second or third trimester, especially for teenagers. Abused women, particularly Hispanic or African-American women, are twice as likely to begin their prenatal care in the third trimester (McFarlane 1993). Pregnant women seen in an emergency room for trauma or assessed for preterm labor should also be assessed for abuse.

Parker's Abuse Assessment Screen (1993) lists three questions:

1. Within the last year, have you been hit, slapped, kicked or otherwise physically hurt by someone? If YES, by whom (circle all that apply): husband, ex-husband, boyfriend, stranger, other, multiple
2. Since you've been pregnant, have you been hit, slapped, kicked, or otherwise physically hurt by someone? If YES, by whom (circle all that apply): husband, ex-husband, boyfriend, stranger, other, multiple
3. Within the last year, have you been forced by anyone to have sexual activities? If YES, by whom (circle all that apply): husband, ex-husband, boyfriend, stranger, other, multiple

Asking these three questions has been shown to be far more successful in identifying abuse than if providers ask questions in their own way; a study using the Abuse Assessment Screen identified 22 percent of women as abused, versus 8 percent identified when providers asked their own questions (McFarlane 1993). A setting in which nurse and client can be alone should be used when asking questions from the Abuse Assessment Screen, and it is also important that the woman understand that the information she provides will be kept confidential.

An abused woman may not admit to abuse the first time she is asked. Prefacing the use of the Abuse Assessment Screen with, "Many women experience abuse, sometimes for the first time during pregnancy," can reassure a woman that she is not alone. Making the questions from the Abuse Assessment Screen part of the woman's comprehensive pregnancy care can relay the message that the nurse cares about women who are abused and is prepared to help them. These actions may be enough to encourage the woman to confide in the nurse at a later time.

▼ Diagnosis

The following nursing diagnoses should be considered for a client experiencing abuse:

- Risk for maternal and fetal injury related to physical abuse
- Knowledge deficit: lack of information related to options for intervention, social services, and legal protection
- Ineffective individual coping related to physical abuse

▼ Planning

On the basis of the nursing diagnoses formulated from the initial assessment, the nurse might develop the following outcome goals:

- The woman and her fetus will not experience injury as a result of abuse during the pregnancy
- The woman will verbalize her understanding of the dangers of her abusive situation and her options for intervention
- The woman will demonstrate effective coping through her behaviors in response to her abusive situation

▼ Intervention

The nursing interventions for the woman who is in an abusive situation are aimed at acknowledging the abuse, ensuring the woman's safety, confirming the legitimacy of her feelings, and empowering the woman to change. If a woman admits to being abused, the following steps may help the nurse to intervene (Furniss 1993):

1. Reassure the woman that she is not alone and that assistance and resources are available to her.
2. Express the belief that violence is not acceptable no matter what the circumstances.
3. Confidentiality must be assured. Many women are afraid that their abuse must be reported and their partner will retaliate. Assure them that their disclosure is private but their abuse is documented on their medical record in case they need it for legal purposes.
4. Documentation should include a description of the abuse with a history of the first, the worst, and the most recent event. Evidence and photographs must be saved with the woman's consent and according to the protocol of the health care setting.
5. Education about the cycle of violence and the likelihood of escalation of the abuse is essential. Women must be given information about options such as shelters for battered women, hot-line numbers, legal protection, and other available services. The national domestic violence hot-line number is 1-800-572-SAFE.

6. Help the woman objectively evaluate her safety in the relationship. It is important to keep in mind that a woman is in most danger of homicide when she leaves her partner or makes it clear that she is ending the relationship (Parker 1993). Besides telephone numbers for a shelter and the police, a plan for quick escape, including a packed bag with extra keys, money, and important papers, needs to be discussed.

CARE FOR THE WOMAN WITH ALTERATIONS IN PREGNANCY

As the knowledge base related to alterations in pregnancy and our ability to manage complications expand, nurses have an ever-increasing opportunity to provide care for women who are experiencing high-risk pregnancies and for their families. The following suggestions may help to improve quality of care as the nurse becomes more aware of the all-encompassing nature of a high-risk pregnancy.

- DO NOT FOCUS ONLY ON THE TECHNOLOGY OF HIGH-RISK PREGNANCY MANAGEMENT. Also, become sensitive to the emotional impact of this experience by talking with women who are experiencing a pregnancy complication. Identify and learn from the emotional challenges, family problems, and social pressures they may face.
- ATTEND GRIEF AND LOSS SUPPORT GROUP SESSIONS FOR PARENTS WHO HAVE EXPERIENCED A FETAL LOSS IN A HIGH-RISK PREGNANCY. Identify the feelings and issues these parents must deal with so that you can understand and be sensitive to their needs when implementing their care.
- ATTEND CONTINUING EDUCATION SEMINARS RELATED TO BATTERING AND SUBSTANCE ABUSE. Learn more about contributing factors, identification, and the nurse's role in management of women experiencing battering or substance abuse. Examine your feelings and discuss with others how you can become more supportive of pregnant women who are facing these problems.

The nurse can provide positive affirmation to a battered woman through active listening and acceptance. Some abused women state that they thought up outrageous explanations for their injuries in the hope that health care providers would challenge them, but more frequently than not they were never challenged. Some providers cut off women when they describe their abuse graphically. These women need an opportunity to tell as much as they want and to have their experience validated. Listening to the woman helps the nurse understand the woman's situation from her point of view and understand the barriers the woman is experiencing in leaving the relationship (Ulrich 1993) (see Improving Your Practice).

It is important to refrain from telling the woman what she should do. She is in a relationship in which her every move and thought is dictated to her. Making decisions for her only reinforces her belief that she is not capable outside her relationship with the abuser. She needs to be recognized for her coping strengths and assisted in identifying the strengths and limitations of her current relationship. In addition, she can be helped by identifying any social support she has besides her partner. If the nurse can find ways during her relationship with the woman to bolster her self-esteem and assist her in learning more about herself, the woman may gradually be able to leave the relationship. The process of leaving can be a lengthy one; the average is 3 to 5 years from the time a woman has admitted she is abused to when she permanently leaves the abusive relationship.

Many materials are available to help prevent abuse during pregnancy and assist nurses with resources for battered women.

Substance Abuse

DESCRIPTION

For several decades the medical profession has been aware of the adverse effects of environmental and chemical substances on the development of the fetus during pregnancy. Even common over-the-counter drugs that are used by pregnant women for analgesia, nausea, or sedation can be teratogenic for the developing fetus. Unfortunately, these drugs are often used because the woman is unaware of their potential effects or because she is unaware that she is pregnant. The use of alcohol and recreational or illicit drugs poses even a greater risk to the woman and her fetus. The use of these teratogenic substances by pregnant women is increasing at an alarming rate, just as in the general public. Alcohol or illicit substances are responsible for an increased incidence of spontaneous abortion, preterm labor, labor and delivery complications, behavioral and neurologic effects that impair the development of the infant, an increased incidence of stillbirths associated with abruptio placentae, and IUGR. The infants of substance abusers often require long-term assessment, evaluation, and intervention (Creasy and Resnik 1994).

▼ **Alcohol.** Alcoholism affects 1 million women in the childbearing age group. Women are drinking more and starting at an earlier age. Alcohol consumption immediately after conception and before awareness of the pregnancy may be of the greatest concern. The risk of teratogenic effects from alcohol increases in proportion to the increase in average daily intake of alcohol. It is probably not the alcohol itself that harms the fetus but rather the breakdown products. Alcoholic beverages contain not only ethanol (grain alcohol) but also lead, congeners, and aldehydes. High levels of these chemicals are distributed to the organs of the fetus, including the liver, pancreas, kidneys, lungs, thymus, and brain. Fetal blood alcohol levels remain high because the fetal liver is immature and is unable to detoxify the alcohol components.

Alcoholism during pregnancy can affect the woman by causing malnutrition, increasing the incidence of infections, and causing bone marrow suppression and liver disease. It is now also recognized that abuse of alcohol during pregnancy can cause a disorder called fetal alcohol syndrome (FAS). The principal features of FAS include (1) growth restriction, including weight, head circumference, and length below the third percentile, and failure to thrive; (2) a variety of facial features, including short palpebral fissures (small eye slits), a broad, depressed nasal bridge, a thin upper lip, ridging under the nose, epicanthic folds, a flattened midface, and ear or eye anomalies; (3) CNS dysfunction, including learning problems, tremulousness, motor incoordination, hyperactivity, irritability, seizures, and below average IQ; and (4) cardiac, renal, and joint abnormalities (Creasy and Resnik 1994). It has been estimated that 11 percent of women who drink moderately (1 to 2 ounces of absolute alcohol a day) during the first trimester of pregnancy have babies with FAS. No minimal safe dosage of alcohol in pregnancy has been determined. Therefore, the recommendation to pregnant women is abstinence. Although chronic alcoholics are at greatest risk for having infants with FAS, moderate drinkers or even occasional binge drinkers are also at risk, depending on the critical times in gestation when the alcohol is consumed.

▼ **Marijuana.** Marijuana is the drug most frequently used by women during pregnancy. Ten to 30 percent of pregnant women are thought to use it at some time. It can be smoked in cigarettes or pipes or even mixed with food and eaten. When smoked, it has a characteristic sweet odor. It results in intoxication and a feeling of being "high." The studies performed to date related to the effect of marijuana on prenatal development have been conducted with animals, and the findings have been conflicting. Although there have been occasional anecdotal reports of malformations and neurobehavioral abnormalities in the fetuses of women who have used marijuana, there is no strong research evidence that marijuana has teratogenic effects. It does cross the placenta and reduces oxygen in fetal blood. Conclusions about the effects of marijuana are not possible at this time, for many of the study samples have been small and often the marijuana use is compounded by alcohol use (Creasy and Resnik 1994).

▼ **Amphetamines.** Amphetamines activate the CNS, producing euphoria. The maternal effects of amphetamines include hypertension, increased uterine activity, abruptio placentae, and preterm labor and birth. The effect of amphetamines on the fetus has not been demonstrated. It is thought that amphetamines are most likely not teratogenic in humans. However, they are thought to result in IUGR and mild neurobehavioral problems in the neonate (Creasy and Resnik 1994).

▼ **Cocaine.** The use of cocaine and crack has increased dramatically in the past few years. Cocaine is in powder form and is inhaled into the nose. Crack is cocaine that is mixed with baking soda and then heated until it reaches a pure rock form, which is smoked in a pipe. Crack is inexpensive but highly addictive. The maternal medical complications resulting from cocaine or crack use include nasal sinus problems, nosebleeds, perforated nasal septum, cardiovascular problems, pulmonary disease, liver damage, seizures, hemorrhagic bronchitis, and death. "Women who use cocaine have an increased incidence of preterm labor and delivery, and have babies with a lower gestational age at delivery, lower birth weights, and an increased incidence of being small for gestational age" (Lindenberg et al. 1991; Peters and Theorell 1991; Creasy and Resnik 1994).

▼ **Heroin.** Heroin is an addictive CNS depressant narcotic that is usually injected intravenously. It alters the woman's perception and causes euphoria. Women who use heroin during pregnancy are at high risk because of the secondary problems it precipitates (e.g., malnutrition, iron deficiency anemia, preeclampsia, placental abnormalities, preterm labor, premature rupture of membranes, and breech position). Studies of the infants of heroin-addicted mothers have demonstrated a high incidence of low birth weight. Both intrauterine growth deficiency and prematurity have been found. These infants often show signs of heroin addiction themselves, such as irritability, seizures, a shrill high-pitched cry, and fist sucking. These symptoms are followed by signs of withdrawal. Infants of heroin-addicted women are usually irritable and difficult to console for several months, which puts them at high risk for mothering disorders or abuse (Creasy and Resnik 1994).

MANAGEMENT

The most important component of the management of substance abuse is recognition of the problem, for drug abuse in pregnancy is one of the most frequently missed diagnoses. The failure to identify substance abuse in the pregnant woman occurs either because it is overlooked in the routine assessment of the woman during her prenatal care, because health care providers lack knowledge about perinatal addiction, because the abusing woman does not seek prenatal care until the third trimester, or because she receives no prenatal care at all (Starn et al. 1993). If she finally does seek prenatal care it is because of anxiety about the delivery or fear of complications resulting from her drug use. The pregnant abuser volunteers little information, and poor compliance with prenatal management is common.

Care for the woman who is a substance abuser can take place in an inpatient or outpatient treatment setting. This care should include routine and high-risk obstetric care, addiction counseling, social service referral, health education related to all aspects of addiction and pregnancy, and psychiatric treatment if necessary. Urine toxicology screening may be done regularly throughout pregnancy to identify the type and amount of drug being used. The pregnant woman is not advised to withdraw from heroin use all at once ("cold turkey"), for this presents a potential risk to the fetus as blood flow to the placenta is decreased. Methadone, a drug used in the treatment of women who are taking heroin, may be used during pregnancy, although its use at that time is controversial. This drug blocks the withdrawal symptoms and craving for heroin. It should be used carefully during pregnancy, for it does cross the placenta. After birth, methadone withdrawal for the infant may be worse than withdrawal from heroin.

Nursing Process

▼ Assessment

The nurse plays an important role in the identification of a pregnant substance abuser, because the nurse is often the member of the health care team who completes the initial assessment interview. A thorough history and assessment of the physical appearance and behaviors of the woman should be performed. The history must include medical, obstetric, social, and substance abuse information (Table 21–11). Examples of the type of questions that may be used when obtaining the substance abuse history include the following (Kaye and Chasnoff 1993):

- How many cigarettes do you smoke daily?
- How often have you taken over-the-counter medications since you've known you were pregnant?
- How often have you taken prescribed medications since you've known you were pregnant? Were the drugs prescribed for you?
- How many times a week do you drink beer, wine, liquor?
- How often did you use cocaine before you knew you were pregnant? How often have you used cocaine since you've known you were pregnant? How much do you use?

It is important to allow adequate time for this initial interview and to establish a trusting relationship with the woman. The nurse's caring, nonjudgmental approach is essential in setting a tone that encourages the woman to admit that she has an abuse problem.

The pregnant substance abuser has a number of characteristics. The woman's physical appearance may be untidy and her hygiene poor; she may have dilated or constricted pupils; she may exhibit track marks, abscesses, or edema of her arms and legs; and her nasal mucosa may be inflamed. If she is an alcohol abuser, she may emit an odor of alcohol. The woman may appear fatigued, drowsy, or lethargic and be either up (elated) or down (depressed). Her weight gain may be poor and she may have a uterine size that does not correlate with her stated gestational age. The pregnant abuser's behavior may be disoriented, and she may be defensive or hostile in her interactions with members of the health care team.

Table 21–11

PRENATAL HISTORY RELATED TO SUBSTANCE ABUSE

MEDICAL HISTORY	SOCIAL HISTORY	OBSTETRIC HISTORY	SUBSTANCE ABUSE HISTORY
Bacteremia	Family history of alcoholism	Spontaneous abortion	Forms of drug use
Hepatitis	Family history of medical problems related to abuse	Preterm labor	Amount
Pancreatitis	Family violence	Abruptio placentae	Duration
Pneumonia	Incarceration	Meconium-stained amniotic fluid	Frequency
Cellulitis	Homelessness	Fetal death	Route of administration
Cirrhosis	Chaotic lifestyle	Low-birth-weight infant	Location of abuse
STDs	No social or family support	STDs	
UTIs	Prostitution	Inactive or hyperactive fetus	
AIDS	Low self-esteem	Poor weight gain	
Heart palpitations	Nonacceptance of pregnancy	Poor nutritional status	
Acute hypertension		Spotting or vaginal bleeding	
Seizures			
Sleep disturbances			
Extreme exhaustion			
Depression			
Suicide attempts			

Data from Kaye, M. E., and Chasnoff, I. J. (1993). Substance abuse in pregnancy. In R. A. Knuppel and J. E. Drukker (Eds.). *High-risk pregnancy: A team approach* (2nd ed.) (pp. 164–168). Philadelphia: W. B. Saunders.

▼ Diagnosis

The following are nursing diagnoses that might be identified from the assessment of a woman who is abusing drugs during pregnancy:

- Altered nutrition: less than body requirements related to effects of use of alcohol or drugs
- High risk for maternal or fetal injury related to detrimental effects of alcohol or drug use
- Altered fetal growth and development related to effects of alcohol or drug use
- Risk for infection related to method of drug administration, poor nutrition, and lifestyle
- Ineffective individual coping related to poor self-esteem and lack of a support system

▼ Planning

The plan of care that is chosen for the woman who is abusing drugs during pregnancy might include the following outcome goals:

- The woman's nutritional status will improve to meet body requirements for pregnancy
- The woman and her fetus will experience no detrimental effects of the substance abuse, and the baby will be delivered safely
- The fetus will not have IUGR or teratogenic defects resulting from the woman's use of alcohol or drugs
- The woman will not develop infections resulting from the substance abuse

- The woman will enter and maintain compliance with an alcohol or drug rehabilitation program

▼ Intervention

The substance-abusing woman may be encountered at any point during her pregnancy. She may be identified in the antepartal period, and interventions can be focused on the improvement of her health status, prevention of complications, management of her addiction, and referral to social or psychological services. Counseling interventions may be initiated by the maternity nurse in collaboration with a psychiatric nurse who works with substance abuse. The intervention might be individual counseling, group support, or family counseling. The nurse's encouragement, support, and positive approach to the woman are important factors in her motivation to be compliant with her care.

However, the woman may not be identified as having a substance abuse problem until she is in labor. At that time interventions must be focused on management of pain and control of withdrawal symptoms of both the woman and her fetus. Because of her high tolerance to narcotic analgesics, the drug-addicted woman is likely to have a low pain threshold. She therefore needs constant, firm, and directive support. Nonpharmacologic pain management strategies (see Chapter 24) or epidural anesthesia is advisable rather than the use of opiate drugs. The staff of the newborn nursery should be notified when the woman is admitted to labor so that they can be prepared for the care of the newborn. During the postpartum period, interventions first focus on stabilizing both the woman's physical condition and the condition of the newborn. The nurse then focuses on establishing a positive mother-infant relationship.

▼ Evaluation

Evaluation of the plan of care for the pregnant substance abuser is based on the woman's nutritional and general health status, the status of the fetus throughout pregnancy and the infant at birth, and the woman's willingness to enter an alcohol or drug rehabilitation program to deal with her substance abuse problem.

Collaborative Process

Health care for high-risk pregnancy often requires a multidisciplinary approach because of the variety of problems that may arise. The health care team can include the physician or nurse-midwife, maternal-newborn and pediatric staff nurses, a pediatrician, a clinical psychologist, a nutritionist, a social worker, the childbirth educator, and home health nurses. Regular communication between these team members is essential if the care needed for the woman and her fetus is to be comprehensive. Many high-risk pregnancy departments plan regular staff meetings to review and plan this care. The woman and her family should also be considered members of the team, for the woman is more likely to be compliant with the care that is needed for a high-risk pregnancy if she has a part in its planning and understands the importance of her care.

Risk Management

The management of risk is particularly relevant in high-risk pregnancy, for the very nature of the pregnancy alterations makes it more likely that risks will also be presented. This management must begin with an awareness by all members of the health care team of the serious nature of many of the complications of pregnancy and a commitment to remain up to date with the theoretical knowledge needed to care for women with those complications. Reviewing and studying textbooks dealing with high-risk pregnancy, attending continuing education conferences, reading professional journal articles related to high-risk pregnancy, and belonging to professional organizations are all ways to maintain the necessary knowledge base.

The nurse working in a high-risk inpatient or outpatient antepartal setting must be sure that her skills are excellent and that she understands the rationale behind each intervention she gives. Consistent use of the nursing process serves as a guide to logical thinking and planning for the woman's care. Risk can also be averted by ensuring frequent communication between and accurate documentation by all the members of the health care team who might be involved in managing a high-risk pregnancy. When many different professionals provide services for the woman, it is easy to assume that an essential component of care has or has not been carried out, thus risking either duplication or omission of an essential intervention. Education of the woman is a final factor that can reduce the risk involved in a high-risk pregnancy, for if she understands the manifestations of her complication and the plan for treatment, she will be more compliant with her care.

Implications for Research

A great deal of medical research has been conducted to answer questions related to high-risk pregnancy. Nursing research is also needed in this area. The following questions are examples of research questions that might be studied:

- What maternal position results in the most consistent and accurate blood pressure readings during pregnancy?
- What nursing interventions are helpful in facilitating compliance with complete bed rest for the high-risk pregnant woman?
- Which method of fetal movement counting (FMC) is preferred and consistently used by women during a high-risk pregnancy?
- Are there differences in maternal role competence in women who experience a high-risk pregnancy?

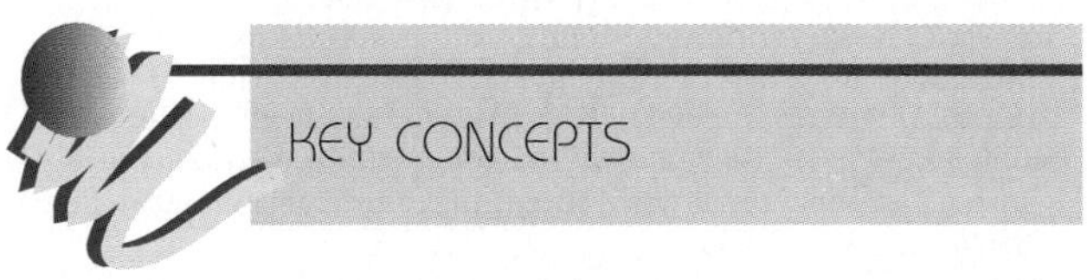

KEY CONCEPTS

- ▼ Pregnancy brings about complex physiologic and emotional changes for women and for those who provide support in their lives. A normal adaptive process must occur in order to ensure a healthy mother and baby. When a pregnancy is identified as high risk these processes are challenged, particularly as the risk of morbidity and mortality increases.
- ▼ Nursing assessment skills are essential to identifying women who are at risk during pregnancy. A thorough history obtained through thoughtful questioning and active listening makes a difference in early recognition and treatment of problems. It allows nursing diagnoses to be made that lead to a plan of care that is individualized. This ultimately decreases risk and improves outcomes.
- ▼ The nursing process of assessment, diagnosis, planning, implementation, and evaluation of a care plan is dynamic and must be ongoing throughout a woman's pregnancy. Communication skills are a critical component of antepartal nursing care in high-risk pregnancies. Open communication between primary providers and between providers and clients should be facilitated.
- ▼ Many conditions require detailed and ongoing education regarding such areas as diet, exercise, recognition of signs and symptoms of potential problems, and compliance with prescribed treatments. Women should be encouraged to listen to their bodies and to recognize and report early warning signs of changes in maternal or fetal condition. This process needs to be validated, and it is often the nurse who promotes this empowerment.
- ▼ Maternal conditions that can complicate a pregnancy or that arise because of pregnancy include incompetent cervix, hyperemesis, hypertensive disorders of pregnancy, Rh isoimmunization, ABO incompatibility, diabetes, anemia, heart disease, infections, eating disorders, trauma or surgery, threats of domestic violence, and substance abuse.
- ▼ Some complications of pregnancy are related to the fetus and include spontaneous abortion, ectopic pregnancy, molar pregnancy, fetal demise, multiple gestation, premature labor, and intrauterine growth restriction.
- ▼ Complications can arise at different times and throughout a pregnancy. The psychological stress of a high-risk designation and the loss of the "perfect pregnancy" fantasy require attention at least as much as the physical needs of the woman. Nurses can help guide families during pregnancy.
- ▼ It is essential to maintain a perspective on the whole woman and not just on her pregnancy and its complications. This may include helping her develop coping strategies to deal with such issues as changes in family role, economic stress, and social isolation such as may occur when bed rest is required for weeks or even months. Caring for women and their families requires a holistic approach to the dynamic process that is pregnancy.

References

Acosta, Y., Goodwin, C., Amaya, M., Tinkle, M., Acosta, E., Jaquez, I. (1992). HIV disease and pregnancy: Part 2. Antepartum and intrapartum care. *Journal of Obstetric, Gynecologic, and Neonatal Nursing,* 21 (2), 97–103.

Adimora, A. A., Hamilton, H., Holmes, K. K. (1994). *Sexually transmitted diseases: Companion handbook* (2nd ed.). New York: McGraw-Hill.

Alexander, G. R., Weiss, J., Hilsey, T. C., Papiernik, E. (1991). Preterm birth prevention: An evaluation of programs in the United States. *Birth,* 18 (3), 160–169.

American College of Obstetricians and Gynecologists (ACOG). (1990). *Prevention of D isoimmunization* (Technical Bulletin 147). Washington, DC: Author.

American College of Obstetricians and Gynecologists (ACOG). (1992). *Cardiac disease in pregnancy* (Technical Bulletin 168). Washington, DC: Author.

American College of Obstetricians and Gynecologists (ACOG). (1993). *Perinatal viral and parasitic infections* (Technical Bulletin 177). Washington, DC: Author.

American College of Obstetricians and Gynecologists (ACOG) (1996). *Hypertension in pregnancy.* (Technical Bulletin 219). Washington, DC: Author.

Arnold, L. S. (1992). Low birth weight and infant mortality: A health policy perspective. *NAACOG's Clinical Issues in Perinatal and Women's Health Nursing,* 3 (1), 1–12.

Beal, M. W. (1992). Acupuncture and related treatment modalities. Part II: Applications to antepartal and intrapartal care. *Journal of Nurse-Midwifery,* 37 (4), 260–268.

Belizan, J. M., Villar, J., Gonzalez, L., Campodonico, L., Bergel, E. (1991). Calcium supplementation to prevent hypertensive disorders of pregnancy. *New England Journal of Medicine,* 325 (20), 1399–1405.

Bowles, B. C., and Williamson, B. P. (1990). Pregnancy and lactation following anorexia and bulimia. *Journal of Obstetric, Gynecologic, and Neonatal Nursing,* 19 (3), 243–248.

Brown, J. E., and Schloesser, P. T. (1990). Prepregnancy weight status, prenatal weight gain, and the outcome of term twin gestations. *American Journal of Obstetrics and Gynecology,* 162, 182–187.

Brustman, L. E., Raptoulis, M., Langer, O., Anyaegbunam, A., Merkatz, I. R. (1989). Changes in the pattern of uterine contractility in relationship to coitus during pregnancy at low and high risk for preterm labor. *Obstetrics and Gynecology,* 73 (2), 166–168.

Burke, M. E., and Vangellow, J. (1990). Anorexia nervosa and bulimia nervosa: Chronic conditions affecting pregnancy. *NAACOG's Clinical Issues in Perinatal and Women's Health Nursing,* 1 (2), 240–254.

Bushnell, F. K. L. (1992). A guide to primary care of iron-deficiency anemia. *Nurse Practitioner,* 17 (11), 68–73.

Campbell, J. (1986). Nursing assessment for risk of homicide with battered women. *Advances in Nursing Science,* 8, 36–51.

Campbell, J. C., Oliver, C., Bullock, L. (1993). Why battering during pregnancy? *AWHONN's Clinical Issues in Perinatal and Women's Health Nursing,* 4 (3), 343–349.

Carson, S. A., and Butler, J. E. (1993). Ectopic pregnancy. *New England Journal of Medicine,* 329 (16), 1174–1181.

Colie, C. F. (1993). Preterm labor and delivery in working women. *Seminars in Perinatology,* 17 (1), 37–44.

Cousins, L. (1991). Etiology and prevention of congenital anomalies among infants of overt diabetic women. *Clinical Obstetrics and Gynecology,* 34 (3), 481–493.

Coustan, D. R. (1991). Management of gestational diabetes. *Clinical Obstetrics and Gynecology,* 34 (3), 558–564.

Creasy, R. K., and Resnik, R. (1994). *Maternal-fetal medicine: Principles and practice* (3rd ed.). Philadelphia: W. B. Saunders.

Cunningham, F. G., MacDonald, P. C., Gant, N. F., Leveno, K. J., Gilstrap, L. C. III. (1993). *Williams obstetrics* (19th ed.). Norwalk, CT: Appleton & Lange.

Department of Health Services, State of California, Maternal & Child Health Branch. (1992). *Sweet success: California diabetes and pregnancy program guidelines for care.* Los Angeles: Author.

Diamond, M. P. (1991). Contraception in diabetic women. *Clinical Obstetrics and Gynecology,* 34 (3), 565–571.

Dyson, D. C., Crites, Y. M., Ray, D. A., Armstrong, M. A. (1991). Prevention of preterm birth in high-risk patients: The role of education and provider contact versus home uterine monitoring. *American Journal of Obstetrics and Gynecology,* 164, 756–762.

Eganhouse, D. J. (1992). Fetal monitoring of twins. *Journal of Obstetric, Gynecologic, and Neonatal Nursing,* 21 (1), 17–27.

Erick, M. (1993). *No more morning sickness: A survival guide for pregnant women.* New York: Plume Books.

Ewton, D. S. (1993). A perinatal loss follow-up guide for primary care. *Nurse Practitioner,* 18 (12), 30–39.

Freund, K. M., Graham, S. M., Lesky, L. G., Moskowitz, M. A. (1993). Detection of bulimia in a primary care setting. *Journal of General Internal Medicine,* 8 (5), 236–242.

Furniss, K. K. (1993). Screening for abuse in the clinical setting. *AWHONN's Clinical Issues in Perinatal and Women's Health Nursing,* 4 (3), 402–406.

Gabbe, S. G., Niebyl, J. R., Simpson, J. L. (1991). *Obstetrics: Normal and problem pregnancies* (2nd ed.). New York: Churchill Livingstone.

Giannini, A. J., Newman, M., Gold, M. (1990). *American Family Physician,* 41 (4), 1169–1176.

Hagay, Z. J. (1994). Diabetic ketoacidosis in pregnancy: Etiology, pathophysiology, and management. *Clinical Obstetrics and Gynecology,* 37 (1), 39–48.

Hare, J. W. (1991). Insulin management of type I and type II diabetes in pregnancy. *Clinical Obstetrics and Gynecology,* 34 (3), 494–503.

Hecht, F., and Soloway, B. (1991). The physical exam in HIV infection. *AIDS Clinical Care,* 3, 4–5.

Herbst, A. L., Mishell, D. R., Stenchever, M. A., Droegemueller, W. (1992). *Comprehensive gynecology* (2nd ed.). St. Louis: Mosby-Year Book.

Hillier, S. L., Nugent, R. P., Eschenkach, D. A., Krohn, M. A., Gibbs, R. S., Martin, D. H., Cotch, M. F., Edelman, R., Pastorek, J. G. 2nd, Rao, A. V., McNellis, D., Regan, J., Carey, J. C., and Klebanoff, M. (1995). Association between bacterial vaginosis and preterm delivery of a low-birth- weight infant. The Vaginal Infection and Prematurity Study Group. *New England Journal of Medicine,* 333 (26), 1737–1742.

Hines, T., and Jones, M. B. (1994). Can aspirin prevent and treat preeclampsia? *MCN,* 19 (5), 258–263.

Holbrook, R. H., Jr., Laros, R. K., Jr., Creasy, R. K. (1989). Evaluation of a risk-screening system for prediction of preterm labor. *American Journal of Perinatology,* 6 (1), 62–68.

Hutti, M. H., (1988). A quick reference table of intervention to assist families cope with pregnancy loss or neonatal death. *Birth,* 15 (1), 33–35.

Imperiale, T. F., and Stollenwerk, A. (1991). A meta-analysis of low-dose aspirin for the prevention of pregnancy-induced hypertension: Up-to-date evidence. *American Journal of Obstetrics and Gynecology,* 158 (4), 898–902.

Institute of Medicine. (1990). *Nutrition during pregnancy.* Washington, DC: National Academy Press.

Institute of Medicine. (1992). *Nutrition during pregnancy and lactation: An implementation guide.* Washington, DC: National Academy Press.

Johnson, J., and Oakley, L. (1991). Managing minor trauma during pregnancy. *Journal of Obstetric, Gynecologic, and Neonatal Nursing,* 20 (5), 379–384.

Jovanovic-Peterson, L., and Peterson, C. M. (1990). Dietary manipulation as a primary treatment strategy for pregnancy complicated by diabetes. *Journal of American College of Nutrition,* 9, 320–324.

Kaye, M. E., and Chasnoff, I. J. (1993). Substance abuse in pregnancy. In R. A. Knuppel and J. E. Drukker (Eds.). *High-risk pregnancy: A team approach* (2nd ed.). Philadelphia: W. B. Saunders.

Keening, C. (1992). Perinatal hypertensive crisis. *NAACOG's Clinical Issues in Perinatal and Women's Health Nursing,* 3 (3), 413–419.

Keohane, N. S., and Lacey, L. A. (1991). Preparing the woman with gestational diabetes for self care. *Journal of Obstetric, Gynecologic, and Neonatal Nursing,* 20 (3), 189–193.

Kitzmiller, J. L., Gavin, L. A., Gunderson, E. (1991). Preconception counseling: Rationale for evaluation and management of diabetes prior to pregnancy. In J. L. Kitzmiller, L. A. Gavin, E. Gunderson (Eds.). *Current obstetric medicine 1.* St. Louis: C. V. Mosby.

Klebanoff, M. A., Shiono, P. H., Carey, J. C. (1990). Outcomes of pregnancy in a national sample of resident physicians. *New England Journal of Medicine,* 323 (15), 1040–1045.

Knuppel, R. A., and Drukker, J. E. (Eds.) (1993). *High-risk pregnancy: A team approach* (2nd ed.). Philadelphia: W. B. Saunders.

Landon, M. B., and Gabbe, S. G. (1991). Fetal surveillance in the pregnancy complicated by diabetes mellitus. *Clinical Obstetrics and Gynecology,* 34 (3), 535–543.

Lenfant, D., Gifford, R., Zuspan, F. (1990). Consensus report: High blood pressure in pregnancy. *American Journal of Obstetrics,* 163 (5), 1689–1712.

Lichtman, R., and Papera S. (1990). *Gynecology: Well woman care.* Norwalk, CT: Appleton & Lange.

Lindenberg, C., McDaniels, A., Gendrop, S., Nencioli, M., Conyhon, D. (1991). A review of the literature on cocaine abuse in pregnancy. *Nursing Research,* 40 (2), 69–75.

Lu, Z. M., Goldenberg, R. L., Cliver, S. P., Cutter, G., Blankson, M. (1991). The relationship between maternal hematocrit and pregnancy outcome. *Obstetrics and Gynecology,* 77, 190–194.

Magee, M. S., Walden, C. E., Benedetti, T. J. (1993). Influence of diagnostic criteria on the incidence of gestational diabetes and perinatal morbidity. *JAMA,* 269 (5), 609–615.

Main, D. M., Grisso, J. A., Snyder, E. S., Chiu, G. Y., Holmes, J. H. (1993). The effect of sexual activity on uterine contractions in pregnancy. *Journal of Women's Health,* 2 (2), 141–144.

Maloni, J. (1993). Bed rest during pregnancy: Implications for nursing. *Journal of Obstetric, Gynecologic, and Neonatal Nursing,* 22 (5), 422–428.

Maloni, J., Chance, B., Zhang, C., Cohen, A., Betts, D., Gange, S. (1993). Physical and psychosocial side effects of antepartum hospital bed rest. *Nursing Research,* 42 (4), 197–200.

Mandeville, L. K. (1992). Diabetic ketoacidosis. *NAACOG's Clinical Issues in Perinatal and Women's Health Nursing,* 3 (3), 514–520.

Martin, J. N., Jr., Blake, P. G., Lowry, S. L., Perry, K. G., Jr., Files, J. C., Morrison, J. C. (1990). Pregnancy complicated by pre-eclampsia with syndrome of hemolysis, elevated liver enzymes, and low platelet count: How rapid is postpartum recovery? *Obstetrics and Gynecology,* 76 (5, part 1), 737–741.

McFarlane, J. (1993). Abuse during pregnancy: The horror and the hope. *AWHONN's Clinical Issues in Perinatal and Women's Health Nursing,* 4 (3), 350–362.

McLean, M., Walters, W., Smith, R. (1993). Prediction and early diagnosis of preterm labor: A critical review. *Obstetrical and Gynecological Survey,* 48 (4), 209–225.

Monahan, P. A., and DeJoseph, J. F. (1991). The woman with preterm labor at home: A descriptive analysis. *Journal of Perinatal and Neonatal Nursing,* 4 (4), 12–20.

Moore, T. R., Reiter, R. C., Rebar, R. W., Baker, V. V. (1992). *Gynecology and obstetrics: A longitudinal approach.* New York: Churchill Livingstone.

Mueller, L. (1991). Second-trimester termination of pregnancy: Nursing care. *Journal of Obstetric, Gynecologic, and Neonatal Nursing,* 20 (4), 284–289.

Murphy, J. M., and Robbins, D. (1993). Psychosocial implications of high-risk pregnancy. In R. A. Knuppel and J. E. Drukker (Eds.). *High-risk pregnancy: A team approach* (2nd ed.) (p. 244). Philadelphia: W. B. Saunders.

Murphy, P. A. (1993). Preterm prevention programs: A critique of the literature. *Journal of Nurse-Midwifery,* 38 (6), 324–335.

Nageotte, M., Casal, D., Senyei, A. (1994). Fetal fibronectin in patients at increased risk for premature birth. *American Journal of Obstetrics and Gynecology,* 170 (1), 20–25.

National Institute of Health (1993). *Management of asthma during pregnancy* (NIH Publication No. 93-3279A). Washington, D.C.: Author.

Newman, V., and Fullerton, J. T. (1990). Role of nutrition in the prevention of preeclampsia: Review of the literature. *Journal of Nurse-Midwifery,* 35 (5), 282–291.

Newman, V., Fullerton, J. T., Anderson, P. O. (1993). Clinical advances in the management of severe nausea and vomiting during pregnancy. *Journal of Obstetric, Gynecologic, and Neonatal Nursing,* 22 (6), 483–490.

Parker, B. (1993). Abuse of adolescents: What can we learn from pregnant teenagers? *AWHONN's Clinical Issues in Perinatal and Women's Health Nursing,* 4 (3), 363–370.

Persson, E. (1994). The threat of AIDS to the health of women. *International Journal of Gynecology and Obstetrics,* 46, 189–193.

Peters, H., and Theorell, C. (1991). Fetal and neonatal effects of maternal cocaine use. *Journal of Obstetric, Gynecologic, and Neonatal Nursing,* 20 (2), 121–127.

Reece, E. A., Homko, C. J., Wiznitzert, A. (1991). Hypoglycemia in pregnancies complicated by diabetes mellitus: Maternal and fetal considerations. *Clinical Obstetrics and Gynecology,* 37 (1), 50–58.

Repke, J. T. (1991). Prevention of preeclampsia. *Clinics in Perinatology,* 18, 779–781.

Riordan, J., and Auerbach, K. G. (1993). *Breastfeeding and human lactation.* Boston: Jones & Bartlett.

Roberts, J. (1994). Hypertension in pregnancy. In R. K. Creasy and R. Resnick (Eds.). *Maternal-fetal medicine: Principles and practice* (3rd ed.). Philadelphia: W. B. Saunders.

Rubin, E., and Farber, J. L. (1988). *Pathology.* Philadelphia: J. B. Lippincott.

Ryan, P. F., Cote-Arsenault, D., Sugarman, L. L. (1991). Facilitating care after perinatal loss. *Journal of Obstetric, Gynecologic, and Neonatal Nursing,* 20 (5), 385–389.

Sacks, D. A., Abu-fadil, S., Greenspoon, J. S., Fotheringham, N. (1989). Do the current standards for glucose tolerance testing in pregnancy represent a valid conversion of O'Sullivan's original criteria? *American Journal of Obstetrics and Gynecology,* 161 (3), 638–641.

Saftlas, A. F., Olson, D. R., Franks, A. L., Atrash, H. K., Pokras, R. (1990). Epidemiology of preeclampsia and eclampsia in the United States, 1979–1986. *American Journal of Obstetrics and Gynecology,* 163 (2), 460–465.

Savitz, D. A., Blackmore, C. A., Thorp, J. M. (1991). Epidemiologic characteristics of preterm delivery: Etiologic heterogeneity. *American Journal of Obstetrics and Gynecology,* 164, 467–471.

Scott, J. R., Wagoner, L. E, Olsen, S. L., Taylor, D. O., Renlund, D. G. (1993). Pregnancy in heart transplant recipients: Management and outcome. *Obstetrics and Gynecology,* 82 (3), 324–327.

Selwyn, B. J. (1990). The accuracy of obstetric risk assessment instruments for predicting mortality, low birth weight, and preterm birth. In I. R. Merkatz, J. E. Thompson, R. D. Mullen, R. L. Goldenberg (Eds.). *New perspectives on prenatal care* (pp. 39–65). New York: Elsevier.

Sibai, B. M., Caritis, S. N., Thom, M. E., Klebanoff, M., McNellis, D., Rocco, L., Paul, R. H., Romero, R., Witter, F., Rosen, M., Depp, R. (1993). Prevention of pre-eclampsia with low dose aspirin in healthy, nulliparous pregnant women. *New England Journal of Medicine,* 329 (17), 13–18.

Smeltzer, S., and Whipple, B. (1991). Women and HIV infection. *Image: Journal of Nursing Scholarship,* 23 (4), 249–256.

Starn, J., Patterson, K., Bemis, G., Castro, O., Bemis, R. (1993). Can we encourage pregnant substance abusers to seek prenatal care? *MCN,* 18 (3), 148–152.

Stone, J., Lockwood, C., Berkowitz, G., Alvarez, M., Lapinski, R., Berkowitz, R. (1994). Risk factors for severe preeclampsia. *Obstetrics and Gynecology,* 83 (3), 357–361.

Surratt, N. (1993). Severe preeclampsia: Implications for critical-care obstetric nursing. *Journal of Obstetric, Gynecologic, and Neonatal Nursing,* 22 (6), 500–507.

Tinkle, M., Amaya, M., Tamayo, O. (1992). HIV disease and pregnancy: Part 1. Epidemiology, pathogenesis, and natural history. *Journal of Obstetric, Gynecologic, and Neonatal Nursing,* 21 (2), 86–93.

Ulrich, Y. C. (1993). What helped most in leaving spouse abuse: Implications for interventions. *AWHONN's Clinical Issues in Perinatal and Women's Health Nursing,* 4 (3), 385–390.

United States Public Health Service (1993). Home uterine activity monitoring for preterm labor. *JAMA,* 270 (3), 369–376.

Villar, J., Farnot, U., Barros, F., Victora, C., Langer, A., Belizan, J. M. (1992). A randomized trial of psychosocial support during high-risk pregnancy. *New England Journal of Medicine,* 327 (18), 1266–1271.

Vomund, S., and Witter, S. (1994). Advanced techniques for the treatment of severe isoimmunization. *MCN,* 19 (1), 18–23.

Weekly, S. J. (1992). Diets and eating disorders: Implications for the breastfeeding mother. *NAACOG's Clinical Issues in Perinatal and Women's Health Nursing,* 3 (4), 695–700.

Wertz, R. W., and Wertz, D. C. (1977). *Lying-in: A history of childbirth in America* (p. 21). New Haven: Yale University Press.

Williams, M. D., and Wheby, M. S. (1992). Anemia in pregnancy. *Medical Clinics of North America,* 76 (3), 631–647.

Windsor, R. A., Li, C. Q., Lowe, J. B., Perkins, L. L., Ershoff, D., Glynn, T. (1993). The dissemination of smoking cessation methods for pregnant women: Achieving the year 2000 objectives. *American Journal of Public Health,* 83, 173–178.

Worcester, N. (1992). The unique role health workers can play in recognizing and responding to battered women. *National Women's Health Network News,* March/April, 1–4.

Worthington-Roberts, B., and Williams, S. R. (1993). *Nutrition in pregnancy and lactation* (5th ed.). St. Louis: C. V. Mosby.

Unit 4

Nursing Care During Childbirth

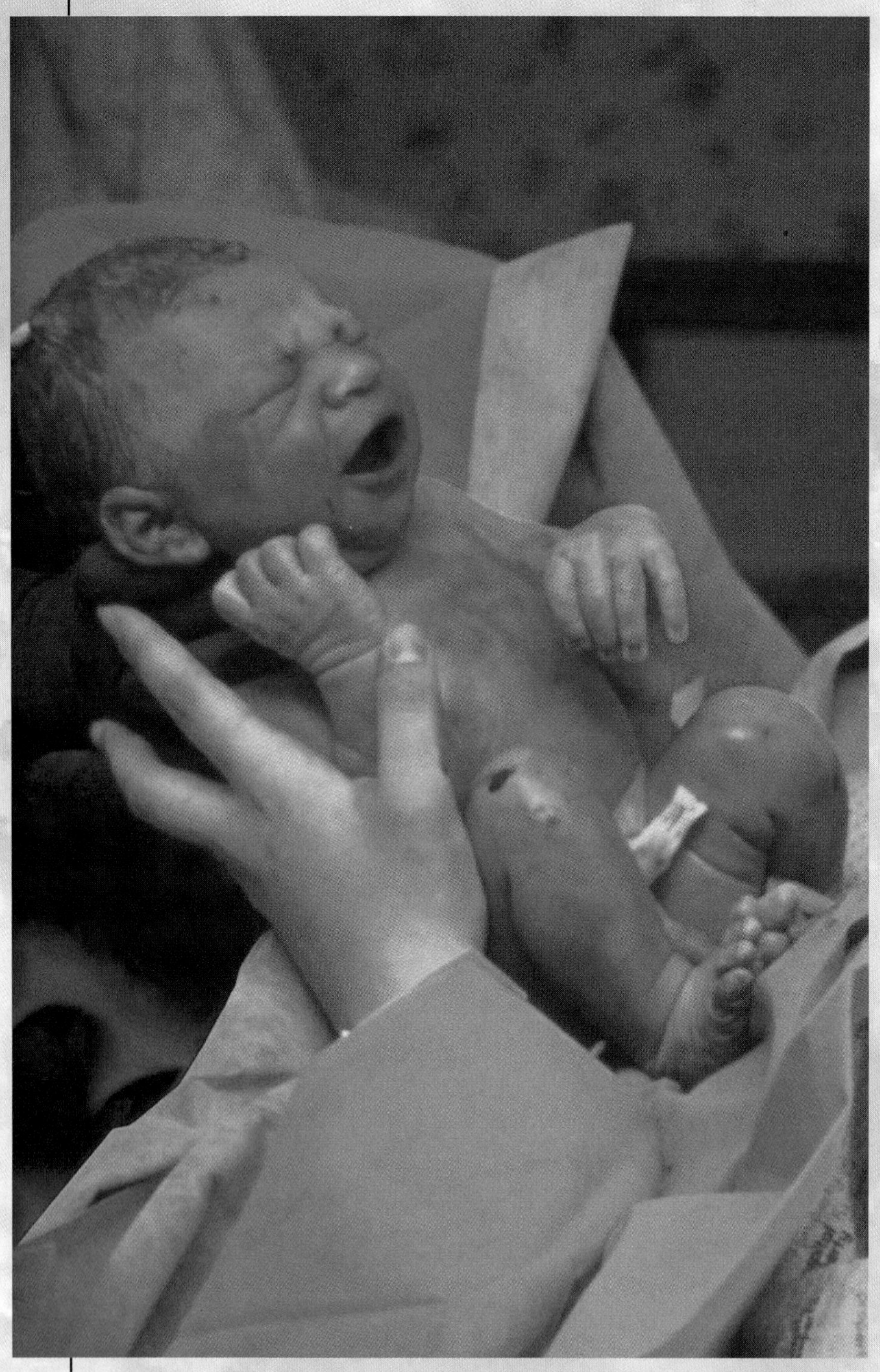

Cradled in his mother's hands moments after birth, this newborn vigorously announces his arrival to his parents and the world. Giving birth has a profound, lifelong impact on a woman; it is the climax of a process that started long before the actual birth event and will continue for the rest of her life.

Trends in Research

THE MEANING OF CHILDBIRTH

> **Pain was unrelated to the woman's feeling of achievement or satisfaction. . . . Other qualities in the psychological domain had more influence on a woman's feelings of a positive birth experience.**

The childbirth experience is consistently described as a significant event of powerful psychological importance in a woman's life. Childbirth can be a developmental task or a time of crisis for a woman with the potential for either personal growth or negative outcomes. Researchers have portrayed the childbirth experience as a test of womanhood, a test of personal competence, a peak experience, and the first act of motherhood.[1]

CONCLUSIONS FROM RESEARCH

Research has shown that the childbirth experience has a dynamic impact on a woman's life.

- Except for those who are unaware because of medication or anesthesia, women have vivid and emotion-laden memories of their childbirth experiences and are often able to recall exact details many years later.[2]
- Variables that influence a woman's perception of childbirth include cultural factors, previous experiences, age, education, socioeconomic status, marital status, self-esteem and self-concept, confidence in her ability to cope during childbirth, expectations for the childbirth experience, accurate knowledge and realistic perceptions of childbirth, attendance at prepared childbirth classes, type of delivery (vaginal or cesarean), support during labor and birth (from partner and nurse), increased level of awareness during labor and birth, environmental conditions of the birthing setting, maternal illness and childbirth complications, and separation from the infant.[1, 3]
- Researchers have found that middle-class and upper-class women find birth satisfying and fulfilling, while women from lower socioeconomic classes are more likely to view birth as an event to be endured to have a baby.[1]
- Each woman's perception of the childbirth experience is intensely personal, and women vary widely in what constitutes a positive, satisfying childbirth experience.[1]
- A woman's expectations of birth have been shown to influence her perceptions of the actual birth experience. For example, a woman who expects birth to be painful most likely will find it so.[1] A woman who has confidence in her ability to cope with labor and delivery will have a more positive childbirth experience.[4]
- Women who were highly satisfied with their childbirth experience have described feelings of personal accomplishment, increased self-esteem, greater self-confidence, and success as a couple.[2]
- Women who perceived that they had the potential to influence events—a feeling of control—had a higher level of childbirth satisfaction and positive psychological outcomes. The perception of personal mastery during the childbirth experience was a key factor in interpretations of the event.[1, 5]
- Women with satisfying birth experiences felt well supported during labor and delivery and had fond memories of their nurses. Participation of the woman's partner during childbirth also had a positive influence on the woman's perception of the birth.[1]
- Pain was unrelated to a woman's feeling of achievement or satisfaction.[1, 6] "A painful birth is just as likely to have a positive evaluation as a pain-free one, reduction of pain [alone] will do nothing to promote a generally positive childbirth experience" (p. 258).[6] Other qualities in the psychological domain had more influence on a woman's feelings of a positive birth experience.[1, 6]

IMPLICATIONS FOR PRACTICE

In addition to providing care that promotes a safe obstetric outcome for the woman and newborn, it is equally important that the nurse provide care that will foster positive psychological outcomes.[2–6] Because of their continued contact with the woman during labor and delivery, nurses, more than any other health care professional, have the opportunity to positively shape the perceived outcomes of the childbirth experience for women.[1]

---

[1]Nichols, F. (1996). The meaning of the childbirth experience: A review of the literature. *Journal of Perinatal Education,* 5 (4).

[2]Simkin, P. (1991). Just another day in a woman's life? Women's long-term perceptions of their first birth experience. Part I. *Birth,* 18 (4), 203–210.

[3]Mercer, R. T., Hackley, K. C., Bostrom, A. G. (1983). Relationship of psychosocial and perinatal variables to perception of childbirth. *Nursing Research,* 32, 202–207.

[4]Lowe, N. (1991). Maternal confidence in coping with labor: A self-efficacy concept. *Journal of Obstetric, Gynecologic, and Neonatal Nursing,* 20 (6), 457–463.

[5]Humenick, S., and Bugen, L. (1981). Mastery: The key to childbirth satisfaction? A study. *Birth and the Family Journal,* 8, 84–90.

[6]Salmon, P., and Miller, R. (1990). Women's anticipation and experience of childbirth: The independence of fulfillment, unpleasantness and pain. *British Journal of Medical Psychology,* 63, 255–259.

–Francine H. Nichols

22 Chapter

The process of childbirth has been compared to an opera . . . where cervical priming (ripening) is the overture to the grand performance by the cervix and uterus. After training and rehearsals, the cervix and uterus are able to act in concert and produce a successful grand finale, delivery. Yet many players and factors in the parturition orchestra are unknown, and remarkably, the director or conductor who starts the event remains unknown.

Ulf Ulmsten (1989)

The Physiology of Childbirth

Mary C. Brucker
Elaine Zwelling

HIGHLIGHTS

- ▼ Phases of Parturition
- ▼ Theories of the Onset of Active Labor
- ▼ Understanding the Process of Labor
- ▼ The Five Ps: Passenger, Passage, Powers, Position, and Psychology of Birth
- ▼ The Stages of Labor
- ▼ Physiologic Responses in Labor
- ▼ Implications for Research

Parturition is the act of giving birth, the climax that occurs at approximately week 40 of gestation. While a great deal is now known about childbirth, much basic scientific information is still missing. Labor is more accurately described as a cascade of endocrinologic and biomolecular phenomena that begin in the final days of pregnancy, rather than the single event of parturition. These phenomena are generally considered physiologic in nature, although the psychological components of labor should never be ignored.

PHASES OF PARTURITION

Parturition is composed of three phases: uterine readiness for labor, uterine contractions of the labor event, and postpartum contractions of uterine involution.

DEFINITIONS

Braxton Hicks contractions—Contractions of the uterus associated with false labor. Although contractions occur, progressive cervical changes are not apparent.

Cardinal movements—The movements the fetus must accomplish to negotiate passage through the maternal pelvis and be born: engagement, descent, flexion, internal rotation, extension, restitution, external rotation, and expulsion (birth).

Crowning—When the biparietal diameter of the fetal head is encircled by the vulvar ring just before birth; if the fetus is in a cephalic presentation, the crown of the head is visualized.

Dilatation—The opening of the cervical os, also called dilation; measured from 0 to 10 cm.

Effacement—The thinning or flattening of the edge of the cervical os; measured from 0 to 100 percent.

Engagement—The entrance of the presenting part of the fetus into the pelvic inlet and the beginning of the mechanism of descent.

Fetal attitude—The relation of fetal parts to one another; a state of either flexion or extension.

Fetal lie—The relationship of the long axis of the fetus to the long axis of the mother; can be horizontal or longitudinal.

Fetal position—The relationship of the presenting part of the fetus to the front, back, or side of the maternal pelvis.

Fetal presentation—The part of the fetal body that appears at the pelvic outlet first; also called the presenting part.

Fontanelles—Soft spots at the top (anterior) and back (posterior) of the fetal head, covered with strong connective tissue, that result from the junction of the suture lines between the unfused bones of the fetal head; allow the bones to override one another and the head to mold during the birth process.

Intensity—Increase in uterine pressure during a contraction; measured in millimeters of mercury on a fetal monitor.

Lightening—A lay term for the engagement of the fetus into the maternal pelvis; derived from the fact that the woman's load feels lighter after the fetus has dropped into the pelvic inlet.

Station—Relationship between the presenting part of the fetus and the midpoint of the pelvis at the level of the ischial spines; measurement of fetal descent.

Suture lines—The areas between the unfused bones of the fetal skull, covered by strong connective tissue, that allow the unfused bones of the fetal head to override one another during the birth process.

Uterine Readiness for Labor

During the first phase, uterine readiness, uterotropins facilitate the body's readiness for labor. Uterotropins are agents that initiate such functions as softening and ripening of the cervix. Cervical softening results from changes in the solubility of collagen and is most likely associated with changes in estradiol, progesterone, relaxin, prostacyclin (PGI_2), prostaglandin E_2 (PGE_2), and prostaglandin $F_{2\alpha}$ ($PGF_{2\alpha}$). The softening of the cervix can be palpated on vaginal examination. Effacement, the thinning or shortening of the length of the cervix, is often pronounced during this period for the primigravida woman. Effacement may be related to cervical ripening, to the weight of the fetus as it engages into the pelvis and acts as a dilating wedge, and to Braxton Hicks contractions (Cunningham et al. 1993).

Uterine Labor Contractions

The second phase of parturition is the one most commonly associated with the term childbirth. Uterotonins, or agents that cause myometrial contractions, are present in this phase, and regular uterine contractions occur. The result of these contractions is active cervical dilatation and expulsion of the infant (Cunningham et al. 1993).

Uterine Postpartum Contractions

The last phase of parturition is the postpartum phase, wherein uterine contractions continue; but the result is involution of the uterus, not expulsion of the contents of conception (Cunningham et al. 1993).

THEORIES OF THE ONSET OF ACTIVE LABOR

During the last few decades, several of the proposed causes of the initiation of labor have been challenged by new information. It currently appears that interrelationships between the mother and fetus play important roles in the initiation of labor, but these relationships are not yet well understood. The role of uterotropins is less understood than that of uterotonins such as oxytocin. The following discussion summarizes the most common theories of the onset of labor. Actual clinical practice questions whether any single theoretic model can explain the total picture. At some time in the future, it will probably be found that a combination of these theories fully explains the onset of labor.

Progesterone Withdrawal

Progesterone suppresses uterine irritability throughout pregnancy by counterbalancing the increased uterine contractility caused by estrogen (Blackburn and Loper 1992; Goff 1993). In lower species, the onset of labor is marked by a sudden decrease in levels of progesterone and an increase in estrogen. Studies of primates have not found that similar hormonal shifts occur before the initiation of labor. However, changes within fetal membranes and decidua as the placenta ages and as term approaches may be associated with increased estrogen synthesis and a decrease in progesterone production (Word 1993). Increased estrogen levels can increase oxytocin in the myometrium. In addition to this traditional view of progesterone withdrawal, there is a suggestion that progesterone withdrawal may be effected in a gene-specific manner by a compound (called transforming growth factor-beta) that not only decreases progesterone but increases oxytocin receptors. Research is currently being conducted in this area. The progesterone withdrawal theory suggests that initiation of labor is related not only to maternal hormones but also to fetal status. Progesterone withdrawal may eventually be viewed as an intermediate modulator in the complex interrelationships.

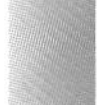

Oxytocin Production

Oxytocin is a hormone released from the posterior pituitary. Oxytocin is not the complete answer to the question of what initiates labor; in fact, oxytocin may be administered in large amounts early in the pregnancy with little or no effect. Progesterone during labor tends to inhibit the myometrial response to oxytocin. It is only after estrogen influences the myometrium that uterine sensitivity to oxytocin evolves in direct response to increased oxytocin receptors. Therefore, oxytocin is of little influence in the first phase of parturition (Blackburn and Loper 1992; Goff 1993). For example, an unripe cervix is unlikely to respond to exogenous oxytocin administration. The level of endogenous oxytocin is increased in the maternal plasma in the expulsive stage of labor, and some studies have indicated that oxytocin may be released with cervical stretching during the dilatation stage of labor (Ferguson reflex). However, this finding has not been consistently duplicated. Pharmaceutical blockage of oxytocin has been suggested as one potential means of tocolysis for the future (Anderson 1989). In summary, oxytocin has influence in the second and especially third phase of parturition, although its role in the first place (as a uterotropin) seems unlikely.

One of the major clinical implications of this physiologic aspect of labor involves the induction of labor. Although the average woman has a normal spontaneous initiation of labor at approximately 38 to 42 weeks' gestational age, there are some circumstances in which it may be advantageous for either the mother or the fetus to initiate labor. (See Procedure 25–3: Induction of Labor by Oxytocin Infusion.) The usual pharmaceutical agent used to induce labor is oxytocin. As mentioned, oxytocin performs best after the oxytocin receptors in the myometrium and decidua have increased. One of the best ways to ascertain whether a woman will respond well to an induction is to perform a pelvic assessment. When a cervix is ripe, it is likely that there are large numbers of oxytocin receptors, and the outcome will be favorable. A Bishop score enables the clinician to assess the cervix and determine the advisability of an induction. This scoring system reflects the common pelvic examination assessments that nurses frequently perform (i.e., dilatation, effacement, station, consistency, and position of the cervix); however, the Bishop scoring format may not be used in all clinical settings. Further explanation of the Bishop scoring system can be found in Chapter 23 (p. 764). Depending on the source, a score of 5 or 6 is usually considered characteristic of a good candidate for induction. It also indicates that even without exogenous influences, it is likely that labor will spontaneously begin soon.

Prostaglandin Production

Prostaglandins are agents that are formed from fatty acids and act as chemical mediators or local hormones; their major effect is apparent near or at the site of production. Prostaglandins are synthesized in every tissue of the human body, including the uterus and the fetus (Word 1993). More than 15 different types of prostaglandins have been identified. Prostaglandins stimulate smooth muscle contraction and probably have been the most studied compounds in relation to initiation of labor in the last 25 years (Blackburn and Loper 1992; Goff 1993).

The most important prostaglandins in the area of reproduction are PGI_2, PGE_2, and $PGF_{2\alpha}$. Evidence links prostaglandins to the initiation of labor. For example, unlike oxytocin, prostaglandins appear to initiate labor at any time during the gestation. A precursor of prostaglandin, arachidonic acid, increases in maternal serum and amniotic fluid during labor. The importance of prostaglandins in the labor process is further enhanced by the findings that women who take high levels of antiprostaglandin drugs (e.g., aspirin, ibuprofen) may have delayed onset of labor. Some of these antiprostaglandins have also been suggested in research to have tocolytic properties (Blackburn and Loper 1992; Cunningham et al. 1993; Word 1993).

In spite of the evidence of the role of prostaglandin in labor, there is a suggestion that it, like oxytocin, may not have a major role in initiation of labor. For example, more than 60 percent of preterm labors begin without a high level of prostaglandin. It is currently hypothesized that prostaglandins may be produced in increased amounts in labor as a consequence of labor. When the forebag decidua is torn from the uterus during early labor (or perhaps during the stripping or artificial rupture of the membranes), the phospholipids that are released produce arachidonic acid, which is then converted to prostaglandins:

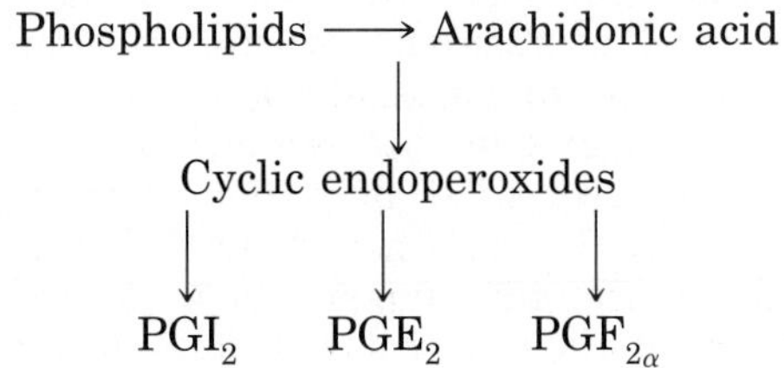

Endothelin Production

Endothelin is a small peptide that is derived from the same family as snake venom. It is a potent vasoconstrictor that causes extreme contractions of smooth muscle. Although sites of production are not known, it has been found at high levels in amniotic fluid, and the amnion has been theorized as a potential site of origin. It is hypothesized that endothelins are produced by the amnion cells. Endothelin attaches to the chorionic vessels and is secreted onto vessel surfaces that enhance uteroplacental circulation. The role of endothelin in parturition is still uncertain, but it is the subject of many current studies (Word 1993).

Estrogen Stimulation

The estrogen stimulation theory acknowledges that estrogen levels rise at 34 to 35 weeks of pregnancy. Estrogen appears to promote oxytocin production, the formation of estrogen receptors in the myometrium, and increased release of arachidonic acid, thus stimulating prostaglandin production. It has been theorized that since estrogen production comes from fetal adrenal precursors, this may be an example of fetal factors having a role in the initiation of labor. Most research in the area concentrates no longer on estrogen stimulation alone but on its relationship to other compounds, specifically prostaglandins (Blackburn and Loper 1992).

Fetal Cortisol

Animal studies emphasize the importance of the fetus in the initiation of labor. This research has shown that the removal of the pituitary gland and adrenal cortex of fetal lambs can delay the onset of labor. As a result of these studies, the fetal cortisol theory is proposed. It suggests that fetal cortisol levels rise to a point at which labor is initiated for unknown reasons. Support of this theory is seen in the clinical findings that anencephalic fetuses tend to be postterm infants. The fetus who is anencephalic has adrenal dysfunctions, which in turn decrease available fetal cortisol (Chamberlain and Hytten 1991; Blackburn and Loper 1992; Cunningham et al. 1993).

Other Theories

Other explanations for the initiation of labor have existed. Among these theories has been the overdistention of the uterus to a set threshold point that leads to synthesis and release of prostaglandins. This has also been termed the stretch theory. Although overdistention and preterm birth are common with multiple pregnancies, some women have triplets of 6 pounds or greater at term.

Infections may be associated with initiation of labor, especially preterm labor. However, it is likely that labor is initiated not simply by the infectious process but probably also by the increased level of prostaglandins that occurs simultaneously as a mediator of an infection. In summary, theories abound regarding both uterotropins and uterotonins. The full truth explaining all the phases of parturition has not yet been discovered. It is anticipated that when it is found, it will be replete with complex maternal and fetal biomolecular and endocrinologic relationships.

UNDERSTANDING THE PROCESS OF LABOR

To understand the process of labor, it is helpful to subdivide the subject into different categories. The traditional way to do this has been to identify the Ps of labor: passenger (fetus), powers (uterine contractions), and the passage (the pelvis and maternal soft parts). Two other Ps have been recognized as potent influences on the course of labor: position (maternal) and psyche (maternal psychological status). These five components work together; they are all interrelated in their influence on the process of labor and birth.

Passenger

BIOLOGIC INFLUENCES

It is well established that the fetus has a role in both the initiation of labor and the process of labor itself, although the exact mechanism is not yet well understood. One of the theories of fetal influence in labor is that a signal may be transmitted from the fetus by the fetal lungs or kidneys through a mediator that is secreted into the amniotic fluid (Cunningham et al. 1993). Whatever the biomolecular events, a pregnancy that terminates during the 38- to 42- week gestation age is likely to indicate a healthy fetus. The same statement may not be true for postterm or preterm pregnancies. For example, fetal demise is often associated with an unripe uterus unresponsive for induction of labor. A fetus with adrenal hypoplasia is frequently associated with a prolonged gestation.

MECHANICAL INFLUENCES

In addition to the biologic influences of the passenger, mechanical influences also exist. How a fetus is positioned within the pelvis can facilitate or impede labor. A fetus should optimally be in an attitude of flexion with the head flexed well on the chest, in a longitudinal lie and a cephalic presentation. This is the ideal clinical picture of fetal position and demonstrates the most common attitude, lie, position, and presentation. These concepts are explained in the following.

Fetal Head

▼ **Bones.** The head is the largest portion of the fetal body, and because it is a firm, noncompliant bony structure, it is the fetal component that is of most significance from an obstetric perspective. Although the shoulders also present a wide diameter, the body of the fetus can be manipulated at the time of birth so that one shoulder is delivered at a time. The fetal head is composed of the face and the skull, which has two frontal bones, two parietal bones, and the occipital bone (Fig. 22–1). At the time of birth, these bones are somewhat flexible because complete ossification has not occurred. This allows some movement and overriding of the bones, so that the fetal head can adapt to the maternal pelvis during the process of labor and birth. This adaptive process is called molding and can often be seen as an elongated head on assessment of the newborn. The molding will disappear within the first few days after birth.

▼ **Sutures and Fontanelles.** Between the bones of the fetal head are membranous spaces called sutures. The suture that runs from anterior to posterior between the parietal bones is called the sagittal suture. It can be easily palpated on physical assessment. The frontal suture is a continuation of the sagittal suture that runs between the two frontal bones. The coronal suture runs in a transverse direction between the frontal and parietal bones, and the lambdoid suture runs in a transverse direction between the parietal bones and the occipital bone. The fontanelles are areas of the head where suture lines intersect. These are wide, membranous areas that can also be palpated during assessment of the newborn (Fig. 22–1). The anterior fontanelle is a diamond shape and is located at the intersection of the sagittal and coronal sutures. It does not close until the baby is about 18 months of age. The posterior fontanelle is triangle shaped and is located at the intersection of the sagittal and lambdoid sutures. It usually closes by 6 to 8 weeks after birth.

▼ **Landmarks.** The fetal head is divided into several designated areas as follows: (1) the sinciput or brow portion of the head; (2) the vertex, or top of the head between the two fontanelles; and (3) the occiput or the back of the head over the occipital bone. Other landmarks of the fetal head are the bregma (anterior fontanelle), the

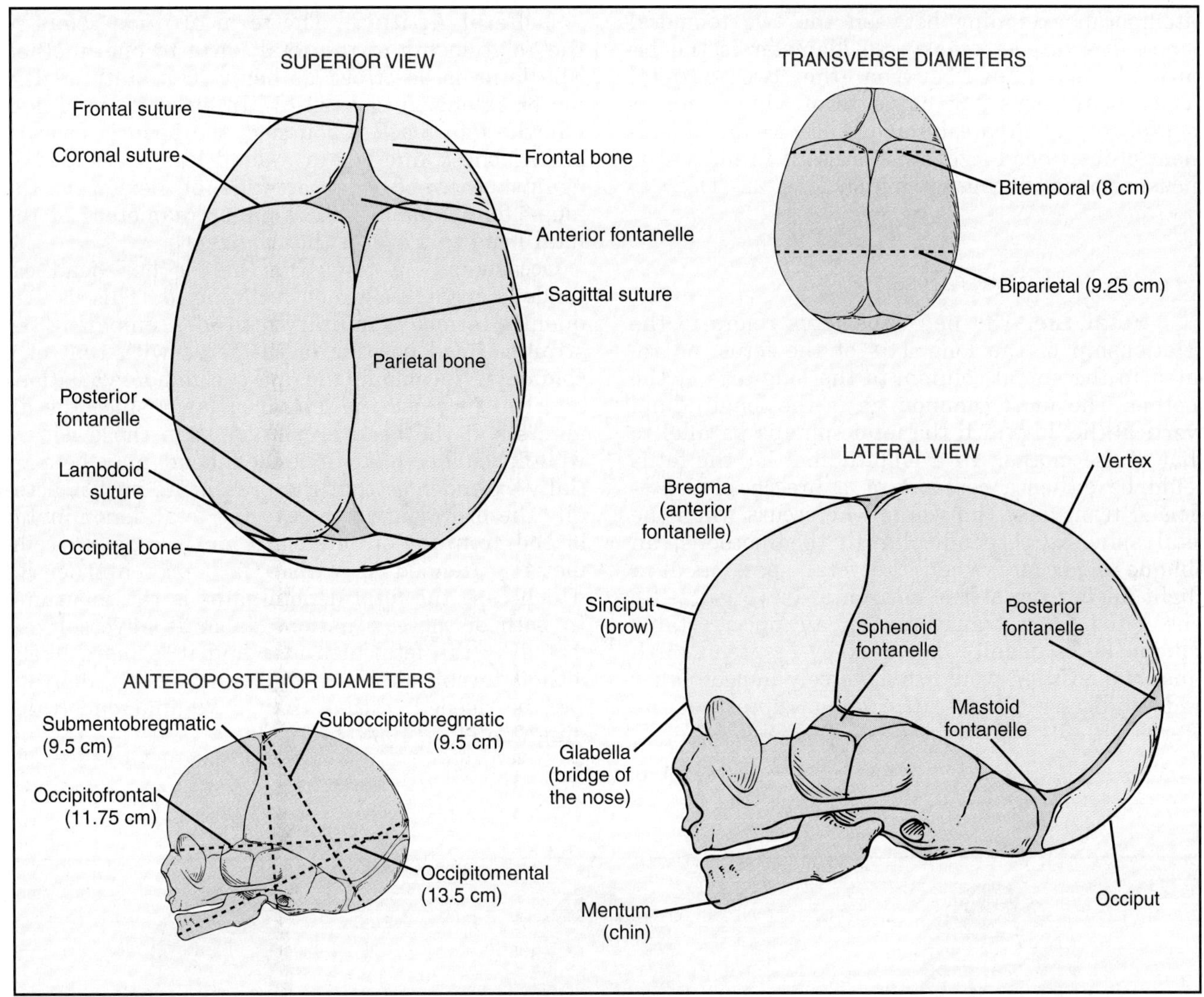

Figure 22–1

An understanding of the placement and relationships of the bones, fontanelles, and sutures of the fetal head as well as the sinciput, vertex, and occiput landmarks can be critical to accurate assessment during the process of labor.

glabella (the bridge of the nose), and the mentum (chin).

▼ **Diameters.** During the labor and birth process, it is desirable that the smallest diameter of the fetal head move through the maternal bony pelvis. There are a number of different diameters of the fetal head, and they vary in length. The diameter that presents through the pelvis depends on the amount of flexion or extension of the head (attitude). There are four anteroposterior diameters of the fetal head:

1. The suboccipitobregmatic diameter is the measurement from the lower edge of the occipital bone to the bregma; it presents through the pelvis when the fetal head is well flexed and averages 9.5 cm at term.
2. The occipitofrontal diameter extends from the occipital protuberance at the back of the head to the bridge of the nose; it presents through the pelvis when the head is straight in a military attitude and averages 11.75 cm at term.
3. The occipitomental diameter is the measurement from just above the posterior fontanelle to the mentum (chin); it presents through the pelvis when the head is extended back and averages 13.5 cm at term.
4. The submentobregmatic diameter is the measurement from the junction of the neck and lower jaw to the bregma (anterior fontanelle); even though small at an average 9.5 cm, this diameter does not promote an easy delivery since it occurs when the head is hyperextended back with a face presentation.

There are also two transverse diameters of the fetal head. The smaller transverse diameter is the bitemporal, extending between the two temporal bones. The largest transverse diameter is the biparietal, extending between the two parietal bones. It averages 9.25 cm at term. This diameter is probably of greatest importance as an assessment of fetal head size. It is assessed in ultrasonic measurements during pregnancy (Fig. 22–1).

Fetopelvic Relationships

Fetal Lie. The lie of the fetus refers to the relationship of the long axis of the fetus, as related to the spinal column, to the long axis of the mother. The most common lie is the longitudinal (vertical) lie, in which the fetal spine is parallel to that of the mother. In a longitudinal lie, the fetus could be either a cephalic or a breech presentation. A transverse (horizontal) lie occurs when the fetal spine is perpendicular to the mother's; an oblique lie occurs when the fetal spine is at a slight angle from a true horizontal lie (Fig. 22–2). The fetus in a transverse or an uncorrectable oblique lie is usually delivered by cesarean birth since the position would so adversely impede labor and could result in a catastrophic rupture of the uterus.

Fetal Attitude. The term attitude refers to the relationship of the fetal parts to one another. The fetus is described as being in a state of flexion or extension (Fig. 22–3). In an attitude of flexion, the fetal back is rounded, the head is forward on the chest, and the arms and legs are folded in against the body. An attitude of flexion is the ideal, for it enables the smaller diameters of the fetal head to traverse the pelvis.

Occasionally a fetus has his or her head extended, or at least not well flexed. This is frequently termed a military attitude, comparing the straight head position of the fetus with that of a soldier. It is among the more common variations and can increase the length of labor since the diameters of the head are larger than those with a well-flexed head. An extended head may be partially extended so that the presenting part is actually the brow (in which case the fetal denominator is the frontum or forehead), or it may be completely extended as with a face presentation (in which case the fetal denominator is the mentum). In both of these situations, labor is adversely affected by the fetal attitudes and it is more likely, although not absolute, that a cesarean delivery will be needed, rather than a vaginal one (Cunningham et al. 1993).

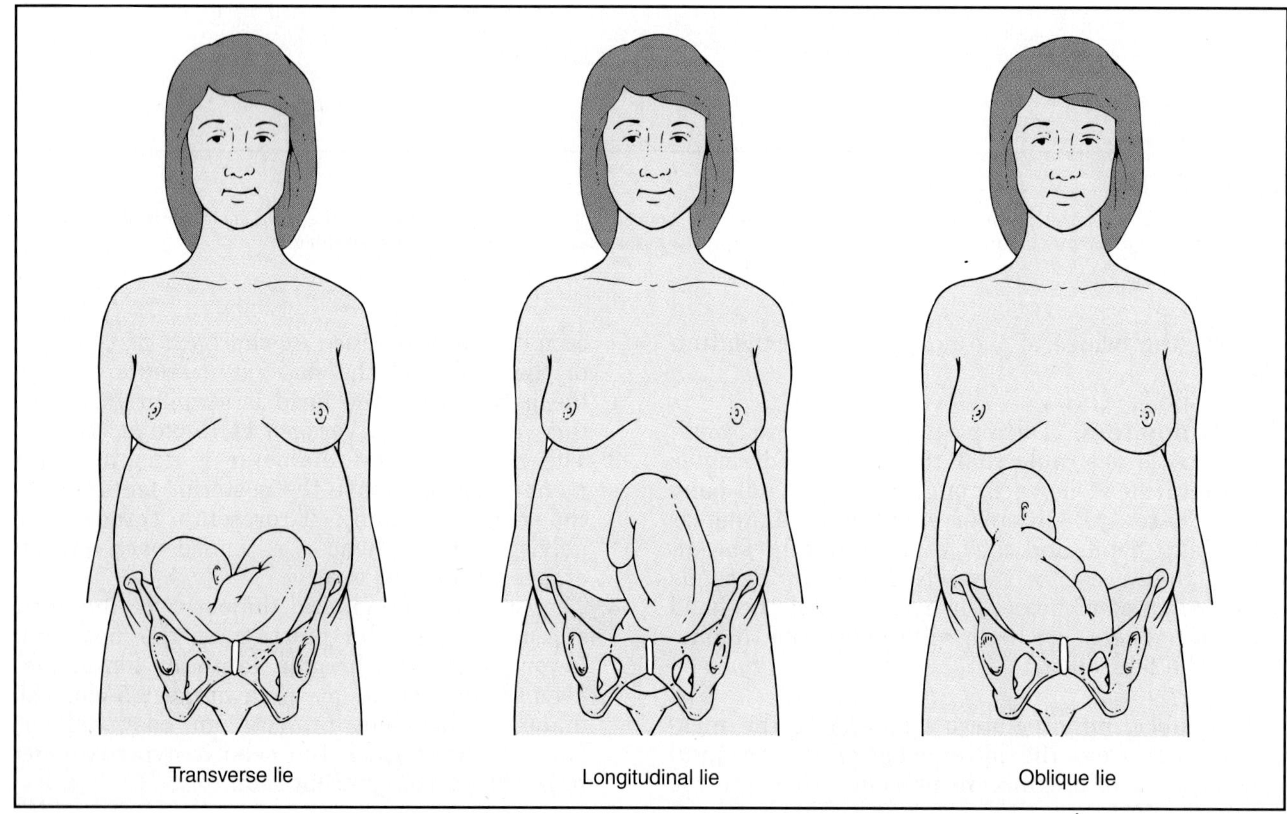

Figure 22–2
The fetal lie represents the relationship of the long axis of the fetus to the long axis of the mother.

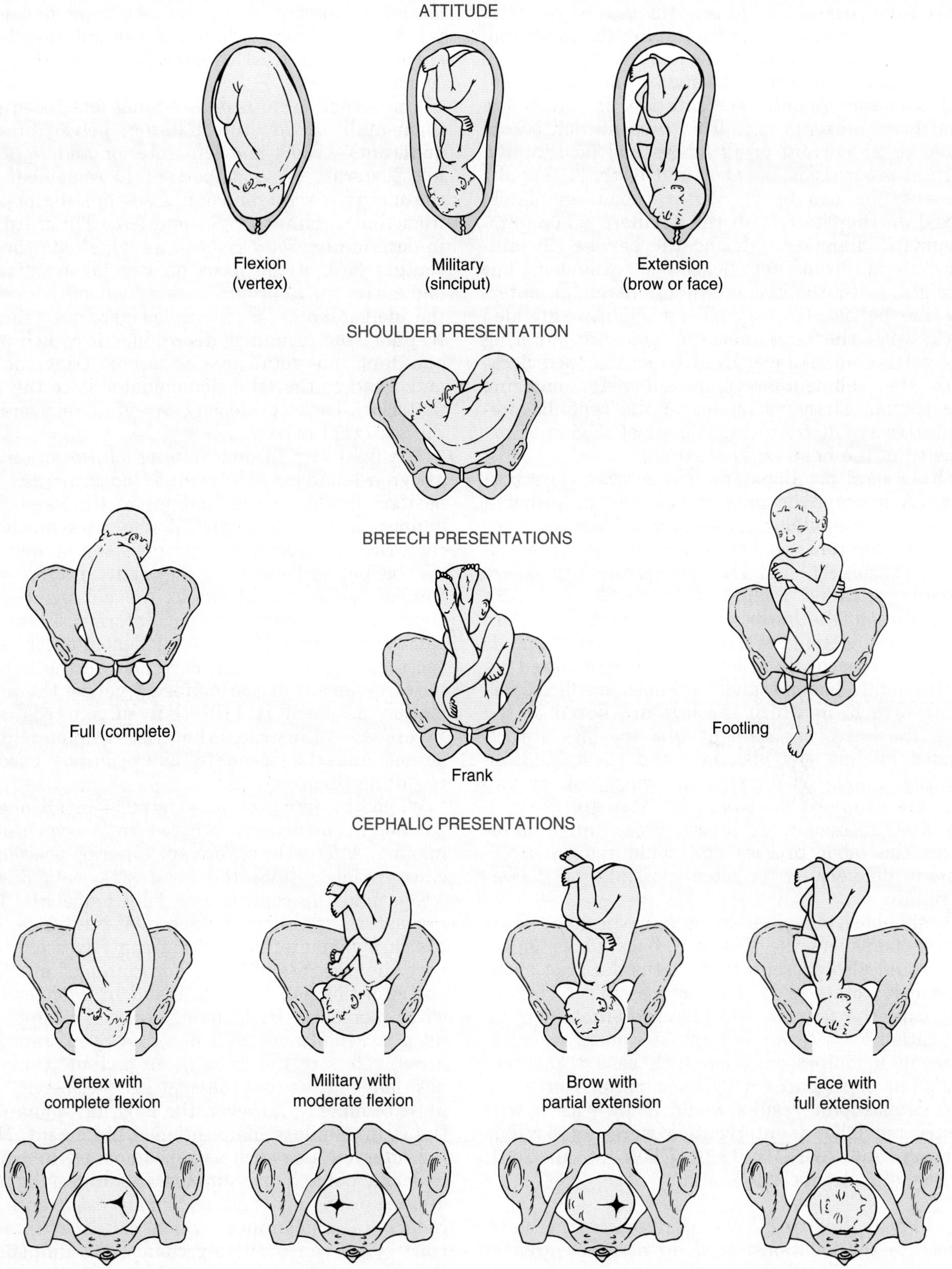

Figure 22–3

Fetal attitude refers to the relationship of the body parts to one another • The desired attitude consists of the fetal head in moderate flexion, fetal arms flexed onto the chest, and fetal legs flexed onto the abdomen • Fetal presentation refers to the fetal body part that enters the maternal pelvis.

Fetal Presentation. The presentation or presenting part of the fetus is the part of the fetal body that enters (or presents to) the maternal pelvis. Figure 22–3 illustrates the various presentations that can occur. The most common presentation is the cephalic presentation, in which the fetal head presents first. This presentation occurs in 95 to 97 percent of all labors and facilitates a normal progression of labor and birth. A cephalic presentation can be (1) vertex (head completely flexed on the chest, with the smallest suboccipitobregmatic diameter entering the pelvis); (2) military (fetal head not flexed or extended, but straight, with the occipitofrontal diameter entering the pelvis); (3) brow (head slightly extended back, with the occipitomental diameter entering the pelvis); or (4) face (head hyperextended back, with the submentobregmatic diameter entering the pelvis). These variations of the cephalic presentation result from the amount of flexion or extension of the head (fetal attitude).

Other fetal positions and presentations are possible. A noncephalic presentation can be either a breech or a shoulder presentation. Because labor may not proceed as easily with these presentations, the breech and shoulder presentations are sometimes called malpresentations. In a breech presentation, the buttocks present first. There are three classifications of the breech presentation: (1) complete breech, in which the legs are flexed up on the fetal abdomen and the knees are flexed; (2) frank breech, in which the legs are flexed at the hips, the knees are straight, and the legs are extended against the abdomen and chest; and (3) footling (single or double), in which one or two legs are extended down and the feet are presenting first. Although the breech presentation influences the labor process and could require a cesarean delivery, it is often possible to deliver vaginally.

A shoulder presentation occurs when the fetus is in a transverse lie. The arm, back, abdomen, or side could also present. If the fetus does not spontaneously rotate or if it is not possible to manually turn the fetus, a shoulder presentation is an indication for a cesarean birth. A woman with her fetus in a malpresentation, such as a transverse lie, often experiences a dystocia pattern of labor, and catastrophic results would occur with a true obstructed labor if intervention were not possible (Cherry and Merkatz 1991; Clark et al. 1991; Creasy and Resnik 1994).

Fetal Position. The position of the fetus refers to the relationship of an assigned area of the presenting part (often called the fetal denominator) to the maternal pelvis. To determine fetal position, the fetal denominator is first identified. For example, when the fetal presentation is cephalic, the occiput is most often used as the fetal denominator to determine position (if the head is extended, the brow or chin is used). When the fetal presentation is breech, the fetal denominator is the sacrum; when the presentation is the shoulder, the fetal denominator is the fetal scapula.

The second step in determining fetal position is to mentally divide the maternal pelvis into four quadrants—right and left anterior and right and left posterior. (It is important to remember that the mother's right and left sides are the opposite from the examiner's right and left.) The third step in determining fetal position is to palpate the presenting part of the fetus on vaginal examination and locate the appropriate fetal denominator. Once the denominator is identified (occiput, sacrum, scapula), the examiner determines in which pelvic quadrant that fetal area is located (right or left) and whether the fetal denominator is to the front (anterior), back (posterior), or side (transverse) of the maternal pelvis.

The final step in determining fetal position is to assign a standard abbreviation indicating the fetal position based on the findings of the vaginal examination. For example, if the presentation is cephalic, the fetal denominator is the occiput, and the occiput is located in the right anterior quadrant of the maternal pelvis; the abbreviation assigned is ROA (right occiput anterior). If the presentation is breech, the fetal denominator is the sacrum, and the sacrum is located in the left posterior quadrant of the maternal pelvis; the abbreviation assigned is LSP (left sacrum posterior). Figure 22–4 illustrates the most common fetal positions and the standard abbreviations used for recording them.

When the fetus, or passenger, is in an optimal position, contractions proceed in a synchronous manner. A fetus in an occiput anterior position facilitates labor since the head acts as a dilating wedge and the contractions help propel the fetus through the smallest diameters of the pelvis. A fetus in a nonanterior position can adversely influence the progress of labor. For example, an occiput posterior position tends to result in a longer labor with increased back pain, especially since the head is usually not well flexed. A deep transverse arrest refers to the fetus in an occiput transverse position that is not navigating the pelvis well. Most commonly, however, the laboring woman's fetus is in a mildly malpositioned placement. Nursing interventions such as repositioning the woman in labor, helping her ambulate, encouraging rocking, or providing ways to reduce pain (and thus reduce catecholamines, which can also interfere with labor) can positively change the influence of the passenger's position on labor.

Synclitism and Asynclitism. One of the most common variations of fetopelvic relationships is a fetal head that is asynclitic, or not parallel to the anteroposterior plane of the pelvis (Fig. 22–5).

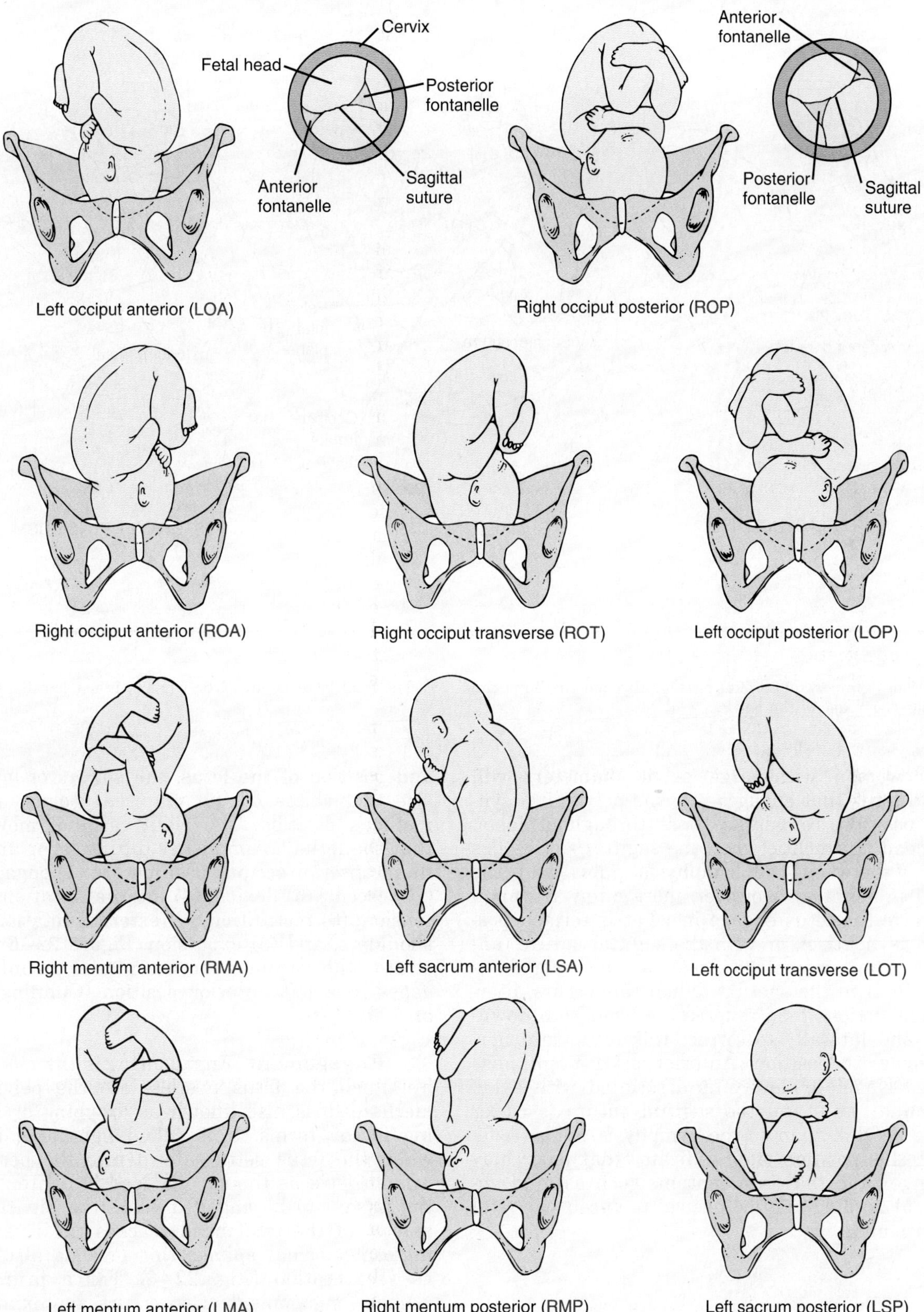

Figure 22–4

Fetal positions refer to how the presenting fetal part is positioned in relationship to the front, back, or side of the maternal pelvis.

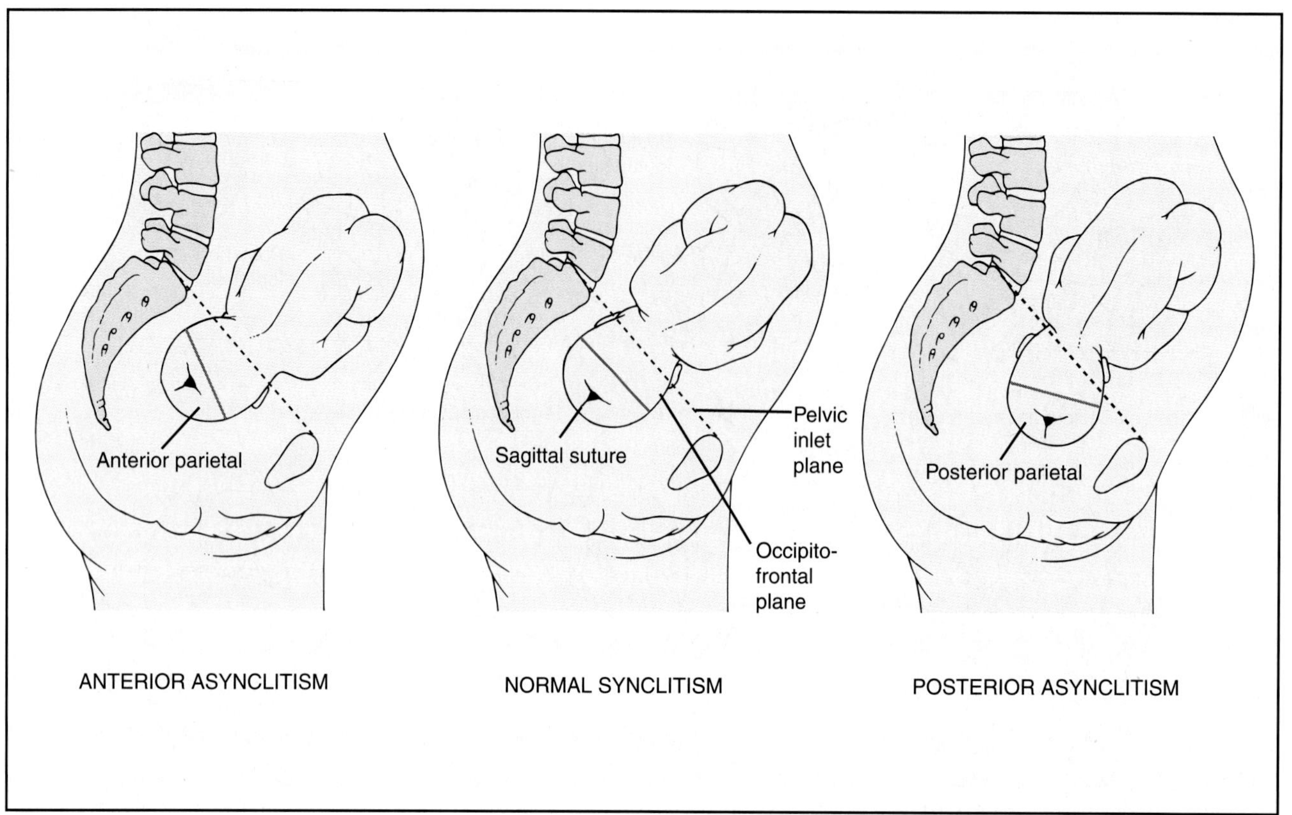

Figure 22–5

Synclitism is important to fetal passage through the birth canal • The fetal head is asynclitic when it is not parallel to the anteroposterior plane of the pelvis.

Many women with large pelvic diameters will have a fetus that engages into the pelvis in a synclitic position, remaining there throughout labor. The head is synclitic when the sagittal suture lies midway between the symphysis pubis and the sacral promontory. However, more often a woman will have the fetus engage in what is termed posterior asynclitism, or with the sagittal suture (anteroposterior diameter) closer to the symphysis pubis than to the sacrum. When this occurs, uterine contractions tend to force the head both downward and laterally to correct this to a more normal synclitic position. Anterior asynclitism (also termed Nägele obliquity) is associated with a lax abdominal wall, and the sagittal suture is closer to the sacrum than to the symphysis pubis. A fetus in this position often indicates that labor may be longer and that interventions such as mild abdominal binding may be needed to encourage fetal repositioning.

Cardinal Movements

The cardinal movements, also called the mechanisms of labor, are a series of adaptations that the fetus makes as he or she moves through the maternal bony pelvis during the process of labor and birth. These movements are influenced by the size and position of the fetus, the powers of labor, the size and shape of the maternal pelvis, and the mother's position. The eight cardinal movements that the fetus accomplishes during labor and birth in an anterior occiput position are (1) engagement, (2) descent, (3) flexion, (4) internal rotation, (5) extension, (6) restitution, (7) external rotation of the shoulders, and (8) expulsion. Figure 22–6 demonstrates the cardinal movements as an infant engages in a left anterior position (Cunningham et al. 1993).

Engagement. Engagement is the mechanism by which the fetus nestles into the pelvis. This mechanism is also known as dropping or lightening in lay terms. It is called lightening because when the fetus settles down into the pelvis, the woman feels as though her load is lighter. The fetus is said to be engaged when the biparietal diameter of the fetal head reaches the level of the maternal ischial spines; this level is also known as zero station (Fig. 22–6). For a primiparous woman, engagement often occurs approximately 2 weeks before labor begins. The woman may report that it is easier to breathe since pressure on the diaphragm and lungs is decreased. Conversely, she may complain of an increased need to urinate or an increased pelvic heaviness. When the examiner

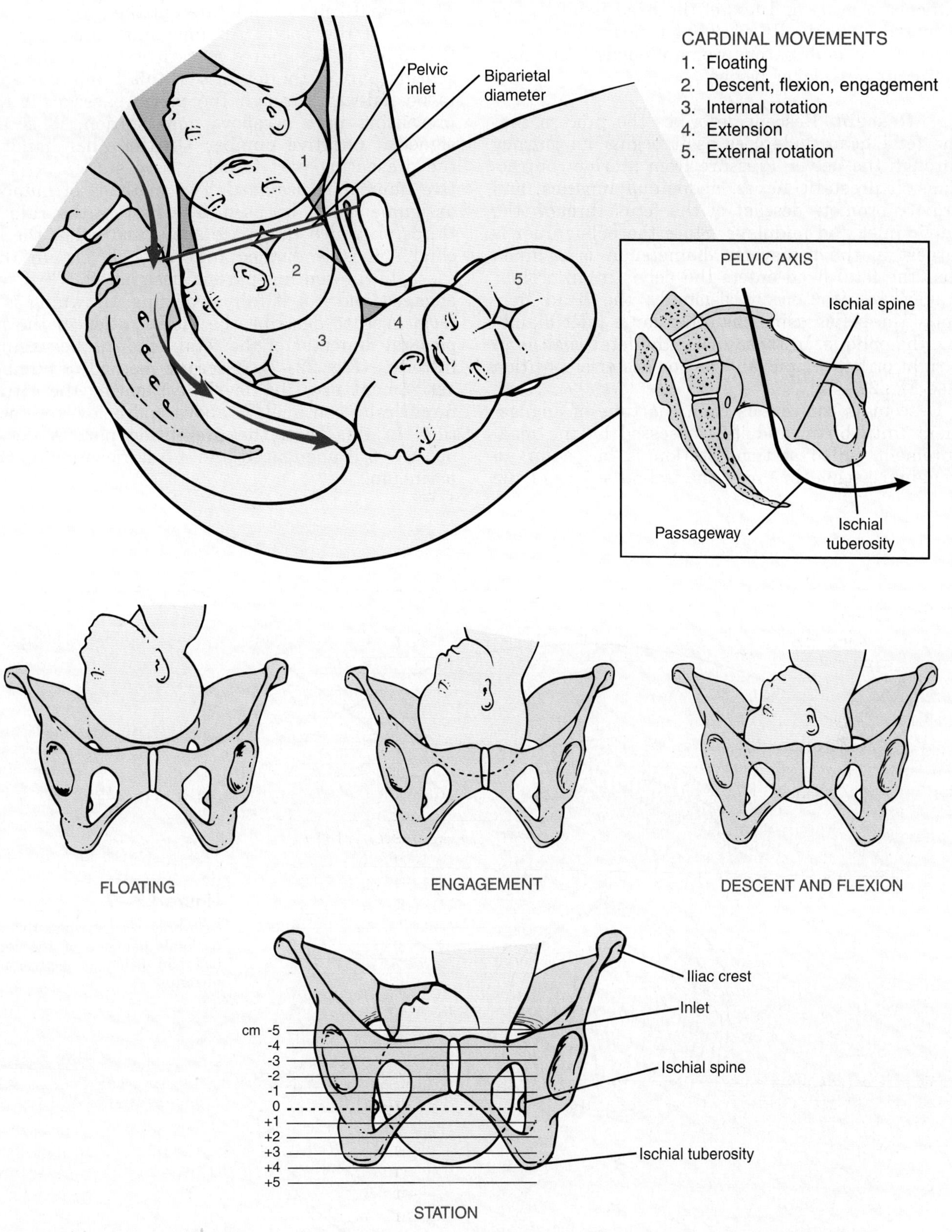

Figure 22–6

The cardinal movements refer to the passage of the fetus as it negotiates the bony pelvis • Fetal station is a measurement of the progress of the descent.

performs the Leopold maneuvers, the head is more difficult to move and less of the head is able to be palpated abdominally after engagement has taken place. For a multiparous woman, engagement may not occur until labor begins.

▼ **Descent.** Descent describes the process that the fetal head undergoes as it begins its journey through the pelvis. Pressure from uterine contractions, hydrostatic forces, abdominal muscles, and gravity promote descent of the fetus through the pelvic inlet and midplane. Since the pelvic inlet is largest in the transverse diameter, it is common that the fetal head enters the pelvis in an occiput transverse position. Occasionally, the head may enter the pelvis using the other large inlet diameter, the oblique. In these cases, the fetal head is in a right or left occiput anterior or posterior position (see Fig. 22–4).

Descent is continuous from the time of engagement until birth, and it is assessed by the measurement called station. Station is based on an imaginary scale that uses the ischial spines of the maternal pelvis as its reference point (Fig. 22–6). The ischial spines are located at the narrowest diameter of the pelvis. An imaginary line between the spines is designated as zero station; if the presenting part of the fetus is at this level, it is said to be halfway through the pelvic passage. If the presenting part is above zero station, it is assigned a negative number. On the other hand, if the presenting part is below zero station, a positive number is assigned. Two methods of number assignment can be used. The first is the rule of thirds, in which the space above and below the ischial spines is divided into three levels. In this case, the presenting part is designated −3 if unengaged and +3 if fully crowning. Crowning is a term used to describe the visualization of the biparietal diameter of the fetal head at the vaginal introitus (Fig. 22–7). A second method of number assignment uses five levels, estimating the actual numbers of centimeters above and below zero station. In this case, the presenting part is designated −5 if unengaged and +5 if crowning on the perineum.

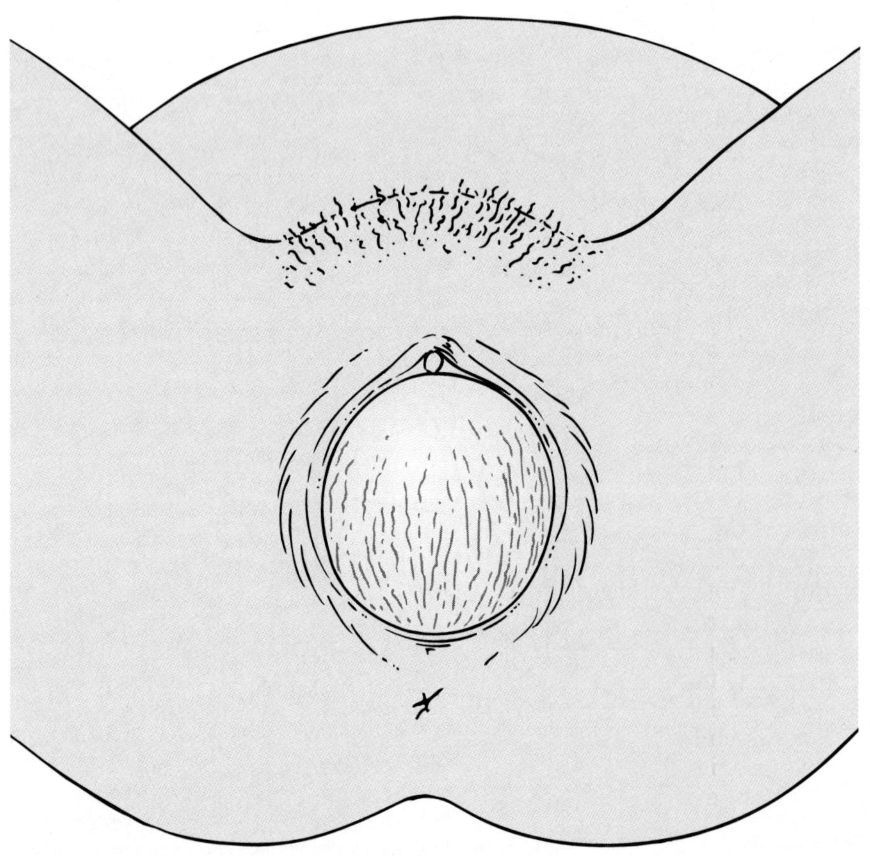

Figure 22–7

Crowning occurs when the biparietal diameter of the fetal head is visible at the vaginal introitus.

Flexion. Flexion is the process of the fetal head's nodding forward toward the fetal chest and occurs as a result of descent, the thickening of the uterine fundus, and increased resistance of the soft tissues. Flexion is advantageous to the fetus as it allows the fetus to enter the pelvis presenting with the smaller suboccipitobregmatic diameter. Engagement, descent, and flexion tend to occur simultaneously.

Internal Rotation. The next cardinal movement is internal rotation. Most commonly, the fetus rotates internally from the occiput transverse position assumed at engagement into the pelvis to an occiput anterior position while continuously descending. It is also possible for the fetus to rotate from the transverse to a posterior position; however, the shape of the pelvis and the pelvic musculature encourage internal rotation to the occiput anterior position. It is in this position that birth of the head occurs. Internal rotation most often takes place in the second stage of labor and is facilitated by the mother's position and expulsion efforts.

Extension. Extension is the cardinal movement that enables the head to be born when the fetus is in a cephalic position. It results from the downward forces of the uterine contractions and the resistance of the pelvic floor muscles. Extension begins after the head has crowned and is complete when the head passes under the symphysis pubis and the occiput, anterior fontanelle, brow, face, and chin pass over the sacrum and coccyx and are born over the perineum.

Restitution. Restitution is the cardinal movement that results in a realignment of the fetal head with the body, after the head is born. It is common that as the head internally rotates to an anterior position before its birth, the shoulders may enter the pelvis in the oblique diameter. This allows the head to turn, but as a result, the neck twists. Restitution occurs when the head is free of pelvic resistance, allowing the head to turn back until it is again at right angles to the shoulders.

External Rotation. The next cardinal movement is external rotation. After the head is born and restitution occurs, the shoulders externally rotate so that they are in the anteroposterior diameter of the pelvis. Since the anteroposterior diameter is the largest diameter of the outlet, it more easily allows the birth of the broad shoulders. The shoulders are born by first delivering the anterior shoulder from under the symphysis pubis and then the posterior shoulder from over the perineum.

Expulsion. Expulsion is the last of the cardinal movements and connotes birth of the entire body. The body usually follows easily after the birth of the head and shoulders. It is common to document the time of birth at the moment of expulsion (birth).

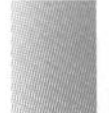

Passage

In addition to the passenger, another factor that influences labor is the passage through which the fetus must pass. The passage consists of both the hard passage, or bony pelvis, and the soft passage, or maternal soft tissue structures.

HARD PASSAGE THROUGH THE MATERNAL BONY PELVIS

Divisions

The bones of the pelvis are described in Chapter 9. The major pelvic bones include the innominate bones (formed by the fusion of the ilium, ischium, and pubis around the acetabulum), the sacrum, and the coccyx. For obstetric purposes, the pelvis is arbitrarily divided into halves—the false pelvis and the true pelvis (see Fig. 9–3). This division is made by an invisible line called the linea terminalis, which extends from the symphysis pubis to the sacroiliac joint. The false pelvis is the wide, broad area between the iliac crests and has no major clinical significance for labor and birth. It does support the uterus and directs the fetus into the true pelvis to engage. The true pelvis is the area below the linea terminalis and is the actual bony passage that the fetus must traverse during labor and birth. The shape of this passage is a curved axis, not a straight passage, because of the diameters and planes of the pelvis (see Fig. 22–6). This means that the fetus must first move down and then up over the sacrum as it descends and has implications for the positioning of women during the expulsion stage of labor.

Planes

The three common planes of the pelvis are the inlet (also termed the pelvic brim), midpelvis, and outlet (see Fig. 9–3). Each plane may be described in terms of diameters—the anteroposterior, transverse, and oblique. However, few of these diameters are measurable directly. Pelvic capacity is usually derived by extrapolation of information that is clinically feasible. The pelvic inlet is at the level of the linea terminalis. It is defined by the superior aspect of the pubis, the iliopectineal lines laterally, and the upper margin of the sacrum and the sacral promontory. For a gynecoid pelvis, the inlet is often "bowl" or heart shaped, with the transverse diameter being greater than the anteroposterior diameter (also called the obstetric conjugate). A roomy inlet allows the fetal head to easily navigate through it (usually in an occiput transverse position), engage, and descend in an occiput transverse or occiput anterior position. The greatest pelvic capacity or diameter is found between the inlet and the midplane.

The midpelvis is often called the cavity or the plane of least dimension since the transverse diameter is measured between the ischial spines (interspinous diameter) and is one of the smallest diameters of the pelvis (see Chapter 9). The anterior portion of the midplane is the posterior aspect of the symphysis pubis, and the posterior portion is the sacrum. Of the three anatomic planes, the midplane is the most clinically significant because of the small transverse diameter. Fetal heads may become impinged on prominent or encroaching spines that diminish the space available. The clinical phenomenon of deep transverse arrest is attributed to the transverse diameter and fetal position.

The pelvic outlet is composed of the area from the inferior margin of the pubic bone to the inner surfaces of the ischial tuberosities to the coccyx. The transverse diameter, between the ischial tuberosities, is called the biischial diameter. It is considered the least important clinically of the three planes, since a pelvis with an adequate inlet and midplane rarely if ever has reduced diameters for the outlet. Moreover, the coccyx has slight mobility, increasing the diameter. In rare situations, the fetal head can cause a break of the coccyx, essentially increasing the available space even more, although at the cost of maternal discomfort. In those situations, pain relief is offered postpartally, and the coccyx generally heals without other intervention.

Assessment of the Pelvis

Various methods have been used to predict the adequacy of a pelvis. Older texts discuss such aspects as assessment of a woman's shoe size or even the length of her fingers. In the late 1920s, Howard Moloy and William Caldwell used the newly popular x-ray method to investigate pelvimetry of women (Steer 1975). They began by devising precise methods for the measurement of critically important (but clinically inaccessible) pelvic diameters. It is from their work that descriptions of the four basic types of the pelvis were derived: gynecoid, android, anthropoid, and platypelloid. It has been estimated that a gynecoid pelvis exists in approximately 50 percent of women. In the other half of the female population, it is most likely that a variation of the other three types of pelvis exists, although not necessarily in pure form.

The pelvic diameters of each of the four types of pelvic shapes are shown in Figure 9–4. It can be demonstrated that each pelvic type influences the course of labor, but controversy exists about the usefulness of clinical pelvimetry. A fetus may be delivered in spite of any of the maternal pelvic types in question. However, it is more likely that an arrest at the inlet may occur with an android or platypelloid pelvis, culminating in an arrest of progress or even an untoward event such as a prolapsed cord. Moreover, arrest of descent is more likely with an anthropoid pelvis than with a gynecoid one. A diagnosis of cephalopelvic disproportion is made when the shape and size of the pelvis, in combination with fetal size and position, are not adequate to allow a spontaneous vaginal delivery. This complication of labor is discussed in Chapter 25.

During the first prenatal examination, a general assessment of the pelvis is made by internal or external palpation. Traditionally, many clinicians also incorporate clinical pelvimetry into the physical assessment they perform. Others, recognizing the effects of progesterone and relaxin on cartilage and joints, wait until the third trimester for increased comfort of the woman and accuracy of findings. Yet others argue that all women deserve a trial of labor and do not assess the pelvis until labor. Pelvimetry techniques include x-ray pelvimetry and computed tomographic pelvimetry to assess the maternal pelvis and ultrasonography to assess the size of the fetus. Prenatal assessment of the pelvis may be beneficial for several reasons:

- Clinical pelvimetry reassures both the health care provider and the woman about the normalcy of the pelvis; this level of security can be psychologically beneficial to both.
- When a minor variation such as an anthropoid hindpelvis exists, it can be discussed and plans can be made for management; anticipatory guidance may be given about backaches in pregnancy, and the probability of back labor can be discussed with strategies for management before the situation actually occurs.
- In the rare instance of an abnormal pelvis such as true android, anticipatory guidance may include the planning for a cesarean birth as well as discussion of normal labor patterns and deviations that may require interventions.

Figure 9–4 lists the most common minimal measurements for the average gynecoid pelvis. Some variations occur among sources, but these are the most commonly accepted measurements. With the exception of the transverse diameter of the midplane (interspinous diameter, between the ischial spines) and the transverse diameter of the outlet (biischial diameter, between the ischial tuberosities), most of the pelvic diameters are not accessible for direct clinical measurement.

Clinical assessment of the inlet and the outlet

of the pelvis can be accomplished indirectly, however, by palpating various pelvic conjugates (diameters) on vaginal examination and extrapolating from data obtained by measurements that are clinically possible. See Chapter 25 for further discussion of pelvic assessment. The conjugates of the pelvis that measure the anteroposterior diameters of the inlet include (1) the diagonal conjugate (measured from the subpubic arch of the symphysis pubis to the sacral promontory), assessed directly on vaginal examination, usually 12.5 cm; (2) the obstetric conjugate (measured from the innermost part of the symphysis pubis to the sacral promontory), estimated from the diagonal conjugate by subtracting 1.5 to 2 cm (Cunningham et al. 1993); and (3) the conjugate vera, or true or anatomic conjugate (measured from the top of the pubis to the sacral promontory) (Fig. 22–8). The transverse diameter of the inlet is the largest but cannot be assessed directly. It corresponds to the linea terminalis. The diameter of the outlet that can be assessed directly is the intertuberous diameter, between the ischial tuberosities. Table 22–1 lists the commonly measured diameters of the pelvis with their variation by type.

SOFT PASSAGE THROUGH MATERNAL SOFT TISSUE STRUCTURES

For normal labor and birth to transpire, the soft tissues of the cervix, vagina, and perineum must stretch to allow passage of the fetus through the axis of the birth canal. Progesterone and relaxin are agents that facilitate the softening and increase the elasticity of muscles and ligaments. During the last few weeks before birth, the cervix ripens. Ripening generally connotes softening, effacement, and increased elasticity of the cervix. It is controlled by estradiol, progesterone, relaxin, PGI_2, PGE_2, and $PGF_{2\alpha}$. These hormones appear to perform several functions either alone or in combination. They can change the solubility of collagen, which in turn weakens the cervical structure and mediates changes in the water and mucopolysaccharide content of the cervix (Blackburn and Loper 1992). Ripening also occurs as a result of Braxton Hicks contractions and the engagement of the fetal head, which serves as a wedge against the cervix.

Already a distensible organ, the fibromuscular vaginal passage becomes even more elastic

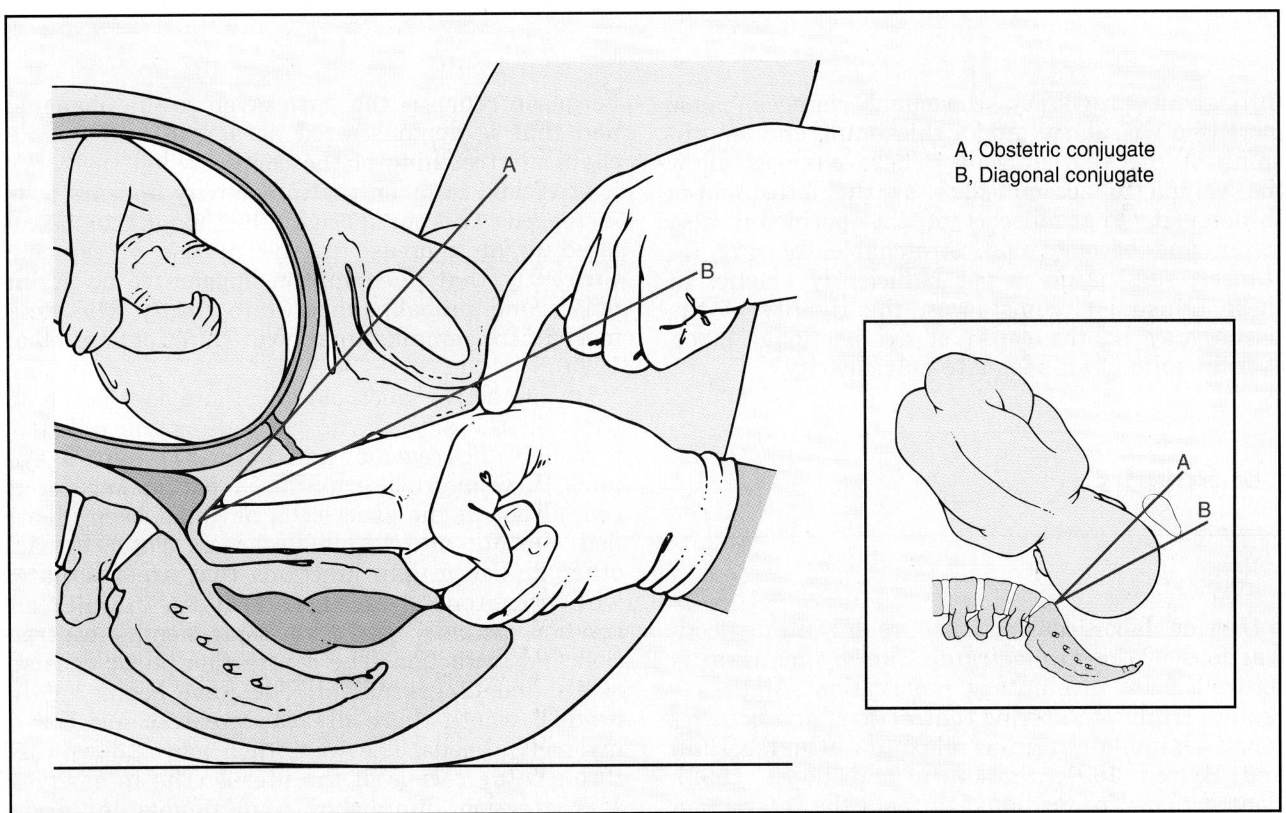

Figure 22–8

The obstetric and diagonal conjugates are the anteroposterior diameters of the pelvis • The obstetric conjugate cannot be measured directly but is the shortest distance through which the fetal head must pass in descending through the pelvic inlet • Measuring the diagonal conjugate and then subtracting 1.5 to 2 cm provides a clinical estimate.

Table 22–1

CLINICAL PELVIMETRY

CLASSIFICATION	GYNECOID	ANDROID	ANTHROPOID	PLATYPELLOID
Pubic arch (subpubic arch)	Wide, adequate 2–2½ fingerbreadths ≥90 degrees	Acute, narrow 1–1½ fingerbreadths ≤90 degrees	Narrow, rounded 1–1½ fingerbreadths ≤90 degrees	Extremely wide 3 fingerbreadths ≥100 degrees
Ischial spines	Blunt, not encroaching	Prominent, encroaching	Prominent, not necessarily encroaching	Difficult to assess
Side walls	Straight or slightly convergent	Slightly convergent	Straight or slightly convergent	Straight
Sacrum	Curved	Straight	Straight	Curved
Inclination	Backward	Forward	Backward	Forward
Length	Average	Average	Average	Average
Diagonal conjugate	≥11.5 cm	≥11.5 cm	≥11.5 cm	≤11.5 cm
Curvature	Slightly curved	Straight	Slightly curved	Flat
Sacrosciatic notch	Average, 3 fingerbreadths	Narrow, 1½–2 fingerbreadths	Wide, 4 fingerbreadths	Average, but shallow
Pubic rami	Wide, flaring	Straight, narrowing	Straight, convergent	Exaggerated flaring

throughout pregnancy. Hormonal changes cause increased vascularity and a thickening and lengthening of the vaginal walls. These changes allow the vagina to accommodate as the fetus moves through it. The muscles of the perineum also soften and become more stretchable. In rare instances, soft tissue is not sufficiently elastic. In these unusual circumstances, the rigidity of the tissue may be the cause of dysfunctional labor, even in spite of an adequate pelvic cavity.

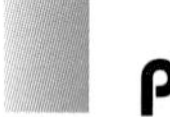

Powers

CONTRACTIONS

Physiology

Uterine labor contractions are essentially contractions of the myometrium. The myometrium is controlled by involuntary innervation. Alpha receptors stimulate uterine contractions and beta receptors stimulate uterine relaxation (Chamberlain and Hytten 1991; Blackburn and Loper 1992). Contractions are mediated through the interaction of actin and myosin. In general, they are produced by spontaneous electromechanical coupling and depend on such agents as prostaglandins, oxytocin, cyclic adenosine monophosphate, mechanical stretch, and energy for the contractile process. The Ferguson reflex is the term given to the phenomenon that is demonstrated as a result of the mechanical stretching of the cervix. When the cervix is stretched in labor, uterine activity appears to be increased. This was originally thought to be related to an increase in the release of oxytocin. Currently, that phenomenon appears to be a simplistic and probably inaccurate theory. The exact mechanism remains unknown (Cunningham et al. 1993).

During active labor, electrical and contractile activity in the smooth muscle cells is controlled by myogenic, neurogenic, and hormonal control systems. A woman's uterus has a pacemaker potential, although the exact cells have not been identified. Smooth muscle bundles come closer to each other and form gap junctions that are associated with synchronous uterine activity. A uterine contraction actually has two components—contraction and retraction. The contraction phase consists of a descending gradient. The wave begins in the fundus, where there are the greatest number of myometrial cells. The wave then moves downward through the corpus of the uterus. The intensity of a contraction diminishes from fundus to cervix. Throughout labor, the upper uterine segment is more active, contracting more intensely and for a longer time than the lower uterine segment. The second part of the contraction is the retraction phase. After the muscle has contracted, it retracts as it relaxes by pulling up the cervix and lower uterine segment. The upper uterine segment becomes thicker in time, while the more passive lower segment becomes thinner. The area that divides the upper and lower uterine segments is known as the physiologic retraction ring (Fig. 22–9). The synchronous nature of contractions is necessary for efficient dilatation and effacement of the cervix.

The issue of adequate nutrition in labor has been raised in regard to the need for energy to accomplish the work of labor. It has been suggested that to labor effectively, a woman needs to be well nourished. It has been reported that women who are dehydrated frequently experience preterm labor that can be stopped by being hydrated. Other scientists and researchers suggest that labor is an intensive physical event, and findings from sports medicine might provide a valuable comparison. Within that context, loading with complex carbohydrates, avoidance of fats, and liberal use of fluids may be of value for labor (Broach and Newton 1988; McKay and Mahan 1988; Newton et al. 1988; Smith et al. 1993). Management of hydration and nutrition in labor is discussed further in Chapter 23.

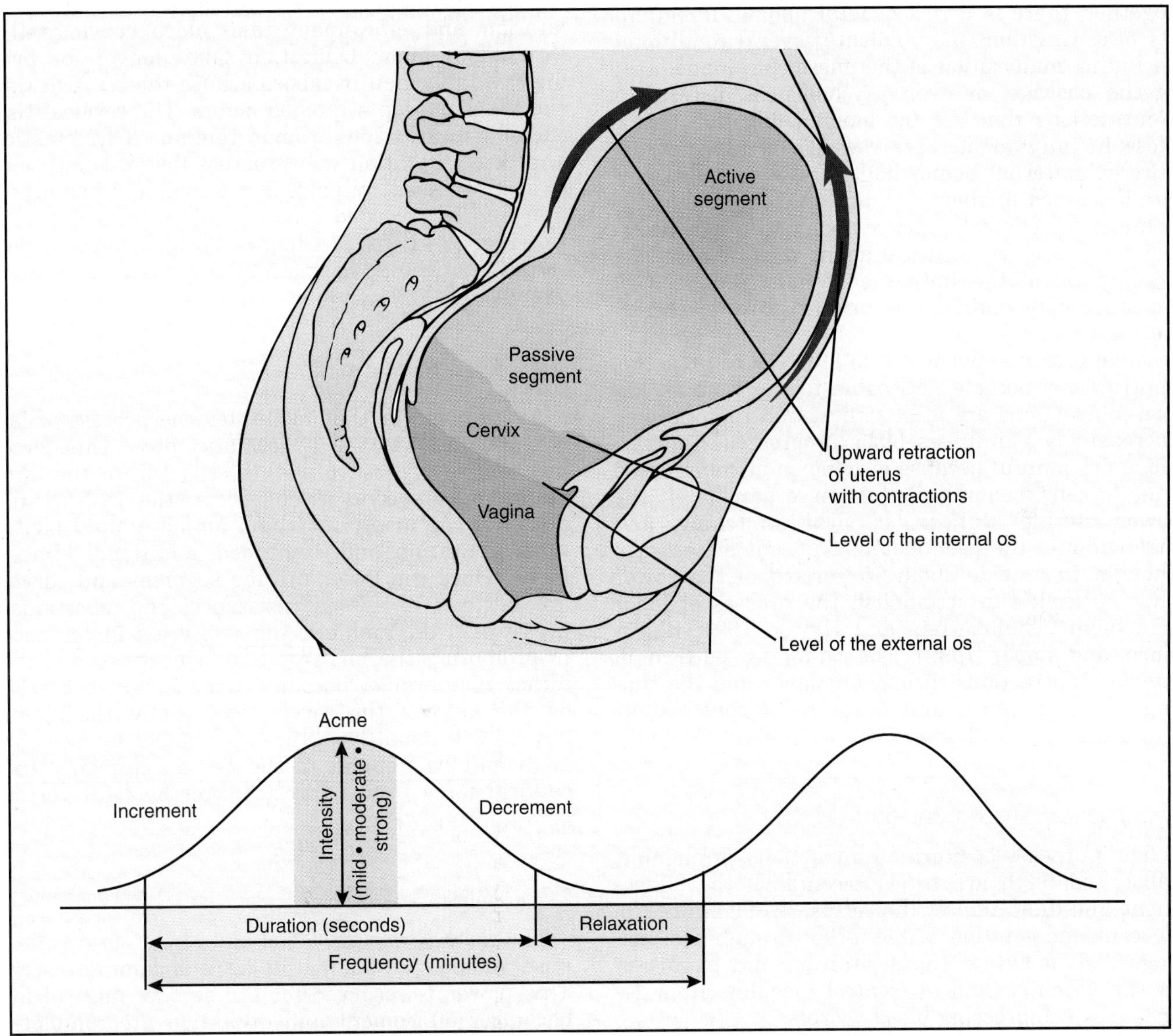

Figure 22–9

Uterine labor contractions consist of both contraction and retraction phases • The upper segment of the uterus is active and becomes thicker as labor progresses • The lower segment of the uterus is passive and becomes thinner • The duration of a uterine contraction includes the increment (ascending portion), acme (peak), and decrement (descending portion) • The relaxation phase is the time between contractions • The interval of a contraction is measured from the beginning of one contraction to the beginning of the next. (Adapted with permission from Cunningham, F. G., MacDonald, P. C., Gund, N. F., Levens, K. J., Gilstrap, L. C. I. [1993]. *Williams obstetrics* [19th ed.] [p. 342]. Norwalk, CT: Appleton & Lange.)

Characteristics

Normal uterine contractions are like waves, composed of an increment (the building up or ascending portion), an acme (the peak), and a decrement (the coming down or descending portion) (Fig. 22–9). Contractions are the primary power needed to accomplish the work of labor and birth. They are intermittent throughout labor, forming a regular pattern interspersed with rest periods. The rest period between contractions is essential, not only for the comfort of the laboring woman but also for the welfare of the fetus. During a contraction, there is a decrease in uteroplacental blood flow, which then rapidly returns to normal between contractions. If contractions are too close together, there is a risk of fetal anoxia. Irregularity of contractions may indicate several conditions, including malposition of the passenger, inadequacy of the passage, or even psychological discomfort. Contractions that are too long in duration or too close in interval increase the risk of uterine rupture or maternal hemorrhage. These complications are discussed further in Chapter 25. Although it is common in clinical practice today to augment labor with a pharmaceutical agent such as oxytocin, recognition of the influence of maternal position on labor may redirect the primary care of the laboring woman.

At approximately 15 to 20 mm Hg of pressure, contractions become noticeable to the woman. Labor contractions are mild at first and then become increasingly painful as labor progresses. Contractions are painful because of hypoxia of compressed muscle cells, compression of nerve ganglia in the lower uterine segment, cervical stretching, and stretching of the peritoneum. The contractions are thought to provide about 75 percent of the power that is needed to accomplish the process of labor and birth (Chamberlain and Hytten 1991; Blackburn and Loper 1992). The changing pattern of uterine contractions throughout labor and the timing of the interval and duration of contractions are discussed in Chapter 23.

Purpose: Effacement and Dilatation

The purposes of uterine contractions throughout labor and birth are to (1) accomplish the effacement and dilatation of the cervix, (2) facilitate the descent and rotation of the fetus through the passages, (3) facilitate the separation and expulsion of the placenta, and (4) control bleeding after delivery by compressing blood vessels.

Effacement is the thinning or shortening of the cervix. Before the latter part of pregnancy, the cervix is about 2 cm long and is firm. As the cervix begins to ripen in the latter part of pregnancy, it may also begin the process of effacement. This is particularly true for primigravida women, who may be 50 percent effaced before labor begins. In multiparous women, effacement may not begin until active labor, so that effacement and dilatation take place concurrently. During labor, effacement is accomplished by the upward retraction of the lower uterine segment as the upper uterine segment becomes thicker. Some effacement must take place before dilatation is possible. By the time the process of effacement is complete, the cervix is completely flat or paper thin, having been pulled up into the lower uterine segment. Effacement is assessed by palpation on vaginal examination and is recorded in percentage ranging from 0 to 100 percent (Fig. 22–10).

Dilatation (or dilation) is the gradual opening of the cervix and is a continued extension of the contraction-retraction process already described. Dilatation and effacement take place concurrently throughout labor. Dilatation takes longer for primigravida women in labor because the cervical tissue has not been stretched before. The cervical tissue of a multiparous woman remains more elastic, and thus dilatation will progress faster. Dilatation is also assessed by palpation on vaginal examination and is recorded in centimeters from 0 to 10 cm (Fig. 22–10). See Chapter 23 for a further description of the assessment of effacement and dilatation.

HYDROSTATIC FORCE

Another power that facilitates the process of labor and birth is the hydrostatic force. This force includes the pressure of the fetus within the amniotic sac. As contractions occur, the hydrostatic action of the membranes and amniotic fluid facilitates dilatation and, if needed, additional effacement. Since the lower uterine segment and cervix are regions of lesser resistance, the additional pressure of the amniotic sac is of great importance in promoting the birth process. The pressure with intact membranes becomes increasingly centered on the area of the cervix. Eventually, the membranes will usually rupture spontaneously and the head will be applied to the cervix, changing the cervical force from hydrostatic to the fetal vertex as a dilating wedge.

ABDOMINAL FORCE

The final power for labor and birth, often called a secondary power, is the intra-abdominal force. This power is reserved for the second stage of labor, after effacement and dilatation are complete. It is commonly referred to as the maternal pushing or bearing down effort. In the expulsion stage, the contractions change in character, and many women begin to experience an involuntary urge to push. When a woman pushes in the second stage, she uses her abdominal muscles by contracting them to provide an auxiliary force to the uterine

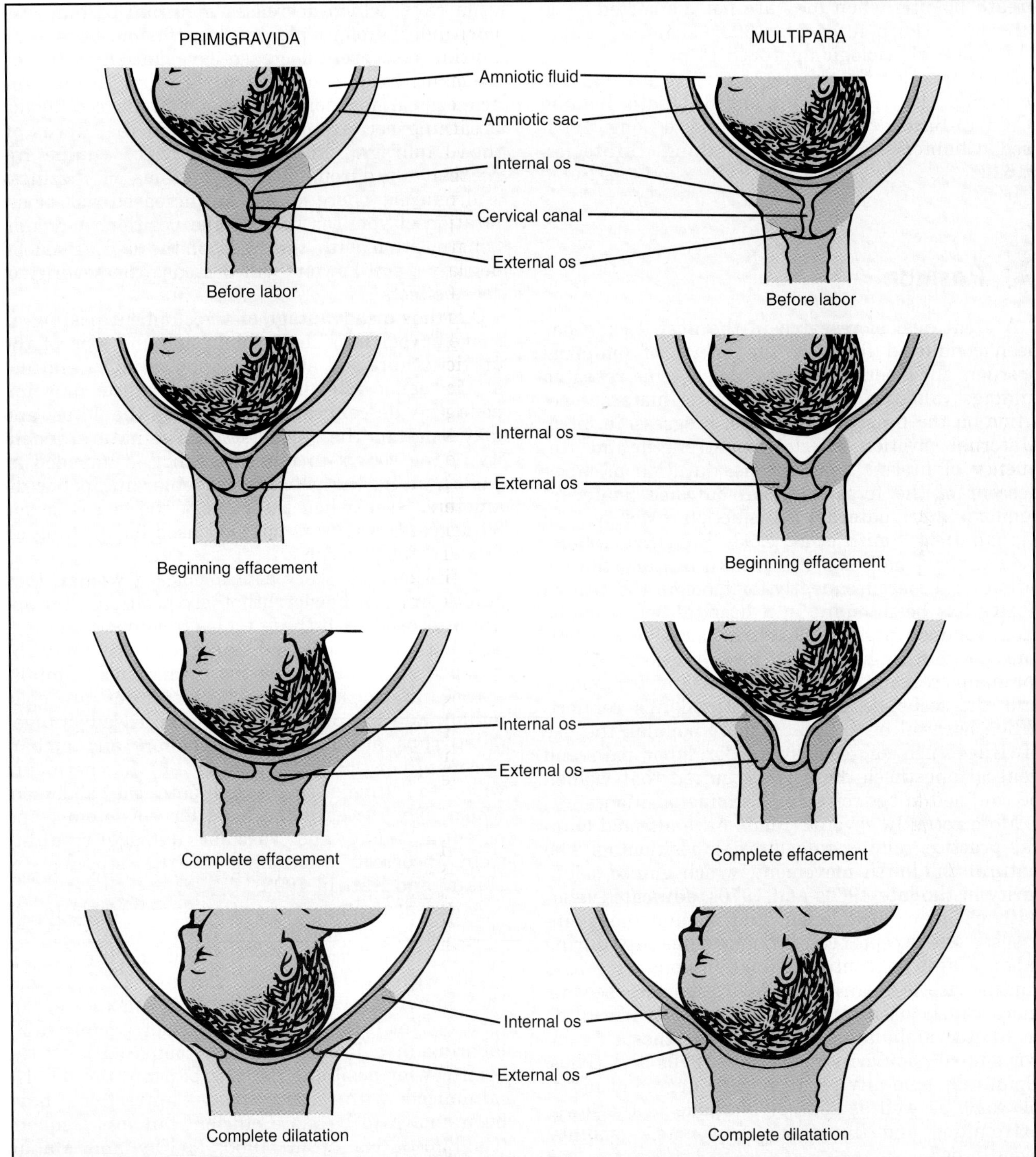

Figure 22–10

Cervical effacement, which is measured from 0 to 100 percent, is the thinning, flattening, or shortening of the cervix as it is pulled up into the lower uterine segment as a result of uterine contractions • Cervical dilatation is the opening of the cervix resulting from uterine contractions and is measured from 0 to 10 cm.

contractions, which increases intra-abdominal pressure to force the fetus through the vagina.

For many years it has been suggested that prolonged breath holding is the way in which a woman should be taught to push. However, evidence has called into question both the efficacy and potential harm of pushing with a closed glottis (also called a Valsalva maneuver) (Burpo 1995). Women have been observed to push effectively by either controlled exhalations or brief breath holding when they are not instructed to do otherwise (Parnell et al. 1993; Thomson 1993). This more physiologic approach to pushing is also termed open glottis, exhale, or gentle pushing, and it avoids the risks of prolonged breath holding (Caldyro-Barcia 1979; Cosner and deJong 1993) (see Chapter 20, Paced Breathing Strategies, p. 612).

Position

A great deal of research in the past decade has been conducted to study the effects of maternal position in labor. The majority of the research findings validates the importance of maternal position on the progress, or lack of progress, in labor. Maternal position affects the strength and frequency of uterine contractions, duration of labor, descent of the fetus, perineal outcome, maternal comfort, and maternal satisfaction (McKay and Mahan 1984; Smith et al. 1993; Biancuzzo 1993a).

In the last half of the twentieth century, the position used most frequently for labor in the United States has been supine in a hospital bed, and the most common position for birth has been a lithotomy position (Fig. 22–11). These positions evolved for many reasons, including the use of technology and the focus on the birth attendant's comfort. When hospital birth became more popular, the use of drugs such as scopolamine for labor pain and general anesthesia for birth required that women be confined to bed, often in a supine position.

More recently, several trends have affected clinical practice related to maternal positioning. The natural childbirth movement, which gained popularity in the late 1960s and 1970s, advocated labor without pain medication and should have increased the acceptance of women's mobility during labor. However, continuous fetal monitoring and routine use of intravenous hydration also became more widely used in the 1970s and often resulted in limited ambulation. Epidural anesthesia for labor gained popularity in the late 1970s and 1980s. Epidurals generally produce some degree of motor blockade as well as sensory blockade in the lower extremities and thus limit a woman's mobility, even in bed.

Maternal positions for labor and birth can be divided into two groups: recumbent and upright. The hands and knees position is a modification of an upright posture. Figure 22–11 summarizes the various positions during labor and birth.

RECUMBENT POSITION

A strictly supine recumbent posture is contraindicated for pregnant women because of the resulting pressure of the uterus on the inferior vena cava, which decreases maternal cardiac output and therefore placental perfusion. This position may severely decrease oxygenation to the fetus, which can lead to hypoxia, bradycardia, and acidosis. In addition, a woman may have difficulty breathing because of pressure from the uterus on the diaphragm. She may experience supine hypotensive syndrome with symptoms of dizziness and nausea. There is also an increased risk of aspiration of vomitus in a supine position. A recumbent position with the head of the bed raised 30 degrees (semi-Fowler) will decrease the severity of these effects.

Another disadvantage of a recumbent position is that the pelvis is less mobile and the axis of the uterus is directed at the symphysis pubis and not at the pelvic inlet. Both of these effects may impede the descent and rotation of the fetus and may lengthen the second stage. The natural mobility of the coccyx in late pregnancy is impeded as well, limiting the potential for enlarging pelvic diameters. Even when the head of the bed is raised 30 degrees, gravity is not well used for pushing efforts in this position.

Traditional delivery tables place a woman in a supine or semi-Fowler lithotomy position. Stirrups are also used with these tables to support the legs so that the lower half of the table may be dropped. This facilitates the attendant's administration of anesthesia, performance of an episiotomy, and use of instrumentation. Disadvantages of stirrups are maternal discomfort and embarrassment; possible tightening of the perineum when the thighs are flexed onto the abdomen, which may increase the need for episiotomy; and potential nerve and vascular damage resulting from incorrect positioning of the stirrups (al Hakim and Katiriji 1993).

A lateral recumbent position is preferable to the semi-Fowler or supine position because oxygenation to the fetus is increased. This position is advised with medical complications of pregnancy that impair placental perfusion to maximize cardiac output. Many women are more comfortable laboring in a lateral position, compared with the semi-Fowler position. The risk of aspiration is also minimized with lateral rest. Contractions have been shown to be more efficient but less frequent (Caldyro-Barcia et al. 1960; McKay and Mahan 1984; Roberts et al. 1983). A lateral maternal position may promote rotation of the fetus from a posterior to an anterior position (Biancuzzo 1993b). A lateral position may also be used for birth, although this is not as commonly seen in the United States as it is in Britain (Lehrman 1985). Advantages of birthing in this position are that the perineum may be less tense and may therefore be less likely to tear. A lateral birth will require an assistant to support the upper leg. A disadvantage of a lateral birth is that maternal participation may be decreased.

POSITION	ADVANTAGES	DISADVANTAGES
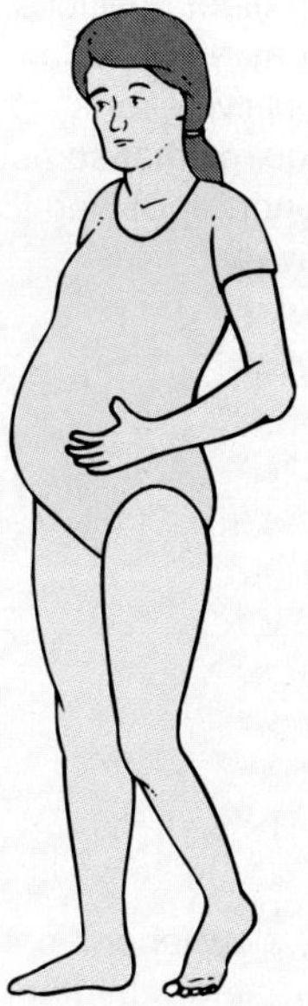 Ambulating	• Utilizes gravity; applies presenting part against cervix • Places fetus in alignment with pelvis; facilitates descent • Enhances effect of contractions and decreases pain • May decrease length of labor • Decreases fetal heart variable decelerations • Relieves backache	• May be tiring • Telemetry required for continuous electronic fetal monitoring • Not possible with regional anesthesia
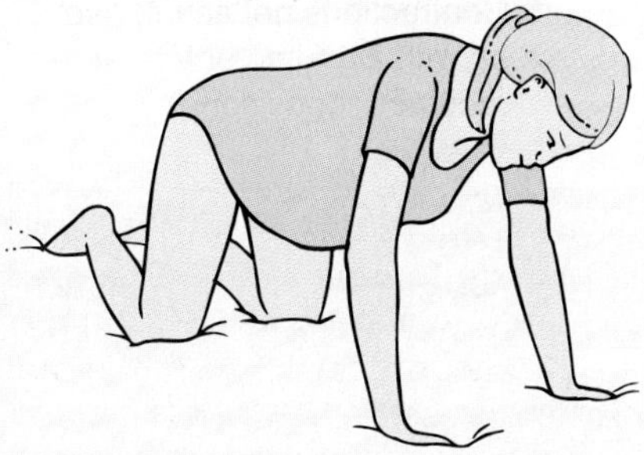 Hands and knees	• Stimulates rotation of fetus from posterior to anterior position • Relieves backache • Relieves rectal pressure • Facilitates pelvic rocking and pelvic mobility • Eliminates weight on inferior vena cava and decreases fetal distress • Relieves pressure on cord if prolapsed • Facilitates delivery, especially in cases of shoulder dystocia, breech position, or persistent occiput posterior position	• May be tiring; causes wrist fatigue • May be embarrassing • External electronic fetal monitor difficult to keep in place • Not possible with regional anesthesia
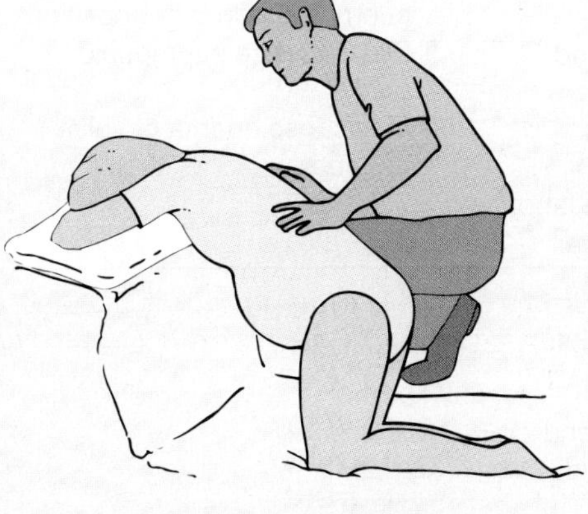 Kneeling and leaning forward with support	• Relieves backache • Facilitates fetal rotation from posterior to anterior position • Enables use of pelvic rocking • Causes less strain on wrists and hands • Allows access to back and sacrum for massage and counterpressure	• External electronic fetal monitor difficult to keep in place • May be tiring • Not possible with regional anesthesia

Figure 22–11

Advantages and disadvantages of various positions for labor and birth.

Continued on following page

POSITION	ADVANTAGES	DISADVANTAGES
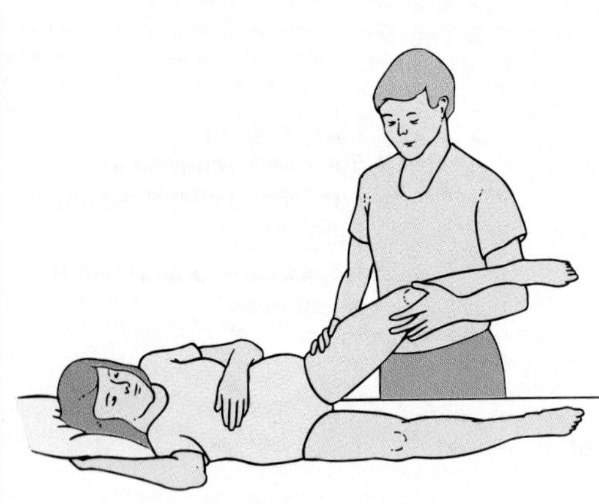 Lateral recumbent	• Provides rest; comfortable • Corrects supine hypotension; facilitates fetoplacental perfusion • Helps to decrease maternal blood pressure • Facilitates less frequent but stronger contractions compared with supine position • Slows rapid labor • Helps to rotate occiput posterior fetus • Decreases back pain • Facilitates interventions (e.g., vaginal examinations, electronic fetal monitoring, regional anesthesia)	• More effective if alternated with other positions • Not as effective for expulsive efforts • Requires that someone support upper leg for delivery
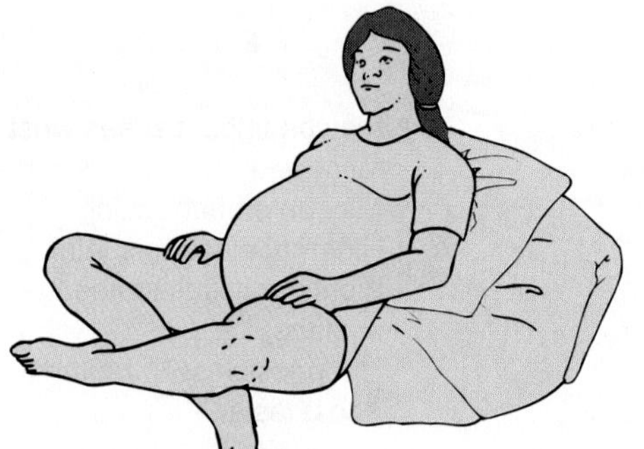 Semi-reclining (30° to 45° angle)	• Promotes comfort; good resting position • Maximizes direction of contractions' force to facilitate descent • Enhances contractions compared with supine position • Shortens labor compared with supine position • May be used with electronic fetal monitor • Facilitates vaginal examination	• May slow labor if not alternated with other positions • May increase back discomfort • Contractions not as intense as with standing or lateral recumbent positions
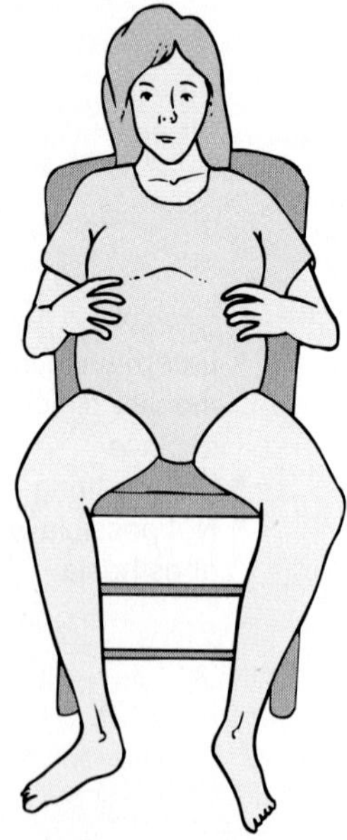 Sitting upright (90° angle)	• Decreases back pain; comfortable • Utilizes gravity • Avoids supine hypotensive syndrome • Shortens labor compared with supine position • May use with electronic fetal monitor • Shortens second-stage labor; increases pelvic diameter • Enhances efficiency for pushing and delivery • Enhances interaction with partner • Allows access to back and sacrum for massage and counterpressure when leaning forward	• Contractions not as intense as with standing or lateral recumbent positions • May slow labor if not alternated with other positions • May increase suprapubic pain • May cause edema of vulva or cervix

Continued on following page

POSITION	ADVANTAGES	DISADVANTAGES
Squatting	• Utilizes gravity • Increases pelvic diameters • Relieves backache • Facilitates pushing efforts in second-stage; increases intra-abdominal pressure • Promotes fetal descent and rotation; may shorten second stage • Enhances interaction between woman, labor partner, and birth attendant	• May impede descent before engagement • May be uncomfortable; tiring • May be embarrassing • May increase risk of uterine prolapse with strenuous bearing down • May increase perineal and cervical edema or lacerations • May increase blood loss
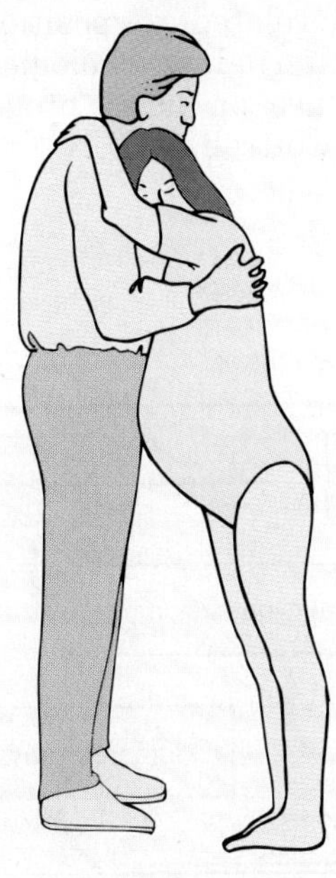 Standing and leaning forward	• Utilizes gravity; applies presenting part against cervix • Places fetus in alignment with pelvis; facilitates descent • Enhances effect of contractions and decreases pain • Promotes comfort; decreases backache because fetus moves forward • May decrease length of labor • Facilitates rest during contractions • May be used with electronic fetal monitor	• May be tiring • Not possible with regional anesthesia • May be difficult to keep external electronic fetal monitor in place • Needs two supporters if used in second-stage
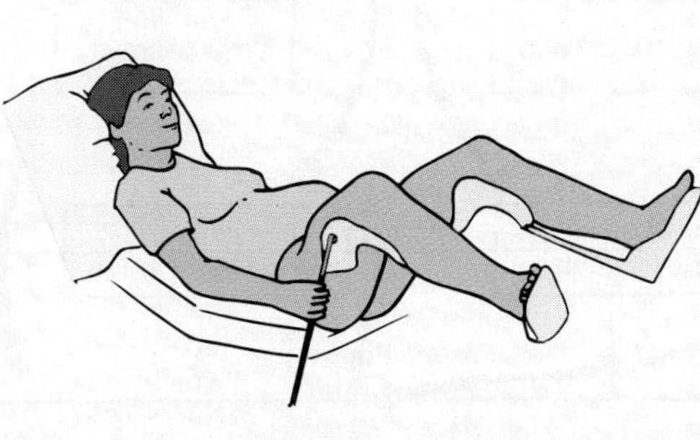 Supine/lithotomy	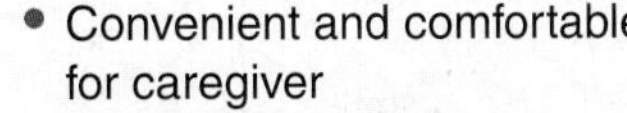 • Convenient and comfortable for caregiver • Restful for some women • Facilitates fetal monitoring and vaginal examination • Facilitates interventions (fetal heart rate, forceps, episiotomy, repair of lacerations) • Facilitates maintenance of asepsis • Facilitates comfort and security for legs for some women through stirrups	• Supine hypotensive syndrome • Increases back discomfort • Contractions less efficient, more painful, and longer in duration • Women may feel psychologically vulnerable or dependent • Decreases maternal participation during birth • Stirrups can promote blood clots or discomfort in legs • Risk of aspiration if woman vomits • Decreases ability to push

UPRIGHT POSITIONS

Upright positions that may be used for labor are sitting, squatting, standing, and ambulation (Liu 1989). The first three may also be used for birth. Gravity is employed with all upright positions, and the uterine axis is in line with the pelvic inlet as well (Biancuzzo 1993a). Birth chairs and stools have been used for centuries to facilitate pushing efforts in the second stage. There are modern versions of the birth stool, and the toilet may also serve as an appropriate and natural place for the second stage to occur. Contractions are more efficient when a woman is sitting compared with lying in bed, but not as efficient as contractions when the woman is squatting or standing. Advantages of sitting are increased comfort, increased maternal participation in birth, shorter second stage, and decreased frequency of neonatal acidosis. Disadvantages include an increase in perineal edema, which has been associated with the birth chair (Knauth and Haloburdo 1988; Shannahan and Cottrell 1989; Waldenstrom and Gattvall 1991).

Squatting is facilitated by the use of a squatting bar or a support person to help a woman maintain her balance. Pelvic diameters are largest in a squatting position. They are increased by more than 28 percent of their supine dimensions. Squatting encourages descent of the fetal head and rotation to an anterior position (Golay et al. 1993) and can facilitate labor progress. Squatting enables a woman to participate in the birth and facilitates massage of her back and sides. Women have also reported increased comfort and an increased urge to push when squatting. Disadvantages of squatting are an increased difficulty in the use of external fetal monitoring, decreased accessibility to and visibility of the perineum for anesthesia administration or instrument use, and increased perineal edema with a prolonged second stage (Cottrell and Shannahan 1986; Knauth and Haloburdo 1988; Shannahan and Cottrell 1989).

The advantages and disadvantages of the various positions during labor are compared in Figure 22–11. The most efficient contractions are measured when a woman ambulates during first-stage labor. Women report enhanced comfort when ambulating; however, it may be fatiguing during long periods. Standing or ambulating improves the alignment of the fetal head in the pelvis; therefore, descent of the head and its application to the cervix are enhanced. These processes are vital to the efficient progress of labor. The hands and knees position has been shown to be helpful in rotating the fetal head to an anterior position, especially combined with pelvic rocking (Andrews and Chrzanowski 1990). Some research has suggested that no single position in first-stage labor is most advantageous but that it is better to use several different positions. The only positions to be avoided are the classic supine or dorsal positions since the supine hypotension syndrome (vena cava syndrome) can occur and result in decreased uterine perfusion. The physiologic effects of the dorsal position can be seen in Figure 22–12.

During second-stage labor, sitting positions have been associated with a shorter length of labor but more perineal lacerations. Lateral recumbent, semi-sitting, and supported squatting positions appear to have advantages related to uterine perfusion. Semi-sitting and squatting have advantages of gravity, and it is easier for the woman to see the birth occur. Some birth attendants do not encourage a semi-sitting or supported squatting position as it decreases their visual fields. Most of the research on positions in labor has focused on the physiologic response of the body to positional changes. However, few studies have noted maternal comfort or desire related to positioning, despite the fact that maternal psychological health is also a major influence on labor progress (Liu 1989; Shannahan and Cottrell 1989).

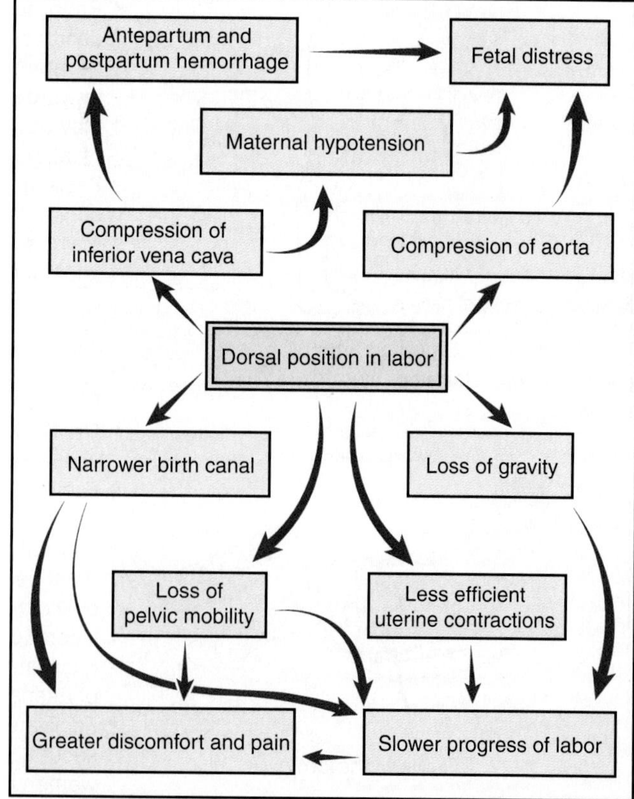

Figure 22–12

The dorsal position in labor can have a number of detrimental physiologic effects.

Psychology of Birth

The woman's emotional status before and during labor is the final influence on the progression of the birth process. If a woman is frightened, anxious, or upset, her psyche can actually alter the normal physiologic process of labor and birth. It is hypothesized that high levels of catecholamines can interfere with the normal progress of labor on a biologic level. It is possible that norepinephrine and epinephrine stimulate both the alpha receptors and beta receptors of the myometrium and interfere with the rhythmic nature of labor, culminating in a pattern of ineffective contractions and resulting in a long labor. Anxiety can also increase pain perception, leading to an increased need for analgesia or anesthesia. This phenomenon is seen clinically with the anxious woman in intense labor who progresses rapidly after some degree of pain relief is achieved (Fig. 22–13).

A number of factors can influence the woman's emotional response to birth. Lack of knowledge, fear of pain, personal or family stress, lack of support of a significant other during labor, degree of self-confidence, feelings of loss of control, negative attitudes about birth, cultural background, and concerns for personal safety can all serve to block the normal physiologic progression of the labor and birth process. The birth environment can have a potential profound influence on labor as well (Albers and Katz 1991; Annie and Groer 1991; Davis-Floyd 1992; Fullerton and Severino 1992). An environment that a woman perceives as friendly and comfortable is one that is more likely to facilitate a healthy birth. Niles Newton (1966), in her classic work with mice, discovered that a

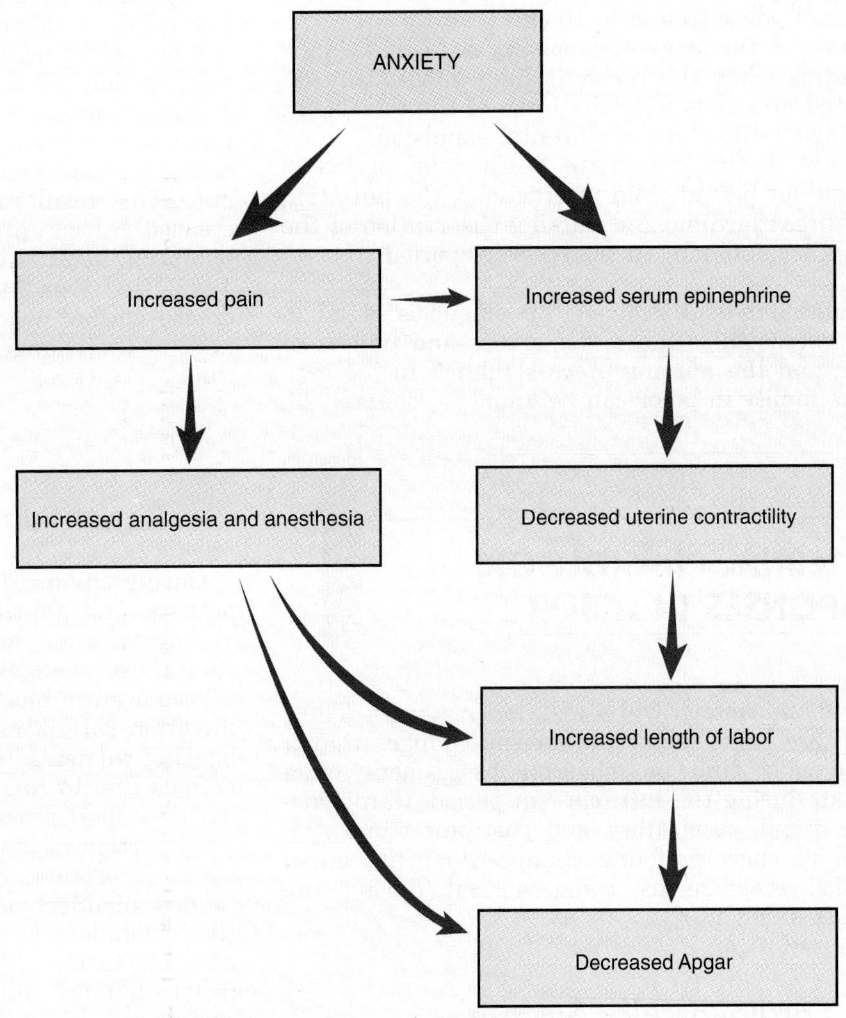

Figure 22–13

The progress of labor and birth can be adversely affected by maternal fear and tension • Norepinephrine and epinephrine may stimulate both alpha and beta receptors of the myometrium and interfere with the rhythmic nature of labor • Anxiety can also increase pain perception and lead to an increased need for analgesia or anesthesia.

healthy mouse in labor was more likely to experience a difficult labor (dystocia) and stillbirths if a single cat hair was introduced into the mouse's otherwise comfortable environment.

THE STAGES OF LABOR

Labor is commonly divided into four stages:

1. Stage 1, the stage of cervical effacement and dilatation. Active contractions occur during this time, and the cervix thins to 100 percent effacement and dilates to 10 cm. Stage 1 is subdivided into three phases: the early phase (also called latent or prodromal) from 0 to 3 cms; the active phase from 4 to 7 cm; and the transitional phase from 8 to 10 cm.
2. Stage 2, the stage of expulsion or birth. Stage 2 begins when the cervix is fully effaced and dilated and ends with the birth of the total baby.
3. Stage 3, the stage of placental expulsion.
4. Stage 4, the immediate postpartum period, a time for parent-child interactions, the initiation of breastfeeding, and nursing observation of the mother and baby in the recovery period.

Additional discussion of the diagnosis of labor, true versus false labor, the stages and phases of labor, and the nursing process related to the care of the family in labor can be found in Chapter 23.

MATERNAL PHYSIOLOGIC RESPONSES IN LABOR

As many women will attest, labor is work. Thus, there are some major physiologic changes that a nurse may find on physical assessment of a woman during the intrapartum period. Cardiovascular, renal, respiratory, and gastrointestinal systems all show profound changes that the nurse should recognize as being normal during the process of labor.

Cardiovascular System

Labor has major influences on the cardiovascular status of a woman. In general, cardiac output, cardiac workload, heart rate, and blood pressure are all increased (Table 22–2). Cardiac output increases as a result of the transfer of maternal blood (300 to 500 mL) from the uterus and placental vascular bed into the maternal systemic vascular system with each contraction. Blood pressure may be elevated and heart rate altered during contractions. Fear and anxiety can cause the release of catecholamines, resulting in transient tachycardia. Therefore, blood pressure and pulse should be assessed between contractions during labor. Hematologic changes may be seen in labor. It is hypothesized that the physical or emotional stress of labor may cause an elevation in white blood cells to 25,000/mm^3 or greater. The physical work of labor may also cause blood glucose levels to decrease. Blood coagulation time may decrease, while plasma fibrinogen levels increase. Peripheral vascular changes may result in maternal flushed cheeks (malar flush) or hot or cold feet during labor.

Position in labor or at birth may further influence the cardiovascular changes. Supine positions can result in decreased cardiac output and stroke volume with increased heart rate as a result of compression of the inferior vena cava and descending aorta. Extended breath holding (Valsalva maneuver) can increase intrathoracic pressure, decrease venous return, and increase venous pressure. This results in increased cardiac output, increased blood pressure, decreased pulse, and potential fetal hypoxia (Blackburn and Loper 1992) (see Fig. 20–7). Anxiety and pain also increase cardiac work and may be a major component of the changes demonstrated with a contraction.

Renal Function

During childbirth, maternal renin, plasma renin activity, and angiotensinogen and fetal renin and angiotensinogen are elevated. It is hypothesized that these changes are needed for control of the uteroplacental blood flow. Although the glomerular filtration rate is increased during labor, the childbearing woman is at risk for urinary tract complications due to increased cardiac output, maternal position, fetal pressure on the bladder, and antidiuretic action of oxytocin. These factors can reduce water excretion either mechanically (e.g., distended bladder) or by iatrogenic water intoxication. Diaphoresis, polyuria, decreased hydration, and increased respirations also affect the electrolyte balance during labor. Proteinuria (trace to 1+) may result from the breakdown of muscle tissue during the work of labor. The laboring woman should be observed closely for bladder distention or inability to void, which can be caused by re-

Table 22–2

PHYSIOLOGIC RESPONSES IN LABOR

	FIRST STAGE	CONTRACTION	SECOND STAGE	THIRD STAGE	FOURTH STAGE	COMMENTS
Cardiovascular System						
Cardiac output and workload	Gradual increase (reports vary—some say no change)	↑ 15%–30%	↑ persists	Brief ↓ after placenta separates	60% ↑ (with ↑ venous return)	↑ with pain, anxiety, physical effort
Heart rate	↑ 10 beats/minute	↑ as starts ↓ with relaxation of uterine contraction	Tachycardia	Drop (↓ pain and anxiety)	Relative bradycardia	
Stroke volume		Reciprocal ↑ Heart rate ↓			↑ (with ↑ venous return)	
Blood pressure	Similar to prelabor value	10–15 mm Hg ↑ of systolic and diastolic	15–25 mm Hg further ↑, especially systolic	Normal	Slight ↑	Change usually seen only in *supine* position
Central venous pressure and femoral venous pressure		↑ with peak of contractions			↑ (with ↑ venous return)	
Renal Function						
Glomerular filtration rate and renal plasma flow	Increased with ↑ cardiac output; polyuria ↓ with supine position, secondary compression of ureters by uterus	↑ Pressure or discomfort or ↓ urge to void	↓ with intra-abdominal pressure; distended bladder may impede descent until it is past ischial spine		Bladder may be hypotonic after delivery and become distended	Potential for bladder distention occurs in one third of women
Proteinuria	May be seen in prolonged labor, especially with anemia		Urethra may be bruised by descent			
Respiratory System						
Rate and rhythm	Altered by pain and anxiety		Altered with urge to bear down	Return to normal unless O_2 deficit		
Functional residual capacity	↓ further to less dilution of inspired air and greater respiration		More rapid general anesthesia induction because of ↑ alveolar concentration			

Continued on following page

Table 22–2

PHYSIOLOGIC RESPONSES IN LABOR Continued

	FIRST STAGE	CONTRACTION	SECOND STAGE	THIRD STAGE	FOURTH STAGE	COMMENTS
			Respiratory System *(cont'd)*			
PCO_2	21–35 mm Hg	By the end of the first stage, mild metabolic acidosis compensated by respiratory alkalosis	16–24 mm Hg	Quickly reversed with compensatory respiratory efforts	↓ O_2 may persist for hours, depending on long or severe labor	
Plasma base deficit	−0.9 to 9.2 mEq/L		−2.3 to 12.3 mEq/L			
pH	7.41–7.54		7.37–7.45			
Hyperventilation	Hypocapnia (↓ CO_2) Alkalosis (↑ pH to 7.68) causes carpopedal spasm and anxiety		Hypoxia with breath holding (↓ O_2 to 87%)			
			Gastrointestinal System			
Emptying time of stomach	Prolonged: retention with apprehension and medication; secretion of gastric juice; absorption *slowed* for solid food; absorption *normal* for liquid		Important role in regurgitation and aspiration			
Peristalsis	Ceases, except for lower colon					
Anorexia	Common				Hunger	
Thirst	Common parotid function					
Nausea and vomiting	Vomiting with beginning of dilatation		Vomiting with passage of head through cervix		Should *not* persist	

Data from Baylor College of Medicine, Midwifery Education Program; Hytten and Chamberlain 1991; Blackburn and Loper 1992; and Cunningham et al. 1993.

laxed bladder tone, analgesia or anesthesia, compression from the fetus, or trauma (Table 22–2).

Respiratory System

When labor begins, there is an increased demand for oxygen. Oxygen consumption is increased with uterine muscle activity. Maternal respiratory rates usually rise with the work of labor, anxiety or pain, or the use of controlled breathing techniques for pain management. Persistent hyperventilation resulting from fear or pain should be avoided. Major changes occur in the acid-base relationships during labor, although these appear to be physiologic and are quickly reversed in the third stage. Among the normal changes are mild respiratory alkalosis apparent in early first-stage labor and mild metabolic acidosis compensated by respiratory alkalosis at the end of stage 1; mild respiratory acidosis during bearing down efforts; and finally metabolic acidosis uncompensated by respiratory alkalosis at the time of birth (Blackburn and Loper 1992) (Table 22–2).

Gastrointestinal System

Before active labor, some women experience diarrhea as a prodromal symptom of impending labor. During active labor, gastric motility is decreased, and the emptying time of the stomach is prolonged. If opioids are administered, the emptying time is likely to be even more prolonged. Thus, food ingested at the onset of labor can remain in the stomach unchanged until labor is over. This not only is uncomfortable for the laboring woman but can increase the occurrence of nausea and vomiting and pose a risk if administration of general anesthesia is necessary. For this reason, women should be instructed before the onset of labor that solid foods be avoided once active labor has begun. Clear liquids are absorbed rapidly, however, so the woman can be encouraged to drink these if no apparent complications exist. Even if the stomach is relatively empty, nausea and vomiting are common normal complaints during the intrapartum period, particularly during the transition phase. In fact, an empty stomach causes increased gastric acidity, which may lead to nausea and vomiting. Some women also experience belching during the transition phase. Nausea and vomiting are generally resolved after birth occurs but may persist because of the side effects of administration of a pharmaceutical agent (Table 22–2).

Implications for Research

The maintenance of the normal physiologic process of labor is an important goal in the care of a pregnant woman and her infant. Research that can identify factors that influence normal labor or show how those factors might be enhanced or altered to maintain labor's normal physiologic progression would be of great value. Examples of research questions for study are as follows.

- What is the difference in uterine contraction pattern (interval, duration, and intensity) when the woman is in the supine, lateral Sims, and upright position?
- Is there a relationship between the woman's position during labor, level of discomfort, and length of labor?
- What factors facilitate the woman's pushing efforts (abdominal force) during the second stage of labor?

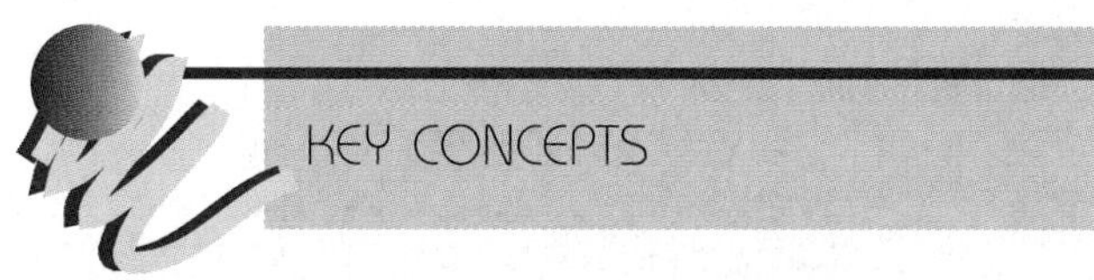

KEY CONCEPTS

- ▼ No single etiologic agent has been found to be the cause of the initiation of labor; the recognized theories of labor initiation are progesterone withdrawal, oxytocin production, prostaglandin production, endothelin production, stretch, estrogen stimulation, and fetal cortisol.
- ▼ Labor probably begins as a result of complex endocrinologic and biomolecular phenomena.
- ▼ Labor can be affected by many factors, including the five Ps: passenger, passage, powers, maternal position, and psychology of birth. These five Ps are particularly influential during the first two stages of labor.
- ▼ The fetal passenger has biologic and mechanical influences on the process of labor. The mechanical influences include the bones, sutures and fontanelles, and diameters of the fetal head; the lie, attitude, presentation, and position of the fetus; and the cardinal movements of the fetus as it moves through the passages.
- ▼ The passages consist of the hard passage (bony pelvis) and the soft passages (uterus, cervix, vagina, and perineum). The divisions, planes, and diameters (conjugates) of the pelvis influence its adaptability to the birth process.
- ▼ The powers of labor consist of the uterine contractions, the hydrostatic force, and the abdominal force.

- Effacement is the thinning of the cervix; dilatation is the opening of the cervix. Both are accomplished by uterine contractions and the pressure of the presenting part of the fetus against the cervix.
- The position of the woman during labor has a definite influence on contractions and the cardinal movements of the fetus. Upright positions are usually more advantageous than recumbent positions.
- The psyche, or emotional status, of the woman during labor can influence the progression of the labor process.
- There are four stages of labor: cervical dilatation, expulsion of the fetus, placental expulsion, and the immediate postpartum period.
- Labor is work, and as such, profound physiologic responses can be observed, especially in the cardiovascular, renal, respiratory, and gastrointestinal systems.

References

Albers, L., and Katz, V. (1991). Birth setting for low-risk pregnancies, *Journal of Nurse-Midwifery,* 36 (4), 215–220.

al Hakim, M., and Katiriji, B. (1993). Femoral mononeuropathy induced by the lithotomy position: A report of 5 cases with a review of literature. *Muscle and Nerve,* 16 (9), 891–895.

Anderson, L. (1989). Oxytocin receptor blockade. *American Journal of Perinatology,* 6 (2), 196–199.

Andrews, C., and Chrzanowski, M. (1990). Maternal position, labor and comfort. *Applied Nursing Research,* 3, 7–13.

Annie, C., and Groer, M. (1991). Childbirth stress: An immunologic study. *Journal of Obstetric, Gynecologic, and Neonatal Nursing,* 20 (5), 391–397.

Biancuzzo, M. (1993a). Six myths of maternal posture during labor. *MCN: American Journal of Maternal Child Nursing,* 18 (5), 264–269.

Biancuzzo, M. (1993b). How to recognize and rotate an occiput posterior fetus. *American Journal of Nursing,* 93 (3), 38–41.

Blackburn, S. T., and Loper, D. L. (1992). *Maternal, fetal, and neonatal physiology.* Philadelphia: W. B. Saunders.

Broach, J., and Newton, N. (1988). Food and beverages in labor. Part II: The effects of cessation of oral intake during labor. *Birth,* 15 (2), 88–92.

Burpo, R. (1995). The pushing ritual of second stage labor. *Journal of Perinatal Education,* 4 (2), 1–5.

Caldyro-Barcia, R. (1979). The influence of maternal bearing-down efforts during second stage on fetal well-being. *Birth and the Family Journal,* 6 (1), 17–21.

Caldyro-Barcia, R., Noriega-Guerra, L., Cibils, L., Hermogence, A., Poseiro, J., Pose, S., Sica-Blanco, Y., Mendez-Bauer, C., Gonzalez-Panizza, V. (1960). Effect of position changes on the intensity and frequency of uterine contractions during labor. *American Journal of Obstetrics and Gynecology,* 80 (2), 284–290.

Cherry, S., and Merkatz, I. (1991). *Complications of pregnancy: Medical, surgical, gynecologic, psychosocial, and perinatal.* Baltimore: Williams & Wilkins.

Clark, S., Cotton, D., Hankins, G., Phelan, J. (1991). *Critical care obstetrics.* Boston: Blackwell Scientific Publications.

Cosner, K., and deJong, E. (1993). Physiologic second-stage labor. *MCN: American Journal of Maternal Child Nursing,* 18 (1), 38–43.

Cottrell, B., and Shannahan, M. (1986). Effect of the birth chair on duration of second stage labor and maternal outcome. *Nursing Research,* 35 (6), 364–367.

Creasy, R. K., and Resnik, R. (1994). *Maternal-fetal medicine: Principles and practice* (3rd ed.). Philadelphia: W. B. Saunders.

Cunningham, F. G., MacDonald, P. C., Gant, N. F., Leveno, K. J., Gilstrap, L. C. III. (1993). *Williams obstetrics* (19th ed.). Norwalk, CT: Appleton & Lange.

Davis-Floyd, R. (1992). *Birth as an American rite of passage.* Philadelphia: Williams & Wilkins.

Fullerton, J., and Severino, R. (1992). In-hospital care for low-risk childbirth. *Journal of Nurse-Midwifery,* 37 (5), 331–340.

Goff, K. (1993). Initiation of parturition. *MCN: American Journal of Maternal Child Nursing,* September/October Supplement, 7–13.

Golay, J., Vedam, S., Sorger, L. (1993). The squatting position for the second stage of labor: Effects on labor and on maternal and fetal well-being. *Birth,* 20 (2), 73–78.

Hytten, F., and Chamberlain, G. (1991). *Clinical physiology in obstetrics.* Oxford: Blackstone.

Knauth, D., and Haloburdo, E. (1988). Effect of pushing techniques in birthing chair on length of second stage of labor. *Nursing Research,* 35 (1), 49–51.

Lehrman, E. (1985). Birth in the left lateral position. *Journal of Nurse-Midwifery,* 30 (4), 193–197.

Liu, Y. (1989). The effects of the upright position during childbirth. *Image,* 21 (1), 14–18.

McKay, S., and Mahan, C. (1984). Laboring patients need more freedom to move. *Contemporary Obstetrics and Gynecology,* July, 90–119.

McKay, S., and Mahan, C. (1988). Modifying the stomach contents of laboring women: Why and how; success and risks. *Birth,* 15 (4), 213–220.

Newton, N. (1966). Parturient mice: Effects of environment on labor. *Science,* 151, 1560–1561.

Newton N., Newton, M., Broach, J. (1988). Physiologic, physical, nutritional, and technologic aspects of intravenous infusion during labor. *Birth,* 15 (2), 67–71.

Parnell, C., Langhoff-Roos, J., Iversen, R., Damgaard, P. (1993). Pushing method in the expulsive phase of labor. A randomized trial. *Acta Obstetricia et Gynecologica Scandinavica,* 72 (1), 31–35.

Roberts, J. E., Malasanos, L., Mendez-Bauer, C. (1983). The effects of maternal position on uterine contractility and efficiency. *Birth,* 10 (4), 243–249.

Shannahan, M., and Cottrell, B. (1989). The effects of birth chair delivery on maternal perception. *Journal of Obstetric, Gynecologic, and Neonatal Nursing,* 18 (4), 323–326.

Smith, M., Ruffin, M., Green, L. (1993). The rational management of labor. *American Family Physician,* 47 (6), 1471–1481.

Steer, C. (1975). *Evaluation of the pelvis in obstetrics.* New York: Plenum.

Thomson, A. (1993). Pushing techniques in the second stage of labor. *Journal of Advanced Nursing,* 18 (2), 171–177.

Ulmsten, U. (1989). Prostaglandins in high-risk obstetrics. In S. A. Brody and K. Ueland (Eds.). *Endocrine disorders in pregnancy* (p. 427). Norwalk, CT: Appleton & Lange.

Waldenstrom, U., and Gattvall, K. (1991). A randomized trial of birthing stool or conventional semi-recumbent position. *Birth* 18 (1), 5–10.

Word, R. A. (1993). Parturition. In B. Carr and R. E. Blackwell (Eds.). *Textbook of reproductive medicine.* Norwalk, CT: Appleton & Lange.

Chapter 23

Promoting a Normal Childbirth

Elaine Zwelling
Catherine E. Ruhl

> The only beneficial forms of care during normal childbirth whose effectiveness is demonstrated by clear evidence from randomized research trials are: emotional and psychological support during labor and birth, maternal mobility and choice of position during labor, agents to reduce acidity of stomach contents before general anesthesia, and fetal acid-base assessment as an adjunct to fetal monitoring in labor.
>
> MURRAY W. ENKIN AND COLLEAGUES (1995)

HIGHLIGHTS

- Preliminary Signs of Labor
- True Labor vs. False Labor
- The Process of Labor: The Four Stages
- Nursing Practice
- Collaborative Process
- Procedure 23–1: Monitoring Women During Labor and in the Immediate Postpartum Period
- Procedure 23–2: Auscultating Fetal Heart Rate During Labor
- Procedure 23–3: Vaginal Examination During Labor
- Procedure 23–4: Identifying the Newborn
- Risk Management
- Implications for Research
- Nursing Care Planning Guide: Normal Childbirth

Most pregnancies, labors, and births are normal events. In the United States, major technologic advances have been developed for the treatment and often cure of diseases that adversely affect perinatal outcomes. However, a major focus in maternity care must be the promotion and support of the normal processes, not simply treatment of disease. For support of normal labor and birth, basic knowledge of physiologic and psychological aspects of childbirth must be appreciated. This chapter describes the stages and phases of labor and the application of the nursing process during the intrapartum period. The advantages and disadvantages of procedures commonly prescribed during labor and birth are also discussed. The nurse's role

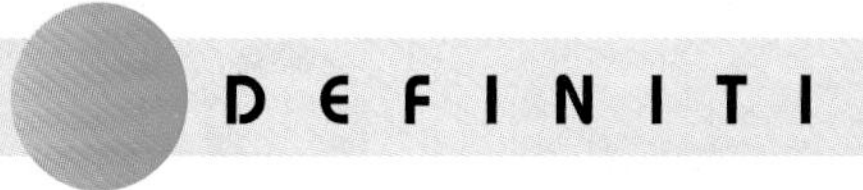

DEFINITIONS

Active phase—The second phase of first-stage labor; dilatation from 4 to 7 cm.

Apgar score—The immediate assessment of the newborn at 1 and 5 minutes after birth; evaluates heart rate, respiratory effort, muscle tone, reflex irritability, and color.

Birth partner—The person (husband, father of baby, mother, family member, friend, or other person) who accompanies the woman during her labor and birth; also called labor companion, coach, or support person.

Birthing room—A single-room concept seen in many hospitals for labor, delivery, and recovery (LDR); in some settings, the room may also be used for the postpartum stay (LDRP).

Bishop score—A system for rating the readiness of the cervix for labor based on the assessment of cervical position, consistency, effacement, dilatation, and fetal station.

Doula—A Greek word referring to an experienced woman who helps other women during childbirth.

Duration—The length of a labor contraction, measured from the beginning to the end of the contraction; recorded in seconds.

Episiotomy—A surgical incision through the perineum made to enlarge the vaginal opening for birth.

False labor—A period of regular or irregular Braxton Hicks contractions that occur toward the end of the pregnancy but do not result in progressive cervical dilatation.

Frequency—Measurement of the interval of labor contractions, from the beginning of one contraction to the beginning of the next; recorded in minutes.

Intensity—Measurement of the strength of a labor contraction at its peak.

Labor—Regular uterine contractions associated with effacement and dilatation of the cervix, resulting in the birth of the baby.

Latent phase—The first phase of first-stage labor; dilatation from 0 to 3 cm.

Spontaneous rupture of membranes (SROM)—The natural breaking of the amniotic sac, either before the onset of labor or during the process of labor.

Transition phase—The third phase of first-stage labor; dilatation from 8 to 10 cm.

throughout the birthing process is to assess the woman's physical status and psychosocial status and the learning needs of the woman and her significant others. The nurse can then provide the care and support needed by the woman and her family to promote a positive labor and birth experience.

THE DIAGNOSIS OF LABOR

Definition of Labor

A major problem exists clinically with the inability to easily diagnose the onset of labor. Labor connotes the beginning of the second phase of parturition (see Chapter 22), when uterotonics are most important and cervical progress is evident in the presence of uterine contractions (Cunningham et al. 1993). The traditional definition of labor, as the period when regular uterine contractions are associated with effacement and dilatation of the cervix, presents many clinical problems. In some facilities, the onset of labor is arbitrarily defined as the time of admission to the birth unit. In other maternity care settings, labor is defined as the time at which a woman's cervix has achieved a dilatation of 3 or 4 cm. Yet other facilities use the woman's self-reporting of the onset of symptoms as the time of onset of labor. Unfortunately, none of these interpretations is entirely adequate, and it remains difficult to obtain an exact time of the onset of labor (Bonovich 1990).

True Versus False Labor

False labor is a common occurrence, particularly although not exclusively among pregnant women. False labor is a period of irregular (but sometimes even regular) contractions that occur without progressive cervical dilatation. The contractions usually do not progress in their frequency, duration, or intensity. These false labor contractions are also known as Braxton Hicks contractions. Although the traditional concept is that these contractions are painless, this is a subjective assessment that is disputed by many women. False labor is frequently associated with contractions that are located more anteriorly in the abdominal area and that decrease with changes in position or activity. Therefore, anticipatory guidance to a pregnant woman should include advice that if she experiences contractions, she should change her activity, obtain adequate nutrition and fluids (in case her contractions progress to become true labor), and observe and record the characteristics of the labor pattern (Varney 1987; Bonovich 1990). A woman in false labor and her support person need education and reassurance. Fatigue and discouragement are common, especially if false labor is lengthy or recurrent. Therapeutic rest may be induced with sedatives. If labor ceases with sedation, false labor may be accurately diagnosed. It is common for women to have periods of false labor, especially during the third trimester. However, because of the risk of preterm labor, women with contractions before term should be assessed immediately to prevent premature birth (Copper et al. 1990; Martin 1990).

In contrast, true labor contractions are rhythmic and regular. The intervals of contractions are constant and decrease in frequency; the duration and intensity increase over time, and they are unchanged by positional or activity changes. True labor contractions are often experienced as first starting in the back and then radiating around to the lower groin area. True labor is usually associated with pelvic pressure, an increase in vaginal discharge, loss of the mucous plug (or "bloody show"), and possibly rupture of membranes. These contractions result in progressive cervical effacement and dilatation. Changes in activity or position do not relieve true labor contractions, and walking may in fact enhance their progression. Table 23–1 compares and contrasts true and false labor.

Preliminary Signs of Labor

▼ **Braxton Hicks Contractions.** Before the beginning of labor, many women find that they experience some prodromal or preliminary signs. These early symptoms could include an increase in Braxton Hicks contractions (the normal contractions of the uterus that occur throughout pregnancy); however, prodromal labor is more frequently associated with subtle signs, such as a low, mild backache.

▼ **Backache.** A low backache could be the result of postural changes by the end of pregnancy or mild early uterine contractions. The backache should be considered suggestive of labor if it seems to come and go at regular intervals, increases in intensity, or is accompanied by feelings of pelvic pressure or cramping.

▼ **Lightening.** The woman may notice that the baby has moved down into the pelvis, an indication that lightening or engagement has occurred. When this occurs, she will notice that breathing is easier and she has less shortness of breath; however, her bladder capacity will be decreased and

Table 23–1

COMPARISON OF THE CHARACTERISTICS OF TRUE AND FALSE LABOR

	FALSE LABOR	TRUE LABOR
Cervical changes	No	Yes
Discomfort	Possible; may range from observation to painful sensations; can be tiring to woman	Generally becomes more uncomfortable as contractions continue; usually is tiring to woman
Location	Often located abdominally	Usually begins in back and radiates to front with fetus in occiput anterior position
Uterine palpation	Uterus is often soft with indentable contractions	Firm uterus when contractions occur
Regularity	Irregular in rhythm and duration	Regular with diminishing interval
Associated events	Often affected by changes in position or activity	Unchanged to any great degree by changes in maternal position or activity; often accompanied by bloody show, bulging of membranes, or rupture of membranes
Response to medications	Often diminishes or stops	May decrease in frequency or intensity somewhat, but contractions will not disappear

she will experience increased urinary frequency. The woman may also notice increased pelvic pressure, vaginal secretions, and leg cramps once lightening has taken place. The shape of the abdomen as the uterus drops forward and a decrease in fundal height measurements also indicate that the baby has dropped.

▼ **Weight Loss.** Weight loss of a few pounds may result from changes in estrogen and progesterone levels, causing electrolyte shifts and the loss of body fluid.

▼ **Diarrhea.** Some women experience a bowel rush and have a mild case of diarrhea, probably associated with prostaglandin release. This may be the body's attempt to empty the bowel before active labor begins.

▼ **Spurt of Energy and Nesting.** Many women describe an unexpected spurt of physical and emotional energy, feeling better than they have in weeks, before labor. This feeling of energy should be ignored and conserved for the work of labor. Some women also experience a nesting instinct, during which they find themselves preparing their home for the newborn with a flurry of activity.

▼ **Bloody Show.** As the cervix ripens and begins to efface, the mucous plug that has sealed the os throughout pregnancy begins to be discharged. This mucous discharge is often termed bloody show because the mucus becomes blood tinged from the rupture of cervical capillaries as the cervix is stretched. Many women notice this discharge before any other preliminary signs of labor have been observed. Bloody show may also be noticed after a routine vaginal examination in the last couple of weeks of pregnancy.

THE PROCESS OF LABOR

Labor has traditionally been divided into three stages that summarize the progress from its onset to its completion. The first and longest stage in the labor process encompasses the period of cervical effacement and dilatation. The second stage involves the period of expulsion of the baby. The third stage is the expulsion of the last of the prod-

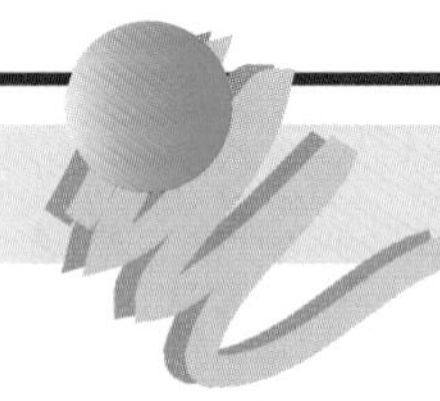

HISTORICAL PERSPECTIVES

EMANUEL FRIEDMAN'S EARLY RESEARCH

Dr. Emanuel Friedman began his descriptive research on labor in the early 1950s and during a period of 20 years defined the phases and length of the stages of labor for nulliparous and multiparous women. His research showed that cervical dilatation and fetal descent follow a predictable pattern and appear as an S curve when plotted on a graph. This kind of graphic analysis of labor is called a partograph and may be used to document events associated with labor relating to labor's progress.

The Friedman curve is the partograph most commonly used in clinical practice in the United States. It provides a basis for decision making about the progress of a woman's labor. The nurse can plot cervical dilatation and fetal descent on the graph, and if labor begins to slow in comparison to the average rate of progress defined by Friedman, the maternal-newborn team can evaluate the data.

Critics of Friedman's descriptions have argued that the childbearing atmosphere of the 1950s with its routine use of medications and forceps and restrictions on ambulation and position changes was markedly different from that of today. It is thought that these differences may have influenced the course of a woman's labor. In addition, Friedman's work revolves around the vague time of initiation of labor. Lacking a single objective parameter, Friedman used the woman's own report of time of onset of labor as the beginning of his division of labor (Friedman 1978). Nevertheless, the work of Friedman and his colleagues is the most universally accepted scientific treatment of labor and is nationally used in eutocia (normal labor) and to diagnose dystocia (abnormal labor) when deviations are apparent.

ucts of conception, the placenta. More recently, a fourth stage of labor has been suggested. Although not commonly found in research studies, the fourth stage of labor encompasses the first hour after birth. This is the time when interactions among members of the new family are important for psychological reasons, and it is also the time frame during which the nurse carefully monitors mother and child for stabilization after the physiologic experience of birth.

The first stage of labor can be further subdivided into three divisions—the preparatory, dilatational, and pelvic divisions. This classification is most often used by nurse-midwives and physicians to describe the progress of the first stage of labor. Labor may also be divided into three phases—the latent, active, and transition phases. This classification is commonly used by nurses in their clinical practice and by childbirth educators to describe the process of labor to expectant parents. Table 23–2 contrasts these two means of classifying the first stage of labor. The length of the total labor process can range from just a few hours to as long as 24 hours. Table 23–3 describes the average length of each phase or stage of labor, cervical status, the characteristics of uterine contractions, a woman's physical and emotional responses, coping strategies, and the nurse's role. The times given for the average length of each phase of labor are based on the research that was done by Dr. Emanuel Friedman (see Historical Perspectives).

The First Stage of Labor

EARLY-PHASE LABOR

Description

The early or latent phase of the first stage of labor begins with the onset of uterine contractions. It is the longest of the three phases, varying considerably in length from less than an hour to many hours.

Some women do not recognize latent labor because the symptoms can be subtle (Bonovich 1990). Contractions of early-phase labor may feel much like the Braxton Hicks contractions that the woman has experienced in late pregnancy, like an intermittent backache, or like menstrual cramps. The contractions are relatively mild and do not

Table 23–2

COMPARISON OF STAGES, DIVISIONS, AND PHASES OF LABOR

STAGES	DIVISIONS	PHASES
First stage • Onset of labor until full dilatation	Preparatory division • Shortening of cervix secondary to changes in cervical collagen and connective tissue; with or without contractions	Latent phase • Period of contractions accompanying softening and effacement
	Dilatational division • Period wherein dilatation proceeds at its most rapid rate	Active phase • Period of acceleration phase, phase of maximal slope, and deceleration phase
	Pelvic division • Usually combined with dilatational division, commences with deceleration phase	Transition phase • Final period of first stage, moving into second stage
Second stage • Full dilatation until birth of child		
Third stage • Birth of child until expulsion of placenta		
Fourth stage • Immediate postpartum period, often defined as approximately 1 hr		

Table 23–3

CHARACTERISTICS OF THE PROCESS OF LABOR

Early (Latent) Phase of First-Stage Labor		
Duration	Average:	Nullipara: 6.4 hr (Friedman, 1978) Multipara: 4.8 hr (Friedman, 1978)
	Range:	<1 hr to many hours
Cervical examination	Dilatation:	0–3 cm
	Effacement:	Varies from uneffaced to 100% effacement
	Position:	Cervix is often posterior, with movement anteriorly as latent labor progresses
	Consistency:	Progressively softens (ripens) as latent labor progresses
	Fetal station:	Usually between −3 and 0 station
	Membranes:	More often remain intact until the active phase
Uterine contractions	Frequency:	Ranges from every 20 min at the beginning of latent labor to every 5–7 min as active labor approaches
	Duration:	15–40 sec
	Intensity:	Mild to moderate (20–40 mm Hg)
Emotions	Elation that labor has begun Relief that pregnancy is at an end Anticipation mixed with doubts and apprehension about labor Discouragement if latent labor is lengthy	
Physical sensations	Thirst, anorexia, nausea, vomiting, diarrhea Uterine contractions usually become more frequent and intense as latent labor progresses; felt in the abdomen as a menstrual cramping sensation and lower back Fetal descent may cause pressure on bladder, creating urge to urinate Fatigue if latent labor is prolonged	
Coping strategies	Ambulation combined with short rests Sleep if fatigued Maintain hydration by drinking at least 250 mL/hr Eat high-carbohydrate, low-fat meals or snacks Frequent urination Practice relaxation and breathing techniques during contractions Warm showers or baths (avoid baths if membranes are ruptured) for pain relief Diversion or entertainment (cards, TV, reading)	
Nurse's role	Make the woman and her family feel welcome and comfortable Use strategies to decrease apprehension Establish a positive relationship Orient the woman and her support persons to the birth environment Assess the client's emotional and physical status Assess progress of labor and fetal status Report findings to the physician or midwife Advise the client on coping strategies whether the client is at home, in the hospital, or at the birth center Review instructions about when to return to the birth site if the client is at home Review the woman's birth plan and develop a collaborative plan of care Teach the client and significant others about the progress of the labor and the fetal status, the normalcy of the physical and emotional changes, and what to expect as labor progresses Facilitate and support use of diversional activities Encourage ambulation if possible	

Table 23–3

CHARACTERISTICS OF THE PROCESS OF LABOR Continued

Active Phase of First-Stage Labor		
Duration	Average:	Nullipara: 4.6 hr Multipara: 2.4 hr
	Range:	Nullipara: 4–6 hr Multipara: 2–3 hr
Cervical examination	Dilatation:	3–7 or 8 cm
	Effacement:	Generally complete effacement is reached during the active phase of labor
	Position:	Anterior
	Consistency:	Soft
	Fetal station:	Usually between −2 and 0 station
	Membranes:	Often remain intact but may spontaneously rupture at any time during the active phase
Uterine contractions	Frequency:	Every 2–5 min
	Duration:	40–60 sec
	Intensity:	Moderate to firm (≥50 mm Hg)
Emotions	Apprehension as contractions become stronger and more frequent Vague fears; concern for self and baby Anxiety about being left alone More serious and introverted Focused on breathing and relaxation	
Physical sensations	Thirst, nausea, vomiting, urinary urgency and frequency Contractions feel more intense and are now painful Pain may radiate from lower abdomen and back to legs Suprapubic or sacral pressure if the fetal presenting part is at or below 0 station Warm, perspiring Facial (malar) flush Fatigue, drowsiness	
Coping strategies	Significant others' attentiveness to the laboring woman's emotional and physical needs Frequent position changes Ambulation Frequent fluids if tolerated Attempt to empty bladder frequently Effleurage, back and leg massage Warm showers, soaks in warm bath if membranes are still intact Hot packs, cold packs Breathing and relaxation techniques Attention-focusing strategies—visualization, music, focal point Mental activity—counting, word repetition, guided imagery Analgesic and anesthetic pain relief if desired	
Nurse's role	Assess the client's emotional and physical status Assess progress of labor and fetal status Report findings to the physician or midwife as appropriate Obtain blood samples as indicated for laboratory analysis Promote coping strategies Do not leave the woman unattended; ensure that the woman has a support person or care provider present if possible Facilitate position changes Promote calm, attentive support for the laboring woman and her significant others Give frequent encouragement, feedback, and praise Facilitate involvement of labor support persons	

Continued on following page

Table 23–3

CHARACTERISTICS OF THE PROCESS OF LABOR Continued

Active Phase of First-Stage Labor *(cont'd)*		
	Keep the client and her support persons informed of labor progress, fetal status, and what to expect as labor progresses Give reassurance of the normalcy of events Provide intravenous hydration if oral fluids are not adequate or tolerated (depending on institutional policy, may need consultation first) Administer analgesics if the client desires (inform of options, benefits and risks) Support the client during administration of anesthesia	
Transition Phase of First-Stage Labor		
Duration	Average:	Nullipara: 1–2 hr Multipara: 30 min–1 hr
	Range:	15 min–2 hr
Cervical examination	Dilatation:	7 or 8–10 cm
	Effacement:	100%
	Position:	Anterior
	Consistency:	Soft
	Fetal station:	Usually at or below 0 station
	Membranes:	Often spontaneously rupture in this phase if they have not previously
Uterine contractions	Frequency:	Every 1–5 min
	Duration:	60–90 sec
	Intensity:	Firm to intense (≥75 mm Hg); multiple peaks
Emotions	Irritability Rejection of support persons Feelings of being out of control, overwhelmed Desire to quit, give up Fearful of being left alone Fearful of the severity of the contractions	
Physical sensations	Continual pain and rectal pressure Thirst, nausea, vomiting Perspiration on upper lip or brow Natural fatigue-induced sleep between contractions (in absence of pharmacologic sedation) Shaking, trembling legs Increased tenderness over abdomen; sensitivity to touch Leg cramps Belching or burping Involuntary urge to bear down Passage of stool Increase in bloody show	
Coping strategies	Same as coping strategies for active phase Cool cloths for face and neck Dorsiflex ankles and change position to relieve leg cramps Sitting on toilet may seem to be a natural position as she progresses through transition and into the second stage	

Table 23–3

CHARACTERISTICS OF THE PROCESS OF LABOR Continued

Transition Phase of First-Stage Labor *(cont'd)*		
Nurse's role	Same as nurse's role for active phase Firm, directive coaching of relaxation and breathing strategies; establish eye contact; breathe with the woman during the contraction Encourage the woman to deal with one contraction at a time Support and encourage significant others Avoid analgesic and anesthetic pain relief if the birth is expected soon (narcotic analgesics may suppress the infant's respirations) Anesthesia, such as an epidural block, may require too much time for placement if the birth is anticipated promptly	
Second-Stage Labor		
Duration	Average:	Nullipara: 1 hr Multipara: 40 min
	Range:	Nullipara: 1–3 hr Multipara: 30 min–1 hr
Cervical examination	Dilatation:	Complete (10 cm)
	Effacement:	Complete (100%)
	Fetal station:	Usually 0 station or lower for primiparas; −1 or slightly higher for multiparas, especially if the membranes are intact
	Membranes:	May be intact or ruptured
Uterine contractions	Frequency:	Varies, usually between 2 and 10 min apart
	Duration:	Varies, usually between 30 and 60 sec
	Intensity:	Moderate to firm (50 mm Hg)
Emotions	Satisfaction and relief at progress of labor Increased sense of control Fearful if pushing is painful or if unprepared Fatigue, exhaustion Excitement that birth is imminent	
Physical sensations	Urge to push (moderate to strong) May feel no urge to push Lull in contractions for even as long as an hour, which provides a chance to rest and mobilize energy Urge to move bowels; rectal pressure; passage of stool Increase in bloody show Warm, perspiring May emphatically state that "the baby is coming" Backache Burning sensation with crowning	
Coping strategies	Continue coping strategies used in first-stage labor Assume positions for pushing that are most comfortable, use gravity, and facilitate descent Drink fluids if tolerated and indicated Active involvement of support persons as in the first stage Use of mirror for observation of progress of pushing and to view birth may be helpful Visualize baby descending and perineal muscles stretching open Touch infant's head as it crowns	

Continued on following page

Table 23–3

CHARACTERISTICS OF THE PROCESS OF LABOR Continued

	Second-Stage Labor *(cont'd)*
Nurse's role	Continue role as described in first-stage labor Suggest alternative positions for pushing as needed Give directive verbal directions for pushing Provide positive feedback and praise Involve support persons in assisting the woman to push in various positions Provide mirror if desired Prepare birth setup for the physician or midwife Prepare infant resuscitation equipment Prepare warm blankets for the infant and mother Maintain awareness of progression of pushing at all times Ensure that the laboring woman is not left alone Notify the pediatrician or neonatologist when birth is imminent if pediatric assistance is needed
	Third- and Fourth-Stage Labor
Duration	Third stage: 5–20 min Fourth stage: 1 hr
Uterine contractions	Frequency: Intermittent Intensity: Mild to moderate cramping
Emotions	Elation, relief, joy Withdrawal, disinterest, numbness Curiosity about the baby and procedures Desire to hold and breastfeed the infant Fear of pain associated with perineal repair or fundal massage Surprise at intensity of uterine cramping after placenta is expelled
Physical sensations	Shivering (due to sudden decrease in intra-abdominal pressure or being cold) Uterine cramping (can be mild, moderate, or intense) Thirst, hunger Fatigue, drowsiness Pain associated with perineal injury Muscle aches in upper body or legs associated with pushing efforts in second-stage labor Sore throat from vocalizations during labor Increased physical energy
Coping strategies	Use relaxation and breathing strategies during periods of discomfort Inform the partner or caregiver of needs Sleep Hold and nurse the baby if desired Share feelings with significant others
Nurse's role	Provide immediate assessment and care of the newborn Document time and method of placental delivery Provide for maternal comfort Administer medication as ordered Promote parent-infant interaction Assess maternal involutional process

usually interfere with the woman's activity. These contractions accomplish the effacement and early dilatation of the cervix (Fig. 23–1).

The latent phase is often a time of excitement and anticipation of the events that lie ahead (Fig. 23–2). The woman may be talkative and enthusiastic. She and her partner should be encouraged to remain at home as long as possible in latent labor, because relaxation and mobility are more easily accomplished there. This period of labor is often used to make last-minute arrangements for children, pets, or the household and to get ready for going to the hospital or birthing center. If latent-phase labor occurs during the night, parents should be instructed to remain in bed and rest or sleep. If spontaneous rupture of the membranes occurs, the woman may be asked to go to the hospital or birthing center to be examined to rule out an umbilical cord prolapse (see Chapter 25).

Unlike false labor, true latent labor is distinguished by the occurrence of cervical changes. As previously discussed, false labor contractions may

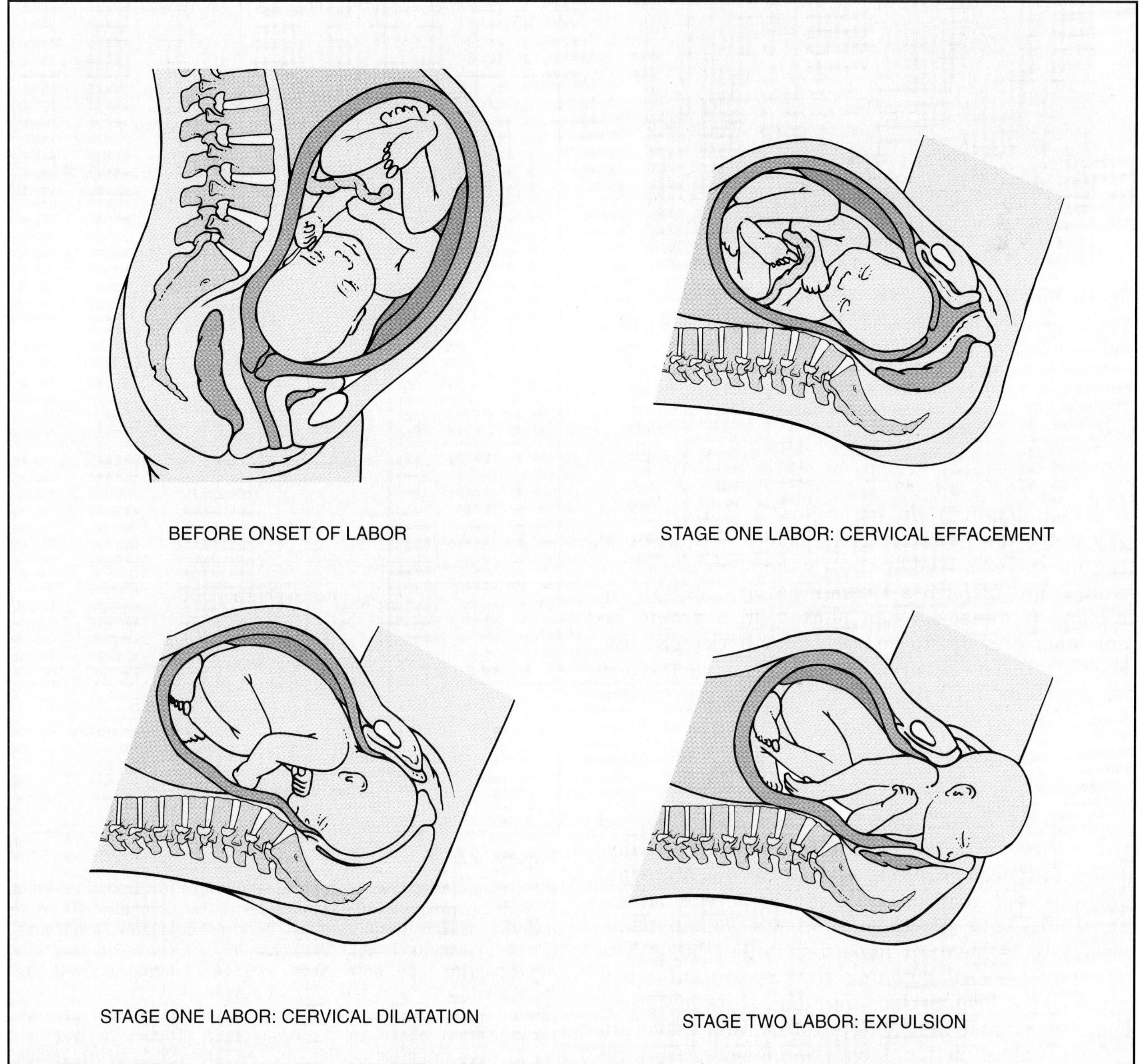

Figure 23–1

The cervix changes throughout first-stage labor and the descent and birth of the baby in second-stage labor • Before the onset of labor the cervix is long, thick, and closed with no effacement and dilatation • Much of the effacement of the cervix takes place in the early or latent phase of labor • Dilatation of the cervix takes place throughout the first stage of labor • Expulsion occurs in the second stage of labor after the cervix is completely dilated, and is accomplished with the woman's pushing effort during contractions.

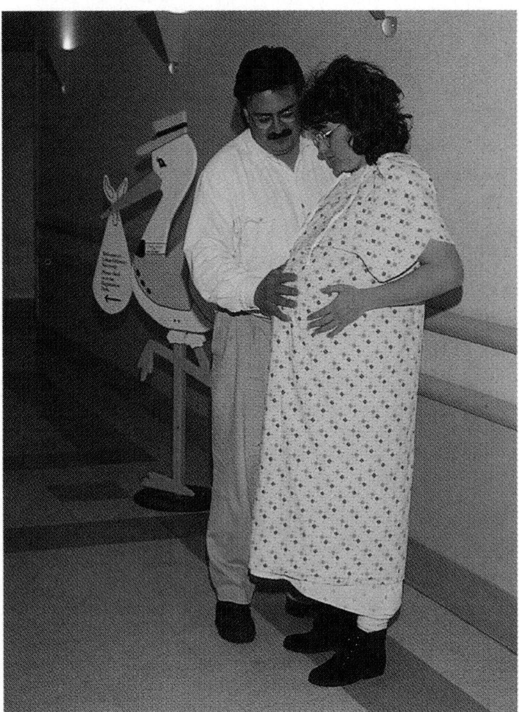

Figure 23–2

Women should be encouraged to stay at home in early labor until contractions are regular at 5-minute intervals, or until membranes rupture • Once the woman is in the hospital, ambulation is often encouraged if membranes are intact • Walking can promote comfort and facilitate the progress of labor.

be irregular, often do not follow a pattern, and may cease for hours or days before the onset of true labor. Latent labor contractions, on the other hand, begin to form a regular pattern and an increasing frequency. When plotted on a graph, latent labor appears to be an almost horizontal line (Fig. 23–3). The S curve described by Friedman is not apparent until the active phase begins (Friedman 1978).

Influences

The progress of latent labor may be influenced by a variety of factors, including the degree of maternal fatigue, hydration, and nutrition. Maternal emotions and attitudes about labor as well as the availability and effectiveness of the woman's support systems have an impact on latent labor. The extent of cervical ripening that is present when latent labor begins also influences its progress. The cervix must first soften, efface, and move anteriorly before active labor commences. A nulliparous cervix usually effaces completely before active labor begins. A multiparous cervix effaces as dilatation occurs, throughout the first stage. Finally, sedation and regional anesthesia may slow or even halt labor if given during this latent phase.

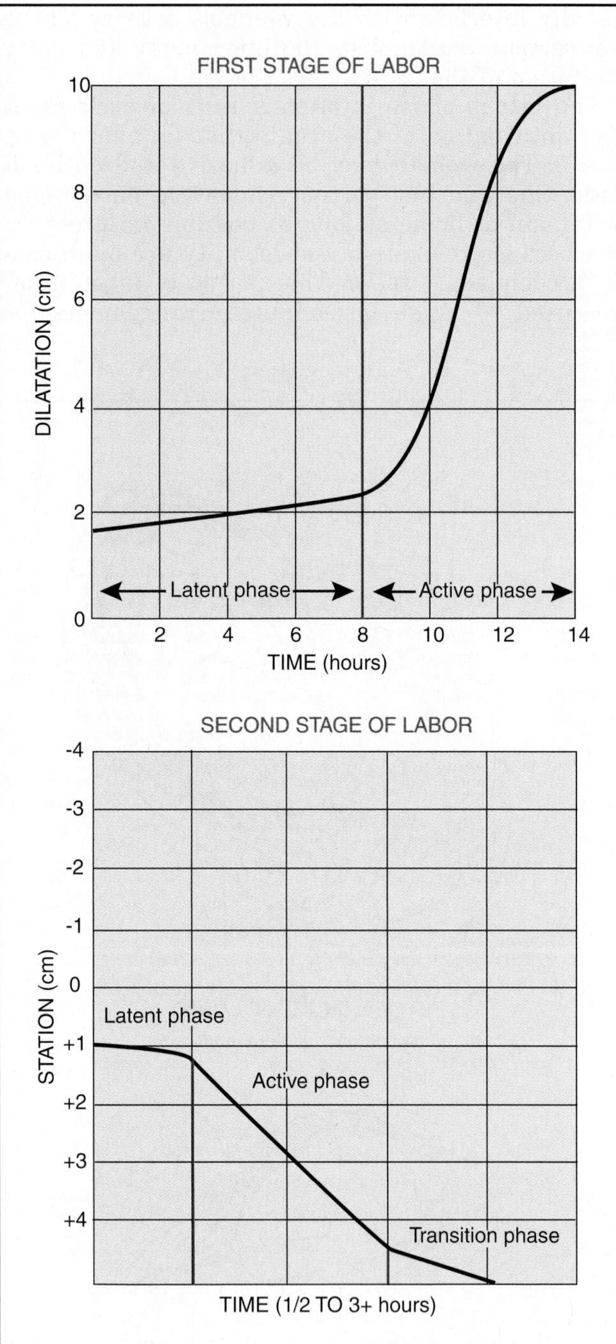

Figure 23–3

First-stage labor curve. This classic illustration from Friedman shows the progress of normal labor as a sigmoid ("S") curve pattern plotted from data on cervical dilatation over time. (From Friedman, E. A. (1978). *Labor: Clinical evaluation and management* (2nd ed.). New York: Appleton-Century-Crofts. Reprinted with permission from Appleton & Lange, Inc.) • Second-stage labor curve: a graph charting normal progress through three phases in the second stage of labor has more recently been proposed by Simkin. The fetal descent through the pelvis is shown as a downward curve when station is plotted over time on the graph. (From Simkin, P., Whalley, J., Keppler, A. (1991). *Pregnancy, childbirth, and the newborn.* Deephaven, MN: Meadowbrook Press. Used with permission from the Childbirth Education Association of Seattle and Meadowbrook Press, Inc.)

ACTIVE-PHASE LABOR

Description

The active phase of the first stage of labor, as defined by Friedman (1978), occurs during the dilatational division and begins when a rate of cervical dilatation of at least 1.2 cm per hour for nulliparas and 1.5 cm per hour for multiparas is achieved. It is completed when the cervix is fully dilated (see Table 23–2). Friedman further subdivided active labor into three phases: the acceleration phase (4 to 5 cm), the phase of maximal slope (5 to 9 cm), and the deceleration phase (9 to 10 cm) (see Fig. 23–3). The most rapid progress in cervical dilatation occurs during the phase of maximal slope. The descent of the fetus in the maternal pelvis has a direct relationship to the dilatation of the cervix (see Fig. 23–1). Descent initially progresses at a slower rate and then occurs more rapidly in a pattern similar to cervical dilatation. Both dilatation and descent should be plotted simultaneously on a labor graph to completely assess the progress of labor. As with dilatation, descent occurs more rapidly for a multipara than for a nullipara.

Contractions in the active phase of labor become intense, frequent, and regular. The woman may experience additional physical symptoms that add to the discomfort of this phase. It is often at this time that she begins to make the decision as to how she will cope with her labor; that is, whether she will fight against the process, decrease her participation through the use of medications or anesthetics, or cooperate and work with the forces of labor. Coping strategies such as relaxation and breathing techniques can be helpful in any of these situations (see Table 23–3). The woman may become increasingly apprehensive as the reality of the work of labor is recognized and she realizes that she cannot influence the frequency or duration of the contractions. She may begin to doubt her ability to accomplish the task ahead. As a result, women in active labor become quiet, introverted, serious, and self-focused. The companionship, support, and coaching of a partner or family member becomes increasingly important (Chapman 1992) (Fig. 23–4).

Influences

In comparison with latent labor, active labor is not as likely to be inhibited by analgesia or anesthesia. In fact, apprehension and pain may increase circulating catecholamines, which may decrease the effectiveness of contractions. When pain is relieved, the subsequent decrease in fear may promote the efficiency of the contractions. Pain relief is not limited to pharmaceutical measures, however. Emotional and physical support provided by significant others and care providers and nonpharmacologic pain relief modalities can also interrupt the effects of pain and fear on effective uterine function. A discussion of nonpharmacologic pain relief measures can be found in Chapter 24.

TRANSITION-PHASE LABOR

Description

Although not described in Friedman's work or other scientific research on phases of labor, transition is commonly accepted as part of labor from a clinical perspective. It corresponds to both Friedman's deceleration phase of active labor and the point at which fetal descent occurs. However, rather than using cervical dilatation as a criterion

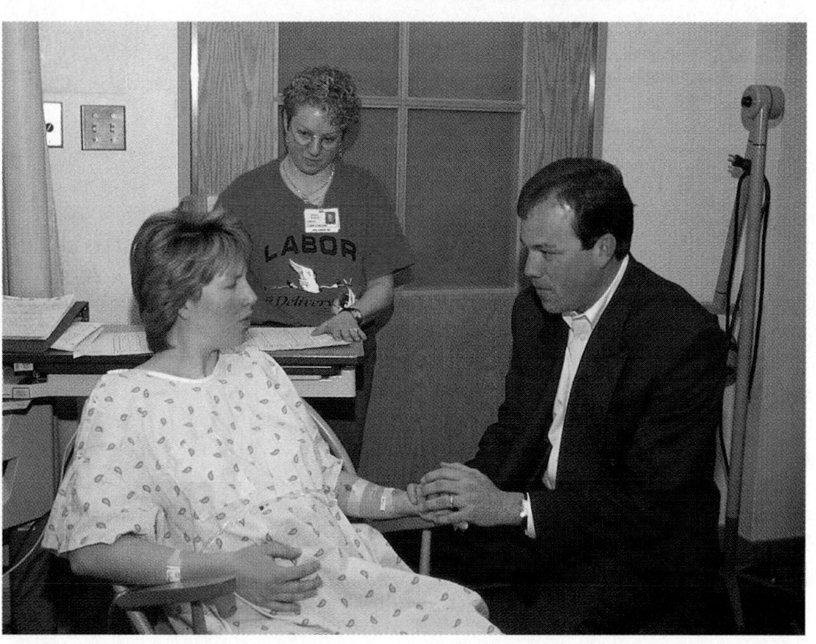

Figure 23–4

Once the woman is in active first-stage labor, she usually needs to begin to use relaxation and breathing techniques to cope with the contractions • She may feel more comfortable sitting up in a chair during some of her labor • A rocking chair allows her to move back and forth, providing distraction and comfort, even when the IV and fetal monitor are attached.

for entry into transition, the transitional point in labor is primarily based on recognition of behavioral signs that are manifested when the woman's labor is moving from first to second stage, hence the term transition. For some rapid labors, this point may occur when the cervix is only 3 or 4 cm dilated; for most labors, the signs of transition begin at approximately 7 or 8 cm of dilatation. In most cases, transition lasts less than an hour but tends to be the most intense part of the labor process. The contractions become close, last longer, and are intense. They may have multiple peaks, and the woman may feel that her pain is continuous. The descent of the fetal presenting part accounts for the signs and symptoms of rectal pressure and a beginning urge to bear down. There may be an increase in bloody show. The membranes may rupture spontaneously during a contraction if they have not ruptured spontaneously or artificially before this time. Additional physical symptoms also add to the woman's discomfort at this time (see Table 23–3). The woman often becomes irritable, is impatient with the labor process, and may panic and feel she can no longer cope. Medication or anesthesia may be requested at this time. The firm, directive support and coaching of the partner and nurse are now essential.

Influences

The final phase of first-stage labor can be affected by several factors. Maternal anxiety, positioning, analgesia, or regional anesthesia could affect the length of transition.

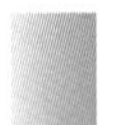

The Second Stage of Labor

Description

The second stage of labor is said to begin when the cervix is completely dilated (10 cm) and ends with the birth of the baby (see Figs. 23–1 and 23–5). Friedman described an average second-stage duration for a nullipara as 1 hour, with the upper limit of normal being 3 hours. Multiparas generally have a shorter second stage, with 40 minutes as the average duration and 1 hour being the upper limit of normal. Many women feel a premature urge to push when they are 8 or 9 cm dilated, especially if the fetal head is at a +1 station. Women who have this premature urge to push often become fully dilated rapidly. Women who do not have an urge but are encouraged to push with an incompletely dilated cervix may actually prolong labor by causing edema of the cervix.

The second stage of labor can be divided into the same three phases as the first stage (see Fig. 23–3). The latent phase begins when the cervix is completely dilated and may last only a few minutes or as long as a half-hour. During this time, there is often a lull in uterine activity and no urge to push. This peaceful interlude preceding the exertion of pushing is thought to be a normal restful interlude, allowing the woman to gain strength and providing the fetus with increased oxygenation. This lull often occurs when the fetal head has not descended enough to distend the pelvic floor and trigger stretch receptors to influence the release of endogenous oxytocin (Anderhold and Roberts 1991; Cosner and deJong 1993; Simkin et al. 1991). When this does occur, a woman feels the urge to push and often comments that it feels as if the baby is pushing on its own.

The active phase of second-stage labor begins when the uterus resumes contracting. It is characterized by increasing vaginal and rectal pressure and an accompanying urge to push. As the woman pushes with contractions, she contracts abdominal muscles to assist the work of the uterus. This increases intra-abdominal pressure and forces the descent of the fetus. The contractions in the second stage of labor often decrease in frequency, shorten in duration, and actually decrease in intensity. Some women state that it "feels good" to push with these contractions, while others find pushing to be uncomfortable (Fig. 23–5). The urge to push is described by many women as being an overwhelming internal force. Although this stage of labor is hard work, many women find renewed energy and excitement in the thought that the birth of their baby is near. This is the period when rapid descent of the fetus usually takes place, resulting in dilatation of the vagina and bulging of the perineum by the presenting part.

The transition phase of second-stage labor occurs as more of the presenting part becomes visible at the pelvic floor and the distention of the tissue causes sensations of extreme stretching and burning in the perineum. If the woman has not been prepared for these sensations, she may be frightened; however, the woman who has had childbirth education will know that these feelings are to be expected and that the pelvic floor muscles have the capability to stretch to allow the birth of the baby. As the fetus reaches the pelvic floor, the perineum begins to bulge outward, the labia separate, and the crown of the fetal head can gradually be seen (Fig. 23–5). After each contraction, the fetal head recedes somewhat until the next contraction, when it will bulge a little farther. As the head descends, the pelvic floor becomes thin and shiny and the anus protrudes. If an episiotomy is necessary, it is done at this time. Episiotomy is discussed in Chapter 25. The physician or nurse-midwife supports the head as it extends and is gradually delivered to control the speed of the delivery and to protect the head and the maternal soft tissues. Delivery of the head is

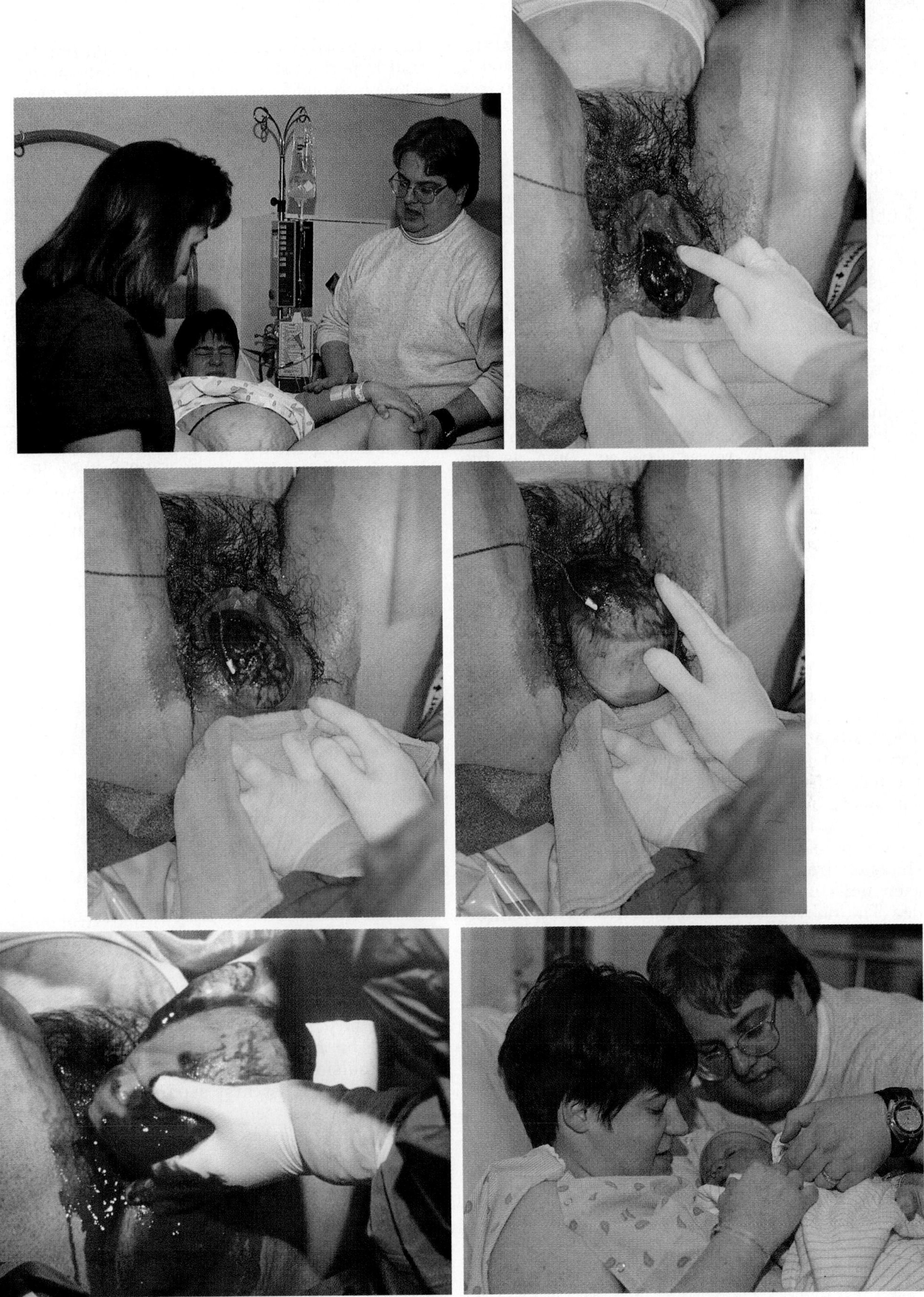

Figure 23–5
Birth sequence shows six views from a normal vaginal delivery.

accomplished best if it occurs between contractions. The woman is asked to blow as the head is delivered, rather than push. This helps facilitate a slow, gentle delivery of the head. After the head is born, the birth attendant palpates around the neck to determine whether the cord is present (nuchal cord). If so, it is slipped over the head; if the cord is too tight around the neck, it must be double-clamped and cut at this time. With the birth of the head and shoulders, the woman experiences a sudden sense of release and a decrease in discomfort.

Figure 23–5 is composed of six photographs taken during a normal vaginal delivery. This birth sequence begins with the mother pushing with a contraction while the father and nurse are actively coaching. As the baby is pushed down the vaginal passageway, the head gradually becomes visible at the vaginal introitus. The physician uses her finger to help retract the perineum as the head descends. As the head begins to crown, the physician uses her hands to support the perineum. The internal fetal scalp electrode is seen still attached to the baby's head. As the birth of the head becomes imminent, the physician places her hands against the mother's anus and applies pressure against the baby's chin to facilitate extension of the head. This is called the Ritgen maneuver.

Once the fetal head is born, it realigns with the body (restitution), and then the entire baby rotates for the birth of the shoulders (Fig. 23–5). The birth attendant supports the head until this occurs and begins to remove the secretions from the baby's face with gauze sponges and to suction the mouth and nose with a bulb syringe. After external rotation has occurred, the birth attendant gently pulls downward to deliver the anterior shoulder from under the symphysis pubis and then pulls upward to deliver the posterior shoulder. The baby's body is then delivered by pulling with gentle traction as the birth attendant carefully supports the body and grabs the feet as they are born. The time of the birth is recorded as the time when the entire body is born. The newborn is placed on the mother's abdomen, where he or she is quickly dried and the Apgar scores are calculated at 1 and 5 minutes. The immediate assessment of the newborn is discussed later in this chapter. Suctioning continues until respirations are established and the baby begins to cry. The cord is usually double-clamped and cut at this time. In many birth settings, the woman's birth partner is given the option of cutting the cord. Controversy exists regarding the best time to clamp and cut the umbilical cord. Some birth attendants believe it is advantageous to delay cutting the cord to allow the transfer of additional placental blood to the newborn's circulation to decrease the occurrence of iron deficiency anemia. However, other practitioners believe that the additional blood volume contributes to polycythemia and hyperbilirubinemia (Cunningham et al. 1993). The physiologic mechanisms (cardinal movements) of this birth process are described in Chapter 22.

After the birth, the parents' first interaction with their newborn is a moment that will always be remembered.

Influences

The duration of the second stage of labor is influenced by many factors. These factors may be organized into five categories: the powers, the passenger, the pelvis, the maternal position, and the psyche, which have been described in Chapter 22. Analgesia and anesthesia may affect a woman's ability to push. If narcotics are given late in the first stage, or if several doses have been administered during the course of labor, a woman may be sleepy and unable to push effectively. Epidural anesthesia may interfere with a woman's urge to push because the sensations of the fetal head on the perineum are blocked. Depending on the strength and type of medication used for an epidural, a woman's ability to move into positions that facilitate descent of the fetus may be limited. The positions used for pushing and the type of breathing used for pushing (i.e., prolonged breath holding versus controlled exhalation) can also influence its effectiveness, as discussed in Chapters 20 and 22. Fear may also influence expulsion. If the woman is frightened of the actual delivery of the baby or the pain she anticipates, she may be reluctant to push. Finally, maternal psychological readiness for birth has been proposed as another factor that can influence the course of the second stage of labor (McKay and Barrows 1991).

The Third Stage of Labor

Description

The third stage of labor begins immediately after the birth of the infant and is completed with the expulsion of the placenta. Before expulsion, the placenta must first separate from the wall of the uterus. This separation is facilitated by a decrease in the surface area of the uterus where the placenta is attached. This decrease in surface area occurs with the birth of the baby. The surface area of the placenta itself is not decreased, and this disparity causes the placenta to weaken its attachment and then separate (Varney 1987). Separation of the placenta takes place in the center first, followed by the peripheral areas. As the placenta separates, a hematoma begins to form at the site of the uterine blood vessels, and the uterus contracts to ligate these uterine vessels. This hematoma facilitates the process of placental separation by adding additional pressure between the uterine wall and the placenta, forcing it to pull away. The fetal membranes are the last portion of the placenta to separate, peeling off the uterine wall as the placenta is delivered. Signs of placental separation are a lengthening of the umbilical cord, a sudden gush of blood, an increase in the level of the uterine fundus, and a change in the shape of the uterus from discoid to globular. In one study, the average duration of third-stage labor was reported to be approximately 7 minutes for both nulliparas and multiparas (Combs and Laros 1991).

The placenta is usually expelled spontaneously, especially if the woman is in an upright position. The birth attendant may place gentle traction on the cord to guide the delivery of the placenta. The woman may be asked to push or bear down at this time (Fig. 23–6). This effort may cause mild discomfort. The placenta is more commonly expelled with the fetal side presenting first. This is called a Schultze presentation. The fetal aspect of the membranes has a glistening appearance. When the placenta is expelled with the uterine side of the membranes exposed, it is termed a Duncan presentation. The uterine side of the membranes has a dark, irregular appearance. These two types of expulsion appear to have little clinical significance. The placenta and membranes are assessed for configuration, completeness, and abnormalities. The umbilical cord should contain two arteries and one vein. Blood samples from the umbilical cord arteries or vein may be drawn promptly after delivery of the placenta and sent for blood gas analysis. The results are one indicator of the infant's condition at birth. An umbilical cord blood sample may be obtained for a Coombs test.

After the delivery of the placenta, the physician or nurse-midwife examines the cervix, vaginal tract, and perineum for lacerations. These are most likely to occur as a result of rapid delivery, malpresentation of the fetus, use of perineal anesthesia, or use of forceps. Lacerations are classified as being of first, second, third, or fourth degree, depending on the tissue involved (see Chapter 25); if present, they are sutured. Other lacerations that can result from a difficult delivery include periurethral tears near the urethral meatus and periclitoral tears near the clitoris. If lacerations are not identified and repaired, profuse bleeding can result.

The contractions of the third stage of labor are of mild or moderate intensity. They most often feel like strong menstrual cramps and are usually overlooked by the woman in her interest in seeing her baby. Some women experience a generalized shivering response during this stage that is thought to be caused by a sudden decrease in intra-abdominal pressure. A range of other physical symptoms may also be experienced.

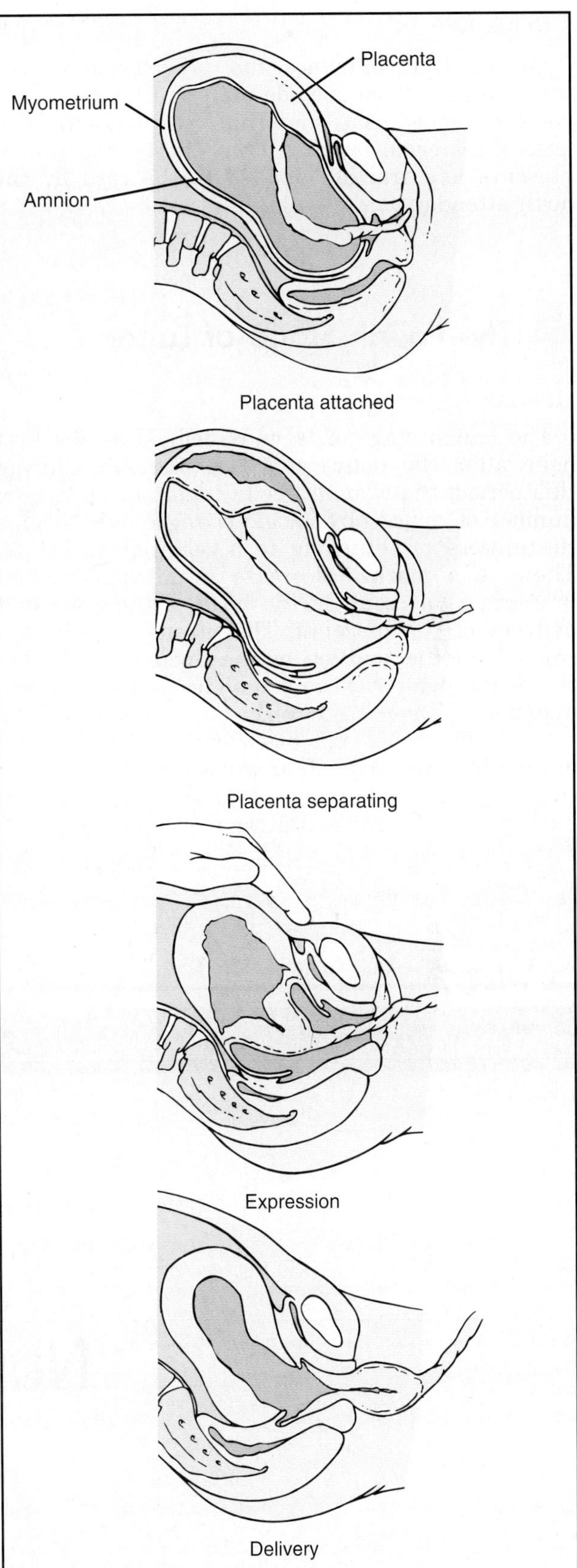

Figure 23–6
Delivery of the placenta.

Influences

Factors that influence the progression of the third stage of labor include maternal fatigue, analgesia or anesthesia, maternal position, effectiveness of maternal bearing down efforts, and fundal pressure and traction applied to the cord by the birth attendant.

The Fourth Stage of Labor

Description

The fourth stage of labor is defined as the first hour after the delivery of the placenta. During this period, the woman's body begins to undergo a number of major physiologic changes as it begins the process of returning to a nonpregnant state. There is a marked decrease in intra-abdominal pressure as a result of the birth of the baby and delivery of the placenta. The uterus is well contracted, in the midline of the abdomen, and between the symphysis and umbilicus. Major hemodynamic changes take place as a result of the normal 250 to 500 mL blood loss at delivery and decreased intra-abdominal pressure. This usually results in a slight drop in blood pressure and moderate tachycardia. Maternal postpartum hemorrhage is the most common complication of the fourth stage of labor; therefore, accurate assessment of excessive bleeding is critical. The woman may initially experience difficulty in urinating because of bladder hypotension from the trauma of birth, so it is important to monitor elimination to prevent urinary retention.

Most women feel only mild discomfort during the fourth stage of labor. In addition to uterine cramping, some women continue to experience the generalized shivering described earlier in the third stage of labor. Women may also feel fatigue, muscle aches, or hunger and thirst. Emotional reactions vary from overwhelming joy and relief to temporary disbelief and withdrawal. The nurse must consider all of these physical and emotional factors as she focuses on monitoring the physical status of the woman and newborn, promotes maternal comfort, provides appropriate education and support, and facilitates bonding of the new family.

Influences

Factors that might influence the fourth stage of labor include immediate complications that might arise (e.g., hemorrhage), the need for repair of lacerations or of the episiotomy, maternal fatigue, maternal analgesia and anesthesia, the condition of the newborn, and the presence and effectiveness of support systems.

Nursing Practice

Nursing Process

The nurse has major responsibilities and accountability during the labor and birth process and in the immediate period after birth. Clinical management depends on an understanding of the normal physiologic and emotional responses in labor and birth, appreciation of and watchfulness for signs of variations and deviations from normal, and individualization so that the experience can be one that is both safe and satisfying for the childbearing family. Using the nursing process helps the nurse formulate a care plan that promotes a positive labor and delivery experience. Beginning at the end of this chapter on page 790, Nursing Care Planning Guide: Normal Childbirth shows how nursing process is applied in creating a plan of care designed to meet an individual's needs.

▼ Assessment

Accurate assessment and nursing diagnosis during the entire process of labor, birth, and recovery are vitally important to ensure the safety of the mother and fetus, plan accurately for the course of labor and birth, and promote a rewarding experience for the entire birthing family. The nurse's management of the process of labor is based on observation and promotion of health. In most hospitals in the United States, the registered nurse is directly responsible for the initial evaluation of a woman who presents at term in labor. The exceptions are larger institutions, which may have obstetric residents or nurse-midwives staffing their triage or emergency department areas. Therefore, although the nurse consults with the birth attendant regarding the management plan, this plan is often based directly on the nurse's assessments. Assessment is an ongoing process from the time of admission to the birth setting until after the baby is born. Knowledge of normal and abnormal physical examination findings is essential for the nurse to provide safe care and recognize deviations from normal. The assessment skills of observation, palpation, and auscultation are used. The following section describes all the assessments used throughout the labor and birth process. The nurse uses assessment tools such as the Obstetric Evaluation Record (p. 791), the Obstetric Admission Record (p. 792), the Labor Flowsheet (p. 794), and the Labor and Delivery Summary (p. 795) to gather and record data essential to the provision of care during labor and birth.

▼ CURRENT LABOR HISTORY

Contractions. Information needs to be obtained about uterine contractions, status of the mucous plug, and membranes (see Questions to Ask About Current Labor). It is important to identify how long the woman has been experiencing contractions, the frequency and duration of the contractions, her perception of the strength of the contractions, and her level of discomfort. The nurse should spend some time with the woman to assess the contractions. By sitting with the woman and placing her hand on the fundus of the uterus, the nurse can quickly determine the characteristics of the contraction pattern and add current information to the woman's report of her contractions.

Skill at recognizing false and true labor is also important in order to advise a woman wisely. Education for the birthing family is an important component of labor triage. A woman who is not in labor and will be sent home needs appropriate information to recognize signs of true labor and reassurance about false labor (see Table 23–1). A woman who is admitted to a labor unit in the earlier part of her labor is usually receptive to education about her current status and anticipatory guidance for the rest of labor.

Questions to Ask About Current Labor

UTERINE CONTRACTIONS

- Time of onset: What was the time of the first contraction and at what time did the contractions become regular?
- Frequency: How often do the contractions occur?
- Duration: How long do the contractions last?
- Intensity: What is the level of pain? Describe the nature and location of the pain.
- Effect on ambulation: Do the contractions become more or less frequent and intense with ambulation?

ADDITIONAL HISTORY

- Bloody show: What was the frequency and amount of discharge?
- Vaginal bleeding: What was the amount, color, and consistency?
- Membranes: Is there leaking or have you experienced spontaneous rupture of membranes? What was the amount, color, consistency, and time of occurrence?
- Fetal activity: Has the fetus moved or kicked since labor began?
- Nutrition, hydration, and sleep: When was the last time you ate, drank, or slept?
- Social support available: Is someone with you?
- General emotional well-being: Are you relaxed? Are you using breathing techniques?
- Transportation: Is transportation to the birth site available?

Bloody Show. In addition to information about uterine contractions, other pertinent history should be obtained. Many women experience a mucous vaginal discharge that may contain blood for several days before the onset of labor. Throughout pregnancy, the cervical canal is plugged with mucus, which is secreted from cervical glands and serves as a barrier to protect the fetus. In the last days of pregnancy, as the cervix softens, this mucus may be passed in varying quantities. When it is tinged with blood from ruptured capillaries in the cervix, it is called bloody show. Some women never notice either the passing of the mucous plug or bloody show. Bloody show must be distinguished from frank vaginal bleeding. The most notable distinction is the mucous quality of bloody show. Many women are surprised at the quantity of mucus and need to be reassured that this is normal.

Spontaneous Rupture of Membranes. It is important to identify whether the membranes of the amniotic sac are intact or have ruptured. If the membranes have ruptured naturally, this is classified as spontaneous rupture of the membranes (SROM). The nurse should ask the woman about the time of rupture, the color and odor of the amniotic fluid, and the amount. This information should be recorded on the admission record. Normal amniotic fluid should be clear, be colorless, and have only a slight musty odor. Any deviation from these norms could indicate amnionitis (a foul odor or thick consistency of the fluid), fetal distress (green or amber fluid indicating the passage of meconium), or hemorrhage from the placenta (wine-colored fluid).

Most women are able to provide this information clearly; however, if the membranes have not ruptured completely but have been leaking amniotic fluid, it may be difficult for the woman to distinguish a leak of amniotic fluid from urinary incontinence. Nitrazine test tape or a Nitrazine cotton swab can be used by the nurse during a vaginal examination to determine whether the membranes have in fact ruptured. The yellow color of the Nitrazine turns a bright blue in the presence of amniotic fluid. Another way to test for amniotic fluid is with a fern test. A sample of vaginal fluid is placed on a slide, allowed to dry, and then viewed under a microscope. If amniotic fluid is present, a fernlike pattern will be viewed. Once it is determined that the membranes have ruptured, it is important to use precaution to prevent the introduction of infection.

In most labors, SROM occurs during active labor. However, the artificial rupture of membranes (AROM), or amniotomy, is often performed on a routine basis by the physician (see Procedure 25–2). The usefulness of this intervention is still debated in the literature, and no consensus has yet been reached.

▼ ANTEPARTUM RECORD

The antepartum record, including such information as gestational age, antepartum complications, prenatal laboratory tests, past obstetric history, medical and surgical history, and social history, should be carefully reviewed when a woman is admitted in labor. Components of Prenatal Health History and Prenatal Laboratory Data (Table 16–2) in Chapter 16 summarize components of the common antepartum chart. An assessment of potentially high-risk factors should also be made. Some birth settings may use a high-risk assessment form for this purpose. Risk Factors in Pregnancy (p. 442) lists high-risk factors that should be identified on admission to labor. Chapters 21 and 25 discuss the complications of pregnancy and childbirth that would place a woman at high risk during her labor.

The nurse should ask the woman whether she has completed a birth plan. This practice is often suggested by the woman's childbirth educator or her care provider to help her identify her desires, expectations, and options for the birth experience. The intent of the birth plan is not to present a list of demands but to share with the labor staff the components of care that are important to her. For example, the woman might identify such things as ambulating during labor, using music to help her relax, having her partner with her at all times, trying the squatting position for expulsion, and nursing her baby as soon after birth as possible as the options that she hopes can be included in her care. If the woman brings a birth plan form with her, it should be attached to her labor record and reviewed by the staff who will be providing her care. If any aspect of the woman's birth plan must be altered, this should be discussed honestly with the woman and her partner.

▼ PHYSICAL ASSESSMENT IN LABOR

Throughout the nursing assessment, it is important to observe the woman's facial expression and behaviors, both during and between contractions, and her response to her significant others. These nonverbal signs can provide invaluable feedback regarding the woman's comfort level and indicate the degree of support she will need throughout the labor and birth. The following physical assessments should be part of the initial admission to the birth setting and should then be carried out at regular intervals as needed throughout the labor process (Procedure 23–1).

Maternal Vital Signs. Blood pressure should be assessed initially and thereafter at intervals designated by institutional protocol. The blood pressure is generally assessed every hour during active labor and more often if it is elevated. The woman's position should be recorded during the initial blood pressure measurement, and subsequent

PROCEDURE 23–1

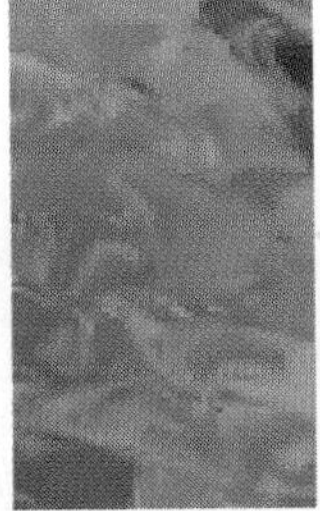

Monitoring Women During Labor and in the Immediate Postpartum Period

▼ PURPOSE

To determine that maternal-fetal status is within normal limits during labor and that maternal status is within normal limits in the immediate postpartum period; to intervene when deviations from normal are noted.

▼ EQUIPMENT

- Thermometer
- Blood pressure cuff
- Stethoscope
- Electronic fetal monitor or fetoscope
- Flashlight or penlight

Monitoring During Labor

1 Assess the following parameters during the first and second stages of labor at regular intervals:

   - Vital signs. Assess and record blood pressure on admission and at least hourly during the active phase of labor (more frequently if blood pressure is elevated). Assess and record temperature, pulse, and respirations on admission and every 4 hours thereafter (more frequently if membranes are ruptured or if deviations from normal are noted).
   - Fetal well-being. To verify fetal well-being, either auscultate and record the fetal heart rate on admission to the birthing unit or place the woman on an electronic fetal monitor for 20 to 30 minutes after admission to the birthing unit. After the initial monitoring period, use continuous or intermittent monitoring, depending on the maternal-fetal risk status. Whether auscultation or electronic fetal monitoring is used, evaluate and record fetal heart rate for low-risk women every 60 minutes during latent first-stage labor, every 30 minutes during active first-stage labor, and every 15 minutes during second-stage labor. For high-risk women, evaluate and record fetal heart rate every 30 minutes during latent

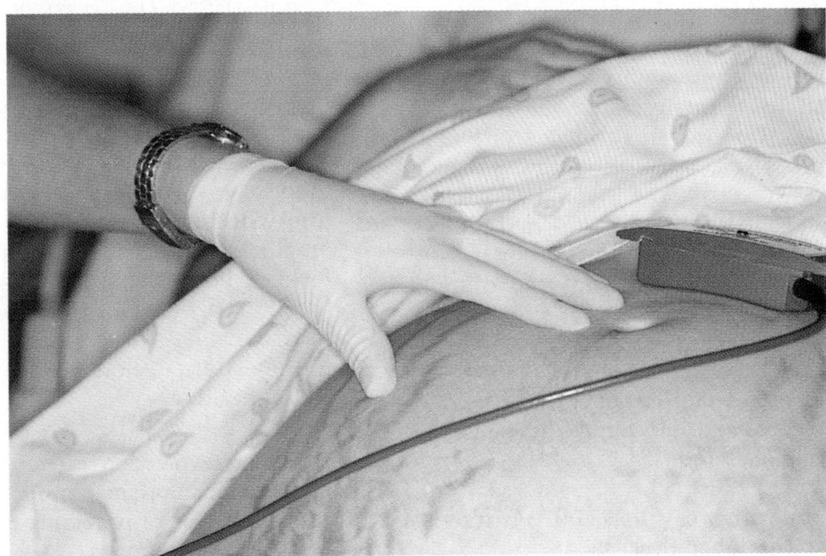

Continued on following page

PROCEDURE 23-1 Continued

first-stage labor, every 15 minutes during active first-stage labor, and every 5 minutes during second-stage labor (American College of Obstetricians and Gynecologists [ACOG] 1995a; Nurses Association of the American College of Obstetricians and Gynecologists [NAACOG] 1990).

- Uterine activity. Assess and record the frequency, duration, and intensity of uterine contractions every 30 to 60 minutes by direct palpation (see text) or through interpretation of electronic fetal monitoring strips. Assess and record the uterine resting tone between contractions by direct palpation.
- Labor progress. Perform a vaginal examination to assess cervical effacement and dilatation, fetal position and station, and status of membranes. Record your findings. Determine whether duration of labor exceeds the normal limits (ACOG 1995b):

Primigravida	
Latent first stage	>20 hours
Active first stage	<1.2 cm dilatation per hour
Second stage	>2 hours
Multipara	
Latent first stage	>14 hours
Active first stage	<1.5 cm dilatation per hour
Second stage	>1 hour

- Intake and output. Assess the woman's intake to ensure adequate hydration. Initiate intravenous fluid administration as needed or before administration of epidural anesthesia. Encourage the woman to empty her bladder frequently during labor, as a distended bladder can impede the descent of the fetal presenting part and slow labor progress. Catheterize the woman with bladder fullness and inability to void due to epidural anesthesia. Evaluate other output measures including vomiting and diarrhea.

An ongoing evaluation of maternal and fetal status during labor ensures that deviations from normal findings are identified and appropriate nursing actions are implemented.

2 Evaluate the following psychosocial parameters throughout the labor process:

- Support system
- Level of understanding of the labor process and procedures related to the care of a woman in labor
- Effectiveness of coping strategies to deal with the labor process and the pain of labor

The psychosocial assessment provides the basis for education of the patient, anticipatory guidance, and provision of supportive care including both pharmacologic and nonpharmacologic measures.

Monitoring in the Immediate Postpartum Period (First Hour After Birth)

1 Assess and record the following parameters every 15 minutes and more frequently if deviations from normal are noted:

- Blood pressure, pulse, and respirations. In the absence of complications, they will return to prelabor values within the first hour post partum.
- Uterus. Palpate the uterus to assess its height, position, and consistency. Place one hand just above the symphysis pubis and apply gentle downward pressure to support the lower segment of the uterus. Place the other hand on the uterine fundus. The uterine fundus should be at the level of the umbilicus or slightly below it and in the midline of the abdomen. The uterus should be firm rather than boggy. If the uterus is boggy, initiate uterine massage to stimulate the uterus to contract.
- Lochia. Assess the color (lochia rubra), the amount (scant, small, moderate, heavy), and whether odor is fleshy (normal) or foul smelling (indicative of infection). Assess lochial flow; report continuous trickle of bright red blood (abnormal) to health care provider. Note presence of clots; report numerous large clots (abnormal) to health care provider.

An ongoing evaluation of maternal status in the immediate postpartum period ensures the identification of potential problems and the prompt initiation of nursing actions.

PROCEDURE 23–1 Continued

2 Assess the following parameters at least once during the immediate postpartum period and more frequently if deviations from normal are noted:

- Temperature. The temperature may remain slightly elevated. Notify health care provider if temperature is greater than 2°F above normal (indicative of infection).
- Perineum. Using a flashlight or penlight, inspect the perineum using the REEDA scale (see Table 23–5). Evaluate redness, edema, and ecchymosis. Confirm that episiotomy or laceration repair is intact and without drainage. Assess for the presence of hematomas and hemorrhoids. Assess the woman's perception of perineal discomfort or pain.
- Bladder fullness. Assess bladder fullness directly by suprapubic palpation or indirectly by fundal location (the fundus is displaced above the umbilicus and to the right by a full bladder). Assess the woman's ability to void spontaneously and the need for catheterization.
- Breasts. Assess status of the nipples. Assist breastfeeding mothers with correct positioning of the infant and latching-on techniques.
- Extremities. Assess the woman's reactivity after anesthesia by evaluating her ability to move her lower extremities.

An ongoing evaluation of maternal status in the immediate postpartum period ensures the identification of potential problems and the prompt initiation of nursing actions.

blood pressures should be measured in the same position if feasible. A supine position is not recommended because of the risk of maternal supine hypotensive syndrome, conversely because the supine position may cause the pressure to be falsely elevated. Blood pressure should not be assessed during a contraction, as that may also cause a false elevation. During labor, normal blood pressure values range from 90 to 140 mm Hg for the systolic pressure and from 60 to 90 mm Hg for the diastolic pressure. Measurements reflecting an increase of greater than 30 mm Hg in the systolic pressure or 15 mm Hg in the diastolic pressure above antepartum baseline values are abnormal. It is important to use an appropriately sized cuff. If the cuff is too small, this may result in an inaccurately elevated finding, potentially causing a woman to be diagnosed as having preeclampsia/eclampsia. A cuff that is too large may cause undue discomfort when inflated.

Temperature should be assessed initially and every 4 hours thereafter. If the membranes are ruptured or the temperature is elevated above 99.6°F, it should be assessed every 1 to 2 hours. The normal range for the temperature is 98.0°F to 99.6°F. Dehydration may be the cause of a slight temperature elevation (99.6° to 100.4°F). If the temperature is above 100.4°F, the woman should be questioned about symptoms associated with upper respiratory, gastrointestinal, or urinary tract infections. Chorioamnionitis, an infection of the amniotic membranes, should also be considered. This condition may occur whether or not the membranes are ruptured, although it is more likely to occur with prolonged rupture of the membranes.

Pulse and respirations should also be assessed initially and every hour thereafter. The normal range for the pulse is 60 to 90 beats per minute; the normal range for respirations is 16 to 24 breaths per minute. Increased pulse and respiration rates may be attributed to anxiety, excitement, or pain. When associated with an elevation of temperature, tachycardia may indicate an infection.

Fetal Heart Rate. Auscultation of the fetal heart rate should be performed promptly on admission and then at regular intervals (Procedure 23–2) if the woman is not being monitored by an electronic fetal monitor. A fetoscope is used for this purpose. Different types of fetoscopes can be used: a head fetoscope, a weighted bell fetoscope, or a Doppler ultrasound stethoscope. Before listening to the fetal heart rate, the nurse needs to perform Leopold maneuvers to determine the position of the fetus (see Procedure 16–1). The fetal heart rate is best heard through the fetal back; therefore, the back needs to be located by palpation. As the fetus descends or changes position throughout labor, the location of the fetal heart rate will also change. Approximate locations for fetal heart sounds are illustrated in Procedure 23–2 and include RSA (right sacrum anterior), ROP (right occiput posterior), ROA (right occiput anterior), LSA (left sacrum anterior), LOP (left occiput posterior), and LOA (left occiput anterior). Figure 22–4 illus-

PROCEDURE 23-2

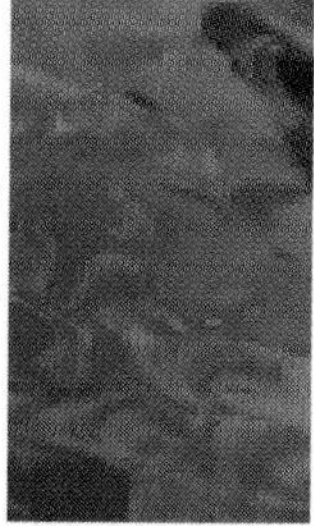

Auscultating Fetal Heart Rate During Labor

▼ PURPOSE

The fetal heart rate is auscultated on admission to the labor suite and at regular intervals throughout labor to assess fetal status and well-being. Frequent assessments detect changes in the fetal heart rate and presence of accelerations and decelerations, all indicators of how well the fetus is tolerating labor.

▼ EQUIPMENT

- Listening device, such as a fetoscope or Doppler ultrasound stethoscope
- Ultrasonic gel

1 Explain the procedure to the woman and her partner, including the reason for and the frequency of the procedure. **Helps to decrease anxiety and improve compliance with the procedure.**

2 Instruct the woman to lie on her back on the bed, with a pillow under her head. Place a wedge under her right or left hip to maintain a slight lateral tilt during the procedure. Lower the head of the bed so that it is flat. **Proper position facilitates location of fetal heart tones. A wedge under the woman's hip displaces the uterus sufficiently to prevent compression of maternal blood vessels and subsequent supine hypotension.**

3 Perform Leopold maneuvers to locate the fetal back (see Procedure 16–1). **Fetal heart tones are best heard through the fetal back. As the fetus changes position during labor, the location of fetal heart tones also changes.**

4 If you are using the Doppler stethoscope, turn it on and gently tap the auscultating end, listening for a resultant sound. Put a small amount of conducting gel onto the Doppler stethoscope. **To ascertain whether the Doppler stethoscope is in working order. The gel enhances the conduction of sound.**

5 If you are using a fetoscope, place the metal band on your head with the diaphragm extending out from your forehead. **The metal band adds bone conduction to facilitate transmission of the sound.**

6 With firm pressure, place the Doppler stethoscope or bell of the fetoscope on the appropriate quadrant of the woman's abdomen. **The heart tones of a fetus in the cephalic presentation are generally heard over one of the two lower quadrants of the maternal abdomen. As labor progresses and the fetus descends into the pelvic cavity, the fetal heart tones may be found midline in the lower abdomen. The position of the baby determines where the heart tones are best heard.**

7 Listen for fetal heart tones and differentiate them from other sounds. **The fetal heart has a characteristic sound similar to that of a galloping horse; count only one beat for each double rhythm. In contrast, blood moving through the uterine vessels or umbilical cord has a soft "swooshing" sound.**

8 Compare the rate of what you are hearing through the fetoscope or Doppler stethoscope with the rate of the maternal heart by palpating the woman's radial pulse. **To confirm that you have located the fetal heart tone rather than the maternal pulse.**

9 Determine the baseline rate by counting the number of beats for 30 to 60 seconds between contractions. Determine fetal response to the stress of contractions by listening for deceleration or acceleration of the fetal heart rate during a uterine contraction and for 30 seconds thereafter. **A**

Continued on facing page

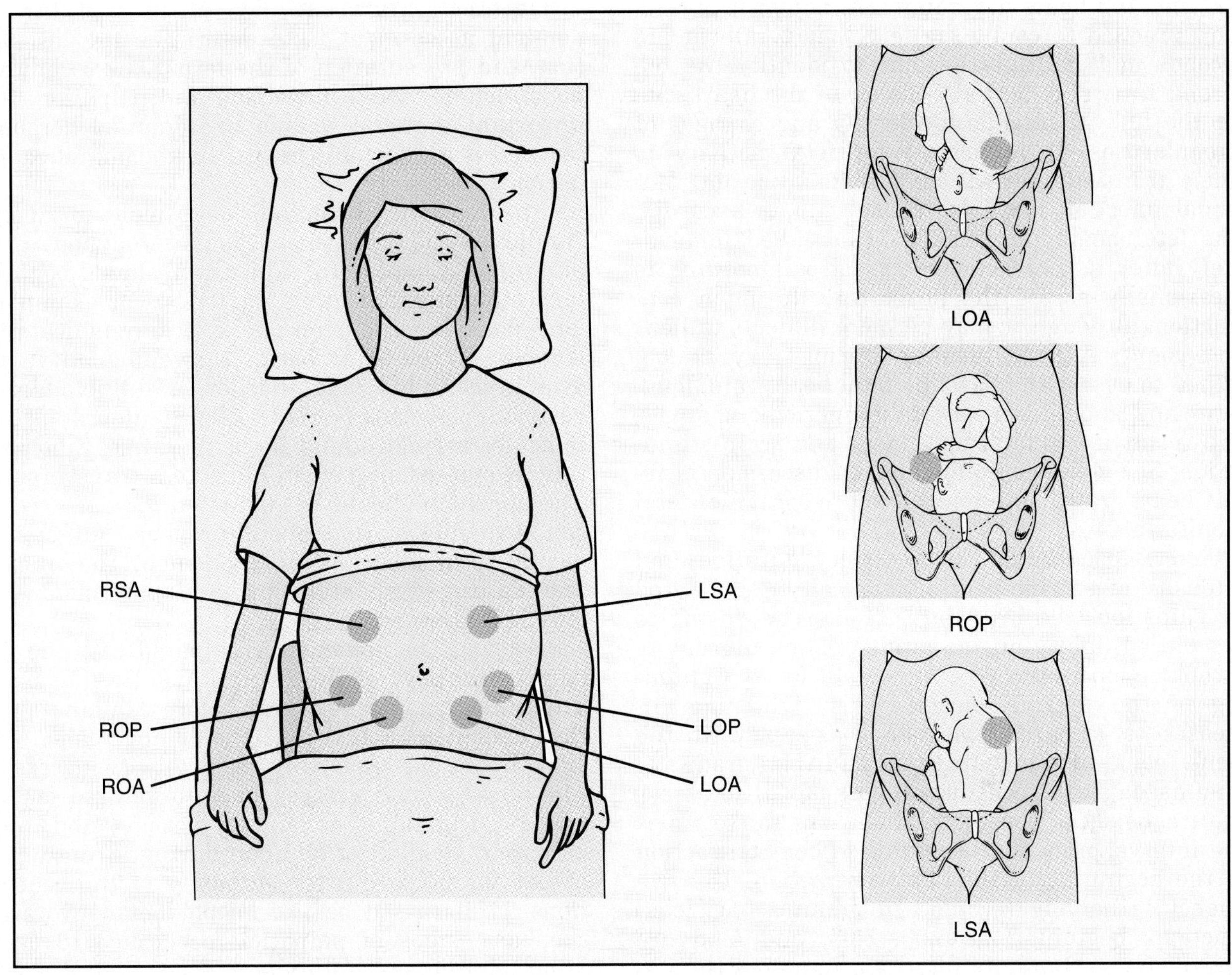

normal baseline fetal heart rate for a full-term fetus is between 120 and 160 beats per minute and is counted between contractions. An acceleration is usually associated with a healthy fetus; a deceleration could indicate fetal stress.

10 Auscultate fetal heart rate at regular intervals. **Current guidelines for frequency of fetal heart rate auscultation during labor (ACOG 1995a; NAACOG 1990) are as follows:**

	Low-risk	High-risk
First stage		
Latent	Every 60 minutes	Every 30 minutes
Active	Every 30 minutes	Every 15 minutes
Second stage	Every 15 minutes	Every 5 minutes

11 Wipe off the woman's abdomen and the tip of the Doppler stethoscope with a clean, dry cloth. **Prevents the gel from getting onto the woman's clothing.**

12 Record the baseline rate, rhythm, and fetal response to uterine contractions. Nursing interventions in response to nonreassuring findings must also be documented. **Repeated findings provide information on fetal status and well-being. If nonreassuring findings are noted, the nurse is obligated to intervene appropriately and place the patient on an electronic fetal monitor to better detect subtle changes in the fetal heart rate.**

trates and describes the relationship of the most common fetal positions to the mother's body during labor and descent.

A normal fetal heart rate is an indicator of fetal well-being. The normal fetal heart rate is between 120 and 160 beats per minute. Although it is common practice to count the fetal heart rate for 15 seconds and multiply by four to identify the 60-second rate, it is better to listen to the heart rate for the full 60 seconds to identify any changes or irregularities. It is normal for fetal activity to cause transient periods of fetal tachycardia. Maternal infection may also cause fetal tachycardia. The fetal heart rate should be assessed immediately after a contraction. It is also important to occasionally assess the heart rate during a contraction, although it may be more difficult to hear and count. A fetal monitor tracing may be obtained to assess the baseline fetal heart rate, long-term and short-term variability, periodic changes, and reactivity to fetal movement and scalp stimulation. See Chapter 26 for further discussion of fetal heart rate assessment and electronic fetal monitoring.

Uterine Contractions. The frequency, duration, and intensity of uterine contractions can be estimated by palpation (see Procedure 23–1). The fingertips are placed lightly on the fundus of the uterus. As a contraction begins, the nurse will feel a tightening of the uterine muscle. This tightening increases to a hard, boardlike consistency at the acme (peak) of the contraction and then gradually diminishes as the contraction goes down. To assess the frequency of the contractions, the nurse times the interval from the beginning of one contraction to the beginning of the next contraction. The frequency is usually recorded in minutes (e.g., contractions beginning at 5:00, 5:03, and 5:06 are recorded as a 3-minute interval). To assess the duration of the contractions, the time is measured from the beginning to the end of one contraction. The duration is usually recorded in seconds (e.g., a contraction lasting from 5:00.00 to 5:00.45 is recorded as 45 seconds). In addition to assessing the intensity of contractions by the woman's description, the nurse should also assess the fundus by palpation during a contraction. During a mild contraction, the fundus is easily indentable. The fundus is slightly indentable during a contraction of moderate intensity. During a strong contraction, the examiner is unable to indent the fundus (e.g., the intensity of contractions is recorded as being mild, moderate, or strong). The frequency, duration, and intensity of contractions can also be assessed by the electronic fetal monitor. If electronic monitoring is used, the transducer is placed on the maternal abdomen at the level of the uterine fundus to measure the frequency and duration of the uterine contractions. The intensity of the contractions is recorded in millimeters of mercury (mm Hg); however, because the transducer is placed externally on the maternal abdomen, it does not accurately reflect the intensity of the contractions. The nurse should continue to occasionally use palpation to assess the contraction's intensity, even if a fetal monitor is being used.

Abdominal Assessment. The purpose of the abdominal assessment is to determine the lie, position, and presentation of the fetus. The techniques used include visual inspection and palpation. It is important that the woman has emptied her bladder and is comfortable before an abdominal examination is done.

Inspection. The abdominal assessment in labor is similar to the assessment done throughout pregnancy (see Chapter 16). The nurse should begin by inspecting the abdominal contours. For example, a long, smooth contour on one side may indicate the location of the fetal back. A swelling above the symphysis pubis may indicate a full bladder. A vertically elongated shape of the uterus usually indicates a longitudinal lie of the fetus; a horizontally elongated shape can indicate a transverse lie. The abdomen should be inspected for scars, which can give information about previous surgery. By visual assessment of the abdomen, the number and nature of spontaneous fetal movements can often be observed.

Palpation. The abdomen is palpated with the flat, palmar surfaces of the fingers, not the fingertips. The hands should be warm before examination of the abdomen. Palpation should be done with smooth motions and only as firmly as necessary. The nurse should proceed in an organized fashion and avoid prodding or jabbing motions. Abdominal palpation should not be done during a contraction except for palpating the intensity of the contractions as discussed before. Leopold maneuvers are the basic steps of palpation performed to determine fetal lie, presentation, and position. The fetal weight may be roughly estimated by attempting to palpate as much of the fetus as possible abdominally and then envisioning the remainder. The sum of the two estimates gives the examiner an approximate idea of the fetal weight. The fundal height is measured with a tape measure (see Chapter 16). The height of the fundus should be compatible with the estimated date of delivery; otherwise, complications such as a baby small for gestational age, hydramnios, or multiple pregnancy should be considered. As the nurse conducts the abdominal examination, it is important for her to share her findings with the woman and her support persons.

Pelvic Examination. A generation ago, assessment of cervical dilatation was done by a rectal examination because of concern about introducing infection into the vaginal tract. Vaginal examinations were avoided at all cost or performed only by the most skilled obstetrician under special circumstances. Today, labor is usually assessed by a vaginal examination (Procedure 23–3), most com-

PROCEDURE 23–3

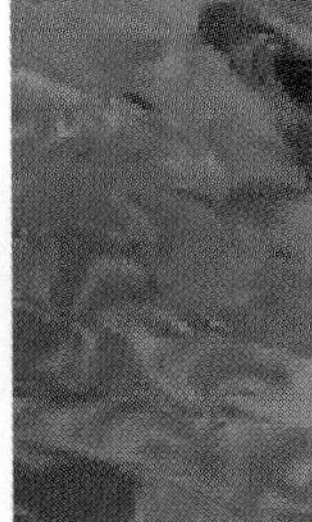

Vaginal Examination During Labor

▼ PURPOSE

Vaginal examinations during labor are performed only when indicated to evaluate labor progress. Performed with use of sterile technique, a vaginal examination during labor can provide information on cervical position, consistency, effacement, and dilatation; fetal presentation, position, and station; and status of membranes.

▼ EQUIPMENT

- Sterile glove
- Sterile lubricant

1 Prepare the woman for examination by explaining the procedure and describing the sensations to expect. **Anticipatory guidance decreases the woman's anxiety and facilitates cooperation during the examination.**

2 Lower the head of the bed. Position the woman so that her knees are flexed. Ask her to separate her legs. Place a wedge under the woman's right or left hip to maintain a slight lateral tilt during the procedure. **Proper position allows the health care provider's easier access to the cervix and enhances the woman's ability to relax during the procedure. A wedge is used in the supine position to prevent compression of the maternal blood vessels and subsequent supine hypotension.**

3 Wash your hands and apply one glove to the examining hand using sterile technique. Using the other hand, apply sterile lubricant to index and middle fingers of gloved hand. **The use of sterile technique decreases the possibility of introducing organisms that may lead to maternal or fetal infection. Lubricant reduces friction between the gloved hand and the vaginal wall during the procedure.**

4 Instruct the woman to relax and to begin slow, rhythmic breathing. **Slow, rhythmic breathing may facilitate the woman's relaxation and comfort during the examination.**

5 Gently insert the index and middle fingers into the vagina until they feel the cervix. The fingers may initially be directed with the palmar surface downward and then rotated upward. Curl the last two fingers inward. Either tuck the thumb in with the last two fingers or keep it above the symphysis pubis. **Directing the palmar surface initially downward enhances the woman's comfort because the posterior surface of the vaginal wall is less sensitive than the anterior surface. Tucking in the thumb or keeping it above the symphysis pubis prevents obscuring the woman's genitalia or irritating the clitoris during the examination.**

6 Assess the following parameters:

- Cervical position
- Cervical consistency
- Cervical effacement
- Cervical dilatation
- Presenting part
- Fetal position as determined by the fetal suture lines and position of the fontanelles (in cephalic presentations) in relation to the maternal pubic bone
- Fetal station as determined by the presenting part in relation to the ischial spines of the pelvis
- Status of membranes

These assessments are the basis for determining labor progress and the relationship of the fetus to the maternal pelvis.

7 To determine dilatation accurately, proceed as follows:

Continued on following page

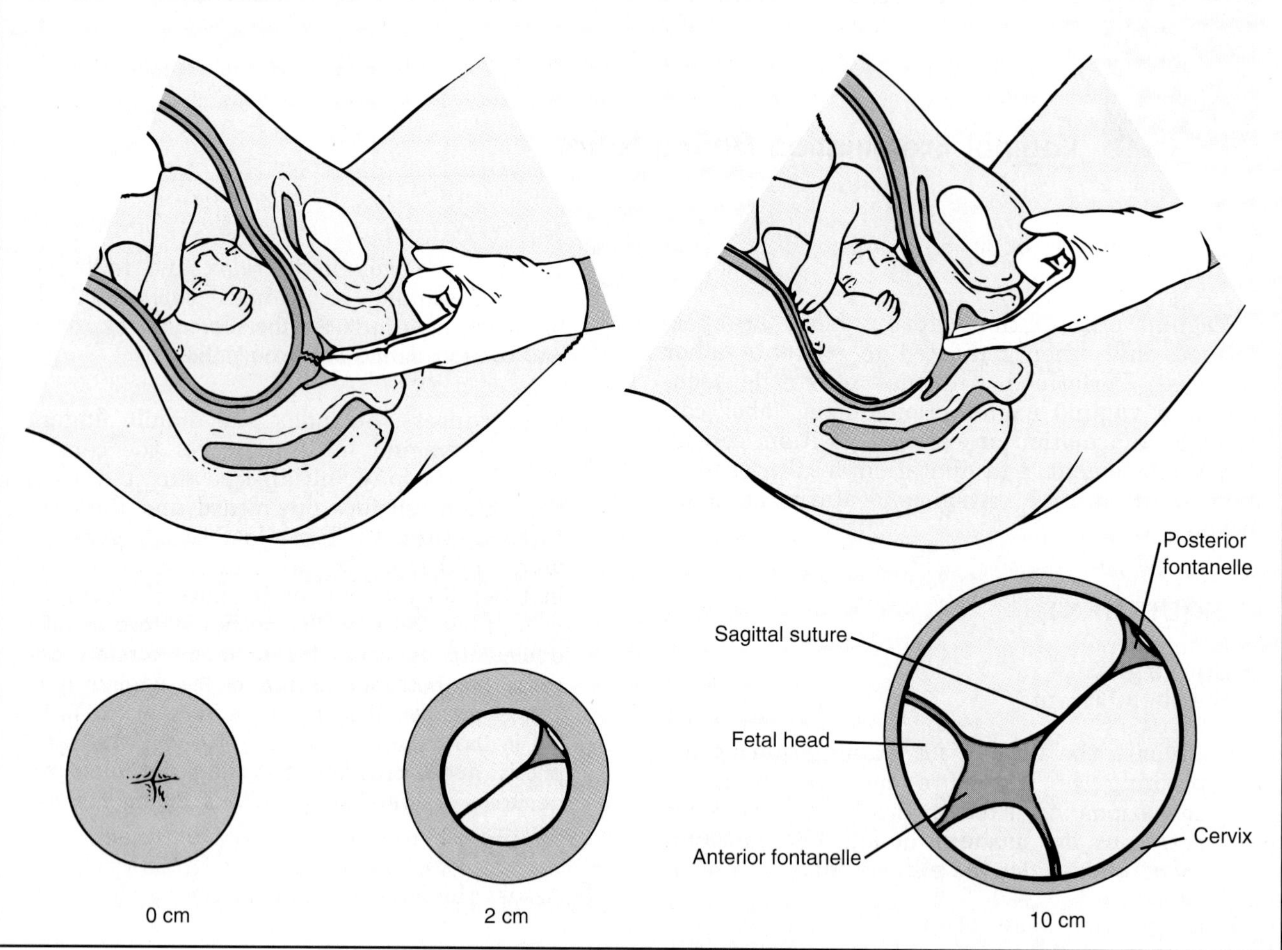

- After inserting fingers into the cervix, determine the internal os of the cervix by curling tip of index finger over upper edge of cervix. **It is important to determine the internal os of the cervix for accurate measurement.**
- Measure the number of fingers of dilatation within the internal os of the cervix by counting across the presenting part with your index finger. **Dilatation proceeds from 0 to 10 cm. You need to know the size of your index fingertip in centimeters. One finger usually equals 1.5 to 2 cm, depending on size of the individual.**
- Measure the number of fingers of cervix on each side of the cervical opening with your index finger and subtract from 10 cm. **This number is used to assess the accuracy of your measurement of dilatation and should equal the centimeters of dilatation. If it does not, repeat measurement of dilatation using the procedure again.**

8 To determine the position of the fetal head, proceed as follows:

- Locate the posterior fontanelle by gently palpating the fetal head. Distinguish the posterior fontanelle, which is triangle shaped, from the anterior fontanelle, which is diamond shaped.
- Determine the relationship of the posterior fontanelle to the maternal pubic bone. If the posterior fontanelle is located just under the maternal pubic bone, the

Continued on facing page

PROCEDURE 23–3 Continued

fetal position is anterior. If the posterior fontanelle is located toward the back of the maternal pelvis, the fetal position is posterior.

The position of the fetal head provides valuable information about the expected progress of labor.

9 After the examination, explain the examination results to the woman and her partner, place a clean pad under the woman's buttocks if needed, and help her to a position of comfort. **Measures to keep the couple involved and keep the woman comfortable enhance the labor experience.**

10 Remove gloves and wash your hands. **Prevents cross-contamination.**

11 Record vaginal examination findings on the fetal monitor tracing and on the labor flow record as follows:

Cervix:	Position	Posterior or anterior
	Consistency	Firm or soft
	Effacement	0% to 100%
	Dilatation	0 to 10 cm
Presenting part:	Cephalic, breech, shoulder, or compound	
Fetal position:	Left, right, anterior, or posterior	
Station:	− 5/5 (floating) to + 5/5 (crowning)	
Membranes:	Intact, bulging, or ruptured spontaneously or artificially	

Recording these results allows comparisons to assess labor progress.

monly performed by a physician, nurse-midwife, or maternal-newborn nurse. Nurses often perform a pelvic examination simply to determine cervical progress. However, a great deal of additional information can and should be obtained with a pelvic examination during labor. This information should include cervical position, consistency, effacement, and dilatation; fetal presentation, position, and station; and the status of the membranes.

There are several important points to consider in regard to pelvic examinations during labor. A digital examination of the cervix should never be performed by any member of the health care team in the presence of frank vaginal bleeding. Such bleeding may indicate a placenta previa or low-lying placenta, and a digital examination might worsen the severity of the bleeding. If the membranes are leaking or ruptured without the onset of contractions, institutional policy may dictate that the cervix be assessed by speculum examination only to decrease the potential for infection.

The cervical examination should be carried out in a gentle but thorough manner. The examiner should be organized in approach so that all aspects of the examination are assessed each time it is performed. Organization also promotes efficiency, which minimizes the amount of time the examination takes and the client's resultant discomfort. Cervical examination is more comfortable when performed between contractions. However, assessment of the cervix during a contraction is occasionally helpful in determining the application of the presenting part to the cervix. The cervix may also be more dilated during a contraction. Similarly, if the membranes are intact and bulging outwardly through the cervix, the cervix may be more dilated before the rupture of membranes. This may account for a difference of 1 to 3 cm. If the fetal head is the presenting part, scalp stimulation can be performed by applying gentle digital pressure against the head with the examining fingers and noting the effect of this pressure on the fetal heart rate. A fetus is termed reactive when the fetal heart rate increases by 10 to 15 beats per minute. This reactivity of the fetal heart rate is considered to be an indication of normal fetal neurologic function.

Pelvic examinations should never be assumed to be the only way in which labor can be assessed. Behavioral signs frequently provide valuable data for the nurse and make a pelvic examination unnecessary. Pelvic examinations always pose two difficulties: the discomfort of the woman and the potential for introduction of infection. Therefore, they should be limited. Before performing an examination, the nurse should consider how important knowing the status of pelvic findings is to the nursing management of the woman at this time. This is the critical "How does it change my management?" question. Examinations should be individualized and not dependent on any rigid time frame (e.g., "women must be examined every 2 hours"). Pelvic examinations should follow a holistic approach to the woman and fetus. The nurse should not only assess the woman's previous labor pattern but also perform Leopold maneuvers to ascertain fetal position (see Procedure 16–1, p. 434). As with any skill, theoretic knowledge and experience make the best practitioner (Bergstrom et al. 1992).

Preparation. The first step in doing a pelvic examination is introduction of the procedure to the woman, explaining the components of the procedure, providing anticipatory guidance, and obtaining her verbal consent. Appropriate language is essential to this process. The woman is positioned so that supine hypotension is avoided and is draped so that modesty is upheld. Family members may be present as she desires. Hands should be washed and a sterile single glove obtained. Controversy exists regarding perineal preparation before an examination. Several agents have been recommended for cleansing of the perineum before an examination as well as for lubrication. No single agent has proved to be associated with decreased intrapartum infections. However, the woman should be asked whether she has any allergies to common detergents or disinfectants that might be used. For the comfort of the woman, most pelvic examinations are performed, or at least begun, between contractions.

External Inspection. As with most examinations, the first part of the examination is to inspect the genitalia. Lesions or masses that may indicate a heretofore unsuspected sexually transmitted disease may be present. Vaginal discharge (e.g., amniotic fluid) can be assessed visually for color and amount. Most practitioners use the index finger and middle fingers of their dominant hand to perform a pelvic examination. The thumb should be tucked securely in the palm of the hand with the other fingers or spread widely away from the two examining fingers. This prevents the examiner from obscuring the genitalia during the examination or irritating the clitoris during the procedure.

Internal Palpation. The first assessment possible often involves the position of the cervix. Following the curve of the vagina, the fingers should slowly and gently slip into the vaginal canal. During early labor, the cervix is often found posteriorly. Therefore, most experienced practitioners begin their examination as far posteriorly as they can comfortably reach. A cervix that is far posterior often is also not well effaced or dilated. As labor progresses, the cervix gradually moves to a more anterior position.

Another component of cervical assessment involves the consistency and length of the cervix. Before active labor, uterotropins have usually influenced the cervix so that it becomes soft and thin. Consistency is described qualitatively in relation to softness or firmness. This is also known as ripening. Effacement, which is the thinning of the cervix, is an estimate based on an assumption that the average, uneffaced cervical canal is 2 cm (0.8 inches) in length. By convention, effacement is described by percentages. An uneffaced cervix is termed 0 percent effacement. When a cervix is estimated to be approximately 1 cm in length, it is usually 50 percent effaced, and so on. When the cervix feels as thin as a piece of paper, it is generally said to be fully effaced, completely effaced, or 100 percent effaced (see Fig. 22–10). Primigravidas frequently do not make considerable cervical progress in labor until their cervices are 100 percent effaced.

Cervical dilatation involves estimation of the cervical opening. Dilatation is usually easiest to assess when the woman is in either early labor (1, 2, or 3 cm) or late labor (9 or 10 cm). In early labor, the examiner is barely able to introduce a finger into the cervical os. In late labor, the examiner tends to subtract from 10 cm. At 10 cm of dilatation, no cervix is palpable. In clinical practice, it is common to hear such terms as "fully" or "complete" to denote 10-cm dilatation; in some locales, 9 cm is termed "rim" to denote the rim of cervix left. Occasionally, especially in the case of an occiput posterior fetus, an anterior lip of cervix is all that is palpable and is charted as such. Since multiparous women have shorter labors, most practitioners suggest that the assessment of cervical dilatation be timed to coincide with a contraction.

The Bishop score is a rating system that may be used with a pelvic examination to evaluate the status of the cervix (Table 23–4). This scoring system includes the cervical components of position, consistency, effacement, and dilatation as well as fetal station. It is most commonly used to evaluate whether the cervix would be responsive to induction of labor. A score of less than 5 indicates that the cervix is not ready for labor and an induction would be unwise.

During assessment of cervical dilatation, several other observations can be made. The fetal presentation and position originally determined by abdominal palpation can be verified. Most fetuses engage and are born in a vertex cephalic presentation (see Chapter 22). A pelvic examination enables the examiner to ascertain the attitude of the head. For example, the examiner can determine if the head is well flexed, if hyperextension is present, or if neither extension nor flexion is present and the head is in a military attitude (fetal head in straight position, not flexed or extended). This information may suggest that because of larger diameters of the head, labor may be increased in length. The position of the sagittal suture helps the examiner to identify the fetal landmarks and, thus, the position. A fetus in an occiput posterior position is not uncommon in labor. These additional assessments can help the nurse facilitate maternal comfort and fetal rotation by changing the maternal positions after the procedure is finished.

Station, which measures the descent of the fetus in the maternal pelvis, may be designated in one of two ways. The level of the ischial spines is al-

Table 23–4

BISHOP SCORE

FACTOR	SCORE 0	1	2	3
Dilatation (cm)	Closed	1–2	3–4	5 or more
Effacement	0%–30%	40%–50%	60%–70%	80% or more
Station*	−3	−2	−1, 0	+1, +2
Consistency	Firm	Medium	Soft	
Position of cervix	Posterior	Midposition	Anterior	

*Based on the rule of thirds (see discussion below).

ways considered zero station and indicates engagement, regardless of which method is used. Some clinicians use a rule of thirds wherein the space above and below the spines is divided into three levels. In this method, a fetus who is unengaged and floating (also known as ballottable) is a −3 station, whereas a fetus whose head is fully crowning on the perineum is a +3 station. The five-level method for station assessment uses the estimation of centimeters above and below the spines. In this method, the fetus who is unengaged and floating is a −5 station, and the fetus who is about to be born is a +5 station (see Fig. 22–6). Variations in between are based on estimates of 1-cm increments. The five-level method is preferred by the American College of Obstetricians and Gynecologists (Cunningham et al. 1993), and more facilities and practitioners use this system. The most important aspect is that all examiners in a given birth facility use the same system and communicate with the same language. To facilitate this communication, the system used (i.e., thirds or fifths) should be recorded as the denominator and the station of the baby's head as the numerator. For example, a nurse might record station as being $-4/5$ or $+3/5$ if the five-level method is used, or $-2/3$ or $+1/3$ if the three-level method is used.

The status of the membranes may also be assessed by pelvic examination. A palpable bag of waters suggests that the membranes are intact or, in the event of a conflicting history of leaking fluid, that a high leak has occurred in the membranes. If the bag of waters is not palpable, it can be suspected that the membranes have ruptured or have been leaking. As discussed earlier in this chapter, a Nitrazine test or a fern test can be done to determine whether there is amniotic fluid in the vaginal canal. Observation should be made for leaking fluid during the examination process. Rarely the situation occurs, especially in association with a malpresentation, that the umbilical cord is palpable. This is an emergency situation, and the nurse should continue to hold pressure against the fetal head to decrease pressure on the cord while simultaneously calling for a physician and placing the woman in a position that also decreases pelvic pressure.

Completion of the Examination. At the completion of a pelvic examination, the woman's perineum and her bed should be cleaned. She should be told the findings of the examination. The examination should also be clearly documented and communicated appropriately. While cervical effacement and dilatation are the most commonly assessed parameters for a woman in labor, a periodic review of the additional aspects of an examination helps the nurse obtain the most relevant information during an examination.

Assessment of the Extremities. The extremities are assessed for edema. Edema in the feet and ankles is normal late in pregnancy. Edema in the face and hands is associated with pregnancy-induced hypertension. Deep tendon reflexes that are brisker than normal and the presence of clonus are also associated with pregnancy-induced hypertension (see Procedure 21–1, p. 645). This complication of pregnancy is discussed in Chapter 21. The legs should be inspected for varicosities. Superficial varices commonly develop during pregnancy. Larger varicosities should be noted and the area near the varicosities inspected for redness, tenderness, warmth, and induration. Such physical findings may indicate the development of thrombophlebitis.

Laboratory Data. Laboratory tests are routinely performed when a woman in labor is admitted to a hospital or birth center (see Laboratory Data). A voided urine sample, often obtained by the clean-catch method, is assessed with a dipstick for protein, ketones, and glucose. A trace of protein in

Laboratory Data

URINE

Test results for protein, ketones, glucose, white blood cells, and nitrites should all be negative. Elevated protein levels could indicate a contaminated specimen, fever, or preeclampsia. Elevated ketone levels could indicate dehydration. Elevated white blood cell and nitrite values could indicate an infection.

HEMATOCRIT AND HEMOGLOBIN

Values less than 32% for the hematocrit and 11 g/L for hemoglobin may indicate iron deficiency anemia or hemorrhage.

WHITE BLOOD CELL COUNT

Values of 4500/mm^3 to 11,000/mm^3 are normal, although values up to 25,000/mm^3 are considered within normal limits for labor, birth, and the early postpartum period because of stress.

SEROLOGIC TESTS FOR SYPHILIS (VDRL)

Samples may be obtained on admission, depending on institutional policy. Results should be nonreactive.

HEPATITIS B SURFACE ANTIGEN

Repeat test if antepartum results are more than 30 days old.

Rh FACTOR AND ABO TYPING

Typing is necessary if it was not done during the antepartum period. If the mother is Rh negative, the baby should be assessed for a titer and the mother given Rh_0 immune globulin (RhoGAM) if necessary.

the urine is normal in pregnancy. More than a trace of protein may be associated with pregnancy-induced hypertension. The presence of ketones in the urine may indicate dehydration. Glucosuria is abnormal, and a history of diabetes should be investigated if it is present. Indicators for white blood cells and nitrites may also be included on the urine dipstick. Positive values indicate possible urinary tract infection. Serologic tests for syphilis (such as a VDRL or RPR test) are routinely done on admission for labor to detect infection that may have developed since antepartum screening. Hemoglobin and hematocrit values below the normal range will reflect anemia or hemorrhage that may have developed late in a pregnancy. Dehydration can cause hemoconcentration, which may falsely elevate the hematocrit value. The ABO blood typing and Rh typing are essential if the client's prenatal record is unavailable or does not include this information. This is essential information if a blood transfusion is necessary.

▼ PSYCHOLOGICAL, SOCIAL, AND CULTURAL ASSESSMENT

It is important that the nurse's assessment of the woman in labor be holistic and include information about her emotional responses, social situation, and cultural background as well as all the physical parameters. The woman's emotional status can be assessed by observation of her behavior in response to the labor process. Her appearance, verbal responses, facial expressions, and body language can give valuable clues to her psychosocial adaptation. The expected behavioral responses to labor and birth are identified in Table 23–3. The woman who is more anxious, fearful, or agitated than expected may have other factors in her life that are influencing her behavior. In this situation, it is important to identify these factors and provide additional understanding and emotional support.

It is also important to assess the woman's coping mechanisms. The nurse should iden-

PROMOTING A NORMAL CHILDBIRTH

Despite the fact that the normal physiologic process of birth remains constant, the nurse should always strive to improve the care of the laboring woman and her family. The stresses and pressures of providing safe care to the woman and her fetus during labor and birth can be balanced with the wonder and joy of the miracle of birth by periodically taking the time to refresh, reflect, and update. The following suggestions will help nurses improve the quality of their clinical practice.

- MAINTAIN AN AWARENESS AND APPRECIATION of the individuality of each woman's labor.
- BE AWARE OF CULTURAL DIFFERENCES related to labor and birth.
- UPDATE YOUR KNOWLEDGE ON INTRAPARTUM RESEARCH TOPICS; stay current by reading professional journals and attending continuing education offerings.
- BECOME REENERGIZED BY MEETING AND SHARING WITH OTHER PROFESSIONALS who work with the same challenges and issues; join specialty professional organizations for perinatal nurses, childbirth educators, or nurse-midwives and attend local, state, or national meetings.
- KNOW YOUR PROFESSIONAL STANDARDS OF PRACTICE. Maintain a current knowledge of the guidelines of the Association of Women's Health, Obstetric, and Neonatal Nurses, the American College of Obstetricians and Gynecologists, and the American Academy of Pediatrics. These form your basis for safe practice.
- ADVOCATE FOR WOMEN'S NEEDS on the basis of your knowledge of safe practice.
- BE AWARE OF YOUR BIASES REGARDING LABOR AND BIRTH. Avoid allowing these biases to interfere with the provision of safe and compassionate nursing care.

tify whether the woman and her partner attended childbirth preparation classes and observe whether they are using relaxation, breathing techniques, or other pain management strategies. An initial assessment of the woman's coping abilities will inform the nurse about the amount of teaching and coaching the nurse will need to provide throughout the labor process. The woman's family situation can also influence her response to labor. If there are social stressors, economic problems, or family crises in her life, these factors are not easily left behind when she arrives in labor. The nurse can provide far better care in labor if these factors are identified. The woman's cultural or religious background can influence her attitudes, values, and customs related to labor and birth. These cultural factors also often shape the woman's behavioral responses to labor. Knowledge of all these components will provide the nurse with the information needed to develop a plan of care that views the woman as a unique individual (see Improving Your Practice).

▼ PHYSICAL ASSESSMENT IN THE IMMEDIATE POSTPARTUM PERIOD

The process of assessment continues throughout the third and fourth stages of labor. This step in the nursing process becomes even more important, for immediately after the birth the nurse is often responsible for the assessment of both the woman and the newborn. When the placenta has been delivered in the third stage of labor, the birth attendant assesses the status of uterine contractility, inspects the placenta and the membranes and cord, and inspects and repairs the episiotomy or any lacerations of the cervix and vagina or perineum. When the third stage of labor is completed, the nurse assumes regular assessments of the status of the woman. These assessments (see Procedure 23–1) should include the following components.

Vital Signs. The blood pressure, pulse, and respirations should return to prelabor values within the first hour post partum if no complications arise. The temperature may remain slightly elevated because of dehydration and physical exertion. If the temperature is greater than 2°F above normal, this may indicate infection, and the nurse-midwife or physician should be notified. The return of blood pressure to prelabor values is due to an increased volume of maternal blood returning to the general circulation from the placental site. If the blood pressure remains elevated, this might be a result of excitement, use of oxytocic drugs, or hypertensive disorders of pregnancy. Vital signs should be monitored frequently during the fourth stage of labor, since excessive blood loss is the most commonly encountered complication. In the event of hemorrhage, blood pressure drops as the pulse rate rises.

Vital signs are usually assessed every 15 minutes during the immediate postpartum period. Women often experience chills and shakes during the fourth stage of labor. When this occurs in the absence of fever, it is attributed to the release of energy or tension built up during labor and birth, the sudden decrease in intra-abdominal pressure, or the difference in internal and external maternal temperature. The exact cause of this phenomenon is uncertain. Education and reassurance are helpful, as are slow relaxed breathing, warm blankets, skin-to-skin contact with the infant, and intake of warm fluids.

Breasts. It is important to observe the degree of eversion of the nipples. Women with flat or inverted nipples may require assistance to help their infants latch on. Education about correct positioning and latching-on techniques is important to the first-time breastfeeding mother. Nursing the infant in the fourth stage of labor promotes bonding, comforts the newborn, and has beneficial effects on uterine contractility because of the natural release of oxytocin stimulated by suckling. Comfort in positioning and warmth facilitate the initial breastfeeding experience. The infant's temperature must also be maintained, and the nose and mouth kept free of secretions. Not all infants nurse immediately, but early attempts at breastfeeding acquaint the newborn with the mother's smell and taste, which will be helpful in subsequent breastfeeding sessions. Chapter 33 provides further suggestions for assisting with initial breastfeeding.

Abdomen. The height, position, and consistency of the uterus should be assessed every 15 minutes for the first hour after delivery. This assessment is made by palpation. The nurse places one hand just above the symphysis pubis and, with gentle downward pressure, supports the lower uterine segment of the uterus. The other hand is placed on the fundus to assess position and consistency. Immediately after delivery, the uterine fundus should be at the level of the umbilicus or one to three fingerbreadths below it and in the midline of the abdomen. If the fundus is above the umbilicus, this may indicate that there are blood clots in the uterus that need to be expelled by fundal massage. This nursing intervention is discussed later in this chapter. If the fundus is deviated to the right and elevated above the umbilicus, this indicates a full bladder, and the mother should be assisted to void. The uterus should be firm, even hard, in consistency. A soft or boggy uterus indicates atonicity, which may be alleviated by massage, expression of clots, and administration of oxytocic agents. Increased blood loss in the fourth stage of labor may indicate retained placental tissue. The placenta and membranes should be examined carefully to ensure that they appear intact, although retained tissue cannot be ruled out even if the placenta and membranes appear intact on inspection. Chapter 29 provides further information on the postpartum assessment of the uterus.

If the nurse suspects that the bladder is full because of the position of the uterus, the length of time since the woman last voided, or the woman's expression of discomfort, the nurse should palpate the bladder to determine whether it is distended. A distended bladder often appears as a bulge just above the symphysis pubis. The woman should be encouraged to void immediately. If she is unable to void, this may be the result of the temporary loss of sensation due to trauma or the effects of anesthesia. Immediate steps must be taken to assist her to void, for a full bladder can prevent the uterus from contracting and can increase the chance of hemorrhage. The first step in assisting the woman to void should be the use of noninvasive interventions to facilitate the relaxation of the urinary sphincter. These interventions include such things as letting the woman hear the sound of running water, pouring warm water over the perineum, or placing a warm towel over the lower abdominal area. If these interventions are not successful, urinary catheterization should be done. It is important to continually assess the bladder during the fourth stage of labor, for it fills rapidly because of the administration of intravenous fluids and the excretion of extra fluid volume as the circulatory system returns to its prepregnant state.

Perineum and Lochia. The perineum is inspected for redness, edema, ecchymosis, discharge from an episiotomy incision or laceration, and approximation. An acronym using the first letter of each of these five parameters is REEDA. The REEDA scale was developed by Davidson (1979) to provide a means of objective postpartum assessment of the perineum. The scale assigns a point value based on the degree to which each observation is present (Table 23–5). If hemorrhoids are present, their number, size, and color should be noted.

In assessment of the perineum, the lochia is evaluated for amount, color, and presence of clots. This assessment is usually done in conjunction with the assessment of the fundus. As the fundus is palpated or massaged, the nurse observes the flow of lochia from the vaginal introitus. The woman's perineal pad is also observed to identify the amount of bleeding that has occurred since the last assessment. The lochia is recorded as being scant, small, moderate, or heavy in amount. If a more accurate assessment of amount is needed because of suspected hemorrhage, the perineal pads can be weighed to estimate blood loss. The color of the lochia during the fourth stage of labor is a dark red color, called rubra.

Lochial flow should be distinguished from bleeding originating from a laceration or episiotomy, which is usually brighter red than lochia and often presents as a continuous trickle of bleeding even though the fundus of the uterus is firm. This bright red bleeding is abnormal and should be reported to the birth attendant. The odor of normal lochia is not unpleasant and is often described as "fleshy," like a normal menstrual flow. A more un-

Table 23–5

REEDA SCALE

CATEGORY	0	1	2	3
Redness	None	Within 0.25 cm of incision bilaterally	Within 0.5 cm of incision bilaterally	Beyond 0.5 cm of incision bilaterally
Edema	None	Perineal, <1 cm from incision	Perineal or vulvar, between 1 and 2 cm from incision	Perineal or vulvar, >2 cm from incision
Ecchymosis	None	Within 0.25 cm bilaterally or 0.5 cm unilaterally	Between 0.25 and 1 cm bilaterally or between 0.5 and 2 cm unilaterally	>1 cm bilaterally or 2 cm unilaterally
Discharge	None	Serous	Serosanguineous	Bloody, purulent
Approximation	Closed	Skin separation 3 mm or less	Skin and subcutaneous fat separation	Skin, subcutaneous fat, and fascial layer separation

pleasant odor could indicate infection. Perineal hygiene, care of sutures, comfort measures, and Kegel exercises should be reviewed with the woman at this time. If the woman is experiencing perineal discomfort, an ice pack can be used to reduce pain and edema.

Extremities. If regional anesthesia has been used, the legs should be assessed for sensation and motor ability. Edema, deep tendon reflexes, and the Homans sign should be evaluated, particularly if the woman has a prenatal history of pregnancy-induced hypertension.

▼ Diagnosis

On the basis of multiple assessments performed during the labor, birth, and recovery process, the nursing diagnoses evolve over time. For the healthy childbearing woman who is progressing well through childbirth, nursing diagnoses should focus on patterns of wellness, health, and teaching needs. Some examples of the more common nursing diagnoses for each stage of labor during a normal childbirth experience are

▼ FIRST-STAGE LABOR

- Knowledge deficit: lack of information related to expected physical changes, symptoms of labor, and options available to the childbearing woman
- Pain related to the process of labor or birth
- Anxiety related to childbirth, pelvic examinations, or obstetric interventions
- Fear related to parenting
- Fluid volume excess related to intake during labor
- Altered nutrition: less than body requirements related to decreased intake during labor

▼ SECOND-STAGE LABOR

- Fear related to birth process, pain, and unknown outcome
- Fatigue related to physical exertion during labor and lack of sleep
- Pain related to fetal descent, crowning, and perineal stretching

▼ THIRD- AND FOURTH-STAGE LABOR

- Risk for infection related to uterine placental site, episiotomy incision, and fatigue
- Urinary retention related to loss of sensation to void and rapid bladder filling
- Ineffective breastfeeding related to maternal knowledge deficit, anxiety, or fatigue

Obviously, many more nursing diagnoses may be apparent throughout the labor and birth process, especially as the nurse performs full physical and psychosocial assessments. These additional nursing diagnoses are inherent in an individualized plan of care.

Planning

Childbirth occurs within a finite time. Although a woman may perceive the time as incredibly long, a nurse in the maternity area is frequently challenged to perform all the necessary components of the professional role. One of the major roles is to use the information obtained from assessment and diagnosis to develop a plan of expected outcomes for the interventions that are anticipated to be needed in a holistic plan of care. The plan should include physical and psychosocial needs and be based on the goals agreed to by the entire health care team, including the woman and her family. The plan for a laboring woman should include labor, birth, and the immediate postpartum period. A plan that is written allows communication among all the members of the team. Some examples of measurable objectives and expected outcomes that are derived from the nursing diagnoses for each stage of labor include the following.

FIRST-STAGE LABOR

The laboring woman will

- Verbalize her understanding of the process of labor and the available options for her care
- Perform paced breathing in conjunction with contractions, demonstrate relaxation of muscles, and use position changes to decrease pain and promote comfort
- Demonstrate decreased fear of pelvic examinations through a relaxed body, decreased facial tension, and verbal confirmation
- Maintain an adequate fluid and calorie intake to meet the energy demands of labor

SECOND-STAGE LABOR

The woman will

- Verbalize decreased fear related to the birth and use effective expulsion techniques
- Conserve energy by resting between contractions, using physiologic pushing techniques with contractions, and maintaining relaxation of her body whenever possible
- Verbalize a decrease in her pain and demonstrate increased comfort through facial expression and body language

THIRD- AND FOURTH-STAGE LABOR

The woman will

- Maintain a normal temperature and show no signs of infection
- Empty her bladder within the first hour after delivery
- Successfully initiate breastfeeding in the first hour after delivery as evidenced by establishing a comfortable position and getting the baby to latch on to the nipple and begin to suck

Intervention

Many interventions can be used for the woman during the process of labor and birth. These interventions need to be derived from the assessment, nursing diagnoses, and plan of care. If interventions are selected in this way, unnecessary interventions can be decreased, if not eliminated. Moreover, interventions need to be assigned an order of priority. The priority may differ, depending on the particular needs of the woman and her family. Identifying a priority of interventions is particularly important since time is frequently of the essence as the normal physiologic events of labor and birth unfold. All aspects of care of the childbearing woman should be recognized and addressed to help determine the ordering of interventions. Safety issues may also be paramount. Interventions should be holistic and include nursing strategies to meet emotional and intellectual needs as well as physiologic needs.

PREPARATIONS FOR BIRTH

Historically, enemas in labor were administered for several purposes. It was proposed that enemas would prevent contamination of the delivery field in second-stage labor and help women avoid the embarrassment of passing stool during pushing efforts. They were also recommended for stimulating uterine contractions during the first stage and for emptying the lower bowel to facilitate descent of the fetal head.

Research addressing the validity of these goals is scant. Romney and Gordon (1981) found no statistical significance in the amount of fecal contamination in the first or second stage between the enema and no enema groups. The enemas administered were a low-volume phosphate type. They also described similar duration of labor and occurrence of neonatal infections for both groups. It was noted that when the enema group did pass stool in the second stage, it was in a liquid form and thus more difficult to contain. Whitley and Mack (1980) found the lowest frequency of fecal contamination for those women who did not receive an enema but did report diarrhea within the 24 hours before their admission to the labor unit. Diarrhea is common in early labor because of prostaglandin stimulation of the bowel. More than half of the women who had no enema and no diarrhea passed stool in the second stage, compared with 38 percent of those who did receive an enema. The authors of both studies recommended selective use of enemas for laboring women based on the history of the amount and nature of stools in the 24 hours preceding labor and the amount of stool palpated on the initial pelvic examination.

In debating the clinical value of enemas, the laboring woman's preference will be the deciding factor. For some women, the embarrassment of receiving and expelling an enema may be equal to or greater than that of passing stool during labor or birth. In addition, contamination may be less of a problem when women are allowed to labor and birth in upright positions. Some women prefer to sit on the toilet during the second stage because it is a more natural position for bearing down efforts and embarrassment is avoided if stool is passed. Women with episiotomies or perineal lacerations may be more comfortable in the first day or two post partum if the lower bowel is relatively empty.

If an enema must be given, the procedure and its rationale as well as the sensations she can expect to feel should be explained to the woman. A small Fleet enema is usually used. The woman is placed on her left side and asked to draw her upper knee up to her chest. The tip of the enema is gently inserted into the anus. It is important that the nurse have a good visual field, for many pregnant woman have hemorrhoids that make insertion more difficult. After the fluid has been inserted, the woman is asked to hold it for several minutes before expelling it. If the membranes are intact, the woman may get up to go to the bathroom. If the membranes have ruptured and the head is not well engaged into the pelvis, the woman should remain in bed and use a bedpan for expelling the enema.

The routine use of perineal shaving or "prep" to prepare the woman for birth is also being questioned today. For many years, either a complete or partial shave of the perineal area was done with the rationale that this would prevent infection, facilitate repair of the episiotomy, and improve postpartum hygiene. These benefits have not been found to be improved with shaving, however, and some physicians and nurse-midwives believe that shaving actually increases the risk for infection. As a result, many birth facilities are now doing a small prep, shaving the pubic hair only at the episiotomy site, trimming the pubic hair with scissors, or doing no prep at all. If the prep is to be done, the nurse should explain the procedure and its rationale to the woman, provide privacy, and position her on her back with her legs drawn up and apart. After applying gloves, the nurse uses a soapy solution to lubricate the area, holds the skin taut, and shaves the pubic hair with firm, short strokes. The soap must be removed after the procedure is completed to prevent burning and irritation. A clean, dry pad should be placed under the woman. The prep procedure is embarrassing to most women. The nurse should be sensitive to this, performing the procedure as quickly as possible and providing emotional support.

▼ PROVIDING HYDRATION AND NUTRITION

Labor and birth require hydration and calorie intake to replenish energy expenditure and promote efficient uterine function and general well-being. Controversy exists over the best method to supply these needs. Adequate nutrition and hydration may be accomplished by oral intake of food and fluids, intake of fluids alone, intravenous hydration, or a combination of methods. The most appropriate means of achieving this goal will be influenced by the risk status of the laboring woman, her desires, the length and nature of the labor, the policies of the care providers, the anticipated level of surgical intervention, and the use of analgesia and anesthesia for pain relief.

Historically, when birth in America moved into the hospital in the 1920s, oral intake for laboring women was limited because of the types of drugs administered for pain relief and the use of general anesthesia for vaginal delivery. These restrictions are still common in many labor units today even when surgical intervention is not planned and analgesics and anesthetics are not used (Ludka and Roberts 1993). The risk of gastric aspiration with general anesthesia in the event of an emergency cesarean birth is often given as the rationale for such restrictions. Gastric aspiration is a rare but potentially life-threatening complication of general anesthesia (Douglas 1988).

However, fasting does not preclude the risk of aspiration because even in fasting, the stomach is never entirely empty. Research has demonstrated that gastric volumes vary widely between any two individuals, as does the time it takes to clear a meal from the stomach (McKay and Mahan 1988). Fasting may also cause what remains in the stomach to be more acidic, therefore making aspiration more dangerous. Antacids have been given in labor to counteract this acidity. This practice is also not without drawbacks, as antacids increase stomach volume and can cause rebound acidity (McKay and Mahan 1988). More research is needed to settle the debate over the safety of oral intake in labor. One large series of studies, reported by Haire and Elsberry (1991), showed no gastric aspiration resulting from general anesthesia in almost 30,000 births. The women in these studies were allowed to eat and drink lightly in labor.

There are a number of reasons for initiating intravenous hydration in labor. Dehydration may be corrected by intravenous hydration when oral hydration is either inadequate or not tolerated because of nausea and vomiting. An intravenous line may be initiated if analgesia is desired by this route. It is necessary when epidural anesthesia is administered. Induction or augmentation of labor with oxytocin (Pitocin) requires an intravenous line for administration of the oxytocin. Intravenous access is recommended when medical complications of pregnancy are present and when a high-risk condition exists that increases the chance of an emergency cesarean section. Intravenous access is also recommended when conditions exist that increase the chance of postpartum hemorrhage. Intravenous access may be maintained through the use of a heparin lock when oral hydration is adequate and not contraindicated.

Intravenous hydration is not without risks. There are the potential adverse effects of the intravenous line itself. There may be difficulty with insertion, pain at the insertion site, and the risks of phlebitis and sepsis. An intravenous line may also convey the sick role to both the client and caregivers. An intravenous line causes partial immobilization of the laboring woman, which decreases the ease of using the bathroom and assuming certain positions that may facilitate labor and birth (Newton et al. 1988). Glucose solutions are commonly used for intravenous hydration during labor but have been shown to have several potential drawbacks. Fetal hyperglycemia and hypoglycemia, fetal hypernatremia, neonatal jaundice, and fetal acidosis have all been associated with the use of intravenous glucose solutions during labor (McKay and Mahan 1988; Smith et al. 1993). The nurse's role includes the administration, monitoring, and documentation of intravenous fluids.

▼ PROMOTING ELIMINATION

The bladder continues to fill throughout labor, particularly if the woman is receiving intravenous fluids. A distended bladder can increase the woman's discomfort with contractions, impede descent of the fetus, and result in decreased bladder tone after birth. The woman in labor may be unaware of a full bladder because of the sensations of pain and pressure she experiences with contractions. For these reasons, the nurse should encourage the woman to void every 2 hours. If the membranes are intact, or if they are ruptured but the presenting part is well engaged into the pelvis, the woman can be encouraged to get up to go to the bathroom to void. Not only is it easier for most women to void on the toilet, but going to the bathroom facilitates a change in position, ambulation, and emotional diversion. If the woman has an intravenous line in place, the pole can be moved right into the bathroom with her. If continuous electronic fetal monitoring is being used, the leads can be disconnected for the short time she is in the bathroom. The nurse can encourage the woman to continue the use of breathing techniques and relaxation with contractions while she is sitting on the toilet. If the membranes are ruptured and the head is not engaged, the woman should remain in bed and void into a bedpan. It helps if the bed is raised so that the woman is sitting up as much as possible. It is also important to provide as much privacy as possible during this time. If the woman is unable to void and it is obvious by observation or palpation that the bladder is full, catheterization may be necessary.

▼ PROVIDING PHYSICAL AND EMOTIONAL COMFORT AND SUPPORT

Physical support during labor includes a number of comfort measures and coaching strategies. Emotional support encompasses such factors as acceptance, understanding, continuous uninterrupted physical presence, and encouragement and praise (Chalmers and Wolman 1993). All these components of the supportive role during labor and birth have been shown to have a major impact on the outcome of the childbirth experience (Hodnett and Osborn 1989a, 1989b; Kennell et al. 1991; Klaus et al. 1992). In fact, one aspect of the childbirth experience that women remember for many years is the nature of the support they received from the nurses who cared for them (Simkin 1991; Bryanton et al. 1994; Mackey and Stepans 1994). The need for the various components of supportive nursing care will change as the labor progresses, for the woman's needs are different in each phase or stage of labor.

Early-Phase Labor. Unless there is a health problem or labor is being induced, health care providers and childbirth educators instruct women to stay at home as long as possible during early or latent labor. Primiparous women are told to come to the hospital or birth center when the contractions have established a regular pattern at a 5-minute interval or if the membranes rupture spontaneously. Multiparous women may be asked to arrive when the contractions are 10 to 15 minutes apart, on the basis of previous labor history. It is advisable for the woman to spend as much of early labor at home as possible, for there she can be more comfortable, be mobile, and find many things to distract and entertain herself. If she arrives at the birth setting too early, she becomes apprehensive and more uncomfortable, and the likelihood of medical interventions increases. Admission to the birth setting is a time of excitement and apprehension, for although the woman is usually eager to give birth to her baby, she may have concerns about the nature of the labor that lies ahead or the interventions she may encounter. The first stressful period in labor often occurs at this time when the reality of the onset of labor is realized.

The nurse's supportive role in early labor includes a number of interventions (see Table 23–3). It is important to make the woman and her family feel welcome, comfortable, and accepted when they arrive at the birth setting. The first few minutes of interaction with the woman can decrease the initial stress she may be feeling and set the tone for her comfort and trust for the remainder of the labor. If the nurse is cold, abrupt, or irritable, the woman will feel defensive and more apprehensive. In addition to all of the assessment activities discussed earlier in this chapter, the nurse should spend as much time as possible with the woman to establish a positive relationship. The woman and her family are usually responsive to teaching at this time, so a major role of the nurse is to identify what they need to know and share that information with them. For example, the nurse should teach the woman and her partner about expected contraction patterns, timing contractions, changes throughout labor that indicate progress (effacement, dilatation, station), coping strategies and comfort measures, expected interventions (intravenous line, fetal monitor), and options for medication and anesthesia. The nurse should encourage the woman to be up and about if possible, either in her room or walking in the hall. Diversional activities should also be encouraged. For example, the nurse might suggest that the woman and her support person play cards, listen to music, or watch television.

If the woman is tense, frightened, or in pain, a soothing back rub might help her relax. If contractions are causing discomfort, the nurse should help the woman relax her muscles during the contraction by using soothing verbal cues (e.g., "Release the tension in your face; relax your arms and hands.") or by gently massaging tense muscles. If the woman has had childbirth preparation, the nurse should remind her to begin slow-paced breathing if needed; if the woman has had no previous preparation, the nurse can begin to teach slow-paced breathing with each contraction. It helps for the nurse to do the breathing with the woman for a few contractions until she feels comfortable with it (see Chapter 20). The nurse should give feedback after each contraction (e.g., "You did very well with that contraction; your muscles were more relaxed."). The nurse should also periodically ask for feedback from the woman regarding the effectiveness of her comfort measures (e.g., "Is the massage helping? Do you like this position? Does it help to have me breathe with you?").

Active-Phase Labor. As the woman moves into active labor, her need for comfort measures and physical and emotional support increases as the work of labor increases and the contractions become painful (see Table 23–3). Physical support includes strategies that will help to relieve discomfort, such as massage, relaxation and visualization, patterned breathing, hydrotherapy, position changes, or use of hot packs or ice packs. These nonpharmacologic methods of pain relief are discussed in Chapter 24. Women should continue to be encouraged to ambulate, for the ability to cope with discomfort decreases with limited mobility. Back rubs at regular intervals, either between or during contractions, help relieve pain that may be caused by pressure from the baby's head on the sacrum. Basic hygiene should not be overlooked in the excitement of labor. The mother should be kept clean and dry. If she is perspiring, her gown should be changed frequently. A cold, moist washcloth can be placed on her forehead or used to wipe her face and hands. The bed should be kept dry, particularly if she is having large amounts of bloody show or her membranes have ruptured and she is leaking amniotic fluid. Oral hygiene, in the form of mouthwash, should be offered regularly to help her feel fresh. Ice chips also help to keep her mouth moist and can usually be offered if all is progressing normally.

The second stressful point in the labor occurs as the contractions in the active phase increase in their intensity and regularity. Attention-focusing strategies, such as a visual focus, counting with breathing, or music, should be encouraged. Verbal coaching during contractions becomes even more helpful to many women in active labor, and although the woman's partner may have been taught to provide this coaching in childbirth classes, the nurse may need to provide additional help at times. The nurse can move in to assist with coaching if needed during a contraction and then step back when the contraction is over. Verbal coaching might include the following: directive cues to remind her how to relax, do a breathing technique, or concentrate on a focus; calling out 15-second intervals so that she is aware how the contraction is progressing; and praise and encouragement about how well she is doing. As the woman becomes more serious and inwardly focused on her labor, the support persons should avoid extraneous conversation and focus only on the woman and her needs. The nurse should also provide support to the woman's partner throughout active labor. This might include teaching, assistance with coaching, a back rub, suggestions for helping the woman, or encouragement to take a break to meet personal needs.

Transition-Phase Labor. Comfort, support, and encouragement become essential during transition, for this is usually the most stressful time in the labor. The woman experiences the most painful sensations, is fatigued, and may feel that she cannot go on (see Table 23–3). Physical comfort measures include those already discussed for early and active labor. Emotional support and coaching are often the critical factors to help the woman through this difficult time. Constant presence is essential so that the woman does not panic and feel abandoned. A calm attitude of the nurse and support person also helps to keep the woman calm. Coaching during a contraction must now be firm and directive (e.g., "Watch me, breathe with me; 1–2–3–4, in–out, in–out; keep going; release the muscles in your face and shoulders."). The nurse or support person should move in close and use firm but gentle touch, either holding her hand or placing the hands on either side of her face or

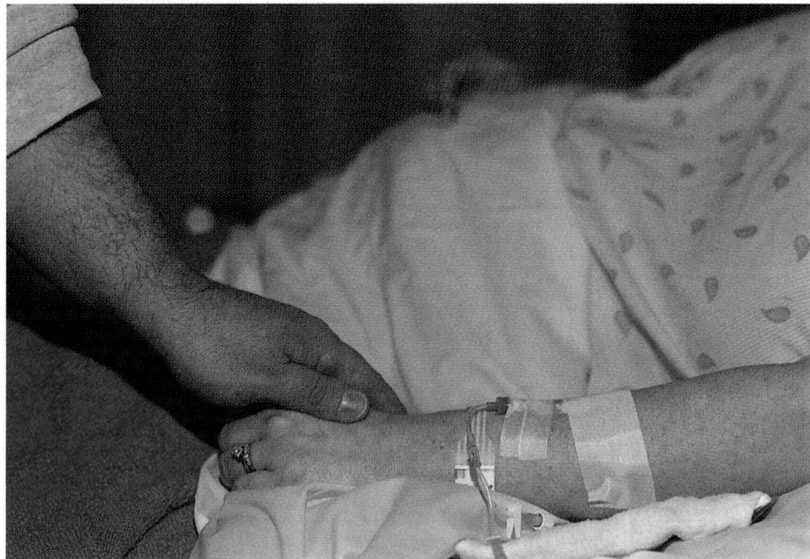

Figure 23–7
The father or other family member can provide emotional support for the woman in labor by just being there with her; holding her hand helps her to know that she is loved and not alone.

shoulders (Fig. 23–7). Establishing eye contact during a contraction is important to keep her focused on what she is being told to do. Encouragement, praise, and reassurance are also helpful. The woman needs to be reminded often that the first stage of labor is almost over, that the contractions will not get any stronger, and that she is doing well. Rather than focusing on how much longer the labor will last, she should be encouraged to focus only on one contraction at a time. Anything the nurse or partner tells her during transition needs to be repeated regularly, for she may have difficulty remembering.

Second-Stage Labor. If the woman experiences a latent phase at the beginning of the second stage and does not initially have an urge to push, she should be allowed to rest and breathe through the contractions for a time. As the urge to push increases, the woman begins her pushing efforts, and the focus of coaching shifts to the work of expulsion. These first few pushing contractions can be stressful, because the initial bearing down sensations that the woman feels may be overwhelming. The nurse or labor partner should provide clear direction as to what she is to do during a contraction (e.g., "Take a couple of slow breaths, in–out, in–out; inhale and slowly blow out the air as you tighten your abdominal muscles and bear down; push, push, keep going; take in another breath."). Encouragement and praise continue to be important, particularly as the baby's head begins to be seen at the vaginal introitus and crowning occurs. The sensations of pressure, stretching, and burning that the woman feels may frighten her at first. She needs to be reminded that these are normal sensations and that her body will accommodate the baby. It is sometimes helpful to encourage the woman by taking her hand to feel the baby crowning at the pelvic floor. This often gives her a sense of the reality of the baby as the cause of her sensations and gives her encouragement to continue. As the head is delivered, the woman should be coached to use blowing to prevent bearing down. This allows the birth attendant to deliver the head more slowly and gently. Physical comfort measures are important in the second stage of labor, for pushing is hard work and the woman is usually warm and perspiring. A cool washcloth after every contraction will feel wonderful. The bed should be kept clean and dry, for bloody show may increase along with the leaking of amniotic fluid.

Third- and Fourth-Stage Labor. After the birth of the baby, the woman needs continual coaching for the delivery of the placenta, the examination of the genital tract, and the repair of the episiotomy or lacerations. The relaxation and breathing strategies used throughout first-stage labor will be useful for these discomforts. The need for emotional support in the third and fourth stages of labor usually decreases. The woman may still need reassurance that everything is going well. If there were aspects of the labor or birth that did not meet the woman's expectations, the nurse should listen, accept her concerns, provide factual information, and offer reassurance. The woman should be praised for her hard work and her accomplishment in giving birth. Physical comfort is provided by helping the woman wash her face and hands, comb her hair, and put on a clean gown. The nurse should wash the perineal area and provide clean peripads as necessary. If the woman is experiencing pain after the delivery, relaxation and breathing techniques can still be used and medication can be administered.

▼ USING AMBULATION AND POSITIONING DURING LABOR AND BIRTH

Ambulation during labor has many benefits. It facilitates progress of labor by stimulating more

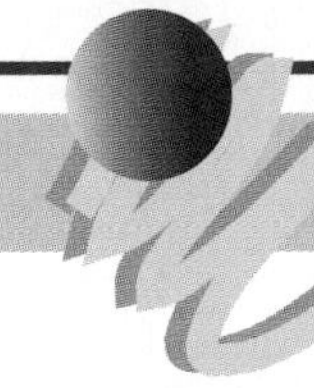

TEACHING GUIDE

MEASURING PROGRESS IN LABOR

TOPIC	*MAJOR CONCEPTS*
Definition of true labor	True labor occurs when regular uterine contractions cause progressive effacement and dilatation of the cervix. Contractions decrease in frequency and increase in intensity and duration. Pelvic pressure may be experienced along with an increase in vaginal discharge, loss of the mucous plug, bloody show, and rupture of the membranes. True labor is not affected by changes in position or activity.
Definition of false labor	In contrast, false labor is a period of irregular contractions that do not progress in their frequency, intensity, or duration. These contractions are also known as Braxton Hicks contractions. There are no cervical changes such as effacement or dilatation. False labor is often stopped by changing position or activity. Teach your client to notify her health care provider if she thinks she is in labor; the health care provider can help evaluate whether the labor is true or false.
Stages and phases of labor	Labor is divided into four stages. The first is called the dilatation stage. This is the longest period (8 to 10 hours), when contractions cause the cervix to efface (thin) to 100 percent and dilate (open) to 10 cm. First-stage labor is subdivided into three phases: (1) early or latent phase, marked by 0 to 3 cm of dilatation; (2) active phase, marked by dilatation from 4 to 7 cm; and (3) transition phase, marked by dilatation from 8 to 10 cm. The second stage of labor is called the expulsion stage. This stage lasts 1 to 2 hours and requires the woman to push with the contractions to expel the baby. The third stage of labor is called the placental stage. This stage lasts about 5 to 10 minutes, during which the placenta separates from the wall of the uterus and is expelled from the uterus aided by the woman's pushing. The fourth stage of labor is composed of the first hour post partum (after delivery), when the woman's body begins to readjust and relax. During this period, the parents may begin to get to know their baby.

Continued on following page

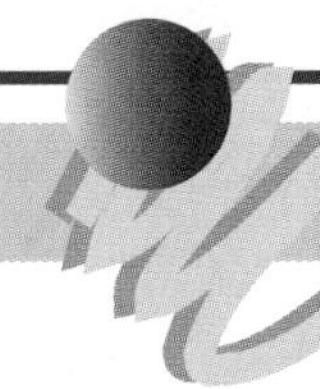

TEACHING GUIDE Continued

MEASURING PROGRESS IN LABOR

TOPIC	*MAJOR CONCEPTS*
How labor progress is measured	During labor, contractions are timed and the woman is examined vaginally to monitor her progress. Progress is measured through • Contraction pattern: The frequency, duration, and intensity of contractions are recorded. At the beginning of labor, contractions are about 5 to 10 minutes apart; they gradually get closer together until a 2-minute interval is established. Contractions last 30 to 45 seconds during beginning labor, gradually increasing to 60 to 90 seconds. The intensity of the contractions also increases from early sensations of pressure or cramping to painful sensations. • Cervical consistency and effacement: The cervix will change from firm to soft consistency and from being long (or thick) to flat (or thin) against the uterus. • Cervical dilatation: The cervix may be closed at the onset of labor and opens to 10 cm by the end of the first stage. • Station: The station charts the fetal movement through the pelvis; zero represents the halfway mark. Above the halfway point, the fetus is at a minus station (−1 to −5); below the halfway point, the fetus is at a plus station (+1 to +5).
Ways to facilitate labor progress	Instruct your client that she can help her labor progress by working with her contractions rather than against them. She should relax her muscles during and between contractions, do paced breathing techniques during contractions, focus on a visual image, walk, change position regularly, listen to music, and communicate with her labor partner and nurse. These actions will help her body work effectively to give birth to her baby.

Continued on facing page

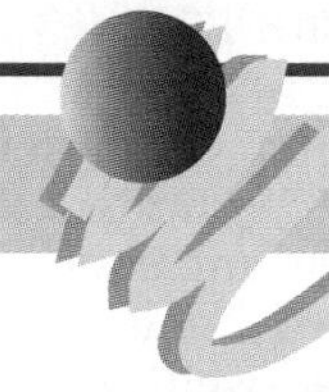

TEACHING GUIDE Continued

Teaching Aids

1. Pamphlets, booklets, or handouts defining true labor, false labor, and preterm labor
2. Pamphlets or handouts explaining the stages and phases of labor
3. Three-dimensional cervical effacement and dilatation chart
4. Bony pelvis model and doll to illustrate station.

Increasing Your Teaching Effectiveness

Your teaching about labor progress will be enhanced by using the following approaches.

1. Identify what your client knows about signs of normal labor; contrast this knowledge with information about false labor and the signs of preterm labor.
2. Ask for frequent feedback and clarification of your client's understanding of these differences. Allow ample time for her questions.
3. Show your client how to time and record contractions, including frequency and duration.
4. Go through the pamphlets and brochures with your client, rather than just handing them to her to take home and read.
5. Encourage your client to examine the three-dimensional cervical effacement and dilatation chart to help her understand how the cervix changes during labor.
6. Encourage your client to examine the bony pelvis model and doll to help her understand the concept of station.

effective contractions, increases the pressure of the presenting part against the cervix to facilitate effacement and dilatation, and promotes rotation and descent. It may promote comfort (although at times it may increase discomfort) and offers diversion and stimulation. Ambulation can be encouraged if the membranes are intact or if the fetal presenting part is well engaged into the pelvis if membranes have ruptured. Many women find it beneficial to walk during early and even active labor. It is the responsibility of the nurse to suggest walking and assist the woman as needed, for the woman in labor may not think of this option. If the woman has an intravenous line inserted, the pole can be taken with her as she ambulates. If electronic fetal monitoring is being used, the leads can be disconnected for short intervals of time if the fetal heart rate and variability are normal. Ambulation should not be used if the woman has had medication or if there is concern regarding maternal or fetal status.

The use of a variety of positions for labor and birth has been studied. The importance of positioning and a brief review of the research related to positions in labor are presented in Chapter 22. It is the nurse's responsibility to become aware of the variety of positions that can be used and the benefits and detriments of each (see Fig. 22–11). The nurse will need to initiate position changes throughout labor, for the laboring woman may not think of altering her position, particularly if she is uncomfortable. It is a good idea to suggest a position change every hour. By moving regularly, the labor is facilitated, the woman can be helped to find positions that promote increased comfort, and muscle fatigue is decreased. Pillows can be used to support various positions and provide comfort.

▼ PROVIDING EDUCATION AND INFORMATION

Teaching, counseling, and support of the need for information during labor and birth should be an ongoing nursing intervention (McNiven et al. 1992; Evans and Jeffrey 1995). During labor, even women who have taken prepared childbirth education classes benefit from reminders of what is normally occurring in their bodies. Often the woman may understand, but her partner or other family members need the teaching. Families should be encouraged to exercise their options during the labor and birth process and voice their choices in ways to individualize the birth experience. When specific interventions are necessary, they should be presented to the woman and explained, and then the woman should be given the opportunity to ask questions before the intervention is performed. Results of interventions or testing should be explained in a way the laboring family can understand. The Teaching Guide: Measuring Progress in Labor gives an example of how to provide information to parents about the process of labor.

▼ ESTABLISHING A POSITIVE ENVIRONMENT

The traditional American model of hospital birth has involved strict distinctions between areas for labor, delivery, recovery, postpartum stay, and nursery. Nursing staff provided task-oriented care with separate staffs for each area. In the past 25 years, birth rooms for labor and birth and in-hospital birth centers, in which all events occur in the same room, have gained acceptance. In-hospital birth centers typically feature a homelike atmosphere, and the limited use of technology may require transfer to a more traditional unit if complications arise or technologic intervention is desired. Out-of-hospital or freestanding birth centers exist in many areas of the United States.

Birth rooms are used for labor and birth and may also be used for the immediate recovery period; in this case, they may be called LDR (labor, delivery, recovery) rooms. In some institutions, these rooms are also used for the postpartum stay, and the infant remains with the mother rather than being relocated to the nursery; in this case, they may be called LDRP (labor, delivery, recovery, postpartum stay) rooms. Birth rooms commonly allow the use of fetal monitoring, and birthing beds in many institutions accommodate the practitioner's use of vacuum extractors or forceps.

Birth rooms and centers offer holistic, family-oriented care that is advantageous to the woman, her family, and the nursing staff. Family involvement and infant bonding are promoted when care is integrated into a single unit with a limited number of nurses involved. This continuity is generally more satisfying to the woman, her family, and the nursing staff, and a more efficient model of care can be provided. In addition, a woman is spared the disruption of transfer to the delivery room, which usually occurs at a critical time in a woman's concentration in the second stage of labor.

Researchers have compared maternal and fetal outcomes for conventional labor and delivery units with outcomes for birth rooms or birth centers. In general, women using birth rooms or birth centers reported increased satisfaction with their birth experience compared with those birthing in traditional units (Bradley et al. 1990). Birth center clients have lower rates of episiotomy and higher rates of intact perineums (Chapman et al. 1986). Cesarean birth rates have been reported to be lower for birth center clients in all but a few studies (Albers and Katz 1991; Albers and Savitz 1991). Infants born in either setting have comparable Apgar scores and rates of morbidity, although two studies have shown increased numbers of neonatal special care unit admissions for those infants born in conventional labor units (Albers and Katz 1991; Waskerwitz et al. 1985).

▼ FACILITATING THE ROLE OF THE BIRTH PARTNER

For many years after birth moved into the hospital in the 1920s, a woman was not permitted to have her husband, a family member, or any support person with her during labor and birth. The strict sterile environment of the hospital as well as the use of a great deal of medication and anesthesia made the presence of a birth partner undesirable. With the natural childbirth movement in the 1950s and 1960s, the importance of a caring person to support the laboring woman began to be recognized as essential to the emotional experience of birth. In most birth settings today, the woman's labor companion is welcomed. Several research studies have now shown that the presence of a continuous support person with a woman in labor can decrease the length of labor, the need for medication, the rate of perinatal complications, and the frequency of cesarean birth (Hodnett and Osborn 1989a, 1989b; Kennell et al. 1991; Klaus et al. 1992).

Although the nurse is ultimately responsible for all aspects of the woman's care throughout labor, the birth partner can be helped to assume some of the coaching and emotional support. Unlike the nurse, who more than likely will have other laboring women to attend to, the birth partner can stay with the woman continuously and offer her uninterrupted attention. If the woman attended childbirth classes, the birth partner more than likely attended them with her and knows the relaxation and breathing pain management strategies she has learned. The partner will therefore have some knowledge of how to coach her through her contractions. The birth partner is likely to be someone who has love for and understanding of the woman and can help to meet her emotional needs. He or she can help to communicate the woman's needs and desires to the nursing staff.

Some parents may decide to hire a doula to provide additional labor support. A doula is a woman who has been trained to provide continuous physical, emotional, and informational support to a woman, before, during, and just after childbirth (Klaus et al 1992, 1993). The role of the doula has evolved during the past decade in response to the increasing demands on the time of staff nurses during labor and birth, often prohibiting the nurse from staying with a laboring woman continuously. The doula role is not an attempt to interfere with the relationship between the woman and her partner or other family members. She is present to be a nurturing, helpful, and objective female supporter so that the family member chosen to be present does not have sole responsibility for the labor. In addition, the doula does not interfere with the role of the nurse but works with the nurse to expand the care being given. The doula is not responsible for any nursing assessments (e.g., maternal vital signs, fetal heart tones), nursing or medical interventions other than labor support, or documentation. The doula does assist with emotional support (e.g., teaching, encouragement, praise), nonpharmacologic pain management strategies (e.g., massage, breathing, position changes), and comfort measures (e.g., hygiene, ice chips).

However, it is important that the nurse not rely on the labor partner or assume that the nurse's presence or support is not still needed. The woman's partner or family member occasionally needs nursing support to help the laboring woman. The labor companion may feel overwhelmed, frightened, or fatigued. The nurse's role is to assess the needs, involvement, and comfort of the labor partner by observing the interaction between the woman and her companion. Some companions readily take an active role in meeting the woman's needs, while others seem to step back and assume an observer role. On the basis of these observations, the nurse will decide the best approach to take in working along with the labor partner and involving him or her in the experience. The nurse either functions as a facilitator to help the labor companion help the woman or steps in to serve a more active role, allowing the labor partner to take a secondary role. Just as continuous teaching is essential for the woman throughout labor, it is also necessary for the labor partner. The nurse should explain everything that takes place. The labor partner's physical and emotional needs also need to be considered. The partner should be encouraged to take an occasional break, eat, and rest. An awareness of emotional needs can be met by occasionally asking, "How are you doing? What are you feeling now? What can I do to help you?" The labor partner needs reinforcement and praise, just as the laboring woman does. By saying, "You are doing such a good job supporting your wife," "Your daughter is lucky to have you with her," or "I really appreciate your help," you can build the labor partner's self-confidence and self-esteem.

Other family members may also be involved throughout the birth experience. Although one primary labor support person is usually involved with the woman during labor, other family members may also be present at the birth setting. These family members can be helped to feel included by keeping them informed of the woman's progress, making it possible for them to see the woman occasionally, or encouraging them to relieve the primary labor partner at intervals. In some birth settings, family members, including the woman's other children, can join the woman and her labor partner for the birth if they desire. Childbirth is an empowering experience for both the woman and her family. The nurse's involvement of the birth partner and other family members, and her response to the woman and her family during the labor and birth, can greatly enhance the impact of this experience.

▼ PROVIDING CONTINUOUS DOCUMENTATION

Documentation of the progress of labor and the events that occur in relation to that progress is an essential component of the nurse's role during childbirth. Documentation is essential not only as a means of recording the important data necessary to guide the plan of care but also as a means of documenting care that is given and creating a legal record of the events of the labor and birth. If the events during the labor or birth and the care given during that time are not recorded, they are not considered by the courts as having taken place. After the woman has been admitted to the birth setting and the initial assessment has been recorded, a continuous record should be initiated. The data that should be recorded at regular intervals include maternal vital signs, fetal heart rate, contraction pattern, results of abdominal and pelvic examinations (cervical status; fetal descent, position, and presentation), status of membranes, laboratory data, hydration, elimination, pain or comfort level, medication or anesthesia, and maternal coping. Records for documentation vary according to the birth setting. A flow chart is usually used, and many settings now also use a labor graph (see Fig. 23–3) to plot the progress of labor. A separate record is usually used for the delivery, which includes information such as the type of delivery, episiotomy, medication or anesthesia, time of birth, sex of infant, newborn assessment, and maternal assessment (see Nursing Care Planning Guide: Normal Childbirth, pp. 790–822).

▼ PREPARATION FOR THE BIRTH

As the birth of the baby becomes imminent, the nurse needs to carry out several activities in preparation. If not already present, the birth attendant is notified. This should be done about 1 hour before the nurse's estimated time of delivery, depending on the rate of labor progress and whether the woman is primiparous or multiparous. If the birth will take place in the labor and birthing room (LDR), the woman will not have to be moved, and a calm atmosphere can be maintained. Equipment or supplies that are not already in the room will be brought in, such as a delivery cart with the sterile delivery pack (including drapes, gown, towels, gloves, scissors, clamps, sutures, perineal prep set, placenta basin, bulb syringe, and baby blanket and cap), radiant-heated infant warmer, newborn suction equipment (including DeLee suction trap, laryngoscope, endotracheal tubes, and bag resuscitation set), infant identification equipment and prophylactic eye treatment, additional light source if needed for good visibility, and items for birth attendants to

Guidelines for Sterile Technique in the Labor/Delivery Suite

All items to be used in a delivery have been sterilized, including linens, instruments, sutures, dressings, and gloves. If there is any doubt as to the sterility of an item, consider it unsterile.

- Doubt sterility if the expiration date is illegible, if sterile gear is left uncovered and unguarded, or if an unsterile person passes too close to sterile items.
- When removing a cover from a table of instruments, do not let the edges that have been hanging down drag along the sterile field. It is best to remove a cover with two people, one on either end to lift and carry it away.
- Do not place items that have fallen below waist level back onto the sterile field. Open a new sterile packet and either flip the item onto the field or let the sterile person grasp it from within the package.

Persons who are sterile touch only sterile items. Sterile persons work over sterile areas and should avoid reaching over unsterile areas.

- When draping an unsterile area, such as a patient's abdomen, sterile persons cover the area closest to them first.
- Do not allow your hands to drop below waist level.
- Never cross your arms and place hands in the axillary area.
- Sterile persons pass "back-to-back."
- Sterile persons stay within a sterile area.
- Do not lean with your elbows on a sterile field.
- Scrub your hands before participating in a sterile procedure.

Persons who are unsterile touch only unsterile items. Unsterile persons never reach over a sterile area.

- Pour water and saline into basins without splashing, reaching over, or touching the basin.
- Assist the surgical team to gown by tying the back of the gown and handing the tie for the front of the gown to the sterile person by holding onto and discarding the paper tab.
- To pass sutures onto a sterile field, pull apart the outer packaging and flip the inner suture pack onto the sterile field without touching or leaning over the table.
- Allow a wide margin of safety around sterile areas and always face the sterile area when passing.
- Never move between two sterile fields.

When cleaning, whether it is the patient or the delivery suite, work from clean to dirty.

- When prepping for a vaginal delivery, start at the top of the symphysis pubis and wipe once downward on the left side toward the rectum. With a second sponge, wipe once downward on the right side. With the final sponge, wipe once down the center.
- For a cesarean birth, scrub with prep solution in a circular motion starting at the incision site and working toward the periphery. Each time the periphery is reached, use a new sponge. Blot the area with a sterile towel. Clean the umbilicus separately with a cotton-tipped applicator or 4 × 4.

Air currents provide mobility for bacteria and dust to move about freely in the air.

- All personnel in the delivery suite wear masks, caps to cover all hair and earrings, and shoe covers.
- Masks must cover the nose and mouth at all times.
- Do not shake, flip, or throw linen, as this will add dust and lint particles to the air.
- Keep doors to the delivery suite closed and avoid needless opening or swinging of the doors.

wear for universal precautions against body substances (gloves, plastic apron, and glasses or goggles). The birthing bed will be adapted for delivery by removing the lower portion and adding stirrups if needed. If additional family members plan to attend the birth, they will be notified and welcomed. They should be asked to wash their hands, but usually they do not have to wear sterile attire.

If the woman must be transferred to a traditional delivery room, the nurse assists in her transfer by labor bed or cart. Once in the delivery room, the woman is helped to move from the cart to the delivery table. If at all possible, the movement of the woman from one place to another should be done between contractions. The equipment for the delivery is usually already in the delivery room, so the nurse needs to check to see that all is ready and in working order. A sterile environment is maintained in a traditional delivery room, so the support person and any other family members must wear scrub suits, disposable shoe covers, caps, and masks (see Guidelines for Sterile Technique in the Labor/Delivery Suite).

Just before the birth, the nurse will cleanse the woman's perineum, pubic area, and inner thighs with a soapy cleansing solution. This is done to remove bloody discharge that may have accumulated during labor. A sterile prep bowl containing several gauze sponges is used for this procedure. A clean sponge is used for each area. The nurse should be careful not to carry material from outer areas to the vaginal orifice. Outer areas are cleansed first, and the vulvar area is cleansed last. If any soapy solution remains after the prep is completed, it is often poured over the vulvar area. When doing the perineal prep or preparing the delivery cart and pack, the nurse should use aseptic technique.

▼ IMMEDIATE CARE OF THE WOMAN AFTER BIRTH

Nursing responsibilities during the third stage of labor include assistance of the woman in the expulsion of the placenta, administration of oxytocic agents, massage of the uterine fundus to aid contractility if necessary, collection of arterial or venous samples from the umbilical cord, and provision of the necessary supplies if suturing is required for repair of an episiotomy or lacerations. When signs of placental separation have occurred, the nurse instructs the woman to bear down just as she did in the second stage of labor. The woman may experience a sensation of cramping and pressure at this time. The level and consistency of the uterine fundus are evaluated by the nurse or birth attendant as soon as the placenta is expelled. Pitocin, a synthetic form of oxytocin, is administered prophylactically in many settings either intravenously (10 units in 500 mL of intravenous fluid or 20 units in 1 L of intravenous fluid) or intramuscularly (10 units) as soon as the placenta is delivered to enhance uterine contractility and minimize blood loss. Oxytocin is the drug of choice for this purpose because it causes intermittent uterine contractions and does not affect the blood pressure. Methergine (methylergonovine maleate), a synthetic ergot preparation, is a stronger agent that is also used to contract the uterus. Methergine is administered intramuscularly. It causes constant uterine contractions and may elevate the blood pressure. It is contraindicated in women who have pregnancy-induced hypertension or are at risk for pregnancy-induced hypertension.

Neither Methergine nor Pitocin should be given by intravenous push (Varney 1987). Some practitioners prefer to consider a woman's risk for postpartum hemorrhage before routinely administering oxytocics. If a woman plans to breastfeed, the oxytocin released from the posterior pituitary, which is stimulated by suckling, will aid in contracting the uterus, and some birth attendants will forgo use of oxytocin. Umbilical cord blood samples are collected for determination of blood type and Rh factor, VDRL (Venereal Disease Research Laboratory) screening for syphilis, and blood gas analysis. After the delivery is completed, the nurse gently cleanses the vulvar area and applies a perineal pad. The woman is helped from the delivery position she has assumed into a more comfortable position in bed, given a dry gown and linen, and given the baby to hold if there are no contraindications. If family members have not been present for the delivery, they are invited to join the woman and her birth partner to see the baby.

The primary nursing function during the fourth stage of labor is regular assessment. These assessments have been discussed earlier in this chapter. Other nursing interventions are also needed in this first hour after delivery. If necessary, the uterine fundus should be massaged at intervals during the fourth stage of labor to prevent hemorrhage. This should be done only if the fundus is above the umbilicus in the first hour after delivery or if it feels soft and boggy. With one hand supporting the lower uterine segment, the other hand is used to gently massage the top, sides, and front of the fundus by moving the flaccid abdominal wall over the fundus. If increased lochial flow results, the massage may be performed with increased pressure to ensure that the uterus is firm and free of large clots. Appropriate education for the woman includes demonstrating fundal massage to the mother so that she may do this herself; giving information about the amount, color, and consistency of lochial flow during the first day post partum; and teaching the importance of emptying the bladder at regular intervals to maintain a well-contracted uterus and prevent complications such as urinary retention. Comfort measures for uterine cramping may be discussed, such as analgesics, warm packs, and ambulation.

Other nursing interventions during the fourth stage of labor include maintenance of fluid balance and nutrition, promotion of elimination, maintenance of comfort and safety, and promotion of hygiene. Many women are hungry after the birth, particularly if they have not eaten throughout labor. If there are no complications from the delivery (e.g., blood loss, general anesthesia), the woman can be offered fluids and light nourishment (e.g., crackers, cookies, Jell-O) immediately and then can begin a regular diet at the next meal. If an intravenous line is in place, it will be maintained until the infusion is completed. This is particularly true if Pitocin has been added to the bag to stimulate uterine contraction. The nurse should continue to monitor intake and output during the fourth stage of labor. The woman should be encouraged to void as soon as possible after delivery, for the bladder may be full if several hours have passed since the last voiding. The status of the bladder can be assessed along with the assessment of the fundus. If the bladder is full, it will displace the uterus upward and to the right of the midline. A distended bladder can prevent uterine contraction, increase bleeding, and contribute to atony and urinary retention.

Most women experience little discomfort during the fourth stage of labor; however, they may begin to notice the sensations of the uterus contracting down in size as it begins the process of involution. These sensations are called afterpains and feel like strong menstrual cramps. Multiparous women may notice more discomfort than primiparous women because the uterus has to contract harder. The nurse can try a number of comfort measures to relieve the pain the woman may experience. The relaxation and breathing used throughout labor can be continued. Helping the woman to void so that the bladder is empty will promote relief. A warm blanket over the abdomen often feels good. A routine order for analgesics will be written by the birth attendant and can be given if other measures do not help. Providing information about the cause of the pain decreases anxiety and promotes an understanding of the physiologic processes behind the discomfort.

The woman may also experience pain from the site of the episiotomy. This usually feels like a burning or throbbing sensation. Ice packs can be applied to decrease pain and edema. Anesthetic sprays or ointments can also be ordered by the physician or nurse-midwife. Application of these agents to the episiotomy site will relieve discomfort. If the woman has hemorrhoids, these may add to the perineal discomfort, for they become tender and edematous as a result of the woman's pushing efforts during the second stage of labor. Many women experience postpartum shivering, although not as a result of being cold. This phenomenon is thought to be related to the sudden decrease in intra-abdominal pressure or a reaction to the stress of labor. Warm blankets usually relieve this discomfort, and it will usually resolve within an hour or so. A final discomfort that may be experienced in the fourth stage of labor is seen in women who have regional anesthesia. As the anesthetic begins to wear off, some women describe a prickly, tingling sensation in the toes, feet, and legs. The nurse should prepare the woman for this sensation before its occurrence and reassure her that it is normal.

The provision of safety is important in the fourth stage of labor. If the woman has had recent analgesic medication, if she has had a general anesthetic, or even if her regional anesthetic makes it difficult for her to move, the side rails of her bed should be raised. The woman may wish to get up to go to the bathroom during this time. This is possible within the first hour after birth if she has not had regional anesthesia. Otherwise, she will need to wait until the anesthetic has completely worn off and she has regained full movement of her legs. Before the first ambulation, the nurse should assess the woman's vital signs and evaluate the labor and birth record to ensure that there are no contraindications. It is a good idea to have her sit on the edge of the bed for a few minutes before getting up, for some women experience dizziness from orthostatic hypotension on rising. It is essential that the nurse accompany the woman to the bathroom, for no matter how well she thinks she feels, she may be wobbly or fatigued as she walks for the first time after the birth. The nurse should carry an aromatic ammonia ampule in case the woman does become dizzy. The nurse needs to stay close by the entire time the woman is in the bathroom and ensure that she returns to bed safely. If the woman has her baby with her during the fourth stage of labor, the nurse (or the labor partner) must stay with her to ensure that the baby is held securely at all times. This is particularly true if the woman is fatigued from a long labor or has had recent medication. The side rails of the bed should be raised to protect the baby.

Another important nursing intervention during this time is the provision of cleanliness and hygiene. Labor is hard work. Perspiration, bloody show, and amniotic fluid make the desire for a bath paramount in the woman's mind after birth. Although a shower or bath is not usually feasible in the fourth stage, the nurse can provide the opportunity for the woman to wash her hands and face, use mouthwash, and comb her hair. The nurse should give perineal care, which not only contributes to the woman's comfort but also prevents infection. Clean perineal pads should be provided as necessary.

The final nursing intervention for the fourth stage of labor is to meet the woman's emotional needs. The woman may be excited and want to talk during this time. This helps her to integrate and accept what has just happened. She may express a great deal of disbelief, for even though she knew for 9 months that she would give birth to a baby, it is an amazing experience to make a transition in a period of about 12 hours from being pregnant to having a baby in her arms. She often has a need to relive the events of the past hours, sometimes in great detail. The nurse can be supportive by showing a willingness to listen and share in the excitement of the birth. Although the nurse has heard "birth stories" many times before, this is only the woman's first (or second, or third) birth experience and she needs to talk about it. If the woman was disappointed about any aspect of her birth experience, she will need to ventilate about that as well. The nurse can be most helpful by showing acceptance and understanding. Not all women are euphoric after their birth. Some women may be more quiet and withdrawn, depending on the amount of anesthesia, the level of their fatigue, the circumstances surrounding the birth, or cultural influences.

▼ IMMEDIATE ASSESSMENT AND CARE OF THE NEWBORN

The nurse who has been caring for the woman during labor and birth is usually responsible for the immediate assessment of the newborn. In some settings, a nurse from the newborn nursery may attend the birth to assume this responsibility. This initial assessment begins at the moment of birth and continues until it is established that the infant is stable. The assessment can take place while the baby is on the woman's abdomen immediately after delivery; in the radiant-heated warmer; or, if there are no concerns about the infant's status, while the infant is being held by the parents. The following components are an essential part of this initial assessment.

Initiation of Respirations. As the infant is delivered, the birth attendant begins the process of establishing a patent airway by wiping secretions from the face and suctioning the nose and mouth with a bulb syringe. The nurse continues this activity as soon as the birth attendant places the newborn in the warmer. The newborn is placed on his or her side in a modified Trendelenburg position to assist with the drainage of mucus. If continuing suctioning is needed, a bulb syringe or DeLee mucus trap is used to remove secretions from the nose or oropharynx (see Procedure 32–1).

Body Temperature. After respirations are established, the second priority is to maintain the newborn's body temperature. The nurse should dry the newborn immediately. Body temperature can then be maintained in several ways. If the newborn is responding well and there are no problems with the initiation of respiration, the newborn can be placed skin-to-skin on the mother's body, with a warm blanket covering him or her. This provides the warmth that is needed and also allows the parents to begin the bonding process. Another option is to place the newborn in the radiant warmer. In this case, the newborn should not be wrapped or covered, for the radiant heat will not penetrate a blanket. In many settings, a stocking cap is placed on the newborn's head to prevent loss of heat.

Apgar Scoring. The Apgar score is the immediate scoring assessment made to determine the initial status of the newborn. It is done in all birth settings at 1 and 5 minutes after birth to assess heart rate, respiratory effort, muscle tone, reflex irritability, and color. The nurse in attendance is responsible for completing and recording this score. The score gives an immediate indication of the infant's adaptation to extrauterine life and signals any need for immediate intervention. A score of 8 to 10 indicates that the newborn is adapting well; if the score is below 8, the newborn may need further suctioning or assistance in establishing respirations. Further discussion of the steps in completing the Apgar score, its advantages and disadvantages, and its significance can be found in Chapter 31.

Umbilical Cord. At the time of birth, the birth attendant places a cord clamp on the umbilical cord before cutting the cord. The nurse should assess the end of the cord stump for the presence of three blood vessels—two arteries and one vein. These vessels can be distinguished easily, for the umbilical vein is seen as being a large vessel, while the two umbilical arteries are seen as much smaller vessels. The purpose of this assessment is a cursory screening for genitourinary abnormalities. The presence of only one umbilical artery usually indicates this complication.

General Assessment. While still in the birth setting, the nurse should conduct a cursory head-to-toe assessment of the newborn. The head should be palpated to feel the fontanelles and sutures, the face should be observed for symmetry, and the mouth should be palpated for an intact palate. The trunk should be inspected for abnormalities, and the back should be inspected for dimples or tufts of hair along the spine. The extremities, hands, and feet should be observed for abnormalities. The genitalia should be observed for abnormalities and the anus inspected for patency. The newborn may be weighed; measurements for length, head circumference, and chest circumference may be taken, although these assessments may be delayed until admission to the newborn nursery. A more complete assessment as well as a gestational age assessment should be conducted once the newborn is transferred to the nursery (see Chapter 31).

Eye Prophylaxis. It is mandatory in all birth settings in the United States that a prophylactic agent be placed in the eyes of the newborn at the time of birth. This preventive treatment is a pre-

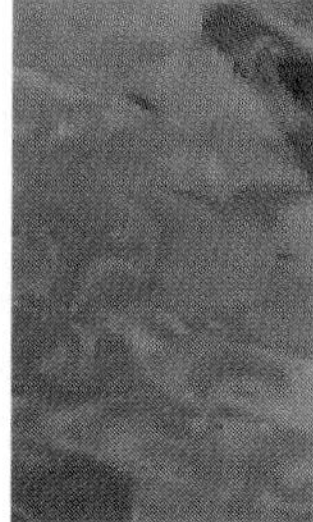

Identifying the Newborn

▼ PURPOSE

To establish accurate identification of the newborn and to ensure that each newborn is given to the right mother. The initial identification of the newborn should always be done *before* mother and newborn are separated.

▼ EQUIPMENT

- Set of four identification bracelets with inserts
- Pen
- Disposable ink pads
- Footprint document

In-Hospital Delivery

1 Prepare equipment and ascertain that the numbers on the identification bracelets match. **Matching the numbers ensures that the correct infant is always given to the correct parent.**

2 At delivery, record necessary information on the bracelet inserts (e.g., mother's name, date and time of birth, sex of baby, and medical record number). **Recording the appropriate information at delivery further ensures accurate matching of parent and infant.**

3 Apply bracelets according to hospital policy. Usually, one bracelet goes around the mother's wrist, one around the baby's ankle and wrist, and the last to a person designated by the mother. When applying the bracelet to the baby, keep your finger under the bracelet while closing the clasp. **Bracelets on the mother and partner that match the ones on the infant allow either person to take or accept the infant from the nursery. Bracelets on the infant should be snug but not too tight. Leaving a gap the width of a finger between the baby and the bracelet allows adequate circulation to the baby's foot or hand while also ensuring that the bracelet is snug enough to stay on the baby.**

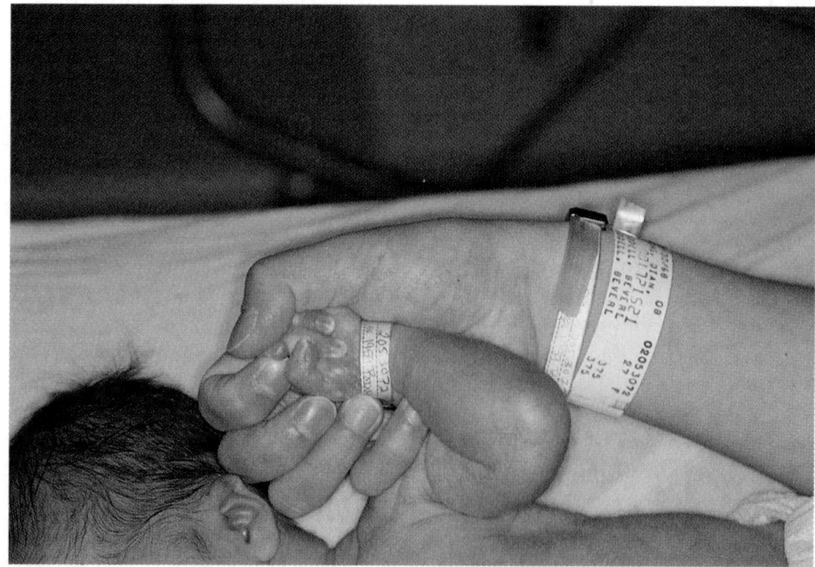

Continued on facing page

PROCEDURE 23–4 Continued

4 Explain the purpose of the identification bracelets to the parents and instruct them not to remove the bracelets until the baby is discharged from the hospital. **Understanding the reason for the bracelets improves parents' compliance with the procedure.**

5 Record the identification bracelet number on the delivery record with the name of the person who applied the bracelets. **In case a question arises, the identification bracelet number and the name of the person who applied the bracelets can be found on this legal document.**

6 If footprints are required, wipe the sole of the baby's foot clean. **The footprint will be more distinct if the foot is clear of vernix, blood, or meconium.**

7 Place the sole of the newborn's foot on the ink pad so that the entire sole is covered. **A print of the infant's entire sole is essential for identification purposes.**

8 Place one hand against the back of the footprint document to provide a firm surface and press the baby's foot onto the paper in the designated spot, being careful not to smudge the print. Repeat with the other foot. **A clear print in which the lines of the foot can be deciphered is essential for identification purposes.**

Out-of-Hospital Delivery

1 Before mother and baby are separated, open blanket and identify sex of infant with parents. **Clarifies any misconception that may have happened in the confusion during an emergency birth.**

2 Follow procedure for in-hospital delivery. **The same precautions should be taken regardless of where delivery has occurred.**

On Postpartum Unit

1 When handing the infant to the new mother in her room or in the nursery, visually confirm that the numbers and names on the identification bracelets match each time. **Ensures that the correct infant is always given to the correct mother.**

2 If someone other than the mother picks up the baby from the nursery or wishes to accept the baby in the hospital room, check to see that this person is wearing an identification bracelet and that the information on the bracelet matches that of the baby's each time. **Ensures that the correct infant is given to the correct individual.**

3 Document this process on the newborn's record. **If a question arises, documentation that this procedure was followed is available.**

4 When picking up the infant from the mother's room or on return of the infant to the nursery by a parent, positively identify the newborn again. **Ensures that the infant received into the nursery is the correct infant.**

5 At the time of discharge from the hospital, check to see that the names and numbers on the identification bracelets match. **Ensures accurate matching of baby and parents at time of discharge.**

caution against ophthalmia neonatorum, an inflammation of the eyes resulting from gonorrheal or chlamydial infection. This infection can be transmitted from the mother to the fetus during the birth process. The agent used for this treatment is usually an antibiotic such as erythromycin or tetracycline. Although silver nitrate has been used as a prophylactic agent in the past, its use is declining because it does not protect against chlamydial infection. The nurse present in the birth setting is usually responsible for the instillation of the eye drops; however, in some settings the treatment may be delayed until the newborn is admitted to the nursery.

Identification. It is important that the infant be identified before leaving the birth setting (Procedure 23–4). The baby and mother are given identical bands so that there will be no mix-up of babies in the nursery. Identification bands are placed on the newborn's wrist and ankle; one band is placed on the mother's wrist. Many birth settings are now also taking footprints of the newborn.

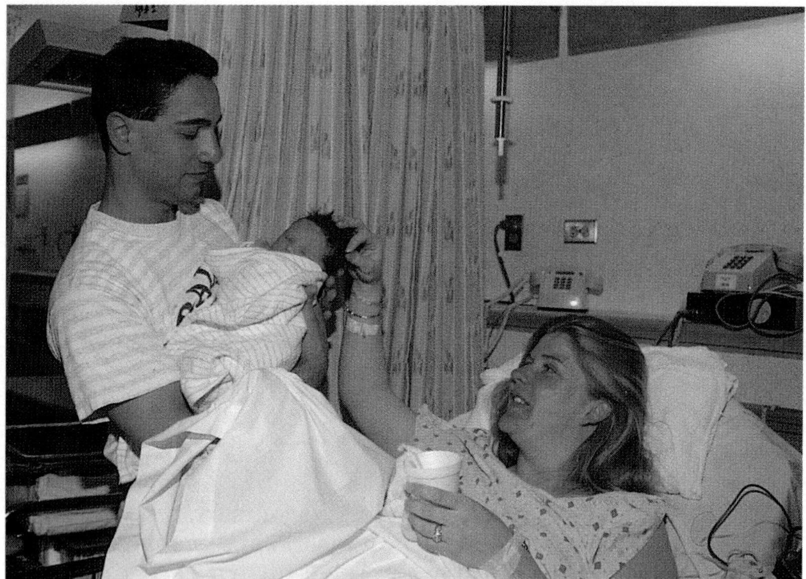

Figure 23–8

Initial evaluation of the newborn can be carried out during third- and fourth-stage labor • The baby should then be wrapped in warm blankets and given to the mother and her partner to hold • It is important to allow time for the promotion of parent-infant interaction immediately after birth.

This becomes part of the infant's record and provides further security. The mother may be fingerprinted as well.

▼ PROMOTING PARENT-NEWBORN INTERACTION

The initial evaluation of the newborn occurs during the third and fourth stages of labor. As soon as possible, the baby should be wrapped in warm blankets and given to the woman and her partner to hold (Fig. 23–8). The nurse may need to provide assistance, for the woman may be fatigued and the partner may be uneasy about holding the baby for the first time. The baby should be positioned so that the woman and her partner have face-to-face contact. The infant experiences a quiet but alert state for the first several hours after birth. If lighting is dimmed, the infant is more comfortable opening his or her eyes, and eye contact will be facilitated. If narcotics are used for analgesia in labor, the newborn may be sleepy and may not exhibit the usual newborn alertness. This first contact with the baby is an excellent time for the nurse to point out the newborn's abilities and features to the woman and her partner. They can be encouraged to unwrap, touch, and examine the baby, although the baby should be unwrapped only for short periods to maintain body temperature. If the woman plans to nurse the baby, breastfeeding can be initiated during the first interaction with the newborn. Chapter 34 provides a further discussion of parent-infant interaction and attachment.

▼ Evaluation

Evaluation of the plan of care for labor and birth is based on the goals and outcomes identified for the woman and her family. It also includes the perinatal and maternal morbidity and mortality outcomes. However, in addition to those essential components, evaluation should also include the more difficult to measure psychosocial outcomes. Level of satisfaction or feelings of mastery of the childbearing experience can influence a woman's perception of the entire event. It is the wise nurse who follows up with visits or phone calls to the childbearing family a few days or weeks after the event to obtain an evaluation from the family as to their feelings regarding the nursing care. No one will argue that the life of the mother and infant are of ultimate importance. In addition, the insight as to satisfaction and suggested changes in nursing care that a new family can provide can change future nursing plans from basic physiologic ones to sophisticated holistic ones.

Collaborative Process

The members of the health care team who are involved in the care of the woman and her family during childbirth include the nurse, the certified nurse-midwife, and the obstetrician. Each of these professionals contributes unique skills that result in a safe, meaningful experience for the family. The nurse is usually the first member of the health care team who meets the woman and her family on arrival at the birth setting. She will admit them to the unit and then provide continual assessment and intervention throughout the entire labor and birth. Nurse-midwives are nurses who have received additional training, enabling them to provide prenatal care for the woman throughout a normal pregnancy, manage the labor, and deliver the baby. The nurse-midwife also attempts to provide continuous attendance for the woman throughout the labor. The obstetrician is a physician with advanced training in maternal-infant care who manages both normal and high-risk pregnancies, labors, and births. The obstetrician may see the woman to assess her progress during the labor and then returns to deliver the baby. The obstetrician also performs a cesarean birth if necessary. These professionals are interdependent, that is, they cannot function safely without the assistance of each other. Collaboration and communication are essential components in working together to ensure a safe outcome for the mother and newborn.

Risk Management

The management of risk throughout the childbirth experience is of foremost concern. Risk management begins when the woman is admitted to the birth setting and continues until she goes home. The management of risk should be the goal of each individual within the system as well as of the entire health care agency, and it is done through collaborative continuous quality improvement. Essential components of risk management include careful and continuous assessment, accurate documentation, frequent communication between members of the health care team, and provision of quality care. The quality of care is influenced by a number of factors, including the availability of resources and the appropriateness, efficacy, efficiency, safety, and timeliness of the care given. To improve quality and decrease risk, nurses who work in the area of labor and birth must understand the importance of these components of their role as a nurse in their area of specialization and as part of the entire organization.

Implications for Research

The nurse has a vital role in developing or contributing to research related to normal labor. Both the psychosocial and physiologic aspects of labor and birth provide a wealth of research opportunities because of the many factors that influence the process. The physical setting for labor and birth, the professional and nonprofessional support available to the birthing woman, and associated routines and procedures have varied throughout history. These factors also vary culturally and even regionally within the same culture. They are dependent on economic, social, and religious influences.

The labor and birth experience varies greatly in the United States. Therefore, setting-specific and region-specific research is valuable. As health care enters a new era in our country, the appropriate use of technology and care providers will be evaluated in terms of quality of care, the patient's satisfaction, and cost effectiveness. Because labor and birth are usually healthy events, they are well suited to research regarding nonphysician care and low-technology approaches. Examples of research questions that might be studied include

- What components of the nursing management of labor and birth influence progress during labor?
- What components of nursing care are most important to the physical and emotional comfort of the woman and her family during labor and birth?
- How can the nurse integrate comfort and support strategies with the assessment, risk management, and documentation aspects of her role?

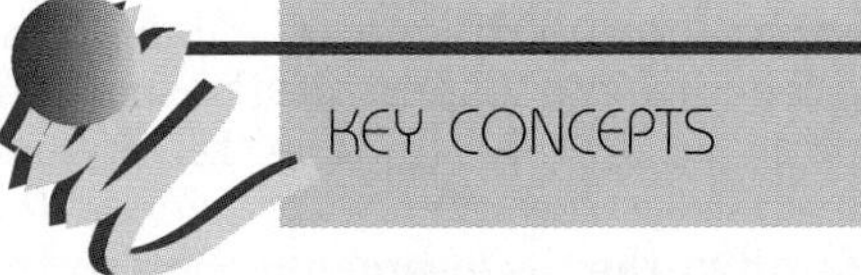

KEY CONCEPTS

- ▼ Most women have normal, healthy pregnancies, labors, and births.
- ▼ Unlike true labor, false labor contractions are usually irregular; do not increase in intensity, frequency, or duration; and do not result in progressive cervical dilatation.
- ▼ Preliminary signs of labor can include Braxton Hicks contractions, backache, lightening, weight loss, diarrhea, a spurt of energy, nesting, and bloody show.
- ▼ Labor can be divided into four stages. The first stage of labor, the effacement and dilatation stage, can be divided into three phases—latent, active, and transition.
- ▼ The latent phase of the first stage of labor is preparatory in nature, both physically and emotionally; contractions are mild and irregular, accomplishing ripening, effacement of the cervix, and dilatation to about 3 cm; the woman is eager and apprehensive emotionally; physical symptoms include low backache, bloody show, and pelvic cramping or pressure; the latent phase varies in length from an hour to many hours.

- The active phase of the first stage of labor averages 4 to 6 hours; contractions are more intense and regular, accomplishing further effacement and dilatation to 7 or 8 cm; the woman becomes serious and introverted emotionally; physical symptoms include pain, nausea, backache, and fatigue.
- The transition phase of the first stage of labor ranges from 15 minutes to 2 hours; contractions are strong and may have multiple peaks; effacement and dilatation are completed; the woman may feel irritable, be overwhelmed, and want to quit; physical symptoms include shaking legs, nausea and vomiting, and an urge to push.
- The second stage of labor is the expulsion stage, from complete dilatation of the cervix to the birth of the baby; during this stage, the woman will push with contractions to move the baby through the pelvis and soft tissues.
- The third stage of labor is the time from the birth of the infant to the delivery of the placenta.
- The fourth stage of labor is the first hour after the delivery of the placenta; postpartum hemorrhage is the major complication of the fourth stage.
- Accurate assessment and diagnosis of labor are important to ensure the safety of the mother and fetus, plan accurately for the labor and birth, and promote a rewarding experience for the entire family; the assessment should include a current labor history, data from the antepartum record, and a complete physical assessment (vital signs, fetal heart rate, contraction pattern, abdominal and pelvic examinations, assessment of the extremities, laboratory data, and psychosocial and cultural data).
- The immediate postpartum assessment includes maternal vital signs; examination of the breasts, uterus, and bladder; evaluation of the perineum and lochia; and assessment of the extremities.
- Enemas may be used to empty the rectum in early labor. The client's preference should be considered in deciding the usefulness of this procedure.
- A perineal prep (shave) may be done to remove pubic hair from the episiotomy site; opinion varies as to the value of this procedure in preventing infection and promoting postpartum comfort.
- Hydration in labor may be accomplished by oral or intravenous fluids or a combination of both. Maternal and fetal status, as well as obstetric risk, should be evaluated in deciding which method is best.
- Urinary elimination should be encouraged throughout labor to promote comfort, decrease pain, and facilitate the descent of the fetus.
- Physical and emotional comfort and support are of primary importance in helping the woman to cope with her labor; physical comfort measures include diversional activities, back rub and massage, relaxation and breathing strategies, visualization, hydrotherapy, hot packs or ice packs, and basic hygiene; emotional support strategies include physical presence, coaching, reinforcement and praise, and teaching.
- Ambulation should be encouraged for as long as possible during labor; there are a variety of possible positions for labor and birth; the client's preference, maternal and fetal status, and obstetric risk determine what positions are used.
- Family involvement and infant bonding are promoted by a single-room concept of labor, birth, and postpartum care.
- The role of the labor partner is an important one and should be encouraged by the nurse; the labor partner can remain with the woman continually and provide emotional support and coaching.
- An important component of the nurse's role during childbirth is continual documentation of the progress of labor and the care that is provided; documentation also serves as a legal account of the events of the labor and birth.
- The nurse prepares for the birth by notifying the birth attendant, organizing the necessary equipment and supplies, preparing family members, and washing the perineal area (wash prep).
- In the third stage of labor, the nursing interventions include assisting the woman in expulsion of the placenta, administering an oxytocic drug, massaging the uterus to facilitate contraction, collecting cord blood samples, and assisting with the repair of lacerations or the episiotomy.
- During the fourth stage of labor, the nurse does fundal massage as necessary to prevent hemorrhage, provides means of pain relief, maintains fluid balance and nutrition, promotes elimination, provides comfort and safety, and provides hygiene.
- The immediate assessment and care of the newborn includes respirations, body temperature, Apgar score, umbilical cord, general body assessment, eye prophylaxis, and identification.

- The first interaction of the parents with the newborn usually occurs in the third or fourth stage of labor. The nurse can facilitate this first encounter by encouraging the parents to hold, touch, and explore the newborn; point out the normal characteristics and capabilities of the newborn; and encourage face-to-face and eye-to-eye contact.
- Team members who are involved with the woman during labor and birth include the nurse, the certified nurse-midwife, and the physician; the labor partner, family members, and a doula can also be important members of the team.

References

Albers, L., and Katz, V. L. (1991). Birth setting for low-risk pregnancies: An analysis of the current literature. *Journal of Nurse-Midwifery,* 36 (4), 215–220.

Albers, L., and Savitz, D. (1991). Hospital setting for birth and use of medical procedures in low risk women. *Journal of Nurse-Midwifery,* 36 (6), 327–333.

American College of Obstetricians and Gynecologists. (1995a). Fetal heart rate patterns. Monitoring, interpretation, and management. *ACOG Technical Bulletin,* 207, 1–7.

American College of Obstetricians and Gynecologists. (1995b). Dystocia and the augmentation of labor. *ACOG Technical Bulletin,* 218, 1–7.

Anderhold, K., and Roberts, J. (1991). Phases of second stage labor. Four descriptive case studies. *Journal of Nurse-Midwifery,* 36, 267–275.

Bergstrom, L., Roberts, J., Skillman, L., Seidel, J. (1992). "You'll feel me touching you, sweetie": Vaginal examinations during the second stage of labor. *Birth,* 19 (1), 10–18.

Bonovich, L. (1990). Recognizing the onset of labor. *Journal of Obstetric, Gynecologic, and Neonatal Nursing,* 19 (2), 141–145.

Bradley, B. S., Tashevska, M., Selby, J. M. (1990). Women's first experience of childbirth: Two hospital settings compared. *British Journal of Medical Psychology,* 63 (part 3), 227–237.

Bryanton, J., Fraser-Davey, H., Sullivan, P. (1994). Women's perceptions of nursing support during labor. *Journal of Obstetric, Gynecologic, and Neonatal Nursing,* 23 (8), 638–646.

Chalmers, B., and Wolman, W. (1993). Social support in labor—a selective review. *Journal of Psychosomatic Obstetrics and Gynaecology,* 14 (1), 1–15.

Chapman, L. (1992). Expectant fathers' roles during labor and birth. *Journal of Obstetric, Gynecologic, and Neonatal Nursing,* 21 (2), 114–120.

Chapman, M. G., Jones, M., Spring, J. E., De Swiet, M., Chamberlain, G. V. P. (1986). The use of a birthroom: A randomized controlled trial comparing delivery with that in the labour ward. *British Journal of Obstetrics and Gynaecology,* 93 (2), 182–187.

Combs, C. A., and Laros, R. K. (1991). Prolonged third stage of labor: Morbidity and risk factors. *Obstetrics and Gynecology,* 77 (6), 863–867.

Copper, R. L., Goldenberg, R. L., Davis, R. O., Cutter, G. R., DuBard, M. B., Corliss, D. K., Andrews, J. B. (1990). Warning symptoms, uterine contractions, and cervical examination findings in women at risk of preterm delivery. *American Journal of Obstetrics and Gynecology,* 162 (3), 748–754.

Cosner, K. R., and deJong, E. (1993). Physiologic second stage labor. *MCN: American Journal of Maternal Child Nursing,* 18 (1), 38–43.

Cunningham, F. G., MacDonald, P. C., Gant, N. F., Leveno, K. J., Gilstrap, L. C. III. (1993). *Williams obstetrics* (19th ed.). Norwalk, CT: Appleton & Lange.

Davidson, N. (1979). REEDA: Evaluating postpartum healing. *Journal of Nurse-Midwifery,* 19 (2), 6–9.

Douglas, M. J. (1988). Commentary: The case against a more liberal food and fluid policy in labor. *Birth,* 15 (2), 93–94.

Enkin, M. W., Keirse, M. J. N. C., Renfrew, M. J., Neilson, J. P. (1995). Effective care in pregnancy and childbirth: A synopsis. *Birth,* 22 (2), 102–103.

Evans, S., and Jeffrey, J. (1995). Maternal learning needs during labor and delivery. *Journal of Obstetric, Gynecologic, and Neonatal Nursing,* 24 (3), 235–240.

Friedman, E. A. (1978). *Labor: Clinical evaluation and management* (2nd ed.). New York: Appleton-Century-Crofts.

Haire, D. B., and Elsberry, C. C. (1991). Maternity care and outcomes in a high-risk service: The North Central Brains Hospital experience. *Birth,* 18 (1), 33–37.

Hodnett, E., and Osborn, R. (1989a). A randomized trial of the effects of monitrice support during labor: Mothers' views two to four weeks postpartum. *Birth,* 16 (4), 177–183.

Hodnett, E., and Osborn, R. (1989b). Effect of continuous intrapartum professional support on childbirth outcomes. *Research in Nursing and Health,* 12, 289–297.

Kennell, J., Klaus, M., McGrath, S., Robertson, S., Hinkley, C. (1991). Continuous emotional support during labor in a U. S. hospital. *Journal of the American Medical Association,* 265, 2197–2201.

Klaus, M., Kennell, J., Berkowitz, G., Klaus, P. (1992). Maternal assistance and support in labor: Father, nurse, midwife or doula? *Clinical Consultations in Obstetrics and Gynecology,* Vol. 4 (December).

Klaus, M., Kennell, J., Klaus, P. (1993). *Mothering the mother.* New York: Addison-Wesley Publishing Co.

Ludka, L., and Roberts, C. (1993). Eating and drinking in labor. A literature review. *Journal of Nurse-Midwifery,* 38 (4), 199–207.

Mackey, M., and Stepans, M. (1994). Women's evaluations of their labor and delivery nurses. *Journal of Obstetric, Gynecologic, and Neonatal Nursing,* 23 (5), 413–420.

Martin, E. (1990). *Intrapartum management modules.* Baltimore: Williams & Wilkins.

McKay, S., and Barrows, T. (1991). Holding back: Maternal readiness to give birth. *MCN: American Journal of Maternal Child Nursing,* 16 (5), 250–254.

McKay, S., and Mahan, C. S. (1988). Modifying the stomach contents of laboring women: Why and how; success and risks. *Birth,* 15 (4), 213–221.

McNiven, P., Hodnett, E., O'Brian-Pallas, L. (1992). Supporting women in labor: A work sampling study of the activities of labor and delivery nurses. *Birth,* 19 (1), 3–7.

Newton, N., Newton, M., Broach, J. (1988). Psychologic, physical, nutritional and technologic aspects of intravenous infusion during labor. *Birth,* 15 (2), 67–72.

Nurses Association of the American College of Obstetricians and Gynecologists. (1990). Fetal heart rate auscultation. *Obstetric, Gynecologic, and Neonatal Nursing Practice Resource,* No. 35.

Romney, M. L., and Gordon, H. (1981). Is your enema really necessary? *British Medical Journal,* 282 (6272), 1269–1271.

Simkin, P. (1991). Just another day in a woman's life? Women's long-term perceptions of their first birth experience. Part I. *Birth,* 18 (4), 203–210.

Simkin, P., Whalley, J., Keppler, A. (1991). *Pregnancy, childbirth, and the newborn.* New York: Meadowbrook Press.

Smith, M., Ruffin, M., Green, L. (1993). The rational management of labor. *American Family Physician,* 47 (6), 1471–1481.

Varney, H. (1987). *Nurse-Midwifery* (2nd ed.). Boston: Blackwell Scientific Publications.

Waskerwitz, S., Fournier, L., Jones, P., Meier, W. (1985). A comparative analysis of newborn outcome in a hospital-based birthing center. *Clinical Pediatrics,* 24 (5), 273–277.

Whitley, N., and Mack, E. (1980). Are enemas justified for women in labor? *American Journal of Nursing,* 80 (7), 1339.

NURSING CARE PLANNING GUIDE

Normal Childbirth

This Nursing Care Planning Guide was developed to be used as a planning tool. You will need to modify and adapt it to individual clients as appropriate.

Performing a complete and thorough assessment is the first step in providing effective nursing care for a client. Major nursing diagnoses used in care that promotes a normal childbirth include

1 Risk for altered maternal tissue perfusion

2 Risk for urinary retention

3 Risk for infection: urinary tract, perineum (episiotomy), uterine placental site (endometritis)

4 Labor pain

5 Risk for ineffective breathing pattern

6 Risk for fluid volume deficit

7 Risk for altered fetal tissue perfusion

8 Risk for fetal injury

9 Risk for maternal fatigue

10 Knowledge deficit: labor, anesthesia, delivery

11 Moderate to severe anxiety

12 Risk for situational low self-esteem

13 Risk for fetal injury: immediate extrauterine adjustment after birth

ASSESSMENT

Assessment of the client during the intrapartum period plays a critical role in facilitating a positive labor and delivery experience. To collect data, use the following Assessment Tools: Obstetric Evaluation Record (p. 791), Obstetric Admission Record (p. 792), Labor Flowsheet (pp. 793–794), and Labor and Delivery Summary (p. 795). In the data collected, identify defining characteristics to use as a basis for formulating nursing diagnoses that are appropriate for your client. Areas requiring special attention in care that promotes a normal childbirth include fetal well-being, labor pain, and anxiety.

Continued on facing page

NURSING CARE PLANNING GUIDE Continued

Assessment Tool

Obstetric Evaluation Record

Date: __/__/__ To:________ by: ☐ walk ☐ w/c ☐ gurney

Time in:________ From: ☐ home ☐ clinic ☐ ________

Evaluation, procedure(s): ☐ **scheduled** ☐ **unscheduled**

☐ NST ☐ Observation ☐ Direct admit* Other

Indication(s)

☐ Patient oriented to unit and call system. Clinical condition, procedures, plan of care explained. Patient verbalizes understanding. Initials

☐ Patient familiar with unit and procedures, denies questions.

NURSE'S NOTES ☐ see OB Evaluation Continuation Sheet

MD/CNM NOTES ☐ see separate progress note

Final Assessment

Plan

MD/CNM

Disposition: ☐ **N/A (direct admit)** ☐ **Admitted*** ☐ **Discharged**

Time discharged or admit decision made:

To: home / Condition:

By: ☐ walk ☐ w/c ☐ gurney ☐ Alone With:

***See Obstetric Admission Record** INIT SIGNATURE

Age	Grav	Term	Preterm	AB	Liv	EDD dates	Gest. (wks)	EDD sono	Gest. (wks)

TIME	BP	T	P	R

ALLERGIES ☐ None	Reaction

DTR's: R L ☐ N/A

Urine albumin ☐ N/A

MISCELLANEOUS

Initial Assessment

Fetal Heart Rate	Uterine activity	Membranes	Other
Baseline:	☐ none	☐ intact by hx	☐ no vaginal bleeding
Variability: ☐ N/A	☐ irritability	☐ ruptured:	☐ normal show
Accelerations? ☐ yes ☐ no	☐ contractions	MO / DAY	☐ fetus active
Decelerations? ☐ yes ☐ no	q ____ min	TIME	☐ see notes
☐ see notes	X ____ sec	**fluid:** ☐ clear	**Assessment**
	mild / mod / firm	☐ no foul odor	**Time:**
	onset: MO / DAY TIME	☐ see notes	**Initials:**

Vaginal exam ☐ not done

CERVIX		CERVIX	
☐ soft ☐ anterior	**dilated:**	☐ soft ☐ anterior	**dilated:**
☐ med. ☐ midpos.	**effaced:**	☐ med. ☐ midpos.	**effaced:**
☐ firm ☐ posterior		☐ firm ☐ posterior	
PRESENTING PART	**station:**	PRESENTING PART	**station:**
☐ vtx (or)		☐ vtx (or)	
COMMENTS		COMMENTS	
Time:	Initials:	Time:	Initials:

NST

☐ **Reactive** Parameters: ≥ ____ FHR accels in ____ minutes *(accelerations ≥15 seconds duration, ≥ 15 BPM amplitude)*

☐ **Nonreactive** (not supine, no recent cigarette)
☐ Unsatisfactory
☐ Decelerations present
Describe in notes

Interpreted by:

Contraction Stress Test

☐ **Negative**
☐ **Positive**
☐ Suspicious
☐ Hyperstimulation
☐ Variable Decels
☐ Unsatisfactory
Describe in notes

☐ Spontaneous
☐ Nipple stimulation
☐ Oxytocin challenge

☐ Reactive
☐ Nonreactive

Interpreted by:

ORDERS ☐ see separate order sheet

Short stay discharge instructions ☐ N/A ☐ See copy attached

☐ Patient verbalizes understanding Instructor Initials:

INIT SIGNATURE INIT SIGNATURE

 Obstetric Evaluation Record Form #5100-1

Courtesy of CSW Forms, Timberon, NM, (800) 284–2815.

NURSING CARE PLANNING GUIDE Continued

Assessment Tool

Obstetric Admission Record

Maternal / Fetal Risks / Problems*
*based on prenatal record, patient interview, current assessment, other

Prenatal Labs	Results	Pending	Not Applicable
Blood type & Rh			
Antibody screen	– / +		
Rubella * immune	– / +*		
Serology	– / +		
HBsAg	– / +		
HIV	– / +		
β strep	– / +		
Chlamydia	– / +		
GC	– / +		

Prenatal care: ☐ yes ☐ no ➤ Began at approx. ___wks gestation

➤ Prenatal record available at admit: ☐ yes ☐ see notes

Maternal Physical/Psychosocial Assessment		
Ht Wt Fundal ht Est fetal wt		
✓ - yes N - see notes N/A - not applicable — - not assessed		
Misc	Prenatal record reviewed	
	Labs reviewed, normal for pregnancy	
Neuro	Alert, oriented X 3, appropriate behavior, speech clear	
	No weakness or c/o dizziness	
	Denies headache or visual disturbances	
Cardiovascular/Skin	SBP is within 30mm Hg, and DBP is within 15mm Hg of early/ pre-pregnancy value. If early value is unavailable, BP < 140/90	
	Skin warm and dry	
	Skin pink	
	Mucus membranes moist	
	Heart rate regular with no irregularities	
	No edema	
	Skin intact, no lesions or bruises	
Resp	Breathing easily. Respirations regular, normal depth	
	Lungs clear bilaterally with good breath sounds to bases	
	No rhinitis, nasal stuffiness or cough	
GI	No nausea or vomiting	
	No epigastric pain resistant to antacids	
	No diarrhea or constipation. Last BM:	
GU	Voiding without c/o difficulty or discomfort	
	Urine clear, not dark. No strong odor	
Psychosocial	Understands, accepts situation, coping well with minimal anxiety	
	Significant other is present, supportive	
	Denies significant life stress (job, finances, social, loss, other)	
	Basic needs (housing, food, clothing) met	
	Pt. feels hospitalization will not cause child care or other problems	
	No evidence of physical/emotional abuse	
	Able to care for self without assistance	
	No communication barriers (cultural, cognitive, sensory, language)	

Primary language: ☐ English ☐ Spanish ☐ ___________

➤ Significant other (S.O.): Name ___________
Relationship ___________ tel. no. ___________
Comments: ___________
Other support: ___________

Birth Preparation and Plans

Prenatal classes attended: ☐ none
☐ Lamaze
☐ cesarean birth
☐ infant care
☐ ___________

Anesthesia/analgesia plans:
☐ none ☐ epidural
☐ IV analgesia ☐ general
☐ local ☐ N/A
☐ spinal
____

Feeding preference:
☐ breast
☐ bottle
☐ undecided
☐ N/A

Patient/family requests: ☐ none (or)___________

Current Medications ☐ none

Medication	last taken	w/ patient	disposition
		Y / N	
		Y / N	
		Y / N	

Substance Use *(tobacco smoking, alcohol, street drugs, etc.)* ☐ none

☐ smokes ____ ppd, last cigarette:___________ ☐ other, see notes

Rest / Intake / Health

Est. sleep in past 24 hrs: ☐

Est. fluid intake in past 12 hrs: ☐

Last oral intake:
fluids mo / day time
solids mo / day time

Recent illness or exposure to communicable disease:
☐ none ☐ see notes

Miscellaneous admission information

Prostheses:
☐ none
☐ contacts
☐ dentures
☐ ___________

☐ ID band on

☐ Allergy band on
☐ N/A *(no allergies)*

Valuables to safe:
☐ yes ☐ no ☐ N/A

Admit information obtained from:
☐ prenatal record
☐ patient
☐ significant other
☐ MD/CNM
☐ ___________

MD/CNM: ___________
notified by: ___________
mo / day time

➤ Infant care provider: ☐ N/A

NOTES

ADMIT NURSE SIGNATURE: mo / day / yr TIME

Obstetric Admission Record Form #5100-2

THE OBSTETRIC ADMISSION RECORD IS INTENDED FOR USE WITH THE OBSTETRIC EVALUATION RECORD

Courtesy of CSW Forms, Timberon, NM, (800) 284–2815.

NURSING CARE PLANNING GUIDE Continued

Assessment Tool

ASSESSMENT SUMMARY		Time			
✓ - yes NN - see nurse's notes/flow sheet — - not applicable or not assessed	Initials				
Safety	Call bell in reach				
	Bed in low position				
	Siderails up				
Psychosocial	Understands, accepts situation, coping well with minimal anxiety				
	Significant other is present, supportive				
	Feels rested				
Neuro	Alert, oriented X 3, appropriate behavior, speech clear				
	No weakness or c/o dizziness				
	Denies headache or visual disturbances				
	DTR's 1+ to 3+, no clonus				
Cardiovascular	SBP ± 30mm Hg of early/pre-pregnancy value				
	DBP ± 15mm Hg of early/pre-pregnancy value				
	Skin warm and dry				
	Skin pink. Peripheral pulses normal				
	Afebrile				
	Mucus membranes moist, good skin turgor				
	Heart rate regular w/ no irregularities, 60–100 BPM (100–120 BPM w/ beta agonist)				
	No c/o chest pain or discomfort				
	No edema of extremities				
	No facial or presacral edema				
	IV site(s): No puffiness, redness, or tenderness				
	IV containers, tubing, sites, current per hospital policy				
Respiratory	Breathing easily. Respirations regular, normal depth				
	Respiratory rate 12–22/minute				
	Lungs clear bilaterally, good breath sounds to bases				
	No rhinitis, nasal stuffiness or cough				
GI	Taking ≥ 50% of diet				
	No nausea or vomiting				
	No epigastric pain resistant to antacids				
	No diarrhea or constipation. Last BM__________				
GU	Voiding without c/o difficulty or discomfort				
	Foley catheter				
	Urine clear, not dark. No strong odor				
	≤ trace protein on urine dipstick				
	Urine output ≥ 120cc/4 hrs (estimated / measured)				
Miscellaneous	Total fluid intake at least 2000cc/24 hrs				
	Maintaining fluid restriction of ≤ ________ cc/24 hr				
	Intake and output appropriate				
	Daily weight ± .5 lb of previous day (or ± .25kg)				
	Labs reviewed, normal for pregnancy				
OB	No vaginal bleeding, uterus non-tender				
	Fetus active				
	Amniotic membranes intact				
	Ruptured, fluid clear (note amt in NN periodically)				
	Ruptured, no odor to fluid				
Membranes ruptured: ___/___ ___:___ AROM / SROM					

Today's Date: / / Admitted: /

Grav	Term	Preterm	AB	Living	EDD dates	EDD sono	Age	Blood Type

RISKS / PROBLEMS / NURSING CONSIDERATIONS

NURSE'S NOTES

INIT.	Signature and title	INIT.	Signature and title

Labor Flowsheet

Form #1100-T12 (Rev. 5/95)

-1-

Portions of Labor Flowsheet. Courtesy of CSW Forms, Timberon, NM, (800) 284–2815.

NURSING CARE PLANNING GUIDE Continued

Assessment Tool

Cervix	Station	Dilation	00 (12MN) 00	15	30	45	01 (1AM) 00	15	11 (11AM) 00	15	30	45	Dilation	Station	Cervix
Consis-tency		9											9		Consis-tency
Ⓕ firm	-3	8											8	-3	Ⓕ firm
Ⓜ medium	-2	7											7	-2	Ⓜ medium
Ⓢ soft	-1	6											6	-1	Ⓢ soft
Position	0	5											5	0	Position
P posterior	+1	4											4	+1	P posterior
MP midposition	+2	3											3	+2	MP midposition
A anterior	+3	2											2	+3	A anterior
	(X)	1 (•)											1 (•)	(X)	
Effacement (%)															Effacement (%)
Examiner															Examiner
CONTRACTIONS: Monitor Mode(s)															Monitor Mode(s)
CONTRACTIONS: Frequency															Frequency
CONTRACTIONS: Duration (sec)															Duration (sec)
CONTRACTIONS: Intensity															Intensity
CONTRACTIONS: Resting Tone															Resting Tone
OPTIONAL															OPTIONAL
FETAL HEART RATE: Monitor Mode															Monitor Mode
FETAL HEART RATE: Baseline															Baseline
FETAL HEART RATE: LTV															LTV
FETAL HEART RATE: STV															STV
FETAL HEART RATE: Accel / Event															Accel / Event
FETAL HEART RATE: Decel															Decel
MATERNAL Position/Activity															MATERNAL Position/Activity
O_2 LPM / Mode															O_2 LPM / Mode
VITAL SIGNS: Temperature															Temperature
VITAL SIGNS: Pulse															Pulse
VITAL SIGNS: Respiration															Respiration
VITAL SIGNS: Blood Pressure															Blood Pressure
L DTR / Clonus															DTR / Clonus L
R DTR / Clonus															DTR / Clonus R
Oxytocin mU/min															Oxytocin mU/min
IV															IV
OPTIONAL															OPTIONAL
OPTIONAL															OPTIONAL
LABS															LABS
LABS															LABS
See NN, Other															See NN, Other
Initials (ø - NO ENTRY)															Initials (ø - NO ENTRY)

Medication - time, med, dose, route

Note: the flowsheet has been collapsed for the purposes of this illustration. The complete form covers 24 hours—12 hours on each side.

Labor Flowsheet Date begun ___/___/___

Assessment Codes

NN - see nurse's notes for description/explanation
→ - no change **NA** - not applicable **ø** - none

UTERINE CONTRACTIONS

Monitor mode
- **P** - palpation
- **T** - tocodynamometer
- **IUC** - intrauterine pressure catheter

Intensity
(palpation)
- **+** - mild
- **++** - moderate
- **+++** - firm

(IUC)
- \# of mm Hg

Resting tone
- **nl** - relaxed (palpation)
- \# of mm Hg (IUC)

MATERNAL POSITION
- **Ⓡ** - right lateral
- **ⓇT** - right tilt
- **Ⓛ** - left lateral
- **ⓁT** - left tilt
- **S** - supine
- **SF** - semi-Fowlers
- **HF** - high-Fowlers
- **SQ** - squat
- **Tr** - Trendelenburg
- **KC** - kneechest

ACTIVITY
- **Sl** - sleep
- **ch** - chair
- **W** - walk

O₂ MODE
- **NC** - nasal cannula
- **M** - simple mask
- **NR** - non-rebreather mask

See NN, Other
- **AS** - See Assessment Summary

FETAL HEART RATE

Monitor Mode
Electronic Fetal Monitoring (EFM)
- **US** - ultrasound
- **FE** - fetal electrode

Auscultation
- **Ⓤⓢ** - ultrasound
- **fts** - fetoscope

Note: if auscultation technique is used, note the FHR, and the presence (+) or absence (ø) of accelerations and decelerations. LTV and STV are not applicable and the type of FHR deceleration cannot be accurately diagnosed by auscultation.

Long term variability (LTV)
- **ø** - absent *(0–2 BPM)*
- **↓** - minimal *(3–5 BPM)*
- **+** - average *(6–25 BPM)*
- **↑** - marked *(>25 BPM)*

Short term variability (STV)
- **ø** - absent
- **+** - present

Note: presence of STV is not diagnostic unless a fetal electrode is used.

Acceleration (Accel)
- **ø** - absent
- **+** - present *(amplitude ≥ 15 BPM above baseline, duration ≥ 15 sec)*

Event
- **FM** - fetal movement
- **SS** - scalp stimulation
- **UC** - uterine contraction
- **NA** - not applicable

Deceleration (Decel)
EFM
- **ø** - absent
- **L** - late
- **E** - early
- **MV** - mild variable
- **V** - moderate variable *(<70 BPM x 30–60 sec, or 70–80 BPM x >60 sec)*
- **SV** - severe variable *(<70 BPM x >60 sec)*

Auscultation
- **ø** - absent **+** - present

Form #1100-T12 (Rev. 5/95) –3–

NURSING CARE PLANNING GUIDE Continued

Assessment Tool

Labor & Delivery Summary

Age	Grav	Term	Preterm	AB	Liv	EDD dates	Gest. (wks)	EDD sono	Gest. (wks)

Risks / problems noted antepartum ☐none

Risks/problems noted intrapartum ☐none

Fetal Heart Rate: ☐severe variable decelerations ☐decreased variability ☐consistent late decelerations ☐bradycardia ☐tachycardia ☐

Labor: ☐prolonged latent / active phase ☐precipitous labor (≤ 3hr) ☐secondary arrest of dilatation ☐ protraction / arrest of descent ☐

Misc: ☐PROM ☐fever ☐see notes ☐ ☐

Presentation: ☐vertex ☐breech ☐

Position:

	Date	Time
Admitted	/ /	
Labor onset ☐N/A	/	
Complete dilation ☐N/A	/	
Delivery of infant	/	
Placenta	/	
☐AROM ☐SROM	/	

Labor Summary *(Optional)*

1st stage	′ ″
2nd stage	′ ″
3rd stage	′ ″
Total Labor	′ ″
ROM X	hrs

Labor

☐spontaneous ☐induced ☐augmented ☐N/A

Induced/augmented w/ ☐AROM ☐prostaglandin ☐oxytocin

Episiotomy/laceration: ☐none ☐2° median episiotomy ☐ Suture:

Fetal monitoring ☐none

Electronic (EFM): external ☐FHR ☐uterus; internal ☐FHR ☐uterus

Auscultation: ☐ultrasound ☐fetoscope

Placenta ☐see notes

Delivery: ☐spontaneous ☐expressed ☐removed manually

Appearance: ☐normal ☐small ☐many calcifications

Other: ☐ to pathology ☐cultured

Amniotic fluid ☐see notes

☐no odor ☐meconium ☐clear ☐

Other procedures: ☐none ☐uterine exploration ☐curettage ☐tubal ligation ☐see notes

Vaginal birth: ☐spontaneous ☐vacuum ☐forceps outlet / low / mid ☐VBAC ☐see notes

Cesarean birth: ☐primary ☐repeat ☐repeat, VBAC trial *Incision:* ☐low transverse ☐

Delivery complications: ☐none ☐hemorrhage ☐see notes ☐

Est. blood loss: cc

INFANT DATA: ☐male ☐female ID band #

Wt: Multiple birth? ☐no ☐yes, birth order: __ of __

☐No trauma, congenital anomalies, or other abnormalities observed, or: ☐see notes

Infant attended at delivery by:

Infant's physician: ☐same, or:

Apgar	1″	5″	10″*
Heart rate			
Resp. effort			
Reflex irrit.			
Muscle tone			
Skin color			
Totals			

**if indicated*

Procedures performed in delivery room

Resuscitation

☐none ☐stimulation ☐free-flow O_2 x ″ ☐naloxone ☐PPV bag/mask x ″ ☐intubation ☐PPV bag/ETT x ″ ☐see resuscitation record

Other

☐naso/oropharyngeal suction on perineum
☐tracheal suction
☐cords visualized ☐clear ☐meconium
☐gastric suction, fluid:
☐
☐erythromycin ½% oint. OU, or:
time: by:
☐Aq Vit. K ___ mg IM in (R / L) lateral thigh
time: by:

Umbilical cord

Vessels: ☐3 ☐2 ☐nuchal x loose / tight ☐

Cord blood to: ☐lab ☐refrig ☐nursery ☐N/A

Meds in labor (PO, IM, SQ, IV): ☐none ☐$MgSO_4$ ☐O_2 ☐oxytocin

OTHER LABOR MEDS	Last dose	OTHER LABOR MEDS	Last dose

Labor/delivery anesthesia Epidural/spinal analgesia: ☐none

NO.	AGENT/MEDICATION	TIME

1=local 2=spinal 3=general 4=epidural bolus 5=epidural bolus + continuous 6=pudendal 7=paracervical 8=caudal ☐see anesthesia record

Output: ☐none ☐urine ☐meconium ☐gastric cc

Intake: ☐none ☐breast well / fair / poor

☐see notes

Disposition: ☐Remains in LDRP room
Transferred: / Time:
☐to regular newborn nursery ☐to NICU
☐with mother to:
☐
Condition:

Delivery room meds: ☐none ☐see OR record ☐$MgSO_4$ drip

☐IV LR / NS / with units of oxytocin/L @ cc/hr

Delivered by: Assistant *(if applicable)*: **Nurse:**

NOTES

Labor & Delivery Summary completed by: **Date:** / / **Time:**

WHITE—MEDICAL RECORD COPY
YELLOW—NEWBORN RECORD COPY
PINK—MATERNAL PHYSICIAN COPY

Labor & Delivery Summary Form #7100

Courtesy of CSW Forms, Timberon, NM, (800) 284–2815.

NURSING CARE PLANNING GUIDE Continued

1

Analysis: ▼ NURSING DIAGNOSIS

***Risk for altered maternal tissue perfusion,* related to**

- Back-lying position during labor that places pressure on the vena cava
- Elevation of blood pressure during contractions
- Blood loss at delivery
- Hemorrhage
- Hypertension
- Preeclampsia
- Hyperactive labor

Defining Characteristics

SUBJECTIVE	*OBJECTIVE*
Preeclampsia	Preeclampsia
Complains of edema	Blood pressure elevated; systolic pressure increases 30 mm Hg; diastolic pressure increases 15 mm Hg
	Protein in urine (albuminuria)
	Edema of face, back of hands, tibial area, feet
Hypotension	Hypotension
Describes dizziness, faintness	Hypotensive blood pressure
	Elevated pulse
	Elevated respiratory rate
	Diaphoresis
	Cool skin, pale
	Decreased sensorium
Hyperactive Labor	Hyperactive Labor
Describes severe pain with contractions	Contractions lasting longer than 1 minute, less than 1 minute of relaxation between contractions, strength >75 mm Hg
	Pitocin IV

Continued on facing page

NURSING CARE PLANNING GUIDE Continued

Client Goal/ ▼ EVALUATION CRITERIA

Client will demonstrate adequate tissue perfusion. / ▼ **Client will evidence normal blood pressure during labor, delivery, and recovery; normal pulse and respirations; normal sensorium; physiologic edema of pregnancy; normal contractions.**

▼ NURSING INTERVENTIONS	Rationale
• Assess blood pressure at admission and every hour in latent and active phases of labor, then every half-hour during transition and delivery.	• Assessing the blood pressure allows detection of hypertension (>140/90), pregnancy-induced hypertension (increase in systolic pressure of 30 mm Hg or greater from baseline level, increase in diastolic pressure of 15 mm Hg or greater from baseline level).
• Assess blood pressure more frequently if it is elevated or if the client is becoming hypotensive. Take every 15 minutes or more often with regional anesthesia or hypotension from blood loss.	• Decreased circulating volume may occur with vena caval hypotension, blood loss or hemorrhage, and uterine rupture. Analgesics can cause vasodilatation with resultant lowering of blood pressure. Regional anesthesia causes vasodilatation in the lower region of the body, with resultant decreased venous return and cardiac output. Pitocin may increase the blood pressure.
• Assess pulse and respirations at admission and then every hour.	• Various conditions result in elevated pulse and respiratory rates. These include anxiety, pain, excitement, blood loss, and shock. Analgesics relax smooth muscles in blood vessels, reducing resistance. Pitocin may increase the pulse.
• Assess for edema; assess pedal and tibial areas, abdominal wall, back of hands, and face.	• There is physiologic edema during pregnancy as a result of restricted circulation from the lower extremities. Edema that occurs on bed rest or in the abdominal wall, the back of the hands, or the face is considered pathologic edema. It often accompanies pregnancy-induced hypertension.
• Regulate and monitor intake, IV fluids, and output.	• Bed rest promotes increased blood flow to the kidneys, with resultant increase in urinary output.
• Test urine for albumin.	• Albumin in the urine occurs as the result of glomerular vasoconstriction, which reduces reabsorption of albumin. Levels greater than +2 indicate kidney involvement; a +1 level typically indicates muscle catabolism with exercise or increased metabolism during labor.
• Assess for hypertensive response to Pitocin administration.	• Oxytocin increases cardiac output and circulating volume because of sodium and water absorption.
• Take temperature at admission, then every 4 hours. Take it more frequently if it is elevated above 99.6°F and every 1 to 2 hours after membranes rupture. Assess skin and mouth for dryness.	• Dehydration may result in elevated temperature and dry skin. The temperature may become elevated as a result of infection such as endometritis, which is more likely to occur after the membranes are ruptured.
• Assess amount of bloody show.	• Bloody show may increase as the cervix dilates. Excess bleeding may indicate placental separation.

Continued on following page

NURSING CARE PLANNING GUIDE Continued

- Assess contractions for frequency, duration, and strength.
  - Contractions are considered hyperactive when the strength is >75 mm Hg as noted by the internal monitor, when the duration is longer than 1 minute, when there is less than 1 minute of relaxation between contractions, and when the uterus does not relax completely between contractions (elevated baseline value). During a contraction, the blood supply to the myometrium is diminished. If contractions are hyperactive, uterine rupture could occur.
- If present, regulate Pitocin IV drip by infusion pump so contractions are not hyperactive.
  - The most common reason for hyperactive contractions is injudicious regulation of IV Pitocin. Pitocin stimulates uterine contractions.

2

Analysis: ▼ NURSING DIAGNOSIS

Risk for urinary retention, related to

- Increased urinary output of fluid retained during the prenatal period
- Decreased adrenal stimulation associated with bed rest
- Dehydration
- Bleeding, hemorrhage leading to decreased circulating blood volume
- Pressure of fetal head on bladder, which reduces sensation and interferes with bladder emptying
- Regional anesthesia

Defining Characteristics

SUBJECTIVE

Describes sensation of full bladder

Describes dysuria, frequency, urgency

OBJECTIVE

Urinary retention, full bladder on palpation

Voids infrequently

Voids small amounts

Output less than intake

Unable to void

Concentrated urine

Symptoms of urinary tract infection (frequency, urgency, dysuria, costovertebral tenderness, elevated temperature)

Continued on facing page

NURSING CARE PLANNING GUIDE Continued

Client Goal/ ▼ EVALUATION CRITERIA

Client will demonstrate normal urinary pattern without retention. / ▼ **Client will evidence bladder emptied regularly, output approximating intake, absence of full bladder on palpation.**

▼ NURSING INTERVENTIONS	Rationale
• Assess intake and output. Note color, concentration, and specific gravity.	• Output typically approximates intake. When output is reduced, urine becomes concentrated, assuming a darker yellow or orange color, and the specific gravity increases.
• Palpate and percuss above the symphysis pubis for bladder distention.	• When the bladder is full, it distends the lower abdomen, just above the symphysis pubis. Palpation and percussion detect the full bladder.
• Facilitate voiding by asking the client to void at regular intervals (every 2 hours), by positioning the client in the upright position or having her ambulate to the bathroom, by running water, or by pouring warm water over the perineum. Disconnect the fetal monitor and take the IV pole if these are in use. If membranes are ruptured and the head is not engaged, the mother should use the bedpan in bed; raise the head of the bed to facilitate voiding.	• All of these measures have been found to promote voiding. A distended bladder retards labor by impeding fetal descent, can lead to uterine atony, and contributes to discomfort; the bladder may be traumatized. If membranes are intact, or if the membranes are ruptured but the presenting part is well engaged, the mother may ambulate to the bathroom.
• Catheterize if unable to void or unable to empty the bladder.	• Emptying the bladder is necessary to avoid trauma and uterine atony.
• Assess for symptoms of urinary tract infection. (See Nursing Care Planning Guide: Healthy Postpartum Woman.)	• Symptoms of urinary tract infection include frequency, urgency, dysuria (cystitis) or costovertebral tenderness, and elevated temperature (kidney infection). (See Nursing Care Planning Guide: Healthy Postpartum Woman).

3

Analysis: ▼ NURSING DIAGNOSIS

Risk for infection: urinary tract, perineum (episiotomy), uterine placental site (endometritis), related to

- Repeated vaginal examinations
- Lapses in aseptic techniques
- Contamination from rectal area
- Ruptured membranes allowing pathogens to ascend to the uterus
- Prolonged labor

Continued on following page

NURSING CARE PLANNING GUIDE Continued

Defining Characteristics

SUBJECTIVE	*OBJECTIVE*
Urinary Tract	Urinary Tract
Describes burning with urination	Distended bladder
	Voids small amounts
	Voids frequently
	Dysuria
	Urgency
	Costovertebral angle tenderness
	Fever
Perineum (Episiotomy)	Perineum (Episiotomy)
Describes discomfort in the perineum	Burning of perineum
	Edema, swelling of perineum
	Laceration of perineum
	Discharge, exudate from episiotomy
	Episiotomy not approximated
	Fever
Uterine Placental Site (Endometritis)	Uterine Placental Site (Endometritis)
Describes foul-smelling lochia	Fever >100.4°F on 2 days post partum
	Elevated pulse
	Uterus larger than expected on palpation
	Dark brown, foul-smelling lochia, but may be odorless

Client Goal/ ▼ EVALUATION CRITERIA

Client will demonstrate absence of urinary tract infection, perineal (episiotomy) infection, uterine placental site infection (endometritis). / ▼ **Client will evidence voiding adequate amounts without symptoms of urinary tract infection, healing episiotomy, perineum without swelling and redness, absence of fever, normal lochia.**

▼ NURSING INTERVENTIONS	Rationale
• Perform vaginal examinations only when necessary. Use aseptic technique.	• Each vaginal examination creates the possibility of introducing microorganisms. Therefore, performing vaginal examinations only when necessary reduces the risk of infection to the lowest level possible.
• Provide perineal care every 4 hours and as needed. Cleanse from front to back. Wear gloves.	• Cleansing of the perineum removes amniotic fluid, bloody show, and any expelled fecal material that harbors microorganisms or provides an environment favorable to the growth of microorganisms. Cleansing from front to back prevents contamination of vagina and urethra with rectal microorganisms.

Continued on facing page

NURSING CARE PLANNING GUIDE Continued

	Standard Precautions advise wearing gloves whenever there is contact with body fluids, especially blood.
• Monitor and describe amniotic fluid.	• With uterine infection, the amniotic fluid becomes a yellowish color and may have a strong odor.
• Administer an enema, if ordered. Wear gloves.	• Historically, enemas were ordered to prevent contamination of the perineum and delivery field and to empty the lower bowel to facilitate descent of the fetal head. A small Fleet enema is usually ordered. If membranes are intact, the mother may ambulate to the bathroom. If membranes are not intact and the fetal head is not engaged, the bedpan should be used in bed. Studies have not found greater fecal contamination when an enema is not administered.
• Shave the perineum, if ordered. Wear gloves.	• Historically, a perineal prep was done to remove pubic hair that was considered to be contaminated. Studies have not found higher rates of infection when perineal preps are not done.
• Change perineal pads frequently. Wear gloves.	• Perineal pads are saturated with warm amniotic fluid and bloody show, both of which are media that enhance the growth of microorganisms.
• Set up the delivery table using aseptic technique. Cover with sterile drapes until time of delivery. Avoid contamination.	• The delivery table is often set up before delivery so it is available and does not interfere with other activities at the time of delivery. Contamination of the instruments introduces microorganisms, increasing the risk for infection.
• Perform the perineal prep at the time of delivery, just before the sterile drapes are applied. Wear sterile gloves; use a sterile solution.	• After the client is placed in the lithotomy, squatting, or other position for delivery, cleansing the perineum with an iodine preparation removes amniotic fluid, blood, or fecal material that could cause an infection.
• Cleanse the perineum after the delivery. Wear gloves. Cleanse from front to back.	• Cleansing after the delivery removes amniotic fluid and blood.
• Apply a perineal sanitary pad; change frequently. Wear gloves.	• The perineal pad absorbs lochia. Lochia contains blood and is moist, both of which provide an environment favorable for growth of microorganisms.
• Apply bed pads (Chux) and change frequently.	• Bed pads (Chux) are placed under the buttocks to collect lochia that is not absorbed by the perineal sanitary pad. An environment of blood fosters growth of microorganisms.
• Take temperature in the recovery room and then every 4 hours.	• When the temperature is elevated above 100.4°F on two occasions, a postpartum infection is suspected.
• Assess perineum/episiotomy for signs of infection. (See *Nursing Care Planning Guide: Healthy Postpartum Woman.*)	• The presence of lochia increases the risk for infection. (See *Nursing Care Planning Guide: Healthy Postpartum Woman.*)
• Instruct the mother to wear slippers when ambulating.	• The floor of the hospital is contaminated. If the feet are not covered with slippers, they become contaminated. The contaminated feet, in turn, can contaminate the bed linens, which can infect the perineum, vagina, and uterus.

Continued on following page

NURSING CARE PLANNING GUIDE Continued

4

Analysis: ▼ NURSING DIAGNOSIS

***Labor pain,* related to**

- Labor contractions
- Cervical effacement and dilatation
- Descent, crowning, and perineal stretching
- Fear of unknown
- Uncomfortable positions during labor
- Full bladder

Defining Characteristics

SUBJECTIVE

Describes pain with contractions

Describes inability to relax

States breathing techniques are not effective

Requests analgesic or regional anesthesia

OBJECTIVE

Contractions increasing in frequency, duration, and strength throughout labor

Cervix effacing and dilating

Fetus descending from −1 to 0 to +1 to +5 station

Perineum stretching

Tense muscles

Grimacing

Grasping and holding on

Breathing techniques ineffective

Holding breath

Unable to concentrate on breathing technique

Unable to relax between contractions

Client Goal/ ▼ EVALUATION CRITERIA

Client will demonstrate tolerance of labor pain. / ▼ **Client will evidence progressing labor, progressing dilatation, descending fetus, frequent bed pad changes, effective breathing techniques, relaxation between contractions, relaxation of tense muscles; client will state that analgesia helps relaxation and takes the "edge" off the pain; client will state that regional anesthesia is effective.**

Continued on facing page

NURSING CARE PLANNING GUIDE Continued

▼ NURSING INTERVENTIONS	Rationale
• During labor, assess discomfort and pain. Observe verbal and nonverbal behavior. Consider cultural variations in expressing reactions.	• Reactions to pain are subjective and individualized. They are based on past experiences, knowledge and acceptance of the situation, and cultural beliefs about pain and childbirth. Some cultural groups express reactions to pain by being quiet and stoic; others react by verbalizing feelings.
• Assist the client in using appropriate breathing and relaxation techniques. Assist with effleurage when appropriate.	• Relaxation and breathing techniques are based on conditioning. The mother concentrates and focuses on a visual object while relaxing muscles and doing a particular breathing technique. In the latent phase, slow-paced breathing is done during contractions. In the active phase, modified-paced breathing is done with contractions (as the contraction begins, slow breathing is done; breathing is accelerated at the peak of the contraction and then slowed again during the decrement of the contraction). In transition, if the urge to push is present, continual blowing is done when the urge to push is felt. Effleurage is an application of the gate control theory, which indicates that pain impulses to the cerebral cortex can be blocked by tactile stimulation. Thus, the effleurage, or stroking of the abdomen, blocks pain impulses.
• Assist with comfort measures. These include 1. back rubs 2. oral hygiene 3. ice chips 4. perineal cleansing 5. changing bed pads 6. changing positions	• Back rubs help the client to relax. Oral hygiene and ice chips refresh the mouth, which is dry from being NPO and from using breathing techniques. Cleansing the perineum promotes comfort by removing the moisture of amniotic fluid. Changing bed pads helps keep the bed dry. A change in position alters areas of pressure.
• Monitor contractions. Note frequency, duration, and strength of contractions at admission, then every hour, then every 15 to 30 minutes in transition. Palpate contractions. Monitor with external or internal monitor.	• Contractions become more frequent, last longer, and become stronger throughout labor. As this happens, the contractions typically become more uncomfortable. Knowledge of contractions and progress of labor is necessary to select appropriate breathing techniques and to decide when analgesia or regional anesthesia is appropriate.
• Point out the beginning and end of contractions to the client. Pace the contraction by informing the client of the passing of 15-second intervals (e.g., 15 seconds, 30 seconds, 45 seconds, 60 seconds).	• As contractions become closer and stronger, it may become more difficult for the mother to determine when a contraction ends. This occurs because the mother remains tense. Stimuli other than contractions (such as touch) can also be interpreted as painful. Defining the contraction and then assisting with the breathing technique and relaxation help the mother to interpret sensations and react more adaptively.
• Assess progress of labor. Note cervical effacement and dilatation, station, and position at appropriate intervals.	• The progress of labor is the basis of decisions about administration of analgesia and anesthesia if these are necessary or requested. If analgesia or anesthesia is administered before labor is well established, contractions can become weaker and less

Continued on following page

NURSING CARE PLANNING GUIDE Continued

effective. Pitocin augmentation might then be necessary. In addition, anesthesia removes sensations/pain, and therefore the mother is unable to "tell" when to push and has difficulty in pushing effectively.

Intervention	Rationale
• Provide information about available analgesics: usual response to analgesics, side effects, and duration of effectiveness. Provide information early in labor when the client is more able to concentrate and comprehend.	• Information is necessary to make decisions. Accurate information enhances understanding; false expectations are minimized when accurate information is provided.
• Administer analgesics on the basis of the client's response to labor and assessment of progress of labor.	• A common analgesic is Demerol (meperidine hydrochloride) given IM or IV. Tranquilizers are sometimes administered in conjunction with Demerol to potentiate its effect. Demerol is a central nervous system depressant that facilitates relaxation during and between contractions; it does not relieve labor pain completely, but it does take the "edge" off the pain. Demerol should not be given within 1 hour of delivery because it is circulated to the fetus. If the fetus is delivered when the greatest amount of Demerol is circulating, the baby's respirations can be greatly depressed after delivery, possibly necessitating the administration of a narcotic antagonist such as naloxone (Narcan) or nalorphine (Nalline); these counteract the depressant effects of Demerol.
• Assist with administration of regional anesthesia if it is desired. Explain the anesthesia and the procedure as it progresses. With regional anesthesia, administer 500 to 1000 mL IV bolus of lactated Ringer's solution just before administering the regional block.	• The nurse opens the sterile equipment, pours the local anesthetic, positions the client, and assists the client in maintaining the proper position. Explanation of the procedure helps reduce fear and anxiety. The most common anesthesia administered during labor is the epidural regional block or a paracervical block. The bolus of 500 to 1000 mL lactated Ringer's solution IV before the block increases the circulating volume, which helps prevent the side effect of hypotension. The main side effect is maternal hypotension, which affects not only the mother but oxygenation of the fetus as well. Fetal bradycardia may result. Therefore, prompt intervention to correct hypotension is essential. Most often, the local anesthetic Marcaine (bupivacaine) or Nesacaine (chloroprocaine hydrochloride) is used; these agents do not diminish fetal heart rate (FHR) variability, and therefore the fetal response to the stress of labor can continue to be evaluated.
• After regional anesthesia, take blood pressure every 1 to 2 minutes for 15 minutes, then every 10 to 15 minutes. If hypotension develops (systolic pressure is below 100 mm Hg or falls 30%), intervene immediately: 1. Turn woman to left lateral position with head flat or displace uterus to the left. 2. Turn up rate of IV fluids. 3. Administer oxygen per mask. 4. Assess FHR variability and whether bradycardia occurs.	• The main side effect of regional anesthesia is hypotension. This results from vasodilatation in the lower body, which reduces venous return. Turning to the side improves venous return and enhances placental circulation. Displacing the uterus takes the weight of the uterus off the vena cava, thereby improving venous return. Increasing the IV flow rate increases the circulating volume. The decreased blood flow to the placenta can affect the fetus; assessing FHR variability indicates the ability of the fetus to adjust to this stressor.

Continued on facing page

NURSING CARE PLANNING GUIDE Continued

- With regional anesthesia, assess redness of large toe or ball of foot.
- Because of vasodilatation, the foot becomes reddened. Noting this indicates correct placement of the anesthesia catheter.
- Assess effectiveness of regional anesthesia as well as return of sensation.
- Regional anesthesia should relieve pain sensation of the uterus and perineum and lower extremities symmetrically on both sides of the body. If the client is turned to one side or the other or is tilted to one side, anesthesia may be more effective on one side than the other. Anesthesia wears off after a time, and sensations will again be felt.
- Encourage the client to void every 2 hours and catheterize if necessary. Palpate above the symphysis to note bladder distention.
- Bladder distention can increase discomfort, increase the risk for trauma to the bladder, and prolong labor. Epidural and caudal blocks interfere with recognizing the sensation of a full bladder. Because of labor sensations or regional anesthesia, the client may be unable to void.
- Assist in administering anesthesia for delivery if the client does not already have regional anesthesia. Assist with reinforcement of regional anesthesia if this is in place. If spinal anesthesia is administered, assess blood pressure and intervene if hypotension occurs.
- Anesthesia during delivery minimizes pain from stretching of the vagina and perineum as well as with an episiotomy. If regional anesthesia has not been administered during labor, a local, pudendal, or spinal block may be used for the delivery. The main side effect of a spinal block is hypotension. A bolus of 1000 mL lactated Ringer's solution IV before administration is necessary to increase circulating volume, which helps prevent hypotension.

5

Analysis: ▼ NURSING DIAGNOSIS

***Risk for ineffective breathing pattern,* related to**

- Anxiety
- Altered breathing patterns
- Hyperventilation
- Upper respiratory tract infection
- Asthma
- Allergies
- Pain of labor

Continued on following page

NURSING CARE PLANNING GUIDE Continued

Defining Characteristics

SUBJECTIVE	*OBJECTIVE*
Describes apprehension with labor	Tense with contractions
Describes pain, discomfort with contractions	Respiratory rate >24 per minute
Describes asthma symptoms	Hyperventilation
Describes allergy symptoms	Inappropriate breathing technique for phase and stage of labor
Describes upper respiratory tract infection symptoms	Upper respiratory tract infection symptoms (nasal congestion, sneezing, nasal discharge, sore throat)
	Allergy symptoms (itchy, reddened eyes; clear nasal discharge; nasal congestion)
	Wheezing

Client Goal/ ▼ EVALUATION CRITERIA

Client will demonstrate effective breathing pattern. / ▼ **Client will evidence normal respiratory rate, absence of upper respiratory tract infection symptoms, absence of allergy symptoms, absence of asthma symptoms, appropriate breathing technique for phase and stage of labor, absence of hyperventilation.**

▼ NURSING INTERVENTIONS	Rationale
• Assess respirations at admission and then every hour.	• The respiratory rate can be altered with anxiety, with pain, and with respiratory conditions. Secretions of respiratory infections and allergies can obstruct the respiratory tract, contributing to increased rate and interference with exchange. Hyperventilation can occur with anxiety of labor. A normal respiratory rate ensures proper oxygenation of blood as well as excretion of carbon dioxide. The enlarged uterus exerts pressure on the diaphragm, potentially restricting expansion of lungs.
• Position the client to favor lung expansion.	• The enlarged uterus exerts pressure on the diaphragm, restricting lung expansion. Positioning on the back with the head elevated, or in the side-lying position in straight alignment, allows expansion of the lungs.
• Teach the appropriate breathing technique for the stage of labor and assist the mother with those techniques.	• The appropriate technique fosters relaxation, expansion of lungs, and proper oxygen and carbon dioxide exchange.
• Administer oxygen per mask at 8 liters per minute if required.	• Administration of oxygen per mask increases inspiration of oxygen, increasing the concentration of oxygen in the blood.

Continued on facing page

NURSING CARE PLANNING GUIDE Continued

- Have the client breathe into a paper bag if hyperventilation occurs.
- Hyperventilation occurs when excessive amounts of carbon dioxide are exhaled. With breathing into a paper bag, a greater amount of carbon dioxide than is present in room air is available for respiration.
- Assess for symptoms of asthma, upper respiratory tract infection, and allergy.
- Infection of the respiratory tract, allergies, and asthma alter respirations.

6

Analysis: ▼ NURSING DIAGNOSIS

***Risk for fluid volume deficit,* related to**

- NPO during labor
- Absence, or reduced rate, of IV fluids
- Rapid breathing
- Hypotension associated with regional anesthesia

Defining Characteristics

SUBJECTIVE

States is thirsty

States mouth is dry

OBJECTIVE

Temperature between 99.6 and 100.4°F

IV fluids running slowly

Mucous membranes dry

Skin turgor reduced

Elevated hematocrit

Concentrated urine, then reduced volume or no output

Client Goal/ ▼ EVALUATION CRITERIA

Client will demonstrate adequate fluid volume. / ▼ **Client will evidence similar intake and output, absence of concentrated urine, normal temperature, absence of dehydration symptoms.**

Continued on following page

NURSING CARE PLANNING GUIDE Continued

▼ NURSING INTERVENTIONS	Rationale
• Assess intake and output.	• During labor, oral fluids are restricted because gastrointestinal motility and digestion are inhibited. Intake and output should be relatively equal.
• Assess urine specific gravity.	• As urinary output decreases, the urine becomes more concentrated and specific gravity increases.
• Assess temperature initially and every 4 hours.	• Dehydration is associated with a slight elevation of temperature. A temperature between 99.6 and 100.4°F may indicate dehydration.
• Provide oral hygiene and hard candy.	• These reduce the discomfort of a dry mouth associated with dehydration.
• Assess mucous membranes and skin tissues for dehydration.	• As dehydration increases, mucous membranes become dry and there is less skin turgor.
• Regulate rate of IV fluids.	• If dehydration symptoms occur, an increase in the IV fluid rate will hydrate the client.
• Assess hematocrit.	• Hemoconcentration, with subsequent elevation of the hematocrit, occurs with dehydration.

7

Analysis: ▼ NURSING DIAGNOSIS

***Risk for altered fetal tissue perfusion,* related to**

- Labor contractions
- Regional anesthesia
- Maternal position
- Pitocin augmentation of labor
- Fetal head does not rotate internally to occiput anterior position

Defining Characteristics

SUBJECTIVE	*OBJECTIVE*
	FHR outside range of 120 to 160 beats per minute
	Persistent late decelerations of FHR
	Prolonged moderate or severe variable decelerations of FHR
	Decreased variability of FHR from baseline assessment

Continued on facing page

NURSING CARE PLANNING GUIDE Continued

Maternal hypotension
Mother positioned on back
Hyperactive, strong uterine contractions

Client Goal/ ▼ EVALUATION CRITERIA

Mother and fetus will demonstrate adequate fetal tissue perfusion. / ▼ **Client will evidence FHR of 120 to 160 beats per minute, absence of late and moderate or severe variable decelerations, normal FHR baseline variability, normal maternal blood pressure, normal uterine contractions; mother positioned on side or in the Fowler or semi-Fowler position.**

▼ NURSING INTERVENTIONS	Rationale
• Perform Leopold maneuvers to determine fetal position and best location to auscultate fetal heart.	• The fetal heart is heard the most distinctly through the fetal back. Therefore, the position of the fetus in utero must be determined to locate the back of the fetus.
• Auscultate FHR by fetoscope, Doptone, or external fetal monitor. Frequency varies by phase and stage of labor; the FHR should be taken or monitored at admission, every hour in the latent phase, every 30 minutes in the active phase, and every 15 minutes in the transition phase of the first stage of labor. In the second stage of labor, the FHR should be taken or monitored every 15 minutes.	• The normal FHR range is 120 to 160 beats per minute. The blood flow to the fetus decreases with each contraction, reducing oxygen flow during the contraction and creating a stress for the fetus. If the fetus adjusts to the stress adaptively, the FHR remains in the range of 120 to 160 beats per minute, exhibits average baseline variability, and has only minor periodic decelerations. Frequency of FHR assessment varies, depending on the phase and stage of labor, because contractions become stronger and closer together as labor progresses, thereby creating greater stress to the fetus as the labor progresses.
• Assess FHR baseline short- and long-term variability.	• Variability of the FHR indicates the ability of fetal nervous systems to regulate the FHR so it remains in the normal range. Average beat-to-beat variability should be 6 to 10 beats per minute.
• Assess FHR for periodic changes.	• The FHR often experiences periodic changes, or changes that occur periodically as the result of some change in circulation to the fetus. Periodic changes are either accelerations or decelerations of the FHR from the baseline level, with a return to the baseline level after the periodic acceleration or deceleration.
• Note FHR and periodic changes when the membranes rupture. Intervene if there could be a cord prolapse. Interventions for possible cord prolapse include the following: 1. Observe at vagina for protruding cord. 2. Elevate the presenting part with a sterile gloved hand. 3. Place mother in Trendelenburg or knee-chest position. 4. If cord is visible, wrap in sterile saline gauze.	• When membranes rupture, the amniotic fluid rushes out through the vagina; the rush of fluid may carry the cord with it, perhaps repositioning the cord so that it is compressed between the fetus and the birth canal. When the cord is compressed, blood flow to the fetus is reduced. A prolonged variable deceleration, with reduced oxygenation of the fetus, may occur if the cord prolapses. Elevating the presenting part reduces the pressure of the fetus on the cord, thereby lessening the degree of cord compression. A Trendelenburg or knee-chest

Continued on following page

NURSING CARE PLANNING GUIDE Continued

position also elevates the fetal presenting part, thereby reducing the degree of cord compression. Saline gauze keeps the cord moist.

- Assess for persistent fetal bradycardia.

- Bradycardia of FHR may occur with fetal hypoxia. The fetal hypoxia could be the result of maternal hypotension from vena caval syndrome or regional anesthesia, chronic pregnancy-induced hypertension, or prolonged hyperactive uterine contractions.

- Assess uterine contractions for frequency, duration, and strength. Intervene to decrease frequency, duration, or strength if needed:
  1. Turn Pitocin drip off or down.
  2. Position in semi-Fowler or side-lying position.
  3. Assess FHR for periodic changes and tachycardia.

- Each contraction presents a stress to the fetus because uteroplacental blood flow is reduced during each contraction. Thus, if contractions are too frequent, too long, or too strong, the restricted blood flow may be detrimental to the fetus.

- Assess maternal blood pressure at regular intervals and after regional anesthesia injection. Correct maternal hypotension:
  1. Turn to side, left lateral.
  2. Turn Pitocin drip off.
  3. Increase IV flow.
  4. Administer oxygen per mask.

- Regional anesthesia, such as epidural, causes vasodilatation in the lower region of the mother's body. With vasodilatation in such a large area, venous return to the heart is greatly reduced. When venous return is reduced, cardiac output and blood pressure are also reduced. With reduced cardiac output, circulatory volume to the mother and fetus is reduced. Turning to the side prevents supine hypotension and increases placental perfusion.

  Stopping Pitocin minimizes the restriction of blood flow that occurs with contractions by lessening the length and strength of contractions. There are also longer periods of uterine relaxation. Increasing the rate of IV fluids increases circulating volume to the mother and placenta. Administration of oxygen increases oxygen saturation of the circulating blood, thereby increasing oxygen available to the fetus.

- Intervene for untreatable variable decelerations:
  1. Turn mother to other side if deceleration does not abate.
  2. Do a vaginal examination to check for prolapsed cord.
  3. Place in knee-chest position if deceleration does not abate or if cord is prolapsed.
  4. Administer oxygen per mask.
  5. Notify the physician.

- A persistent variable deceleration must be corrected so that the cord compression is released and circulation to the fetus is improved. Turning to the sides prevents supine hypotension and improves placental flow. It also changes the position of the fetus and may thereby reduce pressure on the cord. Compression of the cord may occur as a result of a prolapsed cord; a vaginal examination may detect this, and the knee-chest position reduces pressure on the cord. Administration of oxygen increases oxygen saturation of the blood that flows to the fetus.

- Intervene for recurrent late decelerations:
  1. Turn to the side.
  2. Regulate Pitocin and contractions.
  3. Notify the physician.
  4. Administer oxygen per mask.
  5. Correct maternal hypotension.
  6. Assess FHR baseline variability.
  7. Assist with scalp pH if needed.
  8. Prepare for cesarean section.

- Turning the mother to the side prevents supine hypotension and improves placental blood flow. Regulating Pitocin reduces the stress of contractions, which restrict placental blood flow. Administration of oxygen increases oxygen saturation of the blood that flows to the fetus. Maternal hypotension restricts placental blood flow. If late decelerations are not corrected, a cesarean section is done.

  FHR baseline variability is assessed because it indicates the fetal reserves or ability to cope with the stress of reduced oxygenation.

Continued on facing page

NURSING CARE PLANNING GUIDE Continued

The fetal scalp pH indicates the pH of the fetal blood or whether acidosis has occurred as a result of reduced oxygenation. Acidosis occurs with anaerobic metabolism, which is necessary when oxygen for aerobic metabolism is lacking (a pH between 7.20 and 7.25 requires monitoring). If the late decelerations persist and baseline variability is minimal or scalp pH indicates acidosis, a cesarean section is done.

- Intervene for persistent bradycardia:
  1. Turn to the side.
  2. Stop Pitocin.
  3. Administer oxygen per mask.
  4. Correct maternal hypotension.

- Turning to the side facilitates placental blood flow. Stopping Pitocin reduces the stress of contractions. Administering oxygen increases the oxygenation of blood to the fetus. Maternal hypotension as a result of maternal position or regional anesthesia may cause bradycardia. In addition, in second-stage labor, there may be vagal stimulation that occurs with fetal head compression. This may lead to fetal bradycardia.

- Ensure that mother does not lie flat on her back.

- A flat, back-lying position allows pressure of the enlarged uterus to restrict venous return to the heart with resultant hypotension.

- Assess fetal presentation, station, and position. If the position is occiput posterior and the head does not rotate, position mother on her side.

- Malpresentation (face, chin, or brow) may prolong or arrest labor. Occiput posterior position, or failure to rotate to occiput anterior position, may prolong the second stage of labor. Placing the mother on her side facilitates rotation. The longer the labor, the longer the fetus is exposed to the stress of labor. Breech positions and failure to descend or engage allow greater opportunity for cord compression.

8

Analysis: ▼ NURSING DIAGNOSIS

***Risk for fetal injury,* related to**

- Malpresentation
- Breech presentation
- Forceps delivery
- Vacuum extraction
- Scalp electrode
- Precipitous labor
- Prolonged labor
- Cord compression
- Cephalopelvic disproportion

Continued on following page

NURSING CARE PLANNING GUIDE Continued

Defining Characteristics

SUBJECTIVE

OBJECTIVE

Prolonged first stage of labor, slow dilatation

Prolonged second stage of labor, slow or arrested descent

Failure to engage (0 station)

Persistent occiput posterior

Low forceps rotation and delivery

Forceps delivery

Large fetus for maternal pelvis; large fetus on abdominal palpation, pelvic examination with blunt ischial spines, small obstetric diagonal conjugate, flat sacrum

Infant with fractured clavicle

Infant with brachial plexus injury

Infant with cephalhematoma

Infant with caput succedaneum

Client Goal/ ▼ EVALUATION CRITERIA

Client will demonstrate normal labor and delivery with no injury to fetus. / ▼ **Client will evidence normal progression of labor, spontaneous vaginal delivery, and her infant has no injuries.**

▼ NURSING INTERVENTIONS	Rationale
• Assess fetal presentation, position, and station throughout labor.	• Malpresentation, such as face, brow, or mentum, often results in prolonged labor, failure to engage or descend, slow descent, or lack of internal rotation. Breech presentations have a higher risk for cord compression and injury with delivery. A pelvis that is small for the size of the fetus could result in cephalopelvic disproportion with prolonged labor. Prolonged labor subjects the fetus to a greater number of contractions that are stressful to the fetus.
• Assess contractions for frequency, duration, and strength.	• Dilatation, descent, and internal rotation are inhibited if contractions are not of sufficient frequency, duration, and strength. Maladaptive contractions reduce oxygenation and create physical stress to the fetus.
• Administer Pitocin appropriately, if ordered. Assess effect of Pitocin on uterine contractions so contractions are effective but not hyperactive.	• Contractions need to be sufficiently close together, strong, and of sufficient length to dilate the cervix and cause descent. Pitocin IV, administered with a pump, is used to augment labor contractions so they are more effective. Contractions should facilitate progress of labor but not be too frequent, long, or strong.

Continued on facing page

NURSING CARE PLANNING GUIDE Continued

- Assess FHR baseline level and periodic changes. Intervene to correct abnormal occurrences.
- The stress of labor can create reduced variability, late or variable decelerations, and bradycardia.
- Assist with pushing in second stage.
- In the second stage of labor, descent and internal rotation can be enhanced by adding the force of pushing to the force of contractions. Some believe that prolonged pushing of the fetal head on resistive perineal tissues can traumatize the fetus.
- Assist with forceps or vacuum extraction deliveries. Assist with episiotomy.
- The nurse prepares the delivery table and provides the forceps and sutures for the episiotomy repair.

9

Analysis: ▼ NURSING DIAGNOSIS

***Risk for maternal fatigue,* related to**

- Physical exertion during labor
- Lack of sleep
- Anxiety about labor and birth
- Pushing in second stage of labor
- Prolonged labor

Defining Characteristics

SUBJECTIVE	*OBJECTIVE*
Describes feelings of fatigue, exhaustion	Appears pale, drawn
	Eyes droop
	Unable to push effectively
	Muscles tense, unrelaxed
	Signs of moderate anxiety
	Unable to relax between contractions

Continued on following page

NURSING CARE PLANNING GUIDE Continued

Client Goal/ ▼ EVALUATION CRITERIA

Client will demonstrate minimal fatigue. / ▼ **Client will evidence relaxed muscles and relaxation between contractions, will push effectively, and will describe feelings of rest/restoration.**

▼ NURSING INTERVENTIONS	Rationale
• Encourage rest and relaxation between contractions.	• Rest and relaxation conserve energy.
• Monitor progress of labor. Inform client of progress.	• Information about progress conserves psychological energy. Assessing progress allows interventions that enhance progress. The shorter the labor, the less fatigue likely to be experienced.
• Assist with pushing.	• Effective pushing shortens the second stage, thereby reducing fatigue.
• Provide analgesia or regional anesthesia as appropriate.	• Analgesia and anesthesia relax tense muscles so that less energy is used. The more relaxed the mother, the less likely she is to experience fatigue.
• Provide comfort measures. Position comfortably.	• Comfort measures reduce anxiety and tension and aid relaxation.
• Alter environment to foster rest and relaxation.	• Reduction of noise, distractions, and light helps provide rest and sleep.

10

Analysis: ▼ NURSING DIAGNOSIS

***Knowledge deficit: labor, anesthesia, delivery,* related to**

- Lack of information about physical changes of labor
- Lack of information about progress of labor
- Lack of information about options available
- Lack of information about procedures associated with labor and birth

Continued on facing page

NURSING CARE PLANNING GUIDE Continued

Defining Characteristics

SUBJECTIVE	*OBJECTIVE*
Asks questions about labor	First labor
Asks questions about anesthesia	Labor pattern that varies from first pregnancy
	No childbirth education classes
	Only a few childbirth education classes
	Minimal information from health care providers during prenatal period about labor, anesthesia

Client Goal/ ▼ EVALUATION CRITERIA

Client will demonstrate adequate knowledge of labor, anesthesia, delivery. / ▼ **Client will evidence minimal questions, adequate ability to perform breathing techniques, mild to moderate anxiety.**

▼ NURSING INTERVENTIONS	Rationale
• Assess the client's preparation and knowledge of labor and delivery.	• Information establishes educational need. Knowledge allows the client to be aware of alternatives to make an informed choice.
• Orient the client to procedures, such as the fetal monitor.	• Anxiety is typically heightened in an unfamiliar environment and role.
• Explain the process of labor if necessary.	• Knowledge reduces anxiety, allows the client to make informed choices, increases self-control, and contributes to positive feelings about the experience.
• Explain types of analgesia and anesthesia available, including duration and side effects.	• Knowledge reduces anxiety, allows the client to make informed choices, increases self-control, and contributes to positive feelings about the experience.
• Demonstrate breathing and relaxation techniques appropriate for phase and stage of labor.	• Unprepared couples need to learn coping techniques to reduce anxiety. Those who attended childbirth classes typically benefit from reinforcement.
• Explain alternative positions and actions that promote comfort. Allow the client to select the position most comfortable for her.	• Changing position promotes comfort by changing areas of pressure. The client may be unaware of positions that promote comfort in various phases and stages of labor. The clients may vary in their preference, so each should be allowed to select the most comfortable position for herself.
• Clarify inaccurate information and misconceptions.	• Clarification will provide accurate information and allows the client to operate on a sound basis.
• Alter teaching so it is effective for the level of anxiety and phase or stage of labor.	• When one is anxious, perceptions and ability to pay attention are lessened, necessitating a less complex, slower paced instruction.

Continued on following page

NURSING CARE PLANNING GUIDE Continued

11

Analysis: ▼ **NURSING DIAGNOSIS**

***Moderate to severe anxiety*, related to**

- Knowledge deficit about labor and delivery
- Pelvic examinations
- Obstetric interventions such as inserting internal monitor, administering anesthesia
- Absence of support person
- Being left alone, abandonment during labor
- Inability to control reaction to labor

Defining Characteristics

SUBJECTIVE

Moderate Anxiety

Expresses feelings of tension, apprehension, nervousness, concern

Verbalizes expectations of problems

Voices sleeping disturbances, such as insomnia

Severe Anxiety

Expresses feelings of severe apprehension, nervousness, and helplessness

OBJECTIVE

Moderate Anxiety

Voice tremors

Voice pitch changes

Increased rate and quantity of verbalization

Minimal focus of attention; focuses on a particular part of a situation; selective inattention

Able to focus on most of what is happening

Minimal perception

Paces

Hand tremors or shakiness

Increased muscle tension

Rapid pulse

Increased respiratory rate

Irritability

More active reflexes, startle reactions

Face flushed

Localized or generalized sweating

Cheerfulness or laughing with serious matters

Severe Anxiety

False cheerfulness, or laughing with serious matters

Inappropriate verbalizations

Continued on facing page

NURSING CARE PLANNING GUIDE Continued

Intellectualization
Cannot focus on what is really happening
Can follow only simple directions
Inability to focus on reality
Rigid posture
Purposeless activity
Tachycardia
Hyperventilation
Clammy hands and skin
Dry mouth
Diaphoresis
Pallor
Withdrawn

Client Goal/ ▼ EVALUATION CRITERIA

Client will demonstrate reduced anxiety. / ▼ **Client will evidence seeking information, awareness of labor progress, increased attention, ability to follow directions, ability to perform breathing techniques, enhanced ability to learn, mild restlessness, normal pulse and respirations, ability to focus on most of what is happening.**

▼ NURSING INTERVENTIONS	Rationale
• Assess symptoms of anxiety as noted.	• Anxiety is an emotion that occurs as the result of a threat to one's physical self; one's identity, self-concept, self-esteem; or one's relationships. It occurs when something central to one's personality, essential to one's security, is threatened. Symptoms involve cardiovascular, respiratory, skin, gastrointestinal, urinary tract, neuromuscular, verbalization, perceptual/attention, and motor responses. Physiologic responses are mediated through the sympathetic nervous system and are not under voluntary control. The tension and other responses associated with anxiety have a negative impact on the labor process, perhaps prolonging the first phase. Epinephrine is released from the adrenals, which inhibits myometrial contractions. Norepinephrine is also released, which increases uterine activity. This imbalance can cause a dysfunctional labor pattern. In addition, anxiety uses glucose reserves, which reduces the amount available for uterine contractions.
• Assess preparedness for childbirth. Provide information that is lacking.	• Information reduces anxiety associated with the unknown.
• Assess cultural background with its perceptions of childbirth.	• Cultural groups vary in perceptions about childbirth.

Continued on following page

NURSING CARE PLANNING GUIDE Continued

• Assess role of support person. Teach ways to provide support if this is necessary. Explain labor processes and responses to labor as necessary.	• The support person assists the client in maintaining control as well as increases self-esteem by encouragement and reinforcement. When a support person stays, the fear of being alone or feeling abandoned is reduced. Anxiety is also reduced because the client feels the support person will be an advocate. Some support persons may not be aware of activities to assist the laboring mother, such as back rubs or assistance with a particular breathing technique. When the labor process procedures are understood by the support person, the support person's level of anxiety is reduced.
• Orient to the environment, staff, and procedures.	• Information reduces anxiety associated with fear of the unknown.
• Demonstrate breathing and relaxation techniques. "Breathe" with the client at times to reinforce learning.	• Demonstration facilitates learning. Active participation with the learner provides a visual cue that enhances learning.
• Provide for privacy and respect for modesty.	• Modesty is typically a concern to most people. Examinations and procedures in labor and delivery require some exposure and may contribute to anxiety.
• If anxiety is severe, attempt to lower it to moderate or mild levels. This can be accomplished by 1. listening 2. encouraging expression of feelings 3. accepting the client's response 4. answering questions directly 5. modifying the environment (decrease stimulation, provide quiet) 6. staying with the client	• With severe anxiety, most of the energy is directed to relief of the anxiety. Perceptions are greatly reduced. Reducing the discomfort can be accomplished by establishing trust, accepting the client's behaviors, listening, and providing a calm and quiet atmosphere.
• Recognize the client's anxiety.	• Recognition helps the client realize feelings and provides insight.
• Ask the mother to describe the labor situation from her perspective.	• Since anxiety is subjective, description of the situation from the client's perspective allows the nurse to become aware of what is being threatened.
• Tell the client that she will not be left alone and make sure that someone is with her.	• Ensuring the client that she will not be left alone helps lessen fear of abandonment.
• Administer tranquilizers and narcotics or assist with regional anesthesia as appropriate.	• Tranquilizers reduce anxiety and potentiate the effect of narcotics. Anesthesia reduces discomfort of contractions.
• Maintain comfort (provide dry bed pads, assist in changing positions, provide oral hygiene).	• These interventions that maintain comfort let the client know that everything is normal and that the nurse is interested in her well-being.
• Use soothing touch if this is helpful to the client (back rub, massage).	• Touch can aid relaxation. Massage relaxes tense muscles.
• Reinforce information that the labor is progressing normally.	• Knowledge reduces anxiety associated with fear of injury.
• Provide instructions and assist with pushing.	• Active involvement aids coping.
• Encourage rest and relaxation between contractions. Suggest closing the eyes; talk the client quietly through muscle relaxation.	• Rest reduces anxiety and conserves energy.

Continued on facing page

NURSING CARE PLANNING GUIDE Continued

• Encourage and positively reinforce. Inform the client of progress. Point out effective breathing techniques, relaxation.	• Reinforcement helps the client feel positive about the labor experience by recognizing the client's behaviors and efforts.
• Allow the client to see and hold the infant.	• This reduces anxiety associated with fear about the baby's being normal.

12

Analysis: ▼ NURSING DIAGNOSIS

Risk for situational low self-esteem, **related to**

- Request for medication or regional anesthesia when unmedicated birth had been planned
- Inability to cope with labor as anticipated
- Unrealistic expectations of response to labor

Defining Characteristics

SUBJECTIVE	*OBJECTIVE*
Describes expectations of nonmedicated labor	Cries
Describes pain	Grimaces
Requests medication or anesthesia	Tense muscles
Apologizes for behavioral responses to labor	Breathing techniques ineffective
Describes feelings of failure	

Client Goal/ ▼ EVALUATION CRITERIA

Client will demonstrate positive self-esteem. / ▼ **Client will evidence realistic assessment of responses to labor; takes medication/anesthesia as needed.**

▼ NURSING INTERVENTIONS	**Rationale**
• Assess perceptions of behavior during labor from client and significant other.	• The significant other influences evaluations and acceptance of self. In developing the self, feedback from others and one's own perceptions influence the image of the self. Reality is often inconsistent with idealized conceptualizations, and the mother judges herself negatively because she feels she is not "measuring up" to her conceptualizations.

Continued on following page

NURSING CARE PLANNING GUIDE Continued

- Encourage sharing of feelings.
  - The laboring woman often unrealistically feels that she should not behave as she is during labor; she feels that she should be able to cope easily. When this occurs, the mother denies feelings of failure and does not share them for fear of being judged negatively. If she can express the feelings, they can be recognized as normal feelings and she can realize she is not being judged negatively.
- Review progress of labor and alternatives available.
  - Anxiety is lessened if one is aware of what to expect. Expectations can be realistic when there is adequate knowledge and one is better able to set and achieve goals.
- Assist the client in gaining or maintaining control. Review breathing and relaxation techniques; demonstrate them, allow the client to make choices (such as position).
  - When one is allowed to make choices, feelings of control are fostered. When the client is able to perform breathing techniques, there is a sense of control and mastery.
- Provide comfort measures.
  - When the client is the recipient of measures to enhance comfort, she feels valued, that "someone cares."
- Provide positive feedback.
  - Positive comments and feedback from others help to form an image of the self that builds self-esteem.
- Assess the emotional and appraisal support of the significant other. Provide accurate information about common responses to labor and encourage the significant other to provide positive feedback.
  - Feedback is important in the way one judges one's behavior. If feedback is negative, the mother may feel inadequate and suffer lower self-esteem.

13

Analysis: ▼ NURSING DIAGNOSIS

***Risk for fetal injury: immediate extrauterine adjustment after birth,* related to**

- Labor
- Birth
- Need to initiate respirations
- Need to close fetal shunts
- Need to maintain temperature
- Vaginal examinations
- Ruptured membranes
- Exposure to maternal infection
- Internal fetal monitor
- Exposure to microorganisms in utero

Continued on facing page

NURSING CARE PLANNING GUIDE Continued

Defining Characteristics

SUBJECTIVE	*OBJECTIVE*
Does not cry lustily	Does not grimace with stimulation
	Cries weakly with stimulation
	Color pale or cyanotic or cyanotic hands and feet
	Poor muscle tone
	Unflexed position
	Heart rate <100
	Respirations shallow, irregular, with apnea
	Responds with weak cry or without grimace
	Neonatal infection

Client Goal/ ▼ EVALUATION CRITERIA

Infant will demonstrate extrauterine fetal adjustment immediately after birth. / ▼ **Infant will evidence heart rate >100, lusty cry, pink color, resistive muscle tone, normal respirations, absence of neonatal infection; client will appear alert and awake.**

▼ NURSING INTERVENTIONS	Rationale
• Assist with initiating and maintaining respirations: 1. Assess respiratory rate (normal rate, 30 to 60 per minute) 2. Assess for grunting. 3. Assess for retractions. 4. Assess for nasal flaring. 5. Assess for characteristics of normal newborn respirations (abdominal, shallow, nose breathing). 6. Assess for respiratory obstruction. 7. Suction prn. 8. Position on side. 9. Auscultate breath sounds.	• In utero, there is minimal circulation to the respiratory tract, and it is filled with fluid. After birth, the volume of blood circulating to the lungs needs to increase, and the respiratory fluids need to be absorbed or excreted. Some of this fluid, as well as mucus, may obstruct the respiratory tract. Positioning on the side facilitates drainage of fluid to the side of the mouth so that it can be suctioned.
• Assess heart rate and circulation. This can be accomplished by auscultation or by palpating the umbilical cord and by observing the infant's color. Cord blood is sampled for blood type, and a Coombs test is also done.	• After birth, the fetal shunts need to close so that fetal circulation ceases and there is increased blood flow to the lungs. When blood circulates appropriately, tissues are oxygenated and color is pink. Determination of blood type indicates whether there could be a blood incompatibility. Blood incompatibility is associated with an antigen-antibody reaction and hemolysis of red blood cells. The Coombs test indicates whether there are maternal Rh-positive antibodies in the fetal blood.

Continued on following page

NURSING CARE PLANNING GUIDE Continued

• Assist the neonate in maintaining normal temperature: 1. Dry neonate immediately after birth. 2. Place neonate under radiant warmer. 3. Reduce heat loss by conduction (warm crib and linens, warm stethoscope), evaporation (dry neonate), convection (air surrounding neonate warmed by radiant warmer), and radiation (crib away from air conditioner). 4. Double-wrap the neonate and place cap on neonate when removed from radiant warmer. 5. Assess neonate's temperature by skin probe or axillary method.	• After birth, the neonate is exposed to a cooler environment and must increase metabolism (especially of brown fat) to maintain temperature. Heat can be lost by conduction (heat lost to cooler objects in direct contact with the neonate), convection (heat lost to cooler air), radiation (heat lost to cooler objects not in direct contact with the neonate), and evaporation (heat lost by evaporation of moisture).
• Assess neonate's reflex irritability. This is accomplished by stimulation (with catheter or flicking the foot) and observation of response.	• If the neonate's nervous system is adaptive, the neonate will reflexly respond to stimulation by withdrawing the foot and crying, or by crying lustily.
• Assess the neonate's muscle tone. This involves observation for flexed position and notation of resistance to movement of extremities.	• The neonate's muscle tone should be resistive; the neonate should naturally assume a flexed position.
• Assess Apgar score and record at 1 and 5 minutes after birth.	• Apgar scoring assesses the condition of the neonate after birth and the ability of the neonate to adjust after birth. It assesses heart rate, respiratory effort, muscle tone, reflex irritability, and color. Heart rate is assessed by stethoscope or palpation at the umbilical cord; respiratory effort is assessed by observation; muscle tone is assessed by observation and assessment of resistance; reflex irritability is assessed by the reflex response of grimacing or crying with catheter suction or flicking the foot; color is assessed by observation. A neonate receives a score of 0, 1, or 2 for each of these areas. A score of 10 is the highest score possible. Scores of 7 to 10 indicate slight or no distress; scores of 3 to 6, moderate distress; scores of 0 to 2, severe distress.
• Have parents hold neonate. Assist mother with breastfeeding if she wishes to breastfeed at this time.	• Holding the neonate continues the attachment process that began during pregnancy and initiates the "acquaintance" process. Breastfeeding/sucking stimulates production of prolactin and oxytocin, enhancing production of colostrum and subsequently breast milk.
• Complete an abbreviated assessment for gross abnormalities.	• Baseline information is provided for follow-up assessments.
• Note and record voiding or bowel elimination, if it occurs in the delivery or recovery room.	• Voiding indicates ability of urinary tract to function normally. Bowel elimination indicates normally functioning bowel.

Chapter 24

Pain Management During Childbirth

Mary C. Brucker
Elaine Zwelling

> . . . pharmaceutical pain management intervention does play a role in childbirth, but supportive pain management techniques such as labor support, relaxation, controlled breathing and positioning should be the *first approach* used to help laboring women cope with childbirth. Pharmaceutical intervention, when used, should augment supportive strategies rather than become a substitute for them.
>
> SHARRON S. HUMENICK (NICHOLS AND HUMENICK 1988)

HIGHLIGHTS

- The Physiology of Pain in Childbirth
- Pain Pathways
- Understanding Pain Related to Gate Control Theory, Endogenous Biochemical Pain Theory, Fear-Tension-Pain Theory, Cognitive Control of Pain
- Variables Influencing Pain in Childbirth
- Pain Management Strategies
- Nonpharmacologic Modalities Related to Knowledge and Information; Relaxation Techniques; Breathing Strategies; Labor Support; Imagery; Touch and Massage; Application of Heat or Cold; Bathing, Showering, and Jet Hydrotherapy; Biofeedback; Hypnosis; Transcutaneous Electronic Nerve Stimulation; Acupressure, Acupuncture, and Shiatsu
- Pharmacologic Interventions Related to Systemic Medications, Regional Analgesia and Anesthesia, General Anesthesia
- Nursing Practice
- Collaborative Process
- Risk Management
- Implications for Research

It is well recognized that pain is a physiologic component of labor and birth. However, the concept of pain associated with childbirth is usually discussed only in relation to obstetric analgesia and anesthesia. This somewhat narrow treatment of the subject assumes that pharmaceutical agents are the only relief measures invoked for the management of pain in childbirth. Not only is that a misconception, but viewing childbirth pain as an entity treatable only pharmacologically also allows it to be construed as an

DEFINITIONS

Acupressure—The application of pressure with the thumb, index finger, or palm of the hand to an acupuncture point to relieve pain.

Analgesics—Drugs that decrease the perception of pain.

Anesthetics—Pain relief modalities that have the ability to totally block the sensation of pain; regional or general anesthetics.

Biofeedback—The use of monitoring instruments to recognize and alter physiologic processes within the body.

Cognitive dissonance—A difference between what is expected and what is actually experienced.

Endorphins—Morphine-like polypeptides produced in the pituitary gland that are released in response to pain, exercise, or cutaneous stimulation and serve to decrease pain perception.

Epidural block—A regional anesthetic given in active first-stage labor by injection of the agent through an indwelling plastic catheter into the epidural (peridural) space of the spinal column; provides pain relief of the contractions of labor and for delivery.

Local anesthesia—An anesthetic agent injected directly into the muscles and tissue of the perineum for the delivery and episiotomy repair; provides pain relief for the tissues of the perineum.

Nonpharmacologic pain relief—Pain relief based on a variety of methods other than analgesics or anesthetics.

Paracervical block—Regional anesthesia given in first-stage labor by injection of the agent into the cervical tissue; provides pain relief for the contractions of labor but must be followed by another anesthetic for the delivery.

Pharmacologic pain relief—Pain relief based on the use of analgesics or anesthetics.

Pudendal block—Regional anesthesia given immediately prior to birth by injection of the agent transvaginally to the pudendal nerves; provides pain relief for the upper two thirds of the vagina and the perineum.

Regional anesthesia—A nerve block that provides analgesia or anesthesia to one particular area or region of the body; includes paracervical, epidural, spinal, pudendal, and local blocks.

Spinal block—Regional anesthesia given just prior to birth by injection of the agent through the dura into the cerebrospinal fluid of the subarachnoid space of the spinal column; provides pain relief for the birth and perineal repair.

Transcutaneous electrical nerve stimulation (TENS)—Use of a device that emits low-voltage electricity to the body through electrodes placed on the skin to alter pain perception.

unusual or pathologic process. For the nurse or the laboring family to deny that discomfort and pain exist in childbirth is unrealistic. Instead, the nurse, the woman, and her family need to understand the physiologic reasons underlying the experience of pain. Nurses need to recognize that laboring women exhibit individual interpretations and personal expressions of pain. It is important for nurses and expectant parents to explore various strategies for diminishing or managing the pain of labor and birth, so that informed choices can be made regarding the pain relief measures desired. This chapter discusses the nature of pain and the pain experience, theories of pain perception, variables that influence pain during labor and birth, nonpharmacologic and pharmacologic pain management strategies, and the application of the nursing process to the management of pain in childbirth.

THE PHYSIOLOGY OF PAIN IN CHILDBIRTH

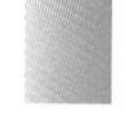

Definition and Characteristics of Pain

Pain is a universal experience; all people experience pain at some point in their lives. Pain is also relative, in that a stimulus that is perceived as painful by one individual may not be painful to another or even to the same individual at another time. Pain is difficult to describe and often difficult to recall when it is over. Pain itself cannot be observed; only the response to the pain stimulus is observed directly. McCaffery and Beebe (1989) stated that pain is whatever the experiencing person says it is, and it exists whenever the experiencing person says it does. This definition implies that each individual is the best judge of his or her pain and that pain should not be discounted by others. Although there may be times when the health care provider questions the amount of pain being experienced by a patient in relation to the identified cause, behavioral responses being demonstrated that are indicative of pain must have either a physical, emotional, or socioenvironmental reason (Jimenez 1988; McCaffery and Beebe 1989).

The nature of pain related to childbirth is unique in several ways. The pain experienced is not the result of illness or abnormal pathology but of normal physiology. Unlike pain resulting from a disease process, pain in childbirth is due to known factors—uterine contractions, cervical stretching, baby descending. This helps to decrease the fear that often exacerbates pain. Although women never look forward to the pain, it is often viewed as a signal that pregnancy is about to end and a baby is about to be born. The fact that the pain experience results in the joy of birth helps to keep the experience in perspective. There is usually a positive outcome. Another characteristic of labor pain that is unique is the fact that it is prescribed by known time limits. Laboring women can be assured that the pain of labor is for a limited duration (approximately 12 hours in length with each contraction lasting approximately 60 seconds) and that when the delivery is over, the pain will be gone. This knowledge helps the woman to cope with the discomfort at hand.

Pain Pathways

The pain pathways that transmit pain during labor and birth can be seen in Figure 24–1. Pain impulses are transmitted along sensory pathways that follow the sympathetic nerves through the cervical plexus, inferior hypogastric (pelvic) plexus, middle hypogastric plexus, superior hypogastric plexus, and lower and lumbar thoracic sympathetic chain and then enter the spinal cord through the tenth, eleventh, and twelfth thoracic nerves and first lumbar nerve. This pathway transmits the pain from uterine contractions in the first stage of labor. The sensory fibers of the genital tract travel through the pudendal nerve to the posterior sacrospinous ligament to the second, third, and fourth sacral nerves. This pathway is responsible for the pain sensations perceived in the second stage of labor (Bonica and McDonald 1995).

Pain in First-Stage Labor

Several physiologic changes that occur during the labor process are thought to be the major ones associated with pain (Oxorn 1986; Jimenez 1988; Bonica and McDonald 1995).

- Cervical stretching and pressure: the cervix, although often characterized by its relative insensitivity to touch or discomfort, has a number of afferent sensory fibers that come together at the posterior cervical plexus. These sensory fibers accompany sympathetic nerves that follow the lumbar sympathetic chain and enter the spinal cord at levels T10 through L1. The stimulation of these nerves with dilatation of the cervix in labor is considered to be the major etiologic agent of pain through this pathway (Fig. 24–1).
- Hypoxia of the uterine muscle: during contractions the blood flow to the uterus is markedly reduced. The hypoxic event may be interpreted physiologically as a painful one. Increasing episodes of hypoxia over time are thought to be the cause of increasing pain as labor progresses.
- Stretching and traction: other physiologic factors that have been postulated as being potentially associated with pain have included traction of internal reproductive organs and ligaments; pressure on urethra, bladder, and rectum; increased intra-abdominal pressure; and stretching of the abdominal peritoneum.

The foregoing factors help in understanding the location of the pain experienced during the first stage of labor. In early labor, discomfort tends to be confined to the back with radiation to the abdomen. As labor progresses and more physiologic changes take place, the discomfort increases. For example, if the infant is in an occiput posterior position, the woman often complains of intense back pain, even to the exclusion of abdominal pain. Figure 24–2 illustrates the areas of the body most commonly associated with pain as first-stage labor progresses (Bonica and McDonald 1995).

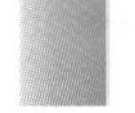

Pain in Second-Stage Labor

The physiologic factors associated with pain in the second stage of labor appear to be associated primarily with distention of the muscles of the vagina, pelvic floor, and perineum. These muscles are innervated predominantly by the pudendal nerve. The two pudendal nerves are located bilaterally and proximate to the sacrospinous ligaments (see Fig. 24–1). Each pudendal nerve is

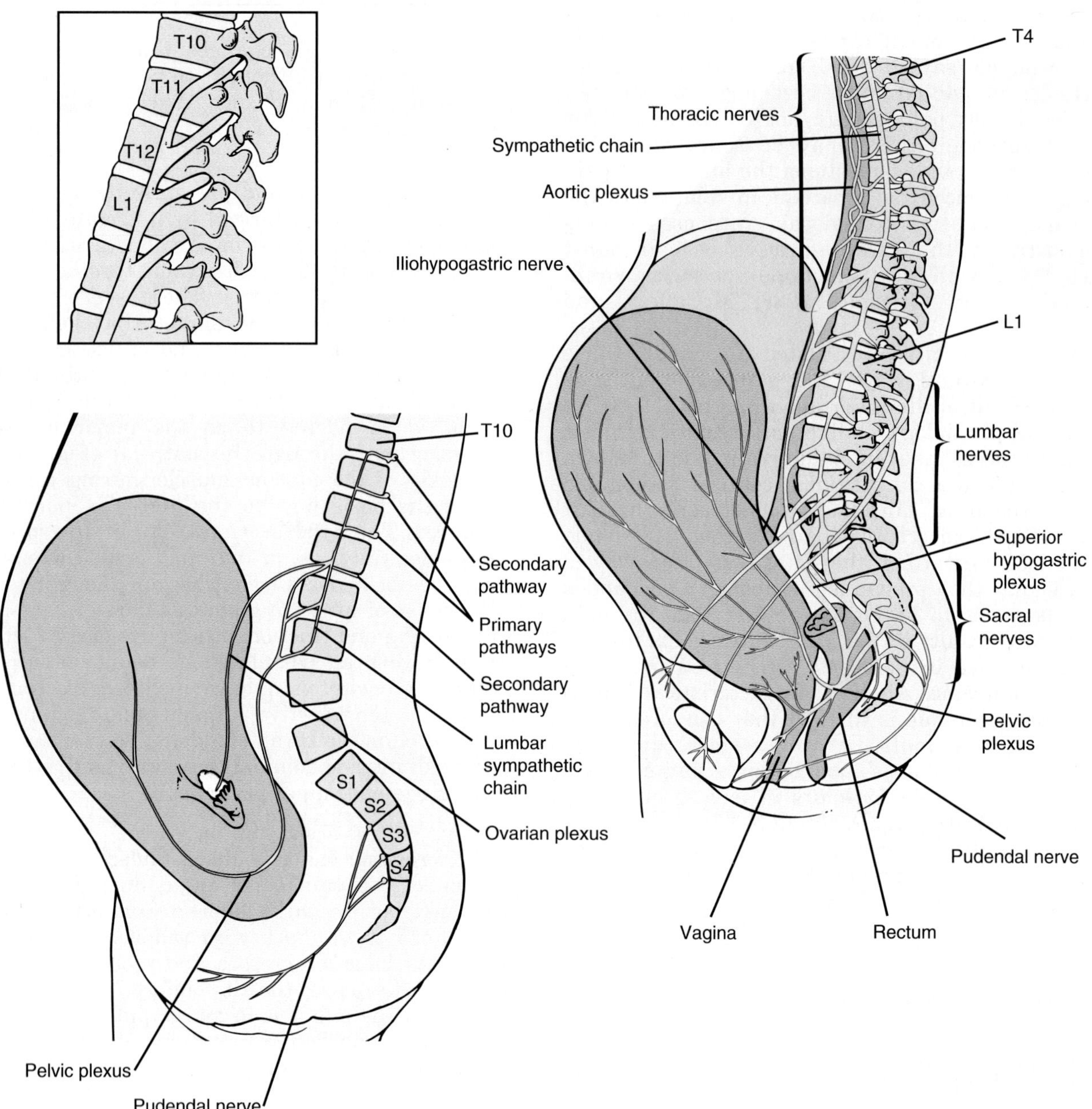

Figure 24–1

Pain pathways related to labor and birth show how sensory (pain) fibers connect the uterus and cervix to the spinal cord • The primary pathways enter at the eleventh and twelfth spinal segments; secondary pathways enter at T10 and L1 • Pathways from the perineum pass via the pudendal nerves to the sacral spinal cord at S2, S3, and S4.

formed from the second, third, and fourth sacral nerves and innervates the pubococcygeal, bulbocavernous, and transverse perineal muscles. The areas and intensity of pain perception in second-stage labor can be seen in Figure 24–2 (Bonica and McDonald 1995).

It has been reported by some women that the second stage of labor is actually less painful. This feeling may be related to satisfaction derived from the physiologic urge to push or bear down that most women experience as the head descends into the vaginal canal after complete cervical dilatation. Not all women find that it feels good to push in second stage, but many state that it is a feeling of relief and accomplishment even if painful. The ability to participate actively in the labor is in sharp contrast to the more passive role experienced in first-stage labor.

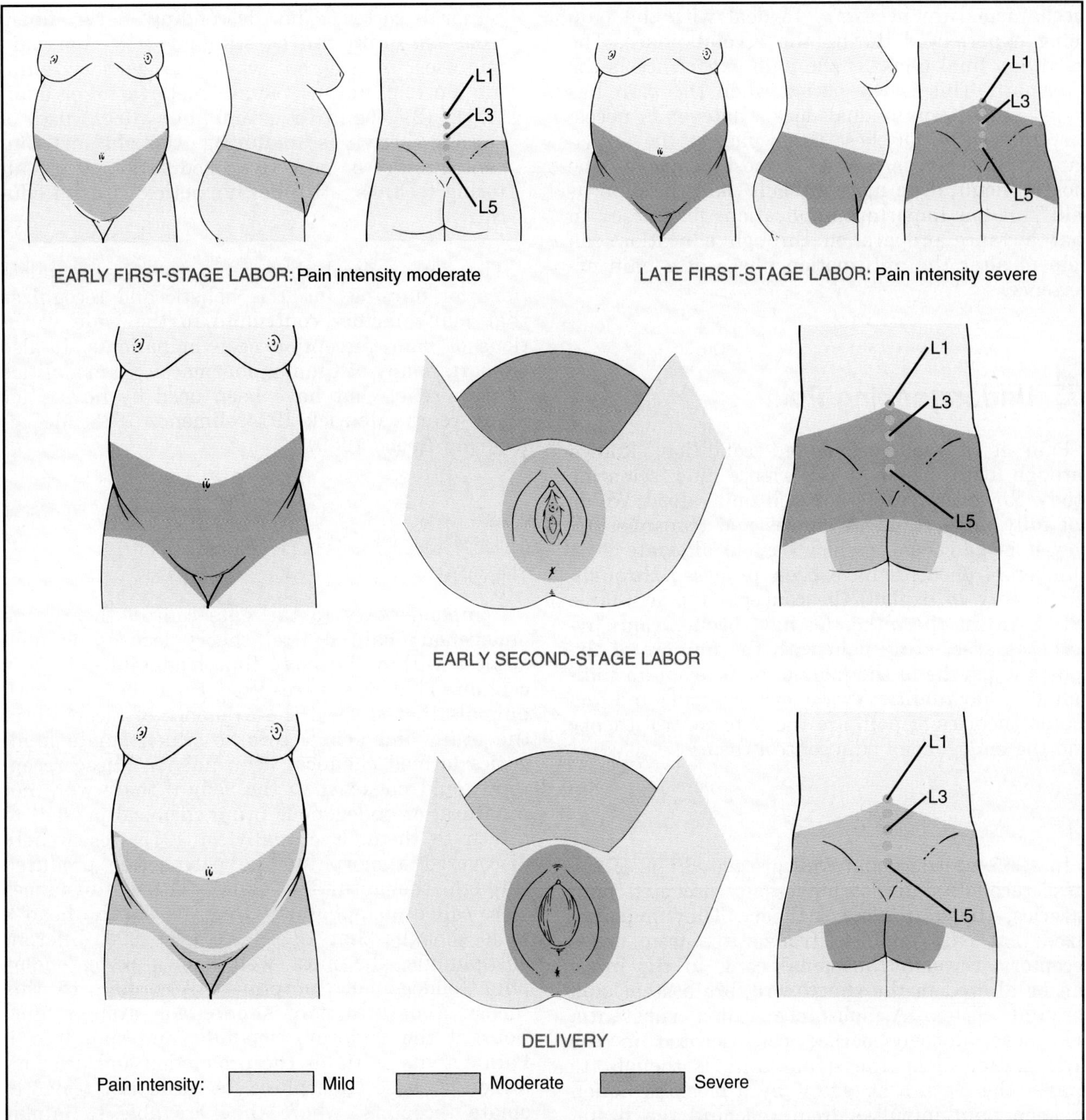

Figure 24–2

The distribution and intensity of pain during first- and second-stage labor progresses in conjunction with the descent and expulsion of the fetus. (Adapted from Bonica, J. J., and McDonald, J. S. (1995). *Principles and practice of obstetric analgesia and anesthesia* [2nd ed.]. Baltimore: Williams & Wilkins.)

Phases of the Pain Experience

There are three phases of the pain experience. The first is the anticipation phase. This period occurs before the actual pain and includes the anticipation, dread, or fear the individual might have in relation to the pain. Examples of the anticipation phase might be a man waiting with an open mouth for the dentist to start the drill, a child watching as the nurse is about to give an injection, and a woman in labor waiting for the next contraction to begin. The second phase of the pain experience is the pain itself. This phase may last a short time (e.g., a labor contraction) and the pain is classified as acute, or the pain may last a long time (e.g., back pain) and is then classified as chronic. The individual uses whatever coping mechanisms are necessary to deal with the pain being experienced during the second phase. The third and final phase of the pain experience is the aftermath. This is the period when the pain has ended and the individual does whatever is necessary to recover. Of these three phases, the anticipation phase is perceived by most people as the most difficult, even more difficult than the pain itself! This has important implications for nurses, in that advance preparation through education can help to alter the anticipation phase of a pain experience.

Understanding Pain

Pain is a well-documented condition, known through both personal experience and scientific study. However, pain is not well understood. We do not fully understand its causes and transmission, how it is perceived, or how best to alleviate it. A number of theories have been proposed throughout history to explain the concept of pain (Jaros 1991). Among these theories have been various hypotheses associating pain with the humors of the body, the psyche of the individual, or even an individual's spirituality. Two more current and accepted theories of pain are the gate control theory and the endogenous pain control theory.

GATE CONTROL THEORY

In 1965, Melzack and Wall presented one of the most recognized if not universally accepted pain theories, the gate control theory. They hypothesized that pain impulses transmitted from nerve receptors, through the spinal cord, to the brain can be altered in the spinal cord, brain stem, and cerebral cortex. A substance called substantia gelatinosa, densely packed cells located in the gray matter along the spinal cord, is thought to trigger the closure of "gates" by a blocking action to keep pain impulses from reaching the brain. The substantia gelatinosa limits the activation of the T cells that are normally responsible for transmitting pain. Several inhibitory mechanisms can be activated to stimulate the substantia gelatinosa to close a gate:

- Stimulation of the skin. Large-diameter afferent nerves (A fibers) are located in cutaneous tissue; stimulation of these nerves can act to block the transmission (i.e., close a gate) of pain impulses along small-diameter nerve fibers (C fibers). This stimulation can be accomplished through rubbing, massage, counterpressure, vibration, or the use of heat or cold.
- Stimulation of the brain stem, thalamus, and cerebral cortex. The descending nerve fibers from the brain can be stimulated to alter pain impulses in several ways: (1) sensory stimulation (e.g., touch, visual, smell, taste, or auditory); (2) cognitive stimulation (e.g., use of specific activities requiring thought or concentration); (3) affective modulation (e.g., altering feelings, attitudes, anxieties through education).

The gate control theory has practical implications for nursing, for it is holistic and recognizes that many factors contribute to the wide variations of pain perception seen in patients. It also supports many of the nonpharmacologic modalities of pain relief that have been used by nurses for many years (Melzack 1974; Jimenez 1988; McCaffery and Beebe 1989).

ENDOGENOUS BIOCHEMICAL PAIN THEORY

Complementary to the gate control theory, the endogenous pain control theory focuses on substances within the body that modulate pain perception. This theory resulted from research with animals that showed the existence of receptors in the brain and spinal cord to which opiate analgesics formed chemical attachments. These receptors would not exist in the body if there were not a natural or endogenous brain chemical present to attach to them. Eventually, in 1975, researchers discovered a morphine-like polypeptide produced through the pituitary gland. These substances were called enkephalins (Greek for "in the head"). It is thought that there are over 200 different enkephalins, the most well known being endorphin (endogenous morphine). According to this theory, a natural pain suppression system functions at the midbrain, medulla, and spinal cord. Pain activity initiates the production and dissemination of these endorphins. In turn, they travel to opiate receptors, where they are able to inhibit pain transmission neurons. Endorphins also cause an individual to feel relaxed, drowsy, or euphoric.

Pain perception, and the need for pharmacologic pain relief, may vary from one individual to another as a result of differences in the amounts of endorphin produced. Endorphin levels have been found to increase in women toward the end of pregnancy and rise markedly during labor and birth. A number of factors can trigger the release of endorphins. Massage, transcutaneous nerve stimulation, acupuncture, exercise, and focused relaxation all are thought to facilitate endorphin release. Suppression of endorphins occurs with the administration of exogenous opiates (e.g., meperidine [Demerol]), perhaps because the exogenous opioids take up all available opiate receptor sites. Endorphin production may also be decreased by such factors as prolonged pain, depression, attitude, recurrent stress, or fear (Jimenez 1988; McCaffery and Beebe 1989).

FEAR-TENSION-PAIN THEORY

An old, simplistic model of pain in labor was described by Dick-Read (1959). He believed that labor pain resulted from the woman's lack of knowledge or her fear, and this fear resulted in excitation of the sympathetic nervous system and activation of contractions of the circular muscle fibers of the uterus, causing the lower portion of the uterus to work in direct opposition to the upper portion. This excessive uterine tension and resultant ischemia were believed to be the source of pain in labor. Dick-Read's theory was not tested through scientific research, although he supplied subjective accounts of many case studies of women who demonstrated differences in pain responses in labor depending on the amount of fear or knowledge they had about the birth process. Although it is scientifically unsupported, the value of the fear-tension-pain model is that it is a concept that women can easily understand and it provides the practitioner with a simple, direct approach that can be used as a basis for the selection of pain management strategies to reduce pain for the woman in labor.

COGNITIVE CONTROL OF PAIN

Pain can be altered through the use of cognitive control, a psychological strategy whereby the individual involves the mind in mental activities other than awareness of the incoming pain sensation. Two types of cognitive control can be used:

1. Dissociation—focusing on a nonpainful aspect of the source of stimulation, for example, focusing on pressure, heat, or tightening, rather than on the pain itself. One type of cognitive dissociation is called sensory transformation. This is the strategy whereby an individual learns to change a pain stimulus into a pleasant feeling. For example, the sensation of a labor contraction can be imagined as being a warm sensation or as being a hug around the baby. This type of cognitive control can increase pain tolerance.
2. Interference—focusing on stimuli outside the source of pain, such as watching television (a passive, distraction technique), counting, using word repetitions, or using controlled breathing (active, attention-focusing techniques) (Jimenez 1988).

VARIABLES INFLUENCING PAIN IN CHILDBIRTH

Physical Variables

In addition to the pain perceived by women related to the general physiologic changes of labor and birth, other physical variables may influence pain perception. Bonica and colleagues (1979) noted that fatigue, malnutrition, and a generally poor physical condition are associated with an increased perception of pain in labor. Fetal position and size can be significant influences on intrapartal pain. A woman with a fetus in an occiput posterior position often reports localized back pain during labor that persists even between contractions. Parity may influence pain in labor. Lowe (1987) found that primiparas may experience greater pain during early labor and less pain during second stage than multiparas. Tension can increase pain. If muscles are tense for prolonged periods, the lactic acid accumulation resulting from hypoxia of the tense muscles increases pain. The activity level of the woman influences her pain perception. If she has nothing to do during a period of pain, the pain is perceived as greater. Having specific activities to perform (e.g., breathing, relaxing, focusing, counting) may help to decrease the amount of pain experienced.

Psychological Variables

Psychological factors are potent influences on the perception of pain in labor. An individual's history of response to pain, level of fear and anxiety, body image, knowledge base, expectation of pain in labor, and current emotional state of mind all can influence personal pain perception (McCaffery and Beebe 1989). Other aspects of distress frequently associated with labor are feelings of helplessness, lack of control, and cognitive dissonance. Cognitive dissonance refers to a difference between what is expected and what is experienced. Thus, a woman expecting not to feel any discomfort may interpret the intensity of the pain as higher than a woman expecting some level of pain, especially if she has learned alternative pain management strategies. Alternatively, women expecting any discomfort to be unbearable may interpret even mild cramping as exquisitely painful. Thus, knowledge and preparation for the birth experience are other factors that certainly influence the psychological responses to pain during childbirth.

Wuitchik and colleagues (1990) found that distress-related thoughts during latent labor were predictive of a longer latent phase, active phase, and second stage of labor. Confidence in the ability to handle labor has also been found to be a significant factor in the amount of perceived pain (Lowe 1989; Wuitchik et al. 1990). Lederman and associates (1978) found that increased maternal anxiety had a significant relationship to increased maternal plasma epinephrine levels, which resulted in decreased frequency of uterine contractions and longer labors.

Sociocultural Variables

Sociocultural factors influence pain perception in labor. A woman's response to pain may result from her cultural background. If she comes from a culture that believes that women are to be stoic during childbirth and would disgrace themselves by making noise or crying out, little behavioral response is observed. On the other hand, if the woman's culture dictates that crying, moaning, or praying relieves pain, she exhibits more verbal responses. Religious beliefs may influence pain response. Some people believe that the pain of childbirth is a result of the curse of Eve, God's punishment of Eve for her sin in the Garden of Eden. In this belief, pain in labor is considered to be a woman's lot to bear in an accepting manner. Another sociocultural factor that can influence pain is the amount of social support the woman has during labor. Sosa and colleagues (1980) found that a supportive companion can decrease the length of labor, the amount of medication used, and complications of childbirth.

Environmental Variables

Environmental influences may be associated with pain perception. Animal studies have suggested the influence of the surroundings on birth outcome. Hostile environments have been associated with higher untoward neonatal outcomes with animals (Newton 1966; Newton et al. 1968). Studies of women using homelike birthing environments have often reported less use of pharmaceutical agents during the childbirth experience than for similar women in traditional hospital environments (Albers and Katz 1991; Fullerton and Severino 1992). The characteristics of traditional hospital birthing facilities are often stressful. The environment is seldom calm. For example, noise and activity levels are high. Staff members can be heard talking or laughing at the desk or in hallways. The paging system can be heard. Sounds from other labor rooms may be audible. Lighting is often bright and not conducive to relaxation. Privacy may be limited, with students, staff, and birth attendants in and out of the room. Another factor that might be considered environmental is the time of day. If the woman is laboring in the middle of the night, her perception of the pain she is experiencing may be greater than if she were laboring during the day. On the other hand, the environment may be more calm in the middle of the night. Despite attempts to make labor rooms more homelike in their appearance, the equipment that is often still visible adds to the stress parents experience from the environment.

PAIN MANAGEMENT STRATEGIES

Since no single factor is the cause of pain in labor, no single management strategy exists to eradicate the pain labor generates. Thus, by recognizing and becoming familiar with a variety of approaches, the nurse can individualize care on the basis of the pain perception of the childbearing couple for whom care is being given. Although most discussions of pain relief begin with the historic advent of anesthesia, the nonpharmacologic pain management strategies for labor and birth are far older and more widely used. Even before the development of anesthesia, warm teas and potions were used as pharmaceutical agents, information about birth was passed from one generation of wise midwives to another, family support was essential, and touch and massage were used in the form of laying on of hands. Today we are fortunate to have available a wide variety of measures for pain relief during childbirth. Pain management strategies may be divided into those that are nonpharmacologic and those that are pharmacologic.

Nonpharmacologic Modalities

KNOWLEDGE AND INFORMATION

One of the most commonly used nonpharmacologic pain management strategies is the acquisition of knowledge and information. The greater a person's understanding of a physiologic process, an illness, or a medical procedure, the less likely the person is to perceive that event as painful. For pregnant women, the most common way to obtain knowledge and information today is through childbirth education classes. As discussed in Chapter

Table 24–1

NONPHARMACOLOGIC METHODS OF PAIN RELIEF

METHOD	ADVANTAGES	DISADVANTAGES	COST
Childbirth Education •Knowledge and information •Pain management skills •Social support	Widely accepted method No physician's order needed Provides education, reduces anxiety, and gives pain management strategies	Time needed to attend series of classes Pain management strategies must be practiced	Varies from no charge to $50 to $150
Relaxation and Paced Breathing •Music	Widely accepted Noninvasive Skills easily mastered with practice Self-initiated and managed	Requires time for learning and practice Requires motivation	Cost of childbirth course
Labor Support	Widely accepted Support persons can be selected by the woman Amount and type of support can be controlled by the woman	Father of baby, partner, family member, or friend may be unwilling or unavailable to provide support Labor nurse may be too busy to provide continuous support	Usually no cost unless a professional doula is hired
Imagery	Noninvasive Easily mastered skill Self-initiated and managed Promotes relaxation	Requires previous practice and motivation to use in labor May be difficult to maintain in labor	None
Acupressure	Widely used with success in Asia for years Noninvasive	Finding a qualified professional is difficult	Variable, depending on treatments; could be integrated into nursing practice
Therapeutic Touch	No devices needed; noninvasive No physician's order needed Nursing background in research and application Self-healing	Not studied well in obstetrics Unknown effect of energy transfer on fetus (two fields involved)	Essentially no cost since it usually is incorporated into nursing care

Continued on following page

20, childbirth education focuses on providing accurate information and pain management skills to the childbearing family. Childbirth education can help to alleviate the cognitive dissonance that may be present for the woman in regard to her expectations about pain in labor. Additional methods of nonpharmacologic methods of pain relief are listed in Table 24–1.

Table 24–1

NONPHARMACOLOGIC METHODS OF PAIN RELIEF Continued

METHOD	ADVANTAGES	DISADVANTAGES	COST
Heat, Cold	Noninvasive Easy to administer No physician's order needed Wide applicability outside obstetrics Provides comfort; self-healing	Could cause localized trauma to tissues	Minimal; moderate costs if purchase ice packs or heating pads
Bathing, Showering, Jet Hydrotherapy	Low cost High satisfaction No physician's order needed	May cause hyperthermia Continuous electronic fetal monitoring is impossible Risk of chorioamnionitis if membranes ruptured	Cost of tub and water (tubs can be rented)
Biofeedback	Wide applicability outside obstetrics No physician's order needed No devices needed after training; noninvasive	Finding a certified biofeedback trainer is difficult Training time is variable	Equipment for training costs several thousand dollars; individual cost is determined by training time
Hypnosis	No physician's order needed No devices needed after training; noninvasive Self-initiated and managed Has been used successfully in obstetrics	Finding a qualified professional hypnotist may be difficult Required time for training and practice Effectiveness for all people is variable	Cost of training by a hypnotist may be expensive
Transcutaneous Electrical Nerve Stimulation (TENS)	Wide applicability outside obstetrics Noninvasive	Constantly need the device Need physician's order Most effective if introduced before pain experience May interfere with continuous electronic fetal monitoring	TENS unit costs approximately $700 to $800 (can be rented)
Acupuncture	Widely used with success in Asia for years	Invasive Needles may cause infection Finding qualified professional	Variable, depending on treatments

Adapted from Brucker, M. (1984). Nonpharmaceutical methods for relieving pain and discomfort in pregnancy. *MCN,* 9, 390–394.

RELAXATION TECHNIQUES

Relaxation has consistently been the most advocated noninvasive technique for reducing muscle tension and pain in childbirth throughout the years. Different types of relaxation techniques (progressive relaxation, autogenic training, meditation, imagery, massage, music, and biofeedback) can be used to reduce childbirth pain (Nichols and Humenick 1988). These are described in detail in Chapter 20. Training and development of the skill are essential for relaxation techniques to be most effective, but one technique that can be easily taught to the unprepared laboring woman and is effective in reducing childbirth pain is progressive relaxation.

BREATHING STRATEGIES

Breathing strategies can be used during childbirth to increase the woman's state of relaxation and thus decrease her perception of pain. Three breathing patterns are commonly used: slow-paced breathing, modified-paced breathing, and pattern-paced breathing. These are described in detail in Chapter 20. To be most effective for decreasing childbirth pain, paced breathing strategies require practice before labor to develop and refine the skill. However, all women can be quickly taught the breathing strategies during labor by a labor nurse. Even when learned during labor, the strategies increase the woman's ability to cope with the pain of uterine contraction.

LABOR SUPPORT

The positive effects of support from a companion during childbirth have been well documented. Women who had support from a companion during childbirth had shorter labors, fewer complications, less distress from pain during labor, and less need for medication; interacted better with their babies following birth; and had higher levels of childbirth satisfaction than women who did not have this type of support during childbirth (Sosa et al. 1980; Butler et al. 1988).

Structured preparation is helpful for the labor companion. Research has shown that as the coach's knowledge and positive feelings toward childbirth increase, so does the confidence level of the laboring woman (Butler et al. 1988). Also, preparation for the role of labor companion enables the labor support person to provide better support and practical help during childbirth.

Not all labor companions are able to provide the same level of support for a laboring woman and not all women want the same type of support. Thus, communication between the woman and her labor companion before the childbirth experience is valuable in planning for the type of support that is most helpful to the woman and best fits with the degree of involvement the labor companion wishes to have. Even if the labor companion does not want to be very involved during labor, the mere presence of the individual who is devoting total personal attention to the laboring woman has been shown to be invaluable in helping the woman cope better during childbirth (Koehn 1992; Enkin et al. 1995). Some expectant parents hire a doula, a woman trained to provide labor support, as an adjunct to the family member and nurse who will be with the woman during labor.

The nurse should assess each situation to determine how best to meet the individual laboring woman's and her companion's needs during childbirth. Most labor companions, even those with structured preparation, benefit from assistance and support from the nurse during the childbirth process. The nurse has the opportunity to enhance the childbirth experience for both the woman and her labor companion through collaboration with them (see Pain Management Strategies for Childbirth).

IMAGERY

Imagery is a commonly occurring function of the mind that involves a temporary shift away from reality activities of the here and now. It is better known as daydreaming or having premonitions. This activity is a normal and necessary part of life. Imagery can be used as a conscious activity for pain management in childbirth (Steffes 1988). Using imagery, the pregnant woman learns to create the images that she wants during the childbirth experience. This could be imagining a pleasant scene, picturing a place in which she felt most relaxed or safe, or focusing on an activity that she likes, such as walking on the beach or taking a hike in the mountains.

As with other nonpharmacologic techniques, for imagery to be most effective in reducing pain, practice is necessary. During practice sessions, the woman tries out a number of imagery approaches and then selects those that work best for her. Laboring women who have mastered the skill of imagery use the images they have developed during practice for coping with labor contractions. The role of the nurse in this situation is to provide support to the woman when she uses imagery and to maintain a calm and quiet environment.

Imagery can also be helpful to the unprepared woman, but the nurse must provide clear, concise instructions. The nurse can use the following sequence of instructions with the unprepared woman during a contraction: close your eyes and relax, visualize a place where you feel most secure and safe, and concentrate on that place and the feelings you have when you are there.

Pain Management Strategies for Childbirth

RELAXATION—THE BASIS OF PAIN MANAGEMENT

- Progressive relaxation
- Massage or acupressure
- Imagery
- Music
- Water therapy
- Therapeutic touch

PACED BREATHING—AN AID TO RELAXATION

- Cleansing breath
- Slow-paced breathing
- Modified-paced breathing
- Patterned-paced breathing
- Expulsion breathing

POSITIONING AND MOVEMENT

- Ambulation or rocking
- Upright or semisitting
- Side-lying

LABOR SUPPORT

- Father of baby
- Family member
- Labor companion or doula

Repeat quietly to the woman during a contraction, "You are safe, you are doing fine." At the end of the contraction, have the woman take a deep breath and relax. Tell her how well she coped with the contraction.

Many different visualizations can be used for imagery during childbirth. They should include positive outcomes only; be gentle and kind, and allow any further interpretation to the woman. Imagery added to the use of relaxation techniques and breathing strategies during labor can provide a powerful means of controlling pain.

TOUCH AND MASSAGE

In 1986, Hedstrom and Newton reviewed the use of touch in labor. They discovered that outside Western cultures, touch is commonly used in labor. It is seen as a method for stimulating contractions as well as providing pain relief, probably through reduction of endogenous catecholamines (Fig. 24–3). Touch also stimulates large-diameter nerve fibers as proposed by the gate control theory and facilitates the release of endorphins (Hedstrom and Newton 1986; McCaffery and Beebe 1989).

One special type of touch is therapeutic touch. It shares the viewpoint of Oriental medicine in its recognition of energy fields of the human body. In Eastern literature, energy fields are called *prana,* a life force that flows through the body. Prana is thought to be in excess in healthy people and deficient in those who are ill or in pain. Based on the classic work of Kriegger (1979), therapeutic touch is the laying on of hands to redirect the energy fields that occur with pain. It has no religious basis but does require the conscious intent of the healer. To use this method, a practitioner must engage in additional study and practice in order to be able to use his or her hands in a therapeutic manner. An individual becomes sensitive to changes in energy fields and learns how to smooth such fields by redirecting or unruffling the energy (Mackey 1995). The efficacy of therapeutic touch is still controversial, although release of endorphins has been postulated as the most likely method of pain relief. Most of the research in the use of therapeutic touch has been performed in medical or surgical areas.

Little research has been done in the area of obstetrics, although individual nurses claim wide use of the technique. For example, some nurses have modified effleurage, the massage technique often used on the abdomen during uterine contractions, in order to redirect energy fields. Kriegger suggested that one side effect of direction of energy toward the head may be increased intracranial pressure or headaches. Thus, the method is not totally without side effects. Therefore, if therapeutic touch is to be performed on a pregnant abdomen, fetal position should first be ascertained so that energy is not inadvertently directed toward the fetal head. More research is needed on the efficacy and safety of therapeutic touch in obstetrics, especially in light of the fact that two energy fields (mother and fetus) are present, not simply one.

APPLICATION OF HEAT OR COLD

The use of heat or cold for relief of discomfort is a fundamental nursing practice. However, this modality is often overlooked for use to relieve pain during labor. Heat can be applied in labor to relieve the back pain caused by a posterior presentation (back labor) or for general backache result-

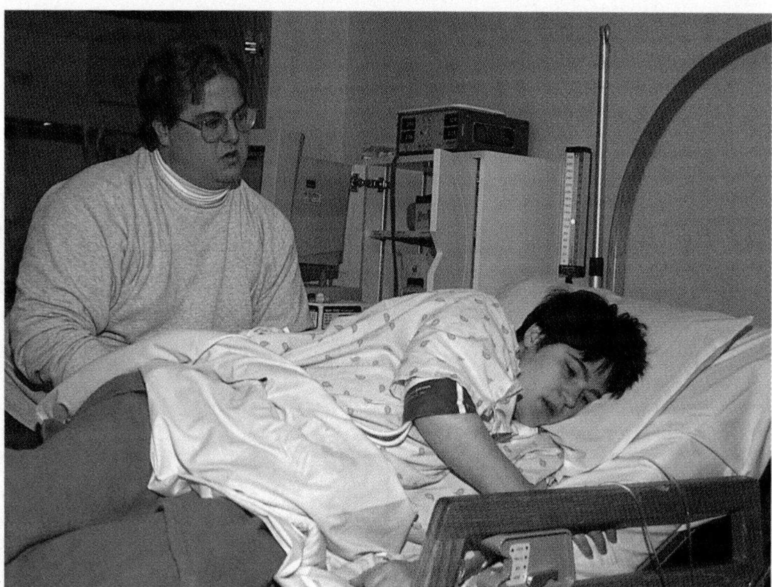

Figure 24–3
A supportive companion can be helpful in relieving pain • This father is giving back massage and counterpressure to relieve back pain during labor.

ing from immobility or fatigue. Superficial heat may relieve pain in labor by reducing muscle spasm caused by ischemia, stimulating large-diameter nerve fibers to cause a gating mechanism against pain (gate control theory), reducing joint stiffness, or causing vasodilatation and increased blood flow to an area of discomfort. Heat may be applied in labor through the application of moist compresses, a hot water bottle, or a moist heating pad (e.g., K-Pad) or by immersion in a tub of warm water (McCaffery and Beebe 1989; Simkin 1995).

The use of cold can help for general comfort if the woman is warm from the work of labor. Cool washcloths can be placed on her forehead or used to wipe face, chest, arms, and hands. Ice can be used against the sacral area of the back to relieve the pain of a posterior position. It can be applied by filling a rubber glove with ice chips or using a chemical cold pack. Superficial cooling may relieve pain by lowering the muscle temperature to reduce muscle spasm, reducing the sensitivity of the skin through stimulation of large-diameter nerve fibers, or reducing inflammation and joint stiffness (McCaffery and Beebe 1989; Simkin 1995).

Heat and cold can be used alternately to produce a better effect. The effects of heating do not last as long as the effects of cold because the increased blood flow rapidly cools the tissues to normal temperature. The effects of cold last longer because the vessels remain constricted after cold application is discontinued and rewarming of the tissue from the inside is delayed along with delayed warming from the outside (McCaffery and Beebe 1989).

BATHING, SHOWERING, AND JET HYDROTHERAPY

Another nonpharmacologic intervention for labor is the use of warm water. Bathing has both hydrokinetic and hydrothermal effects. The warm water allows local vasodilatation, muscle relaxation, and increased velocity of nerve conduction. Therefore, not only can warmth decrease pressure on the abdominal muscles, it can also allow the uterus to contract more efficiently (Aderhold and Perry 1991; Simkin 1995). Pain relief associated with bathing, showering, or jet hydrotherapy (Jacuzzi) has been proposed to be that of a distraction device or stimulation of large-diameter nerve fibers as proposed by the gate control theory or release of endorphins as proposed by the biochemical theory.

An advantage of bathing or showering is that it is associated with a high degree of client satisfaction (Cammu et al. 1994) (Fig. 24–4). A disadvantage is simple environmental risk. A slippery floor or a hot tub of water is a potential risk that needs to be addressed if the method is to be considered. The water should be kept at a temperature of 98° to 110°F (36.6° to 37.8°C) (Simkin 1995). It is also a method reserved for a woman who has a pregnancy at no apparent medical risk, since continuous electronic fetal monitoring is not an option. For a woman using bathing or showering, the fetal heart is monitored by auscultation with a fetoscope or hand-held Doppler device. The water may also cause difficulty in maternal assessments, such as of maternal blood pressure (Aderhold and Perry 1991).

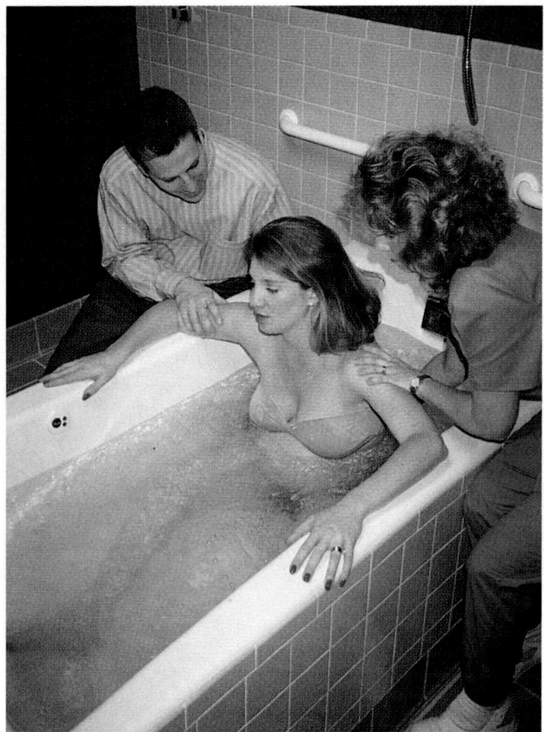

Figure 24–4

The use of a warm bath or Jacuzzi during labor promotes muscle relaxation and pain relief • The woman's partner and maternal-newborn nurse offer support and encouragement. (Courtesy of the Women's East Pavilion, Chattanooga, TN.)

BIOFEEDBACK

In addition to childbirth education and hypnosis, another pain relief method based on relaxation is biofeedback. Biofeedback is based on the concept that individuals can manipulate internal physiologic events (e.g., heart rate, blood pressure) after learning to recognize physical signals of such changes. As with hypnosis, several methods for prenatal training may exist with biofeedback. Most commonly, a machine is used to indicate the level of relaxation. For example, an electrothermal device may measure the warmth of the fingertips. When an individual is more stressed or less relaxed, peripheral perfusion is inhibited and the fingers are cooler. Electromyographic or electrodermal devices can be used to measure muscle tone. Often the area between the eyebrows is used for this measurement. Visually this could be assessed by an individual who may note that a person looks worried, with a furrowed brow (Alexander and Steefel 1995).

During the biofeedback training sessions, relaxation tapes are usually played. These may include imagery or music. Thus, relaxation is a basic component, as with prepared childbirth classes and hypnosis. In prepared childbirth classes the instructor may touch or gently move a woman's leg or arm to assess it for tension. In a biofeedback training session the mechanical device provides that information and it can be interpreted by the trainer. As people become more aware of their body and relaxation responses, eventually they can become relaxed in a shorter time. Eventually they can routinely perform self-initiated biofeedback by recognizing internal signals rather than the biofeedback device.

In the fields of maternal-newborn nursing and obstetrics, little research has been conducted with the biofeedback method of pain relief. In a study by Gregg, 60 women were divided into two equal groups (Basmajian 1989). The group that had biofeedback training prenatally was compared with women who did not receive such education. Those with the training experienced significantly shorter labors and used four to ten times fewer pharmaceutical agents for pain relief. However, in a study by Bernat and associates (1992), prenatal instruction in using a biofeedback technique of temperature control did not decrease stress in labor for experimental subjects compared with control subjects.

Among the advantages of biofeedback is the fact that such training can be used for pain other than childbirth pain. Relaxation can be used for headaches or other muscular discomforts of pregnancy. The disadvantages include the lack of accessibility of a biofeedback trainer and the costs of such training and use of devices. The electric stimulation from the training devices is a minor amount. No studies have suggested that it poses any hazard to the developing fetus (Bernat et al. 1992; Alexander and Steefel 1995).

The relaxation-based nonpharmacologic methods discussed above appear to address pain management by physiologic relaxation to decrease the pain sensations at the origin and recognition of the gate control theory of pain by the use of distractors (e.g., imagery, breathing). Although commonly used, relaxation methods are not the only nonpharmacologic modalities used for intrapartal pain.

HYPNOSIS

Hypnosis in obstetrics has both enjoyed marked popularity and been viewed with cynicism within the last century. The need for antepartal preparation and the emphasis on relaxation are similar to those in childbirth education. Davenport-Slack (1975) failed to demonstrate any differences between two groups of women, one using hypnosis for labor and one having attended prepared childbirth classes, in the areas of length of labor, pharmaceutic agents used, subjective pain reported, and experiential childbirth anecdotes. Jenkins and Pritchard (1993) found significantly shorter labors and less need for analgesics in women who used hypnosis than in women who did not.

Hilgard and Hilgard (1975) noted that hypnosis for labor and birth differed from general use of hypnosis. Successful pain management using hypnosis appears to have eight characteristics:

1. Use of a rehearsal procedure: this is similar to Lamaze preparation wherein the rehearsal helps the individual avoid cognitive dissonance by identifying some of his or her fantasies regarding birth and identify more realistic experiences.
2. Emphasis on relaxation: the use is similar to that in prepared childbirth.
3. Use of symptom substitution: this characteristic is more specific to hypnosis. It enables the woman to substitute another, less noxious symptom for pain.
4. Pain displacement: although prepared childbirth may suggest that a woman focus her attention elsewhere, such as by using a focal point, this step is beyond simple refocusing. In hypnosis, a woman is encouraged to displace the pain outside her body.
5. Direct suggestion of symptom relief: during hypnosis a woman may be told that the pain of labor is diminished.
6. Indirect suggestions such as glove anesthesia: a woman under hypnosis may be given a suggestion that she has diminished sensations in a particular area of her body (e.g., glove), which diminishes pain.
7. Imaginative separation of the uterus from her body: contrary to most imagery espoused by childbirth educators, hypnotists may encourage a woman to dissociate herself from her body or dissociate body parts from herself. This would also relieve the pain sensations associated with childbirth.
8. Posthypnotic suggestions designed to increase confidence: as with prepared childbirth, hypnosis may encourage a woman to increase her self-esteem and control. As prepared childbirth does this with knowledge, hypnosis may also augment confidence with posthypnotic suggestions.

Currently, hypnosis is not a common pain management modality in the United States. Although it has a long history in obstetrics, pharmaceutical methods appear to have displaced hypnosis in popularity as an anesthetic. Prepared childbirth classes have disseminated the use of relaxation methods to expectant couples. Well-trained hypnotists tend to be few in number, costly for training purposes, and difficult to find during the birthing event.

There are definite benefits of the use of positive suggestion and hypnotic techniques for obstetric patients today. There should be increasing use of the combination of hypnosis with pharmaceutical agents. Little scientific research has been conducted in the past two decades on the efficacy of hypnosis in obstetrics compared with other currently used methods. Hypnosis for the reduction of childbirth pain is a safe method of pain relief (Erickson 1994). The efficacy for an individual may be difficult to predict, but when a childbearing family is able to locate and afford a well-trained hypnotist, little can be said against the method as a potential pain relief strategy.

TRANSCUTANEOUS ELECTRICAL NERVE STIMULATION

Transcutaneous electrical nerve stimulation (TENS) is a noninvasive electrotherapy that has been widely used for both acute and chronic pain. A small electrical unit delivers pulsed alternating current to muscles, usually in the area of the pain (Fig. 24–5). It is proposed that the current stimulates large myelinated beta neurons, which in turn

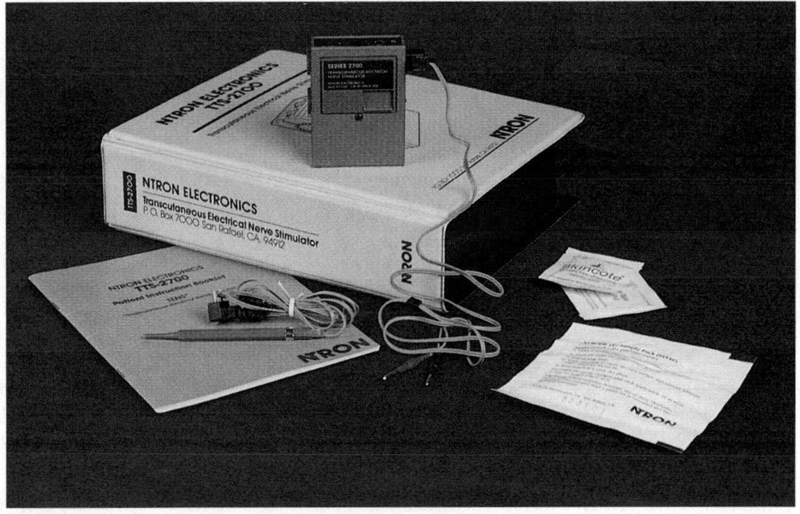

Figure 24–5
The TENS unit provides pain relief by emitting low-voltage electric current that stimulates large-diameter nerve fibers, thus blocking the transmission of pain • For labor pain, the woman increases the intensity of the TENS unit during contractions and decreases the intensity between contractions.

cause hyperexcitation of interneurons in the substantia gelatinosa material of the spinal cord. According to the gate control theory of pain, the excitation of the spinal gating nerves decreases the sensation of pain (McCaffery and Beebe 1989; Simkin 1995).

Although most obstetric studies conducted with TENS in the United States have been in the area of postoperative pain (including pain after cesarean birth), a number of European scientists have researched the use of TENS intrapartally. TENS electrode leads were placed on either the sacrum or inguinal area during labor. Augustinson and colleagues (1977) discovered that 88 percent of women experienced some pain relief with TENS, and Bundsen and associates (1981) discovered that the pain relief was superior if the woman reported that the discomfort was localized in her back. The only side effect of TENS was occasional skin irritation caused by the electrode leads. No fetal complications have been reported, although there have been anecdotal reports of interference of the electronic leads with electronic fetal monitors.

TENS units are obtained only by prescription and are usually distributed through the physical therapy department of a hospital. They are operated by batteries. Some facilities have arrangements for rental of TENS units for short-term usage, such as for labor. Occasionally a woman has a TENS unit that was purchased for some other purpose, for example, chronic back pain. A woman should understand that although TENS therapy may have wide usage, it is a pain management strategy, not a curative treatment. Thus, it is not to be used for pain of unknown origin (McCaffery and Beebe 1989).

ACUPRESSURE, ACUPUNCTURE, AND SHIATSU

Acupuncture has been practiced for centuries in China. This pain relief technique is based on the belief in Oriental medicine that an illness or pain is the result of an imbalance of energy (chi) in the body. To correct the imbalance, needles are inserted into the skin at specific acupuncture points. These points are located along meridians throughout the body that supply organs of the body with energy; 500 to 800 points have been identified. Specific points have been located that are related to organs or areas of the body not even in near proximity to the actual point. These acupressure points are identified by names and numbers that denote the organ association. However, simple study of the complex charts illustrating such points is inadequate for clinical practice, since individual bodies vary in size. Practitioners skilled in Oriental medicine can first identify the point in general and then locate it specifically for an individual by determining the acupoint or tsubo. Stimulation of acupoints by application of needles, massage, electric impulse, and heat or cold has been used for pain management. It is proposed that this pain strategy is based on the release of endorphins and may also be related to the physiology of the gate control theory. Acupressure, in contrast to acupuncture, is the application of pressure instead of needles at the acupoints. Shiatsu is the Japanese modality of acupressure. This practice allows the point to be identified and then massaged in order to repair the imbalance of energy that exists in the body (Jungman 1988; McCaffery and Beebe 1989; Beal 1992).

Three areas have been suggested as the major points for labor augmentation and pain relief in labor (Fig. 24–6). These points are Co4, St36, and Sp6 (Jungman 1988; McCaffery and Beebe 1989):

- Co4, known as the Hoku or Hegu, is found between the first and second metacarpal bones on the dorsum of the hand. Imagine tightly holding and squeezing a woman's hand in labor.
- St36, the Tsusanli or Zusanli point, is found below the tibial tuberosity. It is on the side of the anterior tibial muscle.
- Sp6, the Sanyinchiao or Sanyiniiao point, is found behind the tibia and above the medial malleolus. This is an easily accessible point. Since pregnancy is a state of hypercoagulation, massage of this area should be performed only if there is no evidence of thromboembolic activity.

Stimulation of the Chien-chin acupoint can be helpful in decreasing upper body pain and tension, which in turn helps fatigue that may accompany labor. The Chien-chin is found on either side of the spine at the neck. The Palm point is an acupoint that encourages general relaxation. It can be found in the palm of the hand, close to the insertion of the thumb. For women with pain in their backs, stimulation of the Shen-shu acupressure point, as well as the acupressure point found approximately 5 cm from the anterosuperior iliac spine on a line connecting it to the sacrum, provides relief.

Acupuncture has been used for cesarean births in China, and in the United States its use for chronic pain management is growing. Acupuncture should be performed only by a skilled practitioner, and sterile needles are an essential requirement. Risks of unsterile needles include local abscesses, serum hepatitis, or human immunodeficiency virus (HIV) infection. Acupressure or Shiatsu is slowly being incorporated into nursing interventions by practitioners who have undertaken additional study in the area. Thus, it is becoming more common to find labor and delivery nurses using massage of the acupressure points in order to effect pain relief intrapartally.

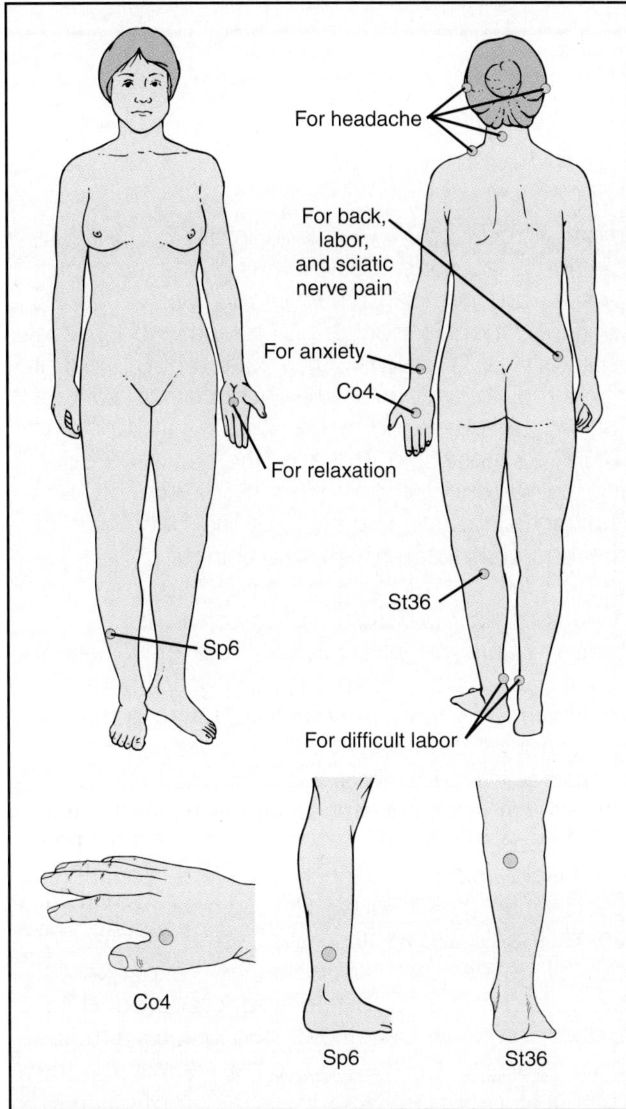

Figure 24–6

Acupressure points that augment labor and promote pain relief include Co4 (Hoku point), Sp6 (Sanyinchiao point), and St36 (Tsusanli point) • The Chien-chin acupoint, which is found on either side of the spine at the neck; the palm point; and the Shen-shu, located 5 cm from the iliac spine, encourage relaxation.

Pharmacologic Interventions

Today, modern obstetrics employs both analgesics and anesthetics for pain relief. Analgesia is achieved with drugs that in some way alter or decrease the perception of pain, while anesthesia totally blocks the sensation of pain. Three categories of pharmacologic pain management exist for the laboring woman: systemic medications (usually analgesics) primarily for use during the first stage of labor, regional anesthesia for use during first- and/or second-stage labor, and general anesthesia for use during second-stage labor. Today general anesthesia is rarely used for a normal vaginal birth; it is reserved for emergency vaginal or cesarean birth.

SYSTEMIC MEDICATIONS

Barbiturates and Amnesic Drugs

Barbiturate drugs, also called sedatives or hypnotics, were at one time popular for use in obstetrics, especially for the treatment of dysfunctional labor patterns. Today, they are used more cautiously, since their association with neonatal depression has been well established. They may still be used occasionally in latent phase labor to allow a woman to sleep before contractions become regular. Another medication less commonly employed today is the amnesic drug. These drugs were most popular in the early and mid-1900s and their effect was known as *twilight sleep*. Twilight sleep involved the combination of an amnesic drug such as scopolamine with a narcotic analgesic such as meperidine. Amnesics did not alter pain perception but allowed the woman to forget the experience by altering her memory. Unfortunately, scopolamine has the property that it can cause excitement or agitation in the presence of pain, and women could experience delirium or hallucinations under its effects. Twilight sleep is rarely used today for labor and birth.

Tranquilizers and Antiemetics

Although anxiety and fear can be altered with childbirth education, supportive friends and family, and effective health care providers, tranquilizer drugs (also called ataractic or relaxant drugs) still have a place in the pharmaceutical armamentarium for labor and birth. The tranquilizer drugs do not decrease pain. In early labor, they provide a mild sedative side effect, allowing the woman to sleep. In active labor they are potent antiemetics and reduce the nausea and vomiting that may accompany labor and delivery. They help the woman to relax by decreasing apprehension and are also used as an adjuvant to narcotics, although their use as a potentiator of narcotics is still controversial (Barash et al. 1992). The most common tranquilizer drugs, the dosage and route of administration, and the effects on the mother, fetus, and labor can be seen in Table 24–2.

Narcotic Analgesics (Opiates)

Narcotic analgesics or opiate drugs are used to decrease pain. The narcotic drug most commonly used in obstetrics is meperidine, which has replaced morphine for pain relief in childbirth because it has less of a central nervous system depressive effect on the fetus. It decreases the woman's perception of pain by interfering with

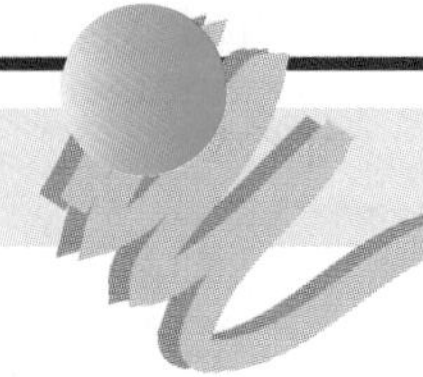

HISTORICAL PERSPECTIVES

THE EVOLUTION OF PAIN MANAGEMENT DURING CHILDBIRTH

In January 1847, a historic event took place in Edinburgh, Scotland. At that time it was not uncommon for women to develop rickets or scurvy as a result of poor nutrition. A pregnant woman, who had a contracted pelvis as a result of these diseases, was found to have a malpositioned fetus. The delivery was difficult and little pain relief was available, aside from the support of those with her.

However, Doctor James Young Simpson was attending this birth. Familiar with the work of the Boston surgeon William Morton, who had used ether for an operation the year before, Simpson felt that it could be of benefit in this case. Using ether, Simpson was able to accomplish an internal podalic version and deliver the baby in a cephalic position. It was the first reported use of obstetric anesthesia.

Simpson quickly realized the potential and the risks of obstetric anesthesia. He experimented with ether, nitrous oxide, and chloroform on himself, his assistants, or any family members who were adventurous enough to agree. As a result of his work, ether and chloroform became the major anesthetic agents in obstetric use for the next hundred years.

Although one might suppose that pharmaceuticals for childbirth would be welcomed wholeheartedly by women and their physicians, some individuals rejected them as unnatural or even in opposition to the Biblical admonishment for Eve to bear children in pain. Both the Catholic Church in Rome and the Anglican Church in England opposed their use for this reason. Thus, it was a major social event when Queen Victoria used chloroform during the birth of her sixth child in 1853, starting a fashionable trend.

Nerve blocks in the form of spinal anesthesia were introduced in Germany in 1898. In 1901, single-dose caudal epidural injections were proposed by the Frenchmen Sicard and Cathelin, working independently. Morphine had been isolated as a drug in the early 1800s, but it took the invention of the hypodermic syringe with a hollow needle, by Alexander Wood in 1853, to make it a feasible analgesic for labor. Morphine and scopolamine provided the first "twilight sleep" in Germany at the beginning of the twentieth century. This combination of drugs proved to be so popular among women that Mrs. John Jacob Astor promoted it in a humanitarian spirit for all laboring women. Twilight sleep was also used as an enticement for women to deliver in a hospital, when hospitals were not usually viewed as maternity sites. Advertising in magazines extolled the virtues of the specific maternity hospitals in which twilight sleep was the norm.

Twilight sleep continued to be commonly used until the 1960s. As women began to voice their desires to have some degree of control over their childbearing experiences, more and more opted to use prepared childbirth in order to be awake and aware. Studies also brought to the lay press some of the neonatal risks involved in pharmaceutical use, causing more women to avoid them. Today, pharmaceuticals are still important agents in the management of childbirth pain; however, nonpharmaceutical pain strategies have come of age. It is not uncommon in the 1990s to meet a laboring woman at the hospital or birthing center doing a breathing technique during a labor contraction and using a TENS unit.

Data from Moir, D. (1978). *Pain relief in labour.* Edinburgh: Churchill Livingstone, and Simkin, P. (1995). Reducing pain and enhancing progress in labor: A guide to nonpharmacologic methods for maternity caregivers. *Birth,* 22 (3), 161–171.

pain impulses at the subcortical level of the brain. The peak effect of analgesia occurs approximately 45 minutes after intramuscular administration but only 5 minutes after intravenous administration. Since the depressant effect in the fetus occurs closely after maternal maximum effect, timing of administration in relation to the progress of labor is important to avoid neonatal depression at birth (McCaffery and Beebe 1989; Steiner and Steiner 1988; Isenor and Penny-MacGillivray 1993). It is usually recommended that meperidine not be given in the last hour of first-stage labor.

Table 24–2

SYSTEMIC MEDICATIONS

DRUG	DOSAGE AND ROUTE	POSSIBLE EFFECTS ON MOTHER	POSSIBLE EFFECTS ON FETUS OR NEWBORN	POSSIBLE EFFECTS ON LABOR
Tranquilizers				
Promethazine (Phenergan)	25–50 mg IM 15–25 mg IV	Decreased tension and apprehension	Minor decrease in beat-to-beat FHR variability; central nervous system depression (respiratory depression, sleepiness, poor sucking, decreased muscle tone, decreased attention, restlessness); appears in breast milk and may cause neonatal drowsiness	May enhance labor if tension interfering with labor progress; may slow if maternal side effects significant
Hydroxyzine (Vistaril)	25–50 mg IM	Drowsiness, sedation Antiemetic		
Diazepam (Valium)	2–10 mg IM 2–10 mg IV	Hypotension		
Propiomazine (Largon)	25–50 mg IM 25–50 mg IV	May lower seizure threshold		
Promazine (Sparine)	50 mg IM 5–10 mg IV	Increased prolactin secretion		
Narcotic Analgesics and Agonist-Antagonists				
Meperidine (Demerol)	50–100 mg IM 25–50 mg IV	Decreased pain Nausea and vomiting	Decreased FHR variability Hypotonia, lethargy	Decreased uterine activity
Fentanyl (Sublimaze)	50–100 μg IM 25–50 μg IV	Respiratory depression	Decreased motor activity	
Nalbuphine (Nubain)	10–20 mg IM or SC, 10 mg IV	Tachycardia Orthostatic hypotension	Decreased alertness	
Butorphanol (Stadol)	1–3 mg IM 0.5–2 mg IV	Drowsiness, sedation Blurred vision Dizziness, "floating" Dry mouth Diaphoresis Hypotension Pruritus	Respiratory depression (decreased Apgar; however Nubain and Stadol have ceiling effect and eventually may become ineffective)	
Narcotic Antagonists				
Naloxone (Narcan)	Maternal: 0.4–2 mg IV Neonatal: 0.1 mg IV (umbilical)	Return of pain Withdrawal symptoms in presence of preexisting narcotic dependency Note: In presence of maternal drug abuse, can precipitate full withdrawal of mother and/or baby	Reverses respiratory depression	

The effect of meperidine on labor has been a topic of controversy (Berg and Rayburn 1992). However, no scientific studies have clearly indicated that it prolongs labor, and several studies have suggested that meperidine may increase uterine activity (Cunningham et al. 1993). Narcotic analgesic drugs, the dosage and route of administration, and effects on the mother, fetus, and labor can be seen in Table 24–2.

Narcotic Agonist-Antagonists

Other types of narcotics are also used for labor and birth. Narcotic drugs exert their therapeutic effect at the receptor site. Two of the major receptor sites are termed mu and kappa. Meperidine is essentially a pure mu agonist. It exerts analgesia via the mu receptor. However, there are a number of agents that exert effect at more than one site, often an agonist at one and an antagonist at another. An example of this type of drug for obstetric pain relief is butorphanol (Stadol). Butorphanol is commonly called a "mixed agonist/antagonist." This drug acts on two different receptor sites—mu and kappa. On the kappa it is an agonist, and thus a woman receives pain relief. However, on mu it is a partial antagonist, occupying the site but not providing the effect of pain relief. Clinically it has been determined that butorphanol and meperidine are essentially equal for pain relief, with similar half-lives. At equal initial doses, both meperidine and butorphanol have equal respiratory depressive effects on the fetus, but butorphanol has a not well understood "ceiling" effect that meperidine does not possess. This effect refers to the fact that although meperidine causes respiratory depression in a direct correlation to dose (dose-related effect), butorphanol has a level of respiratory depression beyond which additional doses have no effect and do not increase the degree of depression. The nurse should be aware that this does not indicate that butorphanol is free of respiratory effects. Moreover, butorphanol has also been implicated with a possible sinusoidal fetal heart rate pattern (Skyken and Petrie 1988; Cunningham et al. 1993).

Some clinicians advocate that these drugs should not be interchanged during the same labor. However, biologic variability is well established with any drug, especially analgesics. Therefore a woman may not obtain great relief with one agent, but might with another drug. Pharmacologically the two drugs can be used during the same labor; however, the nurse should be aware of the fact that the sequencing is important. Meperidine should be administered first. It will saturate the mu receptors. Should a different drug then be desired, butorphanol may be administered. The mu receptors will already be occupied, so there basically is no room for the antagonist occupation and additional pain relief may be obtained by occupying the kappa receptors. This is a logical approach should both drugs be needed. If butorphanol were administered first, it would not only occupy the kappa receptors, but the antagonist would occupy the empty mu receptors as well. Subsequent administration of a mu agonist such as meperidine would have markedly diminished or little additional pain relief for the average woman.

Nalbuphine (Nubain) is another commonly used agonist/antagonist. A major point that a nurse should be aware of with the use of partial narcotic antagonists is that these drugs should not be used in individuals with drug abuse histories. Administration of such agents can catapult a woman into full-scale withdrawal. Dosage, route of administration, and effects on mother, fetus, and the labor are given in Table 24–2.

Narcotic Antagonists

Appropriate administration of narcotics to the laboring woman minimizes the need for narcotic antagonists. However, since all narcotics used intrapartally have the potential to cause neonatal depression, the nurse needs to be aware of treatment of the infant with respiratory depression. Naloxone hydrochloride (Narcan) is a narcotic antagonist. It is the drug of choice for narcotic depression in the newborn. It reverses respiratory depression induced by opiate narcotics by affecting the specific narcotic receptors in the central nervous system. It can be administered to the mother while in labor to decrease neonatal respiratory depression if birth is imminent and a narcotic drug has recently been given, or it can be given directly to the neonate after birth. If it is given during labor, the mother will lose all effect of the narcotic analgesic and experience pain. This medication has a peak effect in 2 minutes with an overall duration of approximately 30 minutes. See Table 24–2 for information on dosage and route of administration.

Two other drugs, levallorphan (Lorphan) and nalorphine (Nalline), are also classified as narcotic antagonists. However, unlike naloxone hydrochloride, they actually can potentiate depression induced by nonnarcotic drugs. Therefore, if the woman received more than simply meperidine during her labor, they can cause the depression to continue instead of resolve. For this reason, these drugs are rarely used. It is interesting to note that narcotic antagonist drugs can also counteract the effects of the body's natural endorphins.

Implications for Nursing Practice

During the prenatal period, women should be given information about systemic medications in order to make informed choices. This information should be provided by the antepartal nurse or childbirth educator. Before the initiation of any pharmacologic pain management strategy, several important issues should be considered. These include maternal preference, maternal size and health status, fetal size and condition, and labor status. Maternal desire concerning pharmacologic pain management is often a problematic area to address. The personal biases of the nurse, nurse-midwife, or physician can be easily conveyed by the manner in which the medication is discussed with the woman. A laboring woman is vulnerable to suggestion. Medications should be offered when needed, but in an unbiased manner so that the woman does not feel pressured into accepting them or guilty if she does desire them. As with any pharmaceutical treatments, medications should be individualized and dosages calculated according to the patient's size, the stage of labor, and the status of the fetus.

Intrapartal medications are prescribed by the nurse-midwife or physician, but most frequently it is the nurse to whom the woman turns for assistance in pain relief, and it is the nurse who administers the medications and monitors their therapeutic benefits and side effects. Therefore, nurses need to be aware of the potential effects of any of the drugs they administer (see Table 24–2). An infant who is preterm or who is in severe fetal distress may be further compromised by neonatal depression secondary to maternal medications. It is important to remember that all medications have the potential of affecting the fetus. Just as systemic analgesics cross the maternal blood-brain barrier to provide analgesic effects for the mother, they also cross the placental barrier and affect the fetus. The effect on the fetus depends on the amount of drug given, its characteristics, the route of administration, and the time in labor when it is given.

Uterine function can also be affected by the administration of analgesics. If medication is given too early in latent labor, contractions may fail to establish a regular pattern or may even stop for a period. If analgesics are given too frequently or too early in active labor, the contraction pattern can be decreased in frequency or intensity. However, dysfunctional labor patterns may be helped or hindered by administration of medication. Therefore, when a pharmaceutical agent is used, it should be individualized to the woman and the labor situation. For systemic drugs, this individualization is accomplished by the choice of medication, dosage, and route. When administering medication during labor, nurses must remember at all times that they are not dealing with one patient but with two.

REGIONAL ANALGESIA AND ANESTHESIA

A variety of regional nerve blocks are available for the management of intrapartum pain. They are called regional blocks because they block pain only in one region of the body. Semantics differ as to whether these blocks are appropriately called anesthetics (since loss of sensation is involved) or analgesics (since loss of consciousness is not involved). Nevertheless, they are popular pharmaceutical methods that are frequently employed as a pain management strategy for childbirth.

Regional anesthesia is achieved by the injection of an anesthetic agent into an area that has direct contact with the nerves being blocked. These drugs work by preventing the initiation and transmission of the nerve impulses, which results in a loss of sensation. Depending on the type of nerve block, the anesthetic agents administered are usually in the "caine" family of drugs. Examples include ester-linked anesthetics such as procaine (Novocain), 2-chloroprocaine (Nesacaine), and tetracaine (Pontocaine) and amide-linked anesthetics such as lidocaine (Xylocaine) and bupivacaine (Marcaine). Ester-linked anesthetics are relatively short acting, may require repeated doses to maintain anesthesia, and do not readily pass into fetal circulation. On the other hand, the amide-linked anesthetics are longer acting but pass more readily into the fetal circulation, so fetal effects are more prolonged. Anesthesia can be accomplished either by a single injection or by introducing a plastic catheter to provide a route for continuous administration of the agent over a longer period.

A major issue in the administration of these anesthetics is use of the correct agent for the desired nerve block. Although when used correctly these drugs rarely cause severe side effects, major hazards can exist when a drug indicated for a spinal block is accidentally substituted for a pudendal block. In addition, it is essential that administration of regional anesthetics be accompanied by a clear understanding of the anatomy of the area of the body being anesthetized, knowledge of the correct procedure, and an awareness of complications that could arise. A list of potential adverse maternal reactions to the anesthetic agents can be seen in Table 24–3. Maternal sensitivity to the anesthetic agent should be determined by first injecting a minute amount of the drug to be used. If an adverse maternal reaction does occur after administration of the block, the woman should be immediately treated with oxygen, atropine, and antihistamine drugs. A regional anesthetic should never be administered unless an intravenous line is in place and equipment for cardiopulmonary resuscitation is available (Steiner and Steiner 1988; Taylor 1993).

Regional Blocks Administered in First-Stage Labor

▼ **Paracervical Blocks.** A paracervical block allows an anesthetic to be administered directly to

Table 24–3

POTENTIAL ADVERSE MATERNAL REACTIONS TO ANESTHETIC AGENTS

MILD	MODERATE	SEVERE
Apprehension	Nausea and vomiting	Respiratory depression
Confusion	Muscle twitching	Bradycardia
Headache	Hypotension	Severe hypotension
Vertigo	Loss of consciousness	Sudden loss of consciousness
Tinnitus	Convulsions	Coma
Metallic taste in mouth		Cardiac arrest
Local toxic effects on tissues		Death
Heart palpitations		

the dilating cervix. Therefore, it is a pain relief modality that can be administered in the first stage of labor to relieve pain resulting from cervical dilatation and vaginal stretching. However, pain relief does not extend to the perineal area, so a paracervical block has to be followed by another anesthetic for the delivery. It is administered by a nurse-midwife or physician, usually in the bed in which the woman is laboring. The anesthetic agent is administered transvaginally to the cervix by use of a long sheathed needle, often in an Iowa trumpet guide, which allows the operator to guide and control bilateral injections into the cervix. These injections are accomplished by placing the sheathed needle first at the 3 o'clock position at the cervix and allowing the needle to protrude only 2 to 3 mm into the vaginal mucosa, to allow injection of several milliliters of the anesthetic. The needle is then repositioned to the 9 o'clock position of the cervix and the injection process repeated (Fig. 24–7). Pain relief is experienced within several minutes after administration of the anesthetic; however, paracervical blocks tend to be of short duration, frequently providing relief for less than 1 hour. The paracervical block is administered when the cervix reaches 4 to 6 cm of dilatation. It may be repeated as long as there is enough cervical tissue present to allow injection of the anesthetic.

Although popular a decade ago, paracervicals are used more judiciously today, or not at all in some areas of the United States, because of their association with fetal bradycardia. Fetal bradycardia has been reported in 10 to 70 percent of cases and is hypothesized to be the effect of transplacental transfer of the anesthetic agent or its metabolites, with a depressant effect on the neonatal heart, or the result of local vasoconstriction resulting from rapid absorption of the agent into the uterine circulation (Table 24–4).

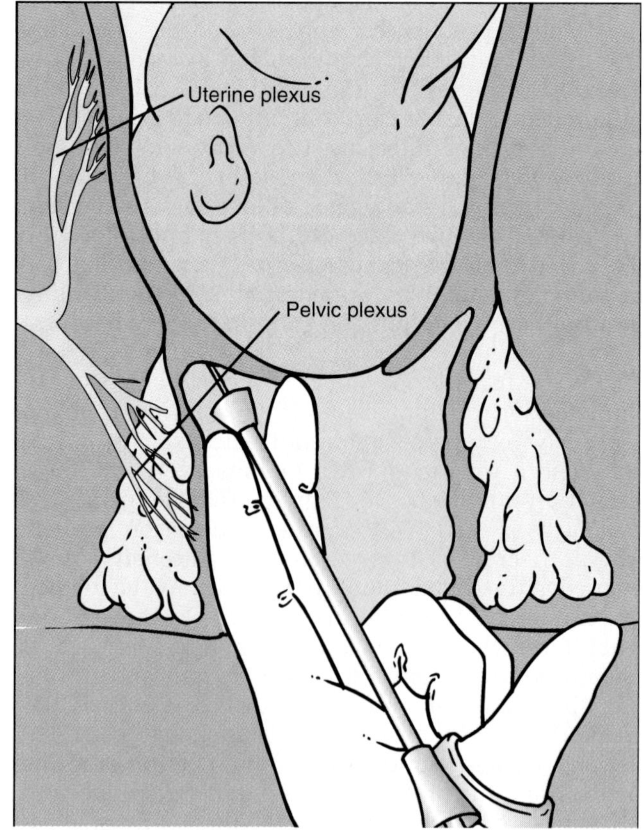

Figure 24–7

The paracervical block involves a shallow injection on each side of the lateral fornices of the vagina at the site of the pelvic plexus • Local anesthesia is used and provides pain relief to the dilating cervix for approximately 1 hour • The needle is protected in a long sheath called an Iowa trumpet guide to help ensure controlled penetration of the vaginal mucosa to only 2 to 3 mm.

Text continued on page 848

Table 24–4

ANESTHETICS FOR LABOR AND BIRTH

ANESTHETIC	DESCRIPTION	ADVANTAGES	DISADVANTAGES	EFFECTS ON FETUS OR NEWBORN	EFFECTS ON LABOR
			Paracervical Block		
Novocain 1% (procaine) Pontocaine (tetracaine)	Agent injected at 3 and 9 o'clock positions of cervix in active phase labor	Relief of pain from contractions Does not interfere with ability to push in second stage	May be "patchy" and not provide complete anesthesia Must be repeated approximately every hour Risk of toxic response to anesthetic Requires electronic fetal monitoring Needs skilled operator to administer	Fetal bradycardia (10%–70% incidence) Decreased baseline and occasional late decelerations	Little effect; may be a transient effect on contractions
			Epidural (Peridural) Block		
Xylocaine 1% (lidocaine) Marcaine 0.125%–0.5% (bupivacaine)	Placement of a catheter into the epidural space for continuous administration of anesthetic drug; active-phase labor through delivery	Complete pain relief for labor and birth Alert and relaxed Dose of drug can be altered to allow for pushing	Administration requires experience and skill High volume of drug required Administration is uncomfortable Slower onset of anesthesia (10–20 min) May be "patchy" and not provide complete anesthesia Risk of maternal hypotension	Usually little, but may occur with rapid absorption of drug or marked maternal hypotension Decreased baseline variability can occur	May disrupt normal labor pattern Depression of contractions may require oxytocin Decreased urge to push may require forceps, vacuum extractor May increase incidence of cesarean section in presence of dystocia

Continued on following page

Table 24–4

ANESTHETICS FOR LABOR AND BIRTH Continued

ANESTHETIC	DESCRIPTION	ADVANTAGES	DISADVANTAGES	EFFECTS ON FETUS OR NEWBORN	EFFECTS ON LABOR
			Epidural (Peridural) Block *(cont'd)*		
			Usually reduces ambulation Risk of accidental spinal block with puncture of dura resulting in respiratory paralysis Risk of toxic response to anesthetic Cost Necessitates electronic fetal monitoring		Increased risk of fetal malpositioning (which may increase poor contractions, use of Pitocin, and operative birth)
			Local Anesthetic		
Nesacaine 2% (chloroprocaine) Xylocaine 1%–2% (lidocaine) Carbocaine 1%–2% (mepivacaine)	Agent injected directly into perineum at time of birth	Minimal amount of anesthesia Quick and easy to administer	Large amounts of solution must be used; resultant distortion of tissue makes more difficult reapproximation for suturing Overdose can occur if insufficient time given to allow anesthetic to "take" before reinjecting Effective only in area where injected Risk of toxic response to anesthetic Requires skilled operator to administer	None	None

Table 24–4

ANESTHETICS FOR LABOR AND BIRTH Continued

ANESTHETIC	DESCRIPTION	ADVANTAGES	DISADVANTAGES	EFFECTS ON FETUS OR NEWBORN	EFFECTS ON LABOR
Pudendal Block					
Nesacaine 2% (Chloroprocaine) Xylocaine 1%–2% (Lidocaine) Carbocaine 1%–2% (Mepivacaine) Marcaine 0.25%–0.5% (Bupivacaine)	Agent injected transvaginally through sacrospinous ligaments to pudendal nerves during late second stage	Decreased vaginal and perineal pain and thus relaxation of tissue and potentially less laceration or need for episiotomy Absence of maternal hypotension Woman able to push in second stage Allows use of low or outlet forceps or vacuum extractor Ease of administration	May not work well 20% of the time because of anatomic variations of site of pudendal nerve Risk of maternal toxicity of anesthetic drug Requires skilled operator to administer	Little	None
Spinal/Saddle Block					
Xylocaine 1% (Lidocaine) Marcaine 0.125%–0.5% (Bupivacaine)	Intradural injection of anesthetic agent into subarachnoid space for delivery	Immediate onset of anesthesia (1–2 min) Relief of pain for delivery and repair of episiotomy or laceration if needed Alert and relaxed for delivery Smaller drug volume needed Can be used for forceps or vacuum or cesarean deliveries	Cannot be given until second stage, just before birth Administration uncomfortable Unpredictable level of anesthesia High incidence of maternal hypotension Possible total or high spinal block Possible postspinal headache	Major potential for fetal bradycardia	Decreased effectiveness of bearing down efforts Oxytocin may be required to stimulate contractions Increased incidence of forceps or vacuum extractor for birth

Continued on following page

Table 24–4

ANESTHETICS FOR LABOR AND BIRTH Continued

ANESTHETIC	DESCRIPTION	ADVANTAGES	DISADVANTAGES	EFFECTS ON FETUS OR NEWBORN	EFFECTS ON LABOR
Spinal/Saddle Block *(cont'd)*					
			Risk of maternal toxicity of anesthetic drug Requires skilled operator to administer		
General Anesthesia					
Nitrous oxide Oxygen Halothane, enflurane, or isoflurane Methoxyflurane Thiopental IV Succinylcholine	Inhalation gas administered through endotracheal intubation just before birth	Total blockage of pain Rapid administration in case of emergency Total uterine relaxation	Loss of consciousness Requires skilled anesthetist Risk of respiratory depression, cardiodepression, or aspiration Hypotension Hepatoxicity Nephrotoxicity Potential postpartum problems: nausea and vomiting, increased uterine atony, hemmorhage	Minimal if given just before delivery	Possible respiratory depression at birth Decreased newborn alertness Birth must occur within 5–7 min from start of anesthesia to decrease potential problem of respiratory depression of baby

Implications for Nursing Practice. The nursing implications related to the use of a paracervical block include close monitoring of the woman and fetus during the procedure and for the remainder of the labor. Because fetal bradycardia is a possibility, fetal heart rate (FHR) should be assessed continuously with the use of an electronic fetal monitor. If bradycardia is observed, the woman should be positioned in a side-lying position to remove the weight of the uterus and fetus from the inferior vena cava. Oxygen should be administered. If the bradycardia does not resolve within 30 minutes, fetal blood sampling should be done and plans initiated for emergency cesarean delivery. To assess for potential toxic response to the anesthetic, maternal blood pressure (BP), pulse, and respiration should be recorded every 5 to 10 minutes.

▼ **Epidural Anesthetic.** An anesthetic agent correctly placed in the epidural or peridural space can provide relief from the pain associated with uterine contractions in the first stage of labor and perineal distention and episiotomy in the second stage. The epidural space lies between the dura and the ligamentum flavum and extends from the base of the skull to the end of the sacral canal (Fig. 24–8; see Fig. 24–1). The anesthetic is administered by a nurse-anesthetist or physician (usually an anesthesiologist). The level of anesthe-

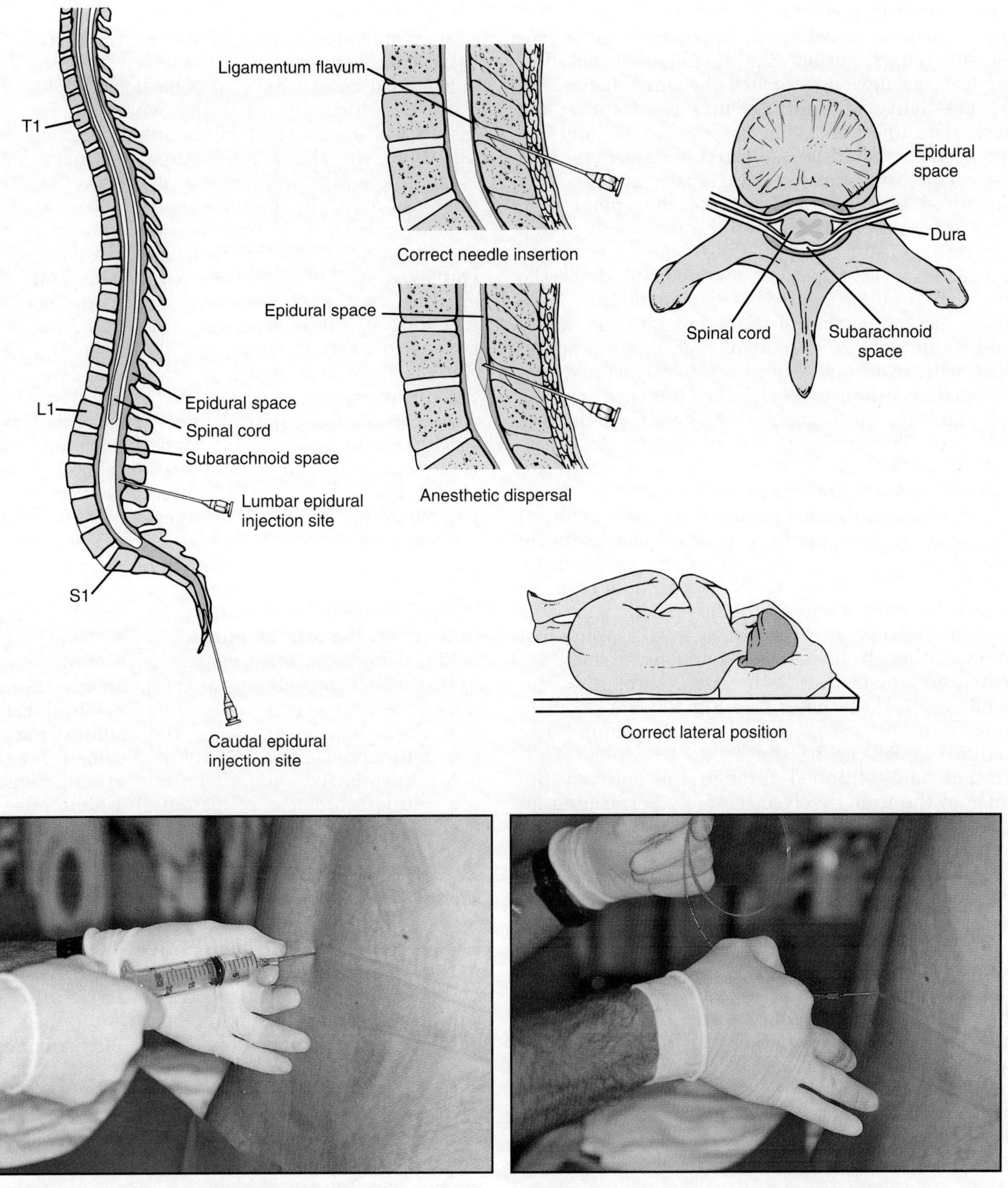

Figure 24–8

Physiology and administration related to epidural anesthesia.

sia that is desired for a lumbar epidural block is from the fifth sacral dermatome (S5) to the tenth thoracic vertebra (T10) for a vaginal birth or the eighth thoracic vertebra (T8) for a cesarean birth. The woman is usually positioned in a sitting or left side-lying position. She should arch, not flex, her back as flexion stretches the dura, increasing the possibility of puncture and resultant spinal block. The injection is made between L2 and L4. The syringe should be aspirated to determine that the needle is in the epidural space and has not punctured the dura and entered the spinal fluid ("wet tap") or entered an epidural vein. If spinal fluid is aspirated, the needle should be removed and insertion attempted at another site. Since the dose for an epidural block is five times that for a spinal block, injection of the agent into the spinal fluid could produce a sudden, high or total spinal block with resultant respiratory paralysis and cardiovascular collapse. Ventilation support may be necessary for the duration of the drug effect. A test dose for sensitivity or allergy to the anesthetic agent should also always be used before full administration of the drug (Taylor 1993).

The dose of the agent used for the epidural anesthesia is dependent on the level of anesthesia desired, the concentration and volume of the drug, and the position of the woman (e.g., mild Trendelenburg or semirecumbent). One injection may be used if delivery is expected within a couple of hours, although it is now common to have repeated administration of the agent through an indwelling plastic catheter (see Fig. 24–8) or continuous infusion using a volumetric pump. The epidural agent can be started at 4 to 6 cm of dilatation and continued through the delivery. Because of the time involved in safely performing an epidural and the time needed for the agent to act (approximately 15 minutes), use of epidural anesthesia with rapid labors or for multiparous women has been questioned in relation to risk and expense (Cunningham et al. 1993; Taylor 1993).

Advantages of epidural anesthesia include the quality of pain relief. Approximately 85 percent of women report being free of pain. The woman is also able to be alert and relaxed. The dose, volume, and type of anesthetic agent can be adjusted throughout the labor process as needed, so that the woman can push in second-stage labor, perineal anesthesia can be provided, and forceps can be used, or cesarean birth can be performed if necessary (Fehder and Gennaro 1993) (see Table 24–4).

There are also disadvantages to the use of epidural anesthesia. Hypotension is the most common important side effect. It can occur because of the blocking of sympathetic tracts by the anesthetic agent. In order to initiate treatment, hypotension must be promptly diagnosed. Therefore, after an epidural injection, the blood pressure should be taken every 2 minutes for at least 20 minutes. It has been demonstrated that hypotension is best corrected by a rapid intravenous infusion of a balanced salt solution, left uterine displacement (placing the woman in a lateral position to relieve pressure on the vena cava), and intravenous ephedrine.

Epidural blocks have also been associated with labor dysfunctions, especially when administered before well-established labor progress (Newton et al. 1995). In the second stage, epidural blocks most frequently impair the maternal desire to push. As a result, they are associated with an increased incidence of high presenting part or failure to rotate internally. In both cases, forceps are employed to remedy the situation, and thus epidural blocks are associated with an increased incidence of midforceps deliveries and forceps rotations (Chestnut 1991; Hawkins et al. 1995). Studies have also shown a significant increase in the incidence of cesarean birth for dystocia in women receiving epidural injections (Morton et al. 1994; Thorpe et al. 1994). Convulsions have also been reported upon administration of an epidural agent. Postspinal headaches could occur in the postpartal period if the injection was intradural.

Contraindications to an epidural injection are maternal hemorrhage, overt hypertension, neurologic disease, bleeding disorders or anticoagulant therapy, allergy to the anesthetic agent, or infections near the site of puncture. The safety of an epidural injection for a woman with mild or acute hypertension (preeclampsia or eclampsia) has been a topic of controversy, with some anesthesiologists and obstetricians suggesting the epidural may be the pain management strategy of choice because of its hypotensive side effect, and others suggesting caution because of potential compromise of uteroplacental circulation by a sudden decrease in blood pressure. Refusal of the epidural by the woman is, of course, an absolute contraindication (Fehder and Gennaro 1993).

▼ **Intrathecal Narcotic Injections.** An alternative to epidural anesthesia in some areas of the United States is the intrathecal narcotic injection. Initially, intrathecal narcotics were used for chronic and postoperative pain management in the late 1970s. Their use for labor began in 1980 with the use of intrathecal morphine. It was observed that a woman could feel her contractions, but not the pain associated with them. It was also noted that the pain relief obtained was not enough for the actual birth. Therefore, intrathecal narcotic injections provide analgesia for the visceral pain of uterine contractions but not anesthesia for the somatic pain of second-stage labor (Manning 1996).

The drug used for an intrathecal injection is not introduced into the epidural space, but into the subarachnoid space. A smaller amount of the drug can be used because of its direct uptake into the cerebrospinal fluid. The drug binds directly to opioid receptors in the dorsal horn of the spinal cord; therefore, there is no motor, sensory, or sympathetic nerve-fiber blockade. Several drugs have been used for intrathecal narcotic injections. Morphine (0.2 to 0.25 mg) is water soluble and moves rapidly in the cerebrospinal fluid to higher central nervous system centers. It remains in the cerebrospinal fluid longer, producing longer-lasting analgesia but potentially greater side effects. It takes effect in 15 to 30 minutes, and pain relief lasts 4 to 7 hours. Fentanyl citrate (25 μg) and sufentanil citrate (10 μg) are lipid-soluble drugs. They are absorbed more rapidly into the central nervous system, producing shorter-acting analgesia but fewer side effects. Analgesic effect takes place in 3 to 5 minutes, and pain relief lasts 1.5 to 3.5 hours. Combinations of the longer-acting morphine and the more rapid-acting fentanyl or sufentanil can be administered (Cunningham et al. 1993; Herpolsheimer and Schretenthaler 1994). A combination of intrathecal narcotic injection for analgesia in early labor and epidural anesthesia for later labor is also being used in some areas (Abouleish et al. 1994; Grieco et al. 1993).

Intrathecal narcotic injections are best administered in active labor, around 5 cm dilatation. If they are given later in the labor, the effect of analgesia may not be as great. If they are given earlier before a good contraction pattern has been established, they may slow down the contractions. Repeated intrathecal narcotic administration is usually avoided, because subsequent injections seem to provide a shorter duration of pain relief. The woman is able to feel the urge to push in the second stage of labor and can participate actively in the birth of the baby. Additional anesthetics, such as local or pudendal blocks, are needed for the birth if episiotomy or surgical repair is required.

Advantages of intrathecal narcotic injections include the ability to achieve pain relief during active labor but not lose mobility or sensation. The disadvantages of intrathecal injections are the possible side effects, which include pruritus, nausea, vomiting, urinary retention, and postdural puncture headache. Pruritus is probably the most common side effect of fentanyl, with an incidence of 80 percent reported in some studies (Barash et al. 1992). It can be treated with 25 to 50 mg of intravenous Benadryl if needed.

Implications for Nursing Practice. When an epidural block is used for pain management during labor, it is essential that the woman be well hydrated before administration. An intravenous line should be started and 500 mL to 1 L of Ringer lactate or Plasma-Lyte should be given to prevent hypotension. The woman should be assisted to lie on her left side or in a supported sitting position for insertion of the epidural catheter. Both maternal and fetal vital signs should be monitored continuously during and after the procedure (Taylor 1993).

Regional Blocks Administered in Second-Stage Labor

▼ **Local Infiltration Anesthesia.** Although a local infiltration anesthetic is given in the second stage of labor, just before the delivery, and for the repair of the perineum if needed, its effectiveness is primarily for the repair. By the time the local anesthetic is injected, the baby's head is usually crowning, which provides some natural anesthesia for the woman as it exerts pressure against the pelvic floor muscles and nerves. The local anesthetic is injected with a long, beveled 22-gauge needle directly into the muscles and cutaneous tissue of the perineum (Fig. 24–9). The anesthetic agents and dosages, advantages and disadvantages, and effects on the mother, fetus, and labor can be seen in Table 24–4.

▼ **Pudendal Block.** The pudendal block is also a pain management strategy for the second stage of labor. It is usually administered by the attending nurse-midwife or physician just before the birth. Pudendal blocks are generally very effective and provide anesthesia for the upper two thirds of the vagina and the entire perineum. Thus, they minimize the discomfort of perineal distention. If an episiotomy is necessary, it can be performed and subsequently repaired with the use of this nerve block. The anesthetic agents are generally the same as those employed for paracervical blocks, and the long needle is again sheathed and guided transvaginally. Unlike the procedure for a paracervical block, the needle is introduced laterally so that, when extended, it passes through the sacrospinous ligament to the pudendal nerve (Fig. 24–9). Since the pudendal artery lies in close proximity to the nerve, the operator needs to aspirate before administration of the drug so that inadvertent intravascular infusion is avoided. The needle is removed and reintroduced on the opposite side to infiltrate the other pudendal nerve in a similar manner.

Although a good pain strategy, a pudendal block has its limitations. Should a woman need to have intrauterine exploration, manual removal of a placenta, or a midforceps delivery, a pudendal block is not sufficient anesthesia and needs to be augmented with systemic medications or alternative anesthetics (Table 24–4).

▼ **Spinal Block.** In contrast to an epidural block, a spinal block involves injection of the anesthetic agent directly through the dura into the cerebrospinal fluid in the subarachnoid space. A spinal block therefore involves an intradural injec-

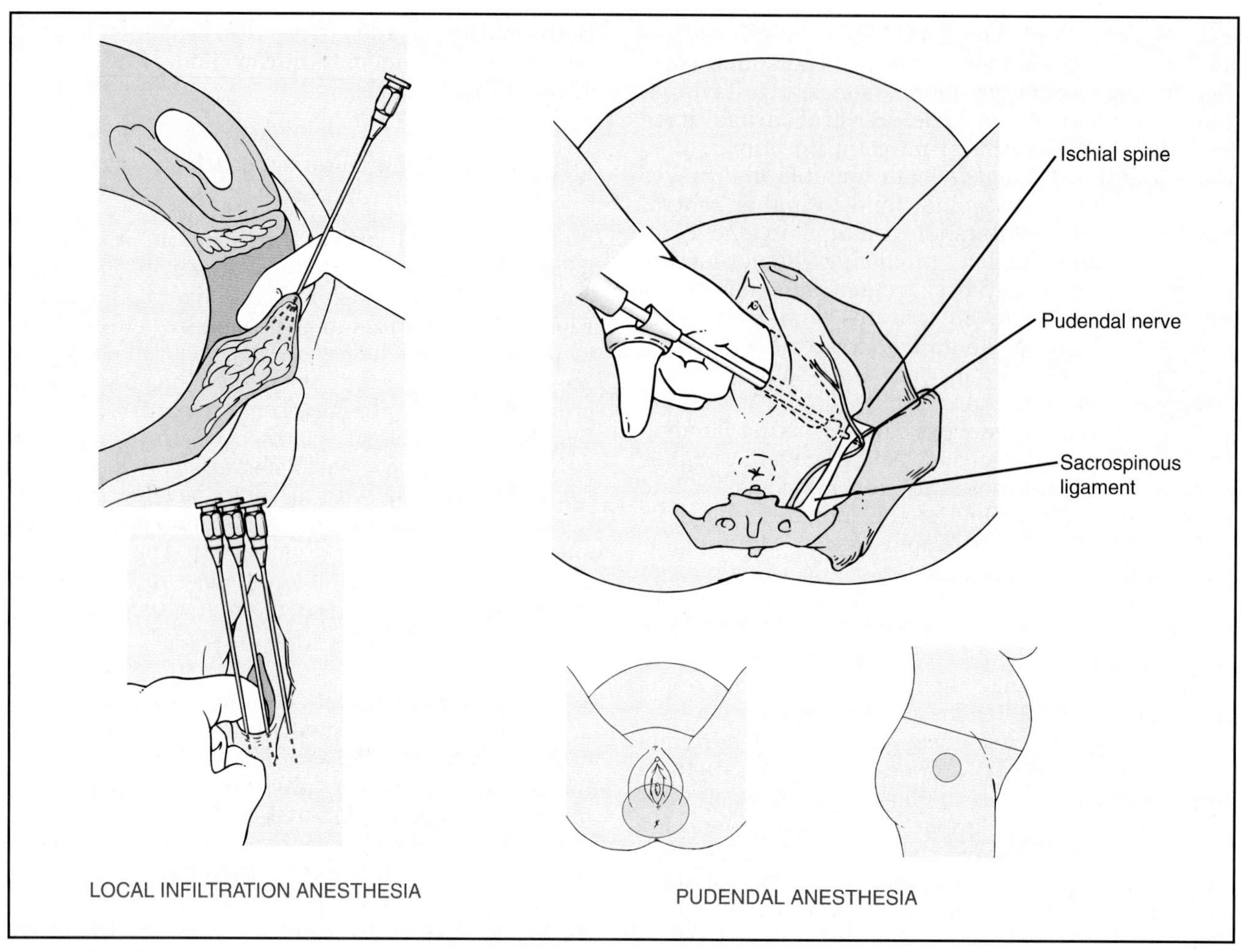

Figure 24–9

Local infiltration anesthesia and the pudendal block are regional forms of anesthesia generally administered during second-stage labor just before birth • Both provide effective pain control to the perineum during the birth and the episiotomy and its repair.

tion (Fig. 24–10). It is administered by a nurse-anesthetist or anesthesiologist just before the delivery in the second stage of labor. Although uncommon today for an uncomplicated vaginal birth, spinal blocks are frequently employed for cesarean birth and allow the woman to remain awake and see her infant at birth. In the case of a vaginal birth, a low spinal block (S1 to T10) or a saddle block (S1 to S4) is used. These blocks provide the anesthesia necessary for the delivery, the episiotomy, and its repair. The spinal block given for a cesarean birth provides blockage to level T6, resulting in anesthesia from the nipple line to the toes (Fig. 24–10).

Complications of spinal anesthesia include maternal hypotension, total spinal block, postspinal headaches, and bladder dysfunction (Table 24–4). The management of hypotension is the same as that discussed for the epidural block and may be of more importance, since the hypotension resulting from a spinal block can be more severe. Hypotension is caused by vasodilatation related to blocking of sympathetic nervous system impulses. If maternal hypotension is marked, the fetus can be compromised as a result of decreased placental blood flow. For paradoxical reasons, the possibility of hypotension resulting from the use of routine ergotamine drugs for postpartum bleeding (ergonovine or methylergonovine) is increased for women who have a spinal block. "The woman with preeclampsia is exquisitely sensitive to the hypotensive effects caused by subarachnoid block. Thus, spinal block is contraindicated in severe preeclampsia" (Cunningham et al. 1993, p. 436). If the complication of a total spinal block occurs (anesthesia level of T4 or above), paralysis of the respiratory muscles results. This is a rare side effect but can be critical. Symptoms of a total spinal block include apnea, absence of blood pressure, dilatation of the pupils, and loss of consciousness. Resuscitative treatment should be initiated immediately.

A spinal headache can result from leakage of spinal fluid at the injection site in the dura. This creates a negative pressure in the spinal column, pulling on central nervous system structures. The

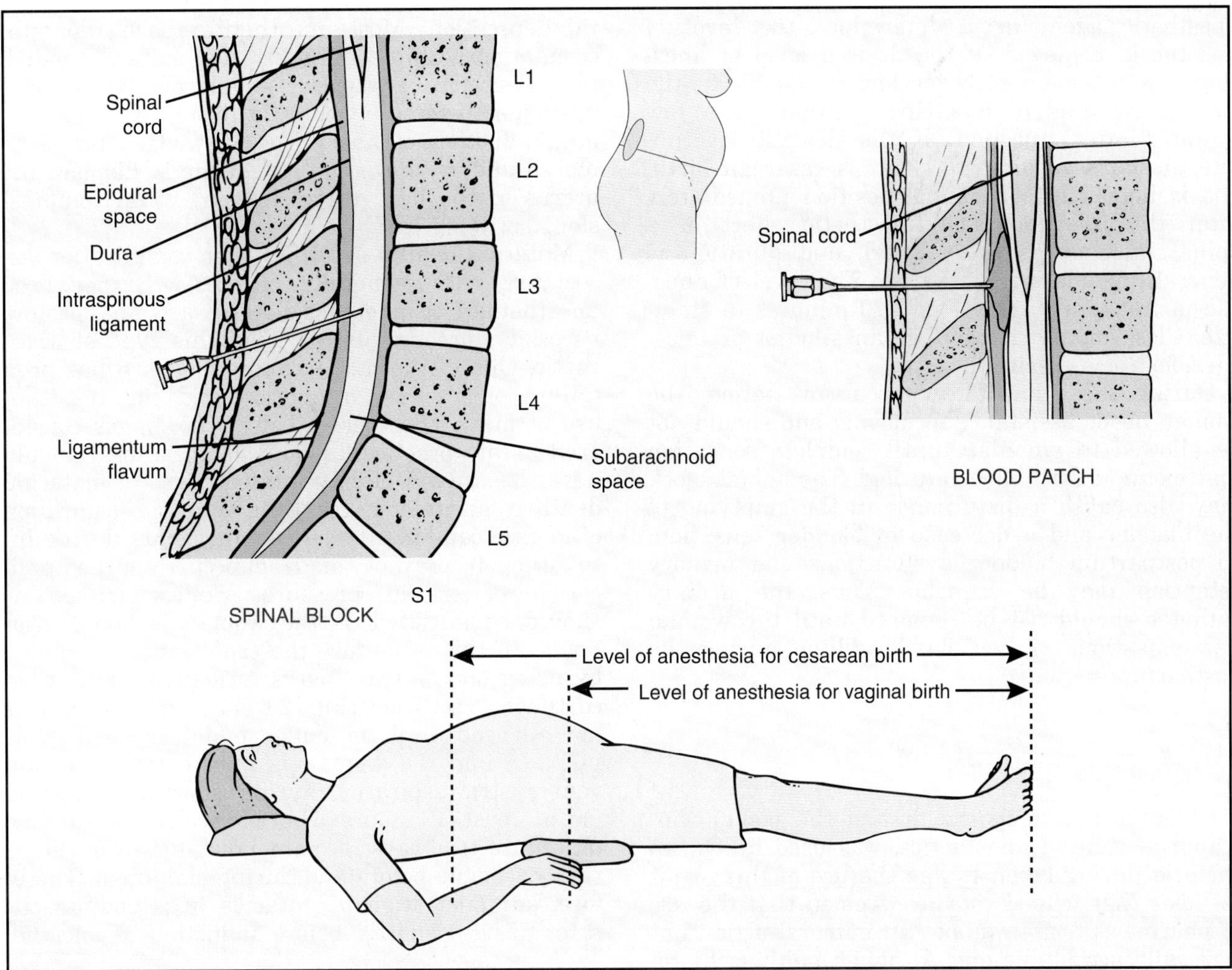

Figure 24–10

The spinal block procedure uses an intradural injection of anesthetic agent into the spinal fluid within the subarachnoid space • This provides anesthesia from S5 to T8 for a cesarean birth • A blood patch to prevent spinal fluid leakage and resultant post-spinal headache is accomplished by injecting 10 to 20 ml of maternal blood into the epidural space at the site of the spinal block injection.

result is a mild to severe headache that usually begins on the second postpartum day and may last for several days to a week, until the puncture site is healed, spinal fluid regenerated, and normal pressure within the spinal column restored. Studies do not support keeping the woman flat in bed for 12 hours after birth as a preventive. Hydration and analgesics may be helpful. Spinal headache may be prevented or treated by the anesthesiologist using a small-gauge needle and placing a blood patch at the site of the dural injection. This is done by injecting 10 to 20 mL of maternal blood into the epidural space at the site of injection. The blood clots and seals the leak, which provides immediate relief (Cunningham et al. 1993) (Fig. 24–10).

Contraindications to spinal blocks are similar to those to epidural blocks. In addition to contraindication for preeclampsia, women with maternal hemorrhage, overt hypertension, neurologic disease, coagulation disorders or anticoagulation therapy, allergy to anesthetic agents, or infections near the site of puncture should not be given this form of anesthesia.

Implications for Nursing Practice. Before administration of the spinal or saddle block, all other necessary activities in preparation for surgery should be performed. The woman should be in the delivery room, a retention catheter should be inserted into the bladder, and shaving of the operative site should be completed. The woman is positioned in either a lateral or sitting position. As with the epidural, she is asked to arch her back to widen the intervertebral space. She needs direction and support from the nurse in order to remain completely still during the injection. The anesthetic should be injected between contractions. The position of the woman immediately after injection, as well as the amount of anesthetic agent used, determines the level of anesthesia achieved. If the desired level of anesthesia is a saddle block or low spinal block, the woman remains in a sitting position for a few minutes after injection; if the desired level of anesthesia is a spinal block for a cesarean birth, she is helped into a supine position immediately after the injection. The anesthetic effect of a spinal injection is fairly rapid, and duration is generally not less than 1 hour. The level of anesthesia frequently takes 10 to 20 minutes to stabilize. Close monitoring by the anesthetist or anesthesiologist is essential.

During the immediate postpartum period, the woman needs assistance in moving and should not be allowed to ambulate until complete sensation and motor ability have returned. The spinal block may also cause a disturbance in the emptying of the bladder and a decrease in bladder sensation, so postpartum bladder dysfunctions and urinary retention may be sequelae. Thus, the urinary catheter should not be removed until the woman has sensations of her bladder filling during the postpartum period.

GENERAL ANESTHESIA

Chloroform, among the first of the popular intrapartal general anesthetics, was used by Queen Victoria during labor. It was the use of this agent in labor that helped convince women that the use of pharmaceuticals was not an immoral action but a socially acceptable one. Although neither chloroform nor even general anesthesia is commonly employed today, the former has its place in history and the latter still has its place in a labor and delivery unit. General or inhalation anesthesia can provide rapid anesthesia, which is needed in an emergency situation, whether it be a cesarean birth, fetal distress, or a placental complication. General anesthesia also results in loss of consciousness, central nervous system depression, and total uterine relaxation.

General anesthesia is initiated with the use of a combination of intravenous and inhalation induction agents and oxygen. The only gas induction agent used in the United States today is nitrous oxide (40 percent). It does not provide true anesthesia but does give analgesia and dissociation. It is usually given with oxygen (60 percent), an intravenous barbiturate induction agent (e.g., thiopental), and a muscle relaxant (e.g., succinylcholine) to allow easier intubation of the trachea. A volatile anesthetic (halothane, enflurane, or isoflurane) can then supplement the nitrous oxide to maintain the anesthesia (Table 24–4). These volatile anesthetics quickly cross the placenta and are associated with neonatal narcosis. When the time for the induction of anesthesia and the birth of the infant increases, so does the risk of neonatal depression. Most anesthetics reach the fetal circulation within 2 minutes after maternal induction. Therefore, anesthesia should not be initiated until just before the baby is to be delivered. Before induction of anesthesia, a wedge should be placed under the woman's right hip to displace the uterus to the left and avoid vena caval compression.

Maternal deaths are the major complication associated with general anesthesia. Experienced anesthetists or anesthesiologists are an absolute necessity for administration of this type of anesthetic. One of the major causes of death has been failure of tracheal intubation and the resultant use of mask anesthesia. This is no longer considered a safe practice, and mask anesthesia should never be used. A closely related cause of maternal death is pneumonia resulting from the aspiration of gastric contents if the woman vomits during intubation. To prevent this from occurring, the application of cricoid pressure (Sellick maneuver) should be initiated as the woman is being intubated. In this procedure the esophagus is occluded by using one or two fingers to depress the cricoid cartilage 2 to 3 cm (Fig. 24–11). The pressure is not released until the cuffed endotracheal tube is in place and the woman is anesthetized. To prevent gastric aspiration during anesthesia, fasting for at least 12 hours before an elective surgical procedure is always recommended; however, this is rarely feasible before and during childbirth. Therefore, administration of antacids (e.g., sodium citrate, Bicitra) shortly before induction of anesthe-

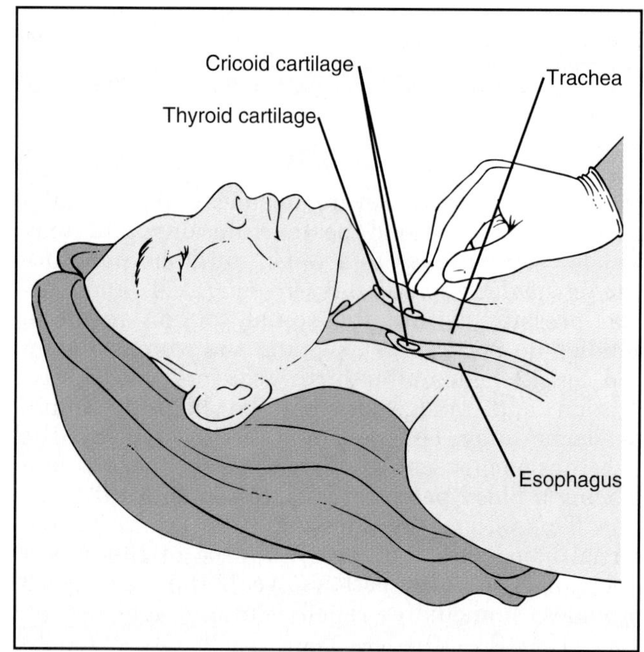

Figure 24–11

Cricoid pressure is applied to depress the trachea against the esophagus, thus preventing regurgitation of gastric contents during intubation and induction of anesthesia.

sia allows the gastric contents to be neutralized and therefore less harmful if aspirated. Extubation should be done only when the woman is conscious. A woman who aspirates may develop symptoms immediately or not until several hours later. This demonstrates the need for close clinical monitoring of the postoperative woman.

Implications for Nursing Practice. Before the administration of general anesthesia, it is important that the nurse obtain a history of the woman that includes information related to any conditions that might affect the use of general anesthesia and information about when and what the woman last ate. If general anesthesia is being considered, the nurse should explain the procedure to the woman so that she knows what to expect. An intravenous infusion line should be started and the woman should receive nothing by mouth. As discussed earlier, an antacid may be ordered to neutralize gastric contents. During the delivery, the nurse should be available to assist the anesthetist and should be prepared to assist in an emergency should it occur. During the immediate postpartum period, close monitoring of respiratory status, hemorrhage, cardiopulmonary status, and level of consciousness is important. General anesthetics may also pose a risk to the nurse. Several studies now indicate that women of reproductive age and pregnant women who commonly work around anesthetic agents are at higher risk for stillbirths, babies with cardiovascular abnormalities, and babies of lower birth weight (Cunningham et al. 1993).

Nursing Practice

Nursing Process

The nursing management of the woman in pain during labor and birth is important, challenging, and rewarding (see Improving Your Practice). The steps of the nursing process enable the nurse to work with the woman and her family to manage the discomforts of labor and birth and make the experience a positive one.

▼ Assessment

One of the difficulties in the study and clinical assessment of pain in labor is the acknowledged interaction of physiologic factors, psychological factors, individual biologic variation, cultural background, and developmental level. As Bonica and colleagues (1979) noted, contractions of the same intensity (e.g., 25 mm Hg) are not uniformly interpreted as painful by all women because of variations in pain perception or tolerance. Even when various factors are recognized as influences, there remains the difficulty of assessing the quantity of pain. When a woman is experiencing an acute episode of discomfort it is difficult for her to interpret the pain objectively, especially since no absolute comparison exists. It is impossible for one woman to compare her labor pain with that of another woman. Retrospective reporting of pain is tainted by the passage of time and does not adequately recognize the changes in intensity of pain during parturition. Many reports on pain in labor use questionable indirect measures, such as the amount of pharmaceutical agents used.

When a woman is admitted to the birth setting in labor, the initial interview and physical assessment contribute information regarding her previous experiences with pain, her current level of discomfort, the physiologic status of her labor, and her desires for pain management. It is important to identify whether she has preexisting physical conditions or allergies that might be affected by

PAIN MANAGEMENT DURING CHILDBIRTH

One of the most challenging experiences in nursing practice is caring for someone who is having pain. Nurses often feel helpless, ineffective, and angry when they do not know how to help someone in pain. The following suggestions should help the nurse who is working with patients who experience pain:

- EXPLORE YOUR OWN ATTITUDES AND FEELINGS ABOUT PAIN. Spend some time thinking about your personal reactions to pain. Does it frighten you? Do you feel helpless in its presence, whether in yourself or in others? Do you feel confident that pain can be managed?
- REMEMBER YOUR OWN PERSONAL EXPERIENCES WITH PAIN. Think about your reactions when you have pain. What kind of coping strategies do you use? What works? What doesn't work? Are there strategies you have found helpful that could be tried with your patients?
- REVIEW THE PROFESSIONAL LITERATURE ABOUT PAIN. Read current articles and research studies about the characteristics of pain and pain management. Be sure you are up to date on the most recent theories or treatment modalities.
- ATTEND A SEMINAR. Watch for seminars or workshops about pain management strategies that are new to you. Participate fully by learning all you can about new methods, personally experience the pain management strategy if possible, and share the information you learn with your colleagues.
- KEEP AN OPEN MIND. Be open to learning about a pain management strategy that you have questioned in the past. Methods of pain management that are not as familiar to our culture work well in other cultures; do not discount something that may sound different without first learning more about it.
- BROADEN YOUR RANGE OF NURSING INTERVENTIONS. Experiment with a variety of nonpharmacologic pain management strategies when caring for women in labor. Be willing to try something new and to try it several times if it does not work the first time.

drug or anesthesia administration, whether she has attended childbirth preparation classes, and her knowledge of the options available for nonpharmacologic and pharmacologic pain management. The initial physical assessment reveals any factors that might contribute to an increase in pain during labor or any concerns regarding maternal or fetal response to methods of pharmacologic pain management.

In attempting to assess a woman's pain during labor, the nurse should begin by observing the woman's nonverbal cues. What does the woman do during a contraction? Does she hold her breath, tighten her fists, move about in bed, vocalize, cry, or wrinkle her face? Or do her face and body remain relaxed, is her breathing unchanged, is she calm, and does she remain quiet during contractions? Although nonverbal cues serve as one indicator of pain, vocalization and body movement in labor may not be directly related to the amount of pain the woman is actually experiencing. The nurse should explore the meaning of the behavior with the woman before making assumptions.

A second means of assessing the degree of labor pain is through verbal communication with the woman. By talking to her between contractions and asking her to describe her pain, the nurse can determine the sensations the woman is experiencing, the location of the pain, whether it is persistent or intermittent, what pain relief measures have been tried, and what has been successful in achieving comfort. It is also important to identify the woman's desires for pain management throughout the labor and birth. This information can help the nurse determine whether the labor is progressing normally and make plans for interventions to help the woman manage her pain. A third means of evaluating pain is by assessment of biophysical measurements such as blood pressure, pulse, and respiration. An increase in any of these measurements can be indicative of increased pain. Nurses' personal experiences with pain may also influence their evaluation of the laboring woman's pain.

Another means of evaluating labor pain is through a standardized pain scale. The McGill Pain Scale is the most popular one. If used intrapartally, it allows the woman to report the intensity and nature of her pain through a 12-point questionnaire. However, the McGill Pain Scale is difficult to administer late in labor when a woman becomes more introverted and less open to interaction. A simpler way to measure the level of pain is through a visual analog scale. This scale consists of a straight line with increments that range from "no sensation" at one end to "the worst pain imaginable" at the other end. The woman is instructed to draw a line across the scale line indicating the degree of her perceived pain. No perfect method of pain assessment exists for intrapartal discomfort. Thus, additional research is needed in the area of pain in labor, especially in the field of psychometrics to measure pain. For the maternal-newborn nurse and the nursing management of a laboring family, the best approach may be the one advocated by McCaffery and Beebe (1989), who suggested that pain exists whenever the woman says it does.

▼ Diagnosis

The nursing diagnoses for the woman experiencing pain during labor or birth might include the following:

- Pain related to the process of labor or birth
- Knowledge deficit: lack of information related to origin and causes of pain and/or types of systemic drugs and anesthetics available
- Risk of maternal injury related to hypotension, decreased motor control, or toxic systemic reaction to administration of regional anesthesia
- Risk of fetal injury related to impaired gas exchange resulting from administration of systemic drugs or anesthetic agents

▼ Planning

The nursing plan is based on a number of factors, including the nature and amount of the woman's pain, the status of her labor, the status of the fetus, the woman's desires and goals for her birth experience, and the analgesic or anesthetic agents used for the labor and birth. Examples of goals and outcomes might include the following:

- The woman will demonstrate decreased pain by verbalizing her comfort and using suggested pain management strategies
- The woman will be able to discuss two nonpharmacologic pain management strategies that she will use to manage pain
- The woman will be able to discuss her desires in regard to the use of systemic drugs and anesthetics for labor and birth
- The woman's vital signs will remain within normal limits and she will show no signs or symptoms of a toxic systemic reaction
- The FHR will remain within 120 to 160, show good baseline variability, and show no ominous periodic changes

▼ Intervention

The nursing interventions for the identification of pain during labor and birth have been discussed in relation to the assessment phase of the nursing process. It is important that the nurse acknowledge the discomfort the woman is experiencing and elicit her involvement in deciding which methods of pain relief to employ. Providing information about any nonpharmacologic or pharmacologic method is an essential component of the nurse's interventions throughout labor. Because many of the nonpharmacologic methods of pain relief are noninvasive, relate closely to many common nursing comfort and support strategies, and do not require a physician's order, they should be used as a first step in the nurse's interventions to help the woman manage pain during labor (see Comfort Measure Checklist for Labor). Coaching the woman in relaxation, massaging her back or extremities, applying ice or heat to her back, helping her use a breathing technique during a contraction, and changing her position are all strategies that should be tried before moving to the use of pharmacologic pain management. It is the responsibility of nurses to learn about any nonpharmacologic methods that are unfamiliar to them so that they are able to make suggestions and teach and support their use.

Before using any method of pain relief, it is important that the nurse first assess the status of the woman (blood pressure, pulse, respiration), the status of the fetus (fetal heart rate, baseline variability, and periodic changes), and the status of the labor (contraction pattern, cervical dilatation, fetal position, station of the fetus). The woman's desire and need for pharmacologic pain relief should also be assessed and validated. If pharmacologic agents are given to a woman too early in labor, the progress of labor may be interrupted. On the other hand, if pharmacologic agents are given too late, pain relief is not achieved, which may increase the mother's ventilation and oxygen consumption and impair neonatal respiratory effort at birth. The nurse needs to reassure the laboring woman that pain relief is available and can have an appropriate role in the childbirth process.

General implications for nursing practice essential to the administration of any method of pain relief include

- Identifying whether the woman is allergic to any drugs; checking the arm band for correct identity
- Asking the woman to empty her bladder before initiation of pain medication or anesthetic and regular assessment for bladder filling or distention after administration
- Explaining the action of the drug, its probable effects on pain perception, and possible side effects; verifying the woman's desire for the drug
- Providing for the woman's safety either by remaining at her side or by raising the bed rails
- Initiating emergency measures in case of adverse maternal or fetal response
- Documenting administration of the medication

COMFORT MEASURE CHECKLIST FOR LABOR

Relaxation

Between contractions ______
During contractions ______

Massage

Face ______
Arms ______
Legs ______
Back ______
Feet ______

Patterned Breathing

Slow paced ______
Modified paced ______
Patterned paced ______

Position Changes

Sitting upright ______
Semireclining ______
Side-lying ______
Standing ______
Walking ______
Hands and knees ______
Squatting ______

Hydrotherapy

Bath/whirlpool ______
Shower ______

Back Labor

Hot packs ______
Cold packs ______
Counterpressure ______
Pelvic rocking ______
Knee chest position ______

Coaching Strategies

Verbal feedback ______
Praise ______
Encouragement ______
Eye contact ______
Physical presence ______
Undivided attention ______
Breathe with woman ______
Call out 15-second intervals ______
Talk her through contraction ______

(drug, dosage, route, time, and site) on the chart and fetal monitor strip

Systemic drugs for labor are administered by either the intramuscular or intravenous route. The intravenous or IV route allows a smaller dosage of drug to be used, results in a more rapid and predictable onset of pain relief, and allows a more predictable duration of effect. The intramuscular or IM route gives a delayed onset of pain relief, requires higher dosages of the drug, and has a more unpredictable pain relief effect. The smallest possible dose of a drug is given so that labor is not impeded and the effect on the fetus is minimal. The power of suggestion often increases the effectiveness of a medication; for example, if the woman believes the drug will help her to relax and manage her pain, that will more than likely be the result. Specific implications for nursing practice include

- Obtaining a drug order or checking the standing order for administration of systemic analgesic drugs; verifying the woman's desire for the drug
- Preparing the correct medication and correct dose; determining the ordered route of administration
- Assessing maternal, fetal, and labor parameters to evaluate the effects of the medication
- Evaluating the effect of the drug on the woman's pain

With the administration of regional or general anesthetics, additional nursing interventions include

- Starting an IV infusion line if not already in place
- Explaining the procedure for administration of the anesthetic, what the woman will feel during the procedure, and the expected pain relief from the anesthetic
- Assisting in positioning the woman for administration of the anesthetic

- Assisting the anesthetist as necessary during the procedure
- Providing emotional support, ongoing information, and assistance with relaxation and controlled breathing throughout the procedure
- Assessing maternal and fetal vital signs every 1 to 2 minutes for the first 15 minutes, then every 10 to 15 minutes; assessing the effects of the anesthetic on the labor process
- And, as before, evaluating the effects of the anesthetic on the woman's pain

▼ Evaluation

The evaluation of the plan of care is based on the identified measurable goals and outcomes and is an ongoing process. If the woman is able to decrease her fear, achieve pain relief, and cope with the labor and birth experience and if the birth takes place without adverse effects on mother or baby, the nursing management of pain has been successful.

Collaborative Process

All members of the health care team work together in the management of pain for the woman in labor. The nurse plays a major role, being the professional who is with the woman continuously throughout labor and birth. The nurse is the one who helps the woman evaluate and cope with her pain; prepares, administers, and monitors the systemic analgesic drugs; and supports the woman while receiving, and then monitors her status after administration of, an anesthetic agent. Nurses who have received advanced training, as either certified nurse-midwives or nurse-anesthetists, may also administer anesthetic agents. Anesthetic agents are also administered by an obstetrician or anesthesiologist.

Risk Management

The management of risk in relation to the administration of pharmacologic pain relief methods is critical. The nurse, as well as all other members of the health care team involved in the administration of drugs or anesthetics, must be diligent in continually assessing the woman and her fetus; explaining the action of the drug or anesthetic, the procedure for administration, the probable effects, and the risks and benefits; obtaining signed informed consent when necessary; using correct technique in administration of the drug or anesthetic; staying with the woman and making provisions for her safety; and documenting accurately the pharmacologic method used and the time, dosage, route, and effects of the drug or anesthetic administered, both on the woman's chart and on the electronic fetal monitor strip.

Implications for Research

Additional research is needed in the area of pain management for childbirth. Although much has been accomplished in the field of pharmacology, nonpharmaceutical modalities have been woefully neglected. Since most nonpharmaceutical remedies are within the realm of nursing management strategies, there is ample opportunity for nurses to explore the effectiveness of these modalities as well as the best modifications for applications during the childbirth process. Another area needing additional research is the measurement of intrapartal discomfort and pain. Examples of research questions that might be developed include

- Which nonpharmacologic pain management strategies are most effective for reducing pain during childbirth?
- What is the degree of satisfaction that women experience for each pharmacologic method of pain relief, both during and after labor?
- Which nursing interventions do women perceive as most helpful in assisting them to cope with the pain of labor?

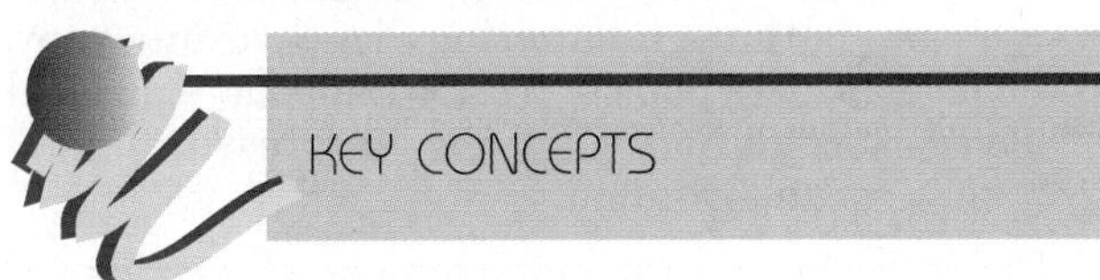

KEY CONCEPTS

- ▼ Pain is a universal experience; it is whatever the person experiencing it says it is, and it exists whenever the person says it does.
- ▼ Pain during labor and birth is the result of normal physiology, results from identifiable causes, has a known time limit, and results in a positive outcome.

- ▼ Pain in the first stage of labor is caused by cervical stretching and pressure, hypoxia of the uterine muscle, and stretching and traction.
- ▼ Pain in the second stage of labor is associated with the distention of the muscles of the vagina, pelvic floor, and perineum.
- ▼ The three phases of the pain experience are the anticipation phase, the actual pain, and the aftermath phase.
- ▼ The gate control theory of pain perception proposes that pain impulses can be blocked along the afferent nerve pathways by a gating mechanism triggered by the substantia gelatinosa along the spinal cord; this gating mechanism can be triggered by stimulation of the skin or stimulation of the brain stem, thalamus, and cerebral cortex.
- ▼ The endogenous biochemical pain theory proposes that a natural pain suppression system functions at the midbrain, medulla, and spinal cord, initiating the release of morphine-like polypeptides called enkephalins that promote relaxation, euphoria, and pain relief.
- ▼ Dick-Read's fear-tension-pain theory proposes that fear of labor and birth causes uterine tension and resultant ischemia, resulting in pain.
- ▼ Theories of cognitive control propose that involving the mind in mental activities can decrease awareness of incoming pain sensations; two types of cognitive control are dissociation and interference.
- ▼ Pain in childbirth can be influenced by physical variables such as fatigue and general health status, psychological variables such as fear or emotional state, sociocultural variables such as expected behavioral responses or religious beliefs, and environmental variables such as noise or privacy.
- ▼ Nonpharmacologic pain management strategies include knowledge and information, relaxation techniques, breathing strategies, labor support, imagery, touch and massage, application of heat or cold, bathing, showering, jet hydrotherapy, biofeedback, hypnosis, transcutaneous electrical nerve stimulation (TENS), acupressure, acupuncture, and Shiatsu.
- ▼ Pharmacologic pain management strategies include systemic analgesic drugs that alter or decrease the perception of pain and anesthetics that totally block the sensation of pain.
- ▼ Systemic drugs used for labor include tranquilizers and antiemetics to promote relaxation and decrease nausea, narcotic analgesics to decrease pain, narcotic agonist-antagonists to provide pain relief and also block respiratory depression, and narcotic antagonists to reverse respiratory depression.
- ▼ Regional anesthetics used in the first stage of labor include paracervical blocks to relieve pain from cervical dilatation and vaginal stretching and epidural or intrathecal anesthesia to block sensation of uterine contractions; regional anesthetics for the second stage of labor include the spinal block for cesarean birth and local anesthetics and pudendal blocks for the repair of the episiotomy in a vaginal birth.
- ▼ The advantages of the epidural for pain management during labor include the fact that it can be administered at 4 to 6 cm in active-phase labor, it provides a high quality of pain relief, and it allows the woman to be alert and relaxed; the disadvantages of the epidural include the possibilities of maternal hypotension, labor dysfunction, inability to push effectively in the second stage of labor, and an increased incidence of forcep deliveries and cesarean birth.
- ▼ General anesthesia is used most commonly when rapid anesthesia is needed in an emergency situation such as cesarean birth, fetal distress, or a placental complication; it provides loss of consciousness, central nervous system depression, and total uterine relaxation.
- ▼ Assessment of a woman's pain during labor can be made through physical assessment, observation of nonverbal cues, verbal communication, or a standardized pain scale.
- ▼ Nursing interventions for the management of pain in labor should include nonpharmacologic as well as pharmacologic strategies.

References

Abouleish, A., Abouleish, E., Cannon, W. (1994). Combined spinal-epidural analgesia in advanced labour. *Canadian Journal of Anesthesia,* 41 (7), 575–578.

Aderhold, K., and Perry, L. (1991). Jet hydrotherapy for labor and postpartum pain relief. *MCN,*16 (2), 97–99.

Albers, L., and Katz, V. (1991). Birth setting for low-risk pregnancies: An analysis of the current literature. *Journal of Nurse-Midwifery,* 36, 215–220.

Alexander, C., and Steefel, L. (1995). Biofeedback: Listen to the body. *RN,* 58 (8), 51–52.

Augustinson, L., Bohlen, P., Bundsen, P., Carlsson, C., Forssman, L., Sjöberg, T., Tyreman, N. (1977). Pain relief during delivery by transcutaneous electrical nerve stimulation. *Pain,* 4 (10), 59–65.

Barash, P., Cullen, B., Stoelting, R. (1992). *Clinical anesthesia* (2nd ed.). Philadelphia: J. B. Lippincott.

Basmajian, J. (1989). *Biofeedback—Principles and practice for clinicians* (3rd ed.). Baltimore: Williams & Wilkins.

Beal, M. (1992). Acupuncture and related treatment modalities. Part II: Applications to antepartal and intrapartal care. *Journal of Nurse-Midwifery,* 37 (4): 260–268.

Berg, T., and Rayburn, W. (1992). Effects of analgesia on labor. *Clinical Obstetrics and Gynecology,* 35 (3), 457–463.

Bernat, S., Wooldridge, P., Marecki, M., Snell, L. (1992). Biofeedback-assisted relaxation to reduce stress in labor. *Journal of Obstetric, Gynecologic, and Neonatal Nursing,* 21 (4), 295–304.

Bonica, J. J., and McDonald, J. S. (1995). *Principles and practice of obstetric analgesia and anesthesia* (2nd ed.). Baltimore: Williams & Wilkins.

Bonica, J., et al. (1979). *Altering the experience of pain.* New York: Pfizer Laboratories.

Brucker, M. (1984). Nonpharmacologic methods for relieving pain and discomfort in pregnancy. *MCN,* 9, 390–394.

Bundsen, P., Peterson. L., Selstorn, U. (1981). Pain relief in labor by transcutaneous electrical nerve stimulation: A prospective matched study. *Acta Obstetricia et Gynecologica Scandinavica,* 60 (5), 459–468.

Butler, M., Luther, D., Frederick, E. (1988). Coaching: The labor companion. In F. H. Nichols and S. S. Humenick (Eds.). *Childbirth education: Practice, research, and theory* (pp. 275–290). Philadelphia: W. B. Saunders.

Cammu, H., Clasen, K., Van Wettere, L., Derde, M. (1994). To bathe or not to bathe during the first stage of labor. *Acta Obstetricia et Gynecologica Scandinavica,* 73 (6), 468–472.

Chestnut, D. (1991). Epidural anesthesia and instrumental vaginal delivery. *Anesthesiology,* 74 (5), 805–808.

Cunningham, F. G., MacDonald, P. C., Gant, N. F., Leveno, K. J., Gilstrap, L. C. III. (1993). *Williams obstetrics* (19th ed.) Norwalk, CT: Appleton & Lange.

Davenport-Slack, B. (1975). A comparative evaluation of obstetrical hypnosis and antenatal childbirth training. *International Journal of Clinical and Experimental Hypnosis,* 23, 266–281.

Dick-Read, G. (1959). *Childbirth without fear.* New York: Harper & Row.

Enkin, M., Keirse, M., Renfrelo, M., Neilson, J. (1995). *A guide to effective care in pregnancy and childbirth* (2nd ed.). New York: Oxford University Press.

Erickson, J. (1994). The use of hypnosis in anesthesia: A master class commentary. *International Journal of Clinical and Experimental Hypnosis,* 42 (1), 8–12.

Fehder, W., and Gennaro, S. (1993). Recent trends in epidural analgesia for childbirth. *Journal of Perinatal Education,* 2 (2), 1–6.

Fullerton, J., and Severino, R. (1992). In hospital care for low-risk childbirth: Comparison with results from the national birth center study. *Journal of Nurse-Midwifery,* 37 (5), 331–340.

Grieco, W., Norris, M., Leighton, B., Arkoosh, V., Huffnagle, J., Honet, J., Costello, D. (1993). Intrathecal sufentanil labor analgesia: The effects of adding morphine or epinephrine. *Anesthesia and Analgesia,* 77 (6), 1149–1154.

Hawkins, J., Hess, K., Kubicek, M., Joyce, T., Morrow, D. (1995). A reevaluation of the association between instrument delivery and epidural analgesia. *Regional Anesthesia,* 20 (1), 50–56.

Hedstrom, L., and Newton, N. (1986). Touch in labor: A comparison of cultures and eras. *Birth,* 13 (3), 181–186.

Herpolsheimer, A., and Schretenthaler, J. (1994). The use of intrapartum intrathecal narcotic analgesia in a community-based hospital. *Obstetrics and Gynecology,* 84 (6), 931–936.

Hilgard, E., and Hilgard, J. (1975). *Hypnosis in the relief of pain.* Los Altos, CA: William Kaufmann.

Isenor, L., and Penny-MacGillivray, T. (1993). Intravenous meperidine infusion for obstetric analgesia. *Journal of Obstetric, Gynecologic, and Neonatal Nursing,* 22 (4), 349–357.

Jaros, J. (1991). The concept of pain. *Critical Care Nursing Clinics of North America,* 3 (1), 1–9.

Jenkins, M., and Pritchard, M. (1993). Hypnosis: Practical applications and theoretical considerations in normal labour. *British Journal of Obstetrics and Gynaecology,* 100 (3), 221–226.

Jimenez, S. L. M. (1988). Supportive pain management strategies. In F. H. Nichols and S. S. Humenick (Eds.). *Childbirth education: Practice, research, and theory* (pp. 97–117). Philadelphia: W. B. Saunders.

Jungman, R. (1988). Relaxation: Acupressure. In F. H. Nichols and S. S. Humenick (Eds.). *Childbirth education: Practice, research, and theory* (pp. 176–183). Philadelphia: W. B. Saunders.

Koehn, M. (1992). Effectiveness of prepared childbirth and childbirth satisfaction. *Journal of Perinatal Education,* 1, 35–43.

Kriegger, D. (1979). *The therapeutic touch.* Englewood Cliffs, NJ: Prentice-Hall.

Lederman, R., Lederman, E., Work, B., McCann, D. (1978). Relationship of maternal anxiety, plasma catecholamines, and plasma cortisol to progress in labor. *American Journal of Obstetrics and Gynecology,* 132, 495–500.

Lowe, N. (1987). Parity and pain during parturition. *Journal of Obstetric, Gynecologic, and Neonatal Nursing,* 16 (5), 340–346.

Lowe, N. (1989). Explaining the pain of active labor: The importance of maternal confidence. *Research in Nursing and Health,* 12, 237–245.

Mackey, R. (1995). Discover the healing power of therapeutic touch. *American Journal of Nursing,* 95 (4), 26–32.

Manning, J. (1996). Intrathecal narcotics: New approach for labor analgesia. *Journal of Obstetric, Gynecologic, and Neonatal Nursing,* 25 (3), 221–224.

McCaffery, M., and Beebe, A. (1989). *Pain: Clinical manual for nursing practice.* St. Louis: C. V. Mosby.

Melzack, R. (1974). *The puzzle of pain.* New York: Basic Books.

Melzack, R., and Wall, P. (1965). Pain mechanisms: A new theory. *Science,* 150, 971–979.

Moir, D. (1978). *Pain relief in labour.* Edinburgh: Churchill Livingstone.

Morton, S., Williams, M., Keeler, E., Gambone, J., Kahn, K. (1994). Effect of epidural analgesia for labor on the cesarean delivery rate. *Obstetrics and Gynecology,* 83 (6), 1045–1052.

Newton, E., Schroeder, B., Knape, K., Bennett, B. (1995). Epidural analgesia and uterine function. *Obstetrics and Gynecology,* 85 (5), 749–755.

Newton, N. (1966). Parturient mice: Effects of environment on labor. *Science,* 151, 1560–1561.

Newton, N., Peeler, D., Newton, M. (1968). The effects of disturbance on labor. *American Journal of Obstetrics and Gynecology,* 101, 1096–1102.

Nichols, F. H., and Humenick, S. S. (1988). *Childbirth education: Practice, research and theory* (opening quotation, p. 96). Philadelphia: W. B. Saunders.

Oxorn, H. (1986). *Oxorn and Foote human labor and birth* (5th ed.). Norwalk, CT: Appleton & Lange.

Simkin, P. (1995). Reducing pain and enhancing progress in labor: A guide to nonpharmacologic methods for maternity caregivers. *Birth,* 22 (3), 161–171.

Skyken, J., and Petrie, R. (1988). Obstetric uses of butorphanol tartrate. *Contemporary Obstetrics and Gynecology,* 33, 95–106.

Sosa, R., Kennel, J., Klaus, M., Robertson, S., Urrutia, J. (1980). The effect of a supportive companion on perinatal problems, length of labor and mother-infant interaction. *New England Journal of Medicine,* 303, 597–600.

Steffes, S. A. (1988). Relaxation: Imagery. In F. H. Nichols and S. S. Humenick (Eds.). *Childbirth education: Practice, research, and theory* (pp. 184–200). Philadelphia: W. B. Saunders.

Steiner, S. H., and Steiner, J. F. (1988). Pharmaceutical pain management strategies. In F. H. Nichols and S. S. Humenick (Eds.). *Childbirth education: Practice, research, and theory* (pp. 291–302). Philadelphia: W. B. Saunders.

Taylor, T. (1993). Epidural anesthesia in the maternity patient. *MCN,* 18 (2), 86–93.

Thorpe, J., Meyer, B., Cohen, G., Yeast, J., Hu, D. (1994). Epidural analgesia in labor and cesarean delivery for dystocia. *Obstetrical and Gynecological Survey,* 49 (5), 362–369.

Wuitchik, M., Hesson, K., Bakal, D. (1990). Perinatal predictors of pain and distress during labor. *Birth,* 17 (4), 186–191.

25 Chapter

> The nurse caring for the critically ill expectant mother must have a thorough understanding of the changes that occur in a pregnant woman's body to be able to recognize the normal as well as the abnormal responses.
>
> MILDRED HARVEY (1992)

High-Risk Childbirth

Nancy J. MacMullen
Mary C. Brucker
Elaine Zwelling

HIGHLIGHTS

- High-Risk Conditions Apparent at the Onset of Labor Related to Malpositions and Malpresentations, Placental Abnormalities, Preterm Labor and Birth, Premature Rupture of Membranes, Postterm Pregnancy, Cord Prolapse
- Procedure 25–1: Maternal-Fetal Transport
- High-Risk Conditions Occurring During First- and Second-Stage Labor Related to Uterine Dysfunctions, Labor Anomalies, Cephalopelvic Disproportion, Rupture of the Uterus, Shoulder Dystocia
- High-Risk Fetal or Neonatal Complications During Labor and Birth Related to Decreased Fetal Oxygenation, Multiple Gestation, Fetal Developmental Anomalies, Intrauterine Fetal Demise
- High-Risk Conditions Associated with the Third Stage of Labor Related to Amniotic Fluid Embolism, Uterine Inversion, Hemorrhage
- Obstetric Interventions Used in High-Risk Situations Related to External Cephalic Version, Induction of Labor, Operative Obstetrics
- Procedure 25–2: Assisting with Amniotomy
- Procedure 25–3: Induction of Labor by Oxytocin Infusion
- Procedure 25–4: Preparation for Cesarean Birth
- Psychological Issues Associated with High-Risk Childbirth
- Risk Management
- Implications for Research

Childbirth is most often a normal, healthy process. It is not wise for a nurse to approach birth as an abnormal event. Such a philosophy influences interpretation of all the profound but normal physiologic and psychological changes during labor and birth as well as the type of care the woman receives. Conversely, it is equally unwise to deny that occasionally deviations

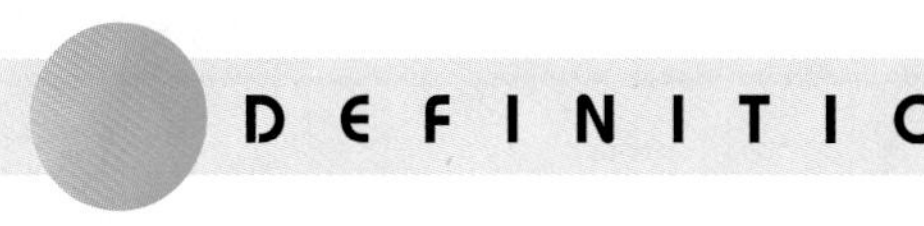

DEFINITIONS

Abruptio placentae—Premature separation of the placenta from the uterine wall; usually results in maternal hemorrhage and fetal compromise.

Amniotic fluid embolism—Infusion of a large amount of amniotic fluid into the maternal circulation; can culminate in respiratory arrest and maternal death.

Cephalopelvic disproportion—A relationship between the fetal head and the maternal pelvis in which either the fetus is too large for the pelvis or the pelvis is too small to allow passage of the fetal head.

Cord prolapse—Condition when a loop of the umbilical cord lies beside or below the presenting part of the fetus.

Dystocia—Abnormal or difficult labor; caused by problems related to the maternal pelvis, maternal soft tissues, or fetus; can refer to abnormal labor pattern when compared with the Friedman curve.

Episiotomy—Surgical incision through the perineum made to enlarge the vaginal opening for birth.

External cephalic version—Manual turning of the fetus in a noncephalic presentation into a cephalic presentation.

Occiput posterior—A position of the fetal head that occurs when the occiput of the head and posterior fontanelle are in the posterior portions of the maternal pelvis and the brow and bregma are in the anterior portion; can be a cause of back labor.

Oligohydramnios—Abnormal decrease in the amount of amniotic fluid.

Placenta previa—Abnormal placement of placenta so that it partially covers the cervix; dilatation results in bleeding, which can be of hemorrhagic proportions.

Polyhydramnios—Abnormal increase in the amount of amniotic fluid.

Postterm pregnancy—A pregnancy that continues for 42 weeks or more from the first day of the last menses in a 28-day cycle.

Premature rupture of membranes (PROM)—Spontaneous rupture of membranes before onset of labor but after 37 weeks' gestation.

Uterine inversion—A turning inside out of the uterus.

from normal can occur that threaten the well-being of the mother or fetus, or both. To ignore signs of complications could mean jeopardizing the health of both mother and baby. Thus, nursing care of the maternal fetal dyad presents an ongoing challenge, especially in the assessment of normal events, awareness of high-risk situations, early recognition of complications, and appropriate intervention when an emergency situation occurs.

High-risk childbirth is included under the generic definition of high-risk pregnancy. Determination of the risk status of a mother and fetus during pregnancy and/or childbirth has been a major task attempted by many researchers. Various risk assessment forms have been developed, but all show evidence of some difficulty in clearly identifying the less than 20% of women whose pregnancies account for more than 80% of all perinatal/maternal morbidity and mortality (Burrow and Ferris 1995; Creasy and Resnik 1994; Merkatz and Thompson 1990). The more risk factors identified, the more sensitive the assessment becomes. However, the more sensitive, the less specific they appear to become, causing an increased number of women to be labeled as "high risk" when ultimately they do not appear to be in such a category. Rather than establishing a general category of "high risk," it seems more reasonable at this time to identify risk factors that increase the likelihood that a woman or fetus/neonate will develop a specific complication of childbirth.

Complications of childbirth may be subdivided in many ways. For the sake of discussion, this chapter addresses complications that are most commonly manifested with each stage of labor. Some complications are apparent at the onset of labor (e.g., preterm labor and birth). Other complications are specific to active labor (e.g., labor dystocias). Still others are more commonly associated with the third stage of labor (e.g., uterine atony). Certain complications are specific to the fetus or neonate and, although potentially life threatening for the fetus, may pose no risk to the mother. An example is any one of a number of congenital developmental anomalies. The incidence of high-risk childbirth is reported according to the specific risk condition. For example, statistics regarding preterm births are specific to that condition. Other childbirth risk conditions are recorded separately.

Complicated childbirth requires sophisticated nursing interventions, including excellent assessment techniques, nursing diagnosis, and holistic plans for interventions that include psychosocial aspects of care. Continual evaluation is an essential component of the process. High-risk labor and birth may also require obstetric interventions, such as labor augmentation/induction or operative birth. If more intensive care is needed and the woman is not being cared for in a tertiary care center, it may be necessary to transport her to

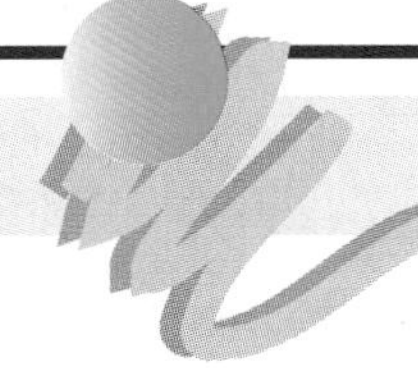

HISTORICAL PERSPECTIVES

BIRTH AS A NORMAL LIFE PROCESS

Complications of childbirth are the exception, not the rule in labor and birth. In 1990 Laurel Thatcher Ulrich received a Pulitzer Prize for writing *A Midwife's Tale: The Life of Martha Ballard Based on Her Diary, 1785–1812.*

Martha Ballard was an American midwife. As Ulrich noted in her critique of Ballard's diary, such a diary had not been unknown. For years it had been ignored because it seemed too commonplace, yet to those interested in life in the Americas, especially in relationship to childbirth, it is a rich source of information.

In less than 6 percent of the births that Martha Ballard attended did she note any complication of childbirth. In the almost 1000 births she attended, she did not lose a single mother at delivery, and only five women died in the immediate post-partum period. These numbers help indicate not only the skill of Martha Ballard but the innate normalcy of birth.

such a center to receive that care (see Procedure 25–1).

HIGH-RISK CONDITIONS APPARENT AT THE ONSET OF LABOR

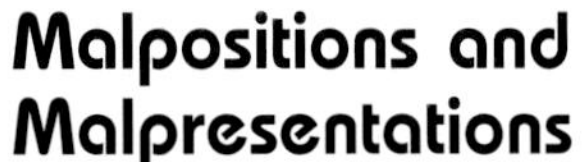

Malpositions and Malpresentations

Malpositions and malpresentations appear to be associated with any factor that prevents the fetus from physically assuming the cephalic presentation. Examples of these factors include preterm labor or prematurity, in which the fetus is so small that it does not nestle well in the pelvis; large pelvic capacities; and lax pelvis musculature, as might be seen in a multiparous woman. Other factors associated with malposition or malpresentation include uterine anomalies, fetal malformations, pelvic tumors, and the placenta obstructing the birth canal (Cherry and Merkatz 1991; Creasy and Resnik 1994; Cunningham et al. 1993).

Malpositions and malpresentations carry a high incidence of risk to both mother and fetus. Labor may culminate with obstruction, since the fetus may not be able to navigate the birth passage. Ultimately, an obstructed labor can result in a ruptured uterus. The intrapartal course also has increased risk for the fetus, since birth trauma is more likely in utero or at the time of birth.

OCCIPUT POSTERIOR

Description

The occiput posterior (OP) position occurs when the occiput of the fetal head and the posterior fontanelle are in the posterior portion of the maternal pelvis and the brow and bregma are in the anterior portion (see Figure 22–4). The posterior position can be right occiput posterior (ROP) or left occiput posterior (LOP). Posterior positions occur in about 15 to 30 percent of all labors and may be related to the shape of the pelvis or cephalopelvic disproportion (Oxorn and Foote 1986). It is difficult to be precise regarding the incidence, since many OP positions rotate anteriorly before anyone is aware that an OP position existed. The posterior position often results in increased back discomfort for the woman due to pressure of the bony portion of the fetal head against the sacrum of the maternal pelvis. This phenomenon is often called back labor. Labor may not progress well because of the inability of the fetus to flex the head, lack of descent, and the uneven pressure of the fetal head on the cervix. In about 70 percent of cases the fetus in a posterior position rotates during labor or during the expulsion efforts of second stage, to allow birth to occur in the anterior position (Biancuzzo 1993a).

Management

Diagnosis of OP position is made by abdominal and vaginal examination. Visual assessment of the woman's abdomen in a supine position should be made to identify any irregular contours that might indicate an OP position. When performing Leopold maneuvers, the examiner is unable to lo-

PROCEDURE 25–1

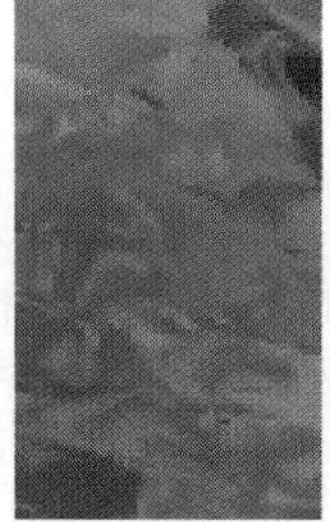

Maternal-Fetal Transport

▼ PURPOSE

A maternal-fetal transport to a tertiary care center is indicated when the condition of either the woman or the fetus warrants more intensive evaluation or intervention than can be provided where the woman is currently hospitalized. When the birth of a compromised neonate is possible, a maternal-fetal transport prevents the transport of a sick newborn soon after birth. Adequate communication and information are imperative for effective maternal-fetal transport.

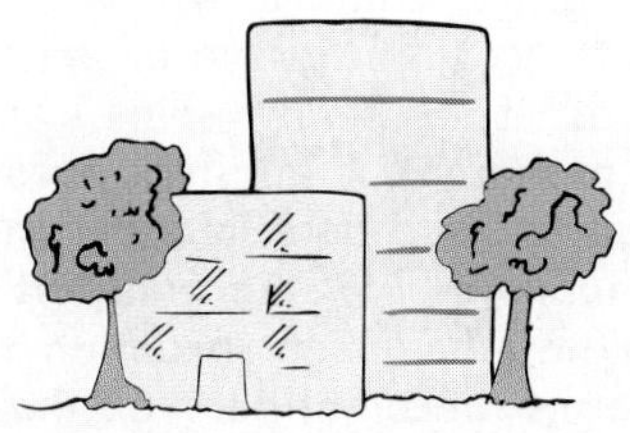

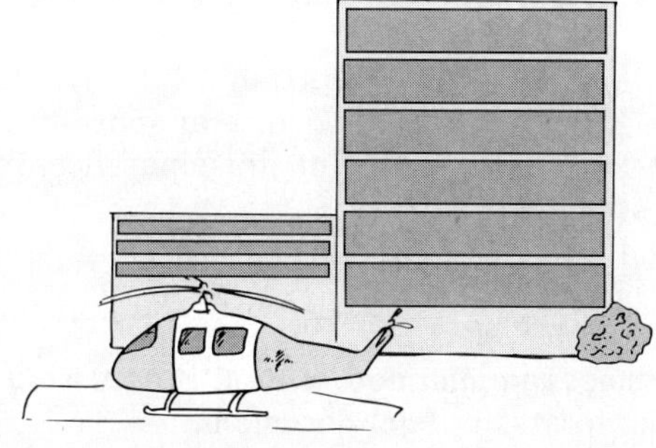

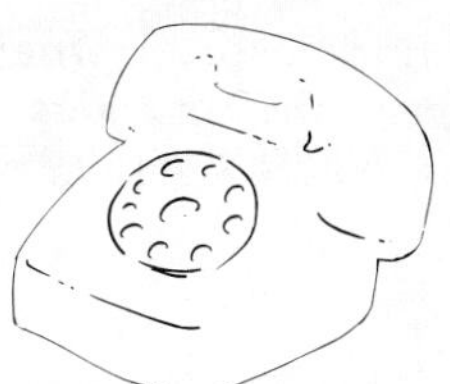

COMMUNICATION

- Provide family with anticipatory guidance
- Facilitate contact between referring physician and receiving physician
- Establish approximate times of transport arrival at referring hospital, departure, and arrival at receiving hospital
- Give up-to-date status report to transport team
- Call receiving hospital when transport team and patient are on their way

INFORMATION

- Photocopy and send client's *complete* chart
- Include sonograms, fetal monitor tracings, and radiographs
- Include signed and witnessed informed consent for transport

PROCEDURE 25–1 Continued

▼ EQUIPMENT

- Consent form
- copy of mother's chart
- transfer form

1 Assess the woman's condition to ensure that she is stable for transport. **Patients in stable condition before transport are less likely to require emergency intervention en route.**

2 Communicate with family and physicians. It is the responsibility of the referring physician to discuss with the receiving physician the status of the woman's condition and to ascertain whether room is available at the receiving hospital. Physicians should also discuss the risks and benefits of transport with the woman and her family. Witness informed consent. **Anticipatory guidance improves the efficiency of the transport and helps to lessen the family's fears and anxieties concerning maternal-fetal transport. Include the following information as you prepare the family for transport:**

- Mode of transportation
- Personnel involved in transport
- Basic discussion of anticipated care at tertiary care center
- Information on family visiting and necessary phone numbers

Witnessing informed consent is necessary because the form is a legal document.

3 Plan for the transport. Obtain estimated times for transport arrival at the referring hospital, departure, and arrival at the receiving hospital. Discuss equipment and personnel needed. Photocopy the woman's chart for the receiving hospital. Also send the consent for transport and other pertinent documents such as sonograms and fetal monitor tracings. **Planning needs ahead of time prevents delays during which the woman's condition could change. The receiving hospital needs all information regarding the patient's diagnosis, care and medications received, and current status. This helps ensure the development of an appropriate plan of care at the receiving hospital.**

4 When the transport team arrives, provide them with an up-to-date report on the woman's status, including maternal vital signs, fetal heart rate, uterine contraction status, medication schedule, and other information relevant to patient diagnosis. Assist in transfer to the stretcher. Document in the woman's chart that a verbal report was given, and record the time of arrival and departure of the team. Ensure that the woman's personal belongings accompany her on transport. **Up-to-date information on the status of the woman helps the transport team anticipate problems that might occur en route. These transfer forms become part of the permanent record.**

5 Call the receiving hospital when the transport team leaves. **This provides the receiving hospital with an estimated time of patient arrival.**

cate the fetal back, while the fetal small parts are easily palpated. Upon vaginal examination, the position of the fontanelles confirms the OP position. OP position and back labor are managed in several ways during the first stage of labor. Frequent maternal position changes should be used to stimulate the fetus to rotate (Biancuzzo 1991, 1993a, 1993b). These are discussed further in the nursing interventions section below. If the fetus does not rotate and remains in a persistent posterior position, labor progress may cease and require augmentation with oxytocin (Pitocin). The delivery of a fetus in a persistent posterior position may be more difficult and require manual rotation, the use of forceps, or cesarean delivery.

BROW PRESENTATION

Description

The presenting part in a brow presentation is the area between the orbital ridges and the bregma (Fig. 22–3). This occurs when the head is straight or extended and results in the largest diameter (the occipitomental) presenting. Brow presentations are rare and occur primarily after labor has begun (Oxorn and Foote 1986). Any factor that interferes with engagement and flexion can cause a brow presentation, especially congenital anomalies such as tumors of the fetal neck or a large number of coils of the umbilical cord around the neck. Brow presentations are also seen more frequently in the multipara owing to lax abdominal and pelvic musculature. If the brow presentation is persistent, labor may be prolonged and maternal or fetal trauma may result.

Management

Diagnosis of brow presentation is made by pelvic examination via palpation of the anterior fontanelle, frontal bones, supraorbital ridges, and

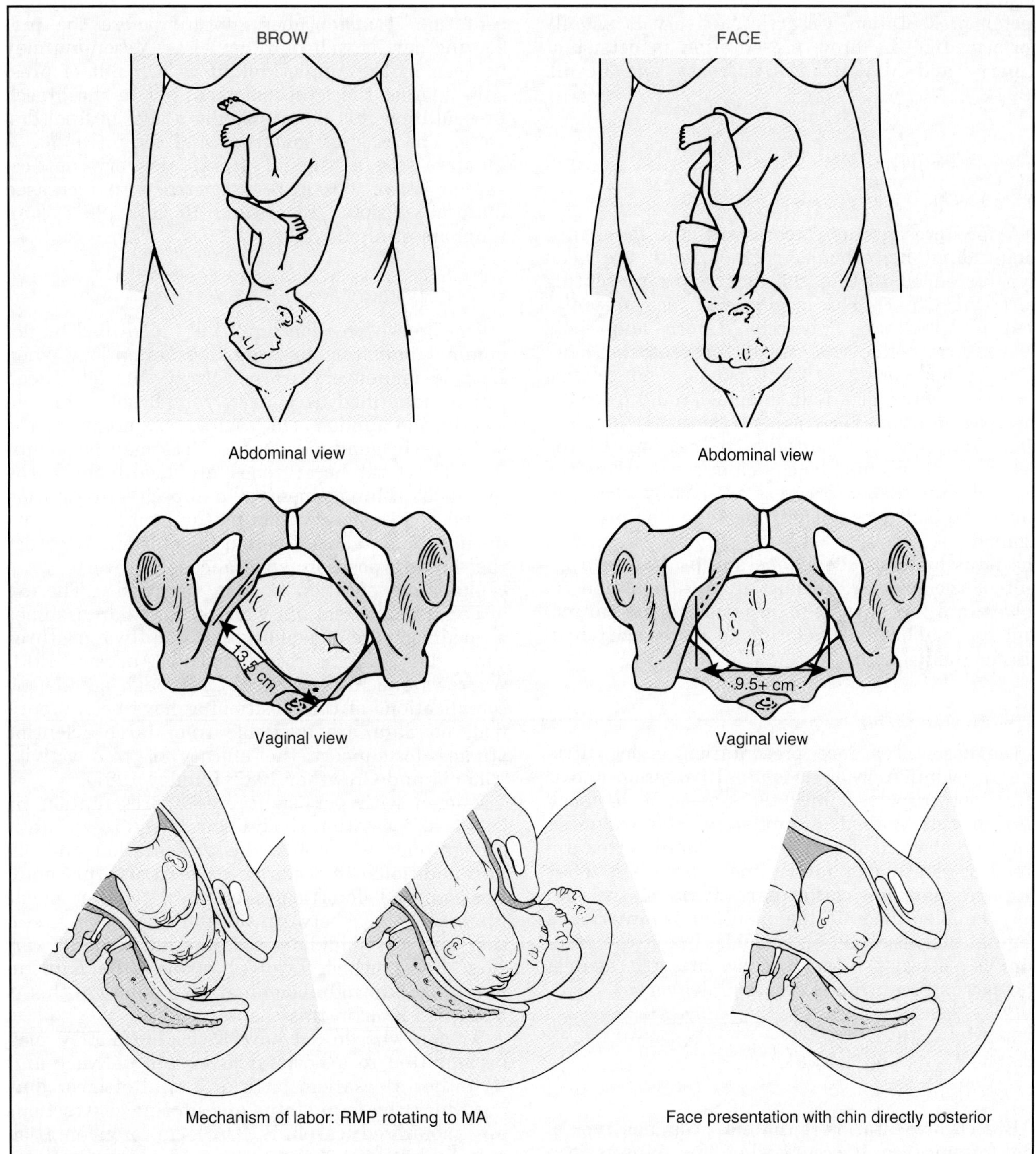

Figure 25-1

The presenting part in a brow presentation is the area between the orbital ridges and the bregma • In a face presentation, the presenting part is the face, often resulting in edema or trauma • During the mechanism of labor, if the right mentum posterior (RMP) rotates to mentum anterior (MA), the vaginal delivery will proceed • However, if the chin is directly posterior, a vaginal delivery cannot be accomplished unless the chin rotates anteriorly.

root of the nose. Diagnosis may be difficult in early labor because of an unengaged presenting part and in late labor because of molding and caput formation. Ultrasonography may be used to confirm the diagnosis. During labor, sufficient time should be allowed to determine whether the fetus' position will convert to a more favorable face or vertex presentation. Cesarean delivery is usually performed if the brow presentation is persistent (Cherry and Merkatz 1991; Creasy and Resnik 1994).

FACE PRESENTATION

Description

A face presentation occurs with the fetus in a longitudinal lie, cephalic position, with the head hyperextended so that the face is the presenting part (Fig. 25–1). The incidence of face presentation is less than 1 percent (Oxorn and Foote 1986). Any factor that might prevent the head from flexing, such as a small pelvis, a large fetus, a preterm fetus, or a fetal anomaly, could lead to a face presentation. Face presentations may be anterior, transverse, or posterior in relation to the pelvis, as determined by the chin (mentum) as the denominator. Labor progress is usually slow, because the face does not provide the same pressure against the cervix as does the occiput. The face of the fetus becomes edematous and bruised as a result of the pressure against it. Although this resolves in a few days, it is upsetting to the parents and has implications relating to increased bilirubin for the neonate.

Management

Diagnosis of a face presentation is by ultrasound examination or abdominal palpation and is often not suspected until the woman is in labor. During the vaginal examination, the examiner notes an absence of a round, even, hard vertex. Instead of identifiable suture lines, there is a softer and irregular presenting part. Parts of the face may be identified. If the mentum is anterior, a vaginal delivery may be possible, but if the mentum is posterior it can become arrested against the sacrum, requiring a cesarean delivery.

BREECH PRESENTATION

Description

Breech presentation is the most common type of malpresentation. It occurs when the fetus is in a longitudinal lie and is presenting with the bottom (breech) first. The four types of breech presentation are defined in Chapter 22 and illustrated in Figure 22–3. Breech presentations occur in 3 to 4 percent of all deliveries and are seen more commonly with preterm infants, multiple gestations, placenta previa, maternal or fetal anomalies, and hydramnios and oligohydramnios. Fetal descent may be prolonged with a breech presentation, because the presenting part does not dilate the cervix as well as the fetal head. There is an increased risk of a cord prolapse with a breech presentation if membranes rupture before the presenting part is well into the pelvis. Meconium may be seen in the amniotic fluid as a result of pressure against the fetal abdomen, but in the breech presentation this is not usually a sign of fetal distress. The risk of maternal and fetal trauma is greater with a vaginal breech delivery, but cesarean delivery is also associated with increased maternal risks (Creasy and Resnik 1994; Cunningham et al. 1993).

Management

The breech position is initially identified by abdominal palpation or vaginal examination. When Leopold maneuvers are performed, the fetal head can be identified as a hard, round, ballotable object in the fundus. On vaginal examination, the soft breech, genitalia, legs, or feet may be identified. The fetal heart tones are heard above the umbilicus. Management of a breech presentation includes close observation by the health care team during the antepartal period to determine whether the breech position spontaneously reverts to a cephalic presentation as term approaches. The use of prenatal exercises in which the woman assumes a modified Trendelenburg position two or three times daily can be recommended (Andrews 1981; Andrews and Andrews 1983). Although no adverse complications of this positioning have been identified, no data are available from large scientific studies to support the efficacy of this activity (Chenia and Crowther 1987; Lumley 1987).

Women with persistent breech presentation by 34 weeks' gestation should be referred to an ultrasonographer to confirm the presentation and obtain additional information on fetal size, placental location, and detection of malformations or pelvic tumors. Women between 36 and 42 weeks' gestation may be candidates for external cephalic version (ECV), which involves turning the fetus in utero via external abdominal manipulation; this is discussed later in this chapter.

Women who do not have a successful ECV may be admitted to a hospital labor and delivery unit for either a cesarean birth or a trial of labor during which the fetal status and uterine contractions are monitored carefully. Oxytocin augmentation may be initiated if there are no contraindications, although its use for a malpresentation is somewhat controversial. A vaginal delivery should not be considered unless the following criteria are met: (1) the pelvis is adequate; (2) the fetus is in a frank or complete breech presentation, with a

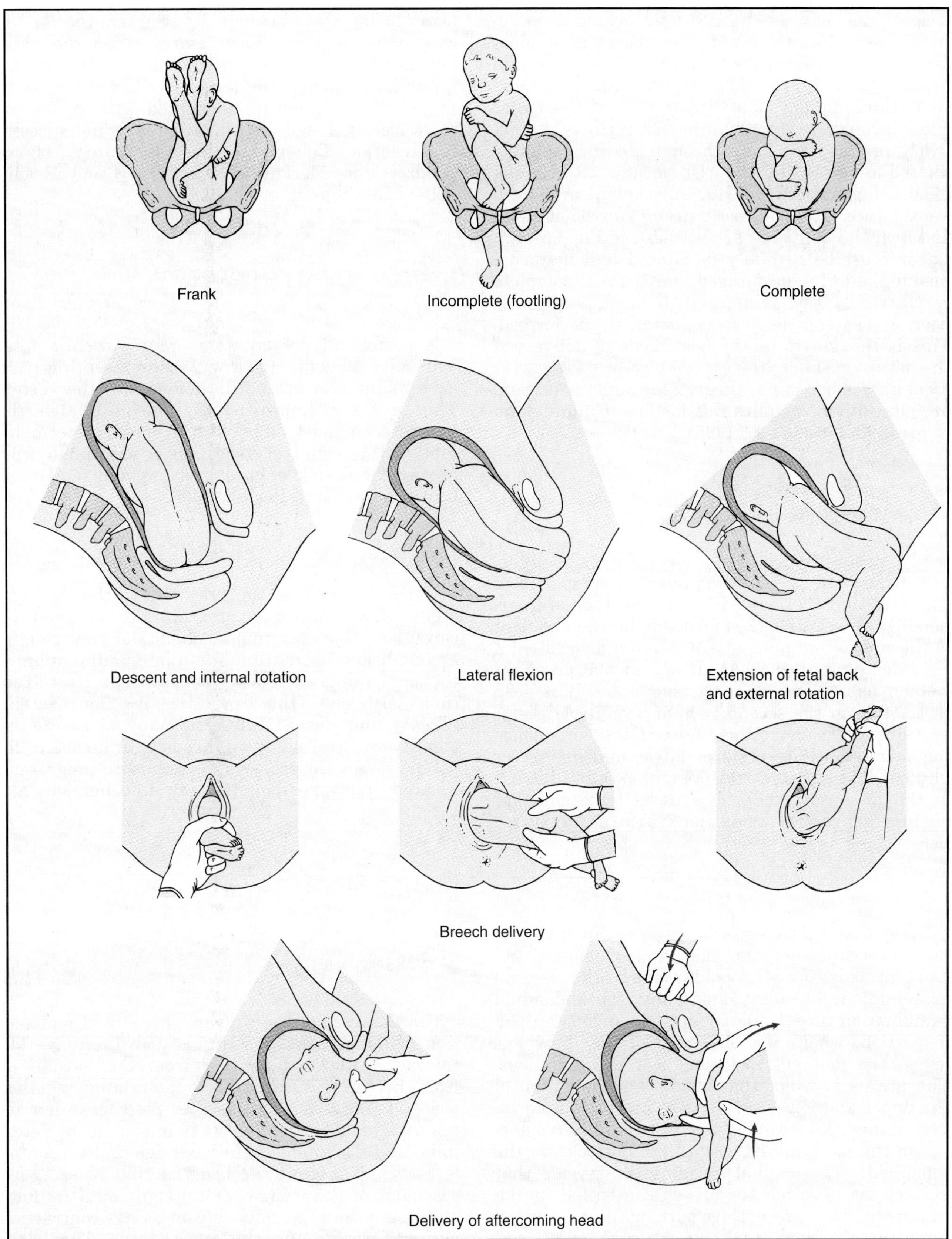

Figure 25–2
The mechanisms of labor in a breech presentation result in the aftercoming head delivering last.

weight less than 3500 g; (3) fetal gestation is between 36 and 42 weeks; (4) the woman is in spontaneous and progressive labor; and (5) skilled staff are available for the delivery and care of the infant (Cunningham et al. 1993). One of the major risks involved in a vaginal breech birth is the delivery of the fetal body through an incompletely dilated cervix, with the risk of the aftercoming head being trapped, causing subsequent prolonged anoxia (Fig. 25–2). Piper forceps can be used to assist in the delivery of the head (see Fig. 25–12). Labor must be carefully monitored and maternal pushing efforts encouraged only when complete cervical dilatation is assured. If labor progress is poor, a cesarean delivery is commonly performed. This is thought to be the best mode of delivery if the fetus is small (under 2000 g) or large (over 3800 g), if labor is not progressing well, or if there are any other complicating factors (Cunningham et al. 1993; Laros et al. 1995).

TRANSVERSE LIE

Description

A transverse lie occurs when the long axis of the fetus and the long axis of the mother are perpendicular (see Fig. 22–2). In this lie the shoulder is the presenting part, and it is often also called a shoulder presentation. About one in 500 pregnant women has a fetus in a transverse lie. It is seen most often in the second twin of a multiple gestation or with a macrosomic fetus. Other predisposing factors include preterm labor, multiparity, or any condition that would prevent normal descent of the fetus into the pelvis. It is impossible for vaginal delivery to take place with a transverse lie.

Management

Diagnosis of transverse lie is determined by visual observation of the maternal abdomen, abdominal palpation (Leopold maneuvers), vaginal examination, and ultrasonography. The abdominal examination reveals an asymmetric abdomen upon inspection, where the long axis of the fetus lies across the mother's abdomen near the umbilicus. The uterus is wider than usual, and palpation of the upper and lower poles of the uterus fails to reveal either the head or the breech. The head is felt in the maternal flank with the buttocks on the other side. The vaginal examination reveals that neither the head nor the breech can be felt by the examiner. The presenting part is high, and in some cases a shoulder, hand, rib cage, or back is felt. Ultrasonography will confirm the diagnosis of transverse lie. It can also detect certain abnormalities of the fetus that may be the associated etiologic factor. Management of the transverse lie should begin before labor starts, when the problem is diagnosed. External version (external manipulation, moving the fetus from a transverse to a cephalic lie) may be attempted with gestations of 35 weeks or more. If the attempt is not successful, cesarean delivery is the only route of choice (Cherry and Merkatz 1991; Creasy and Resnik 1994; Cunningham et al. 1993).

COMPOUND PRESENTATION

Description

A compound presentation occurs when a fetal extremity presents along with the presenting part, such as an arm presenting along with the vertex. This occurs in approximately one in 1000 births and is seen most often with a small preterm infant. A compound presentation is associated with an increased risk of cord prolapse and fetal mortality (Creasy and Resnik 1994).

Management

Early diagnosis is the first step in the management of a compound presentation, followed by careful fetal monitoring. Vaginal delivery can be accomplished with stimulation or manipulation of the presenting extremity to encourage its retraction, although this practice is controversial (Creasy and Resnik 1994). In many cases the extremity will retract spontaneously. In a case of fetal distress, cord prolapse, or failure to progress, a cesarean delivery should be initiated immediately.

Nursing Process

▼ Assessment

Nursing care of the woman with a fetal malposition or malpresentation begins with the nurse obtaining a thorough history from the woman or from her prenatal record to determine whether there are any risk factors that predispose her fetus to a malpresentation. It is important to determine and document gestational age and estimated fetal weight to aid in decision making. Nursing assessment of the woman's vital signs and the fetal status is also important as well as her contraction pattern, if any, and the labor status. The latter can be obtained by either assisting at or performing a vaginal examination. Nursing assessment is ongoing during labor and delivery.

▼ Diagnosis

The nursing diagnoses formulated from the assessment data should be made in collaboration with the physicians and nurse practitioners making the medical diagnoses related to the malpresentation or malposition. Examples of these diagnoses are as follows:

- Risk of injury to the fetus related to birth trauma caused by malpresentation
- Altered tissue perfusion: cardiopulmonary, related to cord compression or prolapse
- Pain related to malpresentation of the fetus
- Anxiety/fear related to uncertainty of the method of delivery and status of self and fetus

▼ Planning

The planned goals for the woman with a malpresentation/malposition during labor might include the following:

- The fetus will be delivered safely
- The woman will verbally describe decreased pain and demonstrate increased comfort as evidenced by a relaxed body and facial expression
- The woman will verbally state less anxiety and fear about the plans for delivery of her infant

▼ Intervention

As with any laboring woman, the nurse initially attempts to determine the fetal position by performing Leopold maneuvers. These findings are communicated to the birth attendant in a collaborative manner so that a plan of management can be made, including the woman as a member of the health care team. The next likely intervention is to prepare the woman for an ultrasound examination to confirm presentation and position. Vaginal examinations may be performed by the nurse or the birth attendant. These are done during labor at judicious times to keep abreast of the woman's labor progress and any changes with regard to position or lie. During this time the nurse continues to assess both maternal and fetal well-being and uterine contractions. Maternal vital signs are taken and recorded appropriately. Electronic fetal monitoring is begun and observed and recorded by the nurse (Oxorn and Foote 1986).

Measures for relief of discomfort may be needed. Distraction, breathing techniques, guided imagery, and position changes are often effective for combatting discomfort. For example, if the fetus is in an OP position and the woman is experiencing back labor, any position that keeps the woman off her back and thus decreases the pressure of the fetal head against the sacrum should be tried (Biancuzzo 1991, 1993a). Examples of effective positions are standing and leaning forward over the bed, sitting and leaning forward against a pillow, lateral side-lying, knee-chest, and hands and knees (see Fig. 22–11). Squatting or flexing the hip and knee joints can bring relief also. The pelvic rock exercise (see Chapter 19) can be used in any of these positions, and decreases discomfort as well as stimulating rotation of the fetus. The application of heat or cold against the sacral area often relieves discomfort. A hot-water bottle or warm washcloths can be alternated with the use of ice. Firm counterpressure to decrease pain in the sacral region can be applied by the nurse or the woman's partner during contractions, and massage can be used between contractions. Counterpressure can be applied against the area when the woman is on her back by placing firm objects such as tennis balls or a rolling pin between the bed and the sacral area.

Intradermal injections of sterile water are an intervention for back pain in labor that have been discussed recently in the literature. These injections consist of four 0.1-mL intradermal injections with a 25-gauge needle. Two injections are placed over the posterosuperior iliac spines and two are placed 2 to 3 cm below and 1 to 2 cm medial to the first points. Sterile water is injected in these areas to form small blebs in the skin. The injections may cause intense stinging for up to 30 seconds, but this discomfort is followed by immediate relief of back pain that lasts for 60 to 90 minutes. The injections can be repeated as often as needed and carry only minimal risks of needle puncture of the skin. Pain relief is thought to result from a rapid increase in endorphin production (Reynolds 1994; Ader et al. 1990; Trolle et al. 1991).

The woman and her family should be continually kept aware of what is happening, and attempts should be made by the nurse to allay their anxiety. Preparations may need to be made for a possible external version or cesarean birth. The nurse is responsible for making certain that the appropriate blood studies are available and that personnel are prepared for the potential surgery.

▼ Evaluation

Evaluation of the plan of care should be based on the success of the stated goals. Evaluation should be continuous so that as assessment data change, diagnoses change, or goals are altered, interventions can also be changed to meet the woman's needs. For example, if attempts to change the fetal position from posterior to anterior by turning the woman from one side to the other have not been successful, more aggressive or more frequent position changes might be tried.

Placental Abnormalities

The two most common placental abnormalities at the onset of labor are placenta previa and abruptio placentae (placental abruption) (Cherry and Merkatz 1991; Creasy and Resnik 1994; Cunningham et al. 1993). Because the placenta is a highly vascular organ, any alteration in its placement or attachment can cause serious hemorrhage with resultant maternal and fetal risks. Bleeding from a placenta previa may occur at any time during pregnancy or labor, whereas an abruption is frequently followed by spontaneous onset of labor.

PLACENTA PREVIA

Description

Placenta previa is an abnormal condition in which the placenta implants early in pregnancy in the lower uterine segment and then covers the os of the cervix either totally (complete placenta previa) or partially (partial placenta previa) as it develops (Fig. 25–3). Marginal placenta previa occurs when the edge of the placenta borders the cervical os, and a low-lying placenta is one in which the placental edge approaches but does not encroach upon the cervical os. Usually a low-lying placenta does not engender the same risks during labor. The classification of placenta previa may change as cervical dilatation begins. For example, what was classified as marginal previa before cervical changes may become partial previa after dilatation has occurred (Pozaic 1991).

The cause of placenta previa is unknown. It occurs in approximately one of every 250 births, although low placental implantations are more frequent in early pregnancy and resolve by the time of delivery (Creasy and Resnik 1994). Several theories are proposed as to the cause. One is that because of previous reproductive tract surgery, the myometrium is scarred and ultimately causes the placenta to implant abnormally. Another theory is that delayed development and implantation of the fertilized ovum causes the abnormal placental implantation. Risk factors for developing placenta previa include increased placental size, a previous uterine scar, multiparity, multiple gestation, advanced maternal age, other previous reproductive tract surgery, and smoking. Once a woman has had a placenta previa, she is more likely to have another one (Creasy and Resnik 1994).

The key symptom that can alert the professional to suspect placenta previa is painless vaginal bleeding in the second or third trimester of pregnancy. The bleeding is usually bright red and the amount varies with the proportion of the degree of separation. Bleeding occurs as the lower segment of the uterus begins to pull upward with cervical effacement and dilatation in late pregnancy, causing the placental villi to tear away from the uterine wall. The bleeding may be scant at first and then become more profuse as more and more of the placenta separates. There is no way that the bleeding from the placenta can be arrested, other than by delivery of the fetus and complete removal of the placenta. The woman is at risk for severe hemorrhage, embolism, or endometritis. The fetus is at risk for prematurity, asphyxia, or hemorrhage.

Management

Clinical diagnosis of placenta previa is reached through an ultrasound examination in which the placenta is localized in relationship to the cervix (Creasy and Resnik 1994; Cunningham et al. 1993). Abdominal examination reveals a soft uterus with the presenting part ballotable above the symphysis pubis. Manual pelvic examinations are contraindicated when major vaginal bleeding is apparent in the third trimester, until a diagnosis is made and total placenta previa is ruled out. This is a general precaution, since digital examination can lead to fatal maternal and fetal exsanguination if total placenta previa is present (Cunningham et al. 1993; Mandeville and Troiano 1992). The placenta may be visualized by means of examination with a sterile speculum. This should be done only with a "double set-up," performed in the birth setting with the personnel and equipment available should a sudden hemorrhage require an immediate vaginal or cesarean delivery.

After the diagnosis of placenta previa is established by ultrasonography, the gestational age is calculated: management depends on the gestation of the pregnancy. If the gestational age is early, an attempt is made to prolong the pregnancy with the intention of optimizing the neonatal outcome. The woman is usually hospitalized to try and avoid preterm labor or hemorrhage, and her mobility is restricted, usually to bed rest at first. Activity may be gradually increased as the pregnancy progresses to term. The hemoglobin and hematocrit values are monitored, and blood replacement or iron therapy is instituted if anemia is present. The pulmonary maturity of the fetus is monitored at appropriate intervals.

Unless an emergency situation arises, delivery is planned for some point after the fetus has reached 36 weeks' gestation and lung maturity is assured. A vaginal delivery would be considered only if the placenta previa were very marginal, the fetal head had descended low enough to act as

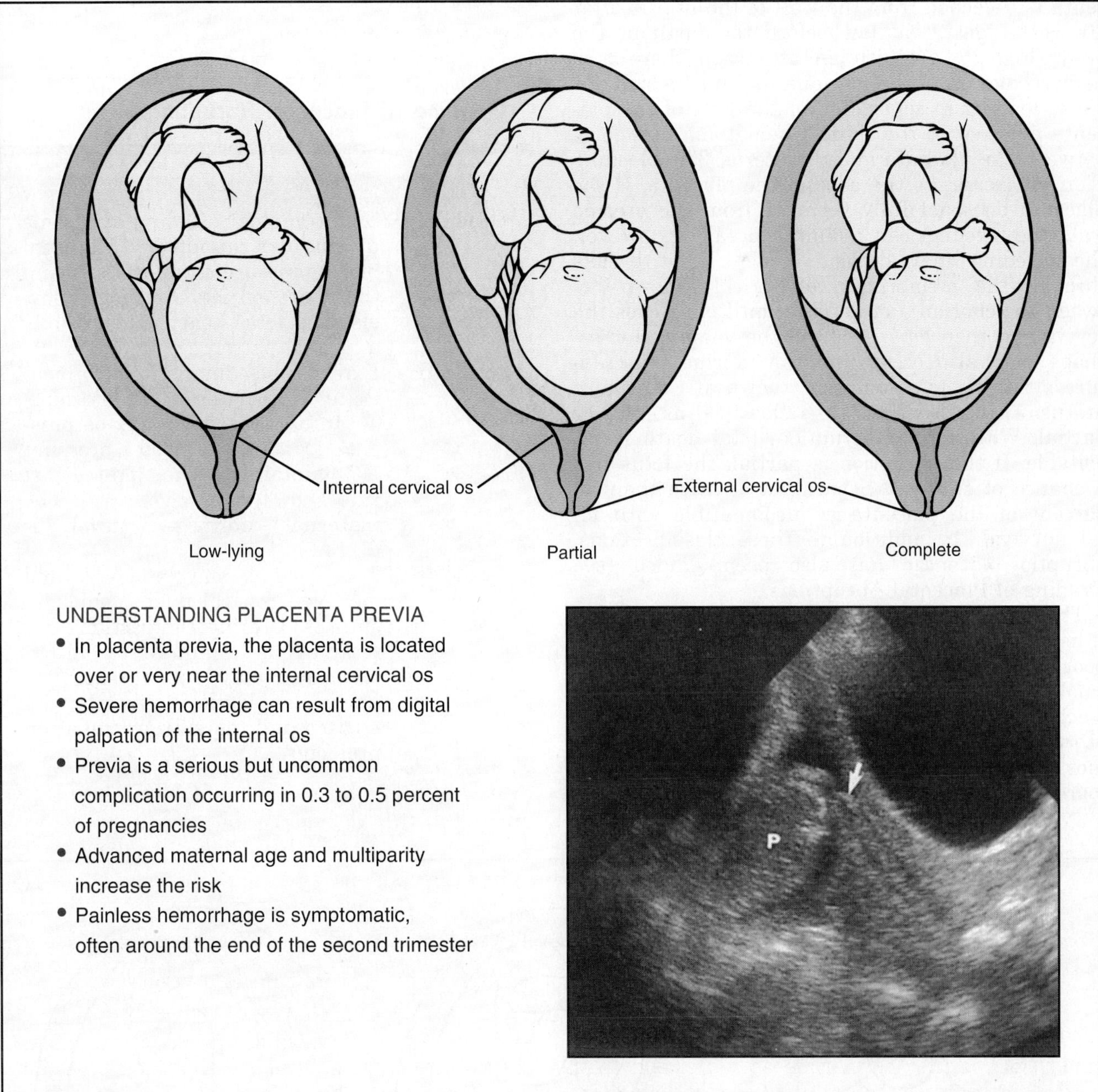

Figure 25–3

Placenta previa can partially or totally cover the cervix, presenting in front of the fetus, or be low-lying in the uterus. The sonogram shows a marginal placenta previa, where the end of the posterior placenta (P) is adjacent to the internal cervical os (*arrow*). Sonogram from Callen, P. W. (1994). *Ultrasonography in obstetrics and gynecology* (3rd ed.) (p. 448). Philadelphia: W. B. Saunders.

a tamponade placing pressure against the placenta, active labor had begun, and no other complications were evident. Vaginal delivery would also be considered if the fetus were dead or had major malformations. In most situations, however, surgical intervention is the delivery method of choice. Close monitoring after the delivery should continue, for the woman has an increased risk for postpartal hemorrhage. This is because the lower uterine segment where the placenta was attached does not have the number of interlacing muscle fibers found in the upper portion of the uterus, and thus is not as efficient in contracting to control bleeding in the early postpartum period (Creasy and Resnik 1994).

ABRUPTIO PLACENTAE

Description

Abruptio placentae is defined as premature separation of a normally implanted placenta. The placenta is detached from the wall of the uterus after 20 weeks' gestation but before the birth of the baby (Fig. 25–4). With an abruption there is a hemorrhage into the decidua basalis, which divides, leading to separation of the part of the placenta adjacent to the split. A hematoma may form between the placenta and the uterus. The bleeding then progresses to the edge of the placenta. If the placenta does not fully separate from the uterine wall, the bleeding can remain concealed. However, the bleeding may become evident if it breaks through the membranes and trickles down between the chorion and decidua until it reaches the cervix and then emerges from the vagina. Hemorrhage may also occur into the uterine musculature, resulting in a condition known as Couvelaire uterus. Abruptio placentae is classified as total or partial. With a total abruption, fetal death is inevitable. If the abruption is partial, the fetus has a chance of survival. Separation of more than 50 percent of the placenta is incompatible with fetal survival. In addition to these classifications, abruptio placentae has also been graded (see Grading of Placental Abruptions).

The cause of abruptio placentae is unknown. It is associated with conditions characterized by poor uteroplacental circulation (e.g., hypertension, smoking, alcohol abuse, cocaine abuse), physical or mechanical factors (e.g., overdistention of the uterus with multiple gestation or polyhydramnios), a short umbilical cord, physical trauma, and increased maternal age and parity. Abruptio pla-

Grading of Placental Abruptions

Grade I: Slight vaginal bleeding and some uterine irritability. Maternal blood pressure is unaffected and there are normal fibrinogen levels. The fetal heart rate exhibits a normal pattern.

Grade II: External bleeding is mild to moderate. The uterus is irritable. Tetanic contractions may be present. Maternal blood pressure is maintained. The fetal heart rate shows signs of distress. The maternal fibrinogen level is decreased.

Grade III: The bleeding may be severe and may be concealed in some instances. Uterine contractions are tetanic and painful. Maternal hypotension may be present. The fibrinogen level is greatly decreased and there are coagulation problems.

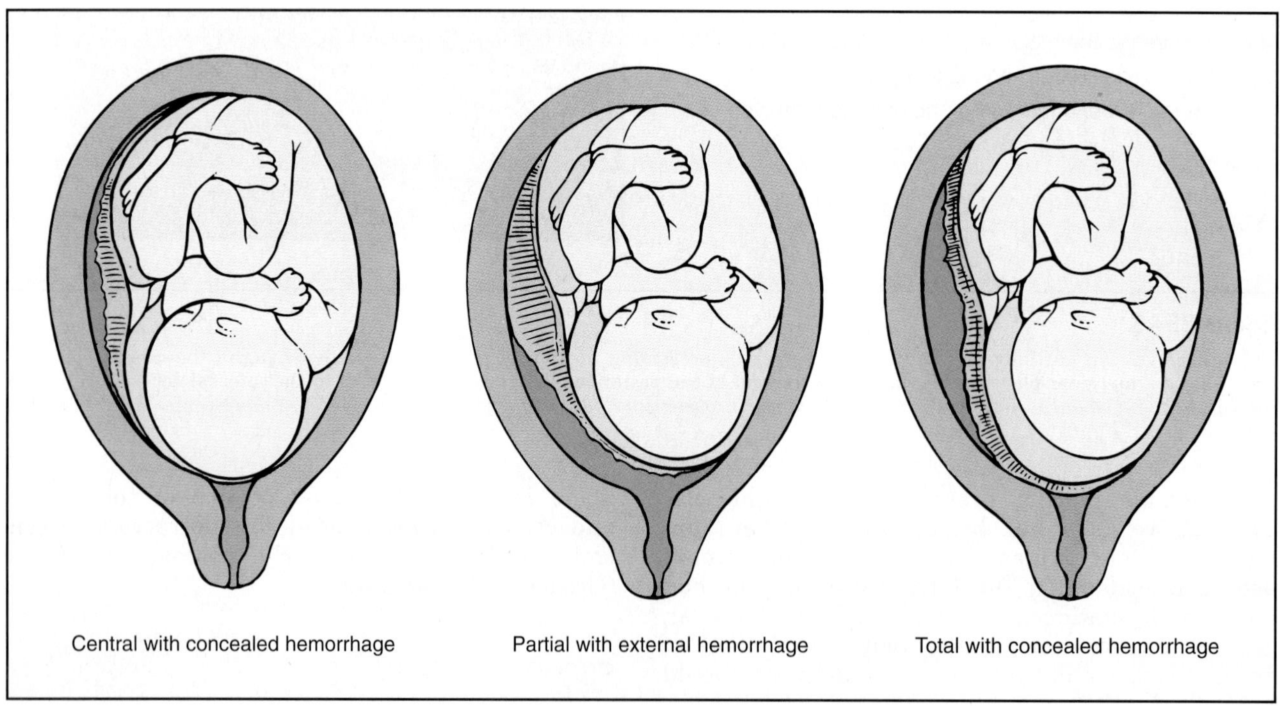

Figure 25–4

The placenta detaches from the wall of the uterus during placental abruption • This usually occurs after 20 weeks of gestation but before term • The resultant hemorrhage may remain concealed, causing great risk to both the fetus and the woman.

centae occurs in one in 75 to 90 births (Cherry and Merkatz 1991; Cunningham et al. 1993; Danforth 1990). It poses serious risks to the woman and fetus. The woman is at risk for the development of shock, cardiac or renal failure, disseminated intravascular coagulation (DIC), and postpartal hemorrhage. The fetal risks relate to preterm birth or intrauterine asphyxia, and perinatal mortality is high because of the sudden onset of a placental abruption.

Unlike placenta previa, the signs and symptoms of abruptio placentae include a small to moderate amount of bright or dark red vaginal bleeding, which is usually associated with acute abdominal pain, uterine tenderness, and high uterine tonicity (often described as a "boardlike" abdomen). Observation of the fetal monitor often reveals increased uterine resting tone, caused by failure of the uterus to relax in an attempt to constrict blood vessels and control bleeding. The uterus may also show a rapid increase in size, particularly if the hemorrhage is concealed.

Management

The diagnosis of abruption may be made by ultrasonography. The location of the placenta is identified and a clot or hematoma may be visualized. Frequently the diagnosis is made clinically and confirmed at delivery with inspection of the placenta. If an abruption is present, there is usually an adherent retroplacental clot with disruption of underlying tissue. The goal of management is to control hemorrhage and deliver the fetus as soon as possible. Coagulation tests are performed to rule out DIC. Fluid and blood replacement are initiated. A vaginal delivery is preferred if the bleeding is minimal, the mother is in stable condition, the labor is progressing, and the presenting part is in the pelvis. Labor may have to be induced if it is not progressing well on its own. A cesarean delivery is performed if hemorrhage is severe, fetal heart tones are present, the presenting part is not in the pelvis, or the cervix is closed or if it is anticipated that birth is not imminent. If the fetus is dead, a cesarean section is performed only if the bleeding is life threatening. A cesarean hysterectomy may be necessary if the bleeding cannot be controlled (Clark et al. 1991).

Nursing Process

▼ Assessment

Nurses' role in the assessment of a placental abnormality is critical, for the data they collect are often used as a basis of medical management or intervention. Data to be collected for the identification of a placental complication include gestational age; history of bleeding; amount and nature of bleeding; pain associated with the bleeding; maternal and fetal vital signs; quality, duration, and frequency of contractions; uterine tone; and pertinent laboratory values, especially hemoglobin, hematocrit, and platelets. Abdominal girth may be measured to assess any increase in uterine size that can occur with concealed hemorrhage.

▼ Diagnosis

The nursing diagnoses formulated from the assessment data should be made in collaboration with the physicians and nurse practitioners making the medical diagnoses related to placental abnormalities. Examples are as follows:

- Altered tissue perfusion: peripheral, related to hemorrhage
- Risk for fetal injury related to decreased placental perfusion
- Fear related to placenta previa/abruptio placentae
- Pain related to abruption

▼ Planning

On the basis of the identified nursing diagnoses, the goals and outcomes that will guide the plan of care should be identified:

- The woman will maintain adequate tissue perfusion as evidenced by stable vital signs and urinary output
- The fetus will maintain a stable heart rate and be delivered safely
- The woman and her family will verbalize their fears and express their emotions related to the bleeding disorder
- The woman will verbally state a decrease in pain and exhibit an increase in comfort as evidenced by body posture and facial expression

▼ Intervention

Nursing interventions for a hemorrhagic complication center on continuous assessment. All maternal and fetal vital signs should be monitored frequently and recorded carefully. The amount and nature of bleeding should be recorded as well as the contraction pattern and cervical status if the woman is in active labor. Urinary output and skin color should be observed. Laboratory values should be monitored closely. The woman should be typed and crossmatched for packed red blood cells. An important component of the nurse's role is to provide the physical comfort, emotional support, and education that are essential for a woman who is hemorrhaging. In addition, nurses should be familiar with potential complications associated with the development of placenta previa or abruptio placentae and be prepared to be involved in the management of these complications. These include hemorrhage, hypotension, hypovolemia, shock, and DIC (Gilbert and Harmon 1993).

▼ Evaluation

The evaluation of the plan is based on the outcome of the identified goals in relation to the nursing interventions that have been implemented. For example, if the vital signs of the woman or her fetus are indicating a change in status, or if the amount of bleeding is increasing, the nurse should immediately revise the plan, notify the physician, and be prepared to initiate further intervention.

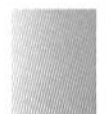

Preterm Labor and Birth

Description

The description, incidence, etiology, risk factors, and signs and symptoms associated with preterm labor are discussed in Chapter 21. Preterm labor that continues to delivery requires additional attention and management and is discussed in this section. A number of factors, such as uterine activity, cervical changes, and patient compliance, determine whether preterm labor can be arrested or whether the woman will progress and deliver prematurely.

Management

The outpatient management of preterm labor during pregnancy is discussed in Chapter 21. If attempts to suppress preterm labor by means of bed rest, hydration, and monitoring of uterine contractions at home are not successful, the woman is then admitted to the hospital for additional monitoring, and tocolytic drug therapy is usually initiated to suppress uterine activity. At this time, hydration is accomplished with intravenous fluids. Continuous electronic fetal monitoring is used to assess fetal status and obtain an accurate assessment of uterine activity. Before tocolytic therapy is begun, the diagnosis of preterm labor should be confirmed, treatable conditions that might be triggering preterm labor should be identified, and maternal or fetal contraindications to labor inhibition should be considered. Regular cervical examinations should be conducted to monitor progressive cervical changes. Urine cultures should be taken to rule out a urinary tract infection, and antibiotic treatment instituted if appropriate (Arias 1993; Creasy and Resnik 1994; Main and Main 1992).

A myriad of pharmaceuticals are used to attain tocolysis. Those most commonly employed today are listed in Table 25–1 (McCombs 1995). Labor-inhibiting drugs currently employed to arrest preterm labor are beta-adrenergic receptor agents, magnesium sulfate, prostaglandin inhibitors, and calcium channel blockers.

▼ **Beta-Adrenergic Agonist.** Beta-adrenergic drugs exert their effect on the myometrial cell through a membrane-mediated mechanism. The interaction of agonist drug and nerve receptor leads to an activation of cyclic AMP–dependent protein kinase, which reduces myometrial contractility by decreasing the effect of calcium on muscle activation. Examples of beta-adrenergic drugs are terbutaline (Brethine) and ritodrine (Yutopar) (McCombs 1995; Rayburn and Zuspan 1992). These drugs are administered intravenously until preterm labor is arrested and are then followed by oral medication if long-term maintenance is possible. A subcutaneous pump may also be used for long-term tocolysis. The pump allows for the administration of continuous low-dose infusions, with intermittent high-dose boluses at times when peak uterine activity occurs (Sala and Moise 1990). Although beta-adrenergic tocolytics are the most commonly used drugs for the management of preterm labor, a major study in Canada suggested that their general use may need to be reevaluated. Findings showed that the average pregnancy treated with such agents was prolonged by less than 48 hours when compared with pregnancies treated with placebos. Thus, the usefulness of the drugs was questioned (Canadian Preterm Labor Investigators Group 1992; Leveno and Cunningham 1992). Maternal side effects of beta-adrenergic drugs can include feelings of anxiety or nervousness, headache, dizziness, tremors, palpitations, tachycardia, hypertension, nausea and vomiting, muscle cramps, and diaphoresis. Beta-adrenergics may also cause maternal pulmonary edema. Fetal tachycardia may be observed. If side effects occur, the dosage of the drug may be decreased in an attempt to prolong therapy.

▼ **Magnesium Sulfate.** In some areas of the United States, magnesium sulfate is used as a tocolytic and is beneficial in that it stops uterine contractions and has fewer side effects than the beta-adrenergic drugs. The action of magnesium sulfate in arresting uterine activity is poorly understood. It is thought that an excess of magne-

Table 25–1

PHARMACOLOGIC AGENTS USED TO TREAT PRETERM LABOR

DRUG	DOSAGE	MATERNAL SIDE EFFECTS	FETAL SIDE EFFECTS
Drugs Inhibiting Uterine Response to Stimulation			
Ritodrine (Yutopar)	150 mg/500 mL IV fluid until response (0.3 mg/mL); dosage 0.05–0.1 mg/min increased to 0.35 mg/min until contractions stop	Cardiac effects: tachycardia, decreased blood pressure, arrhythmia, PVCs, flushing, sweating, increased stroke volume, erythema, palpitations	Increased FHR, cardiac arrhythmia, hypoxia, acidosis, increased serum glucose
	10–20 mg q 2h for 24 hr	Pulmonary effects: shortness of breath, pulmonary edema	Neonatal hypoglycemia, paralytic ileus, tremors, irritability, hypotension
		Nervous system: tremors, headache, nervousness	
		Endocrine effects: hyperglycemia, increased serum insulin and free fatty acids	
Terbutaline (Brethine)	5 mg/500 mL IV fluid for 8–12 hr (0.01 mg/mL); dosage 1–8 mg/min	Same as for ritodrine	Same as for ritodrine
	0.25 mg q 4h SQ for 24 hr		
	2.5 mg q 4–6 hr PO or 5.0 mg q 6–8 hr PO		
Magnesium sulfate	4 g loading dose in 100–250 mL 5% D/W IV at 3–10 mL/min	CNS depression–respiratory depression, paralysis, loss of DTRs, drowsiness, lethargy, blurred vision, slurred speech, confusion	Decrease in FHR variability
	1–4 g maintenance dose IV (2 g/hr) based on serum Mg levels and DTRs	Skeletal and smooth muscle relaxation, generalized hypotonia, and muscle weakness	
		Vasodilatation-flushing, warmth, hypotension, cardiovascular collapse, pulmonary edema, oliguria, thirst, nausea	
Calcium channel blockers (nifedipine)	10–30 mg loading dose, oral or sublingual; 2nd dose may be given in 30 min if contractions persist; 10–20 mg orally q 4–6 hr for maintenance	Facial flushing, mild hypotension, reflex tachycardia, headache, nausea	None reported in clinical studies as yet
Drugs Blocking Release of Production of Uterine Stimulant			
Prostaglandin synthetase inhibitors (indomethacin)	50–100 mg loading dose PO or rectally; 25 mg q 4–6 hr for 24–48 hr maintenance	Nausea, vomiting, dyspepsia	Constriction of ductus arteriosus Decreased GFR and urine output, oligohydramnios

IV, intravenously; SQ, subcutaneously; PO, orally; D/W, dextrose in water; Mg, magnesium; DTRs, deep tendon reflexes; CNS, central nervous system; FHR, fetal heart rate; GFR, glomerular filtration rate.

sium leads to a decrease in the net calcium available for the light-chain phosphorylation of myosin and therefore interferes with muscle contractility. Magnesium sulfate is initially administered intravenously for 12 to 24 hours. The maternal serum level for adequate initial tocolysis is 5 to 8 mg/dL. Long-term therapy can be established with oral magnesium oxide, magnesium gluconate, or magnesium chloride. The desired maternal serum level for maintenance is 2 to 2.5 mg/dL. Magnesium sulfate has less effect on blood pressure and maternal heart rate than beta-adrenergic drugs. Common maternal side effects of magnesium sulfate may include flushing and a feeling of warmth, headache, nausea, diarrhea, dizziness, nystagmus, and lethargy. The most common fetal side effect is hypotonia, lasting for a day or two after birth. The alterations in blood pressure, maternal heart rate, cardiac output and placental blood flow that may be seen with intravenous ritodrine are not seen with magnesium sulfate (Creasy and Resnik 1994; Scheerer and Katz 1990).

▼ **Prostaglandin Synthesis Inhibitors.** Prostaglandin inhibitors or nonsteroidal antiprostaglandins (nonsteroidal anti-inflammatory drugs [NSAIDs]) such as indomethacin (Indocin) have anti-inflammatory, antipyretic, and analgesic actions. These substances inactivate the enzyme cyclooxygenase, which is required to produce the first prostaglandin intermediate PGG_2 from arachidonic acid. All subsequent prostaglandins are derived from this initial step. Therefore, indomethacin is a global inhibitor of prostaglandin synthesis, a substance required for uterine contractility. At the cellular level, indomethacin decreases the gap junction formation and decreases the concentration of intracellular calcium. The calcium decrease leads to an inhibition of myometrial contractility. Therefore, some institutions use NSAIDs as tocolytic agents. Maternal side effects include gastrointestinal symptoms and postpartum hemorrhage. One of the fetal risks of nonsteroidal antiprostaglandins is that of oligohydramnios, secondary to a decrease in fetal urine excretion; there is also a theoretical risk of premature closure of the ductus arteriosus in utero (Creasy and Resnik 1994).

▼ **Calcium Channel Blockers.** Calcium channel blockers are a group of organic compounds that inhibit the influx of extracellular calcium across the cell membrane during the slow, inward current of the action potential. The decreased availability of calcium leads to a decrease of myometrial contractions. These drugs are under study as tocolytic agents but are not in common usage. Other agents under study include a potential pharmaceutical to block the receptor action of oxytocin (Cunningham et al. 1993). It can be anticipated that the investigation and introduction of new tocolytic drugs will be ongoing in the future.

Absolute contraindications to tocolytic treatment for preterm labor include severe preeclampsia, severe abruptio placentae or bleeding from any cause, chorioamnionitis, fetal death, a fetal anomaly incompatible with life, or severe fetal growth retardation. Other contraindications include mild chronic hypertension, mild abruptio placentae, stable placenta previa, cardiac disease, uncontrolled diabetes mellitus, fetal distress, and a cervix dilated more than 5 cm (Creasy and Resnik 1994).

Nursing Process

▼ Assessment

Nursing assessment of the woman with preterm labor begins with the initial collection of data about her pregnancy and history of preterm labor (see Guide to Data Collection: Preterm Labor).

Guide to Data Collection: Preterm Labor

- All criteria pertinent to dating the pregnancy, including last menstrual period and its normalcy; quickening; results of ultrasound testing if available; fundal heights; date the first FHTs were heard
- Subjective data, including the woman's perception of her contractions: degree, location, and quality of pain; when the contractions began, frequency, and intensity; whether the woman has failed to feel contractions
- Objective data, such as an EFM strip and an FHR recording
- Information about the status of the membranes; degree of effacement and dilatation of the cervix; vaginal discharge; sterile vaginal examination
- Urinary status; symptoms of UTI (frequency, urgency, pain); clean-catch urine specimen
- Emotional state and cognitive understanding of the woman and her family

FHT, fetal heart tone; EFM, electronic fetal monitoring; FHR, fetal heart rate; UTI, urinary tract infection.

While the woman is receiving tocolytic therapy the nurse must monitor the uterine contractions, maternal vital signs, and fetal heart rate at frequent intervals (Eganhouse and Burnside 1992; Lynam and Miller 1992). When intravenous tocolytic therapy is being administered, blood pressure, pulse, and respirations should be assessed before each dose increase. Once oral therapy is started, maternal vital signs can be taken before each oral dose. An external electronic fetal monitor may be used to assess uterine activity and fetal status. The woman's cervix is assessed at intervals to detect any changes in effacement or dilatation.

While the woman is on tocolytic therapy, the nurse should auscultate her breath sounds and assess for fluid overload, pulmonary edema (dyspnea, wheezing, coughing, rales, or rhonchi), and cardiac arrhythmias. Deep tendon reflexes should be monitored if magnesium sulfate is being given, to assess for diminished or absent reflexes. Blood samples may be drawn to assess the levels of glucose and potassium in order to identify the development of hyperglycemia and hypokalemia. To assess hydration, the woman should be weighed daily and her intake and output, skin turgor, mucous membranes, and urine concentration assessed and recorded. The physician should be notified at once if any alterations from normal are identified. The woman's physical comfort and emotional status should also be assessed.

▼ Diagnosis

The nursing diagnoses formulated from the assessment data should be made in collaboration with the physicians and nurse practitioners making the medical diagnoses related to preterm labor. Examples are as follows:

- Risk for fetal injury related to preterm birth
- Anxiety and fear related to concern about the health of self and fetus
- Sleep pattern disturbance related to monitoring of fetus and self
- Altered role performance related to hospitalization

▼ Planning

The desired outcome is for the woman's uterine contractions to cease and to avoid or arrest effacement and dilatation of greater than 3 cm. A plan of care directed toward this goal might include the following:

- The fetus will be delivered safely
- The woman will remain on complete bed rest and demonstrate compliance with her medical management
- The woman will express her feelings and fears about her risk for preterm labor and the restrictions on her daily activities
- The woman will demonstrate adjustment of her role within her family by making arrangements for the care of her children and management of the household

▼ Intervention

The nursing care of the woman who is hospitalized for management of preterm labor or who is at risk for preterm delivery is centered on (1) continual maternal and fetal assessment as discussed above, (2) monitoring of tocolytic drug therapy, (3) facilitating compliance with the planned medical management, (4) provision of physical comfort, (5) ongoing education, and (6) emotional support.

Intravenous fluids are started to ensure hydration and serve as a route for the administration of tocolytic drugs. These drugs are usually given by pump infusion. The dosage is gradually increased until uterine activity ceases. The goal is to use the minimal amount possible to maintain uterine quiescence. If contractions have stopped after 12 to 24 hours of intravenous therapy, the tocolytic drug is usually administered orally. If a beta-sympathomimetic drug is being given (ritodrine), a beta-blocking agent such as propranolol (Inderal) should be available as an antidote. If magnesium sulfate is being used, the antagonist is calcium gluconate.

It is important to help the woman to maintain complete bed rest in the left lateral position, as this facilitates fetal circulation, relieves pressure from the fetal presenting part on the cervix, and decreases the incidence of hypotension. However, this is difficult for the woman if she is hospitalized for any length of time. The nurse can help provide the motivation and diversions the woman needs to maintain compliance. Antiembolism stockings should be applied to prevent the blood from pooling in the lower extremities, and passive range of motion of the legs should be effected several times a day.

Continual education regarding the woman's physical status, the tocolytic treatment regimen, and possible side effects of the treatment is essential. The woman and her family also need emotional support to help them deal with the effects of prolonged hospitalization or a preterm delivery and to help relieve fear and anxiety (Lynam and Miller 1992). Referral to other members of the health care team, such as social services or occupational therapy, may be necessary to help the woman meet her psychosocial needs. The following points summarize interventions designed to decrease psychological stressors for the woman on prolonged bed rest and her family:

- Encourage the woman and her family to verbalize fears and anxieties about preterm labor and its sequelae
- Provide clear, concise information on a continuing basis regarding the woman's medical status and her treatment; empower her as a partner in planning her care
- If hospitalization occurs with resultant separation of family and friends, provide opportunities for contact (frequent phone calls, liberal hospital visitation of all family members); discuss the possibilities for child care if there are children at home
- Assess coping style and social support; refer the family to social services for help in meeting social needs; refer to the chaplain to meet spiritual needs
- Arrange tours of the neonatal intensive care unit so that the woman and family will be familiar with the environment where their infant may receive care after birth
- Refer the woman to a support group or hot line for high-risk antepartum women; if she is on bed rest, arrange for a visit from someone who has experienced preterm labor
- Provide diversional activities (television, videos, crafts, reading materials); make a referral to occupational therapy

▼ Evaluation

Evaluation of the effectiveness of the plan for the management of preterm labor is continuous. Careful documentation of all data recorded provides a basis for ongoing management. The woman should be asked frequently about the symptoms being experienced. Validation of the cognitive understanding of the woman and her family regarding her symptoms, the status of the fetus, and the plan for management can be made by talking with them and asking questions to confirm their knowledge. Direct observation of the woman's affect or behavior, as well as asking her questions regarding her feelings, can give clues to her emotional status and fears.

Premature Rupture of Membranes

Description

Premature rupture of the amniotic membranes (PROM) occurs when the membranes spontaneously rupture before labor begins. It is identified by the leaking of amniotic fluid from the vagina in the absence of contractions. PROM occurs in 3 to 18.5 percent of all births (Creasy and Resnik 1994). The term "premature" refers to the fact that the rupture of membranes precedes labor. Among the theories to explain PROM is one suggesting that the spontaneous rupture may be caused by a reduction in membrane strength that occurs because of an ascending bacterial infection (Combs and Kitzmiller 1993). PROM may also be associated with malpresentations and an incompetent cervix.

▼ **Rupture at Term.** Spontaneous rupture of the membranes (SROM) can occur at any time during pregnancy. Approximately 10 percent of pregnancies result in term premature rupture after 37 weeks' gestation. The onset of regular uterine contractions occurs within 24 to 48 hours after rupture of membranes in 80 to 90 percent of women at term (Creasy and Resnik 1994).

▼ **Preterm Rupture.** Spontaneous rupture of membranes before 37 weeks' gestation is referred to as preterm premature rupture of membranes (PPROM). PPROM is responsible for an estimated 30 percent of all preterm births and is a cause of significant maternal morbidity and significant neonatal morbidity and mortality.

There are a variety of clinical risk factors for the development of PPROM, some of which appear to be infectious in nature. These include (1) past or current history of sexually transmitted diseases and (2) nutritional factors, especially lack of copper and ascorbic acid, which are important for stabilization and synthesis of the collagen of which the membranes are composed. Many studies have shown a relationship between smoking and PPROM, although the etiologic role is unclear. Antepartum bleeding (abruptio placentae, placenta previa) is associated with a fivefold risk of PPROM. A questionable risk factor is sexual activity during pregnancy.

The major risks associated with PPROM are prematurity with associated respiratory distress syndrome (RDS) and infection, either maternal (e.g., chorioamnionitis) or neonatal. RDS is a condition in which the lung function of the neonate is compromised. Neonatal infection via chorioamnionitis may lead to sepsis and, if treatment is ineffective, neonatal death (Levine 1991). Other neonatal complications associated with PPROM include pulmonary hypoplasia, fetal distress, fetal deformities, and congenital abnormalities. Maternal risks for PPROM include postpartum endometritis and obstetric interventions such as induction and cesarean delivery.

Management

Diagnosis of premature rupture of the membranes (either term or preterm) is made by carefully collecting a specimen of amniotic fluid by means of speculum examination. According to institutional policy, this examination may be performed by a nurse or by the attending physician or midwife. The most common diagnostic tools are the Nitrazine and ferning tests. The Nitrazine test involves using a strip or cotton swab that changes color if the material being tested is amniotic fluid. Amniotic fluid has a pH of 7.0 to 7.5 and turns the yellow Nitrazine blue. Vaginal secretions have a pH of 4.5 to 5.5 and do not affect the yellow Nitrazine strip or swab. The difficulty with Nitrazine testing is that it is beset by false-positive results. Blood, *Trichomonas vaginalis,* and various other substances may also turn the Nitrazine material alkaline or blue. A ferning test involves use of a microscope. Secretions of the vaginal fluid are obtained by a cotton-tipped applicator and spread on a slide that is allowed to air dry. Salts in the amniotic fluid should allow a ferning pattern. If ferning is not present, the test is considered negative (see Chapter 11). Perhaps the best diagnostic test for rupture of membranes is the simplest. Visualization of fluid emerging from the cervical os may be accomplished by asking the woman to push or cough while she is being examined, and the cervix is visible through a sterile speculum. When fluid can be seen, it is most likely that membranes have ruptured (Arias 1993; Brouillard-Pierce 1993).

Expectant management of term SROM, i.e., waiting up to 24 hours before initiating intervention, has not been linked with increased maternal or perinatal morbidity or mortality. Occasionally labor does not ensue within 12 to 24 hours, and management in these cases is aimed at affecting delivery via induction of labor to avoid maternal or neonatal morbidity. Management also includes excluding cord prolapse and screening for infection, especially by assessing vital signs and evaluating fetal well-being. Administration of prophylactic antibiotics in labor may reduce subsequent endometritis (Cunningham et al. 1993; Creasy and Resnik 1994).

Management of PPROM is based on how early in gestation the rupture occurs. Induction and delivery between 32 and 36 weeks of gestation has been recommended, or a combination of expectant labor management along with antibiotic coverage. Women between 26 and 32 weeks of gestation are usually managed expectantly and are often admitted to a birth site with tertiary neonatal care. These women remain on bed rest with bathroom privileges. Maternal vital signs should be recorded every 4 hours. Daily blood values (white blood cell counts, C-reactive protein, sedimentation rates) and urine values help to determine whether infection is developing. A tocolytic agent may be given if the mother has mild to moderate uterine activity (see discussion of preterm labor). An antimicrobial such as ampicillin may be ordered and administered intravenously for prophylaxis. A betamethasone drug, such as Celestone, may be given daily to accelerate fetal growth and stimulate fetal lung development. Continuous electronic fetal monitoring may be ordered, as well as regular nonstress tests and fetal biophysical profiles. If infection develops or signs of fetal distress occur, delivery should be initiated. Women with PPROM before 26 weeks' gestation generally have a poor fetal outcome. However, tocolysis, antibiotic coverage, and betamethasone administration provide aggressive treatment in the hope of prolonging the pregnancy.

Nursing Process

▼ Assessment

For women who have PPROM, nursing care should begin with an exhaustive assessment. Data to be collected and interpreted include results of tests for rupture of membranes (Nitrazine, ferning); gestational age and criteria for determination; demographic data; gravity and parity; laboratory results, especially urinalysis, white blood cell count, and C-reactive protein; signs of labor; symptoms of leaking or gushing of vaginal fluid; color and odor of fluid; and vital signs, including temperature, pulse, respirations, blood pressure, fetal heart rate, and contraction pattern if present.

▼ Diagnosis

The following nursing diagnoses are examples of those that might be made after the assessment of the woman who presents with PPROM:

- Risk for infection related to a break in the intact amniotic membrane surface
- Anxiety related to concern about the health of self and fetus
- Altered comfort related to leaking amniotic fluid
- Sleep pattern disturbance related to frequent monitoring of the fetus and self
- Altered role performance related to hospitalization
- Knowledge deficit: lack of information related to PPROM, its prognosis and sequelae

▼ Planning

The plan of care that is identified for the woman with preterm premature rupture of the membranes might include the following goals:

- The woman will show no signs or symptoms of infection as evidenced by normal vital signs and laboratory values
- The woman will verbalize an understanding of PPROM and its prognosis, sequelae, and treatment
- The woman will verbalize her anxiety regarding PPROM
- The woman will comply with the medical management of PPROM

▼ Intervention

Nursing interventions for the woman with PPROM include monitoring of vital signs, especially temperature and pulse for elevation. Laboratory values such as elevated white blood cell count, sedimentation rates, or C-reactive protein levels are also monitored. The electronic fetal monitor pattern of the fetus is assessed for tachycardia, which can indicate fetal infection. Color and odor of the amniotic fluid is also assessed: a foul odor can indicate infection. Meconium staining of the amniotic fluid generally gives a greenish or brown appearance that can indicate fetal distress. Ongoing education, as outlined in the discussion of the management of preterm labor, is a necessary component of the nursing plan. Education should involve the woman and her family as appropriate. Emotional support is also important.

▼ Evaluation

The evaluation of the plan of care for a woman with PPROM is based on the identified outcome goals and interventions. For example, if the maternal temperature remains elevated and amniotic fluid continues to leak, interventions other than bed rest will most likely be necessary.

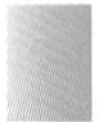

Postterm Pregnancy

Description

A postterm pregnancy is one that persists for 42 weeks or more from the first day of the last menses in a 28-day cycle. It occurs in 7 to 12 percent of all pregnancies (Creasy and Resnik 1994). The etiology cause is unknown, although estrogen deficiency is cited as a possible cause. It is also possible that continued secretion of progesterone, a hormone that functions to inhibit the onset of labor, and the absence of oxytocin or prostaglandins, which stimulate labor, may play a role.

Problems associated with postterm pregnancy primarily affect the fetus. Aging of the placenta results in decreased ability to carry oxygen and nutrients to the fetus. This places the fetus at risk for intrauterine hypoxia. Fetal macrosomia (birth weight greater than 4000 to 4500 g) occurs in 25 percent of postmature infants. Other fetal problems include hypoglycemia, polycythemia, and shoulder dystocia (related to macrosomia). Decreased amniotic fluid (oligohydramnios) is frequently associated with postterm pregnancy. As a result, the umbilical cord may be compressed by the fetus, leading to hypoxia. Meconium aspiration syndrome is seen in 3 to 5 percent of postterm pregnancies. Symptoms include dry, cracked skin; loss of subcutaneous muscle mass; and meconium staining. Although no serious physical problems result for the woman because of postterm pregnancy, there are emotional implications. Women often become impatient when pregnancy continues beyond the expected date of confinement and may feel depressed as fatigue and symptoms of late pregnancy continue to be bothersome. The risks of medical and surgical intervention increase as pregnancy continues past term, for if labor does not begin spontaneously, induction, forceps, or cesarean delivery are often necessary to achieve safe delivery of the infant.

Management

Management of postterm pregnancy centers on careful fetal surveillance. After 41 weeks' gestation, fetal well-being is usually evaluated weekly by biophysical and ultrasonographic evaluations. The woman may be asked to do daily fetal movement counts, and abdominal girth measurements may be made to detect olighydramnios. The cervix may be examined weekly, and induction is initiated if the Bishop score is 5 or greater (Creasy and Resnik 1994; Taffel et al. 1991). If the cervix is unfavorable for induction, twice-weekly fetal testing is commonly performed, including a contraction stress test and amniotic fluid volume determination. If fetal test results are abnormal or oligohydramnios is found, delivery should be accomplished immediately by the safest route for the fetus. During labor, the fetal heart rate should be monitored carefully, and fetal scalp blood pH sampling performed if indicated (Brouillard-Pierce 1993).

Nursing Process

▼ Assessment

The assessment data needed during a postterm labor and birth all relate to the intrauterine status of the fetus and the progress of labor. Continuous electronic fetal monitoring should be used, and once the membranes have ruptured, an internal fetal scalp electrode should be attached. The amniotic fluid should be observed frequently for signs of meconium staining. If there is concern about the status of the fetus, fetal scalp blood sampling should be done to determine the pH. The woman should be assessed regularly by vaginal examination to determine cervical status and fetal descent. The contraction pattern should be closely monitored to determine whether labor is progressing normally or is dysfunctional, or whether surgical intervention is necessary.

▼ Diagnosis

The nursing diagnoses for the woman and her fetus in postterm labor might include the following:

- Impaired fetal gas exchange related to poor placental perfusion
- Risk for fetal injury related to postterm macrosomia
- Anxiety and fear related to concern for fetus and possible surgical delivery

▼ Planning

The plan for nursing care of the woman with a postterm pregnancy is based on the assessment and identified nursing diagnoses. The goals might include the following:

- Adequate oxygenation will be maintained and the infant will be delivered without trauma
- The woman's fears will be identified and addressed and she will be able to cope with the labor and birth

▼ Intervention

In addition to the ongoing assessments discussed above, the woman in postterm labor should be encouraged to stay in the left lateral position as much as possible to facilitate placental perfusion. If there is concern about the fetal response to labor, O_2 should be administered to the woman by mask at 8 to 10 L/min. If labor is not progressing well, preparations should be made for a cesarean delivery. As delivery approaches, the nursery staff should be notified that a postterm infant is about to be born, so that additional personnel can be present to meet the infant's needs. Throughout labor it is important to keep the woman and her family informed about the status of the fetus and the progress of labor. She should be prepared for a possible cesarean delivery. Emotional support is essential in view of the woman's concerns about the fetus and a possible surgical delivery (Campbell et al. 1993).

▼ Evaluation

Evaluation is ongoing throughout the care of the woman in postterm labor, and serves to alter the goals and interventions if necessary. The final evaluation of the plan is based on whether the identified goals are met and on the outcome of the delivery.

Cord Prolapse

Description

Cord prolapse occurs when a loop of cord lies beside (occult or hidden) or below (visible or complete) the presenting part of the fetus. It is noted in one of 239 to 400 pregnancies (Griese and Prickett 1993). Cord prolapse is a grave situation, since compression of the cord between the presenting part and the maternal pelvis decreases or cuts off the blood supply to the fetus. Fetal hypoxia occurs quickly, and if this remains uncorrected, umbilical cord compression leads to central nervous system damage or death of the fetus (Cherry and Merkatz 1991; Cunningham et al. 1993; Danforth 1990). The membranes may or may not be intact with a cord prolapse. If they are intact, the condition is called umbilical cord presentation or a funic presentation. If the membranes are ruptured, the condition is called umbilical cord prolapse.

There are three positions the cord may occupy when prolapsed: (1) occult, (2) complete, and (3) presenting. An occult cord prolapse is hidden, with the cord lying beside the presenting part in the pelvic inlet; it is not visible and usually not palpable. This position is more common than generally thought and can cause fetal death swiftly and

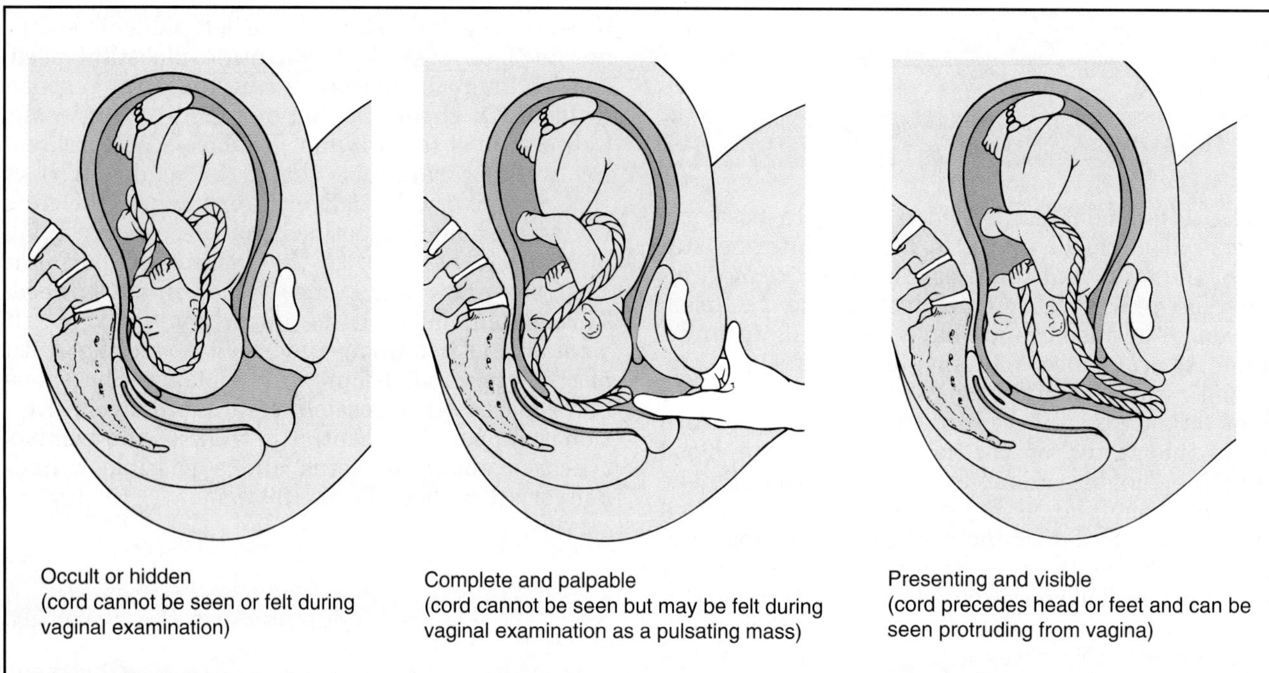

Figure 25–5

A prolapsed cord occurs when the umbilical cord falls in front of the presenting part of the fetus and lies between the fetus and the side of the maternal pelvis • Cord prolapse is very serious, since compression of the cord decreases or cuts off the blood supply to the fetus.

without warning. With a complete cord prolapse, the cord may descend into the vagina. It may not be visible, but it can be felt on vaginal examination. When a cord prolapse is presenting, the cord may be in front of the fetal head, passing through the introitus and out of the vagina, where it becomes easily visible (Fig. 25–5).

Risk factors associated with developing a cord prolapse include an abnormally long cord and a variety of factors associated with the fetus not completely filling the pelvic cavity, such as malpresentation, cephalopelvis disproportion, preterm or low-birth-weight infant, multiple gestation, polyhydramnios, and congenital anomalies. A multiparous woman may be more likely to have a cord prolapse with a pregnancy, since the abdominal muscles may be lax and the fetus may not engage well. Even before the diagnosis is confirmed, cord prolapse should be suspected if abnormal fetal monitoring tracings (bradycardia, severe variable decelerations) occur. Diagnosis is usually made clinically by palpation during a vaginal examination or by visualization of the cord at the vaginal opening.

Management

Management of a prolapsed cord ideally should begin with prevention. If SROM has occurred, the woman should be kept on bed rest until the presenting part of the fetus is engaged. Likewise, artificial rupture of membranes (AROM) should not be attempted until engagement has occurred. If a prolapse does occur, management is then focused on prompt delivery of the fetus by cesarean birth. Oxygen is administered to the woman and the fetal heart rate is monitored continuously. Any prolapsed cord outside the vagina should be kept moistened with saline-soaked gauze at body temperature. This prevents chilling of the cord, which could stimulate a vagal nerve response (Griese and Prickett 1993). If the cord has prolapsed out of the vagina, it should not be replaced into the uterus, for this would cause further trauma and risk infection. While preparations are under way for surgery, oxytocin should be discontinued, and labor may even be halted with tocolytics. The most important strategy is to keep pressure off the cord until delivery can be effected. This is accomplished by placing the woman in deep Trendelenburg or knee-chest position and manually elevating the presenting part with gloved fingers as far out of the pelvis as possible until the infant is delivered. Bladder filling has also been used as a way to relieve pressure on the umbilical cord, by raising the presenting part off the compressed cord (Griese and Prickett 1993). A cesarean delivery should take place as quickly as possible, because fetal survival is directly related to the time elapsed between identification of the prolapsed cord and delivery.

Nursing Process

▼ Assessment

The initial assessment of any woman being admitted for labor and birth should include any information that would alert the nurse to risks for a prolapsed cord. This would include the status of the membranes and the station of the presenting part. Monitoring of fetal heart rate throughout labor also gives important information, for bradycardia accompanied by variable decelerations can be indicative of a prolapsed cord, particularly if there is no improvement with O_2 administration, hydration, or a change in maternal position. If the woman is at risk for a prolapsed cord, careful palpation of the station of the presenting part is important, as is whether the cord can be felt during vaginal examination. The nurse should also include regular observations of the perineum as a part of her assessments. This would be particularly important after SROM.

▼ Diagnosis

Examples of nursing diagnoses that might be identified for a woman with a prolapsed cord include the following:

- Impaired fetal gas exchange related to compression of the umbilical cord secondary to prolapse
- Pain related to labor contractions, manipulation of the cord, and maternal positioning
- Anxiety and fear related to the emergency situation, fetal status, and possible surgery

▼ Planning

The plan of care for the woman with a prolapsed cord might include the following goals:

- Normal fetal gas exchange will be maintained as evidenced by fetal heart rate pattern within normal limits
- The woman will verbally state her understanding of the umbilical cord prolapse and the planned intervention
- The woman will verbally express decreased pain and anxiety
- The woman will deliver a healthy infant

▼ Intervention

Most of the nursing strategies for a prolapsed cord are focused on measures to relieve the pressure of the presenting part of the fetus from the cord and facilitate fetal oxygenation. These include the following:

- Reduce pressure on the cord by placing the woman in the knee-chest or Trendelenburg position
- Place a hand into the vagina to elevate the presenting part and separate the cord from the presenting part and the pelvis
- Assess the fetal heart rate pattern for ominous changes and monitor continuously
- Keep the exposed portion of the cord moist with warmed normal saline; do not attempt to reinsert the cord; assess the cord for pulsation and color
- Administer O_2 at 8 to 12 L/min by mask
- Start intravenous fluids
- Initiate interventions such as bladder filling or real-time ultrasonography as ordered
- Inform the woman and her family of what is happening in regard to the prolapsed cord and the plan for intervention
- Provide constant emotional support

In some hospitals, nurses are being certified to perform real-time ultrasonography to identify fetal heart movements and cord pulsation if a prolapsed cord is suspected (Griese and Prickett 1993). It is also important to provide immediate information and emotional support for the woman and her family while preparing for and awaiting a cesarean birth.

▼ Evaluation

On the basis of the stated goals and the nursing interventions implemented, the evaluation will determine the continued plan of care. For the woman with a prolapsed cord, this evaluation is based primarily on fetal vital signs, and takes place continuously until a cesarean delivery is accomplished.

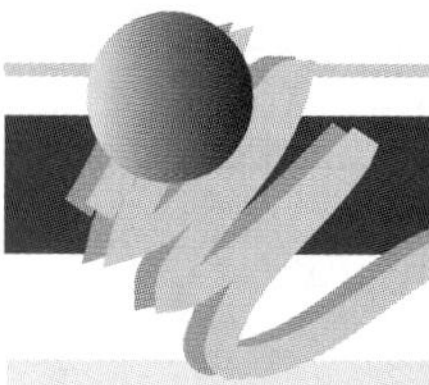

IMPROVING YOUR PRACTICE

CARE FOR CLIENTS DURING HIGH-RISK DELIVERY

Caring for the woman and family experiencing a high-risk delivery is an important but often stressful experience for the nurse. When alterations in the normal childbirth experience are seen frequently, it can be easy to lose one's perspective about birth and difficult to maintain a balance between the physical and emotional care given. The following points will help in providing comprehensive care:

- REMEMBER THAT BIRTH IS A NORMAL PROCESS. The most important components of nursing care are not the ones using high technology but those using high touch, physical and emotional support, teaching, and counseling.
- BEWARE OF ADOPTING NEW TECHNOLOGY SIMPLY BECAUSE IT IS AVAILABLE. Technology should be assessed scientifically with regard to its efficacy and side effects before it is universally adopted.
- BEWARE OF REJECTING NEW TECHNOLOGY SIMPLY BECAUSE IT INVOLVES MACHINERY OR NEW IDEAS. A professional must be open to new ideas and true advances in practice. For certain conditions or complications, high technology can be life saving.
- KEEP CURRENT WITH NEW ADVANCES IN TECHNOLOGY. When high technology is needed, such as electronic monitoring, it should be used correctly. Attend seminars or workshops to familiarize yourself with new procedures or equipment.
- OCCASIONALLY ATTEND A LOW-RISK LABOR AND BIRTH. This will remind you of the normal physiologic process of birth and prevent you from developing the feeling that all births must be high risk.

Bibliography

American College of Nurse-Midwives. (1992). *High technology.* Position paper.

Arias, F. (1993). *Practical guide to high risk pregnancy and delivery.* St. Louis: Mosby–Year Book.

Burrow, G., and Ferris, T. (1995). *Medical complications during pregnancy* (3rd ed.). Philadelphia: W. B. Saunders.

Cherry, S., and Merkatz, I. (1991). *Complications of pregnancy: Medical, surgical, gynecologic, psychosocial and perinatal* (4th ed.). Baltimore: Williams & Wilkins.

Gilbert, E., and Harmon, J. (1993). *High-risk pregnancy and delivery.* St. Louis: Mosby–Year Book.

Harvey, M. (1992). Critical care for the maternity patient. *MCN,* 17 (6), 296–309.

HIGH-RISK CONDITIONS OCCURRING DURING FIRST- AND SECOND-STAGE LABOR

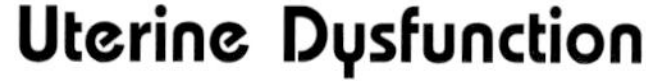

Uterine Dysfunction

Description

Uterine dysfunction is defined as a uterine force insufficiently strong or not appropriately coordinated to efface and dilate the cervix. There are two general types of uterine dysfunction, hypertonic and hypotonic, classified according to when they occur in labor and the nature of the uterine contractions. Uterine dysfunctions can cause a variety of labor abnormalities and often require operative interventions.

Hypertonic Uterine Dysfunction. Hypertonic uterine contractions (also called incoordinate uterine dysfunction) are characterized by an elevated basal tonus or a distorted pressure gradient. This means that the uterus never fully relaxes between contractions; this can be observed on the fetal monitor at levels between 15 and 85 mm Hg (Fig. 25–6). The failure of the uterus to completely relax increases the risk of decreased uteroplacental perfusion or oxygenation of the uterine muscle itself. Hypertonic dysfunction is characterized by frequent, intense, and painful contractions, having no effect on cervical dilatation or effacement. The frequency of contractions may increase while the intensity decreases. The cause of hypertonic dysfunction may be a contracting of the midsegment of the uterus with more force than the fundus, or there may also be incoordinate action of the cornual impulses. This causes asynchronous uterine contractions. Hypertonic uterine dysfunction is a latent-phase disorder sometimes called

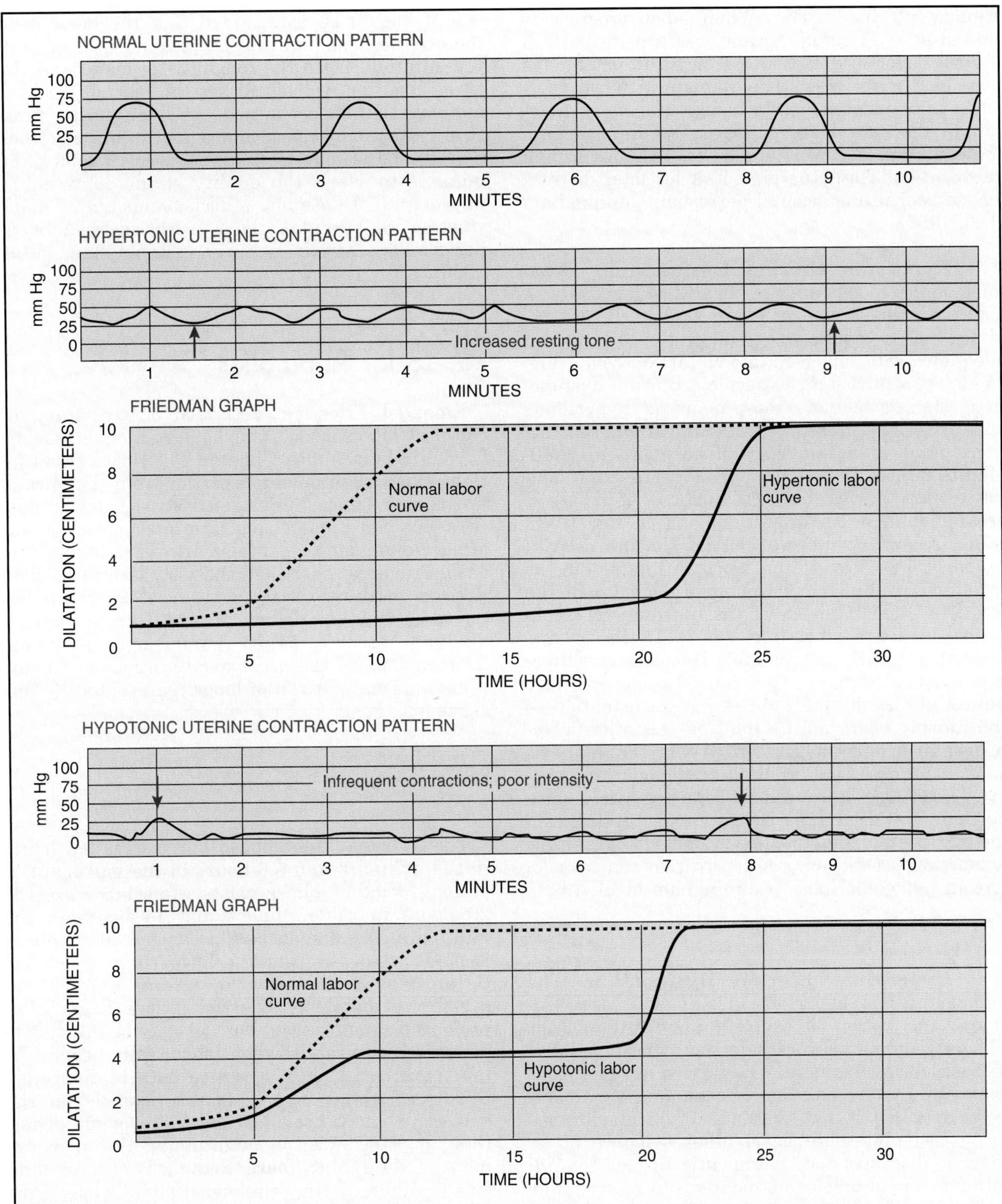

Figure 25–6

Hypertonic uterine dysfunction is suspected when a fetal monitor strip shows frequent contractions without complete relaxation of the uterus; data plotted on the Friedman graph illustrate a prolonged latent phase with no progress of cervical dilatation • Hypotonic uterine dysfunction is associated with contractions that are infrequent and of poor intensity; The Friedman graph shows a decline in the progress of labor in the active phase.

primary uterine inertia. When labor progress is plotted on a Friedman graph over time, a pattern of early labor dysfunction will begin to emerge, as seen in Figure 25–6. The woman with a hypertonic labor pattern becomes discouraged as a result of the slow labor progress and intense pain she experiences. She is at risk for exhaustion and dehydration. The fetus is at risk for fetal distress due to poor uteroplacental perfusion (Cunningham et al. 1993).

Hypotonic Uterine Dysfunction. Hypotonic uterine dysfunction demonstrates only a slight rise in uterine pressure with each contraction, which is insufficient to dilate the cervix at an adequate rate or facilitate fetal descent (Fig. 25–6). In contrast to hypertonic uterine dysfunction, the contractions show no basal hypertonus and a normal pressure gradient. Often, contractions occur at a frequency of only two in a 10-minute period. Hypotonic uterine dysfunction usually occurs during the active phase of labor, at greater than 4 cm dilatation, and is sometimes called secondary uterine inertia. Uterine activity in early labor is within normal limits, but as hypotonic dysfunction develops, a decrease in the frequency and intensity of the contractions is observed in active labor (Fig. 25–6). These contractions are usually not painful. Hypotonic dysfunction may be primary when caused by an intrinsic failure of the myometrium (e.g., overdistention of the uterine fibers due to multiple gestation, polyhydramnios, or grand multiparity) or secondary as a result of excessive sedation or regional anesthesia. It can also be caused by cephalopelvic disproportion. Maternal risks of hypotonic dysfunction include postpartum uterine atony with resultant hemorrhage. Fetal oxygen deprivation can be seen late in hypotonic labor (Cunningham et al. 1993).

Management

Hypertonic Uterine Dysfunction. The management of hypertonic dysfunction rarely includes the option of oxytocin augmentation, for this only serves to exacerbate the hypertonic labor pattern. Assessments may be carried out to ensure that fetal malpresentation or cephalopelvic disproportion (CPD) is not present. If the membranes are intact and there is no other evidence of fetopelvic disproportion, therapeutic rest or the administration of opioids or sedatives (e.g., morphine and meperidine) is appropriate. This will alleviate pain, rest the mother, and arrest the abnormal uterine activity. In many situations, normal uterine activity is established when the woman awakens (Cunningham et al. 1993).

Hypotonic Uterine Dysfunction. To determine whether hypotonic uterine dysfunction exists, it should be ascertained that the labor is in the active phase and that there is no CPD or malpresentation. Once the diagnosis is made and the fetal head is well fixed in the pelvis, an amniotomy can be performed, an intrauterine pressure catheter inserted, and a fetal scalp electrode placed. The woman is observed closely for 30 to 60 minutes to see if the quality of the contractions improves. If it does not, a decision should be made whether to stimulate labor with oxytocin or to perform a cesarean delivery (Cunningham et al. 1993).

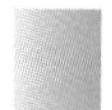

Labor Anomalies

Emanuel Friedman described a partogram, or curve of labor, for normal healthy women (Gabbe et al. 1991) (see also Chapter 23). However, situations exist when deviations occur from the normal progress of labor. As described above, uterine dysfunctions can cause changes in labor patterns, but other circumstances can also arise. For the sake of ease, Friedman described these variations in comparison to the normal curve, now commonly referred to as the Friedman curve (Cunningham et al. 1993) (see Fig. 23–3). A number of additional labor anomalies can occur as alterations in the expected normal pattern of labor represented by this curve.

PROLONGED LATENT PHASE

Description

The average latent phase duration is 8.6 hours in the nullipara and 5.6 hours in the multipara. A prolonged latent phase exists when labor exceeds 20 hours in the nullipara and 14 hours in the multipara. The diagnosis of prolonged latent phase is made when the woman's labor curve shows little progress in dilatation for several hours. There are several problems in arriving at a diagnosis of prolonged latent phase. First, it may be difficult to determine accurately when labor really began. Often there is a lack of objective data to determine this time frame, and diagnosis depends on the subjective data provided by the woman. Thus, there may be error in determining the measurement of the latent phase. Second, it may be difficult to differentiate a prolonged latent phase from false labor and early secondary arrest of labor. It is therefore important to accurately determine the onset of labor and to differentiate false from true labor. There are two common ways to do this:

1. Continuous observation of the woman for 2 hours. Women in false labor have irregular contractions that decrease in frequency and inten-

sity with no cervical change. Women in the latent phase have regular contractions with cervical changes.

2. Therapeutic rest is also used to differentiate false labor from true latent phase. The woman is sedated. Frequently an opioid (e.g., morphine) is used for this function. Women in false labor sleep for a few hours and awake without contractions. Women in latent phase have uterine contractions that increase in intensity and regularity, and also manifest some cervical changes.

The cause of protracted latent phase depends on the parity of the woman. In nulliparas, an unripe cervix is usually the cause of the problem. False labor is the most common cause for the diagnosis of a prolonged latent phase in multiparas. Prolonged latent phase is associated with an increased incidence of subsequent labor abnormalities, the need for cesarean delivery, low Apgar scores, and the need for newborn resuscitation (Chelmow et al. 1993).

Management

Management of the woman experiencing a prolonged latent phase is twofold: therapeutic rest followed by oxytocin stimulation. After careful evaluation of labor status, morphine may be administered intramuscularly. Women will sleep and usually awake in 4 to 5 hours in either active labor or no labor. If labor stimulation is chosen, oxytocin is then begun (Chelmow et al. 1993; Gabbe et al. 1991).

PROTRACTED ACTIVE PHASE

Description

A protracted active phase occurs when the rate of cervical dilatation in the active phase is less than 1.2 cm/hr in nulliparas and 1.5 cm/hr in multiparas. The causes of protracted active phase include fetal malpresentation, CPD, hypotonic contractions, and conduction anesthesia. An occiput transverse or occiput posterior position has also been implicated as the cause (Creasy and Resnik 1994; Cunningham et al. 1993). Diagnosis requires that the active phase of labor be determined accurately. Women with 3 or 4 cm of cervical dilatation may be erroneously diagnosed as having an active-phase disorder when actually they are still in the latent phase.

Management

Management of protracted active phase depends on the cause. Since CPD is a frequent cause of the problem, evaluation of the fetopelvic relationship is necessary. The possibility of an abnormal fetal presentation should be considered. If either of these two situations is established, a cesarean delivery may be necessary. If it is determined that a protracted active phase is the result of inadequate uterine work, oxytocin stimulation is appropriate (Handa and Laros 1993) (see Hypotonic Uterine Dysfunction).

SECONDARY ARREST OF CERVICAL DILATATION

Description

Secondary arrest of labor occurs when the dilatation of the cervix stops for 2 or more hours during the active phase of labor. The major cause of secondary arrest of cervical dilatation is CPD. Other causes are hypotonic uterine dysfunction, malposition of the fetal head, excessive sedation, and regional anesthesia.

Management

Management of secondary arrest should include evaluation for CPD. If this is diagnosed, a cesarean delivery is performed immediately. In women without CPD, a trial labor of oxytocin augmentation for 3 hours may be attempted along with position changes. If there is no progress in cervical dilatation within 3 hours, a cesarean delivery generally is performed.

PROLONGED DECELERATION PHASE

Description

A deceleration phase that lasts more than 3 hours in a nullipara or more than 1 hour in a multipara is prolonged. Diagnosis is established by doing a minimum of two pelvic examinations 3 hours apart in the nullipara and 1 hour apart in the multipara at the end of the active phase. Prolonged deceleration phase is the most frequent of all labor abnormalities. The most common cause is fetal malposition (Gabbe et al. 1991).

Management

The management of prolonged deceleration depends on the characteristics of the descent of the presenting part. If the presenting part is at a high station and if it is accompanied by arrest of descent, the possibility of CPD is great. A cesarean delivery is likely in these cases. However, if the presenting part is below the level of the ischial spines, the possibility of CPD is small and the chances of vaginal birth are good. In this situation, stimulation with oxytocin is feasible.

FAILURE OF DESCENT

Description and Management

In some women the descent of the presenting part does not occur; this is termed failure of descent (Cunningham et al. 1993). The cause of this condition is usually CPD. Failure of descent is often associated with other labor problems such as secondary arrest and protraction disorders. The diagnosis is made by two vaginal examinations 1 hour apart during the second stage of labor. A cesarean delivery is usually performed once the disorder is diagnosed.

PROTRACTED DESCENT

Description

Protracted descent occurs when the maximal slope of descent of the presenting part is 1.0 cm/hr or less in nulliparas or 2.0 cm/hr or less in multiparas. The causes of protracted descent include CPD, hypotonic contractions, excessive sedation, regional block anesthesia, and fetal malposition. Protracted descent also tends to occur with macrosomic infants (Sacks 1993). Diagnosis is established by three pelvic examinations during an observation period of 2 hours.

Management

Medical management depends on the cause of the problem. Regional anesthesia, sedation, and fetal malposition should be ruled out. If none of these factors is present, CPD should be suspected. Excessive sedation and regional block anesthesia problems should be managed by decreasing the agent. Ineffective uterine contractions require oxytocin administration. CPD necessitates cesarean delivery.

ARREST OF DESCENT

Description and Management

Arrest of descent is defined as no progress in pelvic station in the second stage of labor for 1 hour. There are several main causes of this disorder, including fetal malposition, inadequate uterine contractions, and CPD. The diagnosis of arrest of descent depends on a minimum of two pelvic examinations 1 hour apart. It is important to correctly establish descent from caput or molding, which can confuse the practitioner. Abdominal and pelvic examinations are recommended in all cases of suspected abnormalities of descent, to avoid confusion. Abatement of regional anesthesia may be necessary. Oxytocin stimulation may be carried out for inadequate uterine action. Malpositions should be corrected if possible. If not, a cesarean delivery is necessary (Cunningham et al. 1993).

PRECIPITATE LABOR

Description

Precipitate, or rapid, labor is characterized by rates of dilatation and descent greater than 5 cm/hr in nulliparas and 10 cm/hr in multiparas. These labors last less than 3 hours. In most cases, both precipitate dilatation and descent occur simultaneously. The cause of precipitate labor is unclear. Oxytocin stimulation may be a causative factor, although in most cases the situation is spontaneous. Contributing factors include lax resistance of maternal tissues, unusually strong or rapid uterine contractions, multiparity, large pelvis, small fetus in a favorable position, previous rapid labors, and lack of pain sensation to alert the woman to labor progress. The maternal risks of precipitate labor include uterine rupture, lacerations, amniotic fluid embolism, and postpartum hemorrhage. Fetal risks include hypoxia or trauma.

Management

Management of precipitate labor may involve administration of magnesium sulfate or tocolytic agents, although this is rare. If the multiparous woman has a history of precipitate labors, she may be brought into the hospital to have her labor induced and thus observed and carefully managed (Cunningham et al. 1993).

Nursing Process

▼ Assessment

In planning care for the woman with uterine dysfunction, it is important to be certain of the diagnosis. Labor should be evaluated carefully as part of the assessment, and all five "P"s of labor (passage, passenger, pelvis, powers, and psyche) should be considered as possible factors contributing to the dysfunction (see Chapter 22). The essential data to be obtained and documented include cervical dilatation, effacement, and station; and intensity, frequency, duration, and quality of contractions. The data are plotted against time and compared with the Friedman curve. The nurse is often the first member of the health care team to identify a uterine dysfunction. Fetal well-being should be continuously assessed with electronic fetal monitoring. Any ominous fetal heart rate patterns are documented along with the action taken to remedy the problem. Assessment and recording of intake and output provide information about the woman's level of hydration. If the labor is long and membranes have been ruptured for some time, it is important to record maternal temperature and other signs of infection (chills, color or odor of the amniotic fluid). The woman's emotional status and level of anxiety should also be assessed.

▼ Diagnosis

The nursing diagnoses identified on the basis of the assessment data might include the following:

- Altered role performance related to ineffective labor pattern due to incoordinate uterine action
- Pain related to intense uterine contractions associated with hypertonic disorders or prolonged labor
- Impaired gas exchange related to intense uterine contractions or prolonged labor process
- Anxiety and fear related to effect of labor abnormality on self and fetus

▼ Planning

The plan of care for a woman experiencing a uterine dysfunction might include the following goals:

- The woman will establish a normal labor pattern (as determined by the Friedman curve) with efficient cervical effacement and dilatation
- The woman will verbalize decreased or absent pain
- Fetal heart rate and blood gases will be maintained within normal limits
- The woman will verbalize decreased anxiety about herself and her fetus

▼ Intervention

Continuing assessment is an important part of nursing care for the woman with dysfunctional labor. The fetal heart rate and the uterine contractions need to be monitored every hour or more frequently, depending on the stage of labor. An intrauterine pressure catheter and fetal scalp electrode may be placed for more accurate readings. Medications (oxytocin or sedatives) are given in collaboration with a physician or nurse-midwife. Intravenous fluids should be given to prevent dehydration if the labor is prolonged or if operative interventions are planned. Attention to maternal bladder status will prevent a distended bladder that can cause fetal malpositioning and contribute to uterine dysfunction. If the woman is unable to void, she should be catheterized. When a woman is experiencing a hypertonic labor pattern, the nurse should teach or reinforce distractive pain management techniques, maintain a comfortable position for the woman, and promote other comfort techniques such as massage. Changes in maternal position (e.g., squatting, rocking, ambulating) may facilitate correction of fetal malpositions or initiate more effective contractions (Biancuzzo 1991, 1993b). The nurse should continuously explain the labor situation, the diagnosis, and the planned interventions to the woman and her family. She may wish to actively encourage family support and participation in the labor process by giving family members specific comfort techniques to carry out for the woman.

▼ Evaluation

The evaluation of dysfunctional labor is based on the identified goals and the observed results of the selected nursing interventions. For example, if maternal position changes do not facilitate labor progress, additional interventions such as ambulation or oxytocin administration may be necessary. If comfort measures or nonpharmacologic pain management strategies are not relieving discomfort, analgesic medication might be considered.

Cephalopelvic Disproportion

Description

CPD indicates a relationship between the fetal head and the maternal pelvis in which either the fetus is too large for the maternal pelvis or the pelvis is too small to allow passage of the fetal head. It occurs in approximately 5 percent of births. The pelvis may be small because of contractures of the inlet, the midpelvis, or the outlet (see Chapter 9). The fetus may be too large (macrosomic) because of maternal diabetes, genetic influence from large parents, or obesity. Although CPD is a simple concept, it is frequently difficult to diagnose accurately in clinical practice. CPD is a serious cause of abnormal labor, as previously mentioned in the discussion of uterine dysfunctions. There is also a greater risk of abnormal fetal position and presentation due to the attempt of the fetus to adapt to the constricted maternal pelvis (Cunningham et al. 1993; Danforth 1990).

CPD is classified as absolute when there is a disparity between the fetal head and the maternal pelvis despite an optimal fetal head diameter. An abnormally formed pelvis (platypelloid, android) and soft tissue abnormalities (tumors, fibroids) can be causes of absolute CPD. Relative CPD occurs when the fetal head diameter is too large to pass through the pelvis. Abnormal fetal position or presentation is the cause of this type of CPD. The risks of CPD include prolonged labor, PROM, maternal or fetal trauma, uterine rupture, prolapsed cord, and extreme molding of the fetal head.

Management

Awareness of the problem is the key to management. Clinical x-ray or computed tomographic pelvimetry measurements may be taken at the first prenatal visit (see Chapter 22), so that the birth attendant is aware of any discrepancies in pelvic size or shape. Additional pelvimetry or ultrasound examination may be desired at term to assess fetopelvic relationships. These assessments give information about the measurements of the inlet, midpelvis, and outlet of the maternal pelvis, as well as the diameters of the fetal head. If the degree of CPD seems borderline, a trial of labor may be suggested to determine whether vaginal delivery is possible. The disparity created by abnormal positioning or presentation of the fetal part, such as persistent occiput posterior or face presentation, can be corrected by changing maternal positions or, in some cases, by manual forceps rotation. Vacuum extraction with traction may also be an option. When these medical interventions fail, a cesarean birth must be performed (Cunningham et al. 1993).

Nursing Process

▼ Assessment

The nurse should always assess the size of the pelvis, the size of the fetus, and the position and presentation of the fetus when conducting a vaginal examination. Assessment of station is important, for if the fetal head does not engage, a contracted pelvic inlet may be suspected. If the head has engaged but does not further descend, a contracted midpelvis or outlet may be suspected. The presence of an edematous anterior lip of cervix can be indicative of CPD. Documentation of labor progress with a Friedman graph will help the nurse to identify abnormal labor patterns that could be a result of CPD. A hypotonic uterine contraction pattern can be indicative of a contracted pelvis, so it is important to carefully assess the frequency, duration, and intensity of contractions. Continuous electronic fetal monitoring is important if CPD is suspected.

▼ Diagnosis

Nursing diagnoses identified for a woman with a CPD during labor might include

- Pain related to prolonged labor
- Anxiety and fear related to concern for safety of self and fetus
- Risk for infection related to increased vaginal examinations or intrauterine manipulations
- Risk for fluid volume deficit related to hemorrhage due to increased intrauterine manipulation or instrumentation

▼ Planning

The following goals might be formulated based on the assessment data and selected nursing diagnoses:

- The woman will verbalize relief of discomfort or pain
- The woman will verbalize an understanding of CPD and the planned treatment regimen
- Maternal and fetal well-being will be maintained

▼ Intervention

As mentioned previously, the greatest difficulty with management of CPD is an accurate diagnosis. When a high index of suspicion exists for CPD, nursing strategies should concentrate in three areas: education of the woman and her family, correction of any factor that might impede the labor (e.g., fetal malposition, maternal bladder distention, maternal dehydration), and the comfort of the woman. To this end, nursing interventions might include offering distractors or other nonpharmaceutical pain relief remedies, maternal positioning, maternal hydration, pharmaceutical interventions, and continuing support of the woman and her family through education and reassurance.

▼ Evaluation

Evaluation is based on the other components of the nursing process and used to reformulate goals and interventions if necessary.

Rupture of the Uterus

Description

Rupture of the uterus can be a catastrophic event (Clark et al. 1991; Cunningham et al. 1993; Danforth 1990). When it occurs, it places the mother and fetus at high risk for morbidity and mortality. Rupture is defined as an abrupt tearing of the uterus; it can be complete or incomplete. A complete uterine rupture extends through the entire uterine wall, with the entire contents spilling into the abdominal cavity. An incomplete uterine rupture extends through the endometrium and the myometrium without invading the peritoneum. In contrast to a uterine rupture, a dehiscence is the separation of an old scar (e.g., a previous cesarean scar). It tends not to incur any bleeding and is without clinical significance.

A uterine rupture can be further classified as spontaneous or traumatic. A spontaneous rupture is one that occurs during labor owing to a myometrium weakened by a previous scar. A traumatic uterine rupture may be caused by trauma resulting from obstetric instruments or obstetric interventions (Oxorn and Foote 1986). Risk factors for developing a spontaneous rupture of the uterus include having a previous uterine scar, a tumultuous labor, multiparity combined with use of oxytocin, and obstructed labor (such as labor with absolute CPD). Excessive fundal pressure, forceps delivery, violent bearing down efforts, tumultuous labor, and shoulder dystocia can put a woman at risk for a traumatic uterine rupture. Signs and symptoms of uterine rupture include exquisite abdominal pain, vaginal bleeding, lack of progress in labor, palpation of fetal parts outside the uterine wall, rapid onset of fetal distress, progressive signs of maternal hypovolemic shock, restlessness, and anxiety (DeVoe et al. 1992; Jones et al. 1991). The primary maternal risk resulting from a uterine rupture is death due to blood loss and shock. Maternal mortality ranges from 3 to 40 percent, depending on the rapidity with which the rupture is recognized and treatment instituted (Oxorn and Foote 1986). The primary risk for the fetus is also death, resulting from interruption of blood supply and hypoxia.

Management

Management of uterine rupture includes emergency cesarean delivery with repair of the rupture if the woman is undelivered and the symptoms are not severe. If the tear is more severe and cannot be repaired, a cesarean hysterectomy is the appropriate medical intervention. In both instances, hemostasis is the single major consideration.

Nursing Process

▼ Assessment

Assessment data necessary to identify a uterine rupture include maternal and fetal vital signs and the quality and intensity of the uterine contractions if present. Uterine tetany or the sudden absence of contractions can be a symptom of impending uterine rupture. The absence and/or presence of severe abdominal pain and vaginal bleeding is also documented. The woman should be observed for a change in abdominal contour, which may indicate intra-abdominal bleeding.

▼ Diagnosis

The nursing diagnoses for the woman with a uterine rupture might include

- Risk for fluid volume deficit related to hemorrhage secondary to uterine rupture
- Risk for altered fetal tissue perfusion: peripheral related to sudden loss of uteroplacental perfusion
- Pain related to uterine rupture
- Anxiety related to concern over fetus and self

▼ Planning

On the basis of the identified nursing diagnoses, goals for the woman with a uterine rupture might be the following:

- The woman will maintain hemostasis without the development of hypovolemic shock
- The infant will be delivered safely
- The woman will express relief of pain and demonstrate signs of comfort

▼ Intervention

A nursing plan should include cautious assessment of a woman who is predisposed to develop a uterine rupture. For example, women who have a classic uterine scar from a previous cesarean birth are more likely to experience a catastrophic uterine rupture. That rupture is more likely to occur during the third trimester, even before the woman reaches labor. Thus, the woman should be made aware of signs and symptoms of uterine rupture through education about the warning signs of pregnancy.

Labor progress should always be monitored closely to facilitate early identification and treatment of abnormal symptoms, before an obstructed labor might occur. Women with a uterine scar should be monitored particularly closely, and oxytocin should be used cautiously, if ever. Once a uterine rupture is diagnosed, an emergency situation exists. The nurse should continually monitor maternal and fetal vital signs and fluid status. Oxygen is usually administered quickly for both fetal and maternal benefit. A urinary catheter may be inserted and the woman prepared for surgery. Simultaneously, the woman and her family should be kept informed of the situation, the interventions being planned, and the prognosis. Emotional support should be provided.

▼ Evaluation

Evaluation of the plan of care for the woman with a uterine rupture is based on the data being collected, the achievement of identified goals, and the effectiveness of selected nursing interventions.

Shoulder Dystocia

Description

Shoulder dystocia is failure to deliver the fetal shoulders by the usual cardinal movements after the head has been born. The delay in the delivery of the fetal body can result in asphyxia if the umbilical cord is compressed between the body and the maternal pelvis. Less than 1 percent of births are affected by shoulder dystocia, but the risk increases with increased size of the fetus. Shoulder dystocia is associated with maternal obesity, excessive maternal weight gain, a contracted pelvic outlet, macrosomic infants (e.g., infants of diabetic mothers or postterm infants), and a history of shoulder dystocia or macrosomic infants (Cunningham et al. 1993; O'Leary and Leonetti 1990). Labors that manifest an abnormal first-stage labor pattern, a prolonged second stage, protracted descent, arrest of descent, excessive molding of the fetal head, or the need for midpelvic forceps delivery are labors in which shoulder dystocia should be suspected. Shoulder dystocia can result in fetal asphyxia and death or birth injuries such as brachial plexus palsy and fractured clavicle. Maternal complications of shoulder dystocia include lacerations of the birth canal, ruptured uterus, and hemorrhage (Benedetti 1990).

Management

Identification of a macrosomic fetus before the onset of labor is important in the prevention of shoulder dystocia. This can be done by measuring fundal height, palpating crown-rump length, ultrasound, or pelvimetry. The size of the maternal pelvis should also be carefully calculated if a large baby is suspected. The birth attendant employs several methods in the clinical management of shoulder dystocia (Acker 1991; Penny and Perlis 1992; Rubinstein and Schifrin 1992):

- Suprapubic pressure, directed posteriorly to force the anterior shoulder behind the pubic bone and under the symphysis, may be applied by an assistant (Fig. 25–7) at the same time as the birth attendant applies downward traction to the fetal head (Cunningham et al. 1993). The pressure is applied to the fetus' ventral surface. The maneuver slightly decreases the bisacromial diameter, thus dislodging the shoulder.
- The McRoberts maneuver is often used early in shoulder dystocia (Fig. 25–7). The mother's hips are flexed onto her abdomen, which rotates the pelvis anteriorly. This reduces the angle of the symphysis and may disengage the shoulder. The McRoberts maneuver may be performed while the woman is in a dorsal or side-lying position. Squatting is often called a McRoberts position with gravity. Some clinicians believe that use of squatting for birth may reduce the incidence of shoulder dystocia due to pelvic rotation.
- Although shoulder dystocia is a pelvic problem, a birth attendant may cut an episiotomy either in anticipation of the situation or after it is apparent a dystocia exists. An episiotomy is not designed to treat the shoulder dystocia itself, but it can allow additional soft tissue room for manual manipulation that may be needed, such as manual rotation of the shoulders. The shoulders may be rotated to an oblique dimension if the posterior shoulder is at or below the ischial spines in the hollow of the sacrum and/or anteroposterior bisacromial plane. Delivery may be accomplished in the transverse diameter.
- The Wood maneuver of the screw principle advocates rotating the posterior shoulder 180 degrees to the anterior position. Once the posterior shoulder has been delivered in the anterior position, the anterior shoulder will be posterior. The maneuver is repeated to deliver the now posterior shoulder.
- Delivery of the posterior arm may be used to deliver the shoulder. With the anterior shoulder arrested against the symphysis, the birth atten-

dant locates the posterior arm. The attendant flexes the arm, draws it across the fetal chest, and delivers it. Once the arm is delivered, the other shoulder should be delivered easily.

- The Zavanelli maneuver pushes the fetal head back up into the vagina and is followed by a cesarean delivery. This maneuver is extremely difficult to perform and is rarely employed.
- Although fundal pressure has been used in the past as a technique for disengaging the shoulders, it is no longer recommended. It is difficult to ascertain the appropriate amount of pressure and there are negative consequences from too much pressure (uterine rupture, hemorrhage, and impacting the shoulders under the symphysis pubis).

Nursing Process

▼ Assessment

Nursing assessment includes identification of all the parameters described earlier in this chapter related to malpresentations, as well as the factors identified above related to medical management.

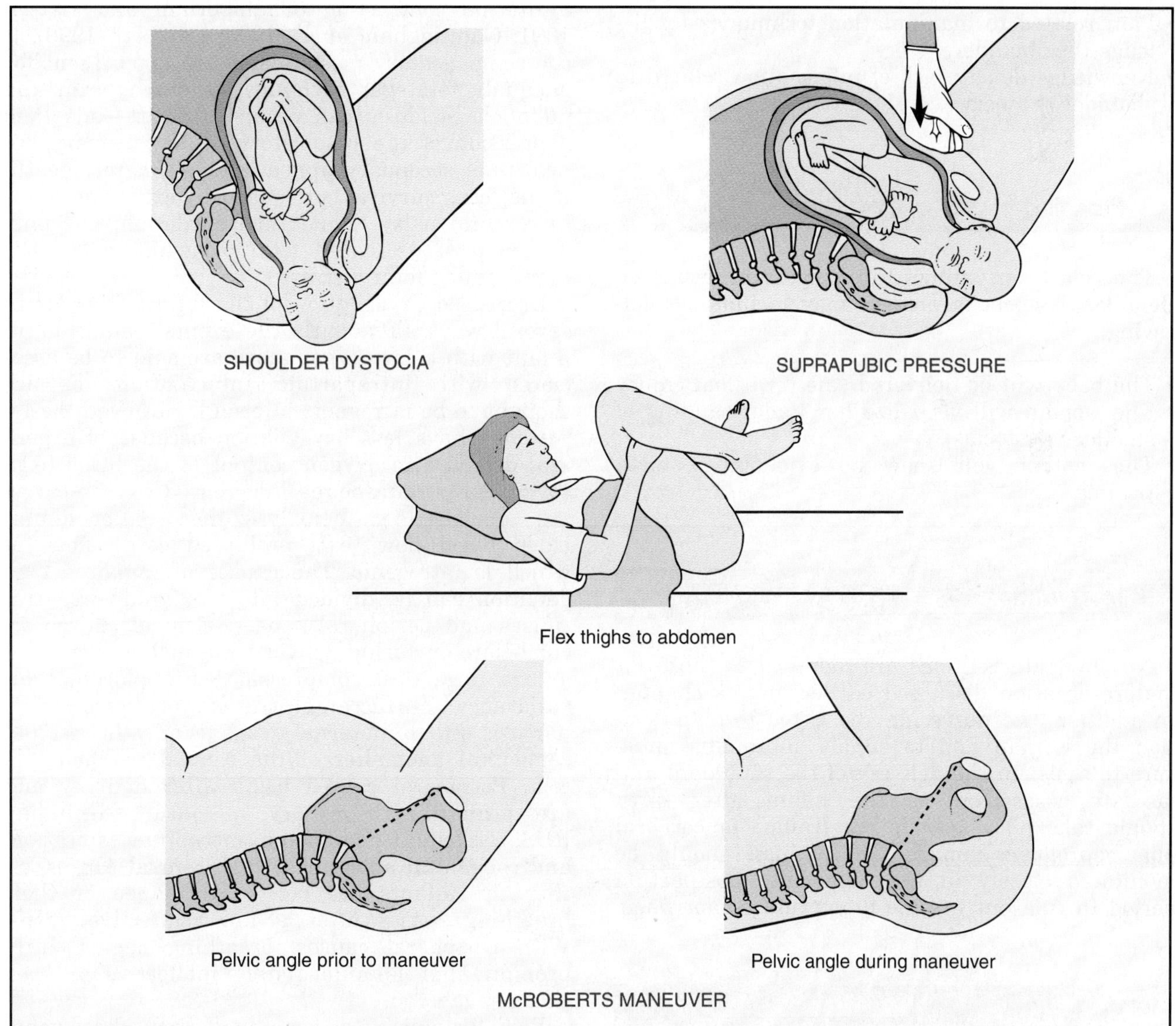

Figure 25–7

Shoulder dystocia describes the failure of the fetal shoulders to deliver according to the usual cardinal movements after the birth of the head • The shoulders become impacted under the symphysis pubis • Suprapubic pressure and the McRoberts maneuver are two of the methods employed by the birth attendant attempting to free the impacted shoulders.

Accurate recording of labor progress and fetal status throughout labor is essential. At the time of birth, the most typical clinical picture to identify is the slow birth of the fetal head, with the emergence of a large, chubby-cheeked baby whose head quickly recedes back against the perineum.

▼ Diagnosis

Selected nursing diagnoses for the woman with a shoulder dystocia might include

- Risk for fetal injury related to the trauma of delivery
- Fear related to uncertainty of delivery outcome
- Pain related to manipulation techniques to dislodge the shoulder
- Knowledge deficit: lack of information related to shoulder dystocia

▼ Planning

The plan for nursing management when a shoulder dystocia is present may include the following:

- The baby will be delivered safely without injury
- The woman will verbalize her understanding of shoulder dystocia
- The mother will show no evidence of birth trauma

▼ Intervention

Nursing interventions are identical to those for malpresentation discussed earlier in this chapter. In addition, the nurse may be asked to help position the woman and to supply suprapubic pressure to assist in the delivery of the shoulders. Immediate assessment of the infant after birth should take place to rule out trauma or cerebral and neurologic damage. The woman should be monitored closely in the immediate postpartum period to rule out uterine atony and hemorrhage.

▼ Evaluation

The evaluation of the plan of care is based primarily on the outcome of the delivery, as evidenced by the amount of trauma experienced by the mother or her infant.

HIGH-RISK FETAL OR NEONATAL COMPLICATIONS DURING LABOR AND BIRTH

Decreased Fetal Oxygenation

Description

Normally, fetal blood supply, oxygenation, and energy requirements are adequate during labor, even with the transient decrease in oxygen supply and increase of carbon dioxide that occurs during a uterine contraction (Chamberlain and Hytten 1991; Cunningham et al. 1993; Danforth 1990). If the compensatory mechanisms are not present for adequate fetal gas exchange, severe hypoxia and metabolic acidosis can occur. Acidosis leads to a depression of the respiratory center, primary apnea, then secondary apnea, and ultimately death. If the fetus survives, prolonged hypoxia can result in cerebral palsy or mental retardation. The phenomenon of decreased fetal oxygenation is commonly called fetal distress.

Decreased oxygenation of the fetus can occur in several ways. Frequently the events leading to an infant with a low Apgar score are said to be associated with intrapartum interventions or are thought to be iatrogenic in origin. However, the fetus may have less oxygenation because of a general decrease in oxygen content of the blood (e.g., severe maternal anemia), decreased oxygen-carrying capacity (e.g., hemolytic disease), or diminished blood flow (e.g., prolapsed cord), none of which is iatrogenic. The causes of impaired oxygenation can be divided into two groups: central causes and peripheral causes. Central causes occur before or during delivery and include perinatal anoxia (e.g., cord compression, uteroplacental insufficiency), intracranial trauma or hemorrhage, narcosis due to maternal drugs or anesthetics, and congenital anomalies of the central nervous system. Peripheral causes begin after delivery and are primarily respiratory in nature, including RDS, congenital pneumonia, meconium aspiration, and congenital anomalies. With central causes, either the infants are born with apnea or their breathing ceases after a few ineffective gasps. With peripheral causes, breathing begins fairly promptly but is immediately ineffective or soon becomes labored.

Risk factors for developing decreased oxygenation during the pregnancy period include maternal disorders related to poor uteroplacental circulation, such as hypertensive disorders of pregnancy, hemorrhage, anemia, or cardiorespiratory disorders. Placental causes include abruption, infection, and infarcts. Umbilical prolapse, compression, and severe knots or entanglements of the cord have also been associated with decreased oxygenation. A vulnerable fetus, such as a preterm fetus, a conceptus with fetal growth restriction, or a fetus with congenital anomalies, is more likely to have impaired oxygenation than a healthy fetus. During the intrapartum period, causes of decreased fetal oxygenation might include a labor with intense and lengthy uterine contractions, prolonged maternal hypotension related to compression of the inferior vena cava or spinal anesthesia, and a difficult second stage.

Signs of fetal distress during labor may include ominous fetal heart rate patterns (see Chapter 26) or meconium-stained amniotic fluid when the fetus is in a cephalic presentation. The resultant neonatal sequelae can include encephalopathy, seizures, disturbances of tone and activity, and damage to the brain stem. Pulmonary hemorrhage and increased incidence of RDS, respiratory complications, acute cardiac failure, and kidney damage are other potential complications.

Management

The medical management of a fetus with decreased oxygenation during labor includes changing the maternal position, usually to a left lateral position to facilitate circulation; administering oxygen by mask, 8 to 10 L/min; continued electronic fetal monitoring; discontinuing oxytocin if it is being used; and obtaining fetal scalp blood samples for the determination of pH, O_2, and CO_2 levels.

Nursing Process

▼ Assessment

Maternal-fetal risk factors that may be of concern should be ascertained from the woman's antepartal history. It is important that the history of intrapartal events and the status of the mother and fetus be carefully documented. Owing to a multitude of medical and legal issues, the terms asphyxia and anoxia should be used judiciously, if at all, in written documentation. Nursing assessment data throughout labor include the electronic fetal monitor tracings, including heart rate, baseline variability, and periodic changes (see Chapter 26); the amount and color of amniotic fluid; and umbilical blood gas values. After birth, the Apgar scores are also important. The type of maternal sedation or anesthesia should be recorded, along with the time of administration and immediate maternal and fetal responses. All pertinent information regarding the course of the labor and birth and the status of the newborn should be shared with the nursery personnel. Nursery staff and/or a neonatologist should be present at the time of birth if decreased fetal or neonatal oxygenation is suspected.

▼ Diagnosis

The nursing diagnoses that might be identified for the woman and her fetus who is experiencing decreased oxygenation include

- Impaired gas exchange related to decreased fetal oxygenation during labor and birth
- Risk for fetal injury related to decreased fetal oxygenation during labor and birth
- Fear related to uncertainty of delivery outcome
- Knowledge deficit: lack of information related to decreased fetal oxygenation during labor and birth

▼ Planning

The specific measurable goals that might be developed to assess the outcome of the plan of care for a woman and her infant experiencing decreased oxygenation may include the following:

- The baby will be delivered safely without injury
- The woman will verbalize her understanding of decreased fetal oxygenation during labor and birth
- The mother will show no evidence of birth trauma

▼ Intervention

The nursing management of fetal distress centers on prevention, continual observation, and immediate intervention if needed. When decreased fetal oxygenation is suspected, continuous internal electronic fetal monitoring is indicated to provide accurate data. All aspects of the fetal heart rate pattern, as discussed in Chapter 26, must be documented frequently. Moreover, the signs and symptoms of labor should be monitored and recorded carefully. It is particularly important that contraction patterns and observations of the amniotic fluid be accurately documented. Prolonged labor, excessive sedative drugs, and deep prolonged anesthesia should be avoided. The woman should be kept comfortable and well hydrated. She should be positioned in the left lateral position to facilitate uteroplacental perfusion, and O_2 should be administered by mask at 8 to 10 L/min. If it is suspected that a cesarean birth may be necessary, preliminary preparations such as the insertion of an intravenous line and urinary catheter can be carried out. It is important that emotional support be given in a calm, caring manner. The woman and her family need to have honest, clear information about the status of the fetus and the possible interventions required.

When there is a high index of suspicion that the infant may have respiratory distress at birth, pediatric personnel should be present for the delivery. Immediate neonatal treatment is based on assessment with the Apgar scores (see Summary of Actions Based on Apgar Scoring). The nursing interventions depend on how severely depressed the infant is at birth. The nurse suctions mucous secretions and administers oxygen. The infant's heart rate and respiratory rate are monitored every few minutes. The appropriate drugs are administered. Equipment should be readily available for intubation. Further discussion of immediate intervention for the high-risk infant is found in Chapter 36.

Summary of Actions Based on Apgar Scoring

APGAR 0–2: SEVERE DEPRESSION

Treatment is aggressive. Laryngoscopy is performed with intubation. If there is no response, metabolic acidosis is suspected and metabolic acidosis should be corrected using sodium bicarbonate via the infant's umbilical vein. External cardiac massage should be initiated.

APGAR 3–6: MILD TO MODERATE DEPRESSION

The infant is warmed and dried. Mucous secretions are removed. Laryngoscopy is performed if meconium is suspected so that suction can be done under direct visualization. Oxygen is given by mask and cutaneous stimulation performed. If narcosis is the cause, an appropriate narcotic antagonist is given. If no improvement is seen, an airway is inserted and the infant is ventilated by mask and bag.

APGAR 7–10: NOT DEPRESSED

The infant is warmed and dried. Mucous secretions are removed, usually by nasal bulb. Cutaneous stimulation can be performed.

▼ Evaluation

The evaluation is directly related to the identified outcome goals. The status of the fetal heart rate, fetal blood gases, and amniotic fluid throughout labor and the Apgar scores at birth will guide the nurse in identifying the continued assessments and interventions needed.

Multiple Gestation

Description

The physiologic cause of a multiple gestation is discussed in Chapter 15 and the management of a multiple gestation during pregnancy in Chapter 21. Several aspects of a multiple pregnancy make it a high-risk situation during labor and birth. Because the uterus is overdistended, the woman is at risk for preterm labor and uterine dysfunction. Abnormal fetal presentations are more likely to occur. For example, in the case of twins, there are a number of positions or presentations that might be assumed (Fig. 25–8). There is also an increased incidence of PPROM, placenta previa, abruptio placentae, cord prolapse, preeclampsia, fetal congenital anomalies, fetal trauma, intrauterine growth retardation, stillbirth, and postpartum hemorrhage (Cunningham et al. 1993).

Management

Prenatal diagnosis of a multiple gestation is the first step in management during the intrapartal period. On occasion, a multiple gestation may not be identified until the intrapartal period, particularly if the woman experiences a preterm labor. This not only adds an increased physical risk due to lack of an awareness of a potential high-risk situation, but also adds emotional and financial stress to a family that had expected one baby. Physical management of the woman with a multiple gestation requires careful maternal and fetal monitoring. For example, if twins are expected, both fetuses should be monitored with continuous electronic fetal monitoring leads. Ultrasound examination should be done to give information about fetal positions and the location of the pla-

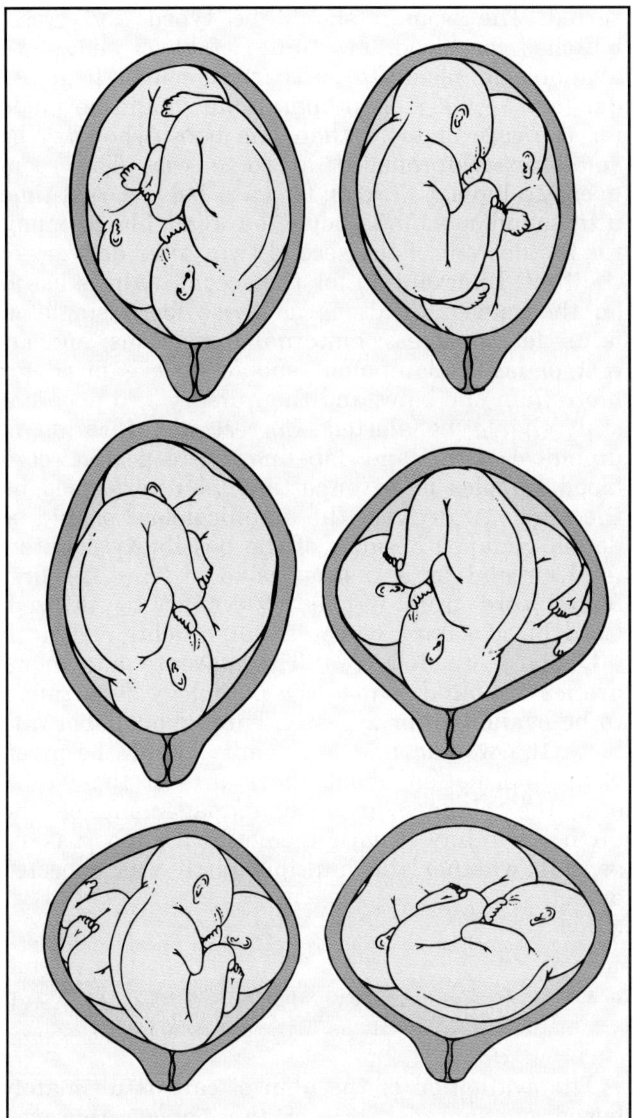

Figure 25–8

Fetuses in a twin gestation can assume any number of different positions that may make the labor and birth more difficult.

centa. A fetogram, a radiograph of the uterine contents, may also be taken to determine fetal positions or anomalies. Analgesia and anesthesia should be carefully planned to provide both comfort for the woman and safety for fetuses that may be preterm or small for gestational age. Regional anesthesia provides a safer alternative than many other analgesics in this situation, but it is important that the woman be placed in the left lateral position to prevent inferior vena caval compression due to the excessively enlarged uterus (Creasy and Resnik 1994).

The method of delivery depends on a number of factors, including maternal and fetal status, additional accompanying risk factors, gestational age, the presentation of the babies, and the availability of anesthesia and neonatal care (Creasy and Resnik 1994). The choice of vaginal or cesarean delivery may not be made until labor is under way and an assessment can be made of labor progress and the risks and benefits of each route of delivery. In most multiple gestation labors a cesarean delivery is planned. This mode of delivery is selected to avoid trauma or fetal hypoxia if the fetuses are preterm or are not in a vertex position. Other indications for a cesarean birth include a breech position or transverse lie of the first presenting fetus, and an increased risk of a prolapsed cord due to monoamniotic twins (twins with one amniotic sac) (Creasy and Resnik 1994).

If a vaginal delivery is planned, it should be determined that the fetuses are not in distress, there is no cephalopelvic disproportion, and the fetal positions will allow a safe delivery with little trauma. It may be necessary to induce labor. Amniotomy of the first sac with or without oxytocin augmentation is the accepted practice, if abnormal fetal presentation that would preclude AROM has been excluded (Creasy and Resnik 1994). Preparations should be ready for an immediate cesarean delivery if labor or vaginal birth is unsuccessful. For either vaginal or cesarean delivery, additional nursing and medical staff should be available to help with the babies and provide assistance in the event of complications. After the delivery, the placentas are examined to determine whether the babies of the same sex are monozygotic or dizygotic.

Nursing Process

▼ Assessment

The nursing assessment of the woman with a multiple gestation in labor should include all the components previously discussed in relation to a complicated labor. The primary addition in a multiple gestation is that the status of more than one fetus should be continually monitored if possible. Continuous external monitoring of each baby should be attempted with an electronic fetal monitor. If membranes are ruptured, an internal fetal scalp electrode can be attached to the presenting fetus. In the immediate postpartum period, the woman should be monitored closely for postpartum hemorrhage resulting from the inability of her overdistended uterus to contract adequately.

▼ Diagnosis

Nursing diagnoses that might apply to the woman experiencing labor with a multiple gestation might include the following:

- Risk of impaired gas exchange related to multiple gestation
- Risk for fetal injury related to positions of multiple gestation
- Anxiety and fear related to status of babies and unknown outcome of labor and birth
- Knowledge deficit: lack of information related to management of labor and birth of multiple gestation

▼ Planning

The plan for the nursing management of a multiple gestation during labor should be based on the available data and the nursing diagnoses. Examples of outcome goals include the following:

- Adequate fetal oxygenation will be maintained in utero and the babies will be delivered safely
- The woman will verbally express her concerns about the status of the babies and her labor and birth
- The woman and her family will ask questions and correctly state the plan of medical management

▼ Intervention

Nursing interventions for a multiple gestation labor and birth center on continual monitoring of the fetuses and the maternal labor pattern and the provision of comfort, education, and emotional support to the woman and her family. If twin fetuses are both in a vertex presentation and the woman has no other contraindications, she may anticipate a vaginal delivery. In this case, additional attempts to use positioning and nonpharmacologic pain relief measures may be necessary owing to the large uterus or the woman's increased anxiety. The woman may have a longer active phase of labor due to poor uterine contractions from overdistention of the uterus. Both babies should be monitored simultaneously when fetal well-being is assessed during labor. The woman and her significant support person need to know that twins, especially the second twin, have a higher potential risk for cord prolapse and fetal distress from a prematurely separated placenta. Therefore, intravenous access is established before delivery in view of the potential for emergency cesarean delivery. Analgesia and anesthesia should be administered and monitored carefully. Documentation of all events is important.

If the woman requires a cesarean delivery, she should be prepared for surgery. An intravenous line should be started and a urinary catheter inserted. The woman should be typed and crossmatched for blood. Two units of blood should be available in case of a postpartum hemorrhage. As delivery approaches, preparations should be made for the care of more than one baby who may be small or compromised in some way. The room needs to have a warmer for each baby. A real-time ultrasound machine should be available to monitor the descent of the second twin after delivery of the first. Intervention for the second twin is based on the same indications as those for a singleton fetus: fetal distress, maternal indications, and arrest of labor. Equipment should be organized for more than one baby, and the nursery and neonatal staff should be alerted. Correct identification of umbilical cords and labeling of respective cord blood samples is an important task performed by the nurse. At delivery the umbilical cord should be double-clamped because of the possibility of interfetal circulation. A method of identifying the first baby's cord from its sibling's must be utilized. Cord blood samples should not be obtained until all babies are delivered. The placenta and membranes are often sent to the pathology department to be evaluated for zygosity. Throughout labor and birth the woman and her family should be given clear information about the status of the babies and the planned medical management of the birth. As in any situation, emotional support is essential, whether the multiple birth was expected or not.

▼ Evaluation

The evaluation of the plan of care is ultimately based on safe delivery of the babies. However, evaluation should be continuous throughout the labor and delivery period, and alterations in the nursing diagnoses or planned interventions should be made quickly if the evaluation so warrants.

Fetal Developmental Anomalies

Some congenital malformations of the fetus can cause complications in the labor and birth process. These include neural tube defects, hydrocephalus, Potter syndrome, and macrosomia.

NEURAL TUBE DEFECTS

Description

A neural tube defect is failure of the neural tube to close in fetal life (Cherry and Merkatz 1991; Cunningham et al. 1993; Danforth 1990). A number of central nervous system anomalies are associated with these types of defects. Anencephaly, absence of the skull vault with complete or partial absence of the brain, is one of the most significant neural tube defects. The brain tissue that exists is not covered and is therefore unprotected. Infants with anencephaly are often delivered without distress, but the condition is incompatible with extrauterine life. Prenatal screening for neural tube defects may be accomplished by assessing the amount of alpha-fetoprotein (AFP) in the amniotic fluid or maternal serum. Elevated levels of AFP may indicate neural type defects. Anencephaly can then be diagnosed by ultrasonography. Polyhydramnios is commonly associated with anencephaly and can cause labor complications resulting from overdistention of the uterus. When polyhydramnios is not present, the pregnancy is often prolonged, resulting in a postdates infant.

Management

Induction of labor may be desired when anencephaly is diagnosed. However, this may be difficult since the distended uterus may not be responsive to oxytocin. If this is the case, intermittent aspiration of amniotic fluid with induction may be necessary (Cherry and Merkatz 1991; Cunningham et al. 1993; Danforth 1990).

HYDROCEPHALUS

Description

Hydrocephalus is a state of progressive ventricular enlargement in association with an increased volume of cerebrospinal fluid. It is a congenital malformation occurring at 6 weeks' gestation and is associated with other anomalies such as spina bifida, myelomeningocele, renal defects, cardiac defects, colon and anal agenesis, cleft lip and palate, and other chromosomal abnormalities. Infants with hydrocephalus have a very large head with a softened skull, resulting in complications during labor due to CPD. Hydrocephalus can be categorized as communicating or noncommunicating. In communicating hydrocephalus the cerebrospinal fluid is able to circulate through the ventricles and into the subarachnoid space without obstruction. In noncommunicating hydrocephalus the cerebrospinal fluid is characteristically blocked by an obstruction in the ventricular system or a blockage from the ventricular system into the subarachnoid space (Smith et al. 1993).

Management

Hydrocephalus may be suspected if the fetal head has failed to engage or if the head is palpable as a large mass during abdominal examination. If the head can be palpated through the cervix on vaginal examination, the suture lines are found to be abnormally separated. Ultrasound examination has made the diagnosis of hydrocephalus during pregnancy a possibility.

Attempts have been made to perform shunt insertion into the ventricles by means of fetal surgery, but to date the results have been disappointing. When hydrocephalus is severe, obstructed labor with potential uterine rupture can occur. To effect vaginal delivery, fluid may be evacuated from the fetal skull. In some cases a cesarean delivery must be performed. Moreover, if the infant is preterm with mild to moderate hydrocephalus, early delivery may be advised with the goal of avoiding brain damage (Creasy and Resnik 1994).

POTTER SYNDROME

Description

Potter syndrome, which is often associated with a breech position, includes such pathologic conditions as a flattened facial appearance with low-set ears, deformed hands, pulmonary hypoplasia, and renal agenesis with a lack of urine production (Clark and Eteson 1991). The lack of urine production is associated with oligohydramnios, an abnormally small amount of amniotic fluid, since fetal urination plays a part in the balance of fluid in utero. Oligohydramnios causes fetal and cord compression, which results in other symptoms such as intrauterine growth retardation, pulmonary hypoplasia, limb abnormalities, a characteristic facial appearance, meconium staining, and hypoxia. The diagnosis of Potter syndrome is made through identification of a uterine fundus that is small for gestational age, a fetal outline that is easily palpated through the abdominal wall, and ultrasound examination. Labor often begins before term and is dysfunctional (Creasy and Resnik 1994).

Management

An intrauterine amnioinfusion may be attempted to relieve pressure on the fetus and cord. If fetal distress is evident during pregnancy or labor, a cesarean delivery is performed.

MACROSOMIA

Description

Macrosomia is usually defined as a weight more than 4000 g (8 pounds, 14 ounces) for an infant at birth. (In some areas, 4500 g is used as the defining weight for macrosomia; 3800 g was the common criterion in the 1970s). Macrosomia occurs in 5 to 11 percent of all births in the general population, but its incidence is much higher in infants of women who are insulin-dependent diabetics (43 percent). If the mother's pelvis is large, a macrosomic fetus will likely cause no problem during labor. However, if the woman has a small pelvis, the large fetus will not be able to accommodate, resulting in CPD. The subsequent maternal and fetal complications have been discussed in the section on CPD.

Management

Management of macrosomia begins with identification before the onset of labor and is similar to the management of CPD as previously discussed. Careful assessments of the size of the maternal pelvis and the size of the fetus should be made. If labor is not progressing as expected and the assessment of the fetopelvic relationship indicates that the pelvis is adequate for the size of the fetus, induction of labor may be initiated. If labor still does not progress, a cesarean delivery is performed.

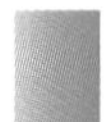

Intrauterine Fetal Demise

Description

Intrauterine fetal demise (IUFD), or death of the fetus before it is born, can occur antepartally after 20 weeks' gestation or intrapartally during labor. In approximately half of antepartal cases, no cause can be found. In other cases, causes found for antepartal fetal death include maternal complications such as preeclampsia, bleeding disorders, and diabetes. Fetal diseases include congenital anomalies, erythroblastosis fetalis, or infection after PROM (Burrow and Ferris 1995; Cherry and Merkatz 1991; Cunningham et al. 1993).

A fetal death occurring in labor is called a term intrapartum death. Fifty percent of these cases have no specific known cause, but contributory problems are reported, including prolonged gestation, PROM, and a tight nuchal cord. Other contributing factors include intrapartum fever, preeclampsia, hypotension, breech presentation, and abnormal glucose tolerance. In the remaining 50 percent of intrapartum deaths, the cause can be determined. These factors include a difficult or traumatic delivery, cord prolapse, fetal congenital anomalies, abruptio placentae, isoimmunization, and ruptured uterus.

Signs and symptoms of fetal demise include cessation of fetal movement, a decrease in the size and tenderness of the woman's breasts, the absence of fetal heart tones, uterine size smaller than dates, failure of uterine growth, a negative pregnancy test, and a decrease in maternal estriols. Diagnosis is accomplished by using ultrasonography to determine the absence of the fetal heart pulsation, the occurrence of fetal skull collapse, and absence of a recognizable fetal internal structure. Fetal demise can also be detected on x-ray examination by the Roberts sign, the appearance of intra-abdominal or intravascular fetal gas, and the Spalding sign, an overriding of the fetal cranial bones.

Since the woman increasingly focuses on the fetus as the pregnancy progresses, her loss upon an antepartal death is very different from that experienced by the rest of the family. This loss also differs from that of the mother who loses a child after birth. The fact that the fetus is still inside the mother's body creates a dilemma that has to be dealt with emotionally, as well as physically, before delivery. Reactions to IUFD include grief for the loss of a wished-for child, anger at the health care system or peer group, and guilt or shame. The woman's body image and self-esteem may also suffer. The death of the fetus may make her feel that her body is inadequate and that she has failed at a basic womanly function. The experience of labor and birth forces the woman to confront the reality of the infant's death, in addition to dealing with the normal stress and pain of the experience (Brown 1992).

Management

Management of IUFD focuses on the termination of the pregnancy because of the risk of the mother developing hypofibrinogenemia from fetal breakdown products. Thromboplastin is released into the maternal bloodstream, activating the extrinsic clotting system and triggering the formation of multiple blood clots. As a result, fibrinogen and factors V and VII are depleted and symptoms of DIC are seen. In most cases of IUFD, labor begins spontaneously within 2 weeks of the fetal death; however, if labor does not begin by 5 weeks after the fetal death, the risk of DIC and resultant hemorrhage is increased. Therefore, if labor has not begun spontaneously by 3 weeks after the IUFD, induction is initiated. Blood coagulation studies are collected at frequent regular intervals. An amniotomy is performed and an intrauterine pressure catheter inserted to monitor contractions (Creasy and Resnik 1994).

Nursing Process

▼ Assessment

In planning nursing care for the woman experiencing a fetal congenital anomaly or a fetal demise, the nurse must first assess what has been diagnosed, when it was diagnosed, and what information the woman and her family have been given regarding the situation. Asking the woman to share her understanding about the anomaly or death can guide the nurse's intervention. The parents' grieving process and the resultant behaviors they exhibit should be assessed continually in order to plan appropriate interventions. It is also important to assess the coping abilities, resources, and support system of the woman and her family.

▼ Diagnosis

The nursing diagnoses formulated for a family experiencing fetal congenital anomaly or fetal loss may include

- Anxiety related to condition of the fetus
- Fear related to the impending labor and birth
- Grief related to fetal anomaly or death
- Knowledge deficit: lack of information related to fetal diagnosis or cause of death

▼ Planning

The plan of nursing care should include the following goals:

- The woman and her family will verbalize an understanding of the anomaly or cause of fetal death
- The woman and her family will express their grief about the loss of their desired infant
- The woman and her family will share in the decision whether to see and hold their infant
- The woman and her family will make provisions for continued support after discharge from the hospital and be aware of community resources available to them

▼ Intervention

To provide effective interventions for the woman experiencing a fetal anomaly or death, the nurse must first be able to confront her own discomfort in dealing with the woman's loss and feel free to express her own sorrow about the woman's experience. The nurse should not be afraid to show her own grief (Stratham and Dimavicus 1992). Before the delivery, factual information should be given to the parents about the situation and the status of the fetus. The parents should be encouraged to ask questions. It is important that the nurse be honest at all times and avoid false reassurances. Parents need to be prepared for the labor and birth experience with the knowledge and coping strategies they need.

After the birth, all hospital staff should be alerted about a fetal demise so that inappropriate encounters are avoided. Provision must be made for continuity of care (e.g., one primary nurse with minimal other staff; a nursing care plan on the chart). Privacy should be provided. A private room can be assigned and parents should be allowed to remain together as much as they wish. They also need to make their own decisions about their care as much as possible to give them a feeling of having some control. See Chapter 38 for a further discussion of the nursing management of perinatal loss.

One intervention that has helped women face the reality of having a child with an anomaly or experiencing an IUFD consists of allowing the woman and her family to express their grief and pain openly. Parents will be encouraged to verbalize their feelings if the nurse is a good listener. The grieving process must be supported. The nurse must be able to recognize denial, accept and understand anger, accept bargaining, support mourning, and reinforce acceptance. Parents need to understand that they may grieve differently and progress through the process at different rates (Ewton 1993; Kowalski 1991).

The options related to the parents' handling of their baby (e.g., seeing and holding the baby, baptism, funeral, memorial service) need to be clearly explained. Viewing the dead infant can help put to rest any negative images the mother or her partner may have fantasized. If the parents choose to see the baby, the baby's appearance should be explained in advance. The baby should be prepared for viewing. The nurse can bathe, dress, and wrap the baby or allow the parents to do this. The nurse should be with the woman and family when they first see their child, to give emotional support and answer questions. Grieving parents should not be avoided. The nurse should stay with them (or nearby) as much as possible and acknowledge the baby's anomaly or death. Mothers of infants with anomalies should be encouraged to hold and feed their infants if possible.

Parents need to be prepared for going home. Before discharge day, the nurse can conduct a "cognitive rehearsal" (e.g., discussion of leaving without the baby, dealing with family and friends, dealing with nursery and baby gifts). Providing a picture of the infant or other mementos (e.g., a lock of hair, articles used in caring for the baby, the baby's record with vital statistics) at the time of discharge helps to preserve memories of the event (Primeau and Recht 1994). A referral should be made for pastoral care or grief counseling. Parents can also be referred to a support group or a social worker in the community. Follow-up phone calls several weeks later let the family know that their loss was also meaningful to others and enables the nurse to assess the coping status of the grieving process (Brost and Kenny 1992; Brown 1992; Lawson 1990; Leon 1992).

▼ Evaluation

The evaluation of the plan of care for parents who experience a loss due to a fetal anomaly or death is based on verbal feedback from parents and direct observation of behaviors. This evaluation may take place throughout the period of hospital care before discharge or a number of weeks later through follow-up phone calls to the parents to assess coping and support.

HIGH-RISK CONDITIONS ASSOCIATED WITH THE THIRD STAGE OF LABOR

Amniotic Fluid Embolism

Description

Amniotic fluid embolism results from the infusion of a large amount of amniotic fluid into the maternal circulation. This infusion usually follows a tear in the fetal membrane that allows the leaking of amniotic fluid into an opening into the maternal circulation. The fluid can enter into the venous system at the site of the placenta or through any area of laceration. AFE can occur during the intrapartal period, resulting naturally from a tumultuous labor or from hypertonic contractions secondary to oxytocin induction. The entry of amniotic fluid into the maternal circulatory system is more easily facilitated by the pressure of uterine contractions. AFE can also appear immediately after the birth in the early postpartal period (Cunningham et al. 1993). It occurs in one in 15,000 to 20,000 pregnancies and is seen more often in multiparas, older women, short tumultuous labors, or cases of oxytocin augmentation (Burrow and Ferris 1995). Emboli from the debris in amniotic fluid (meconium, lanugo, mucus) block pulmonary capillaries. The major symptoms that result are acute respiratory distress, cyanosis, cardiovascular collapse, profound shock, and coma. Failure of coagulation (DIC) and hemorrhage may also occur, resulting from a thromboplastin-like material found in amniotic fluid. These symptoms are so traumatic that many women die within the first hour. The mortality rate of AFE is 80 percent. Fetal mortality rate is also high, and delivery must be facilitated immediately. Risk factors for AFE include a tumultuous labor, multiparity, advanced maternal age, macrosomia, IUFD, and operative birth.

Management

The goal of management of AFE is to reduce the respiratory and cardiac pathology and control hemorrhage. Supportive interventions are instituted immediately to maintain cardiac and respiratory function. Oxygen is a necessary supportive therapy. The woman is intubated and positive end-expiratory pressure (PEEP) may be ordered. Blood gases are drawn periodically. Because DIC is associated with AFE, blood replacement may be necessary as well as other blood products or heparin. A central venous pressure line may be inserted to guard against fluid overload. Cardiopulmonary resuscitation must be instituted immediately in the event of cardiac or pulmonary arrest. Immediate delivery of the fetus is essential, either with forceps if labor has progressed sufficiently or with an emergency cesarean section (Cunningham et al. 1993).

Nursing Process

▼ Assessment

It is essential to recognize the symptoms of AFE, which include respiratory symptoms (e.g., dyspnea, chest pain, cyanosis, or frothy sputum), cardiac symptoms (e.g., sudden hypotension or tachycardia), and sudden massive hemorrhage. These symptoms should immediately signal a critical situation, for they are never seen in healthy women during labor. Once AFE has been diagnosed, maternal vital signs should be assessed and recorded frequently, including the rate and quality of respirations, cardiac rate and quality, blood pressure, and neurologic status. Skin color, vaginal bleeding, and signs or symptoms of shock should also be assessed and recorded. Fetal well-being must be monitored continuously. These assessments govern the management of the entire health care team.

▼ Diagnosis

The nursing diagnoses for the woman experiencing an amniotic fluid embolism might include

- Impaired gas exchange related to blockage of the lungs from AFE
- Altered tissue perfusion: cardiopulmonary, related to AFE
- Risk for fluid volume deficit related to hemorrhage due to DIC secondary to AFE
- Fear for self and baby related to severity of condition

▼ Assessment

The plan for nursing care is based on the previous steps in the nursing process, as well as the plan of medical management:

- The woman will demonstrate an effective respiratory rate and have a normal pulmonary gas exchange
- The woman will demonstrate normal cardiac rate, blood pressure, and skin color
- The woman will show no complications of hemorrhage, hypovolemia, or DIC
- The woman will verbalize an understanding of the complications of AFE

▼ Intervention

AFE is an obstetric emergency of potentially catastrophic proportions (Cherry and Merkatz 1991; Clark et al. 1991). As soon as symptoms are identified and the physician has been notified, an intravenous line should be started. The nurse should immediately administer O_2 and monitor PEEP if ordered. The central venous pressure line should be monitored closely. Additional staff should be called in as necessary to manage the crisis. Continual communication that lets the woman and her family know what is occurring and what to expect is a nursing function of paramount importance. Emotional support is essential for the woman and her family in this critical situation. It may be advisable to enlist the help of a chaplain or clergyman of the family's choice to stay with the family while the crisis is being managed.

▼ Evaluation

The evaluation of an amniotic fluid embolism is based on resolution of maternal respiratory and cardiac crisis, management of hemorrhage, and safe delivery of the fetus.

Uterine Inversion

Description

Uterine inversion is the turning inside out of the uterus. It is a rare but serious condition that occurs in approximately one in 2000 deliveries during the third stage of labor (Cunningham et al. 1993). The cause of uterine inversion is not completely understood, although the condition has been recognized since the time of Hippocrates. It has been theorized that certain risk factors predispose a woman to uterine inversion, including uterine factors (e.g., fibroids, congenital anomalies or weaknesses of the uterine wall, relaxation of the myometrium, disturbances in contractility), placental factors (e.g., adherent placenta, short cord, fundal implantation), and iatrogenic factors (e.g., manual removal of the placenta, improper fundal pressure and massage, traction of the umbilical cord before placental separation, injudicious use of oxytocin, excessive maternal straining in the third stage of labor).

Although uterine inversion is most commonly found during the third stage of labor, it can be first discovered weeks later. Uterine inversion is therefore classified according to the period in which it was discovered. Acute uterine inversion occurs immediately after birth and before the contraction of the cervix. Subacute uterine inversion occurs with the establishment of contraction of the cervix. Chronic uterine inversion occurs when the inversion has been present but has gone unnoticed for more than 4 weeks. Classification of uterine inversion is also based on the degree of inversion. An incomplete uterine inversion occurs when the fundus is not beyond the internal os of the cervix. This may be detected as a result of hemorrhage, inability to palpate the fundus through the abdomen, or the palpation of a cup-shaped mass in the vagina on bimanual examination. Complete uterine inversion occurs when the fundus protrudes through the external os of the cervix and can be visualized as a bluish-gray mass in the vagina. Uterine prolapse occurs when the fundus protrudes through the vulva.

The symptoms of an incomplete uterine inversion may be minor, so that no treatment is carried out until they are recognized several weeks later. Treatment then depends on the symptoms, which are likely to be gangrene, infection, and necrosis. When the inversion is acute rather than chronic, hemorrhage and shock are likely and treatment must be instituted rapidly. Other symptoms likely to occur include severe pelvic pain, extreme fullness in the vagina, tachycardia, hemorrhage, hypovolemia, and shock. Inversion of the uterus should be considered if the shock is out of proportion to the hemorrhage.

Management

The first step in the management of uterine inversion is early diagnosis, because if untreated the cervix can become edematous and constrict the body of the uterus, making reinversion more difficult or impossible (Creasy and Resnik 1994). The second step is the management of hemorrhage or shock so that the woman is stabilized. Reinversion, or manual replacement of the uterus into the pelvis, is the third step in management. A tocolytic drug may be administered to aid in the replacement of the uterus. For reasons of pain relief as well as relaxation, general anesthesia is usually administered while the uterus is being manually replaced. The technique of manual replacement involves the birth attendant placing a hand in the vagina with the fingertips at the uterocervical junction. The uterus is lifted out of the pelvis and directed toward the umbilicus. The fundus is held in position for 3 to 5 minutes, at which time the fundus retracts back from the palm of the attendant's hand. After the uterus has been replaced, oxytocin is administered to stimulate uterine contraction and prevent further inversion. Antibiotics may be ordered to prevent infection. If reinversion is not successful, an emergency hysterectomy is performed.

Nursing Process

▼ Assessment

The routine postpartal assessments discussed in Chapter 29 are critical in the identification of uterine inversion. Observations of the normal and expected physiologic changes in the third and fourth stages of labor alert the nurse to any alterations during this time. Manual palpation of the uterus for consistency, position, and fundal height is critical and should not be taken lightly. Observations of maternal blood flow and degree of discomfort should be carefully recorded. Maternal vital signs should also be recorded regularly. A review of the woman's medical history and labor and birth process should be reviewed to identify risk factors for an inverted uterus.

▼ Diagnosis

The nursing diagnoses formulated for the woman experiencing uterine inversion depend on the degree of inversion, the symptoms resulting, and the period in which it is identified. Examples of potential nursing diagnoses include

- Altered tissue perfusion related to hemorrhage from uterine inversion
- Pain related to uterine inversion
- Anxiety and fear related to symptoms experienced due to an inverted uterus

▼ Planning

The plan of care is based on the assessment and the resultant nursing diagnoses. The plan should be stated in measurable outcomes, such as these examples:

- The uterus will be reinverted and the woman's condition stabilized
- The woman will express relief of fear and pain
- The woman will verbalize an understanding of her condition

▼ Intervention

One of the basic nursing interventions for an inverted uterus is prevention, by developing the habit of "guarding" the uterus when performing fundal massage in the third or fourth stages of labor. To guard the uterus, the nurse should use two hands for uterine massage. One hand is placed immediately above the symphysis pubis and allows the uterus to be stabilized, while the other hand is placed at the fundus to actively massage the uterus.

Once an inversion occurs, the nurse needs to continuously monitor maternal vital signs, administer analgesics or tocolytics as needed, and notify the anesthesia department that general anesthesia may be needed for a reinversion procedure (see Chapter 35). The nurse should observe the woman closely both during the procedure and afterward for signs of hemorrhage, hypovolemia, and shock. Intravenous fluids and oxytocin should be administered as ordered. Fundal massage should be avoided if possible, or applied very carefully. The woman and her family should be told what is happening.

▼ Evaluation

Evaluation of the plan of care is based on accomplishment of the goals. If the uterus is reinverted, hemorrhage is controlled, and the woman is stabilized and comfortable, the plan has been successful.

Hemorrhage

Hemorrhage in the third stage of labor is defined as a blood loss in excess of 500 mL after delivery of the baby and placenta. Hemorrhage is classified as acute or delayed. Acute hemorrhage occurs within the first 24 hours after delivery. Delayed hemorrhage can take place up to 31 days post partum. The causes of postpartum hemorrhage can be classified as follows (Cunningham et al. 1993):

1. Genital tract trauma: large episiotomy; third- or fourth-degree extension of the episiotomy; or lacerations of the vagina, cervix, perineum, or labia
2. Uterine bleeding: atony caused by hypotonic myometrium, general anesthesia relaxation, hypotension and poor perfusion of the myometrium, overdistention (e.g., with twins), prolonged labor, rapid labor, use of oxytocin in labor, previous uterine atony, chorioamnionitis, and high parity; retained placental tissue; or an adherent placenta
3. Coagulation defects: DIC

The three most common causes of hemorrhage immediately after delivery are lacerations of the birth canal, uterine atony, and retained placenta (Burrow and Ferris 1995; Cunningham et al. 1993; Danforth 1990). Other causes include hematoma formation and retained placental fragments. It is important that the woman be carefully assessed during the third stage of labor for indications of hemorrhage. The nurse assesses blood pressure, pulse, vaginal blood flow, and fundal firmness every 15 minutes during the first 2 hours after birth. A soft, or boggy, uterus suggests pooling of blood and possible hemorrhage (Fig. 25–9). Complete descriptions of postpartum hemorrhage and bleeding disorders as well as management are addressed in Chapter 35.

OBSTETRIC INTERVENTIONS IN HIGH-RISK SITUATIONS

When a woman is at high risk for developing a complication during childbirth, or does develop such a complication, modern obstetrics may employ some specific interventions. Among these modalities are induction of labor, augmentation of labor, or operative birth methods. In some cases, childbirth is best induced or augmented so that the process may be closely monitored and so that the process may be shortened for fetal or maternal reasons. Operative birth is undertaken either when the woman is unable to give birth vaginally without assistance, or when for maternal or fetal reasons it is again necessary to shorten the process.

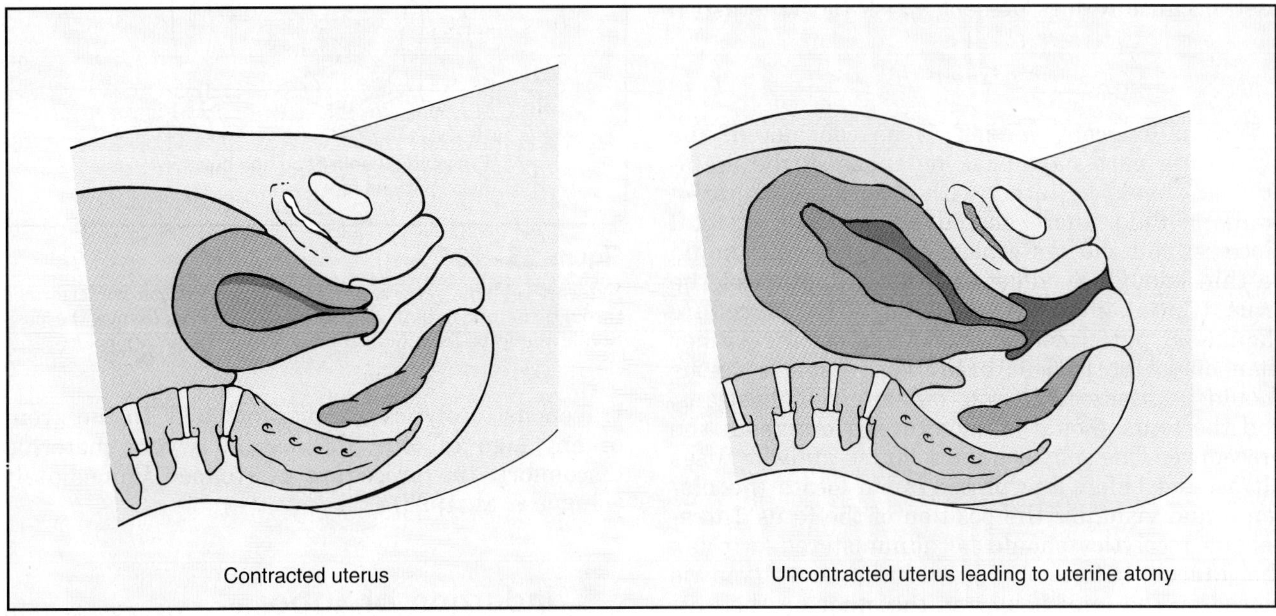

Figure 25–9

The uterus should contract firmly after birth, causing its intertwining muscle fibers to constrict blood vessels so that bleeding is minimal. When the uterine muscles fail to contract efficiently, uterine atony and postpartum hemorrhage result.

External Cephalic Version

Description

External cephalic version (ECV) consists of manipulation of the fetus through the maternal abdominal wall for the purpose of changing fetal position (Fig. 25–10). It is usually done to convert a breech to a vertex presentation, but may also be done to convert a persistent transverse lie (shoulder presentation) to a longitudinal lie (Cunningham et al. 1993). ECV can be performed after 37 weeks' gestation or during early labor. If it is done before that time, the fetus is more likely to spontaneously convert back to its original position.

An advantage of ECV is that it can reduce the risks inherent in malpresentations, particularly the breech presentation. The procedure also helps to avoid cesarean deliveries, but it does not have an effect on the overall cesarean delivery rate (Creasy and Resnik 1994; Cunningham et al. 1993; Laros et al. 1995). The disadvantage of ECV is that the fetus may spontaneously return to the malposition even when conversion is successful. Other risks include antepartum hemorrhage, premature rupture of membranes, preterm labor, or IUFD (Zhang et al. 1993).

A second type, called internal or podalic version, can be performed by an obstetrician for the purpose of turning a second twin to facilitate the birth during a vaginal delivery. The physician's hand is placed into the uterus to grasp the feet of the twin, thus turning it from a cephalic or transverse presentation to a breech presentation. Gentle traction is then exerted to deliver the twin. Internal version is not used as often today as in the past, because it does present a risk to the fetus.

Management

For an external version to be considered, the presenting part should not be engaged, the amniotic sac should be intact with a normal amount of amniotic fluid, there should be no signs of fetal distress, and the maternal abdominal wall should be thin enough to allow accurate palpation of the fetus (Cunningham et al. 1993). The procedure should be performed in the birth setting rather than on an outpatient basis. The woman's status should be assessed to rule out any complications, and the fetus should be monitored throughout the procedure. The physician or nurse-midwife uses ultrasound before the procedure to locate the placenta and visualize the position of the fetus. Intravenous tocolytics should be administered to relax the uterus before the procedure. One hand is placed on the fetal head and the other on the buttocks. The fetus is then rotated either forward or backward until the head is presenting (Fig. 25–10). This position is held in place until the intravenous tocolytics are discontinued. In the event of any sign of fetal distress or severe maternal discomfort, the procedure is stopped immediately (Zhang et al. 1993).

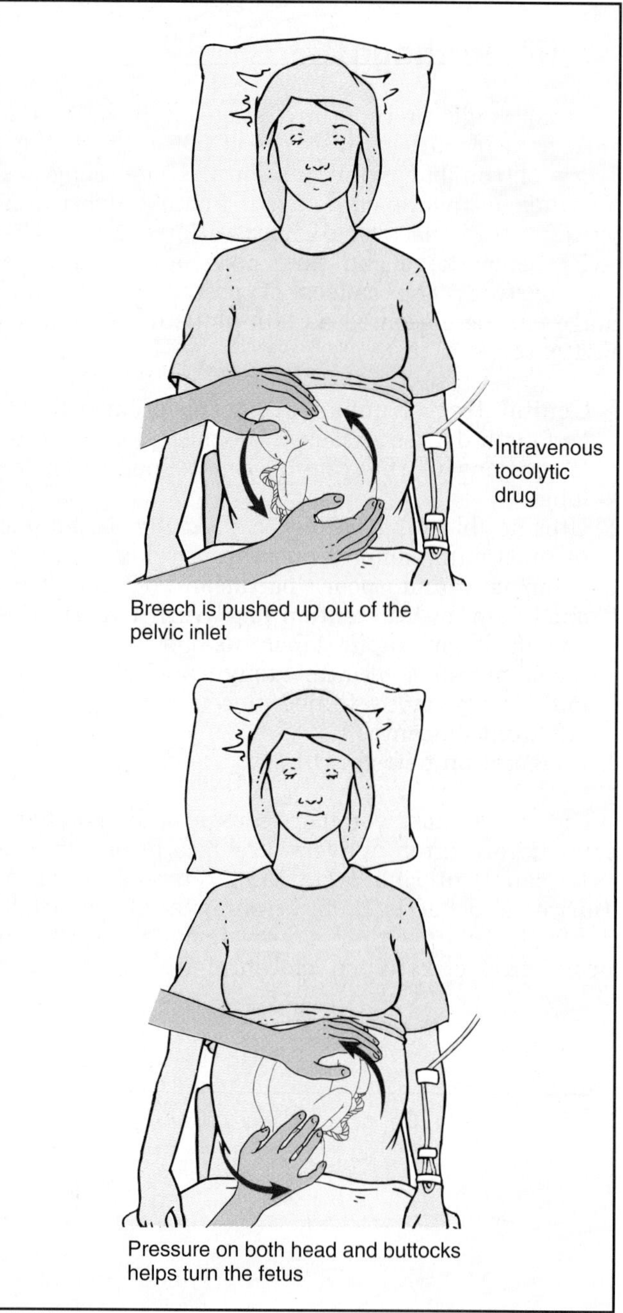

Figure 25–10

External cephalic version is a maneuver that can be performed through the abdominal wall in an attempt to change the position of the fetus from breech to cephalic presentation.

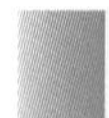

Induction of Labor

Induction of labor is the initiation of labor through mechanical or pharmacologic intervention. It continues to be controversial but is considered to be indicated for a number of obstetric complications that might have serious outcomes for the woman or her fetus if the pregnancy were allowed to continue. Examples of such antepartal complications include preeclampsia, postterm pregnancy, PROM, chorioamnionitis, IUGR, diabetes, fetal macrosomia, oligohydramnios, and suspected fetal jeopardy or demise. Induction may also be recommended because of logistic factors, such as the woman's geographic distance from the hospital, a maternal history of rapid labors, advanced cervical dilatation without signs of labor onset, or a known fetal anomaly that will require specialized pediatric care (Brouillard-Pierce 1993). Induction of labor should be implemented only for medical or obstetric reasons, never as an elective procedure for convenience only (ACOG 1991).

Both maternal and fetal readiness must be assured before induction. Maternal readiness relates to the status of the cervix. If the cervix is not yet ripe (i.e., has not begun to soften, efface or dilate), an induction is not likely to be successful. The Bishop score is used to assess cervical status (Bishop 1968) (see Chapter 23, Table 23–4); a score of 6 or more indicates the likelihood of a successful induction. Fetal readiness is based on the maturity of the fetus. This assessment is critical, for if an induction is initiated before fetal maturity, the delivery of a preterm infant with all the associated problems will result. Methods of confirming fetal maturity include a maternal history taking to verify dates, fundal height measurements, ultrasound evaluation, and amniocentesis to obtain amniotic fluid for the determination of the lecithin-sphingomyelin ratio and the presence of phosphatidyl-glycerol.

Methods to artificially initiate labor have been employed throughout history. Herbs, enemas, acupuncture, and even inflated bags were among the older methods used. Even today, stripping of the membranes, castor oil, nipple stimulation, and advice to engage in sexual intercourse are sometimes suggested as ways to initiate labor (Davis 1984; Mandeville and Troiano 1992). The efficacy of these traditional methods has not been well established. In current obstetric practice, the most common interventions to initiate labor include cervical ripening methods, amniotomy, and oxytocin infusion (ACOG 1991; Day and Snell 1993; Mastrogiannis and Knuppel 1995; Miller and Lorkovic 1993).

PROSTAGLANDIN E_2

Description

When a medical induction of labor is indicated, but the cervix is not favorable, a cervical ripening agent may be used. Extensive research over the past decade has found prostaglandin (PGE_2) gel to be safe and effective for this purpose. PGE_2 softens, effaces, dilates, and relaxes the smooth muscle of the cervix and may even stimulate the myometrium of the uterine fundus. The effectiveness of the gel application depends on the cervical status as determined by a Bishop score (Bishop 1968). With a Bishop score of 4 to 5, the intravaginal and intracervical routes are equally effective, although intravaginal application more frequently produces an onset of labor without the use of oxytocin. With a Bishop score of 1 to 2, the intracervical route is more effective. PGE_2 has been approved by the Food and Drug Administration for intracervical application but not yet for intravaginal application (Miller and Lorkovic 1993). Contraindications to the use of PGE_2 include vaginal bleeding; multiple gestation; malposition; IUFD demise; PID; maternal fever; a vertical uterine scar; and cardiac, pulmonary, renal, or hepatic disease (Mandeville and Troiano 1992; Miller and Lorkovic 1993).

Management

Before the woman is given a cervical ripening agent, an informed consent must be obtained. An assessment of fetal well-being and position as well as maternal cervical status should be made. With the woman in a supine position, PGE_2 gel is applied intracervically with a flexible catheter. The woman is asked to rest in bed for 1 to 2 hours after insertion of the gel, and fetal heart rate and uterine activity are monitored continuously. Maternal vital signs are also monitored every hour. If no adverse maternal or fetal signs are seen during this initial period of time, the woman may get up and walk. If the cervix has begun to show signs of ripening, the woman is sent home and instructed to return the following day for oxytocin induction. If no cervical changes are noted, additional doses of PGE_2 can be given every 4 to 6 hours (Miller and Lorkovic 1993).

AMNIOTOMY

Description

An amniotomy, AROM, is performed by inserting an instrument called an Amnihook into the vagina next to the examining fingers during a vaginal examination (see Procedure 25–2). The cervix must be sufficiently dilated (at least 2 cm) for the amniotic sac to be accessible. The tip of the Amnihook is used to puncture the sac and release the amniotic fluid.

There are several advantages of an amniotomy. The amniotic fluid may be evaluated for the presence of meconium, the initial stool of the fetus that can be expelled in utero as a response to distress. An amniotomy permits the use of internal fetal monitoring and fetal scalp sampling; neither procedure can be utilized when the membranes

PROCEDURE 25–2

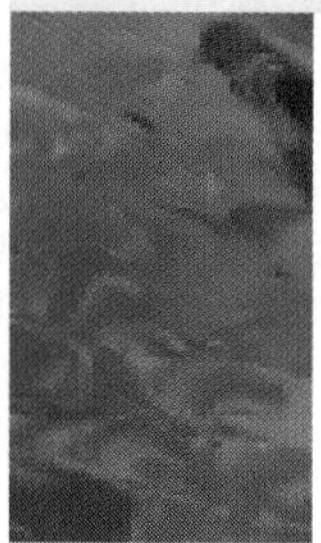

Assisting With Amniotomy

▼ PURPOSE

Amniotomy (artificial rupture of membranes) is performed to induce or augment labor, to insert an internal fetal electrode or an intrauterine pressure catheter for electronic fetal monitoring, or to obtain a fetal scalp blood sample.

▼ EQUIPMENT

- Electronic fetal monitor or Doppler ultrasound stethoscope
- sterile gloves
- sterile lubricant
- Amnihook
- absorbent underpads

1 Prepare the woman for amniotomy by explaining the procedure, including the reason it is being done, and describing the sensations to expect. **Anticipatory guidance will decrease the woman's anxiety and facilitate cooperation during the procedure.**

2 Lower the head of the bed. Position the woman so that her knees are flexed. Ask her to separate her legs and relax them. Place pads under the woman's buttocks to absorb the amniotic fluid after amniotomy. Place a wedge under the woman's right or left hip to maintain a slight lateral tilt during the procedure. **Proper positioning allows the health care provider easier access to the cervix and enhances the woman's ability to relax. A wedge is used when the woman is in the supine position to prevent compression of the maternal blood vessels and subsequent supine hypotension.**

3 Check the fetal heart rate by Doppler or apply the external fetal monitor ultrasound transducer. **Fetal well-being must be confirmed before and after amniotomy.**

4 Assist the woman's health care provider by applying sterile lubricant to his or her gloved hand and opening the sterile package containing the Amnihook. **Lubricant decreases friction between the gloved hand and vaginal wall during the procedure. Sterile technique is essential during amniotomy to prevent potential contamination and decrease the risks of maternal and fetal infection.**

5 Instruct the woman to relax the pelvic floor muscles and to begin slow, rhythmic breathing. **Relaxation of the pelvic floor muscles and slow, rhythmic breathing make performance of the procedure easier and contribute to the woman's relaxation and comfort during the procedure.**

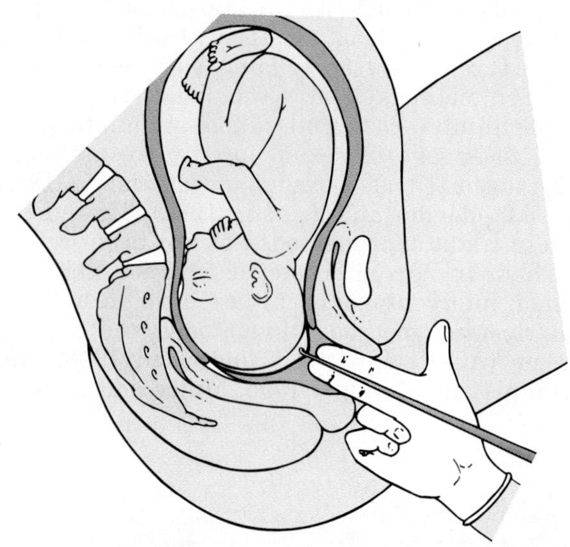

Amnihook ruptures the membranes

Continued on facing page

PROCEDURE 25–2 Continued

6 Place one hand on the uterine fundus and apply gentle downward pressure to maintain contact between the fetal head and the cervix while the woman's health care provider inserts an Amnihook into the vagina next to the examining fingers during a vaginal examination. The health care provider uses the tip of the Amnihook to puncture the amniotic sac, allowing the amniotic fluid to be released. **The risk of prolapsed cord after amniotomy will be decreased if the fetal head is engaged and well applied to the cervix.**

7 Evaluate the color, amount, and odor of amniotic fluid present after amniotomy. Note whether the amniotic fluid is bloody. **The color, amount, and odor of amniotic fluid observed after amniotomy can correlate with fetal well-being. Absent, decreased, or increased amounts of amniotic fluid may indicate fetal stress. (Normal amniotic fluid volume is approximately 1000 ml. The position of the presenting part against the cervix will affect the amount of fluid expelled.) The amniotic fluid should be clear or slightly cloudy and should have no odor. Meconium-stained amniotic fluid (dark green or brown in color) may indicate fetal stress and place the infant at risk for meconium aspiration. Foul-smelling amniotic fluid may correlate with infection. Bloody amniotic fluid may indicate a complication.**

8 Evaluate fetal heart rate after amniotomy. **Fetal well-being must be confirmed after amniotomy to assess fetal tolerance to the procedure.**

9 Change the underpad and help the woman to a comfortable position. **A dry underpad enhances maternal comfort.**

10 Record your findings. **Information regarding the status of membranes and the amount, color, and odor of amniotic fluid is important when assessing fetal well-being and labor progress and in planning for delivery.**

11 Record maternal temperature every 2 hours. **A rise in maternal temperature might indicate an intrauterine infection (chorioamnionitis).**

are intact. Rupture of the membranes facilitates the initiation of labor because the release of fluid allows descent of the presenting part of the fetus, increases pressure from the fetus against the cervix, and causes mechanical irritation from the presenting part to stimulate uterine contractions (Ferguson reflex). With a favorable cervix as determined by a Bishop score, an amniotomy by a physician or nurse-midwife carries a high success rate of inducing labor within 12 to 24 hours (Busowski and Parsons 1995). The contractions after amniotomy do not differ from those with a spontaneous labor and do not carry the risk of hypertonus or uterine rupture as seen with oxytocin induction. Proponents of amniotomy also cite a shortening of the length of labor, but research does not always support this claim. Some studies have shown a decrease in the first stage of labor; others have shown no consistent effect of amniotomy on the length of the first stage (Cunningham et al. 1993).

There are potential disadvantages of amniotomy. During the procedure, bleeding, compression of the umbilical cord, decreased fetal heart rate, decreased uterine perfusion, rupture of abnormal vessels, and prolapse of the umbilical cord (if the presenting part is not engaged) are possible risks. Rupture of abnormal vessels may be avoided by careful examination of the membranes before the amniotomy is performed. The risk of a prolapsed cord may be minimized by waiting to rupture the membranes until the fetal head is engaged in the pelvis. A placental abruption (due to sudden decompression of the uterus from loss of fluid) and AFE (due to sudden decompression and entry of amniotic fluid into the maternal vascular system) are also potential risks. Adverse effects of amniotomy as labor proceeds are compression of the cord vessels and, theoretically, disalignment of the bones of the fetal head and an increase in fetal head compression or molding. Fetal heart rate changes have been reported by some authors, but the significance of these patterns is unclear (Busowski and Parsons 1995).

Amniotomy may potentiate infection of the membranes, chorioamnionitis, especially if delivery does not occur within 12 to 24 hours. This has not been well addressed in the literature, and it may be difficult to distinguish the effect of amniotomy from other variables such as multiple vaginal examinations and the application of indwelling monitoring devices. If labor is not successfully induced by amniotomy alone, oxytocin induction or cesarean delivery may be necessary.

Management

When amniotomy is chosen as the method of labor induction, the woman is admitted to the birth site for the procedure. The procedure should be explained to her as well as the reasons for its use and what she will experience. The woman should be assessed to confirm that (1) the pregnancy is full term, (2) the presenting part is well engaged into the pelvis, (3) the fetal position is identified, (4) there is no indication of placenta previa, and (5) there is no history of herpesvirus Type II. Fetal heart tones are auscultated before, during, and after the amniotomy to rule out occult cord prolapse. If indicated, internal fetal monitoring can be applied when the amniotomy is performed, but this limits the mobility of the woman. The woman should be helped to assume a comfortable position on her back, and a clean pad should be placed under her hips. When the membranes are ruptured, the amniotic fluid should be assessed for amount, color, and odor. The initial amount of fluid will vary and fluid will continue to leak with each contraction. The amniotic fluid should be clear or slightly cloudy; if it appears dark green or brown, it has been stained by meconium; if it is bloody, a placental abruption should be considered. In either case, the fetus should be monitored continuously. The amniotic fluid should have no odor; a foul-smelling odor may indicate infection (AWHONN 1993).

OXYTOCIN

Description

The most common agent for induction of labor is oxytocin, a synthetic hormone. Endogenous oxytocin is released naturally from the posterior pituitary and is discussed in Chapter 22. Synthetic oxytocin has a similar effect in stimulating uterine contractions. It affects the uterine myometrial cells by increasing the excitability of the muscle cell, increasing the strength of contraction, and facilitating the transfer of the contraction from one cell to the next. "The uterine response to oxytocin increases slowly from 20 to 30 weeks of gestation and is unchanged from 34 weeks until term, at which time sensitivity rapidly increases" (ACOG 1991). By 40 weeks' gestation the response to oxytocin varies widely, some women being sensitive to even small amounts. The cervical status is the factor that most greatly influences the amount of oxytocin needed to produce a successful labor induction. If the cervix is ripe, less oxytocin will be needed than if it is still firm, uneffaced, and closed. Oxytocin also has an effect on the cardiovascular and renal systems. Maternal blood pressure may rise and cardiac output and stroke volume are increased. Urinary output may decrease, because oxytocin has an antidiuretic effect (Brodsky and Pelzar 1991; Cunningham et al. 1993).

Oxytocin is contraindicated for women with preeclampsia, overdistention of the uterus, a history of previous major surgery of the uterus, placenta previa, an unripe cervix, CPD, malpresentation or malposition of the fetus, fetal distress, or a preterm infant. The maternal risks of oxytocin induction include hyperstimulation of the uterus, uterine rupture, placental abruption, cervical lacerations, and AFE. Fetal risks include trauma, hypoxia, and hyperbilirubinemia. If the woman is not monitored closely, water intoxication (hypotension, tachycardia, cardiac arrhythmia, shortness of breath, nausea, and vomiting) can occur as a result of the infusion of too much oxytocin and large volumes of the electrolyte solution. There is also a higher incidence of fetal monitoring, epidural anesthesia, and cesarean delivery with oxytocin induction (Cunningham et al. 1993; Lopez-Zeno et al. 1992).

Management

Before the administration of oxytocin, a complete review of maternal history should be conducted and an assessment made to identify risk factors. The procedure for induction should be explained to the woman and her family. A primary intravenous line is started with a physiologic electrolyte solution. The secondary line is then piggybacked with 10 units (10,000 mU) of oxytocin in a 1-L solution of fluids, and the rate is adjusted with a controlled infusion pump device. This allows oxytocin infusion to be discontinued immediately if it becomes necessary. Other intravenous medications should not be administered through the oxytocin line; they may be given through the primary line.

The preferred oxytocin dosage is the minimal amount necessary to maintain an adequate contraction pattern, characterized by three to five contractions in a 10-minute period with resultant cervical dilatation (ACOG 1995b). If contractions are more frequent than every 2 minutes, contraction quality may be decreased. Usually the initial dose ranges from 0.5 mU/min to 1 mU/min (1 mU/min = 6 mL/hr). The dosage is increased gradually by 1 to 2 mU/min at 15- to 60-minute intervals until the desired contraction pattern is established (Table 25–2). Most women require no more than 4 to 8 mU of oxytocin per minute to achieve progressive cervical dilatation.

Fetal heart rate, resting uterine tone, and contraction pattern should be monitored continuously

Table 25–2

OXYTOCIN ADMINISTRATION: DOSAGE AND INFUSION RATES

For use with an IV pump administering 20 gtt/mL; solution is 10 U of oxytocin in 1000 mL of fluid.

DOSAGE (mU/min)	INFUSION RATE (mL/hr)
0.5	3
1.0	6
2.0	12
3.0	18
4.0	24
5.0	30
6.0	36
7.0	42
8.0	48
9.0	54
10.0	60
12.0	72
15.0	90
18.0	108
20.0	120

Adapted from Marshall, C. (1985). The art of induction/augmentation of labor. *Journal of Obstetric, Gynecologic, and Neonatal Nursing,* 14 (1), 22–28.

and maternal blood pressure should be assessed at 30-minute intervals, or when the oxytocin rate is evaluated for dosage maintenance, increase, or decrease. The oxytocin infusion should be discontinued immediately if signs of uterine hypersensitivity or fetal distress occur. With signs of fetal distress, the woman should be placed in the left lateral position and O_2 should be administered by mask. Because the circulating half-life of oxytocin is 3 to 4 minutes, the maternal plasma concentration falls rapidly after the infusion is discontinued. If adverse maternal or fetal symptoms continue, a tocolytic drug may be used to facilitate uterine relaxation. Although rare, uterine rupture and water intoxication should be considered potential complications of induction, and the woman should be periodically assessed for the development of these conditions. Intake and output should be recorded. If a regular labor pattern is not established after 8 to 12 hours of oxytocin infusion, it should be discontinued. Daily or serial induction attempts may then be tried. If labor is not induced after several attempts, a cesarean delivery is performed.

The nurse should remain with the woman at all times and a physician should be present within the birth setting during oxytocin infusion. Induction of labor by oxytocin infusion is described in Procedure 25–3. Accurate, regular documentation should be made in the woman's chart and on the electronic fetal monitor strip. A written protocol for the management of an induction, based on current standards of practice, should be established in every birth setting (ACOG 1991; Brodsky and Pelzar 1991; Satin et al. 1992; AWHONN 1993).

AUGMENTATION OF LABOR

Description

Augmentation of labor is the use of an intervention to promote a more effective labor pattern in a dysfunctional labor that has already started spontaneously. Years ago, oxytocin was administered buccally (with a series of small tablets placed between the upper lip and gum) for augmentation of labor. Today, some clinicians use nipple stimulation, acupressure, or amniotomy for augmentation of the labor process. However, most practitioners use intravenous oxytocin in a manner designed to produce efficient, regular uterine contractions.

Management

Many birth attendants today follow a method of active labor management. With this approach, labor is carefully plotted on a partograph, and any suggestion of slow progress (less than 1 cm/hr of dilatation) based on the evaluation of the graph is cause for intervention with oxytocin, assuming that CPD has been ruled out (O'Herlihy 1993). This active management approach is based on the theory that early intervention in dysfunctional labors, with aggressive use of oxytocin, shortens labor and reduces the incidence of cesarean birth. Higher doses of oxytocin are used with this active management approach. Research is being conducted to determine the safety and efficacy of active management for labor. It has been estimated that currently more than 25 percent of in-hospital parturients receive oxytocin in labor (Mandeville and Troiano 1992). The principles of management outlined above for the induction of labor are followed for augmentation of labor.

Nursing Process

▼ Assessment

The assessment of the woman and her fetus before labor induction is important to rule out any contraindications. The woman's history should be reviewed to identify antepartal complications. The woman's estimated date of confinement and other dating parameters should be confirmed to ensure that the fetus is full term. The position of the fetus should be assessed by performing Leopold ma-

PROCEDURE 25–3

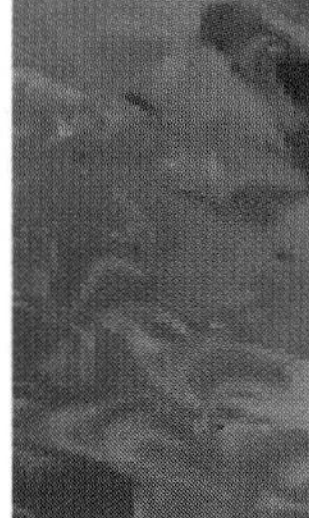

Induction of Labor by Oxytocin Infusion

▼ PURPOSE

To stimulate the onset of uterine contractions in order to facilitate progressive cervical effacement and dilatation and descent of the fetus. The decision to initiate labor using oxytocin is made only after risk factors, cervical readiness, and fetal maturity are evaluated.

▼ EQUIPMENT

- Electronic fetal monitor for continuous monitoring of fetal heart rate and uterine activity
- oxytocin (Pitocin)
- infusion pump

1 Explain the procedure for oxytocin induction of labor to the woman and her partner. Include the following points in your discussion:

- Rationale for oxytocin induction of labor
- Expected maternal response to oxytocin
- Nursing care during oxytocin infusion (frequency of assessment of vital signs, uterine contractions, and fetal heart rate; adjustments in oxytocin flow rate; comfort measures)

An explanation of the procedure for the induction of labor reduces the woman's anxiety and promotes her compliance.

2 Place the woman on the fetal monitor to assess fetal well-being and to establish a baseline for uterine activity. A minimum of 20 minutes of fetal monitoring before induction of labor is essential. Do not start the oxytocin infusion if nonreassuring fetal heart rate patterns are identified. **A baseline of fetal well-being and uterine activity must be established before induction so that the nurse will recognize complications associated with oxytocin administration, such as uterine hyperstimulation and fetal distress.**

3 Establish a primary intravenous line for the infusion of a physiologic electrolyte solution without oxytocin. **A primary intravenous line is essential to maintain the intravenous infusion when the oxytocin infusion is stopped.**

4 Prepare oxytocin solution according to hospital policy or as follows: Add 10 units of oxytocin to 1000 ml of lactated Ringer solution or other physiologic electrolyte solution. Make sure the oxytocin solution is labeled. **Hospital protocols may vary as to oxytocin concentrations used and dosing regimens.**

5 Attach intravenous tubing to the oxytocin solution. Set up an intravenous infusion pump with the oxytocin solution according to the manufacturer's guidelines. **An intravenous infusion pump must be used during oxytocin induction to ensure that accurate volume and dosage of oxytocin are administered to the woman.**

6 Connect a secondary line containing the oxytocin infusion as close as possible to the primary venipuncture site. **An oxytocin infusion is connected as close as possible to the primary venipuncture site to avoid administering a bolus dose of oxytocin, which would occur if the oxytocin were piggybacked distal to the venipuncture site and the primary line infusion rate were increased.**

Continued on facing page

PROCEDURE 25–3 Continued

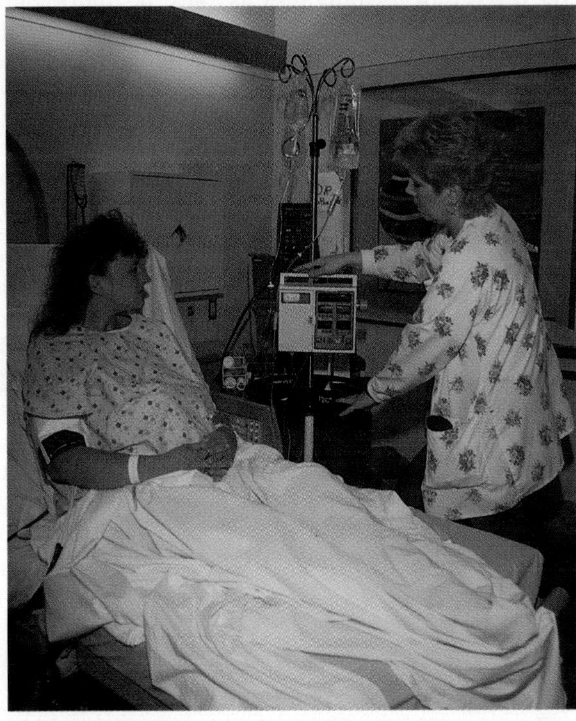

7 Start oxytocin infusion according to hospital protocol or physician's written orders. **The initial dose of oxytocin is usually 0.5 to 1.0 mU/min.**

8 Assess and record the woman's blood pressure and uterine contractions and the fetal heart rate before each increase in oxytocin dosage. Assess and record maternal intake and output. **During oxytocin administration, accurate monitoring of uterine contraction frequency, duration, and intensity and uterine resting tone is essential to evaluate the effect of each oxytocin dosage level and determine the need to increase the infusion rate. An ongoing assessment of the woman's fluid balance (intake and output) is necessary since oxytocin has an antidiuretic effect.**

9 Increase the dosage of oxytocin gradually by 1 to 2 mU/min at the dosing interval specified by hospital policy or physician's written orders until an effective labor pattern is established. **Different oxytocin protocols have been studied and suggest that acceptable dosing intervals may vary from 15 to 60 minutes (ACOG 1995a, 1995b).**

10 Discontinue the oxytocin infusion and notify a physician if maternal or fetal complications develop, including uterine hyperstimulation (contractions closer than every 2 minutes), hypertonic uterine contractions (contraction duration greater than 90 seconds), elevated uterine resting tone (resting tone greater than 20 mm Hg), or nonreassuring fetal heart rate patterns. **Since the half-life of oxytocin is very short (1 to 6 minutes), stopping an oxytocin infusion may quickly reverse the effects of excessive uterine activity and improve fetal oxygenation.**

11 Initiate additional nursing interventions as necessary, including

- Positioning the patient on her left side
- Increasing the primary intravenous fluid rate
- Initiating oxygen via a face mask
- Administering (in some cases) a tocolytic agent, such as terbutaline, to halt excessive uterine activity

Nursing interventions to improve uteroplacental perfusion and fetal oxygenation are indicated when fetal stress results from excessive uterine activity.

neuvers. It is essential that the fetus be engaged into the pelvis; this can be assessed by abdominal palpation and vaginal examination. All maternal vital signs should be recorded and the fetal heart rate assessed. When amniotomy is performed, the fetal response should be assessed and recorded carefully. The amount, color, and odor of the fluid should also be documented. When oxytocin infusion is initiated, continuous electronic fetal monitoring should be used to assess fetal heart rate and the contraction pattern. Maternal urinary output should be measured to assess for fluid retention, fluid deficit, and water intoxication. Vaginal examinations should be made at regular intervals to determine the progression of cervical dilatation, effacement, and station. If signs of uterine hyperstimulation or fetal distress occur, the nurse must discontinue the oxytocin infusion immediately, continue the infusion of the physiologic electrolyte solution, and notify the physician.

▼ Diagnosis

The nursing diagnoses that might be identified for the woman being induced follow:

- Pain related to increased contraction pattern (frequency, duration, and intensity)
- Risk of fetal injury related to amniotomy or decreased placental perfusion from hypertonic contraction pattern
- Anxiety and fear related to apprehension about the induction procedure
- Knowledge deficit: lack of information related to the induction procedure

▼ Planning

The specific goals used to measure the outcomes of these diagnoses might be as follows:

- The woman will remain comfortable during the induced labor through the use of nonpharmacologic or pharmacologic pain relief measures
- The fetal heart rate and variability will remain within normal limits
- The woman will exhibit little anxiety related to the induction procedure
- The woman will ask questions and verbalize her understanding of the induction procedure

▼ Intervention

Accurate preparation of the oxytocin infusion is an important component in the care of the woman being induced (see Procedure 25–3). Constant assessment of the woman and fetus is essential once the infusion has begun. The components of this assessment are discussed above. If any deviations from normal are noted in the contraction pattern or the fetal heart rate pattern, the oxytocin infusion should be discontinued immediately. In case of fetal bradycardia, tachycardia, or decreased baseline variability, the woman should be positioned on her left side and oxygen administered per face mask at 7 to 10 L/min. Nurses caring for women receiving oxytocin must individualize care, since maternal response to oxytocin varies widely. Nursing interventions also include attention to the woman's comfort level. When an amniotomy is performed, the woman should be placed on a bedpan or several Chux pads to collect the fluid. The pads should be changed regularly throughout labor to keep the woman dry and prevent infection. When contractions increase in frequency, duration, and intensity, the woman should be helped to use breathing and relaxation strategies to deal with the discomfort. Contractions may be more painful when oxytocin is being administered, so both nonpharmacologic pain management strategies and pharmacologic agents should be used as necessary. Position changes may help in the management of pain. Education and emotional support throughout any of the induction procedures must be ongoing. Careful documentation of all assessments and interventions is important to the care of the woman being induced.

▼ Evaluation

The evaluation of the plan of care for the woman being induced is based on the identified outcome goals. The desired outcomes are successful induction of the labor, no complications for the woman, and a safe delivery of the infant.

OPERATIVE OBSTETRICS

Occasionally a spontaneous vaginal birth is not possible. Mechanical or physiologic problems can occur that make it difficult for a woman to make the maternal effort needed for second-stage labor. Alternatively, fetal reasons may make it advisable for birth to occur quickly in the presence of a pediatric team ready for resuscitation. In these cases, several common methods of operative intervention are available today: episiotomy, forceps, vacuum extraction, and cesarean delivery.

EPISIOTOMY

Episiotomy, surgical incision of the perineum to facilitate birth, has become a customary procedure in modern obstetrics. It is performed by the physician or midwife as the fetal head distends the perineum immediately before birth (Fig. 25–11). The midline episiotomy is cut through the midline of the perineum. The incision for the mediolateral episiotomy is cut at an angle beginning from the top of the midline of the perineum and slanting laterally and downward toward the ischial tuberosity. A right mediolateral episiotomy is cut to the right of the midline; a left mediolateral episiotomy is cut to the left of the midline. In the United States the midline episiotomy is performed more frequently than the mediolateral episiotomy. The advantages of the former over the latter are that it can be repaired more easily and heals with less pain. The disadvantage of a midline episiotomy is that it may extend into a laceration of the rectal sphincter more frequently than does the mediolateral episiotomy. When the rectal sphincter is torn during birth, this is called a third-degree perineal laceration. When both the rectal sphincter and the anterior rectal wall are torn, this is called a fourth-degree perineal laceration (Cunningham et al. 1993).

An episiotomy may be cut when a difficult delivery of the infant's shoulders (shoulder dystocia) is anticipated. Shoulder dystocia may occur if the size of the infant is large in proportion to the size of the maternal pelvis. In this case an episiotomy would allow the physician or midwife more room for manual maneuvers to free the impacted shoulders of the infant. Episiotomies may be used with forceps to provide more room for their application and, in cases of fetal distress, to shorten the second stage. However, the routine use of episiotomy is not supported by current research.

Historically, episiotomy was advocated by Pomeroy in 1918 as a procedure to prevent undue pressure on the fetal head. It was thought that if the head were allowed to crown slowly as the perineum stretched, the infant might sustain brain damage. However, this idea has never been supported by scientific evidence. Bowe (1981) investigated Apgar scores for infants born over intact perineums as opposed to episiotomy and found them to be lower at 1 minute for the episiotomy group and similar at 5 minutes. This implies that a slow stretching of the perineum is not detrimental to the infant's condition at birth.

A common rationale for episiotomy is that if the perineum is allowed to tear, the edges will be uneven and therefore more difficult both to repair and to heal. Although in some circumstances the edges of a laceration may be more irregular than those of an episiotomy, the idea that a laceration of comparable size to an episiotomy is more painful when healing is not supported by the literature. Researchers have found either no difference in pain and healing time or improved outcomes for those with lacerations (Klein et al. 1992). One reason may be that naturally occurring lacerations often involve less tissue and muscle impairment than do episiotomies. Prevention of pelvic relaxation has also been offered as a rationale for episiotomy. Often, pelvic relaxation is not evident until menopause or later. Researchers have not addressed the effect of episiotomy on long-term pelvic muscle function. Short-term function has been shown to be similar in both groups.

There are several potential complications of episiotomies that indicate the need to question their routine use. Blood loss is frequently increased to more than 500 mL for a vaginal delivery when an episiotomy is performed. Infection may result in increased pain and poor healing, necessitating the use of antibiotics. Necrotizing fasciitis is a rare but potentially life-threatening complication of episiotomy.

Some authors have described an increased risk of rectal injury when episiotomy is performed. The

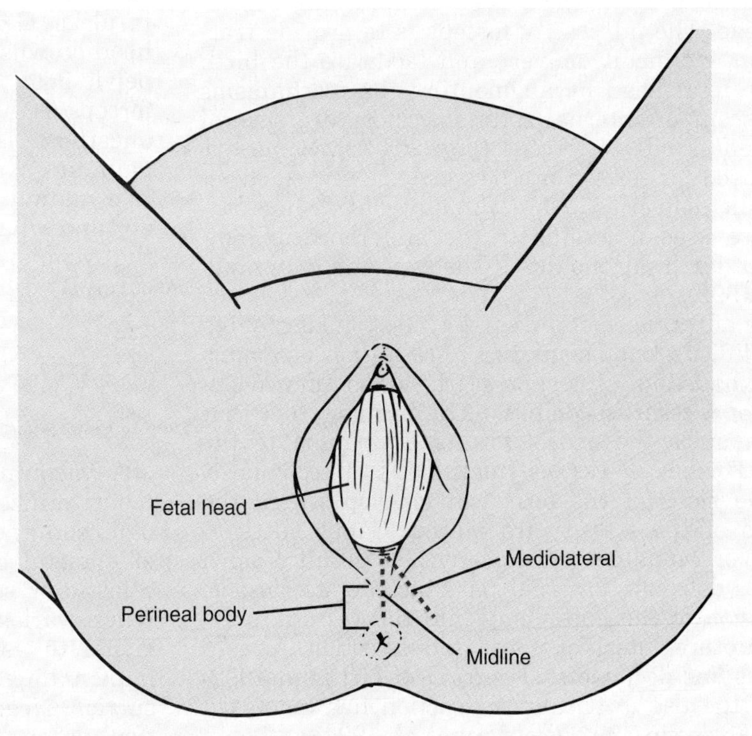

Figure 25–11

An episiotomy is a surgical incision made to facilitate birth as the fetal head distends the perineum • A midline episiotomy is cut through the midline of the perineum • The incision for a mediolateral episiotomy is cut at an angle beginning from the top of the midline of the perineum and slanting laterally and downward toward the ischial tuberosity.

highest risk is for use of both forceps and episiotomy simultaneously for delivery (Fernando et al. 1995; Homsi et al. 1994). Episiotomy may also have a detrimental effect on postpartum sexual function. Women with lacerations but no episiotomy have reported a more prompt resumption of postpartum intercourse and less dyspareunia than those with episiotomies (Klein et al. 1992).

Several studies have evaluated a number of factors that may be associated with perineal outcome. Primiparity, anesthesia use, and very large or small infants are associated with a higher incidence of episiotomy (Nodine and Roberts 1987). Researchers have not found a correlation among perineal outcome and maternal age, prepregnancy weight, weight gain in pregnancy, hematocrit values at term, episodes of prenatal vaginitis, or position used for birth (Nodine and Roberts 1987).

FORCEPS

Description

The invention of forceps has been attributed to the British obstetrician Peter Chamberlen at the beginning of the seventeenth century. Forceps are scissor-like instruments consisting of forged steel blades with a cephalic curve conforming to the fetal head and a pelvic curve conforming to the maternal pelvis. They are composed of several parts: the blades, which can be solid or open (fenestrated), are placed on either side of the baby's head; the shank is the area leading from the blade to the handle; and the handle is used to provide gentle traction. The forceps have a lock at the handle to prevent them from compressing the fetal head. The purpose of forceps is to provide traction in a difficult delivery and facilitate the birth of the fetal head by augmenting the mechanisms of descent or internal rotation. There are several different kinds of forceps (Fig. 25–12). Some are best used for certain procedures (e.g., low or outlet cephalic deliveries or breech deliveries), while others are used according to the preference of individual birth attendants (Gilstrap and Cunningham 1992).

The advantages of forceps include the shortening of a difficult expulsion stage, prevention of maternal exhaustion, protection of the fetus, and avoidance of a cesarean delivery. The primary risk that accompanies the use of forceps is trauma to the baby. Forceps marks, or small areas of ecchymosis on the sides of the face, can develop where the blades of the forceps are placed. Caput succedaneum or cephalhematoma may also result from a forceps delivery. Maternal risks include lacerations, extension of the episiotomy into the rectum, uterine rupture, uterine atony, and infection. Use of forceps has declined (4.3 percent of births in 1992) while the use of vacuum extraction has increased (4.4 percent in 1992) (Ventura et al. 1994).

Management

There are three types of forceps operations: outlet forceps, low forceps, and midforceps (ACOG 1994). Outlet forceps operations require full cervical dilatation with the fetal head on the pelvic floor. The fetal scalp should be visible at the introitus, and the sagittal suture of the fetal head should be in or near the anteroposterior diameter of the pelvis. There should be no more than a 45-degree rotation from an occiput anterior or occiput posterior position. The use of low forceps requires that the leading point of the skull be at a station of +2 or more. Midforceps is the application of forceps when the fetal head is engaged but the leading point of the skull is above +2 station. Midforceps are rarely used today.

Fetal indications for a forceps delivery include fetal distress, fetal malpresentations, large fetal size, and the aftercoming head in a breech presentation. Maternal indications include a prolonged labor, maternal exhaustion with limited maternal reserve, maternal illness, and regional anesthesia. Forceps are contraindicated (1) when the fetal position or station is uncertain, (2) with CPD, (3) with a cervix that is not fully dilated, (4) in an inadequate trial of labor, (5) with inadequate anesthesia or analgesia, and (6) with an inexperienced operator (ACOG 1994; Cunningham et al. 1993).

Forceps must be applied very carefully. One blade is placed on one side of the fetal head, followed by placement of the other blade. The position of the fetus must be known at all times so that the forceps are placed on each side of the head over the ears, not over the soft parts of the face. An episiotomy is made after the forceps are in place. Gentle traction is then applied until the head crowns (Fig. 25–12). Once the head is on the pelvic floor, the forceps are removed. Delivery with forceps is accomplished with regional or general anesthesia, so that sensations of pressure, but not pain, are experienced. The woman should be given information about the procedure of a forceps delivery and what she can expect. After the birth, both the woman and the baby should be examined carefully to identify signs of trauma.

VACUUM EXTRACTION

Description

A vacuum extractor is another type of instrument utilized to assist in delivering the fetus (Johnson and Pace 1993). The instrument consists of a metal or plastic cup connected by a flexible Silastic or rubber tubing to a vacuum pump. The pump varies the strength of the suction with a gauge to assess the force of the suction and a hand pump or floor valve that can interrupt the suction. Negative pressure is exerted with the suction pump, and traction is applied to the fetal

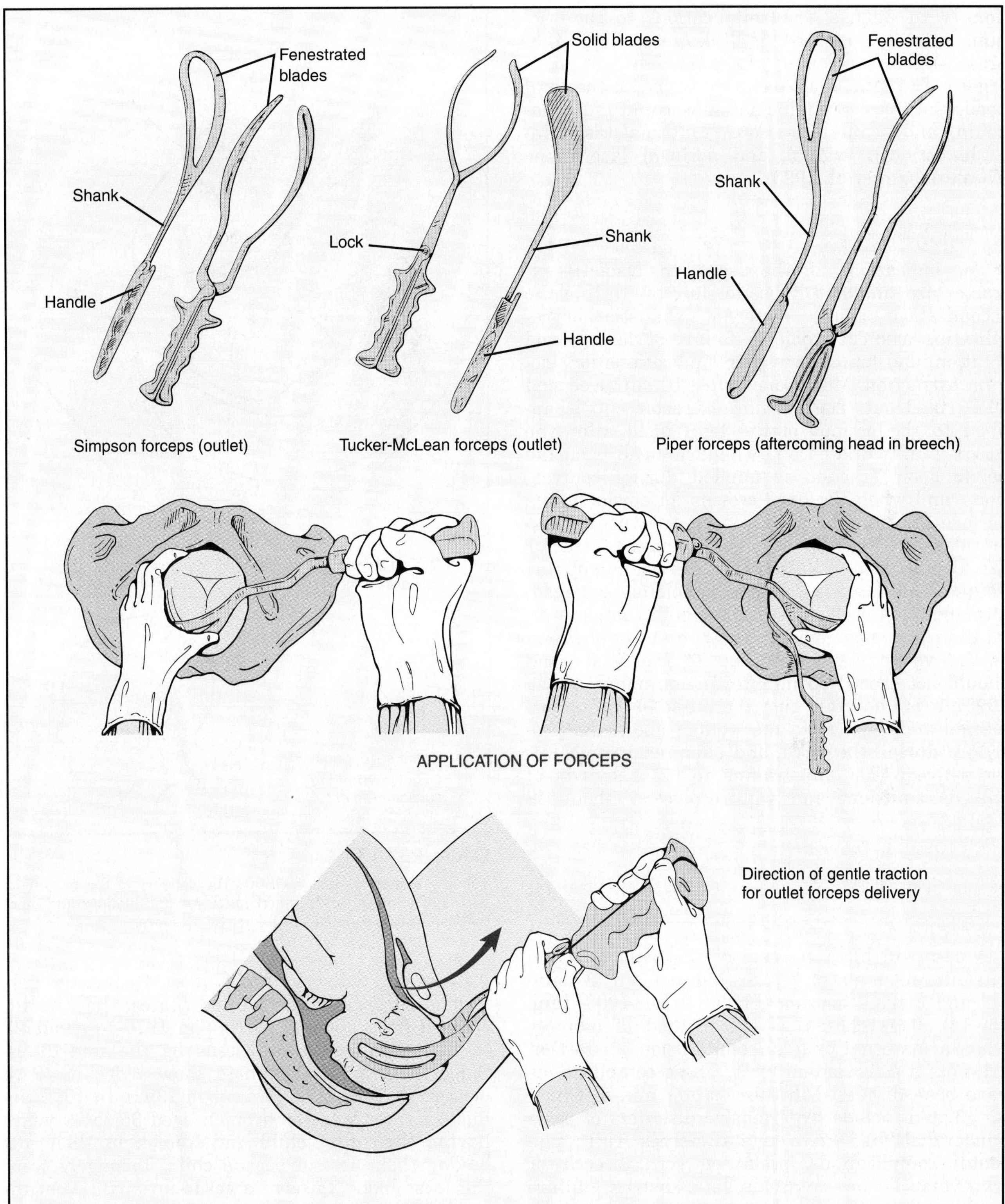

Figure 25–12

Forceps are scissor-like instruments that may facilitate the birth of the fetal head during a difficult delivery.

head. The advantages that the vacuum extractor has over forceps are less damage to maternal tissues, less trauma to the bladder, no absolute need for anesthesia, and more traction on the fetal head with less pressure exerted upon it. Also, a vacuum extractor does not need the additional room in the vagina that forceps require for application, and thus there are fewer associated lacerations with its use. Contraindications to the vacuum extractor include fetal distress, CPD, face presentation, and the aftercoming head in a breech. The fetal risks include trauma to the fetal head, such as cephalhematoma, caput succedaneum, and scalp lacerations. Maternal risks include cervical, vaginal, and perineal lacerations (Cunningham et al. 1993).

Management

The indications for the use of the vacuum extractor are similar to those for forceps. During the second stage of labor, maternal exhaustion or debilitating medical problems, failure of descent and rotation, and fetal distress are indications for vacuum extraction. Membranes must be ruptured and CPD ruled out. The vacuum extractor cup is applied to the occiput of the fetal head after the cervix is fully dilated and when the head is on the pelvic floor. Traction is applied during contractions, and when the head crowns an episiotomy is performed. After the head is born, the vacuum cup is released (Fig. 25–13). The vacuum extractor can also be used when the cervix is not completely dilated and the head is not completely engaged, although it is preferable to have both complete dilatation and engagement. The time of application of the vacuum extractor cup to the fetal head should not exceed 25 minutes (Cunningham et al. 1993). It is important that the nurse provide information and support to the woman about the procedure during the birth, and offer reassurance after delivery that any trauma to the baby's head will be transient and will resolve in about 48 hours.

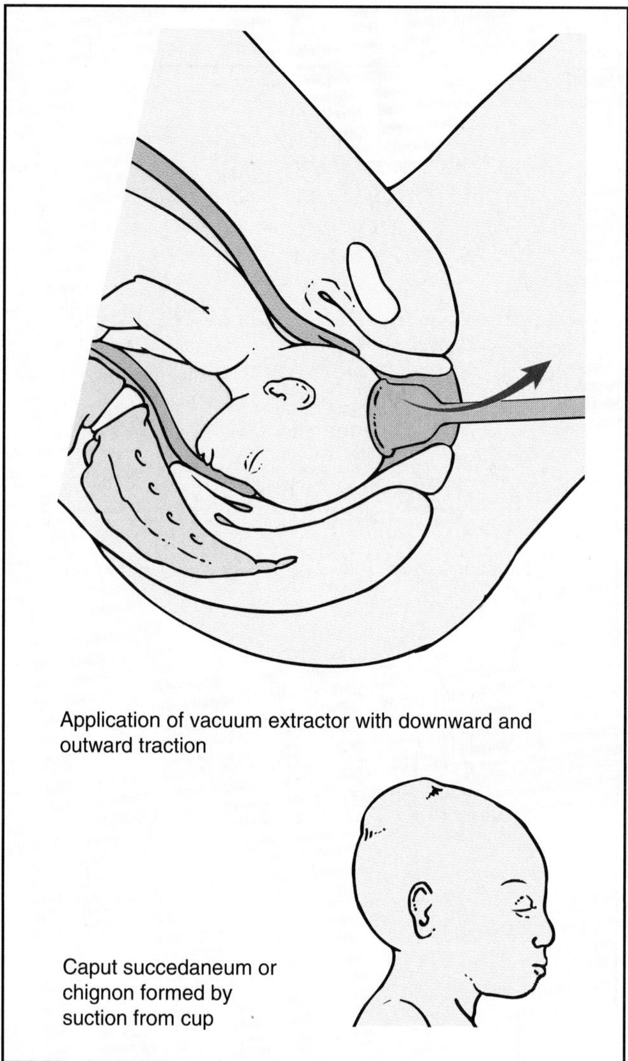

Figure 25–13

Vacuum extractors also facilitate the delivery of the fetal head with less trauma to the maternal tissue and bladder and more traction on the fetal head under less pressure.

CESAREAN BIRTH

Description

A cesarean birth consists of the delivery of an intrauterine fetus or fetuses through an abdominal and uterine incision (Phelan et al. 1993) (Fig. 25–14). It is chosen as the method of delivery when a maternal or fetal complication exists that prevents a safe vaginal birth. These complications have been discussed in this chapter and in Chapter 21 and include hypertensive disorders of pregnancy, diabetes, active genital herpes, CPD, placental complications, prolapsed cord, breech or transverse lie presentations, fetal distress, failure to progress, unsuccessful induction, and repeat cesarean birth. A cesarean birth may be planned (elective) if the complication is recognized during the pregnancy, or unplanned (emergency) if the complication develops suddenly during pregnancy or labor. A primary cesarean delivery refers to the first cesarean that a woman experiences. All following cesarean deliveries are called repeat cesareans.

Cesarean delivery is the most frequently performed surgery in the United States; the rate increased from about 5 percent in 1970 to about 25 to 30 percent in some areas by the mid-1980s. Since then, it has begun to show a decline (22.8 percent in 1989, 22.3 percent in 1992). In 1992 the highest rates were for women aged 35 to 39 years having their first child and women in their 40s having their first or second child. Teenagers were the least likely to have a cesarean birth (Ventura et al. 1994). This dramatic increase in the U.S. cesarean rate resulted from a number of factors, including the now common practice of delivering all breech presentations by cesarean, the increase in diagnosis of fetal distress resulting from routine electronic fetal monitoring, genital herpes, diagnosis of dystocia due to CPD or failure to progress, repeat cesarean deliveries, the increased use of induction and regional anesthesia, and the increase in malpractice lawsuits (Flamm and Quilligan 1995). The significant rise in the cesarean rate since the mid-1970s has caused concern among health care professionals, and a number of professional organizations are now studying ways to reverse this trend. The areas of standard practice being challenged the most are the routine delivery of breech presentations by cesarean, and the routine practice of automatically performing a repeat cesarean delivery once a woman has had a primary cesarean.

Despite the benefits that a cesarean delivery affords to the mother or baby if a complication occurs, there are also disadvantages of cesarean birth. It is a major operation, and because of this it is more costly in terms of hospitalization days and attendant fees than a spontaneous or assisted vaginal birth. Almost 50 percent of women undergoing cesarean delivery incur operative or postoperative complications, some of which are serious or fatal (Meehan et al. 1989). The gross, uncorrected mortality rate for a cesarean birth in the United States and Canada is 30 in 10,000. This is two to four times the rate of vaginal births. One fourth of these deaths are due to anesthesia complications. The national morbidity rate is estimated at 20 percent (Phelan et al. 1993; Taffel et al. 1991). The risks of cesarean birth include the maternal complications of aspiration, fever, wound infection, urinary tract infection, endometritis, wound dehiscence, thrombophlebitis, hemorrhage, atelectasis, and pulmonary embolism. Fetal risks include premature delivery and trauma.

Management

When the decision has been made to deliver the woman by cesarean section, she is prepared for the procedure as for any other major surgery. Procedure 25–4 details the nurse's role in preparing

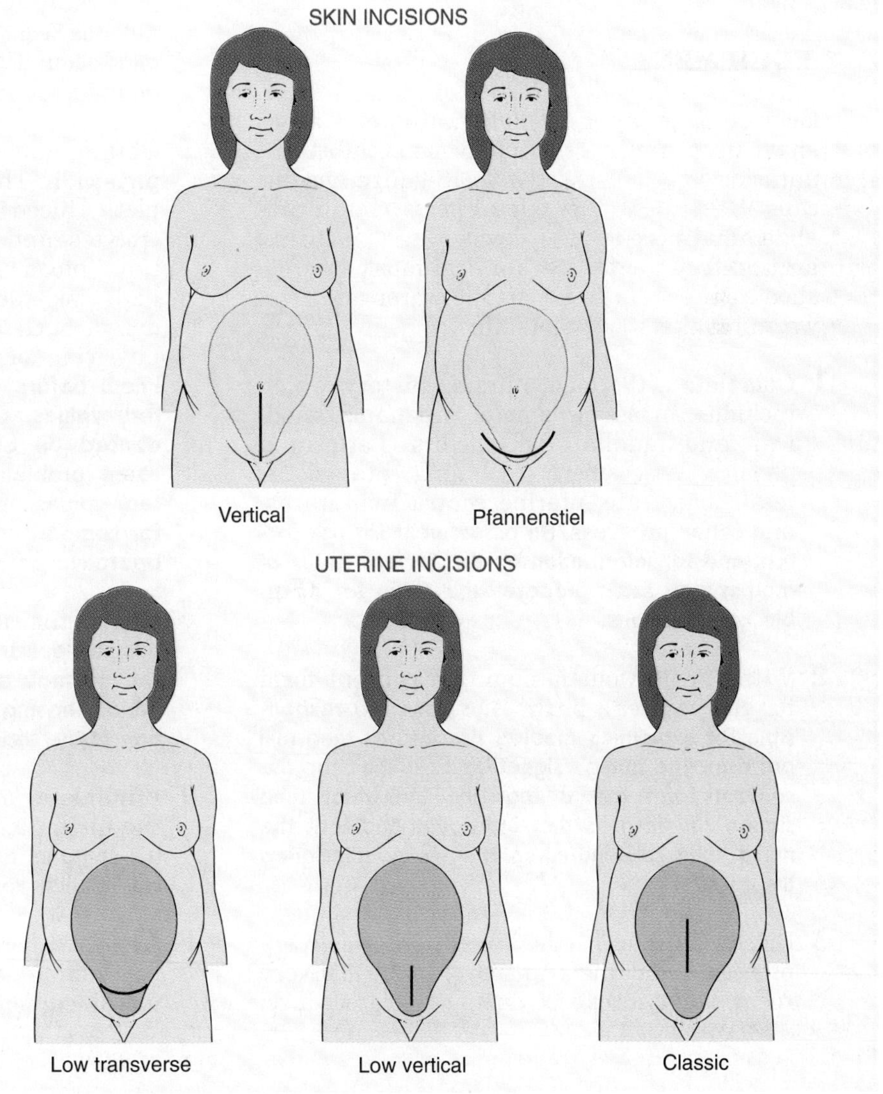

Figure 25–14

Two kinds of incisions are made during a cesarean delivery • First, either a transverse (Pfannenstiel or bikini) or vertical (midline) skin incision is made in the abdomen • Next, a low segment or classic incision is made in the uterine muscle • Low segment incisions can be either vertical or horizontal in orientation.

PROCEDURE 25–4

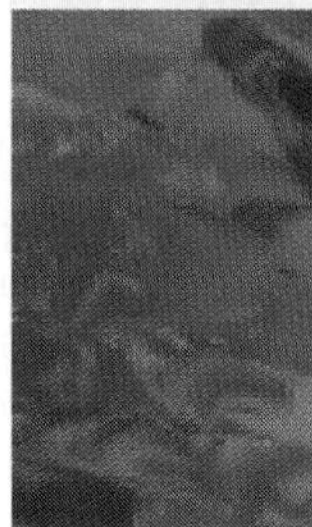

Preparation for Cesarean Birth

▼ PURPOSE

To prepare the woman for the delivery of the baby through abdominal and uterine incisions when maternal factors, fetal factors, or both make vaginal delivery unsafe. To assist the physician and other surgical staff as needed.

▼ EQUIPMENT

- Consent form
- shave prep tray
- antacid
- caps
- abdominal preparation tray
- shoe covers
- warm blankets
- Foley catheter
- intravenous infusion with 18-gauge needle
- fetal heart monitoring device
- surgical mask
- sterile water and saline

1 Complete a thorough nursing history, which includes an assessment of pregnancy, medical, and familial risk factors. Perform a physical assessment, including vital signs, fetal heart rate, uterine contraction status, and labor progress. **An assessment for risk factors and for information on the current status of mother and fetus prepares the team for possible complications.**

2 Witness the woman signing a consent form for the cesarean birth. **Physicians are responsible for explaining medical procedures they will perform. The nurse's signature as witness on the consent form means that the individual who signed the form is that individual and that the nurse was present when the individual signed the form.**

3 Briefly discuss the cesarean delivery process, including transport to the delivery room, what to expect during the procedure, the role of the partner, and the return to the recovery area. Tailor teaching to address the specific concerns of the woman and her partner. **Anticipatory guidance helps ease anxiety.**

4 Start or maintain an intravenous infusion, preferably with a large-bore, 18-gauge needle. **Intravenous solutions hydrate the woman and allow intravenous access for medications and, if needed, blood transfusion.**

5 Obtain laboratory tests ordered by the physician. These will include at least a complete blood count, platelet count, electrolytes, and type and crossmatch for potential blood replacement. If there are high-risk factors, other tests may be ordered, such as clotting studies. Inform the physician of the results. **The physician must know before surgery of any abnormal laboratory values. Certain disease processes as evidenced by abnormal laboratory values could cause problems during the procedure. Laboratory values obtained before surgery are useful for comparison with those obtained in the postoperative period.**

6 Shave the abdominal area. **Depending on hospital policy and the type of incision, the area shaved may extend from the nipple line to the labia. Shaving decreases the risk of contamination at the incision site.**

7 Administer antacid 15 to 30 minutes before the birth. **Antacids decrease the acidity of gastric contents and reduce the complications associated with possible aspiration.**

8 Assist with regional anesthesia by properly positioning the woman and giving her moral support. In emergency situations in

Continued on facing page

PROCEDURE 25–4 Continued

which the woman does not already have regional anesthesia in place, general anesthesia is used. **Proper positioning of the woman facilitates regional anesthesia insertion and provides an opportunity to answer questions and reduce anxiety. General anesthesia, although more hazardous, works more quickly than regional anesthesia and expedites delivery in emergency situations.**

9 Insert a Foley catheter. **An indwelling urinary catheter prevents bladder distention during surgery and enables collection of urine so that the nurse can evaluate urinary output and assess for hematuria.**

10 Position the woman on the delivery table. Place a wedge under her right or left hip to maintain a slight lateral tilt. Check the fetal heart rate. **Placing a wedge under the hip helps maintain placental perfusion. The fetus should be monitored just before the abdominal preparation to ascertain fetal status.**

11 Prepare the woman's abdomen for surgery according to hospital policy. **Scrubbing the maternal abdomen reduces the number of microorganisms on the skin's surface.**

12 Close and tie the gowns of the physicians and scrub nurse; check suction, baby warmer, and other delivery room equipment for proper functioning. Fill basins with sterile water and normal saline and perform initial instrument, sponge, and sharp counts. (Note: Sharps are the suture needles and the blades that are put on the incision knives.) Call nursery staff before surgery. Call neonatal or pediatric medical staff according to hospital policy. **The gowns of sterile personnel should be closed and tied by unsterile personnel. All emergency equipment must be in working order before the start of the procedure in case complications arise during surgery. Basins are used to soak instruments and wet sponges during surgery. A count of instruments, sharps, and sponges is made before, during, and after surgery to make sure all are accounted for. Calling nursery staff before surgery alerts them to the impending birth. Calling neonatal or pediatric medical staff enables them to be present in case the baby has problems.**

13 Prepare necessary paperwork, such as identification bracelets, delivery record, operative record, and preoperative checklists. **Documentation of nursing actions is required to show that care was taken to ensure a safe environment for mother and fetus.**

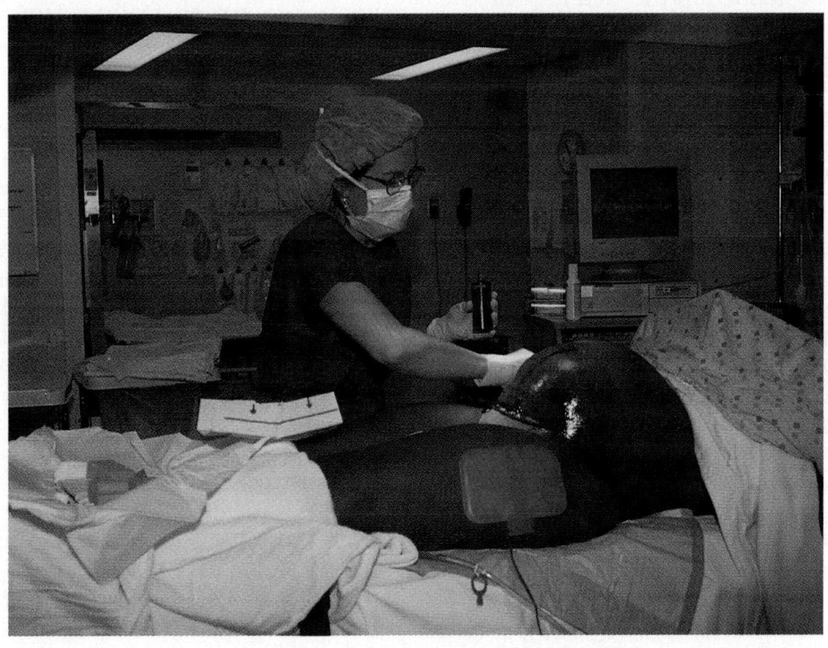

the woman for cesarean birth. Consent forms must be signed. An intravenous infusion line, indwelling urinary catheter, and abdominal/perineal shave preparation are completed. Maternal vital signs and fetal heart rate are monitored regularly. Spinal or epidural regional anesthesia is preferred for the delivery to minimize the effect on the fetus. In the case of an emergency when a rapid delivery is necessary, a general anesthetic is administered.

When a cesarean is performed, the skin incision made into the abdomen is either transverse (sometimes called a Pfannenstiel or bikini incision) or vertical (sometimes called a midline incision). The type of abdominal incision made is determined by the reason for the cesarean, the time factor, the woman's preference, and the operator's skill. It may or may not be the same type of incision that is made in the uterus (Cunningham et al. 1993).

Two types of uterine incisions are used for a cesarean birth, the low segment and the classic incisions (Fig. 25–14). The low uterine segment incision can be either transverse or vertical (Cunningham et al. 1993):

- The low segment transverse incision carries the advantages that it causes less bleeding, is easier to repair, results in fewer adhesions, is less likely to rupture in future pregnancies, and has the potential for an easier subsequent vaginal birth. The disadvantages of the low segment transverse incision are that it takes more time to make and to repair, its size is limited, and it can extend laterally into uterine blood vessels.
- The low segment vertical incision is advantageous in that it can be carried upward if necessary to allow more room for the delivery of the baby. Conditions that may require the incisional extension are placenta previa, a large baby, multiple gestation, a poorly formed lower uterine segment, fetal malposition, and fetal anomaly. There may be more incisional bleeding or an inadvertent upward extension into the upper uterine segment or downward into the cervix. The risk of a rupture with a subsequent labor is increased.

The classic or higher vertical incision in the upper uterine segment was popular in the early part of the twentieth century but is seldom used today. The classic incision becomes necessary if the infant needs to be delivered rapidly. It is also indicated when the development of the lower uterine segment is poor, the placenta is anterior or low-lying, there are extensive lower uterine segment myomas, or varicosities or adhesions are present. The disadvantages of the classic incision include a greater potential for infection, hemorrhage, and uterine rupture.

Figure 25–15 illustrates several of the steps in a cesarean birth sequence. After the proper level of maternal anesthesia has been achieved, the surgeon makes a transverse incision through the skin. The subcutaneous fat is incised with a scalpel and blood vessels are clamped and ligated. Physicians often use their fingers to further separate the fat from the peritoneum. The fascia is incised transversely the full length of the incision; the superior and inferior edges of the fascia are grasped with clamps and elevated by the assistant as the surgeon separates the fascial sheath from the underlying rectus muscles. Immediately after incising the uterus and fetal membranes, the physician inserts his fingers to palpate the presenting part of the fetus. Since this baby was in a breech presentation, the physician first delivers the legs while carefully supporting the baby's body. The aftercoming head is then gently delivered through the incision. Once the baby is delivered, the attendant inserts a finger into the baby's mouth to ensure a clear passage. The nurse assistant immediately uses a bulb syringe to suction the baby as the physician palpates the vessels in the cord before clamping and cutting it. The baby is shown to the parents as soon as possible after being dried, assessed, and identified.

The placenta is delivered, and the repair and closure of the uterus and abdomen begins. The skin is closed with sutures or metal staples. During the postpartum period, the woman must be managed in the same way as any other postoperative patient. It is important that she be monitored closely for surgical complications. At the same time, however, she must be viewed as a postpartum patient and monitored for the progression of the normal involutional process.

The woman undergoing a cesarean birth may experience strong feelings about the delivery. She may express relief after having a long labor. There may be fear if the mother or the fetus is stressed. Feelings of helplessness may occur because the birth plan was altered. There may be disappointment that there was no vaginal delivery, and thus the woman or her partner may feel that she has failed in performing her womanly function. The woman may feel guilty that she in some way was the cause of the need for a cesarean delivery. In addition, the recovery period may necessitate some amount of separation of the mother and infant. It is essential that the woman and her family receive ongoing information and continuous emotional support throughout the cesarean birth experience. In addition to the complication that necessitated the cesarean delivery and the additional medical/obstetric care required, the emotional status of the woman must be recognized and attended to. All attempts should be made to ensure that the cesarean birth experience is a family-centered experience and as meaningful a life event as possible.

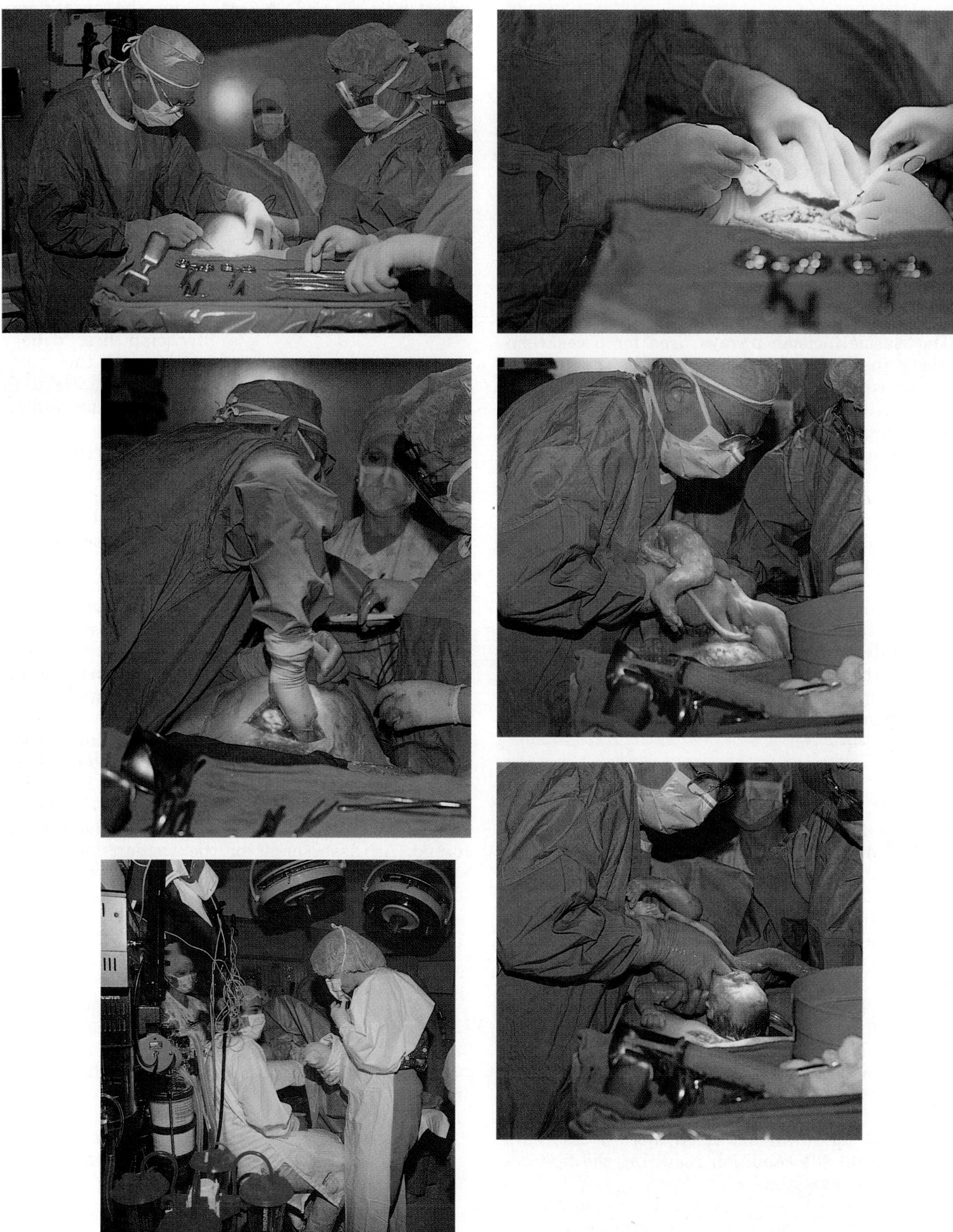

Figure 25–15
Cesarean birth sequence.

VAGINAL BIRTH AFTER CESAREAN

Description

For many decades, the standard of clinical practice was "once a cesarean, always a cesarean." Health care providers believed that once a surgical delivery had been performed, all future deliveries required surgery to prevent the rupture of the uterine scar. This standard is now changing. Many medical studies conducted over the past 30 years support the safety of vaginal birth after cesarean (VBAC). The frequency of VBAC deliveries has continued to increase. In 1992 it was 22.6 percent of births to mothers with a previous cesarean, a rate 20 percent higher than the 18.9 percent rate of 1989 (Ventura et al. 1994).

The classic incision always used for a cesarean delivery in the past has been replaced whenever possible with the low segment uterine incision. There is little risk of uterine rupture with the latter, making labor and vaginal birth a possibility. Other factors such as the dramatic rise in cesarean delivery rates, the soaring cost of health care, and increased consumerism have all influenced the trend toward delivery by VBAC whenever possible (Flamm and Quilligan 1995). VBACs are also encouraged for psychological reasons, as well as the decreased maternal and fetal morbidity and mortality rate associated with a vaginal birth (Abitbol et al. 1993; American College of Nurse-Midwives 1992b; Scott 1991). Studies have indicated that approximately 75 percent of women who attempt a VBAC are successful (Clemenson 1993; Flamm and Quilligan 1995).

Management

Criteria for a vaginal delivery in women who have had a previous cesarean delivery include (1) documentation of one or more earlier low segment incisions, (2) the removal of any previous reason for performing the surgery, (3) informed consent, (4) absence of medical or obstetric complications, and (5) no history of uterine rupture. Contraindications to a VBAC include (1) an upper segment uterine incision, (2) inadequate facilities for performing an emergency cesarean birth, (3) patient refusal, and (4) medical or obstetric complications that preclude labor (ACOG 1995c; Flamm and Quilligan 1995). Since the most common cesarean incision today is the low transverse, most women are eligible for a vaginal birth after a cesarean, assuming that the condition requiring the first cesarean is not repeated.

The woman delivering by VBAC is admitted to the hospital for a trial of labor as soon as she suspects that labor has begun. Blood is drawn for appropriate laboratory studies, intravenous fluids are started, and continuous electronic fetal monitoring is initiated. If oxytocin is given, it should be used with caution, since it has been associated with uterine rupture. The woman's vital signs and contraction pattern should be monitored closely. Her care throughout labor is no different from that for any laboring woman, and her choices of anesthesia can be the same as for any woman. Additional attention should be paid to the woman's anxiety level if she is concerned about a vaginal birth for the first time or the possibility of complications resulting after a previous cesarean birth.

Nursing Process

▼ Assessment

The assessment of the woman having a cesarean birth begins with a thorough nursing history, which includes a review of prenatal events and an assessment for pregnancy, medical, or familial risk factors. This history identifies risk factors that could compromise an operative intervention. The nurse should see that a consent form for surgery is signed. A nursing assessment should then be made, including maternal vital signs, fetal heart rate, uterine contraction pattern, and labor progress, if any. Laboratory results should be obtained (complete blood count, type and crossmatch, electrolytes, and clotting studies) and the physician should be notified of any abnormal values. Monitoring for potential complications should be continued throughout the labor and birth. The knowledge level of the woman and her family regarding the cesarean procedure should be determined. An assessment of the woman's emotional status and coping mechanisms allows the nurse to identify the type of support she and her family will need.

▼ Diagnosis

The nursing diagnoses for the woman experiencing a cesarean birth may include

- Anxiety and fear related to maternal and fetal status and the cesarean delivery procedure
- Knowledge deficit: lack of information related to preparation for cesarean, surgical procedure, anesthesia, and recovery
- Risk for injury related to altered respiratory function
- Pain related to surgical procedure

▼ Planning

Examples of objectives that might be developed to measure the goals and outcomes for the woman delivering by cesarean might include the following:

- The woman will state minimal fear regarding the cesarean delivery
- The woman will verbalize an understanding of all aspects of the cesarean birth process
- The woman will maintain an open airway and experience no alteration in respiratory function
- The woman will verbalize minimal pain during surgery and in the immediate postpartum period

▼ Intervention

The nursing care of the woman delivering her baby by cesarean includes physical, cognitive, and emotional components. The priority given to each of these components depends on whether the cesarean is planned and is not an emergency, or whether it is unexpected and an emergency situation. For example, in an emergency the physical preparation of the woman must be the priority and must be completed quickly so that the baby can be delivered safely. In a planned, ideal situation the educational and emotional components can precede the physical preparation. In many situations the nurse must be adept in carrying out all three components simultaneously. Nursing care planning provides for any eventuality.

Nurses focus their teaching on the needs of the woman and her partner. Knowing what to expect is usually reassuring to the woman and her family. Parents should be informed about the reason for the cesarean, the procedures that will be undertaken in preparation for the delivery, the environment of the delivery room and the staff they will encounter, the options available for anesthesia, the sensations the woman will feel and the discomfort or pain she can anticipate, the role of the support person, the initial contact with the baby, the recovery room experience, and the postpartum recovery period. If time permits, the woman can be taught the deep-breathing and coughing exercises that she will be asked to do immediately after the delivery.

The emotional needs of the parents can be met by identifying their fears or concerns and striving to deal with each of them. It is vital that the nurse present the cesarean delivery experience to the parents as one that is primarily a birth, just as any vaginal delivery would be. If the nurse focuses on the surgical, technical aspects of the experience and negates the normal components of the birth, this will negatively color the parents' view of the experience. Of course, in an emergency situation the focus must be placed on rapid and safe delivery of the infant. When possible, every attempt should be made to make the cesarean birth experience as family centered as it can be. Parents should be given options regarding the father's involvement, the taking of photographs at the time of delivery, the choice of anesthetic, immediate contact with the baby, breastfeeding immediately after birth, and rooming in during the postpartum stay. At the time of the delivery, the father should be welcomed into the delivery room, offered a stool next to the woman's head, and given instructions as to what he can touch and if and when he can move to see the baby. As soon as the baby has been assessed and is stable, the baby should be wrapped warmly and given to the mother and father to hold.

Implementation of the physical components of nursing care involves provision of the appropriate nursing interventions. The nurse monitors the vital signs of both mother and fetus, monitors intake and output, inserts the intravenous line, inserts a Foley catheter, performs a complete abdominal and perineal preparation, and administers preoperative medications. Two units of whole blood should be ordered and be ready for administration if needed. The woman is given nothing by mouth before the delivery, just as for any surgical procedure. If a general anesthetic is to be given, the physician may order a nonparticulate antacid to be given 15 to 30 minutes before the delivery to neutralize the stomach contents in the event of aspiration. If a regional anesthetic is to be given, the nurse will assist by helping the physician as needed and supporting the woman. The newborn nursery personnel should be notified before the delivery so that they are prepared to receive the baby. All equipment in the delivery room (e.g., suction, infant warmer, resuscitation equipment) should be checked before transfer of the woman to ensure that it is functioning properly.

At the time of the delivery, the nurse may need to help position and secure the woman on the operating room table and perform appropriate operating room assignments. Fetal heart rate should be assessed every 5 minutes up until the time the surgery begins. If there are deviations of concern in the fetal heart rate, or if the woman becomes lightheaded or nausous lying on her back, her position should be directed toward her left side by placement of a wedge under her right hip or by adjusting the table to tilt to the left. This will correct the inferior vena cava syndrome and promote better placental perfusion. The anesthetist may also administer O_2 at this time.

The nurse's plan for surgery includes preparation of the preoperative checklist, the birth record, and the operative records. It is essential that accurate documentation of the times of the initial incision, the birth of the infant, and the end of surgery be made. The nurse is responsible for gowning and gloving of the physicians, connecting the suction, administering oxytocin at the time of delivery, assessing the Apgar score, assisting in the care of the infant, recording a correct sponge count, applying the abdominal dressing, and providing emotional support to the parents. The postpartum care of the woman having a cesarean delivery can be found in the Nursing Care Planning Guide in Chapter 35.

▼ Evaluation

Evaluation includes determining whether the goals have been met and whether there has been a safe delivery with a healthy mother and infant. It also involves assessing whether maternal and infant parameters remain within normal limits and determining that there have been no resultant complications from the cesarean birth.

PSYCHOLOGICAL ISSUES ASSOCIATED WITH HIGH-RISK CHILDBIRTH

The psychology of pregnancy recognizes that pregnancy, labor, and birth are potentially, if not universally, stressful periods even under optimal conditions (Mandeville and Troiano 1992). Women who live in poverty or have other environmental or socioeconomic stressors not only may have difficulty with adaptation to pregnancy, but also are more prone to poor health and poor health behaviors. Ultimately, they are more likely to develop complications because of their preexisting poor health. Thus, those women least able to cope psychologically with stress and illness in pregnancy are frequently those most likely to experience such illness. Nurses need to recognize preexisting stressors and, in collaboration with the woman, attempt to identify strategies designed to decrease the stress.

Much has been written about facilitating parental-fetal or parental-infant attachment. However, little has been proved about how high-risk conditions or complications of pregnancy and childbirth influence these interactions. Therefore, although it may be suspected that complications during pregnancy and birth may have untoward effects on parent-child relationships, the consequences of high-risk childbirth remain largely unknown and require future research. Clinicians have noted that many women appear to need to settle issues regarding a complication before they can discuss the more common issues of their pregnancy, birth, and parenting. Nurses need to recognize this preoccupation as normal and to facilitate a woman's understanding so that she can progress in the work of pregnancy and birth.

High-risk childbirth is a field of challenge for nurses today. Care must include identification of risk factors, ways to modify risks, recognition of complications, and appropriate use of nursing interventions incorporating high touch and high technology. Support and education of the woman in crisis remains an essential hallmark of good nursing care.

Risk Management

Risk management for nurses involved in the care of the woman experiencing a high-risk childbirth begins with nurses themselves. They should be well prepared educationally to render quality care to their patients. They can continually add to their education by being active in the appropriate professional organizations. These organizations are the source of standards and practice guidelines that keep nurses abreast of new developments in high-risk care. Educational programs are also available to nurses interested in developing or maintaining their skills.

A second aspect of risk management for a high-risk childbirth situation is frequent and accurate documentation. If there is a doubt whether safe, competent nursing care has been given, precise documentation within the woman's chart will provide the facts about the care given and the rationale for the actions taken. Any review of questions that might arise regarding care is facilitated when there is written evidence. Therefore, charting should be clear, concise, and complete. It may be the only instrument available for mediating a legal dispute. It is important at all times for nurses to maintain regular communication with the members of the health care team.

A trusting relationship with the childbearing woman and her family is the third essential component for solving problems if they do arise. If laboring women have rapport with their nurses, they will be more willing to work with them to solve problems and more likely to trust in their nurses' judgments and actions. Effective and open communication often prevents misunderstandings.

Implications for Research

Further research is necessary to answer clinical questions that arise from caring for women undergoing high-risk childbirth. The following are examples of research questions that are important to the advancement of nursing care:

- Are there better ways of identifying and preventing high-risk labor and birth conditions?
- What components of the nurse's role in caring for a woman with a high-risk labor and birth are most valued by the woman and her family?
- What are the psychological implications for the family experiencing a high-risk childbirth?
- How does a high-risk childbirth affect family member roles and relationships?

High-risk childbirth is a field of challenge for nurses today. Care must include identification of risk factors, ways to modify risks, recognition of complications, and appropriate use of nursing interventions incorporating high touch and high technology. Support and education of the woman in crisis remains an essential hallmark of good nursing care.

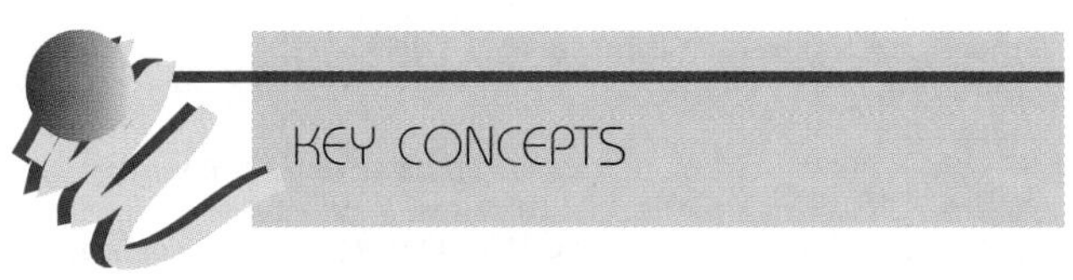

KEY CONCEPTS

▼ Birth is usually a healthy, normal event, but certain conditions may occur that place the woman and/or fetus at an increased risk of morbidity or mortality. Some conditions are associated with maternal risk only; others are associated with only fetal or neonatal risk; and yet others jeopardize the health of both.

▼ Early recognition of conditions that cause a woman or her fetus to be at high risk for specific complications can enable the nurse to carefully monitor the maternal fetal couple during childbirth for signs of those complications.

▼ Early recognition of increased risk, increased awareness, and observation may enable the nurse to more efficiently direct nursing interventions to minimize poor outcomes.

▼ The concept of risk is dynamic. A woman may have certain complications in pregnancy (e.g., second-trimester placenta previa) that are resolved during the antepartal period and she may enter childbirth with no high-risk condition, or she may have an uneventful pregnancy and suddenly develop a complication during labor or birth.

▼ Many high-risk conditions in childbirth are apparent at the onset of labor. These include malpositions or malpresentations, placental abnormalities, preterm labor, and preterm rupture of membranes or cord prolapse.

▼ A few women develop complications after labor has begun, including uterine dysfunctions, labor anomalies, cephalopelvic disproportion, rupture of the uterus, and shoulder dystocia.

▼ Some fetuses or newborns demonstrate complications independent of maternal risk; these can include fetal distress due to decreased oxygenation, multiple gestation, developmental anomalies, and intrauterine demise.

▼ The third stage of labor may be accompanied by complications such as amniotic fluid embolism, uterine inversion, hemorrhage, and bleeding disorders such as disseminated intravascular coagulation.

▼ Among the obstetric interventions commonly employed in treating complications of childbirth are external cephalic version, induction or augmentation of labor, forceps, vacuum extraction, cesarean birth, and VBAC.

▼ When caring for the woman and her family who are either at high risk for childbirth or who have a demonstrated complication of childbirth, nurses need to be aware of their holistic needs. These needs include psychological support and care with not only a recognition of the abnormalities, but an emphasis on the wellness that can always be found in any clinical situation.

▼ It is important for nurses to facilitate a birth experience that is as family centered and positive as possible for parents who have a high-risk childbirth.

References

Abitbol, M., Castillo, I., Taylor, G., Rochelson, B., Shmoys, S., Monheit, A. (1993). Vaginal birth after cesarean section: the patient's point of view. *American Family Physician,* 47 (1), 129–134.

Acker, D. (1991). A shoulder dystocia intervention form. *Obstetrics and Gynecology,* 78, 150–151.

Ader, L., Hansson, B., Wallin, G. (1990). Parturition pain treated by intracutaneous injections of sterile water. *Pain,* 40:133–138.

American College of Nurse-Midwives. (1992a). *High technology.* Position paper.

American College of Nurse-Midwives. (1992b). *Nurse-midwifery care of women planning a vaginal birth after cesarean (VBAC).* Position statement.

American College of Obstetricians and Gynecologists (ACOG). (1991). Induction and augmentation of labor. *ACOG Technical Bulletin,* 157, 1–7.

American College of Obstetricians and Gynecologists (ACOG). (1994). Operative vaginal delivery. *ACOG Technical Bulletin,* 196, 1–7.

American College of Obstetricians and Gynecologists (ACOG). (1995a). Dystocia and the augmentation of labor. *ACOG Technical Bulletin,* 218, 1–7.

American College of Obstetricians and Gynecologists (ACOG). (1995b). Induction of labor. *ACOG Technical Bulletin,* 217, 1–7.

American College of Obstetricians and Gynecologists (ACOG). (1995c). Vaginal delivery after a previous cesarean birth. *ACOG Practice Patterns,* No. 1, August.

Andrews, C. (1981). Nursing intervention to change a malpositioned fetus. *Advances in Nursing Science,* 3, 52–66.

Andrews, C., and Andrews, E. (1983). Nursing, maternal postures and fetal position. *Nursing Research,* 32 (6), 336–341.

Arias, F. (1993). *Practical guide to high risk pregnancy and delivery.* St. Louis: Mosby–Year Book.

Association of Women's Health, Obstetric and Neonatal Nurses (AWHONN). (1993). Cervical ripening and induction and augmentation of labor. *Practice Resource,* 1–7.

Benedetti, T. (1990). Added complications of shoulder dystocia. *Contemporary Obstetrics and Gynecology,* 150–161.

Biancuzzo, M. (1991). The patient observer: Does the hands-and-knees posture during labor help to rotate the OP fetus? *Birth,* 18 (2), 40–47.

Biancuzzo, M. (1993a). How to recognize and rotate an occiput posterior fetus. *AJN,* 93 (3), 38–41.

Biancuzzo, M. (1993b). Six myths of maternal posture during labor. *MCN* 18 (5), 264–269.

Bishop, E. (1968). Pelvic scoring for elective induction. *Obstetrics and Gynecology,* 24 (2), 266–268.

Bowe, N. L. (1981). Intact perineum: A slow delivery of the head does not adversely affect the outcome of the newborn. *Journal of Nurse-Midwifery,* 26 (2), 5–11.

Brodsky, P., and Pelzar, E. (1991). Rationale for the revision of oxytocin administration protocols. *Journal of Obstetric, Gynecologic, and Neonatal Nursing,* 20 (6), 440–444.

Brost, L., and Kenny, J. (1992). Pregnancy after perinatal loss: Parental reactions and nursing interventions. *Journal of Obstetric, Gynecologic, and Neonatal Nursing,* 21 (6), 457–470.

Brouillard-Pierce, C. (1993). Indications for induction of labor. *MCN* September/October Suppl, 14–22.

Brown, Y. (1992). The crisis of pregnancy loss: A team approach to support. *Birth,* 19 (2), 82–88.

Burrow, G., and Ferries, T. (1995). *Medical complications during pregnancy* (3rd ed.). Philadelphia: W. B. Saunders.

Busowski, J., and Parsons, M. (1995). Amniotomy to induce labor. *Clinical Obstetrics and Gynecology,* 38 (2), 246–258.

Campbell, W., Nochison, D., Vintzileos, A. (1993). Prolonged pregnancy. In R. Knuppel, and J. Drukker (Eds.). *High risk pregnancy: A team approach* (2nd ed.). Philadelphia: W. B. Saunders.

Canadian Preterm Labor Investigators Group. (1992). Treatment of preterm labor with the beta-adrenergic agonist ritodrine. *New England Journal of Medicine,* 327, 308–312.

Chamberlain, G., and Hytten, G. (1991). *Clinical physiology in obstetrics.* Oxford: Blackstone.

Chelmow, D., Kilpatrick, S. J., Laros, R. K., Jr. (1993). Maternal and neonatal outcomes after prolonged latent phase. *Obstetrics and Gynecology,* 81 (4), 486–491.

Chenia, F., and Crowther, C. (1987). Does advice to assume the knee chest position reduce the incidence of breech presentation at delivery? A randomized clinical trial. *Birth,* 14 (2), 75–78.

Cherry, S., and Merkatz, I. (1991). *Complications of pregnancy; Medical, surgical, gynecologic, psychosocial and perinatal* (4th ed.). Baltimore: Williams & Wilkins.

Clark, R., and Eteson, D. (1991). Congenital anomalies. In H. Taeusch, R. Ballard, M. E. Avery (Eds.). *Diseases of the newborn.* Philadelphia: W. B. Saunders.

Clark, S., Cotton, D., Hankins, G., Phelan, J. (1991). *Critical care obstetrics.* Boston: Blackwell Scientific.

Clemenson, N. (1993). Promoting vaginal birth after cesarean section. *American Family Physician,* 47 (1), 139–144.

Combs, C., and Kitzmiller, J. (1993). Premature rupture of membranes. In A. Fuchs, F. Fuchs, F., R. Stubblefield. (Eds.). *Preterm birth: Causes, prevention and management* (2nd ed.). New York: McGraw-Hill.

Creasy, R., and Resnik, R. (1994). *Maternal-fetal medicine: Principles and practice* (3rd ed.). Philadelphia: W. B. Saunders.

Cunningham, F. G., MacDonald, P. C., Gant, N. F., Leveno, K. J., Gilstrap, L. C., III (1993). *Williams obstetrics* (19th ed.). Norwalk, CT: Appleton & Lange.

Danforth, D. (1990). *Obstetrics and gynecology* (6th ed.). Philadelphia: J. B. Lippincott.

Davis, L. (1984). The use of castor oil to stimulate labor in patients with premature rupture of membranes. *Journal of Nurse-Midwifery,* 29 (6), 366–370.

Day, M., and Snell, B. (1993). Use of prostaglandins for induction of labor. *Journal of Nurse-Midwifery,* 38 (2), 42S–48S.

Del Valle, G., Joffe, G., Izquierdo, L., Smith, J., Gilson, G., Curet, L. (1992). The biophysical profile and the nonstress test: Poor predictors of chorioamnionitis and fetal infection. *Obstetrics and Gynecology,* 80, 106–110.

DeVoe, L., Croom, C., Youssef, A., Murray, D. (1992). The prediction of "controlled" uterine rupture by use of intrauterine pressure catheters. *Obstetrics and Gynecology,* 80 (4), 626–629.

Eganhouse, D., and Burnside, S. (1992). Nursing assessment and responsibilities in monitoring the preterm pregnancy. *Journal of Obstetric, Gynecologic, and Neonatal Nursing,* 21 (15), 355–365.

Ewton, D. (1993). A perinatal loss follow-up guide for primary care. *Nurse Practitioner,* 18 (12), 30–32, 35–36.

Fernando, B., Leeves, L., Greenacre, J., Roberts, G. (1995). Audit of the relationship between episiotomy and risk of major perineal laceration during childbirth. *British Journal of Clinical Practice,* 49 (1), 40–41.

Flamm, B., and Quilligan, E. (1995). *Cesarean section: Guidelines for appropriate utilization.* New York: Springer-Verlag.

Gabbe, S., Niebyl, J., Simpson, J. (1991). *Obstetrics: Normal and problem pregnancy* (2nd ed.). New York: Churchill Livingstone.

Gilbert, E., and Harmon, J. (1993). *High-risk pregnancy and delivery.* St. Louis: Mosby–Year Book.

Gilstrap, L., and Cunningham, F. (1992). Operative vaginal delivery. *Williams Obstetrics Supplements,* 18 (16), 1–15.

Griese, M. and Prickett, S. (1993). Nursing management of umbilical cord prolapse. *Journal of Obstetric, Gynecologic, and Neonatal Nursing,* 22 (4), 309–311.

Handa, V., and Laros, R. (1993). Active-phase arrest in labor. *Obstetrics and Gynecology,* 81 (5), 758–763.

Harvey, M. (1992). Critical care for the maternity patient. *MCN,* 17 (6), 296–309.

Homsi, R., Daikoku, N., Littlejohn, J., Wheeless, C. (1994). Episiotomy: Risks of dehiscence and rectovaginal fistula. *Obstetrical and Gynecological Survey,* 49 (12), 803–808.

Johnson, P., and Pace, S. (1993). Guide to the use of the vacuum extractor by nurse midwives. *Journal of Nurse-Midwifery,* 38 (2), 88S–94S.

Jones, R., Hagashima, A., Hartnett-Goodman, M., Goodlin, R. (1991). Rupture of low transverse cesarean scars during trial of labor. *Obstetrics and Gynecology,* 77 (6), 815–817.

Klein, M., Gauthier, R., Jorgensen, S. (1992). Does episiotomy prevent perineal trauma and pelvic floor relaxation? *Online Journal of Current Clinical Trials,* Document No 10: July 1.

Kowalski, K. (1991). No happy ending: Pregnancy loss and bereavement. *NAACOG's Clinical Issues in Perinatal and Women's Health Nursing,* 2 (3), 368–380.

Laros, R., Flanagan, T., Kilpatrick, S. (1995). Management of term breech presentation: a protocol of external cephalic version and selective trial of labor. *American Journal of Obstetrics and Gynecology* 172 (5), 1916–1923.

Lawson, L. (1990). Culturally sensitive support for grieving parents. *MCN,* 15 (2), 76–79.

Leon, I. (1992). Commentary: Providing versus packaging support for bereaved parents after perinatal loss. *Birth,* 19 (2), 89–91.

Leveno, K., and Cunningham, F. (1992). Beta-adrenergic agonists for preterm labor. *New England Journal of Medicine,* 327 (5), 349–351.

Levine, C. (1991). Premature rupture of membranes and sepsis in preterm neonates. *Nursing Research,* 40 (1), 36–41.

Lopez-Zeno, J., Peaceman, A., Adashek, J., Socol, M. (1992). A controlled trial of a program for the active management of labor. *New England Journal of Medicine,* 326 (7), 450–454.
Lumley, J. (1987). How to find out if assuming the knee chest position is superior to external cephalic version in turning the breech. *Birth,* 14 (2), 79–80.
Lynam, L., and Miller, M.A. (1992). Mothers' and nurses' perceptions of the needs of women experiencing preterm labor. *Journal of Obstetric, Gynecologic, and Neonatal Nursing,* 21 (2), 126–136.
Main, D., and Main, E. (1992). Pre-term birth. In S. Gabbe, J. Niebyl, J. L. Simpson (Eds.). *Obstetrics, normal and problem pregnancies* (2nd ed.) New York: Churchill Livingstone.
Mandeville, L., and Troiano, L. (1992). *High risk intrapartum nursing.* Philadelphia: J. B. Lippincott.
Marshall, C. (1985). The art of induction/augmentation of labor. *Journal of Obstetric, Gynecologic, and Neonatal Nursing,* 14 (1); 22–28.
Mastrogiannis, D., and Knuppel, R. (1995). Labor induced using methods that do not involve oxytocin. *Clinical Obstetrics and Gynecology,* 38 (2), 259–266.
McCombs, J. (1995). Update on tocolytic therapy. *Annals of Pharmacotherapy,* 29 (5), 515–522.
Meehan, F., Burrke, G., Casey, C., Sheil, J. (1989). Delivery following cesarean section and perinatal mortality. *American Journal of Perinatology,* 6 (1), 90–96.
Merkatz, I., and Thompson, J. (1990). *New perspectives on prenatal care.* New York: Elsevier.
Miller, A., and Lorkovic, M. (1993). Prostaglandin E_2 for cervical ripening. *MCN,* September/October Supplement, 23–30.
Nodine, P.M., and Roberts, J. (1987). Factors associated with perineal outcome during childbirth. *Journal of Nurse-Midwifery,* 32 (3), 123–130.
Nurses Association of the American College of Obstetricians and Gynecologists (NAACOG). (1992). *Appropriate use of technology.* Position paper.
O'Herlihy, C. (1993). Active management: A continuing benefit in nulliparous labor. *Birth,* 20 (2), 95–97.
O'Leary, J., and Leonetti, H. (1990). Shoulder dystocia: Prevention and treatment. *American Journal of Obstetrics and Gynecology,* 162, 5–9.
Oxorn, H., and Foote, W. (1986). *Human labor and birth* (5th ed.). New York: Appleton-Century-Crofts.
Penny, P., and Perlis, D. (1992). Shoulder dystocia: When to use supra-pubic or fundal pressure. *MCN,* 17 (1), 34–36.
Phelan, J. B., Bendell, A., Colburn, V. (1993). Cesarean birth. In R. A. Knuppel, and J. E. Drukker (eds.). *High risk pregnancy: A team approach* (2nd ed.). Philadelphia: W. B. Saunders.
Pozaic, S. (1991). Hemorrhagic complications in pregnancy. In C. Harvey (ed.). *Critical care obstetrical nursing.* Gaithersburg, MD: Aspen.
Primeau, M., and Recht, C. (1994). Professional bereavement photographs: One aspect of a perinatal bereavement program. *Journal of Obstetric and Gynecologic Neonatal Nursing* 23 (1), 22–25.
Rayburn, W., and Zuspan, F. (1992). *Drug therapy in obstetrics and gynecology.* St. Louis: C. V. Mosby.
Reynolds, J. (1994). Intracutaneous sterile water for back pain in labour. *Canadian Family Physician,* 40:1785–1792.
Rubinstein, T. H., and Schifrin, B. (1992). Shoulder dystocia. *Journal of Perinatology,* 12 (1), 74–77.
Sacks, D. (1993). Fetal macrosomia and gestational diabetes: What's the problem? *Obstetrics and Gynecology,* 81 (5), 775–781.
Sala, J., and Moise, K. (1990). The treatment of preterm labor using a portable subcutaneous terbutaline pump. *Journal of Obstetric, Gynecologic, and Neonatal Nursing,* 19 (2), 188–115.
Satin, A., Leveno, K., Sherman, L., Brewster, D., Cunningham, G. (1992). High versus low dose oxytocin for labor stimulation. *Obstetrics and Gynecology,* 80 (1), 111–116.
Scheerer, L., and Katz, M. (1990). Tocolysis for fetal intervention. In M. Harrison, M. Galbus, R. Filly (eds.). *The unborn patient.* Philadelphia: W. B. Saunders.
Scott, J. (1991). Mandatory trial of labor after cesarean delivery. *Obstetrics and Gynecology,* 77 (6), 811–814.
Sisson, M. (1992). Amniotic fluid embolism. *NAACOG's Clinical Issues in Perinatal and Women's Health Nursing,* 3 (3), 469–474.
Smith, J., Christoff, B., Zukowsky, K. (1993). Congenital abnormalities. In S. Mattson, and J. Smith (eds.). *Core curriculum for maternal-newborn nursing.* Philadelphia: W. B. Saunders.
Stratham, H., and Dimavicus, J. (1992). Commentary: How do you give the bad news to parents? *Birth,* 19 (2), 103–104.
Swinnerton, T. (1991). Alternative remedies during labor. *Nursing Times,* 87 (9), 64–65.
Taffel, S., Placek, P., Moien, M., Kosary, C. (1991). 1989 US cesarean section rate steadies—VBAC rate rises to nearly one in five. *Birth,* 18 (2), 73–77.
Trolle, B., Moller, M., Kronborg, H., Thomsen, S. (1991). The effect of sterile water blocks on low back labor pain. *American Journal of Obstetrics and Gynecology,* 164 (5, Part 1): 1277–1281.
Ventura, S., Martin, J., Taffel, S., Mathews, T., Clarke, S. (1994). Advance report of final natality statistics, 1992. *Monthly Vital Statistics Report,* Centers for Disease Control and Prevention/National Center for Health Statistics, 43 (5).
Zhang, Z., Bowes, W. A., Fortney, J. A. (1993). External cephalic version. *Obstetrics and Gynecology,* 82 (2), 306–310.

26 Chapter

FHR patterns can give important insights in the individual fetus into the existence of stress and frequently can help determine in a proper clinical setting the nature and duration of that stress as well as the response to intervention. As with any medical device, the EFM has its strengths and limitations, which must be understood.

BARRY S. SCHIFRIN (1995)

Fetal Monitoring

Deborah Woolley

HIGHLIGHTS

- ▼ Fetal Heart Rate as a Predictor of Birth Outcome
- ▼ Guidelines for Fetal Monitoring During Childbirth
- ▼ Electronic Fetal Monitoring: Instrumentation
- ▼ External Fetal Heart Rate Monitoring
- ▼ Procedure 26–1: External Electronic Fetal Monitoring
- ▼ Internal Fetal Heart Rate Monitoring
- ▼ External Uterine Contraction Monitoring
- ▼ Internal Uterine Contraction Monitoring
- ▼ Antepartum Fetal Heart Monitoring: Indications for Fetal Heart Rate Monitoring, Nonstress Test, Contraction Stress Test, Biophysical Profile
- ▼ Monitor Patterns: Baseline Fetal Heart Rate; Periodic Changes—Decelerations, Accelerations; Nonreassuring Patterns—Loss of Initial and Secondary Acceleration, Prolonged Secondary Acceleration, Biphasic Deceleration, Slow Return to Baseline, Loss of Variability and Decreased Baseline FHR, Changes in the Fetal Heart Rate in the Second Stage of Labor; Correlation Between Electronic Fetal Monitoring and APGAR Scores
- ▼ Nursing Practice
- ▼ Risk Management
- ▼ Implications for Research

Electronic fetal monitoring (EFM) has been described as a window to the womb. It allows the practitioner to assess the well-being of the fetus in the intrauterine environment. Interpretation of fetal monitor tracings and clinical judgment can be enhanced by knowledge of maternal and fetal physiology, understanding of the labor process, and appreciation of maternal and fetal response to labor in normal as well as abnormal circumstances. Experience will also increase the sophistication of a practitioner's interpretation of the data from the electronic fetal monitor. This chapter is an introduction to electronic monitoring of uterine activity and fetal heart rate activity during the antepartum and childbirth periods.

DEFINITIONS

Acceleration—An increase of at least 15 bpm in the fetal heart rate over baseline fetal heart rate that lasts at least 15 seconds and is often associated with fetal movement; considered a sign of fetal well-being.

Baseline fetal heart rate—The most typical fetal heart rate over a 10-minute period or between uterine contractions in labor. The normal baseline rate is 120 to 160 beats per minute (bpm) (ACOG 1995). In full-term (mature) fetus, a baseline rate of 110 to 160 bpm is considered normal (AWHONN 1995).

Contraction stress test (CST)—A test of fetal well-being in which an electronic fetal monitor is applied and the woman is stimulated to have uterine contractions by receiving a dilute dose of intravenous oxytocin (Pitocin). The woman may also use nipple stimulation to induce contractions. The fetal heart rate response to the contractions is assessed; also known as an oxytocin challenge test.

Early decelerations—A decrease in the fetal heart rate that begins and ends at the same time as the uterine contraction, causing a consistent U-shaped waveform that mirrors the contraction on an electronic fetal monitor tracing; thought to be caused by head compression during labor.

Electronic fetal monitoring (EFM)—Continuous monitoring of the fetal heart rate and uterine contractions by an electronic fetal monitor using either external or internal modes.

Fetal bradycardia—A baseline fetal heart rate that is less than 120 bpm.

Fetal heart rate (FHR)—The number of fetal heart beats per minute; traditionally, the normal range is 120 to 160 bpm. The normal range for the mature fetus is 110 to 160 bpm.

Fetal tachycardia—A baseline fetal heart rate that is greater than 160 bpm.

Late deceleration—A decrease in the fetal heart rate that begins after the onset of the contraction and ends after the contraction has ended; caused by compromised uteroplacental perfusion.

Long-term variability (LTV)—The number of oscillations or undulations in the fetal heart rate baseline over 1 minute; usually 2 to 6 per minute.

Nonstress test (NST)—A test of fetal well-being in which the external fetal monitor is used to measure the accelerations of the fetal heart rate; usually in response to fetal movement.

Short-term variability (STV)—The beat to beat interval changes in the fetal heart rate. STV can be measured only by internal/direct fetal monitoring.

Tocodynamometer (Toco)—A pressure-sensitive transducer that is placed over the maternal uterine fundus to record uterine activity. It is held in place by a belt around the abdomen.

Ultrasound transducer—A sending and receiving device that is attached by a belt around the woman's abdomen to obtain and record the fetal heart rate by ultrasound waves.

Variable deceleration—A rapid decrease in the fetal heart rate and a rapid return to baseline that may occur during or between contractions and has a characteristic V-shape; usually caused by cord compression.

FETAL HEART RATE AS A PREDICTOR OF BIRTH OUTCOME

The goal of fetal monitoring is to assist a clinician to identify the fetus who is in danger of asphyxiating (in distress) and intervene in a timely fashion to reduce or relieve that distress. The immediate goal of fetal monitoring is to decrease perinatal mortality. The long-term goal is to decrease the incidence of neurologic impairment (muscular and intellectual) that can follow asphyxia.

Not all obstetric clinicians agree on the manner in which asphyxia manifests itself in a fetal heart rate (FHR) tracing. Despite the efforts that have been put into standardizing the descriptions of FHR changes in labor, two clinicians looking at the same tracing often make different diagnoses regarding the nature and severity of fetal distress indicated by the tracing. The same clinician looking at the same tracing a few months apart may also arrive at a different diagnosis of the fetal status.

Not all babies who exhibit FHR changes indicative of asphyxia have either poor APGAR scores or evidence of long-term neurological impairment. These outcomes suggest that some of the FHR changes thought to indicate asphyxia may instead be the result of a nonasphyctic process. However, it is also quite likely that the "suspicious" or "nonreassuring" tracing prompts interventions that relieve or reduce the asphyxia before any permanent damage occurs. Also, not all babies who have low APGAR scores and/or evidence of long-term neurological impairment have FHR tracings that are suggestive of intrapartum asphyxia.

GUIDELINES FOR FETAL MONITORING DURING CHILDBIRTH

"Well-controlled studies have shown that intermittent auscultation of the fetal heart rate is equivalent to continuous electronic monitoring at specific intervals with a 1:1 nurse-to-patient ratio" (ACOG 1995). Both the American College of Obstetricians and Gynecologists (ACOG 1995) and the Association for Women's Health, Obstetric and Neonatal Nurses (AWHONN 1990; Chez et al. 1991) have adopted standards recognizing the appropriateness of intermittent auscultation in certain circumstances.

For the low-risk woman, the current published ACOG standard is intermittent auscultation (with fetoscope, Doppler, or EFM) every 30 minutes in the active phase of labor and every 15 minutes in the second stage, each preferably during and for 30 seconds after a contraction (ACOG 1995). For the woman with risk factors (high-risk), the recommendation is for the FHR to be recorded and evaluated every 15 minutes in the active phase of labor if auscultation is being used and evaluated every 15 minutes (assuming the recording is done automatically) if continuous EFM is being used.

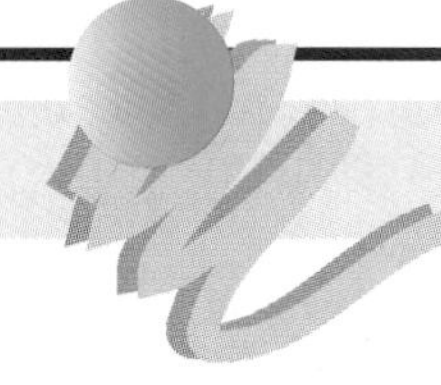

HISTORICAL PERSPECTIVES

FETAL MONITORING

In a general sense, fetal monitoring is composed of any effort made to observe or track the well-being of the fetus. The first such efforts were probably notations of fetal movements, because fetal movements and life are connected in many ancient texts. The modern era of fetal assessment could be said to have started in 1818, when Mayor reported the existence of fetal heart tones, but Mayor apparently did not realize the clinical significance of the ability to hear the fetal heartbeat. Credit for that deduction goes to the Vicomte de Kergaradec, who published his observations in 1821. By 1833, Kennedy compiled a monograph describing the relationships between the common changes in the fetal heart rate and fetal distress. However, such information was not widely disseminated or agreed on until Winkel proposed specific criteria for fetal distress in 1893.

During the next 60 years, experiments revealed much of what we now know about the physiologic mechanisms underlying changes in the fetal heartbeat. However, not until the 1950s, when many of the long-standing problems contributing to maternal mortality had been solved, did fetal assessment become a primary focus of care providers. Only when the mother's survival was more or less ensured could the physicians focus their efforts on the fetus.

Now, some authors are concerned that this emphasis on the fetus has begun to diminish the role of the mother to that of a mere vessel for the fetus. This remarkable shift in focus has occurred in less than 50 years and represents a widening gap between technology and human caring. With the added pressure to reduce costs (often by limiting the number of nurses assigned in a unit), this generation of nurses is faced with the challenge of reconciling these two foci by developing ways to combine the best parts of both and improve the lives of women and their children well into the twenty-first century.

Data from Goodlin, J. R. (1979). History of fetal monitoring. *American Journal of Obstetrics and Gynecology,* 133 (3), 323–352; Rothman, B. (1991). *Labor: Women and power in the birthplace.* New York: W. W. Norton; and Davis-Floyd, R. (1992). *Birth as an American rite of passage.* Los Angeles: University of California Press.

Table 26–1

GUIDELINES FOR MONITORING THE FETAL HEART RATE IN LABOR

RISK STATUS	METHOD OF MONITORING	STAGE/PHASE OF LABOR			
		Admission	Latent	Active	Second
Low risk	Auscultation	Listen during a contraction and for 30 sec after	Every 1 hr	Every 30 min	Every 15 min
	Electronic fetal monitoring	Record × 20–30 min	Same	Same	Same
High risk	Auscultation	Listen during a contraction and for 30 sec after	Listen every 30 min or as often as maternal-fetal status dictates	Listen every 15 min	Every 5 min
	Electronic fetal monitoring	20–30 min	Evaluate every 30 min	Evaluate every 15 min	Every 5 min

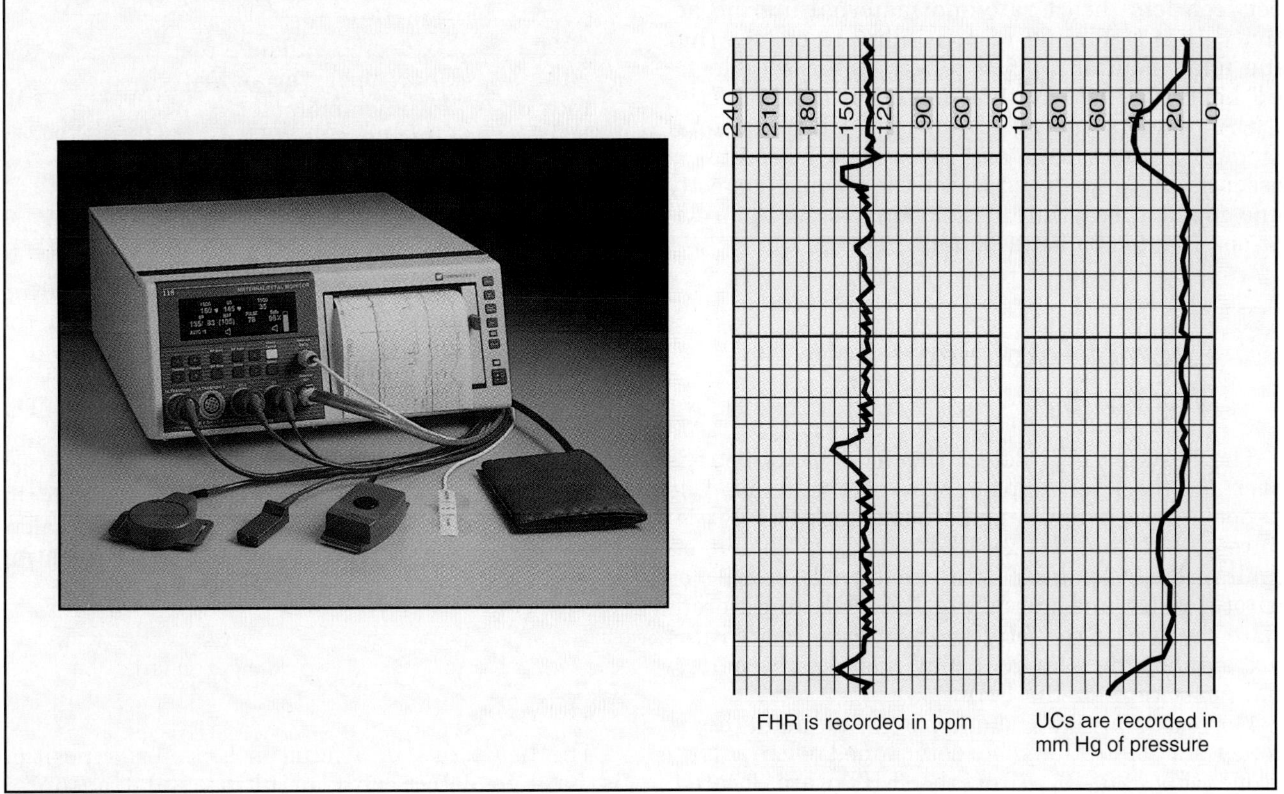

Figure 26–1

The maternal/fetal monitor is an electronic machine that provides a digital reading of the fetal heart rate (FHR) and uterine contractions (UCs) in a window on the unit as well as a paper printout that has recorded both FHR and UC tracings over time • The printout becomes part of the woman's medical record. (Photograph courtesy of Corometrics Medical Systems, Inc.)

During the second stage, the FHR should be evaluated and recorded at least every 5 minutes when auscultation is used and should be evaluated at least every 5 minutes when EFM is used (ACOG 1989, 1995; NAACOG 1990) (Table 26–1).

When feasible, an admission or baseline tracing is recommended. For this procedure, the laboring woman is placed in a comfortable, nonsupine position and the external fetal monitor is applied for 20 to 30 minutes. A normal tracing obtained at this time will be associated with a normal 5-minute APGAR score in 93 to 97 percent of fetuses (Feinberg and Krebs 1989; Ingemarsson and Arulkumaran 1989).

ELECTRONIC FETAL MONITORING: INSTRUMENTATION

The electronic fetal monitor is a two channel monitor that simultaneously records the fetal heart rate and maternal uterine activity. These events are measured and a graphic representation is produced by the monitor (Fig. 26–1). Fetal well-being is determined by looking at the relationship between fetal heart rate and maternal uterine activity. It is a nursing responsibility to ensure that the fetal monitor tracing reflects interpretable fetal heart rate activity and maternal uterine activity. An understanding of how the electronic fetal monitor gathers data and presents information is essential in order to interpret the tracing correctly and make appropriate decisions (also see Abbreviations Related to Fetal Monitoring).

External Fetal Heart Rate Monitoring

The best place to detect the fetal heart beat is over the back or upper chest of the fetus. Use Leopold maneuvers to palpate the back (see Procedures 16–1 and 23–2). The examiner should simultaneously palpate the maternal radial or carotid pulse and auscultate the FHR to differentiate the two. If the fetal and maternal heart rates are similar, the examiner may mistake the maternal heart rate for the FHR.

For external fetal monitoring, the fetal heart tones should initially be determined with a fetoscope (Fig. 26–2). After the FHTs are located, they should be counted for one full minute to detect changes. The fetoscope can be used as needed to validate that the fetal monitor tracing accurately reflects the fetal heart rate.

Abbreviations Related to Fetal Monitoring

AAT	Auscultated acceleration test
AFV	Amniotic fluid volume
bl	Baseline (as in fetal heart rate or uterine tonus)
bpm	Beats per minute
BPP	Biophysical profile
BTBV	Beat-to-beat variability
CST	Contraction stress test
ECG	Electrocardiogram
EFM	Electronic fetal monitoring
FHR	Fetal heart rate (equivalent to FHT)
FHT	Fetal heart tones (used interchangeably with FHR)
FMC	Fetal movement count
FSBpH	Fetal scalp blood pH
FSBS	Fetal scalp blood sample
FSE	Fetal scalp electrode
IUPC	Intrauterine pressure catheter
LTV	Long-term variability
mm Hg	Millimeters of mercury
NST	Nonstress test
OCT	Oxytocin challenge test
STV	Short-term variability
toco	Tocodynamometer
UC	Uterine contraction
US	Ultrasound

After the FHTs are located, the external ultrasound transducer is placed over the point on the abdomen where the auscultated fetal heart beat is loudest (Procedure 26–1). This transducer sends sound waves into the maternal abdomen. The waves reflect off movement of the fetal heart and return to the transducer. The monitor identifies that a cardiac cycle is occurring and, based on the intervals between successive cardiac cycles, calculates the rate at which the fetal heart is beating and marks it on the fetal monitor tracing.

SOURCES OF POOR OR INADEQUATE TRACINGS

The heart rate of a fetus in a posterior position is hard to detect with an ultrasound transducer. Also, a fetus that is very active is hard to monitor, because of movement in and out of the range of the transducer. The heart rate of a fetus of an obese woman may be difficult to locate through

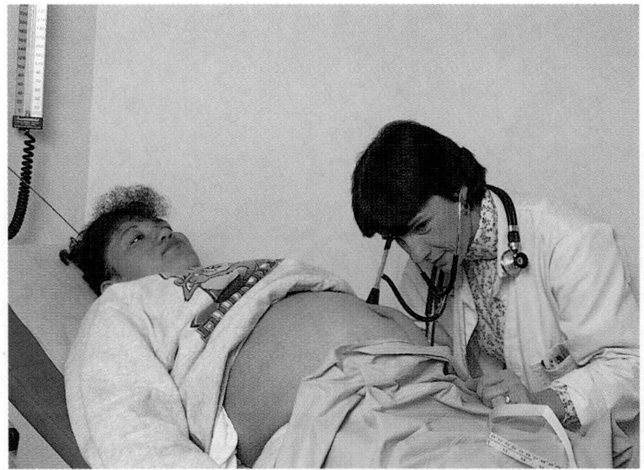

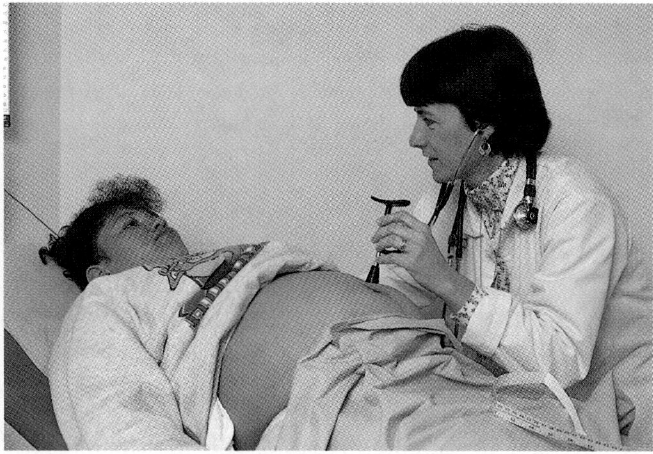

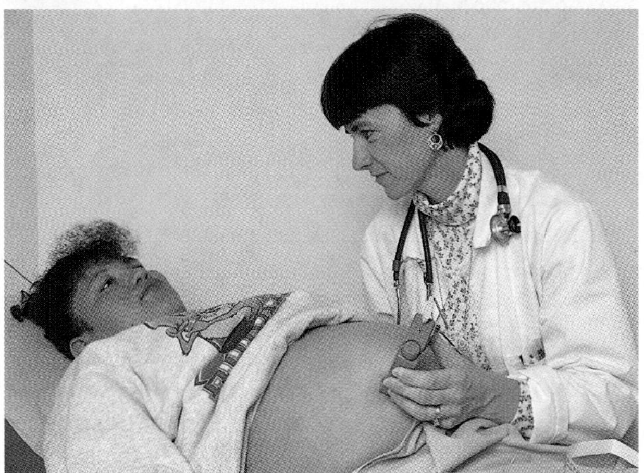

Figure 26–2

The nurse-practitioner auscultates the fetal heart tones with both a DeLee-Hillis fetoscope, which uses bone conduction of the examiner's head to magnify the fetal heart tones, and an ultrasound transducer, which operates by battery and magnifies the sound of the FHR so that both the caregiver and client can hear the fetal heartbeats • Before switching to the transducer, the nurse discusses what she is hearing with her patient.

PROCEDURE 26–1

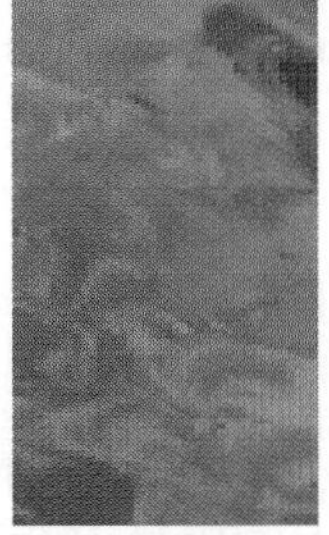

External Electronic Fetal Monitoring

▼ PURPOSE

An external electronic fetal monitor is used when the health of the mother and fetus warrants intensive monitoring or when it is mandated by hospital policy. An external electronic monitor allows the health care provider to assess fetal tolerance to labor by evaluating subtle changes in baseline fetal heart rate, variability, and the presence of accelerations or decelerations. The external electronic fetal monitor also measures uterine contraction frequency and duration, but it is not a reliable indicator of uterine contraction intensity.

Continued on following page

PROCEDURE 26–1 Continued

▼ EQUIPMENT

- Electronic fetal heart monitor
- Ultrasound transducer
- Tocotransducer
- Ultrasound gel
- Belts to hold transducers in place

1 Explain the purpose and function of external electronic fetal monitoring to the woman and her partner. Assure them that while she is being monitored, the woman will still be able to change positions, stand, and walk in the room if the fetal heart pattern allows. **An explanation of the purpose and function of external electronic fetal monitoring and assurance that it will not limit her mobility will reduce the patient's anxiety and promote her cooperation.**

2 Turn on the monitor and press the TEST button. Confirm that the paper speed switch on the back of the monitor is set at 3 cm per minute. **A correct function test ensures that the internal circuitry is calibrated properly and that data obtained during labor are accurate. Setting the paper speed at 3 cm per minute increases the health care provider's ability to interpret the fetal monitor strip accurately.**

3 Record complete patient identification information at the beginning of the monitor strip. Record date and time monitoring is started on the fetal monitoring tracing. Enter the name and credentials of the nurse placing the patient on the fetal monitor. **The fetal monitor tracing is a legal part of the patient's medical record and should include patient identification and ongoing documentation of the patient's status and care provided during the monitoring period.**

4 Perform Leopold maneuvers to determine fetal position and the location of the fetal back (see Procedure 16–1). **Fetal heart tones are best heard when the ultrasound transducer is placed over the fetal back (see Procedure 23–2). As labor progresses and the fetus descends lower in the pelvic cavity, the ultrasound transducer will need to be moved downward and toward the middle of the woman's abdomen.**

5 Place monitor belts under the woman's back so that they are flat against her skin. Position the woman in a semi-Fowler or lateral tilt position. **Belts that are smooth against the back are more comfortable and easily adjusted to maintain steady contact between the transducers and the abdomen. The supine position is avoided to prevent compression of maternal blood vessels and potential supine hypotension.**

6 Connect the ultrasound transducer and the tocotransducer to the fetal monitor. Apply ultrasound gel to the ultrasound transducer. Adjust the volume. **Ultrasound gel is needed to improve conduction.**

7 Confirm the presence of fetal heart tones with a fetoscope or stethoscope (see Procedure 23–2 before applying the ultrasound transducer. **The electronic monitor reliably detects and records pulselike sounds; however, it cannot discriminate between pulselike sounds of similar rate and intensity. Confirming the presence of fetal heart tones with a fetoscope or stethoscope before applying the ultrasound transducer helps ensure that the source of the pulse detected by the electronic monitor is the fetal heart. If any doubt about the presence or rate of fetal heart tones arises during external electronic fetal monitoring, reconfirm the fetal heart rate with fetoscope or stethoscope before relying exclusively on the machinery.**

8 Place the ultrasound transducer on the maternal abdomen over the fetal back. Move the transducer until clear, audible fetal heart tones are heard and the signal light is flashing steadily. Secure the ultrasound device in place with the belt. Confirm that the fetal heart rate is different from the maternal pulse rate by palpating the maternal radial pulse while listening to the rate on the monitor. **A clear heart rate is needed to obtain a fetal monitor strip that is interpretable, that is, without gaps of information. Maternal heart rate may be recorded if the ultrasound transducer is improperly positioned or in the event of a fetal demise.**

Continued on facing page

PROCEDURE 26–1 Continued

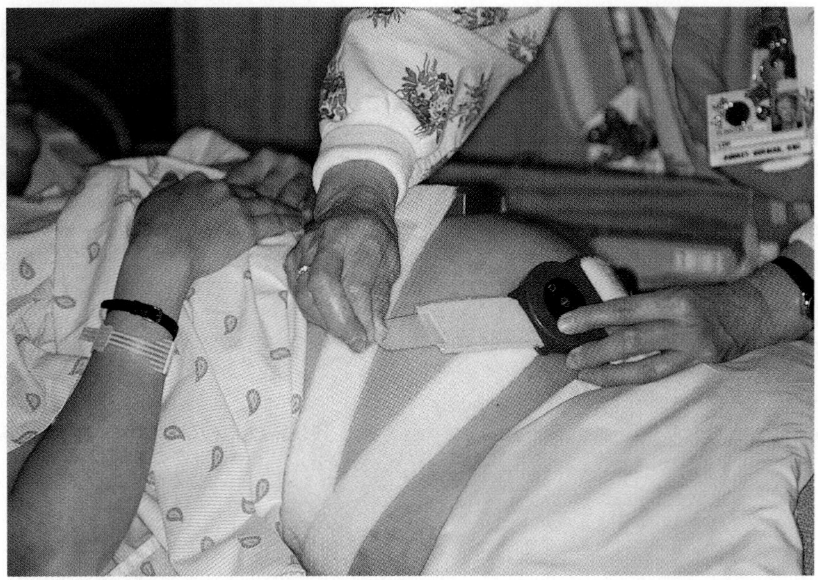

9 Place the tocotransducer on the fundus of the uterus so that the pressure-sensitive button is flush against the maternal abdomen. Secure the transducer in place with the belt. Set baseline uterine activity according to the fetal monitor manufacturer's guidelines. **Since normal uterine contractions originate in the fundus, the fundal region is the best place to position the tocotransducer. When properly positioned, the pressure-sensitive tocotransducer senses changes in the tonus of the maternal abdomen to identify the frequency and duration of contractions. Since it is an external device, it cannot measure the true intensity of contractions.**

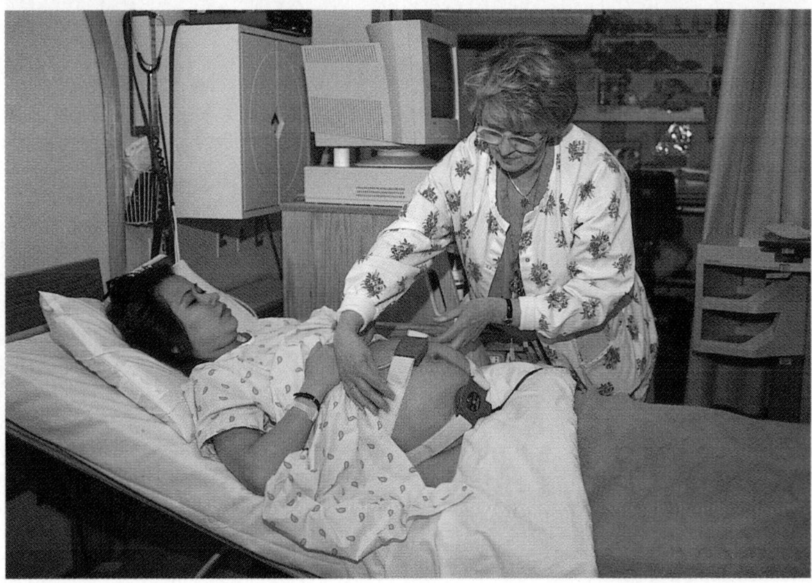

Continued on following page

PROCEDURE 26–1 Continued

10 Evaluate the quality of the tracing to determine whether it is adequate for interpretation. If it is not, reposition the transducers until an interpretable tracing is obtained. **It is the responsibility of the nurse placing the woman on the electronic fetal monitor to obtain a tracing that can be interpreted as reassuring or nonreassuring.**

11 Explain to the woman and her partner what the fetal monitor shows. The top portion depicts the fetal heart rate pattern; the lower half shows contraction frequency and duration. **Explaining the patterns recorded on the monitor promotes the patient's understanding of fetal status during labor.**

12 Evaluate the tracing for baseline rate; long-term variability; accelerations and decelerations; and uterine contraction frequency, duration, and return to resting tonus between contractions. **A systematic review of this information allows the nurse to assess fetal tolerance to labor and to intervene in a timely manner if indicated. The standard of care delineating the frequency of these evaluations (ACOG 1995) is as follows:**

	LOW-RISK	HIGH-RISK
FIRST STAGE		
Latent	Every 60 minutes	Every 30 minutes
Active	Every 30 minutes	Every 15 minutes
SECOND STAGE	Every 15 minutes	Every 5 minutes

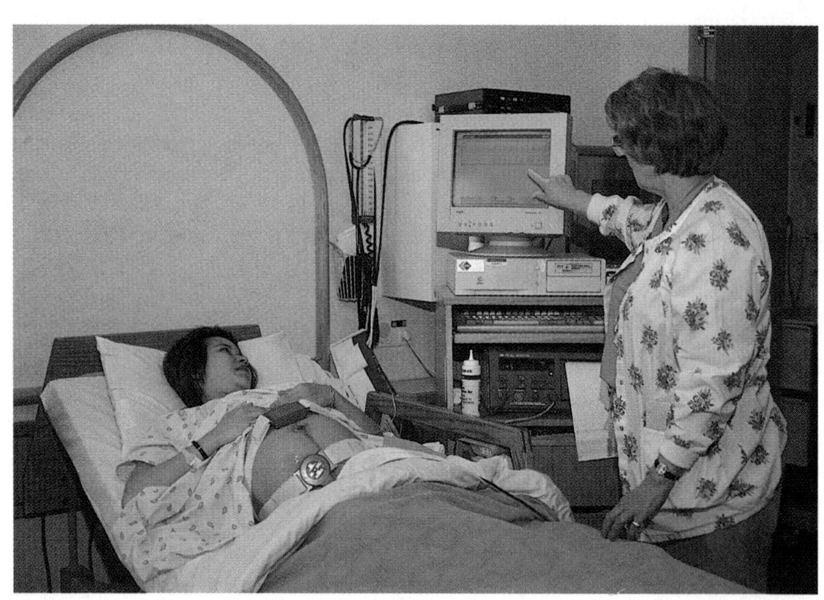

13 Record data at the intervals specified in step 11. **In case the fetal monitor strip becomes separated from the chart, all data and physician/nursing interventions are recorded in the woman's chart as well. Possible findings are**

- Baseline fetal heart rate — Between 120 and 160 bpm is normal
- Long-term variability — Decreased, average, or increased
- Accelerations — Present and are 15 beats above the baseline for 15 seconds
- Decelerations — May be early, late, or variable type
- Uterine contractions — Duration and frequency vary depending on stage of labor but should always return to resting tone between contractions

the thick, maternal adipose tissue. The fetus of a woman who is moving (changing positions, etc.) throughout labor is difficult to monitor continuously because the woman's movements frequently displace the transducer. As the fetus descends and rotates, the ultrasound transducer will have to be relocated to maintain a good quality tracing.

If the quality of the tracing from the transducer is poor, there may be poor conduction between the woman's skin and the surface of the transducer. The application of additional monitor gel generally resolves the problem.

Internal Fetal Heart Rate Monitoring

Direct or internal monitoring is done using a fetal electrode, which is attached to the presenting part, most commonly the scalp. Direct or internal monitoring provides the most accurate means for recording FHR because a consistent measuring point in each cardiac cycle is selected (Fig. 26–3). The scalp electrode consists of a spiral of stainless steel wire that inserts approximately 2 mm under the skin of the presenting part (Parer 1994). The fetal electrode preferentially selects the R wave of the cardiac QRS complex and measures successive fetal RR intervals (i.e., the time in milliseconds between two QRS complexes) of the cardiac cycle.

SOURCES OF POOR OR INADEQUATE TRACINGS

Poor quality tracings may still occur, even with an internal fetal electrode. The attachment of the fetal electrode to the maternal cervix results in little or no perceptible signal. An electrode applied to the presenting part of a dead fetus results in the recording of the maternal pulse. In the absence of fetal cardiac activity, the electrode recognizes and records the maternal pulse. The tracing resembles an FHR pattern and can result in inappropriate clinical decision making.

Fetal monitors can be adjusted so that the paper speed is 1, 2, or 3 cm per minute; 3 cm per minute is the recommended speed used in the United States. The interpretations of tracings obtained at different speeds can be quite different. A 1 or 2 cm per minute paper speed tracing can be difficult to interpret because the tracing is substantially compressed.

External Uterine Contraction Monitoring

The external device used to monitor uterine contractions is the tocodynamometer, or "toco." Its critical feature is a pressure-sensitive, spring-operated plunger on the underside of the transducer.

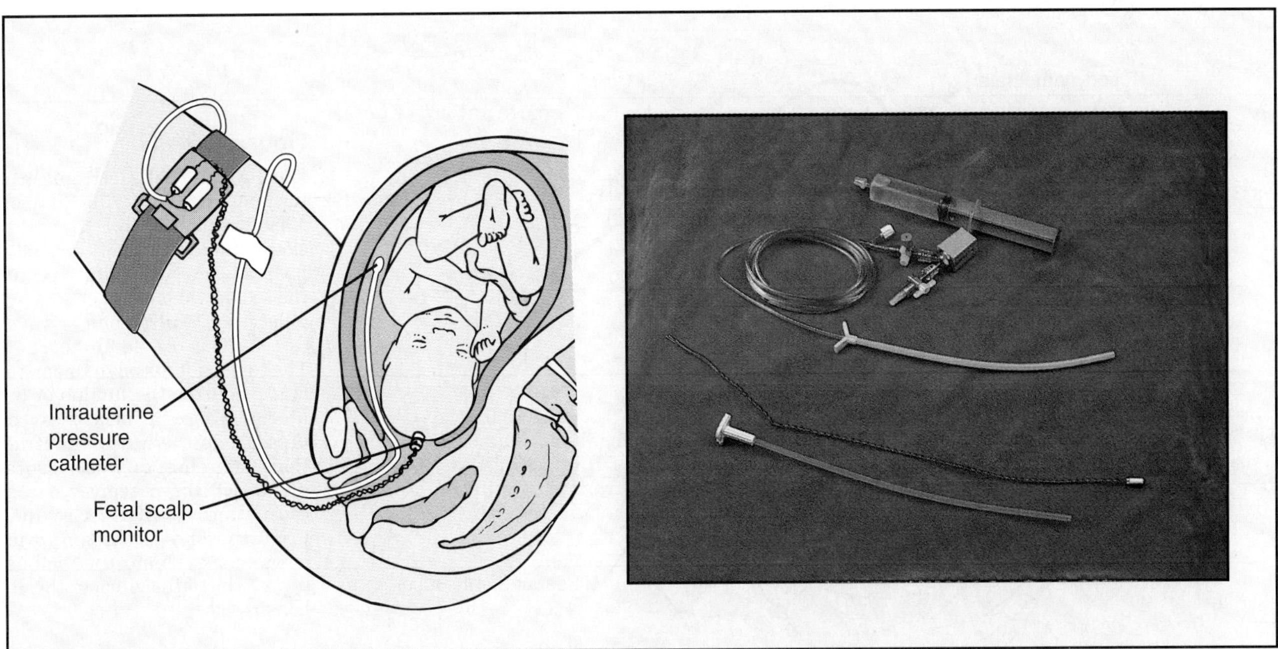

Figure 26–3

Internal electronic fetal monitoring may be used after the membranes have ruptured • The fetal electrode is attached to the presenting part of the fetus (often the scalp) to measure the FHR • The intrauterine pressure catheter (a fluid-filled IUPC is shown above) is inserted between the fetus and the wall of the uterus to measure UCs • Illustrated is the traditional method of securing the leads; however, many care providers tape the IUPC to the mother's lower abdomen where the attachments are less likely to be displaced when she moves.

This plunger is placed against the maternal abdomen over the uterine fundus and stabilized by a belt around the maternal abdomen. When the uterus contracts, the fundus rises and presses against the plunger. This rising and falling pressure triggers the monitor to trace a curve that reflects the presence of a uterine contraction (Fig. 26–4). With a good-quality tracing by external tocodynamometer monitoring of uterine activity, the frequency and duration of contractions can be assessed. Uterine resting tone and contraction intensity cannot be assessed by external uterine monitoring; uterine palpation is the method that must be used for assessment of these features of uterine activity with external monitoring.

SOURCES OF POOR OR INADEQUATE TRACINGS

Any condition that interferes with the ability of the contracting uterus to press against the toco will compromise the accuracy of the tracing obtained. If the belt is too loose, the plunger will not be close enough to the fundus to be depressed by the contracting uterus. If the belt is too tight, the plunger cannot be further depressed, even in the presence of a strong contraction. In either case, the tracing obtained is not an accurate representation of uterine activity.

Other common problems include maternal movement, which can dislodge the toco; and maternal obesity, which interferes with the ability of a contraction to depress the toco button because of the soft, adipose layer between the toco and the uterus. Also, placement of the toco on a part of the uterus other than the fundus causes the tracing to underestimate the uterine activity, because the body of the uterus does not contract as strongly or as early as the fundus. Finally, while the tracing of uterine activity obtained by the external toco provides a fairly accurate picture of the frequency of the contraction, it does not provide reliable information about intensity of contractions. If there is a need for a precise measurement of the intensity of the contractions, an intrauterine pressure catheter should be used.

The belt for the toco must be snug to provide a good external toco tracing of uterine activity. A useful technique is to tighten the belt until the tracing rises to the 50-mm mark (between contractions). Then, reset the baseline tone to 20 mm Hg. Observe the tracing for a contraction or two to see if it correlates with your clinical impression of the frequency and duration of uterine activity.

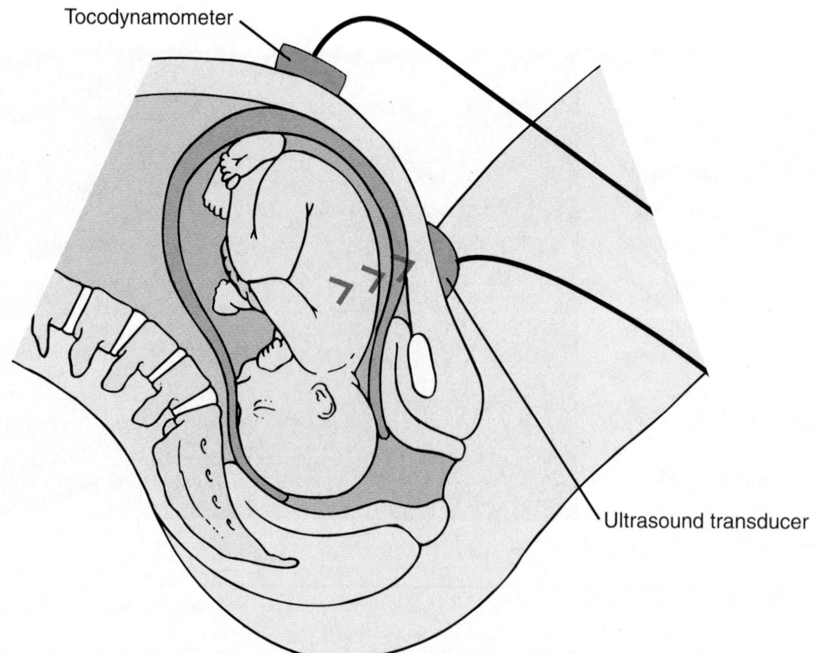

Figure 26–4

During external electronic maternal/fetal monitoring, the ultrasound transducer is placed over the location of the fetal heart tones where it records the reflections or echoes of pulses of ultrasonic waves directed at the fetal heart • The external tocodynamometer is placed over the fundus of the uterus where it measures the pressure of the uterine contractions • The dual measurements let the caregiver assess the pattern of FHR in relation to UCs over specific time windows and evaluate the well-being of the fetus during the labor process.

Internal Uterine Contraction Monitoring

Fetal membranes have to be ruptured before an intrauterine pressure catheter (IUPC) is inserted high into the uterine cavity (see Fig. 26–3). There are two kinds of IUPCs: solid and fluid filled. The solid catheter has a transducer that measures intrauterine pressure built into its tip. The fluid-filled catheter is connected to a disposable transducer located outside the uterus that measures intrauterine pressure. The transducer measures pressure created by the uterine contractions and records it on the uterine activity graph of the monitor paper. With internal or direct monitoring of uterine activity by an IUPC, accurate information is provided about uterine resting tone and uterine contraction frequency, duration, and intensity. Labor is considered to be adequate to cause progressive cervical change and fetal descent when contractions are occurring every 2 to 3 minutes and lasting approximately 40 to 90 seconds, with an intensity of 40 to 90 mm Hg and a normal resting tone of 5 to 20 mm Hg.

SOURCES OF POOR OR INADEQUATE TRACINGS

A major cause of inaccurate readings with an IUPC is incorrect placement of the catheter. If the fetus is deeply engaged at the time of insertion, the catheter may coil in the vagina or around the fetal presenting part instead of being correctly placed into the uterine cavity. It is also possible to perforate the wall of the uterus with the pressure catheter during insertion.

Fluid-filled catheters have an opening on the distal end, which may become obstructed by vernix or mucus. Also, transmission of the pressure may be interrupted by air within the fluid-filled catheter. The catheter can be easily displaced by catching it on bed linens and is commonly pushed out during the expulsive efforts of the second stage of labor.

When a fluid-filled catheter is used, the transducer is external to the uterus, and the transducer should be placed at the level of the xiphoid process or uterine fundus so that it is at the approximate level of the tip of the catheter. The transducer is then opened to air, set at zero, and reclosed. Every subsequent reading of the intrauterine pressure is then measured against this zero point (the height of the transducer). If the transducer is higher than the tip of the tubing (which is inside the uterus), the pressure reading is artificially lowered because the tip of the tubing is lower than the zero point. Conversely, if the tip is higher than the transducer, the pressure recorded is higher than its actual value.

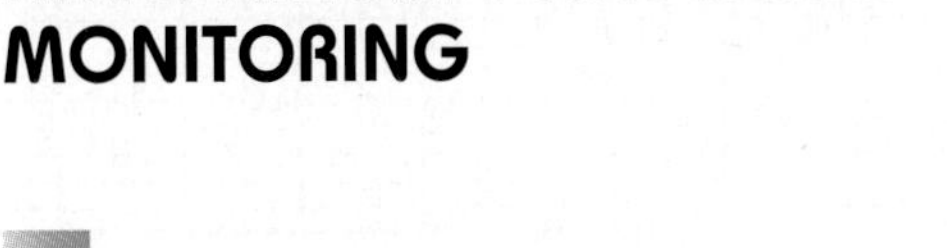

ANTEPARTUM FETAL HEART MONITORING

Indications for Antepartum Fetal Monitoring

The purpose of antepartum fetal heart monitoring is to distinguish a fetus who is healthy from one who is at risk for an adverse perinatal outcome. For the fetus at risk, the evaluations must further discriminate between those conditions that can be improved by intrauterine treatment and those that would best be treated by delivering the fetus and providing treatment after birth. Any maternal or fetal condition that could place the fetus at increased risk of mortality or morbidity is an indication for antepartum fetal heart monitoring (Druzin 1990).

Nonstress Test

A nonstress test (NST) is used to assess the integrity of the fetal central nervous system. The NST is based on the theory that an intact nervous system and a responsive cardiovascular system result in transient accelerations of the FHR in response to fetal activity (Goodwin 1992). For this test, the external ultrasound transducer and the tocodynamometer (toco) are applied to the woman, and a tracing of at least 20 minutes' duration is obtained so that the FHR and the uterine activity can be observed. The woman is positioned in the left lateral position and is asked to press a button every time she feels fetal movement. The monitor records a mark at each point of fetal movement, which is used as a reference point to assess FHR response. A reactive (negative) test result, which indicates a healthy fetus, is defined as two or more accelerations of the FHR with an amplitude of at least 15 beats per minute (bpm) and a duration of at least 15 seconds during a 20-minute period (Devoe 1990) (Fig. 26–5). A nonreactive test result shows no accelerations or accelerations less than 15 bpm or less than 15 seconds in duration for a 40-minute observation window. An unsatisfactory test is one that cannot be interpreted because of poor quality of the FHR tracing.

Some practitioners advocate extending the test-

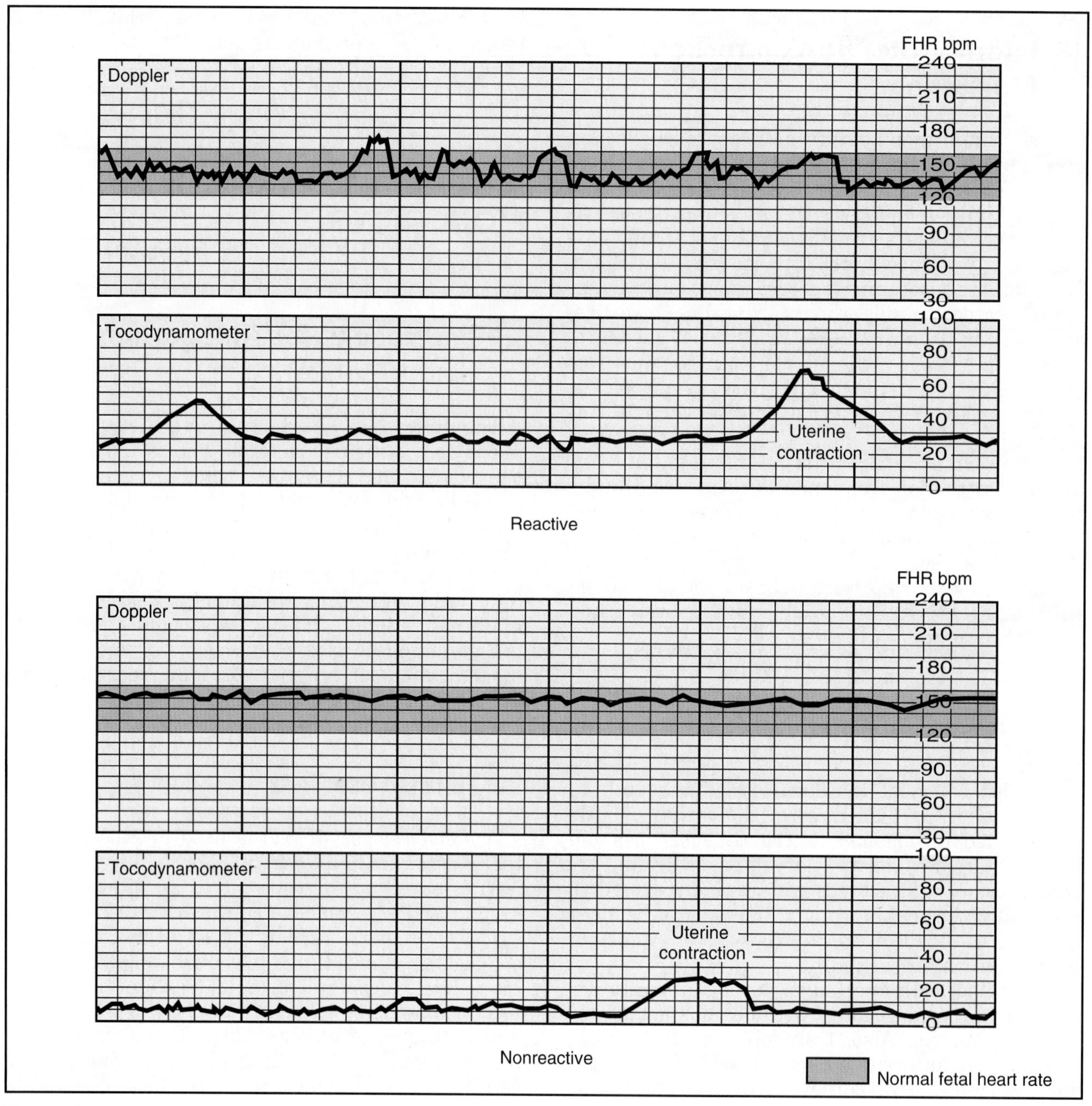

Figure 26–5

Tracings from nonstress tests (NSTs) show two types of results • Reactive results in which two or more accelerations of the FHR record an amplitude of at least 15 bpm and a duration of at least 15 seconds associated with fetal movements • Nonreactive results in which no acceleration of FHR is seen. (Tracings adapted from Parer, J. T. [1983]. *Handbook of fetal heart rate monitoring* [pp. 184 and 186]. Philadelphia: W. B. Saunders.)

ing time for the NST up to 2 hours (Vintzileos, et al. 1987). If the fetus is sleeping, it will awaken during that time. If the fetus is hypoxic, however, the picture on the monitor will not improve. In either event, the care provider will have sufficient data to complete this step in fetal assessment and either discharge the woman or move to the next level of fetal testing.

A fetus will not have accelerations during sleep cycles, so efforts to awaken the fetus by either gentle maternal abdominal manipulation or vibroacoustic stimulation may be useful. However, fetal sleep periods generally do not exceed 40 minutes, so a nonreactive tracing that persists longer than 40 minutes should cause the nurse to consider causes other than sleep. If a reactive tracing cannot be elicited in the recommended time frame, or if spontaneous FHR decelerations are observed, the next level of testing (contraction stress test, biophysical profile) is usually done (Devoe 1990).

Contraction Stress Test

A contraction stress test (CST) differs from the NST in that the fetus is exposed to the stressor of contractions to see if there is adequate placental perfusion under simulated labor conditions. For the test, the external fetal monitor is applied to the woman and a 20- to 30-minute baseline strip is recorded. The uterus is stimulated to contract either by administration of a dilute dose of oxytocin (Pitocin) or by having the woman use nipple stimulation until three palpable contractions with a duration of 40 seconds or more in a 10-minute period have been achieved (Fig. 26–6). Table 26–2 illustrates the possible outcomes.

CST by breast stimulation is more physiologic and less invasive than a CST achieved by using oxytocin through an intravenous line. Preparation

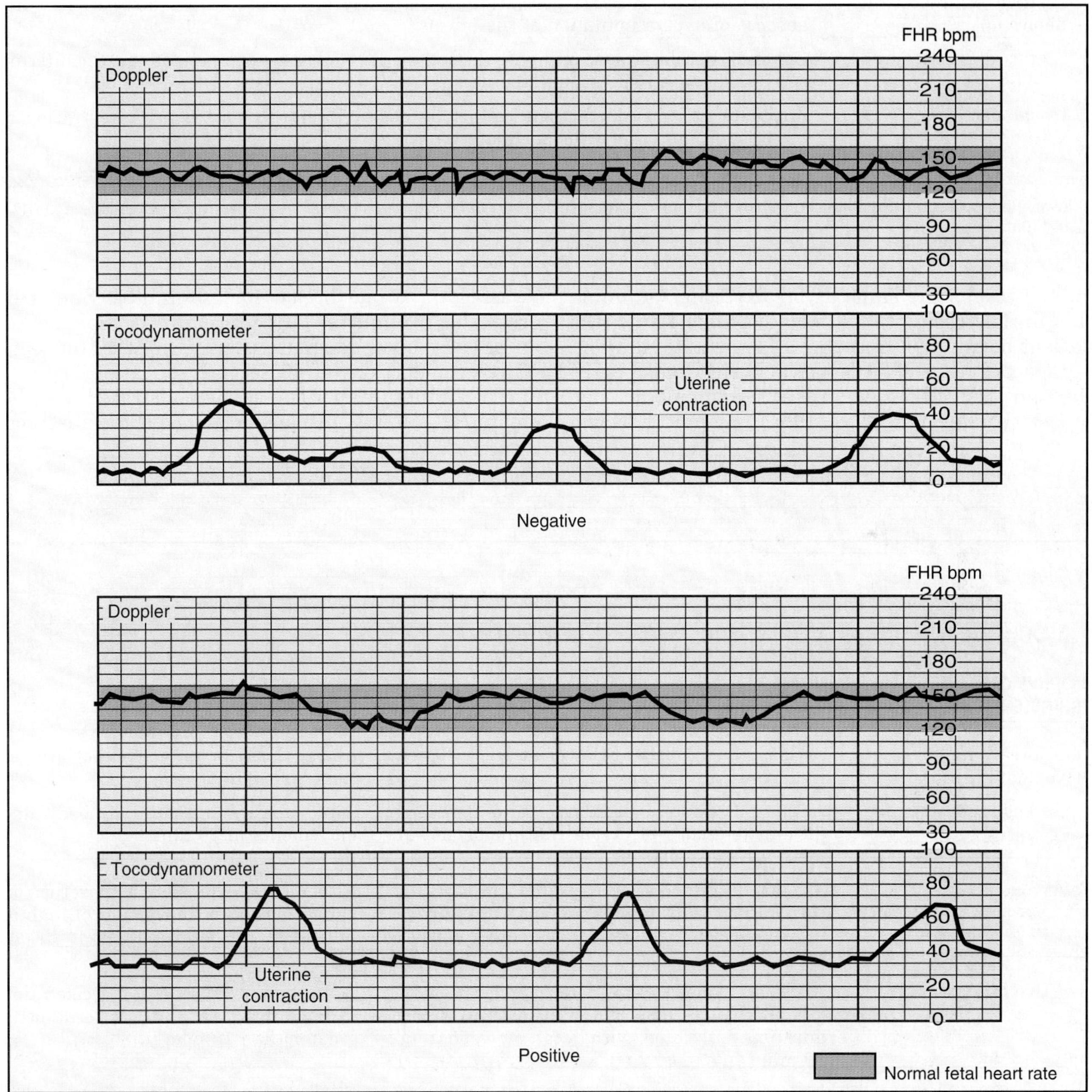

Figure 26–6

Negative results from a contraction stress test (CST) occur when no late or variable decelerations are recorded in response to stimulated contractions, which is a reassuring indication that the fetus can tolerate labor • Positive results occur when late decelerations are recorded with 50 percent or more of the contractions. (Negative tracing adapted from Freeman, R., Garite, T., Nageotte, M. [1991]. *Fetal heart rate monitoring* [2nd ed.] [p. 161]. Baltimore: Williams & Wilkins; positive tracings from Parer, J. T. [1983]. *Handbook of fetal heart rate monitoring* [p. 188]. Philadelphia: W. B. Saunders.)

Table 26–2

CONTRACTION STRESS TEST: FOUR POSSIBLE OUTCOMES

OUTCOME	DEFINITION
1. Negative (reassuring)	Exhibits no late or variable decelerations of the fetal heart rate
2. Positive (nonreassuring, abnormal)	Exhibits late or variable decelerations with 50% or more of the contractions in the absence of hyperstimulation of the uterus
3. Equivocal	Contains decelerations, but with less than 50% of the contractions, or the uterine activity shows a hyperstimulated uterus
4. Unsatisfactory	Adequate uterine contractions cannot be achieved, or the fetal heart rate tracing is not of sufficient quality for adequate interpretation

From Pircon, R., and Freeman, R. (1990). The contraction stress test. *Obstetrics and Gynecology Clinics of North America,* 17 (1), 129–146.

for the test is the same as for oxytocin. Assuming this initial tracing is within acceptable limits, the patient begins the procedure of breast stimulation. In a space that affords privacy, she may gently, through her clothing, stroke the nipple of one breast (Huddleston et al. 1984) or apply a warm washcloth to one breast for 2 minutes. She then rests for 5 minutes. This procedure is repeated as necessary until adequate uterine activity (at least three contractions of 40 seconds' duration or more in a 10-minute period) is demonstrated on the monitor. Nursing responsibilities include instruct-

Table 26–3

BIOPHYSICAL PROFILE SCORING: TECHNIQUES AND INTERPRETATIONS

BIOPHYSICAL VARIABLE	NORMAL (SCORE = 2)	ABNORMAL (SCORE = 0)
Fetal breathing movements (FBM)	At least 1 episode of FBM of at least 30 sec in duration in 30 min of observation	Absent FBM or no episode of greater than 30 sec in 30 min
Gross body movements	At least 3 discrete body/limb movements in 30 min (episodes of active continuous movement are considered a single movement)	2 or fewer episodes of body/limb movements in 30 min
Fetal tone	At least 1 episode of active extension with return to flexion of fetal limbs or trunk; opening and closing of hand considered normal tone.	Either slow extension with return to partial flexion or movement of limb in full extension; fetal movement absent
Reactive fetal heart rate	At least 2 episodes of fetal acceleration of greater than 15 bpm and of at least 15 sec in duration associated with fetal movement in 30 min	Less than 2 episodes of acceleration of fetal heart rate or acceleration of greater than 15 bpm in 30 min
Qualitative amniotic fluid volume	At least 1 pocket of amniotic fluid that measures at least 1 cm in 2 perpendicular planes	Either no amniotic fluid pockets or a pocket less than 1 cm in 2 perpendicular planes

From Manning, F. (1990). The fetal biophysical profile score: Current status. *Obstetrics and Gynecology Clinics of North America,* 17 (1), 147–162.

ing the patient in the procedure, verifying that adequate uterine activity is being achieved and that the FHR is acceptable, and maintaining the woman's privacy throughout.

Uterine hyperstimulation has been noted to occur in up to 55 percent of the women using breast stimulation for CSTs, some of which is associated with fetal bradycardia. Consequently, CST using breast stimulation should always be conducted in a clinical environment where immediate intervention is available for fetal distress.

There are also risks associated with a CST. Because the test involves the stimulation of uterine contractions, a CST is contraindicated in any woman who should not have such contractions: for example, women with threatened preterm labor, placenta previa, multiple gestation and a vertical uterine scar (ACOG 1994).

Biophysical Profile

The biophysical profile (BPP) is the first choice for follow-up fetal evaluation, after an NST. The BPP includes NST, an ultrasound examination that evaluates fetal reactivity, fetal breathing, and fetal tone; the amniotic fluid volume; and the texture (grade) of the placenta (Gebauer and Lowe 1993) (Table 26–3). Fetal biophysical activities that are regulated by the central nervous system (FHR reactivity, fetal movements, fetal breathing movements, and fetal tone) are depressed by acute hypoxia. These indicators go away one at a time and in reverse order of the sequence in which they developed in early fetal life. Specifically, the first indicator to become depressed by hypoxia is the reactivity of the FHR, which first developed in the late second or early third trimester and disappears at a pH of approximately 7.20. Fetal breathing movements are second to be depressed; they first developed at about 20 to 21 weeks and disappear when the pH reaches 7.10 to 7.20. Third are fetal movements, which were first present at about 9 weeks, and fetal muscle tone, which first appeared about 7.5 to 8.5 weeks; these disappear below a pH of 7.10 (Vintzileos et al. 1987).

In addition to acute hypoxia, chronic hypoxia can be detected during a BPP by estimating the amniotic fluid volume. During sustained hypoxia, the fetus protects its vital organs (heart, brain, adrenals) by preferentially shunting blood toward those organs and away from the nonmetal organs (gut, kidney, lungs). If this shunting is maintained, one of the sequelae may be decreased kidney function, decreased urine production, and, consequently, decreased amniotic fluid volume (oligohydramnios). This decrease of the amniotic fluid cushion for the cord can then contribute to the development of variable decelerations. When variable decelerations are seen during an NST/BPP, the decelerations in labor or operative deliveries because of fetal distress increase markedly (Hoskins et al. 1991), even if other BPP components are normal (Vintzileos et al. 1987). Of all the components of the BPP, decreased amniotic fluid is the best predictor of fetal distress in labor as well as of poor perinatal outcome (Gebauer and Lowe 1993).

The last feature assessed during a BPP is the grade or texture of the placenta. Relatively early in fetal life, the placenta is smooth and uncalcified, and it is labeled grade 0. As the cotyledons develop and some calcification takes place, the placenta matures through grade I and is most commonly grade II at term. However, some placentas become excessively aged with much calcification of the cotyledons (Gaffney et al. 1990), to the point that their support of the fetus may be inadequate. This type of placenta, a grade III placenta, should alert the care provider to the increased likelihood of FHR abnormalities and abruptio placentae (see Fig. 25–4) during the intrapartum period (Vintzileos et al. 1987).

MONITOR PATTERNS

A consistent and systematic approach to interpretation of fetal monitor tracings is most likely to result in a thorough and accurate assessment. Basic FHR changes in labor are shown in Table 26–4. The components of FHR assessment are:

- Baseline: rate and rhythm
- Periodic changes
  Decelerations: early, late, and variable
  Accelerations: variable and fixed

Baseline Fetal Heart Rate

Baseline FHR is defined as the typical FHR during a 10-minute period or between uterine contractions in labor. It has two primary features: rate and variability (rhythm).

RATE

The baseline rate is the speed at which the heart is beating. There are three variations:

1. The normal baseline FHR, which has a lower limit of 120 bpm and an upper limit of 150 to

Table 26–4

BASIC FETAL HEART RATE CHANGES IN LABOR

PATTERN	PHYSIOLOGIC MECHANISM	PRIMARY TREATMENT AND EXAMPLE	COMMON CAUSES
Baseline bradycardia	Pressure on fetal head Parasympathetic dominance of fetal heart rate control Fetal hypoxia	Relieve pressure—change maternal position Increase oxygen—administer oxygen	Persistent posterior Fetal CNS maturation Chronic hypoxia
Baseline tachycardia	Increased fetal metabolism Hypoxic sympathetic stimulation of FHR	Slow metabolism—antipyretics Increase oxygen	Fever chorioamnionitis Hypoxia
Decreased variability	Central nervous system depression	Increase oxygen Withhold CNS depressing drugs	Hypoxia Drugs
Increased variability	Stimulation	Decrease or eliminate source of stimulation	Ephedrine Vacuum extractor
Early deceleration	Pressure on the fetal head	Relieve head compression (if indicated)	Descent in second stage
Late deceleration	Uteroplacental insufficiency	Improve circulation to the uterus—change maternal position, administer fluid bolus	Maternal supine position Oxytocin Inadequate placental perfusion
Variable deceleration and fixed acceleration	Compression of the umbilical cord	Decrease cord compression—change maternal position, amnioinfusion	Umbilical cord entrapment or entanglement
Second-stage patterns	Compression of the fetal head Traction on the umbilical cord Maternal valsalva maneuver	Discourage prolonged bearing down efforts (no longer than 5 to 6 sec.). Use open-glottis pushing	Fetal descent Maternal bearing down efforts

160 bpm (ACOG 1995). A baseline of 110 to 160 is considered normal for the mature fetus (AWHONN 1995). An FHR baseline change is one that persists for 10 minutes or longer.

2. Baseline bradycardia, which is an FHR less than 120 bpm. Mild bradycardia is 100 to 119 bpm; severe bradycardia is less than 100 bpm. Common causes of mild baseline bradycardia include postdates pregnancy (postmature fetus) and persistent posterior position. Hypoxia, a congenital heart block, and a prolapsed cord are associated with severe baseline bradycardia.
3. Baseline tachycardia, which is an FHR above 160 bpm. Mild tachycardia is 160 to 180 bpm, and severe tachycardia is more than 180 bpm. Common causes of baseline tachycardia include acute hypoxia, maternal or fetal fever, and betasympathomimetic drugs (Fig. 26–7).

VARIABILITY (RHYTHM)

The second baseline feature is variability, also called rhythm. Variability has two components: short-term variability (STV) and long-term variability (LTV). STV, also called beat-to-beat variability, is a result of beat-to-beat interval changes in the FHR. The most commonly observed range is between 6 and 10 bpm (Cabaniss 1993). STV is commonly charted as present (more than 5 bpm) or absent (less than 5 bpm).

LTV is the oscillations or undulations of the baseline FHR. Average LTV has 2 to 6 cycles per minute (Zanini et al. 1980; Freeman et al. 1991; Cabaniss 1993). An ominous variation, usually associated with fetal anemia, is sinusoidal rhythm, which is characterized by curves of LTV that undulate regularly around a fixed baseline rate with an amplitude of up to 30 bpm and absent STV (Parer 1994).

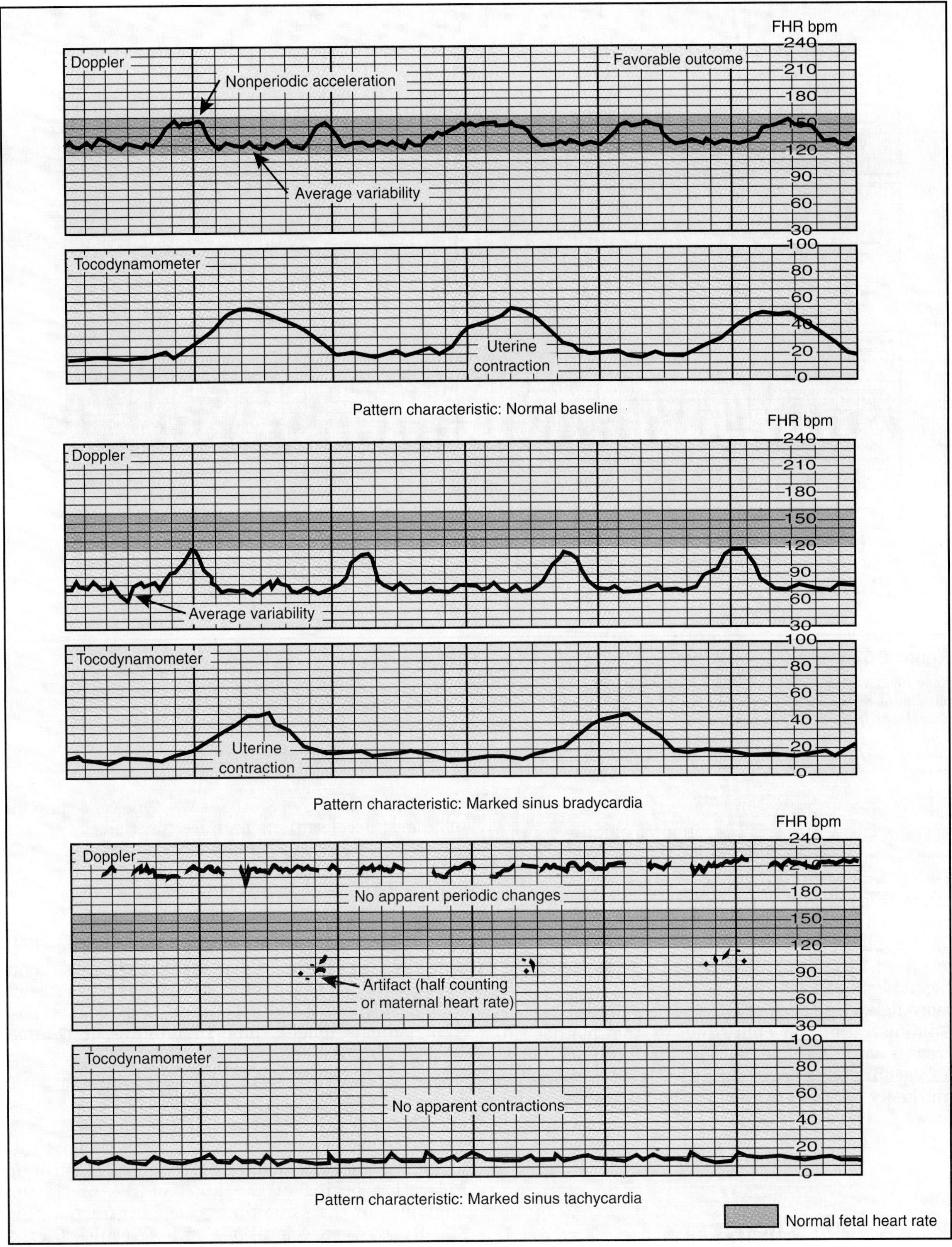

Figure 26–7

A normal baseline FHR ranges from 120 to 160 bpm • Severe baseline bradycardia is shown ranging from 60 to 110 bpm • Severe baseline tachycardia is recorded at 210 bpm. (Tracings adapted from Cabaniss, M. [1993]. *Fetal monitoring interpretation* [p. 7]. Philadelphia: J. B. Lippincott.)

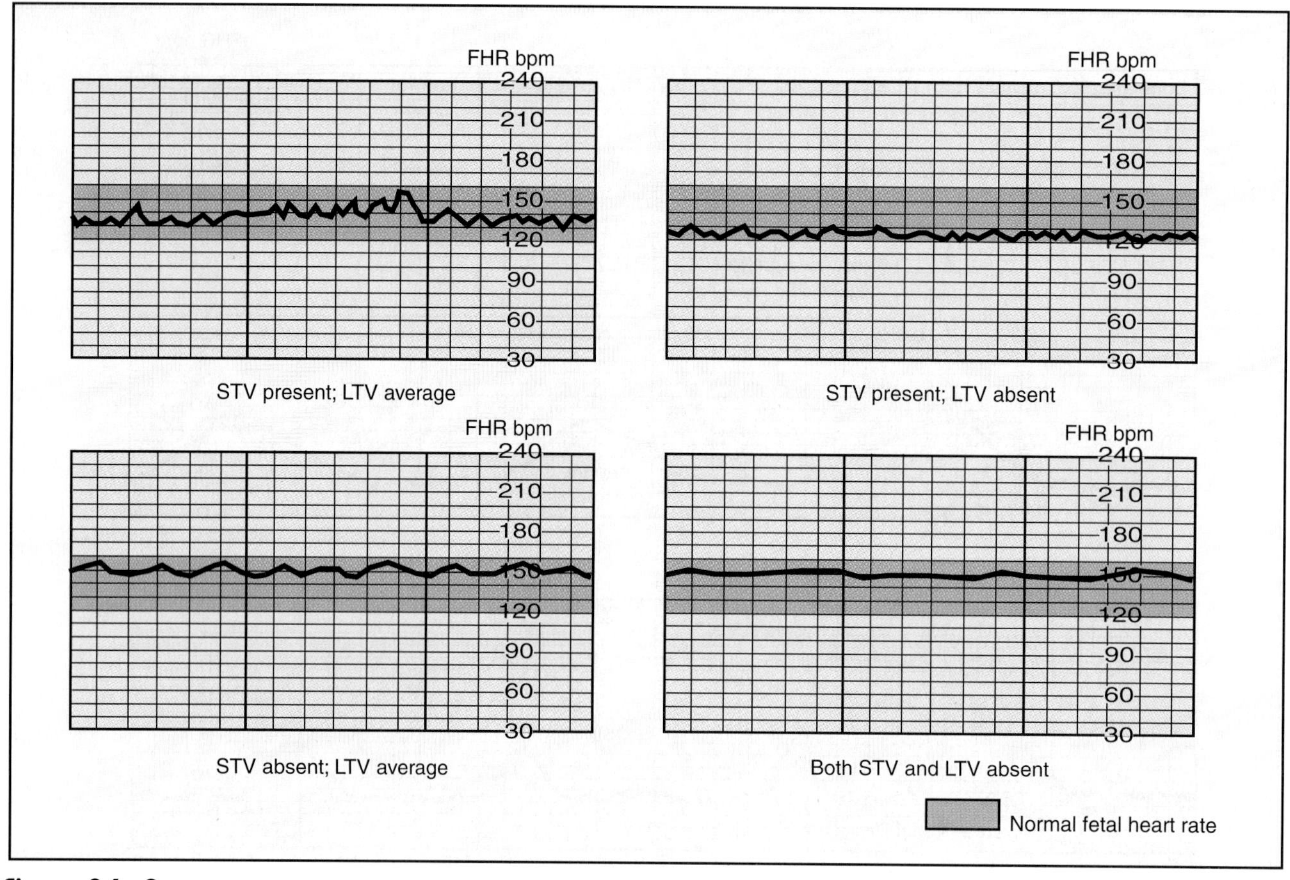

Figure 26–8

Long-term variability (LTV), short-term variability (STV), and combinations and/or absences of each demonstrate the beat-to-beat rhythm of STV and the oscillations of LTV. (Adapted from Zanini, B., Paul, R. H., Huey, J. R. [1980]. Intrapartum fetal heart rate: Correlation with scalp pH in the preterm fetus. *American Journal of Obstetrics and Gynecology,* 136 [1], 43–47.)

Changes in Variability

Fetal sleep cycles cause the variability to decrease temporarily (30 to 60 minutes) (Cabaniss 1993), as do maternal medications such as narcotics (Fig. 26–8). The earliest effect of fetal hypoxia is increased STV and LTV. With persistent fetal hypoxia, STV decreases first, followed by the loss of LTV. When adequate fetal oxygenation is reestablished, LTV reappears first, followed by a more delayed return of STV (Freeman et al. 1991). Administration of ephedrine to the mother increases variability temporarily. The application of a vacuum extractor may increase variability markedly for the duration of time that the suction is on.

Periodic Changes

Periodic changes are brief deviations above or below the baseline that usually occur in relation to uterine contractions or fetal activity (Freeman et al. 1991). There are two types of periodic changes: decelerations and accelerations.

TYPES OF DECELERATIONS

Decelerations are deviations below the FHR baseline that persist for at least 10 to 15 seconds but for less than 2 minutes. A prolonged deceleration lasts longer than 2 minutes. If the deceleration persists longer than 10 minutes, it becomes the new baseline.

Early Decelerations

Early decelerations have a uniform shape, which is a mirror image of the contraction. An early deceleration begins at the start of the contraction and ends at the same time as the contraction (Fig. 26–9). Early decelerations are a result of vagal nerve stimulation caused by fetal head contraction during contractions with descent of the fetal head. Early decelerations are usually within normal FHR baseline range.

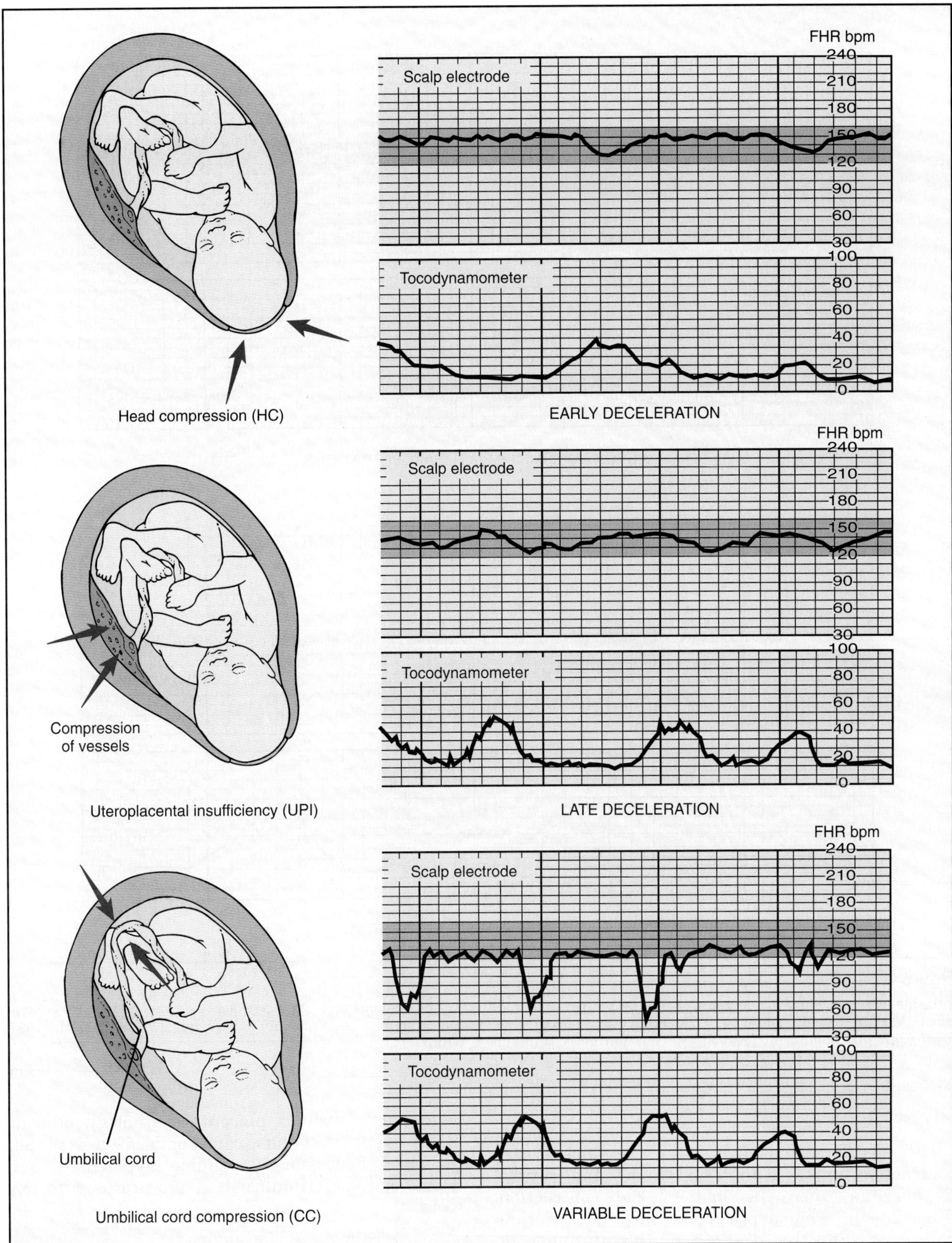

Figure 26–9

Three types of decelerations are demonstrated • Early deceleration caused by head compression (HC) • Late deceleration due to uteroplacental insufficiency (UPI) • Variable decelerations as a result of umbilical cord compression (CC). (Tracings adapted from Cabaniss, M. [1993]. *Fetal monitoring interpretation* [p. 210]. Philadelphia: J. B. Lippincott.)

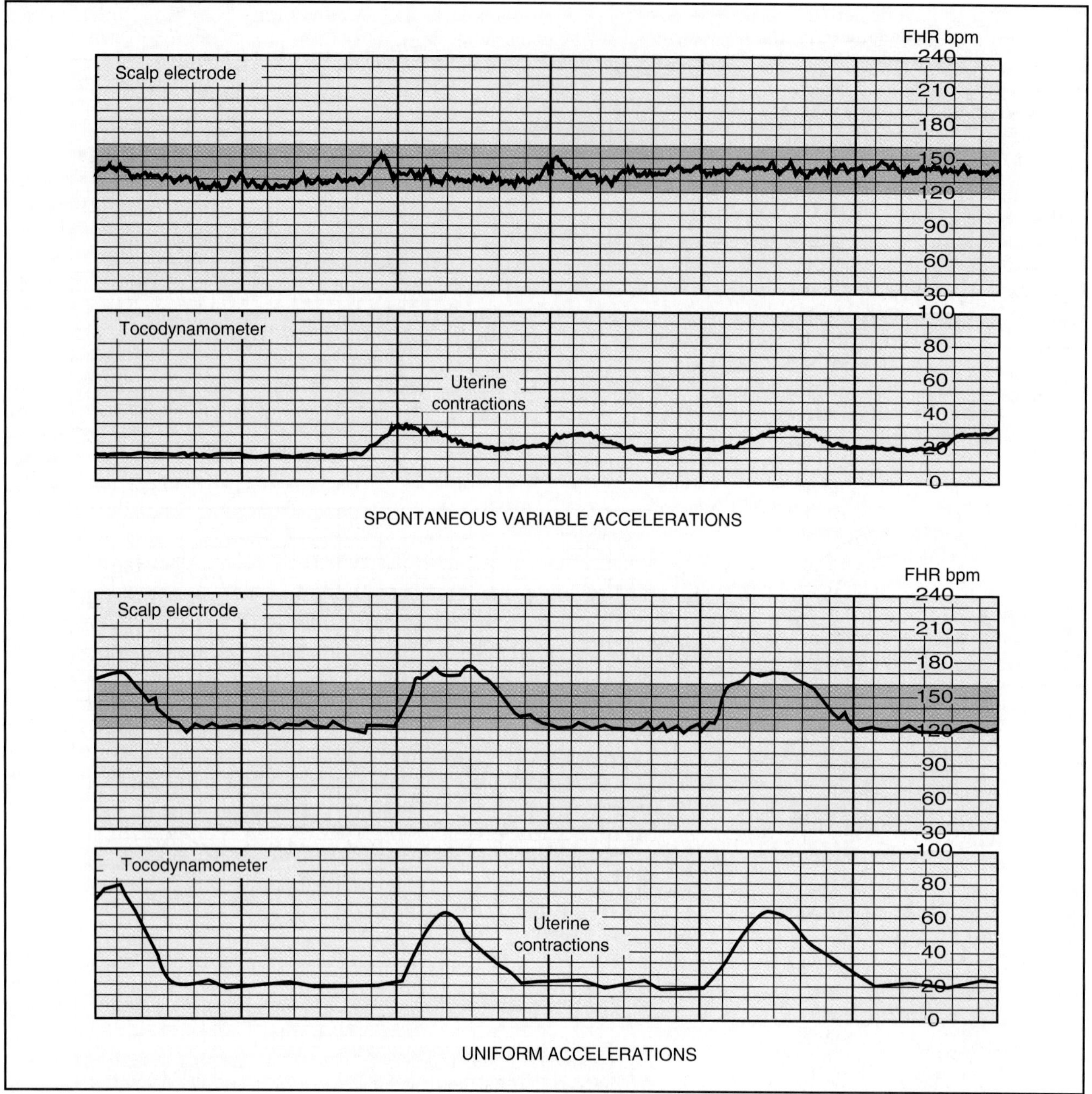

Figure 26–10

Variable accelerations are spontaneous and do not occur in relation to the contractions • Fixed accelerations occur with contractions. (Variable tracing courtesy of Fairfax Hospital; fixed acceleration adapted from Freeman, R., Garite, T., Nageotte, M. [1991]. *Fetal heart rate monitoring* [2nd ed.] [p. 88]. Baltimore: Williams & Wilkins.)

Late Decelerations

Late decelerations begin after the start of the contraction, have a uniform shape, and return to baseline *after* the end of the contraction (Fig. 26–9). The depth of a late deceleration will vary with the strength of the uterine contraction and the severity of fetal hypoxia. Late decelerations are a result of decreased uteroplacental perfusion, which causes a decrease in fetal PO_2. Late decelerations can be caused by a pathologic event, such as placental pathology, or some other event that has compromised uteroplacental blood flow, such as supine hypotensive syndrome or hyperstimulation of the uterus with oxytocin.

Variable Decelerations

Variable decelerations are more angular or V-shaped (i.e., have faster onset and recovery) than the uniform or U-shaped early and late decelerations. The shape of the variable decelerations differs from one deceleration to the next (Fig 26–9). The onset of variable decelerations may or may not have a relationship to the onset of a contraction. Some may even begin between contractions. The mechanism for variable decelerations is compression of the umbilical cord. Movement of the fetus or a contraction of the uterus places pressure on the umbilical cord, which initially causes the umbilical vein to be compressed. This impairs blood flow from the placenta into the body of the fetus and decreases the fetal blood volume. The fetal heart compensates for this drop in the stroke volume by increasing the heart rate to maintain a stable cardiac output. If the compression of the umbilical cord is sufficient to close the arteries, the flow of fetal blood (to the placenta) is impaired, which increases the blood volume in the fetal heart. This increase in pressure causes the fetal heart to decrease its rate of contraction (Berne and Levy 1996), resulting in the variable deceleration. When the compression is released, either by changing the maternal or fetal position or by cessation of the contraction, the processes occur quickly in reverse. The baseline rate usually remains within normal range with variable decelerations.

Repetitive variable decelerations occur with the onset of most if not all uterine contractions. The decelerations are repetitive because the umbilical cord is in a fixed position, such as around the fetal neck or limbs, and it is compressed with each contraction. This type of pattern is likely to increase in severity during the course of labor, particularly with the advent of the second stage, as the fetal body descends and the traction on the umbilical cord increases.

Variable decelerations can be classified as to their severity by observing the amplitude (depth) and duration. Severe variables are characterized by (1) a change in the baseline rate of 60 bpm or more (e.g., a drop from 150 to 90 bpm), or a nadir that is lower than 60 bpm, and (2) a duration of 60 seconds or longer (Parer 1994). Variable decelerations that do not meet these criteria are described as either mild or moderate (Krebs et al. 1983).

ACCELERATIONS

Accelerations are increases in heart rate over baseline FHR, usually in response to fetal movement. Accelerations may be of variable or uniform timing.

Variable Timing

Accelerations that may or may not occur simultaneously with a contraction are called variable accelerations. They are generally associated with periods of fetal movement and are considered a sign of fetal well-being (Fig. 26–10).

Uniform Timing

Accelerations that are consistently associated with the onset of uterine contractions and have a uniform shape that is the same as the curve of the contractions are called uniform accelerations. They are most likely attributable to cord compression that is strong enough to compress the umbilical vein but not the artery (Fig. 26–10). This partial cord compression causes a decreased blood return to the fetal heart, resulting in decrease in the fetal cardiac output. A baroreceptor response causes the compensatory FHR acceleration, as described above. Uniform accelerations are thought to be benign, although they may be predictive of variable decelerations as labor progresses.

Nonreassuring Patterns

These nonreassuring patterns have physiologic and clinical significance and are associated with decreasing fetal well-being (Fig. 26–11). Changes that indicate deterioration in a decompensating fetus usually occur in the following order: loss of initial acceleration (shoulders), followed by slow return of the FHR to baseline rates, loss of secondary acceleration (shoulders), presence of prolonged secondary acceleration (overshoot), biphasic deceleration, loss of variability during the deceleration, and finally, decreased FHR.

LOSS OF INITIAL AND SECONDARY ACCELERATION (SHOULDERS)

The presence of initial and secondary accelerations (shoulders) with a variable deceleration is indicative of the baroreceptor response to the decreased venous return to the heart that accompanies partial cord occlusion. The absence of the small accelerations before and after a variable deceleration most likely has a nonominous interpretation. This is the most commonly seen nonreassuring pattern and it is the least predictive of low Apgar scores (Krebs et al. 1983; Cabaniss 1993).

PROLONGED SECONDARY ACCELERATION (OVERSHOOT)

A 20- to 30-second smooth (without STV) acceleration following a variable deceleration is called an overshoot. It is a compensatory fetal response to hypoxia occurring during a variable deceleration (Cabaniss 1993). An overshoot is an indication of the decreased ability of the fetus to recover from the hypoxia during the variable deceleration. If a severe variable deceleration pattern persists,

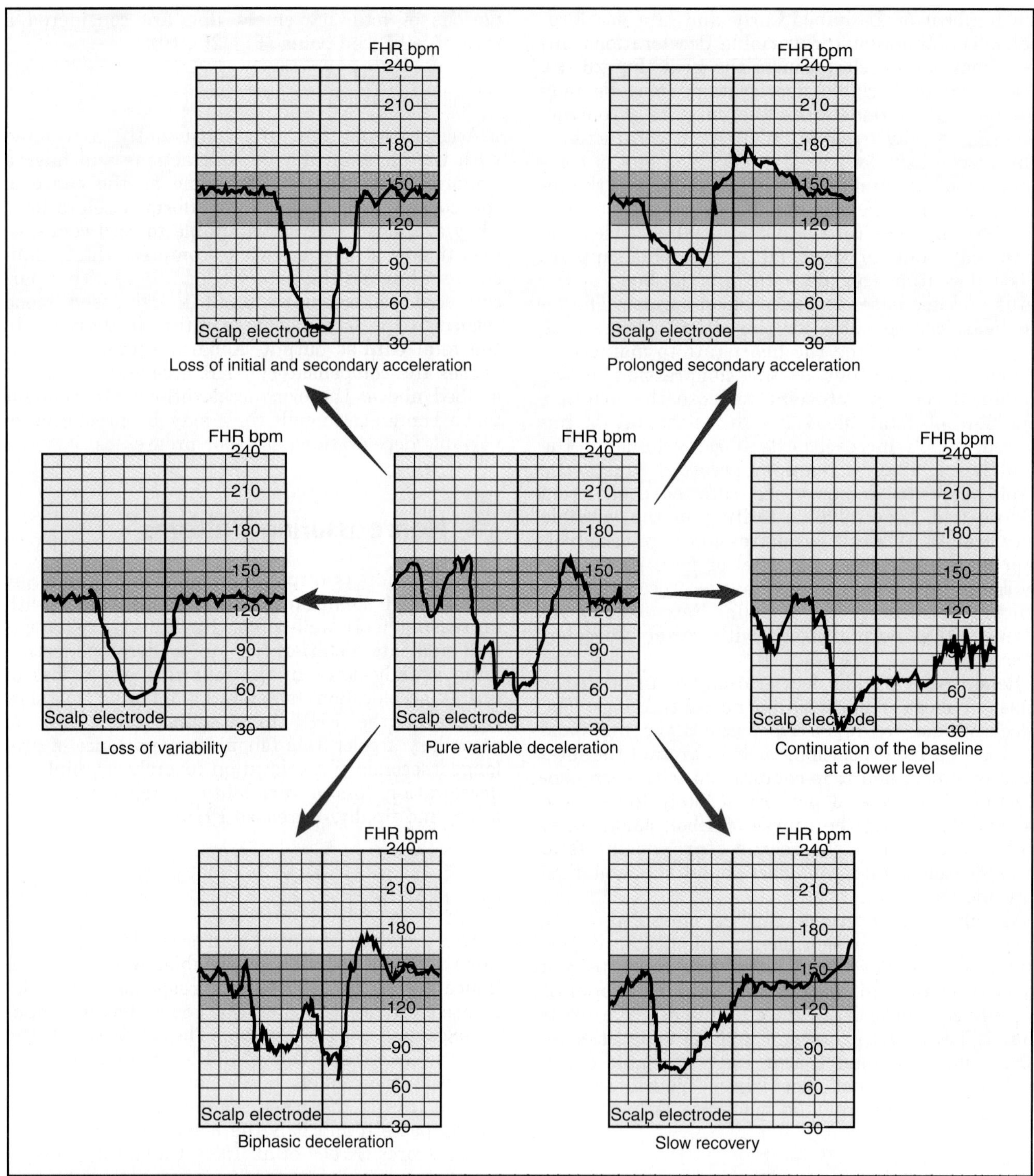

Figure 26–11

Atypical variable decelerations are often accompanied by decreased baseline variability and indicate fetal hypoxia. (Tracings from Krebs, H. B., Petres, R. E., Dunn, L. J. [1983]. Intrapartum fetal heart rate monitoring. VIII. Atypical variable decelerations. *American Journal of Obstetrics and Gynecology,* 145 (3), 297–305.)

fetal hypoxia will progress to acidosis and the overshoots will disappear because the fetus has lost the ability to compensate. Therefore, the loss of the prolonged secondary acceleration should not be mistaken for a sign of improvement in fetal status.

BIPHASIC DECELERATION

The biphasic deceleration is a W-shaped variable deceleration thought to be more ominous than a V-shaped variable deceleration. The biphasic deceleration occurs because a second variable deceleration starts before the FHR has returned to baseline from the ongoing variable deceleration. It is thought to represent the persistence of significant fetal hypoxia beyond the duration of the contraction and may thereby assume the prognostic meaning of late decelerations (Krebs et al. 1983; Cabaniss 1993).

SLOW RETURN TO BASELINE

When biphasic decelerations increase in severity, there is a slow return to baseline FHR.

LOSS OF VARIABILITY

Loss of variability, as discussed earlier, is the most worrisome observation in atypical variables, just as it is with other patterns, and for the same reasons. In the absence of maternal drugs or fetal sleep, STV or beat-to-beat variability is the single most significant indicator of fetal well-being. Loss of STV, regardless of what else is happening, is a nonreassuring pattern.

DECREASED BASELINE FHR

If the variable FHR pattern continues, the fetus further decompensates and is unable to sustain a baseline heart rate in the normal range. The decreased baseline may descend to the level of bradycardia (less than 120 bpm).

CHANGES IN THE FETAL HEART RATE IN THE SECOND STAGE OF LABOR

The more frequent appearance of decelerations is one of the major changes in FHR during the second stage. FHR patterns in the second stage of labor cannot be interpreted appropriately without modification of the guidelines for the FHR pattern interpretation in the first stage. This is primarily because of two physiologic events that are unique to the second stage: descent of the fetus and onset of maternal bearing-down efforts.

With the descent of the presenting part, usually the vertex, increased traction on the umbilical cord may precipitate variable decelerations. Descent through the birth canal also subjects the vertex to greater pressures than are usually present during the first stage of labor. These pressures on the fetal head then stimulate vagal response, which slows the heart rate and produces decelerations that may have characteristics of early or variable decelerations. During the descent of a nonvertex presentation, such as a breech, a wide variety of atypical FHR decelerations may occur. Clearly, the cause of this type of deceleration is a reflex response and not a result of hypoxia.

During the second stage, late decelerations may also appear for the first time when a sudden acute insult, such as maternal hypotension, is imposed on a previously normal fetus. For example, when a woman is turned onto her back to push, a sudden onset of supine hypotension decreases blood pressure and compromises uterine blood flow so that the fetus does not get adequate oxygenated blood. The fetal Po_2 is sensed by the chemoreceptors, which stimulate a vagal response and cause a reflex deceleration. It is also possible that a drop in maternal Po_2 accompanies the apnea associated with maternal bearing-down efforts, and that the drop is more severe during Valsalva-style bearing-down efforts than during mini-pushes or bearing-down efforts that maintain an open glottis (Cosner and deJong 1993: Woolley and Roberts 1995).

There are some characteristic changes in FHR that appear exclusively during the late second stage (Melchior and Bernard 1989).

1. A stable baseline rate in the normal range with repetitive decelerations, usually variable, becoming progressively more severe with each bearing-down effort. A reassuring feature is the return to the previous baseline rate during the short rest between contractions; this indicates recovery of the fetus. This is the most common pattern change during late second-stage labor.
2. A rapid fall in the baseline rate, culminating in prolonged bradycardia. There may be superimposed decelerations during contractions. The tracing will also show decreasing variability, which may terminate in a flat baseline rate.
3. A severe bradycardia baseline (less than 100 bpm with marked accelerations during contractions) may occur. This may often be misinterpreted as a normal baseline with decelerations. However, this pattern is often associated with poor Apgar scores.
4. A normal FHR, with or without decelerations, suddenly slows and develops into bradycardia of less than 90 bpm. This is most commonly seen during the final moments before birth and may reflect the pressures on the fetus that accompany imminent delivery (Piquard et al. 1989).

Correlation Between Electronic Fetal Monitoring and Apgar Scores

Research has shown little correlation between the FHR pattern and the Apgar score. As indicated in earlier sections, many infants who have a nonreassuring or ominous tracing are born in good condition. This is an example of a false-positive finding. However, there are also false-negative findings, that is, infants who receive low Apgar scores in the presence of a normal tracing (Cabaniss 1993).

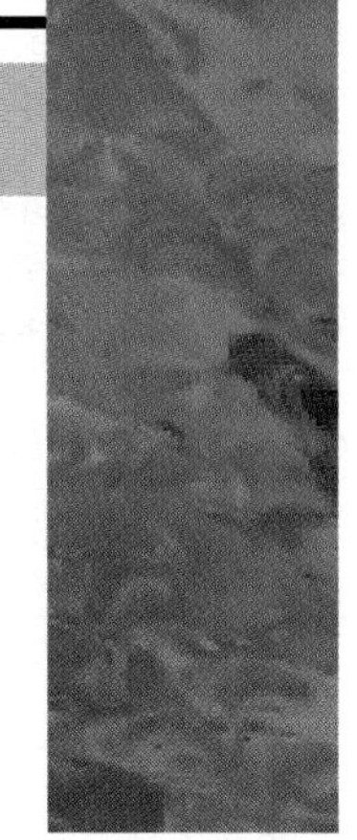

Nursing Practice

Nursing Process

▼ Assessment

The nurse gathers data including but not limited to the following:

- Woman's background data: estimated date of confinement/estimated gestational age; gravidity and parity; history of medical problems; history of obstetric problems; problems with this pregnancy; medications—over-the-counter, prescription, recreational (tobacco and alcohol), illegal
- Labor status: stage and phase of labor; presentation and position of the baby; status of the membranes—intact or date and time of rupture, color and consistency of amniotic fluid; dilatation of the cervix; station of the presenting part; use of Pitocin, analgesia, or anesthesia
- Uterine activity pattern: frequency, duration,

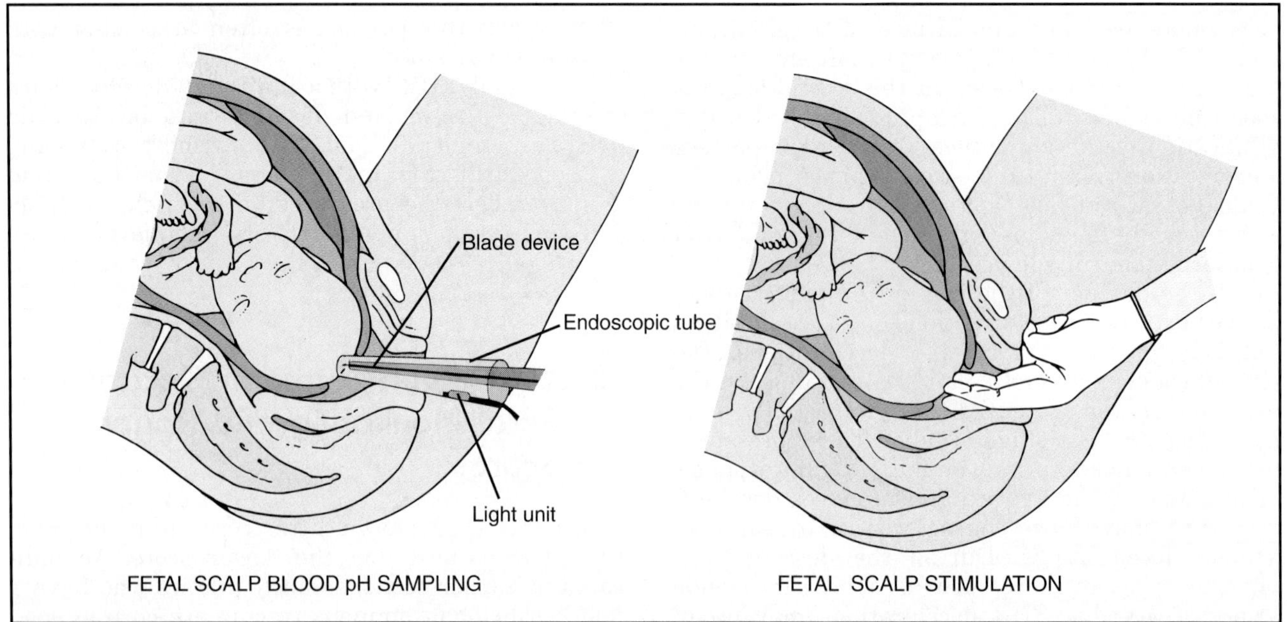

Figure 26–12

Fetal scalp blood pH sampling is done to assess the acid-base condition of the fetus's central circulation • A serendipitous observation arising from this sampling procedure has shown that the pressure or pinching occurring during the sampling often provokes an FHR acceleration • Studies that correlated the presence or absence of an FHR acceleration after scalp stimulation revealed that no acidotic fetus responded to the scalp stimulation with an acceleration.

and intensity of contractions; resting tonus of the uterus; Montevideo units (calculated as mean intensity × mean frequency per 10 minutes = Montevideo units; e.g., a woman having 50 mm Hg contractions every 3 minutes would be exhibiting 150 Montevideo units); 150 to 250 Montevideo units per 10-minute interval indicates adequate uterine activity

This information provides comprehensive assessment data that is the foundation for interpretation of the FHR pattern. The context of each woman's specific clinical situation will also influence the interpretation of the FHR pattern.

▼ ADJUNCTIVE FETAL ASSESSMENT TECHNIQUES

Given that the correlation between the FHR pattern and the infant's status at birth is not perfect, other measures have been added to the clinician's armamentarium for assessment during labor.

Fetal Scalp Blood pH Sampling. Since the primary goal of FHR monitoring is to identify the fetus who may have an acid-base status, one of the major assessment techniques used to improve the sensitivity of monitoring is fetal scalp blood assessment. Small samples of fetal blood taken from the scalp of the fetus correlate reasonably well with the acid-base condition of the central circulation (Fig. 26–12). In general, a value above 7.25 is considered normal, 7.20 to 7.25 is preacidotic, and below 7.19 is acidotic.

A disadvantage of fetal scalp blood sampling is that it is invasive, with potential for both infection and hemorrhage in the fetus and is contraindicated at times of an unknown presenting part, maternal genital infection, maternal HIV, HSV, herpes, maternal or fetal bleeding disorder, and prolonged fetal bradycardia. (Clark and Paul 1982).

Umbilical Cord Blood pH. There is a growing trend to do blood gases analysis of umibilical cord blood samples at delivery. This can be analyzed quickly and accurately, and such samples may assist the pediatric clinicians in the assessment of the acid-base status of the newborn (Parer 1994).

Fetal Scalp Stimulation. One serendipitous observation during fetal scalp blood sampling or vaginal examination was that stimulation of the fetal scalp often provoked an FHR acceleration. In the presence of FHR acceleration after scalp stimulation it has been well substantiated that a fetus who responds to scalp stimulation with FHR acceleration has a pH within the normal range (Clark et al. 1982).

Vibroacoustic Stimulation. Another form of fetal assessment that is even less invasive than scalp stimulation is vibroacoustic stimulation, also known as fetal acoustic stimulation (FAS-Test). It involves the application of a 105 to 110 dB vibration or noise to the maternal abdomen for 3 to 5 seconds. A reactive response is the same as that for the NST, an acceleration in the FHR greater than 15 bpm for more than 15 seconds.

IMPROVING YOUR PRACTICE

ELECTRONIC FETAL MONITORING

Electronic fetal monitoring greatly benefits the high-risk woman and her fetus. Thus, the maternal-newborn nurse needs to understand and be able to apply this tool when necessary. However, experience and comfort with technology should not influence nursing practice based on the normalcy of the events of pregnancy and labor. Skill and commitment to screening and caring for women using a high-touch, low-tech approach should remain a priority. New technology should be used to enhance the nurse's hands and mind, the best instruments that a competent and caring nurse offers to her patient.

- MAINTAIN YOUR THEORETIC BASE. Read accurate information from several points of view. Attend professional seminars related to fetal monitoring.
- REFINE YOUR CLINICAL SKILLS. Organize and attend strip rounds, where you and your colleagues exchange ideas on fetal monitor tracing interpretation and the appropriate associated management options.
- KNOW THE STANDARDS OF PRACTICE published by the Association of Women's Health, Obstetric and Neonatal Nurses and the American College of Obstetrics and Gynecology regarding monitoring during labor.
- ACKNOWLEDGE THAT IT IS IMPOSSIBLE for all women and their families to have a happy ending. Grief work is a desperate need for such families, and maternity nurses are notoriously underskilled in that area. Know the stages of grief and the therapeutic use of self. Most important, know that you cannot fix everything, but with the right skills, you can make it better.
- NEVER FORGET THAT THE WOMAN IN LABOR IS YOUR CENTRAL FOCUS AND RESPONSIBILITY. Respect her needs and wishes. Maintain as normal an experience as possible, no matter how high-risk the pregnancy. Help her to exit the experience feeling good about herself, her baby, and her care.

▼ Diagnosis

The nursing diagnoses related to fetal monitoring during labor might relate to either the mother or the fetus. The nursing diagnoses related to fetal status may be actual (if a problem has been identified) or potential (if no FHR alterations have been identified and the fetal status is stable). The following are examples of those nursing diagnoses that might be appropriate:

- Knowledge deficit: lack of information related to fetal monitoring procedures or status of the fetus
- Fear related to potential fetal injury
- Impaired gas exchange related to fetal risk due to poor placental perfusion
- Risk for injury related to fetal hypoxia

▼ Planning

The plan for the needed nursing care related to fetal status during labor is based on the identified nursing diagnoses. In developing the plan, goals can be identified that will guide the necessary interventions. These goals should be measurable and reflect desired outcomes. Examples of goals might be

- The woman will explain the reasons for the fetal assessment techniques being used, describe what will be done, and verbalize the status of her baby
- The woman will verbalize her feelings and fears related to her baby's status during labor
- The fetal monitor tracing will remain within normal limits, as evidenced by a rate between 120 and 160 bpm, normal baseline variability, and no nonreassuring periodic changes
- The baby will be delivered without injury

▼ Intervention

The nursing interventions for a woman in labor related to fetal status can be broadly categorized into one of two areas: physiologic interventions and active interventions.

▼ PHYSIOLOGIC MANAGEMENT

Physiologic management is in use when "the spontaneous birth process is maintained and encouraged by understanding, supporting and enhancing the body's normal mechanisms of birth" (Simkin 1984, p. 7). Nursing interventions instituted in response to FHR decelerations that could be considered physiologic include

- Changing maternal position, which can improve maternal venous return, assist the fetus to rotate from occiput posterior to occiput anterior position, and relieve cord compression. Upright positions are also associated with more efficient uterine activity (greater intensity, decreased frequency of the contractions). The options include walking, standing, squatting, hands and knees, sitting, and side-lying. Supine position should not be considered unless there is a specific indication for it, because it is associated with supine hypotensive syndrome, and it negatively influences the drive axis of the fetus into the pelvis.
- Administration of oxygen by face mask, generally at the rate of 6 liters per minute. This raises the mother's Po_2 and oxygen saturation, thereby making more oxygen available for transfer to the fetus.
- Verification of the true FHR with a fetoscope/stethoscope, which should be done if there is any doubt as to the accuracy of the FHR being obtained.
- Administration of an intravenous fluid bolus, which can improve both maternal cardiac output (blood pressure) and uteroplacental perfusion. In this situation, a solution such as lactated Ringer's is generally preferable to a dextrose-containing solution (e.g., D_5W) because of the possible adverse response of the infant to a sudden infusion of glucose. On the other hand, use of large or repeated boluses can have adverse effects on the mother's fluid load and so should not be used routinely.
- Discontinuing Pitocin, which should reduce uterine activity and by so doing increase uteroplacental perfusion. If the nurse is in doubt about the need to discontinue the Pitocin, the rule of thumb is to turn it off and consult the birth attendant. The Pitocin can always be restarted, with nothing but a few minutes lost.
- Sterile vaginal examination, which may reveal the cause of the deceleration, such as a prolapsed umbilical cord or precipitous descent of the fetus. It also affords the opportunity to test for the fetus's response to scalp stimulation.
- Physical and emotional support, which will reduce the maternal production of catecholamines and may increase endorphin production, easing both the pain and stress of the labor.

▼ ACTIVE MANAGEMENT

Active management is in use when the caregiver alters the spontaneous birth process through the use of exogenous chemical or mechanical interventions. These interventions usually require a physician's order. Such interventions may be medically indicated (e.g., the use of outlet forceps to

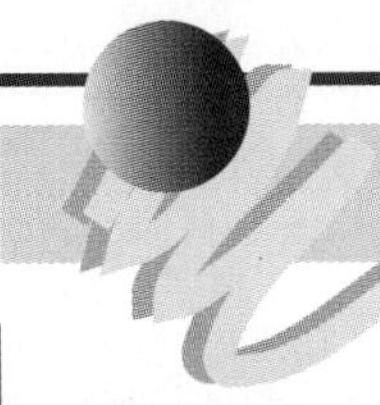

TEACHING GUIDE

THE USE OF THE FETAL MONITOR DURING LABOR

TOPIC	*MAJOR CONCEPTS*
Description of the fetal monitor	The fetal monitor is an electronic piece of equipment that is placed next to the bed to continuously record a laboring woman's contractions and the fetal heart rate during labor.
How the fetal monitor is attached	The fetal monitor can be applied using either external or internal leads. When the woman is monitored externally, a round disk (transducer) is placed around her abdomen over the spot where the baby's heart rate is heard; and a rectangular pressure-sensitive device (tocodynamometer, often referred to as a toco) is placed on the top (fundus) of her uterus to record the contractions. Both of these leads are attached with a belt that goes around the woman's abdomen. When the woman is monitored internally after her membranes have ruptured, a tiny spiral electrode is attached just under the skin of the presenting part of the baby to monitor heart rate. The baby cannot feel this and will not be harmed. To measure the contractions, a small plastic tube filled with sterile water is inserted into the woman's uterus, where it lies between the baby and the side of the uterus.
What the fetal monitoring tracing shows	The baby's heart rate appears as a squiggly line at the left of the paper as it prints out from the monitor; the normal heart rate of a baby in the uterus is 120 to 160 beats per minute. The fetus's heart rate may go above or below this range when a woman has a contraction. This is usually no cause for alarm and a nurse will be monitoring the fetal heart rate closely. Contractions appear as a series of waves along the right side of the monitor paper; they look like hills that will gradually become steeper as labor progresses. Some women and their partners find it helpful to watch the monitor so that they know when a contraction is starting; others prefer not to watch the monitor.
Effect of the monitor on comfort and positioning	Some women find that the fetal monitor is not uncomfortable and are actually unaware of its presence. Others may find that the belt used

Continued on following page

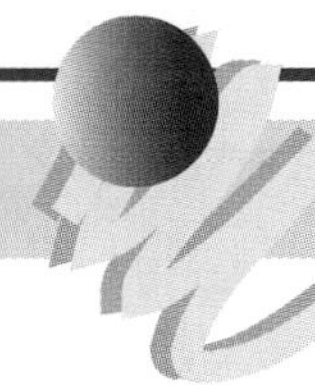

TEACHING GUIDE Continued

THE USE OF THE FETAL MONITOR DURING LABOR

TOPIC	*MAJOR CONCEPTS*
	for attachment of the external leads feels tight; once internal monitoring leads are attached, this discomfort is relieved. The nurse will work with the woman to adjust the monitor leads so that she is able to assume any position she wishes during labor.

Teaching Aids

1. An actual fetal monitor, a poster, or a picture showing the monitor; external and internal leads for monitoring fetal heart rate and uterine contractions.
2. A sample monitor strip showing how the contractions and fetal heart rate will look on the monitor printout.

Increasing Your Teaching Effectiveness

Your success in teaching about the fetal monitor will be enhanced by using the following approaches:

1. Establish a comfortable rapport with the woman and identify her current knowledge about fetal monitoring. Determine whether a support person needs teaching also.
2. Give her the information she needs in a clear, concise manner; use visual aids to increase the clarity of the information you give.
3. Ask her if she has questions; ask her to repeat her understanding of the information you have presented.

deliver an infant in distress), or they may be employed electively (e.g., the use of outlet forceps to deliver every primigravida). Interventions instituted in response to FHR decelerations that could be considered active management include

- Intrauterine resuscitation using subcutaneous terbutaline (a beta-sympathomimetic medication). A standard dose of 0.25 mg intravenous push will reduce uterine activity and thereby improve uteroplacental perfusion. The contraindications to the administration of a beta-sympathomimetic should be considered before the dose is given. These include vaginal bleeding that could be placental in origin and maternal cardiac disease. A physician's order is required before administration of this medication.
- Preparation for an expedited delivery, either instrumental (vacuum extractor, forceps) or surgical (cesarean). The goal is to obtain a delivery with minimal stress by lowering the resistances rather than by increasing the forces. It is important to identify fetal responses to interventions and choose the best compromise between potentially useful and potentially harmful procedures.

▼ COMMUNICATION WITH THE LABORING WOMAN

Communicaton with the woman is a critical feature in facilitation and support of the laboring process. The woman and companions need as much information as possible about the labor condition and the condition of the fetus. In addition to the psychological importance of communication, it may also decrease maternal catecholamine release and thus contribute to improved uteroplacental perfusion.

▼ DOCUMENTATION

The nursing interventions related to fetal monitoring must be thoroughly and accurately documented because they provide a record of the

Table 26–5

NURSING ACTIONS CHECKLIST IN RESPONSE TO ELECTRONIC FETAL MONITORING ABNORMALITIES

ACTIONS	EXAMPLES
*T*hink back (review)	Does the woman's history include any factors predisposing her to a fetal heart rate abnormality in labor? Has anything happened in the labor thus far that suggests a problem is developing?
*T*ests (diagnostic guides)	Are there data in the chart that can help rule out some problems? (e.g., a recent ultrasound examination showing a fundal placenta should rule out concerns of placenta previa in a woman who is bleeding) What maneuvers have you tried to identify the cause of the problem? (e.g., if the variable deceleration disappears when you reposition the woman from her back to her side, then the problem is more likely to be a free-floating cord than an entangled cord)
*T*reatments	Does the problem respond to physiologic interventions (e.g., position change), or do you need to use more active interventions like turn off the Pitocin and administer a uterine relaxant (beta-sympathomimetic)?
*T*each	Tell the mother and family what is happening, and what it means. Tell them what help you need (i.e., turn to your side, put on this oxygen mask). Tell them what they can expect to happen next. Do not overwhelm them with information, but do not conceal essential facts either. Be as encouraging as the circumstances permit while helping them to make reasonably informed judgments every step of the way.
*R*echeck	When are you going to reevaluate the fetal-maternal condition (i.e., look at the monitor strip, repeat a vaginal examination)? Why are you going to check at that time as opposed to some other time? What will be the next step after the reevaluation? (The options are maintain, supplement, or abandon the current plan and develop a new one.)
*R*efer	Do you need another pair of hands? Do you need the judgment of a more experienced professional? Do you need a procedure that you are not qualified to perform (i.e., scalp sampling, ultrasound examination)?
*R*ecord	What did you see? When did it start or stop? What was done about it? What is the condition of the mother and baby now? What is the plan for their immediate management?

woman's care that increases communication with other caregivers, serves as a record for quality assurance review, and documents what occurred in the event of legal action (Eganhouse 1991). The nurse should use the commonly accepted definitions for the FHR patterns and chart the appropriate interpretation (e.g., severe variable with a slow return to baseline) if a monitor tracing is the source of the data. If the FHR change was detected solely by auscultation, the nurse should chart the description of the change in the FHR (e.g., deceleration during a contraction with a nadir of 60 bpm, persisting approximately 10 seconds beyond the end of the contraction) (NAACOG 1990). Interventions should be recorded both in the woman's chart and on the monitor strip. Maternal vital signs, the time and findings of vaginal examinations, spontaneous or artificial rupture of membranes, position changes, administration of medications or anesthesia, administration of oxygen, application of internal leads, procedures, or maternal behavior that might affect the monitor strip (i.e., vomiting, coughing, laughing) should all be recorded on the monitor strip as well as in the chart. While considering each FHR pattern, the nurse may use a short, general checklist such as the one in Table 26–5 to ensure that all necessary steps have been taken.

▼ Evaluation

Evaluation of fetal status is a continual process throughout the intrapartum period (see Fig. 26–13. Short-term evaluation is done after each assessment technique or intervention by evaluating rate, variabilty, and pattern of the FHR. Long-term evaluation is made by periodically looking back over the entire monitor strip to determine changes in fetal status over time. If the status of the fetus remains positive or improves, the plan of care has been successful. If ominous changes occur or persist, the nursing diagnoses, plan, and interventions must be altered in a timely fashion to ensure the safe delivery of the baby.

Risk Management

The use of EFM in and of itself is a means of risk management throughout the antepartal and intrapartal periods for the woman with risk factors so that problems can be indentified and timely and appropriate interventions taken.

When EFM is used, risk management includes ensuring that all nurses have received advanced preparation in EFM and the evaluation of FHR patterns. Application of the monitor must be done correctly, whether external or internal leads are used. Accurate documentation of the observations of FHR and uterine contractions throughout labor, as well as of the nursing interventions that relate to these parameters, is critical for the management of risk.

Implications for Research

The following two questions are timely examples for nursing research related to fetal monitoring and nursing care. When these questions have been examined and implications for nursing practice are identified, other research questions can be examined related to improving care during labor and delivery when EFM is used.

- How does the electronic fetal monitor affect the woman's perception of her labor and her ability to cope?
- How does the use of the fetal monitor affect the nurse's use of physiologic interventions (e.g., ambulation, position changes) and comfort measures throughout labor?

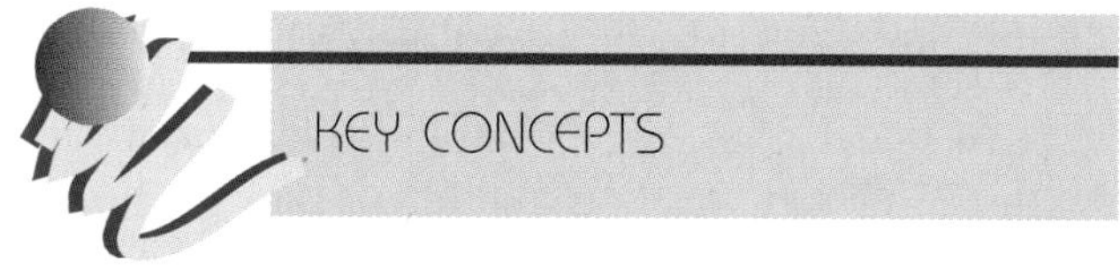

KEY CONCEPTS

- ▼ Neither the EFM equipment nor the nurse's ability to interpret its output is perfect. Good clinical judgment must always be the main guide in the nurse's decision-making process.
- ▼ Intermittent auscultation provides adequate fetal monitoring for women with no apparent medical risk (low-risk women).
- ▼ Continuous EFM has been shown to improve the neonatal outcomes of women with known medical risks (high-risk).

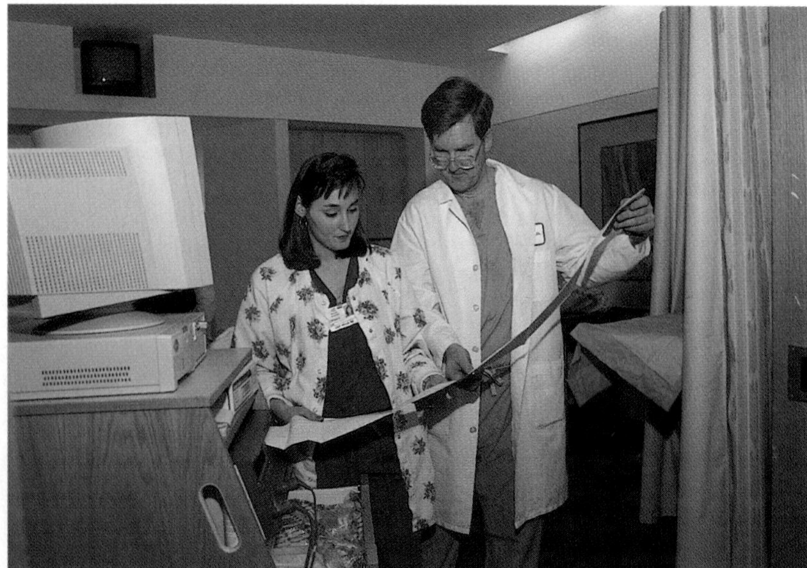

Figure 26–13

A nurse and physician confer about the tracings on a fetal monitoring strip used to interpret the progress of labor and the well-being of the fetus. Since the nurse is with the woman continuously throughout labor, it is important that she alert the physician to any fetal heart rate patterns that are of concern.

- ▼ For those fetuses deemed to be at risk, fetal well-being studies are used to discriminate between those whose conditions can be ameliorated by intrauterine treatment and those who would best be delivered and treated after birth.
- ▼ A consistent and systematic approach to the assessment of the features of the FHR is most likely to result in a thorough and accurate assessment by the nurse.
- ▼ Understanding the basic physiologic mechanism that underlies the FHR pattern must be combined with knowledge of the differential diagnosis for each feature so that the most appropriate interventions can be determined and implemented in a timely fashion.
- ▼ Interventions taken with a woman in labor can be broadly categorized into one of two varieties: physiologic interventions and active interventions (Simkin 1984). Physiologic management is in use when "the spontaneous birth process is maintained and encouraged by understanding, supporting and enhancing the body's normal mechanisms of birth" (Simkin 1984, p. 7). Active management is in use when the caregiver alters the spontaneous birth process through the use of exogenous chemical or mechanical interventions.
- ▼ Selection of nursing actions should consider the philosophy that the goal is to obtain a delivery with minimal stress by lowering the resistances rather than by increasing the forces.
- ▼ There is little correlation between the FHR pattern and the Apgar score. Therefore, the nurse needs to be alert to other measures of infant well-being.
- ▼ When using any test (e.g., FHR monitoring) or combination of tests (e.g., FHR monitoring, vibroacoustic stimulation, fetal scalp blood sampling, umbilical cord blood sampling), nurses need to appreciate that the more tests that are run, the more likely it is that some will turn out "abnormal" just by chance in the absence of any true disorder in the infant.
- ▼ No machine, no matter how sophisticated or expensive it is, can replace the human contact and clinical judgment of a competent and caring nurse. Support the laboring woman—physically and emotionally—to the maximal extent that staffing will allow. In most cases, the nurse, *not* the fetal monitor, is the most critical factor in whether the woman has a positive labor experience and birth outcome.

References

American College of Obstetricians and Gynecologists (ACOG). (1989). *Intrapartum fetal heart rate monitoring: FHR patterns* (Technical Bulletin 132). Washington, DC: Author.

American College of Obstetricians and Gynecologists (ACOG). (1994). *Antepartum fetal surveillance* (Technical Bulletin 177). Washington, DC: Author.

American College of Obstetricians and Gynecologists (ACOG). (1995). *Fetal heart rate patterns* (Technical Bulletin 207). Washington, DC: Author.

Auyeung, R., and Goldkrand, J. (1991). Vibroacoustic stimulation and nursing intervention in the nonstress test. *Journal of Obstetric, Gynecologic, and Neonatal Nursing,* 20 (3), 232–238.

Berne, R., and Levy, M. (1996). *Cardiovascular physiology* (7th ed.). St. Louis: C. V. Mosby.

Blair, E., and Stanley, F. (1988). Intrapartum asphyxia: A rare cause of cerebral palsy. *Journal of Pediatrics,* 112, 515–519.

Burpo, R. (1995). The pushing ritual of second stage labor. *The Journal of Perinatal Education,* 4 (2), 1–5.

Cabaniss, M. (1993). *Fetal monitoring interpretation.* Philadelphia: J. B. Lippincott.

Chez, B., Driscoll, C., Schmidt, J. (1991). *Nursing practice competencies and educational guidelines: Antepartum fetal surveillance and intrapartum fetal heart monitoring* (2nd ed.). Washington, DC: NAACOG.

Cibils, L. (1978). Clinical significance of fetal heart rate patterns during labor. II. Late decelerations. *American Journal of Obstetrics and Gynecology,* 123 (5), 473–494.

Clark, S., and Paul, R. (1982). Intrapartum fetal surveillance: The role of fetal scalp blood sampling. *American Journal of Obstetrics and Gynecology,* 153, 717–720.

Clark, S. L., Gimovsky, M. L., Miller, F. C. (1982). Fetal heart rate response to scalp blood sampling. *American Journal of Obstetrics and Gynecology,* 144, 706–708

Cosner, K., and deJong, E. (1993). Physiologic second stage labor. *MCN: American Journal of Maternal-Child Nursing,* 18 (1), 38–43.

Cottrell, B., and Shannahan, M. (1987). A comparison of fetal outcome in birth chair and delivery table births. *Research in Nursing and Health,* 10, 234–243.

Creasy, R. K., and Resnik, R. (1994). *Maternal-fetal medicine: Principles and practice* (3rd ed.). Philadelphia: W. B. Saunders.

Damus, K., and Merkatz, I. (1993). Fetal movement counting: Which method? *MCN: American Journal of Maternal-Child Nursing,* 18 (6), 314–321.

Davis-Floyd, R. (1992). *Birth as an American rite of passage.* Los Angeles: University of California Press.

Devoe, L. (1990). The nonstress test. *Obstetrics and Gynecology Clinics of North America,* 17 (1), 111–128.

Druzin, M. L. (1990). Fetal surveillance update. *Bulletin New York Academy of Medicine,* 66, 246–253.

Eganhouse, D. (1991). Electronic fetal monitoring: Education and quality assurance. *Journal of Obstetric, Gynecologic, and Neonatal Nursing,* 20 (1), 16–22.

Enkin, M., Keirse, M., Renfrew, M., Neilson, J. (1995). *A guide to effective care in pregnancy and childbirth* (2nd ed.). New York: Oxford University Press.

Feinberg, B., and Krebs, H. (1989). Fetal heart rate patterns. In J. A. D. Spencer (Ed.), *Fetal monitoring: Physiology and techniques of antenatal and intrapartum assessment.* 150–154 Philadelphia: F. A. Davis.

Freeman, R. (1990). Intrapartum fetal monitoring—A disappointing story. *New England Journal of Medicine,* 322 (9), 624–626.

Freeman, R., Garite, T., Nageotte, M. (1991). *Fetal heart rate monitoring* (2nd ed.). Baltimore: Williams & Wilkins.

Gaffney, S., Salinger, L., Vintzileos, A. (1990). The biophysical profile for fetal surveillance. *MCN: American Journal of Maternal-Child Nursing,* 15, 356–360.

Gebauer, C., and Lowe, N. (1993). The biophysical profile: Antepartal assessment of fetal well-being. *Journal of Obstetric, Gynecologic, and Neonatal Nursing,* 22 (2), 115–124.

Goodlin, J. R. (1979). History of fetal monitoring. *American Journal of Obstetrics and Gynecology,* 133 (3), 323–352.

Goodwin, L. (1992). Home fetal assessment. *Journal of Perinatology and Neonatal Nursing,* 5(4), 33–45.

Grant, A. (1989). Monitoring the fetus during labor. In I. Chalmers, M. Enkin, M. Keirse (Eds.), *Effective care in pregnancy and childbirth.* 846–882 New York: Oxford University Press.

Gregor, C., Paine, L., Johnson, T. (1991). Antepartum fetal assessment. A nurse-midwifery perspective. *Journal of Nurse-Midwifery,* 36 (3), 153–167.

Hoskins, I., Freiden, F., Young, B. (1991). Variable decelerations in reactive nonstress tests with decreased amniotic fluid index predict fetal compromise. *American Journal of Obstetrics and Gynecology,* 165 (4,1), 1094–1098.

Huddleston, J. F., Sutliff, G., Robinson, D. (1984). Contraction stress test by intermittent nipple stimulation. *Obstetrics and Gynecology,* 63 (5), 669–673.

Ingemarsson, I., and Arulkumaran, S. (1989). The FHR admission test. In J. A. D. Spencer (Ed.), *Fetal monitoring: Physiology and techniques of antenatal and intrapartum assessment.* 143–146 Philadelphia: F. A. Davis.

Krebs, H. B., Petres, R. E., Dunn, L. J. (1983). Intrapartum fetal heart rate monitoring VIII. Atypical variable decelerations. *American Journal of Obstetrics and Gynecology,* 145 (3), 297–305.

Leveno, K., Cunningham, F., Nelson, S., Roark, M., Williams, M., Guzidk, D., Dowling, S., Rosenfeld, C., Buckley, A. (1986). A prospective comparison of selective and universal electronic fetal monitoring in 34,995 pregnancies. *New England Journal of Medicine,* 315 (10), 615–619.

MacDonald, D., Grant, A., Sheridan-Pereirs, M., Boylan, P., Chalmers, I. (1985). The Dublin randomized controlled trial of intrapartum fetal heart rate monitoring. *American Journal of Obstetrics and Gynecology,* 152 (5), 524–539.

Manning, F. (1990). The fetal biophysical profile score: Current status. *Obstetrics and Gynecology Clinics of North America,* 17 (1), 147–162.

McCaul, J., and Morrison, J. (1990). Antenatal fetal assessment: An overview. *Obstetrics and Gynecology Clinics of North America,* 17 (1), 1–16.

McKinley, J. (1981). From “promising report” to “standard procedure”: Seven stages in the career of a medical innovation. *Health and Society,* 59 (3), 374–411.

McNiven, R., Hodnett, E., O'Brien-Pallas, L. (1992). Supporting women in labor: A work sampling study of the activities of labor and delivery nurses. *Birth,* 19 (1), 3–7.

Melchior, J., and Bernard, N. (1989). Second-stage fetal heart rate patterns. In J. A. D. Spencer (Ed.), *Fetal monitoring: Physiology and techniques of antenatal and intrapartum assessment.* 155–158 Philadelphia: F. A. Davis.

Miller-Slade, D., Gloeb, J., Bailey, S., et al. (1991). Acoustic stimulation-induced fetal response compared to traditional nonstress testing. *Journal of Obstetric, Gynecologic, and Neonatal Nursing,* 20 (2), 160–167.

Mohide, P., and Keirse, M. (1989). Biophysical assessment of fetal well-being. In I. Chalmers, M. Enkin, M. Keirse (Eds.), *Effective care in pregnancy and childbirth.* New York: Oxford University Press.

NAACOG. (1990). Fetal heart rate auscultation. *OGN Nursing Practice Resource.* Washington, DC. Author

Parer, J. T. (1983). *Handbook of fetal heart rate monitoring.* Philadelphia: W. B. Saunders.

Parer, J. (1994). Fetal heart rate. In R. Creasy and R. Resnik (Eds.), *Maternal-fetal medicine: Principles and practice.* Philadelphia: W. B. Saunders.

Pearson, J. (1989). Routine clinical screening for fetal well-being. In J. A. D. Spencer (Ed.), *Fetal monitoring: Physiology and techniques of antenatal and intrapartum assessment.* 54–59 Philadelphia: F. A. Davis.

Piquard, F., Schaefer, A., Hsuing, R., Dellenbach, P., Haberey, P. (1989). Are there two biological parts in the second stage of labor? *Acta Obstetricia et Gynecologica Scandinavica,* 68, 713–718.

Pircon, R., and Freeman, R. (1990). The contraction stress test. *Obstetrics and Gynecology Clinics of North America,* 17 (1), 129–146.

Polzin, G. B., Blakemore, K. J., Petrie, R. H., Amon, E. (1988). Fetal vibro-acoustic stimulation: Magnitude and duration of fetal heart rate accelerations as a marker of fetal health. *Obstetrics and Gynecology,* 72 (4), 621–626.

Rothman, B. (1991). *Labor: Women and power in the birthplace.* New York: W. W. Norton.

Sandmire, H. (1990). Whither electronic fetal monitoring? *Obstetrics and Gynecology,* 76 (6), 1130–1134.

Schifrin, B. S. (1995). Medicolegal ramifications of electronic fetal monitoring during labor. *Clinics in Perinatology,* 22 (4), 838.

Simkin, P. (1984). Active and physiologic management of second stage: A review and hypothesis. In S. Kitzinger and P. Simkin (Eds.), *Episiotomy and the second stage of labor.* 7–22 Seattle: Pennypress.

Spencer, J. A. D. (1989). *Fetal monitoring: Physiology and techniques of antenatal and intrapartum assessment.* Philadelphia: F. A. Davis.

Vintzileos, A., Campbell, W., Nochimson, D. J., Weinbaum, P. (1987). The use and misuse of the fetal biophysical profile. *American Journal of Obstetrics and Gynecology,* 156 (3), 527–533.

Woolley, D., and Roberts, J. (1995). Second stage pushing: A comparison of Valsalva-style with “mini” pushing. *The Journal of Perinatal Education,* 4 (4), 37–43.

Zanini, B., Paul, R. H., Huey, J. R. (1980). Intrapartum fetal heart rate: Correlation with scalp pH in the preterm fetus. *American Journal of Obstetrics and Gynecology,* 136 (1), 43–47.

Unit 5

Nursing Care of Healthy Mothers and Newborns

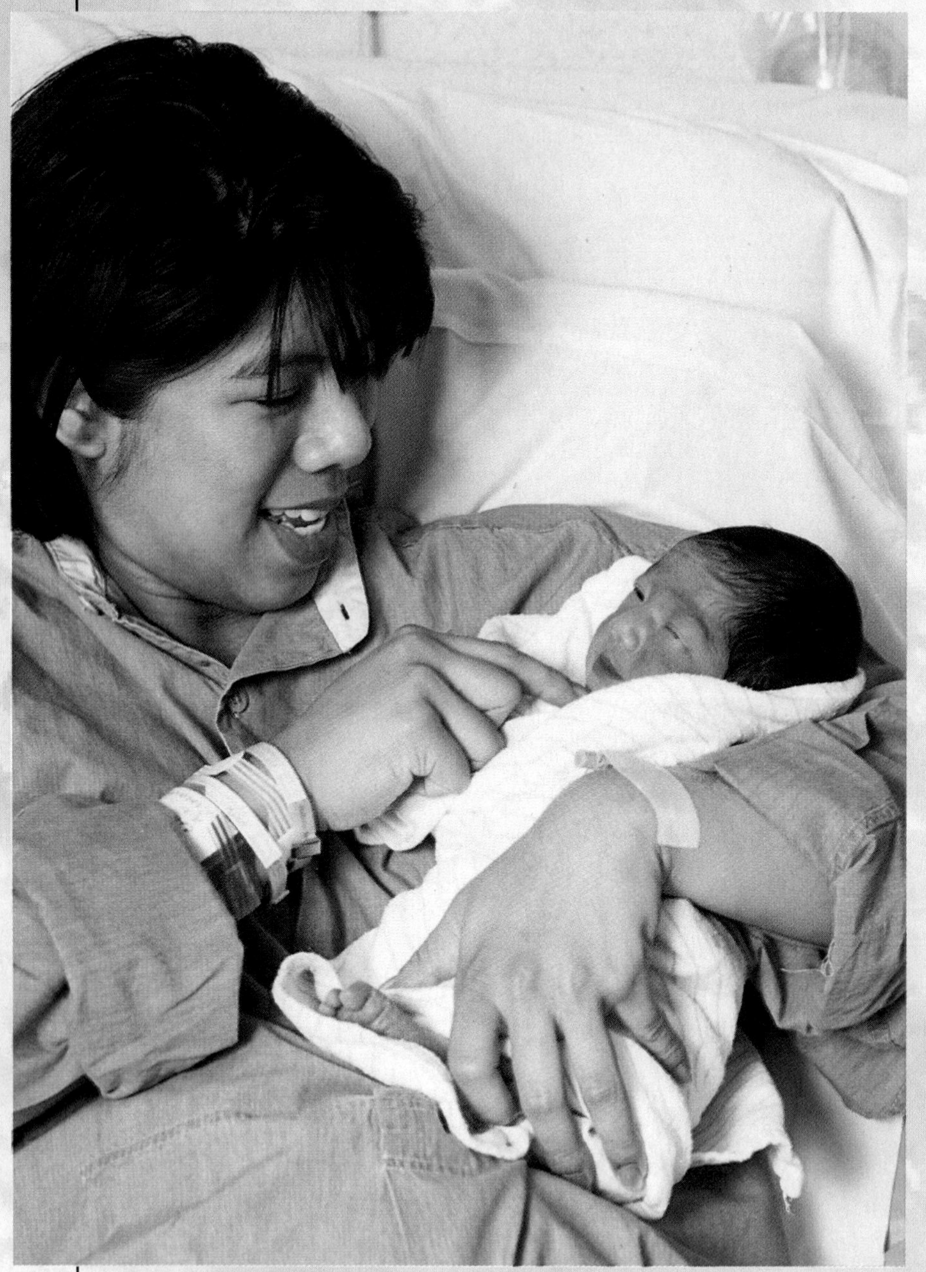

The interaction between each mother and baby is unique. This mother-infant interaction is the foundation from which the attachment relationship evolves. The mother can best develop a positive relationship with her infant if she has a good childbirth experience, is knowledgeable about her infant's behavior and how to communicate with him or her, and has extended contact with her infant during the early postpartum period.

Trends in Research

THE MOTHER-INFANT RELATIONSHIP

Mothering behaviors, nurturing and caretaking, provide the infant with a great deal beyond food and protection. These behaviors provide cognitive stimulation and emotional nurturance within a relationship that also has a regulatory effect on the infant's physiologic status and behavior.[6]

The foundation for the development of a secure attachment relationship between mother and infant is the development of a positive mother-infant relationship. This relationship is also a critical aspect of parenting and strongly influences the physical and emotional health and well-being of the infant.[1]

CONCLUSIONS FROM RESEARCH

- The development of a relationship between the mother and her baby is influenced by many factors: the mother's socioeconomic status, her level of education, her cultural beliefs, how she was mothered as a child, her relationship with her father, and her experiences with past pregnancies as well as with this pregnancy.[2]
- Events surrounding childbirth, such as high levels of stress and anxiety, can have a profound influence on the development of a bond between the mother and the infant and can hinder her postpartum emotional adjustment, her self-image, and her responses to her infant.[2]
- Positive maternal perceptions of the infant are predictors of appropriate maternal behavior, close mother-infant relationships, and normal child development.[3]
- The full-term healthy infant is an active and well-organized participant in the development of the mother-infant relationship and a powerful stimulus that elicits mothering behavior.[2,4]
- The quality of the attachment relationship depends on what the infant brings to the relationship (temperament, internal regulation) and more importantly what the mother brings to the relationship (ego-strength, self-esteem, general sensitivity, capacity for empathy, and childhood memories of her parents and siblings).[5]
- Mothering behaviors, nurturing and caretaking, provide the infant with a great deal beyond food and protection. These behaviors provide cognitive stimulation and emotional nurturance within a relationship that also has a regulatory effect on the infant's physiologic functioning and behavior.[6]
- Mother-infant interaction has a regulatory effect on the infant's physiologic functioning and behavior and influences the following infant neural control systems: behavioral (activity level and state), sucking (nutritive and nonnutritive), sleep-wake cycles, neurochemical, metabolic (oxygen consumption), cardiovascular (heart rate and vasoconstriction), endocrine (growth hormone and corticosterone), and immune (B- and T-cell response).[6]
- The attachment relationship between mother and child starts during early pregnancy and continues for an undetermined time. The existence of a critical or sensitive period after birth is not supported for human maternal behavior.[4]
- Increased mother-infant contact during the first 3 days after birth has been shown to improve mothering behaviors regardless of the exact timing of the contact.[2] However, there are other important factors that also foster and facilitate the mother-infant relationship.[1]

IMPLICATIONS FOR PRACTICE

Clinical practices that foster positive mother-infant interactions are critical to the development of the mother-infant relationship. Improving the clinical and psychosocial elements of the childbirth experience for the woman can have a positive influence on her ability to interact with her infant after the birth.

---

[1]Rutter, M. (1995). Clinical implications of attachment concepts: Retrospect and prospect. *Journal of Child Psychology and Psychiatry and Allied Disciplines,* 36 (4), 549–571.

[2]Sosa, R. A. and Cupoli, J. M. (1981). The birthing process: The effects on the parents. *Clinics in Perinatology,* 8 (1), 197–210.

[3]Priel, B., Gonik, N., Rabinowitz, B. (1993). Appraisals of childbirth experience and newborn characteristics: The role of hardiness and affect. *Journal of Personality,* 61 (3), 299–315.

[4]Walker, L. O. (1992). *Parent-infant nursing science: Paradigms, phenomena, methods.* Philadelphia: F. A. Davis.

[5]Touris, M., Kromelow, S., Harding, C. (1995). Mother-firstborn attachment and the birth of a sibling. *American Journal of Orthopsychiatry,* 65 (2), 293–297.

[6]Hofer, M. A. (1994). Early relationships as regulators of infant physiology and behavior. *Acta Paediatrica,* Supplement 397, 9–18.

Chapter 27

Principles of Family-Centered Maternity Care

Francine H. Nichols
Elaine Zwelling

At the heart of family-centered maternity care are the relationships that develop during the childbearing year. These include relationships among family members, relationships that link the family with society and its support systems, and relationships that occur between childbearing families and those who provide care. Each has important implications for the healthy development of the family unit.

Susan McKay (1988)

A PHOTO ESSAY

Family-centered maternity care is a philosophy of care in which pregnancy and childbirth are viewed as normal life events and are seen within the framework of wellness—rather than illness. It emphasizes health promotion, education, informed decision making, and individualized care based on the needs of all family members. Family-centered maternity care starts during pregnancy with the first contact with the health care provider. It continues with admission to the birthing agency through discharge from the birth setting and into the home. Family-centered maternity care not only encompasses physical care but also emphasizes psychosocial and educational needs of the woman and all family members. The philosophy of family-centered maternity care is reflected in specific actions of the health care team.

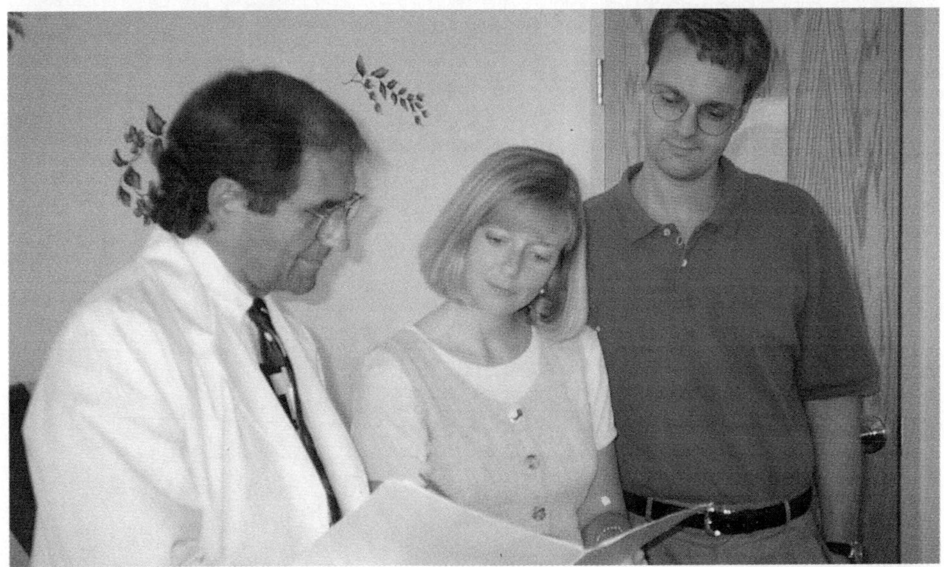

During pregnancy, the health care provider gives comprehensive prenatal care, determines expectant parents' needs and desires for the birth experience, and encourages their participation in childbirth education classes.

A comprehensive program of childbirth education for the expectant parents and their family members is available, and individuals are encouraged to make informed decisions and participate actively in the birth experience.

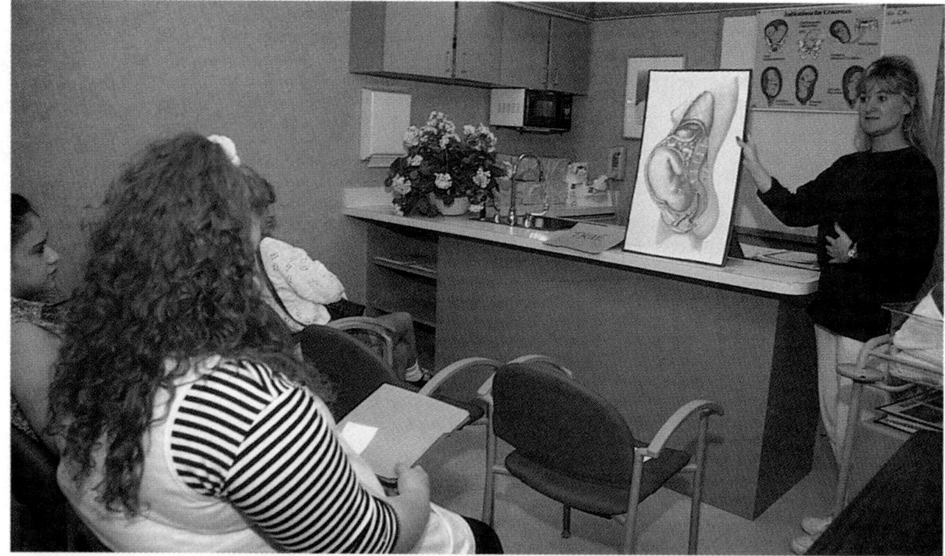

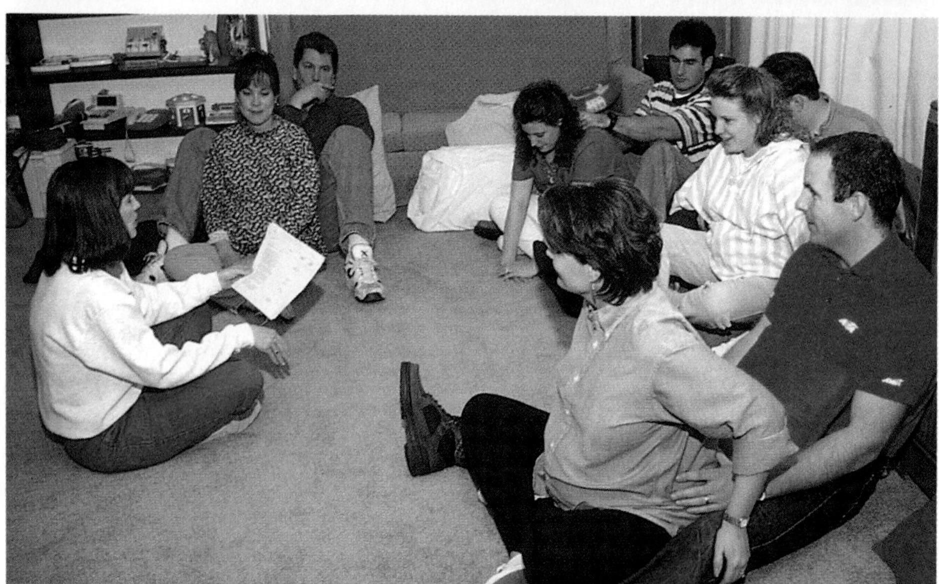

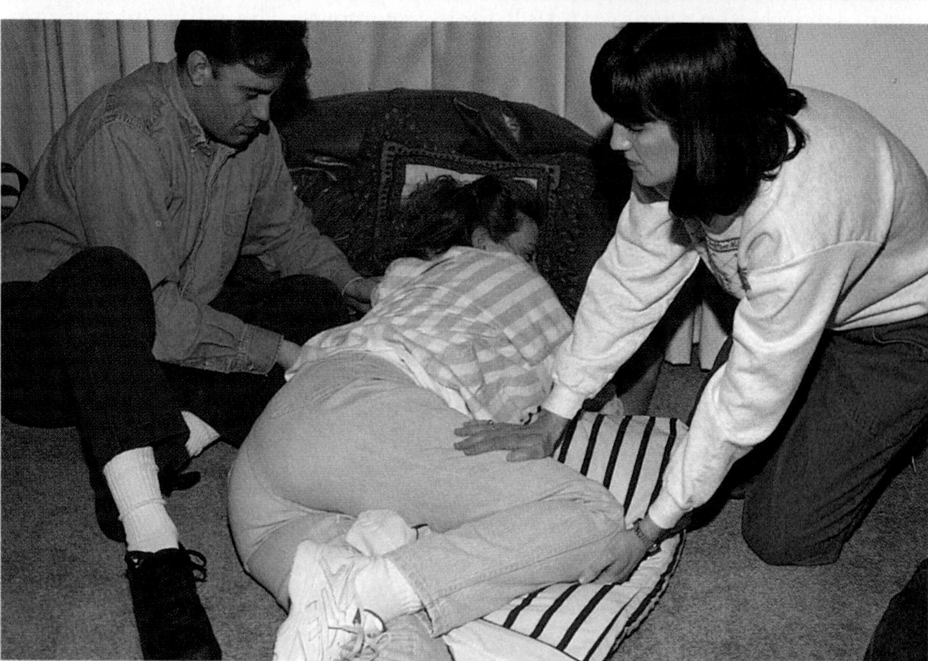

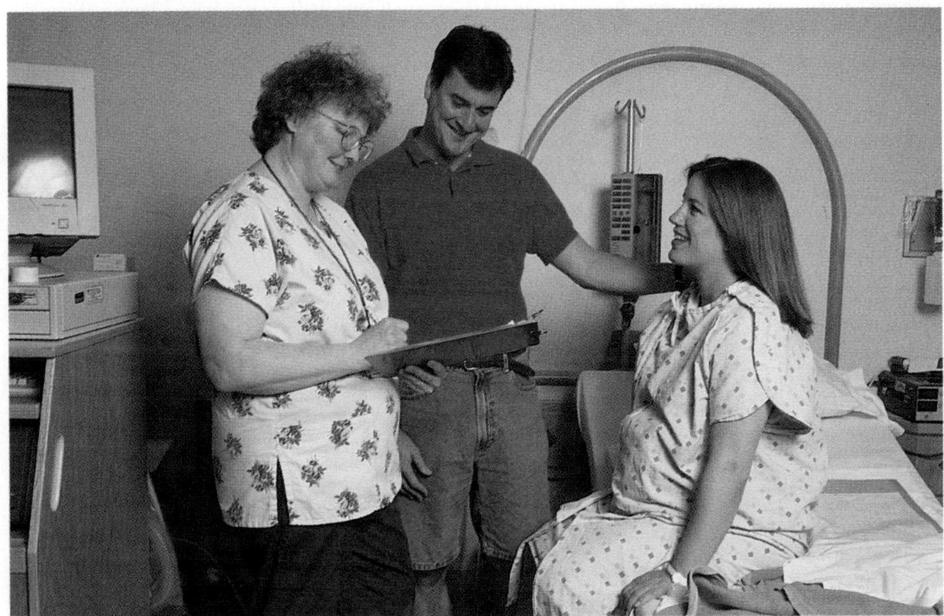

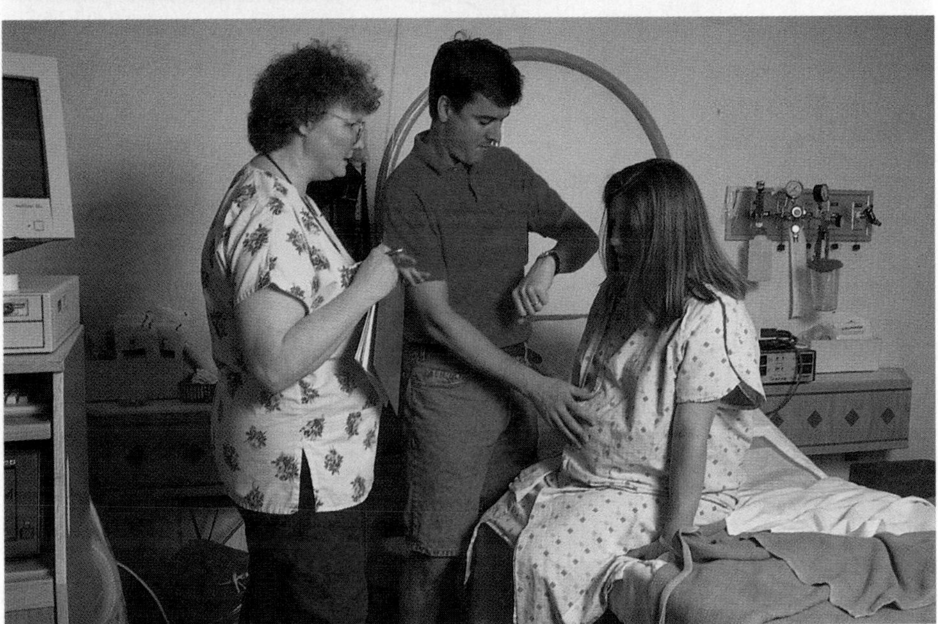

The expectant parents are welcomed into the birthing unit. In addition to assessing physical status, the nurse determines their level of preparation for this birth experience and discusses and clarifies the couple's expectations for this birth experience.

The woman's labor companion and family members or friends of her choice are included during the labor and birth experience. The nurse assists the labor companion in supporting the woman as well as provides direct support to the woman. The woman labors and gives birth in the same room.

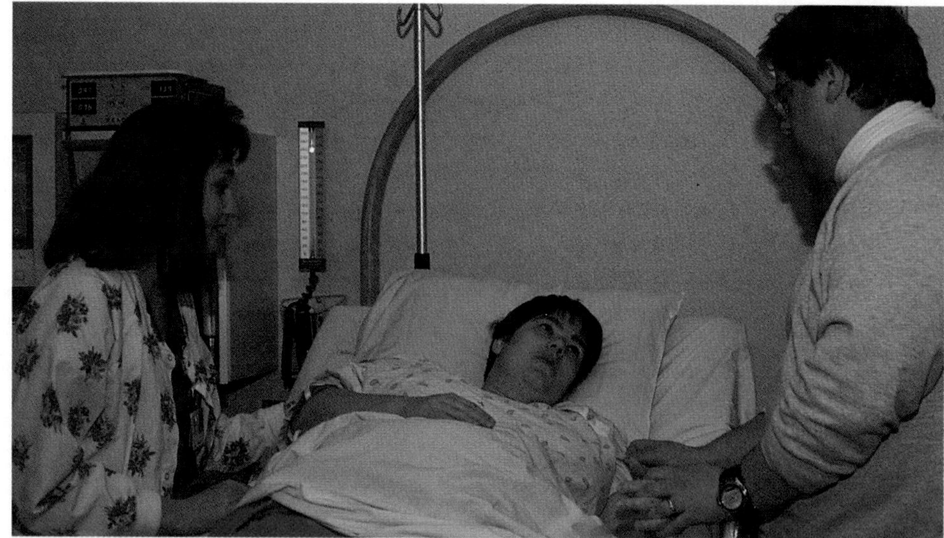

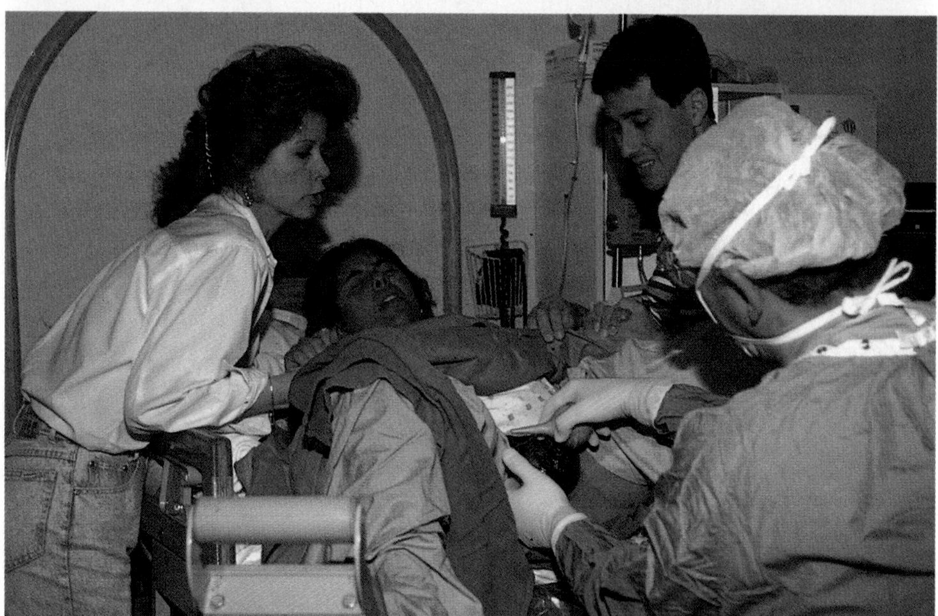

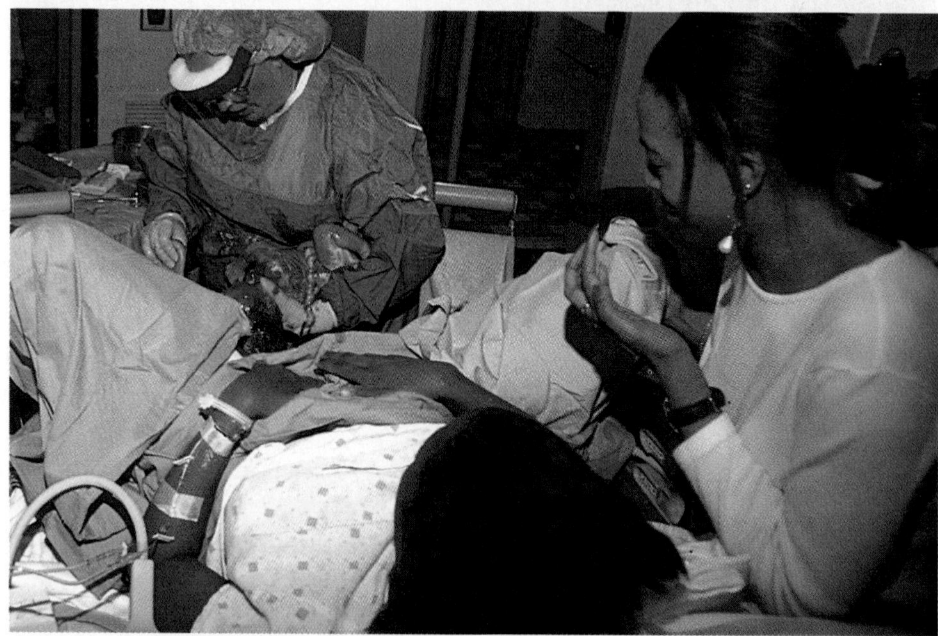

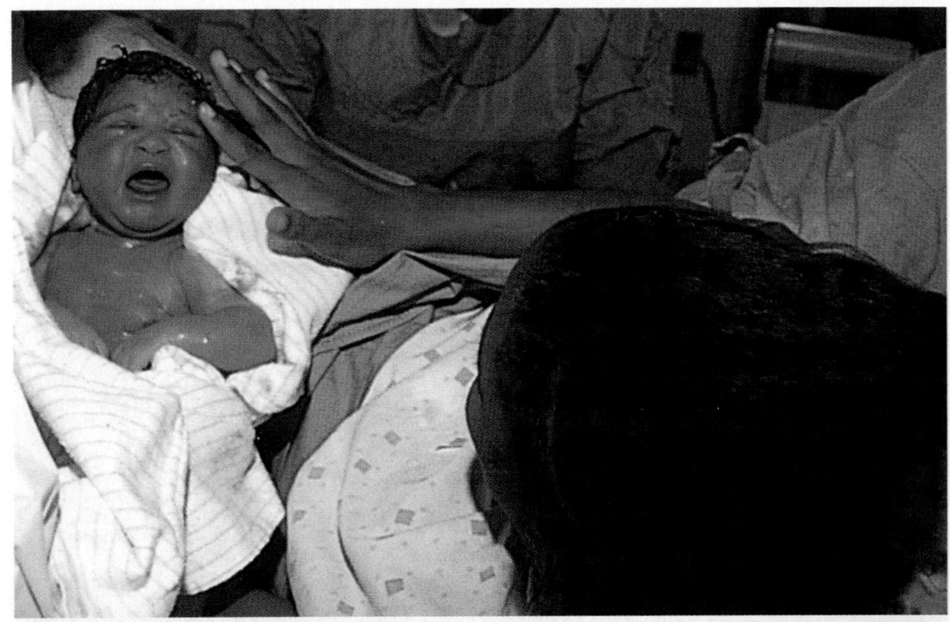

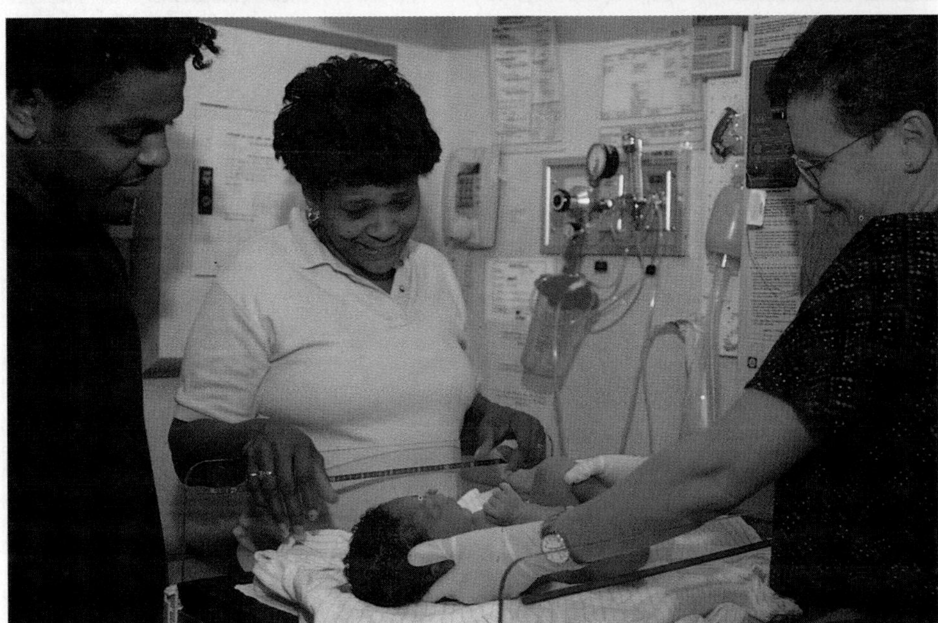

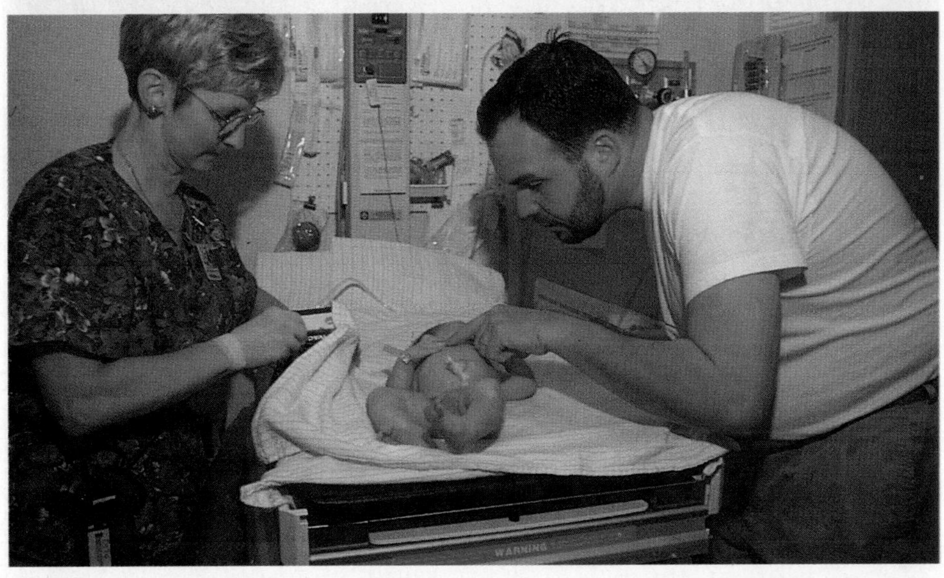

At birth, the mother and her family members are encouraged to touch and interact with the baby. The nurse explains the distinctive characteristics and unique capabilities of the infant to them. These activities form the foundation for mother-infant attachment and positive family relationships.

Unless there are complications that dictate otherwise, the new parents and baby are kept together during the immediate postbirth period. Procedures such as eye prophylaxis are delayed until the new parents have had an opportunity to get acquainted with their newborn.

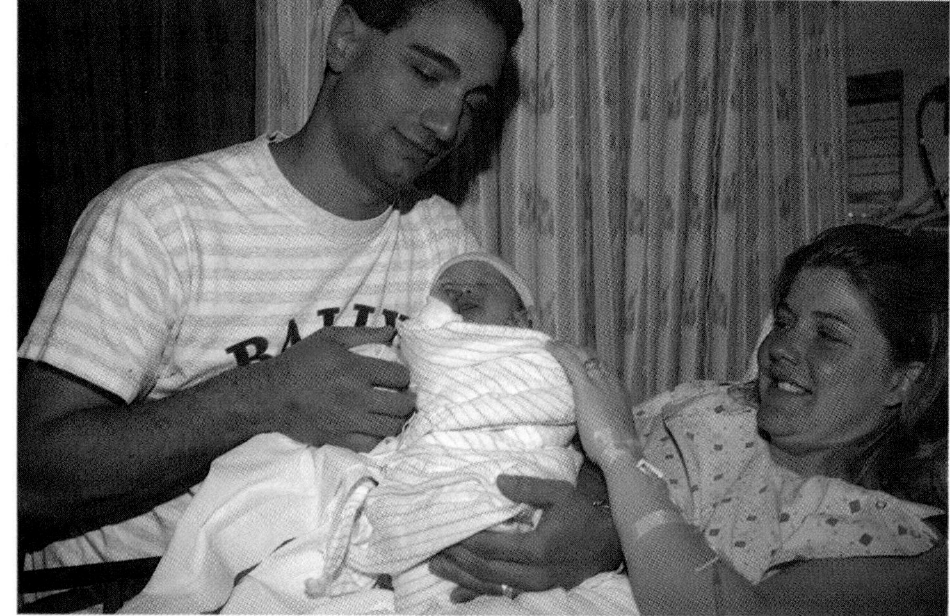

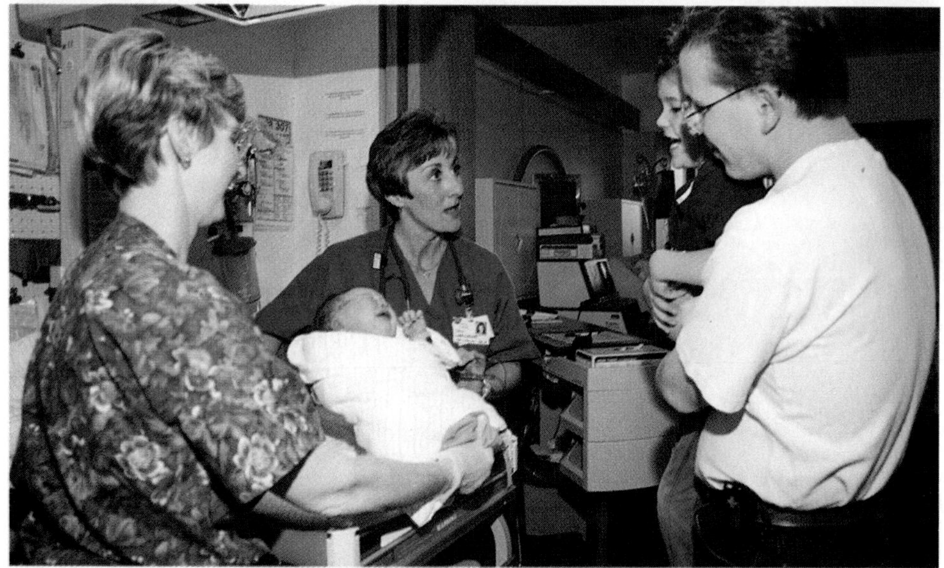

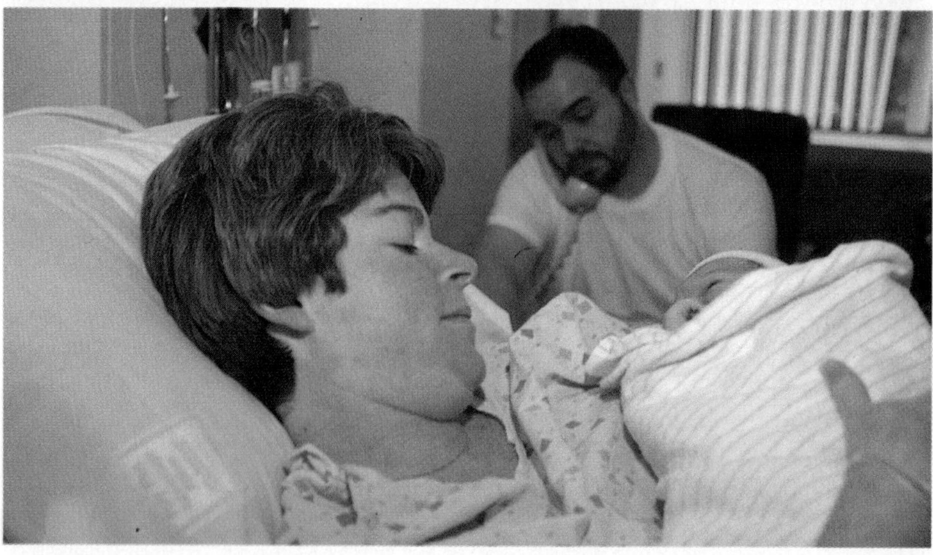

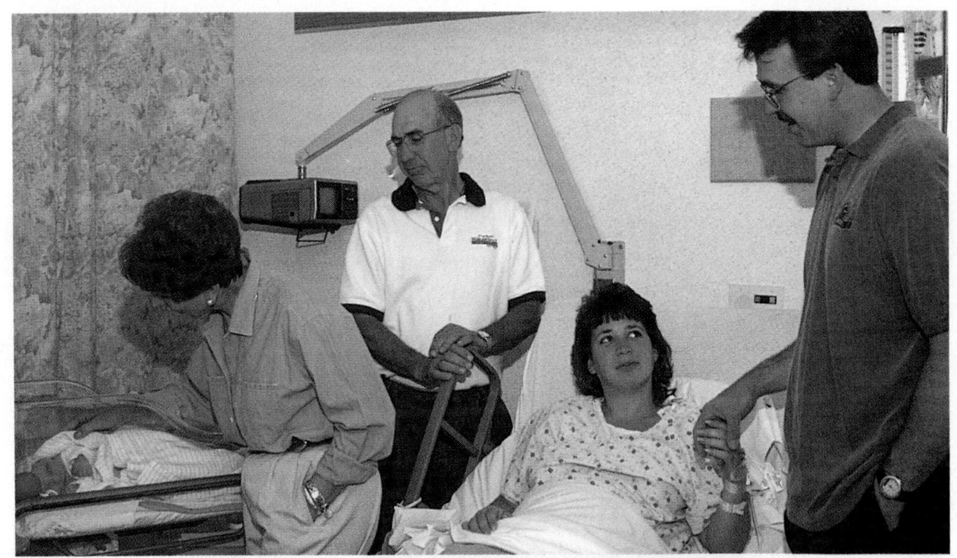

The baby stays in the mother's room at her bedside and is cared for by the same nurse, even if the baby is separated from the mother briefly. Family members and friends are encouraged to visit as the mother desires. Teaching is done at the mother's bedside and includes family members.

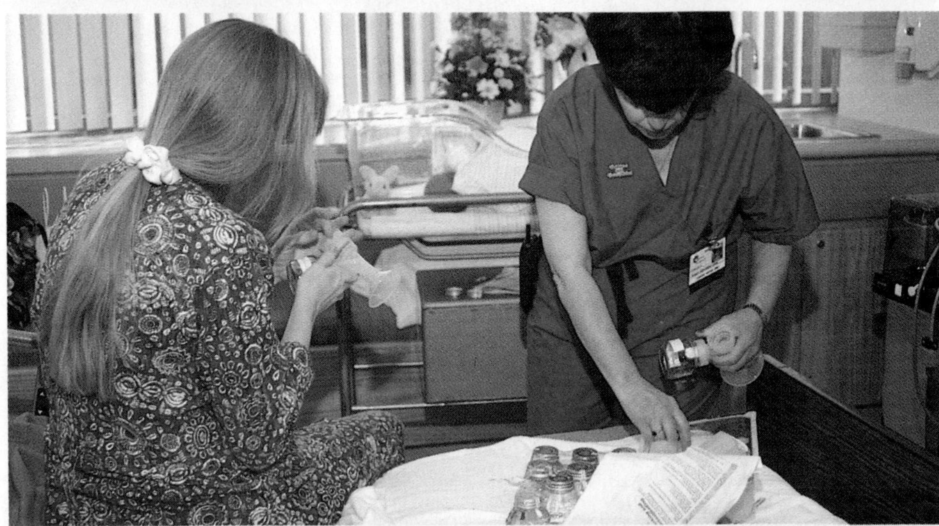

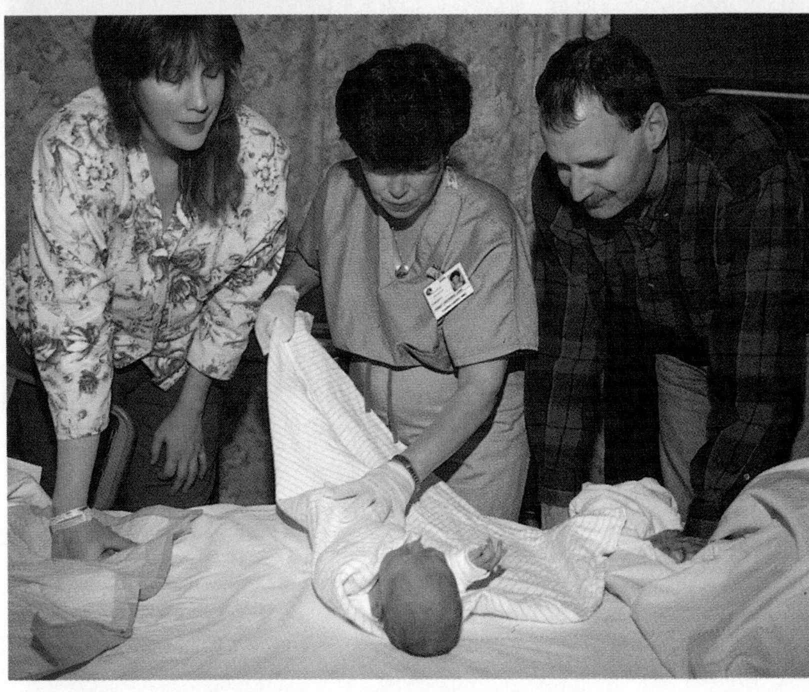

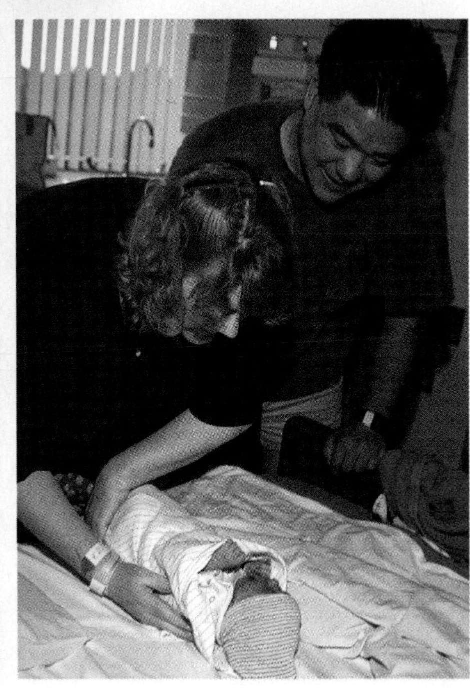

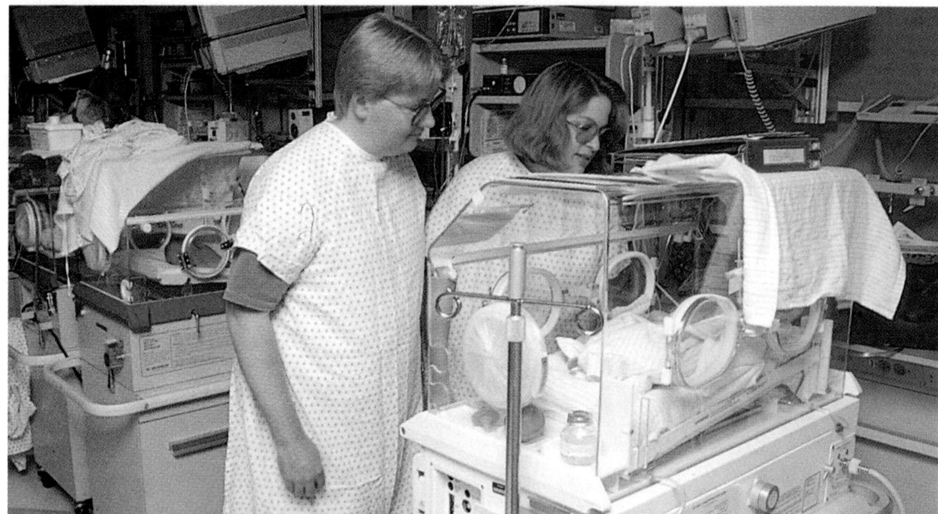

If the baby is in the high-risk unit, parents may visit the baby at any time and are involved in the baby's care.

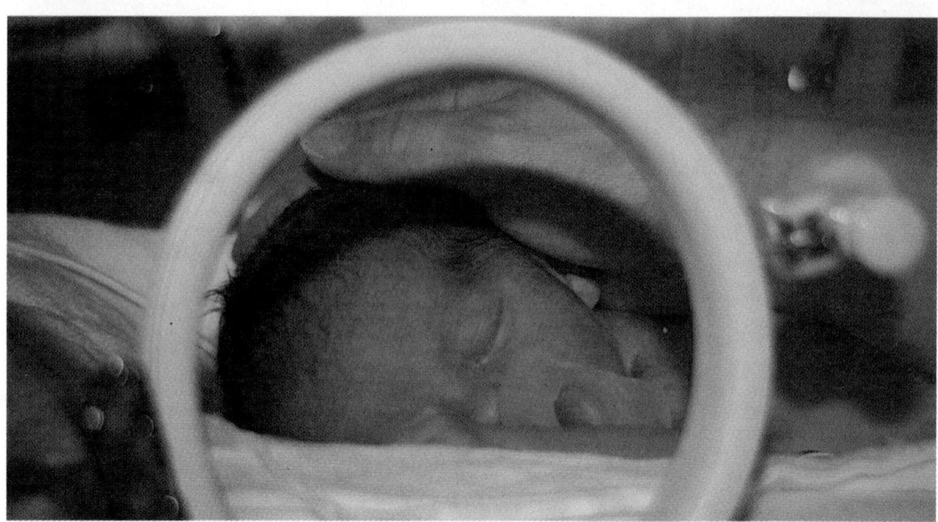

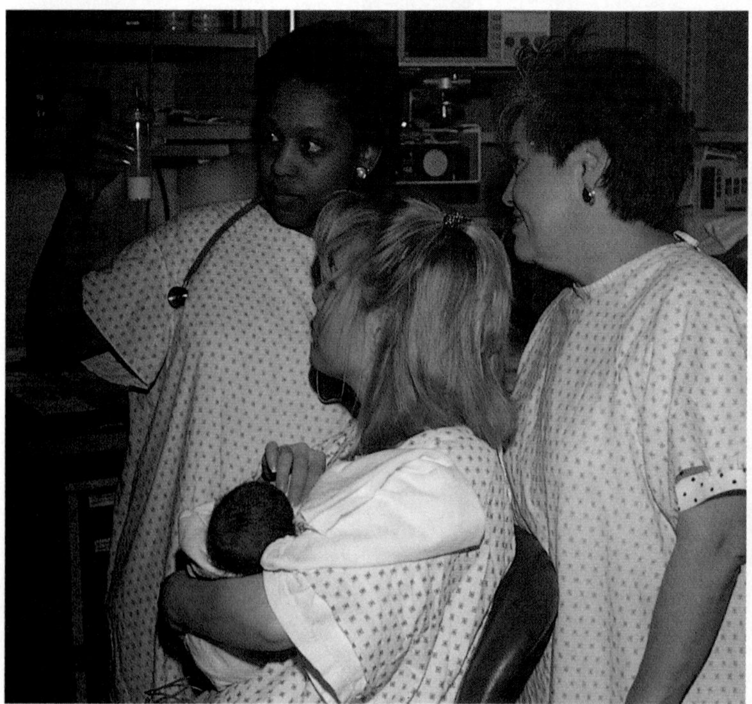

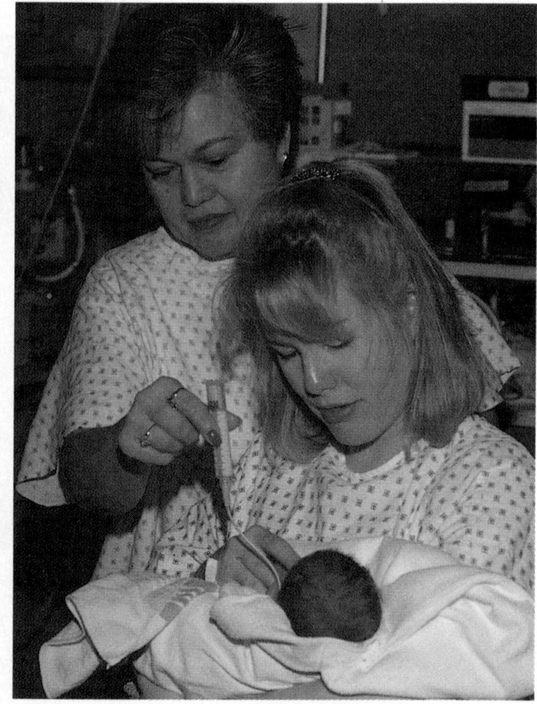

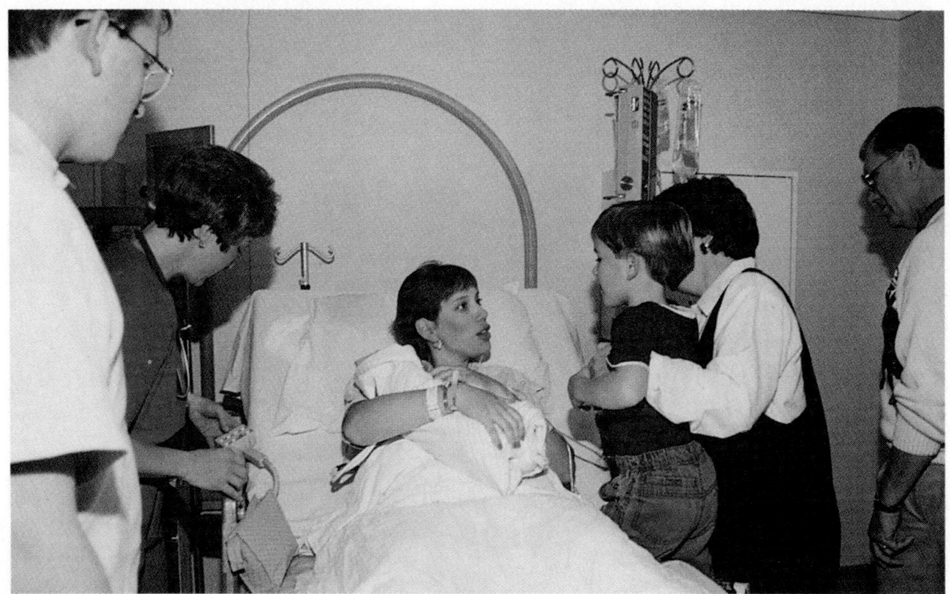

Parents are encouraged to have the baby's siblings visit mother and get acquainted with the new baby.

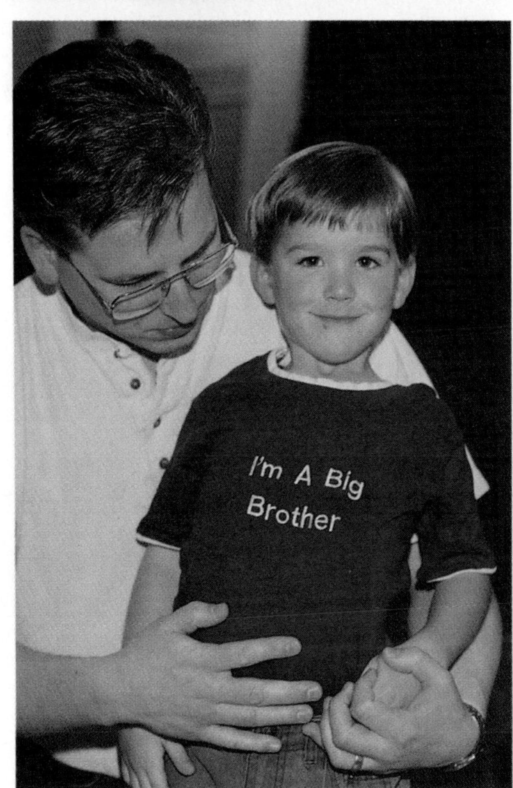

After discharge, care extends into the home. A nurse visits mother and baby at home the day after discharge. A nurse is also available by phone when the mother has questions.

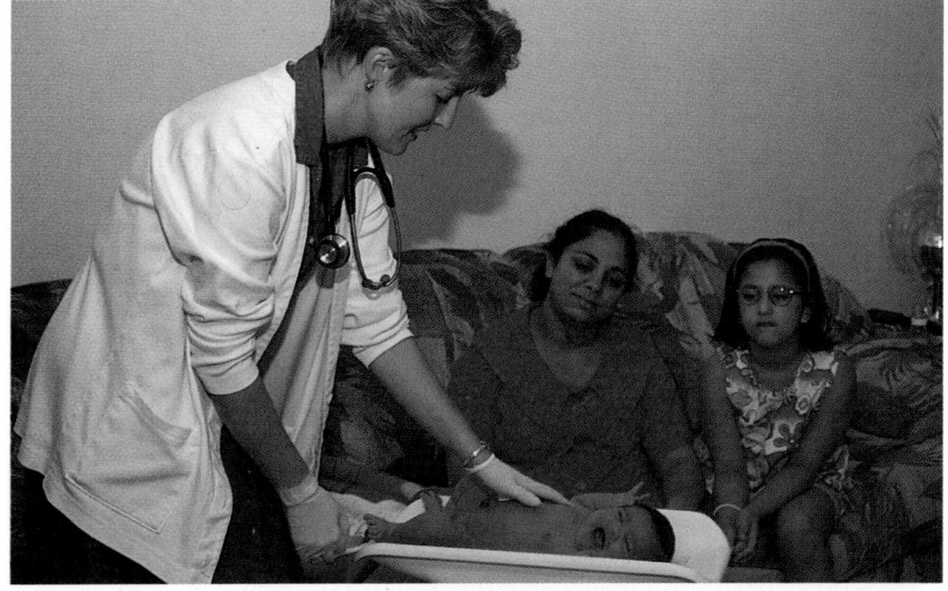

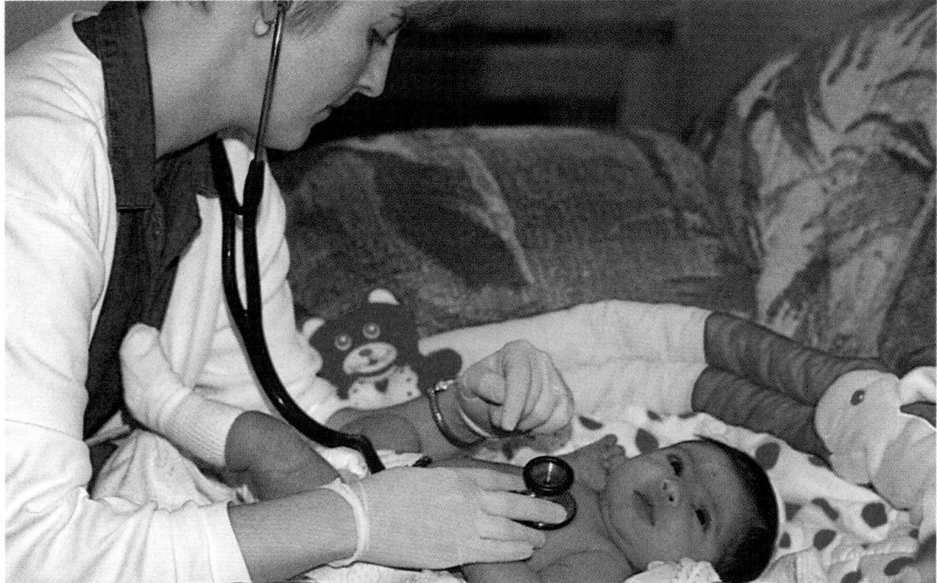

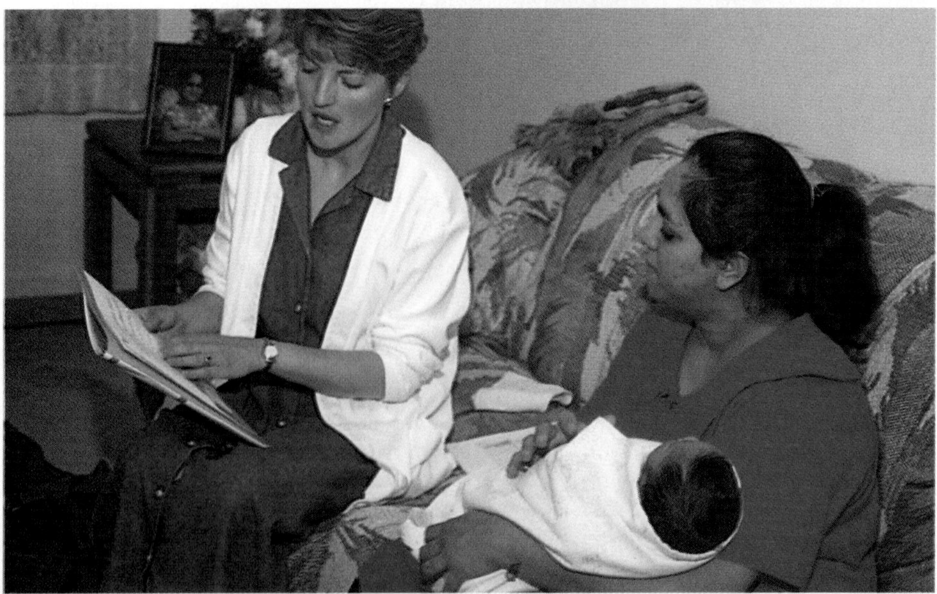

Chapter 28

> The postpartum period is a time of restoration and return to the non-pregnant state.
>
> SUSAN BLACKBURN AND DONNA LOPER (1992)

Postpartum Adaptation

Betty Glenn Harris
Francine H. Nichols

HIGHLIGHTS

- ▼ Physiologic Adaptation Related to the Reproductive System, Cardiovascular System, Hematologic System, Respiratory System, Neuromuscular and Sensory System, Immune System, Renal System, Gastrointestinal System, and Integumentary System
- ▼ Psychological Adaptation
- ▼ Role Adaptation
- ▼ Implications for Research

The postpartum period, also termed the puerperium, is that time after childbirth during which the woman's body is returning to its nonpregnant state. It is a time of profound physiologic, psychological, and social changes. There are marked changes in almost every major organ system after childbirth. Thus, the postpartum period is a time of disequilibrium.

The postpartum period is considered to be the first 6 weeks after delivery (Cunningham et al. 1993). It has also been called the fourth trimester to reflect the time it usually takes the woman to adapt—physically, emotionally, and socially—and to integrate the newborn infant into the family system.

PHYSIOLOGIC ADAPTATION

After delivery, physiologic changes that occurred during the 9 months of pregnancy are reversed. While many of the physiologic changes that occur after delivery are completed before 6 weeks post partum, others require more time (Table 28–1).

DEFINITIONS

Involution—The return of the reproductive organs to a nonpregnant state.

Postpartum period—Also termed the puerperium, the postpartum period is the 6-week period after childbirth during which the woman's body is returning to its nonpregnant state.

Reproductive System

The return of the reproductive organs to a nonpregnant state is termed involution. Reproductive system changes occur rapidly after birth and during the first 7 to 10 days. Daily changes are usually noted during this time. After 7 to 10 days, changes occur at a much slower rate. Involution is typically complete by 6 weeks post partum.

▼ **Uterus.** Three different processes must occur for involution of the uterus to take place normally: the uterus must contract, autolysis of myometrial cells must take place, and the epithelium must regenerate (Blackburn and Loper 1992). Immediately after delivery, strong myometrial contractions cause the uterus to rapidly decrease in size. Within 24 hours, the uterus is a hard globular mass about the same size as at 20 weeks of pregnancy. Within 1 week after delivery, the uterus weighs approximately 500 g, having decreased in size by 50 percent. By 2 weeks after delivery, the uterus has descended into the true pelvis and cannot be felt during abdominal palpation. By 6 weeks (Fig. 28–1), the uterus has decreased in size almost to its prepregnancy size, approximately 60 to 80 g, and uterine involution is complete (Resnik 1994; Guyton and Hall 1996). The uterus will remain slightly larger than its prepregnant state. Multiparous women and women who have overdistention of the uterus during pregnancy (multiple gestation, polyhydramnios, or a large infant), infection, or retention of placental tissue will have a slower involution process.

The decrease in estrogen and progesterone after birth causes autolysis of the endometrium. Necrotic changes occur, and the upper layers of the endometrium are sloughed off in a menstruation-like response. There is a marked decrease in the size of each individual myometrical cell with little change in the total number of myometrial cells. Except for the placental site, the endometrium is fully healed by 3 weeks post partum (Blackburn and Loper 1992).

After delivery, the placental site is thinner than the surrounding endometrium. As the uterus contracts, the placental site becomes smaller, develops a ragged and bumpy texture, and looks like a large desquamating wound (Blackburn and Loper 1992). Blood vessels in the placental site are constricted by muscle fibers in the middle layer of the contracting uterus. During the first several hours after birth, the veins become thrombotic, leaving an area covered with blood clots and fragments of tissues called eschar. Leukocytes rapidly invade the area, protecting against infection and releasing enzymes that break down the degenerating tissues in the area. Healthy endometrium is regenerated and replaces the eschar. Regeneration of the uterine lining begins in 2 to 3 days, but the site will not be completely healed until 6 to 7 weeks after delivery. By 6 weeks post partum, the placental site is less than 2 cm in diameter, a decrease from 4 to 5 cm immediately after birth; by 12 weeks, it has virtually disappeared, leaving no scar that could possibly interfere with the implantation of future embryos. If the process of healing and regeneration at the placental site does not proceed in a normal manner, however, subinvolution may occur and result in severe late postpartum hemorrhage (Resnik 1994).

The position of the uterine fundus is an excellent indicator of uterine involution. By 12 hours after delivery, the uterine fundus is located approximately at the level of the umbilicus. The position can vary slightly to either just above or below the umbilicus. After that, the fundus decreases in size about 1 cm per day (about one fingerbreadth), and by 10 days after delivery, it cannot be palpated abdominally (see Fig. 28–1).

▼ **Lochia.** The postpartum vaginal discharge that is the result of involution and regeneration of the endometrium is called lochia. The color and amount of lochia change as healing occurs. Immediately after birth and until about 2 to 4 days post partum, lochia is composed largely of blood and may include fragments of fetal membranes, lanugo, vernix, or meconium. Called lochia rubra, it is dark red to brownish red in color and has a characteristic fleshy odor.

From 3 to 4 days post partum, bleeding has decreased but plasma is still oozing from the placental site, and white blood cells and fragments of degenerating endometrium are present in the vaginal discharge. The lochia has become brownish in color, thinner in consistency, and more translucent; it is now called lochia serosa. Around 10 to 14 days post partum, lochia becomes thick and white to yellowish in color and is called lochia alba. It is composed largely of mucus and white blood cells. Lochia alba may continue until 3 to 6 weeks post partum, gradually decreasing in amount.

The odor of lochia varies for each individual woman, but at no time should it be offensive. Foul-smelling lochia is characteristic of endometri-

Table 28–1

NORMAL POSTPARTUM PHYSIOLOGIC CHANGES

Reproductive System

Uterus

Fundus is at the level of umbilicus by 12 hours after delivery. Fundal height decreases progressively by 1 cm/day, no longer palpable by day 10

Lochia

Rubra: red, lasts 1 to 3 days
Serosa: pink or brown tinged, lasts 3–10 days
Alba: yellowish white, lasts 10–14 days, can persist up to 3 weeks
Odor of fresh blood
Amount should gradually decrease in first week

Cervix

Edematous immediately after delivery
Easily distensible 4–6 days after delivery
Internal os closed by 2 weeks
External os remains more open than in prepregnant state, appears as a slit

Vagina

Rugae reappear in 4 weeks
Remains slightly larger; near prepregnant size 6–8 weeks after delivery
Normal mucus production returns with ovulation

Perineum

Initial episiotomy healing within 2–3 weeks; may take as long as 4–6 months to heal completely
Hemorrhoids may be present

Menstrual Cycle

Length of time is variable
Lactating women resume menstruation within 12 weeks up to 18 months
Nonlactating women resume menstruation from 6 weeks to within 6 months

Breasts

Vascularity and size increased by day 2 or 3 post partum
Nipples erect when stimulated
If not lactating, engorgement subsides in 24–36 hours

Cardiovascular System

Cardiac output returns to normal in 2–4 weeks
Cardiac load increased

Hematologic System

Prepregnant blood volume returns in 3–4 weeks
Hematocrit rises immediately after delivery, returns to prepregnant level in 4–5 weeks
White blood cell count may increase during first 10 days
Clotting factors elevated, return to normal in 4–5 weeks

Respiratory System

Diaphragm descends, organs return to normal position
Acid-base balance returns by 3 weeks
Basal metabolic rate elevated for up to 14 days

Renal System

Bladder, urethra, meatus edematous
Urinary retention may occur
Increased renal blood flow, glomerular filtration rate, and plasma creatinine levels occur during pregnancy; these usually return to normal within the first 6 weeks post partum

Gastrointestinal System

Motility may be decreased
Normal bowel elimination returns in 2–3 days

Neuromuscular and Sensory Systems

Pregnancy changes resolve rapidly
Headaches and alterations in sleep may occur post partum
Discomfort or pain is common and may affect interaction with the infant and development of the maternal role

Integumentary System

Abdominal skin and musculature is loose and flabby; tone is regained gradually over several weeks, especially if abdominal exercises are done
Skin discolorations fade gradually, although some subtle color changes may persist

Immune System

Immune changes persist for 2–3 months, protecting the mother against infections

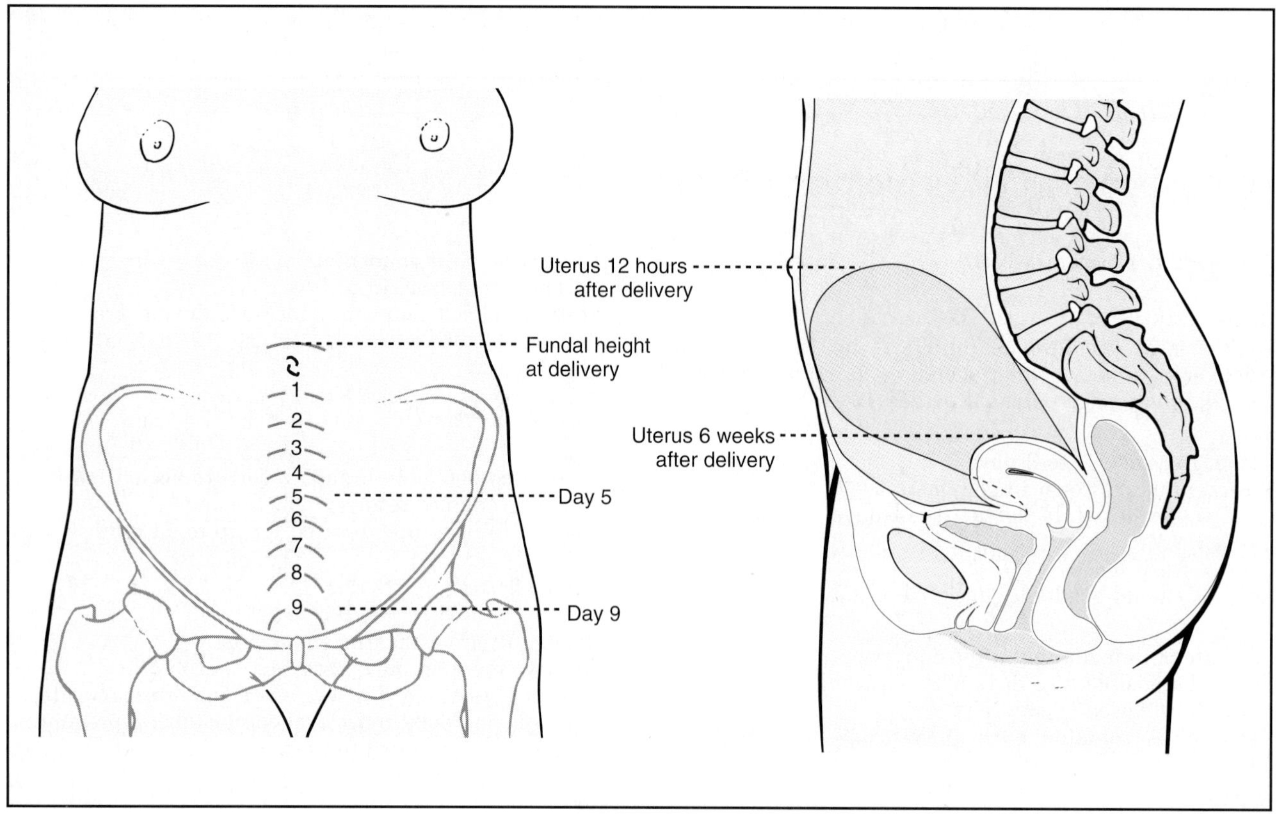

Figure 28–1

Rapid change in the size of the uterus during the first 24 hours post partum. The position of the uterine fundus is an excellent indicator of uterine involution. By 12 hours after delivery the fundus is located approximately at the level of the umbilicus. After that the fundus decreases by about 1 cm per day and cannot be palpated abdominally by 10 days after delivery.

tis, an infection of the uterine lining. The amount of lochia discharged during the postpartum period varies from 150 to 400 mL, with an average of 225 ml (Blackburn and Loper 1992). The amount of lochia varies; multiparous women have greater amounts, and breastfeeding mothers and women who have had cesarean births have lesser amounts. Each individual woman also experiences changes in the volume of lochia throughout the day. Lochia increases with activity and during breastfeeding and decreases at night or on lying down (Blackburn and Loper, 1992).

Cervix. At term, the cervical epithelium is thick and the cervical glands are hypertrophied. The water content of cervical tissues is increased before labor. During labor, further edema and hemorrhage within the tissues are common, and tears may occur. After delivery, the cervix is frequently edematous, ulcerated, and ecchymotic, and small lacerations may be apparent. It is flaccid and has little likeness to its previous nonpregnant state. It is loose, often admitting two fingers, but rapidly becomes thicker, shorter, and firmer. At 1 week post partum, the external appearance of the cervix is similar to its nonpregnant state. However, histologic examination still shows endocervical hypertrophy. At 6 weeks, healing is usually nearly complete, and the cervical opening now has a slitlike appearance characteristic of a woman who has given birth (see Fig. 9–8). There may be evidence of some stromal edema and round cell infiltration of cervical tissues for as long as 3 to 4 months. If a full evaluation of the cervix is indicated, such as for cervical incompetence (see Chapter 21), it should be delayed until 3 to 4 months post partum until complete healing is ensured (Resnick 1994).

Vagina. Immediately after a vaginal birth, the vagina is soft, stretched, and relaxed with loss of tone; it does not have visible rugae. The walls of the vagina appear smooth and may be edematous and bruised with visible small tears or abrasions. Rugae reappear, vascularity and edema decrease, and vaginal tone gradually returns by 3 to 4 weeks. The vaginal epithelium is completely healed by 6 to 10 weeks post partum (Blackburn and Loper 1992)

Perineum. After childbirth, the introitus is typically relaxed, has poor muscle tone, and is gaping open. An episiotomy or repaired vaginal laceration may be present. The tissues of the perineum are frequently edematous, and bruising is visible. Solutions used to cleanse the perineum before birth occasionally cause a tissue reaction that results in redness and edema of the skin. Soreness and pain are common. While all of these phenomena diminish during the first 7 to 10 days and initial healing takes place in 2 to 3 weeks, it can take up to 4 to 6 months for the episiotomy site to completely heal (Backburn and Loper 1992).

▼ **Menstrual Cycle.** After childbirth, expulsion of the placenta removes a major source of estrogen and progesterone, and normal resumption of ovarian function occurs. The return of first menses is extremely variable for individual women. Nonlactating women usually have first menses and ovulate sooner than fully lactating women do. Women who lactated for less than 1 month usually follow the pattern of nonlactating women. Lactating women who introduce supplements (formula or solids) early will have first menses and ovulate sooner than fully lactating women (Blackburn and Loper 1992).

The first menses is usually anovulatory. In lactating women, ovulation usually does not occur before 10 weeks, but it may occur as early as 35 days (Blackburn and Loper 1992). The average time for the first menses of nonlactating women is 7 to 9 weeks. Seventy percent of nonlactating women will have the first menses by 12 weeks (Resnik 1994), and 90 percent will have resumption of menses by 24 weeks (Vorherr 1973).

▼ **Breasts.** During pregnancy, changes occur in the breasts in preparation for lactation. Both ducts and mammary alveoli proliferate, and circulation to the breasts increases. Duct growth is influenced largely by estradiol; alveoli growth is influenced by progesterone (see Chapter 16). Final maturation of the breasts is controlled by prolactin, which increases steadily throughout pregnancy but has its major effect once the inhibiting effect of estrogen and progesterone is removed. After delivery of the placenta, concentrations of estrogen and progesterone decrease, and prolactin promotes final maturation of mammary tissue (Duff 1989).

This final maturation process requires 2 to 4 days. Before that time, the breasts secrete only colostrum, a thick translucent substance that is a precursor to milk. As final maturation is reached, breast engorgement occurs and the breasts usually become enlarged, tight, and tender. This engorgement, while occurring simultaneously with the beginning of the production of true milk, is not caused by the accumulation of milk but by tissue reaction and venous congestion. Engorgement of the breasts will resolve spontaneously in a period of several days (see Chapter 33).

There is disagreement about the effect of pregnancy or lactation on the size and texture of the breasts. For the non-breastfeeding woman, after any puerperal engorgement resolves, her breasts should approximate their prepregnancy size, shape, and texture, provided that she wore a supportive brassiere during pregnancy and does not have significant weight gain. For the lactating woman, support and weight gain are also important, but breastfeeding the infant is also a factor in breast changes after pregnancy.

Cardiovascular System

During pregnancy, an increase in cardiac output occurs, and there is an increase in blood volume with both plasma and red blood cells increasing. After delivery, other changes occur. At birth, there is a further increase in cardiac output, which occurs as vena caval compression is removed and contraction of the uterus leads to a decrease in blood pooling there. Since the pulse rate normally slows immediately after birth, the increased cardiac output is due to increased stroke volume (Duvekot and Peeters 1994b). Cardiac output values return to normal by 2 to 4 weeks (Blackburn and Loper 1992).

Blood volume decreases sharply at delivery, approximately 500 mL for a normal vaginal delivery and 1000 mL in a typical cesarean delivery. In the next 2 to 3 days, blood volume typically increases as 900 to 1200 mL of extracellular fluid is shifted into the maternal circulation. During the next 6 weeks, blood volume decreases as this fluid is eliminated (Bowes 1986; Metcalfe et al. 1986). Because of this transient increase in fluid volume, women with cardiovascular disorders should be carefully observed for fluid overload and cardiac embarrassment during the postpartum period. Blood volume returns to the prepregnant level by 6 to 9 weeks post partum (Duvekot and Peeters 1994b).

Blood pressure in the normotensive woman typically shows minimal change post partum. Some women may experience a transient increase (averaging 5 to 6 mm Hg, systolic) shortly after birth. Blood pressure declines to normal prepregnant levels within the first week (Dennis 1989). Women with hypertensive disease of pregnancy usually have a rapid return to normal prepregnant levels after birth. For those women who have hypertension that was not accompanied by proteinuria, it may require 2 to 3 weeks before their blood pressure returns to normal.

The pulse rate usually decreases in the immediate postpartum period, with rates as low as 50 to 60 beats per minute occurring. The reason for the slow pulse rate is not clear, but the relative state of hypervolemia that occurs after birth is thought to contribute to this phenomenon.

Table 28–2

CHANGES IN BLOOD CELLULAR COMPONENTS DURING PREGNANCY

COMPONENT	CHANGE	PATTERN OF CHANGE
Red blood cells (RBCs)	Increase 33% (450 mL) with iron; increase 18% (250 mL) without iron	Slow, continuous increase beginning in first trimester; may accelerate slightly in third trimester
Hematocrit	Decreases 3%–5% to 33.8% at term (range, 33%–39%)	Decreases from second trimester as plasma volume peaks
Hemoglobin	Decreases 2%–10% to 12.1–12.5 g/dL (range, 11–13) at term	If iron and folate are adequate, little change to 16 weeks; lowest values at 16–22 weeks; slowly increases to term
Reticulocytes	Increase 1%–2%	Gradual increase to third trimester
White blood cells	Increase 8% to 5000–12,000 (up to 15,000 seen)/mm^3	Begins in second month; increase involves primarily neutrophils
Eosinophils	Increase or decrease	Variable
Basophils	Slight decrease	
Platelets	Increase, decrease, or stay the same; usual range, 150,000–400,000/mm^3	Variable
Erythrocyte sedimentation rate	Increases	Progressive

Hematologic System

The increased red blood cell production of pregnancy ceases during the early postpartum period. The hemoglobin level decreases immediately after birth as a result of blood loss. The hematocrit usually remains relatively stable and may even increase slightly the first few days for women who have a vaginal delivery. As extracellular fluid is drawn into the circulation, from day 2 to day 4, the hemoglobin level rises slowly, regaining the values of day 1 by day 9 after delivery. For women with normal blood loss, hemoglobin level and hematocrit should be evaluated on the first postpartum day; values on later days will be inappropriately low. Careful attention to the woman's total physiologic status is necessary to interpret changes in blood components correctly.

Blood composition is altered after birth (Table 28–2). The leukocytosis of pregnancy is exaggerated during labor, and the white blood cell count remains elevated during the early postpartum period. White blood cell values may be as high as 25,000 to 30,000/mm^3 during the immediate postpartum period. The white blood cell count then falls to 6000 to 10,000/mm^3 and returns to normal by 4 to 7 days (Blackburn and Loper 1992). The number of platelets decreases with placental separation. There is an increase in platelets starting about 48 hours after birth, then a gradual return to prepregnant levels (Dennis 1989). Fibrinogen levels are increased for approximately 2 weeks after birth (Dennis 1989). All of these changes create a state of hypercoagulability that persists for 6 to 7 weeks. The hypercoagulability, endothelial damage, and stasis predispose the postpartum woman to thrombus formation (Frisoli 1981).

The risks of both cerebral infarction (stroke) and intracerebral hemorrhage are increased in the

Table 28–2

CHANGES IN BLOOD CELLULAR COMPONENTS DURING PREGNANCY Continued

BASIS FOR CHANGE	INTRAPARTUM CHANGES	POSTPARTUM CHANGES
Erythropoietin stimulated by human placental lactogen, progesterone, and prolactin	Slight increase due to slight hemoconcentration; 50% of increased RBCs lost at delivery	RBC production ceases temporarily; remainder of increased RBCs lost through normal catabolism
Hemodilution		Returns to nonpregnant levels by 4–6 weeks owing to RBC catabolism
Hemodilution	Slight increase due to stress and dehydration	Initial decrease; stabilizes at 2–4 days; nonpregnant values by 4–6 weeks
Increased RBC production		Increases slightly; nonpregnant values by 4–6 weeks
Estrogen	Increase to 25,000–30,000/mm^3	Decrease to 6000–10,000/mm^3; normal values by 4–7 days
	Disappear from peripheral blood	By 3 days, return to peripheral blood
?Hemodilution	20% decrease with placental separation	Increase by 3–5 days with gradual return to nonpregnant levels
Increased plasma globulin and fibrinogen	Increases	Initially 55–80 mm/hr; peaks 1–2 days post partum

From Blackburn, S. T., and Loper, D. L. (1992). *Maternal, fetal, and neonatal physiology: A clinical perspective* (pp. 162–163). Philadelphia: W. B. Saunders.

6 weeks after delivery, but not during pregnancy itself (Kittner et al. 1996).

Thrombus formation is more likely in women after operative delivery or prolonged time positioned in stirrups. Immobilization after anesthesia or bed rest promotes stasis, which favors intravascular clotting. Thrombus formation occurs in approximately 1 percent of vaginal deliveries and 2 to 5 percent of cesarean deliveries.

Respiratory System

Starting shortly after delivery, the respiratory tract rapidly returns to the prepregnant state. This is a result of the loss of progesterone production with separation of the placenta, the immediate decrease in intra-abdominal pressure at birth of the baby, and the increased excursion of the diaphragm. For the first 2 days post partum, as the progesterone levels decrease, there is a rise in Pa_{CO_2} level. By 1 to 3 weeks post partum, anatomic changes in the respiratory system have returned to normal and ventilation has returned to normal (Blackburn and Loper 1992).

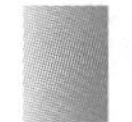

Neuromuscular and Sensory System

The neuromuscular and sensory changes that occurred during pregnancy resolve rapidly during the postpartum period as the woman's hormonal levels return to the prepregnant state. Headaches are common during the postpartum period and often begin to occur about the time of postpartum weight loss. The cause of these headaches is thought to be the rapid changes in fluid and electrolyte balance (Blackburn and Loper 1992).

During the postpartum period, the woman experiences alterations in sleep, which returns to normal by 2 weeks post partum. The amount of rapid eye movement sleep is decreased and the amount of awake time at night increased during the first 3 days post partum (Blackburn and Loper 1992). Having the newborn at the mother's bedside during the night has not been shown to be detrimental to the amount of sleep a mother receives. In fact, Keefe (1988) found that mothers who kept their babies with them at night slept longer than did mothers whose babies were in the nursery, and they also had better quality sleep.

The woman may experience considerable discomfort and pain from a variety of sources during the postpartum period. Sources of discomfort and pain include episiotomy, hemorrhoids, afterpains, breast engorgement, and nipple soreness. The ability of the woman to interact with and care for her infant is influenced by her degree of discomfort and pain; increasing discomfort and pain hinder her ability to interact with her baby and assume the mothering role. The woman's discomfort is highest during the first few days post partum and lasts through the first weeks post partum, although it may last longer if a woman had a complicated childbirth.

Immune System

The changes in the immune system and host defense mechanism that occurred during pregnancy remain altered for 2 to 3 months after delivery (Table 28–3). These changes occurred during pregnancy to protect the fetus from infection and rejection during pregnancy. However, they increase the mother's risk for mycotic, fungal, and other opportunistic infections; increase the risk for colonization with streptococci and staphylococci; and delay the mother's initial response to infection, making accurate diagnosis of infection difficult (Blackburn and Loper 1992).

Renal System

During pregnancy, there is generalized dilation of the urinary tract, with enlargement of the kidneys and dilation of the renal calyces, renal pelvis, and urethra. These changes regress slowly, and most women's urinary system will return to its nonpregnant state of functioning by 3 months post partum. Approximately 10 percent of women will have some permanent enlargement of the kidneys (Resnik 1994).

Renal functioning during pregnancy is characterized by increased renal blood flow, glomerular filtration rate, and plasma creatinine levels. These usually return to normal within the first 6 weeks during the postpartum period. Renal plasma flow may temporarily drop below nonpregnancy levels and usually returns to normal within 1 year (Monheit et al. 1980).

The increased glomerular filtration rate during the early postpartum period combined with the decrease in progesterone, which has an antidiuretic effect, leads to a marked diuresis after childbirth, up to 3000 mL of urine per day. This diuresis typically begins shortly after delivery in women with clinically apparent edema if they are not subjected to the antidiuretic effect of continuing oxytocin administration. For women without clinically apparent edema, diuresis may not begin for 3 to 4 days after delivery. Some women may actually gain weight immediately post partum—possibly owing to a temporary retention of sodium ions and water—before diuresis begins. A transient glycosuria or proteinuria is not uncommon during the first week. Lactosuria, a side effect of lactation, may occur in 60 to 80 percent of women (Frisoli 1981).

Local effects of labor and birth may alter bladder function. Bladder tone and sensation may be decreased from the effects of childbirth, operative vaginal procedures, and the effects of analgesia and anesthesia. Edema and hyperemia of the bladder mucosa and urethra may interfere with free passage of urine, and pain or the fear of pain may interfere with the woman's ability to relax. As a result, bladder function may be decreased. These factors in combination with diuresis frequently lead to distention of the bladder or to incomplete emptying of the bladder. Overdistention further decreases tone and complete emptying of the bladder. Urine retention can lead to the development of bladder infections. In a study of more than 10,000 postpartum women, researchers confirmed bacteriuria in 3.2 percent of the women, most frequently after operative delivery, epidural anesthesia, and catheterization of the bladder (Stray et al. 1989). Frequent assessment of bladder distention is essential during the postpartum period. Catheterization should be used only after other interventions have proved unsuccessful, because catheterization increases the risk for bladder infection.

Gastrointestinal System

The gastrointestinal system, like many other body systems, is affected by pregnancy. There is usually generalized relaxation and hypomotility of the stomach and intestines. This is thought to be caused by the increased progesterone levels that

Table 28–3

ALTERATIONS IN HOST DEFENSE MECHANISMS DURING PREGNANCY

ALTERATION	RESULT	IMPLICATION
	Primary Host Defense Mechanisms	
Increased polymorphonuclear leukocytes (PMNs)	Increased available phagocytes	Protection of mother and fetus from infection
Altered metabolic activity and chemotaxis of PMNs	Delay initial response to infection	Increase risk of colonization; protect fetus and trophoblast from rejection
Decreased natural killer (NK) cells	Delay initial response to infection	Increase risk of colonization; protect fetus and trophoblast from rejection
	Cell-Mediated Immunity	
Decreased T-helper cells	Suppress B-cell function	Increase risk of mycotic, fungal, other opportunistic infections
Increased T-suppressor cells	Alter cell-mediated immunity; decrease graft rejection	Protect fetus from rejection
Altered T-cell function and efficiency	Depress reaction to tuberculin test	Confuse diagnosis of infection in second half of pregnancy
	Antibody-Mediated Immunity	
Suppression of B-cell function	Due to decreased T-helper cells	Increased risk of colonization with streptococci, staphylococci, other organisms
Decreased immunoglobulin G	Due to transfer to fetus and hemodilution	Increased risk of colonization
	Complement	
Increased total complement and C2, C3, C3 split products	Enhance chemotaxis and action of immunoglobulins through opsonization	Augment maternal defenses against bacterial infection; protect fetus from infection
Decreased C1, C1a, B, D	Delay initial activation of complement system	Protect fetus and trophoblast from rejection

From Blackburn, S. T., and Loper, D. L. (1992). *Maternal, fetal, and neonatal physiology: A clinical perspective* (p. 443). Philadelphia: W. B. Saunders.

occur during pregnancy and the relaxant effect of progesterone on smooth muscle.

Changes in gastrointestinal function during the immediate puerperium are an exaggeration of the changes that normally occur during the menstrual cycle. Intestinal transit time is similar during the menstrual cycle and during the postpartum period (Van Thiel and Schade 1986). Decreased motility slows transit time, and relaxation of the abdominal muscles decreases the woman's ability to use her stomach muscles to aid evacuation. The effects of anesthesia and handling of the intestines during a cesarean birth also influence gastrointestinal function. The decreased mobility of a woman after cesarean birth as a result of the surgery or pain further diminishes gastrointestinal function.

Constipation is frequently a problem during the immediate postpartum period. However, this must be evaluated in terms of bowel evacuation during labor and delivery as well as solid food intake during the previous 1 to 2 days. If the woman has had little solid food intake, little solid waste is present, and bowel evacuation will be delayed during the immediate postpartum period. For the woman with severely compromised gastrointestinal function as a result of surgery, the increased slow transit time of stool may cause increased amount of gas and discomfort. Accurate assessment of the woman's gastrointestinal status and the need for implementation of interventions is essential (see Chapter 29).

Integumentary System

Immediately after birth, the abdominal skin and musculature is loose and flabby. For some women, the linea alba is overstretched and thin, permitting separation of the rectus abdominis muscles. The separation is visible as a vertical ridge appearing on the abdomen when the abdominal muscles are contracted and is palpable as a defect (diastasis recti) of varying width between the contracted muscles.

The skin and muscles regain tone in the first weeks of the puerperium, especially if abdominal exercises are done routinely (Frisoli 1981). For some women, regaining and maintaining abdominal tone is difficult, and some women may never fully regain their prepregnancy tone.

On the skin of the abdomen, striae fade and become much less noticeable during several weeks, eventually reaching a silvery appearance. The linea nigra and other pigmentary changes fade, eventually disappearing or becoming much less visible, although some subtle color changes may persist.

PSYCHOLOGICAL ADAPTATION

A wide variety of factors may affect psychological adaptation after childbirth. The factors may be either physiologic or psychosocial in nature. These factors need to be evaluated for each individual woman. Also, the woman's perception of these factors influences how they will affect her.

Prenatal factors that hinder a woman's psychological adaptation after birth are an unwanted pregnancy and a pregnancy judged to be high risk. A high-risk prenatal status is associated with poorer maternal health after childbirth (Mercer and Ferketich 1990). Conventional wisdom indicates that when a pregnancy is unwanted, the mother may have difficulty in adjusting to the mothering role and taking care of the infant after birth. However, little research is available to support this premise. The majority of women who have an unwanted pregnancy adapt to the reality of pregnancy and come to desire the child. In these instances, there is little evidence that the woman's adaptation to the infant or to her new role is adversely affected. For those women who are forced, either by others or by circumstances, to continue an unwanted pregnancy, the outcome is not clear.

Postpartum factors that influence a woman's adjustment after childbirth are her health status and the health status of the infant. Social factors that may influence maternal psychological adaptation include the amount of social support received; length of maternity leave; maternal cigarette or alcohol use; and demographic characteristics, such as education, occupation, race, or age.

Many women experience distressing mood changes after birth called postpartum "blues." This type of psychological problem is normal, usually mild, and transitory in nature. More severe psychological problems after childbirth include postpartum depression and postpartum psychosis (see Chapter 35).

The postpartum blues occur in approximately 60 percent of women in the United States; reported rates in other countries range from 14 percent in Canada to 75 percent in Great Britain (Beck 1991). While there may be wide differences in frequency with which women in different countries experience postpartum blues, it is more likely that the extreme differences are due to the way in which the blues are diagnosed and reported in different areas. Symptoms include feelings of depression, tearfulness, anxiety, changes in concentration or consciousness, irritability, headache, and frequent unpredictable changes of mood. The blues usually appear within 7 to 10 days after birth, most commonly within 3 to 5 days, and persist for a week or less. The cause is unclear but is thought to be related to a change in hormones after birth (Beck 1991). For some women, they may be the result of "responses to the cumulative, rapidly changing priorities that confront women in their efforts to take command of parenting and management of household, family and personal life" (Affonso 1987). Sleep disruption caused by baby care has also been linked to postpartum blues (Beeber 1996).

Postpartum depression arises later, lasts longer, and is more severe than the blues. The profoundly disabling postpartum psychosis is relatively rare. Psychosis during the postpartum period is 15 times more frequent than is psychosis of women who are not in the postpartum period. Postpartum depression and postpartum psychosis require skilled medical treatment and nursing care and appropriate medication (see Chapter 35).

ROLE ADAPTATION

Research has shown that the transition to parenthood is an event of great significance for women and men (Walker 1992). This transition includes cognitive, emotional, and behavioral upsets that are an integral part of all transitions (Golan 1981). Role adaptation involves two specific areas: the adoption of a new social role within the family (e.g., mother or father) and changes in family relationships (Walker 1992).

A substantial amount of descriptive research is available on how the mother or father takes on the social role as parent within the family. In general, fathers have a much easier transition to parenthood than mothers do. Mothers reported more lifestyle changes and a greater degree of crisis in assuming the parenting role. Both first-time mothers and fathers have shown a decline in marital satisfaction during this transition period. Mothers have been shown to anticipate greater involvement in infant caretaking activities and actually have greater involvement in infant caretaking activities than fathers do. Even in the most egalitarian relationships, when fathers anticipated sharing in the care of the infant equally with the mother, their actual involvement in infant caretaking activities was much less than anticipated. An indepth discussion of becoming a parent is presented in Chapter 34.

The transition to the parenting role is influenced by the individual's level of stress and ability to cope, the amount of social support that is available, and the temperament of the infant. There is limited research on the effectiveness of interventions that are used to promote positive adaptation to parenthood (Walker 1992).

Transitional events in family relationships are often found in the area of sexuality for both mothers and fathers and are related to sexual needs, interests, and physiologic changes after childbirth. Women have more worries and concerns about resuming sexual intercourse after birth than men do. Also, women may have decreased sexual interests after childbirth, usually as a result of stress and fatigue. After childbirth, most women resume intercourse between 2 and 8 weeks. Counseling about sexuality and family planning during the postpartum period is critical, yet most women receive insufficient counseling in this area. Many women have also resumed intercourse before their postpartum visit to their health care provider at 4 to 6 weeks (Walker 1992).

Implications for Research

There is a solid basis of descriptive research available on physiologic adaptation during the postpartum period that forms the foundation of nursing care. However, there are still many unanswered questions, and research available on the effectiveness of interventions that are commonly used to promote positive adaptation during the postpartum period is limited.

- What permanent effect do pregnancy and lactation have on the breasts for the woman who breastfeeds? for the non-breastfeeding woman?
- What aspects of role adaptation during the postpartum period are the most difficult for the mother? for the father? for other family members?
- What interventions are most effective for promoting positive role adaptation after childbirth?

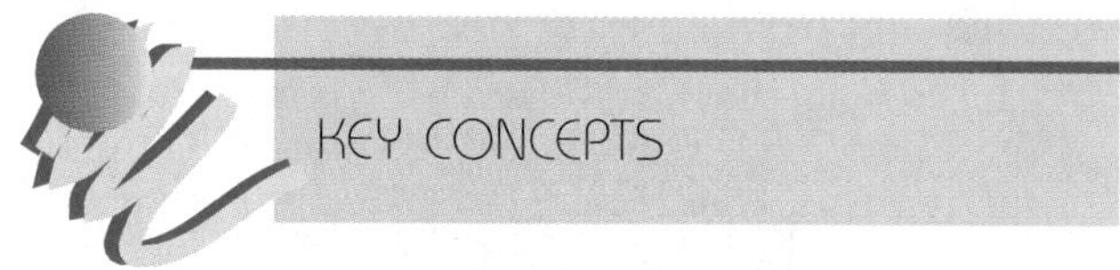

KEY CONCEPTS

- ▼ The postpartum period is a time of profound physiologic, psychological and social changes. There are marked changes in almost every major organ system after childbirth. Thus, the postpartum period is a time of disequilibrium.
- ▼ Three different processes must occur for involution of the uterus to take place normally: the uterus must contract, autolysis of myometrial cells must take place, and the epithelium must regenerate.
- ▼ Shortly after delivery, the fundus is located in the midline about halfway between the umbilicus and symphysis pubis. By 12 hours after delivery, the uterine fundus is located approximately at the level of the umbilicus. After that, the fundus decreases in size about 1 cm per day (about one fingerbreadth), and by 10 days after delivery, it cannot be palpated abdominally.
- ▼ The color and amount of lochia change as healing occurs. Immediately after birth and until about 2 to 4 days post partum, lochia is dark red to brownish red and is called lochia rubra. From 3 to 4 days post partum, lochia becomes brownish in color, thinner in consistency, and more translucent; it is now called lochia serosa. Around 10 to 14 days post partum, lochia becomes thick and white to yellowish in color and is called lochia alba.

- The return of first menses is extremely variable for individual women. The first menses is usually anovulatory. In lactating women, ovulation usually does not occur before 10 weeks, but it may occur as early as 35 days. The average time for the first menses of nonlactating women is 7 to 9 weeks.
- After delivery, there is a further increase in cardiac output, which occurs as vena caval compression is removed and contraction of the uterus leads to a decrease in blood pooling there. The pulse rate normally slows, with rates as low as 50 to 60 beats per minute. Cardiac output values return to normal by 8 to 10 weeks after childbirth.
- Blood volume decreases at delivery, approximately 500 mL for a normal vaginal delivery and 1000 mL in a typical cesarean delivery. In the next 2 to 3 days, blood volume typically increases as 900 to 1200 mL of extracellular fluid is shifted into the maternal circulation. During the next 6 weeks, blood volume decreases as this fluid is eliminated.
- The hemoglobin level decreases immediately after birth as a result of blood loss. The hematocrit usually remains relatively stable and may even increase slightly the first few days for women who have a vaginal delivery. As extracellular fluid is drawn into the circulation, from day 2 to day 4, the hemoglobin level rises slowly, regaining the values of day 1 by day 9 after delivery.
- Starting shortly after delivery, the respiratory tract rapidly returns to the prepregnant state. This is a result of the loss of progesterone production with separation of the placenta, the immediate decrease in intra-abdominal pressure at birth of the baby, and the increased excursion of the diaphragm.
- The neuromuscular and sensory changes that occurred during pregnancy resolve rapidly during the postpartum period as the woman's hormonal levels return to the prepregnant state.
- The changes in the immune system and host defense mechanism that occurred during pregnancy remain altered for 2 to 3 months after delivery. These changes occurred during pregnancy to protect the fetus from infection and rejection during pregnancy. However, they increase the mother's risk for mycotic, fungal, and other opportunistic infections; increase the risk for colonization with streptococci and staphylococci; and delay the mother's initial response to infection, making accurate diagnosis of infection difficult.
- Most women's urinary system will return to its nonpregnant state of functioning by 3 months post partum. Approximately 10 percent of women will have some permanent enlargement of the kidneys. The increased glomerular filtration rate during the early postpartum period combined with the decrease in progesterone, which has an antidiuretic effect, leads to a marked diuresis after childbirth, up to 3000 mL of urine per day.
- Changes in gastrointestinal function during the immediate postpartum period are an exaggeration of the changes that normally occur during the menstrual cycle. Decreased motility slows intestinal transit time, and relaxation of the abdominal muscles decreases the ability of the woman to use her stomach muscles to aid evacuation.
- A wide variety of factors may affect psychological adaptation after childbirth. The factors may be either physiologic or psychosocial in nature. These factors need to be evaluated for each individual woman. Also, the woman's perception of these factors influences how they will affect her.
- Research has shown that the transition to parenthood is an event of great significance for women and men. Role adaptation involves two specific areas: the adoption of a new social role within the family (e.g., mother or father) and changes in family relationships.

References

Affonso, D. D. (1987). Assessment of maternal postpartum adaptation. *Public Health Nursing,* 4 (1), 9–16.

Beck, C. T. (1991). Maternity blues research: A critical review. *Issues in Mental Health Nursing,* 12, 291–300.

Beeber, L. S. (1996). Depression in women. In A. B. McBride and J. K. Austin (Eds.), *Psychiatric-mental health nursing: Integrating the behavioral and biologic sciences* (pp. 235–268). Philadelphia: W. B. Saunders.

Blackburn, S. T., and Loper, D. L. (1992). *Maternal, fetal, and neonatal physiology: A clinical perspective.* Philadelphia: W. B. Saunders.

Bowes, A. A. (1986). Postpartum care. In S. G. Gabbe, J. R. Niebyl, J. L. Simpson (Eds.), *Obstetrics: Normal and problem pregnancies* (pp. 623–643). New York: Churchill Livingstone.

Cunningham, E. G., MacDonald, P. C., Gant, N. F., Leveno, K. J., Gilstrap, L. C. (1993). *Williams obstetrics* (19th ed.). Norwalk, CT: Appleton & Lange.

Dennis, J. (1989). The physiology and management of the puerperium. In A. Turnbull and G. Chamberlain (Eds.), *Obstetrics* (pp. 891–901). New York: Churchill Livingstone.

Duff, J. (1989). The puerperium. In C. J. Pauerstein (Ed.), *Clinical obstetrics* (pp. 179–205). New York: John Wiley & Sons.

Duvekot, J. J., and Peeters, L. L. H. (1994a). Renal hemodynamics and volume homeostasis in pregnancy. *Obstetrical and Gynecological Survey,* 49 (12), 830–839.

Duvekot, J. J., and Peeters L. L. H. (1994b). Maternal cardiovascular hemodynamic adaptation to pregnancy. *Obstetrical and Gynecological Survey,* 49 (12), Supplement, S1–S14.

Frisoli, G. (1981). Physiology and pathology of the puerperium.

In L. Iffy and H. A. Kaminetsky (Eds.), *Principles and practice of obstetrics and perinatology* (Vol. 2, pp 1657–1675). New York: John Wiley & Sons.

Golan, N. (1981). *Passing through transitions: A guide for practitioners.* New York: The Free Press.

Guyton, A., and Hall, J. E. (1996). *Textbook of medical physiology.* Philadelphia: W. B. Saunders.

Keefe, M. (1988). The impact of infant rooming-in on maternal sleep at night. *Journal of Obstetric, Gynecologic, and Neonatal Nursing,* 12, 122.

Kittner, S. J., Stern, B. J., Feeser, B. R., Hebel, J. R., Nagey, D. A., Buchholz, D. W., Earley, C. J., Johnson, C. J., Macko, R. F., Sloan, M. A., Wityk, R. J., Wozniak, M. A. (1996). Pregnancy and the risk of stroke. *New England Journal of Medicine,* 335(11), 768–774.

Mercer, R., and Ferketich, S. L. (1990). Predictors of parental attachment during early parenthood. *Journal of Advanced Nursing,* 15 (3), 268–280.

Metcalfe, J., McNulty, J. H., Ueland, K. (1986). *Burwell and Metcalfe's heart disease and pregnancy: Physiology and management* (2nd ed.). Boston: Little, Brown.

Monheit, A. G., Cousins, L., Resnik, R. (1980). The puerperium: Anatomic and physiologic adjustments. *Clinical Obstetrics and Gynecology,* 23 (4), 973–984.

Resnik, R. (1994). The puerperium. In R. K. Creasy and R. Resnik (Eds.), *Maternal–fetal medicine: Principles and practice* (pp. 140–143). Philadelphia: W. B. Saunders.

Stray, P. B., Solberg, V. M., Torkildsen, E., Lie, S., Velken, M., Aaserud, J., Kierulf, K. A., Blakstad, M., Ulshagen, K., Sandstad, B. (1989). Postpartum bacturia: A multicenter evaluation of different screening procedures and a controlled short-course treatment trial with amoxycillin. *European Journal of Obstetrics, Gynecology, and Reproductive Biology,* 31 (2), 163–171.

Van Thiel, C., and Schade, R. R. (1986). Pregnancy: Its physiologic course, nutrient cost, and effects on gastrointestinal function. In V. K. Rutgi and J. N. Cooper (Eds.), *Gastrointestinal and hepatic complications in pregnancy* (pp. 1–29). New York: John Wiley & Sons.

Vorherr, J. (1973). Contraception after abortion and postpartum. *American Journal of Obstetrics and Gynecology,* 117, 1002.

Walker, L. O. (1992). *Parent-infant nursing science: Paradigms, phenomena, methods.* Philadelphia: F. A. Davis.

29 Chapter

. . . the in-hospital recovery time for new mothers has decreased significantly. In the 1970s, we had a call for shorter lengths of stay because they were safer and more humane. In the 1980s, early discharge programs started as a response to consumer demand and were an alternative to home deliveries. By 1990, however, the push for shorter hospital stays was driven by health maintenance organizations. Most mothers are now discharged 24 hours or less after a vaginal delivery.

KAREN B. HALLER (1996)

Nursing Care of Mothers

Kathy Gill

HIGHLIGHTS

- Factors Affecting Normal Postpartum Adaptation Related to Prenatal and Intrapartum Periods, General Health History, and Cultural and Psychosocial Influences
- The Importance of Historical Data and Assessment Related to Physical, Nutritional, and Psychosocial Assessment
- Normal Laboratory Findings
- Common Problems and Concerns of Postpartum Women Related to Elimination, Episiotomy and Hemorrhoids, Afterpains, Sore Nipples, Breast Engorgement, Regaining Physical Strength, Resumption of Sexual Activity, and Postpartum Blues
- Early Discharge and Postpartum Home Care
- Nursing Practice
- Risk Management
- Implications for Research
- Nursing Care Planning Guide: Healthy Postpartum Woman

DEFINITIONS

Afterpains—Painful uterine cramps during the first few postpartum days that result from normal uterine contrations.

Attachment—The affectionate relationship that develops between parents and the infant during the first year of life.

Bonding—The mutual attraction between the parents and newborn, particularly strong with the mother.

Cultural proscriptions—Behaviors that are taboo or prohibited in a culture, as in the case of new mothers.

Episiotomy—The surgical incision made in the perineum to enlarge the vaginal opening for delivery. There are two types of incision: mediolateral, an incision at a 45-degree angle from the midline; and midline or median, an incision straight in the midline toward the rectum.

Homans sign—Pain in the calf with dorsiflexion of the foot indicating thrombophlebitis or thrombosis.

Living ligature—Smooth muscle fibers of the uterus that contract to close off blood vessels.

Lochia—Postpartum bleeding.

Postpartum blues—Mild, transient mood disturbances beginning on the third postpartum day, lasting for 2 to 3 days; onset coincides with a normal physiologic drop in estrogen and progesterone.

Puerperium—The time after birth, approximately 6 weeks, during which anatomic and physiologic changes of pregnancy resolve. Also called the postpartum period.

Thrombophlebitis—Inflammation of a vein often accompanied by thrombus formation (a clot) resulting from venous stasis, infection, vessel wall trauma, or hypercoagulability.

Thrombosis—An abnormal clot occurring within a blood vessel.

Uterine involution—The normal process whereby the uterus contracts to near its prepregnant size.

The postpartum period is a time of physical restoration and healing, emotional mood swings, and role adjustments as the woman assumes the role of mothering the new infant and redefines her relationships with her family members. During this time, the woman requires rest and support for physiologic regeneration. At the same time, she must develop a relationship with her new baby and learn how to be a nurturing mother; gain competence in performing infant care physical skills, such as feeding, that are necessary to care for the baby; and adapt to changes in roles and responsibilities within the family unit as the new baby is integrated into the family. Becoming a mother is "one of the most emotionally and intellectually demanding, exasperating, strenuous, anxiety-arousing, and deeply satisfying tasks that any human being can undertake" (Kitzinger 1994, p. ix). Other family members—the woman's partner and other children in the family—have special concerns and needs as well as the new baby is incorporated into the family. Roles and responsibilities must be redefined and adjustments made.

The postpartum period provides the nurse with the opportunity to care for the new family during an exciting and rewarding time. In 1996, most mothers were discharged from the hospital within 24 hours of a vaginal birth and within 48 to 72 hours after a cesarean birth. This limited hospital stay presented a challenge.

In response to national concerns related to early discharge, Congress passed the Newborns' and Mothers' Health Protection Act of 1996. This act set a national standard requiring health insurance plans and employer-provided benefit plans that include maternity benefits that provide a minimum of 48 hours of inpatient care following a vaginal delivery and 96 hours of inpatient care following cesarean delivery.

Nursing care is needed that meets the physiologic, psychological, and educational needs of the mother; the growth and development needs of the infant; and the needs of other family members. To achieve this goal, comprehensive prenatal and postpartum programs are needed in outpatient, community, and home settings that provide the crucial nursing care for the postpartum woman and her family (Haller 1996).

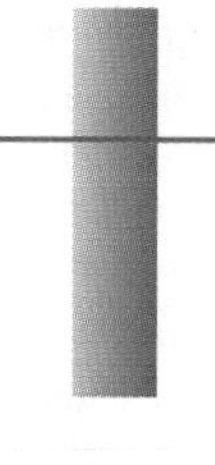

FACTORS AFFECTING NORMAL POSTPARTUM ADAPTATION

The postpartum period is usually a time of uneventful although stressful recovery from the birth process, and it proceeds smoothly for the majority of women. However, conditions may occur in the prenatal period or events may happen during the intrapartum period that can influence the physiologic and emotional recovery of the new mother. The woman's general health status and any preexisting illnesses also affect perinatal outcomes and postpartum recovery.

Prenatal Factors

The presence of pregnancy-related illnesses, such as hypertensive disorders of pregnancy or gestational diabetes, puts the woman at risk during the postpartum period. The development of prenatal complications, such as maternal bleeding, fetal problems, or preterm labor, increases the likelihood that the mother will have a more complicated recovery process.

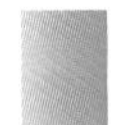

Intrapartum Factors

Cesarean birth, an instrument-assisted birth, and incomplete placental separation are intrapartum complications that have the potential to cause trauma, bleeding, and wound infections during the postpartum period. Uterine involution may be prolonged in cases of overdistention from a multifetal gestation, polyhydramnios, or a large baby. Overdistention of the uterus can also cause hemorrhage during the postpartum period.

The woman who has had a prolonged labor or experienced a difficult birth is likely to be exhausted during the postpartum period. She may have electrolyte and fluid imbalances as the result of the prolonged labor. Return of normal bladder function is often delayed because of bladder trauma, atony, or anesthesia.

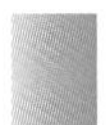

General Health History

General health factors include any preexisting conditions, such as diabetes mellitus or cardiac disease. The woman's medical condition and general health status influence her physical and psychological recovery during the postpartum period (see Chapter 35).

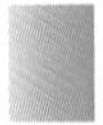

Cultural and Psychosocial Factors

Cultural background can greatly influence how the mother perceives her health status, the postpartum period, and self-care activities. The nurse needs to be familiar with common beliefs and values of differing cultural groups and must also recognize that these beliefs and values vary for each individual within a specific culture. Specific groups may have patterns of self-care for the mother and newborn care that differ from those of the dominant cultural group. These patterns may seem unusual or without scientific basis. However, if they are not detrimental to the patient's safety, these customs can be carried out in the hospital as the woman and her family wish. Dietary and activity proscriptions are common areas of difference from the Western model of care, and these areas should always be discussed with the mother.

SOURCES OF HISTORICAL DATA

The basis for a comprehensive assessment is historical information about the postpartum woman related to pregnancy history, labor and delivery history, laboratory data, infant history, postpartum history, and family history (Table 29–1). The mother's chart contains important information concerning gravida and para status, the length of labor, fetal position, method of delivery, degree of episiotomy, type and amount of analgesia or anesthesia, blood type and Rh factor status, and any complications that may have occurred during the labor and birth.

The woman's prenatal record should be a part of the client's chart. It contains information about length of prenatal care, EDC (estimated date of confinement), baseline vital sign assessments before labor, laboratory studies, and history of any prenatal complications. This information assists the nurse in planning for procedures that may be necessary.

Data obtained from the infant's chart are essential in planning for care. The sex and weight of the infant, difficulties during labor and birth (i.e., fetal distress), choice of feeding method, and presence of any anomalies are important pieces of information in planning for care that promotes bonding.

Laboratory data obtained from the chart include hematocrit and hemoglobin level on admission to the labor and delivery unit; hematocrit 24 hours after delivery to determine the presence of anemia from excessive blood loss during delivery; and the mother's Rh factor, blood type, and rubella status.

Table 29–1

SOURCES OF HISTORICAL DATA

PATIENT'S CHART	DATA
Pregnancy history	• Para, gravida • EDC (estimated date of confinement) • Problems during pregnancy
Labor and delivery history	• Length of labor • Type of delivery • Estimated blood loss • Fetal position • Analgesia or anesthesia • Problems during labor and delivery • Childbirth preparation classes attended
Laboratory data	• Hemoglobin, hematocrit • Rh factor, rubella status, blood type
Infant history	• Sex, weight • Apgar scores • Problems during labor and birth • Feeding method • Presence of anomalies
Postpartum history	• Fundal assessment • Lochia assessment • Perineum assessment • Bowel sounds, elimination status • Lung sounds, respiratory assessment • Homans sign assessment • Maternal response to newborn • Presence of significant other
Family history	• Other children, ages • Occupation • Education level • Type of housing

POSTPARTUM ASSESSMENT

The postpartum assessment is done to detect deviations from normal and to provide a record that accurately depicts the mother's postpartum recovery status. While only a few minutes are required for each component of the assessment, a comprehensive assessment can require considerable time. If used as an opportunity for teaching self-care, the postpartum assessment can serve a dual purpose and promote the woman's return of normal functioning.

The guidelines of the institution direct the frequency of postpartum assessment. After an uncomplicated vaginal birth, a postpartum assessment is usually done twice a day until discharge. Postpartum assessment after a cesarean birth is usually done every 4 hours for 2 days, then twice a day until dismissal.

The postpartum assessment will most likely be done with the woman in bed, where privacy can be maintained. The nurse can follow the mother's lead concerning who she would like to have stay in the room during the assessment. The assessment can be delayed if necessary to allow the mother to calm a crying infant. It is difficult for the mother to listen and respond to the nurse if her infant is hungry, is fussy, or needs to have a diaper change.

Physical Assessment

VITAL SIGNS

During the immediate postpartum period, vital signs are taken every 15 minutes during the first hour after birth, every 30 minutes for the next 2 hours, and every hour for the next 2 to 6 hours. Vital signs are monitored thereafter every 4 hours for the first 24 hours and every 8 to 12 hours for the remainder of the hospital stay. Another common schedule is to check blood pressure and pulse every 15 minutes until they are at predelivery levels. An alteration in vital signs indicates the need for more frequent monitoring. An alteration in vital signs is a signal to the nurse of the need for careful assessment for the underlying cause.

The mother's temperature may be taken every 4 hours while she is awake. Temperatures up to 100.4°F (38°C) in the first 24 hours after birth are often related to the dehydrating effects of labor. Increasing hydration by encouraging oral fluids will help to bring the temperature to a normal reading. Intravenous fluids may occasionally be indicated. A temperature of greater than 100.4°F in any two consecutive readings is considered febrile, and any temperature above 101°F should be reported to the physician. A sustained rise in the temperature for 2 days or a recurrent temperature elevation may be an indication of puerperal sepsis.

During the first week after birth, transient episodes of bradycardia are common. The woman's pulse may be as low as 40 to 50 beats per minute the first 1 to 2 days after delivery. A range of 50 to 70 beats per minute is normal. A weak, thready, or rapid pulse is abnormal and may be a sign of hemorrhage or shock. Particular attention should be paid to the pulse rate when there has been a blood loss of 500 mL or greater during or after delivery.

Blood pressure should be close to measurements obtained during labor. Orthostatic hypotension may be evident during the first 8 hours after birth as the cardiovascular system is readjusting to the nonpregnant state. Feelings of faintness or dizziness are indications that caution the nurse to be aware of the patient's safety. Advise the mother to request help the first few times she gets out of bed.

REPRODUCTIVE SYSTEM

Uterine involution begins immediately after delivery of the placenta. The uterus begins to contract and returns to its prepregnant condition usually in 6 weeks. The fundus is located midway between the symphysis pubis and the umbilicus. At 1 hour post partum, the fundus is firm and contracted at the level of the umbilicus in the midline. Fundal height decreases by 1 cm each day, and the fundus should no longer be palpable by the tenth postpartum day (see Fig. 28–1).

Before the fundal assessment is started, have the mother empty her bladder so that an accurate assessment can be done. The nurse can then assess the bladder for complete emptying as well as accurately assess uterine involution. Have the woman lie flat on her back with the knees flexed. Release the perineal pad to observe for increased bleeding with massage. When palpating the fundus, cup one hand just above the symphysis pubis to support the lower uterine segment. Place the other hand at the level of the umbilicus, gently rolling the outer aspect of the hand down and into the abdomen (Fig. 29–1). If the fundus is boggy (soft), massage gently until firm, observing for increased bleeding or clots. In the medical chart, document fundal position, height, and consistency. If massage is necessary, documentation should reflect the response, such as "uterus boggy, firm with light massage."

It is important to assess the fundus after a cesarean delivery; however, the nurse should splint (support with hand) the low transverse incision while gently palpating the fundus. Uterine involution generally proceeds more slowly after surgery. With a vertical cesarean incision, splint the incision and palpate gently on each side of the incision for firmness and position.

When assessing the fundus, the nurse notes the consistency. A firmly contracting uterus feels firm, much like a strong labor contraction. As blood collects in the uterus and forms clots, the uterine musculature is less able to contract. The fundus rises as the blood collects. A boggy fundus, which may be difficult to locate, is soft and spongy. The position of the fundus is noted to be midline or displaced to the side, which happens if the bladder is full. Fundal height is measured, in relation to the umbilicus, as centimeters or fingerbreadths above or below the umbilicus.

Lochia, the discharge present after birth, consists of endometrial tissue, blood, and lymph. It is red (lochia rubra) the first 1 to 3 days and gradually decreases in amount. Observe the type (rubra, serosa, alba), the amount of bleeding, the presence of any clots, and the odor. Normal lochia has a fleshy odor. Foul-smelling or purulent lochia usually indicates an infection. It is more accurate to observe lochia for clots before fundal palpation. Normally, there may be a few small clots the first 1 or 2 days after birth from pooling of blood in the vagina. Clots larger than 1 cm are considered abnormal and need to be monitored. The cause of such clots, such as uterine atony or retained placental fragments, needs to be determined and treated to prevent further blood loss.

A specified system of measuring lochia should be consistently used on the postpartum unit by all health care personnel (Fig. 29–2). The normal amount of lochia may vary with the individual but should never exceed four to eight pads a day. The average number of pads used is six pads a day (Jacobson 1985). Assessment of lochia volume and early identification of signs of excessive bleeding are critical responsibilities of the nurse (Tables 29–2 and 29–3).

PERINEUM

The perineum is observed for the presence of redness, edema, ecchymosis, discharge, and approximation (REEDA) of the suture line if an episiotomy or laceration is present. Bruising may occur, particularly after a forceps-assisted delivery. The perineum may be edematous after a prolonged second stage. Observe for the presence of a hematoma, which indicates bleeding beneath the surface (Fig. 29–3). This may be associated with a forceps delivery. Observe for the presence of hemorrhoids. Note the number of hemorrhoids, size, and pain or tenderness.

BREASTS

All women, regardless of whether they plan to breastfeed or formula feed, should have their breasts examined every 8 hours. Also at this time, determine if the mother is wearing a bra that provides adequate support. Observe and palpate for nipple soreness, breast tenderness, lumps, engorgement, mastitis, presence of colostrum, and presence of leaking milk. For the breastfeeding woman, note the presence of an erectile nipple that the infant can easily latch on to. A flat or inverted nipple is more difficult for the infant to

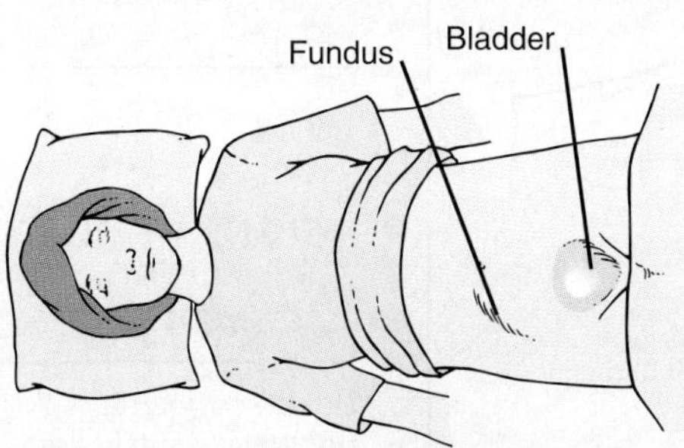

HAVE THE WOMAN VOID BEFORE STARTING ASSESSMENT

- A full bladder displaces the uterus to the side, which causes it to relax and contract poorly, and makes accurate determination of involution of the uterus impossible

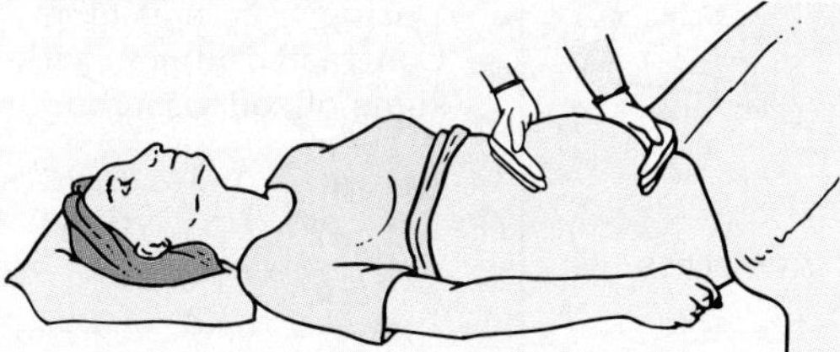

ASSESS THE FUNDUS FOR FIRMNESS FIRST, THEN USE FUNDAL MASSAGE TO ELICIT MAXIMUM FIRMNESS OF THE FUNDUS

- Have the women lie in the supine position with knees flexed
- Lower the perineal pad so that you can determine the amount of lochia flow during fundal massage (see Figure 29-2 on lochia volume)
- Cup one hand against the lower uterine segment just above the symphysis pubis to support uterus and prevent displacement downward
- Cup the other hand against the fundus of uterus and use the flat part of the fingers to gently massage the fundus toward the lower uterine segment

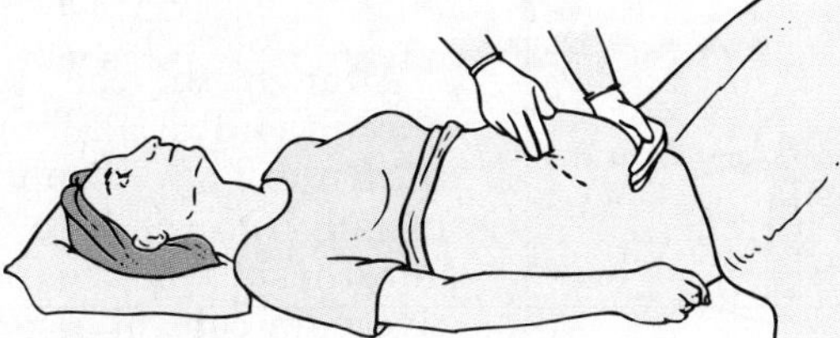

DETERMINE LOCATION OF THE UTERINE FUNDUS FROM THE LEVEL OF THE UMBILICUS BY MEASURING IN FINGERBREADTHS

- Document the consistency of the fundus—boggy (soft), firm with massage, or firm
- Record the location of the fundus—for example, U-1 (one fingerbreadth below the umbilicus)—and note if the fundus is in the middle or displaced to the side
- Record the color and amount of lochia

Figure 29–1

Conducting a thorough assessment of the fundus is an essential part of nursing care.

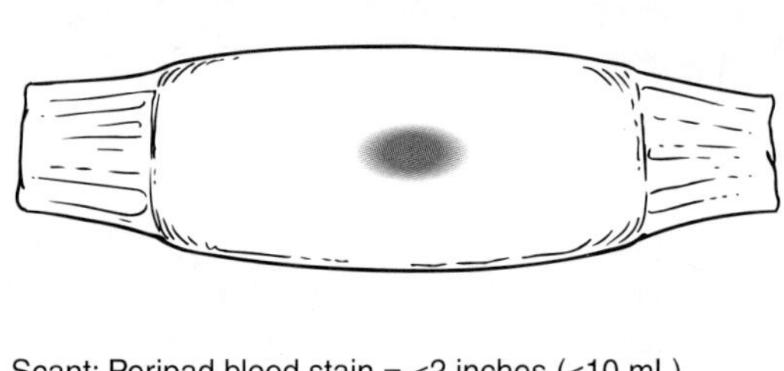

Scant: Peripad blood stain = <2 inches (<10 mL) within 1 hour

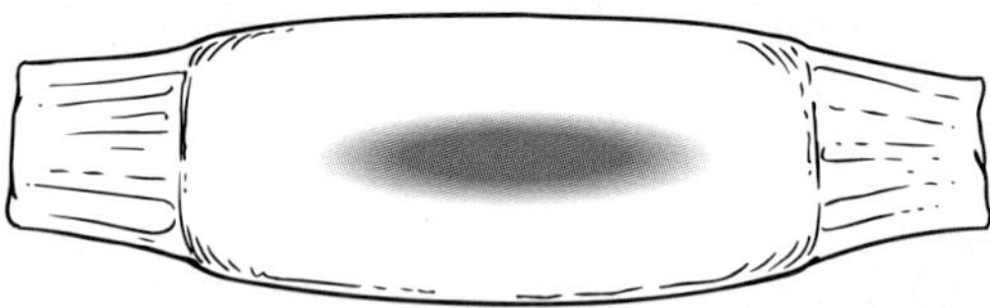

Small: Peripad blood stain = >2 inches but <4 inches (10 to 25 mL) within 1 hour

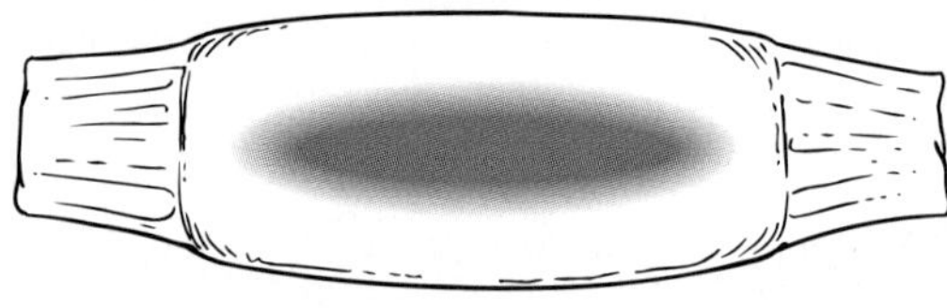

Moderate: Peripad blood stain = >4 inches but <6 inches (25 to 50 mL) within 1 hour

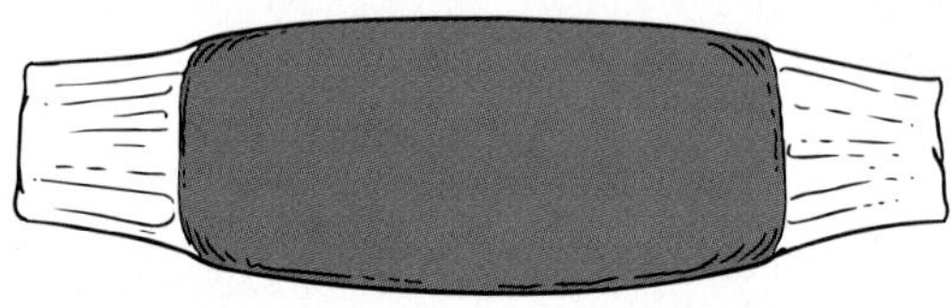

Large: Peripad blood stain = >6 inches to saturated peripad (50 to 80 mL) within 1 hour

Figure 29–2

Lochia volume can be assessed as scant, small, moderate, or large. (Data from Jacobson, H. [1985]. A standard for assessing lochia volume. *MCN: American Journal of Maternal-Child Nursing*, 10 [3], 175; Luegenbiehl, D. L., Brophy, G. H., Artique, G. S., Phillips, K. E., Falk, R. J. [1990]. Standardized assessment of blood loss. *MCN: American Journal of Maternal-Child Nursing*, 15 [4], 241–244.)

Table 29–2

SIGNS OF POSTPARTUM BLEEDING

ASSESSMENT	POSSIBLE CAUSE
Dark red lochia Boggy uterus	Uterine atony, retained placental fragments
Bright red lochia Contracted uterus	Lacerations
Excessive lochia Oozing from episiotomy Contracted uterus with no signs of soft tissue injury	Coagulation defect

grasp and may require intervention for breastfeeding to be successful.

A woman who is not breastfeeding should wear a snug-fitting bra from within 6 hours after birth for 24 hours a day until tenderness subsides. It is important for her to avoid excessive stimulation of the breast and nipples for 1 week. Acetaminophen will usually provide adequate pain relief. It is not necessary to limit fluid intake in nonlactating mothers (Wong and Stepp-Gilbert 1985).

GASTROINTESTINAL SYSTEM

After birth, the woman's abdomen should be auscultated in all four quadrants to determine the return of bowel sounds. Normal bowel elimination usually returns 2 to 3 days post partum. Surgery, anesthesia, and the use of narcotics for postoperative pain control also contribute to a longer period of altered bowel function. After a cesarean birth, bowel sounds are assessed at least every 8 hours until they are active in all quadrants. Ask the woman if she has had a bowel movement and note the occurrence of bowel movements and consistency. It is especially important to assess the return of bowel function after a cesarean birth or a tubal ligation.

RENAL SYSTEM

As diuresis begins after delivery, approximately 3 liters of accumulated fluids and volume is lost. Therefore, it is important to assess the mother's ability to urinate after delivery. The inability to urinate may result from edema of the bladder, urethra, and urinary meatus due to trauma or from the loss of bladder tone. The bladder can be palpated for position and fullness. A suprapubic

Table 29–3

NORMAL PHYSIOLOGIC FINDINGS IN THE IMMEDIATE POSTPARTUM PERIOD

MATERNAL SYSTEM	NORMAL CHANGES
Uterus	Fundal height decreases Consistency firm and contracted in the midline
Lochia	**Color** Rubra: red, lasts 1–3 days Serosa: pink, brown-tinged, lasts 3–10 days Alba: yellowish white, lasts 10–14 days **Amount** Scant: <2-inch stain (<10 mL) on pad in 1 hour Small: >2-inch to <4-inch stain (10–25 mL) on pad in 1 hour Moderate: >4-inch to <6-inch stain (25–50 mL) on pad in 1 hour Large: >6-inch stain to saturated pad in 1 hour
Perineum	Intact: may have ecchymosis, edema, or both Episiotomy: edges well-approximated, without drainage, redness, or edema Hemorrhoids may be present
Breasts	Nipples erect with stimulation Full, heavy on postpartum day 2 or 3
Abdominal incision	Edges well-approximated No drainage or redness
Vital signs	Blood pressure: same as during labor Pulse: 40–80 beats/min Temperature: 36.2–38°C (98–100.4°F) Respiration: 16–24/min
Gastrointestinal system	Bowel sounds return Normal elimination resumes in 2–3 days
Urinary system	Nonpalpable bladder Diuresis
Vascular system	Homans sign absent

bulge noted when the woman is lying flat in bed indicates a full bladder. The fundus will be displaced above the umbilicus and to the side. Before proceeding further with the assessment, have the woman empty her bladder. Voidings should be measured the first two or three times. Urinary output of more than 500 mL usually indicates complete emptying.

CARDIOVASCULAR SYSTEM

The woman's legs are assessed every 8 hours during the hospital stay for the presence of Homans sign. Homans sign is present when there is any discomfort (pain or soreness) in the calf of the leg or increased resistance (compared with the other leg) on forced dorsiflexion of the foot. These findings result from irritability of the posterior muscles of the leg and are indicative of calf vein thrombophlebitis (Sternbach 1989). Both legs are assessed for edema, redness, or increased warmth. Two other signs of calf vein thrombophlebitis that usually disappear promptly on bed rest are swelling of the ankle and coldness of the foot.

To elicit the Homans sign, the nurse asks the woman to extend her leg flat on the bed. The nurse grasps the foot and sharply dorsiflexes it forward (Fig. 29–4). If this causes any discomfort or resistance, the nurse should notify the physician or nurse-midwife that the Homans sign is present.

RESPIRATORY SYSTEM

Respirations are monitored with vital signs. After birth, respiratory rate should return to prepregnancy range. Respirations normally range from 16 to 24 breaths per minute. A lower respiratory rate may be associated with a regional block. Women who have received epidural morphine (Duramorph) for pain control after a cesarean birth or intrathecal anesthesia during labor may be monitored hourly for 24 hours after injection. Respirations that fall below 10 to 12 should be reported to the physician according to the institution's protocol.

Women who have had a cesarean birth or tocolytic therapy should have their lungs assessed more frequently. They are at a higher risk for pulmonary complications due to surgery and the actions of tocolytic medications.

IMMUNE SYSTEM

An important part of the physical assessment includes determining the Rh factor and immunity to rubella of the postpartum woman. Rh factor incompatibility exists in the Rh-negative mother with an Rh-positive fetus. The Rh-negative woman

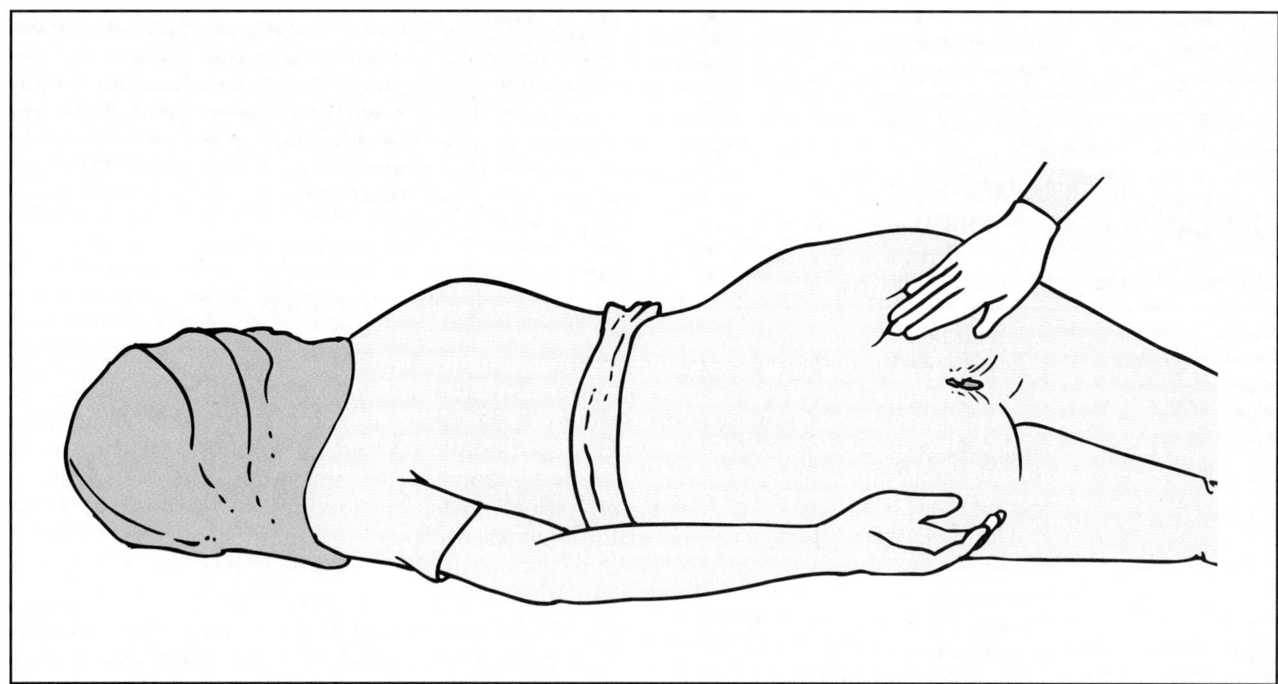

Figure 29–3

For assessing the perineal and anal area, the woman is placed in Sims position and the nurse lifts up the buttock so that the perineal and anal areas can be inspected • The presence of the following should be noted: hemorrhoids (as shown); state of episiotomy or laceration healing (intact perineum shown in figure); and tenderness, hardness, or ecchymosis of areas.

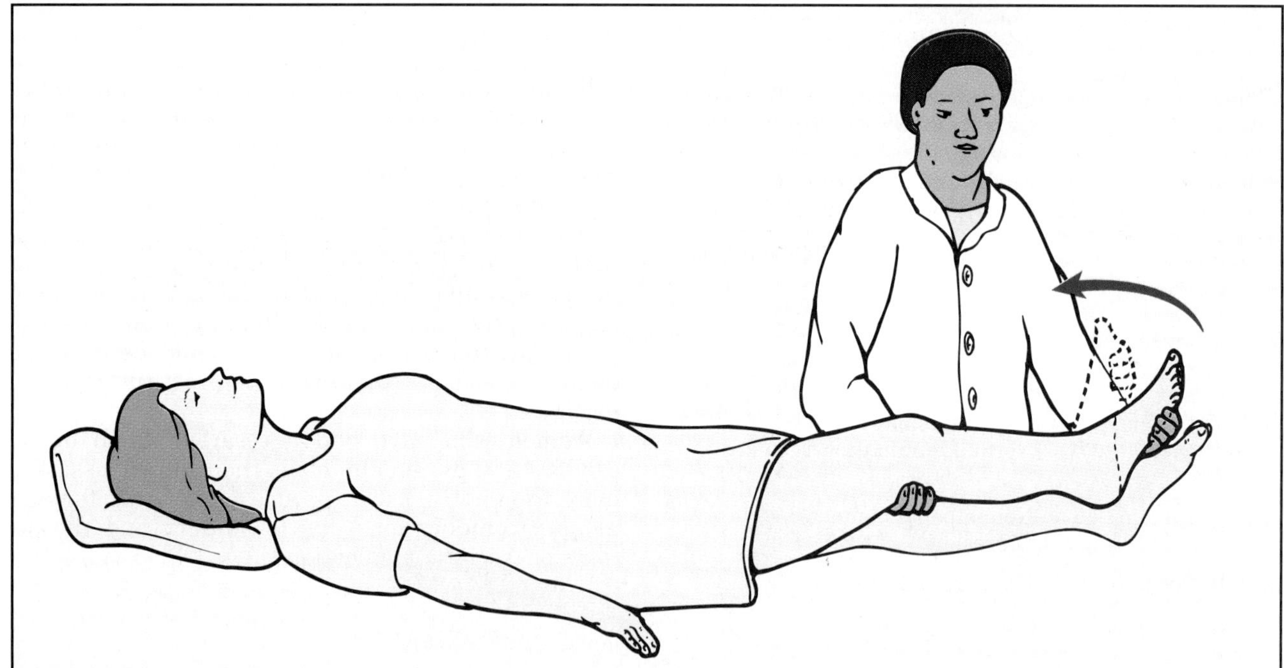

Figure 29–4

In assessing for Homans sign, the woman's knee is flexed slightly and supported underneath with one hand by the nurse • With the other hand, the nurse dorsiflexes the woman's foot • Homans sign is present when there is pain or discomfort in the calf of the leg on dorsiflexion of the foot and may indicate deep venous thrombosis (Data from Sternbach, G. [1989]. John Homans: The dorsiflexion sign. *The Journal of Emergency Medicine,* 7, 287–290.)

who has not been sensitized to Rh-positive fetal red blood cells will have a negative indirect Coombs test result. This woman needs an immunization to prevent sensitization in later pregnancies. The nurse gives 1 unit of $Rh_0(D)$ immune globulin (300 μg) within 72 hours after birth to prevent antibody formation. An interval greater than 72 hours may allow the maternal system to develop antibodies to the fetal cells released in the maternal circulation when the placenta separated. A serum antibody titer greater than 1:16 demonstrates positive maternal sensitization. Sometimes it is not clear whether the mother is already sensitized in later pregnancies. In such cases, $Rh_0(D)$ immune globulin should be given (see Chapter 21 for a detailed discussion of Rh isoimmunization).

A blood sample for a rubella titer is drawn on all women in the antepartum or postpartum period. A woman with a titer of 1:8 or less should receive a subcutaneous rubella virus vaccine (Meruvax II). This stimulates active immunity against the rubella virus. The woman should be counseled to avoid pregnancy for 3 months after receiving the vaccine.

Nutritional Assessment

The goal of the nutritional assessment by the nurse is twofold: to determine the knowledge of the new mother and to determine her nutritional needs. A woman's nutritional needs depend on her prepregnancy weight, her ideal weight for height, and whether she is breastfeeding.

Normal weight loss from diuresis and diaphoresis the first few postpartum days is approximately 5 pounds. Some women may lose their pregnancy weight gain by several weeks after birth, and some women may lose it several months after birth. Women need reassurance that both are normal.

If the mother is breastfeeding, her calorie needs increase by approximately 500 calories per day. The need for fluids may be increased, and prenatal vitamins and iron supplements should be continued. Nutritional counseling is important to breastfeeding mothers and should be provided by the nurse. Contrary to a common belief, breastfeeding does not appear to be a factor in weight loss in the postpartum period (Schauberger et al. 1992). Inadequate maternal nutrition can prevent the success of lactation or impair the health of the mother.

Evaluating the sources of fat in the diet and examining eating patterns are more helpful in promoting good nutrition than is focusing on weight loss and the number of calories consumed. Women who are interested in a weight reduction diet should be referred to a dietitian. The nurse can discuss eating patterns with the new mother and can recommend food groups that will supply the necessary nutrients for repair of tissues and the return of optimal functioning. An observation of foods selected for mealtimes and those eaten can provide the nurse with a basis for starting a discussion on nutrition. The nurse can observe and comment on the positive aspects of the mother's nutritional choices.

Cultural traditions and beliefs may also play a part in the nutritional assessment and nursing care. Individuals from populations that follow traditional lifestyles may have recommendations for or restrictions on certain foods or food groups. These practices should be respected and supported by the nurse. Menu choices can be adapted to fit the desired regimen while still providing nutritionally adequate food. Family members can bring in traditional foods prepared at home to supplement the diet.

Psychosocial Assessment

During the rapid physiologic changes of the postpartum period, psychosocial changes are also occurring with the new mother and her family. An awareness of the normal progression of psychological changes assists the nurse in making an individual assessment of the mother.

NORMAL PSYCHOLOGICAL CHANGES

During the postpartum period, the new mother is adjusting after the birth experience and relinquishing her previous role as a pregnant woman; she must now take on the mothering role. Rubin (1961) identified two phases of regeneration during the postpartum period: Taking-In (first 3 days) and Taking-Hold (3 to 10 days) (Table 29–4). Later research generally supports Rubin's theory but suggests that the length of time of each phase is shorter than what Rubin reported more than 30 years ago. In Rubin's framework, taking-in behaviors existed on day 1 and decreased rapidly, but some taking-in behaviors were present on all three postpartum days; mothers exhibited strong taking-hold behaviors as early as day 1, and these behaviors intensified on days 2 and 3 (Wrasper 1996). While Rubin may have identified longer time frames for these normal emotional stages than what is seen in the majority of most women today, the stages themselves still seem to be true.

During the taking-in phase, the new mother is attempting to integrate her labor and birth experience and fill in the missing pieces. Providing the mother with reassurance about the events of childbirth, providing her with missing information, and clarifying those details she may not have un-

Table 29–4

RUBIN'S PHASES OF REGENERATION DURING THE PUERPERIUM AS INTERPRETED BY MARTELL AND MITCHELL

	PHASES OF REGENERATION	
CATEGORY	**Taking-In (first 3 days)**	**Taking-Hold (3–10 days)**
Energy level	Sleep need, fatigued	Active, may be sleepy or hungry
Time orientation	Past, talks about labor	Present
Interpersonal interests	Self-focused, talkative to others about labor	Others and self, baby, family
Dependent/independent	Dependent, accepting, wants others to meet needs, compliant, needs direction	Independent, initiates activities, tends to organize
Focus of energy	Food, baby's intake	Mothering tasks, regaining body functions
Mood and affect	Passive, euphoric	Active, tends to be anxious, subject to mood swings that stabilize with time, impatient

From Wrasper, C. (1996). Discharge timing and Rubin's concept of puerperal change. *Journal of Perinatal Education,* 5 (2), 13–23.

derstood or may have misunderstood are important. During this time, the new mother will be focused on having her own needs met; food and sleep will be of high priority to her.

During the taking-hold phase, the mother assumes more independence and is ready to begin accepting responsibility for her care and her infant's care. If she is breastfeeding, she may be concerned about her ability to breastfeed her baby and whether she will have enough milk. During this time, involve parents in examining their newborn. Show them the capabilities and reflexes of their newborn, and explain normal newborn characteristics. New parents delight in discovering their newborn's innate abilities and behaviors (see Chapter 34). The newborn's simple grasp of a parent's or sibling's finger can bring big smiles to their faces. All of these activities foster positive parent-infant interaction and promote family adjustment.

Many maternity nurses work with new mothers only the first 24 to 48 hours after birth. It is wise to consider Rubin's research, keeping in mind that changes in our modern society are often reflected in behavior. We may see an alteration in the development of the mothering role as more societal changes occur. Women who are anticipating working after a short postpartum recovery at home have particular needs and concerns with physical recovery, infant care and feeding, and role changes in the family.

CONDUCTING A PSYCHOSOCIAL ASSESSMENT

Immediately after birth, the mother may be tired, sleepy, excited, or hungry. All of these are normal. The nurse takes into account the length of labor and type of delivery when assessing the psychosocial well-being of the mother. The nurse also considers the mother's general attitude, her feelings of competence in caring for her newborn, and the family and community support systems available to her. Since the mother may be fatigued from a long labor, it is useful to make a psychosocial assessment on more than one occasion to avoid incorrectly diagnosing a potential bonding problem. It is normal for the newly postpartum woman to feel that her physical needs must be met before she can respond to her newborn's needs. Some mothers may simply need time to rest and eat before they are responsive to and interested in their newborn. When conducting a psychosocial assessment, observe the problem-solving abilities of the mother. Is she responsive to her crying infant? Does she demonstrate the ability to try different soothing techniques? Also note the presence and quality of social support. Is there a spouse or significant other present? Does she have other family members visit or call? Has she received phone calls from friends? Either extreme—not enough support or too much—can hamper the woman's return to independence.

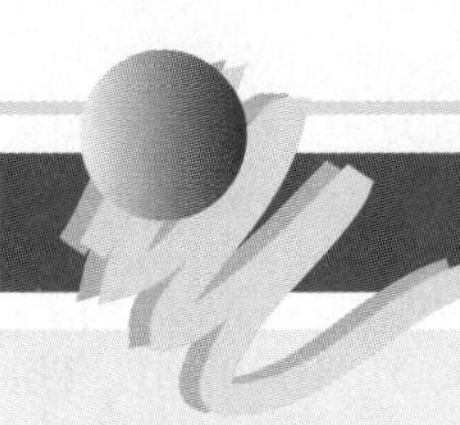

IMPROVING YOUR PRACTICE

CULTURAL INFLUENCES ON MOTHER-INFANT INTERACTION

Typical practices in mother-baby care include breastfeeding immediately after birth, encouraging the mother to be active—walking and resuming self-care activities—early in the postpartum period, and encouraging the mother to be involved in infant care activities. While these practices are seen as normal and beneficial to the Anglo-American population, they are not congruent with the traditional practices among other cultures. You can find out the information needed to provide more culturally sensitive care by determining the answers to the following questions.

- WHAT ARE THE POSTPARTUM AND NEWBORN CARE PRACTICES IN THE MOTHER'S CULTURE? The most effective way to determine this is to simply ask the mother and extended family about traditions and practices in their culture. Often a young woman may not follow all of the proscriptions of her cultural tradition. She may follow some while her parents or other family members are there, then request something different after they leave. It is important to determine which practices the mother believes are important and wants to follow and those that are not essential to her. It is often a challenging time for the mother as she tries to find a blend of traditional cultural practices and other cultural practices that are comfortable for her.
- ARE THERE ANY PHYSICAL RESTRICTIONS OR SECLUSION RITUALS? Activity may be limited in some cultures, and the mother is encouraged to drink only warm liquids and stay covered in bed. This may preclude bathing or showering during the first days to as much as a month after birth. In cultures that follow activity restrictions and ritual seclusion, infants are often kept close to the mother or even share the mother's bed. This can be viewed in a positive way because it increases contact between mother and infant and may actually promote the establishment of lactation.
- WHO SHOULD PROVIDE CARE FOR THE NEW MOTHER AND BABY? In some cultures, for example Southeast Asian, female relatives usually provide care for the mother and baby.
- WHAT IS THE MOTHER'S BELIEF ABOUT BREASTFEEDING? Breastfeeding practices vary among cultures. Some Native American women and Hispanic women may not breastfeed until the third or fourth day, when the milk "comes in." This is because colostrum is believed to be "bad milk." In some Asian cultures, mothers may not breastfeed their babies colostrum because they believe it to be poisonous and may give the baby diarrhea. While this cultural practice does not provide the baby with needed immunologic benefits, it should not be interpreted as an indication of the mother's lack of interest or concern for her newborn. Rather, it reflects the cultural practices and beliefs of the woman and her family.
- WHAT ARE THE MOTHER'S BELIEFS ABOUT EYE CONTACT AND INTERACTIONS WITH THE NEWBORN? Mexican women may believe that *mal ojo* or the evil eye, which may harm her baby, comes from excessive admiration. Women and children are thought to be particularly sensitive to *mal ojo.* Thus, when providing care for a Mexican mother, the nurse should avoid making compliments about the baby's appearance. Ethiopian, Cambodian, and Vietnamese women hold similar beliefs and may worry about their baby's welfare if the nurse makes positive comments about the baby to the mother. In some cultures, the head is considered the "seat of life" and is not touched by anyone other than a close family member. A Southeast Asian mother may be distressed if the nurse touches the baby's head.
- HOW CAN STRATEGIES TO ENHANCE MOTHER-INFANT INTERACTIONS BE ADAPTED TO THE MOTHER'S CULTURAL BELIEFS? After the needed information on cultural beliefs and practices is obtained, the nurse needs to adapt the typical strategies to enhance mother-infant interaction to the mother's cultural belief system. If this is not done, the interventions may be inappropriate or incomplete and may be unlikely to be successful in achieving the desired goal. Cultural practices that are not harmful should not be discouraged and can be allowed to continue. Harmful or potentially harmful practices require careful attention. The concerns and desires of the family should be validated and then a plan developed with the mother and family that ideally honors the mother's cultural beliefs and at the same time accomplishes the needed goals of nursing care. Implementing culturally sensitive nursing care requires an astute, creative, flexible nurse and can be exciting and fulfilling.

The educational level of the mother and her previous experience in dealing with infants also have an impact on her recovery. The nurse can gauge teaching according to the identified needs and background of the mother. This ensures that the mother is learning what is important to her. Many hospitals conduct dismissal classes for new mothers on self-care, nutrition, and infant feeding and care, or provide videos for parents to view on these subjects. While all teaching requires follow-up, videos especially need to be supplemented with direct nurse-to-parent teaching and follow-up.

MOTHER-INFANT INTERACTION

Policies of maternal and newborn health care agencies should be flexible enough to allow adaptation to individual needs and to support the ongoing process of mother-infant interaction. Time for bonding between infant and parents, which is described as the mutual attraction between people at first meeting, should be encouraged (Brazelton 1978). A thorough assessment of mother-infant interaction is critical as a foundation for planning nursing care that promotes the growth and development of the infant (see Chapter 34).

A woman with no experience of handling infants may be fearful and reluctant to handle her newborn or take on physical care. Acceptance of her feelings and acknowledging that many women feel apprehensive can help an unsure mother begin to participate in caring for her newborn. She may be unwilling to give a bath or request assistance with changing a diaper. Gradually, she should become more at ease with her infant and willing to perform aspects of physical care. Some warning signs of potential bonding problems are continued inability or unwillingness to care for the infant, marked depression, excessive physical fatigue, excessive preoccupation with self, evidence of low self-esteem, and lack of support systems. These characteristics may indicate potential physical, emotional, or intellectual difficulties with parenting and caregiving (Ament 1990; Symanski 1992). Referral to public health nurses is an important link to the community that can help these women.

NORMAL LABORATORY FINDINGS

Laboratory findings reflect normal physiologic changes after birth (Table 29–5). Abnormal findings indicate a possible complication and may require nursing intervention. The average blood loss after a vaginal birth is 500 mL. The average blood loss after a cesarean birth is 700 to 1000 mL. The degree of blood loss during birth is reflected in the hematocrit concentration. The hematocrit immediately rises after delivery in response to hemoconcentration. It returns to the prepregnant value within 4 to 6 weeks. A drop in the hematocrit indicates an abnormal blood loss. A drop of less than 10 percent of the predelivery hematocrit requires no further assessment. A hematocrit that has decreased by more than 10 percent of the predelivery value should be repeated 24 hours after delivery.

The white blood cell count, usually an indicator of infection, increases during labor and may stay elevated during the first few days post partum without presence of an infection. Plasma fibrinogen drops to prepregnancy levels after 1 week. During the early puerperium, this accounts for a higher sedimentation rate. Within 4 to 5 weeks after delivery, clotting factors return to normal levels.

Urinalysis may show mild proteinuria (1+) in the early postpartum period. Since this may also be associated with cystitis or pyelitis, the cause of the proteinuria should be investigated. A specimen contaminated with lochia may show slight proteinuria or a change in pH, specific gravity, or bacterial and red blood cell counts. For this reason, a urine specimen needs to be obtained by either the clean-catch midstream technique or catheterization. A clean cotton ball tucked just inside the vaginal introitus will keep the lochia from contaminating the specimen. The diabetic woman or the woman with a prolonged labor and dehydration may have acetone in her urine from fat metabolism.

COMMON PROBLEMS AND CONCERNS OF POSTPARTUM WOMEN

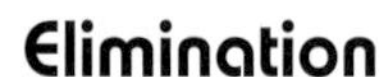

Elimination

Interventions to reestablish normal elimination are essential for most new mothers. The woman should void spontaneously within 4 to 8 hours after delivery. Encouraging voiding early and frequently helps prevent bladder distention. The bladder should be evaluated for distention frequently after birth to determine the need for intervention. The first two voids should be measured and recorded in the intake and output. Voiding

Table 29–5

NORMAL LABORATORY FINDINGS DURING THE POSTPARTUM PERIOD

Hematology	
Hemoglobin	Decreases immediately post partum (500 mL blood loss = 1 g hemoglobin). Average hemoglobin level post partum is 11.5 g/dL. Level stabilizes by 2 to 4 days; return to nonpregnant values by 4 to 6 weeks post partum.
Hematocrit	Rises immediately after birth because of dehydration and a decrease in plasma volume. Returns to nonpregnant values by 4 to 6 weeks post partum.
White blood cell count	Increases in intrapartum and immediate postpartum period, up to as much as 25,000 to 30,000/mm^3. Decreases to 6000–10,000/mm^3, then returns to normal values by 4 to 7 days post partum.
Platelets	Normal range: 150,000–400,000/mm^3 Marked increase 3–5 days after delivery, then gradual return to normal postpartum values.
Urinalysis	
Urine	Mild proteinuria (1+) in early postpartum period Acetone may be present during immediate postpartum period after a long labor; sugar may be present first week post partum

Data from Blackburn, S. T., and Loper, D. L. (1992). *Maternal, fetal, and neonatal physiology: A clinical perspective.* Philadelphia: W. B. Saunders; Cunningham, F. G., MacDonald, P. C., Gant, N. F., Leveno, K. J., Gilstrap. L. C. (1993). *Williams obstetrics* (19th ed.). Norwalk, CT: Appleton & Lange.

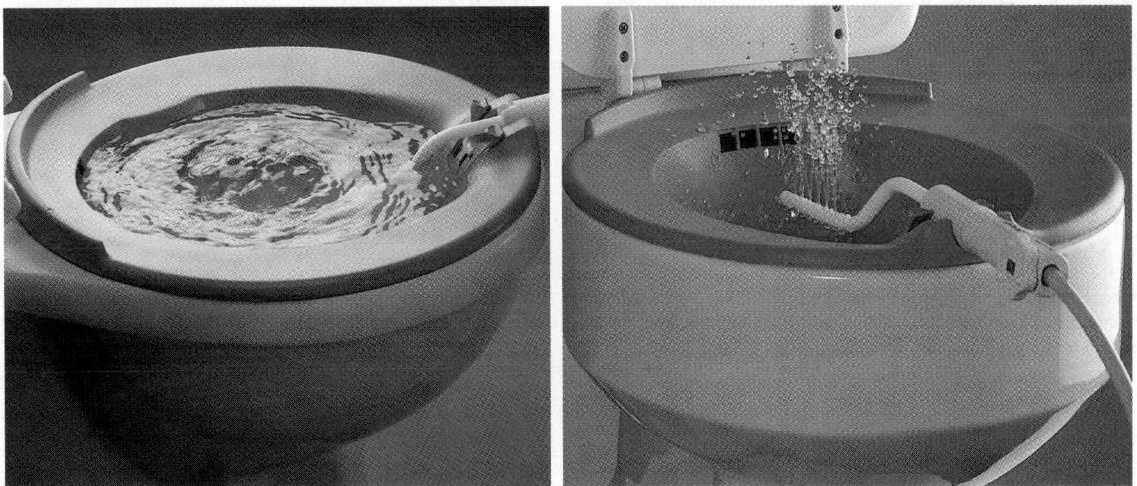

Figure 29–5

A personal whirlpool; sitz bath/bidet system prevents cross-contamination and allows for treatment of postepisiotomy edema, hemorrhoids, and pain in the perineum and anal areas both in the hospital and at home. The system easily connects to a water faucet. Used as a whirlpool sitz bath (*left*) the unit provides continuous waterflow heat therapy at a constant temperature and relief for tender tissues; with the flow-through door open the unit may be used as a bidet (*right*), for self-administered gentle cleansing. (Courtesy Hygenique Plus Whirlpool Sitz Bath/Bidet System, Andermac, Inc.)

less than 100 mL usually indicates incomplete emptying of the bladder. Urinary retention also results in the sensation of urgency soon after voiding. Catheterization may be necessary if this occurs. The dehydrating effects of labor can affect elimination. Ensure adequate intake by encouraging oral fluids after the birth. Regional anesthesia decreases the sensation of the need to void and increases difficulty in voiding (Enkin et al. 1995). Mothers who have had regional anesthesia should be assessed even more frequently for overdistention.

The woman should reestablish bowel elimination and have a soft, formed stool by the second or third postpartum day. Nursing care to facilitate the return of bowel function includes encouraging frequent ambulation, an adequate intake of fluids, and a diet high in fiber. It is not unusual for a woman to be fearful of her first bowel movement, particularly if she has had an episiotomy. Reassurance that this fear is common and that measures to assist her are available will help relieve her anxiety. Stool softeners are usually prescribed and are effective for most women.

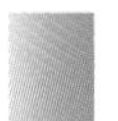

Episiotomy and Hemorrhoids

The assessment of pain from the episiotomy site or from hemorrhoids is an ongoing process. It begins immediately after birth and continues until discharge. The nurse can have the mother rate the amount of pain she has on a scale from 1 to 10, with 1 being "no pain" and 10 being "the greatest amount of pain that can be experienced," to assist the mother in providing a more reliable subjective assessment. With use of the same approach each time, the mother's subjective measurements can be compared across time.

EPISIOTOMY

Ice is applied to the perineum immediately after the birth to reduce swelling and relieve discomfort at the episiotomy site. A chemical ice pack that is activated by folding the ends into the middle can be used. A disposable glove filled with crushed ice and wrapped in a towel is also effective and provides an inexpensive alternative. The perineum needs to be protected from burns due to overexposure to cold. Inspect the perineum for redness or irritation each time the ice pack is replaced, about every 20 minutes. It may be necessary to leave the pack off for 10 minutes before reapplying.

Warm sitz baths and cleansing warm water sprays are also helpful for relieving pain and discomfort due to an episiotomy (Fig. 29–5). These are most helpful after the first few hours post partum. Moist heat increases circulation to the area, promotes healing, and decreases pain. Women who have extensive perineal repair may find sitz baths particularly soothing for a week or two post partum or longer. A sitz bath temperature of 105°F is comfortable for most women, although the mother's personal preference should be followed. Sitting in the bath for about 20 minutes is usually adequate for most women. If the woman uses a sitz bath tub rather than a personal sitz bath system, use caution when assisting her out of the tub; the warmth of the bath may cause sufficient vasodilatation, which increases the risk for dizziness or fainting.

The woman should be taught self-care measures to reduce the risk for infection. This includes teaching her to wipe the perineum from front to back after voiding and defecation. This decreases the risk for contamination with microorganisms from the anus to the vagina. Warm water using a bidet or other irrigator devices should be used to rinse the perineum after elimination. The perineal pad should be changed after each elimination and may be changed in between.

Pain medication may be used for women with deep or extensive episiotomies. Anesthetic ointment or foam is available in a topical form that may be sprayed on a clean pad. Oral pain medication may also be used (Wilson et al. 1993). It is also helpful to teach the mother to tighten her buttocks before sitting and to avoid sitting for prolonged periods.

HEMORRHOIDS

Some women, especially those who had hemorrhoids during pregnancy, may have them after childbirth. Sitz baths two or three times daily, following the same procedure as for episiotomy pain, help in providing relief from discomfort. Avoiding prolonged sitting and altering the sitting position are helpful. Stool softeners or laxatives may be prescribed for women with numerous or large hemorrhoids. Hemorrhoids often disappear within a few weeks after birth. Hemorrhoids are a common concern to many women. Good health habits help the woman to avoid flare-ups. Adequate fluid intake, inclusion of fiber in the diet, and adequate rest and exercise help to establish regular bowel habits and avoid unnecessary soreness. Applying ice packs for 30 to 60 minutes can be used for painful hemorrhoids. Discontinue the ice pack for 1 hour, then reapply if needed. Warm sitz baths are also helpful in providing pain relief. Local anesthetic sprays and ointments, such as Americaine or Epifoam, are often successfully used in treating hemorrhoid pain. Other hemorrhoidal creams may be used, especially those containing hydrocortisone, which decrease swelling. Self-care teaching for the woman with hemorrhoids includes reminding her of daily Kegel exercises.

These promote oxygenation of the area through increased blood flow, which speeds healing. Stool softeners will probably be ordered to prevent further irritation from straining. Encourage the mother to sit with her hips elevated at times and to try to avoid sitting for prolonged periods. This helps prevent further irritation.

Afterpains

Afterpains are a normal occurrence and result from contractions of the uterus as it reduces in size during involution. Afterpains may be especially noticeable during breastfeeding as oxytocin is released in response to the infant's suckling. Multigravida women experience stronger afterpains because of the relaxed structural changes of the uterus from previous births. Women who have had a cesarean birth may feel significant discomfort from afterpains because of the disrupted tissue integrity of the abdominal wall. Afterpains diminish in intensity after a few days.

Women, especially first-time mothers, are often surprised by the painful cramplike contractions they feel after birth. The woman needs information about what is happening and approaches that can be used to diminish the discomfort of afterpains. The mother can be encouraged to empty her bladder just before nursing her baby. This allows the uterus to contract more efficiently and decreases the discomfort of the contraction against a full bladder. Gentle massage against the uterus and lying in a prone position with a small pillow under the abdomen help to decrease the discomfort. Encourage the mother to consult with her physician or nurse-midwife if she experiences severe, unrelieved cramping or unusual uterine tenderness.

Sore Nipples

Breastfeeding mothers may experience nipple soreness in the first few days of nursing, and breasts may become engorged (Gulick 1982). This soreness usually subsides after a few days. The nipples should be observed for redness, cracks, fisures, or bleeding. If a woman experiences extreme soreness, this must be further investigated.

Sore nipples are frequently a result of malpositioning of the infant at the breast. Observe as the mother positions her infant for a feeding. The newborn's head should be in straight alignment with the body, with abdomen flat against the mother. The mouth should be opened wide enough that all of the areola is taken into the mouth. Lips should be flanged outward, and the tongue should be visible just behind the lower lip. Review the proper holding and latch-on techniques with the mother. Review the proper technique to break suction after a feeding (See Chapter 33).

Reassure the mother that this condition is short-lived and correctable. Show her how to stimulate the letdown reflex before her baby latches on. This allows the baby not to have to work so hard to get milk. She should start a feeding session on the least sore side first. Feeding more frequently, about every 2 hours, will actually help her nipple soreness. Her baby will be less frantic to start feeding and will not suck as vigorously. Varying the infant's position during feedings helps distribute the pressure more evenly around the nipple. Demonstrate a variety of positions in which to hold the baby during a feeding.

Self-care teaching includes nipple care and hygiene. Soaps are drying to the skin and should not be used by breastfeeding mothers. The nipple manufactures its own lubrication through the Montgomery glands. Colostrum and breast milk can be expressed and rubbed into the nipple after feedings to heal sore nipples and prevent drying. Anhydrous lanolin may also be lightly rubbed into the nipple.

Many institutions have lactation specialists who visit new mothers before dismissal. They are excellent resources for nursing personnel in troubleshooting problems with breastfeeding. New mothers should always be supplied with phone numbers of the lactation specialist, nursing mothers' support groups, and their health care provider's office for follow-up for breastfeeding problems (see Chapter 33).

Breast Engorgement

Breasts that are enlarged, taut, shiny, and red are said to be engorged. This condition is painful and can be detrimental to breastfeeding. Blood and lymph have backed up behind the milk ducts and prevent the flow of new milk from the alveoli. This condition results from infrequent and delayed breastfeeding. The breasts may be lumpy, firm, and hard to the touch. The nipple is flattened because of pressure behind the areola. Although the duration may be short (24 to 48 hours), it is extremely painful for the mother and difficult for the infant to latch on to the breast.

Observe the mother to ensure that she is using proper breastfeeding technique. Advise her to feed frequently, at least every 2½ hours for 15 to 20 minutes per side. The infant will have an easier time latching on if the mother softens her breasts and expresses some milk before a feeding. Advise her to apply moist heat to both breasts for about 20 minutes before a feeding. This may be in the shower or with warm wet towels. During a feeding, it is helpful to gently massage the breast from

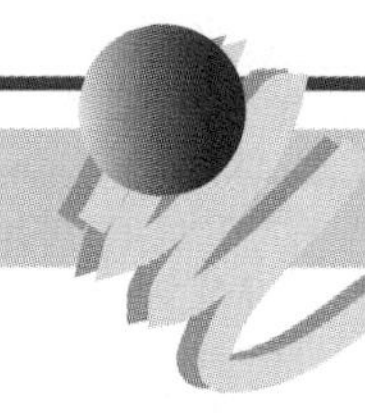

TEACHING GUIDE

STRATEGIES FOR EASING POSTPARTUM ADJUSTMENT

TOPIC	*MAJOR CONCEPTS*
Preparing in advance	Suggest that your client discuss strategies with her partner and develop a plan before the birth of their baby for help and support after childbirth. It is a good idea to prepare and freeze meals in advance. Family members and friends should be advised how they can help after the baby comes. Home projects should be finished before the baby arrives. Suggest that the woman's partner take time off and work shorter days for several weeks after she and the baby come home.
Coping with lack of sleep	Suggest that your client plan to lower housework standards and sleep instead of cleaning. She should rely on her partner to help with household chores while she concentrates on caring for the baby and sleeping. She should nap when the baby sleeps. Partners should take turns being "on call" for the baby. It also helps to post a note on the front door and turn off the bell on the phone when napping. Keeping the baby's bassinet close to the bed facilitates easier breastfeeding at night.
Reducing family workload	Housecleaning and diaper services make great shower gifts and should be suggested. The new mother needs to learn to say yes to offers of help. Making a list of specific chores that others can do helps focus on areas in which friends and relatives may help. Chores should be prioritized and divided among family members. Have groceries delivered. Plan to eat out and order in. Expectations of what should be done and what can be done in a day need to be lowered.

Continued on facing page

the outer areas to the nipple. This helps stimulate the letdown and flow of milk. Between feedings, the mother should wear a supportive bra. She may apply ice in between feedings to decrease the discomfort. Reassurance and support are necessary during this time. It is short-lived but can be very trying for the mother.

If the mother is not breastfeeding, a tight bra or breast binder and minimal breast stimulation will reduce the engorgement that will occur. Lactation-suppressant medications are no longer prescribed on a routine basis because of the risk of cerebrovascular accident and myocardial infarction (Iffy et al. 1986).

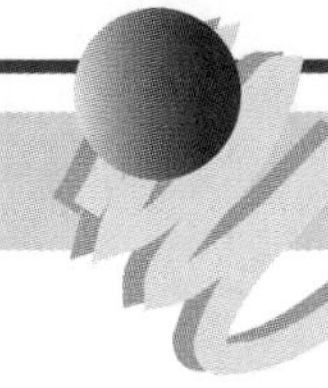

TEACHING GUIDE Continued

Adopting a healthy lifestyle	Advise your client to stay positive, keep a sense of humor, exercise to reenergize, and practice meditation and other relaxation techniques. Eating a nutritious diet is also important. She should be ready to go to bed before the last feeding and rest or sleep whenever she can.
Nurturing relationships	Remind both partners to be extra tolerant and sensitive with one another and take care of each other (with massages and warm baths, for example). They should give each other verbal and practical support. Praise for little things is helpful. Time together to talk about things other than the baby should be planned every day, even if it is only for a brief period. Tickets to events should be purchased ahead of time to ensure that they are taken advantage of.
Finding assistance and support	Support and help with newborns are available from many sources: family, friends, church, professional associates, community health nurses, new parent classes, library books and parenting magazines, and health care providers.

Teaching Aids	**Increasing Your Teaching Effectiveness**
1. Self-assessment checklists	1. Ask the new mother to identify areas where she needs help in the areas of self-care and infant care.
2. Self-care booklets	2. Use every interaction with the mother to talk about self-care, infant care, and family adjustment.
3. Infant care booklets	3. Encourage the parents to identify their resources and strengths.
4. List of community resources	4. Integrate teaching into all aspects of care for the new mother and infant care.

Regaining Physical Strength

Regaining physical strength is a key concern of mothers and an important goal of nursing care. All healthy postpartum women need to learn exercises that promote the resumption of muscle tone and physical strength, contribute to weight loss, and aid in the prevention of constipation.

Before starting an exercise program, the new mother should be taught how to assess for diastasis recti and the exercises for diastasis recti, if needed (Fig. 29–6). This is essential before proceeding to a structured exercise program. There are some simple exercises, such as abdominal breathing and combined abdominal breathing and pelvic rock, that the mother can do in bed starting in the early postpartum period. Other exercises can be added as the woman regains her strength (Fig. 29–7). New mothers will benefit from a postpartum exercise routine both physically and emotionally. The woman should check with her physician or nurse-midwife before starting any strenuous activity or exercise program.

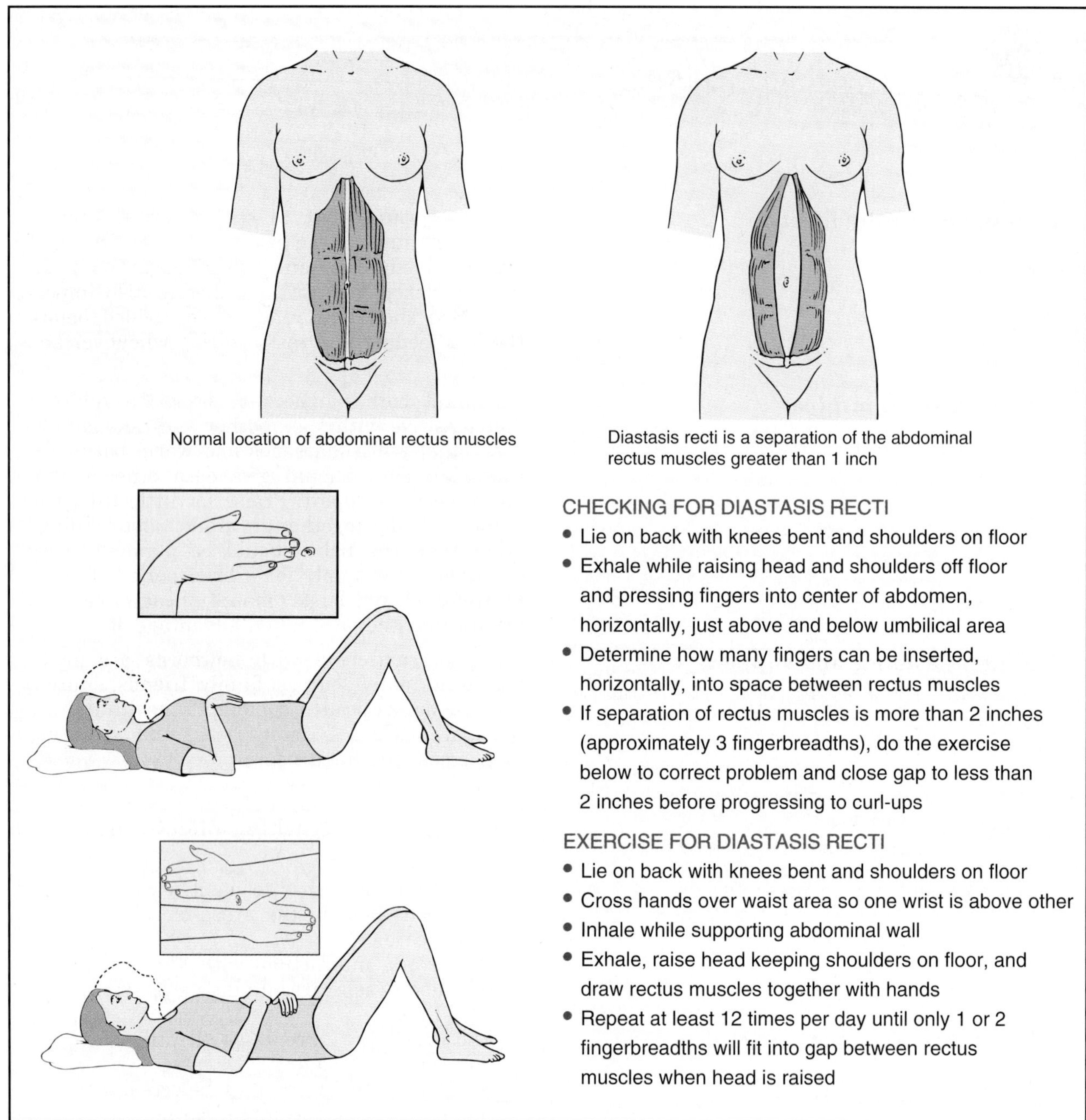

Figure 29–6

The postpartum woman needs to check for diastasis recti before beginning an exercise program • If the rectus muscles are separated by more than 2 inches, she will need to do exercises to correct the problem so that the separation does not increase.

Resumption of Sexual Activity

It is recommended that the woman refrain from sexual intercourse until the episiotomy has healed and lochia has stopped. This usually takes about 3 weeks. The postpartum woman may have a decrease in sexual desire in response to the many physical and emotional changes experienced in the first few weeks after childbirth. This is normal. She may be fatigued from lack of a full night's sleep and be overwhelmed by the newness of caring for an infant. She may be teary and experiencing mood swings. She is also recovering from the significant changes her body experienced during pregnancy. Hormonal changes result in a drying of vaginal wall tissues, which may make intercourse uncomfortable. The breastfeeding woman may experience leaking of milk during sexual stimulation, in response to oxytocin release, that is disconcerting to both her and her partner.

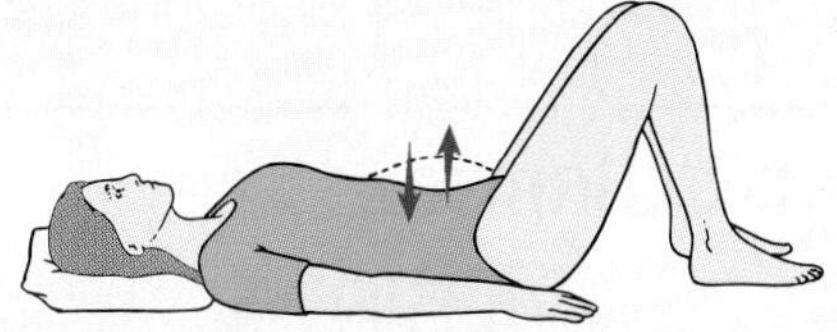

ABDOMINAL BREATHING
- Lie on back with knees bent
- Inhale deeply through nose, keeping rib cage as stationary as possible while allowing abdominal muscles to expand
- Exhale slowly through mouth and tighten abdominal muscles

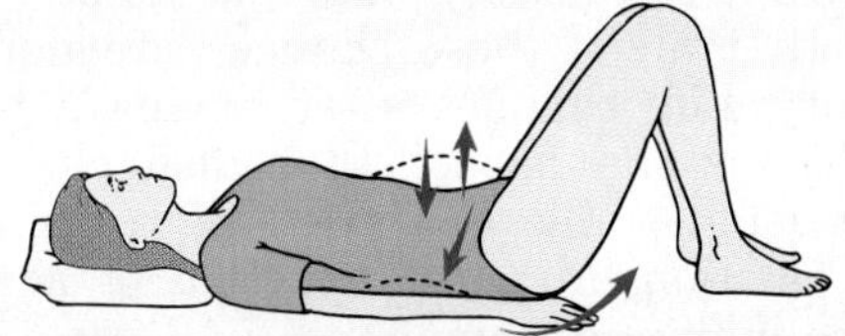

COMBINED ABDOMINAL BREATHING AND PELVIC ROCK
- Lie on back with knees bent
- Inhale deeply, tighten abdomen and buttocks and press lower back flat against the floor
- Hold position for 3 to 5 seconds while exhaling

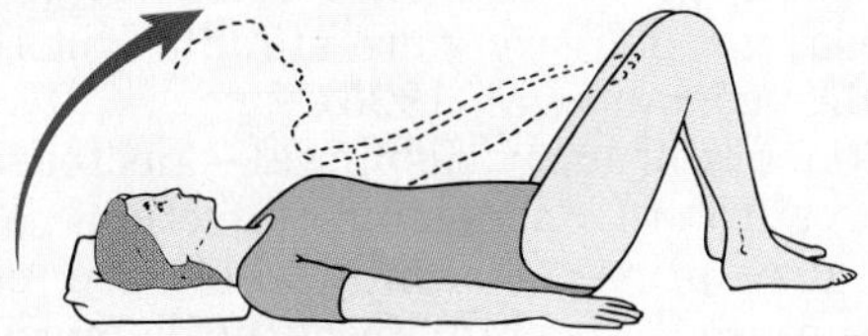

STRAIGHT CURL-UPS
- Lie on back with knees bent
- Inhale, then exhale while bringing head and shoulder forward off the floor and reaching toward knees
- Curl-up only as far as possible while keeping waist on floor
- Inhale and slowly uncurl

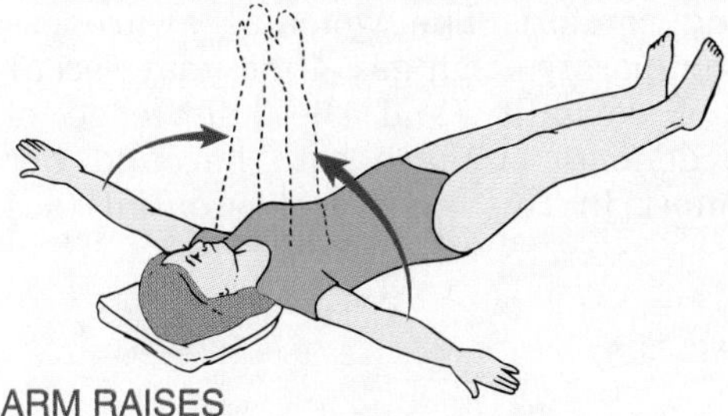

ARM RAISES
- Lie on back with legs extended and arms extended at a 90° angle from body
- Inhale, then exhale and raise arms inward, keeping arms straight, until palms of hands touch
- Inhale and lower arms slowly

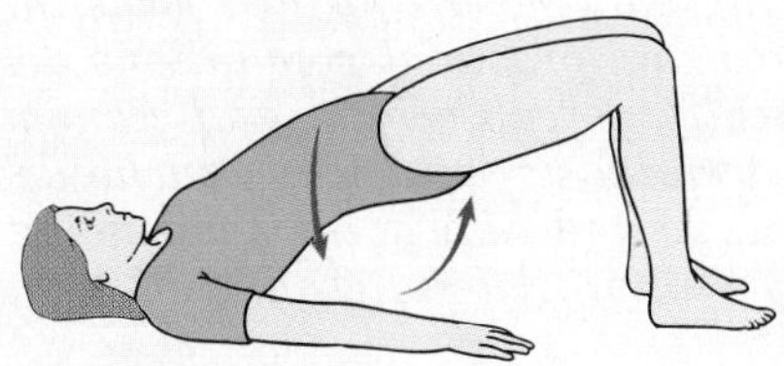

BUTTOCKS LIFT
- Lie on back with knees bent, feet flat on floor, and arms extended along side of body
- Inhale, then exhale and slowly lift buttocks and arch back
- Inhale and slowly return to starting position

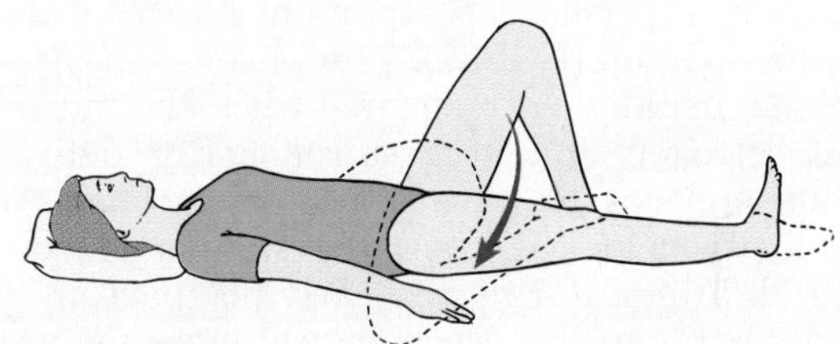

SINGLE KNEE ROLL
- Lie on back with one leg straight and other leg bent at knee
- Inhale, then exhale and slowly swing leg with knee bent over other leg until knee touches floor
- Keep head and shoulders on floor at all times
- Inhale and return to starting position

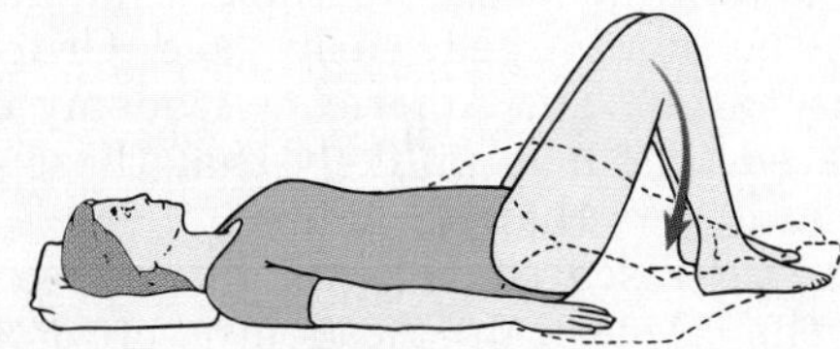

DOUBLE KNEE ROLL
- Lie on back with both knees bent
- Inhale, then exhale and slowly swing both knees over to one side until lower knee touches floor
- Keep head and shoulders on floor at all times
- Inhale and return to starting position

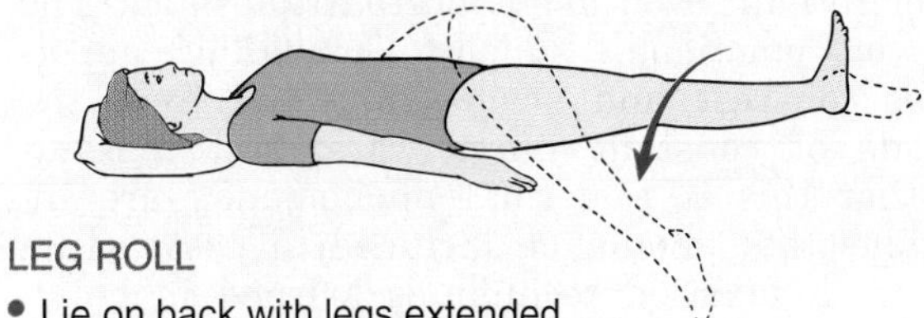

LEG ROLL
- Lie on back with legs extended
- Inhale, then exhale and lift one leg and roll it over other leg to touch floor
- Keep shoulders on floor and leg extended
- Repeat exercise with other leg

Figure 29–7

A postpartum exercise program is important to both the physical and emotional well-being of the new mother.

It is important to reassure both the woman and her partner that all of these changes are normal and temporary. Life changes after having a baby, and sexuality is one aspect that also changes. Couples are usually able to settle into a comfortable sexual relationship after a period of adjustment for both man and woman.

Counsel the woman that pregnancy can occur before the return of menses. Family planning options should be explained thoroughly. Breastfeeding her baby before having sexual intercourse will decrease the occurrence of milk ejection during sexual activity. A vaginal lubricant is often needed and is helpful in decreasing dryness and increasing comfort. The woman's awareness of possible temporary changes that may occur in the area of sexuality and the knowledge of what can be done to enhance both her and her partner's comfort in this area are essential (see Chapter 10).

Postpartum Blues

Postpartum blues are usually described as transient and mild mood disturbances that start on approximately the third postpartum day and usually last 2 or 3 days (Selby 1980). However, some women may experience postpartum blues for several weeks (Gennaro 1988). The onset of postpartum blues usually corresponds with the normal drop in estrogen and progesterone after delivery and thus appears to have a physiologic basis as well as a psychological basis. The woman's level of stress and fatigue during the early postpartum period contributes to the psychological basis for postpartum blues.

Most women, especially first-time mothers, are surprised by the demands a new baby makes on their time and energy. They may be tearful, irritable, anxious, and moody. These mood changes are often surprising and confusing to new mothers. Reassurance that it is not unusual to experience some of these symptoms is helpful for many women. It is important to include the woman's partner in education about postpartum blues. The need for emotional support, providing opportunities for rest and sleep and relief from the demands of constant infant care, and reassurance that this is a normal phenomenon are instructions that should be included in postpartum teaching. Relaxation techniques learned in childbirth preparation classes are helpful coping measures for women overwhelmed by new motherhood. Provide the mother with hot line telephone numbers available in the community. Provide her with strategies that help decrease postpartum blues. Encourage her to contact her health care provider if postpartum blues continue or increase in intensity.

EARLY DISCHARGE

In the early 1800s, women were confined to bed after childbirth for 28 days. In the early 1900s, the usual period of confinement after childbirth was 12 to 14 days (Enkin et al. 1995). The trend toward early discharge that began in the 1980s is now an established occurrence. Stays of 12 to 24 hours or less after an uncomplicated vaginal delivery and 48 to 72 hours after an uncomplicated cesarean delivery were standard in the mid-1990s (Braverman et al. 1995).

The benefits of early dismissal—decreased cost, less exposure to iatrogenic infection, and decreased disruption of family life—are cited by many as reasons to promote early dismissal (Harrison 1990). However, adverse effects of early discharge, such as significantly higher infant readmission rates, have also been cited (Braverman et al. 1995). Braverman and colleagues (1995, p. 724) reached the following conclusion on the basis of a critical review of the literature:

Early discharge with repeated postpartum nurse home visiting may be safe for newborns in carefully selected and prepared populations determined to be medically, psychosocially, and economically at low risk; carefully screened women who desire early discharge and receive intensive home follow-up may have improved maternal well-being and adjustment.

At this time, however, there are a limited number of home visiting postpartum programs, and those that exist are primarily for high-risk mothers and newborns. Criteria for early discharge have been established by the American Academy of Pediatrics (1995) and should be used as guidelines to determine those mothers and newborns who can be discharged early (see Criteria for Early Discharge). The American Academy of Pediatrics stated that it is unlikely that these criteria can be met in less than 48 hours.

Until more research is available on early discharge, the American Academy of Pediatrics and the American College of Obstetricians and Gynecologists (1992) recommend following strict guidelines for early discharge and providing essential postdischarge follow-up (Braverman et al. 1995).

The length of hospital stays for mothers and infants is expected to increase as more mothers elect to stay longer after childbirth with the passage of the Newborns' and Mothers' Health Protection Act of 1996.

Criteria for Early Discharge

GENERAL

- Uncomplicated antepartum, intrapartum, and postpartum courses for both mother and baby
- Knowledgeable family member or other support person is available to assist mother at home
- No unresolved family, environmental, or social risk factors
- Designated source of continuing medical care is identified
- Definitive plan is established for follow-up within 48 hours after discharge

INFANT

- Term infant (38–42 weeks' gestation), single birth, with birth weight appropriate for gestational age
- Vital signs are documented as normal and stable for 12 hours preceding discharge; respiratory rate is below 60 per minute, heart rate of 100 to 160 beats per minute, and axillary temperature of 36.1 to 37°C in open crib with appropriate clothing
- Has urinated and passed at least one stool
- Has completed at least two successful feedings and demonstrates the ability to coordinate sucking, swallowing, and breathing while feeding
- Physical examination reveals no abnormalities that require continued hospitalization
- No evidence of excessive bleeding at circumcision site for at least 2 hours after circumcision
- No evidence of significant jaundice in first 24 hours after birth
- The following laboratory data are available and reviewed as clinically indicated: maternal syphilis, hepatitis B surface antigen, cord or infant blood type, and direct Coombs test
- Plan for performing screening tests in accordance with state regulations is identified

MOTHER

- Vital signs are stable and within normal limits; hemoglobin > 10 g
- Intact perineum without third- or fourth-degree perineal laceration
- Vaginal bleeding is within normal limits
- Has ability to ambulate and void without difficulty
- Has the knowledge, ability, and confidence to provide adequate care for her baby and has received education regarding breastfeeding or bottle feeding; cord, skin, and infant genital care; signs of illness and common infant problems, particularly jaundice; and infant safety

Data from the American Academy of Pediatrics. (1995). Hospital stay for healthy term newborns. *Pediatrics,* 96 (4), 788–790; American Academy of Pediatrics and American College of Obstetricians and Gynecologists. (1992). *Guidelines for perinatal care.* Elk Grove Village, IL: Authors.

Postpartum Home Care

Both the American Academy of Pediatrics (1995) and the American Nurses Association (1996) support the premise that postpartum follow-up care is essential. The American Nurses Association (1996) developed a position paper calling for postpartum home visits by registered nurses for all mothers and newborns who are discharged and the integration of postpartum home nursing care into usual postpartum care after birth.

The purpose of follow-up home care for the newborn infant (American Academy of Pediatrics 1995) is to

- Assess the infant's general health, hydration, and degree of jaundice; identify any new problems; review feeding pattern and technique, including observation of breastfeeding for adequacy of position, latch-on, and swallowing; and obtain information about stool and urine patterns
- Assess quality of maternal-infant interaction and details of infant behavior
- Reinforce maternal and family education in infant care, particularly regarding infant feeding
- Review the outstanding results of laboratory tests performed before discharge

- Perform screening tests in accordance with state regulations and other tests that are clinically indicated
- Identify a plan for health care maintenance, including a method for obtaining emergency services, preventive care and immunizations, periodic evaluations and physical examinations, and necessary screening

The purpose of home care follow-up for the mother is to

- Determine her physical and emotional health status and degree of adjustment in the home environment
- Assess problem areas and reinforce teaching on postpartum care and infant care
- Evaluate the woman's adjustment to her role as mother and the integration of these responsibilities with previous roles
- Determine the need for additional resources and linking mother and baby with needed resources

Appropriate follow-up and referral systems are necessary to ensure a smooth transition from hospital to home. The woman's early and continued contact with her health care provider and her baby's health care provider is critical. Follow-up care can be conducted by phone calls, home visits, and postpartum classes. These may originate from the institution, private home health care agency, physician, or local health department. Self-help and community-based support groups are also available in most cities. A list of health care and community resources should be given to all new parents.

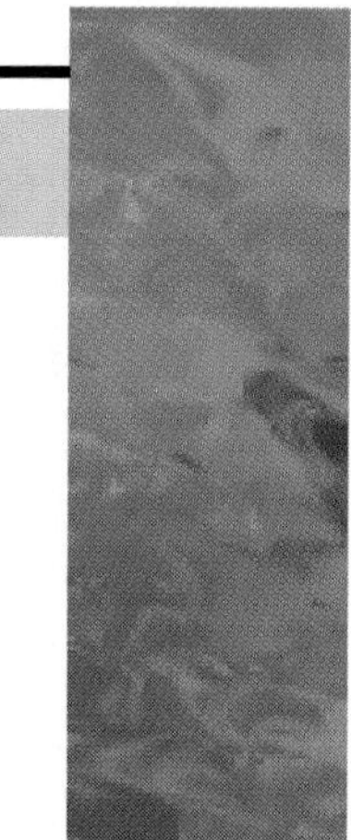

Nursing Practice

Nursing Process

▼ Assessment

The assessment of the mother's physiologic and psychological health status, her ability to care for her infant, and the quality of the mother-infant interaction forms a basis for nursing care. While new mothers have common needs, each new mother has specific individual needs that require identification so that teaching needs can be determined. Beginning on page 1020, the Nursing Care Planning Guide: Healthy Postpartum Woman applies the nursing process to create a plan of care that can be individualized for specific patients. A comprehensive assessment tool, Postpartum Flowsheet, is included within the guide.

Other areas of assessment include support systems that are available to the mother (see Psychosocial Assessment), the number of other children and their ages, adequacy of housing, and community setting. Determining the environment to which the infant will be brought home will assist the nurse in identifying risk factors that may interfere with parenting and infant care. Asking the mother to identify specific concerns that she may have, such as returning to work, will enable the nurse to prioritize specific areas of care and teaching that are needed.

▼ Diagnosis

Major nursing diagnoses to promote health in the postpartum period include

HOLLISTER maternal/newborn RECORD SYSTEM

Education/Discharge Planning

Page 1 of 2

Mother Instruction Given	Care Giver's Initials	Demonstrates Understanding: Date	Demonstrates Understanding: Mother's Initials
Reproductive			
1. Uterine Involution/Cramping			
2. Lochia Progression			
3. Episiotomy Care			
4. Abdominal Incision Care			
5. Return of Menses			
6.			
Breasts			
7. Engorgement			
8. Comfort Measures			
9. Nipple Care			
10. Breast Self-Exam			
11.			
Elimination			
12. Urine Pattern/Signs of UTI			
13. Bowel Pattern			
14. Hemorrhoid Care			
15.			
Daily Living			
16. Hygiene			
17. Nutrition/Fluids			
18. Rest/Sleep			
19. Activity/Exercise			
20.			
Emotions			
21. Mood Changes—Blues			
22. Support			
23. Family Adjustment			
24.			
Sexuality			
25. Physical Changes			
26. Psychological Changes			
27. Resuming Intercourse			
28. Family Planning			
29.			
Follow-Up			
30. When to Call the MD			
31. Medication Instructions ____ ____ ____			
32. Referrals ☐ None ☐ WIC ☐ Social Service ☐ Home Nursing Care ☐ ____			
33. Appointments ☐ OB Date __/__/__ ☐ ____			

Patient Needs/Comments

Initials	Signature (Mother)	Initials	Signature (Care Giver)
Initials	Signature (Care Giver)	Initials	Signature (Care Giver)

Hollister. HOLLISTER INCORPORATED, 2000 HOLLISTER DR, LIBERTYVILLE, IL 60048

EDUCATION/DISCHARGE PLANNING FORM #5716 (Page 1 of 2) 691

MATERNAL RECORD COPY

- Fluid volume deficit related to postpartum hemorrhage
- Altered comfort* related to episiotomy/perineal discomfort, hematoma, bladder distention, hemorrhoids, breast engorgement, nipple soreness, afterpains, headache after regional anesthesia, mastitis
- Risk for infection related to endometritis
- Risk for infection related to urinary tract disturbances
- Altered nutrition: less than or more than body requirements related to intake of nutrients insufficient or exceeding metabolic needs
- Risk for constipation related to pain in the perineum
- Sleep pattern disturbance related to care of infant and rapid physiologic and psychosocial changes

*Although altered comfort is not a current NANDA-approved nursing diagnosis, it is used advisedly here to describe conditions that create discomfort rather than pain.

- Risk for altered tissue perfusion related to thrombophlebitis
- Risk for injury related to exercise
- Altered sexuality patterns related to the birth process and care of the newborn
- Altered family processes related to maternal-infant attachment
- Altered role performance related to the transition to the maternal role
- Risk for altered growth and development related to parenting
- Risk for anxiety related to new roles and health of self and newborn
- Risk for ineffective coping related to postpartum blues or postpartum depression
- Risk for disturbance in self-esteem related to body image

HOLLISTER maternal/newborn RECORD SYSTEM

Education/Discharge Planning

Page 2 of 2

Newborn Instruction Given	Care Giver's Initials	Demonstrates Understanding: Date	Demonstrates Understanding: Mother's Initials	Patient Needs/Comments
Normal Characteristics 34. Appearance				
35. Breathing				
36. Color				
37. Reflexes				
38. Senses				
39.				
Physical Care 40. Bathing				
41. Clothing				
42. Cord				
43. Diapering				
44. Penis (Intact/Circumcised)				
45. Skin/Fingernails				
46.				
Feeding 47. Positioning/Burping				
48. Frequency/Amount				
49. Breast Milk Supply & Demand				
50. Formula Preparation				
51.				
Elimination 52. Urine Pattern				
53. Stool Pattern				
54.				
Behavior/Response 55. Sleep				
56. Awake–Stimulation				
57. Crying–Soothing				
58.				
Safety 59. When to Call the MD				
60. Temperature Taking				
61. Car Seat				
62. Injury Prevention				
63. Immunizations				
64.				
Follow-Up 65. Medication Instructions ______ ______ ______				
66. Referrals ☐ None ☐ ______ ☐ ______				Initials / Signature (Mother) / Initials / Signature (Care Giver)
67. Appointments ☐ Ped Date ___/___/___ ☐ ______				Initials / Signature (Care Giver) / Initials / Signature (Care Giver)

Hollister. HOLLISTER INCORPORATED, 2000 HOLLISTER DR, LIBERTYVILLE, IL 60048

EDUCATION/DISCHARGE PLANNING FORM #5716 (Page 2 of 2) 691

MATERNAL RECORD COPY

▼ Planning

The next step of the nursing process involves setting measurable goals for each nursing diagnosis. These goals serve as the basis for evaluating outcomes of nursing care (see Education/Discharge Planning form).

▼ Intervention

Interventions are based on the nursing diagnosis and are specific to the situation (see Common Problems and Concerns of Postpartum Women). A major intervention for all new mothers is teaching related to expected changes, self-care activities, and infant care. The amount of essential education and discharge planning is significant, and the shortened postpartum stay has decreased the amount of time available for education. Also, the new mother's retention of information can be questioned because it is given at a time when she is usually tired and exhausted after the birth. Use of an education/discharge planning form to document teaching increases the continuity and consistency of care and provides a written document that can be used by other health professionals in providing care. Providing each new mother with clear, easily read, written guidelines that she can refer to at home is also critical in increasing the effectiveness of teaching.

▼ Evaluation

Evaluation is specific to each nursing diagnosis and reflects the degree to which the stated nursing care goal for the mother was achieved. Evaluation is essential in monitoring the effectiveness of nursing care and indicating changes that are needed.

Risk Management

During the postpartum period, the use of three important risk management strategies will decrease injury and problems and improve outcomes for mothers and babies. These strategies are

- Knowledge of risks and possible problems
- Risk assessment
- Complete, accurate, and specific charting

As early discharge of mothers and babies has become the standard, risk management has become even more important. The nurse must be knowledgeable about potential problems, make expert clinical judgments related to safety of discharge and inform the physician or nurse-midwife of any problems, and make certain that the new mother has the information she needs to provide adequate care for the infant at home.

Another area of critical concern in risk management is astute continued observation for signs of excessive postpartum bleeding. Detailed, descriptive charting of the amount of vaginal bleeding and, if needed, notification of the woman's health care provider are critical. If there is any concern about the amount of blood loss, the vaginal pads should be weighed on a gram scale (see Chapter 35) and the results charted each time the pad is changed. Managing risk is an important role of the nurse during the postpartum period.

Implications for Research

Research in the postpartum period is primarily descriptive and has centered on the mother's needs and concerns, the woman's psychological adjustment after childbirth, the mother-infant interaction, and the early parenting experience (Walker 1992). There is limited research that examines the effectiveness of many routine postpartum care strategies currently used. Some of these strategies are clearly effective from a clinical perspective; however, other strategies are used primarily because of tradition. There is a need for research that documents the efficacy of postpartum care practices and that identifies which interventions are the most effective for a specific problem. Research questions that need to be examined are

- How long do healthy mothers and babies need to remain in the hospital?
- Is early discharge with postpartum home care follow-up for healthy mothers and babies as safe as discharging them at the routine time from the hospital?
- What is the most effective intervention for relieving postpartum episiotomy pain?
- How often should routine vital signs and fundal checks be done for healthy mothers? for mothers with complications?
- What are the effects of a self-administered program for routine postpartum medication com-

pared with administration of routine medication under the direct control and supervision of the nurse?

- What is the most effective approach for lactation suppression in the woman who chooses not to breastfeed?

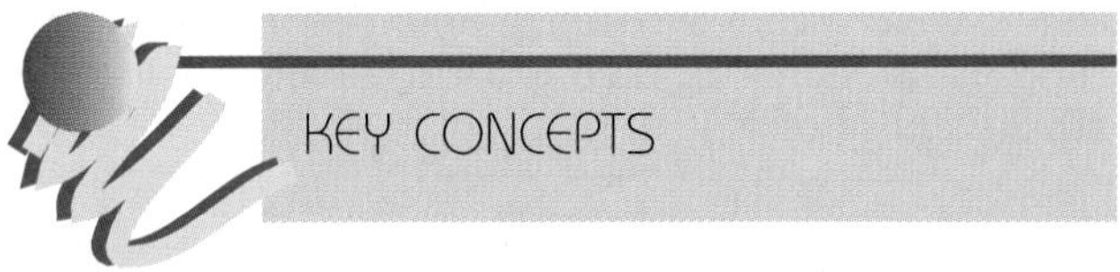

KEY CONCEPTS

▼ The postpartum period is a time of physical restoration and healing, emotional mood swings, and role adjustments as the woman assumes the role of mothering the new infant and redefines her relationships with her family members.

▼ The woman's general health status and any preexisting illnesses also affect perinatal outcomes and postpartum recovery.

▼ Cultural background can greatly influence how the mother perceives her health status, the postpartum period, and self-care activities.

▼ The basis for a comprehensive assessment is historical information about the postpartum woman related to pregnancy history, labor and delivery history, laboratory data, infant history, postpartum history, and family history.

▼ The postpartum assessment is done to detect deviations from normal and to provide a record that accurately depicts the mother's postpartum recovery status.

▼ At 1 hour post partum, the fundus is firm and contracted at the level of the umbilicus in the midline. Fundal height decreases by 1 cm each day, and the fundus should no longer be palpable by the tenth postpartum day.

▼ A specified system of measuring lochia should be consistently used on the postpartum unit by all health care personnel.

▼ All women, regardless of whether they plan to breastfeed or formula feed, should have their breasts examined every 8 hours for nipple soreness, breast tenderness, lumps, engorgement, mastitis, presence of colostrum, and presence of leaking milk.

▼ Normal bowel elimination usually returns 2 to 3 days post partum. Surgery, anesthesia, and the use of narcotics for postoperative pain control contribute to a longer period of altered bowel function.

▼ As diuresis begins after delivery, approximately 3 liters of accumulated fluids and volume is lost. Therefore, it is important to assess the mother's ability to urinate after delivery.

▼ Reva Rubin identified two phases of regeneration during the postpartum period. Research generally supports Rubin's theory but suggests that the length of time of each phase is shorter than what Rubin reported more than 30 years ago.

▼ Policies of maternal and newborn health care agencies should be flexible enough to allow adaptation to individual needs and to support the ongoing process of mother-infant interaction. A thorough assessment of mother-infant interaction is critical as a foundation for planning nursing care that promotes the growth and development of the infant.

▼ The degree of blood loss during birth is reflected in the hematocrit concentration. The hematocrit immediately rises after delivery in response to hemoconcentration.

▼ The white blood cell count, usually an indicator of infection, increases during labor and may stay elevated during the first few days post partum without presence of an infection.

▼ Common problems and concerns of new mothers are related to elimination, episiotomy, hemorrhoids, afterpains, breast engorgement, regaining physical strength, resumption of sexual activity, and postpartum blues.

▼ Until more research is available on early discharge, the American Academy of Pediatrics and the American College of Obstetricians and Gynecologists recommend following strict guidelines for early discharge and providing essential postdischarge follow-up.

▼ A major intervention for all new mothers is teaching related to expected changes, self-care activities, and infant care.

▼ Research in the postpartum period is primarily descriptive and centers on the mother's needs and concerns, the woman's psychological adjustment after childbirth, the mother-infant interaction, and the early parenting experience. There is limited research that examines the effectiveness of many routine postpartum care strategies currently used.

References

Ament, L. A. (1990). Maternal tasks of the puerperium reidentified. *Journal of Obstetric, Gynecologic, and Neonatal Nursing,* 19 (4), 330–335.

American Academy of Pediatrics and American College of Obstetricians and Gynecologists. (1992). *Guidelines for perinatal care.* Elk Grove Village, IL: Authors.

American Academy of Pediatrics. (1995). Hospital stay for healthy term newborns. *Pediatrics,* 96 (4), 788–790.

American Nurses Association. (1996). Home care for mother, infant and family following birth (Position Statement). Washington, DC: Author.

Braverman, P., Egerter, S., Pearl, M., Marchi, K., Miller, C. (1995). Problems associated with early discharge of newborn infants. *Pediatrics,* 96 (4), 716–726.

Brazelton, T. B. (1978). The remarkable talents of the newborn. *Birth and Family Journal,* 5, 187.

Enkin, M., Keirse, M. J. N. C., Renfrew, M., Neilson, J. (1995). *A guide to effective care in pregnancy and childbirth.* Oxford: Oxford University Press.

Gennaro, S. (1988). Postpartal anxiety and depression in mothers of term and preterm infants. *Nursing Research,* 37 (2), 82–84.

Gulick, E. E. (1982). Informational correlates of successful breastfeeding. *MCN: American Journal of Maternal-Child Nursing,* 7, 370–375.

Haller, K. B. (1996). Drive-through deliveries. *Journal of Obstetric, Gynecologic, and Neonatal Nursing,* 25 (1), 9.

Harrison, L. L. (1990). Patient teaching in early postpartum discharge programs. *MCN: American Journal of Maternal-Child Nursing,* 15 (1), 39.

Iffy, L., TenHove, W., Frisoli, G. (1986). Acute myocardial infarction in the puerperium in patients receiving bromocriptine. *American Journal of Obstetrics and Gynecology,* 155, (2), 371–372.

Jacobson, H. (1985). A standard for assessing lochia volume. *MCN: American Journal of Maternal-Child Nursing,* 10 (3), 174–175.

Kitzinger, S. (1994). *The year after childbirth: Surviving and enjoying the first year of motherhood.* New York: Charles Scribner's Sons.

Rubin, R. (1961). Puerperal change. *Nursing Outlook,* 9, 753.

Schauberger, C., Rooney, B., Brimer, L. (1992). Factors that influence weight loss in the puerperium. *Obstetrics and Gynecology,* 79 (3), 424–429.

Selby, J. W. (1980). *Psychology and human reproduction.* New York: The Free Press.

Sternbach, G. (1989). John Homans: The dorsiflexion sign. *The Journal of Emergency Medicine,* 7, 287–290.

Symanski, M. (1992). Maternal infant bonding. *Journal of Nurse-Midwifery,* 37 (2), 675–735.

Walker, L. (1992). *Parent-infant nursing science: Paradigms, phenomena, methods.* Philadelphia: F. A. Davis.

Wilson, B. A., Shannon, M. T., Stang, C. L. (1993). *Govoni & Hayes Nurses' Drug Guide 1993.* Norwalk, CT: Appleton & Lange.

Wong, S., Stepp-Gilbert, E. (1985). Lactation suppression: Nonpharmaceutical versus pharmaceutical methods. *Journal of Obstetric, Gynecologic, and Neonatal Nursing,* 14 (4), 302–310.

Wrasper, C. (1996). Discharge timing and Rubin's concepts of puerperal change. *Journal of Perinatal Education,* 5 (2), 13–23.

Healthy Postpartum Woman

This Nursing Care Planning Guide was developed to be used as a planning tool. You will need to modify and adapt it to individual clients as appropriate.

Performing a complete and thorough assessment is the first step in providing effective nursing care for a client. Major nursing diagnoses used in the care of the healthy postpartum woman include

1. Risk for fluid volume deficit: postpartum hemorrhage
2. Altered comfort*
3. Risk for uterine infection (endometritis)
4. Risk for urinary tract infection
5. Risk for infection: vagina, episiotomy/perineum, breasts (mastitis)
6. Altered nutrition: more than, or less than, body requirements
7. Constipation
8. Sleep pattern disturbance
9. Risk for altered tissue perfusion: thrombophlebitis
10. Risk for injury: exercise
11. Altered sexuality patterns
12. Risk for altered parent-infant attachment
13. Altered role performance: transition to the maternal role
14. Risk for altered growth and development: parenting
15. Risk for moderate anxiety
16. Risk for ineffective individual coping
17. Risk for situational low self-esteem

*Although "altered comfort" is not a current NANDA-approved nursing diagnosis, it is used advisedly here to describe a condition that creates "discomfort" rather than "pain."

NURSING CARE PLANNING GUIDE Continued

ASSESSMENT

Assessment of the healthy postpartum woman plays a critical role in facilitating recovery from the birth process and adjustment to the maternal role. To collect data, use the following Assessment Tool: Postpartum Flowsheet (pp. 1021–1024). In the data collected, identify defining characteristics to use as a basis for formulating nursing diagnoses that are appropriate for your client. Areas requiring special attention in the care of the healthy postpartum woman include comfort, prevention of infection, parent-infant attachment, and maternal role performance.

NURSING CARE PLANNING GUIDE *Continued*

Assessment Tool

Postpartum Flowsheet

Postpartum Graphic Record

Date PP/post-op Day	mo/day/yr Day			mo/day/yr Day			mo/day/yr Day			mo/day/yr Day		
Hour												

Fundal Height	Temperature °C	Temperature °F
	40.0	104
u+3	39.4	103
u+2	38.9	102
u+1	38.3	101
@u	37.8	100
u-1	37.2	99
	37.0	98.6
u-2	36.7	98
u-3	36.1	97

Fundal Height
X - graph as number of fingers above (+) or below (-) the umbilicus

Temperature
● - oral
●R - rectal
●Ax - axillary

Pulse												
Respirations												
Blood Pressure												
Lochia (**L** - light, **M** - moderate **H** - heavy)												
Safety: All siderails up												
Siderails up X ___												
Call light in reach												
Bed in low position												
Initials												
Equipment: IV pump(s)	X	X	X	X	X	X	X	X	X	X	X	X
Auto BP cuff												
Intake & Output: PO												
IV												
8 hr intake												
Urine												
Emesis												
8 hr output												
24 hr Intake/Output	I:	O:		I:	O:		I:	O:		I:	O:	

INIT.	First Initial Last Name	Title	INIT.	First Initial Last Name	Title	INIT.	First Initial Last Name	Title	Any initials on the Flow-sheet should be identified by signature

 Postpartum Flowsheet **Form #4100-SP**

Portions of Postpartum Flowsheet. Courtesy of CSW Forms, Timberon, NM, (800) 284-2815.

NURSING CARE PLANNING GUIDE Continued

Assessment Tool

Postpartum Flowsheet

	Item	Code	Date (Hour)	Date	Date	Date
Hygiene / Activity						
Hygiene	Shower†	S - self, A - assist				
Hygiene	Wash at sink†	S - self, A - assist				
Hygiene	Bedbath/basin at bedside†	S - self, A - assist, T - total care				
Hygiene	Pericare	S - self, A - assist, T - total care				
Hygiene	Oral care	S - self, A - assist, T - total care				
Hygiene	Foley care					
Hygiene						
Activity	Ambulate in hall†	S - self, A - assist				
Activity	Ambulate to bathroom†	S - self, A - assist				
Activity	Transfer to chair†	S - self, A - assist				
Activity	Dangle†	S - self, A - assist				
Activity	Bedrest					
Activity	Bedrest w/ bedside commode	S - self, A - assist				
Activity	Turn q____†	S - self, A - assist, T - total care				
Activity	Cough and deep breathe†	S - self, A - assist				
Activity	Incentive spirometry†	S - self, A - assist				
Activity	No sleep					
Activity	Naps					
Activity	Sleeping most of time					
Activity						
Physical Assessment						
Neuro	Alert, oriented X 3, appropriate behavior, speech clear					
Neuro	No c/o headache, visual disturbance					
Neuro	DTR's 1+ to 3+, no clonus					
Neuro						
Cardiovascular / Skin	SBP ±30mm Hg of baseline/DBP ±15mm Hg of baseline					
Cardiovascular / Skin	Skin warm and dry					
Cardiovascular / Skin	Skin pink					
Cardiovascular / Skin	Temperature ≤ 100.4°F/ 38°C, or ≤______					
Cardiovascular / Skin	Heart rate regular with no irregularities, 50–100 BPM					
Cardiovascular / Skin	No orthostatic dizziness					
Cardiovascular / Skin	No edema					
Cardiovascular / Skin	(-) Homan's sign. No redness, warmth, or pain in extremities					
Cardiovascular / Skin	Abdominal dressing dry, intact					
Cardiovascular / Skin	Abdominal incision: No redness, swelling, or drainage; edges well approximated.					
Cardiovascular / Skin	Incision comfortable or mildly uncomfortable					
Cardiovascular / Skin	IV site(s): No swelling, redness, tenderness, or drainage					
Cardiovascular / Skin	IV containers, tubing, sites, current per hospital policy					
Cardiovascular / Skin						
Cardiovascular / Skin						
Cardiovascular / Skin						
Respiratory	Breathing easily. Respirations regular, normal depth					
Respiratory	Respiratory rate 12-22/min.					
Respiratory	Lungs clear bilaterally w/ good breath sounds to bases					
Respiratory						
	Initials					
	Charge Nurse Initials (if applicable)					

Assessment Codes	
✓ - yes	— - not applicable or not assessed
N - notes (see nurse's notes / Postpartum Graphic Record)	
P - see Pain Assessment	

† - Activity tolerated well (v.s. stable and WNL, no c/o dizziness or other problems).
Note: If activity is not tolerated well, write "N" in square, and document assessment in notes.

Portions of Postpartum Flowsheet. Courtesy of CSW Forms, Timberon, NM, (800) 284-2815.

NURSING CARE PLANNING GUIDE Continued

Assessment Tool

Postpartum Flowsheet

Date / Hour | Date | Date | Date

	Physical Assessment (continued)
GI	Diet
	Taking ≥ 50% of diet
	No nausea or vomiting
	Bowel sounds present, not hypo- or hyperactive
	BM. Description of first BM:
	Passing flatus postoperatively
	No c/o epigastric pain resistant to antacids
GU	Foley catheter, draining clear yellow urine
	Voiding, no c/o dysuria
	Ø signs/symptoms of bladder distension/incomplete emptying
Perineum/hemorrhoids	Episiotomy/repaired laceration: edges well-approximated, no drainage
	Perineum, labia: minimal or no swelling/ecchymosis
	Soft w/ moderate puffiness. Puffiness not increasing
	Soft, very puffy. Puffiness not increasing
	Comfortable or mildly uncomfortable
	Hemorrhoids: Yes / No (circle one)
	Hemorrhoidal discomfort absent or mild
Uterus	Fundal height not increasing, uterus firm
	Uterus midline
	Lochia ≤ moderate (≤ 75-100% of 1 pad q 3°), no large clots
	No foul odor to lochia
	Uterine cramping discomfort absent/mild
Breasts	Method(s) of infant feeding: Breast / Bottle (circle choice(s))
	Breastfeeding, needs minimal/no assist to get babe on breast
	Breasts soft
	Breasts filling
	Breasts full, not engorged. If breastfeeding, good letdown.
	Breasts engorged. If breastfeeding, good letdown.
	Breasts comfortable/mild discomfort
	Nipples: No cracks, blisters. Comfortable/mild discomfort

Psychosocial / Attachment Assessment	
Patient verbalizes that she feels rested	
Baby in room with mother most of the time	
Cuddles baby	**M** - mother, **SO** - significant other†, **B** - both
Talks softly to baby	**M** - mother, **SO** - significant other†, **B** - both
Participates in baby care	**M** - mother, **SO** - significant other†, **B** - both
	M - mother, **SO** - significant other†, **B** - both

Miscellaneous
Care plan/goals reviewed, updated as necessary
Initials
Charge Nurse Initials (if applicable)

Assessment Codes

✓ - yes —- not applicable or not assessed
N - notes (see nurse's notes / Postpartum Graphic Record)
P - see Pain Assessment

† - Significant Other

Name__________ Relationship__________

Comments__________

Portions of Postpartum Flowsheet. Courtesy of CSW Forms, Timberon, NM, (800) 284-2815.

NURSING CARE PLANNING GUIDE Continued

Assessment Tool

Postpartum Flowsheet

	Date	Date	Date	Date
Pain Assessment / Intervention				
Pain related to:				
Intervention: **Ph** - pharmacologic, **O** -other [non-pharmacologic], **B** - both				
Pain after intervention				
Pain related to:				
Intervention: **Ph** - pharmacologic, **O** -other [non-pharmacologic], **B** - both				
Pain after intervention				
Pain related to:				
Intervention: **Ph** - pharmacologic, **O** -other [non-pharmacologic], **B** - both				
Pain after intervention				
Pain related to:				
Intervention: **Ph** - pharmacologic, **O** -other [non-pharmacologic], **B** - both				
Pain after intervention				
PRN Medications				
Comfort Measures / Treatments				
Misc.				
Perineum: Ice pack to perineum				
Perineum: Cool sitz				
Perineum: Warm sitz				
Breasts / Breastfeeding: Ice packs to breasts				
Breasts / Breastfeeding: Air dry nipples 10-15" after nursing				
Breasts / Breastfeeding: Topical(s) used on nipples:				
Breasts / Breastfeeding: Nurse observes good latch-on. Baby's mouth wide open, centered on breast, good grasp of areola				
Initials				
Charge Nurse Initials (if applicable)				

Discharge Checklist		
☐ Self care teaching completed ☐ Baby care teaching completed	Needs rubella vaccine? Y / N	If yes, has it been given? Y / N
☐ Postpartum hematocrit evaluated.	Needs hepatitis vaccine? Y / N	If yes, has it been given? Y / N
☐ Care plan/discharge plan reviewed. Follow up plans finalized.	Needs Rh_o(D) Immune Globulin? Y / N	If yes, has it been given? Y / N
☐ Discharge instructions given	Referral(s) needed? Y / N	If yes, has it been made? Y / N

Assessment Codes

✓ - yes — - not applicable or not assessed
N - notes (see nurse's notes / Postpartum Graphic Record)

Pain
ø - none, **Mi** - mild, **M** - moderate, **S** - severe, **Sl** - sleeping
(Or use 10 point pain scale)
Note: Pain assessment documented by codes should be based on patient's verbal response. Document nonverbal cues and other pertinent information in the nurse's notes.

Portions of Postpartum Flowsheet. Courtesy of CSW Forms, Timberon, NM, (800) 284-2815.

1

Analysis: ▼ **NURSING DIAGNOSIS**

Risk for fluid volume deficit: postpartum hemorrhage, **related to**

- Uterine atony
- Perineal laceration
- Vaginal laceration
- Cervical laceration
- Retained placenta or membranes
- Subinvolution

Defining Characteristics

SUBJECTIVE

Uterine Atony

Complains of dizziness

Perineal, Vaginal, Cervical Laceration

Describes excessive lochia or bleeding

Retained Placenta or Membranes

Describes excessive lochia, an increase after flow was lessening

Subinvolution

OBJECTIVE

Uterine Atony

Soft, boggy uterus

Uterus does not contract and stay firm even with massage

Excessive vaginal bleeding, dark red blood with clots

Elevated pulse

Decreased blood pressure

Increased respiratory rate

Decreased hemoglobin

Less alert and responsive

Cool and clammy skin

Pale color

Perineal, Vaginal, Cervical Laceration

Laceration visible with inspection

Excessive vaginal bleeding, a more continuous flow of blood, bright red blood

Uterus firm and contracted

Retained Placenta or Membranes

Excessive lochia or bleeding, dark red blood with clots

Vaginal bleeding increases after reduction of amount

Subinvolution

Uterine pain with palpation

Uterus larger than expected; not involuting or reducing in size as expected

Greater vaginal bleeding than normal

Continued on facing page

NURSING CARE PLANNING GUIDE Continued

Client Goal/ ▼ EVALUATION CRITERIA

Client will demonstrate adequate fluid volume without postpartum hemorrhage. / ▼ **Client will evidence firm and contracted uterus, normal pattern and amount of lochia, normal pulse, normal respirations, normal blood pressure, normal hemoglobin level.**

▼ NURSING INTERVENTIONS	Rationale
• Assess vital signs: pulse, respirations, blood pressure every 15 minutes in recovery room, then every hour until stable, then every 4 hours, then every shift.	• When excessive blood is lost, signs of shock may appear. The pulse and respirations increase, and blood pressure decreases. The pulse elevates to compensate for decreased volume ejected with each beat. The blood pressure decreases; with lower return of blood to the heart, there is less blood circulated with each beat.
• Assess uterus and fundus for firmness every 15 minutes in recovery room, then every hour, then every 4 hours, then every shift. If fundus is soft, massage until firm. Remain with client, resting hand on fundus; if uterus relaxes, massage. Do not overmassage.	• Assessing the fundus for firmness determines whether the uterus remains contracted. The uterus needs to contract around the large vessels at the placental implantation site, and hemostasis needs to occur or hemorrhage results.
• Assess amount and type of lochia or bleeding on the perineal pad every 15 minutes in the recovery room, then every hour until there is a moderate or lesser amount, then every 4 hours, then every shift. Record number of pads, degree of saturation, and type of lochia.	• Lochia progresses from rubra (dark red) to serosa (pinkish) to alba (yellowish white) in 2 to 3 weeks post partum. The amount is typically assessed by observing the perineal pad.
• Assess fundal height every 15 minutes in the recovery room, then every hour, then every 4 hours, then every shift.	• After delivery, the uterine muscle contracts. In the postpartum period, uterine muscle contraction, autolysis, tissue necrosis, and cell atrophy in the uterine lining lead to reduction in size of the uterus to almost prepregnant size (called involution).
• Assess hemoglobin level and hematocrit. These determinations are typically done in the third trimester, then at admission for labor, and then at 2 days post partum.	• The hemoglobin level and hematocrit fall with hemorrhage. There is typically loss of extracellular fluid, which results in hemoconcentration. Therefore, a drop in hematocrit is abnormal. A drop of $>10\%$ is abnormal.
• Instruct mother about normal pattern of lochia (type and amount) as well as about symptoms to report. Describe the progression from lochia rubra (typically lasting 1 to 2 days) to lochia serosa (typically lasting 2 to 7 days) to lochia alba (typically lasting day 9 until 3 weeks). Describe normal amounts (moderate lochia becomes scant by 3 weeks post partum).	• With knowledge of the normal pattern and amounts of lochia, the client can report abnormal symptoms.
• Start and regulate intravenous fluids with oxytocin (Pitocin) if ordered. Administer whole blood or packed cells if ordered.	• Pitocin is an oxytocic that stimulates uterine contraction. Typically, a fast rate is needed initially in the recovery room to cause the uterus to contract. Blood may be ordered to replace blood that was lost.

Continued on following page

NURSING CARE PLANNING GUIDE Continued

• Administer Ergotrate (ergonovine maleate) or Methergine (methylergonovine maleate).	• These medications are taken orally to stimulate the uterus to contract.
• Assess blood pressure for hypertension.	• Methergine can contribute to elevated blood pressure.
• Elevate the feet if necessary.	• When legs are elevated, venous return is promoted.
• Administer oxygen by face mask if necessary.	• Oxygen per face mask increases blood oxygen levels.
• Have client void as soon as possible after birth, then encourage to void regularly; or insert Foley catheter if client is unable to empty bladder.	• An empty bladder promotes contraction of the uterus. A Foley catheter aids in assessing output, which is an indicator of fluid replacement.
• Educate client about self-administration of iron.	• Iron is necessary to produce red blood cells and may be prescribed if the client is anemic as a result of hemorrhage.

2

Analysis: ▼ NURSING DIAGNOSIS

***Altered comfort,** related to**

- Episiotomy
- Perineal swelling, bruising, lacerations
- Perineal/vaginal hematoma
- Hemorrhoids
- Bladder distention
- Breast engorgement
- Nipple soreness
- Afterpains
- Spinal headache
- Mastitis

Defining Characteristics

SUBJECTIVE	*OBJECTIVE*
Episiotomy/Perineal Swelling, Bruising	Episiotomy/Perineal Swelling, Bruising
States presence of perineal discomfort or pain	Perineal edema
States presence of perineal discomfort or pain when moving, sitting, or walking	Perineal ecchymosis
	Perineal tenderness with movement and touch

*Although "altered comfort" is not a current NANDA-approved nursing diagnosis, it is used advisedly here to describe conditions that typically create "discomfort" rather than "pain." The nursing diagnosis "pain" can apply to these conditions, however, depending on the severity of the condition and the degree of discomfort experienced by the client.

Continued on facing page

NURSING CARE PLANNING GUIDE Continued

	Purulent exudate from episiotomy Suture line not approximated Moves slowly Nonverbal behavior indicates discomfort or pain when moving, sitting, or walking Sits slowly
Hematoma	Hematoma
States severe, relatively constant discomfort or pain in perineum	Firm, tender, bulging mass, bluish red in color, on perineum or in vagina
Hemorrhoids	Hemorrhoids
States presence of dull aching in anal area	Visible hemorrhoids
Bladder Distention	Bladder Distention
States presence of lower abdominal dull discomfort	Lower abdominal bulging noted with palpation Unable to void or voids small amounts
Breast Engorgement	Breast Engorgement
States presence of tenderness in reddened area of breast	Enlarged breasts Tense, hard breasts with palpation Nonverbal behavior indicating discomfort or pain with touching of breasts Veins prominent in breasts Flattened nipple Lumpy breasts
Nipple Soreness	Nipple Soreness
States presence of nipple discomfort or pain with breastfeeding	Cracked nipple Bruised nipple Reddened nipple Nonverbal behavior indicating discomfort or pain with breastfeeding
Afterpains	Afterpains
States feels "cramps" when nursing baby	Nonverbal behavior indicating discomfort or pain when breastfeeding
Spinal Headache	Spinal Headache
Describes discomfort or severe, sharp pain behind eyes, radiating to both temples, and in occipital area States discomfort or pain increases with raising head, sitting, or standing	Nonverbal behavior indicating headache discomfort or pain, especially when sitting, raising head, or standing Holds head, as if uncomfortable or in pain
Mastitis	Mastitis
Describes tenderness in reddened area on breast	Reddened area on breast Hardened area on breast Nonverbal behavior indicating discomfort or pain when reddened area on breast is touched Elevated temperature Enlarged lymph nodes

Continued on following page

NURSING CARE PLANNING GUIDE Continued

Client Goal/ ▼ EVALUATION CRITERIA

Client will demonstrate comfort. / ▼ **Client will evidence healing episiotomy without swelling and bruising; hemorrhoids shrinking in size; absence of lower abdominal bulge; soft, nontender breasts; nipples without cracking, bruising, redness; absence of afterpains; absence of spinal headache; ability to raise head, sit, stand without spinal headache; breasts without reddened, hardened, tender area; absence of elevated temperature; absence of statements of discomfort.**

▼ NURSING INTERVENTIONS	Rationale
Episiotomy/Perineal Swelling, Bruising	
• Assess presence, location, and nature of perineal discomfort.	• These data provide information about healing and subjective experience of discomfort for the client.
• Assess perineum and episiotomy for REEDA (note redness, edema, ecchymosis, discharge and exudate, approximation of suture line). Also assess tenderness and signs of hematoma (tender, firm, bulging area, bluish red in color).	• There may be edema, redness, or bruising of tissues after delivery. If these are assessed, measures to minimize discomfort can be implemented.
• Instruct client in ways to decrease discomfort:	
1. Tighten perineum before sitting, then relax it slowly after being seated.	Gluteal muscle tightening reduces direct pressure on perineum so discomfort is minimized.
2. Apply ice pack to perineum as ordered, particularly in recovery room in first 24 hours.	Ice decreases circulation, promotes vasoconstriction, reduces edema, and promotes a local anesthetic effect.
3. Apply local anesthetic spray.	Local anesthetic spray, such as Americaine, reduces sensation by local anesthetic effect.
4. Use sitz baths (100–105°F) for 15 to 20 minutes three to four times a day.	Heat increases circulation to the perineum, thereby promoting oxygenation and nutrition of tissues. It therefore promotes healing, which reduces discomfort.
5. Cleanse perineal area in recovery room, with morning care, and with each elimination, cleansing from front to back. Some use warm water in a squeeze bottle to rinse the perineum.	Perineal cleansing reduces risk for infection, which causes discomfort. Cleansing from front to back reduces introduction of intestinal tract microorganisms.
6. Change perineal pads frequently.	Changing perineal pads frequently removes lochia, which is a good medium for growth of microorganisms; infection causes discomfort.
7. Wash hands before and after perineal care, elimination, and use of heat.	Cleansing the hands reduces microorganisms, which could be transferred to the perineum.
• Administer pain medication as ordered; assess effectiveness of medication. If epidural, caudal, or saddle block anesthesia was used, assess return of sensation and ability to move.	• Pain medication relieves or reduces discomfort. Sensation of pain and ability to move return within 1 to 2 hours after delivery. When anesthesia "wears off," discomfort or pain in perineal area may be experienced and may require pain medication.
Hematoma	
• Report firm, bulging perineal mass, with severe pain, to physician.	• Hematoma is a collection of blood caused by trauma to a blood vessel. The hematoma may be absorbed if it is a small size; if it is not, surgical evacuation with packing may be required.

Continued on facing page

NURSING CARE PLANNING GUIDE Continued

<u>Hemorrhoids</u>	
• Instruct client in taking a warm sitz bath for 15 to 20 minutes three times a day.	• Sitz baths increase circulation and soothe the area.
• Instruct client in use of local anesthetic spray or rectal ointments or suppositories.	• Local anesthetics relieve pain sensation. Other rectal ointments and suppositories soothe or provide hydrocortisone, which reduces inflammation.
• Reduce constipation by educating client about	• Constipation, with straining, further restricts circulation and aggravates varicose veins in the anal area.
1. adequate fluid intake	Adequate fluid intake promotes softer stool.
2. adequate fiber in diet	Adequate fiber stimulates intestinal peristalsis.
3. adequate exercise	Exercise stimulates peristalsis.
<u>Bladder Distention</u>	
• Assess lower abdomen, just above symphysis pubis, for bulging in recovery room and regularly thereafter. Percuss to note dullness of abdomen and increased tympany over the filled bladder.	• When the bladder becomes filled, it is enlarged; this enlargement can be noted by observing the lower abdomen. Percussion sounds change to tympany with distention.
• Have client void or catheterize before transferring from recovery room to postpartum unit. Encourage voiding (getting up to go to the bathroom, running water). Assess bladder for distention after voiding.	• Ambulating to the bathroom allows voiding in the usual position. The sound of running water often stimulates voiding. If the bladder is emptied, there will not be bladder distention; bladder distention causes discomfort.
<u>Breast Engorgement</u>	
• Assess breasts for engorgement every shift.	• Breast engorgement typically occurs 2 to 3 days after birth. It is due to congestion of blood and lymph as well as increased milk supply. There is discomfort or pain with the engorgement. It typically lasts 1 to 2 days.
• Provide instruction methods to reduce engorgement for those who are bottle feeding.	• Mothers who are bottle feeding may experience engorgement several days after birth when the milk supply increases, even though the breasts were not stimulated.
1. Wear a tight bra or apply a breast binder.	The tight bra or breast binder applies pressure, which reduces congestion and discomfort.
2. Apply ice packs to breasts.	Ice packs reduce circulation and thus congestion and also provide an anesthetic effect.
3. Request ordered analgesics.	Analgesics help relieve pain.
• Provide instruction in methods to reduce engorgement for those who are breastfeeding.	• Engorgement may occur 2 to 3 days after birth when circulation increases and milk "comes in."
1. Wear a supportive bra.	A supportive bra supports the engorged breast and applies pressure, which reduces congestion.
2. Apply moist heat to both breasts for 15 to 20 minutes before each feeding (use a moist washcloth, towel, or heat pack).	Heat to the breasts softens breasts so that the let-down reflex can occur.
3. Nurse baby regularly, every 2 to 3 hours for 10 to 15 minutes per breast.	Regular nursing empties the breast, which decreases engorgement.
4. Massage breasts from outer areas to nipple.	Massage promotes emptying of the breasts.
5. Apply ice packs between feedings.	Ice packs reduce circulation and thus congestion.
6. Express some milk before nursing.	Expressing some milk decreases tension of nipple and makes it easier for baby to latch on.

Continued on following page

NURSING CARE PLANNING GUIDE Continued

Interventions	Rationales
<u>Nipple Soreness</u>	
• Assess nipples for cracking, bruising, and redness. Assess complaints of discomfort or pain. Observe for nonverbal behavior indicating discomfort or pain with latch-on and breastfeeding.	• Nipples can become sore if baby is not positioned appropriately for breastfeeding. The nipple and areola must be in the mouth, with a tummy-to-tummy position. Suction must be released appropriately.
• Instruct client in methods to reduce nipple soreness.	
1. Do not use soap on nipples.	Soap dries the nipple, removing lubrication, thereby increasing the risk for trauma and soreness.
2. Ensure proper positioning of baby at the breast; ensure that nipple and areola are in the mouth, with a tummy-to-tummy position.	Proper positioning decreases pressure and trauma to the nipple.
3. Remove baby from breast appropriately; release suction.	When the suction in baby's mouth is released, removal from the breast does not traumatize.
4. Express some milk before nursing.	Expression of a small amount of milk softens the areola, thereby decreasing discomfort with latch-on.
5. Nurse relatively frequently.	Nursing frequently ensures a less eager baby and a less vigorous, traumatic suck.
6. Nurse the less tender breast first.	Nursing the less tender breast first reduces trauma to the more tender nipple from vigorous suck early in a feeding.
7. Nurse for minimal time for letdown and emptying.	To stimulate letdown, there must be sufficient sucking.
8. Apply breast milk to nipples after feedings.	Application of breast milk to nipples after a feeding provides natural lubrication.
9. Air-dry nipples after feeding.	Air-drying after feedings helps toughen nipples.
<u>Afterpains</u>	
• Encourage client to empty bladder before breastfeeding.	• Afterpains, or uterine contractions, are intensified in multiparas, with breastfeeding, and when ergot or oxytocic preparations are administered.
• Educate client about cause and duration of afterpains.	• Afterpains occur most frequently during breastfeeding when oxytocin is released in response to sucking; oxytocin stimulates release of breast milk but also stimulates uterine contractions. A distended bladder can accentuate uterine cramping.
• Administer analgesics if needed.	• Analgesics relieve pain.
<u>Spinal Headache</u>	
• Assess for spinal headache (discomfort or pain behind eyes, radiating to temples, in occipital area). Assess in recovery room and as needed thereafter for headache aggravated with raising head, sitting, or standing.	• Assessment provides baseline data for interventions. With spinal anesthesia, there may be leakage of cerebrospinal fluid through the dura into the extradural space; this may cause the brain stem to fall onto the base of the skull when upright. This reduces the volume of fluid surrounding the brain.
• Instruct in methods to reduce spinal headache. These include	
1. increasing oral fluids; forcing fluids to approximately 10 8-ounce glasses per day	Fluids help stimulate production of cerebrospinal fluid, replacing that which was lost.
2. encouraging the client to lie flat	Lying flat decreases the pressure and pain.
3. assisting with hygiene, eating, and feeding baby	Lying flat may necessitate assistance with daily and infant activities.

Continued on facing page

NURSING CARE PLANNING GUIDE Continued

4. applying an abdominal binder — An abdominal binder increases intra-abdominal pressure, which also increases pressure in the spinal cord.

5. assisting with "blood" patch if necessary — A blood patch consists of injecting 10 mL of the client's venous blood into the epidural space over the site where spinal anesthesia was administered. It creates a clot that produces pressure and seals off the leak.

Mastitis

- Assess breasts for warm, red, firm, tender area. — Mastitis is an infection of the breasts; it causes discomfort and an elevated temperature.
- Administer analgesics as needed. — Analgesics relieve pain associated with mastitis.
- Administer antibiotics as ordered. — Antibiotics treat the infection of mastitis.
- Instruct client to massage blocked milk duct during nursing. — Massage promotes emptying, thereby minimizing stasis that encourages growth of microorganisms.
- Apply local heat to the reddened, warm area (moist towel, heat pack). — Local moist heat increases circulation, thereby promoting healing.
- Instruct client to wash hands before handling breasts. — Milk ducts open directly onto nipples, so there is easy access for microorganisms.
- Instruct client to apply breast milk to nipple after nursing. — The milk provides a natural lubricant on the nipple.

3

Analysis: ▼ NURSING DIAGNOSIS

Risk for uterine infection (endometritis), related to

- Ascension of microorganisms into uterus
- Introduction of microorganisms with vaginal examinations or insertion of IUPC or fetal electrode
- Membranes ruptured for a prolonged length of time
- Ineffective perineal care
- Trauma with delivery

Defining Characteristics

SUBJECTIVE	*OBJECTIVE*
Describes headache	Elevated temperature, higher than 100°F on 2 days
Describes malaise	Elevated pulse

Continued on following page

NURSING CARE PLANNING GUIDE Continued

Describes backache	On palpation, uterus is larger than expected
States poor appetite	Typically dark brown, foul-smelling lochia, but may be odorless
Experiences pain when uterus is palpated	Elevated white blood cell (WBC) count

Client Goal/ ▼ EVALUATION CRITERIA

Client will demonstrate absence of endometritis. / ▼ **Client will evidence normal temperature and pulse rate, normal-sized uterus (involution progressing), normal lochia without odor.**

▼ NURSING INTERVENTIONS	Rationale
• Assess temperature in recovery room and every 4 hours until stable, then every shift.	• An elevated temperature often accompanies an infection. Dehydration also raises the temperature. Therefore, it is often difficult to determine the reason for an elevated temperature in the recovery room and on the first day after delivery.
• Assess uterine size every 4 hours, then every shift. Assess for tenderness with palpation.	• When endometritis occurs, the uterus may not contract as well, resulting in a larger than expected size.
• Culture the cervix if infection is suspected.	• Culture will identify the amount and type of microorganisms so that appropriate antibiotic therapy can be prescribed.
• Obtain a clean-catch midstream urine specimen.	• A clean-catch midstream specimen is needed to minimize contamination with lochia. There is often a urinary tract infection when the endometrium and therefore the lochia are infected.
• Assist in obtaining blood for WBC count.	• The WBC count is elevated with a left shift differential in an infection.
• Administer antibiotics as ordered.	• Appropriate antibiotics treat the infection.
• Administer intravenous fluids or encourage oral intake as appropriate.	• Fluids provide adequate hydration.
• Administer Ergotrate or Methergine, if ordered.	• These medications stimulate contraction of uterine muscles, which aids emptying of the uterus and involution.

Continued on facing page

NURSING CARE PLANNING GUIDE Continued

4

Analysis: ▼ NURSING DIAGNOSIS

***Risk for urinary tract infection,* related to**

- Overdistended bladder
- Incomplete emptying of bladder
- Trauma to the bladder
- Dilated ureters
- Diuresis post partum
- Caudal or epidural anesthesia with reduced sensation
- Perineal swelling, discomfort
- Inappropriate wiping technique

Defining Characteristics

SUBJECTIVE	*OBJECTIVE*
Describes burning with urination	Distended bladder
	Voids small amounts (<100 mL)
	Voids frequently
	Dysuria with voiding
	Urgency with voiding
	Costovertebral angle tenderness
	Fever

Client Goal/ ▼ EVALUATION CRITERIA

Client will demonstrate absence of urinary tract infection. / ▼ **Client will evidence voiding adequate amounts, absence of bladder distention, absence of symptoms of cystitis or urinary tract infection.**

▼ NURSING INTERVENTIONS	Rationale
• Assess output. Measure first two voidings after birth.	• With trauma, swelling, and decreased distention, there is a tendency toward urinary retention. Urinary retention increases the risk for infection. The client should void at least 100 mL per voiding. Typically, there is diuresis after delivery, so a reduced urinary output is suggestive of urinary retention.

Continued on following page

NURSING CARE PLANNING GUIDE Continued

Nursing Interventions	Rationale
• Note color and appearance of urine.	• Urine may appear cloudy with an infection.
• Assess for bladder distention in recovery room, then every 2 to 3 hours, then every 4 hours. Palpate and percuss. Assess location of fundus, firmness of contraction of uterus, and lochia.	• With trauma and urinary tract changes, the bladder may become distended. In addition, renal plasma flow remains elevated in the first week after delivery, which increases bladder filling.
• Assist with voiding. Assist with ambulation if necessary. Run water, pour warm water over perineum, or have client void in shower or sitz bath.	• Ambulation to the bathroom allows the client to void in the usual position.
• Encourage adequate oral intake.	• Adequate fluid intake hydrates, increases urinary output, decreases concentration, and fosters elimination.
• Obtain urine specimen for culture, clean-catch midstream or catheterized.	• Urine specimen identifies the microorganism so that the appropriate antibiotic can be ordered.
• Administer antibiotics as ordered.	• Antibiotics treat the infection.
• Assess for additional symptoms of cystitis and urinary tract infection. These include 1. frequency 2. urgency 3. dysuria 4. costovertebral tenderness 5. fever	• The symptoms of cystitis include frequency, urgency, and dysuria. The symptoms of a urinary tract infection include costovertebral angle tenderness and fever; they may include symptoms of cystitis as well.
• Encourage a diet high in protein and vitamin C.	• Protein promotes healing and building of new tissues. Vitamin C is necessary for cell wall synthesis.
• Instruct client in Kegel exercises.	• Kegel exercises, done regularly each day, improve tone of the pubococcygeal muscle, preventing or reducing stress incontinence.

Analysis: ▼ NURSING DIAGNOSIS

Risk for infection: vagina, episiotomy/perineum, breasts (mastitis), related to

- Delivery
- Use of forceps
- Lacerations
- Trauma to perineum
- Episiotomy
- Handling of breasts, breastfeeding

Continued on facing page

NURSING CARE PLANNING GUIDE Continued

Defining Characteristics

SUBJECTIVE	*OBJECTIVE*
Vagina	Vagina
Describes pain or pressure in vagina	Malodorous vaginal discharge
	Inflammation of rugae
	Vaginal laceration
Episiotomy/Perineum	Episiotomy/Perineum
Describes discomfort in perineum	Perineal bruising
	Perineal edema, redness, swelling
	Perineal laceration
	Vaginal discharge/exudate
	Episiotomy not approximated
	Elevated temperature
Breasts (Mastitis)	Breasts (Mastitis)
Describes tenderness in reddened area on breast	Reddened area on breast
	Hardened area on breast
	Nonverbal behavior indicating discomfort or pain when reddened area is touched
	Elevated temperature
	Enlarged lymph nodes

Client Goal/ ▼ EVALUATION CRITERIA

Client will demonstrate absence of infection. / ▼ **Client will evidence minimal inflammation and swelling of perineum; absence of perineal or vaginal discharge; episiotomy approximated; healing, soft, nontender breasts.**

▼ NURSING INTERVENTIONS	Rationale
• Observe and assess perineum for signs of infection.	• Symptoms of perineal infection are bruising, swelling, discharge, and episiotomy not approximated.
• Assess WBC count.	• An increase in the WBC count is normal in the first 10 to 12 days after birth; this makes identification of infection more difficult.
• Assess temperature.	• An elevated temperature often accompanies an infection.
• Educate client in how to do perineal cleansing. This includes cleansing from front to back and rinsing with water from squeeze bottle after each elimination.	• Cleansing the perineum reduces the number of microorganisms present. In addition, it removes lochia, moisture that provides an environment favorable for the growth of microorganisms.

Continued on following page

NURSING CARE PLANNING GUIDE Continued

- Instruct client to change perineal pad frequently.
- Changing perineal pads frequently removes blood and moisture, both of which provide a favorable environment for growth of microorganisms.
- Instruct client to wash hands before and after perineal cleansing or changing perineal pads.
- Washing hands reduces microorganisms that can be introduced to perineal pads or the perineum.
- Instruct client in use of sitz bath or apply hot packs for 15 to 20 minutes three times a day.
- Warm heat increases circulation, which promotes healing. It also reduces discomfort.
- Instruct client in Kegel exercises.
- Kegel exercises, 100 times per day, increase circulation to the perineum and aid recovery.
- Instruct client to wash hands before breastfeeding.
- Milk ducts open directly onto nipple. Microorganisms on the hands may be introduced into the breasts through handling associated with breastfeeding.
- Assess breasts for warm, red, firm, tender area.
- Mastitis is an infection of the breasts; it causes discomfort and an elevated temperature. It often occurs as result of stasis of milk or incomplete emptying of milk ducts.
- Instruct client to massage blocked milk duct during feeding.
- Massage promotes emptying, thereby minimizing stasis that encourages growth of microorganisms.
- Apply local heat to reddened warm area (moist towel, heat pack).
- Local, moist heat increases circulation, thereby promoting healing.
- Instruct client to cleanse breasts with only water, not soap.
- Soap dries, which increases the risk for trauma and infection.
- Instruct client to apply colostrum or breast milk to nipple after nursing.
- The milk provides a natural lubricant, thereby decreasing the risk for trauma and likelihood of infection.

6

Analysis: ▼ NURSING DIAGNOSIS

Altered nutrition: more than, or less than, body requirements, related to

More than Body Requirements

- Weight gained during pregnancy
- Altered nutritional needs when breastfeeding
- Altered activities and exercise
- Food preferences

Less than Body Requirements

- Weight gained during pregnancy
- Altered nutritional needs when breastfeeding
- Altered activities and exercise
- Food preferences

Continued on facing page

NURSING CARE PLANNING GUIDE Continued

Defining Characteristics

SUBJECTIVE

More than Body Requirements

States preference for high-calorie foods

Indicates lack of knowledge of requirements for lactation

Less than Body Requirements

Indicates lack of knowledge of requirements for lactation

States desire to lose weight rapidly

OBJECTIVE

More than Body Requirements

Excessive intake of calories

Weight increasing

Exercise reduced

Less than Body Requirements

Inadequate intake of four food groups for lactation

Inadequate intake of calories

Involution not progressing

Perineum not healing well

Weight decreasing

Client Goal/ ▼ EVALUATION CRITERIA

Client will demonstrate nutritional intake adequate for body requirements. / ▼ **Client will evidence adequate amount of calories and nutrients for recovery, adequate amount of calories and nutrients for breastfeeding, resumption of prepregnant weight, ability to relay nutritional requirements.**

▼ NURSING INTERVENTIONS	Rationale
More than Body Requirements and Less than Body Requirements	
• Obtain 24-hour diet recall.	• Baseline data are necessary to assess adequacy of dietary intake.
• Assess whether dietary intake meets nutritional requirements either for recovery and resumption of prepregnant weight or for recovery and breastfeeding. Determine nutritional adequacy of calories, protein, calcium, iron, and vitamins.	• There should be an adequate intake of protein and vitamin C for healing to occur. For lactation, there needs to be an increase of 500 calories per day to provide for production of breast milk.
• Obtain information about dietary preferences, including cultural preferences.	• Dietary intake is influenced by preferences, including cultural practices in relation to food. The client is more likely to obtain dietary requirements if they can be provided in preferred food.
• Obtain information about new daily schedule, who will prepare meals.	• Daily schedule and meal preparation influence intake.
• Assess knowledge level of nutritional needs for lactation.	• The new mother may not have knowledge of requirements for lactation. Mothers should not "diet" but rather have intake adequate for lactation.

Continued on following page

NURSING CARE PLANNING GUIDE Continued

More than Body Requirements

- Assess knowledge of nutritional needs for weight loss. Discuss gradual weight loss of 1 to 1½ pounds per week, exercise pattern, and altered eating patterns as best method of losing, and then maintaining, weight.
- The woman may want to go on a "crash" diet to lose weight rapidly. Exercise assists in weight loss by altering metabolic rate. Weight loss is not sustained if the daily pattern of eating is not altered. When rapid weight loss occurs, weight is typically regained. Adequate protein and vitamin C are needed for recovery.
- Recommend weighing only occasionally.
- Typically, there is a weight loss of about 11 pounds right after delivery. The rest of the weight is often lost by 6 to 8 weeks post partum. Focusing on scale weights places too much emphasis on the weight rather than on altering eating habits long term.

Less than Body Requirements

- Assess postpartum hemoglobin level and hematocrit.
- Hemoglobin level is analyzed to determine anemia after pregnancy. Counseling about foods high in iron as well as iron supplementation, if necessary, is required.

7

Analysis: ▼ NURSING DIAGNOSIS

***Constipation*, related to**

- Decreased activity during labor and after delivery
- Decreased abdominal tone
- Decreased intra-abdominal pressure
- Decreased gastrointestinal motility
- Altered nutrition
- Perineal discomfort

Defining Characteristics

SUBJECTIVE

States stools are hard and difficult to pass

OBJECTIVE

Infrequent bowel elimination

Hard stools

Straining with stools

Continued on facing page

NURSING CARE PLANNING GUIDE Continued

Client Goal/ ▼ EVALUATION CRITERIA

Client will demonstrate normal bowel elimination. / ▼ **Client will evidence normal pattern of bowel elimination and soft stools.**

▼ NURSING INTERVENTIONS	Rationale
• Assess bowel elimination; assess frequency, consistency, difficulty with passage.	• After delivery, there is decreased intra-abdominal pressure and abdominal tone. Gastrointestinal motility remains sluggish. In addition, there is decreased activity and alteration in fluid and fiber intake. All of these contribute to constipation.
• Obtain information regarding knowledge about influences of diet and activity on bowel elimination and clarify as needed.	• The client may lack knowledge about factors influencing bowel elimination.
• Provide information about the role of fiber and liquids in preventing constipation. Teach client which foods are high in fiber, if needed, and number of servings recommended per day.	• Fiber stimulates peristalsis in the gastrointestinal tract. With peristalsis, stool is eliminated before an excess amount of water is absorbed from the stool. Liquid in the diet helps provide a proper consistency to the stool; many advise 8 to 10 glasses a day.
• Assess for hemorrhoids and institute measures to relieve these (see hemorrhoids under Nursing Diagnosis 2, Altered comfort, in this nursing care planning guide).	• Hemorrhoids cause discomfort and may interfere with elimination.
• Obtain information about daily activities and exercise. Devise an individualized exercise regimen with the client.	• Exercise increases peristalsis. Knowledge of the daily schedule as well as of preferences for particular exercises allows the nurse to assist in planning a schedule to which the client is more likely to adhere.
• Instruct client about proper self-administration of medication, if ordered.	• Various stool softeners may be prescribed. These are often wetting agents that lower the surface tension so that the stool is more easily penetrated by water (an example is Colace). Others are a combination of a wetting agent and a chemical that stimulates peristalsis (Peri-Colace). Still others provide bulk, or fiber (Metamucil).

Continued on following page

NURSING CARE PLANNING GUIDE Continued

8

Analysis: ▼ **NURSING DIAGNOSIS**

***Sleep pattern disturbance*, related to**

- Disrupted sleep to feed neonate
- Noise in hospital environment
- Anxiety about learning infant care tasks
- Pain, discomfort

Defining Characteristics

SUBJECTIVE	*OBJECTIVE*
States feelings of fatigue	Difficulty concentrating
States difficulty getting to sleep	Appears fatigued
States is awakened to feed baby	Lack of adequate restful sleep
States concerns about learning infant care tasks	Unable to take naps

Client Goal/ ▼ **EVALUATION CRITERIA**

Client will demonstrate adequate sleep pattern. / ▼ **Client will evidence absence of fatigue, absence of insomnia, feeling refreshed, sleeping 6 to 7 hours per night, taking a nap if necessary, falling asleep readily.**

▼ **NURSING INTERVENTIONS**	**Rationale**
• Obtain information about usual sleep pattern and typical schedule.	• The nurse can assist in adjusting the daily schedule to "fit in" a nap or rest period. Suggestions to aid relaxation just before sleep can be provided (such as quiet time with minimal noise and activity, meditation, soft music, relaxation techniques).
• Recommend a nap or rest period each day.	• Sleep is needed to feel refreshed and restored.
• Recommend positions for sleep that provide adequate support.	• Proper support with pillows for the side-lying position promotes relaxation and aids sleep.
• Educate client about infant care activities.	• Knowledge increases confidence and lessens anxiety over the unknown.
• Assess assistance from others. Schedule assistance so that mother can sleep.	• When others assist with household activities or infant care, the mother is free to relax and sleep.
• Discourage entertaining or frequent visits from others.	• Visiting with friends uses energy and contributes to fatigue.

Continued on facing page

NURSING CARE PLANNING GUIDE Continued

- Encourage restriction of outside activities.
- Encourage client to establish a quiet, relaxing routine before bedtime.

- Outside activities use energy and contribute to fatigue.
- A bedtime routine aids relaxation, so sleep is promoted.

9

Analysis: ▼ NURSING DIAGNOSIS

Risk for altered tissue perfusion: thrombophlebitis, **related to**

- Sluggish blood flow in dilated pelvic veins
- Immobility with bed rest or anesthesia
- Hypercoagulability
- Preexisting varices
- Fetal pressure on pelvic vein

Defining Characteristics

SUBJECTIVE	*OBJECTIVE*
<u>Superficial Thrombosis in Saphenous Vein</u>	<u>Superficial Thrombosis in Saphenous Vein</u>
Describes discomfort and tenderness in lower leg	Warm area over thrombosis
	Bumpy, palpable, hard vein
	Pinkish-red coloration of skin over thrombosis
<u>Femoral Thrombosis</u>	<u>Femoral Thrombosis</u>
Describes discomfort in affected leg	Swelling in leg
Describes malaise	Fever
Describes chills	Shiny, white skin over thrombosis
	Presence of Homans sign
	Diminished peripheral pulse
<u>Pelvic Thrombosis</u>	<u>Pelvic Thrombosis</u>
Describes chills	Temperature swings
Describes pain and tenderness in groin	Pulmonary embolism with sudden chest pain, dyspnea and shortness of breath, cough, pallor, sweating, hypotension

Continued on following page

NURSING CARE PLANNING GUIDE Continued

Client Goal/ ▼ EVALUATION CRITERIA

Client will demonstrate adequate tissue perfusion, absence of thrombophlebitis. / ▼ **Client will evidence normal leg veins without warmth, redness, and tenderness; absence of Homans sign; normal coloration of skin; absence of pulmonary embolism symptoms.**

▼ NURSING INTERVENTIONS	Rationale
• Ambulate early and frequently to prevent thrombophlebitis.	• During pregnancy, there is a shift in the balance between coagulating and fibrinolytic factors to favor clotting. Also, there is decreased blood flow in legs during pregnancy. With thrombophlebitis, there is decreased blood flow and venous return.
• If on bed rest, do leg exercises to prevent thrombophlebitis.	• Inactivity restricts circulation and promotes development of clots.
• If thrombophlebitis occurs, place on bed rest.	• Bed rest discourages dislodgement of the clot and thereby minimizes the risk for pulmonary embolism.
• Apply moist heat or hot packs as ordered.	• Hot packs increase blood flow to legs, thereby minimizing obstruction and development of clots.
• Administer ordered analgesics.	• Analgesics relieve the pain associated with thrombophlebitis.
• Apply support stockings.	• Support stockings provide pressure to vein walls and help improve circulation. They reduce venous stasis.
• Elevate the affected leg.	• Elevating the leg promotes circulation, empties superficial veins, and increases venous return.
• Administer antibiotics as ordered.	• If there is a fever, infection may accompany the thrombophlebitis. An antibiotic will treat the infection.
• Administer heparin, if ordered, by intravenous drip, by heparin lock, or subcutaneously. Explain side effects of heparin.	• Heparin is given to prolong the activated partial thromboplastin time and prevent further development of clots. Knowledge of side effects may result in client's reporting their occurrence; bleeding is the main side effect.
• Assess leg for symptoms of thrombophlebitis. These include	
1. edema (measure circumference of calf), presence of Homans sign	These indicate deep venous thrombosis.
2. redness, heat, tenderness, localized edema	These are symptoms of superficial thrombophlebitis.
3. pallor and coolness of extremity	These are symptoms of femoral thrombophlebitis.
• Assist with, and review, laboratory tests. Prothrombin time, partial thromboplastin time, activated partial thromboplastin time, hemoglobin, hematocrit, aspartate transaminase, and lactate dehydrogenase determinations are often done.	• Review of results indicates effectiveness of treatment.
• Explain the condition and treatments involved, if necessary.	• Knowledge aids compliance and lessens anxiety.

Continued on facing page

NURSING CARE PLANNING GUIDE Continued

10

Analysis: ▼ NURSING DIAGNOSIS

***Risk for injury: exercise,* related to**

- Reduced muscle tone with stretching of abdominal muscles
- Weight gain of pregnancy
- Increased elasticity of tissues
- Relaxation of joints
- Episiotomy discomfort
- Altered activities, schedule

Defining Characteristics

SUBJECTIVE	*OBJECTIVE*
Describes fatigue	Weight has not returned to prepregnant level
Describes altered schedule	Involution progressing; fundal height decreasing daily
Describes discomfort with exercise	Perineum healing
Describes inability to perform at prepregnant level	Abdominal muscle tone diminished
	Activities associated with care of infant

Client Goal/ ▼ EVALUATION CRITERIA

Client will demonstrate absence of injury with resumption of activities and exercise. / ▼ **Client will evidence absence of pain, normal lochia and involution, healing of perineum, absence of injuries.**

▼ NURSING INTERVENTIONS	Rationale
• Educate client about exercises allowed while hospitalized. These include 1. abdominal breathing and pelvic rock 2. combined abdominal breathing and pelvic rock 3. reaching for knees 4. buttocks lift 5. simple knee roll 6. double knee roll 7. leg roll 8. arm raises	• Since recovery is only beginning, relatively easy, relaxed exercises should be done after delivery. Exercise will help restore muscle tone, contribute to weight loss, and help prevent constipation.
• Advise client to do warm-up, stretching, and cool-down.	• These allow stretching, which minimizes injury.

Continued on following page

NURSING CARE PLANNING GUIDE Continued

- Educate client to gradually progress to more strenuous activities as she feels able. Caution against exercises that jog, jar, or bounce.
  - Exercise that jogs, jars, or bounces may injure softened tissues and unstable joints.
- Advise client to stop whenever feeling fatigued or if there is increased lochia.
  - Increases in lochia may occur if exercise is too strenuous.
- Advise client to avoid stretching to point of maximal resistance.
  - Stretching to maximal resistance may increase potential for injury.
- Recommend adequate nutritional and fluid intake.
  - Exercise requires increased calories. Fluid is lost in perspiration and with respiration.
- Instruct client in proper body mechanics, especially for lifting the baby and baby equipment.
  - Proper body alignment minimizes muscle and ligament tension and injury, placing stress on large muscles that can handle it.
- Assist client in planning schedule to allow time for exercise.
  - Activities are altered when care of the infant is incorporated. There needs to be a "sitter" if exercise is done outside the home. Mothers may feel that they should not ask others for assistance with child care.

11

Analysis: ▼ NURSING DIAGNOSIS

***Altered sexuality patterns,* related to**

- Breast tenderness
- Leaking breasts
- Fatigue
- Child care activities
- Decreased vaginal lubrication
- Fear of injury or pain with intercourse
- Decreased desire associated with preoccupation with the new baby
- Recovery from delivery
- Varying sexual desire of husband and wife
- Fear of pregnancy

Defining Characteristics

SUBJECTIVE

Discusses sexual concerns

Shares feelings about alteration in sexual desire

OBJECTIVE

Unable to engage in sexual activity at desired frequency

Continued on facing page

NURSING CARE PLANNING GUIDE Continued

Discusses impact that body changes of recovery and child care activities have on sexual desire

Verbalizes fear of injury or pain with intercourse

Unable to engage in intimate physical activities other than intercourse

Decreased vaginal lubrication

Healing perineum

Client Goal/ ▼ EVALUATION CRITERIA

Client will demonstrate acceptable sexuality patterns. / ▼ **Client will evidence sharing feelings about altered sexual desire, discussing concerns and fears, verbalizing mutual satisfaction.**

▼ NURSING INTERVENTIONS	Rationale
• Obtain information about usual pattern of sexual activity/desire.	• Information about usual pattern provides a baseline for comparison. Desire may decrease with changing energy levels, with body changes of recovery, and with preoccupation with care of the new baby.
• Obtain information about healing of episiotomy, lochia, and leaking of breast milk.	• Most recommend that women refrain from intercourse until the episiotomy has healed and lochia has ceased (typically 3 weeks). With stimulation of sexual activity, oxytocin is released, which also stimulates ejection of breast milk, causing leaking; some couples do not find this appealing.
• Recommend inserting two fingers into vagina to note whether there is discomfort.	• Inserting fingers into the vagina will allow the client to know whether this causes discomfort.
• Recommend use of commercial lubricant such as K-Y jelly.	• The reduction of hormones after delivery results in decreased vaginal lubrication. A commercial lubricant may be used.
• Counsel that pregnancy can occur before return of menses since ovulation occurs before menstruation. It can also occur while breastfeeding. Counsel about contraceptives.	• Unless the baby is solely breastfed and has frequent feedings round-the-clock, ovulation and pregnancy can occur. Therefore, breast feeding is not considered to be a contraceptive.
• Obtain data about feelings associated with changes in sexual activity.	• Verbalizing feelings helps with self-recognition as well as with acceptance by the partner. Communication is essential to resolve concerns.
• Assess feelings about body shape and weight.	• Body image is related to one's identity as a woman. Changes in body shape associated with pregnancy may conflict with the image one has of one's body.
• Discuss ways to enhance physical intimacy through physical contact other than intercourse (hugging, kissing).	• Physical contact provides emotional support and meets needs for affection and attention.
• Encourage client to verbalize fears related to sexual activity. Clarify misconceptions.	• New mothers may fear trauma or pain with intercourse. Both partners may fear pregnancy. Once lochia has ceased, intercourse can be resumed.

Continued on following page

NURSING CARE PLANNING GUIDE Continued

12

Analysis: ▼ NURSING DIAGNOSIS

***Risk for altered parent-infant attachment,* related to**

- New family member
- Need to develop maternal-infant relationship

Defining Characteristics

SUBJECTIVE

Uses negative terms when referring to baby

States baby does not respond to her verbalizations, caretaking

Describes infrequent contact with infant

Expresses generally negative feelings about baby

Voices concern about the baby

OBJECTIVE

Does not talk softly and affectionately, or frequently in high-pitched voice, to baby

Does not consistently recognize baby's cries

Minimal eye contact with infant

Without frequent en face position

Minimal enfolding of infant, does not consistently hold close

Infant does not "alert" to parents' verbalizations

Minimal infant gazing into mother's eyes

Infant does not eat well or gain weight

Infant does not settle well with mother's attempts to settle

Infant does not nestle into mother's arms

Minimal interacting with baby when caretaking

Minimal turning of baby to mother's voice; minimal alerting and widening of eyes

Minimal spontaneous stroking, patting, touching baby

Misinterpretation of baby's cries

Client Goal/ ▼ EVALUATION CRITERIA

Client will demonstrate normal progression with parent-infant attachment process. / ▼ **Client will evidence voicing positive feelings, responding to baby's cries and needs, frequent contact with affectionate touching and verbalizations.**

Continued on facing page

NURSING CARE PLANNING GUIDE Continued

▼ NURSING INTERVENTIONS	Rationale
• Assess mother's attachment behaviors. This includes observation of the following behaviors: 1. Touch—Is it affectionate? Does mom hold baby, cuddle baby, spontaneously stroke, pat? 2. Eye contact—How frequently does mom look at baby? 3. Verbalizations—Does mom talk affectionately to baby? 4. How does mom describe baby? Does she use positive terms? 5. How does mom describe baby's behaviors? 6. Does mom interpret baby's cries appropriately? 7. Does mom meet baby's needs quickly and appropriately? 8. Is there frequent contact, with affectionate touching and verbalization? 9. Can mom interpret baby's cries? 10. Observe mother's behaviors in the context of mothering behaviors considered appropriate for the family's culture.	• Attachment is a mutual positive feeling of attraction that develops in a reciprocal relationship. It begins during pregnancy, progressing over time. Behaviors indicating attachment change over time as well. Attachment is maintained by proximity and interaction; it is facilitated by positive input or feedback from others and the baby. An important part is the acquaintance after birth when the mother "identifies" the baby as a unique individual rather than the envisioned concept initiated during pregnancy. The feelings of attachment, attraction, caring, and love are translated into observable behaviors. Each culture teaches appropriate attachment behaviors involved in the maternal-infant interactions. Thus, while all cultures demonstrate affectionate, caring behaviors between mother and baby, some emphasize relatively constant holding while others do not.
• Assess baby's behaviors during maternal-infant interactions. 1. Does baby seem alert, pay attention? 2. Does baby gaze at mother? 3. How well does baby settle? 4. How well does the baby eat? What is the weight gain pattern? 5. Does baby nestle into mother's arms? 6. Does baby respond to mother's verbalizations? mother's efforts to settle, feed, and quiet the baby?	• The attachment process is facilitated/enhanced by positive input/feedback from others, especially the baby. Attachment is a reciprocal relationship.
• Point out behaviors of baby that indicate positive responses to mother's behaviors.	• A new mother may not notice some behaviors of the baby that indicate a positive response. Attachment is facilitated by positive feedback.
• Assess input/feedback from others. This includes degree of support for mother's caretaking, how others describe the baby, and feedback to the mother about her caretaking.	• Attachment is facilitated by positive reinforcement of others.
• Educate/reinforce maternal caretaking activities.	• Attachment will be fostered when mother is confident in caretaking activities and baby responds positively to those behaviors.
• Assist in providing an environment conducive to attachment. Assess the support network.	• When mother is able to adjust the family's structure and processes to accommodate the new baby as well as to get adequate rest, she feels more positive about mothering and the baby.
• Reinforce appropriate maternal caretaking interaction and behaviors.	• Reinforcement facilitates learning and fosters positive feelings of attachment.

Continued on following page

NURSING CARE PLANNING GUIDE Continued

13

Analysis: ▼ NURSING DIAGNOSIS

***Altered role performance: transition to the maternal role,* related to**

- Inexperience with care of infants
- Conflicting information in literature, media
- Conflicting advice from others
- Physical illness
- Decline in physical strength
- Substance abuse
- Low self-esteem
- Inability to deal with changed expectations of maternal role
- Inability to learn maternal caretaking behaviors
- Lack of maternal role models
- Inadequate social support
- Inadequate resources

Defining Characteristics

SUBJECTIVE

Verbalizes feelings of anger or depression

Verbalizes frustration with maternal role

Verbalizes lack of knowledge about maternal role

Verbalizes uncertainty about maternal role requirements

Voices ambivalence about maternal role

OBJECTIVE

Inappropriate visual, tactile, auditory stimulation of infant

Unresponsive to infant cues

Inability to perform infant caretaking tasks

Refusal to participate in maternal role

Incongruence between mother's and others' expectations of maternal role behaviors

Client Goal/ ▼ EVALUATION CRITERIA

Client will demonstrate adequate transition to maternal role. / ▼ **Client will evidence ability to feed, change, and dress baby; perform cord care; take baby's temperature; bathe baby.**

▼ NURSING INTERVENTIONS	Rationale
• Assess knowledge about infant care tasks (such as taking the temperature, cord care, dressing the baby, elimination, diaper care, bottle feeding or breastfeeding tasks, skin care, sleep-wake patterns).	• Knowledge allows the client to become aware of caretaking behaviors. One must be aware of the behaviors before one is able to demonstrate them.

Continued on facing page

NURSING CARE PLANNING GUIDE Continued

• Assess mother's readiness to learn, and make her as comfortable as possible.	• Immediately after delivery, the mother is often focused on herself. Eventually she will want to perform self-care activities and care of the infant. Learning is facilitated when the mother turns to active interest and when she feels comfortable.
• Clarify any misconceptions.	• Clarification allows the client to operate on sound information.
• Educate client in areas assessed to have a knowledge deficit. Provide rationale for actions.	• The nurse provides information useful in performing infant care tasks. When the rationale is provided, the learner is able to understand the reason for the action.
• Provide appropriate audiovisuals.	• Audiovisuals allow the learner to observe the caretaking tasks and also stimulate not only visual but also auditory learning.
• Demonstrate caretaking tasks.	• Observation of psychomotor tasks allows the learner to observe behaviors required.
• Observe mother during caretaking to assess learning.	• Observation will allow assessment of learning so that reinforcement or additional information can be provided.
• Reinforce appropriate caretaking behaviors by providing verbal feedback.	• When learning is reinforced, it tends to be retained.
• Provide corrective feedback as necessary.	• Feedback allows the learner to alter behaviors.
• Provide appropriate written information, including a phone number to call when questions arise.	• Supplemental information reinforces learning and provides reference at home. When questions arise, the mother can call to obtain answers.
• Teach safety measures involved with care of the infant (such as car seats; locking medications, toxic chemicals; the danger of cords and small objects).	• Parents may not be aware of factors that influence safety of the infant. When aware, parents can avoid exposure to unsafe situations.
• Teach physical, emotional, cognitive growth and development of the infant. Include factors that have a positive influence on growth and development.	• Knowledge of typical growth and development allows parents to assess growth and development of their infant. In addition, it minimizes unrealistic expectations.

14

Analysis: ▼ NURSING DIAGNOSIS

***Risk for altered growth and development: parenting,* related to**

- Period of change
- Individual developmental task of becoming parents
- Family developmental task of altering family structures, processes, and relationships

Continued on following page

NURSING CARE PLANNING GUIDE Continued

Defining Characteristics

SUBJECTIVE	*OBJECTIVE*
Does not state feelings about mothering	Unprepared for physical needs of the baby
Does not share feelings with spouse	Does not make financial adjustments
	Difficulty in noting infant's cues
	Difficulty in meeting infant's needs
	Focuses on own needs rather than the infant's needs
	Daily schedule not altered appropriately
	Fatigued
	Does not spend time with spouse
	Lack of support/help with infant care
	Difficulty in performing parenting skills

Client Goal/ ▼ EVALUATION CRITERIA

Client will demonstrate adequate adjustment to parenting. / ▼ **Client will evidence meeting physical needs of infant, noting and responding appropriately to infant's cues, altering daily schedule appropriately, feeling rested, spending time with spouse, experiencing support with infant care.**

▼ NURSING INTERVENTIONS	Rationale
• Assess relationship of family members with each other.	• Family members need to adjust their own behaviors to accommodate the new family member. Family members meet psychological needs for love, affection, and positive feedback.
• Encourage participation of both parents in infant care.	• When both participate in the care, the family tasks and processes can be altered so that one is not overtaxed.
• Educate client about infant care; assess knowledge, provide appropriate information, demonstrate care, provide reinforcement, and be available to answer questions.	• Anxiety associated with the unknown is lessened with knowledge. In learning role behaviors, there must be knowledge of those role behaviors, then practice with reinforcement and feedback.
• Relay typical emotional reactions to becoming a parent.	• Helps parents to prepare for, and accept, reaction to parenting. Stress and anxiety associated with the unknown can then be reduced.
• Provide references; suggest books about parenting.	• Information can be incorporated into parenting role as needed.
• Suggest parent support groups.	• Parent groups increase knowledge about parenting, help with problem solving, and provide emotional support. In addition, groups can increase self-esteem with mastery of parenting tasks.
• Evaluate social support network.	• The social network can provide instrumental and emotional support. It can relieve parents so that they can spend time with each other.

Continued on facing page

NURSING CARE PLANNING GUIDE Continued

• Discuss alterations in sexual expression, providing recommendations as needed.	• Sexual relationship is important in meeting needs for intimacy/love. The sexual relationship is often altered during recovery because of fatigue or because of infant care.
• Assess family strengths.	• Focus interventions on strengths that will aid adjustment to parenting.
• Assess the parents' perceptions of the infant.	• Parents formulate a conceptualization of "their baby" before birth. Often, the reality is inconsistent with the "idealized" conceptualization. If the perceptions are negative, the parents may have difficulty attaching to, and caring for, their baby.
• Discuss daily schedule, routines.	• Activities need to be adjusted to incorporate infant care.
• Obtain information about the family's perception of stressors.	• The family may not realize what is stressful for them. Once stressors are identified, the nurse can explore, with the family, ways to minimize the stress.

15

Analysis: ▼ NURSING DIAGNOSIS

***Risk for moderate anxiety,* related to**

- Responsibilities associated with motherhood
- Disturbed sleep, fatigue
- Recovery from labor and delivery
- Conflicting advice from others
- Infant's wakefulness
- Incorporating infant care into daily routine

Defining Characteristics

SUBJECTIVE	*OBJECTIVE*
Experiences feelings of temporary apprehension, nervousness, concern	Voice tremors
Verbalizes expectations of problems	Voice pitch changes
Voices sleeping disturbances, such as insomnia	Increased rate and quantity of verbalization
	Narrowed focus of attention
	Inability to focus on most of what is happening
	Narrowed perception

Continued on following page

NURSING CARE PLANNING GUIDE Continued

Paces
Hand tremors or shakiness
Increased muscle tension
Rapid pulse
Increased respiratory rate
Irritability
Overeating or anorexia
More active reflexes, stable reaction
Face flushed
Localized or generalized sweating
Cheerfulness or laughing with serious matters

Client Goal/ ▼ EVALUATION CRITERIA

Client will demonstrate mild anxiety. / ▼ **Client will evidence asking questions or seeking information, increased awareness, increased attending, enhanced ability to learn, only mild restlessness, normal pulse and respirations, ability to focus on most of what is happening.**

▼ NURSING INTERVENTIONS	Rationale
• Assess symptoms of anxiety.	• Anxiety is an emotion that results from a threat to one's physical self, one's identity, one's self-concept, and one's self-esteem or one's relationships. It occurs when something central to one's personality, essential to one's security, is threatened. Symptoms involve cardiovascular, respiratory, skin, gastrointestinal, urinary tract, neuromuscular, verbalization, perceptual/attention, and motor responses. Physiologic responses are mediated through the sympathetic nervous system and are not under voluntary control.
• Assess coping mechanisms being used. These include problem-solving techniques, withdrawal (apathy, lowering aspirations) aggression, compromise (substituting goals), denial, and rationalization. Judge whether they are adaptive or maladaptive.	• One attempts to protect oneself from the threat and therefore uses both task-oriented and ego-oriented mechanisms. Task-oriented mechanisms help to resolve problems or conflicts. Ego-oriented mechanisms are used to protect the psychic self; they become habitual and distort reality to protect.
• If anxiety is severe, attempt to lower the level of anxiety. This can be accomplished by 1. listening 2. encouraging expression of feelings 3. accepting the client 4. answering questions directly 5. not attacking coping mechanisms 6. not forcing 7. modifying the environment (decreasing stimulation, quiet)	• When one has severe anxiety, most of one's energy is directed at relief of the anxiety, the discomfort of it. Therefore, the first goal is to reduce the discomfort. This is accomplished by establishing trust, accepting the client, listening, and providing a calm and quiet atmosphere.
• Recognize the mother's anxiety.	• Recognition helps the client realize feelings and provides insight.

Continued on facing page

NURSING CARE PLANNING GUIDE Continued

• Ask the mother to describe the situation.	• Since anxiety is subjective, description of the situation from the client's perspective allows the nurse to become aware of what is being threatened and of how this client perceives the situation.
• Ask how the mother coped with similar situations in the past. What situation was most similar to this one?	• Allows client to identify actions that were effective and ineffective in the past.
• Assess, with the client, which mechanisms were helpful and which were not.	• Effective mechanisms can be strengthened and ineffective ones eliminated.
• Introduce new coping mechanisms, if necessary.	• Introduction of new mechanisms broadens the array available to cope with situations.
• Promote relaxation. Suggest strategies such as 1. breathing techniques 2. progressive relaxation 3. meditation 4. biofeedback	• Various techniques help one to relax, to consciously respond to stressful situations in a relaxed manner.
• Suggest other techniques that help reduce anxiety in stressful situations, such as 1. assertiveness training 2. time management 3. thought stopping 4. exercise 5. reframing emotional ideas	• Some techniques are helpful in reducing anxiety in particular situations.
• Teach infant care skills.	• Knowledge of role behaviors enhances learning and increases confidence.
• Educate client about growth and development.	• Knowledge of what is normal reduces fear of the unknown and permits realistic expectations.
• Educate client about emotional reaction to parenting.	• When one's awareness of a new situation is enhanced, anxiety about the unknown is lessened.

16

Analysis: ▼ NURSING DIAGNOSIS

***Risk for ineffective individual coping,* related to**

- Postpartum blues
- Postpartum depression

Continued on following page

NURSING CARE PLANNING GUIDE Continued

Defining Characteristics

SUBJECTIVE

Postpartum Blues

States is exhausted

States feelings of sadness

States does not know reason for feeling sad

Describes feelings of loss of control

Postpartum Depression

Describes insomnia or hypersomnia (excessive sleep)

Describes loss of interest and pleasure in usual activities

Describes loss of energy

Describes feelings of worthlessness

Describes suicidal feelings

OBJECTIVE

Postpartum Blues

Cries frequently

Distracted, unable to attend well

Sadness begins 1 to 2 days post partum, lasts several days

Unable to care for self and newborn for a short time

Postpartum Depression

Appears sad

Excessive intake or loss of appetite

Gains weight or loses weight

Sleeps excessive amount of time or unable to sleep or fall asleep

Irritable

Does not participate in or enjoy typical activities

Difficulty concentrating or remembering

Agitated or retarded motor activity

Client Goal/ ▼ EVALUATION CRITERIA

Client will demonstrate effective individual coping. / ▼ **Client will participate in normal activities, have normal amount of sleep in postpartum period, be able to concentrate, have normal intake, have normal postpartum weight loss, not appear sad.**

▼ NURSING INTERVENTIONS	Rationale
Postpartum Blues	
• Assess for symptoms. Note when these occur.	• Symptoms of postpartum blues typically appear several days after birth, lasting anywhere from a few days to a few weeks. They include feelings of exhaustion and frequent crying, without knowing the reason.
• Allow time for mother to reflect, to sort out feelings.	• Time alone allows time to identify feelings and encourages self-awareness.
• Encourage verbalizations about losses, ambivalence about assuming parental role.	• Verbalization of feelings lessens anxiety and facilitates self-understanding. Such verbalizations enhance progression through the prenatal and postpartum tasks associated with assuming the maternal role.
• Explain postpartum blues to significant others.	• Knowledge of postpartum blues helps allay concerns and anxiety.

Continued on facing page

NURSING CARE PLANNING GUIDE Continued

Postpartum Depression

• Assess for symptoms of postpartum depression. Note when this occurs.	• Postpartum depression is suspected with symptoms of sadness, appetite or weight changes, insomnia or hypersomnia, irritableness, loss of interest and pleasure in usual activities, loss of energy, feelings of worthlessness, and difficulty concentrating or remembering. Onset of postpartum depression is 2 to 6 weeks after delivery; the diagnosis normally appears about 3 months after delivery.
• Obtain information about previous stressful events.	• The best predictor of postpartum depression has been found to be exposure to negative or stressful life events in the past.
• Assess for other factors found to be associated with greater risk for postpartum depression.	• The literature indicates that the presence of various factors has been related to greater risk for postpartum depression. These include higher levels of anxiety during the prenatal period than is usual, having external locus of control, and having the characteristic of "learned helplessness."
• Encourage client to share feelings.	• Expression of feelings increases self-awareness.
• Assess social and emotional support.	• Support helps dissipate feelings as well as provides adequate care for newborn.
• Refer to psychiatrist, if necessary	• If postpartum depression is a possibility, professional counseling, with medications, is needed.

17

Analysis: ▼ NURSING DIAGNOSIS

***Risk for situational low self-esteem*, related to**

- Difficulty adjusting to altered body shape
- Weight gained during pregnancy
- Assumption of mothering role
- Addition of new family member
- Temporary alteration of body functions after delivery

Continued on following page

NURSING CARE PLANNING GUIDE Continued

Defining Characteristics

SUBJECTIVE	*OBJECTIVE*
Negative self-appraisal	Difficulty in making decisions
Expresses shame, guilt	Decreased interest in sexual activity
Expresses sense of helplessness	Inability to assume self-care
Expresses feelings of inability to handle events	Inability to follow through or complete infant caretaking tasks
Perceives minimal strength in maternal role	Lack of attention toward parents
	Sensitive to advice about maternal behaviors

Client Goal/ ▼ EVALUATION CRITERIA

Client will demonstrate positive situational self-esteem. / ▼ **Client will evidence positive self-appraisals, adherence to exercise regimen, well-groomed appearance, confidence with infant care, absence of expressions of guilt, ability to make decisions, ability to complete self-care, interest in sexual activity, ability to care for infant.**

▼ NURSING INTERVENTIONS	Rationale
• Obtain information about conceptualizations of mothering behaviors. Point out those that are unrealistic. Clarify distorted perceptions.	• The parenting role is learned. Most of this learning occurs within the family.
• Encourage sharing of feelings about mothering, including negative feelings; accept client's expressions of negative feelings.	• Mothers often unrealistically feel that they should not have any negative feelings about mothering. When these occur, the mother often denies the feelings and does not share them for fear of being judged negatively. If the mother can share those feelings, they can be recognized as normal feelings, and the mother can realize she is not judged negatively.
• Assess the social network for emotional and appraisal support.	• Feedback is important in the way one judges performance.
• Assess/observe the baby's reaction to caretaking.	• One way in which the mother interprets "success" in infant caretaking is by the way the baby responds. If the infant gives positive feedback of eating well, settling, and gaining weight, the mother feels that she is adequate in caretaking.
• Suggest a new parent support group.	• The support group can supply role models, information, help with problem solving, and emotional support.
• Identify maternal role models.	• The new mother can observe maternal role behaviors of the role model.
• Provide opportunities to demonstrate infant caretaking tasks, allowing the mother to practice. Provide positive reinforcement.	• To learn caretaking tasks, the learner observes and then practices the behaviors.

Continued on facing page

NURSING CARE PLANNING GUIDE Continued

• Clarify and validate mother's perceptions of self in the maternal role.	• Clarification of mother's perceptions decreases distortion and contributes to positive self-esteem.
• Work with significant others so that negative statements are minimal and positive reinforcement is increased.	• Positive feedback and reinforcement enhances self-esteem.

30 Chapter

> After the complex physiologic and metabolic transitions in the immediate perinatal period, the human newborn enters an extraordinary phase of rapid postnatal growth and development. . . . The rate of growth in the first year of life is extraordinary. During the first year of life, a typical infant increases in weight by about 200% and in length by about 50%.
>
> JOHN W. SPARKS (1992)

Newborn Adaptation

Mary Lou Moore
Francine H. Nichols

HIGHLIGHTS

- ▼ The Transitional Period After Birth Related to Reactivity, Physiologic Status, Initiation of Respiration, and Circulation
- ▼ Systems Adaptation in the Newborn Related to the Respiratory System, Cardiovascular System, Gastrointestinal System, Hematologic System, Hepatic System, Renal System, Immunologic System, and Neurologic System
- ▼ Thermoregulation
- ▼ Sensory Capabilities Related to Vision, Hearing, Smell, Taste, Touch, Multimodel Sensory Development, Habituation, and Pain Perception
- ▼ Implications for Research

As the baby emerges from a fluid-filled world and the cord that has served as a lifeline for months is cut, a cry is heard, and amazingly a new life begins. This sequence as viewed by the observer is the visible sign of a complex transition to extrauterine life that starts at the instant of birth.

Even more amazing than the changes we see are those we cannot see. Organs receiving only small amounts of blood will now be perfused at far higher levels. Liver function is altered; metabolic processes are reorganized. Moments after birth, nutrition comes through the gastrointestinal tract, and gas exchange occurs in the lungs rather than in the placenta. Probably no 24 hours in a lifetime are as momentous as the first.

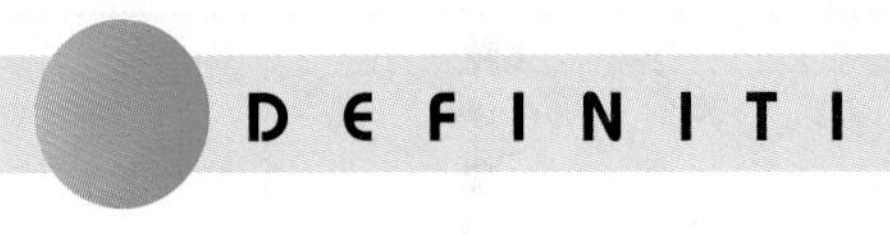

Brown adipose tissue—Often called brown fat, this substance provides the energy for thermogenesis in the newborn.

Habituation—The ability of the infant to "tune out" an incoming stimulus and not respond to it after prolonged exposure to it.

Initial period of reactivity—A period lasting 15 to 30 minutes up to as long as 1½ hours after birth in which the infant is in a state of alertness and responsiveness.

Meconium—The dark "tarry" substance composed of epithelial cells, bile, pancreatic and intestinal secretions, lanugo, and swallowed amniotic fluid that is the infant's first stools.

Period of relative inactivity—A period after the initial active period in which the infant is sleepy, drowsy, and relatively insensitive to both external and internal stimuli.

Second period of reactivity—The third stage of the transitional period that begins at approximately 2 hours and lasts up to 6 hours. During this time, the baby becomes more active, heart rate and respiration fluctuate with activity, the first meconium stool is often passed, and the infant may experience abrupt color changes and have oral mucus.

Transitional period—The period from birth to 6 hours after birth in which the newborn exhibits a typical pattern of physiologic and behavioral changes.

THE FIRST SIX HOURS: A TRANSITIONAL PERIOD

The concept of the first 6 hours of life as a transitional period was first described by Desmond and colleagues (1963). During the transitional period, a healthy full-term newborn exhibits an orderly pattern of changes that include an initial period of reactivity, a period of relative inactivity, and a second period of reactivity (Fig. 30–1).

Initial Period of Reactivity. The initial period of reactivity lasts 15 to 30 minutes to as long as 1½ hours. Immediate physiologic changes during this period involve the respiratory and circulatory systems.

The respiratory and vascular changes occur in a healthy newborn in far less time than reading about them requires. In brief moments, the healthy full-term infant has entered the initial period of reactivity, a period that seems uniquely designed to allow parents and baby to meet for the first time.

This is a magic time for parents. If the mother is planning to breastfeed, the first opportunity for breastfeeding can be provided during this period. Parents should be reassured that if their infant only "licks" and "nuzzles," this is not unusual and in no way suggests that there will be problems with subsequent feeding. This is primarily a time for being with their infant as they begin their extrauterine acquaintance.

Period of Relative Inactivity. After the initial active period, newborn infants enter a period characterized by sleep or drowsiness during which they are relatively insensitive to both external and internal stimuli. This time appears to be a period of recovery after the intense activity of labor, birth, and the immediate postbirth period. This stage may last as long as 1½ hours.

Second Period of Reactivity. The third stage of transition, the second period of reactivity, begins at approximately 2 hours. Both respiratory and heart rates fluctuate with activity, rising as the baby becomes more active. Body temperature also begins to rise. The first meconium stool may be passed at this time. Abrupt color changes, oral mucus, and varied activity are observed during this period. This period may last 2 to 6 hours.

Physiologic Status: Healthy Term Newborn

From a physiologic perspective, a healthy term newborn varies from infants who are even a few weeks older. Nursing assessments that would suggest abnormality in an infant at 3 weeks of age (jaundice, for example) may be within the range of normal for an infant who is 3 days old. Thus, understanding the normal physiologic status of a healthy term infant is essential to neonatal nursing practice (Fig. 30–2).

INITIATION OF RESPIRATION

During intrauterine life, the exchange of gases occurs in the placenta. The alveolar sacs are filled with lung fluid, and blood flow to the lungs is limited, because the lungs are not the site of oxygen and carbon dioxide exchange. Most of the blood circulating in the fetus is diverted from the lungs through the ductus arteriosus, a structure linking

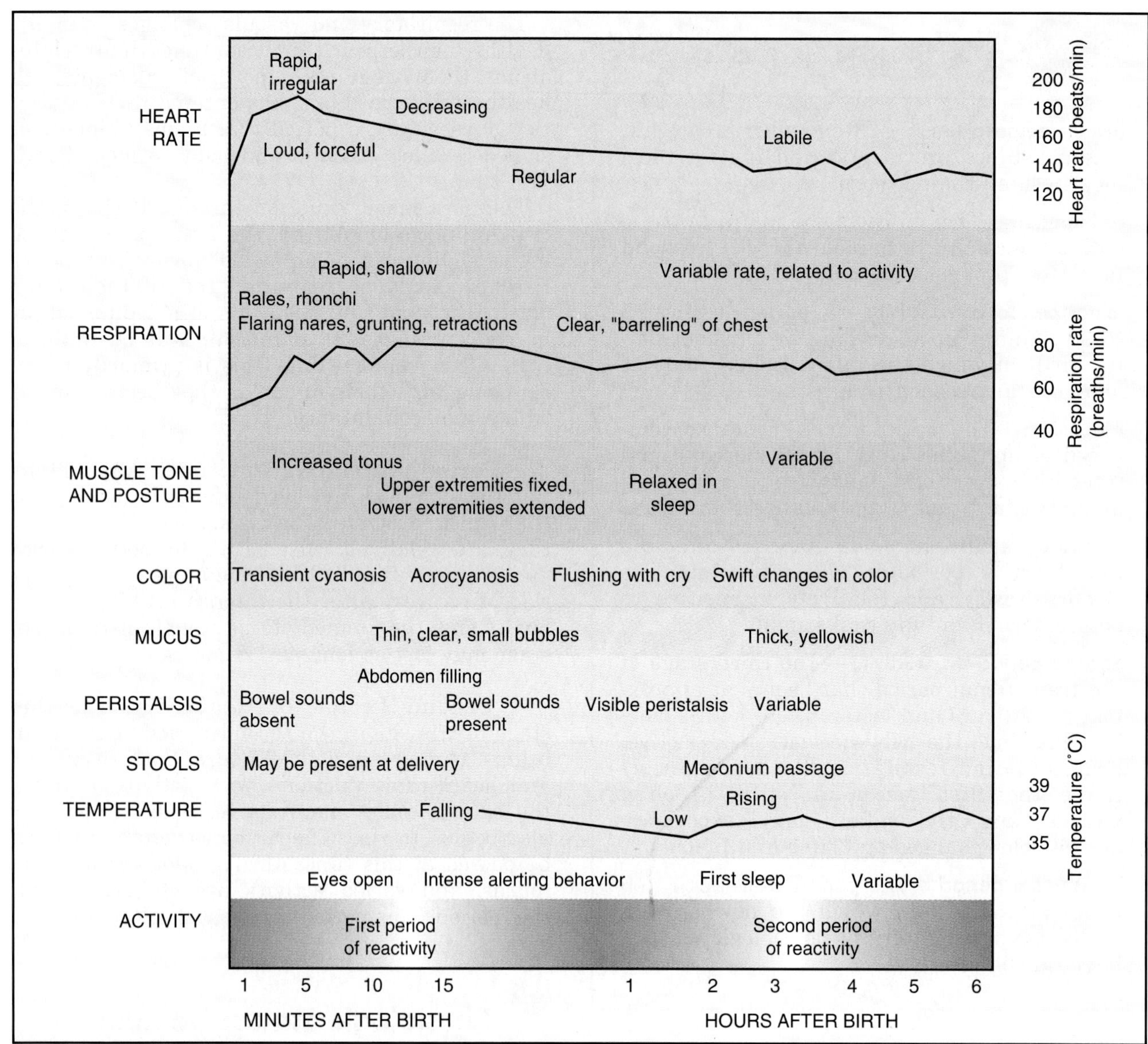

Figure 30–1

In the first 6 hours the infant experiences rapid and fluctuating physiologic changes as he adjusts to his new environment. Also, during this time there are two predictable periods of reactivity. (Based on data from Arnold, H. W., Putnam, N. J., Barnard, B. L., Desmond, M. M., Rudolph, A. J. (1965). *American Journal of Nursing,* 65 (10), 77–80.)

the aorta and the pulmonary artery that is patent in fetal life. Yet within a matter of seconds at the time of birth, the lungs must initiate their lifelong function of exchanging oxygen and carbon dioxide.

Two major categories of stimuli provoke initial respirations: external stimuli and internal stimuli. There are three types of external stimuli: mechanical, sensory, and thermal. Mechanical stimuli involve chest compression and chest recoil as the baby moves down the birth canal. The chest compression stimulates the stretch receptors, which cause the expression of lung fluid. Chest recoil also stimulates stretch receptors, resulting in passive inspiration. Sensory stimuli include sound, light, smell, touch, and pain, which stimulate auditory, visual, tactile, olfactory, and proprioceptive chemoreceptors. Thermal stimuli—the effect of cold on the infant, such as passing from the warm womb into the cool room, and evaporation—influence thermal receptors found all over the body. Internal stimuli are chemical stimuli and include decreased PaO_2, increased $PaCO_2$, and decreased pH. These chemical changes stimulate aortic and carotid chemoreceptors. The chemical stimuli, sensory stimuli, and thermal stimuli all influence the respiratory center in the medulla, resulting in contraction of the diaphragm. These forces all work simultaneously to initiate respiration (Fig. 30–3).

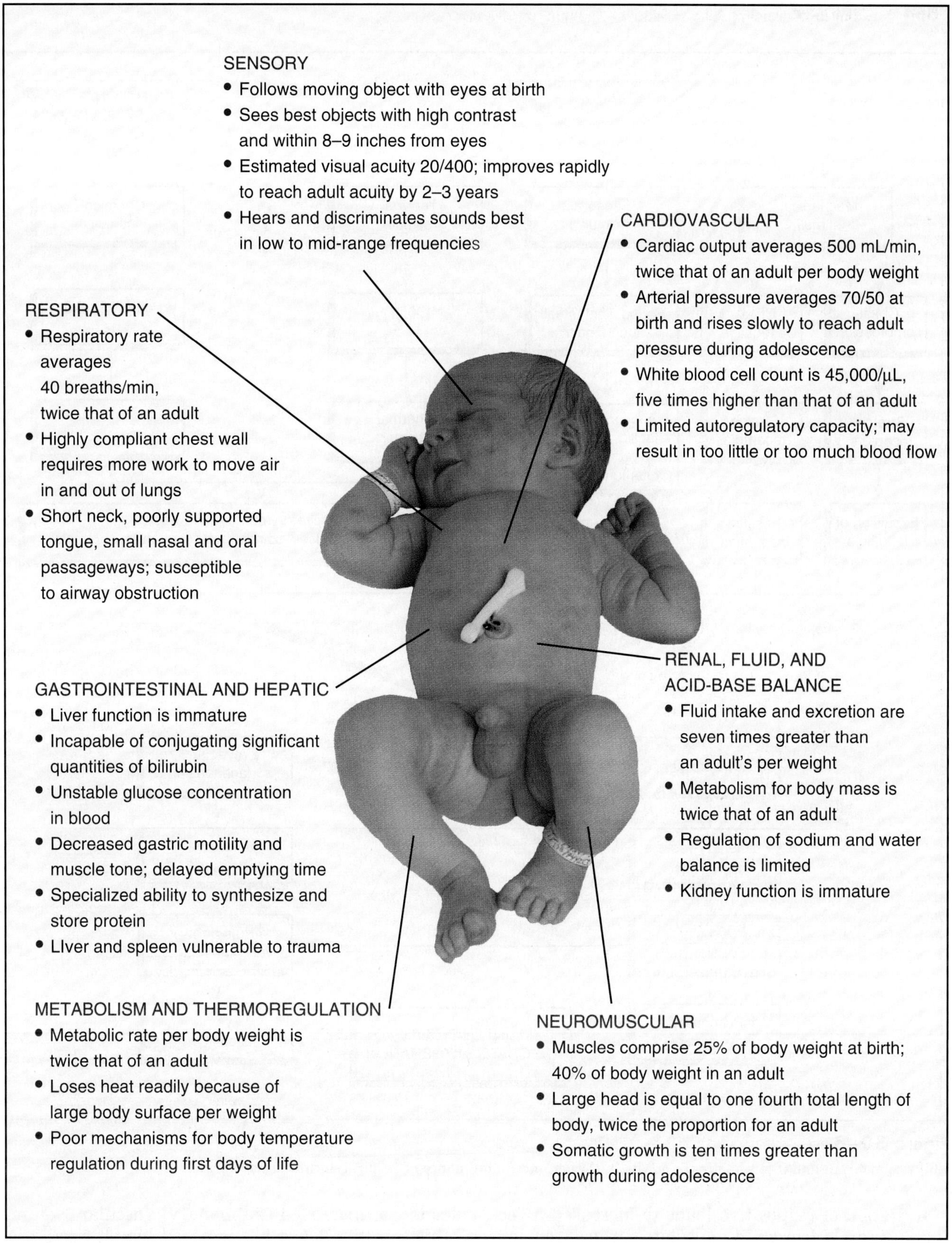

SENSORY

- Follows moving object with eyes at birth
- Sees best objects with high contrast and within 8–9 inches from eyes
- Estimated visual acuity 20/400; improves rapidly to reach adult acuity by 2–3 years
- Hears and discriminates sounds best in low to mid-range frequencies

CARDIOVASCULAR

- Cardiac output averages 500 mL/min, twice that of an adult per body weight
- Arterial pressure averages 70/50 at birth and rises slowly to reach adult pressure during adolescence
- White blood cell count is 45,000/μL, five times higher than that of an adult
- Limited autoregulatory capacity; may result in too little or too much blood flow

RESPIRATORY

- Respiratory rate averages 40 breaths/min, twice that of an adult
- Highly compliant chest wall requires more work to move air in and out of lungs
- Short neck, poorly supported tongue, small nasal and oral passageways; susceptible to airway obstruction

GASTROINTESTINAL AND HEPATIC

- Liver function is immature
- Incapable of conjugating significant quantities of bilirubin
- Unstable glucose concentration in blood
- Decreased gastric motility and muscle tone; delayed emptying time
- Specialized ability to synthesize and store protein
- LIver and spleen vulnerable to trauma

RENAL, FLUID, AND ACID-BASE BALANCE

- Fluid intake and excretion are seven times greater than an adult's per weight
- Metabolism for body mass is twice that of an adult
- Regulation of sodium and water balance is limited
- Kidney function is immature

METABOLISM AND THERMOREGULATION

- Metabolic rate per body weight is twice that of an adult
- Loses heat readily because of large body surface per weight
- Poor mechanisms for body temperature regulation during first days of life

NEUROMUSCULAR

- Muscles comprise 25% of body weight at birth; 40% of body weight in an adult
- Large head is equal to one fourth total length of body, twice the proportion for an adult
- Somatic growth is ten times greater than growth during adolescence

Figure 30–2

Physiologic characteristics of the newborn. Physiologically, the healthy full-term newborn is distinctly different from an adult or even an infant a few weeks older. These unique characteristics influence how the newborn adapts to extrauterine life and what is considered normal. (Data from Blackburn, S. T., and Loper, D. L. (1992). *Maternal, fetal and neonatal physiology: A clinical perspective.* Philadelphia: W. B. Saunders; Polin, R. A., and Fox, W. W. (1992). *Fetal and neonatal physiology.* Philadelphia: W. B. Saunders.

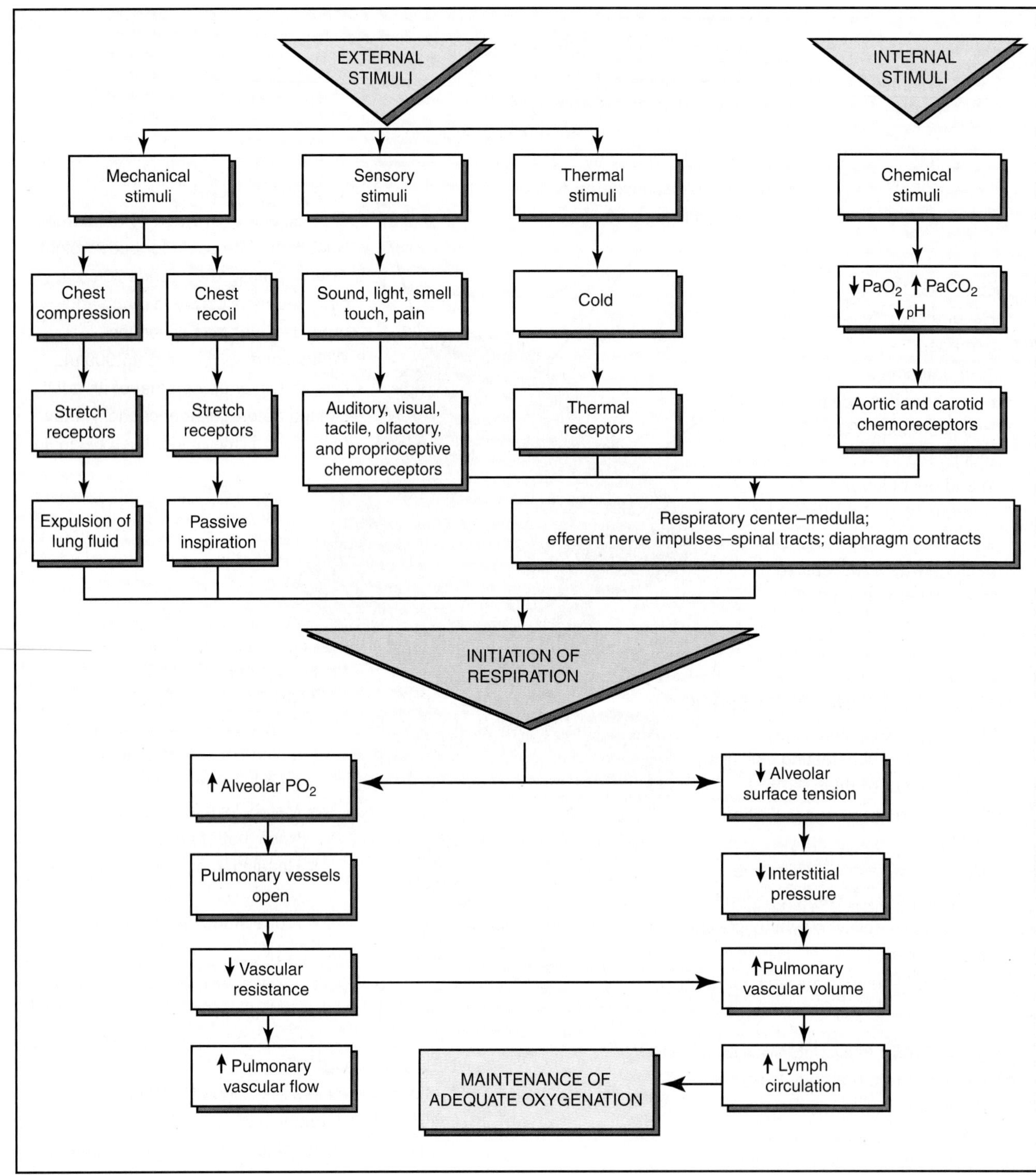

Figure 30–3

Effect of external and internal stimuli on the initiation and maintenance of respiration in the newborn.

Initiation of respiration leads to increased alveolar Po_2 and decreased alveolar surface tension, which allow the lungs to expand more easily. The increased alveolar Po_2 causes the pulmonary vessels to open, resulting in decreased vascular resistance, which leads to increased pulmonary vascular flow. The decreased alveolar surface tension leads to decreased interstitial pressure, which leads to increased pulmonary vascular volume, which in turn leads to increased lymph circulation resulting in the maintenance of adequate oxygenation throughout the body.

The establishment of respirations depends on three basic processes: egress of lung fluid, adequate pulmonary blood flow, and capacity for surfactant production.

UNDERSTANDING THE ABSORPTION OF FETAL LUNG FLUID

- Fetal lungs are filled with fluid (blue) produced by the alveoli that circulates through the amniotic fluid
- Fluid secretion from the alveoli stops during labor, but the air sacs and airways remain filled with fluid
- During vaginal delivery, compression of the fetal chest squeezes out approximately one third of the lung fluid
- After delivery, air (pink) passively enters the lungs as the chest recoils
- The neonate's lungs expand with each breath, forcing the remaining lung fluid into capillaries and lymphatics
- Small residual amounts of fluid are absorbed 6–24 hours following birth; after 24 hours the lungs are filled with oxygen and fluid free

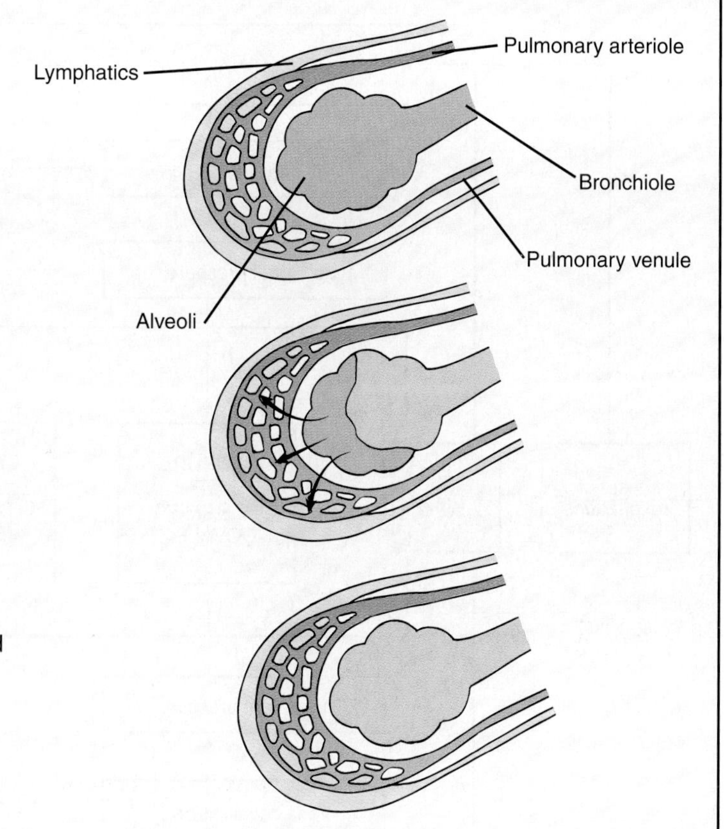

Figure 30–4
The process of absorption of fetal lung fluid after birth.

Egress of Lung Fluid. At birth, the fluid in the terminal air sacs, the alveoli, must be replaced with air. How does this happen? Approximately one third of the lung fluid is expelled through the nose and mouth as the chest is squeezed during vaginal birth. The absence of this "vaginal squeeze" during cesarean birth accounts for a slower removal of lung fluid that is seen in some infants after cesarean births.

The remaining fluid passes through the alveoli into the lymphatics surrounding the lungs during the first few breaths. In healthy newborn infants, the forcefulness of those first breaths is adequate for the passage of lung fluid from the alveoli (Fig. 30–4). Infants with absence of respiratory effort (apnea) or with diminished effort, perhaps due to medications given to the mother, are compromised in their attempt to remove lung fluid.

Adequate Pulmonary Blood Flow. A second factor in respiratory transition involves a five-fold increase in blood flow to the newborn's lungs. In fetal life, only a small blood supply—enough to oxygenate lung tissue—is required. However, from the moment the umbilical cord is cut, the blood supply to the lungs must be sufficient to provide oxygen throughout the body. This is accomplished by the constriction of the ductus arteriosus. Blood from the right ventricle now flows to the lungs, where it can be oxygenated and returned to the left atrium and subsequently to the left ventricle for systemic circulation. The ductus arteriosus normally closes permanently during the first week of life.

Capacity for Surfactant Production. Pulmonary surfactant is a surface-active phospholipid. Because of surfactant, a small amount of air remains in the alveoli at the end of expiration (termed functional residual capacity). This air both decreases the pressure required to distend the lung by preventing the collapse of the alveoli at the time of expiration and prevents wide fluctuations in oxygen and carbon dioxide levels during respiration.

The primary constituent of pulmonary surfactant is lecithin (phosphatidylcholine), which accounts for 64 percent of surfactant; lecithin is also the constituent most important in surfactant function. Pulmonary surfactant is synthesized, stored, and secreted by type II pneumonocytes in the terminal alveoli and bronchioles; these cells become

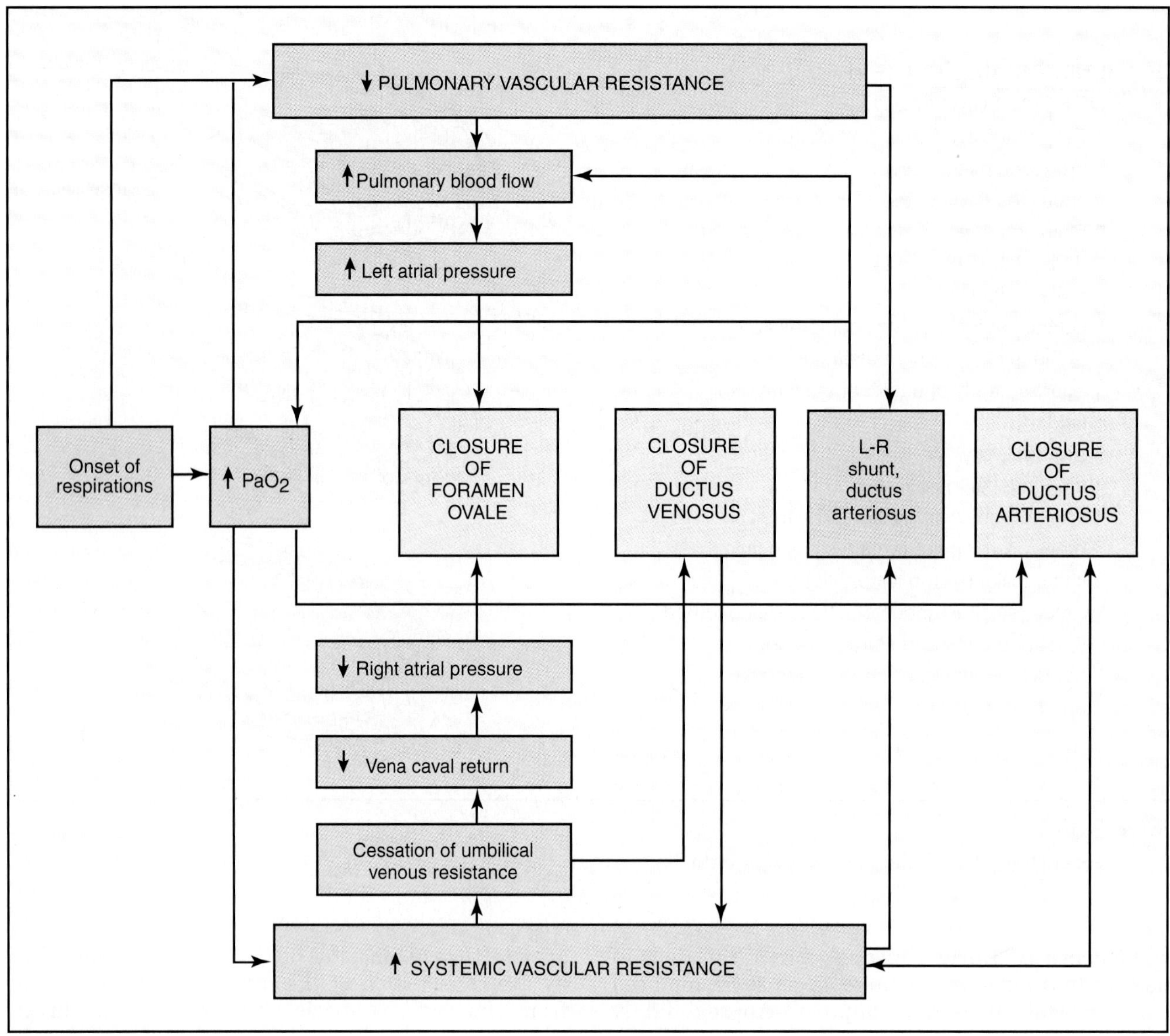

Figure 30–5

The transition from fetal to neonatal circulation is complete at the closure of the foramen ovale, ductus arteriosus, and ductus venosus. (Adapted from Smith, C. A., and Nelson, N. M. (1976). *The physiology of the newborn infant* (4th ed.). Springfield, IL: Charles C Thomas. Courtesy of Charles C Thomas, Publisher, Ltd.)

prominent from 34 to 36 weeks of gestation, which explains the significantly improved pulmonary function in infants born after this period of gestation. Surfactant production is accelerated by certain hormones (including corticosteroids, thyroid hormone, and estrogen) and inhibited by other hormones (including insulin). Perinatal asphyxia also contributes to reduced surfactant synthesis, storage, and release. The implication of surfactant in the care of high-risk newborns is discussed in Chapter 36.

TRANSITIONAL NEONATAL CIRCULATION

The transition from a fetal circulatory pattern, characterized by an essentially single circulation in which blood is shunted away from the lungs and gases are exchanged at the placenta, to a neonatal system of two distinct circulations operating in series in which gases are exchanged in the lung is primarily related to adequate ventilation. Three shunts are involved: the ductus arteriosus, the foramen ovale, and the ductus venosus (Fig. 30–5). In addition, there is a decrease in pulmonary vascular resistance.

The onset of respirations leads to increased Pao_2 (oxygen tension), which results in decreasing pulmonary vascular resistance and increasing peripheral vascular resistance. The changes in the pulmonary and peripheral vascular resistance convert the right-to-left atrial shunt through the foramen ovale into a left-to-right shunt, which closes the foramen ovale. The increased peripheral vas-

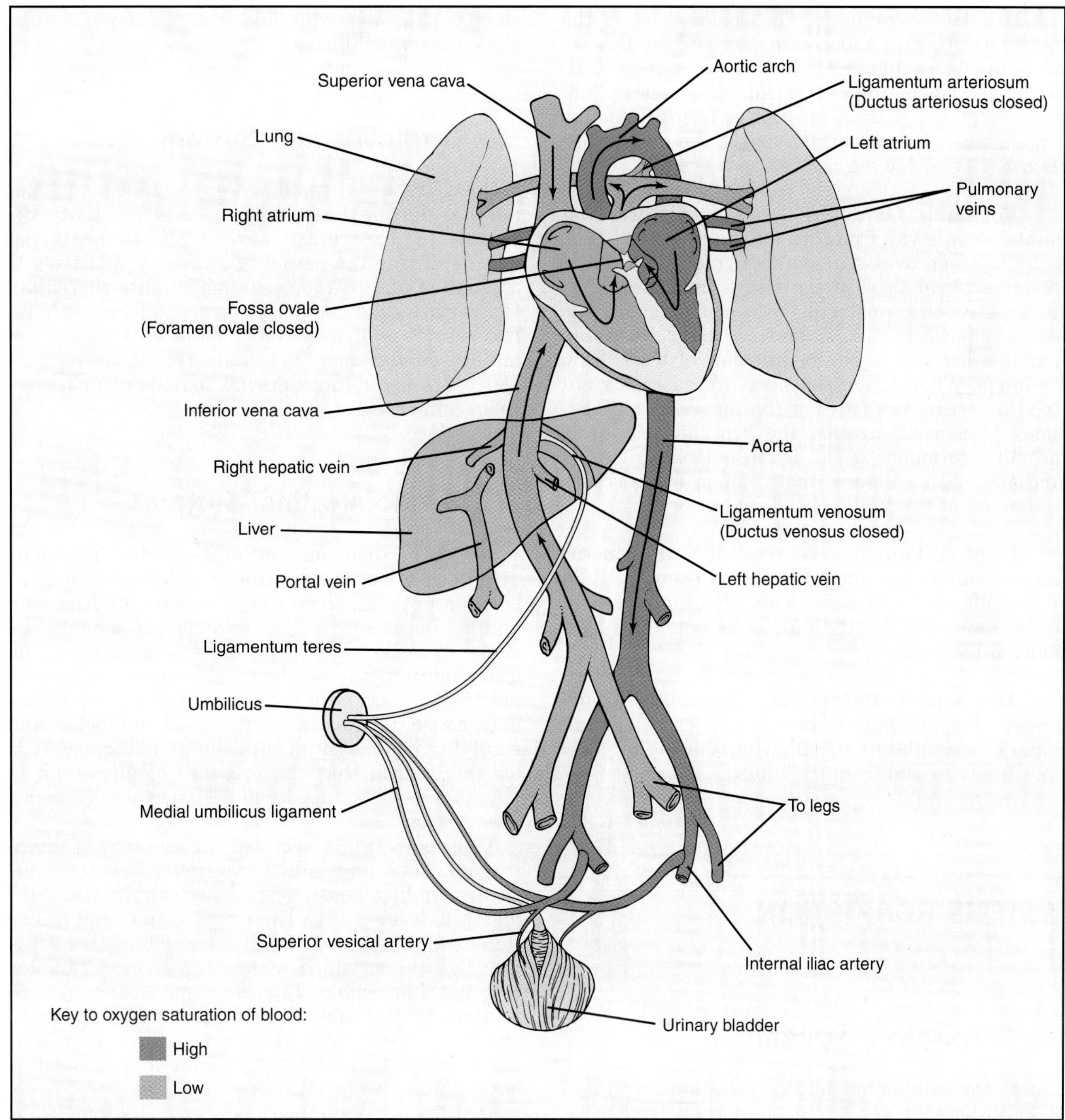

Figure 30–6

Neonatal circulation showing the physiologic changes that occur after birth • The foramen ovale closes and becomes the fossa ovale • The ductus arteriosus closes and becomes the ligamentum arteriosum • The ductus venosus closes and becomes the ligamentum venosum • The umbilical vein becomes the ligamentum teres.

cular resistance leads to a decrease in and finally cessation of umbilical venous return, which causes (1) closure of the ductus venosus and (2) decreasing vena caval return. The decreasing vena caval return leads to decreasing right atrial pressure, which is also a factor in closure of the foramen ovale.

The increased peripheral vascular resistance causes a left-to-right shunt in the ductus arteriosus; closure of the ductus arteriosus follows. The ductus arteriosus is functionally closed within 10 to 15 hours but may remain patent longer in premature infants or infants with persistent hypoxia (Moore 1992).

Ductus Arteriosus. The constriction of the ductus arteriosus, which allows blood to flow to the lungs for exchange of oxygen and carbon dioxide, is described under respiratory changes. Constriction of the ductus arteriosus is mediated by oxygen; when the infant is hypoxic, the ductus has the capacity to remain open or to reopen.

Foramen Ovale. A second structure that shunts blood away from the lungs during fetal life is the foramen ovale, an oval opening between the atria. As blood flow to the lungs increases after the first respirations and the constriction of the ductus arteriosus, the pressure in the left atrium increases because of the return flow of blood from the lungs. When left atrial pressure exceeds right atrial pressure, the valve of the foramen ovale becomes "plastered" against the septum secundum, and the foramen ovale is functionally closed. Anatomic obliteration of the foramen ovale occurs by the end of the first year of life (fossa ovalis).

Ductus Venosus. In fetal life, the ductus venosus shunts umbilical vein blood from the liver to the inferior vena cava. This circulation ceases at the time of birth; the ductus becomes the ligamentum venosum.

Decreased Pulmonary Vascular Resistance. Oxygenation of the lungs leads to pulmonary vasodilatation, allowing blood to flow more freely to and from the lungs.

SYSTEMS ADAPTATION

Respiratory System

After the establishment of respirations, a rate of 30 to 50 breaths per minute is normal for a newborn; rates of 60 to 70 breaths per minute and occasionally as high as 90 breaths per minute for brief periods may occur and are considered normal in the first hour of life. Neonatal breathing is frequently uneven, with brief periods of apnea lasting no longer than 5 seconds and irregularity of both rhythm and depth. This is particularly true during periods of rapid eye movement sleep (see discussion of infant state in Chapter 31). Breathing is most regular when the infant is in a state of deep sleep and least regular during crying, feeding, or motor activity.

Periods of apnea lasting 5 to 15 seconds are characteristic of periodic breathing. Periodic breathing is not associated with either color change or bradycardia, and it is not thought to be associated with illness.

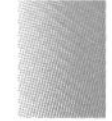

Cardiovascular System

Heart rate is rapid (170 to 180 beats per minute) during the initial period of reactivity, decreases to an average of 120 to 140 beats per minute during the period of inactivity, and rises to a range of 120 to 160 beats per minute thereafter. Heart rate, like respiratory rate, varies with infant state and may fall below 100 beats per minute during deep sleep and rise to as high as 180 beats per minute during periods of motor activity and crying.

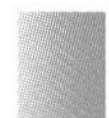

Gastrointestinal System

Secretion, digestion, absorption, and transport are functions of the gastrointestinal tract in newborn infants as they are in older children and adults. In fetal life, gastrointestinal activity includes sucking, swallowing, gastric emptying, and intestinal peristalsis. The meconium in the intestinal tract is normally not emptied; however, anoxia may cause relaxation of the anal sphincter and emptying of meconium into the amniotic sac. It is for this reason that the presence of meconium in amniotic fluid is considered a sign of fetal respiratory distress.

A newborn infant secretes the majority of digestive enzymes and substances necessary to digestion, including pepsinogen, hydrochloric acid, bile, diastase, lactose, invertin, trypsin, and rennin. Little saliva is secreted in the first 3 months. Amylase is lacking, which makes digestion of complex starches impossible. Lipase, important in fat digestion, is minimal. Breast milk contains lipase, and thus the digestion of fat in breast milk is more complete and fat excretion in the stool is lower than with formula feeding.

Structurally, the superior laryngeal sphincter at the proximal end of the esophagus is not firmly closed, and the cardiac sphincter between the esophagus and stomach does not close between swallows. The result is the regurgitation and spitting frequently seen in healthy newborns.

A change in character of the stools is one of the most obvious manifestations of transition in the gastrointestinal tract. Before birth, the intestines are filled with meconium, a dark "tarry" substance that consists of epithelial cells, bile, pancreatic and intestinal secretions, lanugo, and swallowed amniotic fluid. Meconium is usually passed in the first 12 hours after birth, but passage may be delayed as long as 24 to 48 hours. Failure to pass meconium in 48 hours requires evaluation (see

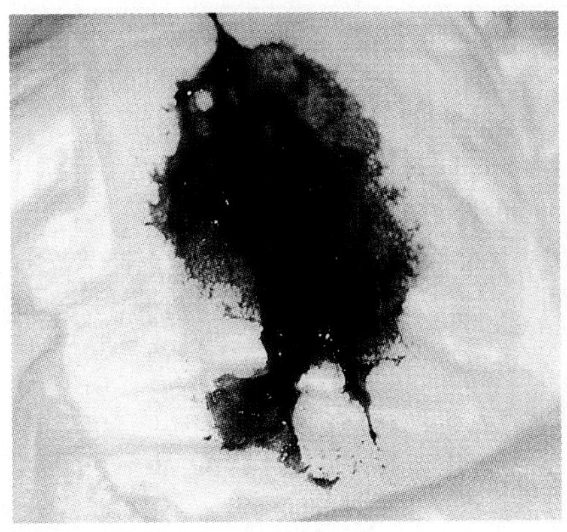
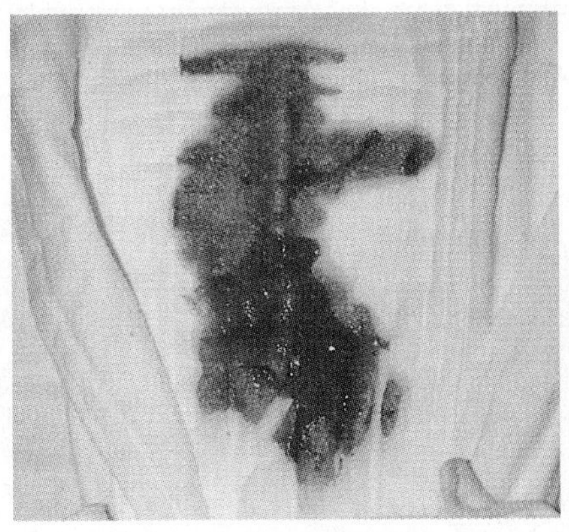
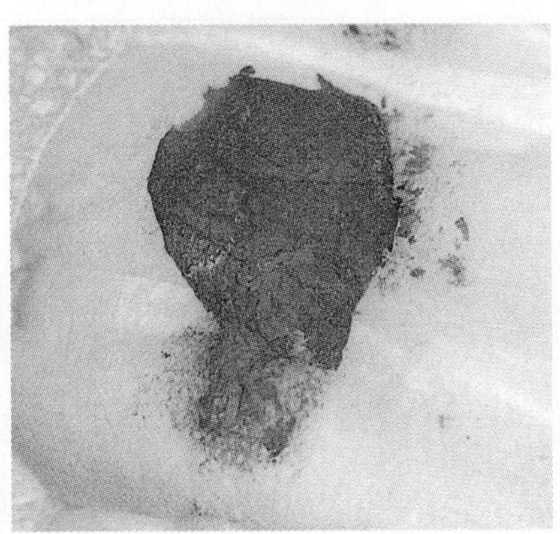

Figure 30–7
The color and consistency of the newborn's stool changes after birth: meconium stool at left, breastfed stool in the middle, and formula-fed stool at right. (Photo of breastfed stool courtesy of Dr. Jan Riordan.)

Chapter 31). By the third or fourth day of life, meconium stools are replaced by transitional stools, which are greenish brown in color and contain both meconium and fecal material. About 2 days later, typical newborn stools are present. These stools vary with the type of feeding. The stools of a breastfed infant are commonly pale to golden yellow in color, soft in consistency, and slightly acidic (pH 4.7 to 5.1). An infant fed formula has a stool that is yellow to light brown in color, firmer than that of a breastfed infant, and more alkaline (pH 6 to 8). The decomposition of protein in formula causes these stools to have a stronger odor. Curds may occur in the stools of both breastfed and formula-fed infants, although they are smaller and less firm in breastfed infants.

Newborns have an active gastroileal reflex that frequently leads to a stool after each feeding. However, there is a great deal of variance in the number of bowel movements in a healthy neonate, from eight to ten each day to one every 2 to 3 days.

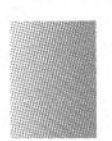

Hematologic and Hepatic Systems

RED BLOOD CELLS AND BILIRUBIN

Jaundice secondary to hyperbilirubinemia of healthy term infants is related to red blood cells (RBCs), to liver function, and to the gastrointestinal tract. Thus, these systems must be considered in relationship to one another.

By the sixth month of fetal life, the bone marrow has become the chief site of blood formation. At the time of birth, most of the marrow space is involved in RBC production. This means that there is little marrow reserve to increase RBC production if any excess hemolysis occurs. The liver and spleen are additional sites of hematopoiesis in the first weeks of life.

Hemoconcentration is a major characteristic of the first hours of life. Hemoglobin concentration rises by as much as 17 to 20 percent in the first 2 hours, then drops slightly but remains elevated until some time between the first and third weeks. Hemoglobin levels range from 17 to 22 g/dL in the term newborn and from 15 to 17 g/dL in the preterm baby. Hematocrit also rises sharply during the first hours of life and then declines slowly; values at 1 week of age are close to values in cord blood (57 to 58 for term newborns; 45 to 55 for preterm infants).

RBCs increase in the first hours to a level of more than 500,000/mm^3 higher than cord blood. The RBCs of the newborn infant are usually larger than those of an older infant; by the end of the second month, cells are close to adult size in term infants.

Fetal RBCs have a life span of approximately 80 to 100 days (adult RBCs have a life span of 120 days). Moreover, cells are increasingly fragile toward the end of this period. Thus, normal destruction occurs during the first days after birth. A byproduct of RBC destruction is bilirubin.

RBC destruction also occurs in fetal life; but while the fetal liver is able to conjugate and excrete bilirubin as early as the second trimester, most fetal bilirubin is excreted across the placenta. Immediately after birth, the liver must conjugate and excrete bilirubin.

The physiologic pathway by which bilirubin is excreted is shown in Figure 30–8. A number of common occurrences and some infrequent occurrences may interfere with this physiologic pathway, resulting in hyperbilirubinemia and neonatal jaundice. Jaundice occurs in 25 to 50 percent of healthy infants born at term and in a higher proportion of preterm infants.

The major causes of increased neonatal bilirubin are physiologic (or pathologic) destruction of RBCs,

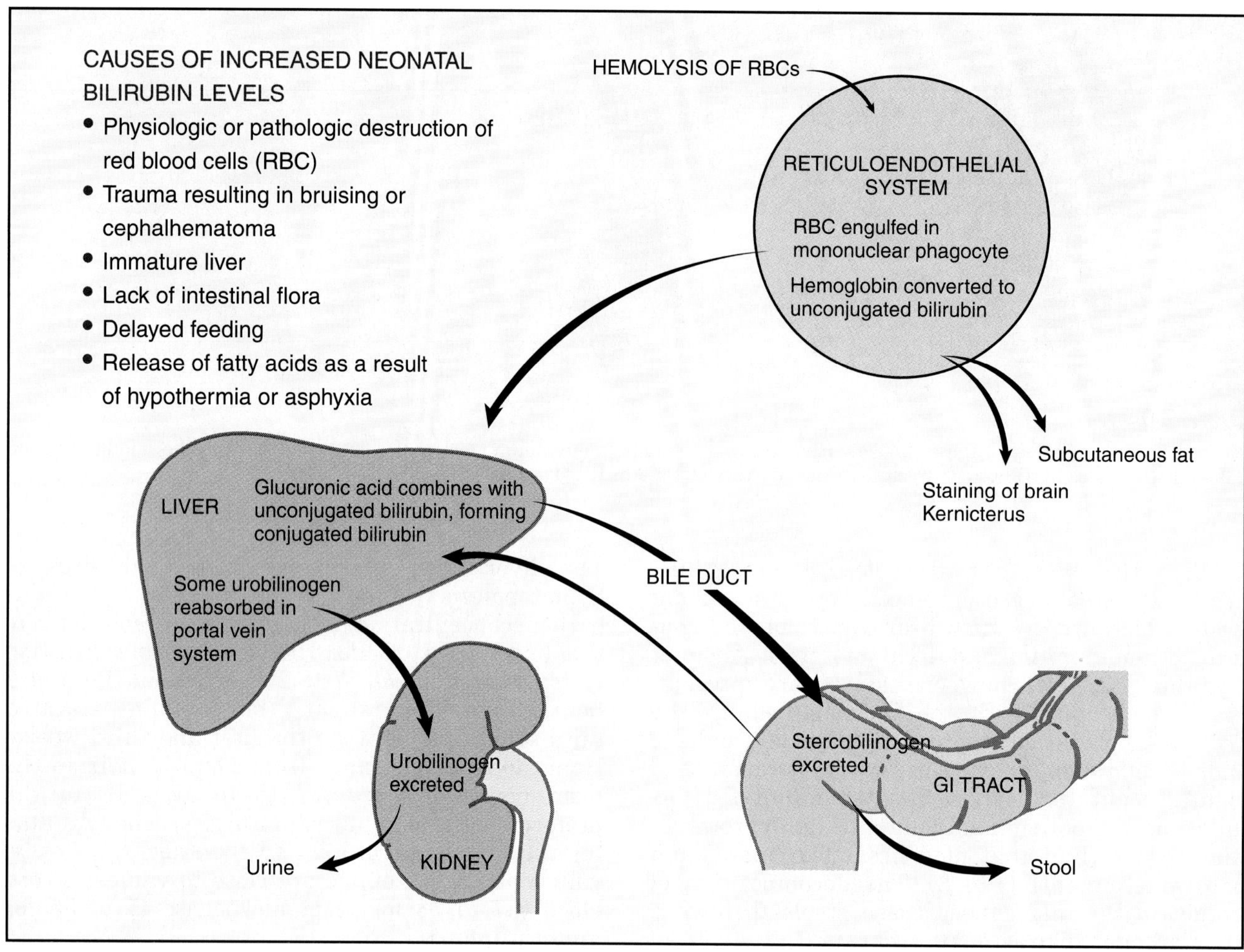

Figure 30–8

The synthesis, transport, metabolism, and excretion of bilirubin.

trauma resulting in bruising or cephalhematoma, liver immaturity, lack of intestinal flora, delayed feeding, and fatty acids as a result of hypothermia or asphyxia. Physiologic jaundice is probably caused by a combination of a number of factors related to the newborn's immaturity.

The clearance of bilirubin in the newborn begins in the reticuloendothelial system, where mononuclear phagocytes clear aging RBCs from the circulation. The hemoglobin is converted to water-insoluble unconjugated bilirubin. To be excreted from the body, this unconjugated bilirubin must be converted to water-soluble conjugated bilirubin. This occurs in the liver, where the bilirubin combines with gluconic acid, forming conjugated bilirubin. The bilirubin is then excreted through both the stool (referred to as stercobilinogen) and the urine (urobilinogen.)

When unconjugated bilirubin is measured in a laboratory test, it is referred to as indirect bilirubin. Conjugated bilirubin is measured as direct bilirubin. Total bilirubin is the sum of measures of direct and indirect bilirubin.

Compared with healthy adults, all neonates could be considered to experience hyperbilirubinemia, because adult bilirubin levels rarely exceed 1 mg/dL. In contrast, neonatal bilirubin levels below 12 mg/dL on the second to seventh days of life are considered within the range of normal; jaundice is visible in the skin at levels from 4 to 6 mg/dL.

Hyperbilirubinemia and jaundice may occur when one or more of the following conditions are present in term newborns. (See Chapter 36 for discussion of jaundice is preterm and sick newborns.)

- Bilirubin is produced at a high rate. The average bilirubin production in the neonatal period is 6 to 8 mg/kg per 24 hours. This rate may be exceeded when there is excessive RBC breakdown, which may occur in certain pathologic processes (see Chapter 36).
- There may be a reduced number of available acceptor proteins (Y and Z proteins) because other substances, such as certain drugs or hydrogen

ions (in infants with acidosis), have already used the binding sites on those proteins.

- The amount of the enzyme glucuronosyltransferase, necessary for conjugation of bilirubin, may be decreased.
- There may be excess beta-glucuronidase, which leads to reconversion of conjugated bilirubin to unconjugated bilirubin in the gastrointestinal tract.
- Delayed passage through the gastrointestinal tract may lead to reconversion to unconjugated bilirubin and subsequent reabsorption.

WHITE BLOOD CELLS

A small increase in white blood cells occurs at birth. After this initial peak, the white blood cell count drops, and leukocytes become markedly less efficient at phagocytosis after the first 24 hours and throughout the first month. The mean number of leukocytes is 18,000 at birth, 12,200 at 7 days, and 11,400 at 14 days. This decrease in number and activity of leukocytes is one factor in the newborn's lowered resistance to infection. White blood cell counts vary widely from infant to infant and even within the same infant from day to day with no apparent reason.

Additional Functions of Hepatic System

Blood coagulation, iron storage, and glucose metabolism are additional functions of the hepatic system.

Important factors in coagulation—prothrombin, factor VII (proconvertin), factor IX (plasma thromboplastin component), and factor X (Stuart-Prower factor)—are synthesized in the liver. Prothrombin levels are low in cord blood. Prothrombin time,* which measures the activity of factors VII and X, may be within normal range or may be low at birth, but it will become most prolonged at 3 to 4 days of life and continue at abnormal levels for 2 to 3 additional days. About 75 percent of term infants and an even larger percentage of preterm infants show this drop in clotting factors. These changes are related to the inability of the baby to synthesize and use vitamin K in the small intestine. The drop in clotting factors means that the infant has a greater risk for hemorrhage than do those infants who have no drop in clotting factors. Giving vitamin K to newborn infants at birth has effectively eliminated hemorrhagic disease of the newborn in healthy term infants (see Chapter 32).

*Factor V (proaccelerin) is also measured in prothrombin time but is of normal levels in the newborn.

The liver is also a site of iron storage. Iron is stored during fetal life, and after birth, iron from the breakdown of RBCs is also stored in the liver. For a baby born at term, iron stores are considered adequate for the first 4 to 6 months of life.

The liver is the organ that stores glycogen, converts glycogen to glucose when serum glucose levels are low, and converts glucose to glycogen for storage. While glycogen is also stored in skeletal muscle, that glycogen is used only for energy in the individual muscle. Only hepatic glycogen is converted to glucose and released into the bloodstream to maintain serum glucose levels.

The need for glucose in the first hours after birth is increased for several reasons: the effort required to initiate breathing, cold stress, muscle activity, and the normal asphyxia of the first minutes of life. At the same time, access to maternal glucose through the placenta has been abruptly interrupted.

After birth, glucose levels drop from 70 to 80 mg/dL to approximately 50 mg/dL. The liver responds to maintain serum glucose in several ways. Glycogen formation is inhibited by changes in hepatic enzymes (as well as by increased production of glucagon by alpha cells and decreased secretion of insulin by beta cells in the pancreatic islet cells). Glycogen stored in the liver during fetal life is mobilized and converted to glucose (glycogenolysis) and used in the first hours, and amino acids and other noncarbohydrates are converted to glucose (gluconeogenesis). (Free fatty acid levels are also increased [lipolysis] in response to norepinephrine, providing additional energy as glycogen stores are depleted.)

As the baby is fed, glucose from milk provides energy and is converted to glycogen. Adult levels of glycogen are found in the liver by the end of the third week of life.

Renal System

At any age, the renal system is a major determiner of both fluid and electrolyte balance. Urine is produced beginning in the twelfth week of gestation, and it is a principal component of amniotic fluid. Just as pulmonary vascular resistance decreases after birth to allow more blood to flow to and from the lungs, so also does the vascular resistance of the renal vessels decrease to allow increased blood flow to the kidneys; a marked improvement in kidney function is seen within a few days after birth. During the first 48 hours after birth, urine output may be 30 to 60 mL. After the third day of life, output is normally between 100 and 300 mL per 24 hours, or approximately 1 to 3 mL/kg per 24 hours.

Kidney function in newborn infants differs from that of older children and adults in several respects. The kidneys of both term and preterm infants have about half the concentrating capacity of the normal adult kidney because of the size of the renal tubules. They function satisfactorily under usual conditions, but they are less able to conserve fluid when the infant is stressed. In an older individual, scanty urine is a fairly reliable sign of dehydration; but because of the newborn's limited ability to conserve water by concentrating urine, urinary output may not decrease. Concentration of urine approaches adult levels at approximately 3 months of age.

In addition to having a limited ability to concentrate urine, newborns are less able to eliminate excess water rapidly because of a decreased glomerular filtration rate. There is limited excretion of solutes in neonatal urine; there is also a limited capacity to reabsorb hydrogen and sodium ions. Urine may initially appear cloudy, because of mucus, and may contain uric acid crystals that are "pinkish."

FLUID AND ELECTROLYTE BALANCE

Fluid and electrolyte balance in newborns is more labile than that of adults not only because of a relatively immature renal system but also because of several other factors. Metabolic rates in the newborn are higher. A newborn produces 45 to 50 calories per kilogram of body weight every 24 hours. The basal metabolic level for adults in the same period is 25 to 30 calories per kilogram. Since metabolism uses water, a higher rate of metabolism uses a proportionately larger quantity of water.

The larger surface area of the newborn in relation to body mass means a higher ratio of water loss through evaporation; the rate of loss per kilogram is twice that of an adult. Evaporative loss is even higher in preterm infants.

The proportion of water in relation to total body mass is greater than at any other period of life—a total of 70 to 75 percent in term infants and 85 percent in infants of 28 weeks' gestation. About 30 to 35 percent of total body weight in the newborn is extracellular water, compared with 25 percent in the older infant and 20 percent in adults. Because of this, the infant has proportionately less reserve; any fluid loss or lack of intake will deplete the extracellular fluid rapidly. In a 24-hour period, an infant excretes about 50 percent of the extracellular water; in the same period, an adult excretes only about 14 percent. A large part of the difference between the newborn and the older infant disappears by the time the baby is 10 days old. The loss of this large proportion of extracellular water accounts for much of the weight loss that occurs in the first 3 days of life.

As might be expected, because of the rapid exchange of water, electrolytes are also exchanged rapidly. Sodium and potassium balances are especially likely to be affected. Any loss of fluids and secretions caused by vomiting, diarrhea, and gastric suction also results in the loss of sodium, chloride, and potassium.

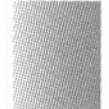

Immunologic System

The role of the immunologic system is to protect the infant from infection and, when infection occurs, to mobilize a defense system that attacks and defeats the invading organisms. Immunologic defenses are both general and specific.

General defenses include the protection offered by the skin and mucous membranes, the process of phagocytosis, and the general inflammatory response system. In newborn infants, there are several portals of entry in the skin and mucous membranes: the vessels of the umbilical stump, the circumcision site, and potential breaks in an epidermis that is more fragile than that of older infants. Phagocytosis, the process by which microorganisms and other cells and foreign particles are ingested, is less efficient. Newborns are less able to concentrate antiinflammatory cells and thereby localize infection; local infections are more likely to become systemic in infants than in older children.

Specific immunologic defenses involve the immunoglobins IgG, IgM, IgA, IgD, and IgE. IgG, IgM, and IgA are more important in the neonatal period. These immunoglobulins contain antibodies to specific bacterial and viral antigens (Table 30–1).

Although the fetus forms low levels of IgG beginning at 20 weeks, most of the IgG present at birth is transferred from the mother across the placenta by 33 weeks' gestation. (An infant born before 33 weeks would have a deficiency of IgG.) IgG protects against those organisms for which the mother has antibodies. Antibodies are commonly present for streptococcus, pneumococcus, meningococcus, and *Haemophilus influenzae;* diphtheria and tetanus; and many viruses, including measles, mumps, and poliovirus. The period of protection afforded by this passive immunity lasts, on the average, approximately 3 months, but the length of protection varies for individual organisms. IgG does not protect the newborn against Group B streptococcal infection and gram-negative organisms such as *Escherichia coli.*

IgM is a large molecule that does not cross the placenta; normal levels of IgM in the newborn are below 20 mg/dL. The fetus is capable of producing IgM; levels of IgM above 20 mg/dL at birth are considered a sign of intrauterine exposure to an antigen.

IgA has two forms. Serum IgA does not cross the placenta and is not normally produced by the

Table 30–1

IMMUNOGLOBULINS IN THE NEONATAL PERIOD

IMMUNOGLOBULIN	SOURCE	PROTECTS AGAINST	DOES NOT PROTECT AGAINST	COMMENTS
IgG	Mother	Streptococcus Pneumococcus Meningococcus *Haemophilus influenzae* Viruses Diphtheria Tetanus	Enteric gram-negative rods	IgG lowest 2–4 months after birth
IgM	Fetus, if exposed to antigen in utero	All infectious agents		Levels above 20 mg/dL in newborn suggest intrauterine infection
Serum IgA	Not detectable in infants at birth	Respiratory and gastrointestinal infections		
Secretory IgA	Breast milk			Produces immunity in mucosal surfaces of intestine

fetus. Secretory IgA occurs in high levels in colostrum, a yellowish fluid that precedes breast milk. Secretory IgA provides immunity on the mucosal surfaces of the intestine and protects against gastrointestinal disease.

Neurologic System

From early in fetal life until the end of the second year after birth, the infant's brain is continuously developing. While all of the neurons of the brain are formed by 26 weeks' gestation, the development, arborization (branching), and myelinization of the brain will not be complete for many months.

Unlike some functions, such as those of the respiratory and cardiac systems, neurologic function undergoes no marked change at birth. A fetus slept and wakened, listened, responded to touch, and was capable of a variety of other neurologic responses before birth. After birth, an infant's ability to console herself or himself with hand to mouth activity, move from one state to another, respond to voices (particularly the voices of mother and father), and many similar behaviors are signs of central nervous system integrity. Neurologic integrity is also evaluated through assessment of neonatal reflexes (see Chapter 31).

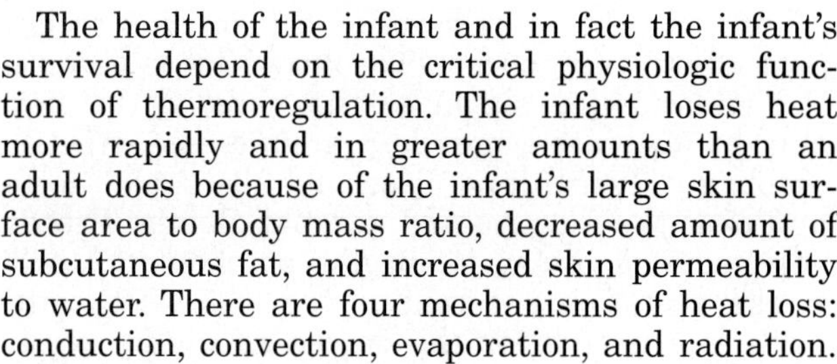

THERMOREGULATION

The health of the infant and in fact the infant's survival depend on the critical physiologic function of thermoregulation. The infant loses heat more rapidly and in greater amounts than an adult does because of the infant's large skin surface area to body mass ratio, decreased amount of subcutaneous fat, and increased skin permeability to water. There are four mechanisms of heat loss: conduction, convection, evaporation, and radiation.

Heat loss through conduction occurs when the baby is on a cold mattress, blanket, scale, or table and heat from the baby's body is transferred to the colder object. In convection, air moves across the baby's skin and heat is transferred to the air. Evaporation of moisture from wet body surfaces or hair dissipates heat along with the moisture. Ra-

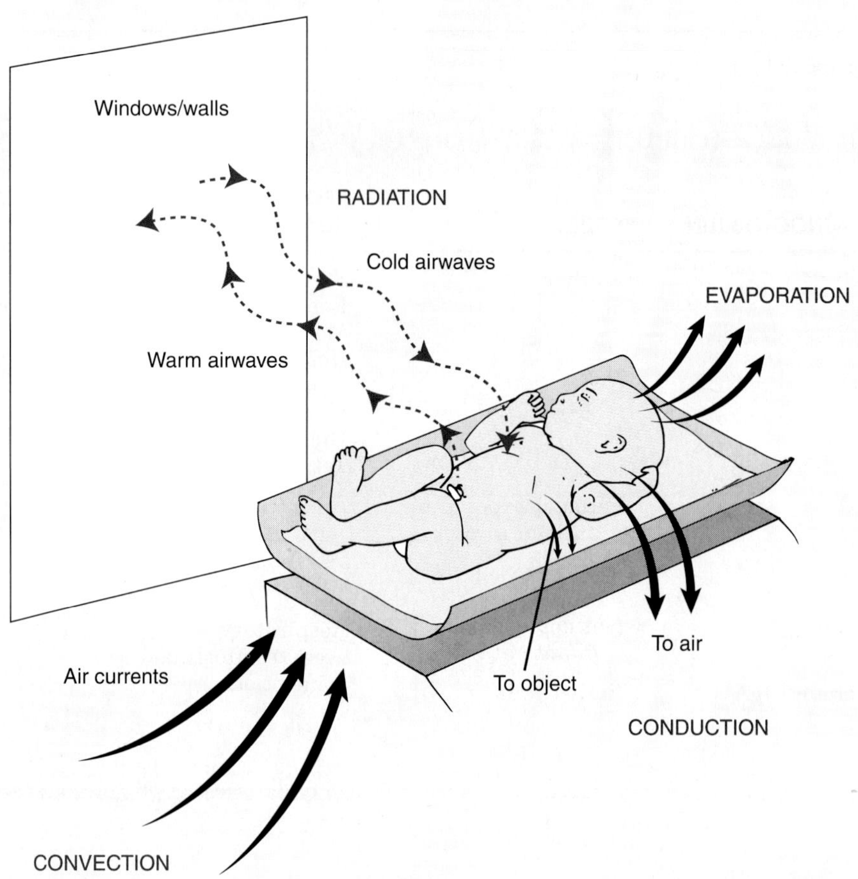

Figure 30–9
Methods of heat loss.

diation occurs when heat from the baby's body radiates to a colder surface, such as a cold incubator wall or outside wall (Fig. 30–9).

Newborns must rely mostly on brown adipose tissue to produce heat, and their ability both to regulate their body temperature and to produce heat is limited during the early neonatal period. The amount of brown fat stores varies with the weight of the infant and the infant's specific genetic makeup. In the term newborn, brown fat accounts for 2 to 7 percent of the infant's weight (Blackburn and Loper 1992). Brown fat is found in the midscapular region at the nape of the neck and at the neck muscles; around the trachea, esophagus, heart, lung, liver, and abdominal aorta; and over the kidneys and adrenal glands. The development of brown fat begins at about 26 to 30 weeks' gestation and continues 3 to 5 weeks after birth, accounting for the decreased ability of the preterm and very-low-birth-weight infant to regulate temperature. Heat loss depends a great deal on the baby's external surroundings. If the external surroundings are cool, the baby will lose heat. If the surroundings are too warm, the baby can easily become overheated. For the newborn, placement in a supportive thermal environment—appropriate temperature, clothing, freedom from drafts—is critical to thermal regulation (Blackburn and Loper 1992).

The provision and maintenance of adequate warmth decreases complications in the newborn and mortality, especially in small babies. Hypothermia leads to increased metabolic rate, which increases oxygen requirements, increases glucose requirements, and increases caloric requirements. These changes can cause the following complications: accentuation of respiratory distress syndrome, hypoglycemia, and loss of weight. Severe hypothermia can cause disseminated intravascular coagulation (see Fig. 30–10).

SENSORY CAPABILITIES AT BIRTH

Mothers and fathers have long reported that their infant could see and hear and was sensitive

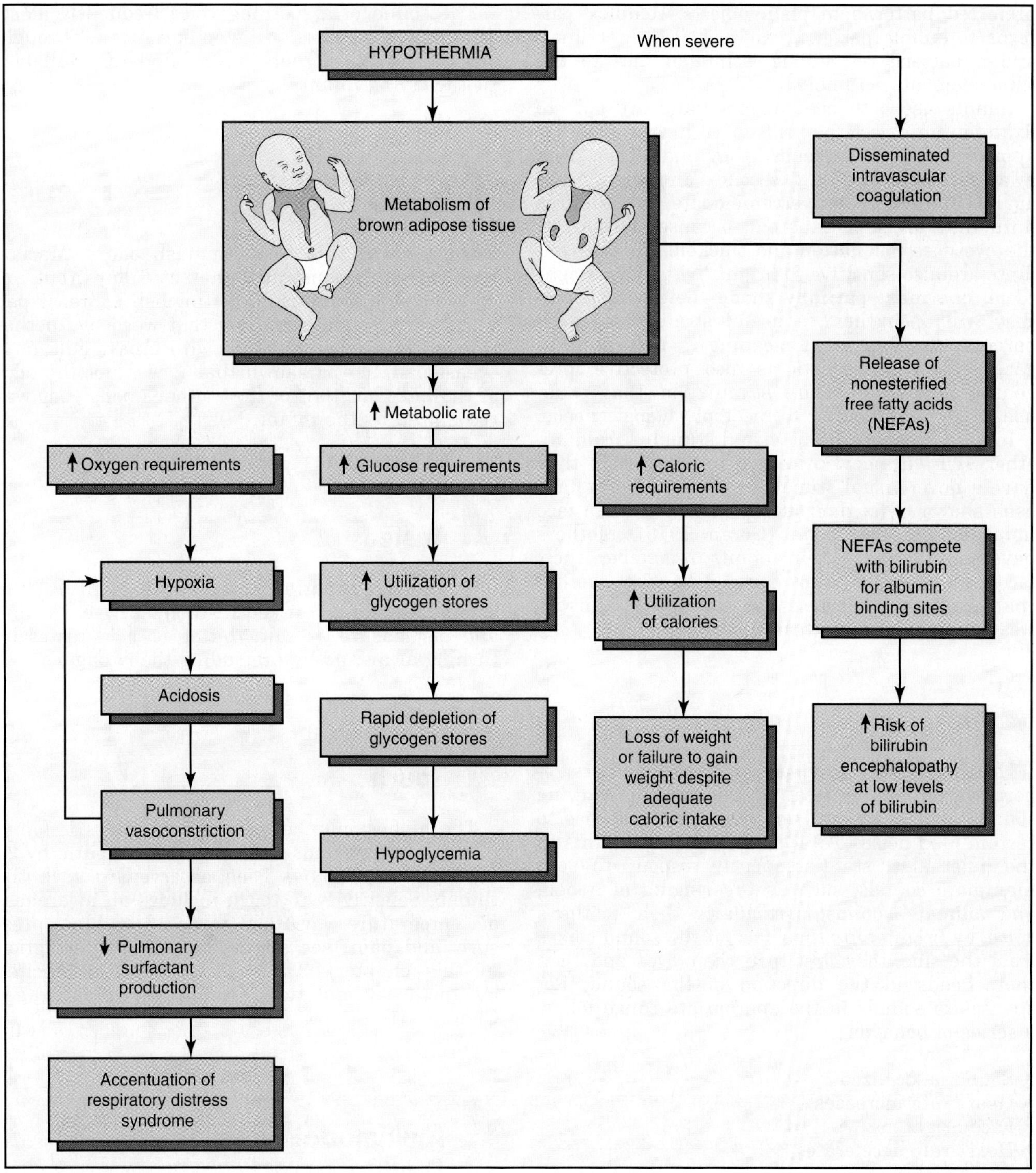

HYPOTHERMIA

When severe

Metabolism of brown adipose tissue

↑ Metabolic rate

↑ Oxygen requirements

Hypoxia

Acidosis

Pulmonary vasoconstriction

↓ Pulmonary surfactant production

Accentuation of respiratory distress syndrome

↑ Glucose requirements

↑ Utilization of glycogen stores

Rapid depletion of glycogen stores

Hypoglycemia

↑ Caloric requirements

↑ Utilization of calories

Loss of weight or failure to gain weight despite adequate caloric intake

Disseminated intravascular coagulation

Release of nonesterified free fatty acids (NEFAs)

NEFAs compete with bilirubin for albumin binding sites

↑ Risk of bilirubin encephalopathy at low levels of bilirubin

Figure 30–10
The effects of hypothermia (cold stress) on the newborn.

to taste. Before the 1960s, however, there was little scientific evidence to support these observations. In the decades of the 1960s and 1970s, a series of creative experiments demonstrated that newborn infants enter life with well-developed sensory capabilities.

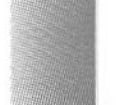

Vision

Fantz (1961, 1963, 1964), in a series of experiments, demonstrated that newborn infants not only could see and distinguish between objects and patterns but showed clear preferences. Infants preferred patterns to plain objects, complex patterns to simple patterns, curves to straight lines, and a pattern resembling a human face to the same elements scrambled.

Infants use both eyes together and are able to fixate on an object that is 8 to 10 inches away for approximately 10 seconds; they may then look away for about 1 to 1.5 seconds and then fixate again. Infants do not accommodate to distances until they are 4 months old, because the lens of the eye does not flatten and thicken. Newborn infants are also sensitive to bright lights; in a bright room, one must partially shade their eyes before they will open them, a useful strategy to teach parents who find great meaning in their infant's gaze. This characteristic is also protective, preventing excessive visual stimulation that could use the energy needed to meet physiologic needs.

Infants distinguish one visual stimulus from another and will show increased interest when they have a novel visual stimulus to view. Infants have been shown to fix their attention on a human face immediately after birth (Goren 1975). Mothers have noticed that their infants remember their faces and will appear puzzled if the mother changes her appearance, for example, begins to wear glasses or stops wearing them.

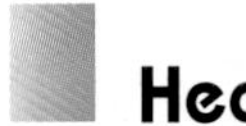

Hearing

Hearing is well developed in utero. Mothers report variation in fetal movement to varying sounds, with high levels of activity in response to certain loud noises. After birth, newborn infants in the quiet alert state frequently respond to both inanimate sounds, such as the ringing of a bell, and animate sounds, particularly their mother's voice, by brightening their face; if the sound comes from the side, they first turn their eyes and then their heads in the direction of the sound. Responses to sounds in the appropriate range follow a series of behaviors:

- Sound is localized
- Heart rate increases
- Face brightens
- Heart rate decelerates
- Breathing slows
- Infant alerts and searches for sound

DeCasper and Fifer (1980) designed a series of experiments in which newborn infants could control the sounds they heard by varying the speed at which they sucked on a nipple. Their findings showed that babies had a preference for a woman's voice over a man's voice, for the voice of the mother over the voice of another woman, but not for the voice of the father over the voice of another man.

The sound of a soothing voice frequently alerts an infant; the infant will stop and listen. Throughout the world, mothers have found that lullabies soothe crying infants.

Smell

Infants are able to distinguish odors. Macfarlane (1975) demonstrated that at 6 days (but not at 2 days), infants could distinguish a breast pad worn by their mothers from that worn by another woman. In further research with breast milk on a breast pad, it was shown that it was not the odor of the milk but that of the mother's body that was recognized by the infant.

Taste

Taste discrimination is present at birth. Infants show pleasure at sweet taste by active sucking and displeasure at salty, bitter, or acid tastes by turning away and by protruding their tongues.

Touch

The highest number of touch receptors is found in the infant's hands and around the mouth; by 24 weeks, the fetus has been observed to suck the thumb. Sensitivity to touch includes an awareness of temperature variation, texture, stroking, pressure, and pain (see discussion of pain perception in this chapter). The rooting reflex is elicited by tactile stimulation around the mouth (see Chapter 31).

Multimodal Sensory Development

Not only are newborn infants able to use individual senses, they can also integrate the input from more than one sense. When an infant hears a sound (a bell or a voice, for example), the infant turns the head and visually searches for that sound. Infants associate particular sights (their mother's face, for example) and sounds (their mother's voice) and will show surprise if their mother's voice comes from an unfamiliar face (their mother's voice behind a mask).

Habituation

Habituation is the term used to describe a lack of response to a stimulus after prolonged exposure to that stimulus. When a visual object or a sound is first presented, the infant may pay attention or respond depending on his or her state; but as the same stimulus is presented several times in succession, the baby will become less responsive. The process of habituation explains why an infant can go to sleep in the midst of ordinary household noise but will be startled by unusual sounds or will show less interest in a visual stimulus after it has been presented several times.

Pain Perception

The ability of newborn infants to perceive pain is an important consideration in planning nursing care. In previous decades, it was suggested that neonates could not perceive pain. Anand and Hickey (1987) reviewed the evidence for neonatal perception of noxious stimuli.

- Sensory receptors are present on all cutaneous and mucous surfaces by 20 weeks' gestation.
- Sensory receptors are present in the spinal cord beginning at 6 weeks' gestation and are complete by 30 weeks' gestation.
- Pain pathways to the brain stem and thalamus are myelinated by 30 weeks' gestation.
- Neurotransmitters for pain are present at 12 to 16 weeks' gestation.
- Behavioral evidence of pain (increased heart rate, fluctuations in transcutaneous partial pressure of oxygen, and sweating of the palms) has been demonstrated in newborns.

Today it is agreed that the anatomic, functional, and neurochemical structures required for pain perception are present in newborn infants and that infants express pain through their behaviors.

Infants make a series of adjustments beginning at the moment of birth. The healthy term infant is uniquely ready from physiologic and behavioral perspectives to begin the adventure of life. Nurses can help parents appreciate these characteristics in their infant and thus foster the best possible development in the weeks ahead.

Implications for Research

Although there is a solid foundation of literature related to the physiologic development and adaptation of the newborn, most of the research was done during the 1960s and 1970s with limited numbers of infants. (For example, the work by Arnold and colleagues (1965) on the physiologic and behavioral characteristics of infants during the first 6 hours was based on 61 infants.) There is a need to validate the research that exists in terms of its appropriateness for infants today.

A major area for research is determination of the basic behavior and physiologic changes during the transitional period (the first 6 hours after birth). These include heart rate, respiration, muscle tone and posture, color, presence of mucus, peristalsis and stools, temperature, and alerting and sleep behaviors. This information is important to identify infants at risk for problems and deviations from normal so that interventions can be enacted as early as possible.

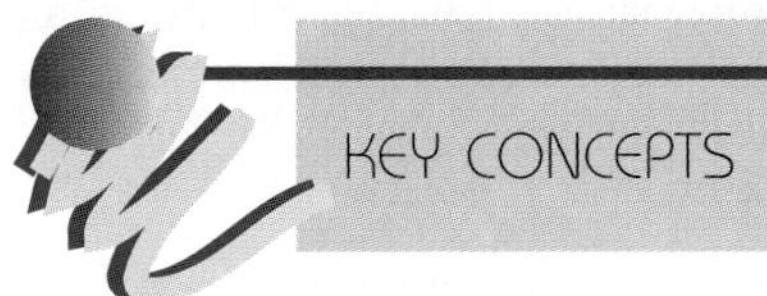

KEY CONCEPTS

- ▼ The first 6 hours of life are a transitional period in which a newborn experiences an orderly pattern of physiologic and behavioral changes.
- ▼ A healthy term newborn differs physiologically from an infant just a few weeks older; assessments that would suggest abnormality in a 3-week-old infant may be within the range of normal for a 3-day-old infant.
- ▼ The two categories of stimuli that initiate respirations are termed external and internal. External stimuli include mechanical, sensory, and thermal stimuli. Internal stimuli are chemical stimuli and include decreased PaO_2, increased $PaCO_2$, and decreased pH.
- ▼ The successful establishment of respirations involves three basic processes: egress of lung fluid, adequate pulmonary blood flow, and capacity for surfactant production.
- ▼ In the fetal circulation, blood is shunted away from the lungs and gases are exchanged in the placenta. The transition to a neonatal circulatory pattern involves the closure of the shunts so that gases are exchanged in the lungs.
- ▼ The characteristics of newborn breathing after respirations are established include a usual rate of 30 to 50 breaths per minute that may vary to 60 to 70 breaths per minute or occasionally reach 90 breaths per minute; breathing is frequently uneven, with periods of apnea lasting up to 5 seconds.
- ▼ Newborn heart rate varies with infant state and may fall below 100 beats per minute dur-

ing deep sleep and rise to as high as 180 beats per minute during periods of motor activity and crying. A range of 120 to 160 beats is considered normal beginning with the second period of reactivity.

- ▼ The character of stools changes during the transition period. Before birth and up to 24 hours to 2 to 3 days after birth, meconium (a dark "tarry" substance) is passed. Transitional stools (greenish brown) are then passed. After that, stools of breastfed babies vary from pale to golden yellow, and formula-fed infants have stools from yellow to light brown.
- ▼ Meconium is usually passed within 12 hours after birth; if meconium is not passed within 24 hours, a problem may exist and further evaluation of the gastrointestinal system is needed.
- ▼ Hemoglobin concentration rises by as much as 17 to 20 percent in the first 2 hours, then drops slightly but remains elevated until some time between the first and third weeks.
- ▼ Jaundice occurs in 25 to 50 percent of healthy infants born at term and in a higher proportion of preterm infants.
- ▼ Laboratory tests refer to unconjugated bilirubin (water insoluble) as indirect bilirubin and to conjugated bilirubin (water soluble) as direct bilirubin. Total bilirubin is the sum of measures of direct and indirect bilirubin.
- ▼ In comparison to adults, all neonates have a high bilirubin level. Adult levels up to 1 mg/dL are usual; in neonates, levels up to 12 mg/dL from the second to seventh days of life are considered normal.
- ▼ The newborn has an increased need for glucose in the first few hours because of the energy needed to initiate breathing, cold stress, muscle activity, and the normal asphyxia of the first minute of life.
- ▼ Urine output during the first 48 hours after birth may be 30 to 60 mL. After the third day of life, output is normally between 100 and 300 mL per 24 hours, or approximately 1 to 3 mL/kg per 24 hours.
- ▼ Fluid and electrolyte balance in newborns is labile because (1) a high metabolic rate uses a large quantity of water and (2) a large surface area in relation to body mass results in a high rate of water loss through evaporation. Because the proportion of water in relation to total body mass is high (70 to 75 percent in term infants, 85 percent at 28 weeks' gestation), fluid loss or lack of intake will affect a newborn much more rapidly than an older infant or adult.
- ▼ The development of the infant's brain begins in early fetal life and continues through the second year of life. All the neurons are formed by 26 weeks' gestation, but branching of neurons and myelinization continue for months after birth.
- ▼ The infant loses heat more rapidly and in greater amounts than an adult does because of the infant's large skin surface area in porportion to body mass, minimal amounts of subcutaneous fat, and high degree of skin permeability to water.
- ▼ The anatomic, functional, and neurochemical structures required for pain perception are present in newborn infants; infants express pain through their behaviors.

References

Anand, K., and Hickey, P. (1987). Pain and its effects in the human neonate and fetus. *New England Journal of Medicine,* 317, 1321–1329.

Arnold, H. W., Putnam, N. J., Barnard, B. L., Desmond, M. M., Rudolph, A. J. (1965). Transition to extrauterine life. *American Journal of Nursing,* 65 (10), 77–80.

Barnard, K., Blackburn, S., Kang, R., Spietz, A. (1978). *Early parent-infant relationships. Series 1, Module 3, The first six hours of life.* White Plains, NY: The National Foundation/March of Dimes.

Burnard, E. D., Todd, D. A., Hindmarsh, K. W. (1982). Beta-endorphin levels in newborn cerebrospinal fluid. *Australian Paediatric Journal,* 18, 258–263.

Daze, A., and Scanlon, J. (Eds.). (1985). *Neonatal nursing.* Baltimore: University Park Press.

DeCasper, A., and Fifer, W. (1980). Of human bonding: Newborns prefer their mothers' voices. *Science,* 208, 1174–1176.

DeCasper, A., and Prescott, P. (1984). Human newborns' perception of male voices: Preference, discrimination, and reinforcing value. *Developmental Psychobiology,* 17 (5), 481–491.

Desmond, M. M., Franklin, R. R., Vallvona, C., Hill, R. M., Plumb, R., Arnold, H., Watts, J. (1963). The clinical behavior of the newly born. I. The term baby. *Journal of Pediatrics,* 62, 307–325.

Fantz, R. (1961). The origin of form perception. *Scientific American,* 204, 66–72.

Fantz, R. (1963). Pattern vision in newborn infants. *Science,* 140, 296–297.

Fantz, R. (1964). Visual experience in infants: Decreased attention to familiar relative to novel ones. *Science,* 146, 668–670.

Goren, C., Sarty, M., Wu, P. (1975). Visual following and pattern discrimination of facelike stimuli by newborn infants. *Pediatrics,* 56, 544–549.

Holmes, D., Reich, J., Pasternak, J. (1984). *The development of infants born at risk.* Hillsdale, NJ: Lawrence Erlbaum Associates.

Johnson, C. C., and Strada, M. E. (1986). Acute pain response in infants; a multidimensional description. *Pain,* 24, 373–382.

Korones, S. (1981). *High-risk newborn infants.* St. Louis: C. V. Mosby.

Macfarlane, A. (1975). Olfaction in the development of social preferences in the human neonate. In *CIBA Foundation Symposium, 33: Parent-infant interaction.* New York: Associated Scientific Publishers.

Owens, M.E., and Todt, E. H. (1984). Pain in infancy: Neonatal reaction to a heel lance. *Pain,* 20, 77–86.

Polin, R., and Burg, F. (1983). *Workbook in practical neonatology.* Philadelphia: W. B. Saunders.

Porter, F. (1989). Pain in the newborn. *Clinics in Perinatology,* 16 (2), 549–569.

Prechtl, H., and Beinlima, O. (1964). *The neurological examination of the full term newborn infant.* London: Heinemann.

Sparks, J. W. (1992). Physiology of growth. In R. A. Polin and W. W. Fox (Eds.), *Fetal and neonatal physiology* (p. 199). Philadelphia: W. B. Saunders.

Tatzer, E., Schubert, M., Timischl, W., Simbruner, G. (1985). Discrimination of taste and preference for sweet in premature babies. *Early Human Development,* 12 (1), 23–30.

Teitel, D. (1988). Circulatory adjustments to postnatal life. *Seminars in Perinatology,* 12 (2), 96–103.

Wolff, P. (1966). The causes, controls, and organization of behavior in the neonate. *Psychological Issues,* 5 (1, Whole No. 17), 7–11.

31 Chapter

> Assessment tools offer the parent-child clinician a systematic and refined method of pinpointing strength, as well as problems, in early development. Assessment tools also help clinicians corroborate or reevaluate clinical impressions of parent and infant needs and coping abilities. . . . Assessment tools do not replace traditional clinical observations and data collection methods. They simply augment the traditional skills and sensitivities that clinicians bring to clients.
>
> LORRAINE O. WALKER, PATRICIA KAY AVANT, KATHERINE M. TAYLOR, AND JOY H. PENTICUFF (1982)

Neonatal Assessment

Mary Lou Moore
Francine H. Nichols

HIGHLIGHTS

- Health History
- Apgar Score
- Assessment of Vital Signs
- Procedure 31–1: Assessing Vital Signs in the Newborn
- Assessment of Growth
- Procedure 31–2: Weighing and Measuring the Newborn
- Maturational Assessment of Gestational Age (New Ballard Score)
- Determining the Relationship Between Infant Size and Gestational Age
- Mortality Risk Assessment
- Physical Assessment
- Assessment of Elimination
- Laboratory Assessment
- Procedure 31–3: Using the Heal Stick Method to Obtain Blood
- Procedure 31–4: Assessing Blood Glucose Level
- Neurologic Assessment Related to Reflexes and Sensory Assessment
- Infant States Related to Behavioral Assessment (Brazelton's Neonatal Behavioral Assessment Scale)
- Follow-up Assessments After Initial Postbirth Period
- Risk Management
- Implications for Research

DEFINITIONS

Apgar score—A systematic evaluation of an infant's adaptation to extrauterine life according to five criteria: heart rate, respirations, reflex irritability, muscle tone, and color.

Brazelton Neonatal Behavioral Assessment Scale (BNBAS)—An assessment tool that can be used to measure certain aspects of infant behavior and identify individual differences in infant behavior. It can be used as a diagnostic tool for neurologic impairment or to teach parents the unique social and interactive capabilities of their newborn. The tool is designed for infants from birth to 1 month of age.

Caput succedaneum—Edema in the tissues of the presenting part that may cross the suture lines of the skull bones.

Cephalhematoma—A collection of blood between the cranial bone and the periosteum that does not cross the suture lines of the skull bones.

Distress/disengagement cues—Behavioral cues that indicate the infant's lack of organization and signal a need for a time-out period of rest and recuperation.

Gestational age assessment—An evaluation of the infant that includes assessment of 11 external physical characteristics and 10 neurologic signs to estimate gestational age of the infant.

Mongolian spots—Areas of dark pigmentation, often mistaken for bruises, that are common in black and other dark-skinned babies. They are typically found on the sacrum or buttocks and disappear of their own accord by early childhood.

Neonatal assessment—An evaluation of the health status of the infant that includes maternal, obstetric, and perinatal history; gestational age assessment; physical assessment; and behavioral assessment.

Stability/engagement cues—Behavioral cues indicating that an infant has good organization and is ready to participate in an interaction.

Assessment of the neonate forms the foundation for making accurate nursing diagnoses and planning and implementing appropriate nursing care. Assessment of the neonate is a critical function of the nurse immediately after birth, on an ongoing periodic basis during the early days after birth, and thereafter as needed during well-baby examinations or if the infant is ill.

The purposes of neonatal assessment are to

- Identify prenatal influences on health status and determine risk status
- Provide baseline information on the infant for use as a reference marker
- Identify anomalies, actual health problems, or potential health problems
- Plan appropriate nursing care for the infant and identify teaching needs of the parents

Neonatal assessment includes evaluation of maternal, obstetric, and perinatal history; gestational age assessment; physical assessment; and behavioral assessment.

HEALTH HISTORY

The beginning of a nursing assessment of any client focuses on that person's health history. When the person is newly born, that history must necessarily focus on the parental preconception period and on maternal and fetal events in the prenatal and intrapartum periods that provide a context for neonatal physical and behavioral assessment. Physical examination of the infant may suggest additional questions related to history. The presence of one or more obstetric risk factors does not automatically lead to a neonatal problem.

Maternal factors that are essential to consider in the assessment of the newborn are summarized in Table 31–1. The relationship between risk factors and neonatal outcome is described in Chapter 36.

TYPES OF ASSESSMENTS

Neonatal assessments can be classified as immediate, subsequent, and ongoing. Immediate assessment includes an Apgar score at 1 and 5 minutes after birth and an initial physical assessment when the nurse notes any obvious problems.

In subsequent assessments within the first hours of life, gestational age is assessed; weight,

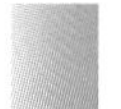

Table 31–1

MATERNAL HISTORY RELATED TO NEONATAL ASSESSMENT

Social and Family History
Absence of prenatal care
Maternal age
Marital status and support systems
Substance abuse
Cigarette use
Exposure to environmental hazards
Family history of genetic disorders
Family history of other disorders
Nutritional History
Inadequate maternal weight gain during pregnancy
Maternal Medical History
Endocrine (diabetes, thyroid disorder)
Cardiovascular (heart disease, hypertension)
Hyperphenylalaninemia
Pulmonary (asthma, pneumonia)
Renal (chronic disease, repeated infections)
Systemic lupus erythematosus
Epilepsy
Hematologic (sickle cell, Rh isoimmunization)
Cancer
Maternal infection
Medications taken during pregnancy
Maternal Reproductive History
Previous perinatal loss, including infant with congenital anomaly
Placental abnormalities
Malformations of cervix, uterus
Maternal Intrapartum History
Precipitous or prolonged labor
Prolonged rupture of membranes
Difficult delivery
Cesarean delivery
Meconium
Analgesia and anesthesia

length, and head and chest circumferences are measured; and complete physical and neurologic assessments are performed. Screening tests for phenylketonuria and hypothyroidism are conducted after the baby has been feeding for 72 hours.

Ongoing assessment includes vital signs (temperature, pulse, and respirations), any changes noted in physical assessment, assessment of behavior (including state), and assessment of parent-infant interaction.

Apgar Score

Dr. Virginia Apgar, an anesthesiologist, devised the Apgar score in the early 1950s to focus systematic attention toward the newborn infant immediately after birth (Apgar 1953). Apgar evaluation should occur precisely at 1 minute and 5 minutes after birth for consistency with established norms. In most birth rooms, a timer is set at birth to facilitate accurate timing of this important assessment. The 1-minute Apgar score indicates the need for resuscitation, although resuscitation efforts are frequently initiated before 1 minute. The 5-minute score is one evaluation of the infant's response to resuscitation. At some delivery sites, a 10-minute Apgar score is also recorded when the infant has required resuscitation.

Apgar scoring is performed by systematically observing the following characteristics; observations are scored as 0, 1, or 2.

1. Assess the infant's heart rate for a full minute through auscultation (at the precordium) or palpation of the umbilical cord pulse at the site where the umbilical cord enters the abdominal wall. Absent heart rate is scored 0. A rate below 100 beats per minute is scored 1; a rate of 100 or above is scored 2.
2. Assess unassisted respiratory rate for a full minute by auscultation and by observing movements of the chest. Absence of respiratory effort is scored 0; effort that is slow, irregular, or shallow is scored 1; regular respiration, accompanied by a strong cry, is scored 2.
3. Assess the infant's response to stimulus (or reflex irritability) by observing behavior when mucus is suctioned from the nares or by gently rubbing the infant's back. If there is no response, the score is 0; a grimace or frown is scored 1; a vigorous cry, sneeze, or cough is scored 2.
4. Assess muscle tone by extending the infant's arm or leg; when the limb is released, it should return to a state of flexion in a term infant. Note also the resistance of the limb to extension. If the limb is limp and flaccid, the score is 0; mild resistance and flexion is scored 1; active motion with spontaneous flexion is scored 2.
5. Note the infant's color. Most newborns are cyanotic to some degree at 1 minute. Acrocyanosis (i.e., cyanosis of the extremities) may persist for several hours. Some observers believe that few babies are pink all over at 1 minute or even at 5 minutes. If the infant is cyanotic or pale all over, the score is 0; if the

body is pink but the extremities are cyanotic, the score is 1; total pink color, including the extremities, is scored 2.

Apgar scoring is summarized in Table 31–2.

Advantages of Apgar Scoring. Apgar scoring directs attention toward the infant at 1 and 5 minutes. The technique is widely accepted, is easily learned, and has clear parameters; it is fast and inexpensive and requires no special equipment.

Disadvantages of Apgar Scoring. Although the parameters are clearly defined, Apgar scoring is a subjective measure, particularly if the scoring is done by a health care provider who thinks that a low score may reflect poorly on caregiving.

Apgar scores were not conceived as a measure of long-term outcome; nor are they good predictors. Even among severely depressed infants with Apgar scores of 3 or less at 5 minutes, fewer than 5 percent will have cerebral palsy (Paneth and Stark 1983). Moreover, Apgar scores do not correlate well even with severe acidosis at the time of birth (Sykes et al. 1982; Silverman et al. 1985).

For nursing practice, these studies suggest that (1) expert neonatal resuscitation is of value even when Apgar scores are low; (2) in most instances, parents can be reassured, even when Apgar scores are low; and (3) some infants with high Apgar scores (higher than 7 at 5 minutes) may subsequently develop acidosis, and thus all newborns should continue to be assessed carefully during the transition to extrauterine life.

Significance of Apgar Scoring. A healthy newborn has an Apgar score of 7 to 10 at both 1 minute and 5 minutes. These infants rarely need resuscitation. A second group of infants, with Apgar scores from 3 to 6, are considered moderately depressed. They frequently need some resuscitation and also require more careful observation during the first days of life. Infants with Apgar scores of 0 to 2 are severely depressed and require intensive resuscitation. (Resuscitation is discussed in Chapter 36.)

Assessment of Vital Signs

Auscultation of heart rate, breath sounds, and bowel sounds (bowel sounds are discussed under assessment of the abdomen) is best accomplished when the infant is in a quiet state, at the beginning of the assessment period. Temperature may also be assessed at this time after the auscultation of heart rate, breath sounds, and bowel sounds. Procedure 31–1 outlines the steps in vital signs assessment.

Temperature. An infant's temperature is assessed by placing the thermometer in the infant's axilla and holding it in place for 5 minutes. The axillary method is considered safer than the rectal method, which may damage rectal tissue. At some birth sites, an initial rectal temperature is taken to assess anal patency. Alternatives for assessment of anal patency include observation of the first stool, digital examination, or insertion of a sterile flexible rubber catheter.

Table 31–2

APGAR SCORING

SIGN	0	1	2
Heart rate	Absent	Below 100	Above 100
Respiratory effort	Absent	Minimal; weak cry	Good; strong cry
Muscle tone	Limp	Some flexion of extremities	Active motion; extremities well flexed
Reflex irritability (response to stimulation on sole of foot)	No response	Grimace	Cry
Color	Blue or pale	Body pink; extremities blue	Pink

From Apgar, V., Holaday, D. A., James, L. S., Weisbrot, I. M., Berrien, C. (1958). Evaluation of the newborn infant—second report. *The Journal of the American Medical Association,* 168 (15), 1985–1988.

PROCEDURE 31–1

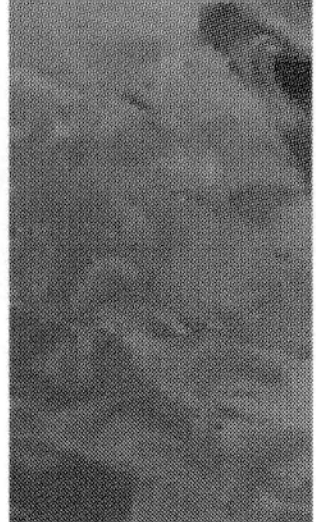

Assessing Vital Signs in the Newborn

▼ PURPOSE

To determine the newborn's respirations, heart rate, and temperature so that abnormalities can be detected and appropriate interventions initiated. Respirations and heart rate are usually measured every hour for the first 4 hours of life and then every shift. Temperature is usually assessed every hour for the first 4 hours of life, every 4 hours for the remainder of the first 24 hours, and then every shift.

▼ EQUIPMENT

- Infant stethoscope
- Doppler device
- Glass thermometer or electronic thermometer
- Probe cover
- Tympanic temperature device

Respirations

1 While the infant is quiet or sleeping, observe and count the respirations for a full minute. Observe the newborn's abdomen rising and falling; palpate the abdomen lightly to determine its rise and fall with each inspiration and expiration. **Counting respirations for 1 minute ensures an accurate assessment because the newborn is a periodic breather (periods of apnea lasting less than 15 seconds are normal). Observing and palpating respirations while the infant is quiet promotes accurate assessment. Palpation aids observation in determining the respiratory rate. Normal respiratory rate varies from 30 to 60 breaths per minute when the infant is not crying.**

2 Observe for normal characteristics of respirations as well as for signs of respiratory abnormalities. **Breath sounds should be clear. Respirations should be shallow and irregular in rate, rhythm, and depth. Respirations should come from the abdomen rather than the chest. Signs of abnormal respirations, including expiratory grunting, nasal flaring, retractions, cyanosis, and seesawing, should be absent.**

3 Record your findings in the newborn's chart. **Respiratory rate and characteristics should be recorded in the chart to facilitate detection of abnormalities and initiation of appropriate interventions.**

Heart Rate and Blood Pressure

1 Auscultate and count, with an infant stethoscope, the newborn's heart rate for 60 seconds at the apex of the heart, which is located to the left of the midclavicular line at

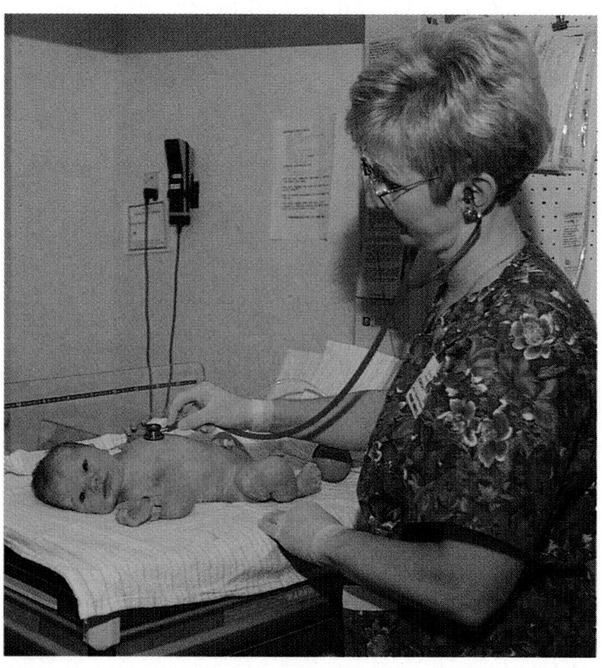

Continued on facing page

PROCEDURE 31–1 Continued

the third or fourth intercostal space. Listen, observe, and count the heart rate (apical pulse rate) when the newborn is quiet or sleeping. If necessary, use a pacifier to soothe a crying infant before assessing heart rate. **The small infant stethoscope allows better contact and more accurate determination of the heart rate and sounds than the larger stethoscope does. Heart sounds are more audible when the newborn is quiet.**

2 Note heart rate and record it in the newborn's chart. **Recording the heart rate facilitates detection of abnormalities and initiation of appropriate interventions. The normal heart rate is 120 to 160 beats per minute.**

3 Listen for heart murmurs or other abnormalities, such as alterations in rhythm. **If a gallop rhythm is heard, heart failure is suspected. Heart murmurs are not unusual in the first days after birth and are usually related to incomplete closure of fetal heart structures.**

Palpating brachial pulse

Palpating femoral pulses

4 Palpate brachial and femoral pulses. **Pulses should be strong, regular, and equal bilaterally.**

5 Blood pressure is not routinely assessed in healthy term newborns. If assessment of blood pressure is necessary, use a correctly sized neonatal cuff (no wider than two thirds of the infant's upper arm). Usually an electronic monitor is used because it is more accurate. **Blood pressure is usually assessed only if an abnormality or problem is suspected or if the infant is ill. The normal range for blood pressure in term infants is 60 to 90 mm Hg for systolic pressure and 40 to 50 mm Hg for diastolic pressure.**

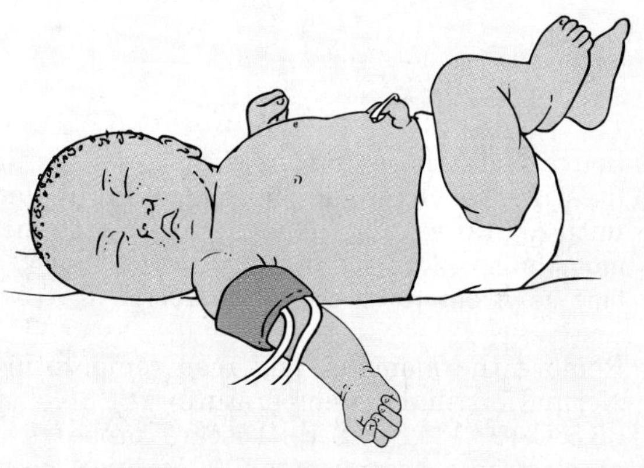

Axillary Temperature

1 Prepare the thermometer. A glass or an electronic thermometer may be used. If an electronic thermometer is used, place a cover on the probe and turn it on. Wear gloves if the neonate has not been bathed. **Gathering and preparing the appropriate equipment facilitates completing the procedure effectively. Placing a cover on the probe prevents cross-contamination. Wearing gloves before the first neonatal bath is consistent with Standard Precautions.**

2 Expose the baby's axilla; if it is moist, pat it dry. **Moisture can interfere with an accurate temperature reading. Friction can raise the temperature.**

Continued on following page

PROCEDURE 31–1 Continued

3 Place the thermometer in the axilla; fold the infant's arm over the chest and hold. **Keeps thermometer in place.**

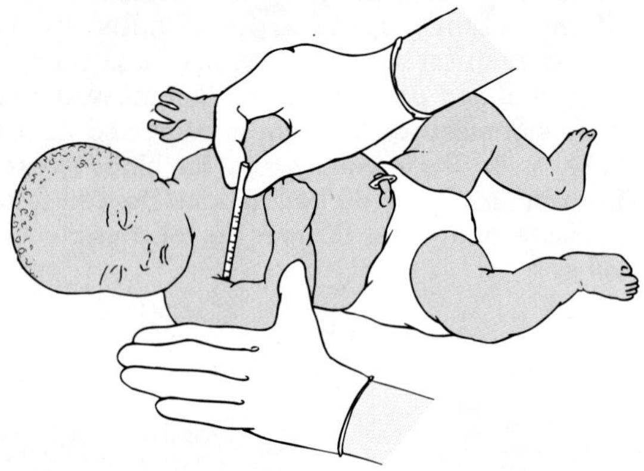

4 Leave glass thermometer in place for 5 minutes. Leave electronic thermometer in place until digital reading appears. **Leaving the thermometer in place for the prescribed amount of time helps ensure an accurate reading.**

5 Remove thermometer and read temperature. Normal axillary temperature is 36.0 to 36.5°C (97.1 to 97.8°F). Discard probe cover of electronic thermometer. **A separate probe cover is used for each infant to prevent the spread of microorganisms.**

6 Record findings in newborn's chart. Record immediately for accuracy. **If temperature is not within the normal range, interventions must be initiated to maintain temperature within the normal range.**

Rectal Temperature

1 Prepare thermometer. If a rectal glass thermometer is used, wipe the cleaning solution off if necessary (use a circular motion, proceeding from the end opposite the bulb to the bulb). Shake down the thermometer. If an electronic thermometer is used, place a cover on the probe and turn the unit on. **Gathering and preparing the appropriate equipment facilitates completing the procedure effectively. Wiping a glass thermometer ensures removal of fecal material and allows better visualization of temperature. Shaking down the thermometer helps ensure an accurate reading. Placing a cover on the probe prevents cross-contamination.**

2 Lubricate the thermometer or probe cover 1.5 to 2.5 cm (0.5 to 1.0 inch). **Lubricating the thermometer or probe cover facilitates insertion by reducing friction.**

3 Place the baby either on the back (while holding legs up) or on the abdomen. The baby must be held securely so that he or she cannot move. **These positions facilitate insertion of the thermometer. Holding the legs firmly ensures that the baby does not sustain injury from the thermometer.**

4 Insert the thermometer into the baby's rectum no more than 0.5 inch. Do not force. **Gentle technique minimizes trauma; the newborn may not have a patent anus.**

5 Hold glass thermometer in place for 5 minutes, holding legs. Hold electronic thermometer in place for 10 to 20 seconds until digital reading appears. (Note: Neonates will often have a stool.) **Leave the thermometer in place for the prescribed amount of time to ensure an accurate reading. Peristalsis or passing a stool may force the thermometer out of the rectum.**

6 Remove thermometer and read temperature. Normal rectal temperature is 36.5 to 37.0°C (97.6 to 98.6°F). Discard probe cover of electronic thermometer. **A separate probe cover is used for each infant to prevent cross-contamination.**

7 Record findings in newborn's chart. **Record route used; temperature varies by route. Recording findings facilitates detection of abnormalities and initiation of appropriate interventions.**

Tympanic Temperature

The tympanic membrane temperature device may be used if the infant's ear canals are

Continued on facing page

PROCEDURE 31–1 Continued

free of vernix and moisture (usually after 24 hours).

1 Attach the probe cover according to manufacturer's directions. **Attaching a probe cover prevents cross-contamination.**

2 Insert the probe into the external auditory canal gently; the probe must occlude the canal. **Gentle insertion prevents injury. The external auditory canal must be occluded to obtain an accurate temperature.**

3 Leave the thermometer in place for 1 second or for the amount of time indicated by the manufacturer. **Leaving the thermometer in place for the prescribed amount of time helps ensure an accurate reading.**

4 Remove the thermometer and read the temperature. Normal tympanic temperature is 36.5 to 37.0°C (97.6 to 98.6°F). Discard probe cover. **A separate probe cover is used for each infant to prevent cross-contamination.**

5 Record findings in newborn's chart. **Note that tympanic route was used; temperature varies by route.**

Normal axillary temperature is 36.0 to 36.5°C (97.1 to 97.8°F) (Blackburn and Loper 1992, p. 680.) If initial temperature is outside the range of normal, further assessment to determine the cause and nursing intervention to maintain temperature in the normal range are essential. In healthy term infants in whom temperature is within the normal range, assess temperature each hour for the first 4 hours of life and every 4 hours for the remainder of the first 24 hours. Routine temperature assessment is not necessary after discharge, although mothers should be taught how to take their baby's temperature in case it is needed at home.

▼ **Heart Rate.** Heart rate is counted for 60 seconds at the apex of the heart, located to the left of the midclavicular line at the third or fourth intercostal space. Immediately after birth, normal heart rate may vary from 100 to 160 beats per minute; after the transition period, the range is 120 to 160 beats when the infant is not crying.

Two heart sounds, a first and a second sound of equal intensity, should be heard. If heart sounds are indistinct, there may be air in the pleural cavity (pneumothorax) or in the mediastinum, in the midchest between the pleurae (pneumomediastinum). Heart failure also results in indistinct sounds. If three heart sounds (a gallop rhythm) are heard, heart failure is suspected. Heart murmurs are not unusual in the first days after birth and are most often related to incomplete closure of fetal heart structures. However, the presence of a murmur, as well as any finding related to heart sounds, should be noted in the infant's health record.

▼ **Respiratory Rate and Breath Sounds.** Respiratory rate varies from 30 to 60 breaths per minute when the infant is not crying. All infants are periodic breathers, with periods of respiration intermixed with brief periods (approximately 5 to 10 seconds) without breathing. No color change accompanies normal periodic breathing. Inspiratory and expiratory periods are approximately equal. Abnormal respiratory signs include expiratory grunting, nasal flaring, and retractions.

Tachypnea, a respiratory rate greater than 180, may be related to respiratory or cardiac disease. However, tachypnea may also be transient. Transient tachypnea is most common in infants after cesarean birth and is believed to be related to the presence of excess fetal lung fluid, which is normally expelled when the infant passes through the vagina. Infants with transient tachypnea rarely have retractions but may have mild cyanosis and occasionally need small amounts of oxygen. Their rapid breathing may interfere with feeding; thus, both the infants and their parents will need extra attention at feeding time. Transient tachypnea is usually limited to the first 24 to 28 hours of life, by which time the excess fetal lung fluid is resorbed.

▼ **Blood Pressure.** Blood pressure is not routinely assessed in healthy term infants. The range of normal for blood pressure in term infants is 60 to 90 mm Hg for systolic pressure and 40 to 50 mm Hg for diastolic pressure.

ASSESSMENT OF GROWTH

Weight. Infants are weighed shortly after birth and each day if they remain in the birth center. The infant is always undressed for weighing, and the scale is covered with a clean disposable pad to prevent cross-contamination and to lessen loss of the infant's body heat to the scale through conduction. In the United States, the average infant weighs 7.5 pounds (3.5 kg) at term. Ninety-five percent of term infants weigh 5.5 to 10 pounds (2.5 to 4.6 kg).

Birth weight is the baseline value for future assessment of weight. A healthy term infant should not lose more than 10 percent of body weight and will usually regain the weight by age 7 to 10 days.

PROCEDURE 31–2

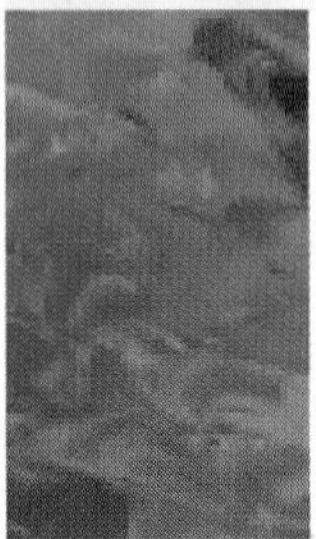

Weighing and Measuring the Newborn

▼ **PURPOSE**

The newborn is weighed to determine whether weight loss after birth is normal and to determine whether nutritional intake is adequate for growth. The newborn is weighed at birth to provide a basis for evaluating further growth and daily thereafter (daily weights are compared with birth weight).

▼ **EQUIPMENT**

- Scale
- Cover sheets
- Paper tape measure

Weighing

1 Place cover sheet (Chux pad or other disposable paper pad) on scale. Wear gloves if newborn has not been bathed. **The cover sheet prevents cross-contamination and lessens heat loss by conduction. Wearing gloves is consistent with Standard Precautions.**

2 Adjust the scale balances to 0, or push the appropriate pads on the digital scales, using a protective barrier on your hand. **Adjusting the scale appropriately ensures an accurate reading. Using a paper towel or other protective barrier prevents cross-contamination.**

3 Place naked newborn supine on scale, holding your hand above the newborn. Compare weight with birth weight. **Newborns should not lose more than 10 percent of birth weight. Newborns regain their birth weight by 7 to 10 days of life and then gain about 1 ounce per day in the first 6 months of life. Holding your hand above the newborn is a protective measure.**

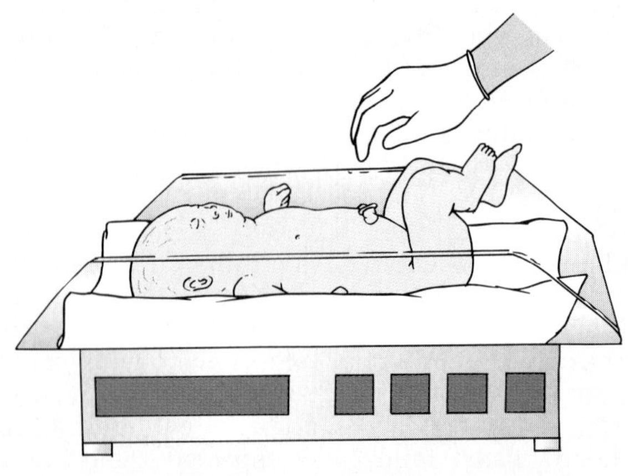

Continued on facing page

PROCEDURE 31–2 Continued

4 Record weight on baby's chart. Weigh baby at the same time each day. **Findings need to be recorded on the chart to determine whether weight loss is normal and to determine whether nutritional intake is adequate for growth. Weighing each day allows comparison of daily weight with birth weight to note whether weight loss is normal or excessive.**

Measuring

1 To measure length, place the newborn in the supine position on the crib mattress, with the head against the top of the crib. Place the paper tape measure beside the infant, with the 0 end of the tape against the top of the crib. Some scales include a built-in ruler for measuring length. Wear gloves if the newborn has not been bathed. **An infant's length is measured from the top of the head to the heel of the extended leg, with the body kept in alignment. The tape must be placed next to the infant to measure the length.**

2 Hold the newborn's head straight with one hand, and extend one leg with the other hand. Watch that the tape measure remains straight. **An infant's length is measured from the top of the head to the heel of the extended leg.**

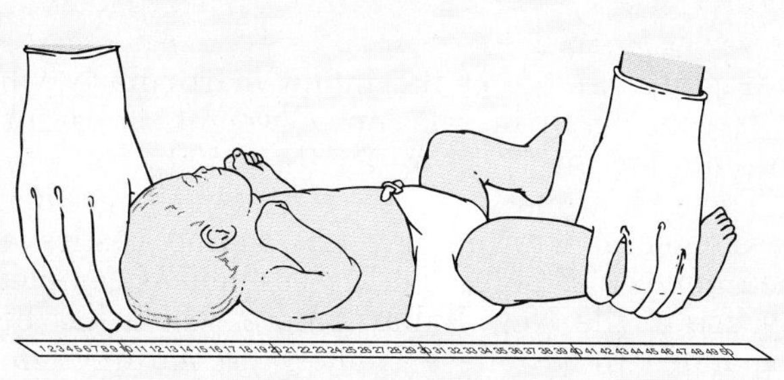

3 Note the length and record it in the infant's chart. Compare your finding with the normal range; most infants are 48 to 53 cm (19 to 21 inches) in length. **Measurements are taken to note abnormalities and provide a baseline value.**

4 To measure head circumference, place the paper tape under the newborn's head. Wrap the tape around the newborn's head, measuring just above the eyebrows so that the largest area of the occiput is included. Record your finding in the infant's chart. **Head circumference of a term newborn is normally 33 to 35.5 cm (13 to 14 inches). The head circumference is approximately 2 cm larger than the chest circumference. Measuring head circumference provides a baseline value for detection of abnormalities, such as hydrocephalus or microcephaly.**

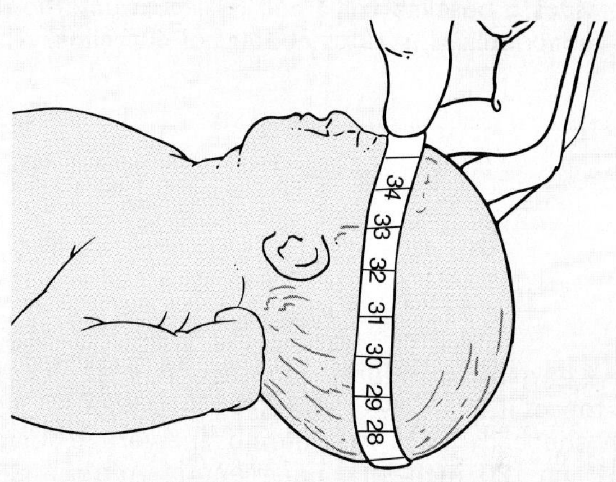

5 To measure chest circumference, place the paper tape under the newborn's chest, at nipple level. Wrap the tape around the chest, at the nipple line. Note the circumference and

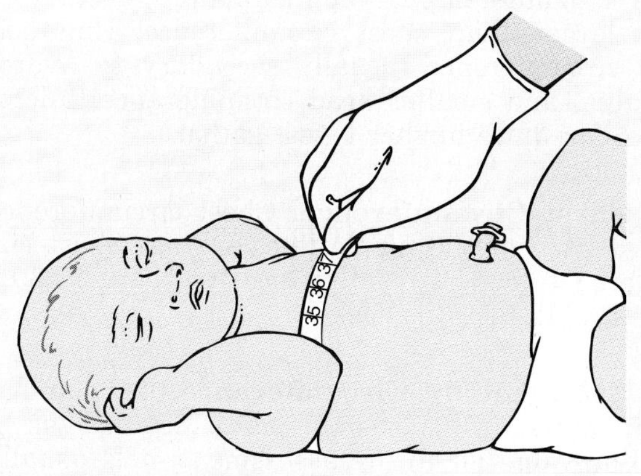

Continued on following page

PROCEDURE 31–2 Continued

record it in the infant's chart. **Chest circumference is measured at the nipple line. Average chest circumference of a term newborn is 30.5 to 33 cm (12 to 13 inches). Recording chest circumference facilitates detection of abnormalities.**

6 To measure abdominal circumference, place the paper tape under the newborn's abdomen, at umbilical level. Wrap the tape around the abdomen, at umbilical level. Note abdominal circumference and record it in the infant's chart. **Abdominal circumferences vary but are typically similar to the chest circumference. Recording abdominal circumference provides a baseline value and facilitates detection of abnormalities, such as abdominal distention.**

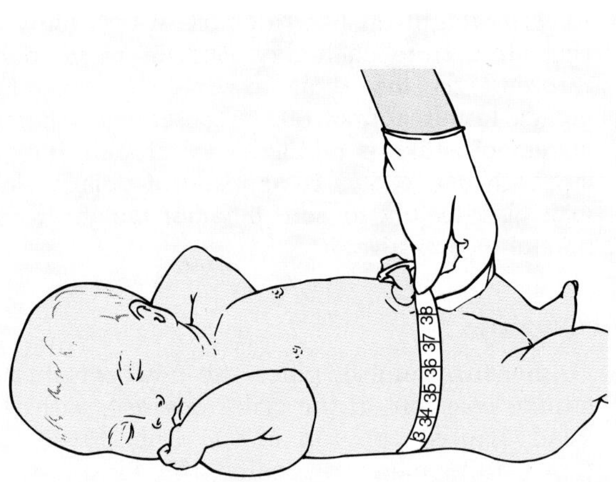

▼ **Length.** An infant's length is measured from the top of the head to the heel of extended legs, with the body kept in alignment. Average length is 51 cm (20 inches); 95 percent of infants measure 48 to 53 cm (19 to 21 inches).

▼ **Head Circumference.** Head circumference in an infant born at term is normally 33 to 35.5 cm (13 to 14 inches). Circumference is measured by use of a tape measure just above the eyebrows, so that the largest area of the occiput is included. Head circumference is approximately 2 cm (0.8 inch) larger than chest circumference. Enlarged head circumference (usually secondary to hydrocephalus) and smaller head circumference (microcephaly) require further investigation.

▼ **Chest Circumference.** Chest circumference is measured at the nipple line. Average chest circumference for the healthy term newborn is 30.5 to 33 cm (12 to 13 inches).

▼ **Abdominal Circumference.** Abdominal circumference is measured and recorded as a baseline value for future assessment; it is usually similar to the chest circumference. Abdominal circumference is measured at the level of the umbilicus. The top edge of the tape is at the lower level of the umbilical cord stump.

ASSESSMENT OF GESTATIONAL AGE

Gestational age of the infant, particularly when it is considered in relation to weight, is essential in planning nursing care for that infant.

The gestational age assessment includes an assessment of external physical characteristics and neuromuscular signs. The assessment is completed by use of the New Ballard Score, which has been expanded to include extremely premature infants for gestational age assessment, particularly neurologic assessment, is influenced by factors including infant health status, medications given to the mother, and infant state. Physical characteristics should be assessed as soon as possible after birth. The physical characteristics are signs of progressive maturity.

After the assessment is completed and scored, the number of points per item are added to obtain a total score. The total score is used to determine an estimate of gestational age in weeks by comparing the infant's score with the maturity rating scale on the New Ballard Score.

MATURATIONAL ASSESSMENT OF GESTATIONAL AGE (New Ballard Score)

NAME ______ DATE/TIME OF BIRTH ______ SEX ______

HOSPITAL NO. ______ DATE/TIME OF EXAM ______ BIRTH WEIGHT ______

RACE ______ AGE WHEN EXAMINED ______ LENGTH ______

APGAR SCORE: 1 MINUTE ______ 5 MINUTES ______ 10 MINUTES ______ HEAD CIRC. ______

EXAMINER ______

NEUROMUSCULAR MATURITY

NEUROMUSCULAR MATURITY SIGN	SCORE -1	0	1	2	3	4	5	RECORD SCORE HERE
POSTURE								
SQUARE WINDOW (Wrist)	>90°	90°	60°	45°	30°	0°		
ARM RECOIL		180°	140°-180°	110°-140°	90°-110°	<90°		
POPLITEAL ANGLE	180°	160°	140°	120°	100°	90°	<90°	
SCARF SIGN								
HEEL TO EAR								

TOTAL NEUROMUSCULAR MATURITY SCORE

PHYSICAL MATURITY

PHYSICAL MATURITY SIGN	SCORE -1	0	1	2	3	4	5	RECORD SCORE HERE
SKIN	sticky friable transparent	gelatinous red translucent	smooth pink visible veins	superficial peeling &/or rash, few veins	cracking pale areas rare veins	parchment deep cracking no vessels	leathery cracked wrinkled	
LANUGO	none	sparse	abundant	thinning	bald areas	mostly bald		
PLANTAR SURFACE	heel-toe 40-50 mm:-1 <40 mm:-2	>50 mm no crease	faint red marks	anterior transverse crease only	creases ant. 2/3	creases over entire sole		
BREAST	imperceptible	barely perceptible	flat areola no bud	stippled areola 1-2 mm bud	raised areola 3-4 mm bud	full areola 5-10 mm bud		
EYE/EAR	lids fused loosely: -1 tightly: -2	lids open pinna flat stays folded	sl. curved pinna; soft; slow recoil	well-curved pinna; soft but ready recoil	formed & firm instant recoil	thick cartilage ear stiff		
GENITALS (Male)	scrotum flat, smooth	scrotum empty faint rugae	testes in upper canal rare rugae	testes descending few rugae	testes down good rugae	testes pendulous deep rugae		
GENITALS (Female)	clitoris prominent & labia flat	prominent clitoris & small labia minora	prominent clitoris & enlarging minora	majora & minora equally prominent	majora large minora small	majora cover clitoris & minora		

TOTAL PHYSICAL MATURITY SCORE

SCORE

Neuromuscular ______

Physical ______

Total ______

MATURITY RATING

score	weeks
-10	20
-5	22
0	24
5	26
10	28
15	30
20	32
25	34
30	36
35	38
40	40
45	42
50	44

GESTATIONAL AGE (weeks)

By dates ______

By ultrasound ______

By exam ______

From Ballard, J. L., Khoury, J. C., Wedig, K., Wang, L., Eilers-Walsman, B. L., Lipp, R. (1991). New Ballard Score, expanded to include extremely premature infants. *The Journal of Pediatrics,* 119 (3), 417–423. Used with permission of Ross Products Division, Abbott Laboratories, Columbus, OH.

Physical Characteristics

The approximate gestational age of a newborn can be determined by an assessment of physical characteristics (Dubowitz 1970).

- *Edema of hands and feet.* A healthy term infant should not have edema of the hands or feet, although edema of the presenting part is not uncommon. Infants with erythroblastosis fetalis (see Chapter 36) or heart failure may have edema at birth, which would affect this assessment.
- *Skin texture.* As infants mature, skin becomes thicker. Some peeling of the hands and feet is common in term infants. Thick, parchment-like skin with cracking is characteristic of infants who are post term. The skin of a preterm infant is thin and smooth, and blood vessels may be visible through it.
- *Skin color.* Skin is red immediately after birth and becomes progressively lighter or paler pink as the baby matures.
- *Skin opacity (trunk).* The thickening of the skin also results in a decreased visibility of blood vessels.
- *Lanugo.* Lanugo, a fine downy hair covering the skin, is absent in very preterm infants (prior to 24 weeks), develops as the fetus matures, and is decreased in term infants (Fig. 31–1).
- *Plantar creases.* Plantar creases on the soles of the feet increase in number and depth as the infant increases in gestational age. By term, creases are clearly visible over the entire foot including the heel (Fig. 31–2).
- *Nipple formation.* The diameter of the areola bud tissue can be measured with a tape measure; in a term infant, the areola is stippled, with the edge raised and the diameter exceeding 0.75 cm. In the preterm infant, the nipple is barely perceptible or just a flat areola with no bud (Fig. 31–3).
- *Ear form and firmness.* Maturity is associated with a well-defined ear with curving of the entire upper pinna. The cartilage extends to the edge of the ear. There is instant recoil when the ear is folded anteriorly. In the preterm infant, the pinna is flat and stays folded (Fig. 31–4).
- *Male genitalia.* The testes normally descend into the scrotum in the eighth month of fetal life. The scrotum is pendulous and has deep rugae in the full-term infant. In the premature infant, the scrotum is empty (testicles have not descended) and faint rugae are present (Fig. 31–5).
- *Female genitalia.* At term, the labia majora should completely cover the labia minora. In the premature infant, there is a prominent clitoris; the labia majora do not cover the clitoris or labia minora (Fig. 31–6).

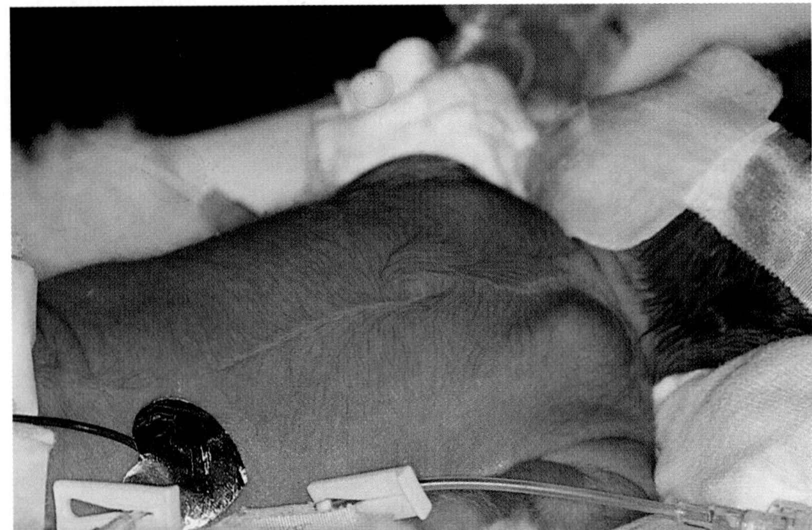

Figure 31–1

Presence of abundant lanugo in a preterm infant.

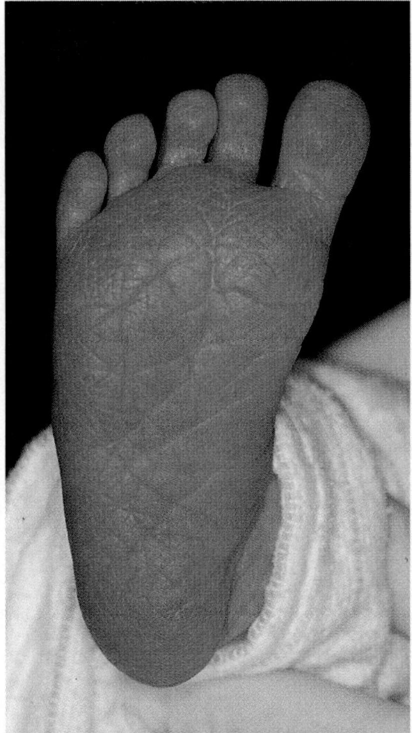
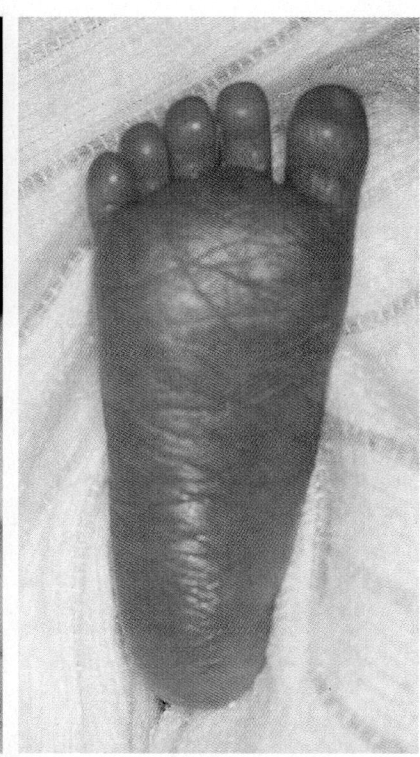

Figure 31–2

Plantar creases • *Left,* Full-term infant • *Right,* Premature infant.

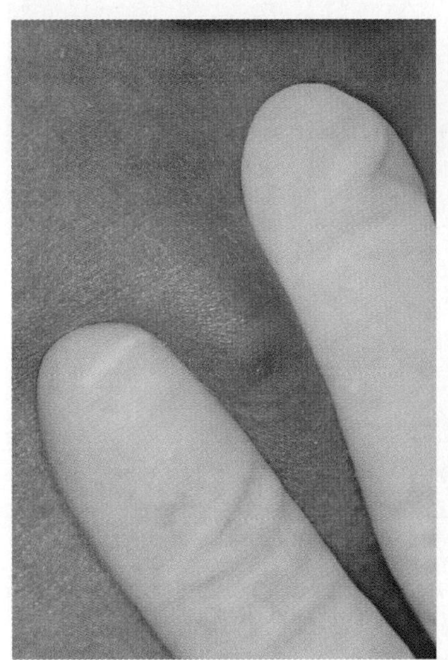
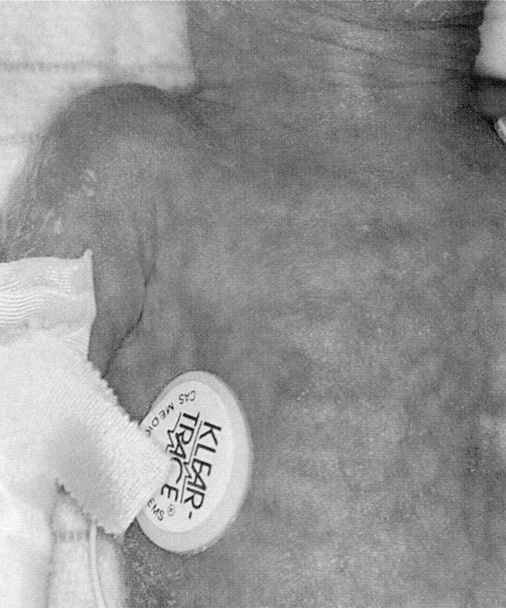

Figure 31–3

Nipple development • *Left,* Full-term infant • *Right,* Premature infant.

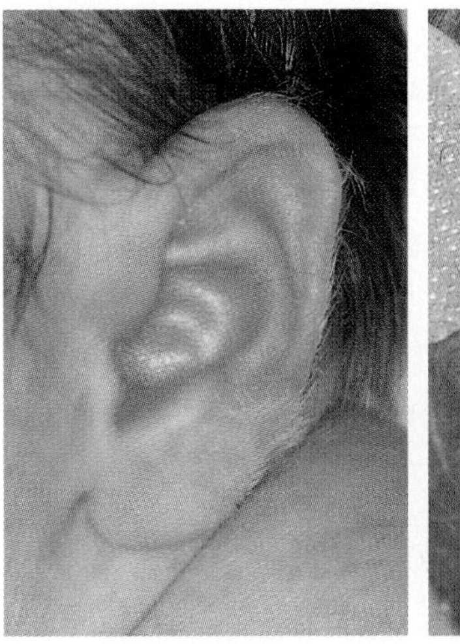

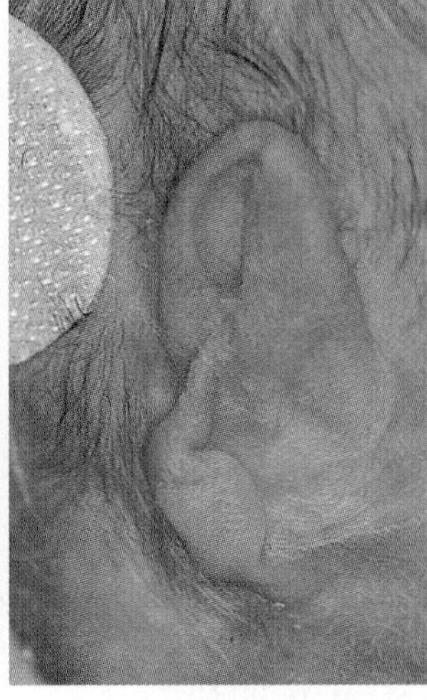

Figure 31–4

Development of the ear • *Left,* Full-term infant • *Right,* Premature infant.

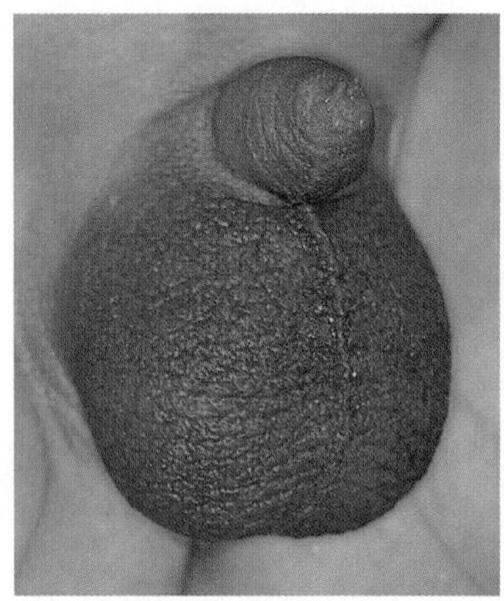

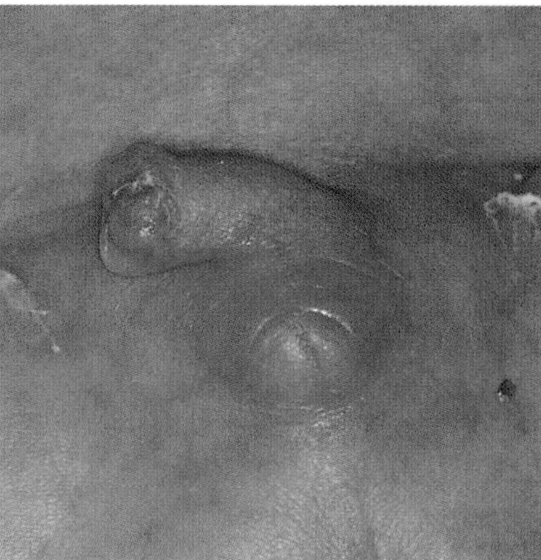

Figure 31–5

Male genitalia • *Left,* Full-term infant • *Right,* Premature infant.

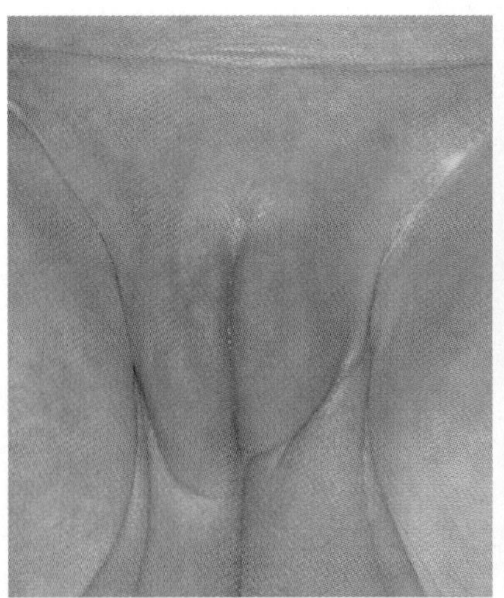

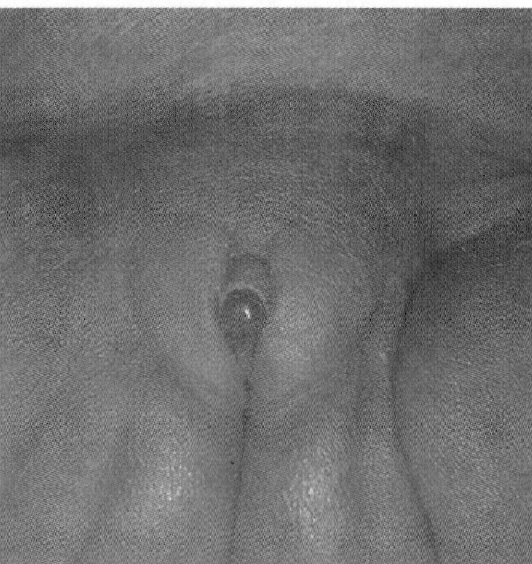

Figure 31–6

Female genitalia • *Left,* Full-term infant • *Right,* Premature infant.

Neuromuscular Characteristics

The number of neuromuscular characteristics assessed depends on the tool used. With the exception of ventral suspension, all assessments are made with the baby in the supine position.

- *Posture.* Observe posture when the infant is quiet, noting the flexion of the arms and legs. The term newborn's arms and legs are flexed; the body has good muscle tone. The premature infant's arms and legs are extended; the body is flaccid (Fig. 31–7).
- *Square window.* Flex the infant's hand to the degree possible. Estimate the angle between the hand and forearm. Be sure not to rotate the wrist. In the full-term infant, there is no angle; you can flex the baby's hand completely against the forearm. In the premature infant, the hand cannot be flexed against the forearm. The degree of the angle is measured against the chart for the New Ballard Score (Fig. 31–8).
- *Ankle dorsiflexion.* Flex the infant's foot to the degree possible. Estimate the angle between the dorsum of the foot and the anterior leg (Fig. 31–9).
- *Popliteal angle.* With the infant's hips on the examining surface, flex one thigh on the abdomen. Attempt to straighten the leg toward the head until you feel resistance. Determine the degree of the popliteal angle (Fig. 31–10).
- *Heel to ear.* With the infant's hips on the examining table, attempt to pull the heel toward the ear until you feel resistance. Observe the distance between the heel and ear.
- *Scarf sign.* Place the infant's arm across the chest with the hand touching the opposite shoulder. Observe the relation of the infant's elbow to the midline of the body (Fig. 31–11).
- *Head lag.* Grasping both arms, pull the infant to a sitting position. Observe the relationship of the head to the trunk.
- *Ventral suspension.* Place the palm of your hand under the infant's chest, with the infant in prone position. Observe posture when you lift the infant from the examining surface.
- *Arm recoil.* Fully flex both arms, hold for 5 seconds, fully extend both arms, and release. Observe the degree of immediate return to flexion.
- *Leg recoil.* With the infant's hips on the examining surface, fully flex both hips, hold for 5 seconds, fully extend, and release. Observe the degree of immediate return to flexion.

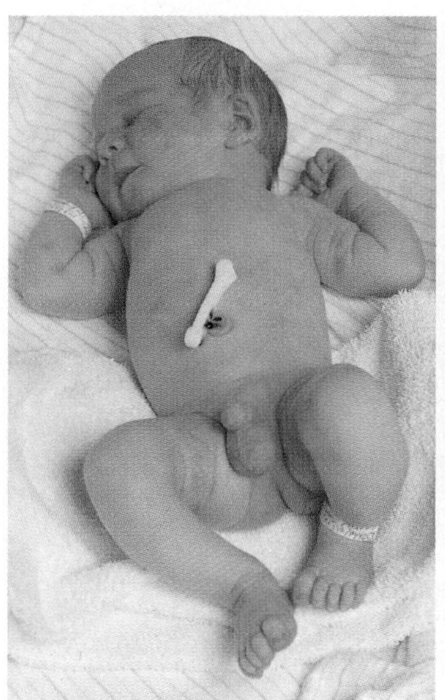

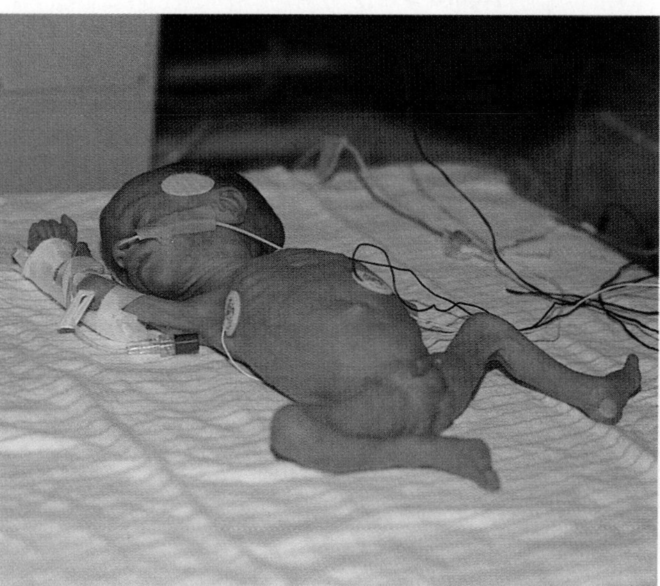

Figure 31–7
Neonate posture • *Left,* Full-term infant • *Right,* Premature infant.

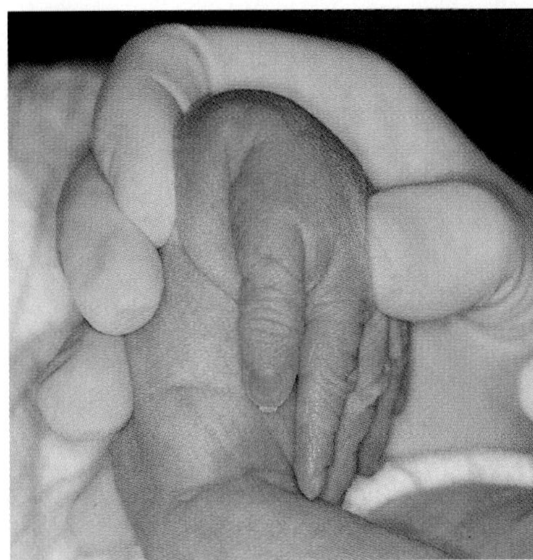
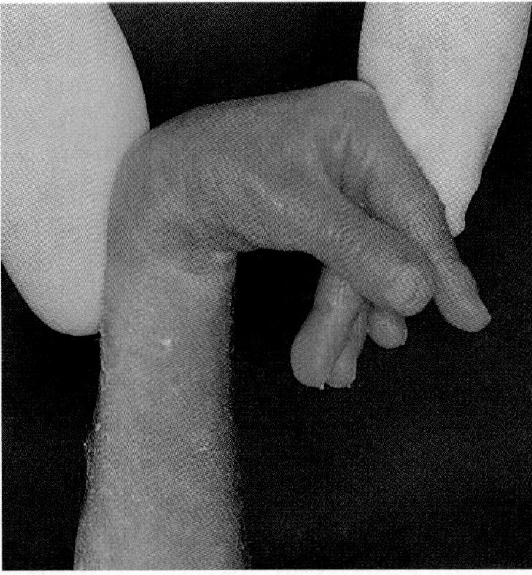

Figure 31–8
Square window • *Left,* Full-term infant • *Right,* Premature infant.

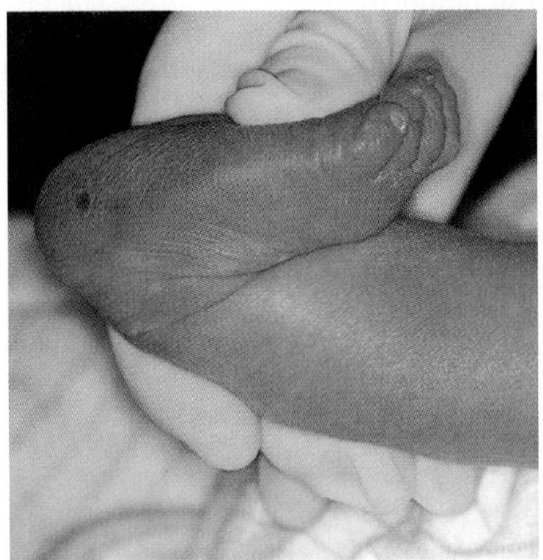
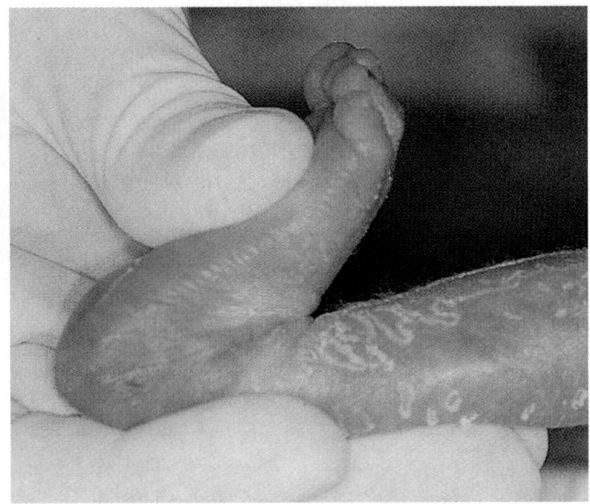

Figure 31–9
Ankle dorsiflexion • *Left,* Full-term infant • *Right,* Premature infant.

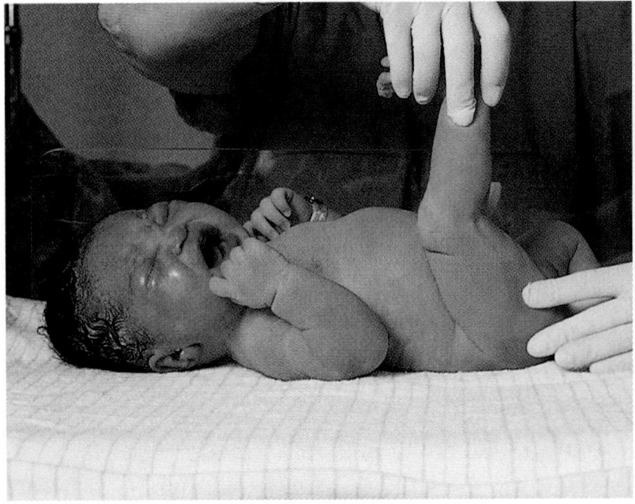
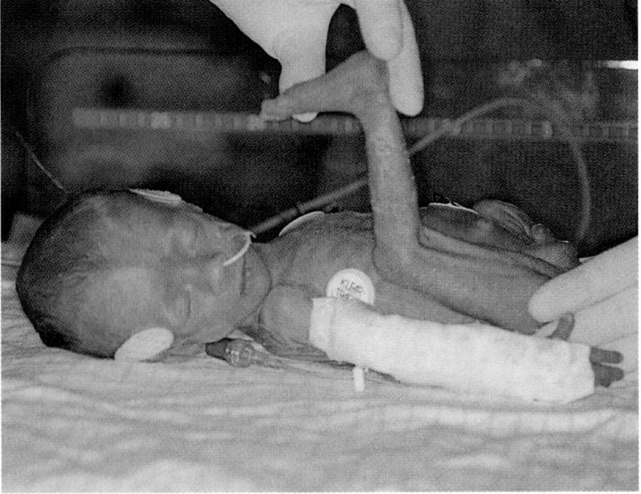

Figure 31–10
Popliteal angle • *Left,* Full-term infant • *Right,* Premature infant.

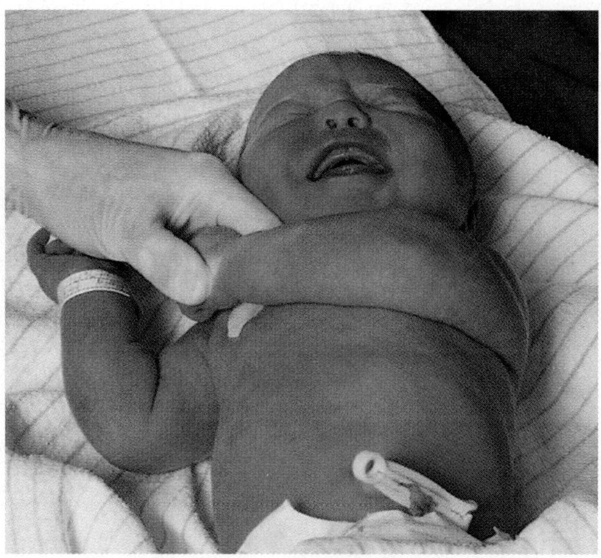
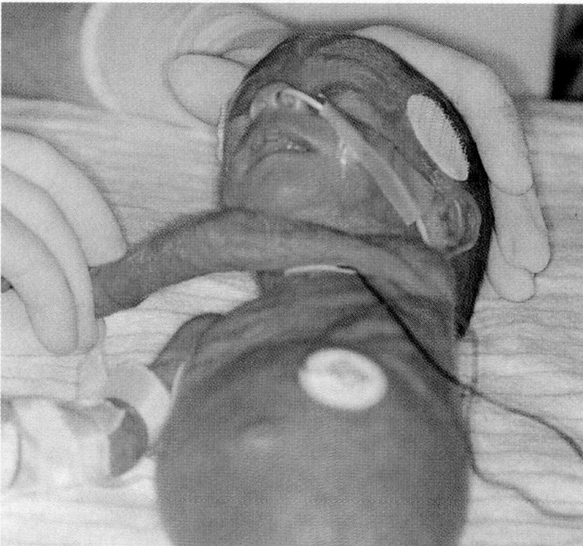

Figure 31–11
Scarf sign • *Left,* Full-term infant • *Right,* Premature infant.

DETERMINING THE RELATIONSHIP BETWEEN INFANT SIZE AND GESTATIONAL AGE

Once gestational age and weight, length, and head circumference have been determined, evaluation of the infant's size in relation to gestational age provides valuable information about the infant's needs. The determination is made by plotting weight, length, and head circumference in relation to the expanded New Ballard Score on the intrauterine growth grids (Fig. 31–12).

An infant is considered appropriate for gestational age if weight, length, and head circumference are between the 10th and 90th percentile on the intrauterine growth grids. Below the 10th percentile, the infant is termed small for gestational age; above the 90th percentile, the infant is large for gestational age (Fig. 31–13).

MORTALITY RISK ASSESSMENT

After physical and gestational age assessments of the infant are completed, determining the mortality risk of the infant is done. While this step is not essential for the healthy neonate, it is an important piece of information for low-birth-weight infants and those with problems. This is done by plotting the infant's birth weight according to gestational age on a mortality risk chart. The common causes of death according to gestational age and birth weight are shown in Figure 31–14.

PHYSICAL ASSESSMENT

An infant should receive several physical assessments in the first 24 to 48 hours of life. The immediate assessment after birth is fairly rapid but thorough to identify major anomalies (particularly those that are life threatening), to determine the effect of labor and birth, and to identify any sign of infectious disease that will require a modification in care.

During the physical assessment the infant should be naked. However, it is essential that the baby be kept warm either by means of a warming device, such as a radiant warmer, or by uncovering the infant's body for only brief periods at a time.

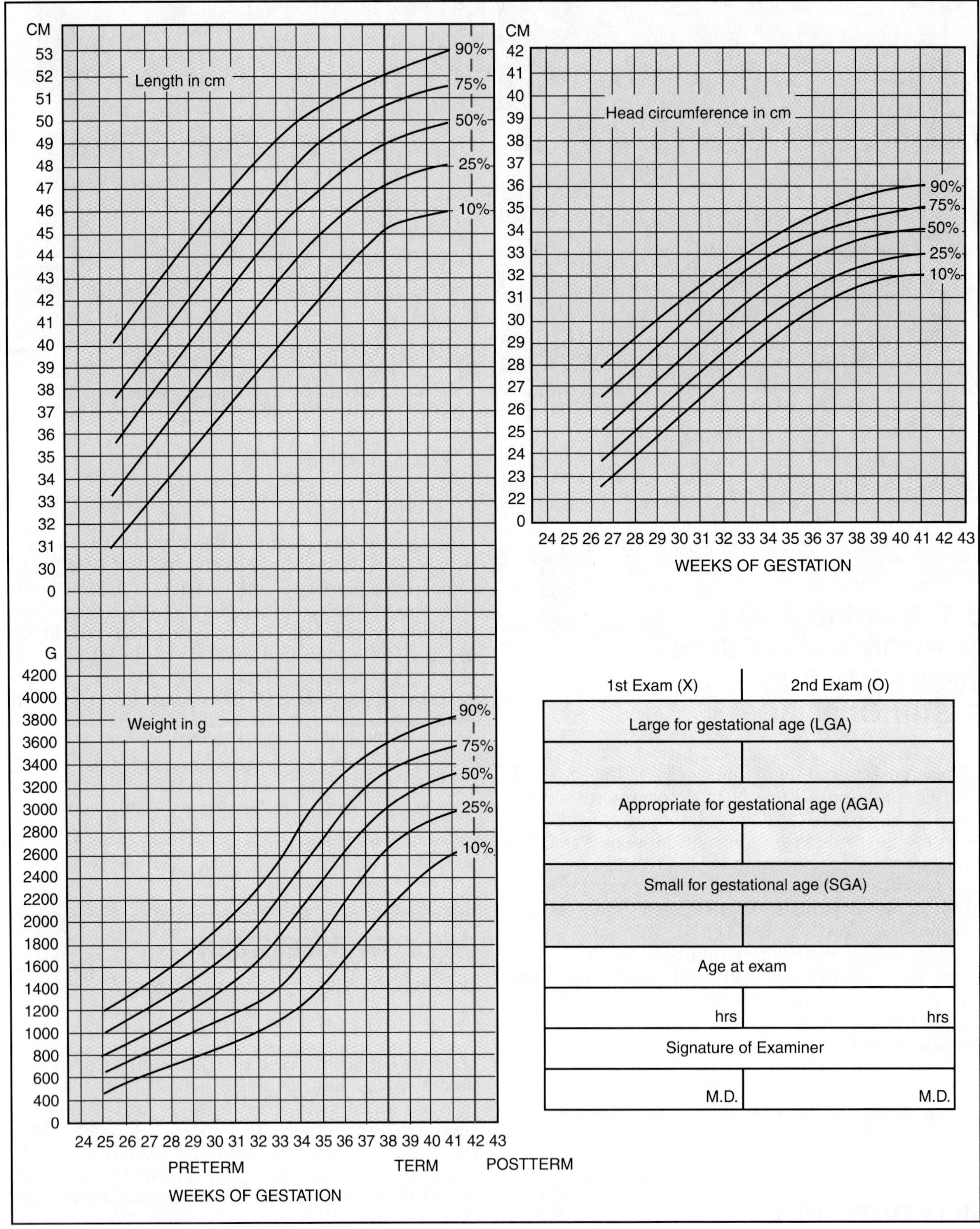

Figure 31–12

Intrauterine growth grids. (Adapted from Lubchenko, L. O., Hansman, C., Boyd, E. (1966). Intrauterine growth in length and head circumference as estimated from live births at gestational ages from 26 to 42 weeks. *Pediatrics,* 37 (3), 403–408. Adapted by permission of PEDIATRICS.)

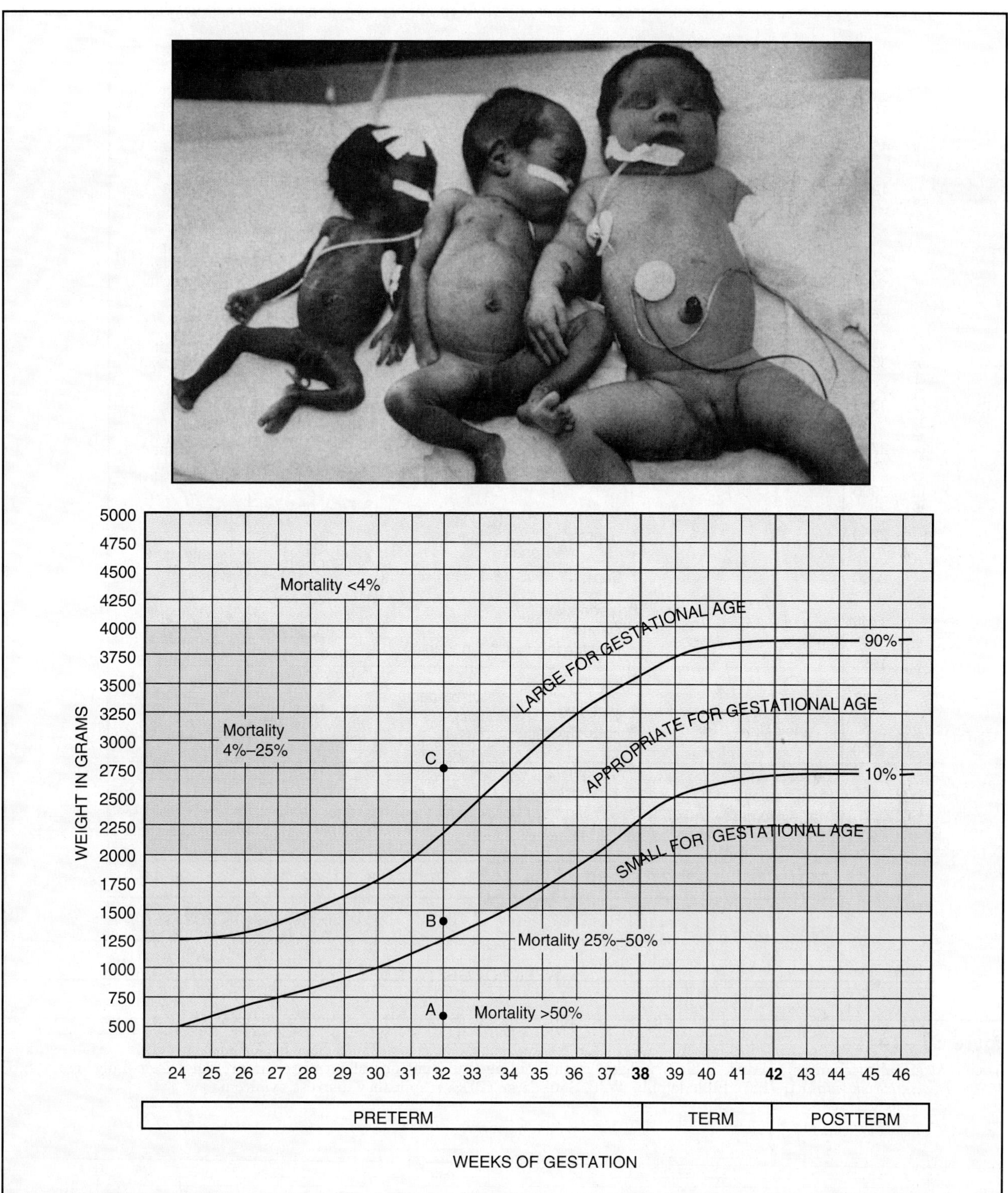

Figure 31–13

Top, Three babies, each born at 32 weeks of gestation, weight 600, 1400, and 2750 g, respectively, from left to right. They are plotted in the growth grid at points A, B, and C. (Photograph from Korones, S. B. [1986]. *High risk newborn infants* [4th ed., p. 118]. St. Louis: Mosby–Year Book. Growth grid modified from Battaglia, F. C., and Lubchenco, L. C.: *Journal of Pediatrics,* 71, 159, 1967.)

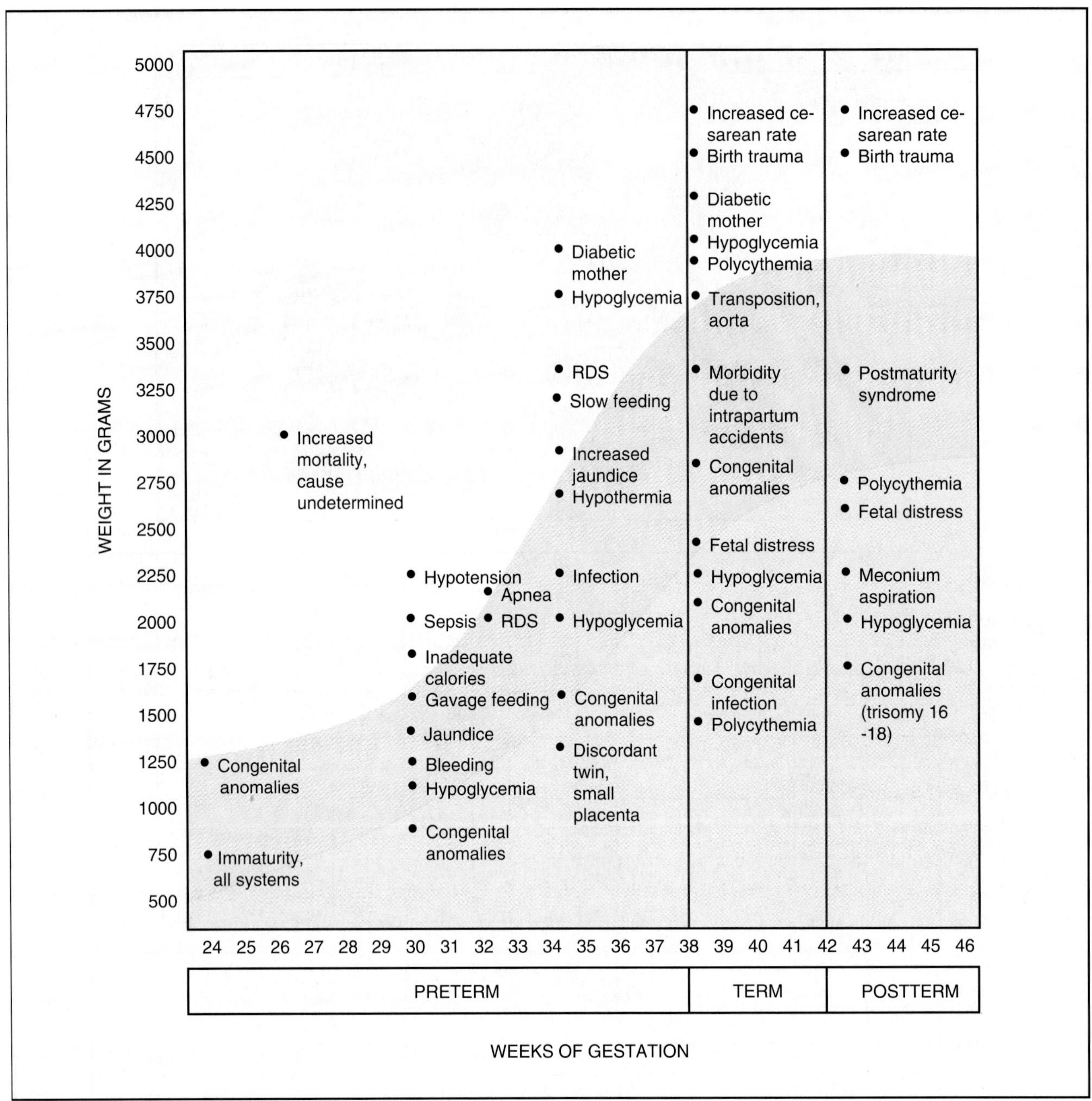

Figure 31–14

Specific neonatal morbidities related to birth weight, gestational age, and pattern of intrauterine growth. (From Lubchenko, L. O. (1976). *The high-risk infant* (p. 122). Philadelphia: W. B. Saunders.) (RDS, respiratory distress syndrome.)

General Assessment

SKIN CHARACTERISTICS

In addition to skin characteristics described in the New Ballard Score (texture, opacity, lanugo), other characteristics should be noted. Vernix caseosa is a cheesy, white material composed of sebum and desquamated epithelial cells that protects the baby's skin in utero. It is most evident in the full-term infant; it does not need to be removed and should be allowed to resolve naturally (Fig. 31–15).

Milia and erythema toxicum are common findings, as are mongolian spots on dark-skinned infants. Milia are tiny cysts that result from the obstruction of the sebaceous glands of the face, particularly those across the bridge of the nose and the chin. They disappear without treatment.

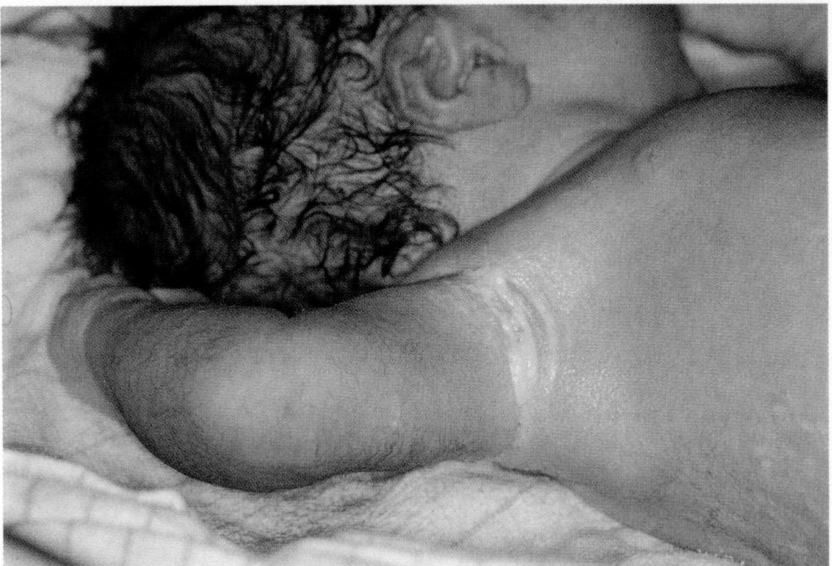

Figure 31–15

Vernix caseosa has a bactericidal property that protects the newborn's skin and does not need to be removed.

The most common skin disorder of infancy, erythema toxicum, is found in 30 to 70 percent of normal term infants (Fig. 31–16). It usually occurs in the first 4 days of life but may appear at any time in the first 2 weeks. A common pattern is for the papule to appear one day, look worse on the second day, and be completely gone by the third, although it may disappear in as brief a time as 2 hours. The cause is unknown and treatment is unnecessary; but the lesions must be differentiated from those of impetigo, which must be treated.

The vesicles of impetigo, which is usually caused by staphylococci in the newborn, are pustular. In impetigo, these vesicles rupture to produce thick, moist, yellow crusts. An antibiotic ointment is prescribed. Healing time is approximately 10 to 14 days.

Mongolian spots, bluish purple areas of skin, are at times mistaken for bruises. They may be present in some dark-skinned babies at the time of birth, usually in the area of the sacrum or buttocks. They disappear of their own accord during early childhood (Fig. 31–17).

A variety of hemangiomas may be seen in newborn infants. Even when they do not pose a threat to the baby's physical well-being, hemangiomas are highly distressing to the baby's parents because they are so obvious. To the extent that they affect the way a mother feels about her baby and the way she treats the infant, they can have far-reaching significance. A port-wine stain (nevus flammeus) is a flat, purple or dark red lesion consisting of mature capillaries that is present at birth. Those port-wine hemangiomas located above the bridge of the nose tend to fade; others do not.

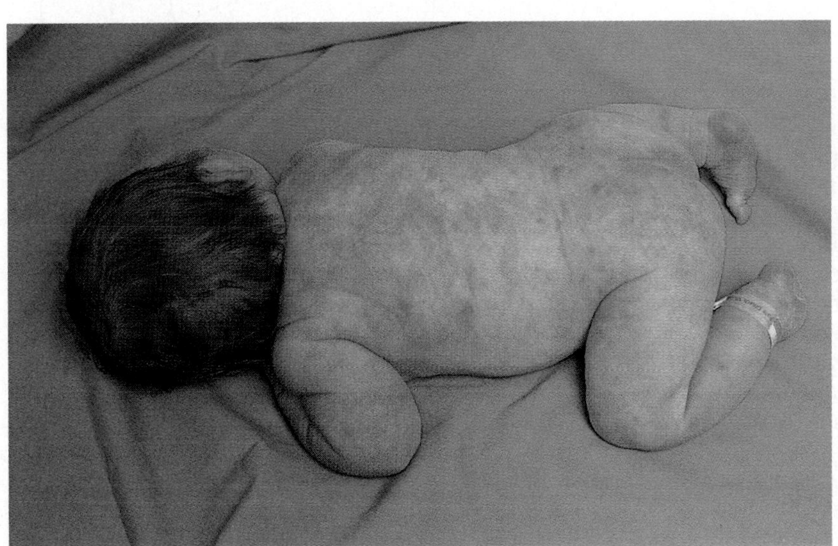

Figure 31–16

Erythema toxicum is most commonly found on the trunk, arms, and diaper area. No treatment is necessary.

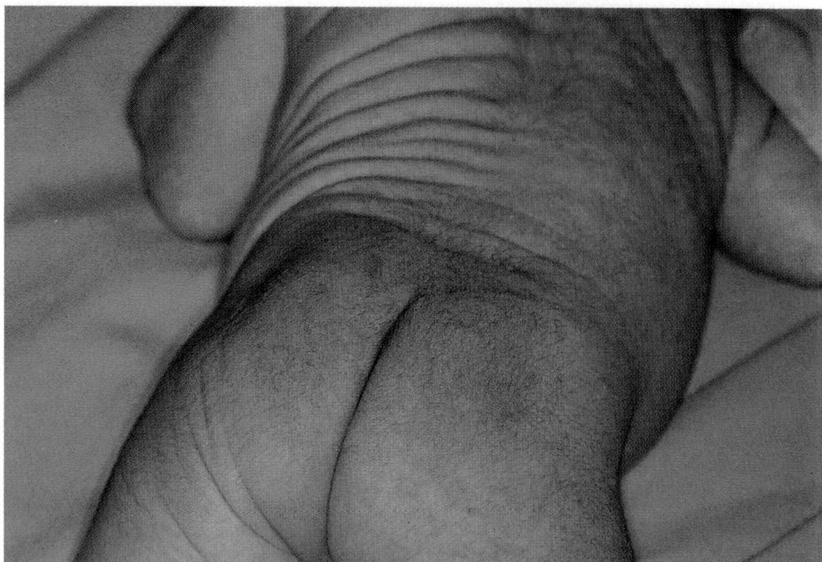

Figure 31–17

Mongolian spot, a pigmented lesion of the skin that is usually blue-gray and irregular and looks like a bruise. It occurs primarily over the sacrum and buttocks.

Since they are level with the surface of the skin, they can be covered with a cosmetic preparation. Strawberry hemangiomas (nevus vasculosus) are elevated areas consisting of immature capillaries and endothelial cells. They may be present at birth or may appear in the first 2 weeks after birth and continue to enlarge for 6 months to a year. After the first birthday, they begin to be absorbed; the process of involution takes as long as 10 years. Half to three fourths of strawberry hemangiomas disappear by the time the child is 7 years old, leaving no evidence that they ever existed. The end result seems to be better if the hemangioma is untreated unless it interferes with normal functioning because of its location. A third type, cavernous hemangioma, consists of dilated vascular spaces with thick walls that are lined with endothelium. They do not regress spontaneously.

COLOR

All infants at birth are normally pink to dark red in skin color, regardless of later pigmentation. This is due to both the higher concentration of red blood cells in the vessels and the thinness of the subcutaneous fat layer, which causes the blood vessels to be close to the surface of the skin. Skin is not fully pigmented at birth in darker-skinned infants; pigmentation develops as the baby matures. If there is a concern about abnormal color, the mucous membranes inside the mouth are assessed for pink color.

Acrocyanosis, blueness of the hands and feet, is associated with immature peripheral circulation and is not uncommon in the first hours of life. Generalized cyanosis, however, is never normal. In infants with dark skin, generalized cyanosis can best be observed by examining the mucosal lining of the mouth, which will be blue.

The relationship between cyanosis and crying is an important observation. The infant may be cyanotic only when crying, which can be a warning of the later, more persistent cyanosis of some types of congenital heart disease.

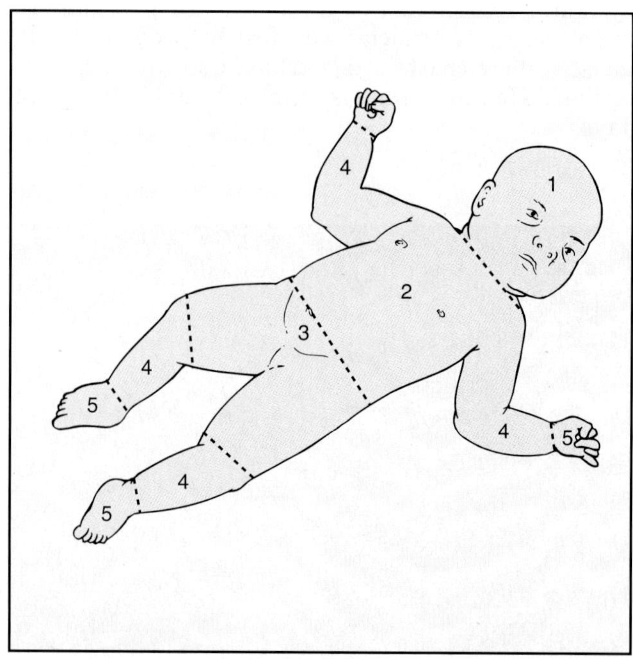

Figure 31–18

Jaundice develops progressively from the head down and from the center of the body out to the extremities.

Harlequin sign is a rare transient color change in which one side of the infant's body (usually the dependent side) is a darker color than the other. Harlequin sign has no known significance.

Sudden cyanosis and apnea may be related to excessive, thick mucus obstructing the upper respiratory tract. For this reason, a bulb syringe should be in each infant's bed, and a suction machine with a supply of catheters should be readily available. Once the obstructing mucus is removed, the infant will be able to breathe without difficulty and will become pink.

Damage to the central nervous system is another cause of cyanosis. The infant may have irregular breathing as well as other signs of central nervous system damage—a high-pitched cry, either rigid or floppy muscle tone, or absence of a Moro reflex. As with infants who are cyanotic because of respiratory distress, crying and oxygen frequently relieve the cyanosis.

Bilateral choanal atresia (occlusion of the posterior nares by either bone or membrane) causes cyanosis because infants are obligate nose breathers; they breathe through their mouths only with great difficulty. Assess this possibility by holding a wisp of cotton in front of each naris; the air movements of respiration can then be easily observed.

Jaundice is found in 25 to 50 percent of infants who have no other health problem. (The physiologic basis of neonatal jaundice is discussed in Chapter 30). Jaundice is yellow in color and is

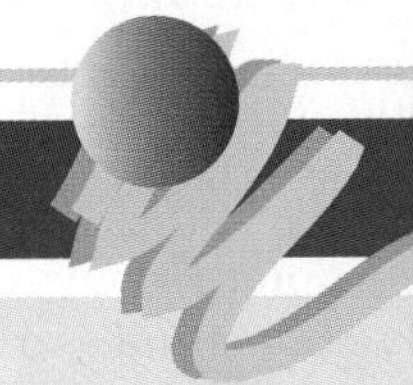

IMPROVING YOUR PRACTICE

PERFORMING NEONATAL ASSESSMENT

Learning how to do neonatal assessment requires a sound knowledge of normal physical findings and behavioral characteristics of the infant and repetitive practice to develop skill in performing the assessment. Conducting an assessment on a wiggling and at times fussy infant is a challenge, especially when you are learning. Following these tips will enable you to complete the assessment more easily.

- REPEATED PRACTICE will increase your facility with instruments, technique proficiency, and especially your confidence.
- PRACTICE ON INANIMATE OBJECTS such as a stuffed animal or doll, before performing an examination on an infant.
- WORK WITH ANOTHER STUDENT OR PEER when doing the examination initially. This will decrease your anxiety and provide a source of validation.
- TIME THE EXAMINATION so that you perform the assessment when the infant is most likely to be quiet. Avoid the time before or after a feeding.
- USE A LOGICAL, SYSTEMATIC APPROACH to decrease the chance of omissions and to proceed more expeditiously.
- KEEP ENVIRONMENTAL INFLUENCES IN MIND. The color of the walls, clothing, and bed linens can affect the appearance of the infant's skin color.
- START THE EXAMINATION WHEN THE INFANT IS QUIET. Count the apical pulse, listen to breath sounds and bowel sounds, and observe the infant's posture first.
- LEAVE INTRUSIVE PROCEDURES AND THOSE REQUIRING HANDLING OF THE INFANT UNTIL LAST, at the end of the procedure.
- WHEN EXAMINING THE EYES, position the infant so that the environmental light does not cause the eyes to close.
- KEEP THE INFANT WARM AT ALL TIMES.
- KEEP A DIAPER POSITIONED OVER THE GENITALIA—especially when examining a baby boy—to decrease unexpected elimination accidents.
- USE STANDARD PRECAUTIONS throughout the examination.
- STOP THE EXAMINATION AND COMPLETE IT LATER if attempts to console or distract a fussy infant do not work.
- FOLLOW THE PRINCIPLES OF GOOD BODY MECHANICS while doing the examination. If you are comfortable, you will be able to conduct the assessment more easily.
- TRY TO RELAX AND ENJOY INTERACTING WITH THE INFANT! Infants are sensitive to the feelings of their caregivers. If you are relaxed and at ease, the baby you are examining will be more relaxed and at ease, making the assessment easier.

From Marchbanks, P. (1987). Newborn assessment: Physical examination. In S. S. Humenick, *Analysis of current assessment strategies in the health care of young children and childbearing families* (pp. 110–128). Laramie, WY: Author.

caused by a high indirect bilirubin concentration. A bilirubin level of 4 to 6 mg/dL is required to cause staining of the skin and sclerae. To determine the presence of jaundice, examine the baby's skin color in natural light. Press your finger over a bone prominence or the tip of the nose to press out capillary blood from the tissues. This is essential to determine the presence of jaundice because the capillary blood will obscure it to some degree. The depth of color and its distribution over the body give a crude estimate of the baby's level of bilirubin and degree of jaundice. Jaundice starts at the head first, spreads to the chest, then the abdomen. The arms and legs followed by the hands and feet are the last to be jaundiced (Fig. 31–18). As a result of brief hospitalization for mothers and their healthy newborns, assessment of jaundice frequently must be made during home or ambulatory visits during the first week. If jaundice is present, bilirubin determination is necessary.

Pallor may be a sign of intracranial hemorrhage, anemia, sepsis, or shock. Pallor is always abnormal and requires further assessment to determine and correct the cause.

Head, Face, and Neck

▼ **Sutures and Fontanelles.** Inspection of the infant's head reveals a diamond-shaped anterior fontanelle; a triangular posterior fontanelle; and the coronal, lambdoid, and sagittal sutures.

The anterior fontanelle is bounded by the frontal and parietal bones of the baby's skull. It is approximately 2.5 to 4.0 cm in width (1.0 to 1.75 inches), or about the width of two fingers. The posterior fontanelle is bounded by the parietal and occipital bones and is less than half the size of the anterior fontanelle (0.5 to 1.0 cm or 0.2 to 0.4 inch). The posterior fontanelle may be closed by birth, but the anterior fontanelle should be open.

While a closed anterior fontanelle is of serious concern to the nurses and physicians who care for the baby (usually being related to microcephaly), it is the open anterior fontanelle that may distress the parents. Parents can be reassured by knowing that (1) the presence of an open fontanelle helped to protect the baby's head during delivery; (2) the fontanelle allowed the baby's brain to grow before birth and will continue to do so for the next 18 months; and (3) the infant's brain is adequately protected by a tough membrane, so there need be no fear of handling the baby and washing the head.

Bulging fontanelles and separation of the sutures are a sign of increased intracranial pressure. Depressed fontanelles indicate dehydration.

A newborn's hair is usually silky; coarse or brittle hair is associated with hypothyroidism.

▼ **Head Shape.** The shape of the infant's head may be affected by molding, by caput succedaneum, or by cephalhematoma, all of which are normal.

Molding is the process by which the bones of the baby's skull override one another during birth, resulting in an asymmetric appearance or even a "misshapen" head. Molding may be pronounced in a long labor but may occur after any labor. While molding is normal, it may be a source of concern to parents who have not been prepared for the possibility or do not understand the reason.

Caput succedaneum is edema in the tissues of the presenting part. Because a caput involves only soft tissue, it may cross suture lines. Caput resolves in a few days after delivery.

Cephalhematoma is a collection of blood between the cranial bone and the periosteum. A cephalhematoma cannot cross suture lines, but more than one cephalhematoma may be present. Blood is absorbed more slowly than fluid, and thus it takes longer for a cephalhematoma to be absorbed (often several weeks) in comparison with caput succedaneum. Thus, differentiating these two conditions is important in providing information and reassurance to parents (Fig. 31–19).

▼ **Face.** Observe the symmetry of the infant's face. Asymmetry, usually related to damage to the facial nerve, may not be observable when the infant is quiet but becomes obvious during crying. The most common cause is intrauterine pressure on the facial nerve.

Infants with fetal alcohol syndrome have characteristic facial changes that may include short palpebral fissures, a hypoplastic philtrum, short upturned nose, hypertelorism, and hypoplastic maxilla.

Infants with bilateral renal agenesis (Potter syndrome) or prolonged oligohydramnios have a characteristic facies in which the nose is flattened and folds appear below the eyes; the ears are frequently low set.

Facial changes are also found in infants whose mothers have ingested a variety of drugs (including warfarin, hydantoin, and valproic acid) and in newborns with chromosome defects. The nursing observation that facies do not appear normal should prompt further investigation.

▼ **Eyes.** Gray-blue or brown in color, eyes may seem to be crossed at times (transient strabismus) in the newborn period. In "normal" strabismus, movements alternate between eyes and are always convergent (i.e., toward the nose). Unilateral or divergent strabismus requires prompt medical attention.

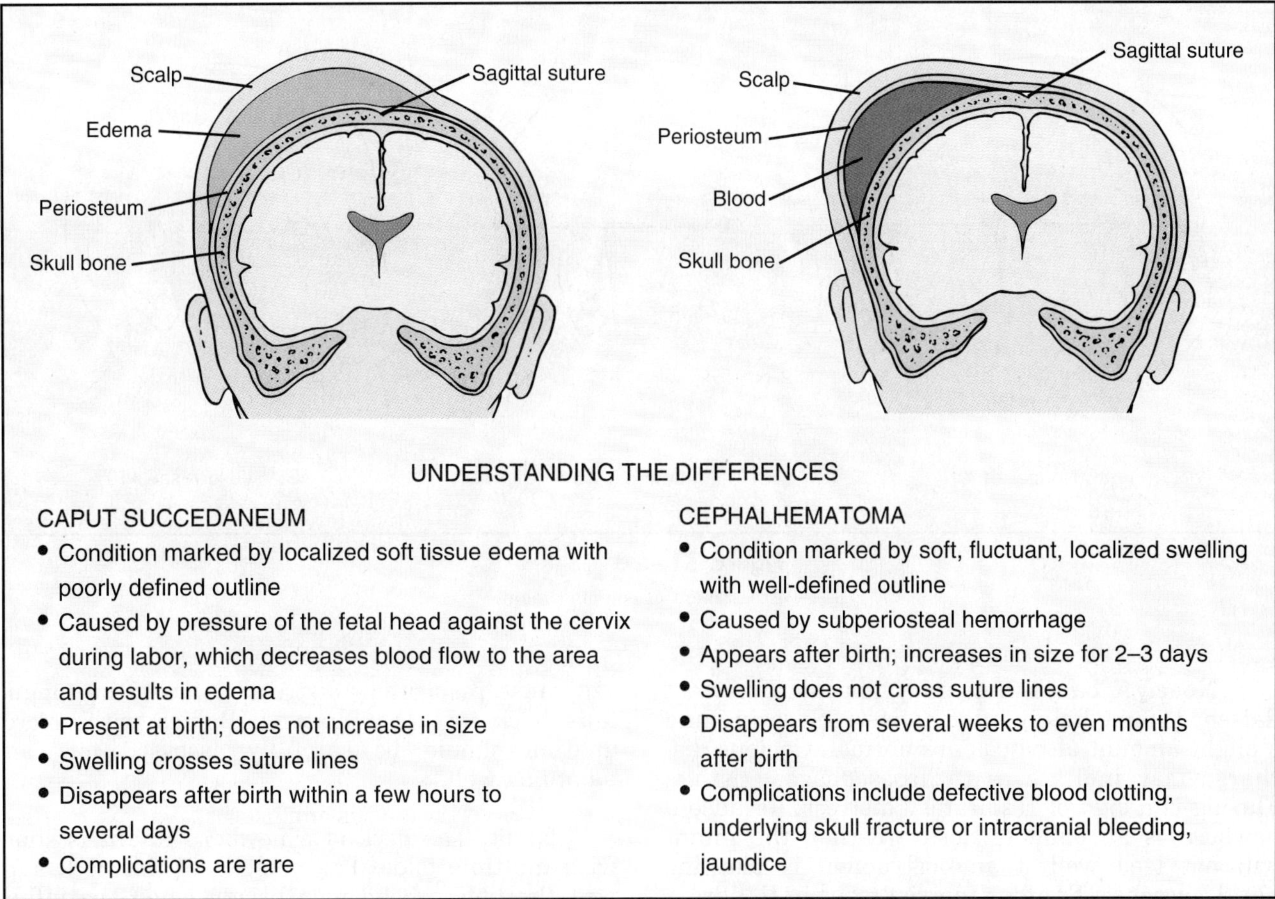

UNDERSTANDING THE DIFFERENCES

CAPUT SUCCEDANEUM

- Condition marked by localized soft tissue edema with poorly defined outline
- Caused by pressure of the fetal head against the cervix during labor, which decreases blood flow to the area and results in edema
- Present at birth; does not increase in size
- Swelling crosses suture lines
- Disappears after birth within a few hours to several days
- Complications are rare

CEPHALHEMATOMA

- Condition marked by soft, fluctuant, localized swelling with well-defined outline
- Caused by subperiosteal hemorrhage
- Appears after birth; increases in size for 2–3 days
- Swelling does not cross suture lines
- Disappears from several weeks to even months after birth
- Complications include defective blood clotting, underlying skull fracture or intracranial bleeding, jaundice

Figure 31–19
Characteristics of caput succedaneum and cephalhematoma.

When the newborn's head is turned, the eyes may occasionally remain in their original position. This characteristic, called doll's eye movement, may be seen in the first 10 days of life.

Infants will close their eyes in response to a bright light; shading the eyes with your hand encourages the infant who is awake to open the eyes and provides an opportunity for interaction and examination.

Subconjunctival hemorrhage, seen either as small patches of red or as a red ring around the cornea, is caused by pressure on the fetal head during delivery. Pressure impairs venous return and causes rupture of capillaries. These small hemorrhages are absorbed in 2 to 3 weeks.

Visual reflexes are the principal means of assessing vision in newborns. Pupils should constrict in response to light (pupillary reflex); if there is no pupillary reflex by 3 weeks of age, it is possible that the infant is blind (Greenman 1963). As noted, newborns close their eyes in response to bright light; therefore, eyes should be examined in subdued light.

Abnormal findings in an eye examination include discharge from the eye, absence of visual reflexes, absence of tears or stagnant tears that flow down the baby's cheek, hypertelorism, opacity of the pupil, and enlarged cornea. Discharge from the eye, usually a sign of conjunctivitis, rarely appears in the first 24 hours.

Absence of tears, or tears that flow down the infant's cheek, may indicate a blocked lacrimal duct. When tears are absent, there may appear to be a film over the infant's eyes because mucus cannot be washed away.

Hypertelorism occurs when the distance between the inner canthi is greater than 3 cm. Hypertelorism may be associated with fetal alcohol syndrome and certain congenital anomalies.

Opacity of the pupil is rare; it signifies congenital cataract and may be associated with cytomegalic inclusion disease or galactosemia. An unusually large cornea or a cornea with a hazy or cloudy appearance indicates congenital glaucoma, a condition requiring immediate medical intervention.

▼ **Ears.** The location of the infant's ears should be noted. The upper part of the ear should be on the same plane as the eye. Low-set ears are associated with certain chromosome anomalies and also with some congenital renal disorders (Fig. 31–20).

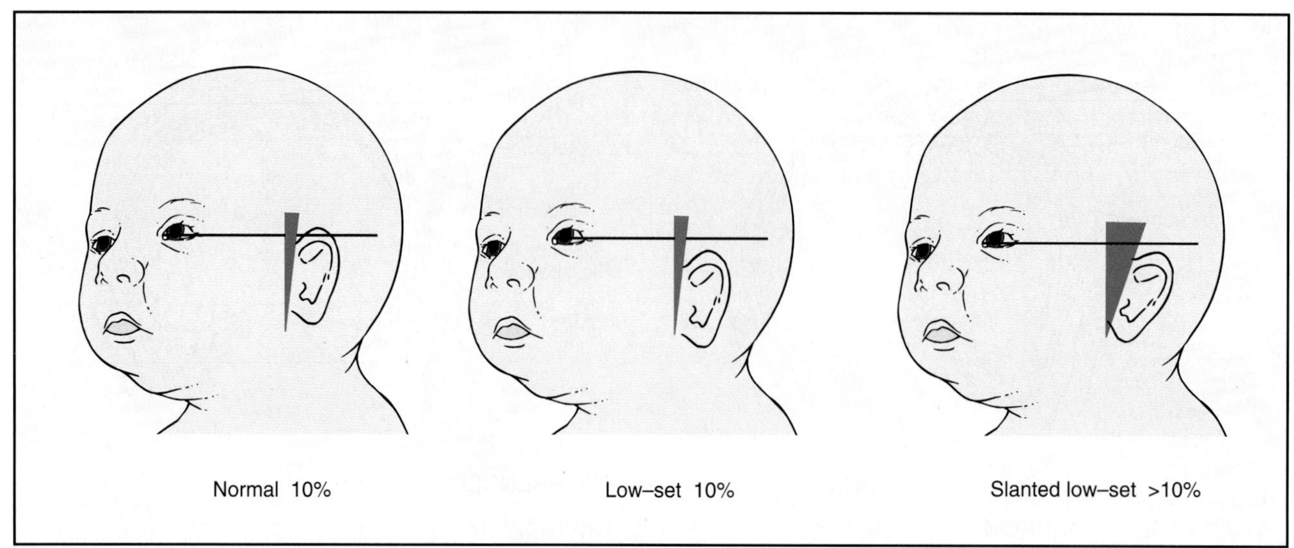

Figure 31–20
Assessment of ear placement.

Nose. A baby's nose may appear somewhat flattened immediately after delivery. Sneezing and a slight amount of mucus are normal. Copious discharge may indicate a tracheoesophageal fistula. Flaring is a sign of respiratory distress. Because a newborn is an obligate nose breather, the infant will not feed well if an obstruction is blocking nasal passages. Snuffles (persistent rhinitis) are a characteristic of congenital syphilis.

Mouth. A sucking blister on the upper lip is normal for a newborn infant, as are epithelial pearls found on the hard palate. Epithelial pearls should be distinguished from thrush, a fungal infection caused by *Candida albicans*. Thrush appears as numerous small white and gray patches in the mouth and on the tongue.

When the infant cries, assess whether both sides of the mouth move symmetrically; movement on only one side of the face indicates injury to a facial nerve in utero, during labor, or during birth.

Cleft lip is readily apparent; the palate should be assessed for evidence of a cleft in both the hard and soft palate by visualizing the palate and by feeling with a gloved finger.

While most infants have some mucus, a large amount of frothy "bubbly" mucus suggests the possibility of esophageal atresia and tracheoesophageal fistula. Infants in whom a tracheoesophageal fistula is suspected should not be fed; feeding will lead to aspiration pneumonia. Failure in an attempt to pass a feeding tube into the baby's stomach suggests a strong likelihood of a tracheoesophageal fistula that should be confirmed by x-ray examination.

Jaw. Newborn infants normally have a receding chin. An abnormally small jaw, micrognathia, can cause respiratory distress, because the tongue falls back into the pharynx. Babies with micrognathia should be carefully assessed for cleft palate as well.

Neck. The neck of a newborn infant is short with multiple folds. The muscles of the neck support the baby's head only briefly when the infant is pulled to a sitting position, but the infant may be able to support the head briefly when prone. By the end of the neonatal period (4 weeks), the infant should be able to hold the chin up and turn the head when prone, but the head will still lag for several weeks when the infant is pulled to a sitting position. Neck muscles should allow the infant to turn the head fully from right to left.

Thorax and Abdomen

Thorax. Breast engorgement is normally found in both male and female infants. During pregnancy, maternal hormones cross the placenta and enter fetal circulation. At birth, when maternal hormones are no longer present, the breasts enlarge and may even secrete fluid resembling colostrum or milk for a period that may last from several days to several weeks. Inspect and palpate the clavicles and shoulders. Clavicles should be intact and shoulders should have full range of motion.

Abdomen. The new baby's abdomen is symmetric and moderately protuberant. Bowel sounds should be auscultated in all four quadrants before palpation is done. Intermittent tinkling bowel sounds should be heard every 10 to 20 seconds.

Bowel sounds may be absent during the first 1 to 2 hours after birth. Palpation of the abdomen is aided by flexing the infant's knees or holding the infant semierect to relax the abdominal muscles. The liver is palpated 2 to 3 cm below the right costal margin. The tip of the spleen is felt at the left costal margin. It may not be possible to palpate the spleen in the first week after birth. Palpate the kidneys by placing one hand beneath the infant's flank and the other below the costal margin and pressing them together. The tip of the left kidney and the lower half of the right kidney should be felt approximately 1 to 2 cm above the umbilicus.

Femoral pulses should be palpated during examination of the abdomen; they should be felt bilaterally and equally. Absent or diminished femoral pulses suggest coarctation of the aorta, a congenital heart defect. Note also the presence of a bulge, which suggests an inguinal hernia.

A small, scaphoid abdomen may indicate a diaphragmatic hernia, in which part of the bowel has herniated through the diaphragm and is in the thoracic cavity. A diaphragmatic hernia requires prompt recognition and prompt surgical treatment.

A distended abdomen is also abnormal. It is an additional sign of a tracheoesophageal fistula. Infection, congenital obstruction of the gastrointestinal tract, and congenital megacolon may also be associated with a distended abdomen. If the abdomen appears distended, marking the area of distention with a wax pencil and measuring abdominal girth will provide a baseline value for future assessment.

When the abdominal muscles are absent, the abdomen has a wrinkled appearance from which the term prune-belly syndrome is derived. The infants, 95 percent of whom are male, may have a number of associated defects including undescended testicles, intestinal malrotation, imperforate anus, dilated and tortuous ureters, hydronephrotic kidneys, and a dilated hypertrophied bladder. Prognosis is related to the degree of gastrointestinal obstruction and the extent of the renal problems.

▼ **Umbilical Cord.** The umbilical cord is bluish white at birth and should contain three vessels—two umbilical arteries and one umbilical vein. The cord begins to dry shortly after birth and usually falls off within 7 to 14 days.

When only two umbilical vessels are present, the possibility of other congenital anomalies is raised. Other abnormalities of the cord include yellow discoloration, which may indicate hemolytic disease; exudate, a sign of infection; and bleeding, which may be due to inadequate clamping of the cord or may be a sign of a bleeding disorder.

Cutis navel describes an umbilical cord that projects beyond the skin. It may seem as if the baby has an umbilical hernia, but a hernia can be returned to the abdomen whereas the cutis navel cannot. No special treatment is required; the navel will slowly invaginate. The presence of an umbilical hernia should be noted.

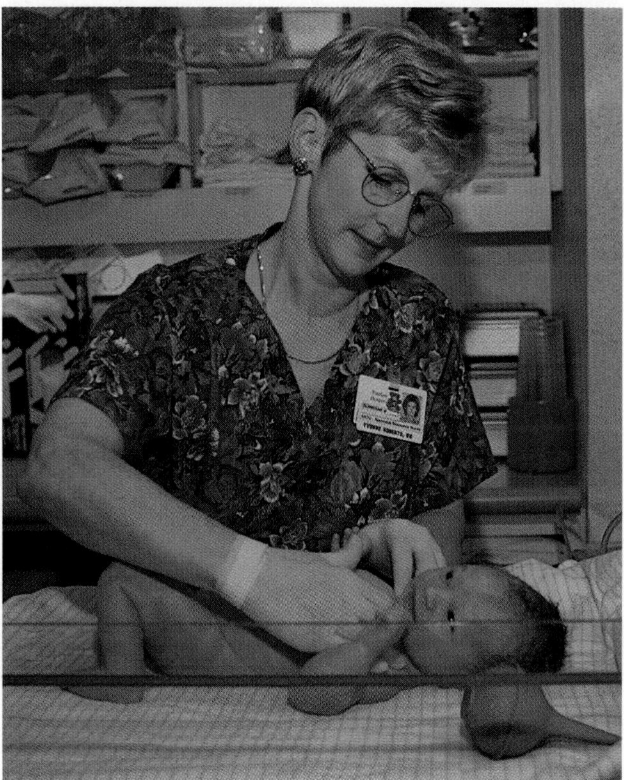

Figure 31–21

Assessment of the clavicles following birth is essential to determine if the clavicles are intact.

Bleeding from the umbilical stump requires prompt attention, as does drainage, which may indicate infection. Note the odor, color, and amount of any drainage.

Genitalia

▼ **Female Genitalia.** The genitalia of a newborn girl are frequently red and swollen; this edema disappears in a few days. There may be a hymenal or vaginal skin tag, which will spontaneously drop off in a few weeks.

A vaginal discharge of thick, white mucus is seen in the first week of life. The mucus is occasionally blood tinged about the third or fourth day, staining the diaper. The cause of this pseudomenstruation, like that of breast engorgement, is the withdrawal of maternal hormones. Excessive vaginal bleeding, however, is not normal and requires further assessment.

Male Genitalia. The foreskin is adherent to the glans penis at the time of birth. The scrotum is frequently swollen; this edema disappears in a few days. Descent of the testicles is described in the assessment of gestational age.

Note the site of the opening of the urethra, which should be at the tip of the penis. In about 1 of every 300 births, the urethra opens on the ventral surface of the penis. This condition is termed hypospadias. Surgical correction is usually made by the time the boy is 2 years old. Infants with hypospadias should not be circumcised, because the foreskin is used in the surgical repair.

Epispadias, the opening of the urethra on the dorsal aspect of the penis, is far less common than hypospadias and is also corrected by surgery.

Ambiguous Genitalia. At times, it is not possible to distinguish sex by observing external genitalia (ambiguous genitalia). Because sex is often the first information given to parents (It's a girl!), the ambiguity of sex characteristics is highly disturbing for new parents. When sex is incorrectly assigned, the potential for long-term emotional stress is significant. In addition, if ambiguous genitalia are secondary to certain forms of congenital adrenal hyperplasia, an autosomal recessive trait in which anorexia, vomiting, diarrhea, loss of weight, and extreme dehydration occur (commonly termed salt losers), the infant is at severe physical risk.

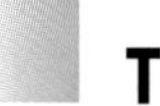

The Back

A major abnormality of the spine, spina bifida with associated meningocele or meningomyelocele, is readily apparent. However, the vertebrae should be palpated for defects in the closure of the vertebral canal (spina bifida occulta) and for abnormal curvature of the spine (Fig. 31–22).

Extremities

Both arms and legs are strongly flexed in a healthy term infant. Muscle tone should be equal bilaterally. Infants who were in a footling breech position in utero may have their legs extended rather than flexed. Note any abnormal position of an extremity, unequal muscle tone, or decreased muscle tone (hypotonia).

Congenital Dislocation of the Hip. The inability to abduct one thigh is an indication of congenital hip dysplasia, in which abnormal development of the hip joint occurs. Dysplasia may be partial (congenital subluxation of the hip), in which the head of the femur is partially dislocated from the shallow acetabulum, or complete (congenital dislocation), in which the head of the femur is completely dislocated from the hip. Congenital subluxation is much more common.

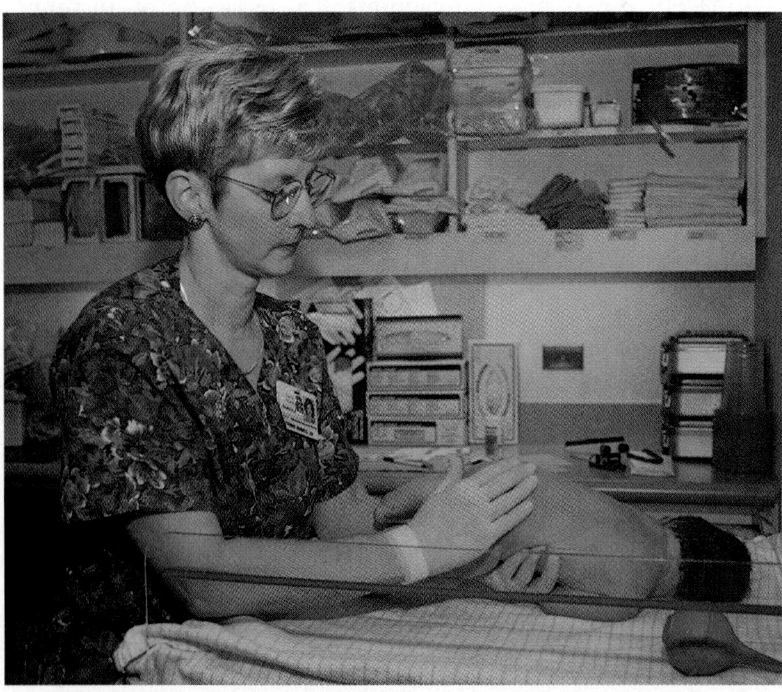

Figure 31–22
Assessment of the back.

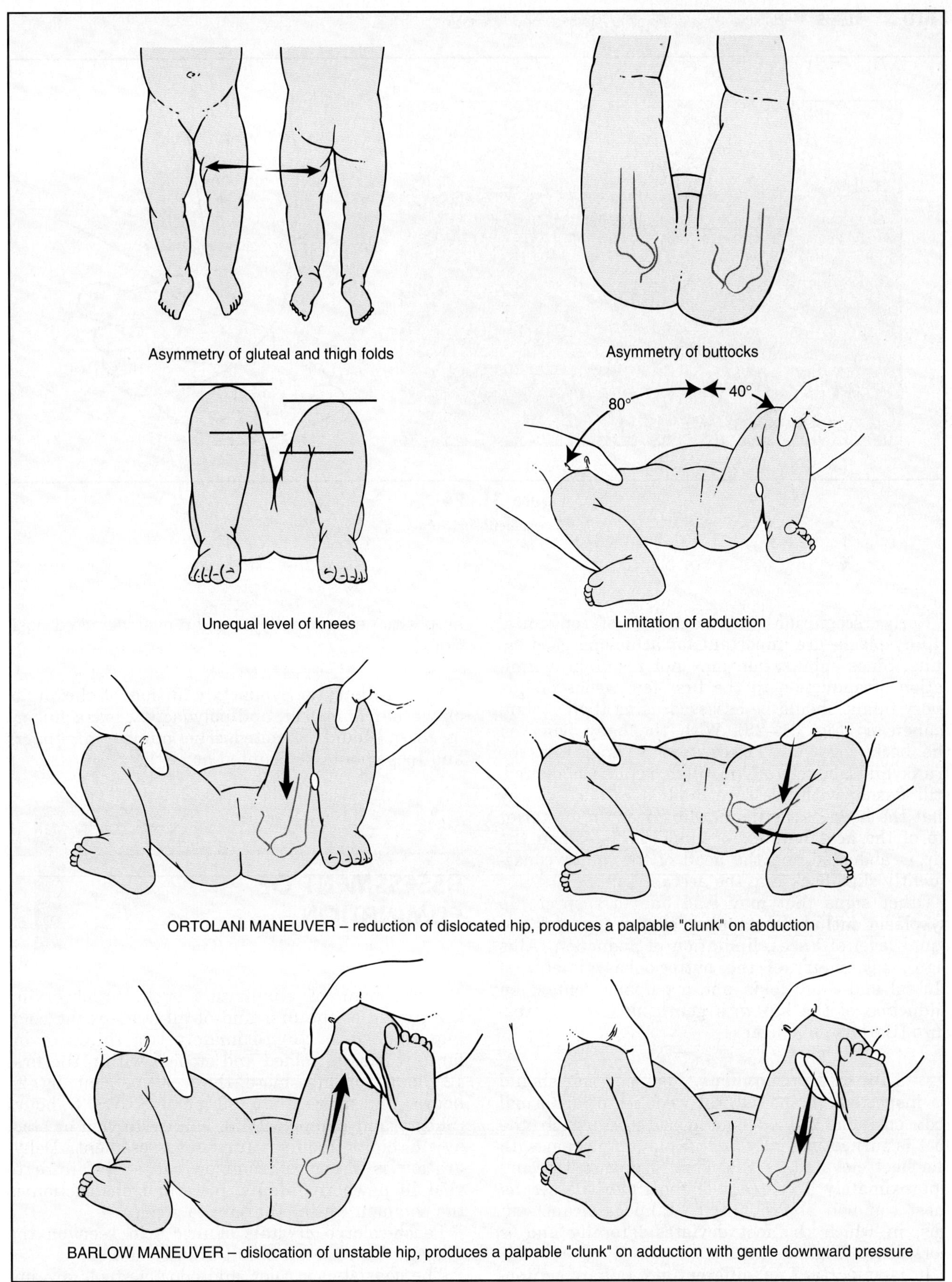

Figure 31–23

Assessment of the newborn for a dislocated or unstable hip includes gluteal and thigh folds, buttocks, knees, abduction, Ortolani maneuver, and Barlow maneuver.

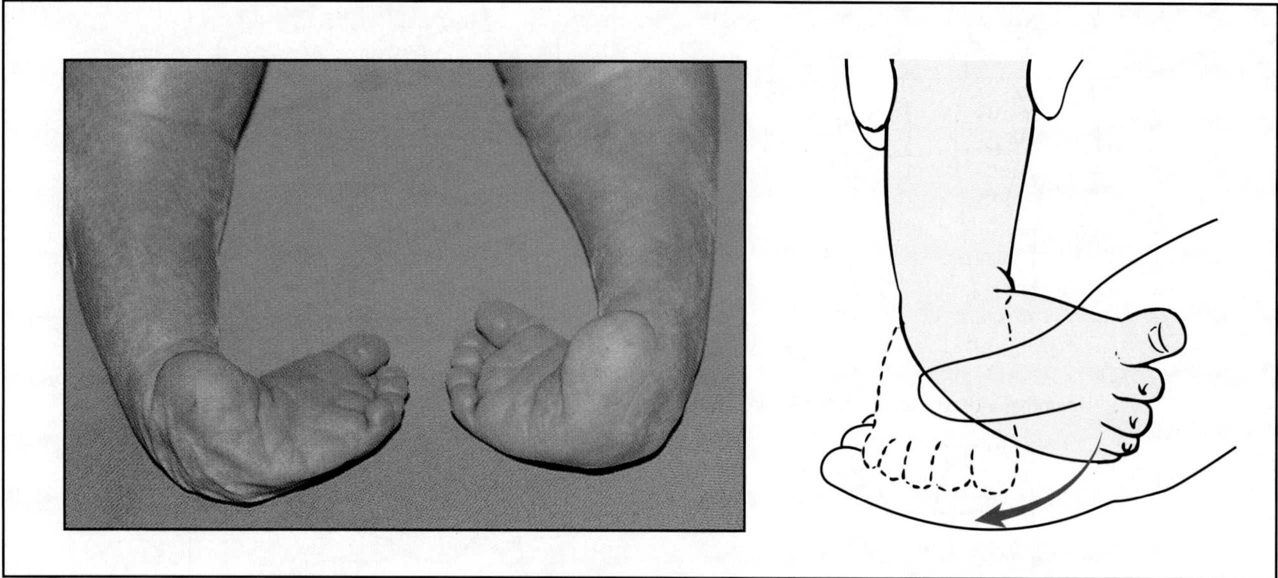

Figure 31–24
Assessment for clubfoot.

Early recognition and treatment of congenital hip dysplasia are important for achieving good results. Since subluxation may not result in a limitation of abduction in the first few weeks of life, every infant should be assessed using the Ortolani maneuver (Fig. 31–23). With the baby lying on the back, legs are flexed at right angles to the trunk and abducted. One thigh is then abducted, still flexed, with pressure applied in such a way that the head of the femur slips over the posterior lip of the acetabulum. A "clunk" is felt when the hip is abducted and the head of the femur consequently slips back into the acetabulum.

Other signs that may lead one to suspect hip dysplasia include shortening of one leg and unequal level of knees, limitation of abduction (Allis sign), asymmetry of the buttocks, asymmetry of gluteal and thigh folds, and a palpable "clunk" on adduction of the hip with gentle downward pressure (Barlow maneuver).

▼ **Talipes Equinovarus.** Foot position should be inspected. Of the several varieties of abnormal foot position, talipes equinovarus, in which the foot is turned medially and in plantar flexion with the heel elevated, is the most frequent; it occurs approximately 95 percent of the time. The second most common abnormality is talipes calcaneovalgus, in which the foot deviates laterally and is dorsiflexed (Fig. 31–24).

It is important to differentiate talipes equinovarus from a foot that appears to be deformed because of the position of the fetus in utero. When the abnormal position of the foot is caused by the position of the fetus in utero, the foot can easily be positioned normally or in an overcorrected position.

▼ **Syndactyly.** Syndactyly, fusion of the digits of the hands or feet, and polydactyly, extra fingers or toes, should be noted. The number of fingers and toes should be counted at birth.

ASSESSMENT OF ELIMINATION

Assessment of elimination includes observing the timing of the first and of all subsequent voidings and stools. Approximately two thirds of infants will have voided and stooled within the first 12 hours of life, more than 90 percent by 24 hours, and more than 99 percent by 48 hours (Sherry and Kramer 1955). Failure to void or stool by 48 hours requires further assessment. Dehydration is the most common cause of failure to void in newborn infants; intestinal obstruction is the common cause of failure to stool.

Peach-colored crystals of uric acid seen on the diaper of a newborn infant are normal.

The consistency, color, and odor of stools are important in evaluating the infant's general condition. Because color changes in the stool can occur shortly after defecation, evaluation has to be made immediately if it is to have meaning.

Stool consistency and color vary in the first days with both age and type of feeding (see Fig. 30–7). The first stools are of meconium, an odorless viscid material that is dark green to black. Meconium stools may last 3 to 4 days. With shortened birth site stays, only meconium stools may be seen before discharge to home.

Meconium stools are followed by greenish brown to yellow transitional stools. In breastfed infants, the next stools are of a golden to mustard color. Initially, breastfed infants may have more frequent stools than bottle-fed infants. However, in subsequent weeks, some breastfed infants may have no stool for several days and yet be perfectly normal. Breastfeeding mothers need to know this. Mothers may also interpret the soft breastfed stool as diarrhea if they do not recognize stool characteristics.

The stools of bottle-fed babies are pale yellow in color. They tend to be more formed, are more frequent after the first days of life, and are more regular than those of breastfed infants.

Abnormal stool characteristics include thick putty-like meconium, small putty-like stools, and diarrhea. Diarrhea is a somewhat nonspecific symptom in newborns. It may be caused by overfeeding. Some infants have diarrhea from certain formulas that will have no effect on other infants. Gastroenteritis causes diarrhea in some babies and can spread quickly from one infant to another. The degree of severity of diarrhea can be estimated by measuring the water margin around the stool if the baby has not voided in the diaper. Aside from the danger of sepsis, diarrhea is always serious because of the newborn's extremely labile water balance.

Signs of intestinal bleeding, either bright red or old blood, can be further assessed by use of readily available chemical tests that can be quickly and easily performed.

LABORATORY ASSESSMENT

Two laboratory tests, one for phenylketonuria (PKU) and a second for hypothyroidism, both of which use the same blood specimen, are required by law. Both conditions, if undetected, lead to severe mental retardation. These tests are the only universally performed laboratory assessments of healthy term newborns. At some birth sites, an initial assessment of hematocrit or of blood glu-

PROCEDURE 31–3

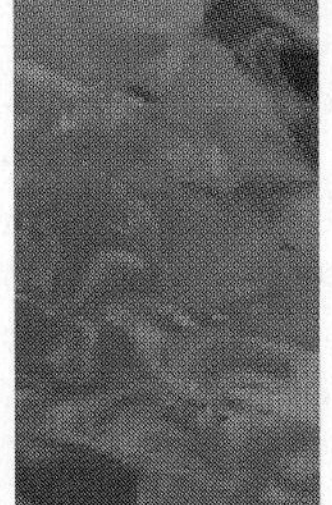

Using the Heel Stick Method to Obtain Blood

▼ PURPOSE

To obtain the newborn's blood for assessment of blood glucose levels, hematocrit, phenylketonuria, or bilirubin level as ordered or when symptoms of hypoglycemia occur.

▼ EQUIPMENT

- Alcohol swab
- Lancet or Tenderfoot capillary tubes
- Dextrostix
- Gloves
- Small, round adhesive bandage
- Sterile 2 × 2 gauze pads

Continued on following page

PROCEDURE 31–3 Continued

1 Wash hands and apply gloves. **Standard Precautions require gloves for contact with blood and body fluids. Washing hands helps prevent cross-contamination.**

2 Warm the baby's heel for 15 to 30 seconds by wrapping the foot in a warm pack (warm a diaper by running it under warm water; do not cover with plastic or use a disposable diaper with plastic). **Wrapping the foot in a warm pack is sometimes helpful to increase circulation to the site (heat causes local vasodilatation and increased blood flow). Application of hot packs can cause thermal burns. Plastic covers prevent heat dissipation and can result in thermal burns.**

3 Choose either side of the heel (either the lateral or medial aspect of the heel) as the puncture site. The lateral aspect of the heel is the preferred heel stick site. **Puncturing the side rather than the middle of the heel prevents damaging the posterior tibial nerve and artery and the longitudinal fat pad, which could interfere with walking.**

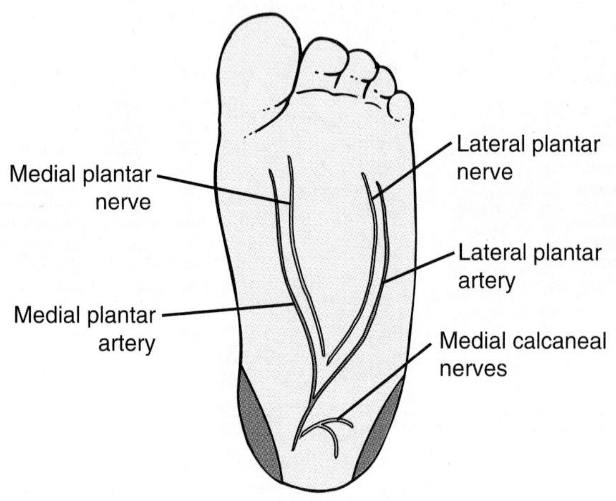

4 Cleanse the site with an alcohol swab. Dry the site with a sterile 2 × 2 gauze pad. **Cleansing the site with alcohol minimizes contamination. Drying the site is important because alcohol can be irritating and can cause hemolysis.**

5 Puncture the heel with the lancet or Tenderfoot to achieve free flow of blood. (Tenderfoot is a small plastic case that houses a needle. When the case is placed on the baby's foot, the needle can be automatically ejected.) **Free flow of blood ensures an adequate sample. Use of Tenderfoot ensures controlled depth of entry and makes optimal penetration possible (i.e., penetration is deep enough to obtain an adequate specimen yet superficial enough to prevent damage to tissues, nerves, and bones and to prevent fibrosis and scarring caused by repeated sampling).**

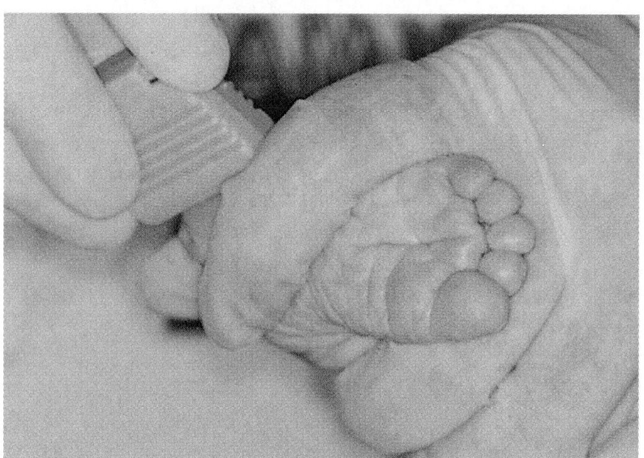

6 Collect blood into capillary tubes, onto Dextrostix, or onto Chemstrip. If necessary, gently apply slight pressure to the foot or ankle above the puncture site to obtain enough blood. **The collection device needed depends on the test being done. Application of slight pressure is sometimes necessary to obtain enough blood.**

7 Cover heel stick site with small circular bandage. **Applying an adhesive bandage creates pressure needed to minimize bleeding, and it protects the site from contamination.**

8 Check the heel stick site frequently for bleeding. **The baby's normal motions, such as kicking and rubbing, can remove the adhesive bandage and cause bleeding.**

PROCEDURE 31–4

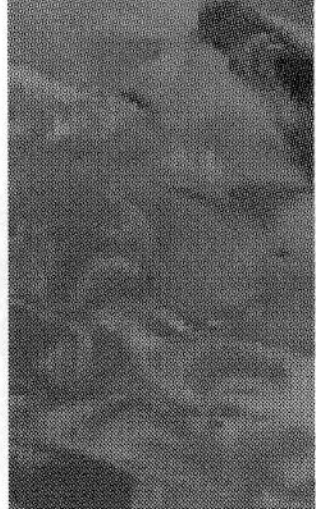

Assessing Blood Glucose Level Using Dextrostix or Chemstrip with Accu-Check II Device

▼ PURPOSE

To assess the newborn's blood glucose level for presence of hypoglycemia when ordered or when symptoms of hypoglycemia are present. Hypoglycemia is diagnosed when blood glucose level is below 30 mg/dL in the first 72 hours or below 45 mg/dL after the first 3 days of life.

▼ EQUIPMENT

- Lancet or Tenderfoot
- Alcohol swabs
- Sterile 2 × 2 gauze pads
- Small, round adhesive bandage
- Cotton balls
- Container of glucose strips (Chemstrip or Dextrostix)
- Gloves
- Accu-Check II device
- Squeeze water bottle

1 To achieve free flow of blood for an adequate sample, follow steps 1 through 5 of Procedure 31–3, Using the Heel Stick Method to Obtain Blood (pp. 1111–1112). **Accurate assessment of blood glucose level requires an adequate sample of the newborn's blood.**

2 Completely cover the treated area of the reagent strip with the blood sample from the newborn's heel. For Chemstrip with Accu-Check II, use the first drop of blood as the sample. For Dextrostix without the Accu-Check device, discard the first drop of blood. **Completely covering the treated area of the reagent strip helps ensure accurate test results. For Chemstrip with Accu-Check II, test results are more accurate if the first drop of blood is used rather than subsequent drops. The first drop of blood is discarded for Dextrostix used without the Accu-Check device, since the first drop is typically diluted with tissue fluid from the stick site.**

3 Leave the blood sample on the glucose strip for exactly 60 seconds. The treated area of the strip will change color during this time. (Note: If the Accu-Check II device is used, press the "time" button to activate the timing mechanism.) **Leaving the blood sample on the strip for the prescribed amount of time helps ensure accurate test results. (With Accu-Check II, three high beeps sound at seconds 57, 58, and 59; one low beep sounds at second 60.)**

4 At 60 seconds, clean blood from the strip. For Chemstrip, use clean cotton balls to wipe away blood completely, leaving no blood on the treated area of the strip. For Dextrostix, use a forceful stream of water from a squeeze bottle to rinse away blood completely from the strip. **Executing the procedure carefully and according to directions is crucial for obtaining an accurate reading.**

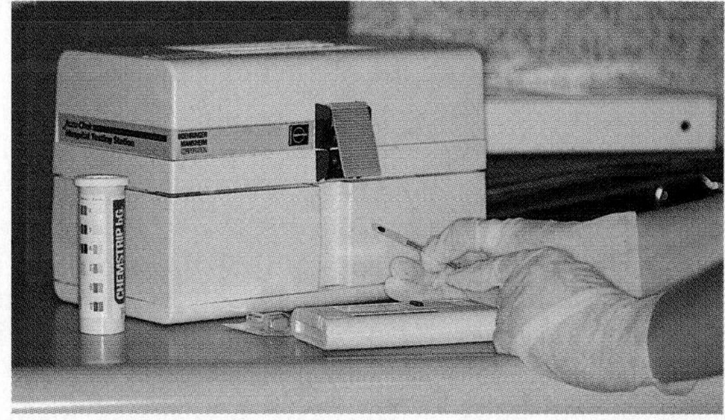

5 Determine blood glucose value. With the Accu-Check II device, insert the Chemstrip into the adapter slot of Accu-Check II before

Continued on following page

PROCEDURE 31–4 Continued

the timer display reads 120 seconds. At 120 seconds, a high beep sounds, and the screen displays a blood glucose value (in mg/dL). For Dextrostix, wait for the amount of time recommended on the container and compare the color of the Dextrostix strip with the colors on the Dextrostix container to ascertain the blood glucose value. **False readings can result from inaccurate timing.**

6 Apply small, round adhesive bandage to heel. **Applying an adhesive bandage creates pressure needed to minimize bleeding, and it protects the site from contamination.**

7 Check the heel stick site frequently for bleeding. **The baby's normal motions, such as kicking and rubbing, can remove the adhesive bandage and cause bleeding.**

cose level is routine. Other laboratory studies are related to symptoms noted in physical assessment, for example, determination of serum bilirubin levels in infants with jaundice.

Phenylketonuria

PKU is an autosomal recessive disease in which phenylalanine, an amino acid, accumulates because of an error in metabolism. Undetected, this accumulation leads to irreversible mental retardation in affected infants. In the United States, PKU occurs approximately once in 14,000 births. Mass screening for the presence of phenylalanine in capillary blood is now required by law in most states.

Because concentrations of phenylalanine may not rise sufficiently to be detected in the first days of life, testing should be deferred until 72 hours. Before 72 hours, the amount of phenylalanine ingested by the baby has not accumulated sufficiently to provide adequate screening. In one study, 16 percent of infants with PKU were missed when screening was done in the first 24 hours, and 2 percent were missed when screening was done between 24 and 48 hours. Screening should be done before 7 days because delays in identifying a baby with PKU and thus feeding with breast milk or a formula other than low-phenylalanine formula will lead to irreversible brain damage. The coordination of birth site discharge and home visit at the appropriate time is an essential nursing responsibility. Thyroid screening is conducted on the same blood sample as PKU screening. When mothers and infants return home before that time, alternative plans for screening are necessary.

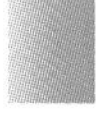

Congenital Hypothyroidism

Congenital hypothyroidism is far more common than PKU, occurring approximately once in 6000 births. Without detection and treatment, both physical and mental growth are affected. If therapy with thyroid hormone is started by 6 weeks after birth, normal development can be expected.

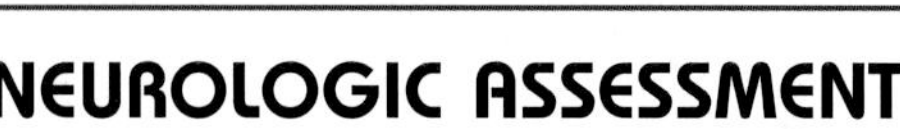

NEUROLOGIC ASSESSMENT

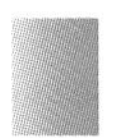

Neonatal Reflexes

Assessment of the reflexes provides valuable information about an infant's neurologic status. Generalized illness and medication given to the mother during labor and birth can affect neurologic status.

▼ **Moro.** The Moro reflex (Fig. 31–25) is elicited by a loud noise such as a hand clap or a slap on the mattress. The baby should respond with (in sequence) extension and abduction of the limbs, followed by flexion and abduction of the limbs, followed by flexion and adduction of the limbs (as if to embrace). The reflex is consistently present by gestational age 34 weeks and disappears at 6 months. This reflex is the most significant single indicator of central nervous system status. A sudden noise or motion may also elicit response. Consistent absence suggests brain dam-

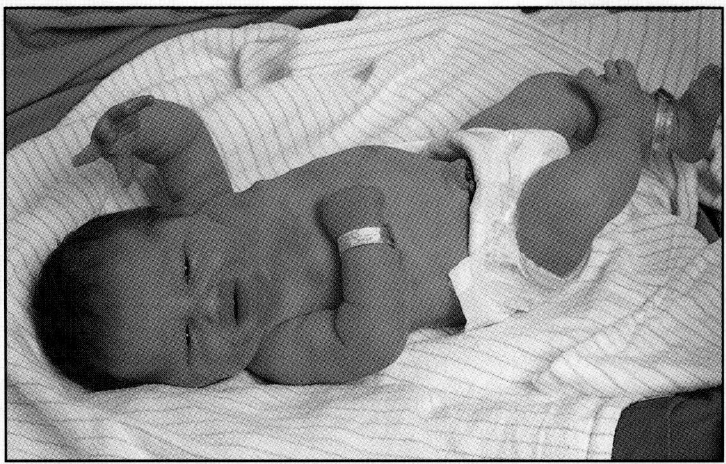

MORO REFLEX

- Elicited by a variety of stimuli - loud noise, sudden movement of the surface the infant is lying on, or the sudden drop of the infant's head backward about 30 degrees into the examiner's hand
- Portions of the Moro reflex are present at 25 to 27 weeks of gestation
- Complete Moro reflex is present at 34 weeks of gestation
- Disappears at approximately 6 months of age

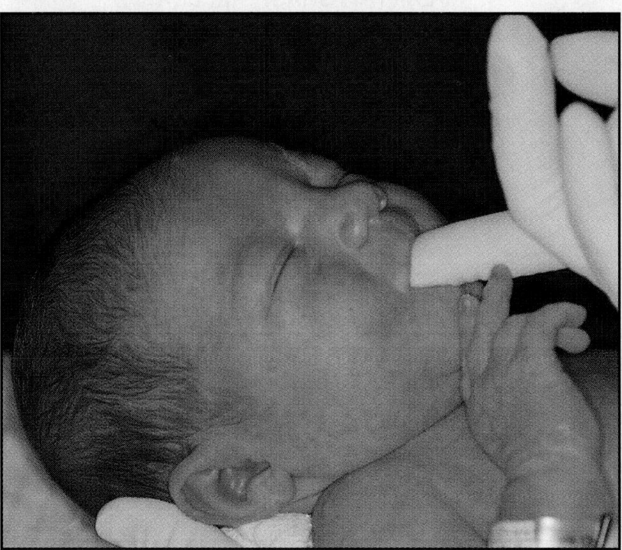

SUCKING REFLEX

- Elicited by stimulating the mucous membranes of the mouth with gloved finger
- Appears at 28 weeks of gestation, weak and uncoordinated suck
- Mature at 34 weeks of gestation, strong and coordinated suck
- Disappears at approximately 4 months of age

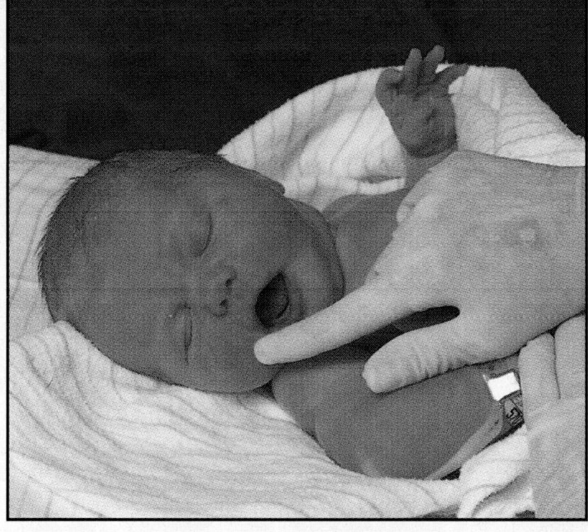

ROOTING REFLEX

- Elicited by stimulating the perioral area with the finger
- Appears at 28 weeks of gestation, immature
- Mature at 34 weeks of gestation
- Disappears at approximately 4 months of age

Figure 31–25

Neonatal reflexes • Moro • Sucking • Rooting

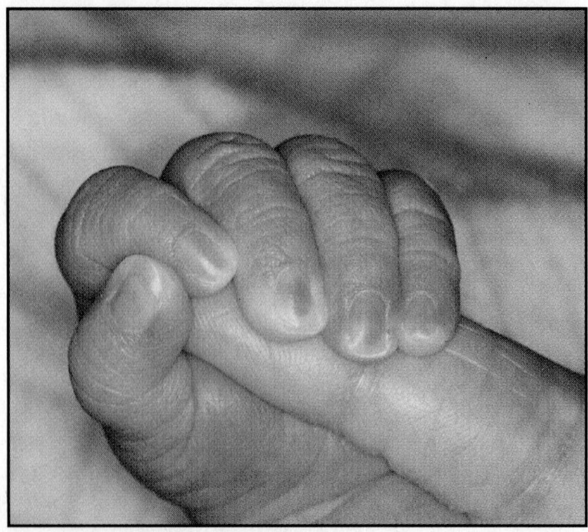

PALMAR GRASP REFLEX

- Elicited by stimulating the palm of the hand by firm pressure
- Appears at 26 to 27 weeks of gestation, immature
- Mature at 34 weeks of gestation
- Becomes inconsistent at 2 months of age when voluntary grasping begins
- Disappears at approximately 6 to 9 months of age

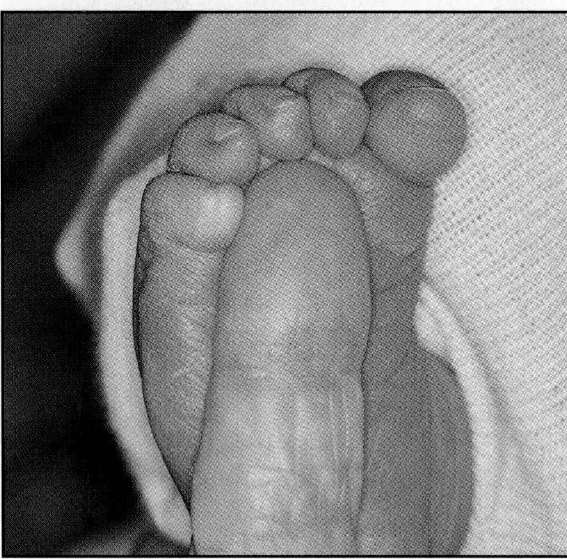

PLANTAR GRASP REFLEX

- Elicited by stimulating the ball of the foot by firm pressure
- Appears at 26 to 27 weeks of geatation, immature
- Mature at 34 weeks of gestation
- Disappears at approximately 6 to 9 months of age

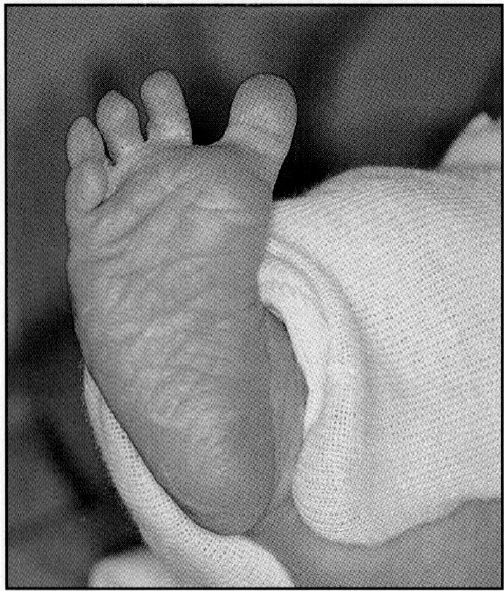

BABINSKI REFLEX

- Elicited by stroking the lateral aspects of the sole of the foot from the heel upward and across the ball of the foot with the fingernail
- Disappears at approximately 12 months of age

Figure 31–25 *Continued*
Palmar grasp • Plantar grasp • Babinski

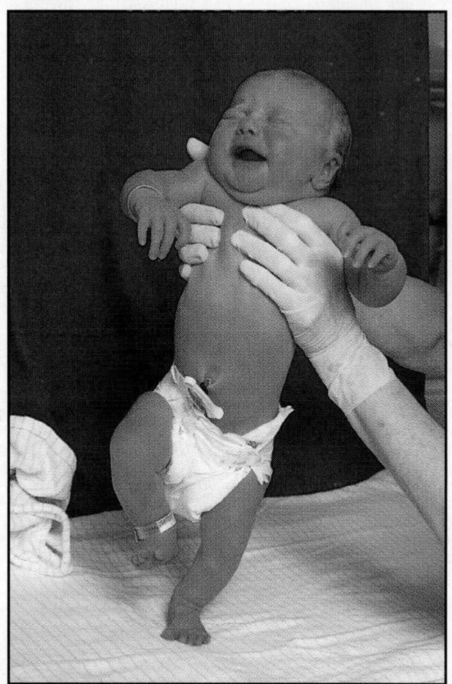

STEPPING REFLEX

- Elicited by holding the infant upright so that the sole of a foot is in firm contact with a flat surface
- Appears at 34 weeks of gestation, immature toe-heel stepping
- Mature, heel-toe stepping, at 38 weeks of gestation
- Disappears at approximately 1 to 2 months of age

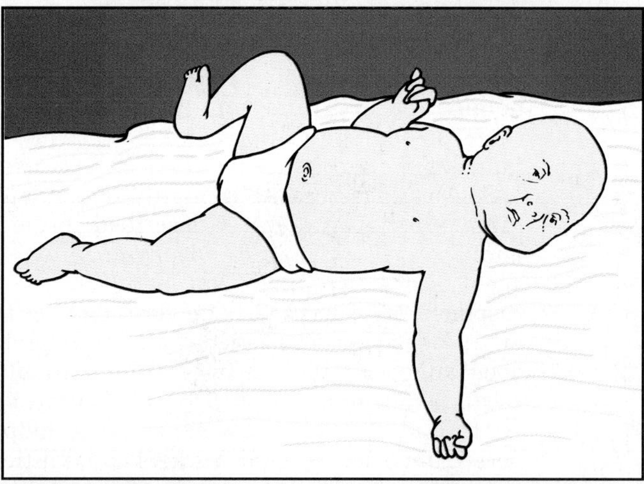

TONIC NECK REFLEX

- Elicited by rotation of the head to one side
- Present as early as 35 weeks of gestation
- Most prominent at 1 month after term
- Disappears by approximately 7 months of age

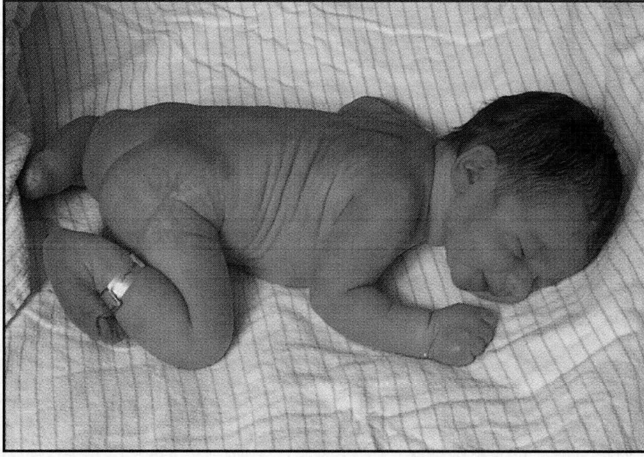

TRUNK INCURVATION (GALANT REFLEX)

- Elicited by gentle stroking of the fingers down the paravertebral area with the infant in prone position
- Appears as early as 24 weeks of gestation
- Disappears by 12 months of age

Figure 31–25 *Continued*
Stepping • Tonic neck • Trunk incurvation

age, a fractured clavicle, or injury to the brachial plexus.

▼ **Sucking.** The sucking reflex (Fig. 31–25) is produced by stroking the lips. It should be reasonably strong by 32 weeks' gestational age and excellent by 34 weeks. It is diminishing by 3 to 4 months. Sucking reflex may be difficult to elicit in a recently fed baby and may be weak or absent in a baby with brain damage.

▼ **Rooting.** Rooting (Fig. 31–25) is elicited by stroking the upper or lower lip or the side of the cheek. The baby turns the mouth and face toward the stimulus and opens the mouth. Rooting reflex is fairly good by 32 weeks' gestational age and is complete at 34 weeks.

▼ **Palmar Grasp.** Pressing the examiner's finger into the baby's metacarpophalangeal groove causes the baby to grasp the finger (Fig. 31–25). Finger grasp is present as early as 26 weeks' gestational age, but gestational age must be approximately 34 weeks before the baby can lift himself or herself off the mattress. Palmar grasp disappears at about 6 to 9 months.

▼ **Plantar Grasp.** Pressure on the plantar surface of the foot causes flexion of the toes (Fig. 31–25). This reflex disappears by about 8 to 15 months.

▼ **Babinski.** Stroking the sole of the foot from the heel to the toe causes the big toe to flex and the other toes to spread (Fig. 31–25).

▼ **Stepping.** The stepping reflex (Fig. 31–25) is elicited by holding the infant erect and supporting the body under the arms; with the soles flat on a surface and the trunk inclined forward, the infant will take regular, alternating steps. At gestational age 34 weeks, the infant may tiptoe; a heel to toe motion appears at 38 weeks. The stepping reflex disappears at 1 to 2 months of age. Failure to step on several occasions suggests neurologic abnormality; stepping with only one foot indicates a unilateral problem.

▼ **Placing.** When the baby is held erect and supported under the arms with the dorsum of the foot drawn against the underedge of the tabletop, the foot is lifted and placed atop the table. The reflex appears consistently at gestational age 35 weeks and disappears at 6 weeks.

▼ **Tonic Neck Reflex.** When the baby is supine and the head is turned to one side, the arm and leg toward which the baby is facing extend, while the opposite arm and leg flex in a "fencing" position (Fig. 31–25). The reflex is incomplete at birth in the normal term infant; it is often more definite in the leg than in the arm. The reflex disappears during the first 7 months, although a partial response may remain until the second or third year. If persistent asymmetry and a full response are easily obtained, a cerebral lesion is suggested.

▼ **Neck Righting.** When the baby's head is turned to one side, the trunk will follow. The reflex appears consistenty by gestational age 34 to 36 weeks and continues to develop. Other righting reflexes develop as the baby grows older.

▼ **Trunk Incurvation.** With the infant in prone position, touching one side of the vertebral column elicits curvature of the spine toward the stimulated side. The reflex is present from 24 weeks of gestation. It is a test of spinal cord integrity.

Sensory Assessment

Sensory development begins early in fetal life. Infants born at term have a sensory capability uniquely suited to their needs. A nursing assessment of sensory development has dual goals of identifying actual or potential problems and of helping parents and family, when it is done in their presence, to appreciate how ready their infant is to relate to them through the senses.

Sensory assessment is highly dependent on the infant's behavioral state (described in detail later) and, in the first hours and days of life, on factors such as obstetric analgesia or anesthesia. Lack of response to stimuli, in the first day or two after birth, does not necessarily indicate a problem but does suggest that the assessment should be repeated in a home or ambulatory clinic visit both for the purpose of assessment and to help parents better understand their infant's capabilities.

Touch is the first sensory modality to develop in utero. The skin is the largest sensory organ of the body; note the infant's response to varying kinds of touch. Touch is frequently a calming sensation for an infant.

Vision can be assessed by showing the infant a red ball or ring within the field of vision and observing the way in which the infant follows the object, turning not only the eyes but also the head. In the quiet alert state (see Infant State), newborns follow an object both vertically and horizontally. A human face is a preferred visual object; a visual stimulus combined with an auditory stimulus is more compelling than a visual stimulus alone. Greenman (1963) studied 127 infants and found that 26 percent followed a 4-inch red ring during the period in which they were in the delivery room. Between a half-hour and 12 hours of age, 56 percent followed the ring; 76 percent followed the ring by 48 hours of age.

Hearing can be assessed by speaking to the infant from first one side and then the other when the infant is in a quiet alert state and watching the infant turn the head to search for the source of the sound. A rattle may also be used. The sources of sound should be approximately 12 inches from the infant's ear. Other behaviors that indicate a response to an auditory stimulus include the initiation or cessation of crying and dilation of the pupils. Loud noises lead to startles; the absence of startles in the first days of life should lead to further evaluation of the infant's hearing.

Taste and smell are not routinely assessed in the neonatal period. Newborn infants have the ability to discriminate between tastes and odors as early as the first day of life.

INFANT STATE: THE FOUNDATION OF BEHAVIORAL ASSESSMENT

The concept of infant state refers to state of consciousness. State is a unifying concept that serves to explain how various behaviors observed in the neonatal period fit together as parts of a whole. Each state is a group of activities that regularly occur together. These activities include a level of sleep; body, eye, and facial movements;

Table 31–3

NEONATAL BEHAVIORAL STATE

STATE	RESPIRATIONS	EYES	FACIAL EXPRESSION	BODY ACTIVITY	RESPONSE TO STIMULI
1 Deep sleep	Regular (briefly)	Closed; no movement	Relaxed	Generally absent; isolated startles	Only intense stimulus will arouse
2 Light sleep	Irregular	Closed; rapid eye movements (REM)	Sucking, mouthing, facial twitching, grimacing, smiling	Low level; some disorganized movement	More easily aroused by external or internal stimuli
3 Drowsy	Irregular	Open or closed; blinking, eyelid flutter	Relaxed	Variable, diffuse, mild startles; reactive to stimuli	Stimuli may lead to state change or delayed response
4 Quiet alert	Regular	Open; bright look; focus on stimuli	Attentive, bright	Minimal	Highly attentive to external stimuli
5 Active alert	Irregular	Open; less bright than quiet alert	Active	Very active	Sensitive to disturbing external and internal stimuli
6 Crying	Irregular	Open or tightly closed	Grimacing	Crying, very active, color change	Highly sensitive to disturbing external and internal stimuli

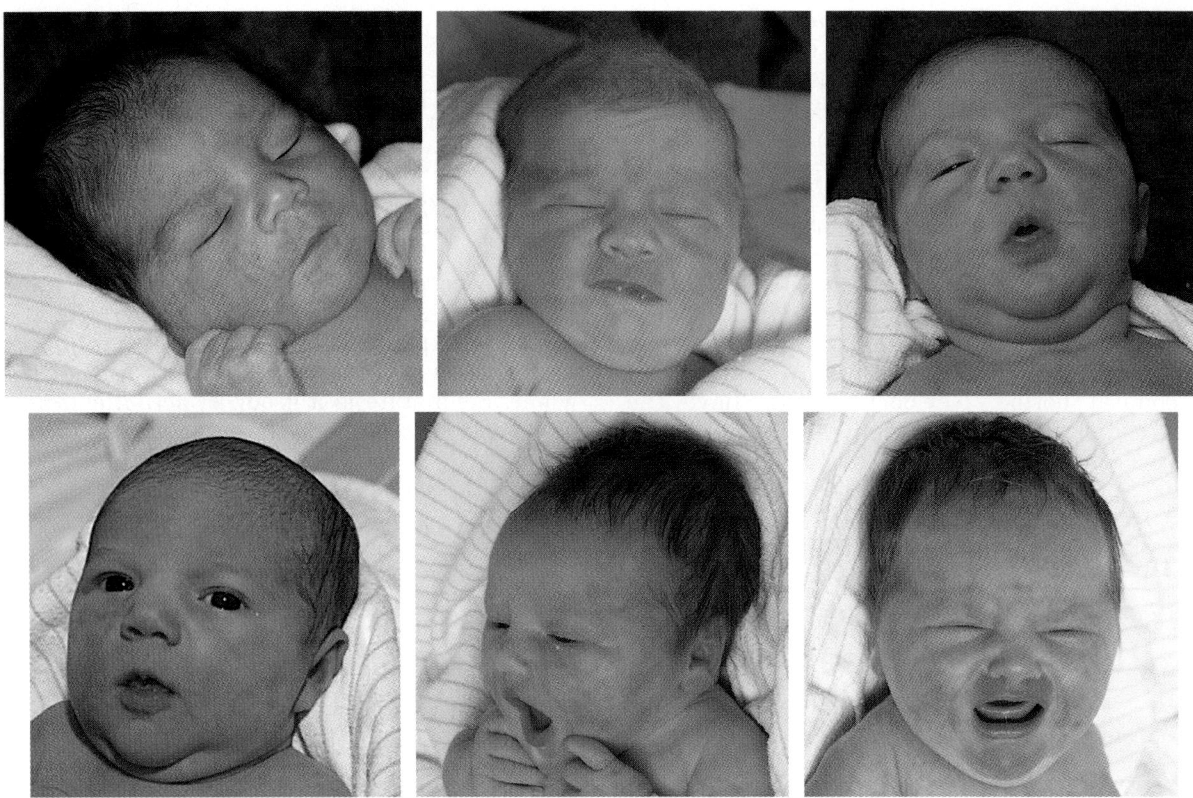

Figure 31–26
Infant states • Deep sleep • Light sleep • Drowsy • Quiet alert • Active alert • Crying

respiration; and responses to both external and internal stimuli. For healthy term infants, six states are commonly described (Wolff 1959). Other researchers in infant development have defined the individual states in a slightly different manner (Prechtl 1964). In the context of six states, two are sleep states: state 1, deep sleep, in which the infant can only rarely be disturbed; and state 2, light sleep, in which the infant is more easily aroused. Although there is individual variation, healthy term infants spend approximately 18 hours a day in the two sleep states.

In state 3, infants are drowsy; they may return to a sleep state or awaken. "Awake" states are state 4, in which the infant is quiet but alert; state 5, characterized by increased activity; and state 6, a state of active crying. An infant's crying is a compelling stimulus for attention. While the initial cry after birth is welcomed by all as a sign of new life, crying in the days after birth can be disconcerting and frustrating to adults, particularly when an infant seems inconsolable. Healthy term infants may cry as much as 3 hours a day, although there is clearly individual variation. Beginning in the second or third week of life, some infants develop periods of inconsolable crying that is commonly described as colic. Helping parents when infants have protracted crying is discussed in Chapter 34. Characteristics of behavioral states are described in relation to respiration, eye movement, facial expression, body activity, and response to stimuli (Table 31–3 and Fig. 31–26).

The concept of state is important to understanding neonatal behaviors, because behaviors are state dependent. For example, an infant will respond to a stimulus, a light or sound, for example, depending on her or his state. In deep sleep, response is likely to be slight, perhaps a blink or a slight stirring. However, in light sleep, the infant may rouse and even move to a drowsy state. In a drowsy state, the infant may startle and open the eyes and perhaps become more alert. If the infant is already in a quiet alert state and a stimulus occurs, the infant becomes even more alert and begins to search for the stimulus, in an active alert state. If crying actively, the infant may not respond to the stimulus at all, or it may catch attention and help bring the infant to a different state. A number of factors can affect infant state, including hunger, degree of hydration, room temperature, position, and the infant's sex.

In assessing the behavior of a healthy term infant, note the ability of the infant to move from one state to another. For example, if the infant is crying, can the infant console himself or herself, perhaps by putting hand to mouth, and move from the crying state to active alert or quiet alert? Does the infant respond to a voice by calming himself or herself? A number of factors affect state and state transition. Infants who are hungry may not console themselves or be consoled except by feeding; a "fussy" baby who is not hungry may be consoled using other approaches. The ability to move easily from one state to another is a sign of state system maturation.

BRAZELTON NEONATAL BEHAVIORAL ASSESSMENT SCALE

Behavioral assessment is not usually a part of routine neonatal assessment. However, awareness of the elements of neonatal behavioral assessment can assist the nurse in overall assessment of infant behavior. The infant's state is a primary consideration in interpreting infant behavior. State varies over the time used to complete the entire examination. The results of this assessment also vary in the first days of life. After an initial period of alertness, healthy term newborns will be more disorganized for 24 to 48 hours (and as long as 3 to 4 days if they have been compromised by medication during birth). Infants subsequently demonstrate organization of behavioral states and thus cortical control and responsiveness (Brazelton 1987).

Brazelton's Neonatal Behavioral Assessment Scale (NBAS) can be used to measure certain aspects of infant behavior and identify individual differences in infant behavior (Brazelton 1973). It can be used as a diagnostic tool for neurologic impairment or to teach parents the unique social and interactive capabilities of their newborn. The scale is designed for infants from birth to 1 month of age.

The NBAS contains 20 reflex (neurologic) items that include infant reflexes, 27 behavioral response items, ratings of the infant's predominant states during the examination and ability to interact, and a description of self-consoling behaviors used by the infant during the examination (Fig. 31–27) (Brazelton 1973).

NEUROBEHAVIORAL CUES

Infants demonstrate neurobehavioral cues that reflect their organizational ability and the readiness for interaction. These behaviors are categorized as distress/disengagement cues and stability/engagement cues and are shown in Table 31–4 (Blackburn and Loper 1992). Stability/engagement cues, such as the infant smiling in Figure 31–27, indicate that the infant has good organization and is ready to participate in an interaction. Distress/disengagement cues, such as the infant yawning in Figure 31–27, indicate the infant's lack of organization and signal a need for a time-

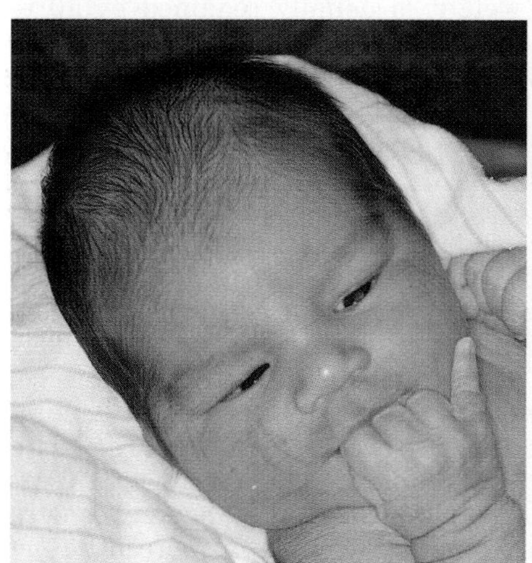
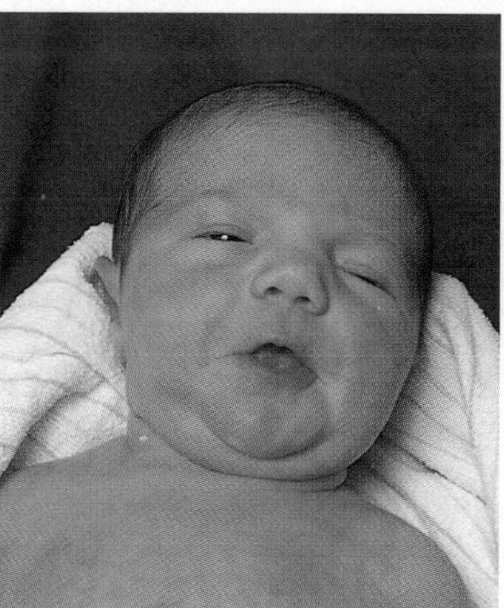
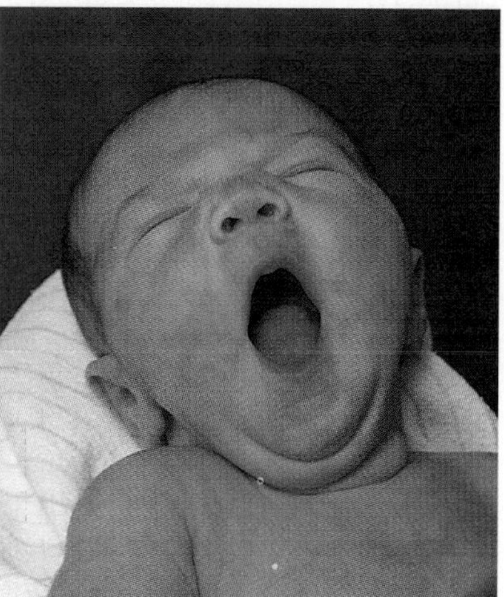

Figure 31–27
Infant behaviors • Self-consoling behavior • Social behavior • Disengagement behavior

Table 31–4

INFANT NEUROBEHAVIORAL CUES

DISTRESS/DISENGAGEMENT CUES	STABILITY/ ENGAGEMENT CUES
Bradycardia, apnea	Facial gaze
Rapid heart or respiration rate	Smiling
Grunting	Vocalization
Stooling	Feeding posture
Mottled skin	Flexion of arms, legs
Dusky color	Eyes alert
Cyanosis	Stable heart rate
Tremor	Stable respiratory rate
Finger splay	Smooth movements
Fingers interlaced	Hand-to-mouth
Arching	Finger folding
Hyperalert face	Smooth state transitions
Facial grimace	Sucking, mouthing
Limb extension	Consolable
Gaze aversion	"Ooh" face
Eyes closed	Alert
Slack jaw	Eye-to-eye contact
Open mouth	Grasping
Tongue thrusting	
Sighing	
Regurgitation	
Jittery	
Flaccid	
Vomiting	
Hand-to-ear	
Worried face	
Rapid state change	
Eyes floating	
Staring	
Hyperextension	
Glassy-eyed	
Tongue protrusion	
Flushed	
Hiccough	
Startle	
Yawn	
Flaccidity	
Sneezing	

From Blackburn, S., and Loper, D. (1992). *Maternal, fetal and neonatal physiology: A clinical perspective* (p. 565). Philadelphia: W. B. Saunders.

out period of rest and recuperation. During a distress period, infants need quiet, reduced handling, and supportive interventions such as swaddling to promote neurobehavioral organization. Parents need information about these neurobehavioral cues of infants so that they can respond to their infants more appropriately. This is especially true for parents of preterm infants or infants who are extremely sensitive to incoming stimuli.

Parents can use the following simple but effective principles when interacting with their infants:

- Be sensitive and alert to the infant's cues.
- Follow the infant's lead when interacting with the infant. If the infant shows engagement behaviors, continue the interaction. If the infant shows distress cues, cease the interaction and provide interventions that support neurobehavioral organization.

FOLLOW-UP ASSESSMENTS AFTER INITIAL POSTBIRTH PERIOD

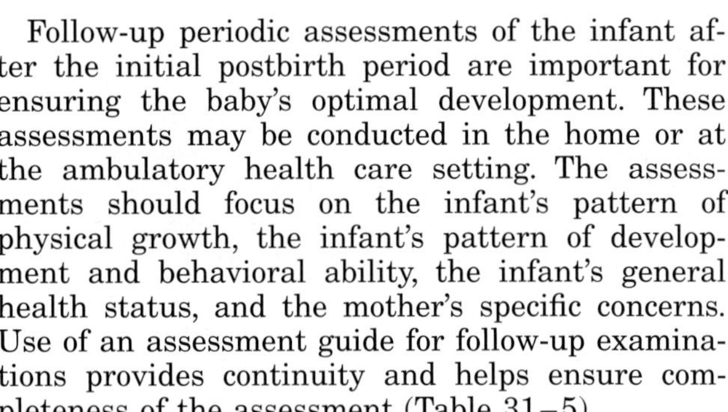

Follow-up periodic assessments of the infant after the initial postbirth period are important for ensuring the baby's optimal development. These assessments may be conducted in the home or at the ambulatory health care setting. The assessments should focus on the infant's pattern of physical growth, the infant's pattern of development and behavioral ability, the infant's general health status, and the mother's specific concerns. Use of an assessment guide for follow-up examinations provides continuity and helps ensure completeness of the assessment (Table 31–5).

Patterns of Growth

Infants may lose up to 10 percent of their birth weight. Birth weight is usually regained by 10 to 14 days. For the next 2 months, infants will gain approximately 1 ounce (28 g) per day. Growth in length occurs also. By the end of 2 weeks, length usually increases by about 1 inch (2.5 cm). Head circumference increases about 1 inch (2.5 cm) by 1 month of age.

Growth is considered normal if it is between the 10th and 90th percentile on a standard growth chart. The consistent use of a growth chart enables both the nurse and the parents to effectively identify the pattern of growth. The pattern of growth is more important than the actual amount of growth because growth is affected by both heredity and environment. For example, infants with parents of small stature may have a pattern of growth that remains at the 10th percentile yet be healthy. Both the rate and pattern of growth are different for breastfed babies as opposed to those receiving artificial formula. Thus, use of a

Text continued on page 1129

Table 31–5

PHYSICAL ASSESSMENT OF THE NEONATE

ASSESSMENT TECHNIQUES	NORMAL FINDINGS	COMMON VARIATIONS	SIGNIFICANT ALTERATIONS/ POTENTIAL ABNORMALITIES
General Appearance			
Observe color.	Pinkish to pale pink (varies with racial background)	Mottling, acrocyanosis (cyanosis of hands/feet), harlequin sign (difference in color along longitudinal axis with one side pale and the other pink), mild jaundice after the first 24 hr	Plethora, pallor, grayness, duskiness, generalized or circumoral cyanosis, jaundice in the first 24 hr, significant jaundice
Observe general tone, activity, and posture initially and throughout examination.	Flexed position with adduction of extremities	Posture reflecting intrauterine position (e.g., breech), tremors with movement or crying	Restricted or asymmetric movement, floppy, lethargic, hypotonic, hypertonic, jitteriness, irritability
Observe and palpate skin.	Smooth, soft, elastic, warm and moist, opaque, presence of lanugo and vernix caseosa (distribution and amount vary with gestation)	Dry and cracked skin on extremities, newborn rash, erythema toxicum (isolated areas of redness around small, raised yellow-white wheals), mongolian spots (dark blue or purplish macular areas generally over the sacrum), milia (small, white sebaceous cysts), telangiectatic nevi ("stork bites")	Rash, pustules, lacerations, excoriation, ecchymosis, hemangiomas, café au lait spots, green or yellowish vernix
	Good turgor with adipose tissue	Desquamation at 2–3 days	Wrinkled or baggy, poor turgor, decreased adipose tissue; dry, cracked, peeling, parchment-like scaling
		Petechiae or edema over presenting part	Scattered petechiae, pitting edema (except over presenting part)
Measure and record weight and length, and plot on growth curve.	Weight (term): 2500–4000 g (5-lb, 8-oz to 8-lb, 13-oz)	Varies with gestational age, loses up to 5%–15% after birth	Low or high birth weight, inappropriate weight or length for gestation (SGA or LGA)
	Length (term: 45–55 cm (18–22 in)	Varies with gestational age	
	Weight and length are appropriate for gestation (10th to 90th percentile)		
Measure and record temperature.	Axillary: 36.5–37°C 97.7–98.6°F		Unstable temperature, hypothermia, hyperthermia

Continued on following page

Table 31–5

PHYSICAL ASSESSMENT OF THE NEONATE Continued

ASSESSMENT TECHNIQUES	NORMAL FINDINGS	COMMON VARIATIONS	SIGNIFICANT ALTERATIONS/ POTENTIAL ABNORMALITIES
Assessment of the Head, Face, and Neck			
Measure and record head circumference, and plot on growth curve.	Occipital-frontal circumference (OFC): 32.6–37.2 cm (13–14.5 in) for term infant	Varies with gestational age	
Inspect and palpate head.	Symmetric and round	Molding (asymmetry of skull bones), caput succedaneum (edematous swelling of the scalp and soft tissues), cephalohematoma (subperiosteal hemorrhage)	Irregularities, depressions, asymmetric, skull fracture
Palpate sutures.	Sutures: present, palpable, and slightly open	Overriding	Fixed, widely spaced, or closed sutures
Palpate and measure fontanelles.	Anterior: diamond-shaped, 3–4 cm long by 1–3 cm wide	Size varies with amount of molding in first days (reevaluate)	Absent anterior fontanelle, presence of a third fontanelle
	Posterior: triangular, 1–2 cm wide	Posterior fontanelle may not be palpable	
	Soft and flat	May bulge with crying	Sunken or bulging
Observe face, nose, and lips.	Face: symmetric at rest and with crying	Transient positional defects due to position in utero	Asymmetric at rest or with crying Micrognathia (small jaw)
	Intact, symmetric nose and lips at midline, no nasal discharge	Sucking blister on upper lip	Flaring of nares, asymmetric, clefts, increased labionasal distance Nasal discharge
	Bilateral patency of nares		Choanal atresia (bone or membranous obstruction)
Observe eyes and measure position.	Position: symmetric, distance between inner aspects equals length of eye (about 2–3 cm)		Close-set or widely spaced eyes (hypertelorism)
	Shape: symmetric	Epicanthal folds in Asian and some non-Asian infants, swollen lids	Asymmetric, short palpebral fissure
	Pupils: round, equal, and reactive to light		Unequal, constricted, poorly reactive or nonreactive to light
	Iris: blue-gray or brown (varies with racial background)	Strabismus (eyes turn inward or outward independent of one another)	Pinkish; clefts
	Sclera: bluish white	Scleral hemorrhages from vaginal delivery	Blue or yellow (jaundiced)

Continued on facing page

Table 31–5

PHYSICAL ASSESSMENT OF THE NEONATE Continued

ASSESSMENT TECHNIQUES	NORMAL FINDINGS	COMMON VARIATIONS	SIGNIFICANT ALTERATIONS/ POTENTIAL ABNORMALITIES
	Cornea and lens: clear and intact		Opacities, cataracts, ulcerations
	Conjunctiva: pale pink, no discharge	Subconjunctival hemorrhage, chemical conjunctivitis	Purulent eye discharge
Observe and palpate ears. Measure position.	Symmetric, with upper part of pinna at or above outer canthus of eye		Asymmetric, low set, excessively small or large, malformed, preauricular or auricular skin tags, sinuses
	Pinna curved with firm cartilage	Amount of cartilage varies with gestational age	
Inspect and palpate mouth.	Mucosa and gums: pink and moist	Epstein pearls, flat or high-arched palate	Clefts
	Intact palates, hard palate is dome shaped		
	Tongue: in midline with free range of movement, proportional in size to mouth	Ankyloglossia (tongue-tie)	Limited movement, thrush, enlarged, small
Inspect and palpate neck, clavicle, and shoulders. Assess mobility.	Neck: short with flexible movement to each side Intact clavicles. Full range of motion of shoulders		Webbing, masses, enlarged lymph nodes or thyroid; fractures, crepitation; limited or no range of movement, torticollis (wryneck)
Assessment of the Chest, Abdomen, and Back			
Observe thorax.	Symmetric, cylindric		Asymmetric or malformed, barrel chest
	Breasts: areola visible and stippled with palpable breast tissue (>1 cm for a term infant)	Amount of breast tissue varies with gestational age; breast engorgement, milky discharge; supranumerary nipples	Mastitis
Measure chest circumference at nipple line.	30–33 cm (12–13 in), should be a 1:1 proportion with OFC		Increased or decreased size, disproportion with OFC
Observe breathing movements.	Predominantly diaphragmatic with symmetric movement of chest and abdomen		Retractions (substernal, intercostal), asymmetric or seesaw movement, use of accessory breathing muscles
Count respiratory rate.	Rate: 40–60/min, irregular or regular (depending on infant's sleep-wake state)	Varies with activity, gestational age, sleep-wake state, temperature, and number of hours since birth	Tachypnea, decreased rate, or apnea

Continued on following page

Table 31–5

PHYSICAL ASSESSMENT OF THE NEONATE Continued

ASSESSMENT TECHNIQUES	NORMAL FINDINGS	COMMON VARIATIONS	SIGNIFICANT ALTERATIONS/ POTENTIAL ABNORMALITIES
		Periodic breathing without bradycardia or color change	Periodic breathing with bradycardia or color change
Auscultate lungs.	Breath sounds: symmetric and clear		Grunting on expiration, rales (crackles—in lung fields) or rhonchi (wheezes—in large air-airways), decreased or unequal breath sounds
Auscultate heart sounds.	Two clear sounds, with S_2 slightly sharper and higher in pitch than S_1	Generally hear functional or benign murmurs over base or left sternal border (all murmurs should be evaluated; may indicate congenital heart defects)	Heart sounds displaced toward the left; distant or muffled heart sounds Murmurs indicating underlying congenital heart defect (note where the murmur is best heard)
Count heart rate.	Rate: 120–160 beats/min, regular rhythm	Rate: 110–120 beats/min, varies with activity, gestational age, sleep-wake state, temperature, and number of hours since birth; irregular beats	Bradycardia or sustained tachycardia; irregular rhythm, arrhythmias
	Point of maximal impulse (PMI): lower left sternal border	PMI visible, thrill (fine vibration) felt in first few hours	Hyperactive precordium
Auscultate bowel sounds (auscultate all four quadrants before palpation).	Intermittent tinkling sounds every 10–20 sec	Absent in first 1–2 hr after birth	Absent, hyperactive
Observe and palpate abdomen.	Symmetric, cylindric, and slightly protruding	Diastasis recti (separation of the rectus abdominis muscle)	Flat, flabby, distention, or localized bulging Masses, visible peristalsis, scaphoid shape (possibly indicating diaphragmatic hernia)
	Liver: in right upper quadrant 1–2 cm below right costal margin, sharp edge		Enlarged liver, round edge
	Kidney: oval structure located in posterior flank, 1–2 cm above umbilicus	Often difficult to palpate	Enlarged or absent kidneys
Inspect umbilical cord and umbilicus.	Cord: Initially white and gelatinous with 2 arteries, 1 vein	Umbilical hernia	Cord: 2 vessels, extrathin cord
	Umbilicus: skin and umbilicus clear and dry		Umbilicus: red, wet, foul odor, meconium staining

Continued on facing page

Table 31–5

PHYSICAL ASSESSMENT OF THE NEONATE Continued

ASSESSMENT TECHNIQUES	NORMAL FINDINGS	COMMON VARIATIONS	SIGNIFICANT ALTERATIONS/ POTENTIAL ABNORMALITIES
Palpate femoral lymph nodes and pulses.	Pulses: bilateral, strong, and regular		Absent, irregular, bounding, weak pulses Enlarged lymph nodes
Record passage and character of stools.	Meconium: dark green, thick, viscous, passed by 24–48 hr after birth	Passage of mucus plug with first stool	Masses, hernias, no meconium passed by 48 hr of age, foul-smelling meconium, diarrhea, mucus, or blood
Determine patency of anus by taking a rectal temperature.	Anus present and patent with wink reflex		Fistulas, imperforate anus
Palpate and inspect spinal column.	Midline, straight, and intact		Asymmetry, scoliosis, masses, sacral dimple, pilonidal dimple with hair tufts, spina bifida
Observe back and buttocks.	Symmetric	Lanugo	Asymmetric skin creases
Assessment of the Genitals and Urinary System			
Confirm urination. Observe stream of urine in the male infant.	Initial urination by 24 hr of age (urination in delivery room may be unnoticed), clear, yellow Full stream	Uric acid crystals (rust color)	No voiding by 24–36 hr, distended bladder, blood-tinged urine Abnormal stream
Note appearance of external genitalia.	Appropriate for given sex		Ambiguous genitalia
Observe genitalia and palpate testes of male infant.	Meatus on tip of penis, glans covered by prepuce		Epispadias, hypospadias
	Scrotum pink to brown, symmetric, and pendulous with rugae	Varies with gestational age Edema and bruising with vaginally delivered breech	Hydrocele
	Testes descended bilaterally	May be partially descended or not descended in preterm infant	Undescended or absent testes
Observe genitalia of female infant.	Labia majora meet in midline	Edema Size of labia varies with gestational age	
	Vagina and meatus present	Hymenal tags, pseudomenstruation, mucous/milky discharge	Absent vagina or meatus
Assessment of the Extremities			
Observe arms and legs for symmetric appearance, size, length, and movement.	Symmetric appearance (legs slightly bowed), size, length; full range of movement	Transient positional deformities (for example, breech legs, frog legs), occasional tremors	Asymmetric appearance, size, or length; restricted range of movement

Continued on following page

Table 31–5

PHYSICAL ASSESSMENT OF THE NEONATE Continued

ASSESSMENT TECHNIQUES	NORMAL FINDINGS	COMMON VARIATIONS	SIGNIFICANT ALTERATIONS/ POTENTIAL ABNORMALITIES
Observe hands and feet	10 intact fingers and toes	Skin tags	Syndactyly, polydactyly, missing digits, absent bones in fingers
	Palmar and plantar creases present	Varies with gestational age	Simian crease (single palmar crease)
	Nails present, intact, and extend to tips	Varies with gestational age	Hypoplasia, dysplasia
	Hands held fisted	Transient positional deformities	Hands held tightly fisted with obligatory thumb in palm
	Full range of motion		Metatarsus varus, clubfeet, positional defects, rocker-bottom feet
Evaluate rotation of hips: Ortolani and Barlow maneuvers.*	Thighs abduct to surface of bed, hips rotate through full range of motion, creases of legs and buttocks are symmetric		Restricted movement Congenital hip dysplasia, or hip click
Palpate peripheral pulses.	Present, symmetric		Absent or asymmetric
	Upper and lower pulses similar in strength		Variation in strength in lower pulses compared with upper pulses

*Ortolani maneuver: Flex knees and hips, placing fingers bilaterally on trochanters with thumbs gripping medial aspect of femurs. Adduct and abduct hips. Jerking motion as femur passes over acetabulum requires further evaluation for congenital hip dysplasia.

Barlow test: Flex hip and knee 90 degrees. Pull the femoral head out of the acetabulum by lateral pressure of the thumb and by rocking the knee medially with the knuckle of the index finger. Palpable or audible hip click requires further evaluation.

Reflex	Examiner's Technique	Expected Infant Response
Assessment of Reflexes		
Rooting*	Stroke side of cheek, lips, or mouth with finger or nipple.	Turns head toward stimulus, opens mouth, and begins sucking
Swallow	Assess with first feed.	Coordinated suck/swallow
Sucking	Insert finger or nipple into mouth.	Sucking movements
Moro (startle reflex)	Hold infant over bed or table in semi-upright position and move head and trunk sharply downward or strike mattress.	Extends and abducts arms accompanied by extension of fingers; may habituate with diminished response after repeated attempts to elicit reflex
Palmar and plantar grasp*	Place finger in palm of hand (palmar grasp) and at base of toes (plantar grasp).	Grasps and holds finger (palmar) or curls toes downward (plantar) for a brief period
Tonic neck reflex or fencing*	Place infant in supine position and turn head to one side.	Extends arm and leg on side head is turned toward with flexion of opposite arm and leg; may not be reliably elicited or complete in newborn period

Continued on facing page

Table 31–5

PHYSICAL ASSESSMENT OF THE NEONATE Continued

Reflex	Examiner's Technique	Expected Infant Response
Stepping or walking	Hold infant upright with feet on flat surface.	Stepping movements with alternating flexion and extension of feet
Pull to sit (traction)	Hold infant supine, grasp arms and pull to sitting position.	Head lags as infant is brought to sitting position, then head is brought up and maintained briefly, with further attempts to right head; note head position and tone of neck and shoulder muscles
Blink (glabellar)	Tap forehead at bridge of nose with finger.	Bilateral blink

*Assess bilaterally.

Technique	Potential Anomalies
Assessments for Specific Congenital Anomalies	
Observe general appearance.	Gross external anomalies
Observe breathing pattern and auscultate chest.	Cardiorespiratory problems, diaphragmatic hernia
Observe breathing with infant's mouth closed.	Choanal atresia
Pass gastric tube or aspirate stomach contents.	Esophageal atresia
Observe appearance of abdomen.	Intestinal atresia (distended), diaphragmatic hernia (scaphoid), omphalocele, gastroschisis
Confirm passage of meconium and observe appearance of anus including wink reflex; perform rectal temperature.	Imperforate anus
Count umbilical vessels.	<3 associated with genitourinary or cardiac anomalies
Measure head circumference and palpate fontanelles.	Microcephaly, hydrocephalus
Inspect and palpate palate.	Cleft palate
Evaluate hips.	Congenital hip dysplasia

From NAACOG OGN Nursing Practice Resource. (August 1994). *Physical assessment of the newborn.* Available from the Association of Women's Health, Obstetric and Neonatal Nurses, 700 14th Street NW, Suite 600, Washington, DC 20005-2019. Reprinted with permission from the Association of Women's Health, Obstetric and Neonatal Nurses.

growth chart that has been standardized especially for breastfed babies is helpful in determining deviations from normal.

Deviation in growth patterns may not be evident at the initial neonatal examination if it occurs before 2 weeks after birth. However, failure to regain birth weight by this time is an indication for further assessment and referral to the infant's health care provider.

Patterns of Development

The infant's pattern of development is evaluated by eliciting infant reflexes and determining whether the infant is capable of performing age-appropriate developmental tasks. Assessment of infant states and the self-consoling ability of the infant as well as other behavioral abilities is important. Again, as with growth, the pattern of development is more important than the rate of development. Assessment of infant temperament as well as of the mother's perception of her infant's temperament is important in identifying teaching needs.

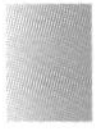

Infant's General Health Status

Assessment of the infant's general health status involves a complete physical examination of the infant and talking with the mother about the baby's health since the infant was last seen. Asking questions about common areas of concern (such as feeding problems, circumcision, sleeping or crying) during the postbirth period can provide you with information that the mother may not have thought to tell you.

Mother's Specific Concerns

Identifying and discussing the mother's specific concerns is critical. Whether the problem actually exists is not the issue; rather, it is important to identify the mother's perceptions and specific concerns so that they can be examined. The information may reveal that teaching or support is needed in some areas, that additional information and follow-up are required, or that an actual problem exists and referral to the infant's health care provider is necessary.

Risk Management

Risk management in the area of neonatal assessment involves the following: accurate and in-depth knowledge of normal physical and neurobehavioral findings in the infant; sound physical and behavioral assessment skills; the expert ability to distinguish normal findings, normal variations, and abnormal findings; complete and accurate recording of findings in the infant's chart; and astute and prompt referral to the infant's health care provider when indicated. The implementation of a comprehensive assessment plan for in-hospital and home care for all infants, with findings charted on a standardized graphic form, further reduces the potential risk from incomplete assessment or inadequate communication of findings. Integration of an individualized teaching plan on infant care and needs, based on the parents' needs and concerns after the assessment of the infant, is essential in minimizing risk.

Implications for Research

While clinical experience has shown the value of conducting neonatal assessments at periodic intervals during the neonatal period for problem identification and wellness promotion, research data on neonatal assessment that can serve as a basis for practice are limited. Research questions that need to be answered are

- What effect does performing physical and behavioral assessments have on parents' knowledge and ability to care for their infant?
- What are the most common variations and abnormal findings detected by physical and behavioral assessments?
- What is the percentage of neonates who have abnormal physical and behavioral examination findings?
- What is the cost savings from early identification and treatment of problems identified through routine neonatal assessment?

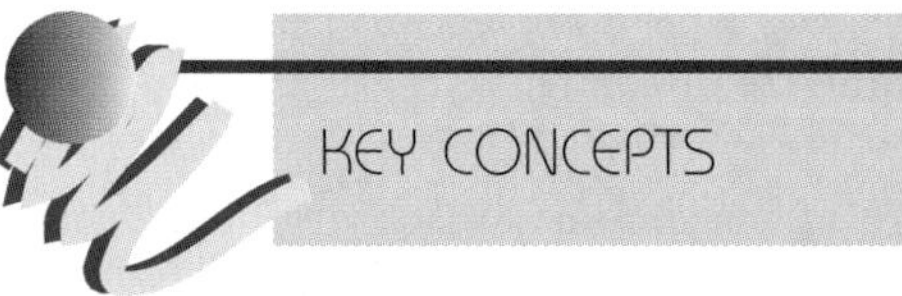

KEY CONCEPTS

▼ Assessment of the neonate is a critical function of the nurse immediately after birth, on an ongoing periodic basis during the early days after birth, and thereafter as needed during well-baby examinations or if the infant is ill.

▼ The purposes of neonatal assessment are to identify prenatal influences on health status and determine risk status; provide baseline information on the infant for use as a reference marker; identify anomalies, actual health problems, or potential health problems; and plan appropriate nursing care for the infant and identify teaching needs of the parents.

▼ The axillary method of taking an infant's temperature is considered safer than the rectal method, which has the potential to damage fragile rectal tissue. Normal axillary temperature is 36.0 to 36.5°C (97.1 to 97.8°F).

▼ Heart rate is counted for 60 seconds at the apex of the heart (called apical pulse); normal range is 120 to 160 beats per minute.

- ▼ All infants are periodic breathers, with periods of respiration intermixed with brief periods (approximately 5 to 10 seconds) without breathing. Normal respiratory rate varies from 30 to 60 breaths per minute when the infant is not crying.
- ▼ The average infant birth weight is 7.5 pounds (3.5 kg). The average length of an infant at birth is 20 inches (51 cm). The average head circumference is 13 to 14 inches (33 to 35.5 cm). The average chest circumference is 12 to 13 inches (30.5 to 33 cm). Head circumference is approximately 0.8 inch (2 cm) larger than chest circumference.
- ▼ Gestational age assessment, especially the neurologic assessment component, is influenced by factors including infant health status, maternal medications, and infant state.
- ▼ An infant is considered appropriate for gestational age if weight, length, and head circumference are between the 10th and 90th percentiles on a standardized growth chart for infants.
- ▼ Examining the baby in the presence of the parents provides an excellent opportunity for explanation and reassurance about the unique characteristics of newborns in general and their infant in particular.
- ▼ Infants demonstrate neurobehavioral cues that reflect their organizational ability and the readiness for interaction. These behaviors are categorized as distress/disengagement cues and stability/engagement cues.
- ▼ Follow-up periodic assessments of the infant after the early postbirth period should focus on the infant's pattern of physical growth, the infant's pattern of development and behavioral ability, the infant's general health status, and the mother's specific concerns.
- ▼ Risk management in the area of neonatal assessment involves the following: accurate and in-depth knowledge of normal physical and neurobehavioral findings in the infant; sound physical and behavioral assessment skills; the expert ability to distinguish normal findings, normal variations, and abnormal findings; complete and accurate recording of findings in the infant's chart; and astute and prompt referral to the infant's health care provider when indicated.

References

Apgar, V. (1953). A proposal for a new method of evaluation of the newborn infant. *Current Researches in Anesthesia and Analgesia,* 40, 340.

Blackburn, S. T., and Loper, D. L. (1992). Maternal, fetal and neonatal physiology: A clinical perspective. Philadelphia: W. B. Saunders.

Brazelton, T. B. (1973). Neonatal behavioral assessment scale. *Clinics in Developmental Medicine,* 50.

Brazelton, T. B. (1987). Behavioral competence of the newborn infant. In G. Avery (Ed.), *Neonatology: Pathophysiology and management of the newborn.* Philadelphia: J. B. Lippincott.

Brazelton, T. B., School, M., Robey, J. (1966). Visual responses in the newborn. *Pediatrics,* 37, 284–290.

Dubowitz, L. (1970). Clinical assessment of gestational age in the newborn infant. *Journal of Pediatrics,* 77, 1.

Greenman, G. (1963). Visual behavior of newborn infants. In A. Solnit and S. Provence (Eds.), *Modern perspectives in child development.* New York: Halmark.

Marchbanks, P. (1987). Newborn assessment: Physical examination. In S.S. Humenick, *Analysis of current assessment strategies in the health care of young children and childbearing families.* Laramie, WY: Author.

The Nurses Association of the American College of Obstetricians and Gynecologists (NAACOG). (1991). Physical Assessment of the newborn. *NAACOG OGN Nursing practice resource.* Washington, DC: Author [now Association of Women's Health, Obstetric and Neonatal Nurses (AWHONN)].

Paneth, N., and Stark, R. (1983). Cerebral palsy and mental retardation in relation to indicators of perinatal asphyxia. *American Journal of Obstetrics and Gynecology,* 147, 960–966.

Prechtl, H. (1974). The behavioral states of the newborn infant (a review). *Brain Research,* 76, 185.

Sherry, S. N., and Kramer, J. C. (1955). The time and passage of the first stool and first urine. *Journal of Pediatrics,* 46, 158.

Silverman, F., Suldan, J., Wasserman, J., Antoine, C., Young, B. (1985). The Apgar score: Is it enough? *Obstetrics and Gynecology,* 66 (3), 331–336.

Sykes, G., Mollay, P., Johnson, P., Gu, W., Ashworth, F., Sterrat, G., Turnbull J. (1982). Do Apgar scores indicate asphyxia? *Lancet,* 1 (February 7), 494–496.

Walker, L. O., Avant, P. K., Taylor, K. M., Penticuff, J. H. (1982). A case study of the use of assessment strategies in clinical practice. In S. S. Humenick: *Analysis of current assessment strategies in the health care of young children and childbearing families* (p. 10). Norwalk, CT: Appleton-Century-Crofts.

Wolff, P. (1959). Observations on newborn infants. *Psychosomatic Medicine,* 21, 110.

32 Chapter

> In family-centered care, the well infant is cared for at the mother's bedside by the same nurse who cares for the mother . . . All infants identified as low-risk are treated as healthy unless proven otherwise . . . Mother-baby nursing is practiced in order to promote mother-infant attachment and facilitate teaching of infant care . . . Basic infant procedures such as venipuncture and heal sticks for hypoglycemia are done in the mother's room if the parents prefer. . . . Newborn exams are conducted at the mother's bedside.
>
> CELESTE PHILLIPS (1994)

Nursing Care of Newborns

Karen Stevens

HIGHLIGHTS

- Assessment of the Newborn
- Maintenance of Life Support Systems Related to Respirations, Circulation, Thermoregulation, and Prevention of Hemorrhage
- Procedure 32–1: Suctioning the Newborn with Bulb Syringe or Catheter
- Procedure 32–2: Thermoregulation of Newborns
- Procedure 32–3: Administration of Vitamin K
- Prevention of Infection Related to Prophylactic Eye Treatment and Umbilical Cord Care
- Procedure 32–4: Instillation of Erythromycin, Tetracycline, or Silver Nitrate Eye Treatment
- Procedure 32–5: Umbilical Cord Care
- Maintenance of Bilirubin Levels, Blood Glucose, and Nutrition
- Maintenance of Elimination
- Positioning, Holding, Bathing, and Dressing the Neonate
- Maintenance of Safety, Rest, and Mobility
- Risk Management
- Procedure 32–6: Nursing Care After Circumcision
- Implications for Research
- Nursing Care Planning Guide: Healthy Full-Term Newborn

DEFINITIONS

Accu-Check II—A device for determining blood glucose level by analysis of blood placed on a Chemstrip.

Acrocyanosis—Peripheral cyanosis of hands and feet.

Central cyanosis—Overall cyanosis, including the central or trunk area of the neonate.

Circumcision—Surgical procedure that removes the foreskin (prepuce) from the penis.

Delee catheter—A plastic catheter used to suction the respiratory tract of the neonate; suction is supplied by the operator or the catheter is adapted to mechanical wall suction, and fluids are collected in a plastic reservoir.

Dextrostix—Chemstrips used to assess the neonate's blood glucose level by comparison of the color strip with a color chart after the strip is saturated with blood.

Hypoglycemia—Neonate's blood glucose level below normal.

Hypothermia—Neonate's temperature below normal levels.

Jaundice—Yellow pigmentation of the neonate's skin occurring as result of bilirubin breakdown or from bile pigments.

Neutral thermal environment—An environment that minimizes the neonate's need to expend calories to maintain heat; an environment that provides for minimal heat loss.

Radiant warmer—Overhead device that warms the baby by radiant heat.

Servomechanism-controlled incubator—Enclosed device that helps maintain a baby's temperature by maintaining constant environmental air temperature.

Skin temperature—Temperature of the neonate's skin, recorded by a probe device placed on the baby's skin.

Thermoregulation—Processes of the neonate that regulate or attempt to maintain body temperature in the normal range.

At the time of birth, the neonate experiences numerous physiologic adaptations. As a result, the neonate requires close observation as well as various nursing interventions to facilitate a smooth, adaptive transition to extrauterine life. The newborn's adjustment is facilitated by individualized nursing care implemented within the nursing process. Beginning on page 1171, Nursing Care Planning Guide: Healthy Full-Term Newborn shows how nursing process is applied in creating a plan of care designed to meet an individual's needs.

ASSESSMENT

Assessment of the neonate affords the opportunity to identify actual or potential problems. Careful assessment helps the nurse to differentiate between normal and abnormal responses. The nurse uses assessment tools such as the Newborn Admission Record (p. 1172) and Newborn Nursery Flow Record (pp. 1173–1174) to gather and record data essential to providing effective care of the newborn. Assessment of factors that influence parents in assuming caretaking and in developing a positive attachment to the neonate allows interventions to assist in parental role attainment. Assessment provides information in relation to parental needs for instruction in child care techniques, in providing a safe environment, in facts about growth and development, and in meeting the psychological needs of the infant. It is important to identify family strengths as well as deficits during assessment so that these can be incorporated into the plan of care. Assessment of parental care and need for education is covered in Chapter 34. Daily assessments and care, while the neonate is on the birthing unit, present an opportune time for education of parents. Assessment of the newborn is discussed in detail in Chapter 31; this chapter focuses on the nursing care of the newborn.

Plan of Care

Goals provide a framework for evaluating the plan that the nurse implements. Overall goals in the care of the normal newborn include providing

- An adaptive physiologic transition from intrauterine to extrauterine life
- A safe environment, with avoidance of trauma, injury, and infection
- Opportunities for developing attachment between parents and neonate
- Instruction to help parents acquire the necessary knowledge, skill, and confidence to care for the neonate

Nursing care includes interventions to promote and maintain the health of the newborn, which includes maintaining the newborn's vital functions, the daily care of newborns, and general routines in newborn nurseries.

The Initial Transition and Stabilization Period

The initial 6 hours after birth have been called the transition or stabilization period because so many physiologic adjustments occur. Typical patterns of behavior emerge during this time. First, there is a period of reactivity in which the newborn is actively "reactive," awake, alert, and often hungry. Because this is the initial transition time, respirations respond to stimuli and are reactive. Respirations may be rapid and may vary. Newborns may have periods of apnea, demonstrate chest retraction, have transient flaring of nares, and have grunting respiration. The heart rate also reacts to stimuli with rapidity and irregularity. While bowel sounds are usually absent for the first 1 to 2 hours after birth, the baby typically displays a strong sucking reflex and may take full advantage of an opportunity to initiate breastfeeding. Most often, this period lasts approximately 30 minutes and therefore typically occurs in the delivery/birthing or recovery room.

Second, there is a sleep period in which the baby's activities diminish, the heart rate and respirations settle down somewhat, and the baby sleeps. The amount of time the baby sleeps varies. Some sleep for a few minutes, whereas others may sleep for 2 to 4 hours. Bowel sounds become audible during this time.

Finally, there is a second period of reactivity. Again, the baby is awake and alert. During this period, which commonly lasts 4 to 6 hours, physiologic responses to internal and external stimuli are variable. Mucus, gastric fluids, and respiratory fluids can obstruct the respirations; the baby responds with gasps, choking, regurgitation, or cyanosis. If this occurs, the nurse intervenes to maintain a clear airway by suctioning the baby. Urine and meconium stools are often passed for the first time. Finally, the baby displays readiness for feeding by sucking, rooting, swallowing, and crying.

After birth, the neonate is assessed. This includes determination of the Apgar score (see Chapter 31). Assessment of respirations, circulation (color), and temperature continues, with appropriate interventions to maintain respirations (such as suctioning, oxygen administration, and positioning) and to maintain temperature (such as use of a radiant warmer or drying the neonate). In many instances, the baby stays with the mother and family for a time before being transported to the normal newborn nursery. During this time, the nurse continues to assess and monitor adaptive functioning.

Many hospitals have observational or transitional nurseries where neonates are typically admitted after delivery. In this nursery, physiologic stabilization of the newborn is ensured by more frequent, vigilant nursing interventions. The delivery nurse gives a verbal report to the nursery nurse. It includes relevant factors about the labor, birth, and neonate that may influence the baby's condition and adaptation.

▼ **Antepartum History.** Any maternal problems that may have influenced the neonate are reported to the nursery nurse, such as hypertensive disorders of pregnancy, maternal illness, infections, diabetes, substance abuse, hypertension, nutritional status, anemia, maternal age, extended date of birth, and number of pregnancies.

▼ **Labor and Birth Information.** A record of labor and birth is usually included in the baby's chart. Relevant information to convey to the nursery nurse includes duration of labor, length of time membranes were ruptured, maternal fever, amount and type of intravenous fluids used in labor, any fetal distress, type of anesthesia, type of delivery (such as cesarean section or vaginal delivery), forceps application, or vacuum extractor use.

▼ **Condition of the Neonate.** Important information typically includes Apgar scores at 1 and 5 minutes, resuscitation or oxygen required, temperature, other vital signs, voiding, and bowel elimination. Any complications are relayed, such as obvious physical abnormalities or abnormal number of cord vessels.

▼ **Parent-Infant Interaction Information.** Any parental desires are relayed, such as circumcision decision and type of feeding desired (breast or bottle/formula). In addition, other pertinent family data may be relayed, such as single mother status, availability of support persons, and living arrangements for the baby.

Assessment on Admission to the Nursery

After the verbal report, the nurse admits the neonate to the observational, transitional, or family-centered care unit. This involves assessing the neonate's current status by taking vital signs (respiration, heart rate, and temperature). Assessment of respirations is most accurately done when the infant is quiet and undisturbed. Therefore, the respiratory rate is usually taken first when the baby is at rest. The rhythm, quality, and character of respirations are also assessed at this time. Next, the apical pulse is assessed. Respirations and apical pulse are usually measured every hour for the first 4 hours and then every shift. Finally, the baby's temperature is taken, usually by the axillary method (see Procedure 31–1: Assessing Vital Signs in the Newborn).

Once the temperature is stable, it is monitored by the axillary method at relatively frequent intervals, such as every 4 hours for 24 hours and then every shift. Controversy exists about method, length of time, and frequency of monitoring the baby's temperature; however, it is a common practice to take vital signs as noted.

Many hospitals place the baby in an open crib under a radiant warmer during the stabilization period, which helps thermoregulation. A skin thermal sensor is placed on the newborn's abdomen (most often), upper thighs, or arm and is secured with a foil-covered foam pad.

The baby is weighed unless this has been done in the delivery/birthing room (see Procedure 31–2: Weighing and Measuring the Newborn).

During the initial stabilization period, the nurse also does a complete physical and gestational age assessment (see Chapter 31). Assessments during the first hours provide a basis for establishing nursing diagnoses, setting priorities for care and parental education needs, and assessing ongoing transition of the neonate to extrauterine life. Once adaptive stabilization is ensured through careful, frequent assessment with appropriate interventions, the baby is typically bathed, dressed, and placed in an open crib without a radiant warmer. In most nurseries, once this transition period has passed and the neonate has been determined to be adapting adequately, the baby can go to the mother's room for feedings and for rooming-in. Physiologic and behavioral adaptations continue.

The remainder of this chapter discusses nursing care necessary to ensure continuing adaptive transition to extrauterine life in each of the important physiologic systems. Underlying these nursing care interventions are scientific concepts from physiology, microbiology, and nutrition.

MAINTENANCE OF LIFE SUPPORT SYSTEMS

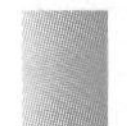

Respiration and Clear Airway

Several factors are necessary to maintain adequate respirations:

- A clear, unobstructed airway
- Adequate breathing efforts
- Functioning nervous and cardiovascular systems
- Thermoregulation (because cold stress increases oxygen needs)

The neonate's airway may become obstructed by respiratory fluids, mucus, or regurgitated feedings. Most respiratory fluids flow by gravity or are propelled to the oropharynx by a cough; fluids then drain out of the mouth or are swallowed. The following nursing interventions are implemented to maintain respirations:

- Assess the neonate's respirations for normality and adaptiveness to extrauterine life (see Table 31–5).
- Position the neonate appropriately.
- Suction the neonate.

Positioning. Immediately after birth the neonate is positioned on the back with his head turned to one side or on the side with a rolled blanket behind the back to maintain the side-lying position. These positions allow secretions to flow by gravity to the mouth and oropharynx.

For sleeping, the American Academy of Pediatrics recommended that "infants should be placed down for sleep in a *nonprone* position. Supine *(wholly on the back)* confers the lowest risk and is preferred. The side is a reasonable alternative which also carries a significantly lower risk than prone" (AAP 1996) (Fig. 32–1).

Since 1992, when the American Academy of Pediatrics issued a statement recommending that infants be placed for sleep in the side or back position, the prevalence of infant stomach sleeping has decreased significantly, from 70% to 27%, and simultaneously the death rate from SIDS has decreased by 15% to 20% during the same period from 1992 to 1995. The current recommendation is for healthy infants only. Gastroesophageal reflux and certain upper airway anomalies that predispose to airway obstruction and perhaps other illnesses may indicate the need for a prone sleeping position. The recommendation for a *nonprone* position is only for sleeping. A certain amount of "tummy time," while the baby is awake and observed, is recommended (American Academy of Pediatrics 1996).

In the past, the side-lying position or positioning on the abdomen was advocated.

Suctioning. When necessary, the nurse suctions the neonate's respiratory tract (oral cavity, respiratory tract, nasal passages) with either a bulb syringe or a catheter (Procedure 32–1). Nurses need to teach parents how to suction their baby by use of a bulb syringe because babies can gasp and choke on fluids or feedings.

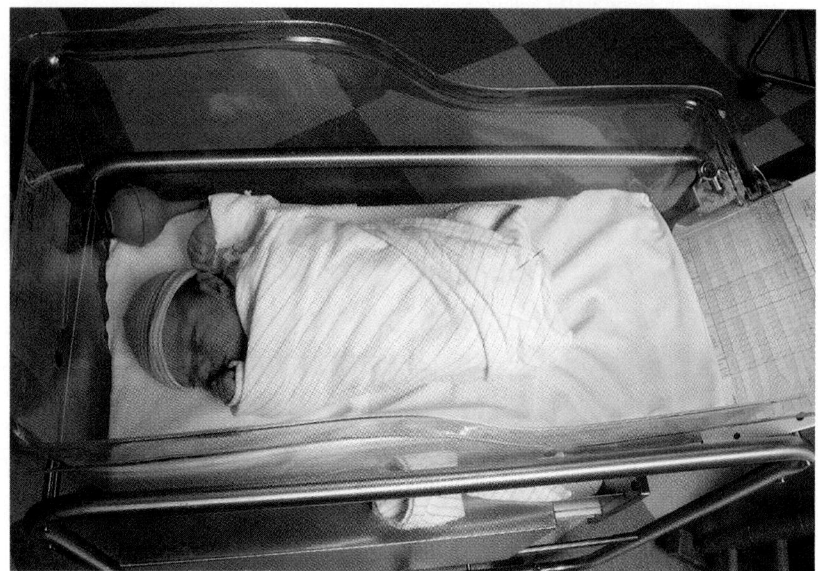

Figure 32–1

For sleep, the infant should be positioned in a nonprone position. Supine *(wholly on the back)* confers the lowest risk of SIDS and is preferred. The side is a reasonable alternative that also carries a significantly lower risk of SIDS than the prone position.

In the past, DeLee catheters were used to suction the newborn as well. With this catheter, suction is supplied by the operator, not by mechanical means. The procedure used to suction with a catheter is followed. Use of the DeLee catheter has decreased substantially since the acquired immunodeficiency syndrome (AIDS) was recognized and concern over contact with body fluids increased. Many now adapt the DeLee catheter so that it can be used with wall suction.

Circulation

As the neonate's circulation changes from fetal to neonatal circulation and fetal shunts close, the nurse should assess the infant for circulatory adaptation (see Chapters 30 and 31). An apical rather than a radial pulse is taken because the neonate's small radial blood vessels are too easily obliterated by the pressure involved in taking a radial pulse (see Table 31–5). Typically, charting conventions involve recording the color of oxygenated tissue as a pink color even though this does not truly describe the color of oxygenated tissue in black, Asian, or Hispanic cultures. The intent is to describe the color of oxygenated tissues. Skin color should not be consistently "too reddish" or "too ruddy" (it is typically red when the baby cries, which is normal, or if polycythemia is suspected). It should not be too cyanotic (bluish), nor should central cyanosis be evident. Central cyanosis refers to general cyanosis of the newborn (even the trunk of the baby may be cyanotic). The normal cyanosis of hands and feet (acrocyanosis) is typically found in the first 8 hours or so as peripheral circulation is established.

Many nurseries do not routinely obtain blood pressure measurements of the neonate. If needed, the blood pressure is obtained by either an electronic monitor or a neonatal cuff. A typical blood pressure at birth is 60 to 80 mm Hg systolic and 40 to 50 mm Hg diastolic.

Thermoregulation

Controversy exists concerning the best method, equipment, and length of time required to most accurately take the neonate's temperature. In the past, rectal temperatures were considered to reflect the "core" temperature and thus were the routine method for taking temperatures. With the advent of radiant warmers and on the basis of research findings, the literature generally recommends axillary temperatures for screening. Because several studies validated that axillary and rectal temperatures typically agree, recommendations have been made for axillary temperatures (Mayfield et al. 1984; Eoff et al. 1974; Schiffman 1982).

Research has not been extensive enough to absolutely determine the preferred method (rectal or axillary), type of thermometer (electronic or glass), or duration required to most accurately reflect the newborn's true temperature. Because of this, policies vary. Many institutions recommend axillary temperatures to avoid the hazard of rectal perforation, which is rare (Morley 1992). Some recommend axillary temperatures with rectal temperatures if thermoregulation problems occur. A few (in the minority now) still recommend rectal temperatures (Morley 1992). Overall, temperatures agree closely, regardless of site (rectal, axillary, skin) (Mayfield et al. 1984; Kunnel et al. 1988).

PROCEDURE 32–1

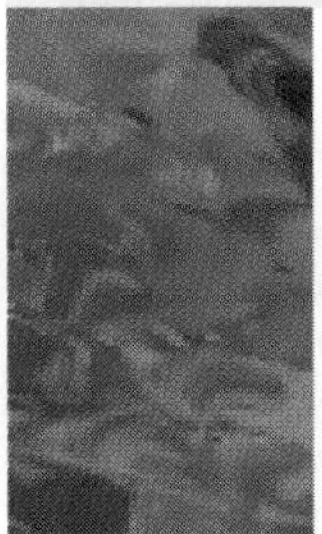

Suctioning the Newborn with Bulb Syringe or Catheter

▼ PURPOSE

To use a bulb syringe or catheter to remove secretions or fluids when they obstruct the newborn's respiratory passages. A catheter rather than a bulb syringe must be used to remove fluids that are lower in the respiratory tract.

▼ EQUIPMENT

For Bulb Syringe Suctioning

- Bulb syringe (each baby has a separate, initially sterile bulb syringe)

For Catheter Suctioning

- French rubber catheters (sizes 10, 12, 14), whistle-tip or two-hole tip, sterile for each baby
- French plastic disposable catheters (sizes 8, 10, 12), finger control, two-hole tip, sterile for each baby
- External suction source (as on radiant warmer)
- Container of sterile water (typically a sterile water feeding bottle)

Bulb Syringe Suctioning

1 Wear gloves. Place infant side-lying in football hold with head down or side-lying in crib. Keep infant warm. **Wearing gloves is consistent with Standard Precautions. Supporting the infant in a side-lying position allows gravity to aid drainage to the side of the mouth. Keeping the infant warm helps maintain his or her temperature.**

2 Compress the bulb to remove the air before inserting the bulb. **Removing the air prevents forcing secretions deeper into the respiratory tract.**

3 Always suction the mouth before suctioning the nares. **Fluids and secretions that could obstruct the respiratory passages may be present in the mouth or the nares or both. If the syringe is placed in the nares first, the infant may experience an inspiratory gasp and may pull mucus farther into the respiratory tract.**

4 Insert the syringe into the space between the cheek and gums or into the nares. Avoid the roof of the mouth and the back of the throat. Release compression gradually to create suction. **Avoiding the roof of the mouth and the back of the throat prevents the gag reflex. The suction created removes the secretions.**

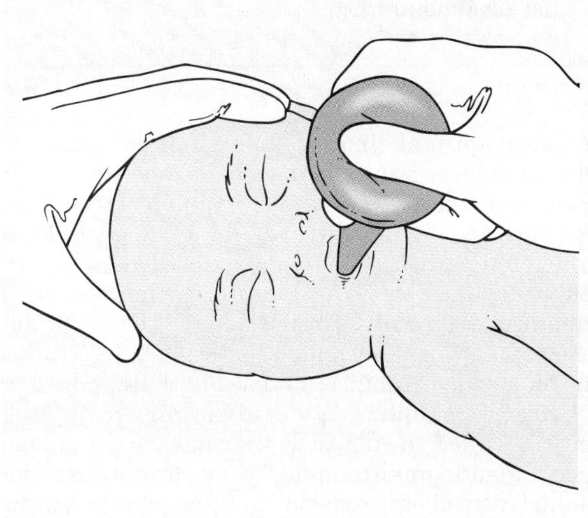

5 Remove the bulb syringe from the mouth or nares. Compress the syringe onto a diaper, a

Continued on following page

PROCEDURE 32–1 Continued

pad, or a tissue. **The bulb syringe needs to be removed to remove the secretions. Compressing the syringe empties the syringe of fluids so that the cycle can be repeated effectively.**

6 Repeat steps 2, 4, and 5 until the cry is clear or until respirations are audibly clear. **Suctioning is no longer needed when the respiratory tract is clear.**

7 Teach parents how to use the bulb syringe. **Parents need to be able to use the bulb syringe to suction the mouth or nares when fluids that could obstruct the respiratory passages are present.**

8 Cleanse the bulb syringe with warm, soapy water and rinse in warm water. **Warm, soapy water cleanses the bulb syringe; warm water rinses the soap away.**

Catheter Suctioning

1 Place the newborn supine in the "sniffing" position (with head slightly forward from neck and with tongue away from pharyngeal wall). Attach catheter to electric suction; set pressure of suction between 40 and 60 mm Hg. **The sniffing position prevents obstruction of the respiratory tract.**

2 Lubricate the tip of the catheter in sterile water by inserting it into a 120-mL (4-oz) infant feeding bottle of sterile water and suctioning a small amount of water through it. **This lubrication process facilitates passage of the catheter. Using sterile water reduces microorganisms and may help prevent infection.**

3 Insert the catheter as follows: orally along the base of the tongue; horizontally into the nares and then raised to advance past the bend in the back of the nares. Insert the catheter 3 to 5 inches. **Inserting the catheter in this way lessens the possibility of laryngeal spasm and reflex apnea by minimizing stimulation of the vagus nerve.**

4 With the catheter inserted, place the thumb over the finger control area to create the suction. **Covering the control area creates a vacuum and the suction.**

5 Rotate the tubing between the fingers while withdrawing it. **Rotating the tubing while withdrawing it prevents adherence of the tubing to the respiratory tract and minimizes trauma.**

6 Limit suctioning to about 10 seconds or less. **Suctioning for 10 seconds or less minimizes the possibility of laryngeal spasm and oxygen depletion by minimizing stimulation of the oropharynx.**

The exact optimal time the thermometer must remain in place has not been documented sufficiently in research either. For example, it may require up to 6 minutes to obtain an accurate axillary temperature (Kunnel et al. 1988).

As noted in previous chapters, the neonate's temperature typically drops some after birth because of heat loss by conduction, convection, radiation, and evaporation; it takes approximately 8 to 12 hours to stabilize. It is important to provide what is called a neutral thermal environment, which is an environment that minimizes the neonate's need to expend calories to maintain heat. This is true when the neonate's temperature is in the range of 36.5 to 37.0°C (97.7 to 98.6°F). If the baby experiences hypothermia, physiologic and metabolic changes to maintain temperature come into play; if excessive, metabolic acidosis, hypoxia, and shock can result (Scopes 1981).

Efforts of nurses are aimed, then, at preventing hypothermia (and hyperthermia as well) by attempting to create the most neutral thermal environment possible. The nurse should assess the neonate's temperature for normality and adaptiveness (see Procedure 31–1). Heat loss is controlled by the four methods (conduction, convection, radiation, and evaporation) by keeping the baby dry, covering the head, wrapping the baby in blankets, keeping the baby's crib away from cold windows or air conditioners, and maintaining the temperature in the nursery and mother's room. Initially, place the unclothed, dry baby under a radiant warmer, both in the birthing room and in the nursery, until the neonate's temperature is stable. This usually requires a pattern or trend of temperature in the normal range (Procedure 32–2). Minimize heat loss during care by doing examinations and activities under the radiant warmer and by postponing the first bath until the baby's temperature is 36.5 to 37.0°C (97.7 to 98.6°F).

While many institutions make a practice of covering the baby's head with a stockinette or knit

PROCEDURE 32–2

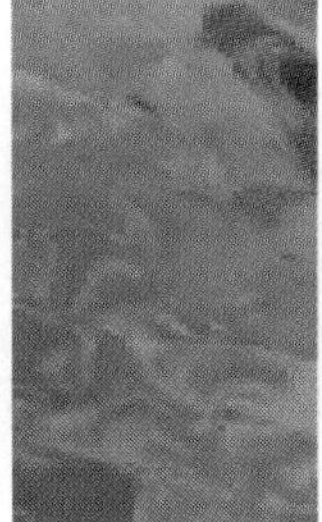

Thermoregulation of Newborns

▼ PURPOSE

To use the overhead radiant warmer or the servomechanism-controlled incubator to help the newborn achieve and maintain a stable body temperature that is within normal limits.

▼ EQUIPMENT

- Thermometer
- Overhead radiant warmer
- Servomechanism-controlled incubator

Overhead Radiant Warmer

1 Make sure the warmer is plugged into an electrical outlet. Turn on the unit to activate (prewarm) the heater before its use with the newborn. The set-point is usually 36.4°C (97.5°F). **The warmer operates by electricity, so it needs to be plugged into an electrical outlet to operate and provide a warm environment. Prewarming provides a warmer environment for the newborn.**

2 Dry the baby well and place him or her in the open crib under the radiant warmer. Babies typically wear only a diaper or are unclothed. **The radiant warmer reduces heat loss by conduction (mattress is warm) and convection (air is warmed). Blankets and clothing can act as a barrier, preventing warming.**

3 Check thermostat setting for accuracy. Servocontrol mode setting is required. **Prevents overheating and underheating.**

4 Apply thermistor probe to baby's anterior abdominal wall between navel and xiphoid process (not over the ribs). The probe must be covered by a small plastic foam disk insulator with a cover shield of aluminum foil. The foam insulator prevents the heat from directly warming the probe, thereby ensuring that the warmer responds to the baby's actual temperature rather than to the probe's temperature. The Association of Women's Health, Obstetric and Neonatal Nurses recommends maintaining skin temperature at 36.5°C (97.7°F). **Sensors in the skin respond to temperature changes. Receptors detect minor changes resulting from peripheral vasoconstriction, vasodilatation, or increased metabolism before a change in deep (core) temperature develops. Therefore, skin temperature accurately indicates the energy exchange between the baby and the environment.**

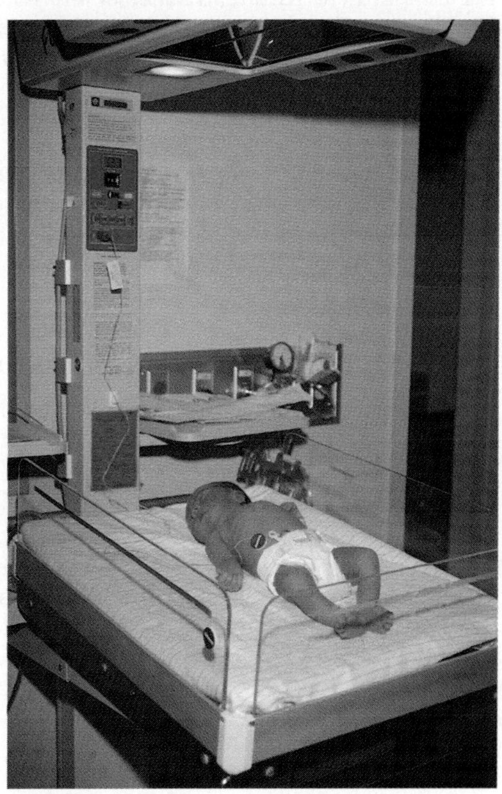

Continued on following page

PROCEDURE 32–2 Continued

5 Check the skin probe frequently to ensure accurate placement. **Prevents misplacement of probe and subsequent overheating or underheating of infant.**

6 Compare the infant's axillary temperature with the skin probe temperature. **The warmer continually indicates the baby's skin temperature from the probe. Comparing the infant's axillary temperature with the skin probe temperature is a way to check the accuracy of the warmer's reading of the infant's temperature. The axillary temperature is often rechecked every 1 to 2 hours to ensure that it stays within normal limits.**

7 Observe the baby for color change, crying, restlessness, or increased respiration rate. **Notes symptoms of cold stress.**

8 When axillary temperature is 37°C (98.6°F), dress the baby and move him or her from under the radiant warmer to an open crib. Recheck infant's temperature in 1 hour. **At 37°C, the temperature has stabilized, and the radiant warmer is no longer needed. Rechecking the temperature ascertains whether the newborn is able to maintain a normal temperature without the radiant warmer. One hour is a logical time to determine the newborn's ability to maintain normal temperature.**

9 Record newborn's temperature. **Documentation of the newborn's temperature is necessary to determine whether interventions are effective in assisting the newborn to maintain a normal body temperature.**

Servomechanism-Controlled Incubator

1 Set the control panel at the level predetermined by agency standards and the manufacturer's recommendations, usually between 36 and 37°C (96.8 and 98.6°F) to maintain a skin temperature of 36.5°C (97.7°F). **Incubator must be set at the proper level to provide an environment that maintains the infant's temperature at a normal level.**

2 Tape a thermistor probe from the control panel to the abdomen, avoiding the bony areas. **Sensors in the skin sense temperature changes before a change in core temperature occurs.**

3 Check the sensor periodically to ensure its attachment. **Prevents overheating or underheating of infant.**

4 Take core rectal or axillary temperature and record as per hospital routine. **Rectal or axillary temperature can be compared with the temperature shown on the probe to check the accuracy of the incubator's operation and recording of skin temperature.**

5 Record skin temperature and ambient temperature within the incubator every 1 to 2 hours. **Temperatures must be monitored periodically to confirm that the infant's body temperature remains stable and within normal limits. Regular temperature monitoring also facilitates the initiation of appropriate interventions when deviations from normal occur.**

Data from LeBlanc, M. H. (1991). Thermoregulation: Incubators, radiant warmers, artificial skins, and body hoods. *Clinics in Perinatology,* 18 (3), 403–421.

cap to prevent heat loss, one study found that the baby's temperature was lower if the head was covered by a stockinette cap (not as low as with an insulated bonnet) under a radiant warmer (Greer 1988).

As mentioned, the neonate is often placed under a radiant warmer right after birth until the temperature is stabilized and again as needed if hypothermia occurs. Many use 36.5°C (97.7°F) as a cutoff temperature; when the baby's temperature is below 36.5°C, treatment for hypothermia begins. The equipment is pictured in Procedure 32–2. The baby is "rewarmed" slowly so that overheating does not occur. This is accomplished by maintaining the ambient temperature 1 to 1.5 degrees higher than the baby's current skin temperature (Brueggemeyer 1993). Once that new skin temperature is reached, the control point is again set another 1 degree higher. Some advocate that measures be instituted before placing the baby under the radiant warmer; if these are effective, a radiant warmer is not needed. These intermediate interventions include keeping the baby away from cold windows and air conditioning, keeping the baby wrapped in two blankets (instead of one), and putting a stockinette cap on the baby.

Some have expressed concern that early mother-infant contact might be detrimental to thermoregulation in that many babies might become hypothermic. However, studies have found that being held by the mother does not typically cause hypothermia; babies who were held had temperatures (whether taken by the axillary or rectal route) similar to those who were placed under a radiant warmer (Britton 1980; Hill and Shronk 1979; Gardner 1979).

According to the standards of the Association of Women's Health, Obstetric and Neonatal Nurses (formerly NAACOG), normal parameters are 36.5°C (97.7°F) to 37.0°C (98.6°F) for an axillary temperature and 36.5°C (97.7°F) for an abdominal skin temperature. The abdominal skin temperature of 36.5°C is considered optimal because oxygen consumption and metabolic rates are minimal when the baby's skin temperature is 36.5°C. (An increase in skin temperature to 37.2°C increases oxygen consumption by 6 percent; a drop to 35.9°C increases oxygen consumption by 10 percent.) The Association of Women's Health, Obstetric and Neonatal Nurses also recommends using axillary temperatures for screening; rectal temperatures are taken only if abnormal deviations occur (NAACOG 1985, 1991). If a baby cannot be rewarmed by the radiant warmer in several hours, a servomechanism-controlled incubator may be used (see Procedure 32–2). The point of control again is the baby's skin temperature, not the temperature

PROCEDURE 32–3

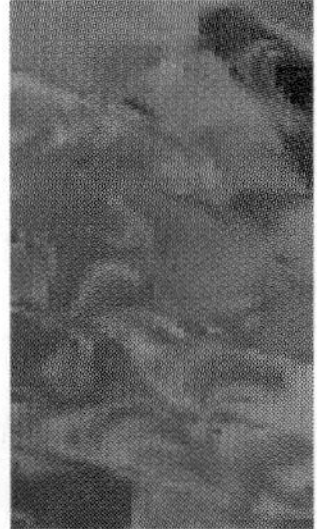

Administration of Vitamin K

▼ PURPOSE

To administer vitamin K one time within 6 hours of birth as prophylaxis for bleeding.

▼ EQUIPMENT

- 1-mL syringe
- 25-gauge ⅝-inch needle
- Ampule of AquaMEPHYTON or Konakion
- Alcohol sponges

1 Check vitamin K order. **A physician's order is required for administration of vitamin K.**

2 Wear gloves. Shake medication to bottom of ampule. Protect fingers and break top off ampule. **Wearing gloves is consistent with Standard Precautions. Shaking medication to bottom of ampule allows medication to flow to large end of ampule where it can be drawn up.**

3 Remove needle cover; maintain sterility. Draw up dosage ordered. **Sterility must be maintained to avoid infection.**

4 Steady the injection leg with one hand. **Restraint ensures placement of needle in appropriate location.**

5 Follow these steps to find the preferred injection site, which is the lateral aspect of the middle third of the vastus lateralis muscle in the baby's thigh:

- Use the baby's greater trochanter and knee as landmarks.
- Visually divide the distance between the landmarks into three equal sections.
- Identify the area that is the middle third of the distance between the landmarks.

The vastus lateralis muscle is the preferred injection site because it is free of major blood vessels and nerves and is big enough to absorb the medication.

Continued on following page

PROCEDURE 32–3 Continued

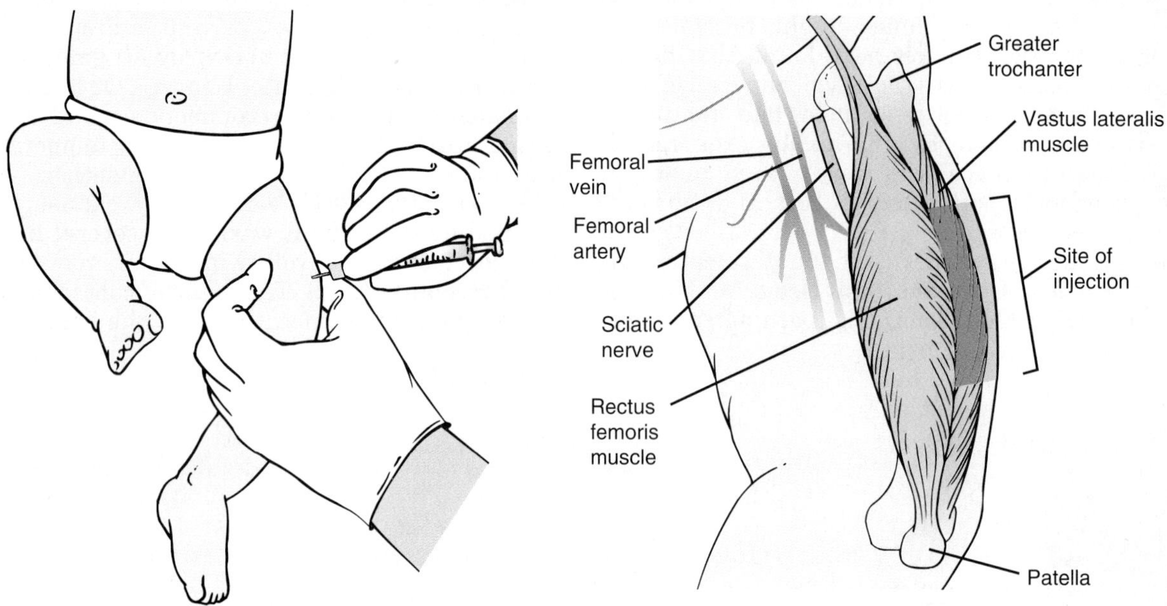

6 Cleanse the injection site with alcohol, holding the thigh between the thumb and forefinger. Insert the needle at a 90-degree angle, aspirate (as you would with any medication), and then slowly inject the medication. Give the injection within 6 hours of birth. **Positioning the needle at a 90-degree angle ensures injection into the muscle rather than the subcutaneous tissue. Injection within 6 hours of birth is recommended so that the newborn receives the prophylactic effect of the medication.**

7 Withdraw the needle, massage the area, apply pressure, and record administration of medication. **Massage hastens absorption. Application of pressure helps prevent bleeding at the site of injection. Recording documents administration.**

8 Observe injection site for bleeding. **Until vitamin K prophylaxis has taken effect, bleeding may occur.**

9 Notify physician if bleeding from any site (i.e., umbilical cord, nose, gastrointestinal tract) occurs after sufficient time for absorption of vitamin K has elapsed. **If the prophylactic dose of vitamin K proves insufficient to prevent neonatal bleeding, additional vitamin K will be administered.**

Vitamin K

Vitamin K is a fat-soluble vitamin. There are approximately seven types of vitamin K, the most significant ones being vitamin K_1 (phytonadione), K_2 (menaquinone), and K_3 (menadione). Vitamin K_1 is naturally found in plants such as green vegetables. Vitamin K_2 is found in animal sources and is synthesized in the colon. For newborns, AquaMEPHYTON and Konakion are the types most frequently used.

Action: Active in clotting, with prothrombin and other clotting factors; increases activity of vitamin K–dependent clotting factors (II, VII, IX, and X).

Dose: 0.5–1.0 mg within 6 hours of birth. May be repeated 6 hours after birth if necessary.

Data from Faucher, M. A., and Jackson, G. (1992). Pharmaceutical preparations. A review of drugs commonly used during the neonatal period. *Journal of Nurse-Midwifery,* 37 (2), 74S–86S.

of the air circulating in the incubator (Scopes 1981).

Parents should be instructed in how to take the baby's temperature, but they need do so only if the baby appears ill.

Prevention of Hemorrhage

It is thought that the gut lacks bacterial flora, which influences the production and synthesis of vitamin K. Vitamin K is necessary, with prothrombin, for clotting. Because the baby has less vitamin K until the bacterial flora is established with feeding (usually about 8 days of life), bleeding is more likely. To compensate for this, the neonate is given a prophylactic injection of vitamin K (Faucher and Jackson 1992).

Injections must be given in muscles large enough to absorb the medication and yet with care taken to avoid major nerves and blood vessels. The preferred site for neonates is the vastus lateralis muscle (Procedure 32–3).

Two types of vitamin K have been used for the neonate, AquaMEPHYTON and Konakion, which promote the formation of clotting factors II, VII, IX, and X in the liver. The usual one-time dosage for the neonate is 0.5 to 1.0 mg intramuscularly into the vastus lateralis muscle (Faucher and Jackson 1992). Side effects may include pain and edema at the injection site or a possible allergic reaction (rash, urticaria). Vitamin K with benzyl alcohol diluents is not recommended because fatal toxic symptoms can result (metabolic acidosis, central nervous system depression, respiratory problems, renal failure, hypotension, seizures, intracranial hemorrhage). Some have investigated administration of oral vitamin K to the mother prenatally since placental transfer has been documented. However, studies found that vitamin K given before delivery was not protective for intracranial hemorrhage in premature infants. Exclusively breastfed babies who were not given vitamin K were found to be at a greater risk for hemorrhage than were formula-fed babies. It is thought that the gut bacteria associated with breastfeeding vary from those with bottle feeding. Breastfed infants have predominantly gram-positive bacilli, *Lactobacillus bifidus.* It has been documented that related bacteria, *Lactobacillus casei,* do not produce vitamin K_2 in the gut. Oral administration of vitamin K has been investigated, but optimal dose and effectiveness have not been determined. Therefore, intramuscular injection continues to be recommended (Faucher and Jackson 1992).

In addition to administering vitamin K, the nurse should observe for bleeding from areas such as the umbilical cord, circumcision site, nose, and gastrointestinal tract and for ecchymosis. On occasion, the prophylactic dose is not sufficient to prevent bleeding. In this case, additional vitamin K is given.

PREVENTION OF INFECTION

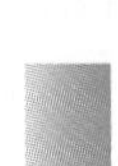

Prophylactic Eye Treatment

Prophylactic eye treatment should be administered to prevent infection of the eye (caused most commonly by gonococci or chlamydiae) that could be acquired as the baby passes through the birth canal (Procedure 32–4). Untreated gonococcal ophthalmia neonatorum can cause blindness or serious damage to the eyes. In addition, chlamydiae can cause inclusion conjunctivitis. There are more than 4 million chlamydial vaginal infections per year; 25 to 50 percent of ophthalmia neonatorum is attributed to chlamydiae (Faucher and Jackson 1992). Various prophylactic agents are used. These include ophthalmic erythromycin 0.5 percent ointment or drops in single-dose tubes or ampules, tetracycline 1 percent ointment or drops in single-dose tubes or ampules, and silver nitrate 1 percent in single-dose ampules.

States have a legal requirement to help prevent infection of the baby's eyes that could be acquired as the baby passes through a potentially infected birth canal. Originally, the concern centered around preventing gonococcal eye infection. This was accomplished by administration of 1 percent silver nitrate (in single-dose ampules) to the eyes one time after birth. Currently, the trend is to administer erythromycin 0.5 percent (Ilotycin) ointment or drops in a single-dose ampule or tube or tetracycline 1 percent ointment or drops in a single-dose ampule or tube to the conjunctival sacs. These medications are effective against other organisms besides the gonococcus (particularly chlamydiae), whereas silver nitrate is not. Prophylactic eye treatment should occur in the first few hours after birth; some indicate within the first hour after birth (National Society to Prevent Blindness 1981). The eye treatment is typically done soon after the baby is admitted to the nursery so that the baby's vision is not obscured by the treatment during first interactions with parents. It is essential that the agent reach all parts of the conjunctiva, which is accomplished by careful manipulation of the lids to spread the agent. The agent must reach the cornea.

Silver nitrate in particular, but other instillations as well, may cause a chemical conjunctivitis (90 percent of the time with silver nitrate). This is

PROCEDURE 32–4

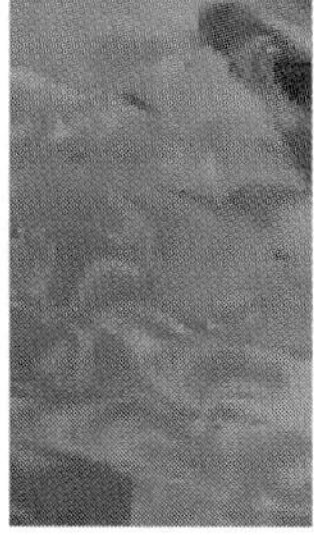

Instillation of Erythromycin, Tetracycline, or Silver Nitrate Eye Treatment

▼ PURPOSE

To administer prophylactic eye treatment one time soon after birth to prevent ophthalmic infections of the newborn.

▼ EQUIPMENT

- Tube of erythromycin eye ointment (0.5%) or tetracycline eye ointment (1%)
- Silver nitrate ampules (1%)

1 Check physician's order. **A physician's order is required.**

2 Wear gloves. **Wearing gloves is consistent with Standard Precautions.**

3 If necessary, clean the eyelids with sterile cotton balls moistened with sterile water. **Allows greater exposure to the prophylactic agent.**

4 If erythromycin or tetracycline ointment is ordered, retract the infant's lower eyelid outward with forefinger to expose the area for instillation of the ointment. Instill a strip (typically 1 inch or 2.5 cm) of ointment along the lower conjunctival sac, starting at the inner canthus and moving to the outer canthus (Faucher and Jackson 1992). Carefully manipulate the lid to spread the ointment. Only one dose per eye and one tube per baby. **Method of administration maximizes absorption of the prophylactic agent, ensuring that it reaches the cornea and all parts of the conjunctiva.**

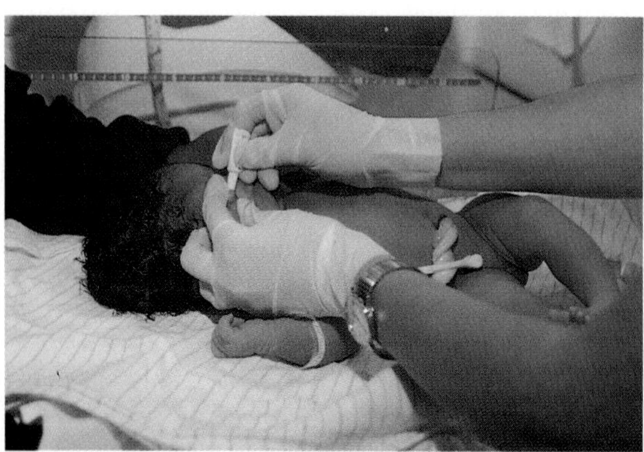

5 Repeat in the other eye. **Both eyes need treatment.**

6 Do not irrigate or rinse the eyes. **Irrigation probably minimizes efficacy and does not seem to decrease occurrence of chemical conjunctivitis (Faucher and Jackson 1992).**

7 Check for side effects such as edema, inflammation, and drainage. Also observe for hypersensitivity. **Edema, inflammation, and drainage may interfere with the newborn's ability to focus. Drainage can be cleansed from the eye. The newborn may be allergic to the medication.**

8 If silver nitrate (1%) is ordered, use a needle to puncture the ampule, which is made of wax, and squeeze the ampule to release the drops. Instill 2 drops in each conjunctival sac. Carefully manipulate the lids. After 1 minute, wipe any excess solution from the eyelids with sterile water. **Lid manipulation spreads the silver nitrate solution. One minute is needed for silver nitrate to be effective. Wiping excess silver nitrate drops from the eyelids removes excess and minimizes irritation.**

9 Chart administration of prophylactic agent. **Charting provides a written record of administration of prophylactic agent as ordered and documents fulfillment of legal requirement to help prevent ophthalmia neonatorum.**

Continued on facing page

PROCEDURE 32-4 Continued

Silver Nitrate (1%)

▼ **Action:** Causes disruption of the microbial cell membrane and death of the organism. Prevents gonococcal eye infection; not effective against chlamydial infection.

▼ **Dose:** 1% silver nitrate in wax ampule (to prevent evaporation and precipitation of the silver caused by glass). Two drops in each eye. Must be administered within 1 hour of birth.

▼ **Side Effects:** Chemical conjunctivitis.

Erythromycin (Ilotycin) Ointment (0.5%)

▼ **Action:** Bactericidal (destroys the bacteria) or bacteriostatic (inhibits growth of the bacteria), depending on the organism. Effective against both *Neisseria gonorrhoeae* and *Chlamydia trachomatis.* No effect on viruses, yeasts, or fungi. Inhibits protein synthesis and bacterial cell multiplication.

▼ **Dose:** At least 0.5-inch (1- to 2-cm) or 1-inch (2.5-cm) ribbon of ointment to conjunctiva of lower eyelids (Faucher and Jackson 1992).

▼ **Side Effects:** None.

Tetracycline (Achromycin or Aureomycin) Ointment (1%)

▼ **Action:** Bacteriostatic for gram-positive and gram-negative organisms, including gonococcus and chlamydia. Inhibits protein synthesis.

▼ **Dose:** At least 0.5-inch (1- to 2-cm) or 1-inch (2.5-cm) ribbon of ointment to conjunctiva of lower eyelids (Faucher and Jackson 1992).

▼ **Side Effects:** None.

Data from Faucher, M. A., and Jackson, G. (1992). Pharmaceutical preparations. A review of drugs commonly used during the neonatal period. *Journal of Nurse-Midwifery,* 37 (2), 74S–86S.

manifested by inflammation and discharge from the eye, commonly starting within the first 24 hours. Treatment includes rinsing the eyes with sterile solution until the condition disappears, which is commonly within a day or so. An infectious conjunctivitis, on the other hand, typically appears later, perhaps 1 to 3 days after birth, and tends to be a more purulent discharge. Eye infections are treated with appropriate antibiotic instillations.

Hygiene During Infant Care

The newborn is susceptible to infections, and the nurse needs to know the ways to prevent infection. Studies have documented that nosocomial infections are possible. Therefore, nurses must be sure to wash their hands. In the past, visitors were also restricted, and cover gowns were worn by staff and fathers while holding babies. A cover gown is a hospital gown worn over a uniform or clothing to protect the baby from contaminated uniforms or clothing. A different gown was worn with each baby held. One study found that babies whose visitors only washed hands and did not wear a gown had a *lower* colonization rate (of umbilical cord) than did babies whose visitors washed hands and wore a gown (Renaud 1983). While practices vary, the trend is to discontinue the use of cover gowns. Another common practice was for nursery nurses to do a complete surgical scrub each day before work. The idea was to decrease skin bacteria and thereby decrease transfer of microorganisms from nurse to baby. Since units have gone to the mother-baby concept with one nurse caring for both the mother and baby, this practice has diminished. Nurses continue to wash hands before touching each baby, however. Typical interventions to prevent neonatal infections include the following:

- Wash hands for 15 seconds before touching a baby. Remove jewelry from hands and arms (NAACOG 1985).
- Keep and use each baby's clothing and equipment only with that baby.

- Clean equipment, such as stethoscopes, after use with one baby before using with another baby.
- Wash hands after caring for one baby and before touching common equipment or supplies used by other babies.
- Observe the newborn for infection of such areas as skin (lesions, rash), cord (moist, discharge, odor), and eye (discharge, purulent); observe for signs of sepsis (hyperactivity, poor feeding).
- Perform appropriate medical asepsis of the umbilical cord (Procedure 32–5) to help prevent infection of the cord (NAACOG 1985). Circumcision care is discussed later in the chapter.
- In the past, neonates were given pHisoHex or hexachlorophene baths to reduce *Staphylococcus aureus* colonization and infection. Once it was discovered that absorption could cause neurologic side effects, these agents were no longer used. Most agencies still rely on one bath, after temperature stabilization, to help prevent infection. There is little literature about the efficacy of routine baths versus daily cleaning or dry skin care, which is merely cleansing the face and diaper area as needed. One study found no difference in colonization rates between routine bathing (bath each morning with soap) and no baths of normal newborns on a family-centered unit (Rush 1986). The same study found that rooming-in was associated with the lowest colonization and that babies born by cesarean section had the highest colonization rates. It was concluded that routine bathing with soap is no more effective than dry skin care. Hand washing continues to provide the best protection against infection (Rush 1986).

Nurses now wear gloves to care for neonates in accordance with current guidelines of the Centers for Disease Control and Prevention (CDC), which require the use of Standard Precautions for contact with body fluids of neonates. This means that gloves and gown need to be worn when touching a baby until the baby's first bath is completed. In addition, it is advocated that gloves be worn for doing cord care. The CDC requires wearing of gloves for changing diapers as well. Others consider oral fluids and regurgitation of the neonate to be potentially infectious since the neonate swallows amniotic fluid in utero. All recommendations are based on the fact that the neonate swallows amniotic fluid in utero, which could therefore potentially infect the baby's initial stools and regurgitations. In addition, the baby's skin had contact with potentially infected amniotic fluid and also retains some vernix. At present, hospitals vary on exact guidelines, but all follow Standard Precautions (see Appendix VI).

BILIRUBIN LEVELS, BLOOD GLUCOSE, AND NUTRITION

Effects of Bilirubin in the Neonate

For several reasons presented in earlier chapters, the neonate has a decreased ability to conjugate bilirubin; often, either physiologic or pathologic jaundice develops. Pathologic jaundice, jaundice within the first 24 hours after birth or persistence of visible jaundice after 1 week of age in term infants or 2 weeks in preterm infants (Blackburn and Loper 1992), is more likely when a large number of red blood cells are hemolyzed (as in blood incompatibilities), in premature infants who have an immature liver, in babies who have cold stress or hypothermia (glycogen is used to maintain temperature rather than for conjugation), and in infections that affect the liver. Since the inability to conjugate bilirubin effectively can result in serious detrimental effects, nursing assessment and interventions are crucial.

The nurse should check the neonate's history to determine the risk for pathologic jaundice. Particularly susceptible infants are those with acidosis, prematurity, hypoglycemia, hypothermia, sepsis, polycythemia, blood incompatibilities; those receiving antibiotic therapy; and those with intestinal obstruction (Blackburn and Loper 1992).

The baby's color is assessed for jaundice (yellow color) by blanching the skin over a bone prominence and visually observing the color. In dark-skinned babies, the yellow color is more difficult to discern because there is often a natural yellow undertone. Therefore, the oral cavity, palate, and conjunctival sacs should be assessed. Visual observation has been shown to be neither precise nor accurate, however (Schumacher 1990).

The bilirubin level is checked in the blood by obtaining a blood sample as explained in Procedure 31–3: Using the Heel Stick Method to Obtain Blood. Most assess the total bilirubin level. While laboratories and institutional guidelines vary, many consider a bilirubin level of 12 mg/dL to be abnormal and institute phototherapy treatment at this level (Sykes and Epstein 1990). Bilirubin can also be assessed by a noninvasive transcutaneous bilirubinometry screening device that gauges whether the degree

Text continued on page 1150

PROCEDURE 32–5

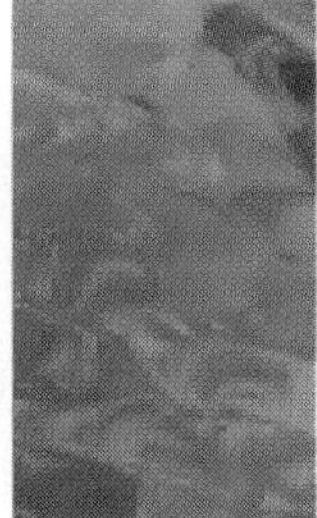

Umbilical Cord Care

▼ PURPOSE

To minimize contamination by microorganisms and prevent infection of the umbilical cord and to foster drying and "falling off" of the cord by applying prescribed preparations two to three times per day.

▼ EQUIPMENT

- Prescribed preparation: triple dye, silver sulfadiazine cream, bacitracin ointment, or isopropyl alcohol
- Cotton-tipped applicator, cotton ball, or alcohol swab
- Gloves

1 If using triple dye for *initial* cord care, open triple dye ampule. Use cotton-tipped applicator to paint the dye, one time, on the cord and on 1 inch of surrounding skin. **Triple dye may be used for initial cord care because it minimizes microorganisms and promotes drying.**

2 For daily cord care, clean umbilical cord and its base with a cotton ball or cotton-tipped applicator moistened with 70% alcohol, at least two to three times per day or use an alcohol swab. Follow these steps:

- Lift cord.
- Wipe around cord, starting at the top and wiping around it.
- Clean base of cord.

Application of 70% isopropyl alcohol minimizes microorganisms and promotes drying. Alcohol swab may be used, but a cotton ball with 70% isopropyl alcohol is typically used. The cotton-tipped applicator may be dipped into the alcohol and used to clean the base of the cord.

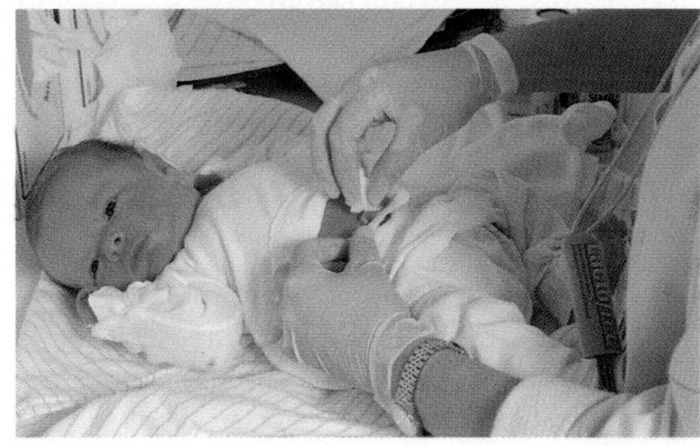

3 Fold diaper below umbilical cord to allow the cord to "air-dry." **Folding the diaper underneath the umbilical cord decreases its contact with potentially wet diaper and also helps drying by exposure to air.**

4 Assess cord each shift or day for symptoms of infection, such as moistness, oozing, discharge, reddened base. **If symptoms of infection occur, notify health care provider; antibiotic treatment is necessary.**

5 Do not give a tub bath until the cord falls off and the area is healed. **Wetness and moistness promote growth of microorganisms.**

6 When cord falls off at 7 to 14 days, assess for bleeding or infection. Explain to parents what to look for and what they should report to the health care provider. **Assesses normal drying and loss of cord. Parents need to know how to distinguish between signs of normal healing and signs of potential problems.**

7 Show parents how to care for umbilical cord. **Baby and mother are usually discharged from hospital 24 to 48 hours after birth. Cord must be cleaned and monitored for infection until it falls off (7 to 14 days after birth).**

Continued on following page

PROCEDURE 32–5 Continued

8 The cord clamp can be removed after the cord has dried (about 24 hours after birth). To remove the cord clamp, clip the circular end of the Hollister umbilical cord clamp with the Hollister cord clamp scissors, then separate the two halves of the cord clamp and remove them. **When the cord is dried and occluded, the clamp can be removed.**

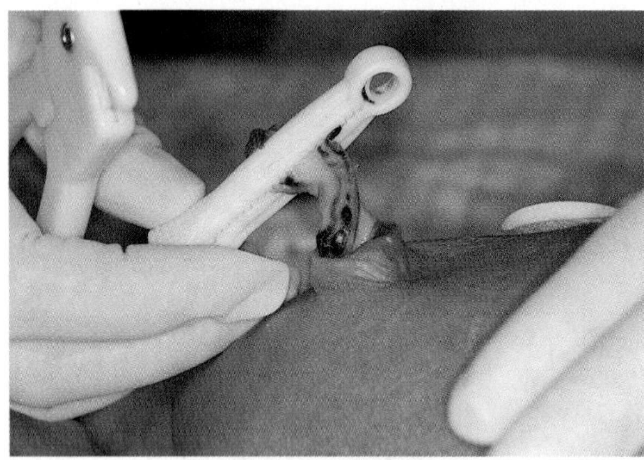

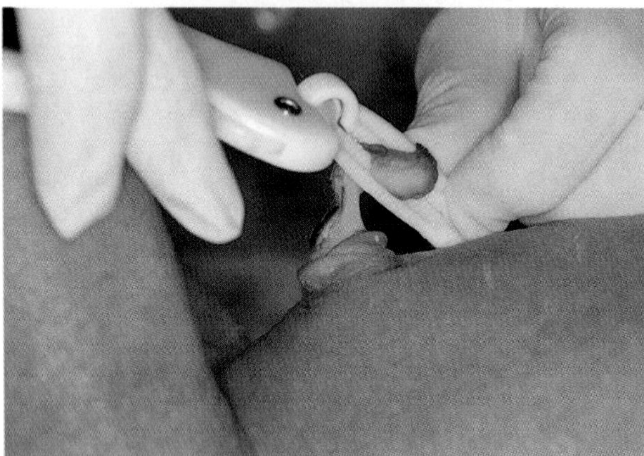

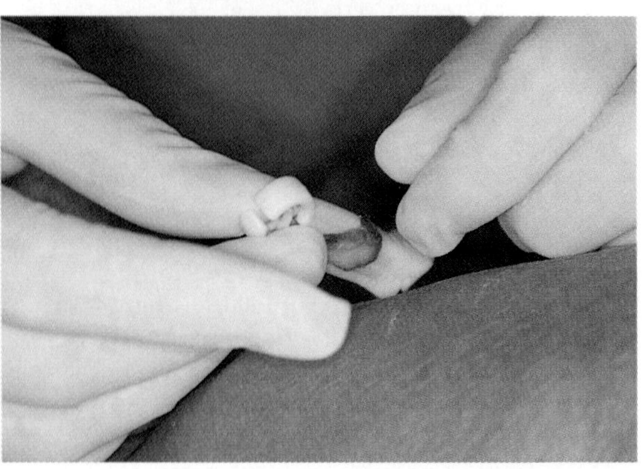

Triple Dye

▼ **Action:** Skin antiseptic killing or preventing growth of microorganisms. Consists of brilliant green, proflavine hemisulfate, and crystal or gentian violet. Oxidizes microbial protoplasm. Effective against *Staphylococcus aureus* colonization.

▼ **Dose:** Paint on cord and 1 inch of surrounding skin with cotton-tipped applicator one time (initial cord care).

▼ **Side Effect:** Bacterial resistance.

Silver Sulfadiazine (Silvadene) Cream (1%)

▼ **Action:** Antimicrobial, broad spectrum. Less effective than triple dye with *S. aureus,* and most effective with gram-negative organisms and group B streptococcus.

▼ **Side Effect:** Bacterial resistance.

Bacitracin Ointment

▼ **Action:** Bactericidal. Inhibits cell wall synthesis. Active against gram-positive organisms.

▼ **Side Effects:** Hypersensitivity. Resistance is rare. Weak effect with *S. aureus* and group B streptococcus.

Isopropyl Alcohol (70%, 90%)

▼ **Action:** Germicidal. Works on bacterial proteins and membrane lipids. Inactive against dried spores. Dries. Used on cord predominantly as a drying agent.

▼ **Side Effects:** Resistance.

Data on pharmaceutical preparations from Faucher, M. A., and Jackson, G. (1992). Pharmaceutical preparations. A review of drugs commonly used during the neonatal period. *Journal of Nurse-Midwifery,* 37 (2), 74S–86S.

Table 32–1

SIDE EFFECTS OF PHOTOTHERAPY

SIDE EFFECT	SPECIFIC CHANGES	IMPLICATIONS
Thermal and other metabolic changes	Increased environmental and body temperature Increased oxygen consumption Increased respiratory rate Increased skin blood flow	Influenced by maturity, calorie intake (energy to respond to thermal changes), adequacy of heat dissipation from phototherapy unit, distance of unit from infant and incubator hood (space for air flow, radiant heat loss), use of servocontrol
Fluid status	Increased peripheral blood flow	Increase fiuid loss May alter uptake of IM medications
	Increased insensible water loss	Due to increases in evaporative water loss, metabolic rate, and possibly respiratory rate Influenced by environment (air flow, humidity, temperature); characteristics of phototherapy unit (heat dissipation, distance from infant); ambient temperature alteration; infant alterations in skin and core temperature, HR, RR, metabolic rate, calorie intake; type of bed (increased with radiant warmer and incubator)
Gastrointestinal function	Increased number, frequency of stools Watery, greenish brown stools	May be related to increased bile flow, which stimulates GI activity
	Decreased time for intestinal transit	Increases stool water loss
	Decreased absorption; retention of nitrogen, water, electrolytes	Increases stool water loss and risk of dehydration
	Altered lactose activity, riboflavin	Temporary lactose intolerance with decreased lactase at epithelial brush border and increased frequency and water content of stools
Altered activity	Lethargy or irritability	May have impact on parent-infant interaction
	Decreased eagerness to feed	May alter fluid and calorie intake
Altered weight gain	Decreased initially but generally catches up in 2 to 4 weeks	Due to poor feeding and increased GI losses
Ocular effects	Not documented in humans, but continued concerns about effects of light versus effects of eye patches	Lack of appropriate sensory input and stimulation Eye patches increase risk of infection, corneal abrasion, increased ICP (if too tight)
Skin changes	Tanning	Due to induction of melanin synthesis or dispersion by UV light
	Rashes	Due to injury to skin mast cells with release of histamine; erythema from UV light
	Burns	From excessive exposure to short-wave emissions from fluorescent light

Continued on following page

Table 32–1

SIDE EFFECTS OF PHOTOTHERAPY Continued

SIDE EFFECT	SPECIFIC CHANGES	IMPLICATIONS
	Bronze baby syndrome	Due to decreased hepatic excretion of bilirubin photodegradation byproducts (especially in infants with elevated direct bilirubin)
Hormonal changes	Alterations in serum gonadotropins (increased LH and FSH)	Significance unclear May also affect circadian rhythms (unclear)
Hematologic changes	Increased rate of platelet turnover	May be a problem in infants with low platelets and sepsis
	Injury to circulating RBCs with decreased potassium and increased ATP activity	May lead to hemolysis, increased energy needs
Psychobehavioral concerns	Isolation/lack of usual sensory experiences including visual deprivation Alteration in state organization and neurobehavioral organization	Impact can be mediated by provision of appropriate nursing care May interfere with parent-infant interaction and increase parental stress

ATP, adenosine triphosphate; FSH, follicle stimulating hormone; GI, gastrointestinal; HR, heart rate; ICP, intracranial pressure; IM, intramuscular; LH, luteinizing hormone; RBCs, red blood cells; RR, respiratory rate; UV, ultraviolet.

From Blackburn, S. T., and Loper, D. C. (1992). *Maternal, fetal, and neonatal physiology: A clinical perspective* (p. 649). Philadelphia: W. B. Saunders.

of jaundice warrants serum bilirubin testing. It is a hand-held battery-powered instrument operating by skin reflection. A photo probe is placed on the neonate's skin, a strobe light transilluminates subcutaneous tissue and is reflected back, and a numeric index is displayed. Transcutaneous devices can be effective for screening but cannot replace serum testing for actual bilirubin values (Schumacher 1990).

The baby should be fed regularly to provide glucose and calories for the conjugation process. Regular feeding helps initiate establishment of gastrointestinal bacteria, which aids conjugation of bilirubin. This often means awakening the baby every 2 hours (if necessary) for breastfeeding or every 3 hours for formula bottle feedings.

In addition, the infant should be observed closely for side effects of phototherapy (Table 32–1). Phototherapy may be done in the hospital or at home (Fig. 32–2). For home therapy, parents need to be instructed on the side effects, correct procedure, and when to call the baby's health care provider. The home health nurse visits the infant to obtain a blood sample, which is sent to a laboratory for evaluation. The duration of phototherapy depends on the measured level of bilirubin.

Blood Glucose Levels in the Neonate

Some newborns may have a decreased ability to regulate and maintain blood glucose level because of immaturity, cold stress, or being an infant of a diabetic mother (see Chapter 30). The diagnosis of hypoglycemia is made when blood glucose levels are below 30 mg/dL in the first 72 hours or below 45 mg/dL after the first 3 days of life. Nursing care for hypoglycemia includes assessing the baby for symptoms of hypoglycemia: jitteriness, tremors, apnea or irregular respirations, lethargy, and poor feeding. A blood specimen by heel stick is also obtained to assess blood glucose level. Heel sticks use either Dextrostix or the Accu-Check apparatus to determine the glucose level (see Procedure 31–4: Assessing Blood Glucose Level Using Dextrostix or Chemstrip with Accu-Check II Device).

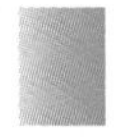

Nutrition in the Neonate

Feeding is vital for the newborn's growth and development. In addition, it helps parent and infant form a close relationship. Parents often place

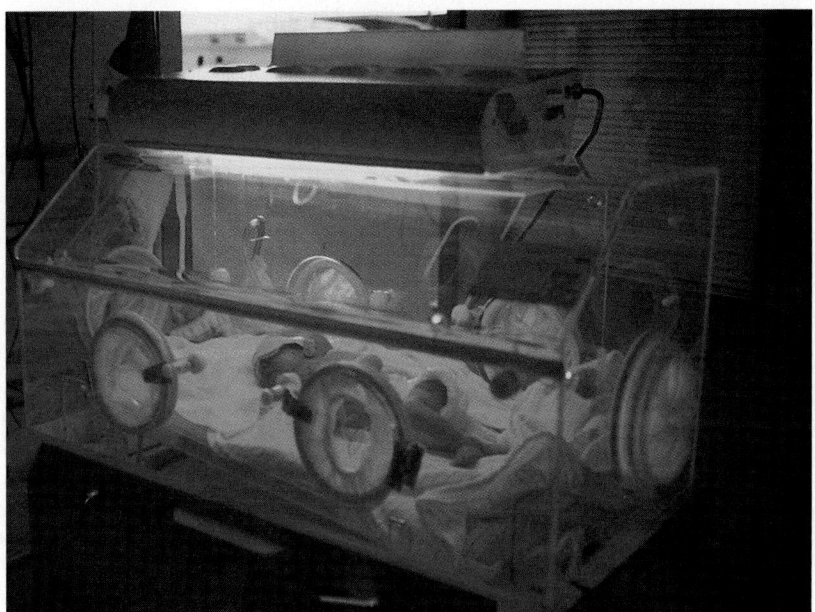

Figure 32–2

Phototherapy, used to treat hyperbilirubinemia, decomposes the bilirubin by photoisomerization • An eye shield provides protection from possible retinal damage related to phototherapy. (Courtesy of Wesley Medical Center, Wichita, KS.)

importance on how well the baby eats and how much weight the baby gains.

The Food and Nutrition Board, the National Academy of Sciences, and the American Academy of Pediatrics provide guidelines concerning nutrition of the newborn. Human breast milk is considered the best source of nutrition for the newborn, but commercial formulas adequately meet the nutritional needs of the newborn (AAP 1993).

ENERGY NEEDS

Infants need a considerable amount of calories, or energy. This is because the infant needs energy for basal metabolism, for maintaining body temperature, for physical activity and digestion of food, and for growth. In the first 4 months, about half of the calorie intake is used for basal metabolism, one third for growth, and about 10 to 15 percent for activity and other needs. During the first 6 months of life, the recommended daily dietary allowance (RDA) for energy is 108 calories per kilogram (or 49 calories per pound). For the second 6 months, it is 98 calories per kilogram (or 44.5 calories per pound) (Food and Nutrition Board 1989). Human breast milk and infant formulas supply approximately 20 calories per ounce (AAP 1993).

CARBOHYDRATES

Newborns typically have small glycogen stores in the liver. In addition, they often have limited gluconeogenesis (or formation of glucose from amino acids and other substrates) and ketogenesis (or formation of ketones from fat). Therefore, it is relatively important that the newborn take in adequate amounts of carbohydrate at fairly consistent intervals (AAP 1993).

Lactose is the primary carbohydrate in milk, and it provides calories in an available form. Human breast milk has more lactose than cow's milk. Therefore, lactose or another simple carbohydrate (such as sucrose, dextrose, or maltose) is added to cow's milk in commercial formulas (AAP 1993).

PROTEIN NEEDS

Protein requirements per unit of body weight for newborns are greater than at any other time in the life cycle. Thus, in the first 6 months, the newborn needs 2.2 g/kg of protein per day and 1.6 g/kg in the second 6 months of life (Food and Nutrition Board 1989).

Even though human breast milk is lower in protein than unmodified cow's milk is, it provides a sufficient amount of protein for the newborn. This is because human breast milk has more lactalbumin in relation to casein, which makes it easier to digest. The amino acids in human breast milk are ideally suited to the newborn. Therefore, commercial formulas often modify the protein in the cow's milk so that the amino acids more closely resemble those in human milk (AAP 1993).

FATS

To acquire adequate calories, newborns need to obtain about 15 percent of their calorie intake from fat. About 45 to 50 percent of the calories in human breast milk and in formulas comes from fat. Besides providing calories, essential fatty acids are required for growth and tissue maintenance. These essential fatty acids are components of cell membranes and are precursors of some hormones. If the infant has an inadequate intake of these essential fatty acids, eczema and growth failure can occur. Because skim and low-fat milks lack essential fatty acids and make it difficult to meet calorie requirements, they should not be fed to infants (AAP 1993). The fat in human breast milk is easier to digest and absorb than is the fat in cow's milk and formulas. Therefore, most commercial formulas remove fat from the cow's milk and then add a fat source (such as corn oil) that is more easily digested and absorbed (AAP 1993).

VITAMINS

Both human and cow's milk provide adequate amounts of most vitamins. Thus, both have adequate A and B complex vitamins. Cow's milk, however, typically lacks sufficient ascorbic acid or vitamin C. For this reason, commercial formulas are fortified with ascorbic acid (AAP 1993). The RDA for vitamin A is 375 g for the first year of life. For the B vitamins, the RDAs for the first and second 6 months of life are as follows:

	First 6 months	*Second 6 months*
Thiamine	0.3 mg	0.4 mg
Riboflavin	0.4 mg	0.5 mg
Niacin	5.0 mg	6.0 mg
Vitamin B_6	0.3 mg	0.6 mg
Folate	25 μg	35 μg
Vitamin B_{12}	0.3 μg	0.5 μg

The requirement for ascorbic acid is 30 mg/day in the first 6 months and then 35 mg/day in the second 6 months (Food and Nutrition Board 1989).

Vitamin K is lower in human milk than in cow's milk. At birth, the newborn's gut is sterile and lacks intestinal flora that is necessary to absorb vitamin K. Since vitamin K is needed for blood coagulation and may be deficient for a time after birth until the intestinal flora becomes established with feedings, an intramuscular injection of vitamin K is given to the newborn to prevent neonatal hemorrhage (AAP 1993; Food and Nutrition Board 1989). The RDA for vitamin K is 5 μg/day in the first 6 months of life and 10 μg in the second 6 months (Food and Nutrition Board 1989). Giving vitamin K supplements to the lactating mother has been investigated, but this supplementation is not recommended because studies found no difference in the vitamin K–dependent clotting factors in either formula-fed or breastfed babies when mothers had these supplements (AAP 1993; Greer et al. 1991).

Vitamin D tends to be somewhat deficient in human milk, but it can be obtained with vitamin supplementation of the infant or by exposure to sunlight. Commercial formulas are fortified with vitamin D (AAP 1993). The RDA for vitamin D is 7.5 μg for the first 6 months and 10 μg for the second 6 months. Breastfed infants not exposed to sunlight should be given a supplement of 5 to 7.5 μg of vitamin D daily (Food and Nutrition Board 1989).

MINERALS

Even though human milk is lower in calcium than formulas, the ratio of calcium to phosphorus is optimal for bones, and breastfed babies receive ample calcium (AAP 1993). The requirement for calcium is 400 mg for the first 6 months of life and 600 mg for the second 6 months of life (Food and Nutrition Board 1989).

Ensuring adequate iron intake requires particular attention because milk of all types is low in iron. Iron in human breast milk is absorbed better (about 50 percent is absorbed) than is the iron in cow's milk and iron-fortified formulas (about 10 percent is absorbed). If the newborn has obtained an adequate store of iron during the prenatal period, the baby will have adequate iron to produce red blood cells for about 4 to 6 months. Therefore, babies who are breastfed human milk, which is lower in iron, will have adequate iron and hemoglobin levels for the first 6 months if they received an adequate store of iron before birth. After 6 months, iron-fortified cereals are included in the diet (AAP 1993). The RDA for iron is 6 mg in the first 6 months and 10 mg in the second 6 months of life (Food and Nutrition Board 1989). It is recommended by the American Academy of Pediatrics (1993) that babies who are formula fed (or those who are weaned from the breast before 6 months of age) receive an iron-fortified formula to ensure adequate iron to prevent anemia.

Many recommend fluoride supplementation for breastfed infants as well as bottle-fed infants who live in areas where the fluoride concentration in the water is low. If the water used for dilution of the formula has adequate fluoride, the baby will receive adequate amounts; but infants whose formula is made with water that is deficient in fluoride will not receive adequate fluoride. Fluoride supplements are available alone or in combination with vitamins. Children who receive adequate fluoride realize a reduction in dental caries (AAP 1993).

WATER

Infants require more water relative to body weight than adults because the baby's kidneys are not as efficient at concentrating urine. Because of this, infants excrete a greater amount of water. In fact, infants excrete about 15 percent of their body weight per day. The RDA for water is approximately 1.5 mL/kcal of body weight (Food and Nutrition Board 1989).

Water needs are met through breast milk or formula. If dehydration is a risk (such as at times when the infant is placed in an environment with a high temperature or suffers vomiting or diarrhea), additional water may be needed (AAP 1993; Clifford and Walker 1983).

CHOOSING BREASTFEEDING OR BOTTLE FEEDING

Many advantages are cited for breastfeeding. Breast milk is considered the "gold standard" for feeding and is considered the best nutrition for the newborn (AAP 1993). Many cite enhanced protection against infections as a benefit of breastfeeding (Holmes et al. 1983). Another advantage of breastfeeding is the prevention or amelioration of diarrhea (AAP 1993; Clifford and Walker 1983). Some believe that the sucking action involved in breastfeeding helps open and drain the pharynx and eustachian tubes. Other advantages of breastfeeding include ease, convenience, and lower cost. Colic has been found to occur less frequently in breastfed than in bottle-fed babies. When it does occur, it is most often thought to be associated with the mother's intake of particular foods, such as garlic and onions, turnips, broccoli, or melons. Contraindications to breastfeeding are uncommon but include serious health problems in the mother, maternal intake of some medicines or illicit drugs, and potential transmission of an illness from mother to newborn (AAP 1993). One of the nurse's primary roles is to assist and support the mother with breastfeeding (see Chapter 33).

There are reasons to bottle feed. These include early return to work as well as the desire to share feedings with the father or others. Some cite previous positive experiences with bottle feeding or previous negative experiences with breastfeeding. Others feel that breastfeeding is immodest and therefore choose to bottle feed. As mentioned, some bottle feed out of necessity as a result of serious health problems or previous breast surgery. Finally, many state that bottle feeding is more convenient (Howard and Weitzman 1992).

COMMERCIAL FORMULAS

Commercial formulas (such as Enfamil, Similac, SMA) are modeled after human milk, but none is identical to it. Because of this, infant formulas have been, and continue to be, changed and improved (AAP 1993). The Infant Formula Act (of 1980 and 1986) mandates adherence to standards developed by the American Academy of Pediatrics. In addition, it mandates quality control, which means formulas must conform to regulations of the Food and Drug Administration (AAP 1993). The following are common adaptations of cow's milk when formulas are manufactured:

- Protein is decreased because cow's milk contains more protein than does breast milk. In addition,

Tips for Safe Preparation of Infant Formula

- Only infant formula should be fed until 1 year of age because cow's milk does not provide adequate nutrition. Infants receiving whole cow's milk have been found to have low iron, linoleic acid, and vitamin E levels. In addition, they have demonstrated high sodium, potassium, and protein levels, which places them at risk for dehydration. The likelihood of iron deficiency anemia also exists (AAP 1993).
- It is important that formulas be diluted properly, if needed, because electrolyte imbalance or water intoxication can occur if they are not (Howard and Weitzman 1992). Parents need to read and follow directions carefully.
- Water used to dilute the formula should be allowed to run for 2 minutes to clear water from pipes that may contain lead.
- The top of the formula can should be washed before opening.
- If water comes from an unsanitized source like a well, it should be boiled for 5 minutes before it is used in the formula.
- Sterilization and boiling of water are not necessary if the city has a safe water supply and bottles are prepared one at a time.
- Preparation involves washing bottles with hot soapy water and a bottle brush or using a dishwasher.
- Partially consumed bottles of formula should be discarded.
- Formula may be fed cold, or it can be warmed slightly under running water, in a bottle warmer, or on the stove. Bottles should not be warmed in a microwave because "hot spots" can occur. The temperature of the formula should be tested before feeding to make sure it is not too hot.
- Bottles with nipples should be inverted to check the flow rate to ensure that the flow is neither too fast nor too slow (Howard and Weitzman 1992).

protein is treated to make it more easily digested (the lactalbumin in breast milk is more easily digested than the protein in cow's milk) (AAP 1993).
- Butterfat is removed and a more digestible vegetable fat is added (such as corn oil) (AAP 1993).
- Lactose or another carbohydrate is added because there is less lactose in cow's milk (AAP 1993).
- Vitamins A, C, D, and E are added. Cow's milk has been found to lack vitamin C and possibly vitamin D (if the mother's intake is inadequate during pregnancy or is inadequate during lactation or the baby has insufficient sunlight exposure) (AAP 1993).
- Iron is added because many believe that the low amount of iron in milk as well as the potential for inadequate iron stores in the newborn puts the infant at risk for anemia (AAP 1993). The American Academy of Pediatrics recommends that all infants receive iron-fortified formula (AAP 1993).
- The American Academy of Pediatrics recommends routine infant supplements of fluoride beginning at 2 weeks of age if the water supply in the area lacks fluoride. The proper fluoride level for water is at least 0.3 ppm. Optimal fluoride levels are 0.05 mg/kg to 0.07 mg/kg of body weight per day (Howard and Weitzman 1992).

If an infant cannot tolerate milk-based formulas, others are available. Soy-based formulas are made by altering the soy protein, adding methionine so that it equals that of casein in cow's milk, and omitting lactose (sucrose, cornstarch, hydrolysates, or a mixture of these are then added). It is recommended that soy formulas be used for the management of lactose deficiencies, for allergy prophylaxis in families with a strong family history, for vegetarian families, and for the management of galactosemia (Howard and Weitzman 1992; AAP 1993).

Some infants will be intolerant of both cow's milk and soy protein milk. Because switching to a soy protein milk introduces a second potential allergen, the American Academy of Pediatrics recommends using a protein hydrolysate formula for babies intolerant of cow's milk formulas. Protein hydrolysate formulas heat treat the protein and enzymatically hydrolyze it. The formula is then fortified with amino acids to compensate for those that were lost in the manufacturing process. Most are free of lactose (another carbohydrate is added), and fats are medium-chain triglycerides, which aid fat absorption (AAP 1993).

Various preparations of formula are available:

- Ready-to-feed formulas, which come in a 32-ounce can, need no preparation and are the most expensive. Once opened, ready-to-feed formulas must be refrigerated and used within 48 hours.
- Concentrated formulas, which come in 13-ounce cans, are diluted 1:1 with water. Concentrated formulas are intermediate in cost. Diluted formula should not be stored more than 24 hours.
- Powdered formulas are made by mixing 1 scoop of formula powder (scoop comes with the formula) with 2 ounces of water. Powdered formulas are the least expensive (Howard and Weitzman 1992).

Research and advances in the development of infant formulas continue. Some project that advances in genetic engineering will make it possible to alter the composition of milk so that "immune milks" can be produced. These will contain polyclonal antibodies against *Salmonella, Listeria,* retrovirus, and human immunodeficiency virus. If nucleotides truly enhance immune function and if formulas can be supplemented with them, the health of infants will truly be improved. The introduction of palm oil in 1988 may allow the production of a vegetable oil blend that more closely resembles human milk (Filer 1992).

Most breastfed babies are put to breast soon after birth. However, for the bottle-fed babies feedings are initiated when the adaptive transition to extrauterine life is ensured. This most commonly occurs right after the initial transition period, or 6 to 8 hours after birthing, once readiness for feeding is determined and vital signs are stable. Nursing interventions to maintain nutrition and weight gain include the following:

- Assess readiness for feedings. Signs of readiness include active bowel sounds, absence of abdominal distention, lusty cry, rooting and sucking reflexes present, normal vital signs (respiration, heart rate), nose breathing, without nasal obstruction.
- Give sterile water feeding. Some institutions advise a bottle feeding, by the nurse, of approximately 10 to 15 mL sterile water to assess normalcy of swallow, patency of nares, and integrity of the gastrointestinal tract. Once that small amount is fed, the remainder of the feeding is finished with either formula or breast milk.
- Ensure the neonate's feedings. Most of the time, the baby is fed by the mother. In this case, the nurse assesses the mother's feeding techniques as well as the baby's feeding behaviors and intervenes appropriately to ensure that the baby is fed at regular intervals (on demand but every 2 to 3 hours for breast babies and every 3 to 4 hours for bottle babies).
- Record infant feedings, infant feeding behavior, and mother's feeding techniques so that appropriate nursing action can ensue.
- Weigh the baby every day and assess weight loss. Most hospitals weigh the baby once a day

(often on night shift) to be able to assess whether the weight loss after birth is normal or too excessive. Weight loss is due to minimal intake at first feedings. While disagreement exists, many consider a weight loss of 5 to 10 percent to be fairly normal. Babies typically regain their birth weight by 7 to 10 days of life and then gain about 1 ounce per day in the first 6 months of life (Bronner and Paige 1992) (see Procedure 31–2).

MAINTENANCE OF ELIMINATION

It is important to understand the characteristics of normal stool and urine (see Chapter 30) as well as to instruct parents about these characteristics so that diarrhea, constipation, and dehydration can be detected and treated.

The nurse should assess and record frequency, color, and amount of urine. Most newborns void within 24 hours. There is concern if a newborn has not voided by 48 hours. Typically, urinary frequency is denoted by a checkmark on the chart flowsheet each time the neonate voids. Amount of voiding is assessed to be normal unless an abnormality is noted in the nurse's notes section of the chart. Since the intake is low the first day or so, urine output is low as well. Assess the diaper for size of the area saturated with urine as well as for color of urine (more yellow color and smaller area saturated indicate more concentrated urine). Many tell parents that the baby should have at least 6 wet diapers a day to be considered well hydrated.

The frequency, color, and characteristics of stools are also assessed and recorded. Most newborns pass a meconium stool within 24 hours. There is concern when the newborn has not passed a stool by 48 hours of life. Characteristics of stools vary if the baby is breastfed or bottle fed. The breastfed baby's stools are more frequent (six per day), have a loose or more "mushy" consistency, and are described as having a golden yellow color as well as a "pleasantly sour" odor. Bottle-fed babies, on the other hand, have fewer stools (four to five a day) that are more formed or have a "pasty" consistency and are described as having a light yellow color and a foul odor. Parents should be instructed about meconium and transitional stools as well.

It is unlikely that breastfed babies will develop constipation, but if this occurs in the first few weeks, it may indicate inadequate milk or fluid supply. Symptoms of constipation include small, hard, firm, infrequent stool, often requiring straining to pass. The newborn typically cries and draws the legs up to the abdomen. Giving additional sterile water may help (Long and Hsia 1992).

Symptoms of diarrhea include loose, watery stool, often green in color and ringed with water. It is typically frequent (ten per day), being forcefully expelled. Diarrhea can be serious, leading to dehydration and electrolyte imbalance. It may be due to overfeeding or to an infection, so careful assessment is necessary. If mild diarrhea is caused by overfeeding, boiled water with 5 percent glucose is fed (Long and Hsia 1992).

Change the baby frequently to minimize contact of stool or urine with the baby's skin. This often means changing with every feeding. Cleanse the diaper area appropriately with each diaper change. For girls, the area is cleansed from the front of the genital area toward the rectum to avoid fecal contamination of the urethra and bladder. Hospitals use either a commercial "wipe" or paper disposable pads that are moistened with water. Each wipe must be used only once to minimize contact of fecal material with the urethral area. For boys, the penis is cleaned first, after which the scrotum and rectal areas are cleaned.

Prevention of diaper rash commonly includes changing and cleaning frequently; it involves keeping the baby dry. Application of baby powder used to be advised because powder absorbs moisture. It has been noted that powder may cake, and more important, it can become dispersed in the air to be inhaled during application. This has been found to be detrimental to the baby's lungs. Therefore, many have returned to advocating application of cornstarch, which also absorbs moisture. It can be purchased inexpensively and should be applied by the hands rather than by "shaking" a container. It is interesting that the commercial market now sells cornstarch in the traditional shaker container. Others advocate barriers or protectants such as zinc oxide ointment, vitamin A and D ointment, or petroleum jelly. There is little research in this area, and varying opinions exist. The principles of promoting dryness and minimizing contact with urine should guide practice. When the rash is severe, some also advise warmth by a 25-watt light bulb placed 18 inches from the diaper area for 15 to 20 minutes several times a day. The rationale is to increase circulation and to promote healing and drying. If the diaper rash continues or becomes more irritated or indurated, an infection of the area should be suspected. In this case, the nurse practitioner or pediatrician can assess the area and prescribe an appropriate antibiotic ointment. This may include nystatin (Mycostatin) or Mycolog cream for monilial infections (Faucher and Jackson 1992).

Teach parents about types of diapers and how to fold and wash diapers, if necessary. Accepted types of diapers have changed over the years, with public and health care opinion varying. In the past, cloth diapers (washed by the mother or provided by a diaper service) were the trend. There are three basic types of cloth diapers: the larger rectangular type, the triangle type, and the prefolded type with extra thickness in the center. Currently, numerous types of disposable diapers are used. Varying diapers for varying weights of babies, those designed for girls and boys (with bulk in front for boys and in back for girls to ensure absorption), and those with a "cutout" for the umbilical cord abound. The environmental controversy about lack of biodegradability of disposable diapers versus the negative effects of detergents used to launder cloth diapers continues, but it seems that the convenience of disposables is winning.

POSITIONING, HOLDING, BATHING, AND DRESSING THE NEONATE

Positioning and Holding the Infant Correctly

While awake, the baby is placed in the side-lying position, with a blanket roll support to maintain the position. This facilitates drainage of mucus, respiratory fluids, or regurgitated feedings. In addition, this position allows minimal pressure on a circumcised penis. The baby's position should be changed from side to side to assist in developing even contours of the head and to change visual stimulation. Many advocate positioning on the right side immediately after a feeding because it is thought that this position promotes gastric emptying into the small intestine. The baby's mattress should be firm, and the crib slats should be narrow enough to prevent the baby's head from entering; paint or stain should be nontoxic because babies suck on and put most things in their mouths.

Hold the baby securely, supporting the head; the baby is unable to maintain an erect head position for more than a few seconds. To pick up the baby, slide one hand under the baby's neck and shoulder and the other under the baby's buttocks. It also helps to grab one leg. There are three main ways to hold a baby (Fig. 32–3). In the cradle hold, the baby is nestled in one's arms with head supported in the crook of the arm, buttocks supported by one hand; the other arm enfolds the baby. This hold is often used for feedings.

In the football hold, the baby's head is held in one hand, the baby is supported by the forearm, and the buttocks are supported on the caretaker's hip. This hold frees one hand for changing the bed, picking up an object, or answering the phone. It is also used for shampooing the hair and for breastfeeding.

Finally, there is the upright or shoulder position in which the baby is held against the shoulder, supported by one hand; the other hand supports the buttocks. This hold is often used for burping the baby.

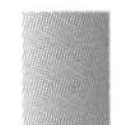

Bathing the Newborn

Bathing the baby allows cleansing and observation as well as promotes comfort. In addition, it is an excellent time for parent-infant socializing. Parents are often anxious about bathing and concerned about bathing "the right way." Since bathing is a psychomotor skill, parents often learn best through demonstration or by viewing a videotape, followed by their own practice. Because bathing is relatively simple and follows a few basic principles, it is important to emphasize these rather than myriad facts. There are often alternative ways to accomplish the task while maintaining the same overall goals. It is not advisable to bathe a baby right after a feeding because the handling may cause regurgitation. Sponge and tub bathing are explained in the Teaching Guide: How to Bathe the Newborn. General points that apply to both methods should be kept in mind:

- Maintain baby's temperature because babies lose more heat than adults do. This is accomplished by bathing quickly, exposing only the portion of the body being bathed at that time, drying thoroughly, and bathing in a relatively warm room free of drafts.
- Cleanse from cleanest to "dirtiest," most contaminated areas. Typically this means eyes, face, and hair first, diaper area last. It also means cleansing from inner to outer canthus of the eyes and from urethra to rectal area.
- The baby's skin is fragile; avoid trauma. This is accomplished by avoiding vigorous cleansing, being gentle, patting dry, using a mild soap without perfume, and bathing only as necessary several times a week (soap and water dry the skin). Most recommend using only water and not soap on the baby's face. Avoid potentially irritating skin applications and lotions as well.
- Newborns often cry during the bath, but as they grow older, the bath becomes a time for fun and socialization with parents.

There is little research about the application of various lotions and oils to the baby's skin. Therefore, recommendations and opinions vary. Some advocate application of baby oil when the baby's skin is dry. Some argue that various preparations can "clog" skin pores and therefore should be

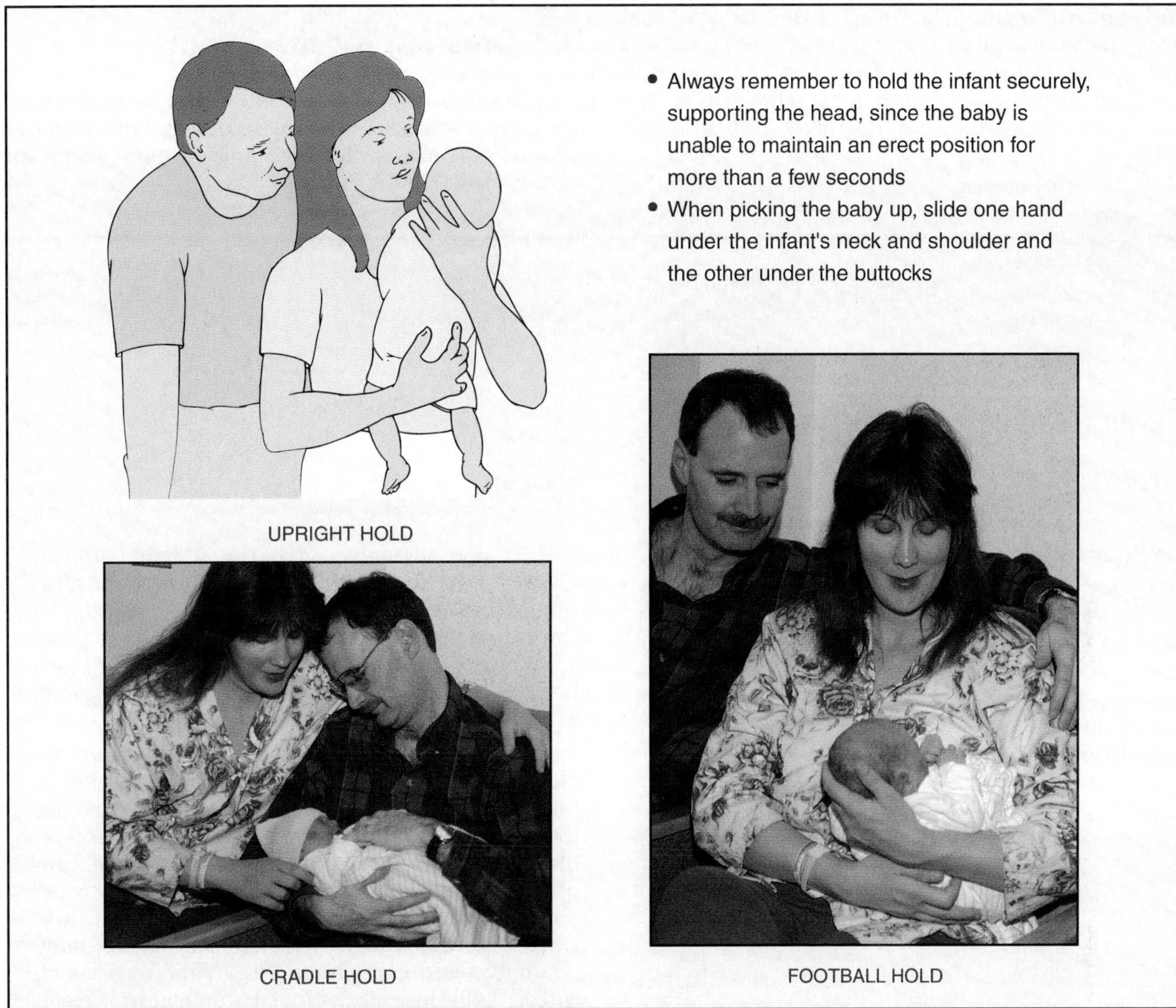

Figure 32–3

Parents should be taught the correct way to hold their newborn • Supporting the infant's head is of utmost importance • In the upright position, parents should keep one hand behind the baby's head and the other on the baby's bottom • When using the cradle hold, the parent's arm supports the baby's head and body • In the football hold, the hand is behind the neck while the rest of the arm supports the baby's body.

avoided. This seems to be a relatively rare occurrence. Since opinions vary, it is wise to keep in mind the underlying reason for advice—the desire to avoid skin irritations or allergies that may occur with exposure to perfumes and other ingredients. Check with your institution's protocol so that you can provide parents with consistent information.

Fingernails and toenails can often be long. To remove excess growth, the nails must grow out far enough from the skin so that skin is not cut by mistake. Before cutting, soften nails by giving the baby a bath. Soon after, when the baby is asleep, use a manicure scissors. Hold the skin back from the nail and cut straight across. If nails remain long, the baby can be scratched during normal hand and leg movements.

Once the umbilical cord has fallen off and the circumcision is healed, which is typically at 2 weeks of age, the baby can be put into the tub for a bath. A commercial baby washbasin/tub or the sink can be used. Until the baby is older, the regular bathtub is not used because it is difficult to bend over the tub and hold the baby. By bathing in the kitchen sink or on the counter or table, the parent's back is spared. Some advise putting a towel on the bottom of the washbasin/tub or sink to avoid slipping. Only several inches of water are needed. Again, check the temperature, as with a sponge bath.

The baby is held at all times. This is accomplished by cradling one arm at the back under the baby's shoulders and grasping the baby's arm with that hand. This leaves the other hand free to wash and rinse the baby. To wash the baby's back, place the noncradling arm across the baby's chest and grasp the baby's arm. Then gently tip or rest the baby forward onto your arm. This leaves the hand that originally held the baby free to wash the back.

Dressing for the Infant

In the hospital, babies wear a T-shirt and diaper and are swaddled in a blanket. At home, babies typically wear a T-shirt, diaper, and gown or

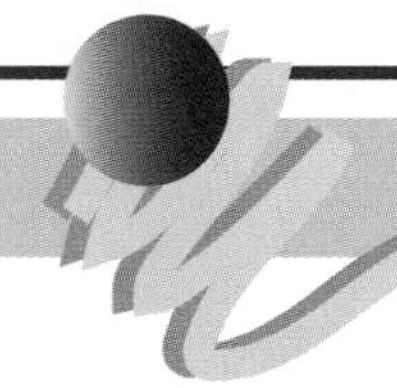

TEACHING GUIDE

HOW TO BATHE THE NEWBORN

TOPIC	*MAJOR CONCEPTS*
When to bathe the baby	It is not advisable to bathe a baby after a feeding because handling may cause regurgitation. Since bathing is thought to be relaxing to the infant, before feeding may be the best time. Sponge bathing is necessary until the cord has fallen off and circumcision, if applicable, has healed (approximately 2 weeks).
Gathering supplies	All supplies should be gathered before the bath is started so that supplies are accessible. Suggest that your client keep supplies together in one place so that they can be easily assembled each time the baby is bathed. Typical supplies include washcloth, towels, mild soap without perfume (examples are Neutrogena and Dove; perfumes can irritate the skin), baby shampoo, cord care items (70% rubbing alcohol, cotton balls or cotton-tipped applicators), clean clothing, diaper, and infant washbasin or sink. The baby should *never* be left alone during the bath.
The environment	The environment should be prepared so that it is warm and disruptions are minimal. Room temperature should be maintained (about 75°) to help the baby maintain body temperature. Suggest that your client minimize disruptions by taking the phone off the hook or ignoring it if it rings.
The bath water	A clean basin or sink should be filled with 2 to 3 inches of warm water; your client can check the temperature with her wrist. The water is used to wet the washcloth and to rinse the baby. When the baby graduates to a tub bath, again only 2 to 3 inches of water should be used in the clean infant tub or sink. A washcloth or towel should be placed in the bottom of the tub or sink to prevent slipping.

Continued on facing page

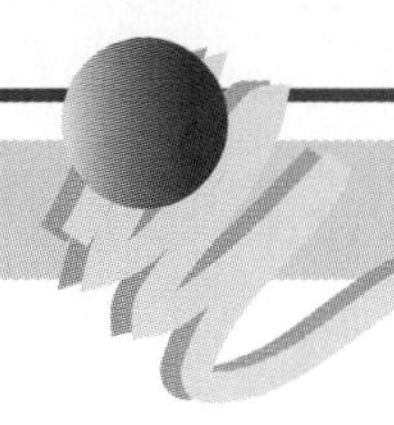

Maintain the baby's temperature

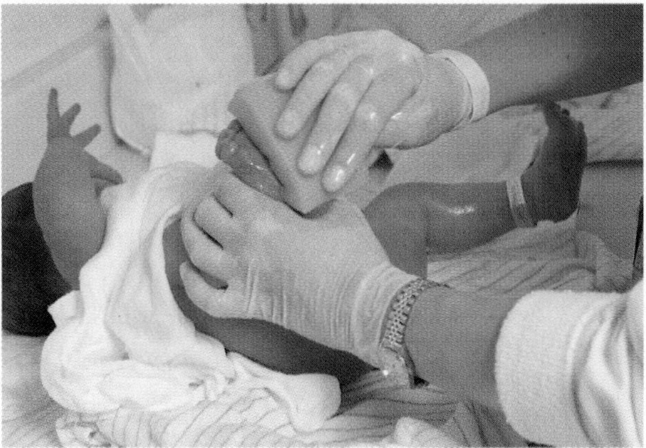

Remind your client that it is important to maintain the baby's temperature because infants lose heat easily. Bathing quickly, exposing only the part of the body being bathed at that time, and drying thoroughly help keep the infant warm.

Cleanse the baby's eyes, ears, and face

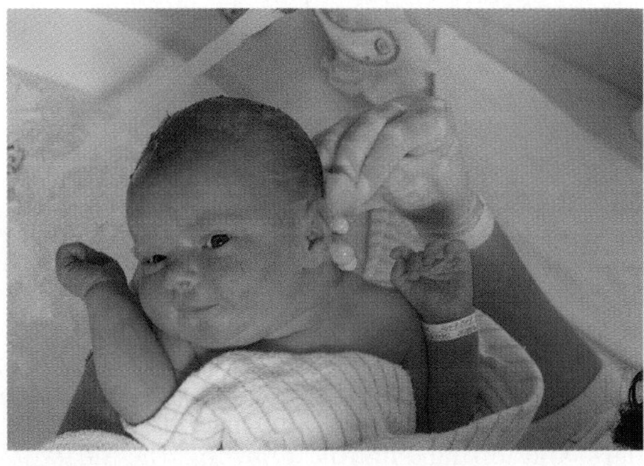

Bathing should start at the eyes and face, generally the cleanest area. Wrapping the washcloth over the index finger and wetting with water (no soap is necessary for the eyes, ears, and face since it could be drying and irritating), gently wipe from the inner to outer corner of one eye. Explain that this will help prevent irritation and infection of the lacrimal duct. The process is repeated on the other eye.

Next, the external ear and behind the ear are cleansed, again with the washcloth over the index finger. A cotton-tipped applicator should not be used because it could be inserted too far and damage the eardrum, or it might push discharge farther into the ear canal. Another part of the cloth should be used for the other ear. Now the baby's face may be cleansed.

Wash the baby's hair

Explain to your client that it is important to wash the infant's hair regularly to avoid cradle cap (or scaling of the scalp). The process is the same for both the sponge and tub bath.

Pick the baby up in a football hold, holding the head over the washbasin and tilted slightly downward. The infant's hair should be rinsed with clean water with a washcloth or cupped hand, allowing the excess to drip into the basin. A small amount of shampoo in the free hand is lathered into the scalp. Teach your client to cleanse and rub the scalp including the soft spots. Then rinse over the basin with washcloth or cupped hand and dry well. A soft brush may be used every day. Should seborrheic dermatitis develop, baby oil may be applied to the scalp a half-hour before the bath.

Continued on following page

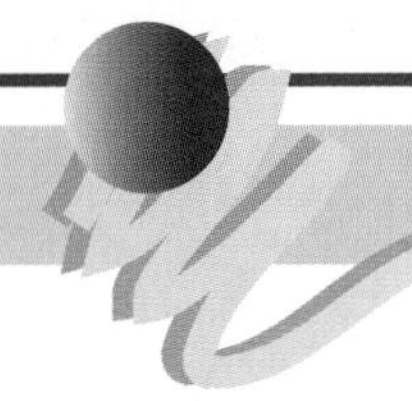

For a tub bath, place and hold the baby in the tub

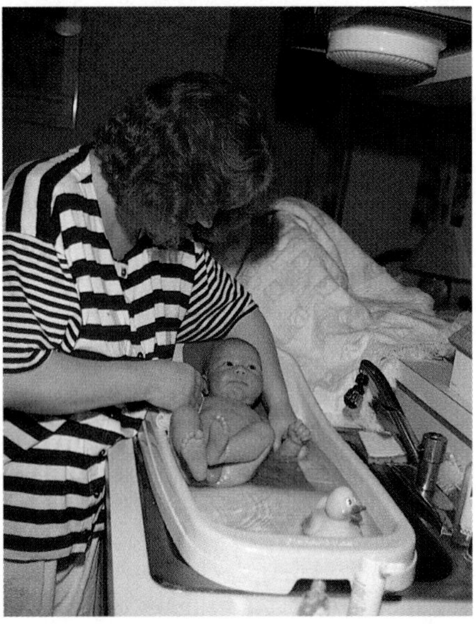

Emphasize to your client that the baby must be held at all times when in the tub. Have your client cradle one arm at the back and under the baby's shoulders, and grasp the baby's arm or thigh with that hand. This will leave the other hand free to wash and rinse the baby.

Wash the baby's neck, chest, arms, and back

For a sponge bath, the blanket is unwrapped and the T-shirt removed; the blanket is then used to loosely cover as much of the infant as possible to prevent heat loss. Each area is soaped, rinsed, and gently patted dry. Explain to your client that the baby's skin is fragile and easily irritated.

The infant's neck should be exposed by placing a hand under the baby's back at the shoulders and lifting slightly, allowing the head to fall back slightly. Formula, breast milk, or lint will often accumulate in the folds of the neck.

Hands and arms are washed by soaping with a washcloth or hand, making sure to gently cleanse the vernix where secretions may collect. The chest should be cleansed and rinsed while being careful to keep the cord dry. Patting dry and putting on a clean T-shirt or wrapping the upper body with a blanket will decrease heat loss.

Soaping and rinsing the baby's neck, chest, and arms with washcloth or hand is done in the same manner for a tub bath. To wash the baby's back, teach your client to place the non-cradling arm across the baby's chest and grasp the baby's arm. Then the baby may be gently tipped forward onto a supporting arm, leaving the other hand free to wash the back.

Continued on facing page

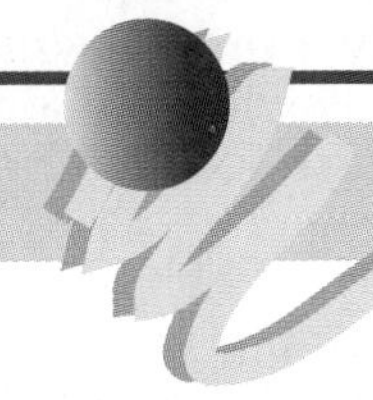

TEACHING GUIDE Continued

Wash the baby's legs

Expose the baby's legs and cleanse with soap and water. Then rinse and pat dry.

Wash the diaper area

For a sponge bath, the diaper should be removed now. Clean from the urethral area back to the rectal area for girls, using a different part of the washcloth each time. For boys, teach your client to cleanse the urethral area of the penis, then down the penis, next washing the scrotum, and finally the rectal area. Using these steps will help avoid fecal contamination of the urethral area. Dry and apply a diaper.

After cleansing the diaper area during a tub bath, the baby may be removed from the tub, patted dry thoroughly, and dressed.

Cord care

Cord care may aid drying of the cord and decreases microorganisms (see Procedure 32–5).

Clothe and wrap in a blanket

When the bath is completed, additional clothing may be needed. The infant may then be wrapped in a blanket if necessary.

Teaching Aids

1. Pictures showing washing of the baby's eyes, ears, face, hair, arms, legs, back, and diaper area
2. Videotape of the bathing procedure
3. Demonstration of the bath; the nurse bathes the baby while the parents observe
4. Parent returns the demonstration or bathes the baby while the nurse observes, provides helpful hints, and provides positive reinforcement

Increasing Your Teaching Effectiveness

Teaching the parents how to bathe their baby will be enhanced by

1. Providing a videotape for home reference
2. Demonstrating the bath with an actual baby
3. Providing a comfortable environment so that parents feel free to ask questions
4. Providing positive feedback and positive reinforcement
5. Providing a phone number for parents to call should they have questions

sleeper. If it is cool, they are wrapped in a blanket. Swaddling in a blanket helps maintain body temperature and provides a feeling of security. Some advise putting one more layer on a baby than the parent is wearing. Dressing at home is dependent on the room temperature as well. A hat or bonnet is needed to minimize heat loss if it is cool or to protect from the sun.

To dress the baby, avoid pulling shirts and gowns over the face and arms. Rather, bunch up the shirt and expand the neck opening; place it over the face first or behind the head first, but keep it bunched and move swiftly over the face before slipping it over the rest of the head. The same idea applies for the arms; bunch up the sleeve, grasp baby's arm, and pull through.

In the hospital, baby clothes are washed separately and autoclaved to prevent cross-contamination. At home, baby's clothes should be washed separately with a mild detergent (such as Ivory) and hot water. Double rinsing helps remove irritating detergent. Many like to add a fabric softener, but some babies may not tolerate clothing washed in a fabric softener. The baby's mattress should be plastic coated, with sheets washed frequently.

MAINTENANCE OF SAFETY, REST, AND MOBILITY

Ensuring the Infant's Safety

Even in the early neonatal period, safety must be maintained. A few general guidelines will serve to highlight safety issues.

- Maintain the neonate on the back or in the side-lying position by placing a blanket roll behind and against the spine. This prevents aspiration of any respiratory fluids or regurgitated feedings and reduces the risk for SIDS.
- Keep one hand on the infant at all times to prevent rolling and falling from changing table or bed. Do not turn away or leave infant alone on changing table.
- Maintain safety during the baby's bath. Do not leave infant in bath water; take baby along if the phone or doorbell rings. Guard against water that is too hot; test water temperature with wrist. Until the infant is able to sit alone, hold onto baby's arm and support baby.
- Use a safe crib and mattress. Crib slats should be narrow to prevent the head from entering (no greater than 2⅜ inches apart). The mattress should be firm, and no pillow should be used to prevent suffocation. Paint or stain should not contain lead and should have a non-toxic coating because babies suck on most objects. Avoid soft-stuffed animals that could suffocate baby.
- Do not position the baby's crib next to a window with a drapery, blind, or shade cord that the baby could grasp and inadvertently wrap around the neck, which could strangle the baby.
- Do not place any overcrib toys with strings that could strangle the baby.
- Avoid small objects and toys that the baby could choke on as well as rattles containing small objects that could choke the baby if the rattle breaks.
- Use appropriate infant car seat (not infant carrier). In many states, this is required by law. The seat is positioned to face the rear of the car until the baby is a year old or weighs 20 pounds (Fig. 32–4). This is considered the time it takes before the bone structure is adequately mineralized and better able to withstand a forward impact in a five-point harness restraint.
- Advise parents to take infant CPR classes.

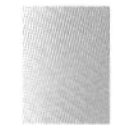

Ensuring the Infant's Adequate Rest and Mobility

Newborns spend between 15 and 20 hours sleeping. Even so, each baby's sleep-activity cycle is unique. It is important that nurses point out infant states to help parents become attuned to their baby's signals and rhythms of activity and sleep. It is not uncommon for some babies to sleep almost continuously at first, awakening only for feedings. Others sleep this deeply only for 12 to 16 hours. Quiet sleep is characterized by regular breathing and no movement except for occasional body jerks. Typically, normal household noises will not awaken a baby in this state. Active sleep is characterized by irregular breathing, fine muscle twitching, or occasional crying out (which does not mean that the baby is awake). Household noises may awaken the baby in this state, but if this

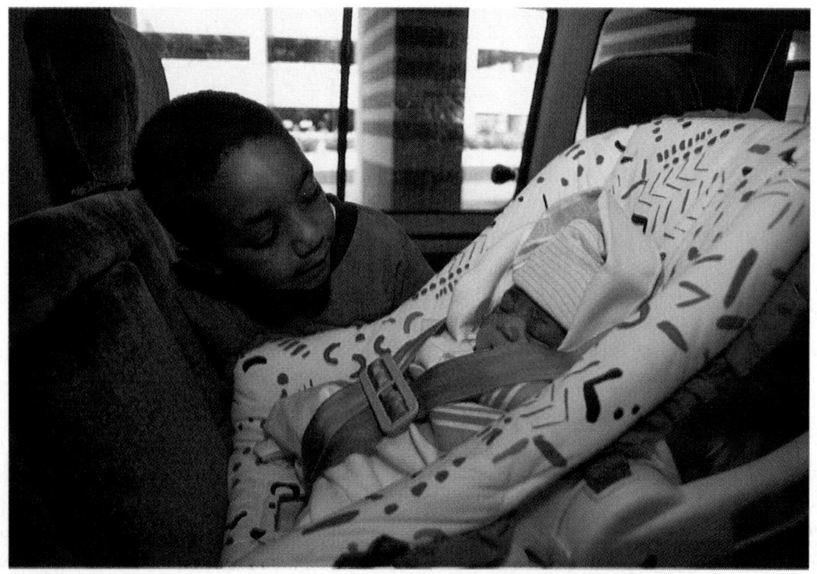

Figure 32–4
The infant's brother happily watches as the car seat is placed in the back seat for the trip home from the hospital • The safety seat is secured with the seat belt and is positioned so that it faces the back of the car's rear seat.

does happen, the baby commonly goes back to sleep quickly. When the baby becomes uncomfortable because of wet diapers, hunger, or feeling cold, the baby cries and becomes actively awake. The cause of crying should be determined and eliminated. Often, moving the baby to an upright position will change the state from crying to quiet alert (Long and Hsia 1992).

Crying is the main means of communication for the baby. As such, cries have varying tones and qualities. The amount of crying varies greatly from 15 to 30 minutes in 24 hours to 2 hours in 24 hours. Studies indicate that the pattern of crying in the early months peaks at about 6 weeks, followed by a decline in crying at about 4 months. Most have crying, fussy periods in the evening hours. Parents attempt to determine and eliminate the cause of the cry. If crying continues after common causes are eliminated, other comforting, consoling measures are tried. These include swaddling, cuddling, rocking, talking to the baby, or using a pacifier (Long and Hsia 1992).

Babies suck at times other than feedings. This is termed nonnutritive sucking and helps the baby feel secure. Sucking is a comforting activity. Controversy exists concerning the advisability of using pacifiers. We do know that sucking a rubber nipple/pacifier requires movements different from sucking the breast. For this reason, some advocate not using pacifiers for breastfed babies. Manufacturers have attempted to produce rubber pacifiers that are shaped to simulate breastfeeding suck. Babies will suck on almost anything from fingers and thumbs to blankets and toys to console themselves.

NURSING CARE WITH CIRCUMCISION

Circumcision is a surgical procedure that removes or excises the prepuce, an epithelial layer covering the penis. The glans of the penis is therefore exposed. For some time, articles and opinions supporting and opposing circumcisions have abounded. The emotional component of the controversy waxes and wanes, depending on current trends.

Male circumcision has been practiced for centuries and continues as a religious rite for the Jewish faith. Pictorials of cave dwellers show them to be circumcised, thus dating the practice from 2800 BC. In addition, Australian aborigines, ancient Aztecs and Mayas, Arabs and Jews, African tribes, North and South American Indians, and Pacific Island peoples have been circumcised. Circumcision evolved from a religious ritual or puberty rite into a routine practice done for "health" reasons in English-speaking countries in the nineteenth century. The cause of diseases was unknown, and theory emerged that masturbation caused many illnesses. To stop masturbation (and many illnesses), circumcision was advocated (Gelbaum 1992).

As science progressed and causes for many illnesses were discovered, new reasons were invented to substantiate the value of circumcisions. During World War I, hygiene prevention of venereal diseases became the rationale. In the 1950s, studies linking penile and cervical cancer with uncircumcised contact were the reason. Current reasons include protecting infants from urinary tract infections and decreasing the risk for AIDS in sexually active men (Gelbaum 1992).

On the other hand, in 1949, Gairdner stated in the British literature that the foreskin was normal, healthy tissue, that the adherence to the glans by common epithelium protects the glans from urine and feces in infancy and childhood. This publication led to discontinuation of payment for circumcision in Britain. Next, a Danish physician, Jacob Oster, conducted a longitudinal study that reported continuous, shared epithelium of the glans and foreskin that separates spontaneously in childhood (Gelbaum 1992; Milos and Macris 1992). In 1975, the American Academy of Pediatrics Ad Hoc Task Force Committee on Circumcision stated that there was no absolute medical indication for routine circumcision. At that time, 85 to 90 percent of American boys were circumcised. In 1983, the AAP and the American College of Obstetricians and Gynecologists agreed with the statement (AAP 1989).

Various controversies have surrounded circumcision. First, proponents claim it is easier to clean and keep clean a circumcised penis. However, a great number of men throughout the world are uncircumcised and they do not appear to encounter problems cleansing the penis. Cleansing is done externally with water until the foreskin separates naturally, and then the foreskin is retracted for cleansing. The foreskin can be retracted at birth in only 4 percent of boys, in 15 percent at 6 months of age, in 50 percent by 1 year of age, and in 80 to 90 percent by 3 years of age. Uncircumcised boys should be taught to gently retract the foreskin only to the point at which resistance is felt. Full retraction probably should not occur until 3 years or older (AAP 1989).

The second controversy is related to whether circumcision of a newborn is *minor* surgery. There are risks. These include pain, hemorrhage, infection, and damage. No actual statistics exist on frequency of these side effects.

The third controversy is the association between circumcision and penile cancer. Penile cancer is a relati ciden rate i circu incid there of th 1992) ated nis. A and 1 certai the a nile c

Anc cumcision of one's partner to the incidence of cervical cancer. Women with circumcised partners have a lower incidence of cervical cancer. Research results are inconclusive in this area, however. Condyloma and human papillomavirus types 16 and 18 have been found to be associated with cancer of the cervix. In addition, herpes simplex virus type 2 has also been associated with cervical cancer. Therefore, the strongest predisposing factors for cervical cancer are a history of intercourse at a young age and multiple sexual partners (AAP 1989).

Some studies have shown that circumcision prevents urinary tract infections. Later research has refuted earlier studies that indicated uncircumcised males had a lower incidence of urinary tract infections. A longitudinal study of 200,000 infant boys found a greater than tenfold increase in urinary tract infections in those that were uncircumcised compared with those that were circumcised (Gelbaum 1992; AAP 1989).

Circumcision is thought to prevent phimosis (opening of foreskin is small and it cannot be retracted). A small percentage of those without circumcision will later require the procedure for treatment of this condition (AAP 1989). Other proponents of circumcision say that uncircumcised boys will be teased. Since the incidence of circumcision is decreasing, this is not as likely to be a problem.

Some proponents of circumcision still claim that the procedure if done early does not cause severe pain and that what pain the infant feels will not be remembered. It is clear now that babies do "feel" the circumcision, since there have been behavioral, cardiovascular, and hormonal changes noted in newborns having a circumcision. It is thought by some that dorsal penile block with 1 percent lidocaine may reduce pain. Experience with this anesthesia is limited, and it has its own risks (AAP 1989). Anesthesia and dorsal blocks are painful when they wear off. Finally, the neonate cannot verbalize memories because the experience occurred in a preverbal period. This does not mean that it was not "remembered."

Only a few males (about 10 percent) will require circumcision later in life, at which time it is more expensive. Some argue that the high cost of adult circumcision should persuade parents to circumcise neonates.

Some proponents favor circumcision because it is thought to lessen the incidence of sexually transmitted diseases. Research in this area is conflicting, however. There has been some association between chancroid, syphilis, human papillomavirus, herpes simplex virus type 2, and uncircumcised status. This research, however, has methodologic flaws. Therefore, evidence of a relationship between circumcision status and sexually transmitted diseases is inconclusive (AAP 1989; Gelbaum 1992; Milos and Macris 1992).

From this discussion, the following appears to be factual:

- Foreskin is normal, healthy tissue.
- Circumcision has risks, pain, and possible error, which can be avoided if circumcision is not done. The complication rate in one study was 0.2 to 0.6 percent. Most complications are minor, however.
- The baby cannot give consent.
- Currently, the American Academy of Pediatrics states that circumcision is not absolutely medically necessary for good health.
- Some insurance companies have stopped covering circumcision, others have not.
- Care of the uncircumcised penis can be easy (Gelbaum 1992; Milos and Macris 1992).
- Properly performed newborn circumcision prevents phimosis and paraphimosis.
- Circumcision may result in decreased incidence of urinary tract infections, but this relationship needs confirmation in prospective studies.
- Evidence concerning a relationship between sexually transmitted diseases and circumcision is conflicting.
- Circumcision is a voluntary, elective procedure. It should be performed only on stable and healthy infants by experienced operators and after informed consent is obtained (AAP 1989).

While most risks of circumcision are minor, they include bleeding, infection, surgical trauma, and pain. Bleeding is the most frequent complication. It is usually minor bleeding or oozing that stops with direct pressure. Occasionally, topical silver nitrate or epinephrine is necessary.

Infection is the next most common complication. Dehiscence of skin edges may occur. Severe infections are rare. Strict surgical asepsis is crucial. Thus, staff and parental hand washing and use of sterile applications are necessary. Some advocate a Neosporin-type dressing prophylactically rather than Vaseline gauze for those done with a Gomco or Mogen clamp. Unit doses should be used.

Surgical trauma can also result. Complications such as damage to the urethral meatus, laceration of penile skin, removal of insufficient skin (can result in phimosis and urinary obstruction), or removal of an excessive amount of skin (can result in denuding of the shaft, or concealed penis) can occur.

It has been demonstrated that pain does accompany the procedure. Increased wakefulness, irritability, and crying as well as increased plasma cortisol levels have been documented. Dorsal penile nerve block adds risk (such as localized bleeding and hematoma). To relieve discomfort, pacifiers, positioning on the side with a looser diaper, and oral acetaminophen have been advocated (Gelbaum 1992; Johnston and Stevens 1990; Myron and Maguire 1991).

The baby should not have eaten for several hours before the procedure because of restraint on the back; should regurgitation occur, aspiration is possible. The procedure is performed by a physician after written consent is obtained and before hospital discharge. The baby is positioned and restrained on a plastic restraint form so movements are restricted (Fig. 32–5). The penis is cleansed with an antiseptic and a sterile drape is applied. There are several methods. Use of the Yellen or Gomco clamp is one method. The prepuce is drawn over the cone part of the clamp, the rest of the clamp is applied, pressure is maintained for 3 to 5 minutes (to reduce bleeding), and the prepuce is cut away (Fig. 32–6).

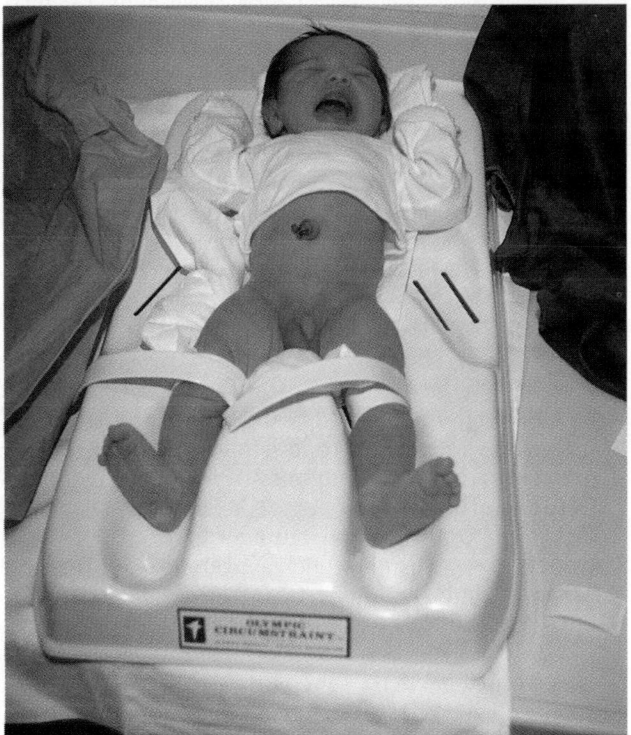

Figure 32–5

The infant is placed on a circumcision board designed to immobilize him during the procedure.

Use of a Plastibell is another method. First, the bell is fitted over the glans. A suture is then tied around the bell's rim, and the excess prepuce is cut away. The plastic rim is allowed to remain in place up to 7 days and to fall off by itself. Rarely, the rim does not fall off within 8 days; in that case, the parents should contact the health care provider, who will remove it. The parents should not attempt to remove it themselves.

After the circumcision, A and D ointment, petroleum jelly, or Vaseline gauze is applied to the penis to keep the diaper from adhering to the site, except when a Plastibell is used. It is reapplied at every diaper change for 24 to 48 hours. The baby is then dressed, wrapped, comforted, and fed. Nursing care after a circumcision is explained in Procedure 32–6. The nurse ensures that consent is obtained, prepares the instruments, identifies and restrains the baby, and comforts him (by lightly stroking his head, giving a pacifier, and talking to him).

Risk Management

Infant abduction from the maternal-newborn health care setting is a concern for parents, all maternal-newborn health care professionals, and agencies' security and risk management administrators. Based on data from 1983 to 1992, it is estimated that 12 to 18 infant abductions, primarily from health care agencies, by non–family members occur each year. The following guidelines for preventing infant abductions were developed by the National Center for Missing and Exploited Children in collaboration with professionals from nursing, medicine, risk management, health care security and safety, and law enforcement (Rabun 1993):

- Every health care facility must develope a written proactive prevention plan for infant abduction.
- Before the removal of a newborn from the birthing room (or within 2 hours of birth), the following should be completed:
  a. Attach identically numbered ID bands to both the infant and mother.
  b. Footprint the baby.
  c. Photograph the baby.
  d. Perform a full, written assessment of the baby.

The footprints, photograph, physical assessment, and documentation of the placement of the ID bands, including their number, must be placed in the baby's medical chart.

- All health care facility personnel must wear conspicuous photo ID cards. A second form of

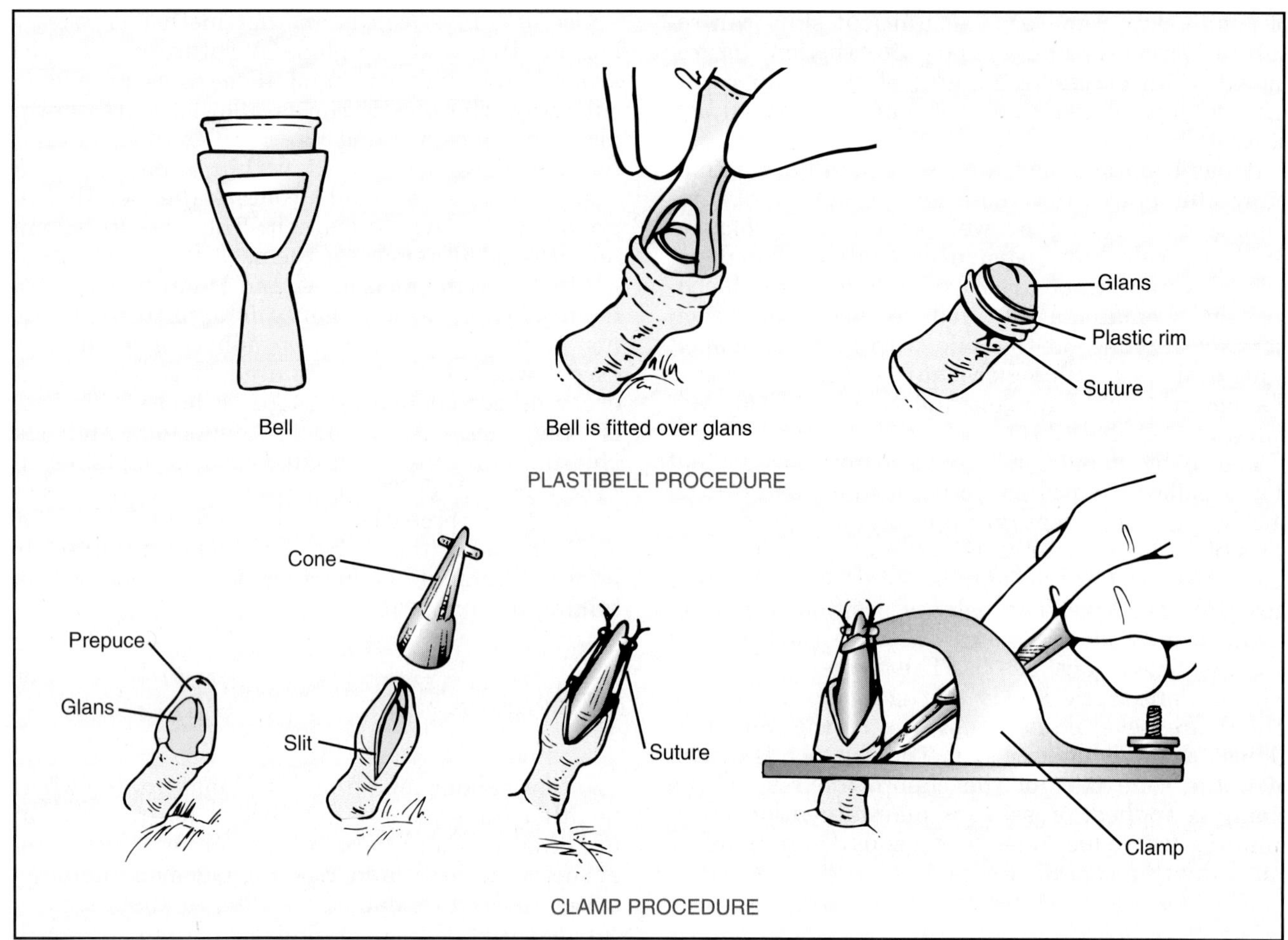

Figure 32–6

Two methods of circumcision are commonly practiced • At the top, the Plastibell is fitted over the glans and a suture is tied around the Plastibell to hold the plastic rim in place when the tip is broken off • At the lower part of the illustration, the procedure is done with the Yellen clamp and scalpel.

identification (color code, etc.) should be used to designate personnel authorized to have direct contact with infants.

- To safeguard the infant while being transported within the health care facility, make sure that
  a. Only an authorized staff member or person with an authorized ID band for that baby is allowed to transport the child.
  b. Infants are taken to mothers or transported one at a time and never grouped together or left without direct supervision.
  c. Babies are never carried; they should *always be pushed in a bassinet.*
- Infants should always be in line-of-sight supervision either by nurses, the mother, or a family member/friend designated by the mother.
- The mother's or infant's full name is not posted where it will be visible to visitors. If necessary, use surnames only. Identifying information on the bassinet may put the family and infant at risk *after discharge.*
- Be alert to unusual behavior such as repeated visiting "just to see" or "hold" infants, close questioning about facility procedures (feeding time, etc.), carrying large packages on the unit, taking staff uniforms or hospital identification, and disturbances in another area of the unit (often done to divert the attention of the health care staff).
- The agency should have detailed procedures for physical security safeguards and procedures to be followed if an infant abduction occurs. If an infant is suspected to be missing, *immediately* call security at the agency and/or other designated authority. Technical assistance in handling ongoing crisis management can be obtained by calling The National Center for Missing and Exploited Children (NCMEC) at 1-800-THE-LOST (1-800-843-5678).

Electronic security measures (infant bracelet alarms, closed circuit television, and access control) can be used to *back up* hospital policy and nursing practices. However, *constant vigilance* and use of *proactive prevention measures* are the keys to preventing infant abductions (Rabun 1993).

PROCEDURE 32-6

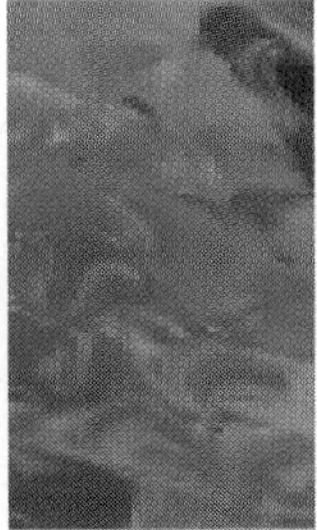

Nursing Care After Circumcision

▼ PURPOSE

To care for the newborn's circumcision, to observe for bleeding, and to prevent infection.

EQUIPMENT

- Sterile 4 × 4 gauze pads
- A and D ointment or Vaseline gauze

1 Assess level of pain (facial expression, body movements, crying). **Assessing for pain allows initiation of interventions to minimize or lessen pain.**

2 Dress, wrap, cuddle, and talk to the baby. **These measures provide comfort after a painful procedure.**

3 Attach diaper more loosely. **A loose diaper decreases pressure and pain at the circumcision site.**

4 Position the baby on his side. **This position minimizes pressure and pain at the circumcision site.**

5 Take the baby to the mother for feeding and comfort right after the circumcision. **The baby will not have been fed for several hours before the procedure, so he will be hungry. The mother will want reassurance that the baby is okay.**

6 Observe the site for bleeding; teach the mother to do this as well. Wear gloves. **Bleeding is the most common complication. Instructions concerning frequency of assessments vary. A common protocol is to assess the site every hour for 8 to 12 hours. Wearing gloves is consistent with Standard Precautions.**

7 If bleeding occurs, apply gentle pressure to the site intermittently with a folded sterile 4 × 4 gauze pad. Wear gloves. If the bleeding is not controlled, notify the physician, who may inject epinephrine or put in a suture. **Pressure decreases bleeding. Wearing gloves is consistent with Standard Precautions.**

8 Assess voiding for amount and adequacy. Instruct the mother to call the physician or midwife if the baby has not urinated within 24 hours. **Swelling or damage may obstruct urine output.**

9 Change diaper. Reapply Vaseline gauze or A and D ointment per physician's order. Wear gloves. If the diaper adheres, squeeze water over the penis to loosen it from the diaper. Use only water to cleanse the area, and squeeze it over the glans. **Frequent changing prevents contamination of the site. Reapplying Vaseline gauze or A and D ointment helps keep the diaper from sticking to the site. Squeezing water over the penis helps remove the diaper without causing more bleeding. Water is used for cleansing because soap may irritate the area and cause discomfort. Wearing gloves is consistent with Standard Precautions.**

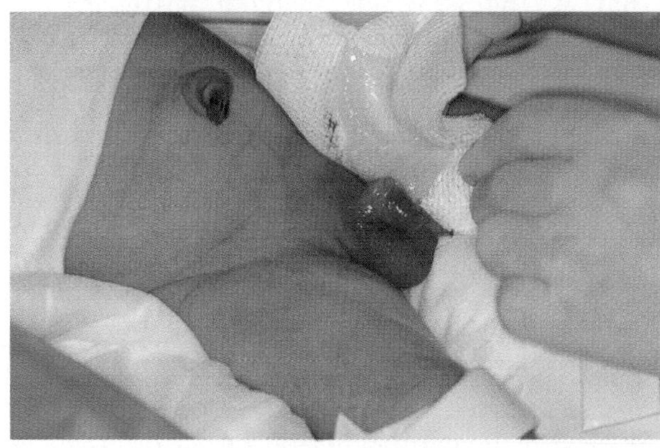

Continued on following page

PROCEDURE 32–6 Continued

10 Observe the site for infection. **Contact with microorganisms may cause infection. A whitish-yellow exudate appears around the glans in 24 hours or so. This is granulation tissue and is part of the healing process. It persists for 2 to 3 days. Symptoms of infection include pus, foul odor, fever, increased redness/swelling/tenderness after healing has started, or no healing within 72 hours.**

11 Show parents how to care for circumcision. **The baby and mother are usually discharged the same day the circumcision is done. Careful observation and care of the circumcision site must continue until healing has occurred (usually about 3 days).**

Implications for Research

Infant care as discussed here is taught to the new parents during increasingly shortened hospital stays after their infant's birth, generally in a self-contained rooming-in environment. It is important that parental knowledge of normal characteristics, growth and development, and caretaking tasks be assessed, after which designated learning needs are met by appropriate, individualized teaching. Follow-up programs should address needs as they occur after discharge, when questions begin to arise and parental anxiety and doubt occur. As the use of neonatal home care increases, documentation through research-based studies should examine the following questions:

- What impact does available nursing guidance after discharge have on the transition to parenting?
- What are the best methods of parental education in the hospital?
- What types of follow-up care best reinforce neonatal care skills?
- What is the effect of evolving obstetric and neonatal care on the normal newborn's transition to extrauterine life?
- What is the effect of evolving obstetric and neonatal care on the assumption of the parental role?

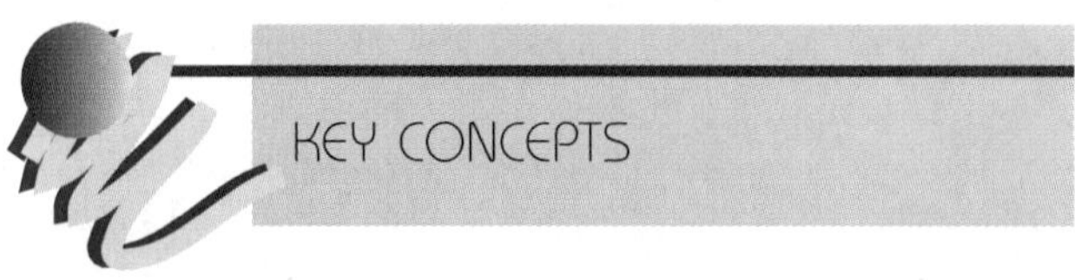

KEY CONCEPTS

▼ Physiologic adaptation of the newborn consists of alterations in physiologic functioning that must occur at the time of birth; the newborn must adjust to extrauterine life by altering physiologic mechanisms that operated in utero. Nursing care can facilitate these adaptive adjustments.

▼ Observational, or transitional, nurseries are nurseries where the neonate is observed/assessed for adaptation to extrauterine life; temperature, heart rate, respirations, and color are assessed at regular intervals and appropriate actions taken to facilitate adaptation.

▼ Nursing care related to the neonate's respirations includes assessment of respirations, proper positioning to facilitate respirations, and suctioning of mucus and respiratory fluids.

▼ Nursing care related to the neonate's circulation includes assessment of the change from fetal to neonatal circulatory patterns. This includes assessment of the apical pulse and skin color, which indicates whether there is adequate oxgenation of tissues.

▼ Nursing care related to the neonate's temperature includes assessment of the neonate's temperature as well as interventions to prevent hypothermia, which is caused by heat loss by conduction, convection, radiation, and evaporation.

▼ Prevention of bleeding in the neonate requires provision of a prophylactic injection of vitamin K (vitamin K is necessary for prothrombin formation and clotting), handling the neonate gently to prevent trauma, and observation for bleeding.

▼ The nurse facilitates prevention of infection in the neonate by following hand washing guidelines, emphasizing hand washing for visitors and parents, keeping each neonate's clothing/equipment separate, properly cleaning equipment used to care for the neonate, administering prophylactic eye treatment that prevents eye infection, and observing the neonate for signs of infection.

▼ CDC guidelines require that the nurse follow

Standard Precautions when caring for the neonate; this requires wearing gloves for contact with the neonate's body fluids until after the first bath.

- ▼ Nursing care related to the maintenance of the normal bilirubin levels in the neonate includes assessing the neonate's color for jaundice, obtaining specimens and assessing the level of bilirubin in the blood, assessing results of the direct Coombs' test, and ensuring that the neonate is fed at regular intervals.
- ▼ Nursing care related to preventing hypoglycemia of the neonate includes assessing for symptoms of hypoglycemia, obtaining and assessing blood sugar levels, and intervening appropriately to treat hypoglycemia.
- ▼ Nursing care related to the nutrition of the neonate includes assessing readiness for feedings, assessing regularity and efficiency of the neonate's feedings, assisting parents with feedings, and weighing the neonate.
- ▼ Nursing care related to maintaining adequate urinary and bowel elimination is accomplished by assessing voiding and bowel elimination patterns, assessing for constipation and diarrhea, and properly cleansing the diaper area.
- ▼ Teaching parents infant care techniques is an important part of nursing care. This includes teaching about feeding techniques, holding the neonate, consoling the neonate, cleansing and diapering, suctioning, positioning, bathing, clothing/dressing, proper skin care, and care of the baby's clothes and linens. In addition, the nurse teaches about normal infant behavior, normal sleep-wake patterns, and normal growth and development patterns.
- ▼ Safety of the neonate is important. Nursing care includes teaching parents about safety involved with positioning the neonate, preventing injuries, maintaining safety during the bath, use of a safe mattress, crib and other infant equipment, use of safe toys, and the proper use of a car seat.
- ▼ Nursing care includes educating parents about crying and other means of infant communication.
- ▼ The nurse ensures that screening texts for certain abnormalities of the neonate are accomplished (such as PKU tests, Coombs' tests, tests for sickle cell).
- ▼ Nursing care includes providing parents with information so that they can make an informed choice regarding circumcision. This includes information about the myths related to circumcision, information about the procedure itself, information about the risks involved, and information about the neonate's responses to circumcision.
- ▼ Rooming in, the practice of having the neonate remain in the mother's room, allows parents to become acquainted with and to learn to care for their baby.
- ▼ Healthy infants should be placed for sleep in a nonprone position. Supine *(wholly on the back)* confers the lowest risk of SIDS and is the preferred position for sleep. Infants with certain medical conditions may still need to be placed prone for sleep.

References

American Academy of Pediatrics. (1993). *Pediatric nutrition handbook.* Washington, DC: American Academy of Pediatrics.

American Academy of Pediatrics (1996). Positioning and SIDS: Update. Press release, November 1996.

American Academy of Pediatrics Task Force on Circumcision. (1989). Report of the Task Force on Circumcision. *Pediatrics,* 84 (4), 388–391.

American Academy of Pediatrics Task Force on Infant Position. (1992). Positions and SIDS. *Pediatrics,* 89 (6), 1120–1126.

Britton, G. R. (1980). Early mother-infant contact and infant temperature stabilization. *Journal of Obstetric, Gynecologic, and Neonatal Nursing,* March/April, 84–86.

Bronner, Y. L., and Paige, D. M. (1992). Current concepts in infant nutrition. *Journal of Nurse-Midwifery,* 37 (2), 43S–58S.

Brueggemeyer, A. (1993). Neonatal Thermoregulation. In C. Kenner, A. Brueggemeyer, L. P. Ginderson (Eds.), *Comprehensive neonatal nursing: A physiologic perspective* (p. 259). Philadelphia: W. B. Saunders.

Clifford, W. L., and Walker, W. A. (1983). Chronic protracted diarrhea of infancy: A nutritional disease. *Pediatrics,* 72, 786–795.

Eoff, M. J. F., Meier, R. S., Miller, C. (1974). Temperature measurement in infants. *Nursing Research,* 23, 457–460.

Faucher, M. A., and Jackson, G. (1992). Pharmaceutical preparations. A review of drugs commonly used during the neonatal period. *Journal of Nurse-Midwifery,* 37 (2), 74S–86S.

Filer, L. J. (1992). A glimpse into the future of infant nutrition. *Pediatric Annals,* 21 (10), 633–639.

Food and Nutrition Board. (1989). *Recommended dietary allowances.* Washington, DC: National Academy Press.

Gairdner, D. (1949). The fate of the foreskin: A study of circumcision. *British Medical Journal,* 2, 1433.

Gardner, S. (1979). The mother as incubator—After delivery. *Journal of Obstetric, Gynecologic, and Neonatal Nursing,* May/June, 174–176.

Gelbaum, I. (1992). Circumcision. To educate, not indoctrinate—A mandate for certified nurse-midwives. *Journal of Nurse-Midwifery,* 37 (2), 975–1135.

Greer, F. R., Marshall, S., Cherry, J., Suttie, J. W. (1991). Vitamin K status of lactating mothers, human milk, and breast-feeding infants. *Pediatrics,* 88 (4), 751–756.

Greer, P. S. (1988). Head coverings for newborns under radiant warmers. *Journal of Obstetric, Gynecologic, and Neonatal Nursing,* July/August, 265–271.

Hill, S. T., and Shronk, L. K. (1979). The effect of early parent-infant contact on newborn body temperature. *Journal of Obstetric, Gynecologic, and Neonatal Nursing,* September/October, 287–290.

Holmes, G. E., Hassanein, K. M., Miller, H. C. (1983). Factors associated with infections among breast-fed babies and babies fed proprietary milks. *Pediatrics,* 72 (3), 300–305.

Howard, C. R., and Weitzman, M. (1992). Breast or bottle: Practical aspects of infant nutrition in the first 6 months. *Pediatric Annals,* 21 (10), 619–631.

Johnston, C. C., and Stevens, B. (1990). Pain assessment in newborns. *Journal of Perinatal and Neonatal Nursing,* 4 (1), 41–52.

Kunnel, M. T., O'Brien, C., Munro, B. H., Medoff-Cooper, B. (1988). Comparisons of rectal, femoral, axillary, and skin-to-mattress temperatures in stable neonates. *Nursing Research,* 37 (3), 162–164, 189.

LeBlanc, M. H. (1991). Thermoregulation: Incubators, radiant warmers, artificial skins, and body hoods. *Clinics in Perinatology,* 18 (3), 403–421.

Long, M. H., and Hsia, L. S. Y. (1992). The role of the CNM in newborn management. *Journal of Nurse-Midwifery,* 37 (2), 8S–17S.

Mayfield, S. R., Bhatia, J., Nakamura, K. T., Rios, G. R., Bell, E. F. (1984). Temperature measurement in term and preterm neonates. *Journal of Pediatrics,* 104 (2), 271–275.

Milos, M. F., and Macris, D. (1992). Circumcision. A medical or human rights issue? *Journal of Nurse-Midwifery,* 37 (2), 87S–96S.

Morley, C. J. (1992). Measuring infants' temperatures. *Midwives Chronicle and Nursing Notes,* February, 26–29.

Myron, A. V., and Maguire, D. P. (1991). Pain perception in the neonate: Implications for circumcision. *Journal of Professional Nursing,* 7 (3), 188–193.

NAACOG. (1985). *Temperature standards.* Washington, DC: Author.

NAACOG. (1991). *Prevention, recognition, and management of neonatal pain.* Washington, DC: The Organization for Obstetric, Gynecologic and Neonatal Nurses.

National Society to Prevent Blindness. (1981). *Prevention and treatment of ophthalmia neonatorum.* New York: National Society to Prevent Blindness.

Phillips, C. (1994). *Family-centered maternity care* (p. 27). Minneapolis: International Childbirth Education Association.

Rabun, J. B. (1993). *For healthcare professionals: Guidelines on Preventing Infant Abductions.* Arlington, VA: National Center for Missing and Exploited Children.

Renaud, M. T. (1983). Effects of discontinuing cover gowns on a postpartal ward upon cord colonization of the newborn. *Journal of Obstetric, Gynecologic, and Neonatal Nursing,* November/December, 399–401.

Rush, T. (1986). Does routine newborn bathing reduce *Staphylococcus aureus* colonization rates? A randomized controlled trial. *Birth,* 13 (3), 176–180.

Schiffman, R. F. (1982). Temperature monitoring in the neonate: A comparison of axillary and rectal temperatures. *Nursing Research,* 31 (5), 274–277.

Schumacher, R. E. (1990). Noninvasive measurements of bilirubin in the newborn. *Clinics in Perinatology,* 17 (2), 417–435.

Schwartz, M. K. (1992). Primary care and differential diagnosis of the newborn. *Journal of Nurse-Midwifery,* 37 (2), 18S–26S.

Scopes, J. W. (1981). Thermoregulation in the newborn. In G. B. Avery (Ed.), *Neonatology* (2nd ed., pp. 171–181). Philadelphia: J. B. Lippincott.

Sykes, E., and Epstein, E. (1990). Laboratory measurement of bilirubin. *Clinics in Perinatology,* 17 (2), 397–416.

Wright, L., Brown, A., Davidson-Mundt, A. (1992). Newborn screening: The miracle and the challenge. *Journal of Pediatric Nursing,* 7 (1), 26–42.

NURSING CARE PLANNING GUIDE

Healthy Full-Term Newborn

This Nursing Care Planning Guide was developed to be used as a planning tool. You will need to modify and adapt it to individual clients as appropriate.

Performing a complete and thorough assessment is the first step in providing effective nursing care for a client. Major nursing diagnoses used in the care of the healthy full-term newborn include

1. Risk for ineffective breathing pattern
2. Risk for altered tissue perfusion
3. Risk for hypothermia or hyperthermia
4. Altered nutrition: less than body requirements
5. Altered nutrition: more than body requirements
6. Risk for bleeding injury
7. Risk for injury: hypoglycemia
8. Risk for injury: physiologic jaundice
9. Risk for infection
10. Risk for constipation or diarrhea
11. Risk for altered urinary elimination
12. Risk for impaired skin integrity
13. Risk for injury
14. Risk for altered parent-infant attachment

ASSESSMENT

Assessment of the healthy full-term newborn plays a critical role in facilitating adjustment to extrauterine life and in enhancing growth and development. To collect data, use the following Assessment Tools: Newborn Admission Record (p. 1171) and Newborn Nursery Flow Record (pp. 1172–1173). In the data collected, identify defining characteristics to use as a basis for formulating nursing diagnoses that are appropriate for your client. Areas requiring special attention in the care of the healthy full-term newborn include respiratory status, circulatory status, thermoregulation, nutrition, and observation for physiologic jaundice.

Continued on following page

NURSING CARE PLANNING GUIDE Continued

Assessment Tool

Newborn Admission Record

Date/time of: **Birth:** ___/___/___ ______ **Admit:** ___/___ ______

Place of birth: ☐hospital (or) ______

Admitted to: ☐regular nsy ☐NICU ☐mother's room ☐ ______

Vaginal delivery: ☐spontaneous ☐vacuum ☐forcep ☐vtx ☐breech

Cesarean: ☐repeat ☐1° for: ______

Apgar: ___1 ___5 Resuscitation: ☐none ☐blowby O_2 ☐see notes

☐male ☐female ID# ______ Feeding: ☐breast ☐formula

Erythromycin ½% oint. OU (or) ______ ☐See L&D Summary
time: ______ by: ______ ☐See medication record

Aq. Vit. K ____mg IM in (R / L) lateral thigh ☐See L&D Summary
time: ______ by: ______ ☐See medication record

Mother's name:

Age	Grav	Term	Preterm	AB	Liv

Maternal Labs ☐ see maternal record	Results	Pending	N/A		Results	Pending	N/A
Blood type & Rh				β strep	− / +		
Antibody screen	− / +			Chlamydia	− / +		
Serology	− / +			GC	− / +		
HBsAg	− / +						
HIV	− / +						

PHYSICAL ASSESSMENT Time:

Weight: ______	Gest. age by dates: ______ wks	T ______
Length: ______	Gest. age by exam: ______ wks	P ______
Head circ.: ______	☐AGA ☐SGA ☐LGA	R ______

✓ - findings consistent w/ given parameters **N** - see notes **—** - not assessed

Alert, lusty cry		Skin intact	
Good muscle tone, not jittery		No bruising/hematomas	
Moves all extremities well		No skin lesions	
Reflexes normal, symmetrical		No skin tags	
Strong suck		No unusual pigmentation	
Anterior fontanel flat, soft		Heart tones normal, ø murmur	
Molding: ☐none ☐mild/mod ☐marked		Regular cardiac rhythm	
No caput		Femoral pulses present, equal	
Eyes clear, not red, ø drainage		Abdomen soft, not distended	
Red reflex present bilaterally		Normal bowel sounds	
Ears normal, not low set		Anus patent	
Face, neck normal		Genitals normal for gest. age	
Palate intact		If ♂, both testes ↓	
Breathing easily		3 vessel cord	
Lungs clear		Spine normal, closed	
Good equal breath sounds		Extremities normal, 5 digits ea	
Thorax normal		Joints/range of motion normal	
Skin pink			

Newborn Problems/Risks ☐None

Admission notes

Admit signature: ______

Newborn Discharge Record

Procedures: ☐Circumcision ☐Hepatitis vaccine ______

Labs: Type/Rh ______ ☐N/A ☐Pending; Coombs ______ ☐N/A ☐Pending; Bilirubin ______ ☐N/A ☐Pending

PKU test done or pending? ☐yes ☐N/A ☐see notes

Discharge wt: ______ Baby has: ☐voided ☐stooled ☐see notes

☐Feeding established ☐breast *(note feeding aids)* ☐formula ☐see notes

☐Basic baby care demonstrated by mother/______ ☐see notes

Follow up w/______ in ___ days

Parent(s) to obtain follow up ☐bilirubin ☐PKU

Referral(s): ☐none (or) ______

Other discharge instructions: ☐routine ☐see notes ☐see attached

Discharged / transferred to: ☐home (or) ______

Accompanied by: ☐mother (or) ______

Date: ______ Time: ______ Condition: ______

Discharge notes / Follow-up considerations ☐None

Discharge Signature: ______

 Newborn Admission & Discharge Record Form #8200

Courtesy of CSW Forms, Timberon, NM, (800) 284-2815.

Continued on facing page

NURSING CARE PLANNING GUIDE Continued

Assessment Tool

Newborn Nursery Flow Record

Complete Summary using specific codes as given, or general codes:

- ✓ - assessment consistent with given parameters
- **N** - see notes
- — - not applicable or not assessed

Risks / Problems ☐ none

	Assessment Summary													
	Date / Time	/ /	/	/	/	/	/	/	/	/	/	/	/	/
Neuro	Alert, lusty cry													
Neuro	Good muscle tone, moving all extremities well													
Neuro	Strong suck													
Cardiovascular / Skin	**P** - completely pink, **A** - centrally pink, acrocyanosis													
Cardiovascular / Skin	Jaundice: **ø** - none **sl** - slight **mod** - moderate													
Cardiovascular / Skin	Mucus membranes moist													
Cardiovascular / Skin	Skin intact, no bruises													
Cardiovascular / Skin	No lesions													
Cardiovascular / Skin	No cardiac murmur													
Cardiovascular / Skin	Regular cardiac rhythm													
Respiratory	Breathing easily. No grunt, flare, or retract.													
Respiratory	Lungs clear. Good equal breath sounds bilaterally.													
GI	Abdomen soft, not distended													
GI	Normal bowel sounds													
GI	Taking feeds well													
GI	Retaining feeds													
GU	Circumcision: no bleeding, swelling, drainage, or odor. Circumcision date / time:													
Family (**M** - mother, **SO** - significant other)	Cuddles baby													
Family	Talks softly to baby													
Family	Participates in baby care													
Miscellaneous	Anterior fontanel flat													
Miscellaneous	Eyes clear, no redness or drainage													
Miscellaneous	Umbilical cord drying, no purulent drainage or odor. No redness around cord.													
	Initials													

DATA SUMMARY — Use area below to record weights and other miscellaneous data

Date	Time	Weight
	@birth	
/		
/		
/		
/		
/		

Date	Time	
/		
/		
/		
/		
/		
/		

Date	Time	
/		
/		
/		
/		
/		
/		

Date	Time	
/		
/		
/		
/		
/		
/		

 Form #8100

Portions of Newborn Nursery Flow Record. Courtesy of CSW Forms, Timberon, NM, (800) 284-2815.

Continued on following page

NURSING CARE PLANNING GUIDE Continued

Assessment Tool

Newborn Nursery Flow Record ____ of ____

Complete flow sheet using numerical values where appropriate, specific codes as given, or general codes:
✓ - yes **N** - see notes — - not applicable or not assessed **ø** - no or none

Definitions: ***good latch:*** *babe facing breast, babe's mouth opened wide, tongue down, approximately one inch of areola in mouth, lips flanged*
good suck: *suck strong & quiet, rhythmic movement of jaw and muscles in front of ear, continuous sucking or with mild stimulation, no cheek dimpling*

Flow sheet Part 1		/ /	/	/	/	/	/	/	/	/	/	/	/	/
	Date / **Time**													
Vital signs	Temperature													
	Apical pulse													
	Respiratory rate													
	Blood pressure													
	BP mean													
Miscellaneous	Blood sugar													
Environment	Open crib													
	I - incubator **R** - radiant warmer													
	Mode: **S** - servo **M** - manual													
	Servo control temperature													
	Skin probe temperature													
	Air temperature in incubator													
Activity	**A**-awake, quiet **C**-crying **S**-asleep													
	In mother's room													
	In nursery													
	To mother, identification check													
Breastfeeding	Feeding: **O** - observed, **R** - reported													
	Time to latch ≤ 5 minutes* Left/Right													
	Feeding time ≥ 10 minutes* L/R													
	Good latch L/R													
	Good suck L/R													
	Staff assistance ≤ 5 minutes* L/R													
	Audible swallowing ✓-yes **ø**-no													
Intake *(other)*														
Output	Urine													
	Stool													
	Gastric													
Treatments	Cord care w/													
*CHART THE FEEDING AT EACH BREAST. USE THE GENERAL CODES (✓, N, —, ø) OR NOTE THE NUMBER OF MINUTES.	Initials													

 Form #8100

Portions of Newborn Nursery Flow Record. Courtesy of CSW Forms, Timberon, NM, (800) 284-2815.

Continued on facing page

NURSING CARE PLANNING GUIDE Continued

1

Analysis: ▼ NURSING DIAGNOSIS

***Risk for ineffective breathing pattern,* related to**

- Prenatal or intrapartum stressors (such as pain medications, cord compression)
- Excess mucus or respiratory tract fluid
- Cold stress (increases oxygen needs, which contributes to acidosis)
- Respiratory acidosis
- Ineffective airway clearance

Defining Characteristics

SUBJECTIVE	*OBJECTIVE*
Absence of crying	Acrocyanosis
	Central cyanosis
	Gagging or choking
	Persistent alteration in respirations (<30/min, >60/min)
	Abdomen immobile with respirations
	Pronounced thoracic/chest movement with respirations
	Sternal/intercostal retractions
	Grunting
	Nasal flaring

Client Goal/ ▼ EVALUATION CRITERIA

Client will demonstrate effective breathing patterns. / ▼ **Client will evidence a patent airway, normal respiratory rate, absence of acrocyanosis and central cyanosis, normal characteristics of newborn respirations, absence of retractions, absence of grunting and nasal flaring.**

▼ NURSING INTERVENTIONS	Rationale
• Assess gestational age.	• Surfactant develops in the third trimester. When birth occurs before adequate surfactant is present, there is greater likelihood for development of respiratory distress syndrome.

Continued on following page

NURSING CARE PLANNING GUIDE Continued

• Differentiate periodic breathing pattern from apnea.	• Periodic breathing is a normal characteristic of the newborn. It consists of periods of apnea lasting 5 to 15 seconds, and it more commonly occurs in rapid eye movement (REM) sleep or during motor activity. Treatment consists of tactile, sensory stimulation that increases inspired oxygen. Apnea lasting longer than 20 to 30 seconds may be associated with changes in heart rate and cyanosis; it may require further intervention.
• Assess and observe respiratory rate as frequently as needed. Typical frequency is every 15 minutes for four times, then every hour until stable, then every shift.	• Respirations below 30 or above 60 breaths per minute indicate inadequate ability to expand lungs. Respiratory rate varies with stimulation and activity, but consistently remains within these parameters.
• Observe for characteristics indicating normal respirations. Characteristics of normal respirations are shallow; irregular in rate, rhythm, and depth; nose breathing; abdomen moves with inspiration and expiration; thoracic area remains relatively immobile with respirations; periodic breathing; color indicates oxygenation.	• Normal newborn respirations do not require intercostal and sternal muscles if pressure to expand lungs is normal. Periodic breathing is manifested by apneic periods of 5 to 15 seconds. It can be converted to normal breathing by tactile stimulation or increasing inspired oxygen.
• Observe for symptoms indicating that respirations are abnormal. Characteristics of abnormal respirations are persistently abnormal rate, retractions, grunting, nasal flaring, or central cyanosis.	• Symptoms of respiratory distress appear when the lungs are unable to initiate exchange of oxygen and carbon dioxide. To accomplish transition to extrauterine breathing, lung fluid must be replaced by air, blood flow to the lungs must increase appropriately, and surfactant must be adequate.
• Auscultate breath sounds. Breath sounds should be symmetric, without rales or rhonchi.	• Breath sounds should be equal bilaterally. Persistent rales may indicate respiratory distress syndrome or pneumonia. Rhonchi may indicate aspiration.
• Position on side with blanket roll behind back.	• Side positioning allows secretions to flow by gravity to the side of the mouth or pharynx to avoid respiratory obstruction. Suctioning is facilitated.
• Clear airway as needed. Suction as needed with bulb syringe or wall suction/catheter. Keep bulb syringe in infant's crib at all times.	• Removal of fluid or mucus clears the airway. Bulb syringe removes upper respiratory tract fluid; suction catheter removes respiratory fluid lower in respiratory tract.
• Assess color for cyanosis.	• Central cyanosis indicates inadequate respirations or circulation.
• Maintain newborn's temperature.	• Chilling leads to increased oxygen consumption and to tachypnea. In addition, it can create apnea. It also leads to decreased surfactant production and respiratory acidosis. Hyperthermia also increases the metabolic rate and oxygen consumption. (It may increase oxygen consumption by 6 percent.)
• Have emergency respiratory resuscitation equipment available.	• Equipment must be available to provide respiratory assistance should this be necessary.
• Provide tactile stimulation if necessary.	• Touch provides sensory stimulation, which activates respiratory muscles.

Continued on facing page

NURSING CARE PLANNING GUIDE Continued

2

Analysis: ▼ NURSING DIAGNOSIS

***Risk for altered tissue perfusion*, related to**

- Persistent fetal circulation; shunts not closing
- Respiratory distress (contributing to decreased oxygen-carrying capacity)
- Hemolysis of red blood cells associated with Rh factor and blood incompatibility
- Excessive amount of red blood cells (RBCs)

Defining Characteristics

SUBJECTIVE

OBJECTIVE

Tachycardia

Rales

Tachypnea

Absence of peripheral pulses

Cool, clammy skin

Absence of bowel sounds

Absence of bowel elimination

Absence of urine elimination

Decreased capillary filling

Poor feeding

Vomiting

Symptoms of respiratory distress

Client Goal/ ▼ EVALUATION CRITERIA

Client will demonstrate adequate tissue perfusion. / ▼ **Client will evidence absence of central cyanosis, heart rate of 120 to 160 beats per minute, normal respirations, bowel sounds, normal bowel elimination, normal urine elimination, absence of vomiting, feeding well, normal peripheral pulses.**

Continued on following page

NURSING CARE PLANNING GUIDE Continued

▼ NURSING INTERVENTIONS	Rationale
• Assess apical pulse rate as frequently as needed. Typical frequency is every 15 minutes for four times, then every hour until stable, then every shift.	• Normal apical pulse is 120 to 160 beats per minute. The pulse varies with stimulation and activity but consistently remains within these parameters. A heart rate consistently below 100 beats per minute indicates severe asphyxia. A heart rate above 160 beats per minute may indicate normal adjustment or recent asphyxia.
• Observe color for cyanosis. Blanch skin on trunk and extremities periodically to assess capillary fill time.	• Normal color indicates adequate respiratory efforts and circulation that provides for normal gas exchange. It means that the ductus arteriosus closes and an increased amount of blood can flow to the lungs for oxygenation. The foramen ovale also closes so that blood flows to the lungs rather than being shunted away. The ductus venosus closes so that blood is no longer shunted away from the liver to the inferior vena cava. Cyanotic color indicates inadequate circulation and tissue perfusion. Acrocyanosis is normal until circulation adjusts. Central cyanosis is not normal. Capillary fill time, centrally, is typically 3 seconds. Peripheral fill time may be slightly longer because of sluggish peripheral circulation. The newborn has elevated RBC and hemoglobin levels, which contribute to a reddish coloration. Newborns with an excess amount of RBCs may have polycythemia (which may lead to development of thrombus) and have a persistent reddish coloration.
• Assess for brachial, radial, femoral, popliteal, and dorsalis pedis pulses.	• Presence of pulses with equal amplitude and quality indicates absence of obstruction. Obstruction between right and left subclavian arteries leads to stronger pulse in right arm. Diminished strength of pulses in lower extremities is related to coarctation of aorta, hip dysplasia, or thrombus formation. Bounding pulses are related to patent ductus arteriosus.
• Auscultate heart sounds and report murmurs for evaluation.	• Murmurs may indicate a shunt that has not closed completely; they are usually transient and typically systolic. The foramen ovale typically closes 1 to 2 hours after birth, the ductus arteriosus 3 to 4 days after birth. Patent ductus arteriosus may occur with hypoxia, congestive heart failure, prenatal or birth asphyxia, polycythemia, and hypoglycemia.
• Auscultate breath sounds.	• With inadequate tissue perfusion, fluid may accumulate in the lungs, resulting in rales.
• Note intensity of cry.	• Initial lusty cry increases oxygenation in lungs, allowing necessary chemical changes to convert from fetal circulation. The heart rate may increase to 170 or 180 but then returns to normal range of 120 to 160. If the infant cries, circulation and tissue perfusion are adequate.

Continued on facing page

NURSING CARE PLANNING GUIDE Continued

• Obtain heel stick sample of blood for hematocrit. Assess hemoglobin level and hematocrit.	• A low hemoglobin level (15 g/dL) indicates reduced oxygen-carrying capacity. Low levels may be associated with blood loss, hemolysis, reduced RBC production, or anemia. An elevated hematocrit (>60) may be associated with polycythemia. To meet tissue needs, adequate oxygen is necessary. Normal hemoglobin is 15 to 20 g/dL; normal hematocrit is 43 to 60 percent. Hematocrit below 43 percent reduces oxygen-carrying capacity.
• Note blood group and Rh factor of mother and newborn. Note results of Coombs' test.	• This assessment identifies whether mother is Rh-negative and whether newborn could suffer from Rh factor or blood incompatibility. Blood incompatibility is associated with antigen-antibody reaction and hemolysis of RBCs. With hemolysis, hemoglobin levels drop, oxygen-carrying capacity is reduced, and tissues are inadequately perfused. Coombs test indicates whether there are maternal Rh-positive antibodies in fetal cord blood.
• Assess bowel sounds and bowel elimination.	• With inadequate perfusion, the bowel may not function normally, resulting in absence of bowel sounds and elimination.
• Assess urine output.	• With inadequate perfusion, the kidney may be unable to function normally, resulting in decreased urine output.
• Assess feeding behaviors and note if vomiting occurs.	• With inadequate perfusion to the gastrointestinal tract, the newborn may be unable to feed or digest well, and vomiting may occur.

3

Analysis: ▼ NURSING DIAGNOSIS

***Risk for hypothermia or hyperthermia,* related to**

Hypothermia	Hyperthermia
• Large body surface in relation to body mass	• Excessive clothing
• Minimal insulating fat and limited brown fat	• Overwarming
• Thin epidermis with proximity of blood vessels to skin (permitting loss of heat to cooler environment)	• Inability to sweat
• Exposure to a cold environment from a warmer intrauterine environment	• Dehydration
	• Inadequate intake of fluids

Continued on following page

NURSING CARE PLANNING GUIDE Continued

- Inability to shiver
- Decreased metabolic rate
- Inadequate clothing

Defining Characteristics

SUBJECTIVE	*OBJECTIVE*
Hypothermia	Hypothermia
Restless	Axillary temperature <97.7°F
	Increased activity (restless, agitated, hyperactive)
	Poor appetite, poor feeder
	Decreased heart rate
	Cold stress symptoms (drop in skin temperature; increased activity; pallor or mottling; cool skin, hands, feet)
	Symptoms of respiratory distress
Hyperthermia	Hyperthermia
Restless	Axillary temperature >99.5°F
	Perspiration on face, head
	Apnea, seizures
	Tachypnea
	Flushed skin, becoming dry
	Tachycardia

Client Goal/ ▼ EVALUATION CRITERIA

Client will demonstrate normal body temperature. / ▼ **Client will evidence axillary temperature of 97.7 to 98.6°F; absence of increased activity; absence of perspiration, apnea, seizures, cold stress symptoms, respiratory distress; normal skin temperature; normal heart rate; adequate intake.**

▼ NURSING INTERVENTIONS	Rationale
Hypothermia	
• Dry newborn. Place stockinette cap on infant's head. Dress and wrap in warm blankets.	• This reduces heat loss by evaporation and conduction. The newborn's head is relatively large in relation to the body, and therefore a large amount of heat can be lost from the head. The crib and air currents are typically cooler than the newborn.
• Place newborn on prewarmed mattress or in parent's arms. Warm colder objects coming in contact with the newborn (stethoscope, scale, hands).	• This minimizes heat loss by conduction (heat loss to cooler objects in contact with the newborn).
• Maintain environmental and room temperature. Maintain controlled heat source at 98.6°F.	• This reduces heat loss by convection (heat loss to cooler air).

Continued on facing page

NURSING CARE PLANNING GUIDE Continued

• Position crib away from cold air conditioner, cold walls, or cold window. Maintain radiant warmer at 98.6°F. Position crib away from heater and sunlight.	• Positioning minimizes heat loss by convection (heat loss to cooler air) and radiation (heat loss to cooler objects that are not in direct contact with the newborn).
• Adjust clothing in relation to room temperature.	• Correct clothing allows appropriate heat loss.
• Cover newborn as much as possible when changing diaper, providing care, or bathing/cleansing. Postpone first bath until body temperature is stable.	• Covering reduces heat loss by convection, evaporation, and radiation.
• Assess axillary temperature. Typical frequency is every hour in the first 4 hours, then every 4 hours in the first 24 hours of life, and then every shift.	• Normal axillary temperature is 97.7 to 98.6°F.
• Observe for symptoms of cold stress. These include drop in skin temperature as determined by skin probe; increased activity; poor eating; pallor or mottling; cool skin, hands, and feet; flexed position.	• The newborn attempts to maintain temperature by vasoconstriction, increasing muscle activity, metabolizing brown fat, and increasing metabolism in general. A flexed position decreases body surface through which heat can be lost to the environment. Cooling leads to peripheral vasoconstriction and accompanying pallor or mottling.
• Assess for symptoms of respiratory distress. These include apnea, central cyanosis, grunting, retractions, nasal flaring, bradycardia, and abnormal respiratory rate.	• Increased metabolism requires extra oxygen, so respiration is necessary to help maintain temperature. When respiratory distress occurs, increased water is lost by evaporation and less oxygen is available for metabolism.
• Feed on regular schedule.	• Calories are needed to support the increased metabolic rate that helps maintain temperature. For every 1.8°F increase in body temperature, metabolism and fluid needs increase approximately 10 percent.
• Assess heart rate.	• With alteration in temperature, the heart rate often decreases.
<u>Hyperthermia</u>	
• Assess for symptoms of hyperthermia. These include restlessness, perspiration on head or face and later on chest, apnea, seizures, temperature above 99.5°F, increased respiratory rate, and increased heart rate.	• Heat is lost by peripheral vasodilatation and insensible water loss. Vasodilatation is associated with evaporative water losses, cerebral ischemia, and dehydration.
• Assess for symptoms of dehydration. These include sunken fontanelles, elevated temperature, poor skin turgor, and delayed or decreased voiding.	• A temperature above 99.5°F is hyperthermic. Dehydration may occur with overheating because of increased insensible water loss.
• Note infant's clothing and covering.	• Overdressing and covering are associated with overheating and prickly heat.
• Assess feeding behaviors.	• With hyperthermia, a newborn often feeds poorly.

Continued on following page

NURSING CARE PLANNING GUIDE Continued

4

Analysis: ▼ **NURSING DIAGNOSIS**

Altered nutrition: less than body requirements, **related to**

- High metabolic rate and calorie requirement
- Poor sucking, feeding
- Inadequate or depleted glucose stores

Defining Characteristics

SUBJECTIVE

Cries at intervals

OBJECTIVE

Regurgitation (relaxation of sphincters)
Infrequent stools
Distention of stomach
Crying at frequent intervals
Poor suck; dribbles or gags
Sleepy at feeding times
Weight loss
Does not settle or sleep for 2–3 hours after feeding
Dehydration symptoms
Less than 6 wet diapers a day
Inadequate intake
Jitteriness with hypoglycemia

Client Goal/ ▼ **EVALUATION CRITERIA**

Client will have nutrition adequate for body requirements. / ▼ **Client will evidence regaining birth weight by 10 days of life and then gaining 1 to 2 ounces per day in the first 6 months, absence of dehydration symptoms, settling after feedings, at least six wet diapers a day, and absence of hypoglycemia.**

▼ **NURSING INTERVENTIONS**	**Rationale**
• Initiate sterile water feeding of approximately 10 mL sterile water. Then feed glucose water, breast milk, or formula depending on protocol.	• Some advocate an initial sterile water feeding to assess sucking, swallowing, and gag reflex and to assess whether there is a gastrointestinal abnormality (such as esophageal atresia).

Continued on facing page

NURSING CARE PLANNING GUIDE Continued

Intervention	Rationale
	Early feeding provides fluid and calories for the newborn, who has a high metabolic rate. Formula and breast milk have a greater sustained effect than glucose water and, therefore, are associated with reduced risk for hypoglycemia. Early feedings help the newborn maintain temperature by providing calories for metabolism.
• Assess readiness for feeding. Signs of readiness include rooting, sucking, hand-to-mouth activities, alert state, nose breathing, stable heart rate and respirations, and presence of bowel sounds.	• Newborns need to be able to breathe through the nose to be able to suck. Rooting and sucking reflexes are necessary for feeding. Newborns with respiratory distress use available energy and activity to breathe. Hypothermia is associated with increased metabolism and therefore increased calorie needs.
• Weigh shortly after birth and daily thereafter. Compare daily weight with initial baseline weight and determine percentage of weight loss. Weigh at checkup and compare with growth chart.	• Weight shortly after birth establishes a baseline value. Newborns typically lose 5 to 10 percent of birth weight in the first 3 to 4 days of life because of minimal intake, high metabolic rate, and water loss. Calorie requirement is approximately 50 to 54 calories per pound. Newborns regain birth weight by 10 to 14 days of life and then gain 3 to 5 ounces a week or 1 to 2 ounces a day in the first 6 months of life.
• Correctly position nipple in newborn's mouth.	• Newborns have difficulty transferring feedings from front of mouth to pharynx. Therefore, the nipple should be well inside the mouth, with the tongue under the nipple. Sucking with this position will compress the bottle nipple or the lactiferous sinuses so that suction can propel milk into the pharynx for swallowing. (See Chapter 33, Breastfeeding.)
• Note and record amount and frequency of infant feeding. Feed on demand within appropriate parameters.	• Hunger varies. Approximately 6 to 8 feedings a day for bottle-fed babies (every 3 to 4 hours) or 8 to 12 feedings a day (every 2 to 3 hours) for breastfed babies should meet nutritional requirements and replace fluid losses. Breast milk is digested more rapidly and readily. Therefore, breastfed babies are often ready to eat every 2 to 3 hours.
• Note and record infant feeding behaviors.	• Newborns need to learn to suck for feedings. Many are sleepy, do not have a vigorous suck, do not have good suction, gag, or dribble formula or breast milk. Observation determines the cause of difficulty so that appropriate interventions can follow.
• Assess and record frequency, amount, and color of urine.	• Fluid loss with minimal intake decreases extracellular fluid and decreases urine output. Because of inactivity of the kidneys, urine output is reduced. Fluid requirement is approximately 1 to 2 ounces per pound per day. Many state that the newborn should have at least six "wet" diapers per day, which would indicate adequate fluid intake.

Continued on following page

NURSING CARE PLANNING GUIDE Continued

• Observe and record frequency, color, and characteristics of stools. Assess for constipation or diarrhea.	• First stools are meconium. Then characteristics vary if the baby is breastfed or bottle fed. The breastfed baby's stools are more frequent, have a loose or more "mushy" consistency, are a golden yellow color, and have a "pleasantly sour" odor. The bottle-fed baby's stools are fewer, are firmer with a "pasty" consistency, are a light yellow color, and have a foul odor. Symptoms of constipation include small, firm, infrequent stools that often require straining to pass. Symptoms of diarrhea include loose, watery, frequent stools, often green in color and mingled with water, that are forcefully expelled. The cause includes overfeeding or infection.
• Observe for symptoms of gastrointestinal abnormalities. These may include intestinal obstruction, cystic fibrosis, or tracheoesophageal fistula.	• Signs may include abdominal distention, abnormal stool, absence of stool, excessive mucus, choking, and refusing to feed.
• Observe for signs of hypoglycemia.	• Signs of hypoglycemia include tremors and irritability. Hypoglycemia occurs with blood glucose levels of less than 45 mg/dL. With limited intake and high metabolic rate, the newborn may use glycogen stores and available glucose, thereby developing hypoglycemia.
• Feed iron-supplemented formula if ordered.	• The liver stores iron that is needed to produce RBCs. Iron is stored during fetal life. If iron stores are thought to be adequate and the likelihood for development of anemia is minimal, iron-supplemented formula is unnecessary.
• Assess for dehydration. Symptoms include sunken fontanelles, elevated temperature, poor skin turgor, and delayed or decreased voiding.	• Minimal intake predisposes to dehydration.
• Assess parents' knowledge about feeding.	• Assessment allows the nurse to educate the parents when knowledge deficit is present.
• Assess mother's knowledge about preparation of infant formula if baby is bottle fed and mother's diet if baby is breastfed.	• Education ensures proper preparation of formula and cleaning of bottle/nipples as well as appropriate dilution of formula. Mother's dietary intake is assessed for adequacy to provide calories, fluid, and nutrients for breast milk.

Continued on facing page

NURSING CARE PLANNING GUIDE Continued

5

Analysis: ▼ **NURSING DIAGNOSIS**

***Altered nutrition: more than body requirements,* related to**

- Overfeeding
- Addition of solid foods too early

Defining Characteristics

SUBJECTIVE	*OBJECTIVE*
Cries frequently	Gains >1 ounce/day or >7 ounces/week

Client Goal/ ▼ **EVALUATION CRITERIA**

Client will have nutrition adequate for body requirements. / ▼ **Client will evidence gaining 1 ounce a day or 7 ounces a week.**

▼ **NURSING INTERVENTIONS**	**Rationale**
• Weigh newborn. Compare with growth chart.	• Weight gain of more than 7 ounces per week or greater than 85th percentile is considered excessive.
• Assess amount and frequency of feedings. Include assessment of solid food intake.	• When the newborn cries, it is easy to assume that hunger is the reason. With bottle feedings, it is easier to overfeed.
• Assess parents' feeding behaviors.	• Education about demand feedings and behavioral cues may aid in proper frequency and amount of feedings. Explain other techniques to settle the newborn if there is a knowledge deficit in this area.
• Educate about proper time to introduce solid foods.	• Most advocate introducing solid foods at 4 to 6 months.

Continued on following page

NURSING CARE PLANNING GUIDE *Continued*

6

Analysis: ▼ **NURSING DIAGNOSIS**

***Risk for bleeding injury,* related to**

- Minimal vitamin K
- Gastrointestinal tract without bacterial flora, which inhibits absorption of vitamin K

Defining Characteristics

SUBJECTIVE	*OBJECTIVE*
	Bleeding from circumcision
	Oozing cord; bleeding from cord
	Ecchymosis
	Hematuria
	Blood in stools
	Bleeding from injection site
	Bleeding or bruising with handling

Client Goal/ ▼ **EVALUATION CRITERIA**

Client will remain free from injury. / ▼ **Client will evidence absence of bleeding.**

▼ **NURSING INTERVENTIONS**	**Rationale**
• Administer vitamin K injection intramuscularly (see Procedure 32–3).	• The newborn's gastrointestinal tract lacks bacteria, which facilitate absorption of vitamin K. Vitamin K is necessary to form prothrombin, which is required for clotting. When feeding is established, bacterial flora is present in the gastrointestinal tract.
• Assess newborn for signs of bleeding. Assess stools, urine, injection site, circumcision site, and skin for bleeding.	• Bleeding can result from lack of vitamin K.
• Handle newborn gently, reducing trauma.	• Gentle handling will reduce the likelihood for trauma, which could lead to bruising or bleeding.

Continued on facing page

NURSING CARE PLANNING GUIDE Continued

7

Analysis: ▼ NURSING DIAGNOSIS

***Risk for injury: hypoglycemia,* related to**

- Minimal intake after birth
- Sleepiness
- Inability to suck well or vigorously
- High demand for glucose right after birth (to initiate breathing, to maintain temperature)

Defining Characteristics

SUBJECTIVE	*OBJECTIVE*
Sleepy, lethargic, weak, high-pitched cry	Poor suck Jitteriness Tremors (spontaneous or with stimulation) Hypotonia Weak, high-pitched cry Poor feeding Seizures

Client Goal/ ▼ EVALUATION CRITERIA

Client will demonstrate absence of hypoglycemia. / ▼ **Client will evidence a normal blood glucose level; feed well; demonstrate absence of jitteriness, tremors, hypotonia, weakness, high-pitched cry, seizures.**

▼ NURSING INTERVENTIONS	Rationale
• Check blood glucose level by Dextrostix or by Chemstrip with Accu-Check II device (see Procedure 31–4).	• Blood glucose levels are obtained. Hypoglycemia is diagnosed when blood glucose level is below 30 mg/dL in the first 72 hours or below 45 mg/dL after the first 3 days of life.
• Assess for symptoms of hypoglycemia.	• Symptoms of hypoglycemia include jitteriness, tremors, apnea, listlessness, hypotonia, poor feeding, weak high-pitched cry, and seizures.

Continued on following page

NURSING CARE PLANNING GUIDE Continued

- Feed at regular intervals.

- The liver stores glycogen and converts it to glucose. After birth, the glucose supply that was obtained through the placenta is interrupted. Glycogen stores are mobilized, but formation of glycogen for storage is inhibited by changes in hepatic enzymes. Feeding at regular intervals provides glucose for metabolism and for conversion to glycogen.

8

Analysis: ▼ NURSING DIAGNOSIS

***Risk for injury: physiologic jaundice,* related to**

- Immature liver (inability to produce enzymes needed for conjugation)
- Conditions that cause hemolysis (cephalhematoma, polycythemia)
- Rh factor or ABO blood group incompatibility
- Infections in utero that affect liver functioning
- Asphyxia
- Hypothermia (increased metabolism results in free fatty acids that dislocate bilirubin)
- Hypoglycemia (increased metabolism results in free fatty acids that dislocate bilirubin)

Defining Characteristics

SUBJECTIVE

Lethargy

OBJECTIVE

Jaundice after the first 24 hours of life, typically the second or third day of life

Serum bilirubin level does not increase faster than 5 mg/dL in 24 hours

Serum bilirubin level not higher than 12 mg/dL for term infants

Hypotonia

Diminished rooting and sucking

Client Goal/ ▼ EVALUATION CRITERIA

Client will demonstrate absence of injury from elevated bilirubin level. / ▼ **Client will evidence bilirubin levels within physiologic range, absence of hypotonia without diminished rooting and sucking.**

Continued on facing page

NURSING CARE PLANNING GUIDE Continued

▼ NURSING INTERVENTIONS	Rationale
• Assess color for jaundice. Blanch skin over bone prominence at sternum, forehead, and knees. In dark-skinned babies, check oral palate and conjunctival sacs because skin naturally has a yellow cast. Daylight is the best light in which to see jaundice. Perhaps use a transcutaneous device to assess jaundice.	• Jaundice color occurs when bilirubin is deposited in the skin. It occurs with hyperbilirubinemia or elevated bilirubin levels. Hemoglobin breaks into heme, globin, and iron. The heme portion breaks down to bilirubin. In the first hours of life, the hemolysis or breakdown of RBCs is great because of a shorter life span of the newborn's RBCs, the fragility of RBCs, and the amount of blood received at birth before the cord is clamped. Unconjugated bilirubin most often binds to albumin (indirect) and then travels to the liver where it is conjugated (it becomes water soluble). It then passes to the intestine, where it is converted to urobilinogen by bacteria and excreted in the stools. Conjugated bilirubin is called direct bilirubin. The sum of direct and indirect bilirubin measurements is the total bilirubin level. Normal total bilirubin level is less than 12 mg/dL on days 2 to 7 of life. Jaundice is visible when bilirubin is 4 to 6 mg/dL. Jaundice is most often physiologic, but it may become pathologic when levels become too elevated. A transcutaneous device to measure bilirubin illuminates the skin and measures color intensity at forehead, sternum, upper right abdomen, heels, and upper and lower back. It is not accurate at all times; some advocate its use only for screening.
• Assess for conditions associated with greater risk for pathologic jaundice.	• Conditions with a greater rate of hemolysis lead to greater breakdown of RBCs and therefore a higher bilirubin level. Those at risk include newborns with bruises, cephalhematoma, and polycythemia. An infant born early has a less mature liver and therefore has less ability to produce enzymes necessary for conjugation. With asphyxia, bilirubin is less able to bind to albumin. With hypothermia and hypoglycemia, the excess free fatty acids dislocate bilirubin from albumin. With infections in utero, the liver may be less effective with conjugation. The most common cause of pathologic jaundice is hemolysis associated with Rh factor or ABO blood group incompatibility.
• Assess bilirubin level in blood. Obtain blood specimen by heel stick.	• Pathologic jaundice occurs in the first 24 hours of life; the serum bilirubin level increases faster than 5 mg in 24 hours, or the bilirubin level is higher than 12 mg/dL in term infants and 14 mg/dL in preterm infants. Physiologic jaundice occurs when there is no jaundice in the first 24 hours of life. Jaundice typically appears at days 2 to 3 of life; the bilirubin levels peak at days 2 to 4 and then decrease. Peak levels may go to 10 to 12 mg but should not increase faster than 5 mg/dL per 24 hours.
• Feed at regular intervals.	• Feedings provide glucose for conjugation and glucuronic acid. They also increase bacteria in the gut, which aids conversion to urobilinogen.

Continued on following page

NURSING CARE PLANNING GUIDE Continued

9

Analysis: ▼ **NURSING DIAGNOSIS**

Risk for infection, **related to**

- Deficiency of neutrophils (used in phagocytic response)
- Deficiencies of specific immunoglobulins. The newborn receives some passive immunity (IgE) but is deficient in IgM, which is stimulated by exposure to infections, such as with gram-negative enteroorganisms and some viruses.
- Deficiencies of IgA in bottle-fed newborns. IgA may protect surfaces of respiratory, urinary, and gastrointestinal tracts.
- Exposure to microorganisms from a relatively large number of portals of entry (umbilical cord, circumcision site, skin breaks with internal fetal monitor or forceps, delicate epidermis, diaper rash)
- Lack of normal intestinal flora until feedings are established

Defining Characteristics

SUBJECTIVE	*OBJECTIVE*
Crying	Skin rash
Listless, lethargic	Diaper rash
	Cracking skin
	Diarrhea
	Umbilical cord moist, with discharge and odor
	White curdy patches on oral mucosa
	Low temperature
	Respiratory infection symptoms
	Poor feeding
	Purulent discharge from eyes

Client Goal/ ▼ **EVALUATION CRITERIA**

Client will demonstrate absence of infection. / ▼ **Client will evidence normal temperature, absence of diarrhea, absence of skin irritation and rashes, absence of respiratory infections, absence of eye infection.**

Continued on facing page

NURSING CARE PLANNING GUIDE Continued

▼ NURSING INTERVENTIONS	Rationale
• Assess gestational age.	• IgG antibodies can be transferred in utero in the last trimester. If the newborn is early, this passive immunity is reduced. Typically, IgG antibodies may protect against infection with gram-positive cocci like pneumococci, streptococci, meningococci, and *Haemophilus influenzae;* toxins such as diphtheria and tetanus; and some viruses.
• Assess mother's history for factors predisposing newborn to infection.	• Signs may include maternal fever in weeks before delivery; membranes ruptured longer than 24 hours; prolonged labor; foul-smelling amniotic fluid; diagnosis of herpes simplex, gonorrhea, chlamydial infection, group B streptococcus infection, cytomegalovirus infection, or toxoplasmosis.
• Do arm and hand scrub with appropriate preparation before working in nursery. Wash hands before handling each newborn (15 to 30 seconds). Have parents and others wash hands before caring for newborn.	• Proper hand washing helps protect newborn from exposure to pathogens. Iodophor preparations are effective against both gram-negative and gram-positive organisms. Washing hands prevents transfer of organisms to newborn.
• Maintain separate equipment and supplies for each newborn.	• This helps prevent cross-contamination.
• Screen visitors for illnesses and ask them to wash hands before handling newborn. Advise client to stay away from crowds until the infant is 1 month of age.	• This helps prevent exposure to pathogens. The newborn may be more susceptible to infection. As newborn matures, the immune system is more able to respond.
• Assess newborn for symptoms of infection.	• Symptoms of umbilical cord infection include red, moist cord with discharge and odor. Skin infection would be evidenced by a rash. Diaper rash may become infected with increased irritation, redness, and discharge. Symptoms of sepsis include hypoactivity and poor feeding. Symptoms of eye infection include purulent discharge from eye. An infected circumcision site might have signs of redness, discharge, and an inability to heal. Thrush is evidenced by white patches on mouth mucosa that cannot be removed and tend to bleed when touched.
• Administer prophylactic eye treatment.	• Erythromycin eye ointment (or other eye treatment) prevents gonococcal and chlamydial infection of the eye.
• Expose umbilical cord to air by folding diaper below and T-shirt above the cord stump. Apply alcohol to cord stump according to protocol.	• These procedures facilitate drying through exposure to air; minimize contact with the moist diaper; minimize moist medium, which fosters bacterial growth; enhance drying; and minimize exposure to microorganisms.

Continued on following page

NURSING CARE PLANNING GUIDE Continued

- Monitor laboratory values. Laboratory tests may include a white blood cell (WBC) count; serum levels of IgG, IgM, and IgA; blood cultures; and cultures of lesions.
- A WBC count does not increase when the newborn has an infection. It may drop in sepsis. Elevated IgM may be present at birth in response to an infection acquired in utero. IgE levels increase in the third trimester as mother transfers passive immunity to infections to which she has been exposed and is immune. Blood cultures aid in diagnosing sepsis and in identifying causative organisms. Cultures of rashes (vesicles or lesions) identify microorganisms and help differentiate erythema toxicum (vesicles or lesions that are a local inflammatory response, are of no consequence, and contain eosinophils).
- Administer appropriate topical, oral, or parenteral antibiotics.
- Appropriate antibiotic treatment will eradicate the organism and cure the infection.
- Wash newborn's clothes separately, using hot water, mild detergents, and double rinses.
- This prevents infection from contact with contaminated clothing and minimizes irritation.
- Instruct client in treatment of upper respiratory tract infection. Symptoms include poor feeding, breathing difficulty, nasal congestion, and cough.
- Cold may result in otitis media or lower respiratory tract infection. Treatment includes increased fluid intake (helps liquefy secretions), raised head area of mattress 30 degrees to increase chest capacity, and use of vaporizer to humidify air (helps liquefy secretions).
- Administer hepatitis B immune globulin (HBIG) and hepatitis B virus (HBV) vaccine according to protocol if mother has hepatitis B surface antigen (HBsAg), core antigen (HBcAg), or e antigen (HBeAg).
- Immunization decreases risk for getting hepatitis B or becoming a carrier.

10

Analysis: ▼ NURSING DIAGNOSIS

***Risk for constipation or diarrhea,* related to**

Constipation

- Allergies
- Inadequate fluid/milk intake
- Inactive bowel at birth
- Diet and medications of lactating mother

Diarrhea

- Gastrointestinal infection
- Overfeeding

Continued on facing page

NURSING CARE PLANNING GUIDE Continued

Defining Characteristics

SUBJECTIVE	*OBJECTIVE*
<u>Constipation</u>	<u>Constipation</u>
Straining with stools	Absence of meconium stools
Perspiration with passing stools	Absence of transitional stools (yellowish color)
Cries	Abdominal distention
	Stools change to firm, hard, infrequent stools
	Vomiting
<u>Diarrhea</u>	<u>Diarrhea</u>
Cries	Stools change to frequent, watery, forcefully expelled stools
	Watery ring on diaper
	Anal irritation

Client Goal/ ▼ EVALUATION CRITERIA

Client will demonstrate normal bowel elimination. / ▼ **Client will evidence anal patency, soft undistended abdomen, meconium to transitional to breastfed or bottle-fed stools, absence of diarrhea, absence of constipation.**

▼ NURSING INTERVENTIONS	Rationale
<u>Constipation</u>	
• Check record for passage of meconium in utero or at delivery.	• The rectal sphincter may relax in utero, causing passage of meconium.
• Auscultate bowel sounds.	• Bowel sounds normally occur within 1 to 2 hours after birth.
• Monitor and record passage of meconium.	• Once feedings are initiated, bowel action commonly follows. Most pass the first stool within 48 hours. If not, intestinal obstruction is suspected.
• Percuss abdomen for distention. Note if vomiting occurs.	• Abdominal distention and vomiting suggest intestinal obstruction. The higher the obstruction, the sooner vomiting occurs after birth. Partial obstruction is characterized by intermittent obstruction. Failure to pass a stool may indicate imperforate anus.
• Assess for symptoms of necrotizing enterocolitis (NEC) or Hirschsprung disease.	• Symptoms of NEC include abdominal distention and tenderness, poor feeding, vomiting, and blood in stool (positive Hematest result). In NEC, there are ischemic attacks to the intestine, which lead to systemic shock and hypoxia. In Hirschsprung disease, there is aganglionic megacolon with absence of parasympathetic nerves in muscles and submucosa of rectosigmoid colon that inhibits passage of stools. Symptoms include constipation, vomiting, and fluid and electrolyte imbalance.

Continued on following page

NURSING CARE PLANNING GUIDE Continued

- Assess frequency, amount, character, and odor of stools.
- Stools vary. They progress from meconium to transitional to breastfed or bottle-fed stools. Breastfed stools are looser and golden or mustard in color; they are more frequent at first (with every feeding) and then occur every couple of days. Bottle-fed stools are firmer, less frequent (one to two times per day at first and then every 2 to 3 days), and pale yellow.
- Assess feeding behaviors.
- With constipation, the newborn may feed poorly and vomit.

Diarrhea

- Assess for diarrhea.
- Symptoms include frequent, watery stools that are forcefully expelled. Often there appears to be a "ring of water" on the diaper. Diarrhea may be caused by overfeeding or infection. It can lead to fluid and electrolyte imbalance.
- If diarrhea is present, assess for dehydration; assess skin turgor, fontanelles.
- Excess fluid loss with diarrhea can lead to dehydration.
- Assess feeding behaviors.
- Diarrhea may occur when the newborn is overfed.

11

Analysis: ▼ NURSING DIAGNOSIS

Risk for altered urinary elimination, related to

- Immature kidneys at time of birth
- Low glomerular filtration rate at birth
- Limited tubular reabsorption, which can contribute to acidosis or electrolyte imbalance
- Limited or minimal oral intake
- Excessive regurgitation
- Increased insensible water losses
- Renal anomaly

Defining Characteristics

SUBJECTIVE

OBJECTIVE

Absence of urine output/dry diapers

Minimal saturation of diapers, infrequent voiding/less than 6 wet diapers in 24 hours

Sunken fontanelles

Poor skin turgor

Continued on facing page

NURSING CARE PLANNING GUIDE Continued

Client Goal/ ▼ EVALUATION CRITERIA

Client will demonstrate normal pattern of urinary elimination. / ▼ **Client will evidence voiding at least six times a day, each diaper saturated with urine, normal fontanelles, normal skin turgor.**

▼ NURSING INTERVENTIONS	Rationale
• Monitor and record initial voiding and then frequency of voiding.	• Normal kidney function may not be established until 24 hours after birth. Commonly, output is scanty until oral intake increases. The newborn voids 2 to 6 times a day in the first few days, totaling about 30 to 60 mL. As intake increases, output increases. With renal anomaly, urine output may be absent.
• Monitor intake.	• Fluid intake contributes to amount of urine output.
• Note degree of saturation of diapers.	• Larger urine output will lead to greater saturation of diapers.
• Note color of urine.	• Concentrated urine is darker in color. The presence of peach crystals indicates urates and uric acid crystals, which means that fluid intake needs to be increased.
• Assess for dehydration; assess skin turgor and fontanelles.	• Symptoms of dehydration include poor skin turgor and sunken fontanelles.
• Palpate for bladder distention.	• Distention may occur with bladder or urethral anomalies.

12

Analysis: ▼ NURSING DIAGNOSIS

***Risk for impaired skin integrity,* related to**

• Skin contact with ammonia in urine	• Moist diaper area in contact with skin
• Skin contact with stools	

Continued on following page

NURSING CARE PLANNING GUIDE Continued

Defining Characteristics

SUBJECTIVE	*OBJECTIVE*
Cries at intervals and is not hungry	Rash/lesions in diaper area
Cries when diaper area is cleaned	Inflammation/erythema in diaper area

Client Goal/ ▼ EVALUATION CRITERIA

Client will demonstrate normal skin integrity. / ▼ **Client will evidence normal skin in diaper area.**

▼ NURSING INTERVENTIONS	Rationale
• Assess diaper area for erythema, inflammation, and rash.	• Early recognition of irritation allows interventions to prevent worsening of irritation or development of infection.
• Teach parents how to prevent or minimize diaper rash.	• Various actions help prevent diaper rash by minimizing contact of irritating substances with the skin. Diapers should be changed frequently with gentle cleansing (with nonirritating, nonperfumed soap or water). There is little if any research about which preparation is more effective in preventing diaper rash. Some advocate a protective coating of petroleum jelly or A and D ointment. Some advocate use of cornstarch, which absorbs moisture. Others state that cornstarch cakes and may contribute to fungal infections. Most state that powder should not be used because it becomes dispersed in the air and can be inhaled. Exposure of diaper area to heat by 25-watt bulb placed 24 inches from diaper area for 15 minutes several times a day will aid in drying and healing. The newborn should not be left unattended and must be prevented from moving toward, and touching, the bulb.
• If using cloth diapers, use nonirritating detergent. Follow interventions to minimize diaper rash.	• Some detergents are irritating. Some infants are allergic to disposable diapers.
• Instruct parents to contact health care provider if diaper rash worsens or persists.	• Prescription medications may be needed, especially if secondary infection develops.
• Reinforce teaching concerning prescribed medicated topical ointments or creams.	• Repetition and reinforcement facilitate learning.

Continued on facing page

NURSING CARE PLANNING GUIDE Continued

13

Analysis: ▼ NURSING DIAGNOSIS

***Risk for injury,* related to**

- Lack of safety measures

Defining Characteristics

SUBJECTIVE	*OBJECTIVE*
	Choking on small objects, toys
	Strangling from overcrib toys, from drapery cords, or between slats of crib
	Suffocation from stuffed animal, pillow, soft mattress
	Aspiration from fluids
	Injury from falls
	Drowning in bath water

Client Goal/ ▼ EVALUATION CRITERIA

Client will remain free from injury. / ▼ **Client will evidence absence of injury.**

▼ NURSING INTERVENTIONS	**Rationale**
• Maintain newborn in side-lying position.	• This position prevents aspiration of mucus and respiratory fluids or regurgitation.
• Keep one hand on infant at all times to prevent rolling and falling from changing table or bed.	• This helps prevent injury from falling.
• Maintain safety during bath. Do not leave infant in bath water (take baby along if interrupted). Test water temperature. Until the infant is able to sit alone, hold onto baby's arm.	• Attention to safety measures during the bath prevents slipping into water, prevents burns, and prevents drowning.
• Use a safe crib and mattress: firm mattress, no pillow; crib slats narrow; painted or stained without lead; no stuffed animals.	• Use of a safe crib avoids suffocation, strangling, and lead poisoning.
• Place crib away from window.	• Blind, shade, or drapery cords could strangle baby.

Continued on following page

NURSING CARE PLANNING GUIDE Continued

• Do not place overcrib toys with strings.	• Strings could strangle baby.
• Do not place small objects, toys, or rattles in crib.	• Small objects could choke baby.
• Use appropriate car seat. Do not use infant carrier in car.	• Use the appropriate, approved car seat. Position baby to face the rear of the car until the baby is 1 year old or weighs 20 pounds, when bones are mineralized and better able to withstand a forward impact.
• Advise parents to take infant CPR classes.	• CPR training allows parents to have knowledge necessary to resuscitate the newborn should this be necessary.

14

Analysis: ▼ NURSING DIAGNOSIS

***Risk for altered parent-infant attachment,* related to**

- Dysfunctional family relationship
- Parental illness
- Lack of external resources
- Unrealistic expectations of newborn or spouse
- Lack of knowledge about parenting
- Inability or unwillingness to assume parenting role
- Poor problem-solving techniques
- Daily stressors

Defining Characteristics

SUBJECTIVE

Nonverbal behavior does not indicate attachment (minimal gazing at newborn, few smiles, little touching, touches newborn roughly)

Verbalizes frustration with parenting role

Frequently identifies negative characteristics of newborn

Frequently attaches negative meanings to characteristics or behaviors of the newborn

Verbalizes resentment toward the newborn

Frequently verbalizes dissatisfaction or disappointment with the newborn

OBJECTIVE

Responds inappropriately to baby's cries

Does not place newborn en face, ensuring eye contact

Handles baby roughly

Incongruent verbal and nonverbal behavior

Inappropriate caretaker behaviors

Inappropriate visual, tactile, or auditory stimulation of newborn

Growth and developmental lag in newborn

Frequent accidents or illnesses of newborn

Minimal parental attachment behaviors

Inattention to newborn's cries and needs

Continued on facing page

NURSING CARE PLANNING GUIDE Continued

Client Goal/ ▼ EVALUATION CRITERIA

Client will demonstrate adequate parent-infant attachment behaviors. / ▼ **Client will evidence adequate parenting tasks and parental attachment behaviors.**

▼ NURSING INTERVENTIONS	Rationale
• Inform parents about newborn care and routines in hospital.	• Knowledge decreases anxiety, especially about condition of newborn. Anxiety decreases ability to concentrate and attend to tasks/interactions.
• Give newborn to mother and father to hold right after delivery. Suggest they touch and examine the newborn.	• Various behaviors that foster attachment or emotional bonding between parent and child have been identified. These include touch, type of talking, eye-to-eye contact, type of physical contact, and proximity. Attachment is a process that develops in time. It begins in utero and continues after birth with acquaintance.
• Point out behaviors and responses of the newborn to parental interactions.	• Immediately after birth, the newborn is typically alert and able to interact with visual fixation and eye-to-eye contact. Varying behavioral states are accompanied by different behaviors and types of crying. As parents talk to and hold the newborn, noting characteristics, the newborn may "attend," "alert," and gaze into the parent's face.
• Explain behavioral capabilities of newborn if parents are unaware.	• Parents may not be aware of all of the newborn's capabilities. Explain interactional capabilities of newborn. Examples may include ability to follow with eyes to midpoint; distance of visual ability; shapes, colors, and patterns the newborn prefers.
• If mother wishes to breastfeed, inquire whether she wishes to breastfeed soon after delivery and assist if she does.	• Close body contact facilitates attachment. Mother can feel that she is meeting the infant's needs. As the infant latches on and sucks, the mother receives positive reinforcement for her caretaking/feeding, which contributes to forming an attachment bond.
• Assess strengths, demographic factors (such as age, socioeconomic status, cultural group), and support network that foster development of parenting skills and emotional attachment. Assess mother's physical status for conditions that may influence ability to interact with newborn.	• An adolescent mother may need resources to support her development as a person as well as to support her development as a new mother. Single mothers may also need various resources to adjust to parenting. Cultures with "familialism" as a value may be able to provide supportive information, direct assistance, and emotional support. Physical discomfort may distract the mother from acquaintance with her new infant and interfere with the attachment process.

Continued on following page

NURSING CARE PLANNING GUIDE Continued

- Act as a role model for parenting behaviors and identify other role models within the parents' social network. Assist client in learning caretaking skills.

- Parenting behaviors are learned. Most parents have little education or experience in parental tasks.
  Parenting behaviors are learned by observation, imitation, and practice. Feedback helps the parents to evaluate their behavior and modify behaviors accordingly. Feedback comes from the newborn (baby settles, baby is satisfied with feeding, baby attends), the other parent (complementary parental role behaviors are learned in interaction with each other), and other significant role models. Parents enter parenting with expectations of their own as well as expectations of each other's parenting behaviors. Once the newborn arrives, the reality of parenting is often inconsistent with expectations. Parents then negotiate and modify their behaviors as a parent. If parents feel that caretaking tasks are effective, emotional attachment is enhanced.

- Assess infant's condition and interactional responses.

- Parents develop expectations about the perfect infant they will have. Once the infant is born, a type of grief occurs, or a sense of loss of this idealized image. The nurse can assist with reconciliation of differences between fantasy and reality.

- Provide for rooming in and privacy, but be available to support as needed.

- Parents need to have privacy to become acquainted with the newborn and to "practice" caretaking behavior, asking for assistance as needed. Parents need not feel helpless if the nurse is available to assist as needed. They can assume independent parenting behaviors as they are able.

- Provide experiences in which parents can demonstrate caretaking skills and ask for information as needed, giving reinforcement as appropriate. Provide phone number for client to take home.

- Learned parenting behaviors require practice time. Feedback assists learning and modification of behaviors. Reinforcement when mastery of caretaking activities occurs enhances self-esteem and attachment.

- Refer client to appropriate support groups.

- Support groups can provide role models, information/advice, direct assistance, emotional support, and recognition of feelings. La Leche League can provide support for breastfeeding, for example.

- Assess and record behavioral indicators of attachment.

- These behaviors include type of touching, type of body contact, type and amount of talking to the newborn, responses to infant cries and behaviors, extent of eye contact, type of words used to describe the newborn (positive or negative "feelings"), and amount of contact with the newborn. Recognize that attachment is a process; as such, behaviors indicating attachment will change in time. Also recognize that different cultures demonstrate varied attachment behaviors. The type of attachment behavior deemed to be appropriate is learned from the culture.

Chapter 33

Breastfeeding

Marsha Walker

Lactation and breastfeeding exist within the constraints of each culture in which the physical function and the behavior are practiced. Just as the breastfeeding course flows and ebbs in a mother's life, so also has it experienced flows and ebbs in different cultures through the years. While clearly playing an important beneficial role in the health of women and infants, the importance of breastfeeding *as a human behavior* is reflected in society over time by how it is practiced—when, where, and for how long—and under what circumstances it is not allowed.

JAN RIORDAN (1993)

HIGHLIGHTS

- Trends in Breastfeeding
- Importance of Breast Milk and Breastfeeding Related to Nutrients and Immunology
- Initiation and Maintenance of Lactation
- Nursing Implications in the Prenatal Period Related to Planning and Education, Breast and Nipple Assessment, Maternal History, and Breast and Nipple Preparation and Care
- Nursing Implications in the Perinatal Period
- Nursing Implications in the Postnatal Period Related to Follow-up, Early Breastfeeding Problems, Early Infant Behaviors, and Care for the Preterm Mother and Infant
- Expressing, Storing, and Transporting Breast Milk
- Implications for Research

Breastfeeding and breast milk protect infants against disease and allergy (Host et al. 1988) and promote the proper growth and development of the brain. Breastfeeding has major health benefits for women as well, including decreased risk for breast and ovarian cancer and osteoporosis. Thus, breastfeeding is a major public health concern. Currently, the *Healthy People 2000* national health goals for breastfeeding are targeted at a 75 percent initiation rate and a 50 percent continuation rate at 5 to 6 months by the year 2000 (Table 33–1). The nurse is an important member of the health care team that will cause this to happen.

One important way to promote, protect, and support breastfeeding is to identify and remove cultural and institutional barriers to the choice and continuation of breastfeeding. The nurse requires the knowledge and clinical skills based on current, accurate, and research-based information to support breastfeeding mothers. Nursing care is critical to successful lactation outcomes for both healthy and sick newborns. Thousands of high-risk neonates born each year are admitted to the newborn intensive care unit (NICU), often for prolonged periods. Initiating and maintaining lactation in high-risk situations requires the close ongoing support of knowledgeable

DEFINITIONS

Alternate massage—A technique to sustain the infant's sucking at breast that increases the volume and fat content per feed. The breast is massaged and compressed during each pause between sucking bursts.

Breast shells—Plastic devices worn during pregnancy or between breastfeedings to evert flat or retracted nipples. Use during pregnancy has not been shown to be beneficial.

Colostrum—The first food the infant receives from the breast. The yellowish fluid is present in the breasts from the fourth month of pregnancy and contains immunoglobulins for disease protection.

Engorgement—Swelling and distention of the breast, usually in the early days after delivery, due to edema, vascular congestion, and the increased production of milk.

Feeding cues—Signs of feeding readiness in the infant demonstrated by rapid eye movements under the eyelids, sucking movements of the mouth and tongue, hand-to-mouth movements, body movements, and small sounds.

Flat or retracted nipple—Identified when the nipple fails to protrude when it is compressed for breastfeeding.

Foremilk—The milk obtained at the beginning of a breastfeed. The high water content serves to hydrate the baby and supply water-soluble vitamins.

Hindmilk—The milk obtained after the milk ejection reflex has occurred and nearer to the end of a feeding. Fat content is two to three times that of foremilk.

Latch-on—The act of attaching to the breast by drawing in of the nipple and part of the areola into the baby's mouth.

Letdown or milk ejection reflex—A reflex initiated by sucking at the breast that triggers the pituitary gland to release oxytocin into the bloodstream. When oxytocin reaches the myoepithelial cells surrounding the milk-making glands and collecting ducts, it causes them to contract and eject milk from the breast.

Mastitis—Inflammation or an infective pro-cess in the breast.

Nipple shields—Rubber, silicone, or latex coverings for the nipple-areola with a firm nipple sometimes used for latch-on difficulties or sore nipples.

Nonnutritive sucking—Characterized by two sucks per second, drawing in no milk.

Nutritive sucking—Characterized by one suck per second, a drawing in of the nipple-areola, and milk transfer from the breast to the baby's mouth.

Supplemental feeding devices—Devices other than bottles with artificial nipples. These may include dropper, spoon, cup, feeding tube attached to a syringe, or commercial feeding tube devices.

nurses who believe in the value of breast milk and breastfeeding for these infants and their families.

Given the critical role of hospitals, UNICEF and the World Health Organization (WHO) launched the Baby Friendly Hospital Initiative to motivate hospitals to remove institutional barriers to breastfeeding. The Baby Friendly Hospital Initiative is a voluntary implementation of the Ten Steps to Successful Breastfeeding (WHO 1989). Institutions that adopt and apply these guidelines qualify for an award of public recognition from WHO. These steps serve as a guide for the creation and implementation of research-based protocols on maternity units and promote an optimal start to breastfeeding.

Assessment is the foundation of the nursing process and the basis for choice of interventions to promote desired outcomes. An understanding of milk production, milk transfer, and breastfeeding techniques is central to attaining effective breastfeeding. It is the goal of this chapter to provide recommendations for clinical practice based on the anatomy and physiology of lactation and research-based assessments and interventions.

TRENDS—WHO IS BREASTFEEDING?

Breastfeeding trends throughout the world have shown cyclic variations for many years. In the United States, there was a dramatic decline in breastfeeding during the 1930s and 1940s, lasting until the early 1970s, when only 22 percent of infants in hospitals were breastfed. The last two

Table 33–1

HEALTHY PEOPLE 2000 HEALTH STATUS OBJECTIVES ON BREASTFEEDING

Objective: Increase to at least 75% the proportion of mothers who breastfeed their babies in the early postpartum period and to at least 50% the proportion who continue breastfeeding until their babies are 5 to 6 months old. Baseline: 54% (1988) and 56% (1993) during early postpartum period, and 21% who are still breastfeeding at 5 to 6 months (1988).

Special Population Targets

Mothers Breastfeeding Their Babies	Baseline 1988 (%)	Baseline 1993 (%)	2000 Target (%)
During Early Postpartum Period			
Low-income mothers	32	NA	75
Black mothers	25	31	75
Hispanic mothers	51	56	75
American Indian/Alaskan Native mothers	47	51	75
*At Age 5 to 6 Months**			
Low-income mothers	9		50
Black mothers	8		50
Hispanic mothers	16		50
American Indian/Alaskan Native mothers	28		50

*There has been little progress among women breastfeeding 5 to 6 months post partum.

Note: The definition used for breastfeeding is exclusive use of human milk or the use of human milk with a supplemental bottle of formula or cow's milk.

From Department of Health and Human Services (1996). *Healthy People 2000: National health promotion and disease prevention objectives. Healthy People 2000 review 1995.* Hyattsville, MD: Author.

Ten Steps to Successful Breastfeeding

Every facility providing maternity services and care for newborn infants should

1. Have a written breastfeeding policy that is routinely communicated to all health care staff.
2. Train all health care staff in the skills necessary to implement this policy.
3. Inform all pregnant women about the benefits and management of breastfeeding.
4. Help mothers initiate breastfeeding within a half-hour of birth.
5. Show mothers how to breastfeed and how to maintain lactation even if they are separated from their infants.
6. Give newborn infants no food or drink other than breast milk unless it is *medically* indicated.
7. Practice rooming-in—allow mothers and infants to stay together—24 hours a day.
8. Encourage breastfeeding on demand.
9. Give no artificial teats or pacifiers (also called dummies and soothers) to breastfeeding infants.
10. Foster the establishment of breastfeeding support groups and refer mothers to them on discharge from the hospital or clinic.

From the World Health Organization (1989). Protecting, promoting and supporting breastfeeding: The special role of maternity services. A joint WHO/UNICEF Statement. Geneva: Author.

Table 33–2

CHANGES IN PERCENTAGE OF BREASTFEEDING MOTHERS* FROM 1984 TO 1993

	IN HOSPITAL	2 MONTHS	4 MONTHS	6 MONTHS
1984	52.1	35.9	22.9	16.7
1987	47.6	31.5	18.6	13.1
1990	43.5	27.9	15.8	10.4
1993	45.2	27.6	14.9	10.7

*Exclusive breastfeeding with no supplements in the hospital.

Used with permission of Ross Products Division, Abbott Laboratories, Columbus, OH 43216 from *Breastfeeding trends.*

decades have shown a considerable improvement (Table 33–2). Another 10.7 percent of mothers practice partial breastfeeding in the hospital with formula supplements.

There are also clear differences across the country, with higher rates on the West Coast and the lowest rates in the South East. Ethnic variations exist throughout the United States; black mothers record the lowest breastfeeding rates, white mothers have the highest, and Hispanic mothers are in-between. Of low-income women participating in the Special Supplemental Food Program for Women, Infants, and Children (WIC), 34.2 percent breastfeed in the hospital and only 9.2 percent are breastfeeding at 5 months (Fig. 33–1).

IMPORTANCE OF BREAST MILK AND BREASTFEEDING

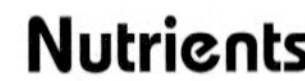

Nutrients

Breast milk is a highly specialized, complex fluid uniquely suited to the needs and metabolic capacity of a growing infant. In addition to protein, fat, lactose, vitamins, minerals, and trace elements, breast milk contains hormones and dozens of enzymes that have both regulating and disease protective effects that are not found in infant formulas (Akre 1989).

Colostrum, the first or early milk, is present in the breasts by the second trimester of pregnancy. It is a yellowish fluid secreted in amounts of 10 to 100 mL/day with a mean of about 30 mL. It is a high-density, low-volume food with less lactose, fat, water, and water-soluble vitamins than the mature milk it will evolve into. It contains more protein, fat-soluble vitamins (E, A, K), and more of some minerals such as sodium and zinc. The composition of colostrum is in keeping with the nutritional requirements, nutrient stores, and metabolic immaturity of a newborn (Table 33–3).

Colostrum has a laxative effect on the newborn, encouraging the expulsion of bilirubin-laden meconium. This reduces the uptake of bilirubin from the reservoir present in meconium and decreases the systemic load of circulating bilirubin. It is therefore unwise to diminish colostrum's effects by supplementing with sugar water or formula. The common practice of following colostrum feeds with water until the milk "comes in" or because the baby is large or small can increase the likelihood of high bilirubin levels, low infant intake, weight loss, and maternal engorgement with sore nipples (Riordan and Auerbach 1993). Breast milk is present in the breasts from the third to fourth month of pregnancy (Whitworth 1988). It changes composition and increases in amount during the course of the lactation. Breast milk composition also varies during a feeding; a two to three times higher fat content is present at the end of a feeding (hindmilk). This is due to the triggering of the milk ejection reflex several times in the course of a feed, and it is one of the reasons that time limits at breast are discouraged.

Components of breast milk have a high bioavailability and are not required in as high amounts as in infant formulas. The fat in breast milk is well absorbed and is high in long-chain polyunsaturated fatty acids. These are important in brain development, nerve myelination, and retinal growth. Infant formulas contain little to none of these. Lactose is the major carbohydrate in human milk; it is important to brain growth and promotes calcium and iron absorption. It encourages the colonization of the intestine with *Lactobacillus bifidus.* These bacteria inhibit growth of pathogenic bacteria, fungi, and parasites by creating an acidic environment. The *bifidus* factor present in breast milk contributes to this condition and can be interfered with by food supplements given to the newborn during the early days. Seventy percent of the iron in breast milk is absorbed by the baby. Only 10 percent of iron in infant formula is absorbed, which is why large amounts of iron are added. This favors the development of pathogenic gut bacteria. Formula (unlike breast milk) does not contain lactoferrin, which prevents iron from being available to intestinal bacteria.

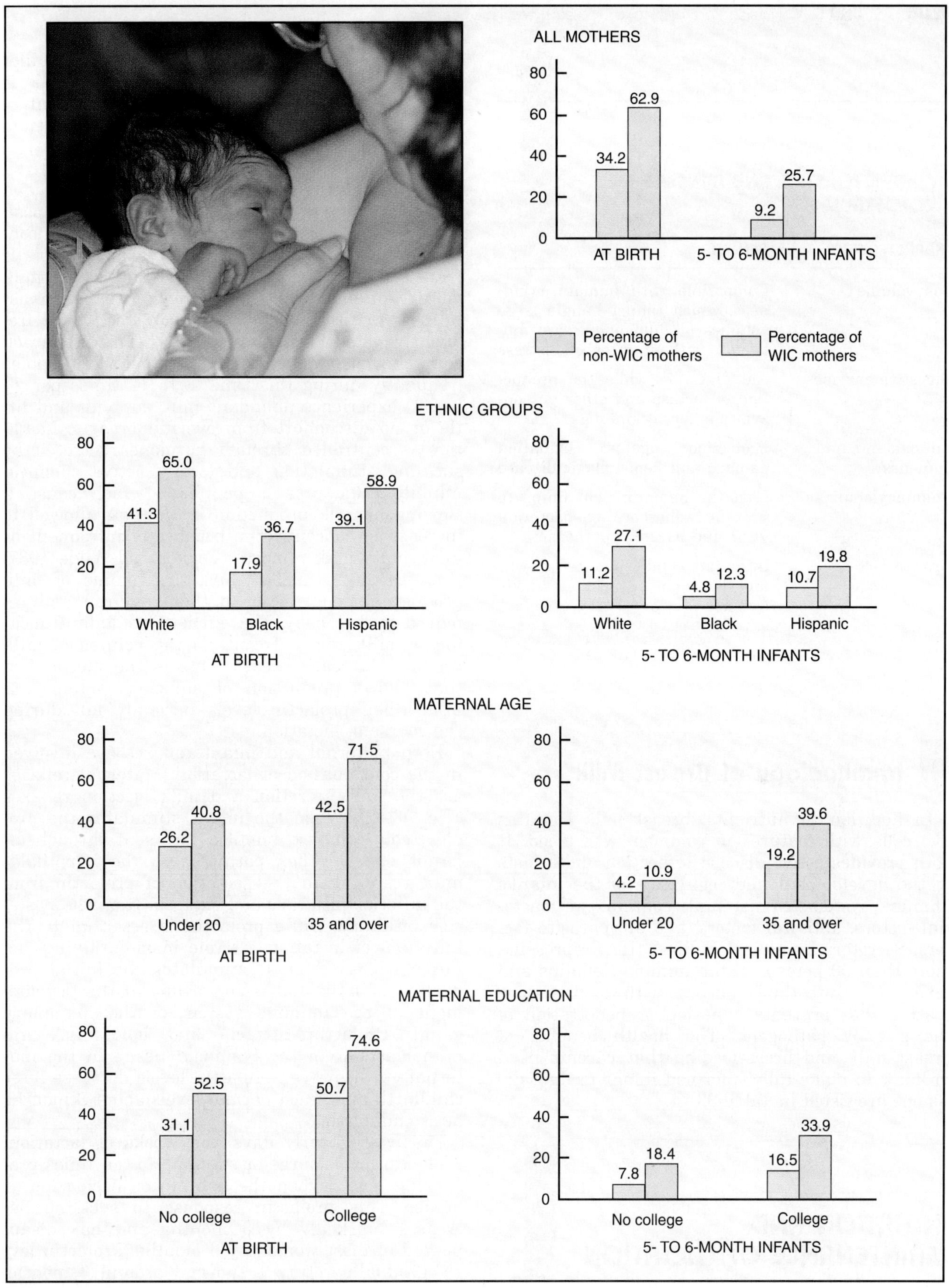

Figure 33–1

WIC mothers who breastfeed at birth and after 5 to 6 months determined by ethnic group, maternal age, and maternal education. WIC = Women, Infants, and Children. (Data from the 1989 Ross Mothers' Survey, Ross Laboratories, Columbus, OH.)

Table 33–3

CHARACTERISTICS AND BENEFITS OF COLOSTRUM

CHARACTERISTIC	BENEFIT
Low volume	Compatible with immature kidneys, which cannot handle large volumes of fluid and excess nutrients without metabolic stress
Digestive enzymes	Aid digestion while the production of lactase and other gut enzymes is just beginning
Antioxidants and quinones	Protection against oxidation damage and hemorrhagic disease
Immunoglobulins	Coat the immature gut lining to prevent adherence of bacterial, viral, and parasitic pathogens
Growth factors	Stimulate and enhance growth and development of infant's body systems

Immunology of Breast Milk

In addition to nutrients, breast milk contains live cells with features in common with blood. It both provides active disease protection and assists in the development and regulation of the infant's immune system. Breast milk contains antibacterial factors, antiviral factors, and antiparasite factors. Secretory immunoglobulin A (IgA) represents more than 90 percent of the immunoglobulins and covers the intestinal mucosa with a protective coating that prevents adhesion or penetration of the gut by pathogens. The health benefits of breast milk and breastfeeding that parents need to know to make fully informed infant feeding decisions are listed in Table 33–4.

INITIATION AND MAINTENANCE OF LACTATION

After birth, with the expulsion of the placenta and rapid drop in progesterone, lactation is initiated. The cells lining both the alveoli and smaller ductules secrete milk continuously. The milk is stored in the alveoli and small ducts adjacent to the cells that secrete it, compressing and flattening the cells.

The breasts fill with milk, which is colostrum until about 30 hours after birth. Between 30 and 40 hours, there is a rapid change in milk composition; a sharp increase in lactose and citrate concentrations marks the beginning of lactogenesis II (Kulski and Hartmann 1981). This rise in milk volume often occurs before any noticeable breast fullness or discomfort from engorgement and frequently after the mother has been discharged from the hospital. Mothers who feed their babies frequently during this time (8 to 12 times per 24 hours) experience abundant milk supplies and little or no discomfort from overfull breasts. Lactation is controlled through hormones secreted by suckling stimulation and locally active chemical inhibitors (suppressor peptides), which cause a slowing in milk production if they are allowed to increase in concentration because of infrequent or inadequate milk removal (Peaker and Wilde 1987; Prentice et al. 1989). Thus, the volume of milk produced is equivalent to that required and removed by the baby. The efficiency of infant sucking or milk removal controls the volume of milk produced in each breast. This is the mechanism that allows production of sufficient volumes of milk when prolactin levels normally fall during the course of lactation.

Both maternal and infant reflexes are involved in the continuation of lactation. Maternal reflexes are the milk secretion and milk ejection reflexes (Fig. 33–2). When the infant stimulates the nipple-areola complex, impulses are sent through afferent neural reflex pathways to the hypothalamus, resulting in the secretion of prolactin from the anterior pituitary and oxytocin from the posterior pituitary. While prolactin is essential to the initiation of lactation, its role in maintaining lactation is less clear. It stimulates the initial production of milk and is important in the development of the immune system of the mammary gland. Prolactin attracts and holds IgA immunoblasts from the lymphoid tissue in the maternal gut. However, prolactin levels decrease after childbirth and reach normal levels about 3 months after childbirth.

During the early days and weeks of lactation, prolactin levels surge or spike up to ten times presucking levels when the baby feeds each time at breast. This prolactin response to suckling decreases markedly by 3 months and has disappeared in most women by 6 months. Prolactin levels gradually return to normal around 3 months post partum in lactating women but continue to show normal diurnal variation of increasing levels during sleep. Even though prolactin levels fall and the response to suckling decreases in time, suffi-

Table 33–4

HEALTH BENEFITS OF BREAST MILK AND BREASTFEEDING

GENERAL AREA	COMMENTS
Nutrition	No excesses or deficiencies Protein correct proportion of casein to whey, nonallergenic Fatty acids profile promotes optimal central nervous system development
Acute diseases of infancy	Threefold to fourfold decrease in risk for gastrointestinal diseases 60% decrease in risk for ear infections 80% decrease in risk for pneumonia Fourfold decrease in risk for meningitis Decreased risk for sudden infant death syndrome Decreased risk for necrotizing enterocolitis
Chronic childhood diseases	Insulin-dependent diabetes mellitus is 2% to 26% higher in formula-fed infants Sixfold decrease in risk for childhood lymphomas Fourfold to fivefold decrease in allergic symptoms
Cognitive development	Improved cognitive development with higher scores on mental development tests
Women's health	Women who have breastfed have half the risk for development of premenopausal breast cancer compared with women who have never breastfed; breastfeeding increases lumbar spine density by 1.5% per breastfed child, decreasing the risk for osteoporosis
Economic	Families who do not breastfeed will spend approximately $1000 to formula feed a baby during the first year

Adapted from Walker, M. (1993). A fresh look at the risks of artificial infant feeding. *Journal of Human Lactation,* 9, 97–107.

cient milk is still produced to sustain good growth in infants up to 8 months of age. Prolactin release occurs only in response to direct stimulation of the nipple.

Once lactation is well established, milk yield is not dependent on high levels of prolactin. Suckling becomes the primary stimulus. Martin (1983) pointed out that the frequency and duration of breastfeeding significantly affect milk production (prolactin) mechanisms during the first 2 weeks of lactation but that this no longer holds true at 35 to 40 days post partum. A high milk yield in the first week post partum can be predictive for the long-term success of lactation. There appears to be a critical time early in lactation during which the ability of the breast to produce the quantities of milk that will be required in later weeks or months is established in response to sucking frequency. This makes it extremely important that proper feeding techniques be established and that no restrictions be placed on the frequency and duration of feedings.

Suckling also stimulates the release of oxytocin from the posterior pituitary. It causes a contraction of the myoepithelial cells surrounding the alveoli and results in the movement of milk from the alveoli into the collecting ducts of the breast. This promotes milk transfer from mother to baby. Some women feel the milk ejection reflex (letdown) as a heaviness or tingling in the breast and may complain that it is somewhat painful. Milk can be sprayed many inches from the breast or can drip from the breast not being used. Some women never feel milk being ejected, but they notice a change in the baby's suckling rhythm and pattern. Milk ejection usually occurs within a minute or two after suckling begins, although oxytocin can be released without tactile stimulation by the baby, hand expression, or a breast pump. Sights, sounds, and odors that a mother associates with her infant are enough to elicit this reflex (Cobo et al. 1967; Drewett et al. 1982). There is an increased blood flow to the breasts and a rise in their temperature; these rises in ductal pressure end shortly after the feeding episode stops. Oxytocin release also causes uterine contractions to help complete the organ's involution. These "afterpains" can be uncomfortable, especially for the multipara. Mothers require an explanation of this and reassurance that the pains are temporary. Pain relief medications may be helpful if the contractions are extremely strong.

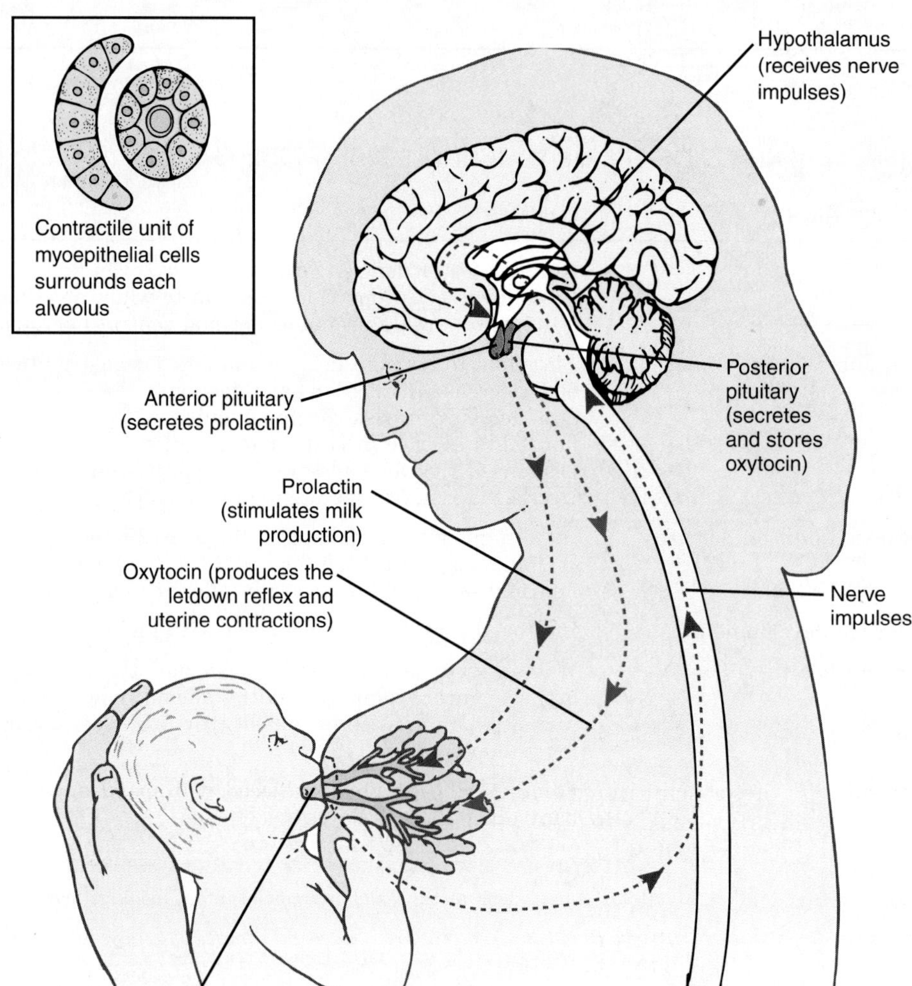

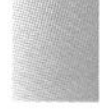

Figure 33–2

The physiologic process of breast milk production is cyclic • It begins with the physical stimulation of nerve impulses that initiate hormone production in the pituitary gland to release prolactin, which in turn stimulates milk production, and oxytocin, which produces the letdown reflex as well as uterine contractions.

In humans, little milk can be removed in the absence of the milk ejection reflex. Therefore, it becomes important to allow women to breastfeed under comfortable, nonrestricting circumstances because the milk ejection reflex is sensitive to disturbances during the early neonatal period. While the milk ejection reflex may be delayed by such stressors as minor pain, anxiety, and embarrassment, sometimes the milk ejection reflex truly will not release milk, as when the breasts have become overfull and the resulting extreme back pressure prevents oxytocin from contracting the myoepithelial cells. Early and frequent breastfeeding prevents overfullness (painful or secondary engorgement). Moist heat, pumping, or hand expression of some milk will drop this internal pressure and allow the reflex to operate.

Both prolactin and oxytocin affect a mother's emotions, mood, and physical state. They are both currently being referred to as the mothering hormones and are involved in the natural state of a postpartum woman.

The Infant's Contribution to Breastfeeding

Initiation and maintenance of lactation are also dependent on the behaviors the infant brings to the process. Within 60 minutes, most infants from unmedicated labors are capable of actively searching for the nipple, opening the mouth wide, and attaching to the nipple (Widstrom et al. 1987).

Several infant reflexes are involved when a baby feeds at breast. Presence of the rooting reflex allows the infant to find and attach to the nipple by orienting in the direction of a touch to the cheek or lips. As a teat is formed and drawn into the mouth, the sucking reflex is triggered when the palate is touched (Ardran et al. 1958). In a coordinated nutritive cycle (when milk is flowing), the suck-swallow-breathe pattern is seen in which breathing appears to be continuous and uninterrupted. Breathing may be interrupted by swallowing when the sucking mechanism is not as well coordinated. Sucking forms a rhythmic pattern with bursts of suck cycles followed by pauses (Shrago and Bocar 1990).

In normal, healthy, full-term infants, these feeding reflexes are strong and capable of allowing the baby to obtain sufficient nutrition from the breast when not interfered with. Common causes of decreased efficiency in early breastfeeding often come from obstetric analgesia, other oral objects placed in the baby's mouth that interfere with the learning process after birth (pacifiers and artificial nipples), separation, delay in going to breast, scheduled or limited feedings, poor positioning, and use of supplemental water or formula.

Barriers to Breastfeeding

Numerous factors can impede both the initiation and duration of breastfeeding. Societal barriers include attitudes toward women's roles, in which a greater value is placed on a woman's independence and career than on mothering, and attitudes toward sexuality, in which exposure of the breasts is deemed inappropriate. Sometimes mothers are advised to reduce contact with their baby to avoid spoiling the baby or causing dependency. Given misinformation and without role models in friends or relatives, mothers may lack the confidence necessary to be successful at breastfeeding. Lack of support in the workplace, where maternity leave is often short and facilities are unavailable for pumping and storing milk, does not encourage breastfeeding. Media promotion of formula sends the message that formula and breast milk offer the same nutritional components but that formula is easier to use.

Health care barriers begin with nonconducive hospital routines or protocols that include lengthy separations; lack of continuous rooming-in; test feeding with liberal use of sterile water, glucose water, or formula; scheduled feedings; inconsistent or contradictory advice; professional ambivalence that projects a message that formula and breast milk are the same; heavily medicated labor and delivery; and lack of follow-up to encourage the new mother to make the feeding choices with research-based data (Lawrence 1994).

Family barriers include lack of support of mother's effort, constant doubt about the adequacy of the milk supply, emphasis on the baby's sleeping through the night, lack of help with household chores, insistence that formula supplements be given when the baby cries, and a father's attitude regarding sexuality and his role as a parent.

Economic concerns may provide additional barriers to breastfeeding for low-income and minority women in the form of late initiation of prenatal care; misinformation due to language or cultural differences; a desire to follow the perceived American bottle-feeding model; and free formula distribution through the WIC program, which may be understood as a government endorsement of bottle feeding.

Infant Feeding Choices and Duration of Breastfeeding

A number of factors influence infant feeding choices and the duration of breastfeeding. Statistics show that ethnicity plays a role; more white mothers breastfeed than black or Hispanic mothers do. Highly educated women also tend to breastfeed more often than do those with less education (see Fig. 33–1). The factors that influence infant feeding choices also vary according to socioeconomic status.

Factors that have been identified as affecting the rate and duration of breastfeeding care include supplemental feedings with sugar water or formula, the time breastfeeding is initiated, the type of delivery, early introduction of solid foods, and insufficient milk supply. Mothers may request formula if they think their infant is not getting enough nourishment or may interpret formula bottles in the newborn nursery as a recommendation to augment breastfeeding. Established feeding patterns are often followed after discharge from the hospital, and the addition of supplements may shorten the duration of breastfeeding.

Early termination of breastfeeding has been linked to late initiation of breastfeeding after birth. Mothers who breastfed within the first 10 hours after birth were more likely to continue breastfeeding during the hospital stay than were mothers who breastfed 11 or more hours after birth. Newborns should be left undisturbed with the mother until the first breastfeed is accomplished, usually within an hour after birth.

Medication during delivery can affect the baby's breastfeeding ability and delay establishment of breastfeeding by several hours or days (Matthews 1989). In addition, lower rates of breastfeeding are seen in cesarean section mothers. This may occur because of the mother's discomfort after delivery or limited contact with the baby in the hospital.

The early introduction of solid foods may also interfere with continued breastfeeding. There is no nutritional or developmental advantage to introducing baby foods within the first 4 months of life.

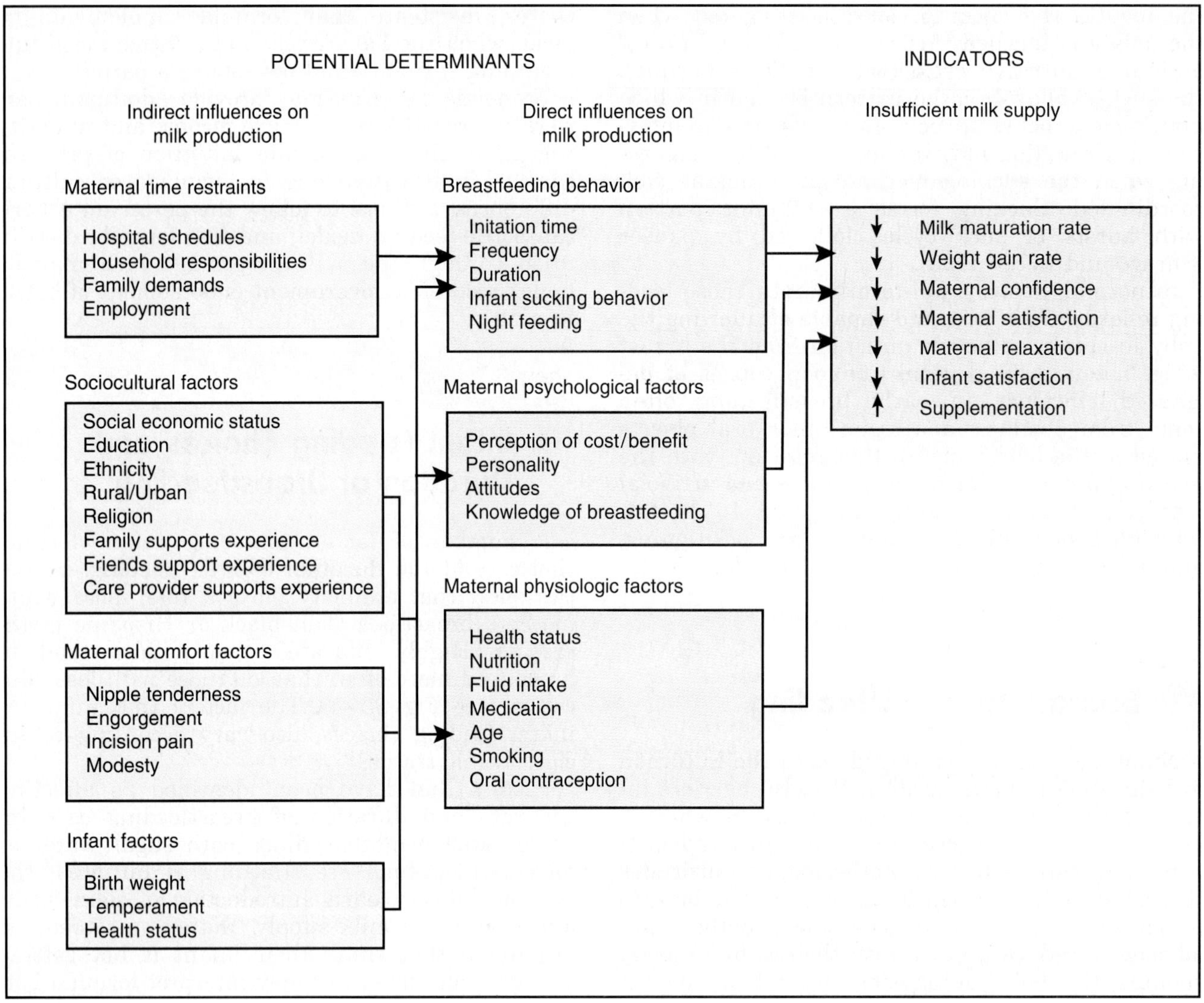

Figure 33–3

Factors contributing to insufficient milk supply. (From Hill, P. D., and Humenick, S. S. [1989]. Insufficient milk supply. *Image,* 21, 145–148.)

Beginning of solid foods signals the start of the weaning process. To prevent premature weaning from the breast, solid foods need not be offered a breastfed baby until 6 months of age and the use of sterile or sugar water should be discouraged.

Worldwide, real or perceived insufficient milk supply is the major reason given for early weaning from the breast. Many factors contribute to this situation including misunderstanding of how lactation works, incorrect management techniques with rules limiting frequency and duration of feedings, minor problems with nipples and sucking that can be easily prevented or corrected, unnecessary supplemental feedings suggested by health care providers and family or friends, misinterpretation of infant behavior, breast surgery, or, rarely, insufficient glandular tissue (Fig. 33–3).

NURSING IMPLICATIONS

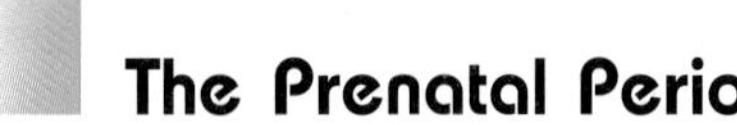

The Prenatal Period

Preparation for breastfeeding may include discussions with health care providers, prenatal breastfeeding classes, reading materials, videos, or simply observing other breastfeeding mothers. Little is necessary to physically prepare for breastfeeding; mothers should not be overwhelmed with lists of rules and regulations regarding special diets or breast preparation rituals, and they should not be given the impression that breastfeeding is complicated. Many problems can be prevented by proper prenatal education that corrects misconceptions and identifies potential areas of concern. Responsibilities of the nurse during this time include the following:

- Ask the mother what she knows about breastfeeding.
- Identify and correct misconceptions about breastfeeding.
- Perform a prenatal breast and nipple assessment.
- Record elements in the maternal history that might have an impact on successful breastfeeding.
- Acknowledge the mother's feelings and concerns about breastfeeding.

HOW DOES THE MOTHER INTEND TO FEED HER BABY?

Decisions about feeding are often made before pregnancy and are influenced by many factors. Jones (1987) found that when mothers were asked their reason for choosing to breastfeed, most stated that it was best for the baby. When all rea-

Table 33–5

MYTHS ABOUT BREASTFEEDING

MYTH	REALITY
Small breasts are an indicator of potential low milk supply.	Size of the breasts is determined by the amount of fat and is not related to the quantity of functional breast tissue.
Breastfeeding will cause the breasts to sag.	Heredity, age, and pregnancy affect the shape of the breasts, not lactation.
A mother will be tied down if she breastfeeds.	Parenthood requires some form of time commitment to the child, and changes will need to be made in the previous lifestyle no matter how a baby is fed.
A mother cannot return to paid employment if she is breastfeeding.	Breastfeeding can successfully continue. Employment is not a reason to avoid breastfeeding.
Nursing will expose the breasts.	Breastfeeding can easily be done discreetly.
Women with fair skin or red hair will get sore nipples.	Skin and hair color have no influence on or predictive value regarding sore nipples (Hewart, R. J. and Ellis, D. J. [1987]. A comparison of the effectiveness of two methods of nipple care. *Birth*, 14, 41–45.)
A special diet is necessary for breastfeeding.	Mothers eat about the same as when they were pregnant. There are no special foods to avoid that might produce gas in the baby.
Fathers will feel left out.	Fathers do not need to give a bottle to share in parenting. They learn and enjoy other parenting methods.
A mother may be too nervous or high-strung.	This does not affect the ability to breastfeed.
The grandmother, other family members, or friends could not breastfeed because of low milk supply, sore nipples, or other problems.	These situations usually reflect poor management and are not hereditary or the norm.
Infant formula is equivalent to breast milk; babies will do just as well.	The two are not the same. Parents should receive balanced information on both the benefits of breastfeeding and the side effects of artificial feeding. Lawrence (1994) states, "Parents have the right to hear the data. They can make their own choice. Fear of instilling guilt is a poor reason to deprive a mother of an informed choice."

sons concerning the health and well-being of the baby were combined, they accounted for more than 90 percent of all reasons and were termed infant centered. The mothers who preferred bottle feeding gave reasons for rejecting or avoiding breastfeeding, not because they considered bottle feeding positively. Many thought it would be more convenient and allow them to go out more often. Bottle feeding was considered less embarrassing. These reasons were termed mother centered.

Seventy-eight percent of the breastfeeders and 26 percent of the bottle feeders thought that feeding method made a difference to the well-being of the baby. Adair (1983) found that lower income, less educated women rely more on personal networks (friends and relatives) as major sources of information; higher income, more educated women use reading materials to a greater extent. Health professionals did not appear to play a large role in the choice. Numerous studies have tried to discover the major sources of influence in feeding choice. They have found that these sources vary by ethnic background. Baranowski and coworkers (1983) found that the male partner was the most important influence for Anglo-Americans, the mother's mother for Hispanics, and close friends for black women. Bryant (1982) also found that Anglo-Americans viewed husbands and friends as having an important impact on feeding decisions and rarely consulted their mothers. For Puerto Ricans and Cubans, the mother's mother was the key support person within the family, although husbands were responsible for other decisions.

IDENTIFY AND CORRECT MISCONCEPTIONS ABOUT BREASTFEEDING

Identifying and correcting myths or misconceptions about breastfeeding allows women to base their feeding decisions on current and accurate information (Table 33–5).

PERFORM A PRENATAL BREAST AND NIPPLE ASSESSMENT

Primary caretakers such as the maternal-newborn nurse practitioner or nurse-midwife have considerable prenatal contact with women and are in a position to begin breastfeeding care early on. Breast changes can be confirmed by asking the mother if her breasts have enlarged or become tender. This establishes breast tissue changes in response to pregnancy hormones and is one of several markers that are indicators of adequate milk-making potential. Prenatal assessment will enable the care provider to formulate necessary interventions to promote successful breastfeeding (Table 33–6).

RECORD ELEMENTS IN THE MATERNAL HISTORY THAT MIGHT HAVE AN IMPACT ON SUCCESSFUL BREASTFEEDING

Identification of potential problems allows either prenatal correction or the time to create a feeding plan for successful breastfeeding.

- Previous breastfeeding experience
- History of diseases and medications (diabetes, arthritis, multiple sclerosis, asthma, seizures, depression)
- Hormone imbalances (thyroid disease; Sheehan syndrome, which is a severe postpartum bleed)
- Findings from the breast and nipple assessment
- Smoking
- Drug abuse

DISCUSS BREAST AND NIPPLE PREPARATION AND CARE

Up to 10 percent of pregnant women who intend to breastfeed can have inverted or non-protractile nipples (Fig. 33–4). For many years, these women were told to prepare their breasts by stretching the areola vertically and horizontally with both their index fingers (called Hoffman exercises), pulling and rolling the nipples between the thumb and index finger, or wearing breast shells. No clear evidence has shown that any nipple preparation treatments have an effect on the length or protractility of nipples (Alexander et al. 1992). A more effective approach is to concentrate on the interventions in the early postpartum period. Mothers should avoid rubbing their nipples with towels because this friction removes keratin layers and does not serve to toughen nipples. Soap is unnecessary on the nipples because it dries the skin and removes the natural secretions of the glands of Montgomery. Creams, lotions, and ointments are not necessary on the nipple or areola; they have not been shown to prevent or cure sore nipples. They have the potential to change the pH of the areola and block nipple pores. Creams are best avoided unless a medical condition warrants the use of medicated preparations.

The Perinatal Period

Labor, delivery, and the immediate postpartum management of the mother and newborn can have early and lasting effects on breastfeeding. The hospital experience strongly influences the initiation and duration of breastfeeding. Hospital staff have a pivotal role in removing constraints to breastfeeding (Chute 1992). Because hospital stays are short, all contacts with the mother be-

Table 33–6

PRENATAL BREASTFEEDING ASSESSMENT CHECKLIST

BREAST	INTERVENTION
Markedly hypoplastic (small); asymmetric (one breast much smaller than the other); scars from breast surgery (altered nipple sensation, nipple autotransplantation, augmentation, reduction mammaplasty (Neifert, M., Seacat, J., Jobe, W. [1985]. Lactation failure due to insufficient glandular development of the breast. *Pediatrics*, 76, 823–828; Neifert, M., DeMarzo, S., Seacat, J., Young, D., Leff, M., Orleans, M. [1990]. The influence of breast surgery, breast appearance and pregnancy-induced breast changes on lactation sufficiency as measured by infant weight gain. *Birth*, 17, 31–38)	Observe after delivery for initiation and maintenance of lactation. Encourage early frequent feedings for optimal supply. Do frequent weight checks of the infant. Use supplemental feeding devices if necessary.
Skin thickening or dimpling of breast or nipple	May be rare early sign of neoplasm; refer the mother to her physician.
Lumps, cysts, fibrocystic disease	Benign forms rarely cause problems. Mother can massage breast during feedings to promote adequate drainage as needed.
NIPPLE AND AREOLA	
Look for firmness or suppleness of the breast tissue behind the nipple	The baby may be hindered in taking enough tissue into the mouth if tissue is not supple. Avoid overfilling of the breasts after delivery by frequent feedings. The mother can use a breast pump before feedings to form a teat if necessary.
Check for nipple protrusion, flattening, or retracting by compressing the areola between the thumb and forefinger just behind the base of the nipple (pinch test); this mimics the action of the nipple when the baby is at breast	Flat nipples can contribute to soreness if the infant cannot latch on and form enough of a teat to draw into the mouth. This can lead to decreased milk intake and low milk supply. Little can be done prenatally to correct this; but after the baby's birth, several techniques have been shown to be successful.

come teachable moments. The nurse-patient relationship becomes a growth-fostering experience so the mother feels empowered and confident in her ability to breastfeed her baby. The following 13 interventions form the nucleus of breastfeeding care to be provided by the nurse (Walker 1995)(Fig. 33–5).

1. Infants should be placed at breast immediately after delivery or as soon as possible thereafter. This should take place in the labor, delivery, and recovery room; the labor, delivery, recovery, and postpartum stay room; the delivery room; or the recovery room.

This intervention facilitates the organized sequence of prefeeding behaviors, which develop in a predictable way during the first hours of life. Infants placed between their mother's breasts demonstrate spontaneous sucking and rooting, hand-to-mouth activities, and body movements that culminate in latching and sucking at breast. Feeding problems can develop when the feeding reflex system has been disturbed by separation, improper positioning, or delays in going to the breast.

Encourage uninterrupted skin-to-skin contact for the first hour after birth, especially if the mother has received labor analgesia or anesthesia. Do not separate until after the first attachment at breast has occurred (Righard and Alade 1990).

Brief separation combined with the use of labor medications decreases the chances of correct latch and suck in the immediate postpartum period. Some pain medications used during labor and given 1 to 3 hours before delivery can delay effective breastfeeding by several hours to several days (Sepkoski et al. 1992; Crowell et al. 1994).

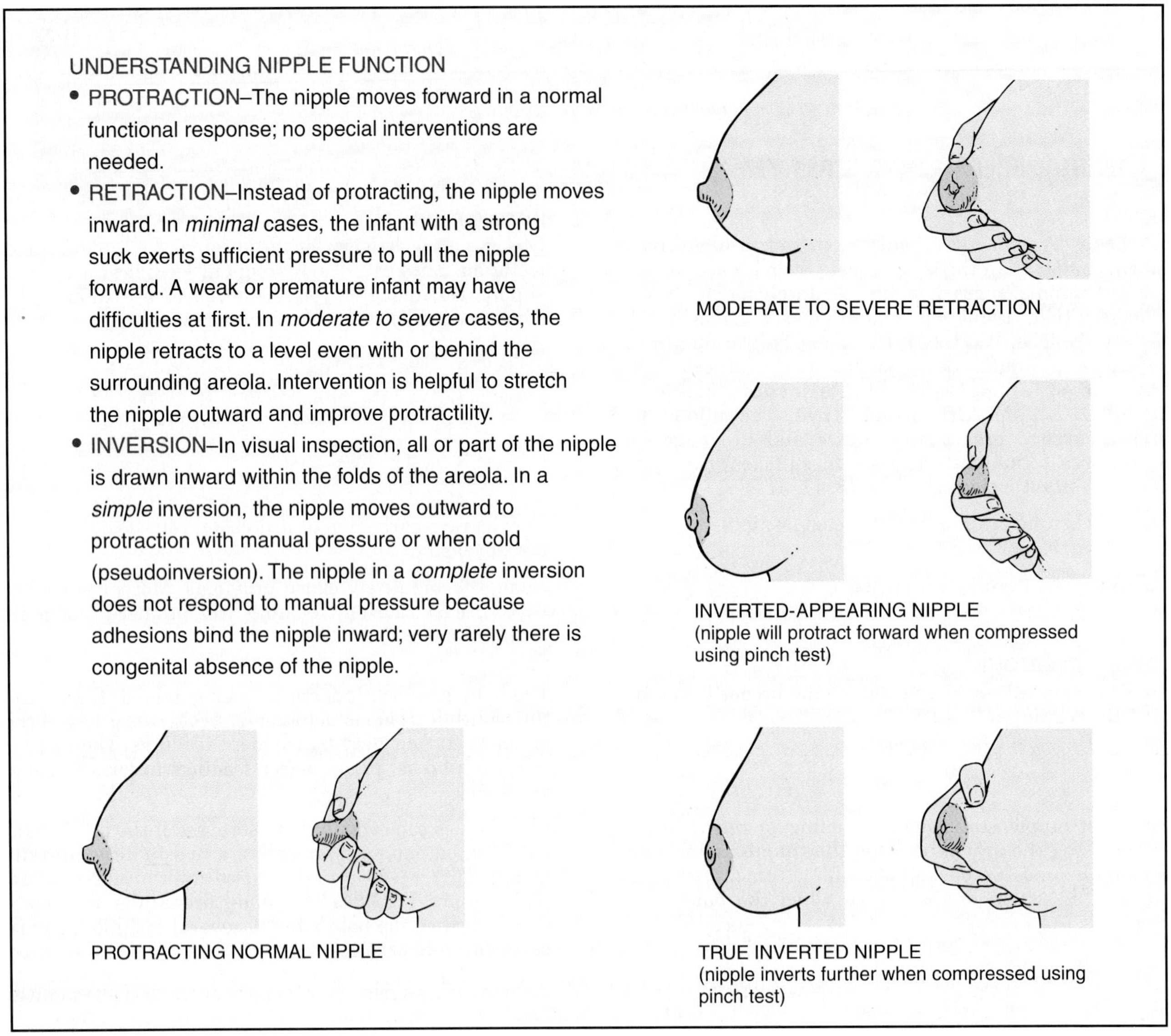

UNDERSTANDING NIPPLE FUNCTION

- PROTRACTION–The nipple moves forward in a normal functional response; no special interventions are needed.
- RETRACTION–Instead of protracting, the nipple moves inward. In *minimal* cases, the infant with a strong suck exerts sufficient pressure to pull the nipple forward. A weak or premature infant may have difficulties at first. In *moderate to severe* cases, the nipple retracts to a level even with or behind the surrounding areola. Intervention is helpful to stretch the nipple outward and improve protractility.
- INVERSION–In visual inspection, all or part of the nipple is drawn inward within the folds of the areola. In a *simple* inversion, the nipple moves outward to protraction with manual pressure or when cold (pseudoinversion). The nipple in a *complete* inversion does not respond to manual pressure because adhesions bind the nipple inward; very rarely there is congenital absence of the nipple.

MODERATE TO SEVERE RETRACTION

INVERTED-APPEARING NIPPLE
(nipple will protract forward when compressed using pinch test)

PROTRACTING NORMAL NIPPLE

TRUE INVERTED NIPPLE
(nipple inverts further when compressed using pinch test)

Figure 33–4

Characteristics of protracted, retracted, and inverted nipples. (Data from Riordan, J. [1990]. *A practical guide to breastfeeding.* Boston: Jones & Bartlett Publishers.)

Uninterrupted contact after birth decreases crying and startling in newborns, reduces blood pressure, and stabilizes temperature and respirations faster than when the infant is left alone in a bassinet.

Cesarean-born infants should be put to breast as soon as possible, either in the operating room or recovery room. Avoid delaying the first breastfeed if possible. Method of delivery does not alter the physiologic principles of lactation.

A low-grade fever in a cesarean or vaginally delivered mother should not interrupt breastfeeding. In the absence of other symptoms, a low-grade fever does not pose a danger to the breastfed baby. Many women who have had epidural anesthesia exhibit low-grade fevers as a side effect.

Keep the baby in bed with the mother as much as possible. Constructing the environment for comfort and positive outcomes greatly increases the success of breastfeeding. Try a lateral Sims position with the mother's back supported against the guardrail and cushioned with a pillow. Place the baby on the side facing the mother pulled in very close. The mother may prefer to sit up in bed and breastfeed. Have her rest her feet against either the footboard or a rolled up bath blanket and pillow (Fig. 33–6). Teach the father or other helper how to aid the mother in positioning so that help is available whenever it is needed.

2. Each breastfeeding mother should be shown how to breastfeed, including positioning, latch-

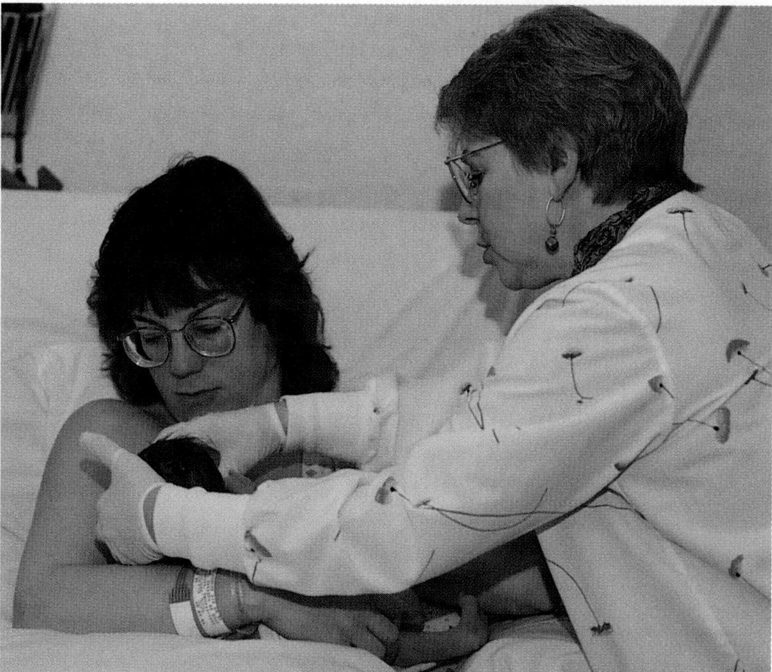

Figure 33–5

The lactation consultant not only reinforces the correct positioning of the newborn to breast but observes the infant's sucking ability, offers suggestions to improve the nursing practice for long-term success, and provides encouragement to all members of the new family.

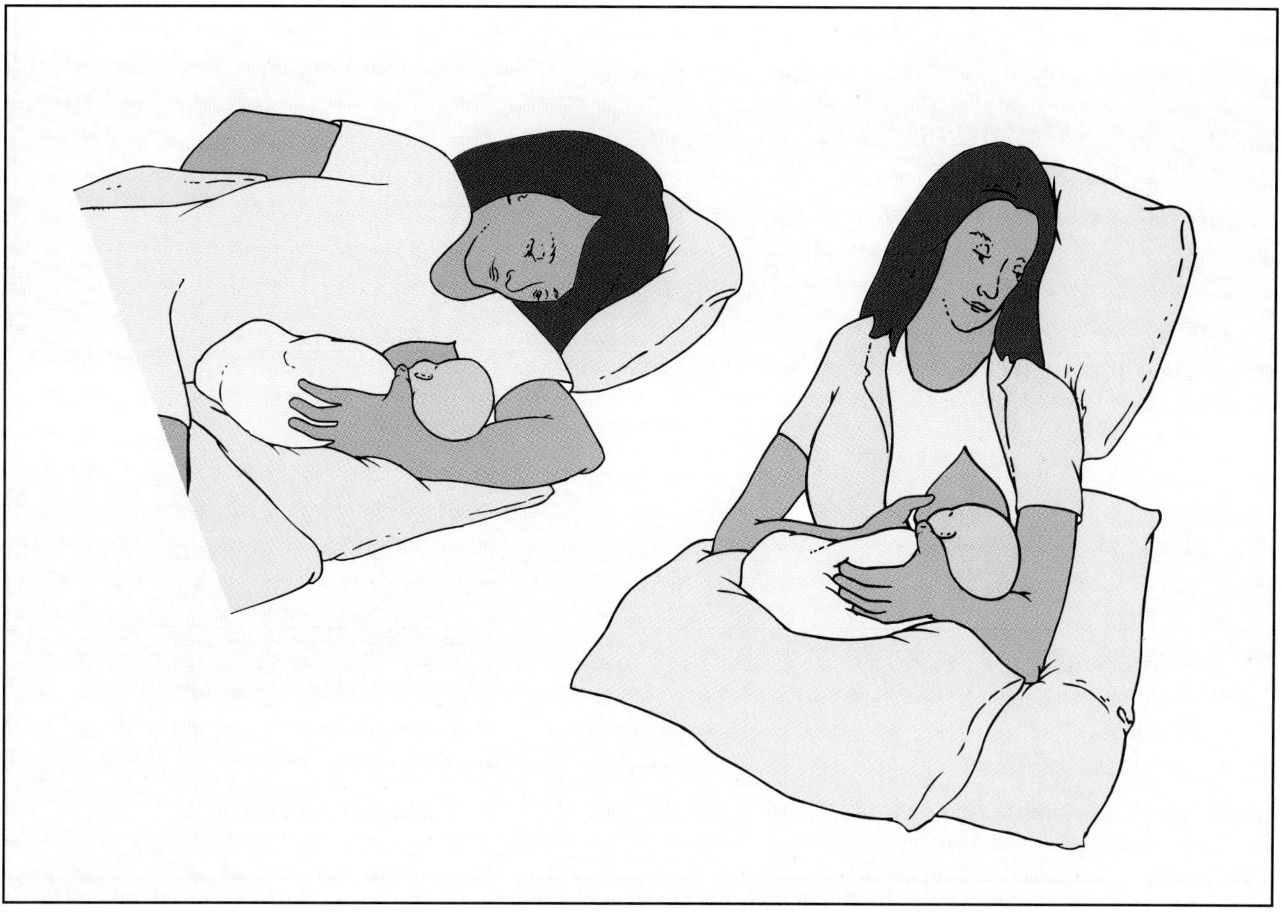

Figure 33–6

Comfort when breastfeeding is important to success, particularly for mothers who have experienced a cesarean delivery.

on, and how to tell when baby is swallowing milk. This should be taught to both primiparous and multiparous mothers, evaluated on each shift, and reviewed before discharge.

Lack of role models usually means that mothers need to be taught the art and skill of breastfeeding. Poor positioning can compromise an infant's ability to feed effectively. Proper head, neck, and trunk alignment is important to smooth feeding performance. The head and neck will be in neutral alignment, with overall body position one of slight flexion, including the hips. Proper positioning during feedings affects respiratory mechanisms, oral-motor control, swallowing, and the development of head and neck postural responses.

Explore one to four feeding positions, using what works best (cradle, football or clutch, cross-cradle, or side-lying) (Fig. 33–7). Proper positioning and attachment to the breast avoids nipple trauma, ensures adequate milk intake, and pro-

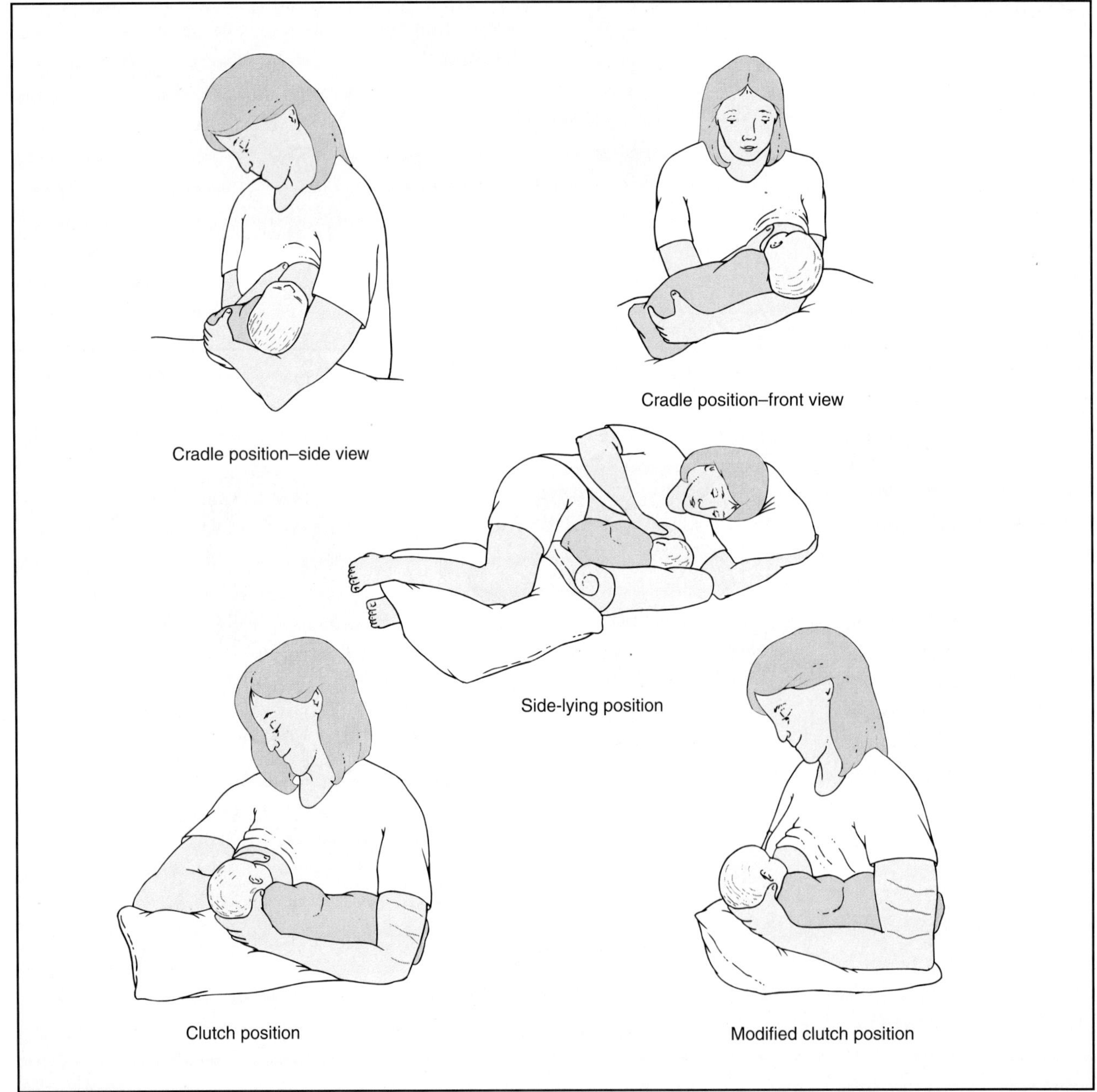

Figure 33–7

Three basic positions are recommended for successful breastfeeding • The cradle position • The clutch or football hold • The side-lying position.

vides positive feedback experiences to the mother (Renfrew 1989). Mothers should be instructed to

- Bring the baby to the level of the breasts. Do not lean over or push the breast sideways to the baby.
- Turn the baby completely on the side, facing the mother with the arms embracing the breast on either side.
- Bring the baby in as close as possible with the legs wrapped around the mother's waist and the tip of the nose touching the breast.
- Center the baby's mouth directly in front of where the nipple points. Avoid moving the breast sideways to the baby.
- The mother should hold the breast with four fingers under it for support and thumb on top. All fingers will be away from the areola.
- Bring the baby's lips to the nipple (Fig. 33–8); when the baby opens the mouth to its widest point, draw the baby the rest of the way onto the breast.
- Avoid tilting up the nipple or squeezing the areola and pushing it into the baby's mouth.
- Avoid pushing on the back of the baby's head. Pushing on the occiput may cause extension of the neck, biting of the nipple, and an aversion to being held close to the breast. Pushing on the back of baby's head will not cause the baby to latch on or feed faster.

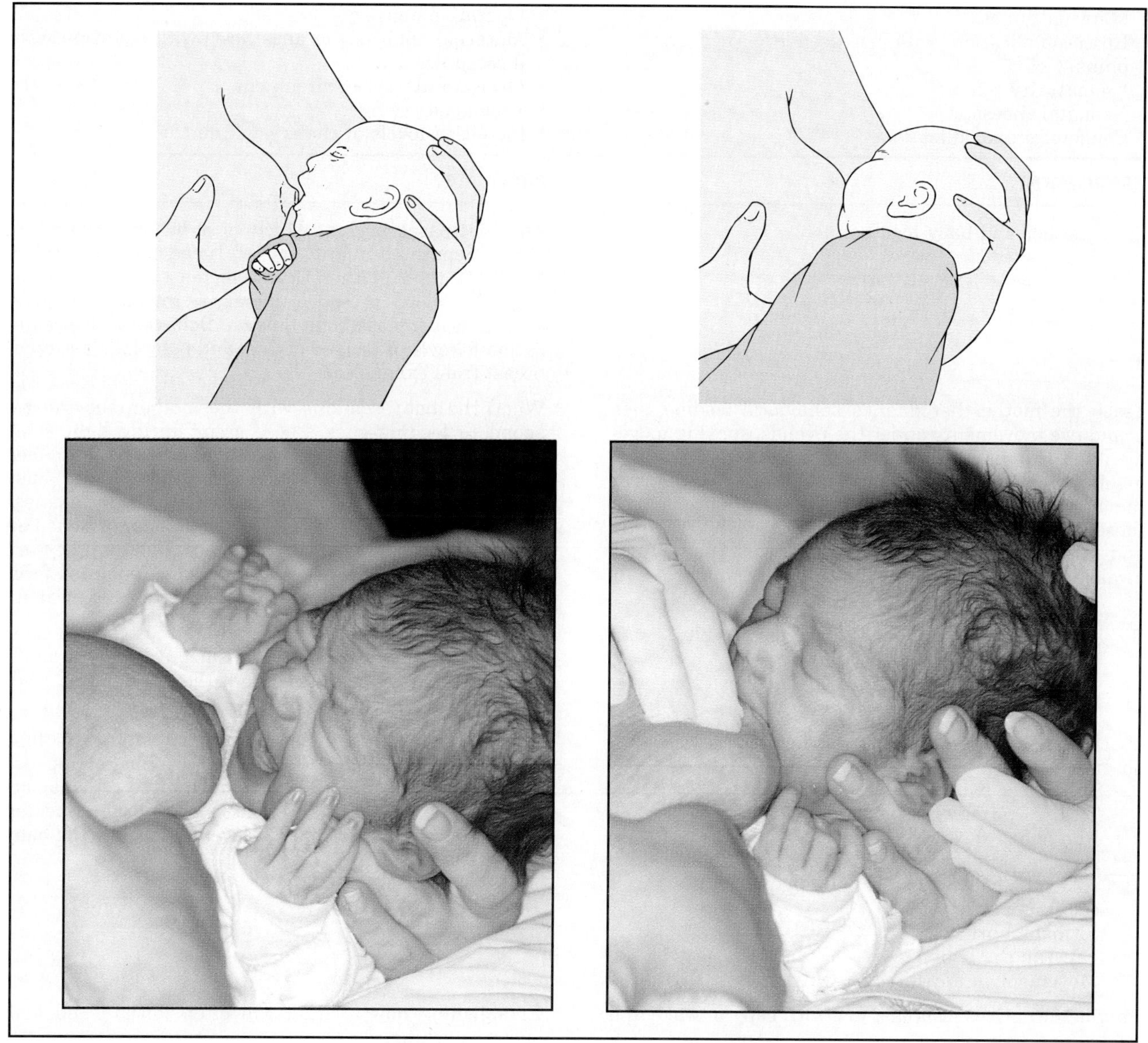

Figure 33–8

Initiation of breastfeeding requires the correct latch-on • Offer the nipple to an infant with open mouth • The infant latches on by grasping the breast • When the infant is finished sucking, the mother may insert her finger at the side of the baby's mouth to release the suction.

Table 33–7

BEDSIDE PROBLEM SOLVING: SLEEPY BABY

Problem Description

- Baby does not wake or fuss on a regular basis to indicate hunger
- Baby falls asleep at breast after a few sucks
- Baby sucks sporadically at breast, wakes when put down, but continues to feed poorly
- Baby asleep for the second side

Contributing Factors

Some conditions that affect baby's state and response to the feeding situation are

- Maternal illness
- Birth complications with increased levels of endorphins
- Prematurity
- Neonatal illness
- Congenital anomalies
- Operative delivery
- Maternal analgesia or anesthesia with resulting state disorganization
- Overstimulating environment
- Prolonged crying
- Increased levels of cholecystokinin

MANAGEMENT	RATIONALE
Keep mother and baby together.	This decreases crying, which is a behavioral sign of stress. Separated infants cry ten times more than when kept with their mother. Crying increases cortisol levels, increases blood pressure, increases intracranial pressure, and increases body tension. Behavioral disorganization follows prolonged crying, and baby falls asleep at breast from exhaustion.
Teach the mother her infant's behavioral feeding cues (rapid eye movements under the eyelids, sucking movements of the mouth and tongue, hand-to-mouth movements, body movements, and small sounds). Instruct the mother to put her baby to breast when she sees these cues as many times as possible during the day and a few times at night when she hears the baby or awakens. Keep the baby with the mother at night.	When the baby remains with the mother, she can respond to feeding cues. These occur during light sleep and indicate times when the baby is most likely to feed well. These feeding cues are easily missed in a busy nursery. Babies do not need to come to full awakeness and cry as a cue to feed. Sleepy babies cannot be fed on a schedule of every 2 hours or every 3 hours. They are likely to be in a deep sleep state at the appointed feeding times and overhungry when they finally do awaken.
Suggest skin-to-skin contact as much as possible.	Mothers can respond immediately to these subtle cues. This helps to repattern baby to suck at breast if artificial nipples have been used or if the mother was medicated during labor and delivery.
Teach alerting techniques to use when feeding cues are observed: • Talk to the baby with variable pitch • Tickle or stroke the palms or soles • Rub baby's face • Put the baby's hand to the baby's mouth • Allow the baby to smell a nursing pad with colostrum on it • Sit baby upright • Unwrap the baby • Movement in any direction with uneven rhythms	These activities stimulate the trigeminal nerve (fifth cranial nerve), which is the sensory arm for rooting and sucking. The trigeminal has input into the reticular activating system—the alarm clock of the brain. Sucking action decreases above 80°F. Movements allow the baby to awaken.
Provide incentives at breast to entice baby to wake and feed: • Dropper of colostrum or D_5W • Feeding tube devices or butterfly tubing taped to breast and connected to a 10-mL syringe	Establishing flow of fluid will often initiate and help sustain sucking.

Continued on facing page

Table 33–7 *Continued*

BEDSIDE PROBLEM SOLVING: SLEEPY BABY

MANAGEMENT	RATIONALE
• Gavage tubing taped to breast • Syringe, periodontal syringe used to deliver boluses at breast	
If the baby is overstimulated and is shutting out the noise and light by sleeping, modify the environment: • Quiet, dim room • Gentle walking • Pat baby's back at the rate of the heartbeat, gradually slowing the patting to 72 per minute • Feed the baby for short periods with time-outs • Avoid talking to baby or rubbing the baby's head while at breast • Avoid jiggling the baby • Tug back gently on the nipple to induce a suck as long as the nipples are not sore • Use alternate massage if baby dozes at breast between sucking bursts	Environmental modification helps supply behavioral organization to a disorganized or dysmature baby.
Avoid pacifiers, artificial nipples on bottles, and nipple shields. If baby needs additional fluids, use a device as above or a cup to avoid nipple confusion.	Artificial nipples do not lengthen and compress the way a human nipple-areola does. Artificial nipples are a strong stimulus in a baby's mouth, which causes the oral structure to conform to a rigid shape. Use of artificial nipples weakens a baby's suck as the baby decreases sucking pressures to slow fluid flow.
If baby refuses the second breast at a feeding, suggest that the mother offer it after about an hour or when she sees feeding cues again.	Cholecystokinin levels usually fall after this, and baby may start to cycle into a lighter sleep state.

Courtesy of Lactation Associates, 254 Conant Road, Weston, MA 02193.

- Teach the mother how to know when the baby is swallowing milk. Swallowing indicates that nutritive sucking is occurring and that milk is being received by the baby. Nutritive sucking is characterized by bursts of sucking followed by a pause. Swallowing follows nutritive sucking. The ratio of sucks to swallows in a newborn is several sucks per swallow, gradually changing to a ratio of 1:1 when the milk lets down and increasing toward the end of a feeding to 2:1 or 3:1 (Wolf and Glass 1992). Swallowing can be heard as a puff of air from the nose, which is the exhalation segment of the suck-swallow-breathe cycle. As milk volume increases in amount and pressure, swallows can be heard as milk passes through the throat. If in doubt, place a stethoscope on baby's throat to confirm swallowing (Vice et al. 1990).
- Teach the mother how to break suction before removing the baby from the breast. The mother should place a clean finger in the side of the baby's mouth to break the suction before removing the baby from the breast.

3. Keep breastfeeding mothers and babies together during their hospital stay, including at night.

Physiologically and psychologically, the newborn infant and postpartum mother are an interdependent unit. Keeping the two together promotes synchronization of sleep-wake patterns, allows flexible feeding options, and enhances adjustment to the maternal role.

Encourage and facilitate the mother's and baby's remaining together during their short hospital stay. Unlimited access to the baby decreases neonatal feeding problems (Yamauchi and Yamanouchi 1990). Inform the family that mothers and babies who experience rooming-in show a higher frequency of breastfeeding, better baby weight gain on day 7, reduced need for supplements, lower bilirubin levels, decreased infant crying, and increased milk production and duration of breastfeeding; rooming-in also helps offset the effects of labor medications on breastfeeding, and it does not decrease the amount of sleep a mother gets.

Mothers do not sleep longer or better when their babies are returned to the nursery at night (Keefe 1987). Average amounts of sleep are 4 to 5 hours at night, irrespective of whether the baby is in the mother's room (Keefe 1988). Another 2 hours of sleep can be obtained by dozing or napping during the day. The nurse can modify the mother's environment during the day by limiting visitors, decreasing visiting times, discouraging the use of the telephone and television, and minimizing disruptions to allow mothers to increase the amount of sleep they get by napping and dozing.

4. Breastfed infants should be put to breast 8 to 12 times each 24 hours, including cesarean-born infants. Infant behavioral feeding cues should be used if the baby cannot initiate sufficient feedings because of sleepiness.

Feeding frequency is based on the composition of the milk, the emptying time of the stomach, the physiologic mechanism of milk production, and the needs of the infant for frequent contact. Breastmilk is digested in 60 percent of the time required for infant formula.

Inform mothers that breastfed babies need to be fed 8 to 12 times each 24 hours. Scheduled or limited feedings create hunger and crying in infants and can lead to maternal insufficient milk supply. Infants do not necessarily feed every 2 or every 3 hours, but they may bunch or cluster their feeds several times within a few hours. Feedings are erratic at first; a baby may take one breast at a feed, fall asleep, and wake 45 to 60 minutes later for the other side. Babies are not using their mothers as pacifiers if they feed frequently, and infrequent feeds do not cause a baby to become independent. Sleep is not an indicator of getting enough milk, and infrequent feeds do not prevent sore nipples.

Teach mothers five infant behavioral feeding cues to use with a sleepy baby or one who cannot initiate enough feedings to gain weight: rapid eye movements under the eyelids, sucking movements of the mouth and tongue, hand-to-mouth movements, body movements, and small sounds. These feeding cues occur before the demand (crying) for food. Waking a baby from a sound sleep, which can happen with scheduled feeds, often results in failed feeding attempts. These feeding cues are external indicators of changing sleep and internal feeding readiness.

Avoid wrapping the baby with arms pinned to the sides or covering the baby's hands with undershirt cuffs. Wrapping the baby like this or covering the hands prevents hand-to-mouth movements, which are important to signal hunger and provide self-calming. Teach mothers the technique of alternate massage for use with sleepy babies or babies who feed poorly at breast. The breast is massaged and compressed with each pause between sucking bursts. This prompts more sucking, increases the volume and fat content of each feed, enhances milk production, increases infant intake, prevents milk stasis, and provides mothers with a simple technique to help baby get more milk. Additional suggestions for sleepy babies and reluctant nursers are found in Tables 33–7 and 33–8.

5. Time limits for breastfeeding on each side should be avoided. Babies are offered both breasts at each feeding but may feed only on one side at each feeding in the early days.

Historically, limiting the time a baby could feed at breast in the early days was thought to prevent sore nipples (Millard 1990). No evidence supports this practice, especially since it leads to engorgement, decreased milk intake, low milk supply, and early abandonment of breastfeeding.

Teach correct positioning and latch techniques to the mother. Nipple trauma is most frequently caused by physical or mechanical problems of attaching the baby to the breast (Hill and Humenick 1993) (Table 33–9). Observation during feedings often reveals the source of the problem. Assess for other contributors to sore nipples, such as flat or inverted nipples that may make latching on to the breast difficult and contribute to poor breastfeeding performance.

Recommend that the mother leave the baby on the first side until the baby is done, then burp and offer the other side. Restricting time on the first side so that the baby will take the second side can create low-fat feeds, slow weight gain, fussiness, gas, rapid gastric emptying, and high lactose load to the intestines. Babies are done when they will no longer suck and swallow when the breast is compressed or when they come off the breast by themselves (Righard et al. 1993).

6. Nipple shields or bottle nipples should not be used to cover a mother's nipple with the intention of causing latch-on, to prevent or manage sore or cracked nipples, or when mothers have flat or inverted nipples. Because the shield forms an artificial barrier between the baby's mouth and mother's breast, it has the potential to alter both the sucking dynamics of the baby and stimulation to the breast for milk production (Woolridge et al. 1980).

Text continued on page 1224

Table 33–8

BEDSIDE PROBLEM SOLVING: RELUCTANT NURSER

Problem Description

- Baby may latch to the breast only after many attempts
- Baby may exhibit rapid side-to-side head movements and may or may not latch to breast
- Baby may completely refuse to latch to breast, either falling asleep or aggressively pushing away with an arched body
- Baby may have a one-sided preference

Contributing Factors

- Poor positioning at breast
- Interruption in the organized sequence of prefeeding behaviors immediately after birth
- Drug-induced interference, which prolongs the period of state disorganization in the newborn (epidural, Stadol, Nubain, Demerol)
- Fetal history of breech presentation, extension in utero, protracted labor, cervical spine pain or damage, precipitous delivery, dislocated hip, fractured clavicle, asymmetric positioning in utero with right-sided preference
- Vacuum extraction; forceps delivery; shoulder dystocia with misalignment of head, neck, and shoulders
- Cephalhematoma
- Hypertonia (jaw clenching, pursed lips, neck and back hyperextension, tongue retraction or elevation)
- Infrequent feeds leading to an overhungry baby, excessive or prolonged crying resulting in behavioral disorganization
- Interference with imprinting on the breast from separation, artificial nipples, pacifiers, nipple shields
- Excessive pressure on occipital region of baby's head from pushing the head forward into the breast
- Vigorous or deep suctioning or intubation may cause swelling or discomfort in the mouth or throat with resulting clenched mouth, tongue thrusting, neck extension, or pushing away from the breast
- Short or tight lingual frenulum

MANAGEMENT	RATIONALE
Check positioning of baby at breast: • Baby completely facing mother with head, neck, and spine aligned • Mouth in front of where nipple points • Baby brought to breast and held close • Mother does not lean forward, maneuver breast sideways, compress areola and insert into baby's mouth, or tilt nipple up at latch-on	Poor positioning increases the number of latch attempts needed before obtaining milk, which can frustrate both mother and baby. Improper positioning increases the chances that the baby will not attach to the breast, leading to sore nipples, engorgement, insufficient milk production, and slow weight gain.
Positioning may vary, depending on symmetry of baby. Babies with a right-sided preference may need to be held in a football hold on the right breast and in a cradle or prone position for the left breast. Some babies do better when the mother is in a side-lying position. Breech babies may feed better sitting upright in the football hold. Babies with delivery trauma such as a cephalhematoma may be more comfortable and feed better when held with the affected side up. Babies with a fractured clavicle may feed better in a football hold if the weight of the breast is kept off the chest or in a cradle hold with the affected side up.	Positioning in utero and delivery events influence breastfeeding patterns. Several different positions may need to be explored to find one that is satisfactory.
Allow the baby time on the mother's breast immediately after delivery. Let baby seek and find the nipple before removing the baby from the mother's chest.	This provides the opportunity for the prefeeding sequence of behaviors to occur, which increases the likelihood of proper attachment to the breast.
Keep the mother and baby together. Place baby skin-to-skin on mother's chest. Instruct the mother to feed her baby on cue: when the baby stirs at breast, when she sees rapid eye movements under the eyelids, when she	This reestablishes or repatterns the initial sucking sequence that may not have occurred immediately after delivery. With the baby in close, the mother can feel the infant's feeding cues and place to breast before the baby

Continued on following page

Table 33–8 *Continued*

BEDSIDE PROBLEM SOLVING: RELUCTANT NURSER

MANAGEMENT	RATIONALE
sees movements of the tongue and mouth, when baby exhibits hand-to-mouth movements, or when the baby makes small sounds.	becomes overhungry and when the baby is most likely to latch on.
An alternative technique is to place mother and baby in a bath, allowing baby to repattern in the warm water. To keep baby warm and soothed, a helper can gently pour warm water over baby's back as the baby creeps to the breast and attaches.[1]	
Place a warm towel over baby's neck, massage the baby's shoulders and arms. This is helpful after a precipitous delivery, forceps delivery, or vacuum extraction. It is also soothing to a high-tone baby.	Baby may be in pain from overriding cervical vertebrae. This helps relax the cervical structures and decrease tone in a high-tone baby.
For rapid side-to-side head movements, touch the midline of baby's upper lip with a dropper of colostrum or D_5W. Move baby onto the breast as the baby follows the dropper to the nipple. When the mouth is wide open, place a few drops of water or colostrum on the tongue to elicit sucking and swallowing.	The dropper acts to provide external control and food incentives to attach and suck at breast.
An arching baby can be placed either in the football hold or with the mother lying on her side. The mother can also use a sling to help position the baby in flexion. If this does not calm the baby, place the baby on a receiving blanket; have two adults pick up the corners of the blanket and rock the baby from side-to-side like a hammock. Then put baby to breast.	These techniques help to flex the back and hips to avoid arching and jaw clenching.
Provide latch and sucking incentives to the baby, which can include • A periodontal syringe placed in the side of the baby's mouth, which delivers a small amount of colostrum or sugar water with each suck until baby demonstrates rhythmic suck and swallow at breast • A syringe or soft clinic dropper can be used to elicit sucking • Butterfly tubing attached to a 10-mL syringe and taped to the breast can provide these incentives as well as a supplement if needed	Incentives help prevent pulling away from the breast before the baby latches on or swallows.
A baby who is crying hard or has been crying for a time may not be able to organize himself or herself to feed. Allow this baby to suck on a finger or place the tubing on a finger and allow baby to suck a little colostrum or sugar water by finger feeding before putting the baby to breast. Avoid pacifiers, bottles, and nipple shields. If baby will not suck on a finger, place some colostrum or sugar water in a 28-mL medicine cup and have the baby sip from the cup until she or he calms down and has a little food in the tummy.	
If the baby will not open the mouth wide enough for painless latch-on or clenches the jaw, hold the baby's jaw between your thumb and index finger and move the jaw a small amount from side to side.	This helps inhibit jaw clenching.

[1]Harris, H. (1994). Remedial co-bathing for breastfeeding difficulties. *Breastfeeding Review,* II (10), 465–468.
Courtesy of Lactation Associates, 254 Conant Road, Weston, MA 02193.

Table 33–9

BEDSIDE PROBLEM SOLVING: SORE NIPPLES

Problem Description

- Initial sensitivity or soreness at latch-on
- Discomfort that subsides with onset of milk ejection reflex or when baby begins swallowing; this pain is aggravated by engorgement
- Pain or discomfort periodically during a feeding or throughout the entire feeding
- Periodic sharp pain in one or both nipples after feedings

Nipple may
- Blanch (vasospasm) on removal from baby's mouth
- Have horizontal or vertical red or white stripe
- Be asymmetrically stretched when removed from baby's mouth
- Be fissured, cracked, or bleeding
- Be cratered or scabbed over
- Be blistered

Contributing Factors

- Transient latch-on pain may occur from lack of established keratin layer on nipple epithelium
- Unrelieved negative pressure, which is present until the milk ejection reflex occurs and is relieved by the periodic swallowing of the baby
- Manipulation of the nipple-areola, such as squeezing it, tilting it up, pointing it down, pushing it into the baby's mouth
- Mother leaning down over the baby to "insert" the breast into baby's mouth

Pain during a feeding may be attributed to
- Nipple-areola not in baby's mouth symmetrically or not in far enough
- Baby's lower or upper lip curled under rather than flared out
- Baby's tongue behind lower gum and pinching or biting the nipple
- Baby with tongue-tie
- Breast pushed sideways to the baby rather than baby's mouth centered over where the nipple points naturally
- Nipple confusion (mouth configured for feeding on an artificial nipple)
- Disorganized or dysfunctional sucking pattern
- Flat or retracted nipples
- Baby's mouth not opened wide enough

MANAGEMENT	RATIONALE
Suggest that the mother initiate the milk ejection reflex or express drops of colostrum before putting baby to breast.	Colostrum/milk flow prevents traumatic sucking by causing swallowing at the start of the feeding.
Review and correct positioning: • If in the cradle hold, baby completely faces the mother, is held close with legs wrapped around the mother's waist	Proper positioning and latch techniques prevent or alleviate many of the problems with sore nipples.
• Four fingers are under the breast and the thumb is on top with all fingers off of the areola • The baby is brought to the breast with the mouth centered over where the nipple points	If the mother pushes the breast sideways to the baby, she can cause vertical cracks on either side of the nipple.
• The baby's lips should touch the nipple; when the mouth opens to its widest point, the baby is drawn the rest of the way onto the breast	Baby must be brought close to the breast to facilitate enough of the areola's being drawn into the mouth, rather than just the nipple tip.
• If the baby does not open wide enough, or if the nipple feels pinched, the mother can use the side of her index finger under her breast to gently pull down on the chin; this also rolls out the lower lip; some babies who do not open wide enough may benefit from sucking on an adult's finger before feeds	This technique helps baby draw in the portion of the breast needed to effect milk transfer with no pain.
The mother can massage and compress the breast to initiate milk flow if the baby does not begin sucking. If	Milk flow regulates sucking and alleviates unrelieved negative pressure when the baby is not swallowing peri-

Continued on following page

Table 33–9 *Continued*

BEDSIDE PROBLEM SOLVING: SORE NIPPLES

MANAGEMENT	RATIONALE
the baby pauses for long periods between sucking bursts, the mother can add the technique of alternate massage (squeezing the breast when baby pauses, alternate with the sucking bursts).	odically. Alternate massage provides milk incentives to start the suck-swallow sequence.
Avoid extension in the baby's back or neck; align head and trunk. The mother can use the football hold or prone infant positioning for a high-tone baby.	Extension causes jaw clenching with the tongue moving behind the lower gum.
The mother should avoid depressing the top of the breast or areola under the baby's nose to create an airway. A properly positioned baby should have the tip of the nose touching the breast and can breathe without assistance. The mother should also avoid the scissors hold on the areola, which compresses it and flattens an inverted nipple.	This action pulls the nipple and areola out of the mouth and contributes to nipple sucking and blisters.
The baby should be fed on cue 8 to 12 times each 24 hours. Avoid trying to lengthen time intervals between feeds or feeding the baby a bottle in the nursery at night (de Carvalho, M., Robertson, S., Klaus, M. H. [1984]. Does the duration and frequency of early breastfeeding affect nipple pain? *Birth*, 11, 81–84).	Feeding frequently avoids frantic overhungry pulling at breast. Full, firm breasts make latch-on more difficult and painful.
Breastmilk can be applied to the nipples after each feeding. Avoid creams, lotions, oils, and ointments unless they are medically indicated.	Some preparations have the ability to slow the healing process.
Avoid pacifiers (especially the flavored or scented ones as well as the orthodontic ones), artificial nipples on bottles, and nipple shields. Use alternative devices for supplemental feeds if needed (cup, syringe, dropper, feeding tube devices).	This prevents incorrect patterning of mouth conformation. Artificial nipples do not elongate and compress like a human nipple. Their use weakens a baby's suck as the baby decreases sucking pressure to slow milk and regulate milk flow.
Avoid squeezing the areola and pushing it into the baby's mouth. Baby's head should not be pushed into the breast.	Squeezing the areola changes and distorts its shape, stresses the skin, and contributes to cracks. Pushing the baby's head into the breast can cause reflexive neck extension and superficial nipple sucking.

Courtesy of Lactation Associates, 254 Conant Road, Weston, MA 02193.

Avoid recommending the use of a nipple shield. Shield use can decrease milk production by 22 to 58 percent, depending on the thickness of the shield. Inherent risks in the use of shields include addiction to the nipple shield for baby or mother, faulty sucking, decreased milk production, and assumption by the mother that the baby is getting enough milk. Use other means of assisting baby to latch on to the breast. No studies show that shields decrease nipple pain or promote healing.

The problems for which shields are used can require considerable amounts of time to manage. Refer the mother who is using a shield or wishes to use a shield to the hospital lactation consultant or one in the community for follow-up.

7. Routine use of nipple creams, ointments, or any other topical preparations should be avoided unless therapy has been prescribed for a dermatologic problem. Creams do not significantly affect the intensity or duration of nipple soreness.

Avoid the routine use or recommendation of topical applications of creams, oils, or other preparations to the nipple. Limited data are available on

Comparison of Nipple Shields and Breast Shells

NIPPLE SHIELDS	BREAST SHELLS
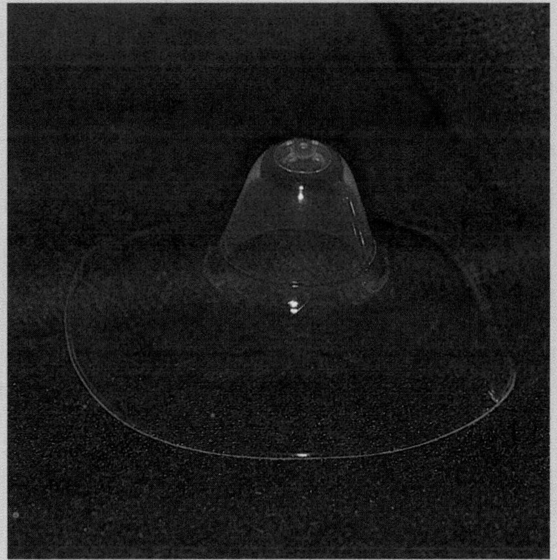	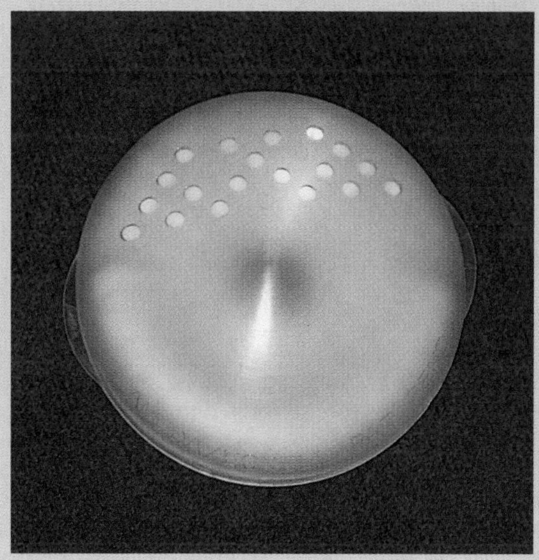
Primary Reason for Using	
Inverted nipple	Inverted nipple
Description	
Shape similar to rubber nipple	Plastic dome-shaped device
Disadvantages	
Abrades nipple tissue; prevents nipple from getting adequate stimulation (hence milk supply decreases); frequently a baby who has nursed with a shield refuses to nurse without it. Multiple studies have documented the detrimental effects of nipple shields.	Usually none, but can sometimes be too tight
Comments	
Should be used only as a last-resort management strategy. Referral should be made to a lactation consultant for follow-up.	Has been shown to be ineffective prenatally in everting flat nipples. Can be used post partum between feedings.

Adapted from Biancuzzo, M., (1994). *Breastfeeding the healthy newborn: A nursing perspective.* p. 47. White Plains, NY: March of Dimes Birth Defects Foundation.

the effectiveness of this practice. Use of topical preparations can delay the mother's seeking early help for sore nipples and may allow the condition to progress into a severe problem or early termination of breastfeeding.

Mothers should also refrain from using sunlamps or hair dryers on nipples. These devices remove an excessive amount of moisture from the skin. Their use could worsen the condition of the skin and make it more vulnerable to damage.

Application of expressed breast milk to the nipples after each feeding in the early days seems a reasonable approach. Breast milk is bacteriostatic and may provide some protection to damaged skin, minimizing bacterial counts and normalizing skin pH.

8. Pacifiers, especially scented or flavored ones, should not be given to breastfeeding infants in the hospital or during the learning stage of breastfeeding.

Displacement of sucking from the breast to a more powerful reinforcer may change and weaken an infant's suck. If effective sucking is changed or weakened, then appropriate stimulation to the breast is compromised. This can lead to insufficient milk and low infant weight gain (Newman 1990).

Avoid pacifier use during the hospital stay. Pacifier use can cause the baby's mouth to conform to the shape of the rigid object, which interferes with the baby's ability to remove milk from the breast. This improper mouth conformation may also cause nipple pain and damage from a tightly closed mouth that has difficulty opening wide. Limited milk removal and nipple pain can lead to insufficient milk and early weaning (Righard and Alade 1992). Pacifier use has also been implicated as a risk factor for acute otitis media. Displacement of sucking at breast (with its immune factors) to pacifier sucking (with no disease protection) may pose health hazards to infants, especially those who are the most environmentally compromised (Victora et al. 1993).

If the baby is fussy, rather than using a pacifier, consider the following:

- Observe breastfeeding to make sure that the baby is swallowing.
- Ensure that the mother knows when the baby is swallowing.
- Check that the baby is being fed 8 to 12 times each 24 hours.
- Eliminate visitors, television, and other distractions that prevent frequent, effective breastfeeding or that limit mother-baby contact.
- Encourage skin-to-skin contact of mother and baby with comfort sucking.
- Do not tell the mother that a frequently feeding or fussy baby is "using her as a pacifier." This creates an adversarial situation between the mother and baby and implies that the mother is more of an object than a person.
- Instruct the baby's father and grandparents to avoid pacifier use.
- Differentiate fussiness from the pain and consequences of birth trauma, such as a fractured clavicle or cephalhematoma.
- Advise the mother to put the baby in a sling at home to settle the baby.
- Consider giving mothers a sling rather than a commercial discharge pack that may contain a pacifier.
- Avoid night pacifier use.

9. Sterile water, glucose water, or formula should not be given to breastfed babies unless it is ordered by a physician for a specific problem. Bottles should not be placed in the infant's bassinet or opened and placed at the mother's bedside. In the hospital, supplemented breastfed infants can lose significantly more weight if they satisfy their hunger with low-calorie water (Glover and Sandilands 1990). Sugar water, at 6 calories per ounce, decreases breastfeeding frequency, allowing baby less opportunity to consume higher calorie colostrum at 18 calories per ounce. Glucose water does not lower bilirubin levels. Early and frequent feeds at breast help prevent lowered blood glucose levels. The higher protein levels in colostrum have a more stabilizing effect on blood glucose levels than does sugar water.

Facilitate early and frequent breastfeeding without restrictions to length. Encourage 24-hour rooming-in and nighttime feedings. Use alternate massage to increase the infant's intake. Early and frequent breastfeeding accelerates intestinal peristalsis, shortens gut transit time, and promotes stool output, which minimizes reuptake of bilirubin from the intestine. Decreased number of feedings or skipped night feeds contribute to calorie deprivation, dehydration, increased bilirubin levels, decreased blood glucose levels, impaired milk production, engorgement, slow weight gain, nipple confusion, and sore nipples.

Exercise careful consideration before using any formula in a breastfed infant, especially if there is a history of allergy in the family. Some infants who are exclusively breastfed develop allergic symptoms to cow's milk after their first challenge with it because of previous sensitization in utero, through their mother's milk, or in the hospital nursery.

Caution parents not to feed bottles of water to a fussy, ill, or hungry baby or to stretch intervals between breastfeedings. Use of water as a feeding supplement puts infants at an increased risk for oral water intoxication and hyponatremic seizures. Rapid ingestion of large volumes of fluids with little or no solutes can cause brain swelling and acute neurologic disturbances (Keating et al. 1991).

10. If a baby consistently feeds poorly in a period of two to three feedings, consider regular breast pumping to stimulate milk production. Expressed milk/colostrum can be fed to the baby by cup, dropper, or feeding tube device. The rapid pace of the hospital stay puts performance pressures on the staff, mother, and baby to hurry and establish in 24 hours or less what may take more like 36 to 48 hours or more. Hasty attempts to push the baby onto the breast, insertion of the breast into a baby's sensitive mouth like a bottle, and use of artificial nipples to ensure fluid intake may upset nature's intended sequence of learning how to feed.

There is a wide range of timing in babies for the acquisition of effective feeding skills. Maternal labor analgesia and anesthesia can delay effective breastfeeding by several hours to many days. Modify the postpartum environment to provide quiet, private time for calm attachment to the breast. Discourage visitors other than the father or significant other. Keep the baby in bed with the mother, skin-to-skin, to help repattern correct infant feeding sequences at breast. Turn off the television and unplug the telephone. Avoid unnecessary separation of the mother and baby.

If the mother is too ill to breastfeed the baby, use alternative feeding devices rather than artificial nipples (Table 33–10). This helps avoid nipple confusion. The father or other helper can feed the baby by dropper, cup, or feeding tube device. Consider the use of an electric breast pump that expresses both breasts simultaneously. Feed the baby any colostrum or milk obtained after pumping.

If the baby has not attached to the breast or shown much interest in feeding by the time a mother is halfway through her stay in the hospital, have her use an electric breast pump to help elongate the nipples, entice baby to breast, and stimulate the breasts if the baby is unable to do so. This helps avoid painful engorgement and low milk supply after the mother returns home.

11. Breastfeeding teaching, assessment, and documentation should be done on each shift during each contact with the mother to accomplish the necessary teaching in a short time (Shrago 1992). The length of hospital stay is now determined externally, rather than by the patient's recovery progress; therefore, nurses must squeeze assessment and teaching tasks into a compressed time that is not related to the patient's status or needs.

Care paths can be used to identify critical components of intervention and care that must occur to achieve a predetermined length of stay. Their use views patient care on a continuum, rather than as a series of discrete tasks. A path sequences major interventions to achieve teaching objectives and patient outcomes within the anticipated length of stay and states expected patient outcomes. It ensures consistency in patient care and eliminates duplication or omission of information. A time frame is constructed such that objectives are met on each shift or in designated times to avoid information overload at discharge. It is a systematic plan of care so that each nurse has responsibility for a part of the total patient education plan (Zander 1987; Zander 1991).

12. Before leaving the hospital, breastfeeding mothers should be able to

    - Position the baby correctly at breast
    - Latch the baby to breast properly
    - State when the baby is swallowing milk
    - State how many times each 24 hours the baby should be fed
    - Describe feeding cues that indicate when it is time to feed the baby
    - State how many wet diapers and how many bowel movements the baby should have each day during the first 2 weeks at home
    - Determine when a disposable diaper is wet
    - State how much weight the baby should be gaining at home
    - List indications for calling the pediatrician or family physician
    - State when and who to call for help with breastfeeding

A mother who can demonstrate the acquisition of these behaviors will be adequately instructed in the fundamentals of breastfeeding. Provide each breastfeeding mother with these ten topics formatted as a checklist. This helps the mother organize what she needs to learn while in the hospital as well as focus where she needs help with unmet skill attainment.

Provide an individualized feeding plan. Because new mothers have difficulty remembering verbal instructions, providing individualized written guidelines will help bridge memory gaps. Include an instant photograph of her baby properly positioned at breast and instructions for the baby's father or helper to assist with breastfeeding at home.

13. Mothers should be given names and telephone numbers of community resources to contact for

Table 33–10

BEDSIDE PROBLEM SOLVING: ALTERNATIVE FEEDING METHODS

Problem Description

A full-term breastfed baby who
- Cannot latch to the breast
- Latches only periodically
- Needs supplements
- Has a cleft lip or palate
- Has a dysfunctional or disorganized sucking pattern
- Is already nipple confused
- Can feed at breast but cannot satisfy all nutritional needs there
- Fights the breast and will benefit from some milk to help settle before feedings at breast
- Is sleepy and may arouse when first fed by cup or tube before being put to breast

Growing preemies on the maternity unit who
- Cannot latch to the breast
- Gag when a gavage tube is placed
- Are being breastfed but whose mothers cannot be present for all feedings
- Cannot obtain all the milk they need at breast
- Are nipple confused
- Are from a no-bottle protocol unit
- Have episodes of oxygen desaturation and bradycardia when fed by bottle
- Are so stressed by bottle feedings that they cannot obtain sufficient amounts of milk
- Spit up during or after many bottle feedings
- Shut down during bottle feedings
- Have a chronic inability to coordinate sucking, swallowing, and breathing

Contributing Factors

- Delay in going to breast
- Separation of mother and infant
- Failure to imprint on the breast
- Use of artificial nipples, pacifiers, nipple shields
- Prematurity
- Sedated infant from labor and delivery medications

MANAGEMENT	RATIONALE
For latch difficulties, consider the following techniques to provide a latch-on incentive. These techniques can also be used to construct the environment for all feeds to be done at breast until the baby no longer needs the extra help.	These devices can be used to start the baby sucking at breast. They can also be used to deliver supplements or incentives before and after breastfeeding attempts. The goal is to conduct as much and as many of the feedings at breast.
Dropper can be used to place a drop or two of colostrum/milk or glucose water into the side of baby's mouth at latch-on. For rapid side-to-side head movements, touch the midline of the upper lip, lead the baby to breast, and place a drop of milk into baby's mouth. Droppers can also be used for finger feeding to calm the baby before a feed or deliver supplement after breastfeed attempts. A finger is drawn by the baby into the mouth, and a soft clinic dropper full of milk is placed next to it. Milk is drawn out of the dropper when the baby sucks correctly. Milk is not pushed into baby's mouth. For a baby who chews on the finger, squeeze the dropper gently to deliver a couple of drops of milk; reward the sucking attempts each time with a drop of milk until the baby is sucking the milk out of the dropper by himself or herself.	

Continued on facing page

Table 33–10 *Continued*

BEDSIDE PROBLEM SOLVING: ALTERNATIVE FEEDING METHODS

MANAGEMENT	RATIONALE
Tube feeding devices (either commercial ones or butterfly tubing with the needle removed, hooked up to a 10-mL syringe[1]) can be used as an incentive or to deliver supplement at breast while the baby learns to breastfeed. These are taped over the areola and can be regulated by the height at which they are hung and the size of the tubing. If the baby cannot yet latch to the breast, supplements can be delivered by finger feeding with the tubing taped to a finger.[2]	
Syringes, such as a tuberculin syringe or periodontal syringe, can be used in much the same way as the dropper. The periodontal syringe has a curved tip and can rest in the corner of the baby's mouth while at breast so supplement can be given for sucking rewards and incentives. Check the tip of the periodontal syringe; some are rough or sharp.	
Cup feeding can be used for babies unable to feed at breast or who can obtain only a portion of their needs at breast. Cups are good for nipple-confused babies and babies who are unable to feed at breast because they have become dependent on finger feeding. Cup feeding can be used for both term and preterm babies as an interim measure until baby is fully established at breast.[3–8] Cup feeding instructions are as follows: • Cross baby's arms over the chest and wrap securely. • Sit the baby upright, supporting the baby's head and neck with one hand. • If the mother or nurse wants both hands free, the baby can be placed in her lap with her knees elevated so the baby is facing her. • Place a bib or little towel under baby's chin. • Fill the cup half full. A 28-mL plastic medicine cup can be used and compressed as needed for a better fit of the rim on the mouth. • Place the rim of the cup between the baby's upper and lower lips. • Elevate the cup so that milk touches the lips. The baby's cupped or grooved tongue will often rest under the cup, which may help the baby hold the cup better. • Keep the milk in touch with the baby's lips but do not pour it into baby's mouth. The baby will sip and swallow at his or her own pace. Hold the cup securely but do not press down on the baby's jaw. • Leave the cup in place when the baby pauses. Each time the cup is removed, the baby must reorganize movement patterns and the mouth, which can prolong the feeding and frustrate the baby.	Little energy is expended by cup feeding and the baby can pace feeding to avoid apnea, bradycardia, oxygen desaturation, spitting up, and general distress that can occur during bottle feedings. Avoiding an artificial nipple prevents weakening the baby's suck. A baby decreases sucking pressure to prevent choking and to control the rapid flow of milk from an artificial nipple.

Continued on following page

Table 33–10 *Continued*

BEDSIDE PROBLEM SOLVING: ALTERNATIVE FEEDING METHODS

MANAGEMENT	RATIONALE
• Avoid tilting the baby's head back to drain milk from the bottom of the cup. • If needed, jaw stability can be provided by slipping a finger under baby's chin to prevent the jaw from dropping down too far. • The Dancer hand position can be used to completely stabilize the head and jaw. The baby can be propped on a pillow elevated in the mother's lap. Her free hand forms a U under the baby's jaw with the thumb on one cheek and the index finger on the other. The baby's jaw rests in the area between these two fingers.	

[1]Edgehouse, L., Radzyminski, S. G. (1990). A device for supplementing breastfeeding. *MCN,* 15, 34–35.
[2]Bull, P., Barger, J. (1987). Fingerfeeding with the SNS. *Rental Roundup,* Summer.
[3]Lang, S. (1994). Cup-feeding: An alternative method. *Midwives Chronicle and Nursing Notes,* 107, 171–176.
[4]Jones, E. (1994). Breastfeeding in the preterm infants. *Modern Midwife,* 4, 22–26.
[5]Musoke, R. N. (1990). Breastfeeding promotion: Feeding the low birth weight infant. *International Journal Gynecology Obstetrics,* 1(Suppl), 57–59.
[6]Armstrong, H. C. (1987). Breastfeeding low birthweight babies: Advances in Kenya. *Journal Human Lactation,* 3, 34–37.
[7]Muhudhia, S. O., et al. (1989). Postnatal weight gain of exclusively breastfed preterm African infants. *Journal Tropical Pediatrics,* 35, 241–244.
[8]Minchin, M. (1987). Premature babies: Why breast is best. *New Generation,* September, 36–37.
Courtesy of Lactation Associates, 254 Conant Road, Weston, MA 02193.

help with breastfeeding. Such resources could include

- Hospital outpatient programs (Gillerman and Beckham 1991)
- Home visiting programs sponsored by the hospital, insurance carriers, Visiting Nurse Association, public health nurse (Serafino-Cross and Donovan 1992)
- Warm lines or hot lines for telephone help
- Lay breastfeeding support groups such as La Leche League or Nursing Mothers Councils
- Lactation consultants
- Breastfeeding clinics
- Parent support services
- WIC programs, peer counselors, neighborhood health centers

The need for home support is greater than ever. Women who are supported breastfeed longer, show enhanced breastfeeding competency, and become empowered with breastfeeding success.

Provide all breastfeeding women with support sources in the community. Early detection of problems, quick intervention, and health promotion activities are benefits from close follow-up. Rather than addressing ongoing difficulties or a weaning situation at a 2-week check, breastfeeding questions or problems are handled quickly, preserving lactation.

Do not give breastfeeding mothers commercial discharge packs containing infant formula and related items. Eliminating this practice supports the physiologic process of lactation, has positive benefit, and can increase the probability of breastfeeding success (Wright et al. 1996).

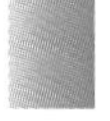

The Postnatal Period

New nursing mothers are discharged from the hospital at precisely the time they need the most help with breastfeeding. Fear, fatigue, and anxiety often accompany the mother. Continuation of breastfeeding care must be ensured during the transition home and for the period the mother lactates. Nurses in the outpatient or community setting provide this ongoing support. Depending on the practice setting, the nurse's responsibilities may include

- Initiating a follow-up telephone call on the day after discharge and periodically thereafter
- Conducting a home visit 24 to 48 hours after discharge
- Recognizing and preventing early breastfeeding problems
- Intervening with therapeutic guidelines for breastfeeding problems
- Assessing early infant behaviors
- Initiating or providing breastfeeding care for preterm mothers and infants
- Assisting with the selection of breast pumps and providing guidelines for their use

BREASTFEEDING COUNSELING AFTER DISCHARGE

Many hospitals, pediatric offices, and clinics routinely call new families after discharge to provide breastfeeding help and answer questions common to breastfeeding.

Question: How many times each 24 hours should the baby feed at breast?

Eight to 12 feeds is the normal range. Less than this may indicate underfeeding; more may indicate ineffective infant feeding behaviors. Sleepy babies may feed less than eight times each 24 hours; hungry, inefficient feeders may go to breast more than 12 times.

Question: How many wet diapers and bowel movements should the baby have each 24 hours?

Diaper counts range from two wet diapers and one bowel movement at day 1 to four to five wet diapers and three to four bowel movements at day 4 to eight wet diapers and three or more bowel movements at day 7. If the parent indicates a decreased diaper count, a home visit may be necessary for feeding observation. Possible solutions include increasing the number of feeds and use of such techniques as alternate massage and feeding on cue.

Question: Are the mother's nipples sore?

Sore nipples are an indicator that baby may not be positioned correctly at breast, which increases the chances of poor milk transfer from breast to baby. The nurse may discuss correct positioning or suggest a home visit. Sore breasts may indicate unrelieved engorgement. Increasing the number of feeds, using alternate massage, or pumping the breasts will relieve engorgement.

In addition, a home or office visit at 48 hours after discharge for a weight check is advised. Weight checks ensure adequacy of intake and identify problems early. The nurse is able to check positioning, latch-on, milk transfer, diaper count, and feeding cues for a sleepy baby.

EARLY BREASTFEEDING PROBLEMS

Engorgement

Breast changes after delivery are best viewed on a continuum from normal fullness to secondary or pathologic engorgement. Thirty to 40 hours after delivery, a major change occurs in both the composition and quantity of milk secreted. At the end of the first 2 days, the metabolic capacity of the breasts increases; this is noted by the mother as a feeling of breast fullness by the third day post partum. This normal fullness is the result of a large amount of fluid diverted to the breasts, resulting in lymphatic and vascular congestion and fluid accumulation in the breast tissue. Paralleling this is the increased volume of milk in the alveoli, lactiferous ducts, and lactiferous sinuses. This breast fullness is a positive sign of lactogenesis and is followed with continued frequent feedings (8 to 12 each 24 hours). The swelling (edema) dissipates by the end of the first week or so. This type of breast fullness is sometimes called physiologic or normal engorgement. Absence of this is an indicator of a possible pathologic process and needs immediate attention to discover factors delaying milk production.

Secondary or pathologic engorgement is often the result of mismanaged breastfeeding. The breasts change from normal fullness to gross enlargement. The breasts are hard and hot to the touch, the skin is shiny and taut, and there are lumps or blocked areas of the breast where milk cannot drain. Areolar engorgement, nipple flattening, and severe pain accompany breast engorgement. This type of milk stasis can be caused by infrequent feedings; a baby who feeds ineffectively; skipped feedings; long delays between feeds; poor positioning; temporary overproduction of milk; separation with no or infrequent pumping; interrupted breastfeeding with insufficient or no pumping; and the use of supplements or pacifiers that displace, change, or weaken the suck. If this type of engorgement is allowed to persist, it can lead to sore nipples as the areola and nipple become distorted, no latch-on, little or no milk transfer, decreased milk production (both acute and long term), slow weight gain, and mastitis.

Interventions include prevention and treatment by frequent feeds; alternate massage; proper positioning and latch-on; assessment for milk transfer; avoidance of limits of frequency and duration of feeds; avoidance of bottles, pacifiers, or nipple shields; and avoidance of long intervals between feedings. The breasts should be pumped with a large electric pump if there is an interruption or delay in baby latching to the breast or if baby cannot temporarily keep up with the amount of milk being produced. The baby will catch up in a day or two. Failure to pump milk allows the growing volume of milk to exert back pressure on the milk-secreting glands, slowing and stopping their activity. The longer milk stays in the breasts without removal, the higher the level of suppressor peptides that provide local control of milk synthesis. This down-regulates the quantity of milk and can lead to atrophy and shut down of milk-secreting glands and insufficient milk supply by 4 to 6 weeks.

Cold packs can be placed on the breasts between feedings to reduce edema. Warm compresses or immersing the breasts in a bowl of hot water for about 3 minutes before feedings and using breast massage will enhance the milk ejection reflex and improve milk flow. Pain medication such as acetaminophen can enhance maternal comfort. Do not limit maternal fluid intake. The amount of fluid a woman drinks does not reduce engorgement or affect milk supply.

Plugged Milk Ducts

Areas of the duct system that transport milk through the breast may occasionally become blocked. Precise causes are not known, but the obstruction is usually a local accumulation of milk and shed cells that impede or interrupt the flow of milk. Factors associated with these blockages include poor or inadequate drainage of a section of the breast. This may occur from skipped feedings, engorgement, a blocked nipple pore, or an inefficiently nursing baby. A mechanical blockage could occur from a tight-fitting bra, restrictive clothing, or straps from baby carrier packs.

The affected area may feel like a hard pea and be tender to the touch under reddened skin. If this blockage persists, milk may back up into a lobe of the breast and a large area may experience little or no milk drainage. Mothers of multiples with an abundant milk supply may commonly experience blockages. Interventions include

- Frequent breastfeeding beginning on the affected side
- Thorough drainage of each quadrant of the breast at each feeding
- Warm compresses or immersing the breast in a bowl of hot water with massage of the affected area before each feeding
- Massage of the affected area while the baby is feeding
- Sometimes changing the baby's position at breast is helpful

Improvement can be seen by the end of a feeding or within 24 to 48 hours. Unsuccessfully treated blockages can lead to mastitis.

Mastitis

Mastitis is an infectious process in the breast. Mothers generally present with symptoms of fatigue, chills, and aching; a red, hot, tender section of the breast; and fever of 101°F (38.5°C) or higher. The infection is usually unilateral and frequently in the upper outer quadrant. While the infectious process may raise the sodium and chloride levels in the milk, the milk remains safe and nutritious. Mastitis is most likely to occur during the first several weeks after delivery. About one third of cases have been found to occur after 6 months (Riordan and Nichols 1990). The sixth postpartum week was the most common time of mastitis (Foxman et al. 1994). Factors associated with lactation mastitis include stress, fatigue, obstructed milk ducts, cracked or fissured nipples, engorgement, and abrupt changes in the number of feeds. In the week before the mastitis, mothers were more likely to have experienced fatigue (fewer hours of sleep each day, fewer daytime naps), stress, cracked nipples, and plugged milk ducts (Riordan and Nichols 1990; Foxman et al. 1994). Women who had experienced mastitis with a previous child were twice as likely to have mastitis.

The offending organisms are usually *Staphylococcus aureus, Escherichia coli,* and less frequently *Streptococcus.* Standard antibiotic treatment is typically a penicillinase-resistant penicillin (cloxacillin, dicloxacillin, oxacillin) or a cephalosporin (such as cephalexin or cefaclor) given for 10 to 14 days. All of these antibiotics are compatible with breastfeeding (see Appendix V). Chronic or recurring mastitis is sometimes seen when antibiotic treatment is not prescribed or is not continued for a full 10 to 14 days, when the organism is resistant to the antibiotic, or when there is continued reinfection acquired from the baby or another carrier in the household. At this point, a culture and sensitivity test should be done on the breast milk, the areolar skin, and the baby's nasopharynx and oropharynx to determine the actual organism, what it is most sensitive to, and the source of continued reinfection. Treatment includes

- 10 to 14 days of antibiotics
- Bed rest
- Frequent nursing starting on the affected side
- Breast massage before and during each feeding to thoroughly drain any blockages (or use of a breast pump if the baby is unable to do this)
- Moist heat, increased fluids, and increased vitamin C are helpful

It is important that breastfeeding continue on the affected side, because failure to do so increases the risk for abscess formation and relapse. Some mothers are maintained with 500 mg daily

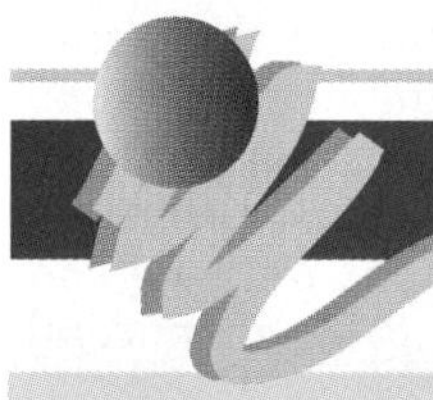

IMPROVING YOUR PRACTICE

THE NURSE'S RESPONSIBILITY RELATED TO MEDICATIONS AND THE BREASTFEEDING MOTHER

The nurse must be knowledgeable about the effect of drugs on lactation, the onset and peak duration of the drug's action, and the contraindications to taking specific drugs by the breastfeeding mother. The nurse is also responsible for teaching the mother about the therapeutic and adverse effects of the drug and serving as the woman's advocate with health care professionals who prescribe drug treatment. You can improve your practice related to medications and the breastfeeding mother by following these guidelines.

- KNOW THE RISKS AND BENEFITS OF DRUGS AND THEIR EFFECT ON BREASTFEEDING MOTHER AND INFANT. When necessary, remind the physician who is prescribing a drug that the woman is breastfeeding her infant. Encourage the mother to alert her dentist and other health care professionals that she is breastfeeding. If the physician recommends discontinuing breastfeeding because of a medication, ask about the perceived risk of the drug on lactation and to the infant. Also, consult the American Academy of Pediatrics comprehensive list of drugs, entitled Transfer of Drugs and Other Chemicals Into Human Milk (see Appendix V).
- DETERMINE THE DRUG'S ONSET, PEAK, AND DURATION OF ACTION. This will help you to establish an appropriate schedule for the administration of the drug. The drug should be administered so that its peak effect is after the mother breastfeeds her baby. Sources of information are the American Academy of Pediatrics comprehensive list of drugs (See Appendix V; the University of California at San Diego (UCSD) Medical Information, (900) 288–8273; and the Lactation Fax Hotline, Pharmasoft Publishing; call (806) 358–8138 for instructions.
- TEACH THE MOTHER THE RISKS OF DRUGS DURING LACTATION. This should include birth control pills and other birth control methods (Norplant, Depo-Provera); prescription drugs; over-the-counter drugs; other drugs such as alcohol; caffeine use and smoking; and illegal drugs. These are the major areas of concern for most lactating women. While some of the drugs listed in this section may be definitely contraindicated, others are safe only if used in moderation, and some are safe and do not interfere with lactation.

The nurse plays a critical role in promoting successful breastfeeding by being knowledgeable about the effects of drugs on lactation and on the infant and by educating breastfeeding mothers about a drug's effect on her and her infant.

Adapted from Biancuzzo, M. (1994). *Breastfeeding the healthy newborn: A nursing perspective.* pp. 47–48. White Plains, NY: March of Dimes Birth Defects Foundation.

of erythromycin for chronic bacterial disease of the breast during the entire lactation period. If family members are identified as asymptomatic disease carriers, they are also treated.

Breastfeeding Practices and Jaundice

Physiologic, pathologic, and breastfeeding jaundice are discussed in Chapter 32. Breastfed infants do not produce more bilirubin than artificially fed infants do (Maisels 1988), even though they are reputed to have higher bilirubin levels. Several studies have shown that the more sugar water that is given to breastfed infants, the higher their bilirubin levels, the less breast milk they consume, and the less they stool (Nicoll et al. 1982; de Carvalho et al. 1981; Kuhr and Paneth 1982). Calorie deprivation and decreased stooling lead to bilirubin reabsorption and increased bilirubin levels. Therefore, preventive measures should include

- Early frequent breastfeeding with alternate massage if necessary to sustain sucking and swallowing
- No bottles of sterile or glucose water. Glucose water contains 6 calories per ounce; colostrum has 18 calories per ounce. Displacing colostrum

and breast milk intake with sugar water reduces calorie intake by two thirds, which increases the likelihood of intestinal bilirubin reabsorption. Supplementing with water or dextrose in water does not lower bilirubin levels (Nicoll et al. 1982).

- Phototherapy is often used when bilirubin levels reach 15 to 20 mg/dL (American Academy of Pediatrics 1994). Phototherapy lights can be brought to the home to avoid readmission. Fiberoptic blankets can also be used at home; these wrap the baby in phototherapy lights and make breastfeeding easier since the eyes do not need to be covered and therapy can continue during feedings

Early exaggerated jaundice while breastfeeding is frequently an outcome of poor breastfeeding management or follow-up (lack-of-breastfeeding jaundice)(Auerbach and Gartner 1987). Breast milk jaundice or late-onset jaundice is seen in only a small percentage of breastfed infants. The baby is 5 to 7 days old before this diagnosis is considered. Speculation abounds as to the agent in some mothers' milk that would prolong jaundice, but no definite cause has been identified. The bilirubin levels may show two peaks, at 3 to 4 days and again at 10 to 21 days. Babies with late-onset jaundice have other forms of disease ruled out and present as healthy, vigorous, and gaining weight appropriately. Treatment is generally just observational unless bilirubin levels reach 25 mg/dL, when phototherapy or temporary interruption of breastfeeding is considered (Oski 1992).

Choices of interventions and nursing responsibilities at this point are: to initiate phototherapy; secure home phototherapy services (lights or blanket); monitor bilirubin levels with the physician; explore the use of intermittent phototherapy, 1 hour of every 4 (Lau and Fung, 1984); consider placing the baby in natural light, unclothed, at a window but not in direct sunlight; and explore alternating feedings at breast with commercial baby milk.

If breastfeedings are alternated with commercial baby milk feedings, then at every other feeding the mother will pump breast milk when the baby receives artificial milk. This pumped breast milk can be frozen for later use; expressed mother's milk that has been heated to 56°C for 15 minutes can be used in place of commercial baby milk. This alters whatever is in the breast milk that contributes to prolonged jaundice. This is especially important to discuss in allergic families.

Breastfeeding may be interrupted for various periods. The mother will be advised to pump her breasts 8 to 12 times each 24 hours to maintain her milk supply. Choosing this option can produce undesired outcomes. Interrupting breastfeeding can reduce continued breastfeeding by 50 percent, increase emergency room visits, increase sick visits, and alter the parents' perception of their child to one of special vulnerability (Kemper et al. 1989, 1990). Care should be taken to explain that the infant is not sick; that the elevated bilirubin levels are not an indication of a serious ongoing condition; and that once the levels drop to normal, the baby has recovered.

EARLY INFANT BEHAVIORS

Much of the neonate's behavior is reflexive. Reflexes are protective and enhance survival until the brain matures and assumes control over behavior. Temperament styles vary from a quiet, nondemanding, placid baby to a high-activity, high-needs infant. An infant who is crying is signaling a need (food, comfort, help with behavioral organization). Neonates do not ask for more than what they need. Thus, parents should respond to these cries. They cannot spoil a newborn or make the baby overdependent on the parents.

Breastfed babies need 8 to 12 feedings each 24 hours. A breastfed baby who cries after feedings and is unable to settle may indicate that not enough milk has been taken. If a mother describes this type of behavior, she may assume that she has insufficient milk and start supplementing with bottles of commercial baby milk. The nurse should intervene with a feeding observation and work toward improving breastfeeding techniques. If the baby is receiving sufficient milk at breast but is just fussy, the mother can be encouraged to wear baby in a sling, which is soothing and provides easy access to the breast. Infants cry more and are more wakeful during the late afternoon and evening. This is a time when babies will bunch or cluster several feedings into a short period. Experienced breastfeeding mothers feed the baby a lot during this time to prepare baby for a longer stretch of sleep at night.

Each baby differs in the number of hours of sleep experienced, but all will get as much sleep as they need. Sleeping is not an indication that baby is getting enough milk. Babies tend to have short periods of sleep interrupted by fussing and crying. This is normal during the day and night and should not be construed as an infant sleep disorder. A breastfed neonate who is sleeping several 4- or 5-hour stretches each 24 hours may be at risk for reduced milk intake and slow weight gain. Behavioral feeding cues should be taught or reviewed to ensure sufficient milk production and an adequate number of feedings.

BREASTFEEDING CARE FOR THE PRETERM MOTHER AND INFANT

Preterm birth is a bewildering and frightening crisis that occurs in approximately 7 to 10 percent of U. S. births. What and how to feed these babies presents a challenge to both mothers and health professionals. A baby born before 37 weeks' gestation is premature. A very-low-birth-weight baby is an infant weighing less than 1500 g (3 pounds, 5 ounces). A baby weighing between 500 g and 1000 g is sometimes called a micropreemie. Preterm infants are not simply smaller versions of term infants. They are born into a world in which they are not equipped to survive on their own. The degree of prematurity influences not only how these babies are fed but also the nature and number of prematurity-related problems they may encounter.

Mothers should be encouraged to provide milk for their babies. During the first 4 weeks of lactation after a preterm birth, mother's milk contains higher levels of protein, sodium, chloride, magnesium, fat, and IgA (an important immunoglobulin) (Butte et al. 1984). The immune system of human milk helps protect preemies from sepsis (Goldman et al. 1994), necrotizing enterocolitis (Lucas and Cole 1990), and rehospitalization (Malloy and Graubard 1994). Preemies at 8 years of age who were fed breast milk in the NICU, even by gavage, showed an 8-point IQ advantage over those not fed breast milk (Lucas et al. 1992).

Larger, more mature preemies who can consume 180 mL/kg per day may be able to grow appropriately without needing their milk fortified. However, if the baby cannot consume this much milk, calcium and phosphorus are generally added to the mother's milk. Some units use a commercial fortifier containing bovine milk protein and numerous other ingredients, without analyzing the mother's milk before fortification. This could lead to overnutrition or undernutrition. Polberger and Lonnerdal (1993) recommended analysis of the mother's milk to provide individualized fortification to better meet the needs of each preemie. While the goal of preemie nutrition in most units is to support the same growth rate as if the baby were still in utero, this may not always be possible. Improved weight gain has been seen by using hindmilk or fortified hindmilk, which is known to have two to three times the fat content of foremilk (Valentine et al. 1994). Care must be taken in supplementing human milk with additives; some may adversely affect the absorption of other nutrients or interfere with the antiinfective properties of the milk. Adding regular or premature formula to breast milk reduced lysozyme activity by 41 to 74 percent. Human milk fortifier reduced activity by 19 percent. All cow's milk formulas increased *E. coli* growth (Quan et al. 1994).

Given the importance of breast milk to this population of infants and the repeated statements by preterm mothers that breastfeeding was the only thing they could uniquely do for their baby, then the 30 to 70 percent breastfeeding failure rate before the baby leaves the hospital becomes an important issue (Ehrenkranz et al. 1985). Major system barriers to successful breastfeeding for this population include

- Inconsistent and conflicting information
- Detrimental nursery practices
- Lack of a single, knowledgeable source of help
- Inadequate follow-up after discharge

To address these issues, many NICUs have a clinical nurse specialist or lactation consultant who coordinates breastfeeding care in the unit.

Helping Mothers Breastfeed Preemies

Begin preliminary breastfeeding activities as soon as baby is stable in units with skin-to-skin (kangaroo) care. This type of care decreases crying; increases weight gain; stabilizes vital signs and temperature; and results in earlier discharge, higher milk yields, and earlier and longer breastfeeding (Anderson 1991). The baby has self-regulatory access to breastfeeding and can often avoid using bottles by moving directly from gavage to breast. In units without kangaroo care, mothers begin holding their infant in a breastfeeding position, allowing nuzzling of the nipple, and hand express small amounts of breast milk so that the baby tastes and associates mouth movements with nourishment. The baby can also be put to breast for practice after the breast has been pumped, with no expectation of milk intake.

In units with a no-bottle protocol, practice sessions occur at breast as soon as the baby is stable and tolerates short periods outside the isolette. Stine (1990) recommended the following supplementation after breastfeeding by gavage:

- None if the baby breastfeeds well with swallowing for 5 minutes
- Half the usual volume if baby breastfeeds for less than 5 minutes
- Full feed if the baby did not breastfeed

Finger feeding or cup feeding can be used after breastfeeds to deliver any needed supplement. This reduces the problems associated with the fast flow of milk from artificial nipples.

If the baby latches to the breast but cannot sustain sucking for a full feeding, consider using a supplemental nutrition system or a similar device made from a syringe and length of No. 5 tubing. The supplemental nutrition system is a plastic bottle for holding milk; two lengths of tubing emerge and are taped to each areola (Fig. 33–9). The baby feeds from the breast while the supplement is delivered, which helps avoid artificial nipples, stimulate milk production, nourish the baby, and assist the baby in learning how to feed at breast. The baby can be positioned in the football (clutch) hold or a transitional hold (across the lap with the opposite hand holding the baby's head).

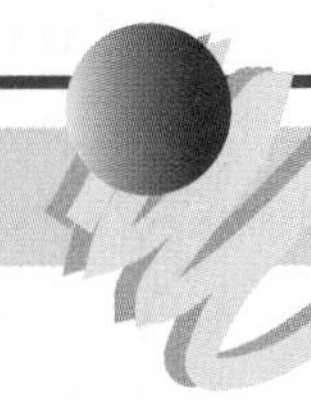

TEACHING GUIDE

GOING HOME BREASTFEEDING FOR PRETERM INFANT

TOPIC	*MAJOR CONCEPTS*
Planning for discharge	Advise your client to secure help with other children and household responsibilities for the first 2 weeks at home. She should also keep the phone number of the lactation consultant or other health care professional knowledgeable about breastfeeding preterm infants. Suggest that she call or arrange for an appointment regarding breastfeeding help, as needed.
Number of feedings	The infant should be fed on cue 8 to 12 times per 24 hours or more often if needed. Short feedings increase the efficiency of feedings (baby sucks better and does not get as tired). Frequent feedings increase assurance that baby is getting adequate milk (Newell et al. 1993).
Watch for cues that infant may be hungry	The preterm infant may sleep a lot and may not give distinct hunger signs. Parents should watch for other cues of the preterm infant that may indicate the baby is hungry: rapid eye movements under closed lids, sucking movements of mouth and lips, stretching of body parts, and little sounds that baby makes. The infant should be fed when these cues are noticed. In time, mother or caregiver will be able to identify the unique subtle cues of baby that indicate hunger.
Use alternate massage	Breast massage increases the fat content and volume of breast milk (Stutte et al. 1988). Breast milk is readily available to the infant, which promotes sustained sucking. Increased calories in hindmilk help increase weight gain.
Avoid overstimulation of infant	Preterm infants can easily become overstimulated because their immature nervous systems have difficulty dealing with multiple sensory inputs. This can have a negative impact on their ability to breastfeed. The infant needs a quiet, calm environment with minimal stimulation. Activities should be avoided during breastfeeding that may overstimulate the infant, such as rubbing the head or other body parts, singing, jiggling, bright lights, loud noises, and areas of high activity level.
Periodic increase in frequency of nursing	The infant will have rapid growth spurts. During these times, the infant will want to nurse more frequently. Frequency of feedings

Continued on facing page

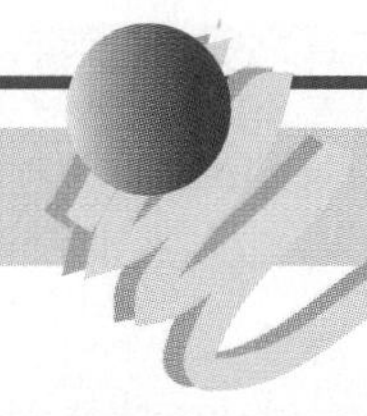

TEACHING GUIDE Continued

GOING HOME BREASTFEEDING FOR PRETERM INFANT

TOPIC	*MAJOR CONCEPTS*
	should be increased according to the infant's needs. The increased frequency of feedings will increase milk production to meet the infant's increased requirements.
Weighing infant	The infant should be weighed weekly for 4 weeks after discharge, starting the next morning after discharge. The infant should be weighed unclothed at about the same time of morning before a feeding. The baby's health care provider should be asked for guidelines regarding adequate weight gain. If the baby does not have adequate weight gain, the baby's health care provider and lactation consultant should be contacted for help.

SPECIAL PROBLEMS

Low milk supply

The Medela Supplemental Nursing System (SNS) may be used as follows until adequate milk supply is established:

- Start with both lines of the SNS pinched closed; breastfeed infant on both breasts using alternate massage.
- When infant no longer swallows with breast compression on either side, open the SNS tubing.
- As infant leaves more milk in the SNS at the end of feeding, reduce amount of supplemental feeding gradually until the baby is entirely breastfeeding.

The SNS maximizes breast stimulation, increases milk supply, and provides sufficient calories for growth.

Infant mostly bottle feeding at discharge

Shortly after arrival at home, the infant should be breastfed; then the infant should be breastfed one to two times per hour for 3 to 5 hours. At the next feeding, the baby should be given breast milk or formula by bottle. For the next 2 to 3 days, breastfeeding should be followed by a supplemental bottle after each feeding. When the infant takes only half the supplement, the supplemental bottle may be offered at every other feeding. When the infant takes only half of that supplement, the supplemental bottle may be offered every third feeding until supplements are no longer necessary. Monitor weight gain weekly until breastfeeding is totally established.

Adapted from Walker, M. (1992). Breastfeeding the premature infant. *NAACOG'S Clinical Issues in Perinatal and Women's Health Nursing: Breastfeeding,* 3, 620–633.

The mother will use alternate massage on each breast at each feed until the baby no longer needs help in sustaining sucking and swallowing. Overstimulation should be prevented by decreasing lights and noise and by not stroking or talking to the baby during the feeding. If the baby does not open the mouth wide enough, pull down very gently on the chin.

Before discharge, some units have a parents' room where they stay with the baby to learn parenting skills and refine breastfeeding techniques. Other units admit the mother and baby to the

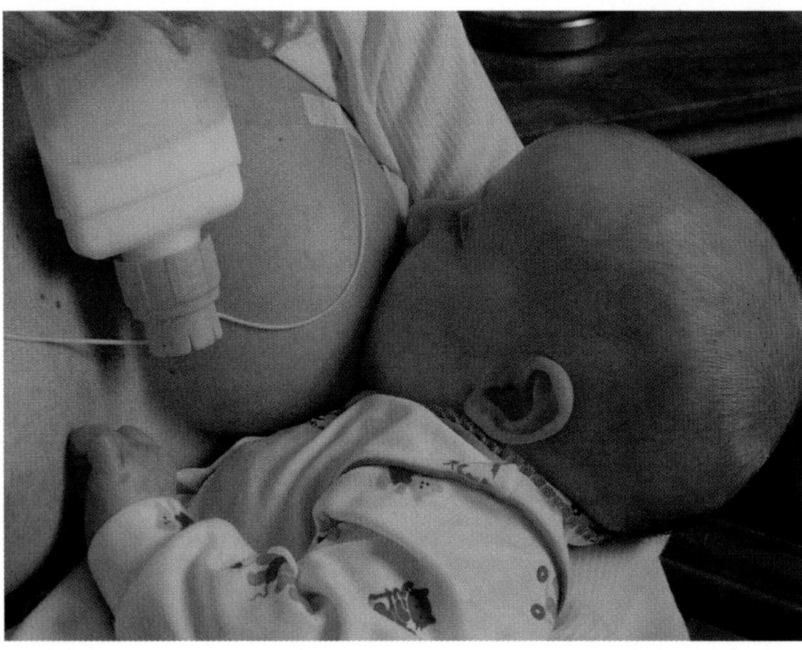

Figure 33–9

The supplemental nutrition system allows the mother to nurse her infant while the supplement is delivered, helping to avoid artificial nipples, stimulate milk production, nourish the baby, and assist the infant in learning how to feed at the breast. (Photo courtesy of Medela, McHenry, IL.)

regular postpartum floor for a couple of days to establish breastfeeding and increase the mother's confidence in her caretaking ability. Written feeding plans for discharge should be created (Walker 1992)(see Teaching Guide). Emphasis in the feeding plans should be placed on maintaining an abundant milk supply, how to judge the adequacy of intake at each breastfeeding, how to ensure intake of optimal amounts of milk at each feed, how to know the baby is swallowing, and how to know the baby is getting enough (Kavanaugh et al. 1995).

EXPRESSING, STORING, AND TRANSPORTING BREAST MILK

Prematurity generally involves a delay before the baby can feed at breast. Therefore, mothers must initiate and maintain their milk supply with a breast pump. Most mothers obtain the best results with a piston-type intermittent-pressure electric breast pump (Fig. 33–10). These pumps are capable of pumping both breasts simultaneously, which increases prolactin levels, increases milk yields, and decreases pumping time by half (Neifert and Seacat 1985).

Milk expression should begin as soon after delivery as possible and continue eight or more times each 24 hours. Mothers will need to rent a pump for use after discharge. Lists of pump stations in the community can be obtained from the manufacturers. Pumps are available from pharmacies, medical supply companies, breastfeeding counselors, and lactation consultants. Written pumping instructions that are provided to mothers generally include the following:

- Begin pumping as soon after delivery as possible with an electric breast pump whose collection kit pumps both breasts simultaneously.
- Colostrum and milk can be pumped into Vol-u-feeders at first, which fit on some pump kits to avoid transfer of milk into other containers.
- Pump at least eight times each 24 hours.
- Wash hands and nails thoroughly before each pumping session, taking care not to touch the insides of the collection kit.
- Some units use a sterile collection kit for each pumping session while the mother is in the hospital. Others use one for each day, which is washed after each use. The nurse is responsible for proper care of the pump and collection kits to ensure bacteriologically safe milk. The outside of the hospital pump should be cleaned with antiseptic solution daily and cultured monthly (Wilks and Meier 1988).
- Encourage mothers to stimulate the milk ejection reflex before beginning to pump as well as to massage each quadrant of the breast thoroughly while pumping. This reduces the likelihood of sore nipples and blockages in the breast. For many mothers, this also shortens pumping times and increases the amount of milk pumped at each session (Auerbach and Walker 1994).
- Milk should be stored in sterile, airtight containers with the name of the infant, date, and

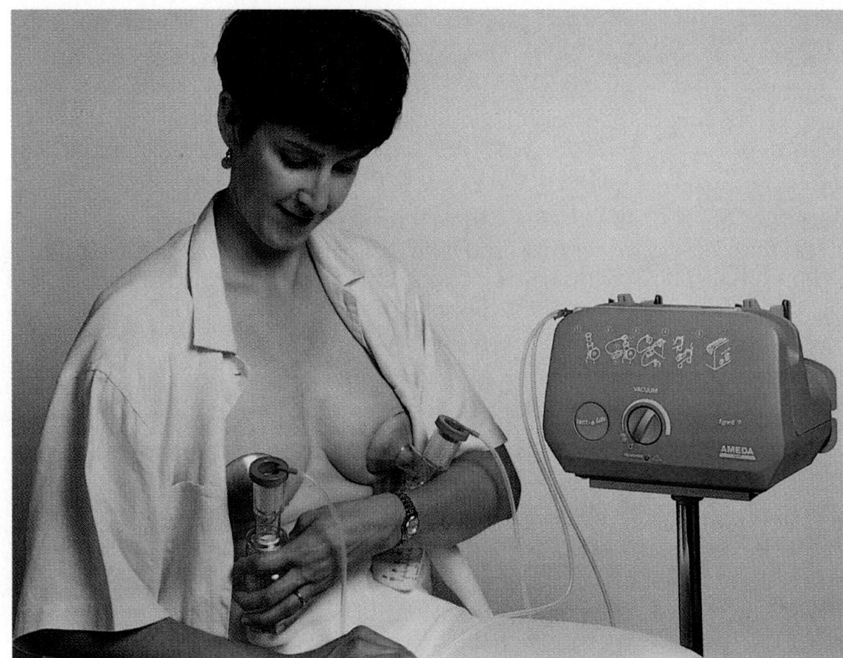

Figure 33–10

The breast pump allows the mother to breastfeed even when she needs to be away from her infant as well as to continue to stimulate the production of milk if the baby is unable to nurse for a given time. (Photo courtesy of Ameda/Egnell, Cary, IL.)

time of milk expression on the label. Containers can be made of glass, polycarbonate (clear, hard plastic), or polypropylene (cloudy, hard plastic). Use of polyethylene soft bags for milk storage for preterm infants is discouraged (Human Milk Banking Association of North America 1993).

- Mothers must be referred to a source of breastfeeding support in the community if there is no out-patient lactation program in the hospital.

Implications for Research

A large body of research supports the advantages and benefits of breastfeeding to the infant and mother (Department of Health and Human Services 1984). The importance of breastfeeding as a public health issue is underscored by the health status objective for the year 2000 on breastfeeding (Department of Health and Human Services 1995), which has goals of a 75 percent breastfeeding rate for all mothers in the early postpartum period and a 50 percent breastfeeding rate at 5 to 6 months. Research is needed on the most effective ways to achieve these goals:

- What approaches are the most effective for increasing the breastfeeding rate of all mothers in the early postpartum period?
- What approaches are the most effective for increasing the rate of continued breastfeeding until 5 to 6 months?
- What approaches are the most effective for increasing the breastfeeding rates of special populations (black, Hispanic, and American Indian/Alaskan Native mothers)?
- What interventions in the hospital are the most effective in promoting the initiation of breastfeeding?

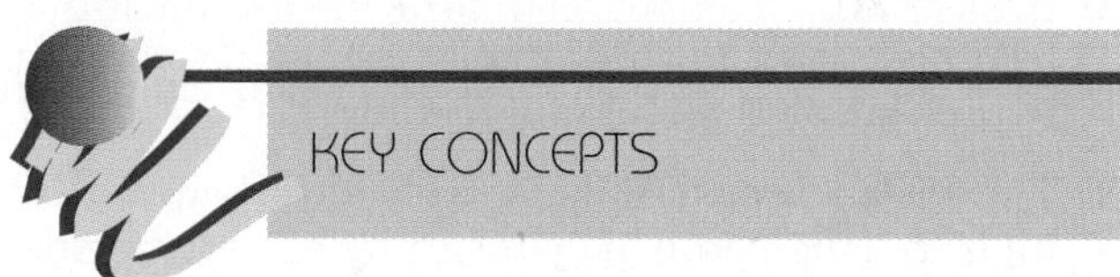

KEY CONCEPTS

- ▼ Breastfeeding is a public health issue of documented importance to infants and mothers.
- ▼ Breastfeeding is a health-promoting behavior compatible with government health goals for the nation.
- ▼ Cultural and medical barriers to breastfeeding exist in numerous settings, which are being addressed through programs designed to promote, protect, and support breastfeeding.
- ▼ The nurse's role is critical to successful lactation outcomes for both healthy and high-risk infants.
- ▼ Women have the right to be fully, not partially, informed regarding all aspects of providing or not providing breast milk for their infant.
- ▼ Breastfeeding and breast milk protect infants against disease and allergy and are central to

the proper growth and development of the brain.

- ▼ Breastfeeding has major health benefits for women as well, including decreased risk for breast and ovarian cancer and osteoporosis.
- ▼ Given the critical role of hospitals, UNICEF and the World Health Organization launched the Baby Friendly Hospital Initiative to motivate hospitals in removing institutional barriers to breastfeeding.
- ▼ In the United States, there was a dramatic decline in breastfeeding during the 1930s and 1940s, lasting until the early 1970s, when only 22 percent of infants in hospitals were breastfed. The last two decades have shown a considerable improvement.
- ▼ Currently, the *Healthy People 2000* national health goals for breastfeeding are targeted at a 75 percent initiation rate and a 50 percent continuation rate at 5 to 6 months by the year 2000.
- ▼ Breast milk is a highly specialized, complex fluid uniquely suited to the needs and metabolic capacity of a growing infant. In addition to protein, fat, lactose, vitamins, minerals, and trace elements, breast milk contains hormones and dozens of enzymes that have both regulating and disease protective effects that are not found in infant formulas.
- ▼ Colostrum has a laxative effect on the newborn, encouraging the expulsion of bilirubin-laden meconium.
- ▼ Breast milk composition also varies during a feeding; a two to three times higher fat content is present at the end of a feeding.
- ▼ The fat in breast milk is well absorbed and is high in long-chain polyunsaturated fatty acids. These are important in brain development, nerve myelination, and retinal growth. Infant formulas contain little or none of these.
- ▼ Breast milk contains antibacterial, antiviral, and antiparasitic factors. Secretory IgA represents more than 90 percent of the immunoglobulins and covers the intestinal mucosa with a protective coating that prevents adhesion or penetration of the gut by pathogens.
- ▼ The major sources of influence in feeding choice vary by ethnic background: the male partner for Anglo-Americans, the mother's mother for Hispanics, and close friends for black women.
- ▼ Skin and hair color have no influence or predictive value regarding sore nipples.
- ▼ One of several indicators of adequate milk-making potential is breast changes and enlargement during pregnancy.
- ▼ Flat nipples can contribute to soreness if the infant cannot latch on and form enough of a teat to draw into the mouth.
- ▼ Creams, lotions, and ointments are not necessary on the nipple or areola; they have not been shown to prevent or cure sore nipples.
- ▼ Uninterrupted contact after birth decreases crying and startling in newborns, reduces blood pressure, and stabilizes temperature and respirations faster than when the infant is left alone in a bassinet.
- ▼ Infants should be placed at breast immediately after delivery or as soon as possible thereafter.
- ▼ In the absence of other symptoms, a low-grade fever does not pose a danger to the breastfed baby. Many women who have had epidural anesthesia exhibit low-grade fevers as a side effect.
- ▼ Proper positioning and attachment to the breast avoids nipple trauma, ensures adequate milk intake, and provides positive feedback experiences to the mother.
- ▼ Swallowing indicates that nutritive sucking is occurring and that milk is being received by the baby.
- ▼ Mothers do not sleep longer or better when their babies are returned to the nursery at night.
- ▼ Breastfed babies should be fed 8 to 12 times each 24 hours. Scheduled or limited feedings create hunger and crying in infants and can lead to maternal insufficient milk supply.
- ▼ Time limits for breastfeeding on each side should be avoided.
- ▼ Nipple trauma is most frequently caused by physical or mechanical problems of attaching baby to the breast.
- ▼ Nipple shield use can decrease milk production by 22 to 58 percent, depending on the thickness of the shield.
- ▼ Use of nipple creams does not significantly affect the intensity or duration of nipple soreness.
- ▼ Avoid use of sunlamps and hair dryers on the nipples; they remove an excessive amount of moisture from the skin.
- ▼ Avoid the use of pacifiers, especially scented or flavored ones. This displaces sucking from the breast and increases the chances for improper latch-on, poor milk transfer, weakened suck, slow weight gain, and illness.
- ▼ Sterile water, glucose water, or formula should not be given to breastfed babies unless it is medically indicated.

- ▼ Maternal labor analgesia and anesthesia can delay effective breastfeeding by several hours to many days.
- ▼ Avoid giving mothers commercial discharge packs from baby milk companies. They have no therapeutic benefit and decrease the probability of breastfeeding success (Snell et al. 1992).
- ▼ Decreased diaper counts during the first week necessitate a visit and feeding observation.
- ▼ Sore nipples are an indicator that baby may not be positioned correctly at breast.
- ▼ Milk production is under both endocrine and autocrine control. It is during the early days that frequent feedings, which drain the breasts, increase the quantity and sensitivity of prolactin receptors in the breasts.
- ▼ Mastitis is most likely to occur during the first several weeks after delivery.
- ▼ The populations at an increased risk for bilirubin deposition into the brain are preterm babies; babies with ABO incompatibility or hemolytic diseases; and babies who have experienced acidosis, anoxia, asphyxia, hypothermia, or infection (Newman and Maisels 1990).
- ▼ The more sugar water given to breastfed infants, the higher their bilirubin levels at day 3.
- ▼ An infant who is crying is signaling a need.
- ▼ Preterm birth occurs in approximately 7 to 10 percent of U. S. births.
- ▼ A baby born before 37 weeks' gestation is preterm.
- ▼ Preemies who were fed breast milk showed an 8-point IQ advantage at age 8 years.
- ▼ The immune system of human milk helps protect preemies from sepsis, necrotizing enterocolitis, and rehospitalization.
- ▼ Emphasis in preemie feeding plans should be placed on maintaining an abundant milk supply, how to judge the adequacy of intake at each breastfeeding, how to ensure intake of optimal amounts of milk at each feed, how to know the baby is swallowing, and how to know the baby is getting enough.

References

Adair, L. S. (1983). Feeding babies: Mothers' decisions in an urban U.S. setting. *Medical Anthropology,* 7, 1–19.

Adcock, W., Burleigh, A., Scott-Heads, J. (1988). Hind milk as an effective topical application in nipple care in the post partum period. *Breastfeeding Review,* 13, 68.

Akre, J. (Ed.). (1989). Infant feeding: The physiologic basis. *Bulletin of the World Health Organization Supplement,* 67, 1–108.

Alexander, J. M., Grant, A. M., Campbell, M. J. (1992). Randomized controlled trial of breast shells and Hoffman's exercises for inverted and non-protractile nipples. *British Medical Journal,* 304, 1030–1032.

American Academy of Pediatrics, Provisional Committee for Quality Improvement and Subcommittee on Hyperbilirubinemia. (1994). Practice parameter: Management of hyperbilirubinemia in the healthy term newborn. *Pediatrics,* 94, 558–565.

Anderson, G. C. (1989). Risk in mother-infant separation. *Image: Journal of Nursing Scholarship,* 21, 196–199.

Anderson, G. C. (1991). Current knowledge about skin-to-skin (kangaroo) care for preterm infants. *Journal of Perinatology,* 11, 216–226.

Ardran, G. M., Kemp, F. H., Lind, J. (1958). A cineradiographic study of breast feeding. *British Journal of Radiology,* 31, 156–162.

Auerbach, K. G., and Gartner, L. M. (1987). Breastfeeding and human milk: Their association with jaundice in the neonate. *Clinics in Perinatology,* 14, 89–107.

Auerbach, K. G., and Walker, M. (1994). When the mother of a premature infant uses a breast pump: What every NICU nurse needs to know. *Neonatal Network,* 13, 23–29.

Baranowski, T, Bee, D. E., Rassin, D. K., Richardson, C. J., Brown, J. P., Guenther, N., Nader, P. R. (1983). Social support, social influence, ethnicity, and the breastfeeding decision. *Social Science in Medicine,* 17, 1599–1611.

Bowles, B. C., Stutte, P. C., Hensley, J. H. (1988). Alternate massage in breastfeeding. *Genesis,* 9, 5–9, 17.

Bryant, C. A. (1982). The impact of kin, friend and neighbor networks on infant feeding practices. *Social Science in Medicine*, 16, 1757–1765.

Butte, N., et al. (1984). Longitudinal changes in milk composition of mothers delivering preterm and term infants. *Early Human Development,* 9, 153–162.

Chute, G. E. (1992). Promoting breastfeeding success: An overview of basic management. *NAACOG's Clinical Issues in Perinatal and Women's Health Nursing: Breastfeeding,* 3, 570–582.

Cobo, E., DeBemal, M. M., Gaitan, E., Qumtero, C. A. (1967). Neurohypophyseal hormone release in the human. II. Experimental study during lactation. *American Journal of Obstetrics and Gynecology*, 97, 519–529.

Crowell, M. K., Hill, P. D., Humenick, S. S. (1994). Relationship between obstetric analgesia and time of effective breastfeeding. *Journal of Nurse-Midwifery,* 39, 150–155.

de Carvalho, M., Hall, M., Harvey, D. (1981). Effects of water supplementation on physiologic jaundice in breast-fed babies. *Archives of Disease in Childhood,* 56, 568–569.

de Carvalho, M., Robertson, S., Klaus, M. H. (1984). Does the duration and frequency of early breastfeeding affect nipple pain? *Birth,* 11, 81–84.

Department of Health and Human Services. (1984). *Report of the Surgeon General's workshop on breastfeeding and human lactation* (DHHS publication HRS-D-MC 84-2). Washington, DC: U. S. Government Printing Office.

Department of Health and Human Services. (1995). *Healthy people 2000: National health promotion and disease prevention objectives* (DHHS publication [DHS] 91-50213). Washington, DC: U. S. Government Printing Office.

Drewett, R. F., Bowe-Jones, A., Dogterom, J. (1982). Oxytocin levels during breastfeeding in established lactation. *Hormonal Behavior*, 16, 245–248.

Ehrenkranz, R. A., Ackerman, B. A., Mezzer, J., Bracken, M. B. (1985). Breastfeeding and premature infants: Incidence and success. *Pediatric Research,* 19, 99A. (Abstract 530).

Foxman, B., Schwartz, K., Loman, S. J. (1994). Breastfeeding practices and lactation mastitis. *Social Science in Medicine,* 38, 755–761.

Gillerman, H., and Beckham, M. H. (1991). The postpartum early discharge dilemma: An innovative solution. *Journal of Perinatal and Neonatal Nursing,* 5, 9–17.

Glover, J. (1995). Supplementation of breastfeeding newborns: A flow chart for decision-making. *Journal of Human Lactation*, 11, 127–131.

Glover, J., and Sandilands, M. (1990). Supplementation of breastfeeding infants and weight loss in hospital. *Journal of Human Lactation,* 6, 163–166.
Goldman, A. S., Chheda, S., Keeney, S. E., Schmalstieg, F. C., Schanler, R. J. (1994). Immunologic protection of the premature newborn by human milk. *Seminars in Perinatology,* 18, 495–501.
Hartmann, P. E., and Prosser, C. G. (1984). Physiological basis of longitudinal changes in human milk yield and composition. *Federation Proceedings,* 43, 2448–2453.
Henrikson, M., Wall, G., Lethbridge, D., McClurg, V. (1992). Nursing diagnosis and obstetric, gynecologic, and neonatal nursing: Breastfeeding as an example. *Journal of Obstetric, Gynecologic, and Neonatal Nursing,* 21, 446–456.
Hill, P. D., and Humenick, S. S. (1993). Nipple pain during breastfeeding: The first two weeks and beyond. *Journal of Perinatal Education,* 2, 21–35.
Host, A., Husby, S., Osterballe, O. (1988). A prospective study of cow's milk allergy in exclusively breastfed infants. *Acta Paediatrica Scandinavica,* 77, 663–670.
Human Milk Banking Association of North America. (1993). *Recommendations for collection, storage, and handling of a mother's milk for her own infant in the hospital setting.* West Hartford, CT: Author.
Jones, D. A. (1987). The choice to breastfeed or bottlefeed and influences upon that choice: A survey of 1525 mothers. *Child Care, Health and Development*, 13, 75–85.
Kavanaugh, K., Mead, L., Meier, P., Mangurten, H. H. (1995). Getting enough: Mothers' concerns about breastfeeding a preterm infant after discharge. *Journal of Obstetric, Gynecologic and Neonatal Nursing,* 24, 23–32.
Keating, J. P., Schears, G. J., Dodge, P. R. (1991). Oral water intoxication in infants, an American epidemic. *American Journal of Diseases of Children,* 145, 985–990.
Keefe, M. R. (1987). Comparison of neonatal nighttime sleep-wake patterns in nursery versus rooming-in environments. *Nursing Research,* 36, 140–144.
Keefe, M. R. (1988). The impact of rooming-in on maternal sleep at night. *Journal of Obstetric, Gynecologic, and Neonatal Nursing,* 17, 122–126.
Kemper, K., Forsyth, B., McCarthy, P. (1989). Jaundice, terminating breastfeeding, and the vulnerable child. *Pediatrics,* 84, 773–778.
Kemper, K., Forsyth, B. W., McCarthy, P. L. (1990). Persistent perceptions of vulnerability following neonatal jaundice. *American Journal of Diseases of Children,* 144, 238–241.
Kesaree, N., Banapurmath, C. R., Banapurmath, S., Shamanur, K. (1993). Treatment of inverted nipples using a disposable syringe. *Journal of Human Lactation,* 9, 27–29.
Kuhr, M., and Paneth, N. (1982). Feeding practices and early neonatal jaundice. *Journal of Pediatric Gastroenterology and Nutrition,* 1, 485–488.
Kulski, J. K., Hartmann, P. E. (1981). Changes in milk composition during the initiation of lactation. *Australian Journal of Experimental Biological and Medical Science*, 59, 101–114.
Lau, S. P., and Fung, K. P. (1984). Serum bilirubin kinetics in intermittent phototherapy of physiological jaundice. *Archives of Disease in Childhood,* 59, 892–894.
Lawrence, R. (1994). *Breastfeeding: A guide for the medical profession* (4th ed.). St. Louis: C. V. Mosby.
Lucas, A., and Cole, T. J. (1990). Breast milk and necrotising enterocolitis. *Lancet,* 336, 1519–1523.
Lucas, A., Morley, R., Cole, T. J., et al. (1992). Breast milk and subsequent intelligence quotient in children born preterm. *Lancet,* 339, 261–264.
Maisels, M. J. (1988). Neonatal jaundice. *Seminars in Liver Disease,* 8, 148–162.
Malloy, M. H., and Graubard, B. (1994). Predictors of rehospitalization among very low birth weight infants (VLBW). *Clinical Research,* 41, 791A.
Martin, R. H. (1983). The place of prolactin in human lactation. *Clinical Endocrinology*, 18, 295–299.
Matthews, M. K. (1989). The relationship between maternal labour analgesia and delay in the initiation of breastfeeding in healthy neonates in the early neonatal period. *Midwifery,* 5, 3–10.
Millard, A. V. (1990). The place of the clock in pediatric advice: Rationales, cultural themes, and impediments to breastfeeding. *Social Science in Medicine,* 31, 211–221.
Mobbs, E. G. (1989). Human imprinting and breastfeeding—Are the textbooks deficient? *Breastfeeding Review,* 14, 39–41.
Mosher, C., Cronk, P., Kidd, A., McCormick, P., et al. (1992). Upgrading practice with critical pathways. *American Journal of Nursing,* 92, 41–44.
Neifert, M., and Seacat, J. (1985). *Milk yield and prolactin rise with simultaneous breast pumping* (abstract). Washington, DC: Ambulatory Pediatric Association Annual Meeting, May 7–10.
Newell, S. J., Chapman, S., Booth, I. W. (1993). Ultrasonic assessment of gastric emptying in the preterm infant. *Archives of Disease in Childhood,* 69, 32–36.
Newman, J. (1990). Breastfeeding problems associated with the early introduction of bottles and pacifiers. *Journal of Human Lactation,* 6, 59–63.
Newman, T. B., and Maisels, M. J. (1990). Does hyperbilirubinemia damage the brain of healthy full term infants? *Clinics in Perinatology,* 17, 331–358.
Nicoll, A., Ginsburg, R., Tripp, J. H. (1982). Supplementary feeding and jaundiced newborns. *Acta Paediatrica Scandinavica,* 71, 759–761.
Niemela, M., Uhari, M., Hannuksela, A. (1994). Pacifiers and dental structure as risk factors for otitis media. *International Journal of Pediatric Otorhinolaryngology,* 29, 121–127.
Oski, F. A. (1992). Hyperbilirubinemia in the term infant: An unjaundiced approach. *Contemporary Pediatrics,* 9, 148.
Peaker, M., Wilde, C. J. (1987). Milk secretion: Autocome control. *News on Physiological Sciences*, 2, 124–126.
Polberger, S., and Lonnerdal, B. (1993). Simple and rapid macronutrient analysis of human milk for individualized fortification: Basis for improved nutritional management of very-low-birth-weight infants? *Journal of Pediatric Gastroenterology and Nutrition,* 17, 283–290.
Prentice, A., Addey, C. V. P., Wilde, C. J. (1989). Evidence for local feedback control of human milk secretion. *Biochemical Society Transactions,* 17, 122.
Provisional Committee for Quality Improvement and Subcommittee on Hyperbilirubinemia, American Academy of Pediatrics. (1994). Practice parameter: Management of hyperbilirubinemia in the healthy term newborn. *Pediatrics,* 94, 558–565.
Quan, R., Yang, C., Rubinstein, S., Lewiston, N. J., Stevenson, D. K., Kerner, J. A. (1994). The effect of nutritional additives on anti-infective factors in human milk. *Clinical Pediatrics,* June, 325–328.
Renfrew, M. J. (1989). Positioning the baby at breast: More than a visual skill. *Journal of Human Lactation,* 5, 13–15.
Righard, L., and Alade, M. O. (1990). Effect of delivery room routines on success of first breast-feed. *Lancet,* 336, 1105–1107.
Righard, L., and Alade, M. O. (1992). Sucking technique and its effect on success of breastfeeding. *Birth,* 19, 185–189.
Righard, L., Flodmark, C. E., Lothe, L., Jakobsson, I. (1993). Breastfeeding patterns: Comparing the effects on infant behavior and maternal satisfaction of using one or two breasts. *Birth,* 20, 182–185.
Riordan, J., and Auerbach, K. G. (1993). *Breastfeeding and human lactation.* Boston: Jones & Bartlett Publishers.
Riordan, J., and Nichols, F. (1990). A descriptive study of lactation mastitis in long-term breastfeeding women. *Journal of Human Lactation,* 6, 53–58.
Sepkoski, C. M., Lester, B. M., Ostheimer, G. W., Brazelton, T. B. (1992). The effects of maternal epidural anesthesia on neonatal behavior during the first month. *Developmental Medicine and Child Neurology,* 34, 1072–1080.
Serafino-Cross, P., and Donovan, P. R. (1992). Effectiveness of professional breastfeeding home support. *Journal of Nutrition Education,* 24, 117–122.
Shrago, L. C. (1992). The breastfeeding dyad: Early assessment, documentation, and intervention. *NAACOG's Clinical*

Issues in Perinatal and Women's Health Nursing: Breastfeeding, 3, 583–597.

Shrago, L., and Bocar, D. (1990). The infant's contribution to breastfeeding. *Journal of Obstetric, Gynecologic, and Neonatal Nursing,* 19, 209–215.

Snell, B. J., Krantz, M., Keeton, R., Delgado, K., Peckham, C. (1992). The association of formula samples given at hospital discharge with the early duration of breastfeeding. *Journal of Human Lactation,* 8, 67–72.

Stine, M. J. (1990). Breastfeeding the premature newborn: A protocol without bottles. *Journal of Human Lactation,* 6, 167–170.

Stutte, P. C., Bowles, B. C., Morman, G. Y. (1988). The effects of breast massage on volume and fat content of human milk. *Genesis,* 10, 22–25.

Valentine, C. J., Hurst, N. M., Schanler, R. J. (1994). Hindmilk improves weight gain in low-birth-weight infants fed human milk. *Journal of Pediatric Gastroenterology and Nutrition,* 18, 474–477.

Vice, F. L., Heinz, J. M., Giuriati, G., Hood, M., Bosma, J. F. (1990). Cervical auscultation of suckle feeding in newborn infants. *Developmental Medicine and Child Neurology,* 32, 760–768.

Victora, C. G., Tomasi, E., Olento, M. T., Barros, F. C. (1993). Use of pacifiers and breastfeeding duration. *Lancet,* 341, 404–406.

Walker, M. (1992). Breastfeeding the premature infant. *NAACOG's Clinical Issues in Perinatal and Women's Health Nursing: Breastfeeding,* 3, 620–633.

Walker, M. (1995). *Hospital breastfeeding policies and protocols: A model for the short stay.* Weston, MA: Lactation Associates.

Walker, M., and Driscoll, J. (1989). Sore nipples: The new mother's nemesis. *MCN: American Journal of Maternal-Child Nursing,* 14, 260–265.

Whitworth, N. S. (1988). Lactation in humans. *Psychoneuroendocrinology,* 13, 177–188.

Widstrom, A. M., Ransjo-Arvidson, A. B., Christensson, K., et al. (1987). Gastric suction in healthy newborn infants: Effects on circulation and developing feeding behavior. *Acta Paediatrica Scandinavica,* 76, 566–572.

Wilks, S., and Meier, P. (1988). Helping mothers express milk suitable for preterm and high-risk infant feeding. *MCN: American Journal of Maternal-Child Nursing,* 13, 121–123.

Wolf, L. S., and Glass, R. P. (1992). *Feeding and swallowing disorders of infancy: Assessment and management.* Tucson, AZ: Therapy Skill Builders.

Woolridge, M. W., Baum, J. D., Drewett, R. F. (1980). Effect of a traditional and of a new nipple shield on sucking patterns and milk flow. *Early Human Development,* 4, 357–364.

World Health Organization (1989). Protecting, promoting and supporting breast feeding: The special role of maternity services. A joint WHO/UNICEF statement, Geneva: Author.

Wright, A., Rice, S., Wells, S. (1996). Changing hospital practice to increase the duration of breastfeeding. *Pediatrics,* 97 (5), 669–675.

Yamauchi, Y., Yamanouchi, I. (1990). The relationship between rooming-in/not rooming-in and breastfeeding variables. *Acta Paediatrica Scandinavica,* 79, 1017–1022.

Zander, K. (1987). Critical paths: Marking the course. *Definition: Center for Case Management,* 2 (3).

Zander, K. (1991). Care maps: The core of cost/quality care. *The New Definition,* 6, 9–11.

Chapter 34

Parenting the Healthy Infant

Lynda L. Harrison

> Babies, it turns out, for thousands of years have been signaling with their bodies and their faces, sending messages to parents which parents react to, but with rare exceptions hardly any parent ever knows consciously that they're getting a signal and responding to it.
>
> BETH AND JOHN GALL (1991)

HIGHLIGHTS

- Historical and Cultural Factors Affecting Parenting
- Concepts of Bonding and Attachment
- Effects of Parental Perceptions on the Development of Parent-Infant Attachment
- Assessment of Early Parent-Infant Relationships
- Assessing Parents' Perceptions of Their Infants
- Nursing Practice
- Families with Special Needs
- Implications for Research

The first few months of an infant's life are considered by many to be a critical period for the formation of positive parent-child relationships. There are numerous factors that influence the development of motherliness and fatherliness and a couple's transition to parenthood after the birth of a healthy newborn. Appropriate nursing intervention during the early neonatal period can help to establish positive parent-child interaction patterns that will have long-lasting effects on the health of the child, parents, and family.

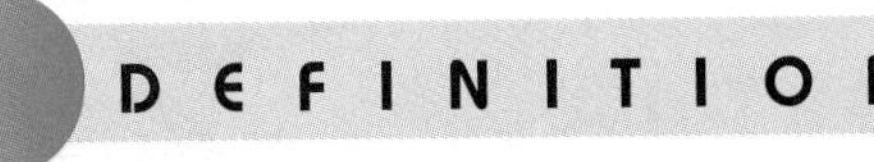

DEFINITIONS

Adaptive parenting behaviors—Behaviors that facilitate the development of positive parent-infant attachment.

Bonding—A parent's feeling of closeness toward the newborn infant that is facilitated by early physical contact between parent and infant (Campbell and Taylor, 1979).

Competency motivation—An intrinsic motive to cope effectively with the environment.

Early contact—Interaction between parent and newborn infant during the first few days after birth.

Infant-parent attachment—A behavioral system that develops during the first year of life by which the infant develops a trusting relationship with his or her caregiver.

Infant temperament—A characteristic style by which an infant responds to the animate and inanimate environment.

Maladaptive parenting behaviors—Behaviors that interfere with the development of positive parent-infant attachment.

Parent-infant attachment—A reciprocal process by which parents develop synchronous and loving relationships with their infants.

Parental role attainment—The process of acquiring the parenting role.

Reciprocity—Rhythmic cycles of attention and nonattention during synchronous mother-infant interactions (Brazelton et al. 1974).

Sensitive period—The period in the early weeks after birth when parents develop close attachments to their infants.

Taking-hold phase—The phase in the process of maternal role attainment during which mothers attempt to master their new maternal roles (Rubin 1967a, 1967b).

Taking-in phase—The first few days after childbirth during which mothers focus primarily on meeting their own needs.

HISTORICAL AND CULTURAL FACTORS AFFECTING PARENTING

Social, cultural, and historical factors affect the nature of parenting roles and the quality of parent-child relationships. Okagaki and Divecha (1993) reviewed several theories that have been developed to explain how parental beliefs and behaviors are influenced by cultural values and traditions. Although parents in all cultures share basic goals for their children, the strategies for achieving these goals vary across cultures. Parental attitudes are also influenced by which of two basic parent needs children are expected to satisfy (economic security or love and affection). A cultural value that is commonly held among ethnic minority families in the United States is "a strong emphasis on family and group identity. In contrast, Anglo-American culture emphasizes the individual and individual achievement" (Okagaki and Divecha 1993, p. 38). Nurses need to be aware of cultural values that might influence the attitudes, behaviors, and expectations of their clients. It is also important that research about parenting and family development focus more on cross-cultural comparisons. Marc Bornstein, editor of a book entitled *Cultural Approaches to Parenting,* warns that "to discuss or reach conclusions about the growth of perception, cognition, communication, emotion, personality, or social interaction outside of a cross-cultural developmental framework is perilous" (Bornstein 1993, p. 5).

Historical changes have influenced parenting from the ancient Greek and Roman cultures to contemporary Western cultures (Bigner 1985; Stendler 1950; Sunley 1955). In ancient times, the family was viewed as the core element of society, and fathers were considered the family leaders. Children had few rights; child sacrifices and slavery were common. During the Middle Ages, children were reared in extended families, and most societies were based on rural lifestyles. Parents were relatively indifferent to the special needs of their children, devoting their primary energies to meeting basic survival needs. Because the infant mortality rate was high, parents were often reluctant to develop close attachments to their infants. During the Renaissance (1400–1600), wealthy parents frequently sent their babies to live with other women or wet nurses for the first 2 years of life. Artistic works produced during this period, however, suggest an increased interest in childhood and an increased focus on families rather than a focus only on individual adults (Bigner 1985).

During the Colonial period (1600–1800), parents were influenced by a predominantly Puritan religious orientation and became increasingly involved in shaping their child's development. Between 1800 and 1860, mothers began to assume increased responsibilities for discipline as well as religious and moral instruction, which had previously been considered the father's duties. In 1815, the first maternal associations were developed in the United States, focusing on providing parent education (Hamner and Turner 1985). An increased focus on early child development was noted during this period as parents were encouraged to use persuasion and reward rather than physical punishment in disciplining their children.

Mothers continued to be viewed as the child's primary caregivers during the early twentieth century as men were preoccupied with capitalism and industrialism. In 1912, the federal government established the Children's Bureau to focus on promoting the welfare of American children (Hamner and Turner 1985). Their well-known serial publication *Infant Care* was revised six times between 1914 and 1976 and was distributed to more than 60 million people (Hamner and Turner 1985). Increasing numbers of parenting books and articles were published beginning in the early twentieth century. Bigner (1985) noted that there have been wide swings in the types of parenting advice offered in these publications. Stendler (1950) reviewed childrearing practices advocated in three popular women's magazines from 1890 to 1950 and noted that in the 1890s, the articles stressed the importance of mother love and advocated flexible and permissive child care routines. In the 1900s, writers began to advocate the use of punishment rather than rewards as a means of discipline (Stendler 1950). By 1910, the magazines advocated more restrictive parenting and strict scheduling of infant routines.

This restrictive approach was encouraged by behavioral psychologists such as J. B. Watson, who warned against the dangers of excessive "mother love" (Bigner 1985). Stendler (1950) noted that by 1910, "love, and particularly the physical manifestation of it was discouraged in most of the articles on 'Infant Discipline' . . . baby's strength was needed for rapid growing, and picking the baby up deprived him of his strength. Still another reason for discouraging physical contact with the baby was the belief that postnatal conditions for the infant should closely approximate prenatal conditions, and since the infant was not handled in the uterus, he should not be handled after birth" (p. 128).

Stendler (1950) suggested that even though the field of child psychology had its origins in the 1880s, there was no scientific evidence to account for the change in childrearing advice noted in the women's magazines. One reason for the shift in promoting stricter feeding schedules may have been the campaign to reduce infant mortality by ensuring adequate infant nutrition. Magazine writers may have then advocated their own personal opinions, suggesting increased regimentation in other aspects of infant care.

Another change in childrearing attitudes noted between 1935 and 1945 was largely due to the influence of freudian psychology and the emphasis on the importance of early infancy and the importance of secure mother-infant attachments. Literature published during this period stressed the importance of early cuddling and handling to foster emotional security in the infant (Bigner 1985). The classic work of Benjamin Spock (*The Common Sense Book of Baby and Child Care*) was first published in 1946 and emphasized the importance of the parenting role. This book has been published in 26 languages, and more than 30 million copies have been distributed (Spock 1989).

As more women entered the workforce after World War II, fathers began to assume increased responsibilities for childrearing (Bigner 1985; Hamner and Turner 1985). It is estimated that 60 percent of women with preschool children are currently in the labor force (Dawson and Cain 1990). The changing roles of women and men in Western societies have had a significant influence on parenting and childrearing. Mothers and fathers are faced with the challenge of balancing multiple roles and promoting the optimal development of their children. Daycare centers are providing care to increasing numbers of infants and preschool children. In 1988, 13.3 million children in the United States who were younger than 5 years were in some type of child care arrangement (Dawson and Cain 1990). Parents need guidance in assessing the quality of various daycare facilities and selecting the program that best meets their needs.

The inauguration of the War on Poverty in 1964 resulted in an increased number of federally funded programs to promote positive parenting among low-income families. Programs such as Head Start and Home Start focused on helping parents create effective home environments to promote child development (Hamner and Turner 1985). Head Start programs continue to provide important services to low-income preschool children and families.

Articles and books containing childrearing advice have continued to flourish and often contain conflicting information that can be confusing for parents. Boukydis (1986) suggested that the extensive literature and media resources on parenting have replaced the "oral transmission of parenting lore and the experimental base for learning parenting in the extended family" (p. 5).

Auvenshine and Enriquez (1985) identified the following trends in contemporary American society that are influencing parenting and family life:

- Decreasing family size and an increased number of older first-time parents
- Decreasing marriage rates, increased number of adolescent and single-parent families
- Increasing rates of divorce and remarriage
- Decreasing availability of extended family members in geographic proximity
- Increasing education and career opportunities for women
- Technologic advances in obstetric care (e.g., artificial insemination, surrogate parenthood, in vitro fertilization)

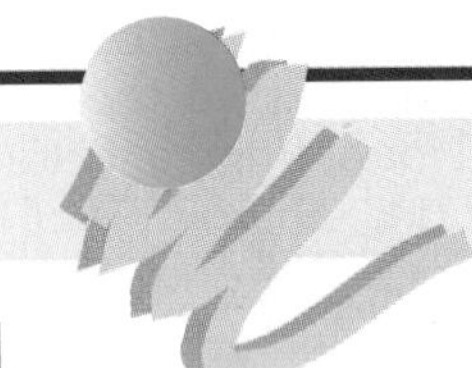

HISTORICAL PERSPECTIVES

SOCIAL SUPPORT FOR FAMILIES

Ancient times
Children had few rights; father was the family leader.

Middle Ages
Most children were reared in extended families; families focused energies on survival; high infant mortality rates.

Renaissance (1400–1600)
Increased interest in childhood and increased focus on families.

American Colonial period (1600–1800)
Puritan influence; increased maternal influence.

Early 1900s
Children's Bureau established to promote child welfare; emphasis on physical punishment and strict scheduling.

1900–1935
Influence of freudian psychology resulted in increased recognition of early mother-infant attachment.

1960–1970
War on Poverty resulted in new programs for families: Maternal-Child Health Infant Care Project; Medicaid EPSDT (Early and Periodic Screening, Diagnosis, and Treatment for children in poverty); Head Start (assists preschool poor children to increase learning skills and readiness for school).

1974; 1980s
Child Abuse Prevention and Treatment Act defined child abuse and neglect and established National Center on Child Abuse and Neglect. In 1988, Public Law 100-294, The Child Abuse Prevention, Adoption, and Family Services Act, consolidated and expanded abuse and violence prevention efforts. State governments passed laws mandating health professionals to report suspected abuse. Child abuse and domestic violence became widely discussed in public forums. Emergency shelters and other resources were established in many communities. Need for support of parents was more widely recognized.

1986
Amendments to the Education for All Handicapped Children Act (P.L. 94-142, passed in 1975) expanded coverage for high-risk children from birth. The act encouraged states to identify infants with disabilities and to provide special services as early as possible. Consolidated in 1991 to Individuals with Disabilities Act.

1993
Family and Medical Leave Act provides employees with up to 12 weeks of unpaid leave per year to care for newborn infant or a newly adopted child, foster child, or child with serious illness. Applies to public and private employers with 50 or more employees.

Trends 1990–2000
Decreasing family size and increasing number of older first-time parents; increased numbers of adolescent and single-parent families; increased divorce rates; decreased availability of extended family support.

Challenges and opportunities
As hospital stays shorten and families are geographically spread, education needs for new parents increase. Opportunities can be created for home mother-baby care visits; new mother or new parent groups led by nurses (similar to childbirth education classes); providing health supervision and teaching to daycare facilities (diaper hygiene, common symptom recognition, accident prevention); providing consultant services for parents selecting in-home child care or daycare; providing respite care for parents with homebound ill children.

Another trend that has had a profound effect on a substantial percentage of parents in the United States is the increasing proportion of families living in poverty. Many of these families are chronically poor and live in concentrated inner-city neighborhoods where they are exposed daily to violence, drugs, and danger. Garbarino and Kostelny (1993) noted that childhood poverty has increased 25 percent since 1979 and suggested that poverty has a negative effect on parenting because it decreases family resources and precipitates mental health problems. Parents living in poverty face significant challenges as they attempt to serve as buffers of stress for their children. Garbarino and Kostelny (1993) described the difficulties faced by such families (p. 216):

. . . parental adaptations to dangerous environments may produce child rearing strategies that impede normal development as in the case of a mother who does not allow her child to play on the floor because there is poison on the floor to kill the rats. . . . Likewise, the parent who prohibits the child from playing outside for fear of shooting incidents may be denying the child a chance to engage in social and athletic play.

Social, cultural, and historical forces will continue to influence the ways in which parents enact their parenting roles. An awareness of these forces can help nurses understand the factors that influence parenting behaviors and plan effective strategies for promoting culturally relevant childrearing practices.

CONCEPTS OF BONDING AND ATTACHMENT

Attachment between a parent and child is generally defined as an enduring affectionate bond that is reciprocal and gradual in development during the child's first year of life (Bowlby 1969; Campbell and Taylor 1979; Klaus and Kennell 1982). Rubin (1977) used the term binding-in to describe the gradual process of development of the mother-child relationship (or attachment), which she suggested takes place during the first 12 to 15 months of the child's life. Robson and Moss (1970) noted that mothers may not develop feelings of close attachment until several weeks after the infant's birth. Tulman (1981) emphasized the importance of the reciprocal interaction between parent and infant in the development of their attachment to one another. This interactional concept of parent-infant attachment recognizes that infants are active partners in the interaction process from birth. According to Tulman (1981, p. 13):

The behavior of one of the individuals triggers a response in the other person. This in turn acts as a stimulus for the other person and leads to further development of the behavior into a more complex pattern. In this interactional process, modification of responses occurs as the behavior is shaped into a pattern.

Brazelton and colleagues (1974) used the term reciprocity to describe the rhythmic cycles of attention and nonattention during synchronous mother-infant interactions. According to these researchers, this reciprocity forms the roots of parent-infant attachment. Yarrow (1972) also viewed attachment as an interactional concept in which reciprocity is central.

Although Klaus and Kennell (1982) have used the terms attachment and bonding interchangeably, other writers have suggested that the two terms represent different concepts. According to Campbell and Taylor (1979, p. 3), for example:

Bonding is primarily unidirectional (parent-infant), rapid (within the first hours or days after birth), and facilitated or optimized by physical contact. Attachment, on the other hand, is reciprocal (mother-infant), develops gradually during the first year of life, and is influenced by psychological variables such as the quality, timing, and pacing of adult-child encounters.

Early attachment research was focused primarily on the infant-to-parent attachment relationship (Ainsworth and Wittig 1969; Bowlby 1969), but more recently there has been increased emphasis on parent-to-infant attachment (Campbell and Taylor 1979; Klaus and Kennell 1982). Although most research and literature related to attachment has been focused on the relationship between the biologic mother and her child, it is recognized that the concept also applies to the relationship between fathers and infants and between adoptive parents and their children.

Infant-to-Parent Attachment

Bowlby, one of the earliest writers in the field of infant attachment, viewed attachment as a behavioral system. Infant attachment or signaling behaviors were identified as those which served to initiate and maintain proximity between the mother and infant (e.g., crying, smiling, and cooing). According to Bowlby (1969), secure attachment helps the infant develop a sense of security identified by Erikson (1950) as "basic trust." Bowlby (1969) suggested that the first 6 months of life constituted a sensitive period during which the infant must develop a trusting relationship with the caregiver.

Ainsworth has conducted extensive empirical research on infant-to-parent attachment and has developed a laboratory procedure (the Strange Situation Procedure) to assess the quality of an infant's attachment to his or her parent. This procedure has been validated and used by many researchers with children between the ages of 12 and 18 months. It involves observations of the child's behaviors during specific interactions with the mother and with an examiner who is not familiar to the child. Three general patterns of infant-to-parent attachment have been identified by use of this procedure: avoidant, ambivalent, and secure (Ainsworth et al. 1978). Avoidant infants show little distress during separation, treat the stranger like the mother, and avoid proximity to or interaction with the mother during reunion episodes. Ambivalent infants resist contact with a stranger and are often angry or resistant to the mother on reunion. Once contact with the mother is initiated, however, they seek to maintain it. Securely attached infants, in contrast, seek proximity and contact with the mother, especially during reunions, but also explore the environment and express an interest in the stranger. Although Ainsworth recognized the reciprocal nature of the attachment relationship, the Strange Situation Procedure provides a measure only of infant behavior and does not specifically assess the nature of parent-child interaction patterns. Ainsworth and colleagues (1978) have, however, reported significant positive relationships between maternal responsiveness to the infant as early as 3 months of life and subsequent security in infant-to-mother attachment as measured by the Strange Situation Procedure. Mothers who were sensitive to the infant's cues and who met the infant's needs promptly fostered the development of secure attachment relationships. Mothers who failed to respond to their infants or who responded inappropriately fostered the development of avoidant or ambivalent attachments. This observation suggests that parental sensitivity and responsiveness may be key indicators of a parent's attachment to his or her infant and may affect the infant's subsequent attachment to the parent. Other studies have shown that secure infant-to-parent attachment patterns at age 12 to 18 months are related to the child's adaptive problem-solving ability at age 2 years and to social competence at age 3 years (Matas et al. 1978; Waters et al. 1979). Thus, preliminary data suggest that the quality of a child's early attachment relationship with the parents has long-term effects on child development.

Parent-to-Infant Attachment

Robson and Moss (1970) were among the first researchers to systematically assess the process of a mother's attachment to her infant as opposed to the infant's attachment to the mother. Since then, there has been considerable research to explore the nature of the parent's attachment to the infant and the factors that affect its development (Campbell and Taylor 1979; Curry 1982; Klaus and Kennell 1982; Mercer 1981). Many factors that have been identified as affecting the develop-

Factors Affecting Parent-Infant Attachment

PARENTAL VARIABLES

- Age
- Self-concept (including concepts of masculinity and femininity)
- Relationships with significant others
- Attitudes toward parenting
- Knowledge related to parenting and infant care
- Expectations of infant
- Illness
- Perceptions of infant
- Mother's physical health during pregnancy
- Parent's satisfaction with his or her interactions with infant
- Perceptions of the birth experience

SITUATIONAL VARIABLES

- Presence of other stressors or crises
- Support systems
- Whether pregnancy was planned or unplanned
- Experience surrounding pregnancy, labor, and early postpartum period
- Quality and quantity of parent-infant contact in early newborn period

INFANT VARIABLES

- Temperament and behaviors
- Physical characteristics
- Illness

ment of a parent's attachment to the infant are related to parental, situational, and infant variables.

The results of several studies suggest that parents begin to develop attachments with their infants during the prenatal period (Cranley 1981; Weaver and Cranley 1983). Cranley (1981) defined maternal-fetal attachments as "the extent to which women engage in behaviors which represent an affiliation and interaction with their unborn child" (p. 65). Cranley (1981) reported that mothers who experienced increased stress and less social support during pregnancy had lower maternal-fetal attachment scores.

Klaus and Kennell (1982) have reported a number of studies suggesting that there is a relationship between early or extended contact between mothers and infants and subsequent maternal attachment behavior. This research was stimulated by observation that there was a high rate of child abuse and neglect among parents of premature infants who had been separated from their infants for prolonged periods after the infant's birth (Klein and Stern 1971). Mothers who had extended contact with their infants immediately after birth and during the first 3 days after delivery (as opposed to the more limited contact permitted by most routine hospital practices) have demonstrated more attachment behaviors up to 2 years after delivery (deChateau 1977; Klaus et al. 1972; Klaus and Kennell 1982; Ringler et al. 1975).

On the basis of the early contact studies, Klaus and Kennell (1982) have proposed the existence of a sensitive period immediately after birth when the parent is particularly ready to bond with the infant. This theory has been criticized because it fails to recognize the adaptability and potential for growth inherent in human beings (Tulman 1981). These early-contact studies have also been criticized for their small sample sizes, the lack of valid measures of attachment, and the failure to differentiate the effects of the amounts and timing of initial contact. For example, many of these studies used frequency counts of parental affectionate behaviors (e.g., kissing, en face positioning, holding, smiling) and the length of time the mother breastfeeds her infant as indices of parent-infant attachment. Such measures fail to assess the reciprocal nature of parent-child interactions, the sensitivity of the parent to the infant's cues, or the ability of parents and infants to adapt to one another. Other studies have failed to identify a relationship between early or extended parent-infant contact and subsequent parent-to-infant attachment (Curry 1982; Siegel et al. 1980; Svejda et al. 1980; Taylor et al. 1979). Thus, the hypothesis of a sensitive period for development of parent-infant attachment has yet to be proved or disproved (Goldberg 1983).

It is possible that early contact is one of many factors that may facilitate the development of parent-infant attachment, particularly for those who are at risk for the development of maladaptive parent-child relationships. For example, O'Conner and coworkers (1980) found a lower frequency of inadequate parenting among low-income primiparous mothers who were randomly assigned to room-in with their infants after delivery compared with a control group who had contacts with their infants only for feeding during the postpartum hospital stay. Similarly, Norr and colleagues (1989) found higher attachment scores among a group of medically indigent mothers who roomed-in with their newborns, compared with a control group of mothers who did not experience rooming-in. Because it is relatively easy to provide parents with the opportunity to have early contact, hospital practices that promote this practice (e.g., rooming-in, birthing rooms) should be encouraged. However, it is also important to respect individual differences in parents' levels of interest in early or extended contact. Some mothers may need extra contact or rooming-in. Parents should realize that the absence of such early contact will not necessarily hinder the development of positive parent-infant attachment. Goldberg (1983) noted, for example, that "the emphasis on 'early bonding' has already created an expectation on the part of many parents that if they do not have this experience they have somehow failed and will never be fine parents . . . it is important to emphasize that the parent-infant relationship is a complex system with many fail-safe or alternative routes to the same outcome. Its success or failure does not hinge on a few brief moments in time" (p. 1379).

The Process of Parental Role Attainment

The term maternal role attainment was first described by Rubin (1967a, 1967b) to refer to the process of acquisition of the mothering role. The process of parental role attainment develops simultaneously with parent-infant attachment (Moore 1983). Rubin (1963) also identified states in the progression of maternal touch as the mother becomes acquainted with her new infant, from fingertip to palmer touch and finally to enfolding the infant close to the mother's body (Fig. 34–1). Martell and Mitchell (1984) studied 20 mothers of full-term infants during the first 3 days post partum and found that the mothers exhibited few taking-in behaviors, although the number of taking-hold behaviors increased from day 1 to day 2, peaking on the second postpartum day.

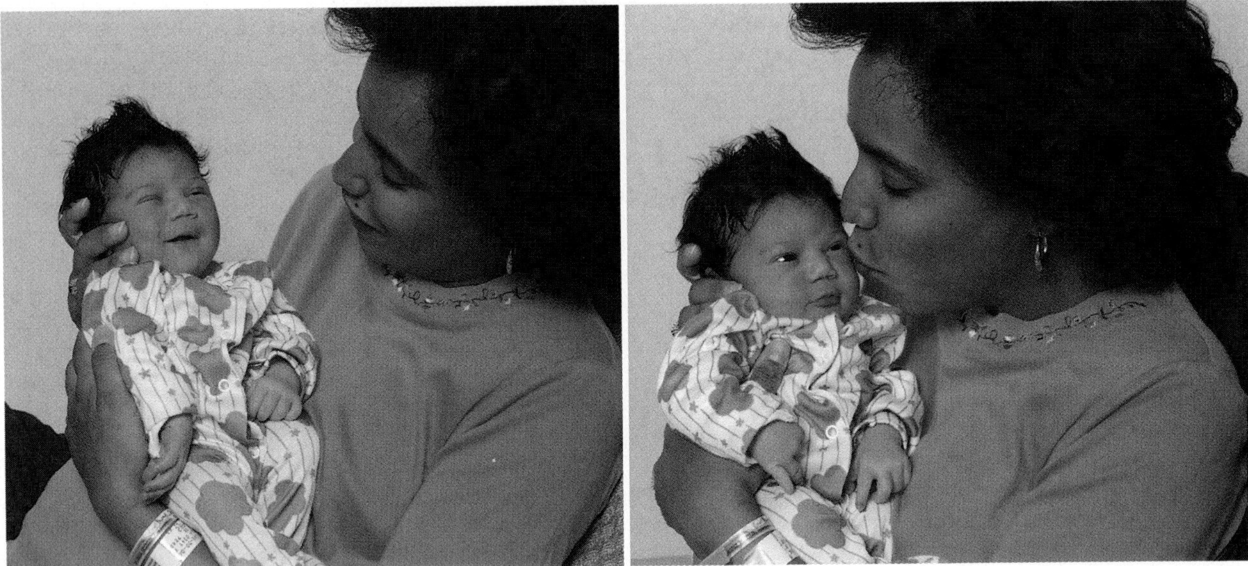

Figure 34–1
The process of parental role attainment develops simultaneously with parent-infant attachment • It is seen in the progression from maternal touch as the mother becomes acquainted with her new infant to the final enfolding of the infant close to the mother's body.

Bocar and Moore (1987) identified four stages in the process of parental role acquisition. The *anticipatory* stage occurs before delivery and involves learning about the role from multiple sources. Prospective parents need realistic information and often benefit from interactions with other new parents. The *formal* stage begins after delivery when parents assume responsibility for their infant's care. During this stage, parents are interested primarily in mastering practical child care tasks. They often lack self-confidence and may become easily overwhelmed and confused with conflicting advice about child care. During this stage, parents need concrete demonstrations and suggestions as well as acknowledgment that they are the "experts" in relating to their infant. Once parents develop confidence in their ability to meet their infant's basic needs, they are ready to progress to the *informal* role acquisition stage. Through informal interactions with their peers, parents in the informal stage "begin to modify the rigid rules and directions they sought out during the formal stage" (Bocar and Moore 1987, p. 5). During the final stage of role acquisition (the *person* stage), parents further modify their behaviors to evolve their own unique parenting styles.

Father-Infant Attachment

As mentioned before, most parent-infant attachment research has been focused on mothers and infants. Some researchers, however, have studied the process of father-to-infant attachment. Greenberg and Morris (1974) found that fathers experienced increased self-esteem after the births of their infants and used the term engrossment to describe the father-infant attachment relationship (Fig. 34–2). Parke (1979) has conducted a number of studies illustrating that fathers have unique ways of interacting with their infants, which differ from typical maternal interactions, although both are equally sensitive in their abilities to identify and respond to the infant's needs. Several studies have demonstrated that presence at delivery or early and extended father-infant contact during the newborn period increases subsequent paternal caregiving and attachment behaviors (Bowen and Miller 1980; Rodholm, 1981).

Effects of Parental Perceptions on the Development of Parent-Infant Attachment

An important determinant of the quality and quantity of interaction between a parent and infant is the parent's perceptions of the infant's characteristics and behaviors (Goldberg 1979; Johnson and Grubbs 1975; Klaus and Kennell 1982). Milliones (1978), for example, reported that mothers who perceived their infants as difficult to care for were less responsive to the infant's cues and spent less time interacting with them.

The interaction between parents and infants during the early days and weeks after birth has been described as an acquaintance process

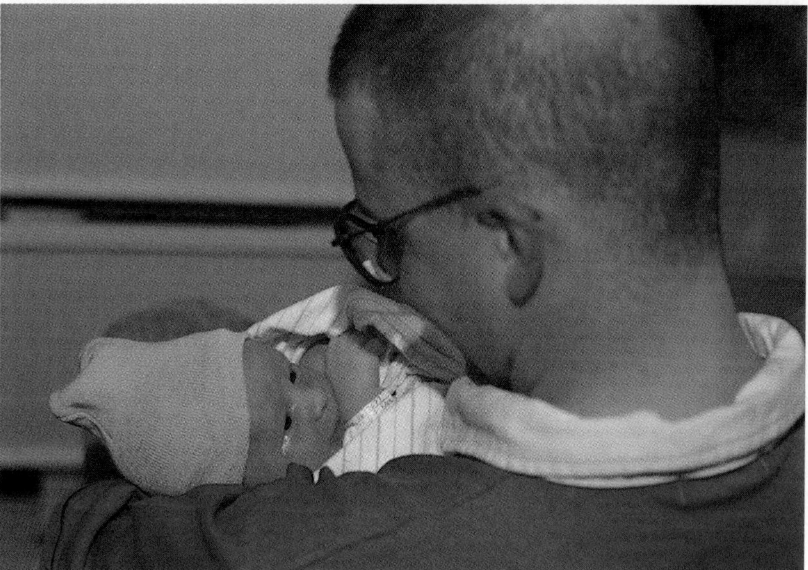

Figure 34–2
Greenberg and Morris have termed the father-infant attachment relationship "engrossment," which is clearly demonstrated here as father and son become acquainted shortly after birth.

(Kennedy 1973). During this acquaintance process, parents attempt to "get to know" their babies and compare the real infant with the infant they expected or fantasized during the pregnancy (Kennedy 1973). If there are discrepancies between reality and the parents' expectations of the infant, the development of early parent-infant attachment may be delayed because the parents must first accept the loss of their fantasized child.

The temperament of the infant has a great effect on parental perceptions and on parent-infant interaction patterns. Thomas and coworkers (1968) conducted a study to identify temperament differences among children. Three general types of infant temperament were identified: easy, difficult, and slow to warm up. Thomas and Chess (1980) proposed that the "goodness of fit" between a parent and child affects the quality of their relationship. If a child's temperament is very different from that of the parent, it may be difficult for the child to develop satisfying interaction patterns. Parents need to understand that an infant's behavior is, to a large extent, determined by his or her temperament and is not necessarily a result of something the parents have or have not done. It is also important for parents to learn which parenting behaviors are most effective with children of different temperaments and to learn how to recognize and respond to their infant's cues.

Goldberg's (1979) application of the competency motivation model provides a framework for understanding the influence of parents' perceptions of their infants on subsequent parent-child interaction patterns. Competency motivation is an intrinsic motive to cope effectively with the environment. "Behavior that enables the organism to cope effectively with the environment gives rise to feelings of efficacy that strengthen competence motivation" (Goldberg 1979, p. 215). The individual's perception is a key variable in whether he or she will respond competently to environmental stimuli, and it is the way in which the individual will determine the adequacy of her or his response. When parents perceive their behaviors as successful in meeting the needs of their infants, they perceive themselves as competent and effective caregivers, and the development of parent-infant attachment is facilitated. Infants who are most likely to promote feelings of competence in their parents are those who are readable, predictable, and responsive. Perceptions of incompetence, on the other hand, lead to feelings of helplessness and tend to make the parent less effective in initiating satisfying interactions with the infant. The development of parent-infant attachment is thus inhibited.

ASSESSMENT OF EARLY PARENT-INFANT RELATIONSHIPS

A number of tools have been developed to help nurses systematically assess the quality of early parent-infant interactions. Nurses in a variety of settings are in key positions to promote positive interactions and to identify and help resolve early problems in the developing parent-infant relationship. Because parent-infant attachment is a reciprocal process, it is important to evaluate the behaviors of both parents and infants in interaction with one another. This section thus reviews strategies to assess parenting behaviors as well as infant behaviors and temperament. In addition, a means for assessing a parent's perceptions of his or her infant is described.

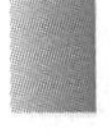

Assessment of Parenting Behaviors

Assessment of parenting behaviors must always be individualized, although assessment tools can provide useful guidelines in this process. It is important to assess parent-child interactions on a number of different occasions, because single observations may be misleading. Cultural differences in parenting styles must also be considered.

A key indicator of parent-infant attachment is the degree of sensitivity or responsiveness on the part of the parent to the infant's cues and needs. Does the parent recognize when the infant is hungry or needs comforting? Are the parent's behaviors effective in soothing the infant? Other indices that have been used frequently as measures of parent-infant attachment are parental behaviors that convey affection and a desire for contact with the infant: smiling, eye-to-eye contact (or en face position in which the parent's and infant's eyes meet in the same plane of rotation), kissing, close holding, affectionate stroking or touching, talking to the baby, and expressing positive feelings about the baby (Fig. 34–3). Finally, it is important to assess the parent's attitude toward the infant, parental self-concept, existing support systems, and the extent to which the parent is able to fulfill her or his personal needs. All parents need to have their own physical and emotional needs met to have the energy to nurture a new baby.

Table 34–1 was developed by Cropley (1986) to identify adaptive and maladaptive mothering be-

Text continued on page 1259

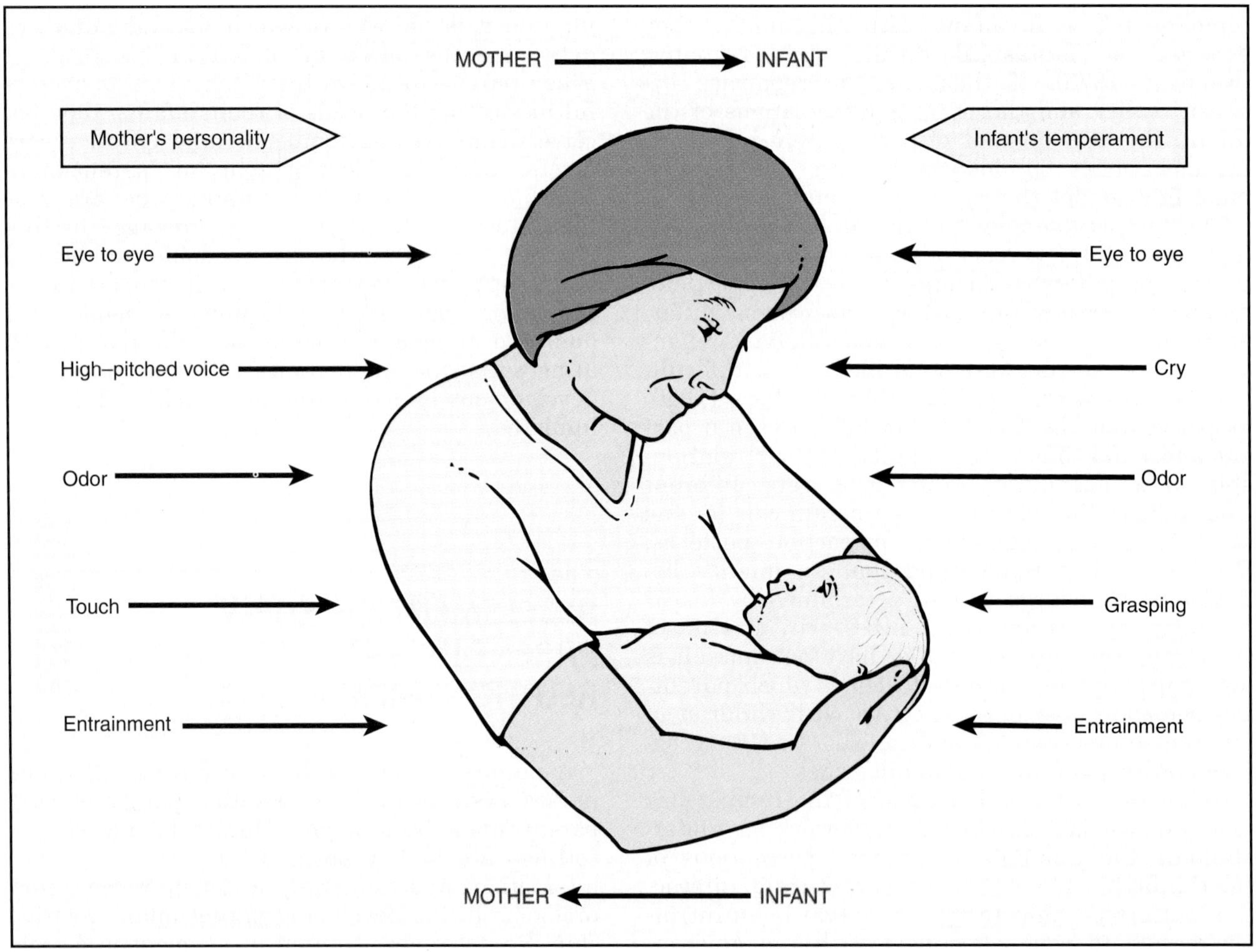

Figure 34–3

Smiling, eye-to-eye contact in which the parent's and infant's eyes meet in the same plane of rotation is called the en face position • Such eye-to-eye contact triggers vocal and physical communication and leads to entrainment or the reciprocal sharing of physical and emotional cues between parent and infant as attachment progresses.

Table 34–1

POTENTIAL ADAPTIVE AND MALADAPTIVE MOTHERING BEHAVIORS

TIME/SITUATION	ADAPTIVE	MALADAPTIVE
Delivery	Attempts to position head to see infant as soon as delivered and while infant is on warming table	Does not position head to see baby Stares at ceiling
	When shown infant: Smiles Keeps eyes on infant, looking at all parts exposed Attempts en face position Uses fingertip touch on face and extremities Asks to hold baby Partially opens blanket to see more of infant Talks to baby Asks questions about baby	When shown infant: Frowns Stares at baby without expression Does not assume en face position Turns head away Does not touch baby Does not ask to hold baby Declines offer to hold baby If infant is placed in her arms, lies still and does not touch or stroke face or extremities May not look at infant Does not talk to baby Asks few or no questions
	Makes positive statement about baby: "She is so cute." "He is so soft!"	Makes no comments or makes only negative statements: "She looks awful." "He's ugly."
	May cry out of joy or relief that infant is normal or of desired sex	May cry, appearing unhappy or depressed
	May smile and cry at the same time; to differentiate from crying out of disappointment, must note facial expressions and verbal statements	When asked why she is crying, states being disappointed in baby
	Expresses satisfaction with or acceptance of sex of infant. "We really wanted a girl, but it is more important that he is healthy." "I can't believe a boy at last!"	Expresses dissatisfaction with sex of the baby. "Not another girl. I should have known better than to have tried again for a boy." "I don't even want to see him." May use profanity when told sex
	Predominant affect—appears pleased and happy	Predominant affect—appears sad, angry, or expressionless
	Suddenly decides she wants to breastfeed	Suddenly decides against breastfeeding
First week	Initially uses fingertips on head and extremities Progresses to using fingers and palm on infant's trunk Eventually draws infant toward her, holding infant against her body	Uses fingertip touch, without progressing to using palm on trunk or drawing infant toward her body
	Snuggles infant to neck and face	Does not hold infant to neck and face
	Makes spontaneous movements: kissing, stroking, rocking	Makes few or no spontaneous movements with infant
	Attempts to establish eye contact by moving infant, assuming en face position, or shielding infant's eyes from light	Does not use en face position or attempt to establish eye-to-eye contact
	Handles and holds baby at times other than when giving direct care	Handles baby only as necessary to feed or change diapers
	Talks to infant	Does not talk to infant
	Smiles at baby frequently—changes affect appropriately, such as when infant cries	Rarely smiles at baby *or* smiles all the time without change in affect

Table continued on following page

Table 34–1

POTENTIAL ADAPTIVE AND MALADAPTIVE MOTHERING BEHAVIORS Continued

TIME/SITUATION	ADAPTIVE	MALADAPTIVE
	Makes many specific observations of infant: "Her eyes look like they might turn brown." "One foot turns in just a bit."	Makes no observations Makes few observations that are either general or negative
	Discusses infant's characteristics, attempting to relate them to others in the family: "He has my ears, but his daddy's chin." "She really doesn't look like either of our baby pictures, she just looks like herself."	Does not discuss infant's characteristics in relation to characteristics of family members
	With a positive affect and affectionate manner, uses animal characteristics to describe baby: "She is just like a cuddly little kitten." "His hair feels like down."	In a negative or hostile manner, uses animal characteristics to describe baby: "She looks awful, just like a drowned rat." "He looks just like an ape to me."
	Asks questions about caring for infant after discharge	Asks no questions about care
	By the time infant is discharged, has obtained basic supplies for caring for infant	Has made no plans for obtaining basic supplies
First few weeks	If infant remains hospitalized after mother is discharged:	
	Calls every 1–2 days	Calls less frequently than every other day, or not at all
	Visits minimum of twice a week	Visits less frequently than twice a week, or not at all
	Visits minimum of 30 minutes	Visits less than 30 minutes
	Asks specific questions about infant's condition	Asks nonspecific questions Asks very few questions Asks inappropriate questions
	Spends most of visit looking at and handling infant	Spends most of visit observing unit activities and other infants (this may be normal behavior first 1 or 2 visits); has little or no interaction with infant during visits
	Becomes involved with care when encouraged and supported by staff	When encouraged by staff to participate in care, refuses, terminates visit, or does only minimal care
	Although visits are frequent and last longer than 30 minutes, makes statements about missing infant, e.g., expresses that she misses baby at home or that she wishes she could visit more often and stay longer	Makes no statements about missing infant *or* States she misses baby at home and wishes she could visit more often, but comments are not validated by frequent or lengthy visits
	Expresses reluctance to terminate visit	Leaves nursery with little hesitation
	Waits until infant is asleep before leaving; touches or talks to baby just before leaving; may stand outside window and look at baby before leaving unit	Frequently asks nurse to complete feeding or to change or settle infant
First months	Holds infant close to her body	Does not hold infant securely against body
	Supports infant's trunk and head in position of comfort	Head and body of infant are not well supported

Table continued on facing page

Table 34–1

POTENTIAL ADAPTIVE AND MALADAPTIVE MOTHERING BEHAVIORS Continued

TIME/SITUATION	ADAPTIVE	MALADAPTIVE
	Muscles in arms and hands are relaxed and conform to curvature of infant's body	Shoulder, arm, and hand muscles appear tense
	During feedings, holds infant in well-supported position against her body	Holds infant away from body during feedings, or props infant or bottle
	Positions during feeding so eye-to-eye contact can occur	Position during feeding prevents eye-to-eye contact
	Minimizes talking to infant during sucking	Continues talking to infant during feeding, even though infant is distracted and stops sucking
	Refers to infant using given or affectionate name	Refers to infant in impersonal way, e.g., "the baby," "she," or "it"
	Plays with infant at times unrelated to direct care	Handles infant mainly during caretaking activities
	When infant is in infant seat, playpen, or crib, frequently interacts with the baby	Leaves infant for long periods in infant seat, playpen, or crib, interacting only after baby becomes fussy
	Places infant, when awake, in an area where the baby can observe and interact with others	Leaves infant, when awake, alone for long periods in bedroom or isolated area
	Occasionally leaves infant with someone else	Frequently leaves baby with someone else *or* Refuses to leave baby with someone else
	Uses discretion in selecting baby-sitter and provides baby-sitter with instructions on baby's routines, likes, and dislikes	Does not use good judgment in selecting baby-sitter; provides inadequate or no instructions for care
	Provides infant with routine well-baby care	Fails to provide infant with well-baby care, seeking medical assistance only after problems arise *or* Keeps all appointments and makes additional phone calls or additional visits to physical or emergency department for imagined or insignificant problems
	Carries out medical plan for management of specific problems or conditions, e.g., thrush, anemia, or an ear infection	Fails to carry out or is inconsistent in carrying out medical plan for specific problems
	Remains close to infant during physical examinations and attempts to soothe if the baby becomes distressed	Remains seated at a distance from the examination table; does not soothe infant during examination; frequently arranges for someone else to take infant for medical appointments
	Makes positive statements about mothering role	Makes negative statements about mothering role

From Cropley, C. (1986). Assessment of mothering behaviors. In S. H. Johnson (Ed.), *Nursing assessment and strategies for the family at risk: High-risk parenting* (2nd ed., pp. 22–24). Philadelphia: J. B. Lippincott.

Assessment Tool: Mother-Infant Screening Tool

	A	B	C	D
TACTILE	**Mother** Holds infant close to her body	Holds infant on forearm	Holds infant away from body	Does not hold infant
	Infant Curls up close to mother	Keeps some distance	Moves away when touched	Stiffens up when held
	Mother Comfortable touching infant, strokes head or face	Looks comfortable, pats infant's back	Tentative when touching infant	Avoids touching infant
	Infant At ease, turns toward mother's touch	Looks at ease	Looks tense	Cries when touched
VISUAL	**Mother** Establishes eye contact	Looks at infant's face	Does not look at infant's face	Does not look at infant
	Infant Establishes eye contact	Looks at mother's face	Does not look at mother's face	Does not look at mother
	Mother Smiles and makes faces in play	Smiles	No special facial expressions	Looks unhappy
	Infant Laughs or big smile	Smiles	No special facial expressions	Looks unhappy
AUDITORY	**Mother** Talks to infant in soothing or playful way	Talks to infant in calm way	Talks but just gives directions	Does not talk to infant
	Infant Makes happy sounds, coos and goos	Makes ah-ah sounds	Cries	Does not talk
	Mother Understands meaning of infant's cries	Differentiates most of infant's cries	Seldom differentiates infant's cries	Never differentiates infant's cries
	Infant Exhibits different cries	Usually exhibits different cries	Seldom exhibits different cries	Never exhibits different cries
FEEDING	**Mother** Shows signs of pleasure during feeding—smiles rocks, sings	Looks content during feeding	Acts unsure during feeding—stops and starts	Agitated or irritable
	Infant Shows pleasure in being fed—smiles, coos	Looks content during feeding	Restless during feeding	Agitated—cries during feeding
	Mother Looks pleased after feeding	Looks satisfied after feeding	Looks uneasy after feeding	Looks agitated after feeding
	Infant Looks happy after feeding	Looks satisfied after feeding	Looks restless after feeding	Looks agitated after feeding

TOTAL SCORE
Mother
Infant
DATE

From Reiser S. L. (1981). A tool to facilitate mother-infant attachment. *Journal of Obstetric, Gynecologic, and Neonatal Nursing,* 10, 294–297.

haviors at four different points in time during the first few months of an infant's life and to describe the parent's responses to milestones in the infant's life. Cropley (1986) defined adaptive behaviors as "those which are indicators of maternal-infant attachment and meet both the infant's and mother's needs" and maladaptive behaviors as "those which indicate a lack of maternal-infant attachment and result in unmet infant and/or mother's needs" (p. 21).

Reiser (1981) developed a screening tool that can be used to rate eight infant and eight maternal behaviors on a 4-point scale (see Mother-Infant Screening Tool). This tool is relatively easy to administer, and the total scores can be used to assess changes in the developing attachment relationship, although further research is needed to determine its reliability and validity. Reiser (1981) suggested that two or more behaviors in the C or D categories suggest the need for further evaluation or intervention.

Murphy (1986) developed an Observation Guide for Fathering Behaviors to assess adaptive and maladaptive fathering behaviors. The frequency of behaviors in each category (always, usually, or rarely adaptive) is summed to obtain a numerical score on the tool. Although the items in the tool identify passive paternal involvement in child care as maladaptive behavior, Murphy (1986) acknowledged that such a lack of involvement may be adaptive for some families. Nurses should assess the "fit" between maternal and paternal role expectations when assessing fathering behaviors. It is also important to ask parents whether they are experiencing a conflict between their role expectations and present parenting responsibilities. The results of several studies suggest that fathers often participate less in infant care than they expected and that fathers' participation often lags behind mothers' expectations (Humenick and Bugen 1987; Rustia and Abbott 1990). Rustia and Abbott (1990) observed 53 couples for 2 years after the birth of their first infant and found that in the early postpartum period, mothers expected more help from fathers with infant care than they received. By the end of the first year, fathers assumed increased responsibility for child care, although most of their activities were play oriented. Mothers assumed primary responsibility for caretaking activities such as diapering, feeding, and dressing. Rustia and Abbott (1990) found that it took nearly 2 years for couples to agree on a mutually acceptable pattern of child care and suggested that nurses should help new fathers with paternal role attainment.

Table 34–2 lists some of the other tools that have been developed to aid in assessing early parent-infant relationships. Not all of the tools have been tested to establish their validity and reliability, but they do provide guides that can be useful for nursing practice.

Measures of Infant Behaviors and Temperament

The infant's behavior and temperament have significant effects on the developing parent-infant relationship. Helping parents to understand their infant's behaviors and to perceive them realistically is one way to promote a healthy parent-infant acquaintance process and the development of optimal attachment. Two tools that can be used by nurses as guides for assessment and parent education in this area are the Carey-McDevitt Infant Temperament Questionnaire and the Brazelton Neonatal Behavioral Assessment Scale (BNBAS). In the Carey-McDevitt Questionnaire, parents are asked to rate their infants on a series of items related to nine categories of infant temperament: activity, rhythmicity, adaptability, approach, sensory threshold, intensity, mood, distractibility, and persistence. Parental responses to this questionnaire can be used by the nurse as a basis for teaching parents how to interact with their infants in the most effective and satisfying ways.

The BNBAS (Brazelton 1984) is used to evaluate a neonate's innate capabilities and his or her responses to inanimate and animate stimulation. The scale measures 27 infant behaviors that are organized into the following seven clusters: orientation, habituation, motor maturity, range of state, state regulation, autonomic stability, and reflexes. For the scale to be used reliably for research, the examiner must be trained in its administration, but nurses without special training can use the scale as a guideline for newborn assessment and parent education. The Mother's Assessment of the Behavior of Her Infant (MABI) scale is a modification of the BNBAS that can be used by mothers to assess their infants' behaviors (Field et al. 1978). The results of several studies suggest that mothers of both full-term and preterm infants are able to assess their infants' behaviors accurately with use of the MABI scale (Field et al. 1978; Harrison et al. 1991). Field found that asking teenage mothers to assess their babies weekly for 6 weeks using the MABI scale promoted positive parent-infant interactions.

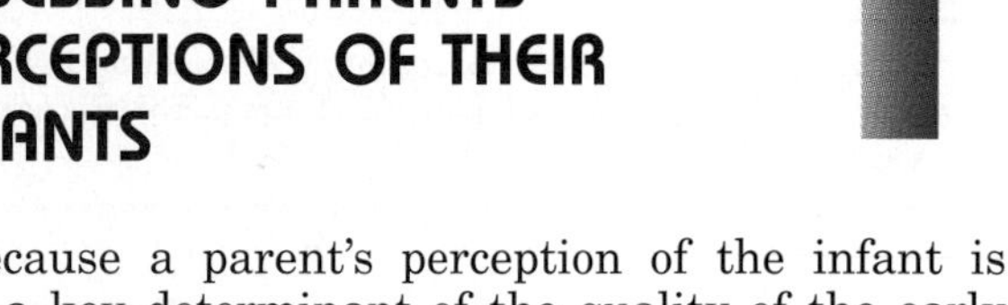

ASSESSING PARENTS' PERCEPTIONS OF THEIR INFANTS

Because a parent's perception of the infant is also a key determinant of the quality of the early parent-infant relationship, assessment of this perception can help the nurse to identify potential

Assessment Tool: Observation Guide for Fathering Behaviors

	Fathering Behavior		Frequency			
		Adaptive Behavior	always adaptive	usually adaptive	rarely adaptive	Maladaptive Behavior
father-child interaction	touches child	freely, gentle	○	●	○	rare, rough
	holds child	close, relaxed	○	○	●	distal, unrelaxed
	talks to child	appropriate	●	○	○	inappropriate
	listens to child	attentive	○	●	○	inattentive
	plays with child	active	●	○	○	passive
	posture	relaxed	○	●	○	rigid
	facial expression	expressive	●	○	○	inexpressive
	eye contact	frequent	●	○	○	infrequent
	response to cues	prompt	○	●	○	delayed
	knowledge of child's habits	knowledgeable	○	●	○	not knowledgable
	participation in physical care	active	○	○	●	passive
	protects child	aware, active	○	●	○	unaware, inactive
	disciplines child	initiates, reasonable	○	●	○	passive or inappropriate
	teaches child	initiates	●	○	○	no initiation
	reinforces child	active	●	○	○	passive
role gratification	initiates activity	active	○	●	○	passive
	verbally expresses pleasure	frequent	●	○	○	infrequent
	appears gratified	frequent	●	○	○	infrequent
growth potential	seeks information	active	●	○	○	passive
	response to teaching	positive	●	○	○	negative
family support	aware of own needs	aware, expressive	○	●	○	unaware, inexpressive
	verbally supports mother	active	○	○	●	passive
	verbally supported by mother	active	○	○	●	passive
	speaks of other children	frequent	●	○	○	infrequent

From Murphy, C. (1986). Assessment of fathering behaviors. In S. H. Johnson (Ed.), *Nursing assessment and strategies for the family at risk:* High-risk parenting (2nd ed., p. 53). Philadelphia: J. B. Lippincott.

Table 34–2

OTHER TOOLS FOR ASSESSING EARLY PARENTING (ARRANGED ALPHABETICALLY BY TITLE)

NAME OF TOOL	VARIABLES ASSESSED	WHERE PUBLISHED OR AVAILABLE
Assessment of Maternal-Infant Sensitivity (AMIS)	Reciprocity on mother-infant interaction during a feeding; assesses both maternal behaviors and infant behaviors (reliability and validity have been tested)	Price, G. M. (1983). Sensitivity in mother-infant interactions: The AMIS scale. *Infant Behavior and Development,* 6, 353–360.
Categories of Adaptive and Maladaptive Mothering and Infant Behaviors	Maternal and infant behaviors (not tested for reliability and validity)	Harrison, L. L. (1976). Nursing intervention with failure to thrive family. *MCN: American Journal of Maternal-Child Nursing,* 1, 111–116.
Home Observation for Measurement of the Environment (HOME)	Characteristics of the child's physical, social, and emotional environment in the home (reliability and validity have been tested)	Caldwell, B. M., and Robert, H. B. (1970). *Home Observation for Measurement of the Environment.* Available from Dr. Caldwell at Child Development Research Unit, University of Arkansas at Little Rock, 33rd & University Avenue, Little Rock, AR 72204.
Maternal-Fetal Attachment Scale	Mother's attachment to her fetus; subscales measure roletaking, differentiation of self from fetus, interaction with fetus, attributing characteristics to the fetus, and giving of self (reliability and validity have been tested)	Cranley, M. (1981). Roots of attachment: The relationship of parents with their unborn. *Birth Defects Original Article Series,* 17 (6), 59–82. March of Dimes Birth Defects Foundation.
Maternal-Infant Observation Scale	Maternal attachment behavior observed during a feeding session	Avant, P. K. (1982). A maternal attachment assessment strategy. In S. S. Humenick (Ed.), *Analysis of current assessment strategies in the health care of young children and childbearing families* (pp. 171–178). Norwalk, CT: Appleton-Century-Crofts.
Mother-Infant Interaction Assessment	Maternal behaviors during a feeding session (reliability and validity have been tested)	Funke-Furber, J. (1978). *Reliability and validity testing of indicators of maternal adaptive behavior.* Alberta, Canada: University of Alberta.
Mothering Behaviors Observation Guide	Maternal attachment behaviors (reliability and validity have been tested)	Harrison, L. L. (1982). *Teaching parents about their premature infants: Effects on attachment and perceptions.* University of Tennessee, Knoxville. Unpublished doctoral dissertation.
Nursing Child Assessment Satellite Training Project (NCAST) feeding and teaching scales	Maternal behaviors related to sensitivity, response to distress, and growth fostering; also assesses infant's clarity of cues and responsiveness (reliability and validity have been tested)	Kathryn Barnard, RN, PhD, University of Washington College of Nursing, Seattle, WA.

Table continued on following page

Table 34–2

OTHER TOOLS FOR ASSESSING EARLY PARENTING (ARRANGED ALPHABETICALLY BY TITLE) Continued

NAME OF TOOL	VARIABLES ASSESSED	WHERE PUBLISHED OR AVAILABLE
Nursing Inventory for Assessing Early Father-Infant Interaction	Paternal attachment behaviors (reliability and validity have not been tested)	Weiser, M. A., and Castiglia, P. T. (1984). Assessing early father-infant attachment. *MCN: American Journal of Maternal-Child Nursing,* 9 (2), 104–106.
Observation Guide for Maternal Behavior	Critical attachment tasks, e.g., identifies infant's physical condition, includes infant in the family, changes behaviors in response to infant's behavior (reliability and validity have not been tested)	Cropley, C. (1986). Assessment of mothering behaviors. In S. H. Johnson (Ed.), *Nursing assessment and strategies for the family at risk: High-risk parenting* (2nd ed., pp. 36–37). Philadelphia: J. B. Lippincott.
Paternal-Fetal Attachment Scale	Father's attachment to the fetus (an adaptation of the maternal-fetal scale)	Weaver, R. H., and Cranley, M. S. (1983). An exploration of paternal fetal attachment behavior. *Nursing Research,* 32 (2), 6.
Perinatal Assessment of Mother-Baby Interaction	Warning signs suggesting the potential for child abuse and neglect or other maladaptive parenting behaviors (reliability and validity not described, but authors report that a group of mothers at high risk for child abuse or neglect was successfully identified by perinatal screening procedures)	Gray, J., Cutlier, C., Dean, J., Kempe, C. H. (1976). Perinatal assessment of mother-baby interaction. In R. E. Helfer and C. H. Kempe (Eds.), *Child abuse and neglect: The family and the community.* Cambridge, MA: Ballinger.
Post Partum Self-Evaluation Questionnaire	Factors related to maternal adaptation: quality of relationship with husband; mother's perception of father's participation in child care; gratification from labor and delivery experience; satisfaction with life circumstances; confidence in ability to cope with tasks of motherhood; satisfaction with motherhood and infant care; support from parents; support from friends and other family members (reliability and validity have been tested)	Lederman, R. P., Weingarten, C. T., Lederman, E. (1981). Post partum self evaluation questionnaire: Measures of maternal adaptation. *Birth Defects Original Article Series,* 17 (6), 201–231.
Prenatal Assessment of Parenting Guide	Perceptions of complexities of mothering; attachment; acceptance of child by significant others; ensuring physical well-being; problem areas in the woman's life situation (reliability and validity have not been tested fully)	Josten, L. (1981). Prenatal assessment guide for illuminating possible problems with parenting. *MCN: American Journal of Maternal-Child Nursing,* 6, 113–117.
What Being the Parent of a New Baby Is Like (WPL)	Parents' beliefs about themselves and their perceptions of the parenting experience; subscales measure centrality of infant in parent's life, change experienced by parent, and evaluation of parenting performance (reliability and validity have been tested)	Pridham, K. F., and Chang, A. S. (1989). What being the parent of a new baby is like: Revision of an instrument. *Research in Nursing and Health,* 12, 323–329.

problem areas, such as an incorrect or negative perception of the infant. Broussard developed the Neonatal Perception Inventory (NPI) to measure a parent's perception of her or his infant compared with her or his conception of the "average" infant (Broussard and Hartner 1971). The NPI is a six-item scale describing infant crying, spitting, feeding, elimination, sleeping, and predictability behaviors. Values of one through five are assigned by the parent to each item, with lower values representing more desirable behaviors. One set of items refers to "Your Baby," and the other to the "Average Baby."

The NPI score is obtained by measuring the discrepancy between the parent's ratings of his or her infant and the average baby. Mothers who perceive their infants as average or worse than average are considered to have negative perceptions. Broussard administered the inventory to a large group of primiparous mothers on two occasions: 2 to 4 days after birth (NPI 1) and 4 to 6 weeks after delivery (NPI 2). Negative NPI 2 scores were found to be predictive of subsequent emotional problems in the children on follow-up studies when the children where 4½ and 10 to 11 years old (Broussard 1979). Palisin (1980) replicated Broussard's study and did not find a significant relationship between NPI 2 scores and subsequent psychiatric assessments of the children. Even though the NPI may not be a valid predictor of the child's subsequent emotional development, it could be useful to nurses in identifying parents who perceive their infants negatively. Intervention could then be directed toward learning the reasons for the parent's negative perceptions and correcting any misconceptions the parent might have.

Nursing Practice

Nursing Process

▼ Assessment

Assessing the early interactions between parents and their new infant enables the nurse to diagnose actual or potential problems related to parenting. The limited amount of contact between nurses and parents during the postpartum hospital stay (generally only 24 to 48 hours) makes it difficult to identify parenting problems in all but the most overt situations. Clinic nurses or public health nurses may have more opportunity to develop ongoing relationships with parents and to identify actual or potential parenting problems.

▼ Diagnosis

Five potential nursing diagnoses related to parenting that might be considered include

- Altered parenting related to the state in which a nurturing figure experiences an inability to create an environment that promotes the optimal growth and development of another human being
- Family coping: potential for growth related to effective managing of adaptive tasks by family member involved with the health challenge, who now is exhibiting desire and readiness for enhanced health and growth in regard to self and in relation to the client

- Knowledge deficit: absence or deficiency of cognitive information related to disease management procedures and self-care practices recommended to restore health or maintain wellness
- Parental role conflict related to the state in which a parent experiences role confusion and conflict in response to crises
- Risk for altered parenting related to the state in which a nurturing figure is at risk to experience an inability to create an environment that promotes the optimal growth and development of another human being

▼ Planning

After identifying the appropriate diagnosis, the nurse needs to establish priorities and plan appropriate interventions to promote parent-infant attachment. Although the nurse should begin to assess parental reactions to the fetus during pregnancy, the focus of the intervention discussed in the following section is the early postpartum period. Interventions should be appropriate for the parent's stage of role acquisition (Bocar and Moore 1987). An interdisciplinary approach to intervention is generally recommended, because young families have contacts with a variety of helping professionals. Nurses need to coordinate their interventions with other service providers such as social workers, physicians, and parent educators.

▼ Intervention

General intervention strategies that might be used after the child's birth are helping parents to integrate the birth experience (Konrad 1987); helping parents meet their own needs; helping parents develop successful infant care skills and satisfying interactions with their infants; promoting realistic parental perceptions and expectations of infant behavior; providing parents with education and anticipatory guidance, for example, demonstrating the newborn's reflexes to the parents (Fig. 34–4); and initiating group parenting classes

▼ HELPING PARENTS TO INTEGRATE THE BIRTH EXPERIENCE

Several writers have suggested that mothers need to review their performance and experiences during labor to reconcile differences between what they expected and what actually occurred (Konrad 1987; Mercer 1981; Rubin 1961). Such a review can be equally helpful to fathers and may be particularly important if parents feel embarrassed or guilty about how they acted during labor and delivery. The opportunity to discuss their experiences with a nurse can help prevent long-lasting problems with decreased self-esteem that might interfere with early parenting (Bocar and Moore 1987).

▼ HELPING PARENTS MEET THEIR OWN NEEDS

Parenthood in today's society is a role fraught with joy and fulfillment as well as frustration and difficulty. It is important for all parents to have

HELPING PARENTS SUCCEED WITH PARENTAL ROLE ATTAINMENT

During the early, formal stages of parental role acquisition, avoid overwhelming parents with too much information or with conflicting sources of advice about infant care. Parents need concrete demonstrations and suggestions during this period. It is also important to

- DEVELOP A TRUSTING, SUPPORTIVE RELATIONSHIP WITH PARENTS, in which you serve as a resource person rather than an expert with all the answers.
- ACKNOWLEDGE AND ENCOURAGE POSITIVE PARENTING BEHAVIORS. Focus on the family's strengths.
- ACCEPT PARENTS "WHERE THEY ARE." Base your teaching on the needs identified by the parents.
- WHEN DEMONSTRATING INFANT CARE SKILLS, using a doll rather than the parent's own baby may decrease the chances that parents will feel inadequate by observing your deft handling of their infant (Bocar and Moore 1987, p. 10).
- BE AWARE THAT PROBLEMS WITH PARENTING MAY BE COMPLEX and avoid offering simplistic solutions (Egeland and Erickson 1990, p. 34).
- ENCOURAGE PARENTS TO FILL OUT A SLEEP/ACTIVITY RECORD OF THE INFANT'S BEHAVIORS AND ACTIVITIES DURING A 24-HOUR PERIOD so that they can develop a more realistic understanding of the baby's behavioral patterns and the effect of the infant on family activities.

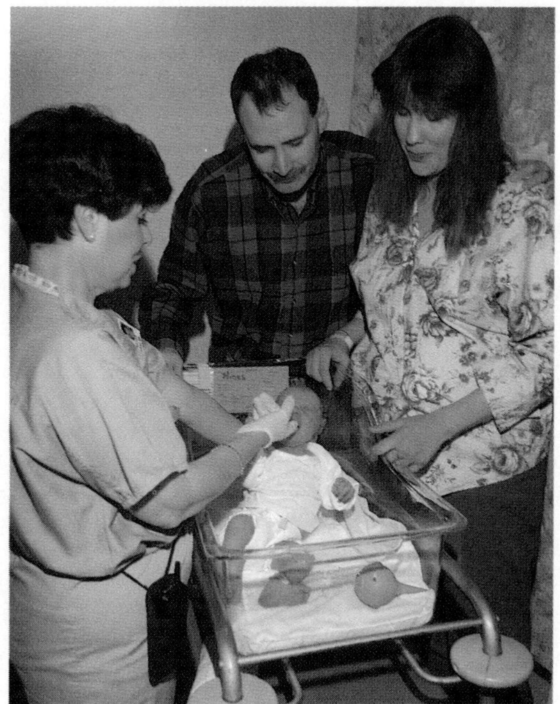

Figure 34–4

The nurse provides parents with education and anticipatory guidance when demonstrating care skills and the infant's reflexes.

time to meet their own needs in addition to meeting the many needs of their new infant. This is often difficult in today's society when many families live far away from the support of extended families. Nurses can help parents plan ways to meet their needs for growth and fulfillment as individuals and as a couple. Such planning might include identifying various support systems within the community, such as baby-sitting resources, or helping parents identify individual goals and ways to achieve them.

▼ HELPING PARENTS DEVELOP SUCCESSFUL INFANT CARE SKILLS AND SATISFYING INTERACTIONS

Early and extended contact between parents and their newborn provides an opportunity for development of confidence in parenting skills. Nurses can help parents by providing individual or group teaching about infant care. As with all teaching interventions, it is necessary to begin by assessing the parent's needs for and interest in teaching. Some hospitals have a variety of parent education films available on closed-circuit television so that parents can view films of particular interest at a convenient time. If written teaching materials are used, it is important to ensure that they are culturally relevant and appropriate for the parent's literacy level. Role modeling by the nurse is another strategy for demonstrating skills, such as feeding, bathing, diapering, and calming a distressed infant. Parents sometimes feel inadequate when they compare their own infant care skills with those of an experienced nurse. In teaching parents, therefore, it is important for nurses to identify and reinforce positive and successful parenting behaviors frequently to enhance parental confidence and self-esteem. Comments such as "he really seems to enjoy the way you hold him" can be encouraging to an insecure parent.

Early home visits by a community health nurse can help parents develop confidence in their parenting skills, particularly if the mother and baby were discharged from the hospital soon after delivery or if the initial nursing assessment identified potential maladaptive parenting problems. Home visits allow the nurse to better assess environmental factors that may influence the early parent-infant relationship. Many questions and concerns do not arise until parents leave the hospital and confront the realities of their new roles. Home visits provide an opportunity for parents to discuss these concerns in a comfortable, nonthreatening environment. The results of several studies have confirmed the benefits of home visits to new parents (Hardy and Street 1989; Olds et al. 1988). For example, Olds and colleagues (1988) evaluated a comprehensive program of prenatal and postpartum nursing home visits for socially disadvantaged primiparous women. Compared with a control group, women who received the home visits had more favorable pregnancy outcomes, less dysfunctional caregiving, and fewer subsequent pregnancies. In addition, mothers who received the home visits were more likely to return to school or seek employment.

After assessing the infant's individual responses or temperament, the nurse can help parents identify effective interaction strategies. For example, the BNBAS or the MABI scale may indicate that the baby has difficulty in habituating to or shutting out noxious environmental stimuli. The parents of such an infant might then be advised to decrease environmental stimuli by using soft voices when talking to the infant and eliminating extraneous noise and light. The BNBAS and MABI scale can also be used to help parents identify measures that are effective in consoling the infant when he or she is irritable. Because it takes approximately 30 minutes to administer the BNBAS, the nurse may use only some of the items (e.g., those related to orientation, habituation, and consolability) as a basis for parent education.

▼ PROMOTING REALISTIC PERCEPTIONS AND EXPECTATIONS

As discussed previously, unrealistic or negative parental perceptions or expectations of the infant

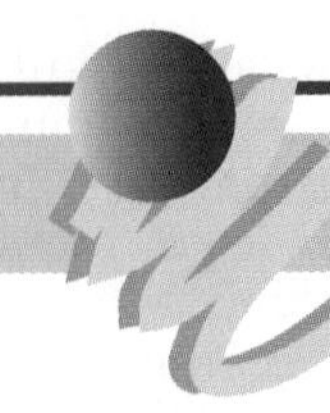

TEACHING GUIDE

PROMOTING POSITIVE PARENT-INFANT RELATIONSHIPS

TOPIC	*MAJOR CONCEPT*
Emotional reactions after the birth of an infant	Many women go through a period of emotional distress beginning 2 to 3 days after delivery, which is probably due to hormonal changes (Porter 1985). However, Bocar and Moore (1987) caution that overemphasis on hormonal influences may increase mothers' feelings of oversensitivity and dependency. Both parents may feel overwhelmed with the recognition of their new responsibilities. During the early weeks after delivery, it is common for parents to feel inadequate, lack self-confidence, and be unusually sensitive to comments about their parenting behaviors (Bocar and Moore 1987). Explain to your clients that parents will experience highs and lows—both joys and disillusionment during the process of developing an attachment to their infant. "Contradictory and ambivalent feelings are normal, and all feelings are legitimate" (Bocar and Moore 1987, p. 7). The process of parent-infant attachment takes time and evolves as both parents and infant become acquainted and comfortable with one another.
Needs to readjust family roles after the birth of a new infant	Parents may experience a discrepancy between role expectations and actual behaviors. Fathers sometimes participate less than they expected to during the early months. But by the end of the first year, fathers often assume increased responsibility, especially in play activities (Rustia and Abbott 1990). It may take up to 2 years for couples to agree on a mutually acceptable pattern of child care (Rustia and Abbott 1990).
Need for parents to receive physical and emotional support to focus their energies on parenting tasks	Some parents try to be "superparents," taking on new parenting responsibilities without relinquishing previous responsibilities. Encourage parents to identify friends and family members who can assist them. Parents may need to examine and readjust their priorities.
Need for parents to meet their own needs to meet infant's needs	Parents who have supportive relationships with other adults and feel a sense of personal fulfillment will be better able to meet their infants' needs. Encourage your clients to spend some time with the spouse or partner, away

Continued on facing page

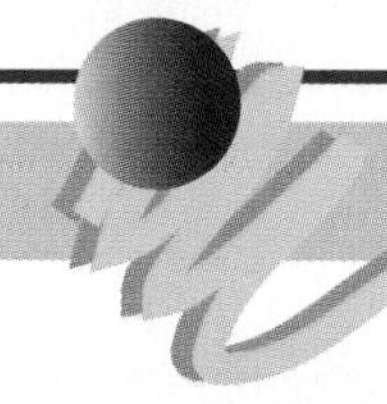

TEACHING GUIDE

PROMOTING POSITIVE PARENT-INFANT RELATIONSHIPS Continued

TOPIC	*MAJOR CONCEPT*
	from the infant; ask friends and family members to assist periodically with child care; evaluate their individual long-term goals related to work, school, and family roles.
Infant care skills	It is sometimes overwhelming to hear conflicting advice from multiple sources (family, friends, media) about infant care. There is usually no single best way to feed, bathe, hold, or diaper an infant. Parents will need time to identify specific "techniques" that work best for them. Observing others (e.g., nurses, friends, family members who have had experience with infant care) demonstrate infant care skills, and then practicing these skills, will help your clients become comfortable in meeting their infant's basic needs for "nourishment, protection, and daily hygiene care" (Bocar and Moore 1987, p. 5). As parents become more comfortable with infant care skills, they can replace the fantasy of the "perfect" parent with more realistic expectations and their own unique parenting styles. They will soon be the "experts" in caring for their baby.
Promoting optimal infant development	Realistic expectations of infant development and awareness of how to promote optimal development can enhance parent-infant attachment. The *Washington Guide to Promoting the Development of the Young Child* provides useful guidelines for understanding and promoting development in the areas of motor activity, feeding, sleep, play, language, and discipline.
Dealing with the infant's crying	Many infants go through a period of irritability starting when they are 4 to 6 weeks old. Some infants develop "colic" and have daily episodes of inconsolable crying during the first 3 months of life. By observing their infants closely, parents can learn to identify the meaning of different infant cries (e.g., hunger, fatigue, wet diaper, or the need for holding or attention). By asking parents how they feel when their infant cries, the nurse can identify potential problems and assess the need for supports or anticipatory guidance. Crying is the infant's most effective means of communicating his or

Continued on following page

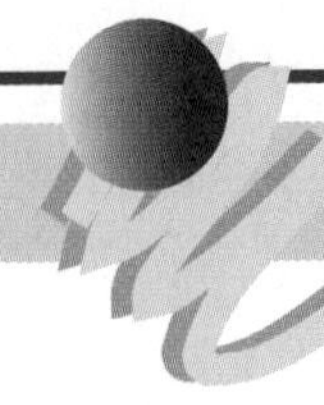

TEACHING GUIDE

PROMOTING POSITIVE PARENT-INFANT RELATIONSHIPS Continued

TOPIC	*MAJOR CONCEPT*
	her needs. By responding readily to the infant's cries, parents promote the development of a satisfying reciprocal attachment relationship. There may be times when parents experience extreme frustration with the infant's crying behaviors, or the "end of the rope syndrome" (Bishop 1980). It is helpful to identify friends or relatives who can provide some relief for the parents by assisting with infant care at these times.
Factors affecting parent-infant bonding and attachment	The attachment relationship between parent and infant is influenced by characteristics of the parents, the infant, and the environment (Barnard 1986). Attachment is a reciprocal process in which parents and infant continually influence each other. The development of attachment is enhanced if parents are attentive to the infant's behaviors and maintain close physical contact through touch, eye contact, and talking or singing to the infant (Porter 1985, p. 7). Factors in the infant that may influence attachment are the baby's temperament, sleep and activity patterns, crying behaviors, responsiveness to parents, and the clarity of cues indicating the infant's needs (Barnard 1986; Porter 1985). The BNBAS and MABI scales can be used to help parents identify the individual characteristics and behaviors of their baby.

Teaching Aids

1. *Falling in Love with Your Baby, Getting to Know Your Newborn,* and *Parenting Insights*—Pamphlets available from Johnson & Johnson Baby Products Company, Grandview Road, Skillman, NJ 08558 (1-800-526-3967).
2. *From Pregnancy to Parenthood* and *Your Marvelous Newborn*—Available from Ross Laboratories, Columbus, OH 43216.
3. Hack, M. (Producer), and Rambasek, P. (Director). (1975). *Amazing Newborn* (film). Available from Polymorph Films, 118 South Street, Boston, MA 02111 (1-800-223-5107).
4. *Keys to Caregiving*—A program made up of six videotapes, an 80-page study guide, and five booklets for parents about newborn behavior. The program is designed to help nurses aid parents in adjusting to their parenting role. Available from Nursing Child Assessment Satellite Training, The University of Washington, WJ-10, Seattle WA 98195 (206-543-8528).
5. *Washington Guide to Promoting the Development of the Young Child*—An excellent resource identifying expected tasks and suggested activities for promoting development in areas of motor behavior, feeding, sleep, play, language, and discipline for infants and young children. Useful as a guideline for parent education. This guide is available from Nursing Child Assessment Satellite Training, The University of Washington, WJ-10, Seattle, WA 98195 (206-543-8528).

can have adverse effects on parent-infant attachment. After assessing the parent's perceptions and expectations, the nurse can plan interventions to either correct misconceptions or reinforce positive or realistic perceptions. The results of several studies indicate that demonstrating the BNBAS to parents enhances parents' knowledge about infant behavior and appropriate responses and enhances maternal-infant sensitivity (Anderson 1981; Golas and Parks 1986; Poley-Strobel and Beckman 1987). Demonstrating the infant's individual characteristics and responses to the parents is generally more effective than merely telling parents about their infant's behaviors (Anderson 1981).

▼ ANTICIPATORY GUIDANCE

Providing parents with anticipatory guidance about situations they are likely to encounter during the early weeks at home can also promote parent-infant attachment. The results of several studies have identified informational needs of new parents that can help nurses provide meaningful guidance and education. Martell and coworkers (1989) studied the information needs of 42 women at 3 days postpartum (28 multiparas and 14 primiparas). All of the mothers had been discharged between 6 and 8 hours after delivery. These mothers were most interested in teaching related to health threats, infant care, and feeding. They were less interested in information about their own sexuality or family changes. Hiser (1987) interviewed ten multiparous women in their homes 10 to 14 days post partum and found that the mothers in this study expressed worries about meeting the needs of everyone at home, finding time for themselves, being a good mother, and their weight. They were particularly interested in learning about infant safety, health, growth, and development; reactions of siblings; cord care; and maternal tension and fatigue (Hiser 1987). The results of these studies can help nurses plan appropriate teaching programs for new mothers at different phases of the early postpartum period.

Although parents may feel comfortable with infant care in the hospital, they need to know about changes they might encounter during the early weeks at home related to such aspects of infant care as feeding and elimination patterns. Bishop (1980) reported that new mothers frequently express concern about their infants having either constipation or diarrhea. The nurse might help parents to understand the normal variability in infant elimination and to identify signs of problems in this area. Many infants go through a period of irritability starting about 4 to 6 weeks after delivery. Helping parents anticipate ways to deal with such a situation will enable them to cope with it more effectively. Finally, helping parents understand general patterns of infant growth and development will help them to have realistic expectations of their infants and plan appropriate infant stimulation activities. Bishop (1980) recommended that all parents receive anticipatory guidance about what she called the "end of the rope syndrome," which occurs "when the infant's crying or need for constant attention seems overwhelming or when some other thing has gone wrong in the home and the mother (or father) has no energy left for coping" (p. 218). Bishop (1980) recommended that nurses help parents develop contingency plans for how they will handle such situations.

Bocar and Moore (1987) suggested that interventions should also be based on the parent's stage of role acquisition. The anticipatory stage occurs before delivery and involves collecting information about the parenting role from multiple sources. Prenatal education classes can help parents prepare for the role changes that will occur after delivery. The formal stage of role acquisition encompasses the early postpartum period when parents first assume responsibility for their infant's care. During this stage, parents are interested primarily in mastering practical child care tasks. They may lack self-confidence and become overwhelmed and confused with conflicting advice about infant care. During this stage, parents need specific, concrete demonstrations and suggestions as well as acknowledgment that they are the "experts" in relating to their infant. Once parents develop confidence in their ability to meet the basic needs of their infants, they are ready to progress to the informal role acquisition stage. During this stage, parents are better able to process multiple sources of information about child care.

Helping parents to anticipate the role changes involved in the transition to parenthood helps them to adjust to their new roles and develop satisfying relationships with their infant. Multiparas need guidance about how to help siblings adjust to the new baby. Parents need reassurance that it takes time to become acquainted with their new infant and develop close feelings of attachment. Many parents feel guilty when they do not experience feelings of warmth and attachment immediately after delivery.

Anticipatory guidance can also help parents identify resources they might use to help them during the early months at home with their new infant. Such resources might include friends, neighbors, extended family members, helping professionals, and parent education or support groups.

▼ GROUP PARENTING CLASSES

Group parenting classes can be an effective forum for providing both education and support to ease the transition to parenthood. Parents benefit from the opportunity to meet others who share

Table 34–3

CURRICULUM FOR WORKING MOTHERS GROUP

SESSION	OBJECTIVES	CONTENT
One	To build atmosphere conducive for sharing ideas/feelings To begin exchange of ideas and information about employment and parenting	Labor and delivery experience Worries/concerns regarding return to work Myths about working mothers Overview of child care: Types of child care Advertising for child care
Two	To exchange ideas/information about finding child care To begin self-assessment of working parents	Child care issues: Telephone screening Interviewing techniques Contracts Maintaining relationship with provider Danger signs Working out transitions between work and home Self-assessment: type E woman
Three	To assess environmental conditions that foster stress To continue self-assessment of reactivity to stress, personal strengths/weaknesses, and resources and demands	Coping strategies: Which ones predict success? The importance of setting priorities Self-assessment: vulnerability to stress
Four	To increase confidence in the parenting role To understand and promote family adjustments To discuss changing one's environment as a coping strategy	Comparison of experiences Common concerns of all new parents Stumbling blocks during the transition back to work Families of origin as models for family behavior Role negotiation: Who does what at home and work?
Five	To develop strategies for maintaining well-being To address issues related to termination of the group To summarize personal resources and environmental demands to arrive at one's personal coping style	Identifying long- and short-term goals Finding choices when there seem to be none Career planning: pacing work involvement Day-to-day happiness The art of balancing Time-management strategies

From Collins, C., and Tiedje, L. B. (1988). A program for women returning to work after childbirth. *Journal of Obstetric, Gynecologic, and Neonatal Nursing,* 17 (4), 246–253.

similar experiences, and group teaching often enables the nurse to reach more families than would be possible with individual teaching. Parenting classes can be conducted in a variety of settings: hospitals, schools, homes, churches, or other community facilities. Participation can be enhanced by providing arrangements for child care and meeting at convenient times and locations. While serving as a public health nurse, the author developed an education/support group for mothers living in an inner-city apartment building. Volunteers provided child care, and the group meetings were held in the group members' apartments. Each session included a presentation by the nurse on a topic identified by the parents, followed by a discussion of the selected topic or other areas of concern to group members. Mothers evaluated the group favorably and were able to learn from the experiences of other group members.

Collins and Tiedje (1988) developed an innovative group program for working mothers. The program consisted of a series of six 2-hour sessions held in the group leader's home. Each group included four to six participants, and mothers were welcome to bring their infants to the meetings. Table 34–3 illustrates the objectives and content for each session. Collins and Tiedje (1988) suggested that nurses planning such groups should incorporate structured content as well as unstructured time to focus on the particular concerns of group members. In a formal evaluation comparing 18 mothers who participated in the group program with 13 mothers who did not participate, Collins and colleagues (1992) found that group participants had higher scores on marital satisfaction 1 year after delivery.

Thayer (1987) described a program in which a pediatric nurse practitioner and pediatrician co-led a series of three evening parent classes. Classes focused on child development, adjustment to parenting, child temperament, child care, discipline, and management of illness. Class sizes varied from 5 to 20 participants, although 10 parents seemed to be the optimal number for cost effectiveness and parent satisfaction. During the past 20 years, there has been a tremendous increase in the number of professional-supported self-help groups focusing on children and families.

▼ Evaluation

Evaluation is a key component of the nursing process. Nurses can use a variety of strategies to determine whether their interventions are effective in promoting positive parent-infant interaction. Ongoing assessment of parent-infant interaction with one of the assessment tools described can help nurses identify changing interaction patterns. It is also helpful to ask parents to describe their perceptions of their infants and of their parenting experiences. Active listening and focused observations enable the nurse to accurately evaluate interventions and revise the nursing care plan as needed.

FAMILIES WITH SPECIAL NEEDS

Adoptive Parents

Adoptive parents may have special needs for information on child care and reassurance that they are adequate parents. Walker (1981) suggested that adoptive parents need preparation for parenthood classes similar to those that are readily available to most biologic parents. Adoptive parents who have only minimal information about their child's genetic and social background may have special concerns about the child's growth and development. These parents may also be anxious about how others evaluate their parenting skills, particularly if they fear that the adoption agency could take their child away from them. With all of the publicity about the possibility of a sensitive period for attachment during the period immediately after delivery, these parents also need reassurance that they can develop close attachments to their children through the processes of caregiving and acquaintance. Watkins and Fisher (1993) described the conflicts experienced by many adoptive parents as they develop attachment relationships with their infants: "Healthy attachment requires that parents be able to bear feelings of rage and anger at the child's helplessness, dependency, and needfulness, at the demands of the child, her lack of gratitude, and the changes her presence has made in their lives. Adoptive parents are frequently reluctant to admit experiencing these ordinary mixed feelings about being a parent because they fear that in the eyes of others this admission might compromise their 'suitability' for parenthood—and it could!" (p. 15). Adoptive parents must also deal with several issues that are not faced by biologic parents, such as relationships with birth parents, disappointment about infertility, and for some, issues related to becoming a multiracial family (Watkins and Fisher 1993). In addition, there is an element of social stigma surrounding adoption and a prevailing social attitude that blood ties are essential for optimal parenting (Bartholet 1993). Nurses need to be sensitive to the many issues confronting adoptive parents so they can provide appropriate support to these parents in their transition to parenthood.

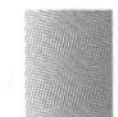

Parents of Twins

The principle of monotropy described by Klaus and Kennell (1982) specified that it is difficult for a mother to form a close attachment to more than one baby at a time. Parents of twins may experience special demands as they establish attachment relationships to two infants simultaneously (Fig. 34–5). Gromada (1981) reported that it often takes months or even years for the mother to form an individual attachment to each twin and noted that many mothers first develop an attachment to the twins as a unit. Once a mother has established this attachment, she is ready to distinguish the infants' individual characteristics. Identifying differences in the infants' appearances and behaviors helps parents develop distinctive attachments to each twin (Allen et al. 1976). Anderson and Anderson (1987, 1990) interviewed ten mothers of twins 1 month after delivery and found that parents were reluctant to discuss their infants' similarities. However, they were able to clearly differentiate their infants on the basis of physical characteristics and behaviors. Parenting literature

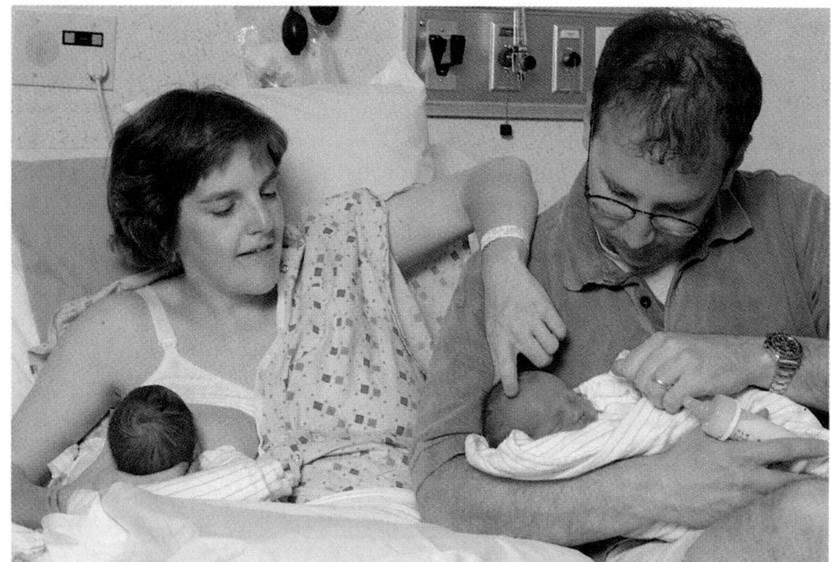

Figure 34–5

Parents of twins must establish attachment relationships with two infants simultaneously • Many mothers first develop an attachment to the twins as a unit before being able to distinguish the infants' individual characteristics.

that advises parents not to compare their twins may actually jeopardize parent-twin interaction (Anderson and Anderson 1987). Some mothers experience a delay in attachment to the second-born twin. Parental responses to the infant may be influenced by the placement of twins in the family (e.g., first-born or second-born) as well as by the time the parents had to prepare for the birth of twins. Nurses should observe the parents' interactions with each baby. Differences in the interaction patterns may be a clue to attachment difficulties.

Single Parents

There are a number of factors contributing to the rising frequency of single parenthood in our society: the high divorce rate, the increased occurrence of unmarried mothers who decide to keep their babies, and the increasing numbers of adoptions by single parents (Tankson 1986). Mercer (1990) reported that there were 933,013 infants born to unmarried women in 1987, representing a 40 percent increase above the number reported in 1980 (p. 199). The types of problems encountered by single-parent families vary according to factors such as socioeconomic status, cause of single parenthood, and sex of the parent. Role strain, financial insecurity, and social isolation are common stressors. Most single-parent families are headed by mothers, although Mercer (1990) pointed out that there are increasing numbers of such families headed by grandmothers. Important nursing interventions with these parents include helping them to determine priorities, identify resources, and develop problem-solving skills.

Nonmarried Lesbian Mothers

Mercer (1990) noted that increasing numbers of women who are openly lesbians are electing to have foster children, adopt children, or bear children after artificial insemination. Johnson and coworkers (1987) reported that approximately 1.5 million parents are gay or lesbian, and up to one third of lesbians are mothers. Mercer (1990) interviewed 18 lesbian mothers about their decision making and preparation for motherhood and found that most had spent several years before making the decision to become pregnant preparing themselves financially and emotionally. Because these women were creating families considered abnormal by the predominant culture, they needed to prepare themselves for parenting with limited social support and possible hostility from extended families, neighbors, health care providers, schools, and other institutions. Mercer (1990) identified the need for clinicians to provide culturally sensitive care to lesbians. Health care providers should not assume that all mothers are heterosexual. Clients need to feel comfortable talking with nurses and other health care providers about their lifestyles and sexual orientations so that they can receive appropriate support and guidance (Mercer 1990).

Adolescent Parents

Teenage parents face numerous challenges as they attempt to accomplish the developmental tasks of adolescence and parenthood simultaneously. An adolescent pregnancy is associated with a high risk for both physical and psychological complications among mother and infant. Although it is not possible to discuss adolescent pregnancy comprehensively in this book, several problems commonly encountered by adolescent parents are identified.

A major cause of the increased risk for physical complications of adolescent pregnancy is inadequate prenatal care. Thus, an important nursing goal is early identification of teenage pregnancies and provision of prenatal care that is both accessible and acceptable. Helping the pregnant adolescent to make decisions about whether to keep the infant or consider placing the infant for adoption and helping her develop a realistic understanding of the situation are important nursing strategies. Unmarried adolescent mothers who choose to keep their babies need considerable assistance and support as they attempt to accomplish their own developmental tasks and also meet the needs of their infants. Prenatal and postpartum education/support groups can help such mothers develop realistic expectations and coping strategies. Home visiting programs have also been effective in helping adolescent parents learn how to interact positively with their babies (Ware et al. 1987). Many schools have developed programs for pregnant adolescents that provide child care for the infant while the mother attends school so that she can continue her education.

Families of adolescent parents also need assistance in adjusting to the role changes that are precipitated by the infant's birth. Smith (1983) studied adolescents who continued to live with their families after the infants were born and noted that the families reacted in one of three ways to the birth of the infant: role blocking, role binding, and role sharing. Role blocking referred to the mother's failure to assume the maternal role. Role binding involved the "complete assumption of the maternal role by the adolescent" (p. 50). Role sharing was the pattern observed most frequently and occurred when the adolescent and family members shared the tasks associated with child care. Smith (1983) suggested that the pregnant adolescent and her parents could benefit from anticipatory guidance about the role changes and development tasks that accompany adolescent parenthood. Chapter 39 provides a more in-depth discussion of the special needs of adolescent parents; other resources include Barnes (1987), Corbett and Meyer (1987), Rosenheim and Testa (1991), and Williams (1991).

Implications for Research

Nurse researchers have initiated studies addressing many issues related to positive parent-infant attachment. The results of such research will provide future nurses with a scientific basic for their interventions with parents and young children. Some of the unanswered questions related to the promotion of positive parent-infant attachment include

- Are there different patterns of parent-to-infant attachment corresponding to the different patterns of infant-to-parent attachment?
- Are parental sensitivity, reciprocity, and responsiveness to the cues and needs of infants key indicators of parent-infant attachment?
- How can parental sensitivity, reciprocity, and responsiveness be measured? What are cultural differences in patterns of attachment?
- How does mother-infant attachment differ from father-infant attachment?
- Is there a sensitive period for the development of parent-infant attachment? What nursing interventions help parents develop positive and realistic perceptions of their infants?
- What are the most effective ways to help parents cope with the transition to parenthood and develop positive attachment relationships with their infants?

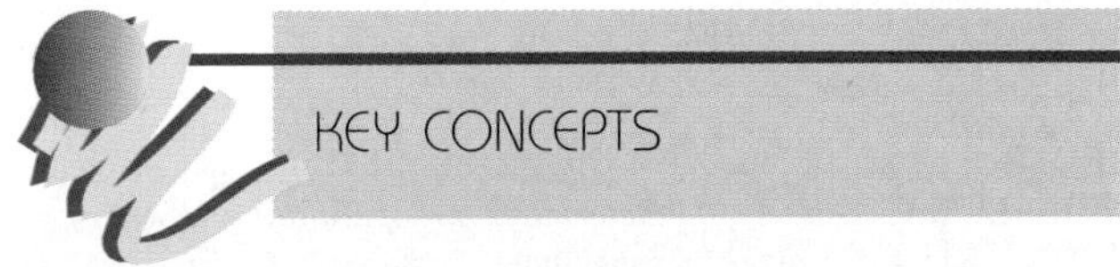

KEY CONCEPTS

- ▼ Social, cultural, and historical factors affect the nature of parenting roles and the quality of parent-child relationships.
- ▼ Attachment between a parent and child is an enduring affectionate bond that is reciprocal and gradual in development during the child's first year of life.
- ▼ Parental, situational, and infant variables affect the development of parent-infant attachment relationships.
- ▼ An important determinant of the quality and quantity of interaction between a parent and infant is the parent's perceptions of the infant's characteristics and behaviors.
- ▼ A key indicator of parent-infant attachment is the degree of parental sensitivity or responsiveness to the infant's cues and needs.
- ▼ The limited amount of contact between nurses and parents during the postpartum period makes it difficult for nurses working on postpartum units to identify parenting problems in all but the most overt situations.
- ▼ Nurses need to coordinate their interventions with other service providers such as social workers, psychologists, and parent educators.

- ▼ General nursing intervention strategies that might be used to promote positive early parent-infant relationships include helping parents integrate the birth experience, helping parents meet their own needs, helping parents develop infant care skills, promoting realistic perceptions and expectations, and providing parent education.
- ▼ Adoptive parents may have unique needs for information and support.
- ▼ Parents of twins may experience special demands as they establish attachment relationships to two infants simultaneously.
- ▼ Role strain, financial insecurity, and social isolation are common stressors experienced by both heterosexual and homosexual single parents.
- ▼ Important nursing interventions with adolescent parents include helping the adolescent make decisions about placing the infant for adoption and helping her develop a realistic understanding of her situation.

References

Ainsworth, M. D. S., and Wittig, B. A. (1969). Attachment and exploratory behavior of one-year-olds in a strange situation. In B. M. Foss (Ed.), *Determinants of infant behavior IV* (pp. 111–136). London: Methuen.

Ainsworth, M. D. S., Blehar, M. C., Waters, E., Wall, S. (1978). *Patterns of attachment—Psychological study of the strange situation.* Hillsdale, NJ: Lawrence Erlbaum Associates.

Allen, M., Greenspan, I., Pollin, W. (1976). The effect of parental perceptions on early development in twins. *Psychiatry,* 39, 65–71.

Anderson, A., and Anderson, B. (1987). Mothers' beginning relationship with twins. *Birth,* 14 (2), 94–98.

Anderson, A., and Anderson, B. (1990). Toward a substantive theory of mother-twin attachment. *MCN: American Journal of Maternal-Child Nursing,* 15, 373–377.

Anderson, C. (1981). Enhancing reciprocity between mother and neonate. *Nursing Research,* 30 (2), 89–93.

Auvenshine, M. A., and Enriquez, M. G. (1985). *Maternity nursing: Dimensions of change.* Monterey, CA: Wadsworth.

Barnard, K. (1986). *Nursing child assessment satellite training instructor's learning resource manual.* Available from NCAST, University of Washington, WJ-10, Seattle, WA 98195.

Barnes, A. S. (1987). *Single parents in black America: A study in culture and legitimacy.* Bristol, IN: Wyndham Hall Press.

Bartholet, E. (1993). *Family bonds: Adoption and the politics of parenting.* Boston: Houghton Mifflin.

Bigner, J. J. (1985). *Parent-child relations: An introduction to parenting* (2nd ed.). New York: Macmillan.

Bishop, B. (1980). *The maternity cycle: One nurse's reflections.* Philadelphia: F. A. Davis.

Bocar, D. L., and Moore, K. (1987). *Acquiring the parental role: A theoretical perspective.* Lactation Consultant Series. Franklin Park, IL: La Leche League International.

Bornstein, M. H. (1993). Approaches to parenting in culture. In M. H. Bornstein (Ed.), *Cultural approaches to parenting* (pp. 3–22). Hillsdale, NJ: Lawrence Erlbaum Associates.

Boukydis, C. F. Z. (1986). *Support for parents and infants—A manual for parenting organizations and professionals.* New York: Routledge & Kegan Paul.

Bowen, S. M., and Miller, B. C. (1980). Paternal attachment behavior as related to presence at delivery and preparenthood classes: A pilot study. *Nursing Research,* 29 (5), 307–311.

Bowlby, J. *Attachment and Loss: Attachment* (Vol. 1). (1969). New York: Basic Books.

Brazelton, T. B. (1984). *The neonatal behavioral assessment scale* (2nd ed.). Philadelphia: J. B. Lippincott.

Brazelton, T. B., Koslowski, B., Main, N. (1974). The origins of reciprocity: The early mother-infant interaction. In M. Lewis and L. Rosenblum (Eds.), *The effect of the infant on its caregiver.* New York: John Wiley & Sons.

Broussard, E. R. (1979). Assessment of the adaptive potential of the mother-infant system: The neonatal perception inventories. *Seminars in Perinatology,* 3, 91–100.

Broussard, E. R., and Hartner, M. S. S. (1971). Further considerations regarding maternal perception of the first-born. In J. Hellmuth (Ed.), *Exceptional infant—Studies in abnormalities* (Vol. 2). (pp. 432–439). New York: Brunner/Mazel.

Campbell, S. B. A., and Taylor, P. M. (1979). Bonding and attachment: Theoretical issues. *Seminars in Perinatology,* 3, 3–13.

Collins, C., and Tiedje, L. B. (1988). A program for women returning to work after childbirth. *Journal of Obstetric, Gynecologic, and Neonatal Nursing,* 17 (4), 246–253.

Collins, C., Tiedje, L. B., Stommel, M. (1992). Promoting positive well-being in employed mothers. *Health Care of Women International,* 13 (1), 77–85.

Corbett, M., and Meyer, J. H. (1987). *The adolescent and pregnancy.* Boston: Blackwell Scientific Publications.

Cranley, M. (1981). Roots of attachment: The relationship of parents with their unborn. In R. P. Lederman and B. S. Raff (Eds.), *Perinatal parental behavior: Nursing research and implications for newborn health.* Birth Defects Original Article Series, 17 (6), 59–75.

Cropley, C. (1986). Assessment of mothering behaviors. In S. H. Johnson (Ed.), *Nursing assessment and strategies for the family at risk: High-risk parenting* (2nd ed.). Philadelphia: J. B. Lippincott.

Curry, M. A. (1982). Maternal attachment behavior and the mother's self-concept: The effect of early skin-to-skin contact. *Nursing Research,* 31, 73–78.

Dawson, D. A., and Cain, V. S. (1990). Child care arrangements: Health of our nation's children, United States, 1988. In *Advance Data, 187. Washington, DC: Vital and Health Statistics of the National Center for Health Statistics,* United States Department of Health and Human Services.

deChateau, P. (1977). The importance of the neonatal period for the development of synchrony in the mother-infant dyad—A review. *Birth and the Family Journal,* 4 (1), 10–22.

Egeland, B., and Erickson, N. F. (1990). Rising above the past: Strategies for helping new mothers break the cycle of abuse and neglect. *Zero to Three—Bulletin of National Center for Clinical Infant Programs,* 11 (2), 29–35.

Erikson, E. H. (1950). *Childhood and society.* New York: W. W. Norton.

Field, T. M., Demkpsey, J. R., Hallock, N. H., Shuman, H. H. (1978). The mother's assessment of the behavior of her infant. *Infant Behavior and Development,* 1, 156–167.

Gall, B., and Gall, J. (1991). *Elegant parenting: How to do it right the first time* (p. 8). Ann Arbor, MI: General Systematics Press.

Garbarino, J., and Kostelny, K. (1993). Neighborhood and community influences on parenting. In T. Luster and L. Okagaki (Eds.), *Parenting—An ecological perspective* (pp. 203–226). Hillsdale, NJ: Lawrence Erlbaum Associates.

Golas, G. A., and Parks, P. (1986). Effect of early postpartum teaching on primiparas' knowledge of infant behavior and degree of confidence. *Research in Nursing and Health,* 9, 209–215.

Goldberg, S. (1979). Premature birth: Consequences for the parent-infant relationship. *American Scientist,* 67, 214–220.

Goldberg, S. (1983). Parent-infant bonding: Another look. *Child Development,* 54, 1355–1382.

Greenberg, M., and Morris, N. (1974). Engrossment: The newborn's impact upon the father. *American Journal of Orthopsychiatry,* 44, 520–531.

Gromada, K. (1981). Maternal-infants attachment: The first step toward individualizing twins. *MCN: American Journal of Maternal-Child Nursing,* 6, 129–134.

Hamner, T. J., and Turner, P. H. (1985). *Parenting in contemporary society.* Englewood Cliffs, NJ: Prentice-Hall.

Hardy, J. B., and Street, R. (1989). Family support and parenting education in the home: An effective extension of clinic-based preventive health services for poor children. *Journal of Pediatrics,* 115, 927–931.

Harrison, L. L., Sherrod, R. A., Dunn, L., Olivet, L., Jeon, J. (1991). Effects of hospital based instruction on interactions between parents and preterm infants. *Neonatal Network,* 9 (7), 27–33.

Hiser, P. L. (1987). Concerns of multiparas during the second postpartum week. *Journal of Obstetric, Gynecologic, and Neonatal Nursing,* 16, 195–203.

Humenick, S. S., and Bugen, L. A. (1987). Parenting roles: Expectation versus reality. *MCN: American Journal of Maternal-Child Nursing,* 12, 36–39.

Johnson, S. H., and Grubbs, J. P. (1975). The premature infant's reflex behaviors: Effect on the maternal-child relationship. *Journal of Obstetric, Gynecologic, and* Neonatal Nursing, 4, 15–21.

Johnson, S. R., Smith, E. M., Guenther, S. M. (1987). Parenting desires among bisexual women and lesbians. *Journal of Reproductive Medicine,* 32, 198.

Kennedy, J. C. (1973). The high-risk maternal-infant acquaintance process. *Nursing Clinics of North America,* 8, 549–556.

Klaus, M. H., and Kennell, J. H. (1982). *Parent-infant bonding* (2nd ed.). St. Louis: C. V. Mosby.

Klaus, M. H., Jerauld, R., Kreger, N., McAlpine, W., Steffa, M. K., Kennell, J. (1972). Maternal attachment: Importance of the first post-partum days. *New England Journal of Medicine,* 286, 460–463.

Klein, M., and Stern, L. (1971). Low birth weight and the battered child syndrome. *American Journal of Disease of Childhood,* 122, 15–18.

Konrad, C. J. (1987). Helping mothers integrate the birth experience. *MCN: American Journal of Maternal-Child Nursing,* 12, 268–269.

Martell, L. K., and Mitchell, S. K. (1984). Rubin's "puerperal change" reconsidered. *Journal of Obstetric, Gynecologic, and Neonatal Nursing,* 13, 145–149.

Martell, L. K., Imle, M. K., Horwitz, S., Wheeler, L. (1989). Information priorities of new mothers in a short-stay program. *Western Journal of Nursing Research,* 11 (3), 320–327.

Matas, L., Arend, R., Sroufe, L. (1978). Continuity of adaptation: Quality of attachment and later competence. *Child Development,* 49, 547–556.

Mercer, R. T. (1981). A theoretical framework for studying factors that impact on the maternal role. *Nursing Research,* 30, 73–77.

Mercer, R. T. (1990). *Parents at risk.* New York: Springer Publishing.

Milliones, J. (1978). Relationship between perceived child temperament and maternal behaviors. *Child Development,* 49, 1255–1257.

Moore, M. L. (1983). *Realities in childbearing* (2nd ed.). Philadelphia: W. B. Saunders.

Murphy, C. M. (1986). Assessment of fathering behaviors. In S. H. Johnson (Ed.), *Nursing assessment and strategies for the family at risk: High-risk parenting* (2nd ed., pp. 41–60). Philadelphia: J. B. Lippincott.

Norr, K. F., Roberts, J. E., Freese, U. (1989). Early postpartum rooming-in and maternal attachment behaviors in a group of medically indigent primiparas. *Journal of Nurse-Midwifery,* 34 (2), 85–91.

O'Conner, S., Vietze, P. M., Sherrod, K. B., Sandler, H. M., Altmeier, W. A. (1980). Reduced incidence of parenting inadequacy following rooming-in. *Pediatrics,* 66 (2), 176–182.

Okagaki, L., and Divecha, D. J. (1993). Development of parental beliefs. In T. Luster and L. Okagaki (Eds.), *Parenting—An ecological perspective* (pp. 35–68). Hillsdale, NJ: Lawrence Erlbaum Associates.

Olds, D. L., Henderson, C. R., Taltelbaum, R., Chamberlin, R. (1988). Improving the life-course development of socially-disadvantaged mothers: A randomized trial of nurse home visitation. *American Journal of Public Health,* 78, 1436–1445.

Palisin, H. (1980). The neonatal perception inventory: Failure to replicate. *Child Development,* 51, 737–742.

Parke, R. D. (1979). Perspectives on father-infant interaction. In J. D. Osofsky (Ed.), *The handbook of infant development* (pp. 549–590). New York: John Wiley & Sons.

Poley-Strobel, B. A., and Beckman, C. A. (1987). The effects of a teaching-modeling intervention on early mother-infant reciprocity. *Infant Behavior and Development,* 10, 466–467.

Porter, L. (1985). *The West Virginia Model Program on Parenting Enhancement with High-risk Adolescents.* Unpublished manual. Available from West Virginia University, School of Nursing, Morgantown, WV 26506.

Reiser, S. L. (1981). A tool to facilitate mother-infant attachment. *Journal of Obstetric, Gynecologic, and Neonatal Nursing,* 10, 294–297.

Ringler, N. M., Kennell, J. H., Jarvella, R., Navojesky, B. J., Klaus, M. H. (1975). Mother-to-child speech at 2 years—Effects of early postnatal contact. *Journal of Pediatrics,* 86, 141–144.

Robson, K. S., and Moss, H. A. (1970). Patterns and determinants of neonatal attachment. *Pediatrics,* 77, 976–985.

Rodholm, M. (1981). Effects of father-infant postpartum contact on their interaction 3 months after birth. *Early Human Development,* 5, 79–85.

Rosenheim, M. K., and Testa, M. F. (1991). *Early parenthood and coming of age in the 1990s.* New Brunswick, NJ: Rutgers University Press.

Rubin, R. (1961). Puerperal change. *Nursing Outlook,* 9, (12), 753–755.

Rubin, R. (1963). Maternal touch. *Nursing Outlook,* 11, 828–831.

Rubin, R. (1967a). Attainment of the maternal role: Part 1, Processes. *Nursing Research,* 16 (3), 237–245.

Rubin, R. (1967b). Attainment of the maternal role: Part II, Models and referrents. *Nursing Research,* 16 (4), 342–346.

Rubin, R. (1977). Binding-in in the postpartum period. *Maternal-Child Nursing Journal,* 6 (2), 67–75.

Rustia, J., and Abbott, D. A. (1990). Predicting paternal role enactment. *Western Journal of Nursing Research,* 12 (2), 145–160.

Siegel, E., Bauman, K. E., Schaefer, E. S., Saunders, M. M., Ingram, D. D. (1980). Hospital and home support during infancy: Impact on maternal attachment, child abuse and neglect, and health care utilization. *Pediatrics,* 66, 183–190.

Smith, L. (1983). A conceptual model of families integrating an adolescent mother and child into the household. *Advances in Nursing Science,* 6 (1), 45–60.

Spock, B. S. (1989). *Dr. Spock on parenting.* New York: Pocket Books.

Stendler, C. B. (1950). Sixty years of child training practices: Revolution in the nursery. *Journal of Pediatrics,* 36, 122–134.

Sunley, R. (1955). Early nineteenth century American literature on childbearing. In M. Mead and M. Wolfenstein (Eds.), *Childhood in contemporary cultures.* (pp. 150–167). Chicago: University of Chicago Press.

Svejda, M. J., Campos, J. J., Emde, R. N. (1980). Mother-infant bonding: Failure to generalize. *Child Development,* 51, 775–779.

Tankson, E. A. (1986). The single parent. In S. H. Johnson (Ed.), *Nursing assessment and strategies for the family at risk: High risk parenting;* (2nd ed., pp. 262–275). Philadelphia: J. B. Lippincott.

Taylor, P. M., Taylor, F. H., Campbell, S. B. G., Maloni, J.,

Dickey, D. (1979). Effects of extra contact on early maternal attitudes, perceptions, and behaviors. In P. M. Taylor (Chair), *Early contact and rooming-in: Effects on bonding and attachment.* Symposium presented at the meeting of the Society for Research in Child Development, San Francisco, March.

Thayer, M. B. (1987). An effective teaching system in an office setting. *Pediatric Nursing,* 13, 48–49.

Thomas, A., and Chess, S. (1980). *The dynamics of psychological development.* New York: Brunner/Mazel.

Thomas, A., Chess, S., Birch, H. G. (1968). *Temperature and behavior disorders in children.* New York: New York University Press.

Tulman, L. J. (1981). Theories of maternal attachment. *Advances in Nursing Science,* 3 (4), 7–14.

Walker, L. (1981). Identifying parents in need: An approach to adoptive parenting. *MCN: American Journal of Maternal-Child Nursing,* 6, 118–123.

Ware, L. M., Osofsky, J. D., Elberhart-Wright, A., Leichtman, M. L. (1987). Challenges of home visitor interventions with adolescent mothers and their infants. *Infant Mental Health Journal,* 8 (4), 418–428.

Waters, E., Wippman, J., Sroufe, L. A. (1979). Attachment, positive affect, and competence in the peer group: Two studies in construct validation. *Child Development,* 50, 821–829.

Watkins, M., and Fisher, S. (1993). *Talking with young children about adoption.* New Haven: Yale University Press.

Weaver, R. H., and Cranley, M. S. (1983). An exploration of paternal-fetal attachment behavior. *Nursing Research,* 32, 68–72.

Williams, C. W. (1991). *Black teenage mothers: Pregnancy and child rearing from their perspective.* Lexington, MA: Lexington Books.

Yarrow, L. J. (1972). Attachment and dependency: A developmental perspective. In J. L. Gewirtz (Ed.), *Attachment and dependency* (pp. 81–96). Washington, DC: V. H. Winston.

Unit 6

Nursing Care of Mothers and Newborns with Special Needs

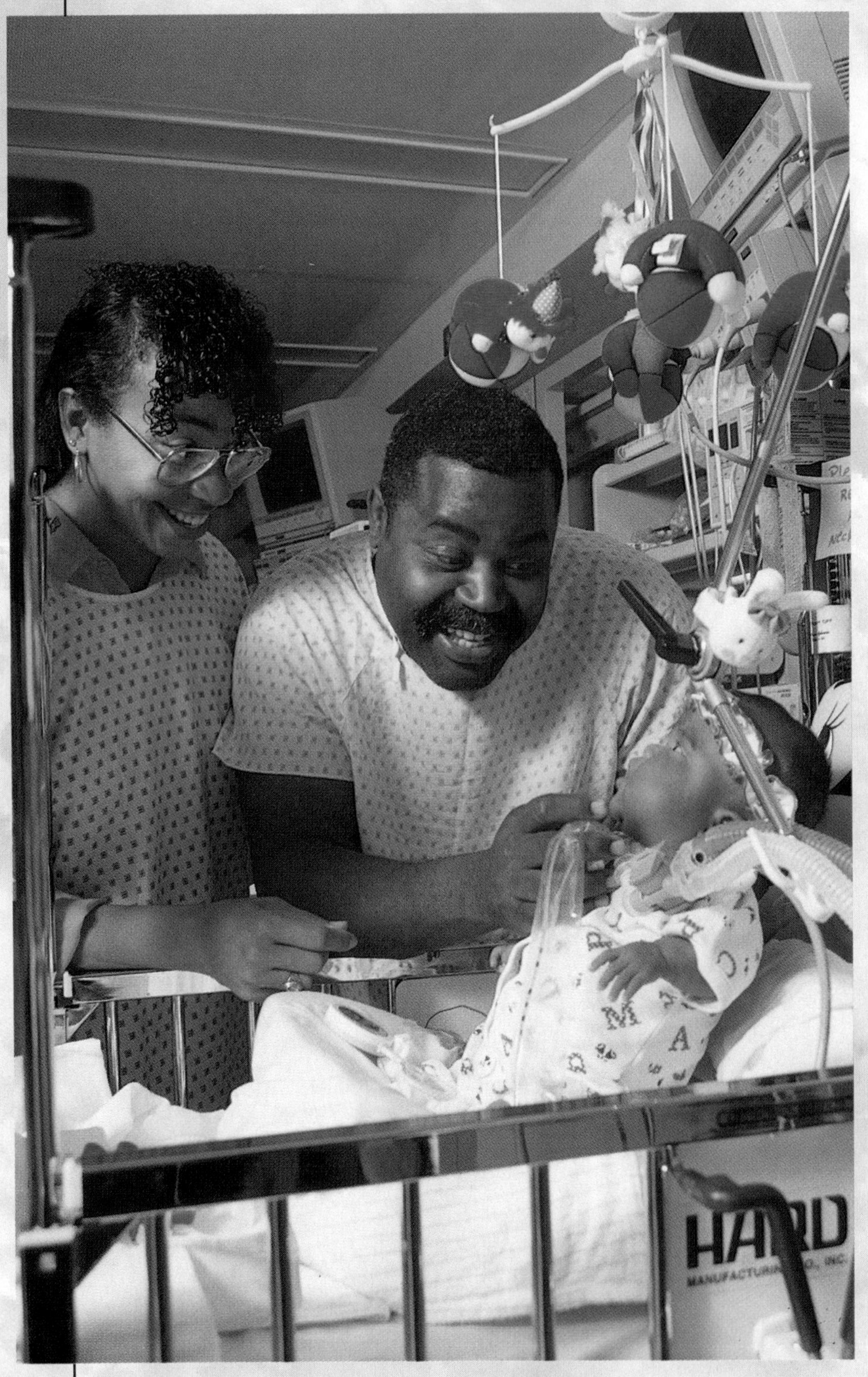

Enhancing parent-infant attachment is an important goal of both newborn intensive care and developmental supportive care for high-risk infants. Parents' attachment to their high-risk infant can be promoted by helping them understand their baby's behavioral cues and learn how to respond appropriately. Involving parents in the care of their infant will promote their confidence and ability to care for and nurture their baby. Parents who are involved in their infant's care in the hospital are more comfortable in caring for their baby at home. Secure attachment between parent and infant is essential for the infant to achieve full social, emotional, and intellectual potential.[2]

Trends in Research

DEVELOPMENTAL CARE FOR HIGH-RISK INFANTS

Environmental factors and care practices in the neonatal intensive care unit (NICU) can contribute to the physiologic instability of the high-risk infant, hinder the infant's recovery from illness, adversely affect the infant's growth and development, and interfere with parent-infant attachment.[1]

Care for high-risk newborns has improved dramatically over past years because of increased knowledge, sophisticated technology, and expert neonatal intensive care. However, the risk of crippling problems for the most immature babies—from 23 to 26 gestational weeks—who survive today, approximately 35 percent, remains the same as it was for the most immature survivors in the mid-1960s.[1]

CONCLUSIONS FROM RESEARCH

Research has shown that environmental factors and supportive care play an important role in the high-risk neonate's development.

- Environmental factors and care practices in the neonatal intensive care unit (NICU) can contribute to the physiologic instability of the high-risk infant, hinder the infant's recovery from illness, adversely affect the infant's growth and development, and interfere with parent attachment.[1]
- At birth the preterm infant's visual system is the least mature, the auditory system is more mature, and the tactile system is the most mature.[2] In the NICU the preterm infant's visual and auditory systems are bombarded with potentially harmful stimuli while the tactile system does not receive enough stimulation.
- High-risk infants in NICUs are constantly exposed to levels of noise that are known to cause hearing loss in adults, can cause physiological instability, and may affect auditory development. Thus, the intensity of environmental noise from equipment, alarms, voices, and other sources that reaches the infant should be reduced to the lowest level possible.[1]
- Prolonged exposure of preterm infants to bright light may contribute to visual problems (retinopathy). Constant lighting alters the rhythmic release of growth hormone that normally occurs with cyclic (day and night) lighting and has the potential to interfere with neonatal growth. Therefore, lighting in the NICUs should be reduced to the lowest level that is needed for accurate clinical observations and should mimic normally occurring day and night cycles.[1,3]
- Incubator air has been found to contain traces of oils, metals, and other residues. Thus, the opening of vials, swabs, or containers in the incubator that produce vapors or odors should be avoided.[1]
- All care procedures and handling should be done in a manner that minimizes stress and maintains the infant in an organized and stable condition.[3,4]
- Outcomes of developmentally supportive care for high-risk infants are better health and growth, lower morbidity, better-organized behavior at discharge, shorter hospital stays, and better development during the first year.[5]

IMPLICATIONS FOR PRACTICE

Research findings show that optimal infant outcomes require both developmental care and complex physiologic care. These findings also provide direction for modifying the environments of high-risk infants and improving neonatal intensive care practices.

[1]Graven, S. N., Bowen, F. W., Jr., Brooten, D., et al. (1992). The high-risk infant environment: Part I. The role of the neonatal intensive care unit in the outcome of high-risk infants. *Journal of Perinatology,* XII (2), 164–172.

[2]Graven, S. N., Bowen, F. W., Jr., Brooten, D., et al. (1992). The high-risk infant environment: Part II. The role of caregiving and the social environment. *Journal of Perinatology,* XII (3), 267–275.

[3]Oehler, J. M. (1993). Developmental care of low birth weight infants. *Nursing Clinics of North America,* 28 (2) 289–301.

[4]Becker, P. T., Grunwald, P. C., Moorman, J. (1993). Effects of developmental care on behavioral organization in very-low-birth-weight infants. *Nursing Research,* 42 (4), 14–20.

[5]Als, H., Lawhon, G., Brown, E., et al. (1988). Individualized behavioral and environmental care for the VLBW preterm infant at high risk for bronchopulmonary dysplasia and intraventricular hemorrhage. Neonatal intensive care unit and developmental outcomes. *Pediatrics,* 317, 1123–1132.

—Francine H. Nichols

Chapter 35

Alterations in the Health Status of Postpartum Mothers

Jan L. Kabler
Marjory K. Waterman
Sharon L. DuMenil

. . . The ramifications of a postpartal crisis are most serious. Family integrity may be disrupted, and the integration of the new family member may be hindered. If the crisis is continued from the antepartal or intrapartal periods, the neonate may be experiencing physiological aftereffects. The mother herself may be in grave danger, and her psychological well-being may be compromised. In all, while a postpartal crisis may physiologically affect only the parturient, the long range effects may be staggering not only on her but on the entire family.

Carole Ann Miller McKenzie (1983)

HIGHLIGHTS

- Early Postpartum Hemorrhage Related to Uterine Atony, Lacerations, Hematoma, Coagulation Disorders, Uterine Inversion, Placenta Accreta, Placenta Increta, and Placenta Percreta
- Procedure 35–1: Identifying and Caring for Women with Early Postpartum Hemorrhage
- Late Postpartum Hemorrhage Related to Retained Placental Fragments
- Thrombophlebitis and Thrombosis Including Pulmonary Embolism
- Procedure 35–2: Identifying and Caring for Women with Thrombophlebitis
- Postpartum Infection Related to Perineal and Vaginal Infections and Reproductive Tract Infections Including Endometritis, Parametritis, Peritonitis, Urinary Tract Infections, Cesarean Birth Incision Infections, Breast Engorgement, and Mastitis
- Procedure 35–3: Identifying and Caring for Women with Postpartum Infection
- Postpartum Affective Disorders Related to Postpartum Blues, Postpartum Depression, and Postpartum Psychosis
- Procedure 35–4: Identifying and Caring for Women with Postpartum Psychological Complications
- Implications for Research
- Nursing Care Planning Guide: Cesarean Birth Postpartum Woman

DEFINITIONS

Disseminated intravascular coagulation (DIC)—A coagulation disorder characterized by decreased platelets and fibrinogen and increased fibrin degradation products that may be due to a complication of pregnancy.

Endometritis—Infection of the lining of the uterus.

Hematoma—A tumor-like mass produced by bleeding from an injured blood vessel into the surrounding tissue.

Inversion of the uterus—A condition in which the uterus turns partially or completely inside out.

Mastitis—Inflammation of the breast.

Parametritis—Pelvic cellulitis, when the infection process extends beyond the endometrium into the broad ligaments.

Peritonitis—An extension of the infectious process into the peritoneum by gradual progression or the rupture of a pelvic abscess.

Placenta accreta—An abnormal adherence of the placenta to the endometrium in which the chorionic villi attach to the myometrium.

Placenta increta—An abnormal adherence of the placenta to the endometrium in which the chorionic villi attach into the myometrium.

Placenta percreta—An abnormal adherence of the placenta to the endometrium in which the chorionic villi attach through the myometrium.

Postpartum blues—A common transient mood change in the early postpartum period characterized by insomnia, tearfulness, anxiety, poor concentration, and a mild depressive affect.

Postpartum depression—A psychological disorder that is nonpsychotic in nature. Although the symptoms are similar to postpartum blues, they remain more persistent, lasting 2 weeks to 1 year or more.

Postpartum hemorrhage—Loss of 500 mL or more of blood after childbirth.

Postpartum (or puerperal) infection—Maternal temperature elevation to 100.4°F (38°C) or higher on two successive postpartum days, not including the 24 hours after birth.

Postpartum psychosis—Psychotic mood disorder occurring within 3 weeks post partum. It is characterized by delusions, hallucinations, and debilitating confusion.

Subinvolution—Slower than expected return of the uterus to its prepregnancy status after childbirth.

Thrombophlebitis—Inflammation of the wall of a vein; precedes the formation of a clot.

Uterine atony—Failure of the uterine muscle to contract after birth.

The postpartum period is typically considered a joyful time when the new parents learn new skills and new roles as the infant is integrated into their family. The mother's body undergoes dramatic changes as it adapts to the events and stresses of delivery. Despite the magnitude and complexity of these processes, the postpartum period proceeds without incident most of the time. However, when a postpartum complication does occur, it may compromise expected outcomes. The nurse's astute vigilance for any deviations from the normal is essential to prevent a catastrophic event. The maternal-newborn nurse caring for the postpartum patient experiencing a complication has the opportunity to help the patient and her family in promoting a positive outcome for all involved.

POSTPARTUM HEMORRHAGE

Modern obstetric practices have greatly reduced the high mortality once associated with obstetric hemorrhage. Despite medical advances, postpartum hemorrhage remains among the leading causes of maternal morbidity and mortality, accounting for approximately 25 percent of obstetric deaths (Cruikshank 1986).

A healthy pregnant woman can usually tolerate

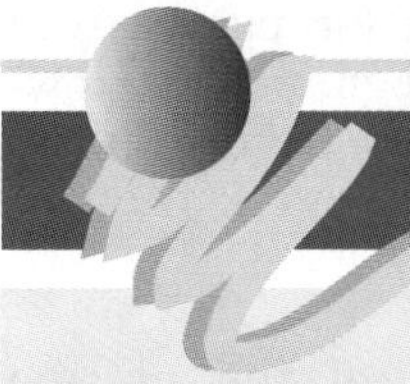

IMPROVING YOUR PRACTICE

IDENTIFYING THE PATIENT AT RISK

Complications of the postpartum period have known predisposing factors that help identify the patient at risk. Prompt identification of actual as well as of potential complications during the postpartum period can have a positive influence on the patient's outcome. A thorough familiarity with the patient's antepartum and intrapartum course, coupled with a sound knowledge base, allows the nurse to quickly identify complications and implement appropriate interventions to benefit the patient.

- BE AWARE OF THE RISK FACTORS THAT PREDISPOSE A PATIENT TO POSTPARTUM COMPLICATIONS. The use of a risk assessment system may guide your judgment.
- IN GENERAL, THERE ARE THREE CATEGORIES OF ASSESSMENT. Medical risk factors include known medical complications that occurred before pregnancy or are diagnosed during the pregnancy. Obstetric risk factors include conditions of past pregnancies as well as of the current pregnancy, such as placenta previa or previous postpartum hemorrhage. Psychosocial risk factors include socioeconomic and psychological status as well as psychological disorders.
- GOOD RECORD KEEPING AND HISTORY TAKING ARE ESSENTIAL IN DETECTING THE PATIENT'S RISK.
- ASTUTE OBSERVATION, ONGOING SYSTEMATIC ASSESSMENT, AND INTERPRETATION OF THE RESULTS WILL IDENTIFY THE PATIENT AT RISK IN A TIMELY MANNER.
- DISCUSSION OF THE IDENTIFIED RISKS WITH THE HEALTH CARE TEAM IS THE FIRST STEP IN DEVELOPING A PLAN OF CARE. Prompt ongoing communication is essential as the condition of the patient changes.
- REHEARSING FOR THE UNEXPECTED AND BEING FAMILIAR WITH MEDICAL MANAGEMENT TECHNIQUES allow the nurse to feel more comfortable with the system and to anticipate the physician's needs, thereby saving time and possibly preventing life-threatening sequelae.
- FINALLY, WHEN THE CRISIS CAUSED BY AN ACUTE POSTPARTUM COMPLICATION HAS RESOLVED, THE NURSE IS THE PRIMARY SOURCE TO PROVIDE POSTPARTUM TEACHING, ANTICIPATORY GUIDANCE, AND FOLLOW-UP on actions that are health promoting for the patient and her family. This may include teaching stress management techniques, counseling a mother who is having doubts about returning to work, or telephoning discharged patients to ascertain recovery progress.

From Dauphinee, J. D. (1992). Risk assessment. In L. K. Mandeville and N. H. Troiano (Eds.), *High-risk intrapartum nursing* (pp. 31–39). Philadelphia: J. B. Lippincott.

the typical 300- to 500-mL blood loss of delivery. Postpartum hemorrhage is defined as blood loss that exceeds 500 mL after delivery (ACOG 1991). The hemorrhage is considered to be severe (Hayashi et al. 1984) if it results in

1. hypotensive response with a decrease of 30 mm Hg in systolic or diastolic blood pressure
2. decrease in hemoglobin concentration by 3 g percent
3. blood loss greater than 1000 mL

Postpartum hemorrhage is further classified as immediate or early if it occurs within 24 hours after delivery or delayed or late if it occurs more than 24 hours after delivery.

Primary causes of postpartum hemorrhage include uterine atony (the most common cause); perineal, vaginal, or cervical lacerations; and retained placenta or membranes. Other less frequent causes include hematoma, subinvolution, and coagulation disorders including disseminated intravascular coagulation (DIC).

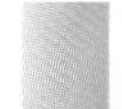

Early Postpartum Hemorrhage

The greatest threat of bleeding occurs during the first hours after birth. Blood loss in the immediate period after birth can occur rapidly with dire consequences if it is undetected by the nurse. At term, blood flows through the placental site at the rate of 600 to 700 mL per minute (Assali et al. 1953). If the amount of blood loss is underestimated, serious hypovolemia may develop before hemorrhage is recognized. Pulse and blood pressure may change only moderately until blood loss is significant (Akins 1994). Complications from bleeding are related to shock and loss of vital blood components. The nurse's role in identifying and caring for women with early postpartum hemorrhage is described in Procedure 35–1. **The most important thing to remember is that frequent, accurate assessment and documentation of blood loss is a priority in postpartum care.**

UTERINE ATONY

Description. After delivery, the uterine musculature normally contracts around the large vessels at the placental implantation site. This action works in combination with normal blood clotting mechanisms to decrease bleeding. If this does not occur, the result is uterine atony, a condition identified by the presence of a soft, boggy uterus that will not contract and stay firm even with massage and medication. There is the presence of a moderate blood flow after delivery of the infant and placenta. Blood loss occurs primarily because of the lack of adequate constriction of the maternal vessels at the placental site. Uterine atony is responsible for up to 90 percent of cases of postpartum hemorrhage (Druelinger 1994).

Factors placing a woman at risk for postpartum hemorrhage can often be identified before delivery (see Predisposing Risk Factors for Uterine Atony). Women with a history of previous postpartum hemorrhage are at increased risk for postpartum hemorrhage with subsequent pregnancies. However, **two thirds of postpartum hemorrhage occurs without any predisposing risk factors** (Cohen 1991).

Predisposing Risk Factors for Uterine Atony

- Prolonged labor
- Rapid or precipitous labor and delivery
- Operative or traumatic delivery
- Uterine overdistention from multiple gestation, polyhydramnios, or macrosomia
- High parity
- Retention of placental fragments or amniotic membranes
- Medications during labor (oxytocin, magnesium sulfate, inhalation anesthesia)
- History of postpartum hemorrhage, uterine surgery, or uterine rupture
- Maternal exhaustion

Management. Management of the uterine atony is directed toward firming the soft, boggy uterus. Initially, the uterus is massaged to control the bleeding. If fundal massage is ineffective, bimanual massage or compression is initiated. Figure 35–1 illustrates this technique.

Simultaneously, oxytocin (Pitocin) is administered intravenously to promote constriction of the relaxed uterine vessels and decrease bleeding. If intravenous Pitocin is not successful, further pharmacologic therapy may include the administration of ergot preparations such as ergonovine (Ergotrate) or methylergonovine (Methergine). Clinical applications have also proved prostaglandin E vaginal suppositories (Hertz et al. 1980) and prostaglandin F (Hayashi et al. 1984; Hayashi 1992) to be relatively successful in promoting uterine contraction when oxytocin and ergot preparations have not reduced bleeding.

LACERATIONS

Description. Perineal, cervical, or vaginal lacerations are often associated with a trauma during the birth process. Possible causes include the delivery of a large infant, a rapid delivery, or an operative delivery using forceps or the vacuum extractor. In many cases, a perineal or vaginal laceration is visible on inspection of the affected area; however, a cervical or deep vaginal laceration may be detected only upon internal visualization by the physician. Although blood loss associated with lacerations is not usually life threatening, it can be serious enough to result in symptoms of volume deficit, require fluid or blood replacement, and prolong the recovery period.

Management. When bleeding persists in the presence of a firmly contracted, intact uterus, hemorrhage from lacerations of the cervix, vagina, or uterus should be suspected. When the laceration is suspected to be relatively small, some physicians take an expectant approach, hoping that the body's clotting mechanisms will control the bleeding. More severe lacerations or lacerations that continue to bleed may require surgical repair of the affected tissue.

HEMATOMA

Description. Hematomas resulting from the birth process can occur at any site along the reproductive tract. A hematoma occurs when blood

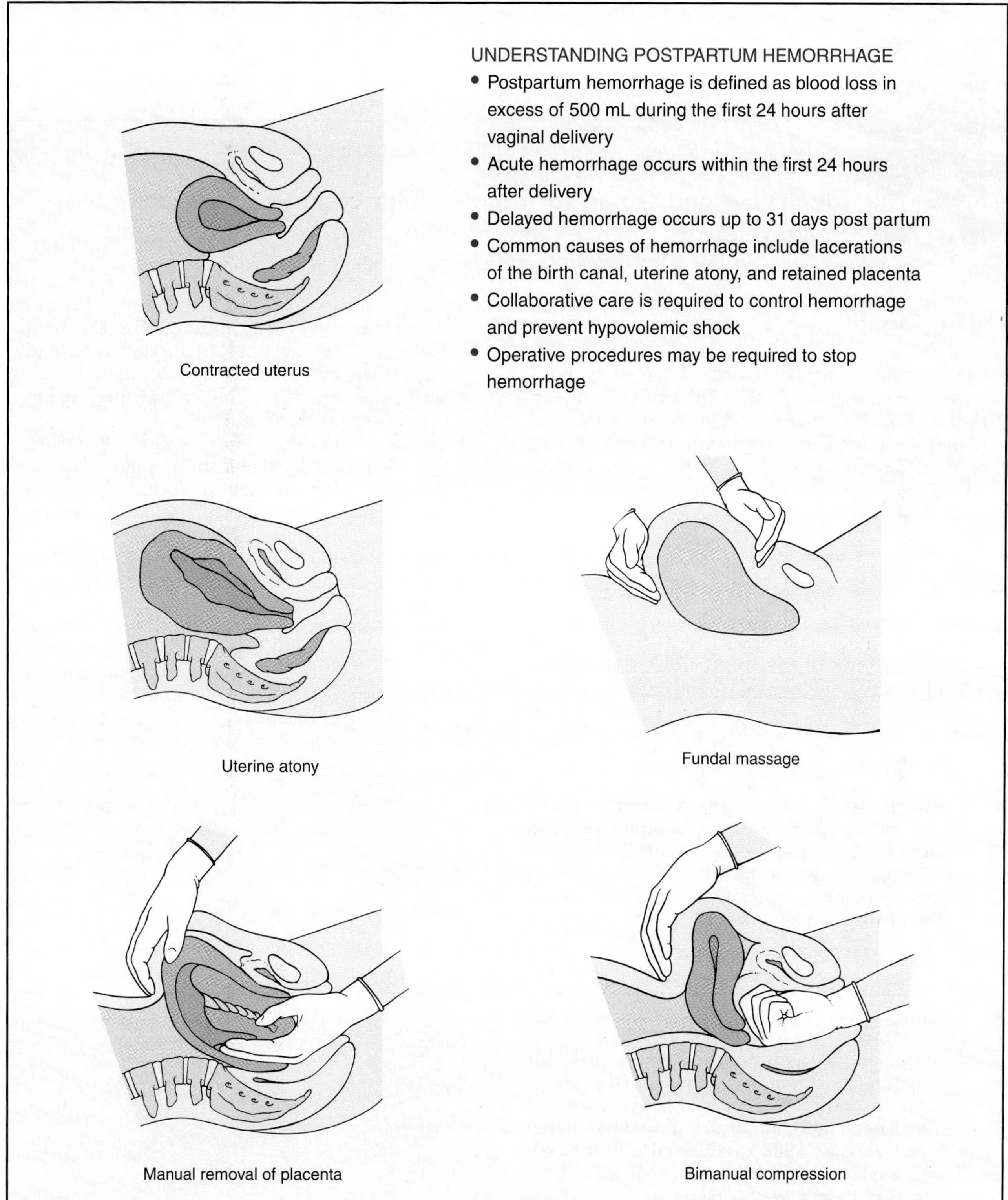

Figure 35–1

Uterine atony occurs when the intertwining muscle fibers of the uterus fail to contract efficiently after delivery, and is the most common cause of postpartum hemorrhage • Fundal massage, manual removal of the retained placenta, and bimanual compression of the uterus are among the therapies used to control hemorrhage during third-stage labor.

PROCEDURE 35–1

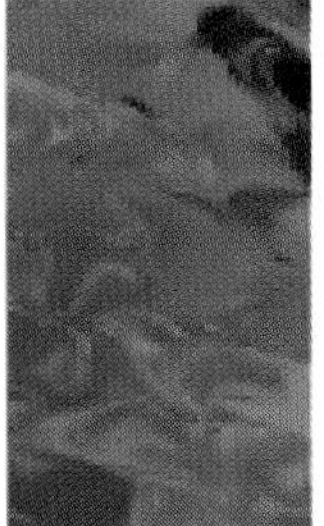

Identifying and Caring for Women with Early Postpartum Hemorrhage

▼ PURPOSE

All women must be assessed for early postpartum hemorrhage (PPH). The presence of certain risk factors, however, puts some women at higher risk for this complication. Identification of risk factors before delivery is a key component of the nursing role, as is prompt diagnosis and intervention post partum.

▼ EQUIPMENT

- Blood pressure recording device
- Peripads
- Underpads
- Gloves
- Gram scale to weigh pads
- Intravenous access with 18-gauge catheter
- Oxygen source with face mask
- Foley catheter
- Light source

1 Anticipate PPH from the woman's history and intrapartum course. **Numerous risk factors place a woman at increased risk for PPH, including uterine overdistention, precipitous or prolonged labor, medications that relax the myometrium, and high parity.**

2 Obtain and record the woman's blood pressure and pulse at least every 15 minutes for the first hour after delivery, then every 30 minutes for the next hour. Notify the physician if the woman is tachycardic or hypotensive. **Overt hypotension and signs of shock associated with PPH will not be seen until the woman has lost almost one third of her blood volume (1500 to 2000 mL). Tachycardia and orthostatic blood pressure changes will be observed before overt hypotension.**

3 Evaluate the amount of vaginal bleeding every 15 minutes for the first hour after delivery, then every 30 minutes for the next hour. The terms scant, small, moderate, and large (as defined here) can be used to describe the amount of blood loss after delivery (Luegenbiehl et al. 1990):

Scant	Peripad blood stain <2 inches (<10 mL) within 1 hour
Small	Peripad blood stain >2 inches <4 inches (10 to 25 mL) within 1 hour
Moderate	Peripad blood stain >4 inches but <6 inches (25 to 50 mL) within 1 hour
Large	Peripad blood stain >6 inches to saturated peripad (50 to 80 mL) within 1 hour; a saturated peripad holds approximately 80 mL of blood

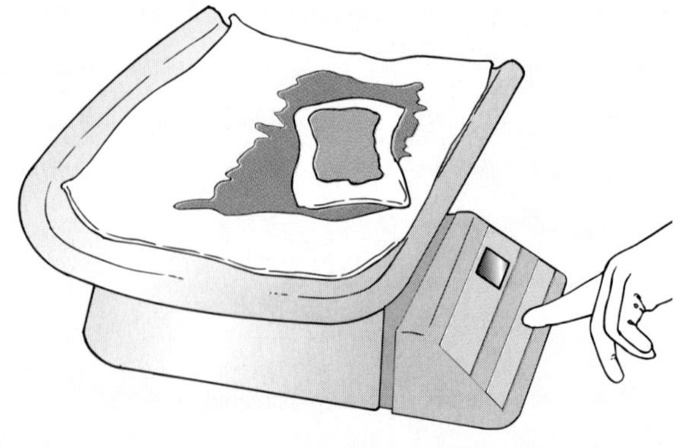

Continued on facing page

PROCEDURE 35–1 Continued

PPH is most likely to occur during the first hour after delivery of the placenta. Blood loss may be more accurately quantified by weighing peripads: 1 g = 1 mL of blood.

4 Assess for uterine atony at least every 15 minutes for the first hour after delivery, then every 30 minutes for the next hour. If the uterus is soft or difficult to locate, begin external uterine massage. (Place one hand above the symphysis pubis to support the uterus and prevent uterine inversion; use the other hand to massage the uterine fundus.) Note the passage of blood clots. **Dark red vaginal bleeding with clots and a soft, boggy uterus usually accompany uterine atony or retained placental fragments. External uterine massage usually stimulates the uterus to contract. If external uterine massage is ineffective, the physician might choose to initiate bimanual compression.**

5 If the uterus remains soft after external uterine massage or if the fundus is located above the umbilicus, evaluate the woman for bladder fullness. Ask her to void to empty her bladder. If she is unable to void, catheterize according to the physician's order. **A full bladder interferes with uterine contraction in the postpartum period.**

6 Administer pharmacologic agents used in the treatment of uterine atony according to the physician's orders. **Oxytocin, the ergot alkaloids (Methergine and Ergotrate), and prostaglandins are used in the treatment of uterine atony. Each agent differs in mode of administration and potential side effects.**

7 If vaginal bleeding continues despite a well-contracted uterus and an empty bladder, notify the physician or certified nurse-midwife to examine the woman for the presence of a perineal, vaginal, or cervical laceration. **A continuous trickle of bright red blood, despite a well-contracted uterus, can indicate a laceration of the lower genital tract.**

8 Initiate intravenous fluid replacement and obtain laboratory studies as ordered by the physician. Administer blood products as needed. **A comparison of the postpartum hemoglobin level and hematocrit with values of the sample drawn on admission can help estimate the severity of the blood loss. Rapid infusion of intravenous fluids or blood products with one or more large-bore catheters is used to correct hypovolemia and to replace the blood loss associated with PPH.**

9 If the woman's condition warrants, administer oxygen by face mask. Insert a Foley catheter. Position the woman with her legs elevated at a 30-degree angle. **Supplemental oxygen is administered to increase oxygen to peripheral tissues. A Foley catheter monitors urine output, which reflects intravascular volume status. Positioning the patient as described facilitates venous return and promotes oxygenation of vital organs.**

10 Prepare the woman and her partner for uterine exploration or surgical intervention as indicated. Transfer the woman to the operative area. **Surgical measures used to control PPH include repair of lacerations, evacuation of hematomas, ligation of uterine arteries, and hysterectomy. Preparing the woman by answering her questions and explaining the medical and nursing interventions helps alleviate her fears and decrease tension.**

escapes from damaged vessels into the surrounding tissue (Fig. 35–2). In addition to the usual symptoms of a postpartum hemorrhage, physical indications of a hematoma include a firm uterus with bright red blood noted at the vagina, increasing perineal or pelvic pain, rectal pressure, and difficulty voiding. A vulvar hematoma is seen as a bulging, bluish swelling that is painful to palpation. Vaginal or peritoneal hematomas are more difficult to diagnose because they are not readily visible. In these cases, initial symptoms may be only the patient's complaints of increasing pain or pressure and subtle changes in vital signs. Bleeding may appear minimal although a substantial amount of blood may be hidden in the paravaginal or pararectal spaces.

▼ **Management.** Management of hematomas depends on early diagnosis and treatment to prevent morbidity and mortality. The patient who complains of severe pain in the perineal or rectal area in the early puerperium should be carefully

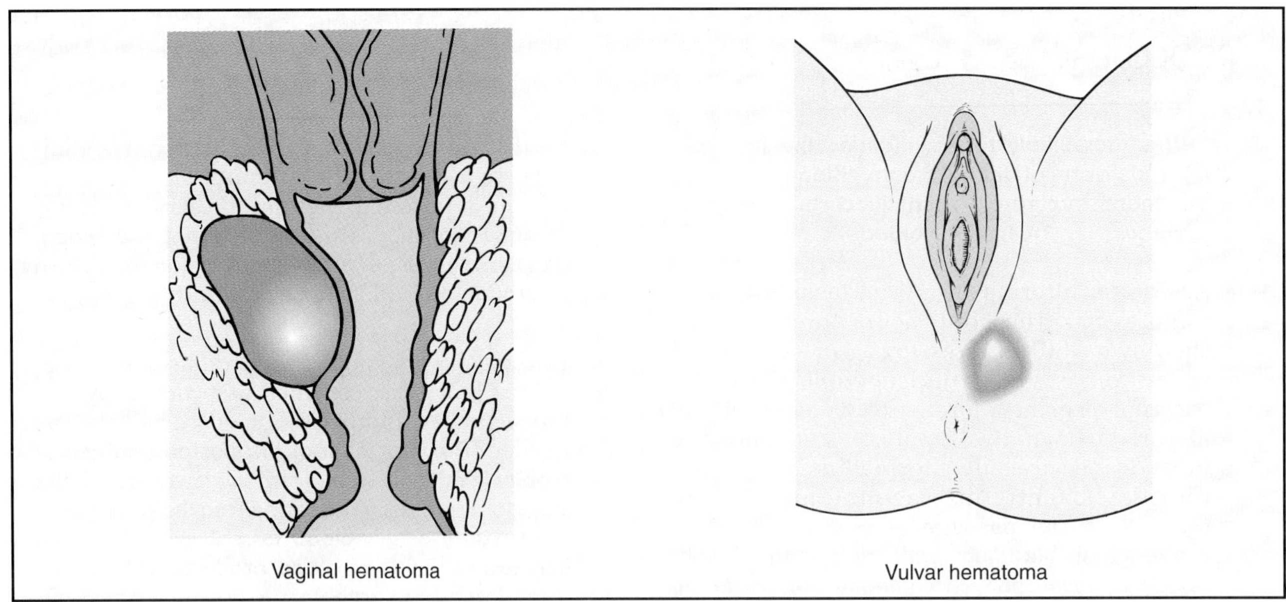

Figure 35–2

Hematomas resulting from injury to a blood vessel may occur anywhere in the reproductive tract • A hematoma is often difficult to detect because bleeding can be hidden and the development can be gradual.

examined for the presence of a hematoma. Hematomas are typically small and, other than discomfort of the patient, usually result in minimal sequelae. Application of ice to the perineum may help decrease this discomfort as well as possibly slow the bleeding into the tissues. Analgesics may be administered for pain. Hematomas do not usually require medical intervention, although if the hematoma continues to expand or becomes very large, surgical evacuation may be required. Blood transfusions and the administration of antibiotics may be indicated.

COAGULATION DISORDERS

Description. Although control of bleeding after delivery is primarily dependent on contraction of the uterine musculature around the large placental site vessels, maternal clotting mechanisms are also critical in reducing maternal blood loss. If a coagulation disorder exists, the patient may not bleed excessively immediately after delivery but may bleed heavily several hours later. Moreover, there may be more bleeding than expected from episiotomy sites, incisions, injection sites, or the bladder.

DIC is among the most common blood clotting disorders that occur after delivery. In DIC, the blood clotting mechanism is drastically altered, with an acceleration of the coagulation process and activation of the fibrinolytic system. Although rare, it may occur as a complication of a severe postpartum hemorrhage or infection or fetal demise. Other coagulation disorders that may affect the postpartum period include idiopathic thrombocytopenia purpura and von Willebrand disease.

Management. Management of the patient with a coagulopathy involves determination of the cause of the coagulation disorder. Monitoring of the patient includes careful evaluation of vital signs, amount of bleeding, and laboratory values. Blood products including fresh-frozen plasma, platelets, or cryoprecipitate may be administered.

UTERINE INVERSION

Description. Uterine inversion is a rare but serious complication in the immediate postpartum period. It occurs in approximately 1 per 10,000 births (Still 1994). It may be complete, when the fundus has passed completely below the cervix, or incomplete with the fundus above the cervix. Predisposing conditions for an inversion of the uterus include poorly contracted uterus, open cervix, birth of a large infant, and a pulling (such as traction on the umbilical cord) or pushing force on the fundus.

Clinical signs of uterine inversion include profuse bleeding accompanied by abdominal pain. A physician must be notified immediately. On abdominal examination, the fundus cannot be palpated; on inspection, the uterus may appear as a bluish gray mass in the vaginal vault or be visible at the perineum.

Management. Prompt response to the management of uterine inversion is necessary to decrease bleeding and prevent shock. Medical treatment includes repositioning of the uterus and fluid replacement. Patients must be carefully monitored after the repositioning of the uterus because inversion of the uterus can recur. Surgical intervention is occasionally required if manual replacement cannot be accomplished. Hysterectomy may be necessary.

PLACENTA ACCRETA, INCRETA, AND PERCRETA

Description. Placenta accreta refers to an infrequent but dangerous situation when the chorionic villi of the placenta adhere abnormally to the endometrium. The result is that the placenta fails to separate from the uterus. The entire placenta or only a part of it may be involved. Three types of abnormal attachment exist:

- Placenta accreta—superficial attachment of chorionic villi to the myometrium
- Placenta increta—invasion of the chorionic villi into the myometrium
- Placenta percreta—invasion of the chorionic villi through the myometrium

Placenta accreta is the most common condition. Identified risk factors for abnormal placental attachment include multigravida, uterine scar, placenta previa, uterine infection, and a history of previous retained placenta (Herbert and Cefalo 1984).

Management. Placenta accreta is suspected when placental separation is delayed for longer than 30 minutes or when manual separation is required and is difficult. With a diagnosis of placenta accreta, quick action is necessary because hemorrhage with placenta accreta can exceed 4000 mL (Druelinger 1994). All attempts of placental removal will cease and the patient will be prepared for surgery. Hysterectomy may be necessary.

Late Postpartum Hemorrhage

Late postpartum hemorrhage, occurring 24 hours after birth, happens infrequently. The patient may not present until 1 to 2 weeks post partum. Patients most commonly present with complaints of heavy, bright red bleeding. Late postpartum hemorrhage may cause the rapid onset of shock (Luegenbiehl 1991). The most common cause of late postpartum hemorrhage is retained placental fragments. Other causes of late postpartum bleeding include subinvolution of the uterus, infection, or recurrent hemorrhage from lacerations of the episiotomy (Luegenbiehl 1991). Client teaching before discharge must be explicit about what is normal and abnormal bleeding and the importance of reporting abnormal bleeding promptly.

RETAINED PLACENTAL FRAGMENTS

Description. In contrast to other postpartum complications, subinvolution due to retained placental fragments is typically diagnosed after the postpartum patient has been discharged. With this condition, the uterus fails to undergo the normal involution process. As the tissue fragments slough, the uterus has no stimulus to contract, and heavy bleeding results. The uterus is painful to palpation and larger than expected. Bleeding is uncharacteristic for the length of time post partum (i.e., the patient who has been having lochia serosa or alba reports a sudden change to lochia rubra).

Management. Treatment of delayed postpartum bleeding from retained placental fragments depends on the condition of the patient. Initial treatment focuses on assessment and stabilization of the patient's hemodynamic status. Ergot preparations are administered, and the patient may require admission for curettage. In patients without heavy bleeding, outpatient treatment of oral ergot medication (methylergonovine) may be considered.

Nursing Process

▼ Assessment

Nursing care of the woman with postpartum hemorrhage begins with assessment. Physical assessment of all postpartum patients includes monitoring of vital signs, fundal location and firmness, bladder status, intake and output, and blood loss. Those caring for postpartum patients must be attuned to the factors or events that place a woman at risk for postpartum hemorrhage. Prompt intervention when deviations occur can minimize complications from postpartum hemorrhage.

▼ Diagnosis

Nursing diagnoses that relate to the patient with postpartum hemorrhage may include

- Altered tissue perfusion: peripheral, related to hemorrhage
- Fear related to postpartum hemorrhage
- Pain related to alteration in comfort

▼ Planning

On the basis of the identified nursing diagnoses, the goals and outcomes that will guide the plan of care should be identified:

- The woman will maintain adequate tissue perfusion as evidenced by stable vital signs.
- The woman and her family will verbalize their fears related to the bleeding.
- The woman will verbally state a decrease in pain and exhibit an increase in comfort as evidenced by body posture and facial expression.

▼ Intervention

Nursing interventions begin with careful assessment of the postpartum patient. The most obvious indication of postpartum hemorrhage is the visible evidence of the bleeding. The effect of this bleeding may be further evidenced by changes in vital signs, laboratory values, or level of consciousness. As blood loss increases, vital signs may change, with the pulse and respirations increasing while the blood pressure drops. However, normal vital signs may persist until excessive blood loss has occurred. Other signs of hemorrhagic shock, including changes in skin color, may also occur.

Because of the increased total blood volume with pregnancy, a blood loss of up to 500 mL during the delivery process is usually well tolerated in a healthy woman with minimal change in vital signs. Subtle changes in vital signs may indicate hypovolemia caused by a steady trickle of bleeding instead of a large gush.

Sources of postpartum bleeding can often be identified by the color and character of the blood and the consistency of the uterus (Table 35–1). Dark red vaginal bleeding with clots and a soft, boggy uterus usually accompanies uterine atony or retained placental fragments. Bright red vaginal bleeding with a firm, contracted uterus suggests that bleeding is more likely due to a laceration.

Table 35–1

IDENTIFYING CHARACTERISTICS OF POSTPARTUM BLEEDING

	UTERINE ATONY OR RETAINED PLACENTAL FRAGMENTS	LACERATIONS
Color	Dark red with clots	Bright red
Uterus	Soft, boggy	Firm, contracted

During the postpartum period, routine monitoring of vital signs includes assessment of temperature, pulse, respirations, and blood pressure. These vital signs may reflect hypovolemia and developing shock. Significant changes in vital signs may not occur until 30 to 50 percent of total body fluid has been lost. Other late indicators of large blood loss include changes in capillary refill and cyanosis of mucous membranes.

It is suspected that the assessment of blood loss after delivery is often inaccurate and underestimated by as much as 50 percent (Cunningham et al. 1993). Accurate estimates are further complicated by the fact that blood loss can be concealed, as in the case of a hematoma or vaginal laceration. One practice that enables the nurse to objectively measure blood loss is to count and weigh perineal pads (see Procedure 35–1). Any clots or tissue should be carefully evaluated by the nurse and saved for the physician's inspection.

Actions to be taken by the nurse when postpartum hemorrhage is suspected include prompt reporting and collaborative implementation of measures to control the hemorrhage and its sequelae. In the event of a boggy uterus, uterine massage and administration of oxytocic agents are indicated to promote the contraction of uterine muscles. The uterus should be massaged with one hand while the second hand is placed above the symphysis pubis to prevent uterine inversion.

Oxytocic drugs have proved effective in the control of postpartum hemorrhage; however, certain precautions need to be observed when they are used. Intravenous oxytocin should never be administered in a bolus because profound hypotension, cardiac arrhythmias, and cardiac arrest may result (Kelly 1976). Ergot preparations may produce vasoconstriction and hypertension. For this reason, they are not typically given to hypertensive patients or patients with pregnancy-induced hypertension.

If bleeding continues, efforts may be needed to avert shock. Placing the patient in the Trendelenburg position is not recommended. Trendelenburg position has been shown to impede cardiac function and interfere with cerebral circulation and respiratory efforts (Luegenbiehl 1991). Positioning the patient with legs elevated at a 30-degree angle will facilitate venous return and promote oxygenation of vital organs without the dangers of the Trendelenburg position. Oxygen may be administered by face mask to supplement blood oxygen levels.

A full bladder can further impede contraction of the uterine musculature. To avoid this possibility, the bladder should be emptied frequently. If the patient is unable to void, an indwelling catheter helps promote uterine involution as well as monitors kidney perfusion.

The rapidly occurring events may be frightening to the patient and her family. It is imperative that the nurse take time to alleviate fears by answering questions and explaining the medical and nursing interventions.

Finally, the nurse caring for the patient with continued blood loss must be prepared for the possibility of surgical intervention to control the hemorrhage.

▼ Evaluation

The evaluation of the nursing care is based on the identified goals in relation to the nursing interventions. For example, vital signs, vaginal bleeding, physical status, laboratory values, and urinary output will stabilize as vaginal bleeding decreases. The patient and her family will verbalize understanding of what has occurred as well as understanding of treatment of the postpartum hemorrhage.

THROMBOPHLEBITIS AND THROMBOSIS

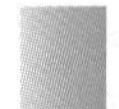

Thrombophlebitis

Thrombophlebitis is a condition in which a clot forms in a vessel wall secondary to an inflammation of the vessel wall or a partial obstruction of the vessel. Thrombosis is the formation of blood clots inside a blood vessel. All postpartum patients are potentially at risk for development of thrombophlebitis because of increased blood clotting factors in the postpartum period; however, less than 1 percent of postpartum patients actually have this complication. There are three types of thrombophlebitis: superficial, femoral, and pelvic. Superficial thrombophlebitis is seen more frequently during the postpartum period than during pregnancy. It is more common in women with preexisting varices. A marked reduction in complications of thrombophlebitis in recent times may be attributed to early postpartum ambulation, decrease in traumatic births, and better health of pregnant women. Factors associated with the development of thrombophlebitis during pregnancy or post partum include advanced maternal age; multiparity; obesity, heart disease, hemorrhage, or anemia; use of oral contraceptives before pregnancy; preexisting varices or history of venous thrombosis; fetal head pressure on pelvic veins for a prolonged period; immobility related to bed rest and anesthesia; hypercoagulability in pregnancy and the early postpartum period; and employment requiring sitting for long periods. Any one or more of these factors may contribute to the development of thrombophlebitis. The nurse's role in identifying and caring for women with postpartum thrombophlebitis is outlined in Procedure 35–2.

▼ **Description.** The saphenous vein is most commonly affected by superficial thrombophlebitis. The patient experiences tenderness and pain in the affected lower extremity; the thrombus may be palpable, feeling bumpy and hard to the touch; and the skin over the area may be warm and pinkish red in color. The patient may experience a slight elevation in pulse rate; however, it is unusual to have a marked increase in either pulse or temperature.

Femoral thrombophlebitis is characterized by pain, fever, and swelling of the affected leg. These symptoms are due to clot formation in the veins of the leg, making return circulation difficult. This condition usually develops about ten days post partum, although it may occur as late as the twentieth day. The patient typically experiences malaise accompanied by chills and fever. The affected area soon becomes stiff and painful, and in approximately 24 hours, the leg becomes swollen. The discomfort may prevent sleep. Skin over the affected area may appear shiny and white. Physical examination often reveals the presence of a Homans sign and diminished peripheral pulses. These initial symptoms may persist for a week, at which time the pain gradually decreases and the patient begins to feel better. Femoral thrombophlebitis may last 4 to 6 weeks. Long term, the affected leg may remain permanently enlarged and be a source of continuing trouble to the patient.

Pelvic thrombophlebitis is a major complication of the postpartum period characterized by severe chills and dramatic temperature swings. This condition typically occurs approximately 2 weeks after delivery, long after the patient has been discharged from the hospital. Pelvic thrombosis is more common in patients undergoing a cesarean birth than a vaginal birth because of decreased mobility and increased chance of pelvic infection (Dorman 1991). The thrombi form in the dilated pelvic veins; but without associated thrombophlebitis, there may not be any clinical signs or symptoms. Sometimes the first sign of pelvic thrombophlebitis is the occurrence of pulmonary embolism.

▼ **Management.** Superficial thrombosis is readily treated with analgesia, rest, elastic support stockings, and hot packs. Should symptoms not clear quickly, or if deep venous involvement is suspected, further measures are indicated.

PROCEDURE 35-2

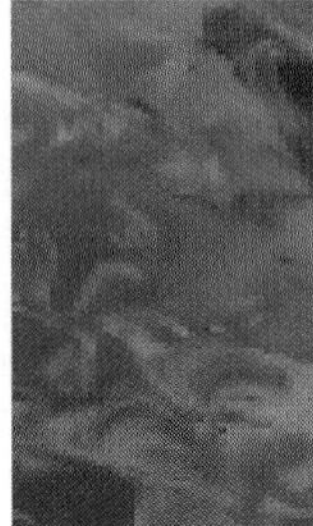

Identifying and Caring for Women with Thrombophlebitis

▼ PURPOSE

All women should be assessed for thrombophlebitis every shift during the postpartum period. The presence of certain risk factors, however, places some women at higher risk for development of this condition. When postpartum thrombophlebitis is diagnosed early, prompt intervention may help prevent complications and a worsening of the condition. Education of the patient is a large component of the nursing role.

▼ EQUIPMENT

- None

1 Identify women at risk for thrombophlebitis. Encourage early ambulation after delivery to prevent thrombophlebitis. **Factors that place a woman at increased risk for development of thrombophlebitis in the postpartum period include advanced maternal age, multiparity, obesity, immobility related to anesthesia, and varicosities. For these women, preventive measures such as early ambulation and the wearing of support hose might be warranted. Early ambulation after delivery decreases the occurrence of thrombophlebitis.**

2 Obtain and record vital signs. Check for the presence of Homans sign by extending the woman's leg, supporting it under the knee, and dorsiflexing the woman's foot. Pain in the calf or behind the knee is the Homans sign (see Fig. 29–4). **Women with thrombophlebitis might demonstrate a slight increase in pulse rate. In more severe cases, a fever is usually present. The presence of Homans sign may indicate a deep vein thrombosis. It is important to differentiate what might be Homans sign from the muscle tenderness often felt by women after a long labor. Further testing is needed to diagnose thrombophlebitis when the Homans sign is present.**

3 Inspect lower extremities from the groin to the foot, noting color, presence of edema, and warmth or coolness. Evaluate the woman's complaints of tenderness and pain in the affected extremity or groin. **Redness, heat, tenderness, and localized edema are indicative of superficial involvement. Pallor and coolness of the extremity suggest femoral thrombophlebitis.**

4 Place the woman on bed rest and elevate the affected extremity. Apply heat to the affected area according to the physician's orders. **Elevating the legs above heart level empties the superficial veins and increases venous return. Heat application relieves pain and promotes circulation.**

5 Administer analgesic agents to relieve the pain associated with thrombophlebitis as needed. Nonpharmacologic pain measures include elevating the legs and changing position at least every 2 hours. **Inflammation and arterial spasm contribute to the pain.**

6 Start anticoagulant therapy according to the physician's orders. Review laboratory results including clotting times. **Therapeutic anticoagulation is achieved when the activated partial thromboplastin time is 1.5 to 2.5 times normal.**

7 Administer antibiotics as ordered. **A fever is usually indicative of deep vein thrombosis; antibiotics are used to control infection.**

8 Apply support hose and gradually increase the woman's ambulation. **Support hose and**

Continued on facing page

PROCEDURE 35–2 Continued

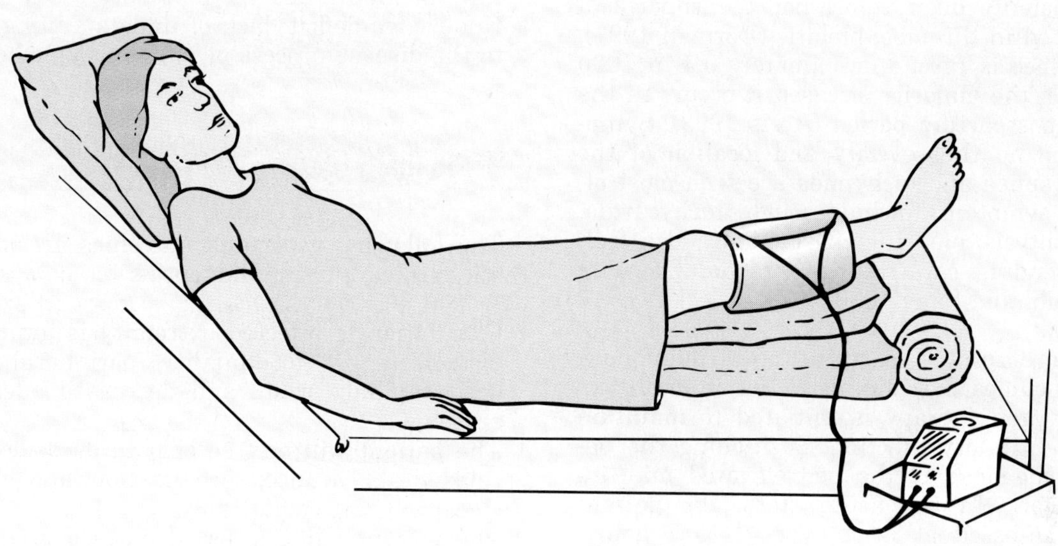

ambulation improve venous blood flow in the lower extremities.

9 Provide education as follows:

- Instruct the patient to avoid rubbing or crossing her legs and to avoid constrictive clothing in the acute phase of the disease.
- Instruct the patient to avoid activities that might contribute to venous stasis, such as prolonged standing or sitting and crossing of the legs.
- Review the importance of taking anticoagulant therapy as ordered and keeping appointments with the physician on a regular basis to monitor therapy.
- Inform the patient that both warfarin and heparin are compatible with breastfeeding.

Document all education provided to the patient. **Education of the patient is critical, because the woman with thrombophlebitis must demonstrate responsibility for performing self-care. If she is unable to assume responsibility, she may need the services of a visiting nurse after discharge from the hospital.**

Femoral thrombophlebitis is treated with bed rest, elevation of the affected leg, analgesia, and administration of intravenous heparin to prevent further thrombus formation. A "cradle" is often used to protect the affected part from the pressures of bed linens. Moist heat applied continuously to the area over the affected vessels often helps alleviate the patient's discomfort. If the patient experiences fever, a broad-spectrum antibiotic may be ordered. Typically, once treatment is started, the pain is relieved and temperature returns to normal. In severe cases that are unresponsive to the traditional treatment, surgical intervention may be indicated to remove the thrombus.

Patients experiencing pelvic thrombophlebitis may feel discouraged, depressed, and physically ill. Their treatment is similar to that of patients with femoral thrombophlebitis—antibiotic and heparin therapy and bed rest. The purpose of anticoagulation therapy is to prolong the activated partial thromboplastin time by 1.5 to 2.5 times the normal level (normal = 25 to 42 seconds). Acute symptoms of pelvic thrombophlebitis subside in 7 to 14 days; at that time, treatment may be reduced to lower doses of heparin or warfarin for a period of 4 to 6 weeks. After resolution of the acute symptoms, the patient may be maintained on self-administered medication with clotting studies monitored on an outpatient basis.

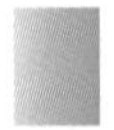

Pulmonary Embolism

Description. Pulmonary embolism is caused by the migration of thrombi formed in the legs; the majority are from sites above the knee. The source is usually deep veins, not the superficial veins involved in thrombophlebitis (Dorman 1991). The occurrence is rare, approximately 0.4 in 1000 deliveries. In the majority of cases, it occurs in the immediate postpartum period (Arias 1993). Symptoms depend on the severity and location of the embolus; dyspnea and tachypnea are seen most often. Other symptoms include cough, tachycardia, rales, hemoptysis, pleuritic chest pain, and a feeling of impending catastrophe or doom (Dorman 1991; Benrubi and Sang 1990).

Management. Treatment of a pulmonary embolism includes the administration of an anticoagulant. Oxygen therapy is initiated to maintain adequate ventilatory function. Positioning the patient with the head of the bed elevated may increase comfort. In the acute state, the patient should be assessed at least every 1 to 2 hours. Frequent assessments will include respiratory rate, breath sounds, and general condition for signs of increasing hypoxemia. Signs of respiratory distress include tachypnea, tachycardia, restlessness, cool and clammy skin, cyanosis, and the use of accessory muscles to breathe. Diagnostic studies may include chest radiography, lung scans, pulmonary angiography, and electrocardiography. Laboratory tests may include blood gas analysis, prothrombin time, partial thromboplastin time, and complete blood count with differential.

Nursing Process

▼ Assessment

Assessment of the patient with thrombophlebitis and thrombosis includes visualization and palpation of the affected area. The quality of peripheral pulses and the presence of Homans sign should be assessed. Vital signs including temperature need to be monitored. Laboratory tests are necessary to monitor clotting times.

▼ Diagnosis

Nursing diagnoses that relate to the patient with pulmonary embolism may include

- Altered tissue perfusion: peripheral, related to decreased blood flow
- Pain related to alteration in comfort caused by the inflammatory process of thrombophlebitis
- Anxiety related to changes in ability to perform activities of daily living, decreased ability to care for infant, and the disease process
- Knowledge deficit: lack of understanding related to the disease process of pulmonary embolism

▼ Planning

The following goals and outcomes are based on the identified nursing diagnoses:

- Circulation to affected extremity is improved as evidenced by good-quality peripheral pulses, good capillary refill, and decreased edema and erythema.
- The patient will be free of pain as evidenced by relaxed appearance, verbalization, and ability to sleep and rest comfortably.
- The patient will express decreased anxiety and be supported by her family.
- The patient will verbalize an understanding of treatment and procedures.

▼ Intervention

Thrombus formation decreases blood flow and venous return, thereby altering perfusion in the affected area. Careful explanations and instructions should be given to the patient to maximize compliance with treatments and therapy. Bed rest is encouraged to minimize the risk of dislodging the clot and creating emboli. The feet and lower legs should be periodically elevated above the level of the heart to empty the superficial veins and increase venous return. The patient is instructed to avoid rubbing the affected area; such action could also cause the clot to dislodge. She is also cautioned to avoid constricting clothing and crossing or propping her legs, because such restriction of circulation impedes blood flow.

The nurse needs to assess the extremity for color, presence of edema from groin to foot, and symmetry. The calf circumference should be measured and recorded. These symptoms provide a means of distinguishing between superficial and femoral or pelvic thrombophlebitis. Redness, heat, tenderness, and localized edema are indicative of superficial involvement; pallor and coolness of the extremity suggest femoral thrombophlebitis. Assessment revealing the presence of Homans sign indicates the possibility of a deep vein thrombosis.

Typically, heparin anticoagulation therapy is administered by continuous intravenous drip, heparin lock, or subcutaneous routes. While warfarin derivatives may also be ordered, heparin is often preferred initially because of its prompt, predictable antagonist action toward clot formation and prevention of further clotting. Since heparin is not excreted in breast milk, it is considered safe for breastfeeding mothers. The nurse should review laboratory work ordered to determine effectiveness of therapy.

Elastic support hose may be ordered to decrease the tendency to venous stasis. Care must be taken to apply the hose properly to prevent any tourniquet-like effects. Once the acute phase has passed, progressive ambulation may be initiated to increase venous return. Support hose may continue to be used intermittently when ordered by the physician.

Pain is the result of the inflammatory process as well as the arterial spasms occurring during the acute phase of thrombophlebitis. Nursing interventions are directed at assessing the degree of discomfort and implementing appropriate actions based on findings. The degree of pain experienced by the patient is directly related to the extent of arterial involvement, degree of hypoxia, and extent of edema. The nurse should palpate the leg while cautioning the patient not to rub the affected area. Measures initiated to reduce discomfort may include bed rest, elevation of the extremity, and changes in position. All treatments, procedures, and nursing interventions should be clearly explained to foster the patient's sense of control and decrease her anxiety.

Another intervention directed at reducing discomfort is administration of medications as ordered, such as analgesics, antipyretics, and antiinflammatory drugs. Moist heat applied to the extremity serves to increase circulation and relax muscles.

Nursing care directed at reducing the patient's anxiety is based on the assumption that complications alter postpartum expectations and plans for discharge. The patient may have a lengthy hospital stay or be readmitted, causing separation from infant and family, increased cost, and the potential for reduced income. It is important that the patient and family, if appropriate, be involved in developing the plan of care. The nurse should review instructions and restrictions and encourage questions and discussion. Thorough explanations of the interventions serve to reduce fear of the unknown. Allowing the mother to actively participate in her baby's care as well as her own may reduce anxiety as she discovers she is capable of self-care and baby care. If the infant has been discharged, encourage visits as permitted by policy to minimize the mother's feelings of separation and anxiety.

Initial assessment of the patient's knowledge and understanding of the disease process serves to identify patient needs. When the nurse is aware of the patient's level of understanding, appropriate teaching and instruction may be instituted.

The nurse should provide information regarding nursing and medical management, diagnostic tests, and signs and symptoms indicating change in status. Medications need to be reviewed with emphasis on their actions, possible side effects, and interactions with other drugs and diet.

The patient needs to be aware of symptoms of excessive or spontaneous bleeding as a result of medication therapy. Safety measures such as the use of a soft-bristled toothbrush or safety razor should be recommended to avoid trauma that could lead to bleeding or infection. The patient should be instructed to report physical changes, such as increased pain, tenderness, fever, or swelling, to the physician or nurse.

▼ Evaluation

The evaluation of the plan of care for a postpartum patient with thrombophlebitis is based on the identified outcome goals and interventions. Nursing assessment of the affected extremity should reveal good-quality peripheral pulses, good capillary refill, and decreased edema and erythema. The patient will verbalize relief of pain and will be observed to appear rested and relaxed. Finally, the patient will verbalize an understanding of treatment and procedures.

POSTPARTUM INFECTION

Postpartum or puerperal infection is defined as the development of inflammatory processes in the postpartum period as a result of a bacterial invasion. The infectious process may remain localized in the reproductive or genital area, urinary tract, or breasts; or it may progress, resulting in metritis, endometritis, peritonitis, or parametritis. Such infections are a major cause of maternal death, ranking second only to postpartum hemorrhage. **The diagnosis of puerperal infection is based on a maternal temperature elevation to 100.4°F (38°C) or higher on two successive postpartum days, not including the 24 hours after delivery.** Other than infection, perinatal events that may cause an elevated temperature

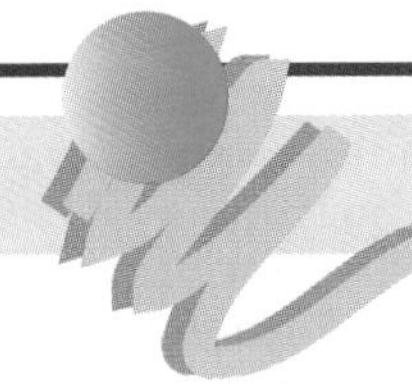

HISTORICAL PERSPECTIVES

PUERPERAL INFECTIONS

1646 First puerperal epidemic is recorded in the Hôtel Dieu in Paris.

1774 Thomas Kirkland of Ashby, England, wrote his *Treatise on Childbed Fevers* about the concept of contagion in puerperal infection.

1821 A 20-month puerperal epidemic at the Allgemeines Krankenhaus in Vienna took the lives of 829 of 5139 mothers (almost one in six).

1843 Oliver Wendell Holmes wrote *The Contagiousness of Puerperal Fever,* which emphasized the physician's role as a carrier of infection.

1853 The Louisiana State Medical Society flatly rejected puerperal sepsis as a contagious disease.

1856 During a 10-day period, 31 of 32 patients succumbed after childbirth at the Maternité in Paris.

1861 Ignaz Philipp Semmelweis wrote *The Cause, Concept and Prophylaxis of Childbed Fever.*

1871 Of 376 new mothers in New York's Bellevue Hospital, 9% died of childbed fever.

1876 Joseph Lister published a series of papers in *Lancet* regarding antisepsis and the reduction of postoperative pyemia.

1895 Dry heat and steam were used for sterilization of instruments.

1927 Sloane Hospital for Women in New York was ordered closed after 15% of the 163 new mothers contracted streptococcal infection; 9 mothers died.

1929 Alexander Fleming discovered penicillin.

1933 In the United States, there were 2.5 maternal deaths from sepsis for each 1000 live births.

1941 Penicillin was introduced as treatment for infection.

Data from Mickal, A. (1994). Historical notes on infection in obstetrics and gynecology. In J. G. Pastorek (Ed.), *Obstetric and gynecologic infectious disease.* New York: Raven Press; and Speert, H. (1980). *Obstetrics and gynecology in America: A history.* Baltimore: Waverly Press.

include dehydration and breast engorgement. Procedure 35–3 outlines the nurse's role in identifying and caring for women with postpartum infection.

Many factors clearly predispose women to the development of postpartum infection (see Risk Factors Associated with Postpartum Infection). While antepartum risk factors are important, intrapartum factors are more directly related to the potential for development of postpartum infection. There are three main intrapartum factors that contribute to the majority of infections. The first is the introduction of harmful bacteria into the genital or urinary tract through vaginal examinations and procedures. The second factor is trauma during delivery that compromises tissue integrity. Trauma can lead to hematoma formation, with the hematoma providing an excellent medium for growth of opportunistic or nosocomial organisms. The third factor that predisposes the woman to infection is hemorrhage. Both hemorrhage and tissue trauma increase the risk for infection by providing multiple portals of access for contaminants. In addition, excessive blood loss decreases the body's ability to resist pathogens.

The most common pathogens responsible for postpartum infections are those that inhabit the lower genital tract and bowel; however, pathogens may also be exogenous in nature. After birth, portals of entry for bacterial invasion include the placental site, the perineum, the episiotomy, an incision or laceration, the vagina, the urinary tract, the breasts, and the lymphatic system along the uterine veins. Common organisms include *Streptococcus, Escherichia coli,* staphylococci, *Clostridia, Klebsiella,* and *Neisseria gonorrhoeae.* Most infections are caused by a combination of anaerobic bacteria. Cultures may be done to identify the infective organism and plan appropriate care. sing the nursing process, the nurse can provide optimal care to the postpartum woman. The Nursing Care Planning Guide: Cesarean Birth Postpartum Woman (pp. 1310–1330) shows how the nursing process can be applied to the postpartum woman who has experienced a cesarean birth.

PROCEDURE 35–3

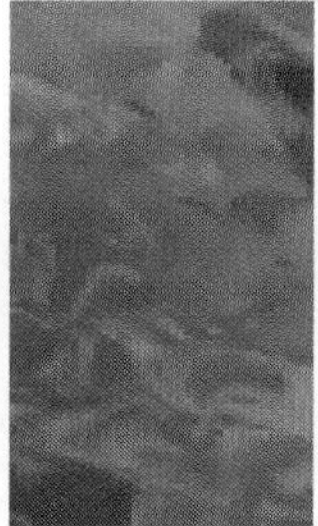

Identifying and Caring for Women with Postpartum Infection

▼ PURPOSE

All women should be assessed for postpartum infection. The presence of certain risk factors, however, makes some women more likely to experience this complication. Early detection and intervention can help prevent worsening of the condition.

▼ EQUIPMENT

- None

1 Identify factors that predispose the woman to the development of a postpartum infection. **Numerous risk factors predispose a woman to postpartum infection, including prolonged rupture of membranes, traumatic or operative delivery, labor longer than 24 hours, anemia, postpartum hemorrhage, and diabetes.**

2 Obtain and record the woman's temperature in the first hour after delivery. Recheck temperature according to hospital policy. Notify the physician of temperature above 100.4°F (38°C). Administer antipyretics as ordered. **Temperature elevations in the postpartum period may be due to dehydration or infection. Antipyretics, whether pharmacologic or nonpharmacologic (e.g., cool cloths), reduce fever.**

3 Observe the woman for signs and symptoms of a postpartum infection, including

- Elevated temperature
- Increase in pulse rate
- Foul-smelling lochia
- Complaints of pain or tenderness at site of infection
- Infection site that is red and warm to touch
- Drainage of pus or blood, or separation of incision site
- Malaise, chills, backache, headache

Signs and symptoms of postpartum infection vary with its location and the infective organisms.

4 Obtain laboratory tests as ordered by the physician. Laboratory tests may include culture and sensitivity, complete blood count, and chest radiograph. Review all laboratory findings and report abnormalities to the physician. **Cultures are done to identify the infective organism so that appropriate antibiotic therapy can be initiated. The white blood cell count normally increases in the postpartum period. To identify an abnormality, look for upward trends or for an increase of more than 30 percent in the white blood cell count during a 6-hour period. (Normal values may be as high as 25,000/mm^3 to 30,000/mm^3 on the first postpartum day. On the second postpartum day, normal values decrease, ranging from 6,000 to 10,000/mm^3. Values return to normal 4 to 7 days post partum [Blackburn and Loper 1992, pp. 162–163].) A chest radiograph is obtained to rule out pneumonia or pulmonary tuberculosis.**

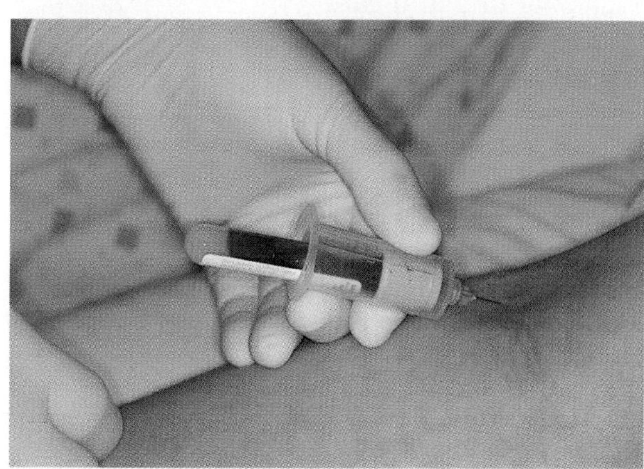

5 Start antibiotic therapy according to the physician's orders. **Antibiotic therapy based on culture and sensitivity reports is the recommended treatment of postpartum infections.**

Continued on following page

PROCEDURE 35–3 Continued

6 Ensure adequate fluid and nutrient intake. Monitor intake and output. **Adequate fluids, nutrition, and rest are therapeutic measures that contribute to the return to a healthy state. Continuous monitoring of intake and output gives the nurse information needed for determining whether the patient is dehydrated, well hydrated, or overhydrated (fluid overload).**

7 Encourage ambulation balanced with adequate bed rest. Administer analgesics as needed. **Ambulation, to promote circulation, respiratory clearing, and a feeling of well-being, should be balanced with bed rest so that the woman does not get fatigued. Analgesics reduce fever and provide some relief for muscle aches.**

8 Instruct the woman in proper pericare techniques, wound care, disposal of contaminated items, and importance of hand washing. **Infection control measures are essential to prevent the spread of infection.**

9 Assess the need for a breastfeeding mother to pump her breasts and discard milk to maintain lactation until she can resume breastfeeding. **Maternal condition or the specific type of antibiotic ordered might prevent breastfeeding or feeding the baby mother's breast milk in a bottle. Pumping must be done early and on a regular basis to initiate and maintain lactation.**

Risk Factors Associated with Postpartum Infection

ANTEPARTUM

- Preexisting infections, chronic diseases
- Anemia
- Poor nutritional status
- Diabetes
- Lack of prenatal care
- Low socioeconomic status
- Obesity

INTRAPARTUM

- Prolonged rupture of membranes (more than 24 hours)
- Maternal exhaustion or stress
- Frequent vaginal examinations
- Chorioamnionitis
- Intrauterine fetal monitoring
- Intrauterine manipulation
- Traumatic delivery, lacerations of reproductive tract
- Operative delivery
- Retained placental fragments, manual removal of placenta
- Hematomas, postpartum hemorrhage
- Improper aseptic technique
- Inadequate or improper perineal care

Perineal and Vaginal Infections

Description. Despite that the genital area is a highly vulnerable site for bacterial invasion after birth, infections of perineal wounds, including episiotomy incisions and repaired lacerations, are relatively uncommon (Cunningham et al. 1993). The most common problem is a localized infection of an episiotomy or repaired perineal laceration.

Symptoms of an episiotomy infection may include elevated temperature, localized pain and warmth at the affected area, and burning on urination. The area may become red and edematous, with seropurulent discharge. If a laceration of the vulva becomes infected, the entire vulva may become edematous. Any infection of the perineum, vulva, or vaginal area is a source of significant discomfort and anxiety to the patient. Such localized infections rarely lead to severe physical reactions if care and treatment are prompt and appropriate. A rare but frequently fatal complication of perineal and vaginal wound infections is necrotizing fasciitis.

Management. Treatment of an infected perineal wound involves removing sutures and opening the wound for drainage. Broad-spectrum antibiotics are administered. Analgesics help with pain relief. Urinary retention is treated with the use of an indwelling catheter. If dehiscence of the episiotomy results from the infection, surgical repair will be necessary at a later date.

Reproductive Tract Infections

ENDOMETRITIS

▼ **Description.** Endometritis, or infection of the lining of the uterus, remains the most frequent cause of postpartum infection (Druelinger 1994). Aerobic and anaerobic bacteria invade the lesion, usually the placental site, and may spread to involve the entire endometrium. Early endometritis occurs within 48 hours of delivery. In its mildest form, the patient may experience few symptoms other than a temperature elevation to 101°F (38.4°C). The temperature elevation may be present for several days and subside. Symptoms of more virulent infections include chills, high fever (up to 104°F) with concurrent rise in pulse rate, malaise, loss of appetite, headache, backache, and generalized discomfort. The patient may experience severe and prolonged afterpains, and attempts to palpate the uterus may be painful. In addition, the uterus remains unusually large and may not descend below the umbilicus as expected. The lochia may be decreased or copious, dark brown in appearance, and foul smelling. In some cases of endometritis, especially when the causative factor is hemolytic streptococcus, the lochia may be odorless.

The single most important risk factor for the development of postpartum endometritis is nonelective cesarean birth after the onset of labor or rupture of membranes (Druelinger 1994). Other risk factors include prolonged labor, prolonged rupture of membranes, increased frequency of vaginal examinations, internal fetal monitoring, lower socioeconomic status, and anemia.

▼ **Management.** Management of the postpartum woman with a suspected endometritis begins with careful assessment of risk factors, history, and presenting complaints. Palpation of the uterus and assessment of the lochia may confirm signs and symptoms of infection. Vital signs including temperature are monitored. Treatment includes the use of a broad-spectrum antibiotic.

PARAMETRITIS

▼ **Description.** Parametritis, or pelvic cellulitis, is an extension of the infectious process beyond the endometrium into the broad ligaments. The infection is usually unilateral in nature and frequently limited to the base of the broad ligament. However, it may be bilateral and extend to the pelvic wall and umbilicus.

Parametritis typically does not occur until the second postpartum week. The patient with parametritis presents with a high, persistent fever (102 to 104°F), malaise, chills, and lethargy. She may experience marked pain and tenderness over the affected area, which may become swollen and hard and may progress to a pelvic abscess. If an abscess forms, the skin over the area becomes red, edematous, and tender. The patient's lochia may remain red and heavy. Laboratory findings include an elevated leukocyte count and positive blood and urine cultures.

▼ **Management.** Management of the patient with parametritis includes careful monitoring of vital signs including temperature, the affected area, and lochia, and laboratory test results. Treatment includes the use of intravenous antibiotics. The woman with parametritis should be watched closely for signs of peritonitis. Surgical drainage of the abscess may be necessary.

PERITONITIS

▼ **Description.** Peritonitis, an infection of the peritoneum, may occur as a result of gradual progression or by the rupture of a pelvic abscess. The patient with pelvic peritonitis is seriously ill with symptoms similar to those of a patient with surgical peritonitis. The patient experiences a high fever (102 to 104°F), pronounced tachycardia, rapid or shallow respirations, excessive thirst, marked anxiety, and constant and severe abdominal pain. The infectious process may be complicated by paralytic or mechanical ileus, causing abdominal distention, nausea, and vomiting. While this is an uncommon condition, peritonitis can be severe and life threatening.

▼ **Management.** Assessment of the postpartum woman with peritonitis includes vital signs, intake and output, and laboratory test values. Antibiotic therapy is initiated. The gastrointestinal tract may be decompressed by continuous nasogastric suction. Fluids and electrolytes need to be replaced. Analgesics may be given for pain. Surgical drainage may be necessary.

URINARY TRACT INFECTIONS

▼ **Description.** Urinary retention after vaginal birth is not uncommon. Several factors contribute to the urinary retention, including the varying degrees of stretching and trauma to the base of the bladder with vaginal birth; the use of regional anesthesia; the increased capacity and decreased sensitivity of the puerperal bladder; and the use of oxytocin infusion after birth, which induces potent antidiuresis until the oxytocin is stopped, when there is rapid diuresis. The bladder, traumatized from childbirth, provides optimal conditions for the development of a urinary tract infection after catheterization. The insertion of the catheter introduces residual urine and bacteria into the bladder. Initial symptoms include dysuria, frequency, and urgency. The woman may have an elevated temperature and pain. Bacteriuria is present.

Management. Management of the woman presenting with the symptoms of a urinary tract infection begins with urine culture. Treatment includes the use of antibiotic therapy. The patient should be instructed to rest and to obtain adequate fluid and nutrition. The temperature should be monitored.

CESAREAN BIRTH INCISION INFECTIONS

Description. Abdominal incision infections after cesarean birth have been reported to range from 3 to 15 percent. With the use of prophylactic antibiotics, the frequency is approximately 2 percent or less (Cunningham et al. 1993). The most common symptom is fever usually occurring about the fourth day. Erythema and drainage of the wound may be present. Risk factors for abdominal wound infections include obesity, diabetes, corticosteroid therapy, immunosuppression, anemia, and poor hemostasis with hematoma formation (Cunningham et al. 1993).

Management. Treatment includes the use of antibiotic therapy. Cultures of any drainage identify the organism causing the infection. Surgical drainage may be necessary.

BREAST ENGORGEMENT AND MASTITIS

Description. At 48 to 72 hours post partum, there may be an elevation of temperature corresponding with breast fullness. The temperature rarely exceeds 39°C and is brief in duration, typically lasting 4 to 16 hours (Calhoun and Brost 1995). A transient breast fullness is an indication of increased milk production. If the breastfeeding woman is mismanaged by delayed or restricted breastfeedings, the breast fullness may progress to breast engorgement (Auerbach et al. 1993). In the woman who is not breastfeeding, the signs and symptoms gradually disappear within 2 days if the breasts are not stimulated.

Engorgement, usually starting on the second day, is a combination of two factors: (1) congestion and increased vascularity, which is physiologic; and (2) accumulation of milk (Lawrence 1994). With moderate to severe engorgement, the breasts become full, hard, tense, tender, and hot. The woman may complain of throbbing and aching pain and not be able to find a comfortable position.

Mastitis, an infectious process of the mammary glands, is thought to be a relatively rare condition. One study estimated the frequency to be as high as 33 percent in women who breastfed long term (Riordan and Nichols 1990). It seldom occurs within the first week post partum. Initial symptoms include localized breast tenderness and an influenza-like muscle aching, fatigue, and headache. These initial symptoms are soon followed by a fever and tachycardia. A hard, reddened, painful area appears on the breast. It is almost invariably unilateral. Table 35–2 compares the signs and symptoms of breast fullness, engorgement, and mastitis. About 10 percent of women with mastitis will have development of an abscess (Cunningham et al. 1993). Factors related to development of mastitis include stress, plugged

Table 35–2

COMPARISON OF SIGNS AND SYMPTOMS OF BREAST FULLNESS, ENGORGEMENT, AND MASTITIS

CHARACTERISTICS	BREAST FULLNESS	ENGORGEMENT	MASTITIS
Onset	2–4 days	Gradual, immediately postpartum	Sudden, after 10 days
Site	Bilateral	Bilateral	Unilateral
Swelling	Generalized	Generalized	Localized
Heat	Occasional	Generalized	Localized
Pain	None–rare	Generalized	Localized, intense
Body temperature	<38°C	<38.4°C	>38.4°C
Maternal symptoms	Feels well	Feels well	Influenza-like symptoms

Adapted with permission from Auerbach, K. G., Riordan, J., Countryman, B. A. (1993). The breastfeeding process. In J. Riordan and K. G. Auerbach, (Eds.), *Breastfeeding and human lactation* (p. 227). Boston: Jones & Bartlett; and Lawrence, R. A. (1994). *Breastfeeding: A guide for the medical profession* (4th ed., p. 261). St. Louis: C. V. Mosby.

ducts, cracked or fissured nipples, constriction caused by a tight bra, abrupt change in frequency of feedings, engorgement, and stasis of milk.

Management. Management of engorgement for the breastfeeding woman includes early, frequent, and unlimited breastfeedings. Warm compresses to the breast and the judicious use of pumping are indicated if the breast becomes engorged. The woman can use hand expression or an electric pump. To avoid traumatizing the distended breast tissues, an electric pump should be set on intermittent minimal pressure for no more than 10 minutes (Auerbach et al. 1993). If the woman is not breastfeeding, comfort techniques include support with a binder or bra, cold packs on the breast, and mild analgesics for pain. If the woman is very uncomfortable, warm showers and gentle massages followed by cold packs may be used; however, suppression of lactation may be delayed. Routine use of drugs to suppress postpartum lactation is no longer recommended (Cunningham et al. 1993).

Management of mastitis includes the use of antibiotics, the application of moist heat, increased fluids, and bed rest. Breastfeeding should not be interrupted. Symptoms are relieved within a few days, but the woman should be instructed to finish the complete antibiotic therapy to prevent recurrence. If an abscess forms, it may require needle aspiration or surgical aspiration.

Nursing Process

Assessment

Postpartum infections may be difficult to diagnose and treat in the early stages because many postpartum patients experience some degree of abdominal pain and a 1-day fever. On the other hand, there are some infected patients who do not have a temperature elevation. Patients with a low-grade fever of 100.4 to 101.5°F (38 to 38.6°C) should be assessed before antibiotic therapy is prescribed. In the absence of other signs of infection, fever may subside within 24 hours, and antibiotics may not be needed. Patients with persistent, high, or fluctuating temperatures need to be thoroughly examined with attention directed to the genital tract, urinary tract, lungs, veins, and breasts. Laboratory tests may include cultures of blood, vagina, cervix, endometrial cavity (aerobic and anaerobic), and urine; complete blood count; and chest radiography. The complete blood count may indicate normal white blood cells, or it may reveal an elevation with a left shift differential indicative of an infectious process. The sedimentation rate and red blood cells will be markedly increased if an infection is present. However, in the presence of anemia, hematocrit, hemoglobin level, and red blood cells are decreased.

Diagnosis

Nursing diagnoses that relate to the patient with postpartum infection may include

- Risk for infection related to bacterial presence in the body and the trauma associated with the birth
- Pain related to inflammation secondary to the infectious process
- Risk for altered parent-infant attachment related to limited contact with the infant, secondary to the infectious process

Planning

The plan will be developed on the basis of assessment and the identified nursing diagnoses. Examples of measurable outcomes include

- The infectious process will be identified and treated promptly, thereby avoiding more serious complications.
- The woman will express relief of pain.
- The woman will exhibit attachment behaviors during mother-infant interactions.

Intervention

Nursing care for the postpartum patient includes careful review of the antepartum, intrapartum, and postpartum history to identify factors that may place the patient at increased risk for development or spread of infection. It is imperative that strict hand washing policies be observed by physicians, staff, patients, and visitors to prevent the spread of infection. Proper disposal of linens, dressings, and other contaminated supplies is extremely important. The patient should be instructed to perform perineal cleansing after urination and defecation and to frequently change perineal pads to minimize the moist medium favorable to bacterial growth.

Vital signs should be monitored closely for elevations that may accompany infections. Fluctuation in vital signs indicates an alteration in the patient's status and requires further assessment. Potential signs of a developing infection are foul-smelling lochia; an extremely tender uterus;

subinvolution of the uterus; or incisional redness, edema, drainage, or separation. The patient's intake and output should be monitored, noting the presence of nausea, vomiting, or diarrhea. At least 2400 to 3000 mL of fluid per 24 hours is needed to prevent dehydration, enhance circulating volume, and replace lost fluids.

The nurse should encourage the patient to maintain a semi-Fowler position in bed to promote the flow of lochia and uterine drainage. Early ambulation is encouraged to increase circulation, promote respiratory clearing, and provide a feeling of well-being. Ambulation must be balanced with adequate rest periods so that the patient does not become fatigued. The patient may be instructed in performing fundal massage to promote uterine involution and contractility.

All laboratory studies and results should be reviewed with the physician. Blood administration may be ordered to increase the oxygen-carrying capacity of a circulation system that has been compromised by anemia or hemorrhage. Oxygen may be administered to promote healing and enhance oxygenation, particularly if pulmonary compromise exists. Patients with peritonitis or sepsis may need to be transferred to an intensive care unit for appropriate monitoring.

Inflammation, fever, or chills associated with postpartum infections will cause the patient discomfort. The nurse's role is to assess the location and type of discomfort and initiate appropriate comfort measures. The patient's position should be changed frequently to reduce muscle fatigue and promote relaxation. Instruction in specific techniques, such as the application of heat, back rubs, and adequate rest and nutrition, and techniques that direct the patient's attention and promote a positive attitude may enhance the patient's comfort. If the mother is breastfeeding, she should be encouraged to continue if her condition permits. If breastfeeding is contraindicated, instruction in the use of a manual or electric breast pump will relieve the discomfort of engorgement and promote adequate milk supply. Administration of analgesics and antipyretics aids in reducing discomfort associated with infection. The use of sitz baths and heat lamps provides some comfort in the case of localized perineal infections.

Any alteration in the patient's physical status may potentially interfere with the mother's ability to attend to her infant's needs. If contact with her infant is reduced, maternal-child bonding may be impaired. The partner may also experience anxiety due to concern for the mother's well-being. This anxiety could interfere with the parent's ability to bond with the infant.

Parents expect a normal, uncomplicated postpartum period. Illness due to an infection may result in separation of the patient from her family, creating a feeling of isolation and depression. Such separation may depress and anger the mother. The nurse should be sensitive to the family's needs and provide every possible opportunity for maternal-infant contact. Pictures of the infant may facilitate attachment if the mother and infant require separation for an extended period. If anger or depression occurs, advise the patient that her feelings are normal and that she will be able to more fully participate in caring for her infant as her infection resolves. Encouraging the father and other family members to provide care for the infant may reassure the mother that the family is bonding with the infant. When possible, the mother should be encouraged to feed her baby; such participation enhances her outlook and promotes bonding. The nurse should observe maternal-infant interaction to identify behaviors that may interfere with the bonding process.

Evaluation

Outcome is evaluated on the basis of the accomplishment of the identified goals. The expected outcome for the postpartum patient with an infection is resolution of the infection and healing of the affected areas.

POSTPARTUM AFFECTIVE DISORDERS

The birth of a baby is a dynamic and potentially stressful period for the woman and her family. Major psychological changes, role changes, and interaction with a complex health care system can overwhelm the healthiest women. However, the majority of women undergo the physiologic and psychosocial changes of the early puerperium and adjust to motherhood while continuing their daily activities. Mood changes accompanying childbirth have been identified since the time of Hippocrates (Unterman et al. 1990). Postpartum psychiatric disorders are generally divided into three main conditions—postpartum blues, postpartum depression, and postpartum psychosis—although some professionals identify the symptoms as a continuum (Dunnewold and Sanford 1994; Hansen 1990). Indeed, although the symptoms of postpartum blues and postpartum psychoses are somewhat easily defined, the symptoms of postpartum depression are more elusive.

Despite ongoing efforts, research has failed to establish a definitive cause-and-effect relationship for postpartum psychological complications. There is disagreement in the literature on whether postpartum psychological complications are unique to the postpartum period or only symptoms triggered by the events of childbirth.

Possible causes that have been identified for postpartum psychological complications include biologic factors, such as hormonal changes, chemical imbalances, and genetic predisposition; psychological factors, such as poor ego development, lack of or low self-esteem, and life experiences; and environmental or sociocultural factors, such as problems with the marital relationship, lack of support systems available to the patient, and the patient's perception of being unable to meet others' expectations.

The effects of postpartum psychological complications range from mild depression-like symptoms to actions that may interfere with maternal-infant attachment and marital relationships, render the mother unable to care for herself or her infant, or result in maternal actions that may lead to self-injury or harm to the infant. The nurse's role in identifying and caring for women with postpartum psychological complications is described in Procedure 35–4.

Possible Causes of Postpartum Psychological Complications

BIOLOGIC FACTORS

Sudden changes in hormone levels after birth
Chemical imbalances (imbalances of neurotransmitters that affect emotions and mood)
Genetic predisposition to depression

PSYCHOLOGICAL FACTORS

Poor ego development
Inadequate self-esteem
Life experiences

SOCIOCULTURAL FACTORS

Problems with marital relationship
Lack of support systems
Patient's perception of being unable to meet others' expectations

PROCEDURE 35–4

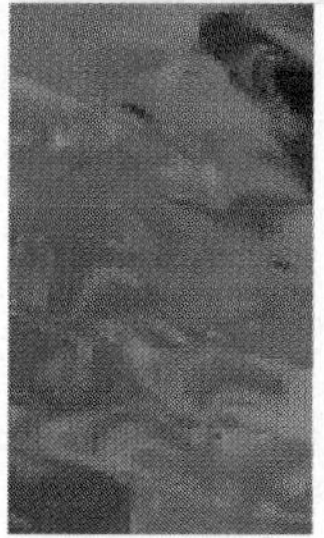

Identifying and Caring for Women with Postpartum Psychological Complications

▼ PURPOSE

All women should be assessed for postpartum psychological complications. Early detection and intervention might prevent an escalation of psychological problems. Educating the patient and her family about the emotional responses possible during the postpartum period prepares them to recognize and report changes that may be associated with postpartum psychological complications.

▼ EQUIPMENT

- None

1 Assess mother's interaction with her infant, including attachment, emotional responses,

Continued on following page

PROCEDURE 35–4 Continued

and caretaking behaviors. **Psychological complications may interfere with the maternal-infant attachment process as well as with a mother's ability to provide appropriate newborn care.**

2 Facilitate positive mother-infant interaction and provide the new mother with positive reinforcement:

- Show the mother how the baby responds to her voice.
- Point out familial characteristics of the baby.
- Educate the mother on the sleep-wake cycles of the baby and on the best times to interact with the baby.
- Encourage eye-to-eye contact between mother and baby.
- Encourage maternal touch and stroking of infant.

Facilitating positive mother-infant interaction and providing positive reinforcement will promote the desired behaviors.

3 Evaluate mother's perceptions of the maternal role and how that role fits with her other roles. Discuss with the mother and her partner what they expect the next few weeks to be like at home. **The new mother and her family need support and educational guidance with role transition to new parent as well as with integration of the new role into other roles, including spouse and career.**

4 Assess the mother's individual coping skills and the adequacy of her family support system by having her identify those persons who are available to provide support. **Lack of adequate emotional support or dysfunctional family relationships could interfere with maternal adjustment during the postpartum period.**

5 Observe the mother for signs and symptoms of psychological complications, including

- Alterations in sleeping and eating
- Extreme fatigue
- Tearfulness, irritability, mood swings, anxiety behaviors, agitation
- Detachment from reality, thought disturbances, hallucinations
- Feelings of helplessness, inability to cope with activities of daily living

Individual manifestations of depression or psychosis vary.

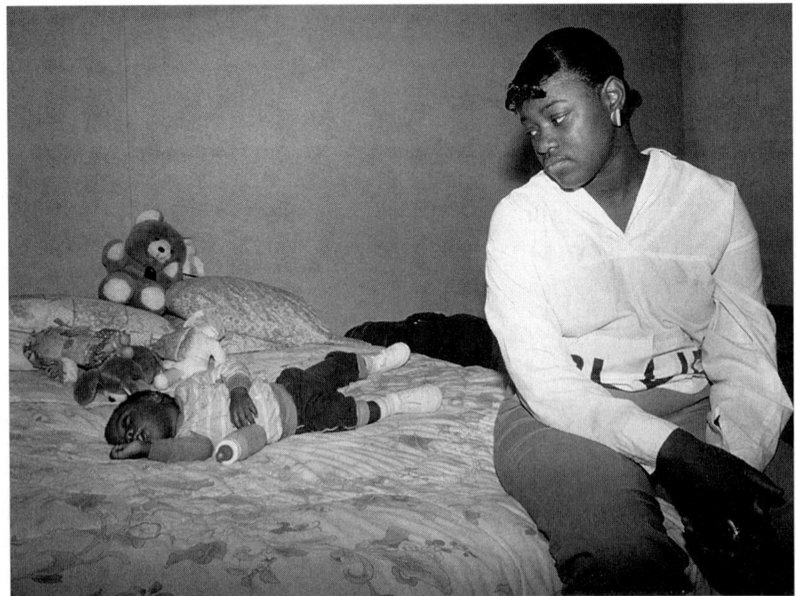

Mother and infant in a homeless shelter. The lack of adequate resources and emotional support can lead to postpartum psychological complications and interfere with mother-infant attachment. (Photo copyright Shooting Back from Hubbard, J. (1991). *Shooting back: A photographic view of life by homeless children* (p. 74). San Francisco, CA: Chronicle Books.)

Continued on facing page

PROCEDURE 35–4 Continued

6 Initiate appropriate referrals on the basis of individual needs:

- Psychiatric consultation: to diagnose the disorder and make recommendations for further care
- Professional counseling: to provide ongoing support and measures to cope with depression
- Social services: to coordinate referrals at discharge and assist with the mother's immediate financial needs
- Public health nurse: to assess the home environment and provide nursing care after discharge
- Community support groups: to provide opportunities to share experiences with families in similar situations so that the mother does not feel isolated and alone
- Mental health clinics: to provide ongoing psychological follow-up

A multidisciplinary approach is needed to ensure appropriate therapy for the mother and her family.

7 Document in nurse's notes the woman's affect (e.g., flat, elated, withdrawn) and whether appropriate maternal-infant interactions are observed. Document that education was provided to the patient regarding signs and symptoms of postpartum blues; signs and symptoms of postpartum depression; when to call her doctor; and the importance of exercise, communication with family, getting sleep, and eating a balanced diet. **Education about signs and symptoms of postpartum blues and depression prepares the patient and her family to recognize and report changes that may be associated with postpartum psychological complications. Healthy lifestyle behaviors promote a state of positive well-being.**

Postpartum Blues

Description. Postpartum blues are experienced by as many as 50 to 80 percent of all postpartum women. In general, the new mother experiences the symptoms within 2 to 4 days after giving birth. The symptoms include insomnia, tearfulness, fatigue, anxiety, irritability, poor concentration, and mild depressive affect. Typically transient, the duration of symptoms is 2 to 3 days (Horowitz et al. 1995).

Management. Given the frequency of occurrence, the blues are considered normal by many professionals. However, many women are confused by their feelings of sadness during what they thought would be a joyful and fulfilling time. An explanation by the nurse about the normalcy of the new mother's feelings may allay her fears. Nurses need to dispel the popular myth that equates becoming a mother with happiness and to give women permission to speak about any negative feelings they may be experiencing (Beck et al. 1992; Beck 1995). Brief supportive psychotherapy focusing on the woman's feelings is an appropriate nursing intervention. Educating the family members about the symptoms and duration of postpartum blues is essential because they will be the ones interacting with the woman after her dismissal from the hospital (Ugarriza 1992).

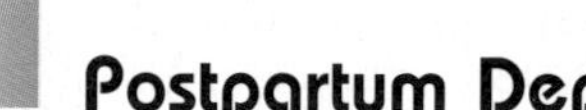

Postpartum Depression

Description. Postpartum depression is a psychological disorder that is nonpsychotic in nature with an insidious onset. The symptoms, similar to depression unrelated to a postpartum status, include tearfulness, mood swings, despondency, feelings of inadequacy, inability to cope with the care of the baby, and increasing guilt over the birth and performance as a mother. Generalized fatigue and complaints of ill health are typical along with irritability, impaired concentration, and poor memory (Ugarriza 1992). The symptoms of postpartum depression are more persistent than those of postpartum blues. Onset is unclear but likely to occur 2 to 6 weeks after birth. It is reported to occur as frequently as in 10 to 20 percent of new mothers (Boyer 1990).

Management. Management of postpartum depression is first geared toward identifying the woman who is suffering from the disorder. Women generally downplay their symptoms. Most women are not being seen by professionals after the 6-week postpartum period is completed. Women and their families need education about postpartum depression (Martell 1990).

Postpartum Psychosis

Description. Postpartum psychosis, a much rarer and more disturbing disorder than postpartum blues or depression, occurs in 1 to 2 per 1000 women and is rare in the absence of a history of a previous psychiatric illness. It results in severe changes in cognitive processes, emotions, and behavior. Symptoms can include hallucinations, delusions, disorganization, marked emotional lability, bizarre or violent behavior, and mania (Horowitz et al. 1995). Onset is usually within 3 weeks.

Management. Management of postpartum psychosis may require hospitalization. Treatment may include the administration of antidepressants or other medications and professional psychiatric counseling involving both the patient and her family.

Nursing Process

Assessment

Differentiating the symptoms of postpartum blues, normal postpartum adjustment, and a postpartum affective disorder can be difficult (Dunnewold and Sanford 1994). Assessment of the postpartum woman needs to include inquiry about appetite, sleep, guilt, performance, social interaction, and somatic complaints as well as mood (Ugarriza 1992). The symptoms of a postpartum affective disorder are more extreme than the normal postpartum adjustment and worsen over time if untreated. Table 35–3 compares the postpartum affective disorders.

Assessment must be ongoing; the community health nurse or the pediatric nurse who sees the mother at well-baby visits has a responsibility to assess for symptoms of postpartum disorders.

Diagnosis

Nursing diagnoses that relate to the patient with postpartum affective disorders may include

- Individual ineffective coping related to the woman's feelings of anxiety and depression
- Ineffective family coping: compromised, related to family's reaction to the woman's feelings of anxiety and depression
- Knowledge deficit: lack of understanding related to normal postpartum emotions, psychological complications, treatment plan, and support
- Altered family processes related to postpartum psychological complications, as evidenced by the woman's inability to function effectively in the role of mother or spouse

Planning

The plan of care is based on the nursing assessment and the resultant nursing diagnoses. The plan should be stated in measurable outcomes as in the following examples.

- The woman will verbalize feelings and thoughts and will develop the skills needed by a new mother to cope effectively with the activities of daily living.
- The woman and her family will adapt to the changes brought about by the postpartum period and the complications experienced, use support systems appropriately, and realistically plan for the future.
- The woman and her family will interact with each other, support one another, and be able to perform the activities needed to care for each other as appropriate to their role.

Intervention

Given the many changes that occur in the postpartum period, it is vital that the emotional status and responses of the mother be carefully assessed. How successfully a woman reacts to her new role is directly influenced by her past experiences, coping mechanisms, sociocultural background, perception of what those close to her expect from her, and availability of help when she leaves the hospital.

The new mother and her family need emotional support and anticipatory guidance, coupled with postpartum teaching, to learn to adapt to and cope with their new roles. This may include suggested strategies for coping with the sleeplessness and frustration that often accompany the integration of a neonate into the family. With an awareness of emotional responses possible during the postpartum period, the postpartum patient and her family will be better prepared to recognize and report changes that may be associated with postpartum psychological complications. The patient experiencing postpartum psychological complications may

Table 35–3

COMPARISON OF POSTPARTUM BLUES, POSTPARTUM DEPRESSION, AND POSTPARTUM PSYCHOSIS

	POSTPARTUM BLUES	POSTPARTUM DEPRESSION	POSTPARTUM PSYCHOSIS
Frequency	50%–80%	10%–20%	1–2 per 1000 postpartum women
Symptoms	Insomnia, tearfulness, fatigue, anxiety, irritability, poor concentration, mild depressive affect	Worsening of "blues" symptoms	Symptoms of "blues" plus hallucinations, delusions, disorganization, marked emotional lability, bizarre or violent behavior, mania
Onset	2–4 days after birth	Insidious, 2–6 weeks after birth	Within 3 weeks
Duration	Transient, 2–3 days	More persistent, 2 weeks–1 year or longer	Improvement within 2–3 months with treatment
Treatment	Education, anticipatory guidance, support	Identification of depression, alleviation of symptoms	Psychotherapy, antidepressants

need to be referred to a professional counselor who can promote the development of additional coping skills. Other possible referrals may be to community support groups, public health nurses, social services, and mental health clinics.

As previously noted, most postpartum patients have some educational needs. The patient and family experiencing a postpartum psychological complication are no exception. Instruction for these patients varies, depending on the severity of the illness, the treatment required, and the patient's and family's reaction to the illness. Education may include a review of symptoms and their causes, if known; a review of prescribed medication, including dosages, actions, compliance requirements, and side effects; and an explanation of options available, such as social service referrals and support groups, to provide further assistance.

The entire family is affected by the presence of a postpartum psychological complication. Problems that may occur include decreased communications, inadequate parenting, behavioral problems with older children, and marital discord.

The patient may often be able to verbalize feelings of depression or confusion to a nurse, while she may be hesitant to discuss these same issues with a family member. Concrete recommendations for the mother may help her better adjust to her new role and improve the family dynamics. Possible recommendations may include alternatives for child care so that she may obtain more rest, suggestions as to how to get more sleep, techniques for stress and time management, and suggestions as to how to better delegate responsibilities.

When a problem has been identified, the family will benefit most if everyone is involved in working toward a solution. This includes encouraging the family, as well as the postpartum patient, to openly discuss concerns, fears, and expectations. In these discussions, the nurse must be attuned to any suggestion that suicidal ideation or a plan for suicide exists. If this is assessed to be present, it must be reported to a physician immediately for follow-up. The nurse can be instrumental in increasing family understanding of the changes that the newly assumed roles require. In cases of severe alterations in family processes, referral for professional counseling may be required.

▼ Evaluation

Outcome is evaluated through assessment of the patient's ability to discuss the situation, become self-directing and assume self-care, demonstrate stable emotional status, and participate fully in family and community activities. Through assessment of patient and family, the nurse determines their understanding of any complication that has occurred, treatment plan, and need for follow-up care. Assessment of family dynamics, including communication patterns and interpersonal relationships, shows the family's adaptation to their new roles. Family members will exhibit a feeling of self-respect and use support services as appropriate to their needs.

Implications for Research

Despite advances in health care technology and knowledge, many questions related to postpartum complications remain unanswered. Most research on postpartum complications has a physical focus, with little attention given to the emotional or the cognitive components of physical complications. Nursing research could contribute in these areas. Research questions that could be explored and answered by nurses include the following:

- Is there a relationship between an identified high-risk pregnancy and the development of postpartum depression?
- How does a postpartum complication affect a woman's emotional response to her infant?
- How does a postpartum complication affect a father's emotional response to his infant?
- Is there a correlation between the severity of the mother's complication and bonding with her infant?
- Is there a higher frequency of infection in emergency deliveries, whether vaginal or operative?

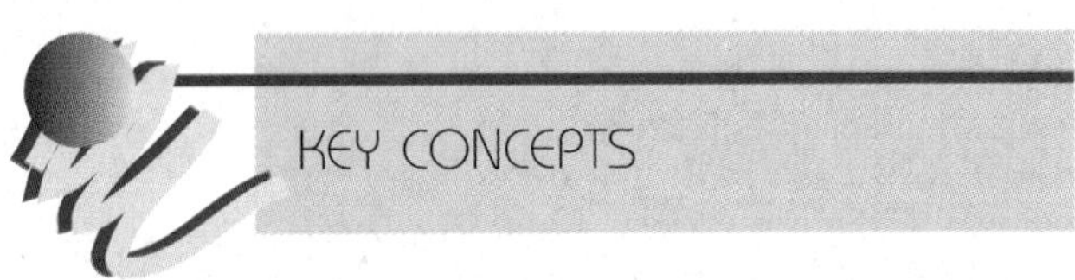

KEY CONCEPTS

- ▼ Despite the magnitude and complexity of the birth process, the postpartum period proceeds without incident most of the time. However, when a postpartum complication does occur, it may compromise expected outcomes. It is essential that the nurse be aware of any deviations from the normal to prevent a catastrophic event.
- ▼ Despite medical advances, postpartum hemorrhage remains among the leading causes of maternal morbidity and mortality. It accounts for approximately 25 percent of obstetric deaths.
- ▼ Primary causes of postpartum hemorrhage include uterine atony; perineal, vaginal, or cervical lacerations; and retained placenta or membranes.
- ▼ The first hours after birth pose the greatest threat of hemorrhage. Blood loss in the immediate period after birth can occur rapidly with dire consequences if it is undetected.
- ▼ Uterine atony identified as a boggy uterus accounts for up to 90 percent of postpartum hemorrhage. Treatment is directed toward firming the soft, boggy uterus with the use of massage and medications.
- ▼ Although there are identifying factors that place a woman at risk for postpartum hemorrhage, two thirds of postpartum hemorrhage occurs without any predisposing risk factors.
- ▼ Uterine inversion is a rare but serious complication that causes profuse bleeding. Prompt response is necessary to prevent shock.
- ▼ With late postpartum hemorrhage, the patient may not present until 1 to 2 weeks post partum with profuse bleeding. The most common cause is retained placental fragments.
- ▼ Careful assessment of postpartum bleeding is essential to identify the woman who is at risk for postpartum hemorrhage. As blood loss continues, there may be changes in vital signs, although normal vital signs may persist until an excessive blood loss has occurred.
- ▼ Although all postpartum patients are potentially at risk for development of thrombophlebitis due to increased blood clotting factors in the postpartum period, less than 1 percent of postpartum women actually develop this condition. A marked reduction in thrombophlebitis in recent times may be attributed to early postpartum ambulation, decrease in traumatic births, and improved health status of pregnant women.
- ▼ Postpartum infections are a major cause of maternal death, ranking second only to postpartum hemorrhage. The most common pathogens responsible for postpartum infections are those that inhabit the lower genital tract and bowel.
- ▼ Postpartum infections may be difficult to recognize in the early stages because many postpartum patients experience some degree of abdominal pain and a 1-day fever. To add confusion, there are some infected patients who do not have a temperature elevation.
- ▼ The birth of a baby is a dynamic and potentially stressful period for the woman and her family. Major psychological changes, role changes, and interaction with a complex health care system can overwhelm the healthiest women. However, the majority of women undergo the physiologic and psychosocial changes of the early puerperium and adjust to motherhood while continuing their daily activities.
- ▼ Postpartum blues are experienced by as many as 50 to 80 percent of all postpartum women. The symptoms include insomnia, tearfulness, fatigue, anxiety, irritability, poor concentration, and mild depressive affect.
- ▼ Assessment of the postpartum woman should include emotional responses; inquiries are

made about appetite, sleep, guilt, performance, social interaction, and somatic complaints as well as mood.

- ▼ How successfully a woman reacts to her new role is directly influenced by her past experiences, coping mechanisms, sociocultural background, perception of what those close to her expect from her, and availability of help in the early postpartum period.

References

Akins, S. (1994). Postpartum hemorrhage: A 90's approach to an age-old problem. *Journal of Nurse-Midwifery,* 39 (2 Suppl.), 123S–126S.

American College of Obstetricians and Gynecologists (ACOG). (1991). Diagnosis and management of postpartum hemorrhage (ACOG Technical Bulletin 143). *International Journal of Gynecology and Obstetrics,* 36, 159–163.

Arias, F. (1993). *Practical guide to high-risk pregnancy and delivery* (2nd ed.). St. Louis: C. V. Mosby.

Assali, N. S., Douglass, R. A., Baird, W. W., Nicholson, D. B., Suyemoto, R. (1953). Measurements of uterine blood flow and uterine metabolism IV: Results in normal pregnancy. *American Journal of Obstetrics and Gynecology,* 66, 248–253.

Auerbach, K. G., Riordan, J., Countryman, B. A. (1993). The breastfeeding process. In J. Riordan and K. G. Auerbach (Eds.), *Breastfeeding and human lactation.* (pp. 215–252). Boston: Jones & Bartlett Publishers.

Beck, C. T. (1995). Screening methods for postpartum depression. *Journal of Obstetric, Gynecologic, and Neonatal Nursing,* 24 (4), 308–312.

Beck, C. T., Reynolds, M. A., Rutowski, P. (1992). Maternity blues and postpartum depression. *Journal of Obstetric, Gynecologic, and Neonatal Nursing,* 21, 287–293.

Benrubi, G. I., and Sang, L. (1990). Postpartum emergencies. In G. I. Benrubi (Ed.), *Obstetric emergencies.* (pp. 171–182). New York: Churchill Livingstone.

Blackburn, S. T., and Loper, D. L. (1992). *Maternal, fetal, and neonatal physiology: A clinical perspective.* Philadelphia: W. B. Saunders.

Boyer, D. B. (1990). Prediction of postpartum depression. *Clinical Issues in Perinatal and Women's Health Nursing,* 1, 359–368.

Calhoun, B. C., and Brost, M. C. (1995). Emergency management of sudden puerperal fever. *Obstetric and Gynecology Clinics of North America,* 22 (2), 357–367.

Cohen, W. R. (1991). Postpartum uterine hemorrhage. In S. H. Cherry and I. R. Merkatz (Eds.), *Complications of pregnancy, medical, surgical, gynecological, psychosocial and perinatal* (4th ed. pp. 1132–1141). Baltimore: Williams & Wilkins.

Cruikshank, S. H. (1986). Management of postpartum and pelvic hemorrhage. *Clinical Obstetrics and Gynecology,* 29, 213–219.

Cunningham, F. G., MacDonald, P. C., Gant, N. F., Leveno, K. J., Gilstrap, L. C. III. (1993). *Williams obstetrics* (19th ed.). Norwalk, CT: Appleton & Lange.

Dauphinee, J. D. (1992). Risk assessment. In L. K. Mandeville and N. H. Troiano (Eds.), *High-risk intrapartum nursing* (pp. 31–39). Philadelphia: J. B. Lippincott.

Dorman, K. (1991). Acute pulmonary insults during pregnancy. In C. J. Harvey (Ed.), *Critical care obstetrical nursing.* (pp. 73–89). Gaithersburg, MD: Aspen Publishers.

Druelinger, L. (1994). Postpartum emergencies. *Emergency Clinics of North America,* 12 (1), 219–237.

Dunnewold, A., and Sanford, D. G. (1994). *Postpartum survival guide.* Oakland, CA: New Harbinger Publications.

Hansen, C. H. (1990). Baby blues: Identification and intervention. *Clinical Issues in Perinatal and Women's Health Nursing,* 1, 369–374.

Hayashi, R. H. (1992). Postpartum hemorrhage and puerperal sepsis. In N. F. Hacker and J. G. Moore (Eds.), *Essentials of obstetrics and gynecology* (pp. 289–307). Philadelphia: W. B. Saunders.

Hayashi, R. H., Castillo, M. S., Noah, M. L. (1984). Management of severe postpartum hemorrhage with a prostaglandin F analogue. *Obstetrics and Gynecology,* 63, 806–808.

Herbert, W. N., and Cefalo, R. C. (1984). Management of postpartum hemorrhage. *Clinical Obstetrics and Gynecology,* 27, 139–176.

Hertz, R. H., Sokol, R. J., Dierker, L. J. (1980). Treatment of postpartum uterine atony with prostaglandin E vaginal suppositories. *Obstetrics and Gynecology,* 56, 129–130.

Horowitz, J. A., Danato, E., Solon, L., Von Metzsch, G., Gill, V. (1995). Postpartum depression: Issues in clinical assessment. *Journal of Perinatology,* 15 (4), 268–278.

Kelly, I. V. (1976). Postpartum hemorrhage. *Clinical Obstetrics and Gynecology,* 19, 595–605.

Lawrence, R. A. (1994). *Breastfeeding:* A guide for the medical profession (4th ed.). St. Louis: C. V. Mosby.

Luegenbiehl, D. L. (1991). Postpartum bleeding. *NAACOG's Clinical Issues,* 2 (3), 402–409.

Luegenbiehl, D. L., Brophy, G., Artigue, G., Phillips, K., Flack, R. (1990). Standardized assessment of blood loss. *MCN: American Journal of Maternal-Child Nursing,* 15 (4), 241–244.

Martell, L. K. (1990). Postpartum depression as a family problem. *MCN: American Journal of Maternal-Child Nursing,* 15, 90–93.

McKenzie, C. A. (1983). Postpartal crises. In K. W. Vestal and C. A. McKenzie (Eds.), *High risk perinatal nursing.* (p. 258). (quote) Philadelphia: W. B. Saunders.

Mickal, A. (1994). Historical notes on infection in obstetrics and gynecology. In J. G. Pastorek (Ed.), *Obstetric and gynecologic infectious disease.* (pp. 3–10). New York: Raven Press.

Riordan, J., and Nichols, F. (1990). A descriptive study of lactation mastitis in long-term breastfeeding women. *Journal of Human Lactation,* 6, 53–58.

Speert, H. (1980). *Obstetrics and gynecology in America: A history.* Baltimore: Waverly Press.

Still, D. K. (1994). Postpartum hemorrhage and other problems of the third stage. In D. K. James, P. J. Steer, C. P. Weiner, B. Gonik (Eds.), *High risk pregnancy.* (pp. 1167–1181). Philadelphia: W. B. Saunders.

Ugarriza, D. N. (1992). Postpartum affective disorders: Incidence and treatment. *Journal of Psychosocial Nursing,* 30 (5), 29–32.

Unterman, R. R., Posner, N. A., Williams, K. N. (1990). Postpartum depressive disorders: Changing trends. *Birth,* 17, 131–137.

NURSING CARE PLANNING GUIDE

Cesarean Birth Postpartum Woman

This Nursing Care Planning Guide was developed to be used as a planning tool. You will need to modify and adapt it to individual clients as appropriate.

Performing a complete and thorough assessment is the first step in providing effective nursing care for a client. Major nursing diagnoses* used in the care of the cesarean birth postpartum woman include

1. Risk for maternal injury
2. Risk for ineffective breathing pattern
3. Pain
4. Risk for infection: endometritis, incision infection, cystitis, nephritis
5. Constipation
6. Urinary retention
7. Altered nutrition: less than body requirements
8. Knowledge deficit: cesarean birth
9. Anxiety: moderate to severe
10. Risk for situational low self-esteem

ASSESSMENT

Assessment of the cesarean birth postpartum woman plays a critical role in facilitating recovery from the birth process and adjustment to the maternal role. To collect data, use the Assessment Tool: Postpartum Flowsheet in the Nursing Care Planning Guide in Chapter 29 (p. 1020). In the data collected, identify defining characteristics to use as a basis for formulating nursing diagnoses that are appropriate for your client. Areas requiring special attention in the care of the cesarean birth postpartum woman include maternal well-being and prevention of infection.

*These nursing diagnoses focus on alterations with cesarean birth. The nursing diagnoses in the Healthy Postpartum Woman Nursing Care Planning Guide also apply in most instances.

Continued on facing page

NURSING CARE PLANNING GUIDE Continued

1

Analysis: ▼ NURSING DIAGNOSIS

***Risk for maternal injury,* related to**

- Aspiration of gastric contents
- Positioning during anesthesia
- Misplacement of surgical sponges
- Bladder injury during surgery
- Injury from jewelry, contact lenses, dentures
- Excessive blood loss

Defining Characteristics

SUBJECTIVE

Complains of incisional pain

OBJECTIVE

Vomiting with aspiration of gastric contents; respiratory distress

Asymmetric breath sounds

Urine not draining into Foley drainage bag

Legs not maintained on operating table

Bloody urine draining from catheter

Hypertension after epidural anesthesia

Sponge or instrument count incorrect

Hypertension

Hypotension and symptoms of shock associated with blood loss

Signs of thrombophlebitis (red, warm area on legs)

Significant drop in hematocrit

Uterine atony and excessive blood loss

Client Goal/ ▼ EVALUATION CRITERIA

Client will demonstrate minimal maternal injury. / ▼ **Client will evidence normal breath sounds, urine draining into Foley drainage bag, absence of blood in urine, normal blood pressure, absence of signs of thrombophlebitis, normal blood loss.**

Continued on following page

NURSING CARE PLANNING GUIDE Continued

▼ NURSING INTERVENTIONS	Rationale
• Determine time and content of last meal/intake.	• Gastrointestinal peristalsis diminishes when labor starts. If the client ate after labor started, digestion will not occur. There is then danger of vomiting and aspiration. General anesthesia is contraindicated for this reason.
• Note intake and urinary output during labor.	• Minimal urinary output indicates dehydration or possible urinary retention. With urinary retention, introduction of Foley catheter, and surgery, there is the possibility of trauma and urinary tract infection.
• Transport with side rails up. Assist in transfer to operating table. Position appropriately for anesthetic administration and then for surgery.	• The client is typically transferred by stretcher to the operating room. If epidural anesthesia was administered in the labor room, the client may be unable to move easily or to detect temperature extremes in the lower extremities. Proper positioning is essential for correct anesthesia placement. Without sensation in the lower extremities, it is essential to protect the lower extremities and fasten the leg strap securely.
• Insert Foley catheter, maintaining asepsis.	• A Foley catheter is inserted to ensure emptiness of the bladder. This lowers the risk of trauma to the bladder.
• Ensure drainage flow of Foley catheter. Do not allow kinks in tubing, place bag lower than bladder.	• If tubing is kinked, the bladder will not empty. If the drainage bag is not lower, there will not be sufficient force for the flow of urine into the catheter drainage bag.
• Obtain urine specimen for culture when the Foley catheter is inserted.	• The culture notes the presence or absence of urinary tract infection before surgery.
• Assess urinary output during surgery and in the recovery period. Note whether there is blood in the urine.	• Monitoring urinary output ensures emptying of the bladder. Blood in the urine may indicate trauma to the bladder. Urinary output is an index of circulating blood volume.
• Assess for untoward reactions to anesthesia. Assess blood pressure and other symptoms of hypotension. Assist with administration of intravenous (IV) bolus and IV fluids if necessary.	• The most common anesthesia is epidural or caudal regional anesthesia. A larger dose than that administered for vaginal delivery ensures higher level and deeper anesthesia. The main side effect is hypotension that occurs as the result of vasodilatation in the lower region of the body. A bolus of IV fluid helps minimize the risk of this side effect by increasing the circulating volume. Treatment of hypotension involves increasing the rate of IV fluids to a rapid rate (increases circulating volume), administering oxygen per mask, and tilting the uterus or turning the client to the side (takes pressure of uterus off the vena cava so blood can return to the heart to be circulated).
• Administer atropine, if ordered.	• Atropine is sometimes given subcutaneously to dry respiratory secretions that may accumulate with general anesthesia.
• Administer 30 mL of antacid before surgery, if ordered.	• Some authors believe that administration of an antacid alters the pH of gastric contents. Then, if

Continued on facing page

NURSING CARE PLANNING GUIDE Continued

aspiration should occur, the gastric contents would cause less trauma to the lungs.

• Keep accurate instrument and sponge counts.	• Counting ensures that no instruments or sponges are mistakenly left in the abdomen.
• Assess blood pressure and pulse. Assess blood loss by counting bloody sponges.	• Hypertension may indicate eclampsia, for which magnesium sulfate may be required. Hypotension and tachycardia may indicate dehydration or hypovolemia. If there is excessive blood loss, the decreased circulating volume may result in hypotension and symptoms of shock. Compensatory vasoconstriction shunts blood to vital organs, resulting in cool, clammy skin. Counting the number of sponges and lap sponges indicates the amount of blood lost.
• Assess dressing for excessive bleeding.	• Oozing is not expected unless there is a drain.
• Assess lower extremities for signs of thrombophlebitis. These include redness, warmth, and the possible presence of Homans sign.	• The cesarean client is at greater risk for thrombophlebitis than is the client with a vaginal delivery. Plasma losses, alteration in clotting factors, and immobility contribute to this risk.
• Encourage ankle and leg exercises in early recovery. Ambulate early.	• Exercises and ambulation improve circulation, promote venous return, and reduce stasis or pooling of blood in the lower extremities. Thrombophlebitis is more likely to occur with stasis and pooling of blood in the lower extremities.
• Hydrate the client with IV fluids.	• IV fluids are necessary to provide adequate circulating volume, which is reduced by blood loss during surgery. The physiologic edema of pregnancy, which returns fluid to the circulation post partum, provides some fluid replacement. Many advocate 3 liters of IV fluid during surgery and the recovery period.
• Monitor postoperative hemoglobin level and hematocrit.	• Typically there is hemoconcentration post partum, so a drop in hematocrit is significant. If there is a significant drop in circulating volume, blood replacement may be necessary.
• Assess uterine fundus for firmness. Gently palpate fundus. Administer oxytocin in IV fluids.	• The uterus must remain contracted to prevent hemorrhage. Oxytocin added to the IV fluids stimulates uterine firmness. The uterus is more tender after a cesarean than after a vaginal delivery, so palpation needs to be more gentle.

Continued on following page

NURSING CARE PLANNING GUIDE Continued

2

Analysis: ▼ NURSING DIAGNOSIS

***Risk for ineffective breathing pattern,* related to**

- Narcotics
- General anesthesia
- Postoperative pain interfering with respiratory expansion of lungs
- Immobility, inactivity

Defining Characteristics

SUBJECTIVE	*OBJECTIVE*
Describes difficulty with deep breathing	Abnormal respiratory rate, depressed rate
	Dyspnea
	Sputum
	Asymmetric breath sounds
	Inactive, minimal ambulation
	Maintains one position in bed; little movement
	Difficulty with deep breathing and cough

Client Goal/ ▼ EVALUATION CRITERIA

Client will demonstrate effective breathing pattern. / ▼ **Client will evidence normal respiratory rate, normal breath sounds, deep breathing and coughing, adequate ambulation.**

▼ NURSING INTERVENTIONS	**Rationale**
• Assess respiratory rate and depth.	• Narcotics are central nervous system depressants and can reduce respirations. Inactivity reduces the respiratory rate. When there is discomfort, depth of respirations is often restricted.
• Assess lung sounds.	• Breath sounds may be diminished for 24 hours after surgery, and rales or secretions should not be

Continued on facing page

NURSING CARE PLANNING GUIDE Continued

present. Absence of lung sounds may indicate consolidation or lack of air exchange, possible atelectasis, or pneumonia.

- Note symptoms of respiratory distress or infection, such as sputum or dyspnea.
- With presence of fluid in the respiratory tract, dyspnea may occur. With infection, there may be sputum and fever.

- Have client turn every 1 to 2 hours. Encourage semi-upright position.
- Turning lessens the possibility of pooling of lung secretions in one portion of the lungs to create infection or obstruction. The semi-upright position increases the vertical chest diameter and prevents abdominal organs from pressing on the diaphragm.

- Have client complete deep-breathing exercises every 2 hours.
- Deep breathing improves the depth of respirations and expands the lungs. In addition, the greater expansion clears secretions from the bronchioles. If the client can "raise" these secretions (productive cough), the deep breathing has been effective in clearing the respiratory tract.

- Hydrate the patient with IV fluids and then oral fluids.
- Hydration liquefies respiratory tract secretions so that they can be expectorated.

3

Analysis: ▼ NURSING DIAGNOSIS

***Pain,* related to**

- Bladder distention
- Flatus, abdominal distention
- Incisional pain
- Hemorrhoids
- Breast engorgement
- Nipple soreness
- Afterpains
- Spinal headache
- Mastitis

Defining Characteristics

SUBJECTIVE

Bladder Distention

Describes presence of lower abdominal, dull discomfort

OBJECTIVE

Bladder Distention

Lower abdominal bulging noted with observation and palpation

Unable to void or voids small amounts

Continued on following page

NURSING CARE PLANNING GUIDE Continued

Flatus, Abdominal Distention

Describes discomfort with distended abdomen

States is not passing flatus, or only minimal flatus

States no bowel movement

Incisional Pain

Describes incisional pain

Describes pain that is aggravated by movement

Flatus, Abdominal Distention

Distended abdomen noted by observation and percussion

Minimal, or sluggish, bowel sounds

Absence of bowel movement

Incisional Pain

Abdominal incision

Grimaces with movement

Nonverbal behavior indicates pain with movement, sitting, walking

Nonverbal behavior indicates pain, tenderness when incisional area is touched

Guarding of incision

Restricted movements

For care planning information about pain associated with hemorrhoids, breast engorgement, nipple soreness, afterpains, spinal headache, and mastitis, see Nursing Diagnosis 2, Altered comfort, in the Healthy Postpartum Woman Nursing Care Planning Guide.

Client Goal/ ▼ EVALUATION CRITERIA

Client will demonstrate comfort. / ▼ **Client will evidence absence of lower abdominal bulge, voiding of adequate amounts, minimal abdominal distention, absence of statements about incisional pain or will state incisional pain is lessened.**

▼ NURSING INTERVENTIONS	Rationale
Bladder Distention	
• Assess lower abdomen just above the symphysis pubis for bulging. Percuss to note dullness of abdomen and increased tympany over the filled bladder.	• A Foley catheter is typically in place for 6 to 8 hours after surgery to ensure output and emptying of the bladder. When it is removed, voiding may be difficult and retention may occur.
• Encourage voiding (assist in ambulating to bathroom, run water). Assess bladder for distention after voiding.	• Ambulating to the bathroom allows voiding in usual position. The sound of running water or pouring water over the perineum often stimulates voiding. If the bladder is emptied, there will not be distention.
• Ambulate early and frequently.	• Activity increases the need for oxygen. When there is an increased need for oxygen, the respiratory center is stimulated to encourage respirations.
• Administer pain medication 30 minutes before ambulation.	• The analgesic reduces incisional pain so that the client participates in breathing exercises and ambulation.
• Obtain sputum specimen if necessary.	• The sputum specimen is cultured to identify pathogens, and appropriate antibiotic treatment can be ordered if necessary.

Continued on facing page

NURSING CARE PLANNING GUIDE Continued

• Administer antibiotics if ordered.	• Antibiotics eradicate the infection.
Incisional Pain	
• Assess presence, location, and nature of incisional discomfort. Assess for complications.	• These data provide information about the subjective experience of discomfort for this client. Complications such as paralytic ileus, wound infection, and wound dehiscence may cause discomfort.
• Assess incision for healing.	• If the incision is approximated, dry (without bleeding or exudate), with minimal redness, healing is progressing.
• Provide information about wound healing and typical regression pattern of pain.	• Information helps reduce anxiety associated with fear about the unknown.
• Assess blood pressure and pulse.	• Pain may be associated with anxiety; blood pressure and pulse are elevated with anxiety.
• Assist with measures that reduce discomfort. This includes	
1. repositioning to comfortable position (side, back)	Certain positions lead to less tension and pressure on the incision, lessening incisional pain.
2. demonstration and encouragement of relaxation and deep-breathing techniques, effleurage	When one is relaxed, without tense muscles, pain perception is lessened. Effleurage distracts from painful sensations.
3. reduction of stimulation in the environment	Unpleasant noise and activity heighten tension rather than relaxation.
4. provision of back rubs	Back rubs enhance relaxation.
• Administer pain medication as ordered every 3 to 4 hours, progressing from intramuscular and subcutaneous to oral routes. Assess effectiveness of pain medication. Explain action of analgesic, time factors, restrictions.	• Analgesics relieve pain and enhance relaxation. Pain is most severe at first; therefore, intramuscular narcotics are most effective at this time. As pain lessens, oral analgesics become effective. Knowledge of typical effect aids in developing realistic expectations. Knowledge of time restrictions, with reasons, allows client to comply with orders.
• Encourage the client to use the football hold with pillows while feeding the baby. Administer pain medication, if necessary, before infant feedings.	• The football hold minimizes pressure on the incision. The pillow helps support the infant and protects the incision. Pain medication before feedings lessens pain during the maternal-infant interaction, facilitating maternal-infant attachment. Pain medications ordered should be safe even with breastfeeding.
• Assist with feedings and infant care as needed.	• The incisional discomfort makes activity associated with infant care more difficult and even aggravates pain. Activities and movements are often restricted, necessitating assistance with handling the infant.

Continued on following page

NURSING CARE PLANNING GUIDE Continued

4

Analysis: ▼ NURSING DIAGNOSIS

***Risk for infection: endometritis, incision infection, cystitis, nephritis,* related to**

- Ascension of microorganisms into uterus
- Membranes ruptured >6 hours before cesarean delivery
- Exposure to microorganisms during surgery
- Trauma to bladder
- Foley catheter
- Urinary retention after Foley catheter removed

Defining Characteristics

SUBJECTIVE	*OBJECTIVE*
Endometritis	Endometritis
Describes headache	Elevated temperature >100°F on 2 days
Describes malaise	Elevated pulse
Describes backache	Uterus larger than expected on palpation
States poor appetite	Dark brown, foul-smelling lochia, but may be odorless
Experiences pain when uterus is palpated	Elevated white blood cell count
Incisional Infection	Incisional Infection
Describes incisional pain	Incision reddened
	Incision not totally approximated
	Incisional exudate
Cystitis/Nephritis	Cystitis/Nephritis
Describes burning with urination	Foley catheter
	Distended bladder
	Voids small amounts (<100 mL)
	Voids frequently
	Dysuria with voiding
	Costovertebral angle tenderness
	Fever

Continued on facing page

NURSING CARE PLANNING GUIDE Continued

Client Goal/ ▼ EVALUATION CRITERIA

Client will demonstrate absence of uterine, incisional, urinary tract infection. / ▼ **Client will evidence normal temperature and pulse rate, normal-sized uterus (involution progresses), soft uterus without tenderness, normal lochia without odor, normal white blood cell count, voiding of adequate amounts, absence of bladder distention, absence of symptoms of cystitis and urinary tract infection.**

▼ NURSING INTERVENTIONS	Rationale
• Assess abdominal dressing or incision for redness, edema, approximation, exudate.	• There is commonly a sterile dressing for the first 24 hours after surgery to help protect the incision. A wet dressing may indicate wound dehiscence, loss of suture, or infection.
• Note whether there is an operative drain. Note moisture on the dressing and change the dressing as ordered or needed.	• If there is an operative drain, the dressing will become moistened. A drain is inserted to allow moisture to be removed and healing to occur from inside to the skin. Moisture is an excellent medium for bacterial growth. Bacteria can travel by capillary action through the wet dressing.
• Assess temperature every 4 hours until stable, then every shift.	• The temperature is often elevated with infection because the metabolic rate increases.
• Assess pulse every 4 hours and then every shift.	• Tachycardia often accompanies infection; the metabolic rate increases.
• Note white blood cell count.	• Leukocytosis accompanies infection as a mechanism to "fight" the infection.
• Assess uterine fundal height and uterine tenderness every 4 hours, then every shift.	• The uterus may remain larger than expected for the stage of involution, and the uterus may be tender with palpation if there is an infection. With a cesarean section, the fundus may remain at the level of the umbilicus for up to 5 days because incisional healing occurs before placental site healing. Because of this, lochia may increase. With delayed involution, the likelihood of infection increases.
• Assess lochia for amount, color, and foul odor every 4 hours, then every shift.	• With uterine infection, the lochia is often a brownish color, has a foul odor, and is greater in amount.
• Encourage semi-Fowler position.	• Semi-Fowler position promotes flow of lochia, reducing pooling that fosters bacterial growth.
• Remove incisional dressing after 24 hours.	• Removal of the dressing promotes drying.
• Culture the lochia if infection is suspected.	• Culture identifies the amount and type of microorganisms so that the appropriate antibiotic can be prescribed.
• Administer Ergotrate or Methergine if ordered.	• These medications stimulate contractions of uterine muscles, which aids emptying of the uterus and involution.
• Encourage a diet high in protein, vitamin C, and iron.	• Protein is needed for tissue growth, vitamin C is needed for collagen function, and iron is needed for hemoglobin formation.

Continued on following page

NURSING CARE PLANNING GUIDE Continued

• Encourage warm showers daily.	• Showers are commonly allowed on the second day after surgery. They promote hygiene and may stimulate circulation and wound healing.
• Maintain medical asepsis with Foley catheter. Provide perineal cleansing.	• Contamination of the catheter or collection bag introduces microorganisms. Lochia and moisture are excellent media for bacterial growth. Bacteria can easily ascend the catheter.
• After Foley catheter is removed, assess output. Measure first voidings.	• With the trauma of surgery, there is a tendency to urinary retention, which predisposes to infection. The client should void at least 100 mL at each voiding.
• Note color and appearance of urine.	• Urine may appear cloudy if there is an infection.
• Assess for bladder distention. Assess location of fundus, firmness of uterine contractions, and amount of lochia.	• With trauma and urinary tract changes, the bladder may become distended. In addition, renal plasma flow remains elevated in the first week after delivery, which increases bladder filling. When the bladder becomes distended, it often displaces the uterus to the side, relaxing uterine muscle contraction and thereby increasing lochia.
• Assist with voiding. Assist ambulation to void.	• Ambulation to the bathroom allows the client to void in the usual position.
• Encourage adequate oral intake.	• Adequate fluid intake hydrates, increases urinary output, decreases concentration of urine, and fosters elimination.
• Assess for symptoms of cystitis and nephritis.	• The symptoms of cystitis include frequency, urgency, and dysuria. The symptoms of nephritis include costovertebral angle tenderness and fever.
• Instruct the client in Kegel exercises.	• Kegel exercises, 100 times a day, improve muscle tone of the pubococcygeal muscle, preventing or reducing stress incontinence.
• Administer appropriate antibiotics. Prophylactic IV antibiotics are often administered (often penicillin with gentamicin), typically one dose after the cord is clamped, and then two or more doses 6 hours apart.	• The prophylactic antibiotic reduces the risk of endometritis as well as incisional infection.

Continued on facing page

NURSING CARE PLANNING GUIDE Continued

5

Analysis: ▼ NURSING DIAGNOSIS

***Constipation*, related to**

- Change in intra-abdominal pressure during surgery
- Reduced gastrointestinal motility
- Initial bed rest
- Inactivity
- Altered fluid and nutritional intake
- Flatus
- Incisional discomfort

Defining Characteristics

SUBJECTIVE	*OBJECTIVE*
States absence of flatus	Infrequent bowel elimination
Describes discomfort with abdominal distention	Hard stools
Describes concern to have a bowel movement	Straining with stools
	Absence of flatus or minimal flatus
	Abdominal distention
	NPO for a time
	Altered diet
	Ambulates infrequently
	Absent to minimal bowel sounds

Client Goal/ ▼ EVALUATION CRITERIA

Client will demonstrate normal bowel elimination. / ▼ **Client will evidence flatus, ambulating, active bowel sounds, bowel movement.**

Continued on following page

NURSING CARE PLANNING GUIDE Continued

▼ NURSING INTERVENTIONS	Rationale
• Auscultate bowel sounds in all four quadrants every 4 hours.	• With handling of the bowel during surgery, peristalsis ceases for up to 24 hours after surgery. On the second day, bowel sounds become faint. By the third day, bowel sounds are active.
• Assess abdominal distention. Palpate and percuss the abdomen.	• When gas forms in the bowel and is not expelled with peristalsis, it accumulates, causing distention.
• Note passing of flatus.	• When flatus is passed, it indicates that gastrointestinal motility has returned.
• Avoid very hot or very cold oral fluids, straws, and carbonated beverages.	• Some believe that all of these contribute to the formation and accumulation of gas and, therefore, abdominal distention.
• Hydrate with oral fluids once bowel sounds are present.	• Hydration helps prevent excessive absorption of fluid from the stools, which contributes to constipation.
• Encourage leg exercises, turning, and ambulation.	• After the first 24 hours, progressive ambulation stimulates gastrointestinal motility, peristalsis, and expulsion of flatus. Leg exercises tighten abdominal muscles, which improves gastrointestinal motility.
• Instruct the client to include fiber in the diet (fresh fruits and vegetables, whole grains).	• Roughage provides bulk in the stool, which stimulates peristalsis.
• Administer stool softeners or cathartics as ordered.	• Stool softeners soften the stool by minimizing absorption of water from the stool, stimulating peristalsis.
• If there is abdominal distention and minimal passage of flatus, insert rectal tube.	• At times, inserting a tube into the rectum stimulates peristalsis and facilitates the passage of flatus.
• Administer a hypertonic Fleet enema if ordered.	• The enema promotes peristalsis, expulsion of gas, and elimination of stool.

6

Analysis: ▼ NURSING DIAGNOSIS

***Urinary retention,* related to**

- Foley catheter for 6–24 hours
- Inactivity
- Handling of bladder during surgery
- Diuresis post partum
- Incisional discomfort
- Inactivity

Continued on facing page

NURSING CARE PLANNING GUIDE Continued

Defining Characteristics

SUBJECTIVE	*OBJECTIVE*
Describes burning with urination	Foley catheter
	Distended bladder after removal of Foley catheter
	Voids small amounts (< 100 mL) after Foley catheter is removed
	Voids frequently
	Dysuria with voiding
	Urgency with voiding
	Costovertebral angle tenderness
	Fever

Client Goal/ ▼ EVALUATION CRITERIA

Client will demonstrate normal urinary elimination, without infection. / ▼ **Client will evidence voiding of adequate amounts, absence of bladder distention, absence of symptoms of urinary tract infection.**

▼ NURSING INTERVENTIONS	Rationale
• Maintain sterile, closed urinary system.	• This prevents introduction of bacteria, which can ascend to the bladder.
• Provide perineal care and instruct client in perineal care. Change perineal pads frequently.	• Cleansing the perineum removes moisture and blood, which are excellent media for the growth of microorganisms. When the client is able, she performs perineal care with each voiding.
• Ensure that Foley drainage bag is dependent and tubing is not kinked.	• If drainage tubing is kinked, urine remains in the bladder, which increases the risk for infection. If the drainage bag is not dependent, there can be urinary reflux and urine cannot drain from the bladder.

For additional applicable nursing interventions, refer to Nursing Diagnosis 4, Risk for urinary tract infection, in the Healthy Postpartum Woman Nursing Care Planning Guide, and to Nursing Diagnosis 3, Pain related to bladder distention, in this nursing care planning guide.

Continued on following page

NURSING CARE PLANNING GUIDE Continued

7

Analysis: ▼ NURSING DIAGNOSIS

***Altered nutrition: less than body requirements,* related to**

- NPO after cesarean birth
- Reduced gastrointestinal motility after cesarean birth
- Inactivity after cesarean birth

Defining Characteristics

SUBJECTIVE	*OBJECTIVE*
Describes lack of knowledge of four food groups	NPO
Describes lack of knowledge of requirements for healing	Absent or minimal bowel sounds
Describes lack of knowledge of requirements for breastfeeding	Not passing flatus, then passes flatus
	Difficulty tolerating clear, full liquids
	Abdominal distention
	Breastfeeding

Client Goal/ ▼ EVALUATION CRITERIA

Client will demonstrate nutritional intake adequate for body requirements. / ▼ **Client will evidence gastrointestinal motility; will resume normal bowel sounds; will tolerate clear liquids, full liquids, regular diet; will take in adequate amount of calories and nutrients for recovery; will take in adequate amount of calories and nutrients for breastfeeding; will resume prepregnant weight; will be able to relay nutritional requirements.**

▼ NURSING INTERVENTIONS	Rationale
• Assess bowel sounds every 4 hours.	• After surgery, peristalsis ceases for a time. Therefore, bowel sounds are absent. Auscultation allows the nurse to determine the presence and strength of bowel sounds.

Continued on facing page

NURSING CARE PLANNING GUIDE Continued

- Assess abdomen for distention. Palpate and percuss.
- When peristalsis ceases or is minimal, gas develops and accumulates, contributing to abdominal distention.
- Once bowel sounds are returning and flatus is passed, start oral fluids. Start with clear liquids, then progress to full liquids and regular diet.
- When peristalsis is returning, the client is able to tolerate fluids. Clear liquids provide fluids and require little digestion. Full liquids require more digestion and gastrointestinal motility. The progression allows time for the gastrointestinal tract to resume normal activity.
- Administer analgesics before ambulation
- Analgesics relieve pain so that the mother can ambulate more easily. Ambulation and activity stimulate peristalsis. The sooner peristalsis returns, the sooner an adequate nutritional intake can be consumed.

For additional applicable nursing interventions, see Nursing Diagnosis 6, Altered nutrition: less than body requirements, in the Healthy Postpartum Woman Nursing Care Planning Guide.

8

Analysis: ▼ NURSING DIAGNOSIS

***Knowledge deficit: cesarean birth,* related to**

- Unplanned cesarean birth
- Lack of knowledge about cesarean procedures
- Lack of retention of information from childbirth education classes
- Lack of knowledge about reason for the cesarean birth
- Lack of clear memory about previous cesarean birth

Defining Characteristics

SUBJECTIVE

States inexperience with cesarean procedures

Asks questions about reason for cesarean birth, preoperative care, the procedure itself

Describes concern about safety and outcome of cesarean birth

OBJECTIVE

First cesarean procedure

Symptoms of anxiety

Continued on following page

NURSING CARE PLANNING GUIDE Continued

Client Goal/ ▼ EVALUATION CRITERIA

Client will demonstrate adequate knowledge of cesarean birth. / ▼ **Client will evidence moderate anxiety, ability to attend to information, minimal number of questions about procedures, compliance with instruction, verbalization of understanding of cesarean procedures.**

▼ NURSING INTERVENTIONS	Rationale
• Assess learning needs.	• Instruction and teaching should add to, supplement, or clarify information the client already has available. This information provides the baseline level for development of a teaching plan.
• Assess level of anxiety (see anxiety nursing diagnosis). Intervene to reduce anxiety.	• Assessment provides information that influences interventions to either lower anxiety or maintain it at an acceptable level. As the level of anxiety increases, the ability to attend and learn is reduced. Therefore, interventions to reduce anxiety enhance the ability to learn.
• Provide information in simple terms. Include rationale for action.	• When anxiety is increased, the ability to understand is hampered. In addition, the client can often respond only to selected parts of the environment. When the rationale is provided, the learner is able to understand the reason for the action and comply.
• Encourage the client to ask questions.	• Misconceptions and concerns can be clarified if questions are asked.
• Review procedures as they occur.	• Review helps the client to recall what was previously explained, facilitating clarification and understanding.
• Provide information about preoperative, operative, and postoperative routines and procedures.	• The client needs to understand what will occur. Information about postoperative procedures, such as leg exercises, deep breathing, and early ambulation, increases understanding and facilitates compliance.
• Provide information regarding possible complications after a cesarean birth (fever, uterine infection, urinary tract infection, bleeding, abdominal distention).	• If the client knows possible complications, there is greater likelihood of compliance with actions to prevent them.
• Provide information related to self-care after the cesarean birth, such as perineal care, Foley catheter, and hygiene.	• Providing information about self-care allows the client to become independent as soon as possible.
• Review activity and exercises after cesarean birth.	• The client should not lift objects heavier than the infant for 2 weeks. When the infant is picked up, the client should bend at the knees. Once abdominal discomfort has lessened (approximately 3 to 4 weeks post partum), an exercise program can be initiated.
• Provide information about resuming sexual intercourse and explain contraception as needed.	• As soon as the client is comfortable after lochia has ceased, intercourse may be resumed. Information about contraception allows the client to select an acceptable method.

Continued on facing page

NURSING CARE PLANNING GUIDE Continued

- Plan home management with the client, assistance with housework, infant sleeping arrangements, and support person availability.
- The cesarean client needs more assistance than does a client who delivered vaginally. Stairs are difficult and should be avoided for a time. Low infant cradles would be difficult. Household chores create greater discomfort, and the client should not lift more than the weight of the infant.
- Demonstrate methods to relieve discomfort at home, such as how to get out of a flat bed.
- To exit a flat bed, the client turns on her side, uses her arms to lift herself to a sitting position, and then pushes on the bed to lift herself up.
- Review symptoms that warrant reporting to the physician after discharge.
- Symptoms of fever or heavier blood flow warrant reporting to the physician.
- Provide appropriate written information, including a phone number to call when questions arise.
- Supplemental information reinforces learning and provides a reference at home. When questions arise, the client can call to obtain answers.

9

Analysis: ▼ NURSING DIAGNOSIS

***Anxiety: moderate to severe,* related to**

- Cesarean surgery
- Unfamiliarity with cesarean preoperative and postoperative routines
- Concern for safety of fetus
- Concern for own safety
- Fear of pain
- Fear of the unknown
- Unmet expectation of vaginal delivery
- Threat to physical self and infant
- Threat to self-esteem

Defining Characteristics

SUBJECTIVE

Moderate Anxiety

Expresses feelings of tension, apprehension, nervousness, concern

Verbalizes expectations of problems

Verbalizes concern for self and fetus

Experiences fear of the surgery

OBJECTIVE

Moderate Anxiety

Voice tremors

Voice pitch changes

Increased rate and quantity of verbalization

Narrowed focus of attention; focuses on a particular part of the situation; selective inattention

Able to focus on most of what is happening

Continued on following page

NURSING CARE PLANNING GUIDE Continued

	Narrowed perceptions
	Hand tremors or shaking
	Increased muscle tension
	Rapid pulse
	Increased respiratory rate
	Irritability
	More active reflexes
	Face flushed
	Localized or generalized sweating
Severe Anxiety	Severe Anxiety
Experiences feelings of severe apprehension, nervousness, helplessness	False cheerfulness or laughing
	Inappropriate verbalizations
	Intellectualization
	Cannot focus on what is happening
	Can follow only simple instructions
	Denial—does not want to talk about it
	Rigid position
	Purposeless activity
	Tachycardia
	Hyperventilation
	Clammy hands and skin
	Dry mouth
	Diaphoresis
	Pallor
	Withdrawn

Client Goal/ ▼ EVALUATION CRITERIA

Client will demonstrate mild or moderate anxiety. / ▼ **Client will evidence asking questions or seeking information, increased awareness, increased attention, mild restlessness, normal pulse and respirations, ability to focus on most of what is happening, ability to follow instructions.**

For applicable nursing interventions, refer to Nursing Diagnosis 15, Risk for moderate anxiety, in the Healthy Postpartum Woman Nursing Care Planning Guide, and to Nursing Diagnosis 12, Moderate to severe anxiety, in the Normal Childbirth Nursing Care Planning Guide.

Continued on facing page

NURSING CARE PLANNING GUIDE Continued

10

Analysis: ▼ NURSING DIAGNOSIS

***Risk for situational low self-esteem*, related to**

- Cesarean birth: loss of experiencing vaginal birth
- Addition of infant to family

Defining Characteristics

SUBJECTIVE

Describes expectation of vaginal delivery

Voices concern for safety during cesarean procedure

Feelings of failure

Feelings of disappointment

Unmet expectations

Negative self-appraisal in response to cesarean birth

Negative verbalizations about cesarean birth

Expresses shame or guilt and evaluates self as inadequate

OBJECTIVE

Symptoms of anxiety

Difficulty in making decisions

Client Goal/ ▼ EVALUATION CRITERIA

Client will demonstrate positive self-esteem. / ▼ **Client will evidence expressions of expectations and feelings about cesarean birth, have mild to moderate level of anxiety, verbalize understanding of reason for cesarean birth, refer to cesarean delivery as a birth, relay similarities between vaginal and cesarean births.**

▼ NURSING INTERVENTIONS	Rationale
• Obtain information about the mother's conceptualizations of pregnancy, labor, and delivery.	• The "self" is formed by developing perceptions of one's body (body image) and of one's characteristics, personality, and behavior. These perceptions, or concepts of one's self, come from observation of role models, with internalization of behaviors that are valued. In addition, they come from feedback, or input from others. The mother forms conceptualizations of childbirth and the mothering role as well as of how she believes she should behave during these experiences. When one's behavior is not

Continued on following page

NURSING CARE PLANNING GUIDE Continued

consistent with expectations and conceptualizations, there can be feelings of failure, and one's self-concept suffers.

Intervention	Rationale
• Encourage verbalizations of feelings.	• When one verbalizes feelings, awareness is increased and anxiety reduced.
• Provide information about cesarean procedure or reinforce previous learning. Refer to the cesarean delivery as a cesarean birth.	• With review, previous learning is reinforced. Information lessens anxiety associated with fear of the unknown. Referring to the cesarean delivery as a birth increases awareness that there is, indeed, a birth as there is with a vaginal delivery.
• Point out similarities between vaginal and cesarean births.	• Awareness of similarities heightens feelings of normalcy. Then, the cesarean birth will not seem as different or as unnatural.
• Encourage the significant other to be present for the cesarean birth.	• The significant other can emotionally support the mother. In addition, it allows participation in childbirth.
• Assist with strategies that help to restore self-esteem; care of infant to ease transition to parenting, normalizing the cesarean birth.	• Normal self-care and infant caretaking activities performed successfully will enhance self-esteem.
• Assess the emotional reaction to the cesarean birth.	• Even though all proceeds normally and there is a healthy outcome, there may be a feeling of guilt associated with the loss of expected childbirth experience.

For additional applicable nursing interventions, refer to Nursing Diagnosis 13, Risk for situational low self-esteem, in the Normal Childbirth Nursing Care Planning Guide, and to Nursing Diagnosis 17, Risk for situational low self-esteem, in the Healthy Postpartum Woman Nursing Care Planning Guide.

Chapter 36

Alterations in Health Status of Newborns

Jan L. Kabler
Paula M. Delmore

> Having a child born too soon is a unique terror, one part irrational guilt that you somehow caused this event to happen, two parts uncertainty as to the role you can play in this vulnerable infant's care, and three parts anxiety that you will lose your dream child.
>
> JANINE JASON AND ANTONIA VAN DER MEER (1989)

HIGHLIGHTS

- Assessment of the Newborn for Gestational Age and Birth Weight
- Procedure 36–1: Gavage Feeding
- Conditions Related to Preterm Infants, Including Respiratory Distress Syndrome; Pulmonary Interstitial Emphysema; Pneumothorax; Pulmonary Hemorrhage; Bronchopulmonary Dysplasia; Patent Ductus Arteriosus; Intraventricular Hemorrhage; Necrotizing Enterocolitis; and Special Considerations for Renal Conditions, Retinopathy, Skin, and Neurobehavioral Development
- Procedure 36–2: Neonatal Transport
- Conditions Related to the Postterm Infant
- Special Clinical Conditions Related to Newborns, Including Jaundice; the Infant of the Diabetic Mother; the Infant Exposed to Human Immunodeficiency Virus; and the Infant Exposed to Substance Abuse
- Conditions Related to Congenital Anomalies, Including Omphalocele and Gastroschisis, Esophageal Atresia and Tracheoesophageal Fistula, Anorectal Agenesis, Hirschsprung's Disease, Duodenal Atresia, Diaphragmatic Hernia, Potter's Syndrome, Polycystic and Multicystic Dysplastic Kidney Disease, Ambiguous Genitalia, Anencephaly and Myelomeningocele, Hydrocephaly, Cleft Lip and Palate, Talipes Eqinovarus, Syndactyly, Polydactyly, Trisomy 13, Trisomy 18, Trisomy 21, Turner's Syndrome, Phenylketonuria, Galactosemia, Congenital Hypothyroidism, Maple Syrup Urine Disease, and Cardiac Disorders
- Risk Management
- Support for the NICU Nurse
- Implications for Research
- Nursing Care Planning Guide: Healthy Preterm Newborn

DEFINITIONS

Acrocyanosis—Bluish discoloration of the hands and feet in the newborn; also termed peripheral cyanosis. Considered normal immediately after birth but should not persist for longer than 24 hours.

Agenesis—Absence or failure of development of any organ or part.

Anomaly—A deviation from the normal, usually from a congenital or hereditary origin.

Apnea—Respiratory pause greater than or equal to 20 seconds in length, associated with bradycardia and cyanosis.

Bradycardia—A heart rate less than 80 to 100 beats per minute in the newborn.

Congenital—Condition present at birth.

Hydrocephalus—Excessive cerebrospinal fluid within the ventricular and subarachnoid spaces.

Hypoxia—Decreased amount of oxygen in the organs and tissues.

Jaundice—Yellow discoloration of the skin and sclera related to excess bilirubin in the blood; mainly due to functional immaturity of the liver in the neonate.

Microcephaly—A head circumference below the 10th percentile for gestational age.

Pneumothorax—Accumulation of air in the pleural space.

Retraction—A drawing in of the chest during inspiration; often associated with respiratory distress.

Tachycardia—A heart rate greater than 180 to 200 beats per minute in the newborn.

Tachypnea—Respirations of greater than 60 breaths per minute in the newborn.

Umbilical artery catheter—A radiopaque catheter placed in one of the umbilical arteries through which parenteral fluids may be delivered or blood samples withdrawn.

Although the majority of infants are born healthy, there are those infants who are born at risk with increased chances for morbidity or mortality. Nurses are challenged to meet the needs of families who experience the birth of a high-risk infant. Although the nurse may be busy stabilizing the infant, a team member needs to be designated to care for the parents. Keep parents informed of the progress of their infant at all times. They must be provided with explanations of all procedures.

The parents will be grieving for the loss of their vision of a perfect baby. Provide the family with opportunities to ventilate their feelings. Involve other members of the health care team, such as social workers and chaplains. Critical care nurses can become so overwhelmed by the demands and responsibilities of their job that they appear uncaring to parents (Rushton 1991). It is important to balance technology with the emotional needs of parents (Fig. 36–1).

Despite the high-tech environment of the neonatal intensive care unit (NICU), the nurse must not forget the needs of high touch. Involve parents in the care of their sick newborn. They must be provided with opportunities to interact with and become attached to their infant (Fig. 36–2).

This chapter provides the background for assessment, planning, and implementation of nursing care for the neonate with special needs. It is divided into two parts. The first part examines problems of the neonate related to gestational age and weight. The second part describes congenital anomalies that can be recognized in the newborn period.

Neonatal assessment includes evaluation of gestational age and birth weight to determine which infants should be observed more closely. The infant not born at term or at the appropriate weight for gestational age is at increased risk for morbidity and mortality. The following terms are used to classify the newborn according to gestational age:

- Preterm: Born before the end of week 37, regardless of weight
- Term: Born between the beginning of week 38 and the completion of week 41
- Postterm: Born at the onset of week 42 or anytime thereafter

After the newborn's weight is plotted on the growth curve according to gestational age, the newborn is classified as follows (see Fig. 31–13):

- Small for gestational age (SGA): The infant's birth weight is below the 10th percentile, or 2 standard deviations below normal
- Large for gestational age (LGA): The infant's birth weight is above the 90th percentile, or 2 standard deviations above the normal
- Appropriate for gestational age (AGA): The in-

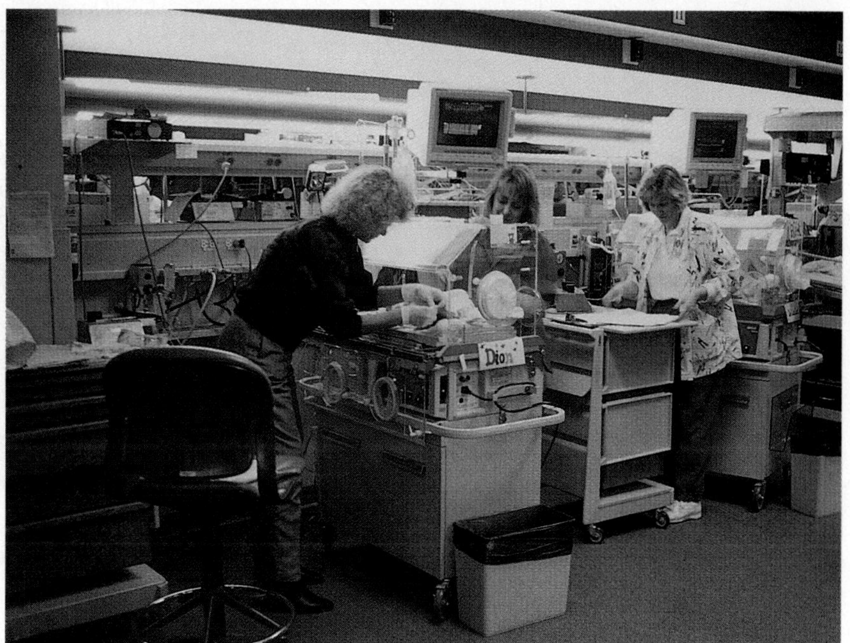

Figure 36–1
The high-tech environment of the neonatal intensive care unit (NICU) may be intimidating to parents. Orienting them to equipment and providing information about their infant's status is comforting and can decrease anxiety. (Courtesy of Wesley Medical Center, Wichita, KS.)

fant's birth weight falls between the 10th and 90th percentiles

- Low birth weight (LBW): The infant's birth weight is 2500 g or less
- Very low birth weight (VLBW): The infant's birth weight is 1500 g or less

SMALL-FOR-GESTATIONAL-AGE INFANT

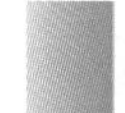

Description

SGA is related to maternal factors such as low socioeconomic status, malnutrition, or high-altitude residence. Maternal smoking, use of alcohol, and use of illicit drugs are associated with the birth of newborns who are SGA. Maternal illness such as hypertension, chronic cardiovascular or renal disease, advanced diabetes, or preeclampsia may retard fetal growth, resulting in the birth of an infant with SGA. In addition, chromosome disorders, congenital abnormalities, and intrauterine infections are associated with SGA infants.

The appearance of the SGA newborn depends on when the malnutrition or insult occurred. When the insult occurs early in the gestational period and is sustained throughout the pregnancy, the newborn appears symmetric, with body parts in proportion to each other. They are considered hypoplastic. Because they are affected early in the gestational period when there is a rapid proliferation of cells as the organs and body structures are formed, there are fewer cells being developed. Because the organs contain cells that are normal in size but fewer in number, the organs are smaller. Since there are fewer cells, the growth retardation is irreversible. These infants frequently have experienced an early intrauterine nonbacterial infection, such as rubella or cytomegalic inclusion disease, or have congenital malformations.

Growth restriction occurring later in gestation may be associated with maternal conditions of preeclampsia, chronic hypertension, and chronic renal disease. This late growth restriction causes hypotrophic intrauterine growth restriction with cells that are smaller in size but without a decrease in the number of cells. These infants have appropriate-sized heads and body length with reduced chest and abdominal circumferences. The brain and heart are larger in proportion to the overall body weight, whereas the liver, spleen, adrenal, and thymus are diminished. With optimal maternal nutrition or adequate postnatal nutrition, the growth restriction may be reversible (Korones 1986).

Management

Optimal management of the SGA infant begins in the antenatal period with a detailed maternal history to determine the presence of any risk factors.

In the antepartum period, fetal tolerance to labor is assessed by the use of fetal monitoring. It is not unusual for growth-restricted infants to be hypoxic before labor. Many are undergrown as a re-

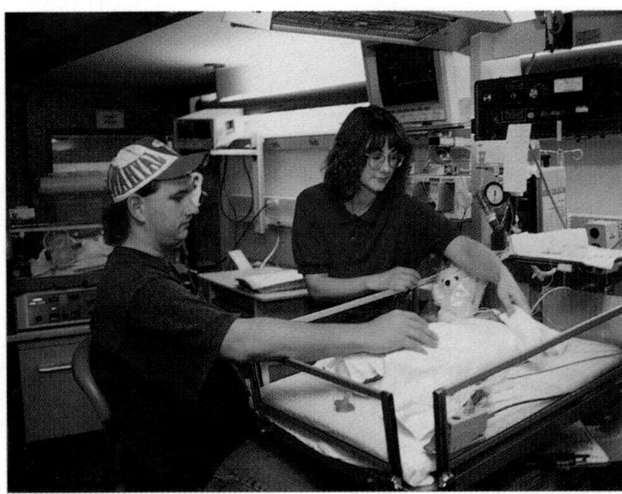
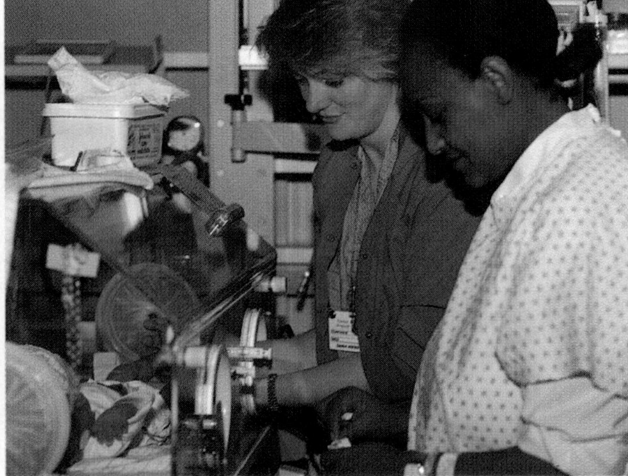

Figure 36–2

The nurse can promote parent-infant attachment by involving both mothers and fathers in the care of their infant. (Photo at left courtesy of Wesley Medical Center, Wichita, KS.)

sult of placental insufficiency. Because of this hypoxia, not only are they unable to tolerate the asphyxia of normal birth, but they are also unable to compensate for it after birth (Korones 1986). Polycythemia in the SGA infant may be a response to chronic fetal hypoxia.

Physical examination of the infant begins immediately after birth. Identification of any abnormalities or variations from normal is essential to provide optimal care. The SGA infant is at high risk for hypothermia because of a large body surface area in relation to weight, lack of subcutaneous tissue, and limited brown fat stores. The SGA infant also has decreased glycogen stores, which increases the risk for hypoglycemia and hypothermia. Almost two thirds of SGA infants become hypoglycemic. Early initiation of an intravenous dextrose solution or feeding by breast, bottle, or gavage is necessary to treat or prevent hypoglycemia (Procedure 36–1).

Gestational age assessment as described in Chapter 31 is one part of the physical examination. However, gestational age assessment according to physical characteristics may be misleading. Because the SGA infant achieves neurologic maturity, the neurologic examination may be more accurate than the physical examination. Physical characteristics common to the SGA infant include decrease in amount of breast tissue; diminished amount of skinfolds; skin that is loose, dry, and scaling; decrease in amount of adipose tissue; diminished muscle mass, especially in extremities; smaller than average length, weight, or head circumference; and a wide-eyed and alert facial expression.

After the SGA infant has been stabilized, laboratory testing to assess for any infections may include complete blood count (CBC) with differential and platelets, TORCH titer (for toxoplasmosis, other agents, rubella, cytomegalovirus, and herpes simplex), urine culture for cytomegalovirus, or determination of bilirubin level. A chromosome analysis may be performed if congenital anomalies are present. Screening for drugs in the newborn's urine or stool is indicated by maternal history. An ultrasound examination or computed tomography (CT) scan may be ordered to rule out hydrocephalus.

Nursing Process

▼ Assessment

The maternal, prenatal, and intrapartum history is thoroughly reviewed by the nurse receiving the SGA infant. The infant is then assessed for gestational age and physical maturity as described in Chapter 31. The infant is examined for any abnormalities. The nurse is responsible for monitoring vital signs, especially the temperature for elevation or hypothermia, and the respiratory rate and pulse for elevation. Routine physical assessments are also performed. A ruddy appearance, cyanosis, jaundice, or apnea may be signs of polycythemia. Laboratory values such as serum hemoglobin and hematocrit are analyzed for indications of polycythemia; platelet counts, CBC with differential, and blood cultures are monitored for signs of infection. The blood glucose level is monitored for hypoglycemia. The infant's weight is monitored daily.

PROCEDURE 36–1

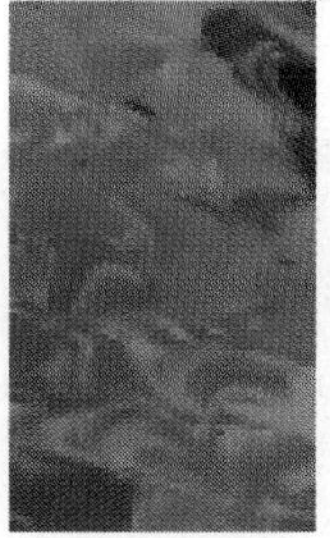

Gavage Feeding

▼ PURPOSE

To provide either breast milk or formula to those infants unable to feed orally.

▼ EQUIPMENT

- Pediatric stethoscope
- Gastric tube (6 to 8 French for oral feedings, 3.5 to 5 French for nasogastric feedings)
- Breast milk or formula
- Tape
- Blanket roll
- Syringe
- Suction equipment
- Infusion pump

1 Select the appropriate size tube. For nasogastric tubes, measure (with the tube itself) from the tip of the infant's nose to the earlobe and either to the distal end of the xiphoid process or to a point midway between the distal end of the xiphoid process and the umbilicus (Weibley et al. 1987). Mark the tube at the measured point with tape. For orogastric tubes, follow the same steps but use the mouth as the initial landmark. **The smallest bore tubing that will deliver the feeding but not occlude the naris should be selected for nasogastric feedings. Using these steps to measure the tube before its insertion helps ensure that the tube will be long enough to reach the infant's stomach.**

2 Place the infant in a supine position and gently insert the catheter through the nose or mouth, with the head in a slightly extended position, until the tape marker is positioned at the orifice. If the infant should begin to cough, gag, or turn cyanotic, remove the tube immediately. If regurgitation occurs, suction the airway until it is clear and then resume tube placement. **Slight ex-**

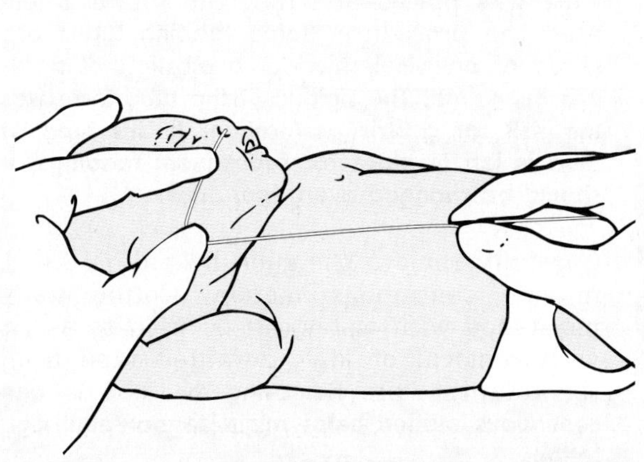

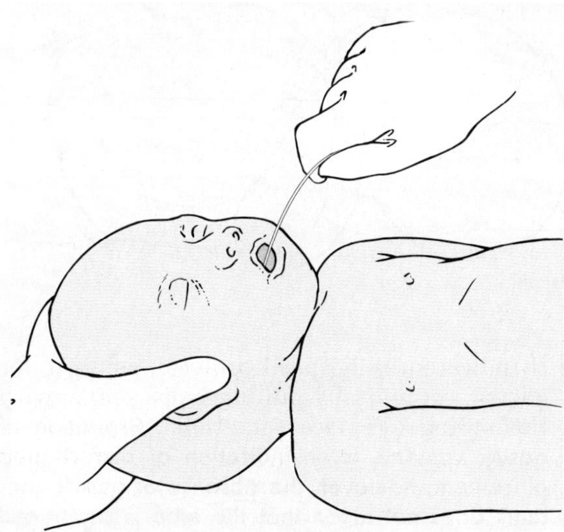

Continued on following page

PROCEDURE 36–1 Continued

tension promotes entry of the tube into the esophagus. Hyperextension or underextension may decrease air entry.

3 Secure the orogastric or nasogastric tube in place by taping it to the infant's cheek. Limit the amount of tape to the minimum required to ensure security. A pectin barrier may be placed under the tape if there are concerns about skin integrity. **Removing adhesives can result in epidermal stripping. This loss of skin integrity may lead to increased risk for infection, increased water loss, and thermal instability.**

4 Before each feeding, check tube placement by using a syringe to inject 0.5 to 1.0 mL of air into the tubing while listening with a stethoscope over the epigastric area for a "swoosh." **Correct tube placement is critical to avoid delivery of the feeding into the lungs.**

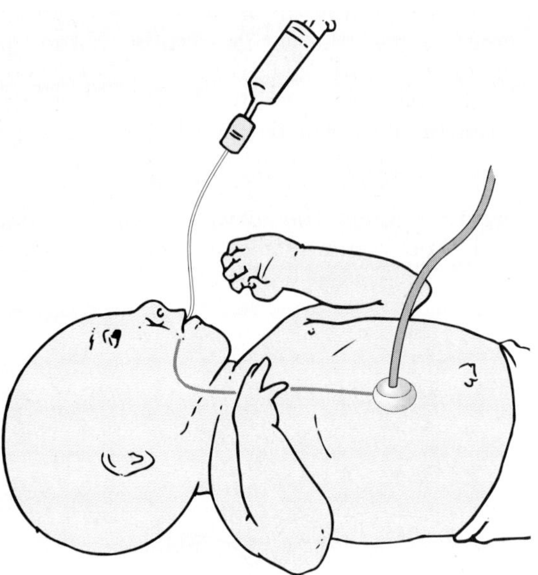

5 If indicated by hospital protocol, aspirate for gastric contents by pulling back gently with the syringe; replace secretions. **Aspiration of gastric contents is an indication of correct tube placement; however, the absence of gastric contents does not mean that the tube is positioned improperly. Routine aspiration of gastric contents can cause irritation of the stomach lining.**

6 The infant may be held by a parent or nurse during the feeding or placed in the prone or right lateral position with the head of the bed slightly elevated. **Elevation of the bed reduces the risk for gastroesophageal reflux. Oxygenation can be affected by the infant's position; therefore, the position that best supports adequate oxygenation should be considered. The infant may be supported or nested into position with blanket rolls. Having parents hold the infant during the feeding promotes parental attachment.**

7 Deliver the prescribed amount of breast milk or formula by the method designated by the physician. Feedings can be delivered on either a continuous or an intermittent schedule by either gravity flow or an infusion pump. **There are no reports that convincingly support one method over another. Clinician preference and the infant's ability to tolerate the feeding without physiologic compromise (such as apnea, bradycardia, or gastroesophageal reflux) most often determine the method of choice.**

8 Offer the infant nonnutritive sucking during gavage feeding. **Research indicates that nonnutritive sucking may improve the sucking reflex and promote weight gain.**

9 Document the date and time the feeding tube was placed and how the infant tolerated the procedure. **Some feeding tubes are made of polyvinyl chloride, a plastic that hardens over time. The rigidity of the tube increases the risk for gastric perforation. If this type of tube is left in place for subsequent feedings, it should be changed every few days.**

10 Carefully remove the tube by pulling on it in one continuous motion. Cotton balls moistened with water can be used to assist with removal of any unwanted tape from the infant's skin. **Removing the tube in one continuous motion helps minimize potential agitation.**

▼ Diagnosis

Nursing diagnoses for the SGA infant might include the following:

- Altered nutrition: less than body requirements related to a high metabolic rate with low or rapidly depleting glycogen stores
- Hypothermia related to decreased subcutaneous tissue and glycogen stores
- Impaired gas exchange related to intrauterine hypoxia
- Risk for infection related to intrauterine infection

▼ Planning

The plan of care that is identified for the SGA infant might include the following goals:

- The infant will have a blood glucose level of greater than 40 mg/dL.
- The infant will not lose more than 8 percent of birth weight.
- The infant will take breast milk or formula without fatigue and will gain weight.
- The infant will maintain an axillary temperature between 36.4 and 36.9°C.
- The infant will show no signs of respiratory distress or tachycardia.
- The infant will show no signs or symptoms of infection as evidenced by normal vital signs and laboratory values.

▼ Intervention

The SGA infant is at risk for meconium aspiration if there is meconium in the amniotic fluid before birth. During birth, the infant's nose, mouth, and pharynx are suctioned while the head is on the perineum before the delivery of the shoulders. Then immediately after birth, before the infant is stimulated to inhale, if meconium is present, intubation is initiated for suctioning of the airway. It is mandatory that stimulation be kept to a minimum so that breathing is not initiated before suctioning is completed; this prevents any meconium from being drawn into the lungs. Although there is debate about whether the infant with light meconium-stained amniotic fluid should be intubated for suctioning, most agree that the stressed infant with thick meconium will benefit from airway suctioning at birth (Bloom and Cropley 1990). As soon as the airway is clear, the infant is dried with warm blankets to prevent hypothermia. After the head is dry, a cap is placed on the head to prevent heat loss. The nurse provides the assessments of the SGA infant as discussed before.

If the infant is stable after birth, the mother should be given the infant to hold and feed. If the mother is breastfeeding, she should be assisted with positioning and latch-on. Early feeding of the newborn is important to prevent hypoglycemia.

To decrease metabolic requirements of the unstable SGA infant, nursing care may include feeding by gavage (see Procedure 36–1), maintaining a neutral thermal environment, ensuring adequate rest, and decreasing stimuli to the infant by offering a pacifier and clustering care. Protect the infant from heat loss by preventing drafts, and avoid the use of cold equipment such as scales. Ongoing education should include informing the parents of the infant's progress. Emotional support to the parents is important.

▼ Evaluation

Evaluation of the plan of care is based on the stated goals. Evaluation is continual, and nursing interventions are adjusted according to the outcomes of the evaluation. For example, if the infant's axillary temperature falls below 36.4°C, the infant may be wrapped in a warm blanket with the head covered or be moved back into the warmer. The temperature is then monitored frequently until it is stable.

PRETERM INFANT

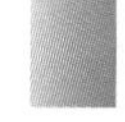

Description

An infant born before the end of 37 weeks' gestation is considered preterm. Infants born before 30 weeks of gestation and with a birth weight below 1500 g have the highest morbidity and mortality rate. Infants born after week 37 and with a birth weight above 2500 g are the most likely to survive.

Most preterm infants are born with a birth weight that is appropriate for gestational age. However, some experience intrauterine growth restriction and are born SGA. Many preterm infants of diabetic mothers are born LGA.

Although it is usually difficult to determine the cause of prematurity, there are a number of associated factors: maternal chronic hypertension, preeclampsia, maternal infections, premature rupture of membranes, placenta previa, abruptio placentae, multiple gestation, and cervical incompetence.

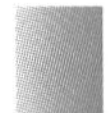

Management

Ideally, the focus of management of the preterm infant is prevention. All pregnant women should have early prenatal care that includes risk screen-

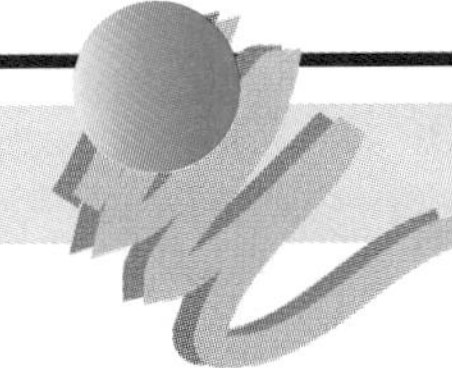

HISTORICAL PERSPECTIVES

REGIONALIZATION OF PERINATAL CARE

The need for specialized care and equipment for the preterm infant was recognized around the turn of the century. By the 1920s and 1930s, centers for the care of preterm infants were developed. Neonatal care based on isolation, thermal stability, proper nutrition, and specialized nursing care was the standard of care by the 1940s and 1950s. The first newborn intensive care units followed in the 1950s and 1960s.

In 1971, the American Medical Association issued a policy statement, Centralized Community or Regionalized Perinatal Intensive Care 1, favoring the development of regionalized perinatal health care. The statement called for the development of centrally operated special care facilities, the training of personnel, and the formation of guidelines. The March of Dimes provided financial and administrative support for the formulation of guidelines in 1973. The goal of regionalized perinatal care is to provide quality care for all pregnant women and newborns with the assurance of reasonable cost-effectiveness.

A comprehensive regional perinatal care system provides patient care, education, evaluation and research, and administration. Patient care includes outpatient and inpatient services, consultation and referral, and transportation. Education includes education of the patient, education to professionals and institutions, and public health information for the prevention of disease. Evaluation and research of maternal and neonatal outcomes, of current therapy and techniques, and of the system itself is an important component of the program. Administration includes analysis of the cost-effectiveness of the program and resource allocation, consultation services, and program development and management.

The majority of regionalized perinatal care programs use a three-level system. A level I program is generally a community hospital and the usual focus of the patient's entry into the system. The common physician leadership at a level I hospital is the primary care physician or a specialist. A level II unit is generally in a large community hospital with at least 2000 deliveries per year. They provide diagnosis and treatment of selected high-risk pregnancies and neonatal problems. The physician leadership is generally a specialist or subspecialist. A level III center is usually located at a large medical center or university. They not only provide diagnosis and treatment of most perinatal problems but are involved in conducting research. They provide outreach education and administration to the community. The physician leadership is a subspecialist.

The past decade has brought new challenges to the regional care system. A competitive atmosphere has developed in the health care system. With the growth of knowledge and technology, there has been a proliferation of services. To remain competitive, hospitals are expanding the services they offer. As the health care system continues to change, the challenge is to continue to offer quality perinatal health care. The future emphasis of perinatal care is on preventive health care with a focus on education. There is a need to ensure that health care is accessible to all while being economically efficient for the provider.

ing for preterm labor. All women should be taught the signs of preterm labor for early recognition if it should occur. Early interventions for preterm labor are more successful in postponing delivery of a preterm infant.

After delivery, early assessment and vigilant monitoring for complications of prematurity are of the utmost importance. Because of the lack of organ development in preterm infants, they have difficulty maintaining extrauterine homeostasis. Some infants with prematurity require more intense nursing care or access to technologies not available at the hospital in which care is being provided. In these instances, trans fer to an institution that provides these services offers the infant the best chance for survival (Procedure 36–2). This method of providing regionalized care for sick infants has been practiced for the past 25 years (see Historical Perspectives).

The most common problems encountered with preterm infants include

- Respiratory distress
- Hyperbilirubinemia
- Metabolic disturbances
- Fluid and electrolyte imbalance
- Infection
- Nutritional deficits and feeding problems
- Ineffective thermoregulation
- Cardiovascular disturbances
- Hematologic disturbances

Respiratory distress in the preterm infant is common because of the immature lungs. In addition, the preterm infant is frequently exposed to other maternal factors during the pregnancy that put the infant at risk for asphyxia at birth.

Respiratory distress may be present at birth or soon thereafter (Fig. 36–3). In the first 3 to

PROCEDURE 36–2

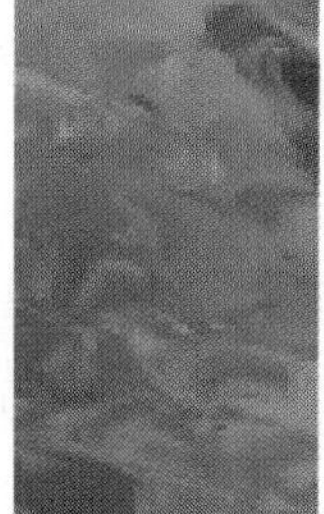

Neonatal Transport

▼ PURPOSE

Neonatal transport to a tertiary care center is indicated when the condition of a neonate warrants more intensive evaluation or intervention than can be provided where the infant is currently hospitalized. Adequate communication and information are imperative for effective neonatal transport.

▼ EQUIPMENT

- Consent form
- Copy of maternal chart
- Copy of baby's chart including x-ray films
- Transfer form
- Tube of mother's blood
- Information about the receiving hospital for parents

1 Assess the neonate to ensure that he or she is stable for transport. A thorough risk assessment includes review of maternal history and delivery; the neonate's vital signs, neurologic status, color, and muscle tone; blood glucose evaluation; weight and measurement; anomalies; and gestational age assessment. **A neonate in stable condition will handle the stress of a transport better and be less likely to require emergency intervention en route.**

2 Communicate with family and physicians. It is the responsibility of the referring physician to ascertain that room is available at the receiving hospital, to communicate with the receiving physician regarding the baby's history and status, and to discuss transport with the parents. The nurse may witness informed consent for transfer and give parents

Continued on following page

PROCEDURE 36–2 Continued

information on the receiving hospital including unit phone numbers and local motels. **Open, frequent communication between nurse, physician, and parents helps to decrease uncertainty and confusion, thereby improving the efficiency of the transport. Witnessing informed consent is necessary because the form is a legal document.**

3 Plan for the transport. Estimate times of transport arrival at referring hospital, departure, and arrival at receiving hospital. Discuss equipment and personnel needed. **Planning needs ahead of time prevents delays during which the condition of the baby could change.**

4 Provide the receiving hospital with a photocopy of the maternal record and of the neonate's complete chart, x-ray films, and a tube of the mother's blood. **The receiving hospital needs all information regarding the neonate's stay to develop an appropriate plan of care and provide continuity of care.**

5 When the transport team arrives, give an up-to-date report on the baby's status. Document in the chart that a verbal report was given and the time of arrival and departure of the team. **Up-to-date information on the status of the newborn helps the transport team anticipate problems that might occur en route. The transport records become part of the baby's permanent record, so accurate documentation regarding all aspects of the transport is important.**

6 Allow parents contact with their baby and provide parental support. **Parents will be grieving the loss of an ideal birth outcome and be fearful about their baby's condition. For some parents, it may be their last opportunity to see their baby alive.**

7 Call the receiving hospital when the transport team leaves. **This provides the receiving hospital with an estimated time of arrival.**

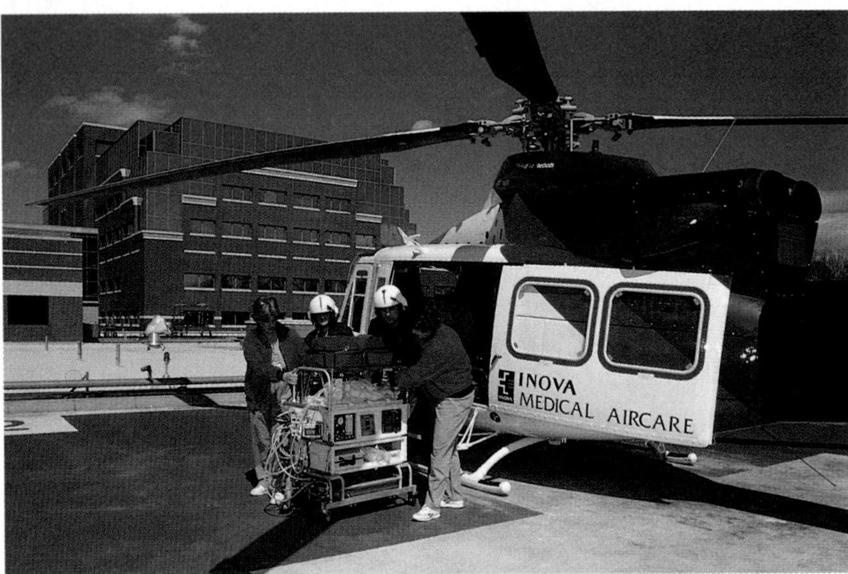

6 hours after birth, respiratory distress may become progressively worse. Symptoms include tachypnea, audible expiratory grunt, intercostal and sternal retractions, nasal flaring, and cyanosis. One of the goals of management of respiratory distress syndrome (RDS) is to prevent the complications that can accompany it.

Respiratory Distress Syndrome

▼ **Description.** Despite the growth of knowledge and technology, respiratory failure remains the leading cause of infant morbidity and mortal-

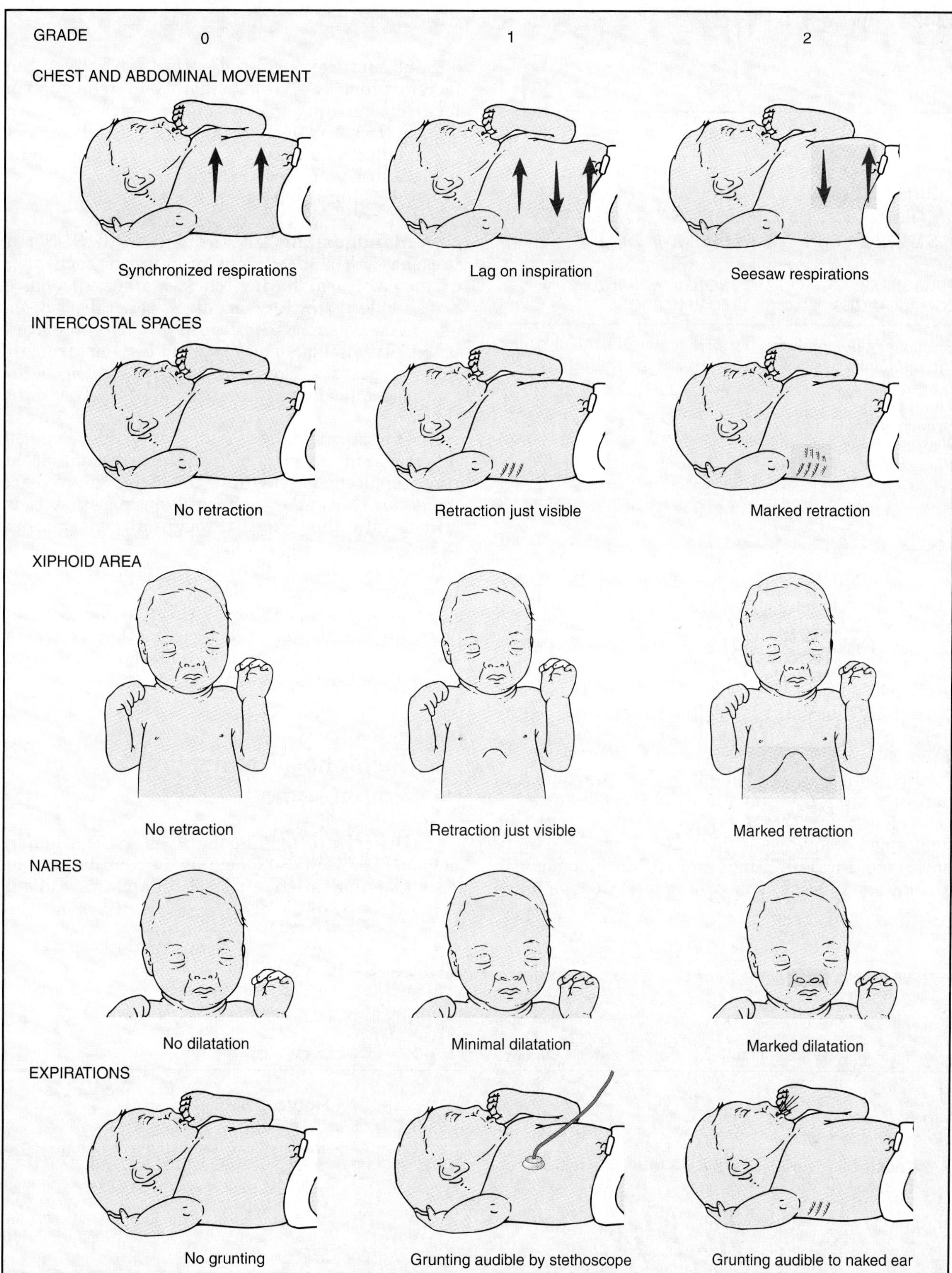

Figure 36–3

The Silverman-Anderson Index is used to assess respiratory distress in the neonate. (Adapted from Silverman. W., and Anderson, D. (1956). A controlled clinical trial of effects of water mist on obstructive respiratory signs, death rate and necropsy findings among premature infants. *Pediatrics,* 17(1), 1–10. Adapted by permission of PEDIATRICS.)

Table 36–1

PULMONARY AND NONPULMONARY COMPLICATIONS OF RESPIRATORY DISTRESS SYNDROME IN THE PRETERM INFANT

PULMONARY COMPLICATIONS	NONPULMONARY COMPLICATIONS
Pulmonary hemorrhage	Intraventricular hemorrhage
Intrapulmonary interstitial emphysema	Necrotizing enterocolitis
Bronchopulmonary dysplasia	Patent ductus
Pneumothorax	Sepsis

ity in the NICU (Krause and Youngner 1992). Approximately 10 percent of preterm infants will experience RDS, also known as hyaline membrane disease (Urrutia 1991). Use of mechanical ventilation has increased the survival rate of affected neonates, but pulmonary and nonpulmonary complications have increased the morbidity of the preterm infant. Complications of RDS are listed in Table 36–1.

RDS in the preterm infant is due to a combination of factors. Anatomic and functional lung development in the fetus occurs in stages, with the final stage occurring in the third trimester. The final stage includes lung growth, development of ventilatory muscle strength, development of alveoli, and maturation of the surfactant system. Surfactant provides alveolar stability by reducing surface tension during exhalation, which keeps the alveoli from collapsing. The remaining volume of gas results in a residual lung volume that minimizes subsequent respiratory work during inspiration (Boeckling 1992).

▼ **Management.** The neonate with RDS may present with clinical signs of cyanosis, tachypnea, or apnea. Nasal flaring, chest wall retraction, or an audible expiratory grunt is generally present as an early sign (see Resuscitation of the Newborn). Treatment usually includes supplemental oxygen, positive pressure support, or intubation and mechanical ventilation (Fig. 36–4). The aim of therapy is to support the neonate until the disease runs its course with the subsequent development of surfactant. The infant may benefit from surfactant replacement therapy. In surfactant replacement, an exogenous surfactant preparation is instilled into the lungs through an endotracheal tube.

There is evidence that the use of maternally administered corticosteroids may enhance fetal lung development (Jobe 1986). With pregnancies of less than 34 weeks' gestation, the mother is treated with an intramuscular injection of corticosteroids 24 to 48 hours before delivery.

Pulmonary Interstitial Emphysema

▼ **Description.** Pulmonary interstitial emphysema (PIE) is a complication of ventilation support. Overdistention of the distal airways and sub-

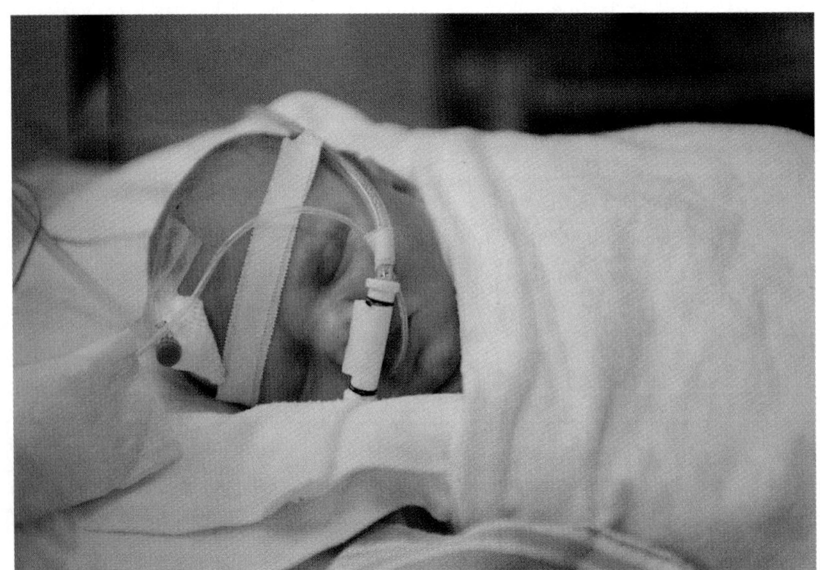

Figure 36–4

Infants with respiratory distress syndrome are often managed with nasal continuous-positive airway pressure (NCPAP). This infant also has an orogastric tube in place to maintain gastric decompression. Intravenous fluids are administered through a scalp IV line. (Courtesy of Wesley Medical Center, Wichita, KS.)

Resuscitation of the Newborn

The decision to initiate a resuscitation is not determined by the Apgar score (American Heart Association and American Academy of Pediatrics 1990). The infant is assessed immediately after birth, and interventions should be started immediately. The evaluation is based on respirations, heart rate, and color. Neonatal resuscitation requires all involved health care providers to work together as a team. The American Heart Association and American Academy of Pediatrics have detailed a systematic approach to neonatal resuscitation (Bloom and Cropley 1990). The guidelines are described here briefly; see *Textbook of Neonatal Resuscitation* for more detail (Bloom and Cropley 1990).

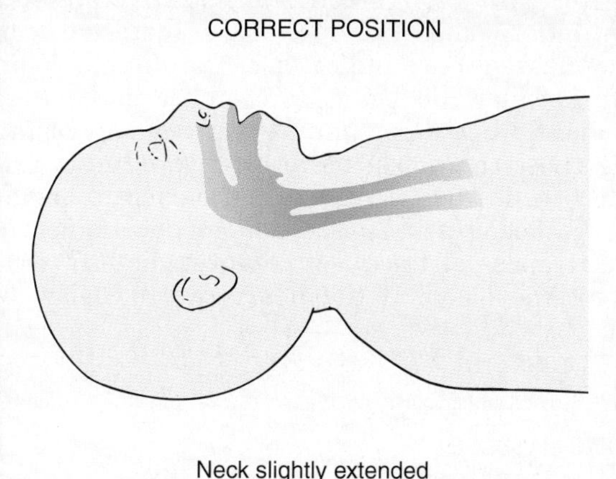

INITIAL STEPS

1. Prevent heat loss
   Place the infant under a radiant heat source and quickly dry the body and head to remove amniotic fluid. The act of drying provides gentle stimulation, which may help initiate or stimulate breathing.
2. Open the airway
   Position the infant on his or her back or side with the neck slightly extended in a "sniffing position." Suction the infant's mouth and then nose to clear the airway.
3. Initiate breathing
   Provide tactile stimulation to initiate breathing by slapping or flicking the soles of the feet or rubbing the infant's back.
4. Evaluate the infant
   Monitor and evaluate respiratory effort, heart rate, and color.

INCORRECT POSITION

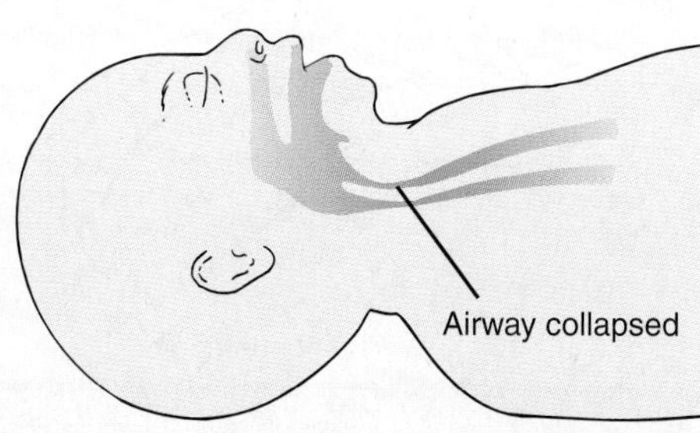

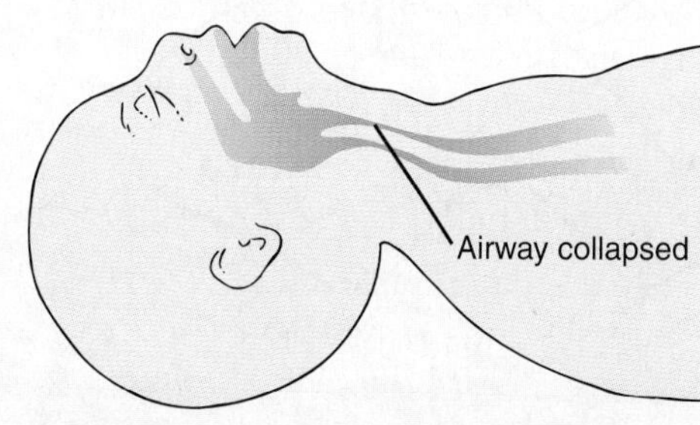

Continued on following page

Resuscitation of the Newborn Continued

If the infant has spontaneous respirations after gentle suctioning of the airway and the heart rate is above 100 beats per minute, the infant is receiving adequate oxygenation. When respirations are adequate and the heart rate is above 100 beats per minute, the infant should be pink in color. If central cyanosis is present in the infant, free-flow oxygen should be given. If the infant has a heart rate above 100 beats per minute but the respirations are shallow and irregular, position the infant properly and increase stimulation.

If the infant is apneic or has gasping respirations after stimulation or the heart rate is below 100 beats per minute, positive-pressure ventilation by bag and mask can be given. The anesthesia bag used for neonatal resuscitation should have a pressure gauge. Ventilation should be given at a rate of 40 to 60 breaths per minute at pressures of 15 to 20 cm H_2O (normal lungs). An initial pressure of 30 to 40 cm H_2O may be necessary to inflate collapsed alveoli.

After 15 to 30 seconds of positive-pressure ventilation, chest compressions (external cardiac massage) are indicated if the infant's heart rate is below 60 beats per minute or between 60 and 80 beats per minute and not increasing. The chest compressions are delivered at a rate of 120 times per minute. The heart rate should be checked every 30 seconds to determine the effectiveness of the chest compressions in circulating the blood. If the heart rate is below 80 beats per minute, ventilation and chest compressions continue. When the heart rate is above 80 beats per minute, chest compressions are no longer needed. Ventilation continues, and the heart rate is checked periodically.

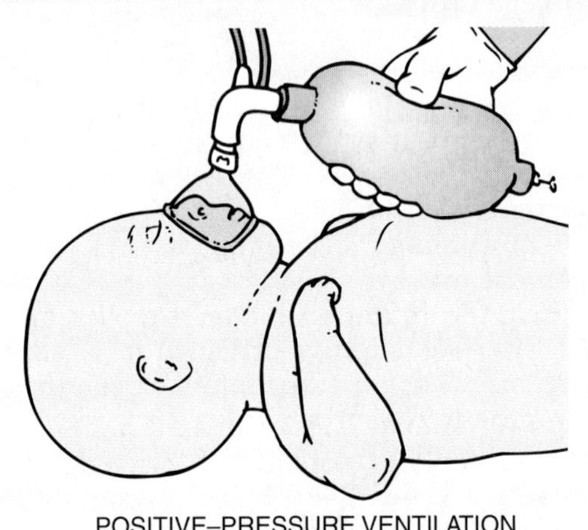
POSITIVE–PRESSURE VENTILATION

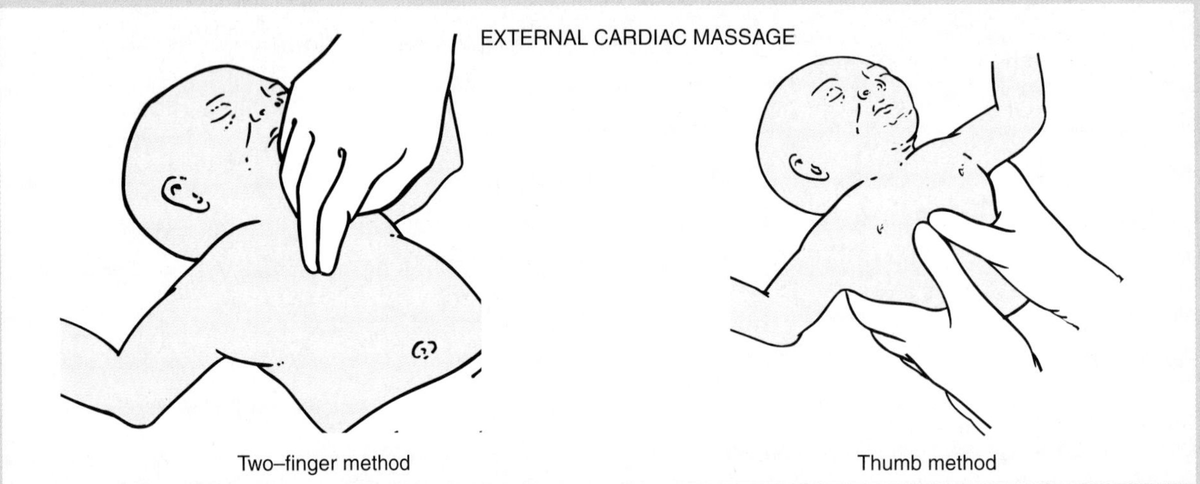

EXTERNAL CARDIAC MASSAGE

sequent rupture of the ductus allow air to leak into the connective tissue that surrounds the airways. PIE may involve one lobe, one lung, or both lungs. Diagnosis can be made only by x-ray examination. Clinical signs may include increased oxygen requirements and carbon dioxide retention. Predisposing factors (Thibeault 1986) include RDS, lung immaturity, pulmonary anomalies, overzealous resuscitation at birth, intubation of a bronchus followed by positive-pressure ventilation, iatrogenic needle puncture of a lung, transient tachypnea of the newborn, inhomogeneity of alveolar ventilation, and assisted ventilation.

The mortality rate for these infants is greater than 50 percent. For those infants who survive, the development of bronchopulmonary dysplasia is frequent (Whitsett et al. 1994).

▼ **Management.** Ideally, management of PIE begins with prevention. Peak and mean inspiratory pressure should be monitored carefully. Unilateral PIE may be treated by positioning the infant with the affected side down for 24 to 48 hours (Whitsett et al. 1994). With unilateral PIE, selective intubation of the nonaffected lung has been successful. High-frequency ventilation may be used as a form of mechanical ventilation with PIE. High-frequency ventilation reduces pressure fluctuation in the distal airways and causes less stretching of injured tissue (Mammel and Boros 1996).

Pneumothorax

▼ **Description.** Pneumothorax, the result of alveolar rupture from overdistention, is frequent in infants with PIE (Martin et al. 1993). Air is forced from the alveolus into the interstitial space. It may be related to mechanical ventilation. Signs and symptoms include the chest becoming barrel shaped with overdistention, diminished breath sounds on the affected side, grunting, cyanosis, tachypnea, retractions, oxygen desaturation, hypotension, and bradycardia.

▼ **Management.** Pneumothorax is a medical emergency. A serious pneumothorax may result in acute respiratory and cardiac decompensation. Cardiopulmonary resuscitation may be necessary as well as evacuation of the air by needle aspiration. Chest tubes are inserted to remove fluid and air from the pleural space and to allow the collapsed lung to reexpand. The chest tubes are then attached to a closed drainage system connected to suction.

Pulmonary Hemorrhage

▼ **Description.** Pulmonary hemorrhage may occur in ill infants with RDS, intrapartum asphyxia, infection, hypothermia, and surfactant therapy (Martin et al. 1993). The infant may present with symptoms that include bradycardia, apnea, slow gasping respirations, and blood-tinged secretions from the trachea.

▼ **Management.** Management of pulmonary hemorrhage begins with immediate attention to maintaining a patent airway. Suctioning must be done carefully to avoid further bleeding. Treatment includes the use of mechanical ventilation employing extra positive end-expiratory pressure. Blood transfusion may be indicated.

Bronchopulmonary Dysplasia

▼ **Description.** Bronchopulmonary dysplasia (BPD), or chronic lung disease, is a complication of RDS. The tiny preterm infant exposed to intubation, mechanical ventilation, and supplemental oxygen is more at risk for developing BPD than is the more mature neonate. Chronic lung disease is characterized by pulmonary fibrosis, bronchiolar metaplasia, emphysema, and interstitial edema (Haywood et al. 1993).

▼ **Management.** The ideal treatment of BPD is prevention. The prevention of prematurity and, secondly, the prevention of RDS would decrease the number of infants at the highest risk for developing BPD. Exogenous surfactants given as prophylaxis or treatment for RDS may decrease BPD in the preterm infant. If the preterm infant develops RDS, the goal is to limit the amount of iatrogenic tissue injury. The dilemma is to provide adequate oxygenation to prevent hypoxic damage while limiting complications related to hyperoxia. Intubation and mechanical ventilation are used cautiously to prevent trauma and injury.

Once BPD is present, management includes enhancing the healing process to restore normal function as much as possible and controlling complications from damaged lung tissue. Treatments include oxygen therapy and the use of diuretics, bronchodilators, and steroids.

Patent Ductus Arteriosus

▼ **Description.** At birth, with the initiation of respirations, circulation adapts from fetal to neonatal in response to an increase in systemic blood pressure, lung expansion, and the shift in pressure gradients from the right side of the heart to the left. With the rise in blood oxygen concentrations, there is closure of the ductus arteriosus.

In the preterm infant, patent ductus arteriosus (PDA) is a common complication. The ductus is not as responsive to the increased oxygenation content and does not close. The increased pulmonary vascular resistance related to hypoxia and immaturity causes blood to shunt from left to right and bypass the pulmonary artery as it passes through the ductus to the aorta. The result is systemic circulation of mixed blood. Increasing carbon dioxide levels lead to an increase in pulmonary vascular resistance.

The infant may present with bounding peripheral pulses, hyperactive precordium, widened pulse pressure, and a continuous murmur. The murmur is best heard at the upper left and middle sternal border.

Management. Management of PDA depends on the severity of the symptoms. In the preterm infant with respiratory distress, untreated PDA may prolong the use of the ventilator. Early intervention to close the shunt may shorten the duration of respiratory support (Heymann et al. 1993). Medical treatment may include fluid restriction. Calorie intake should be watched closely. The hemoglobin level and hematocrit should be monitored. A drop in hemoglobin level may impair cardiac function by the increase in cardiac output to maintain peripheral oxygenation. Digitalis is not used in the very small preterm infant because it has little benefit and the risk for toxic effects is high (Heymann 1989). Indomethacin, a prostaglandin inhibitor, can close the ductus in some preterm infants. Indomethacin is highly nephrotoxic, so blood urea nitrogen and creatinine levels should be monitored closely. If medical management is not successful, surgical closure is performed.

Intraventricular Hemorrhage

Description. Intraventricular hemorrhage is associated with increasing arterial blood pressure and birth asphyxia. The intraventricular hemorrhage occurs when the fragile blood vessels in the brain rupture. It occurs in 30 to 50 percent of infants with a birth weight less than 1500 g. With the use of real-time ultrasonography, intraventricular hemorrhage can be visualized. Intraventricular hemorrhage is categorized from grade I through grade IV, depending on the size of the bleed. In grade I, bleeding is confined to the germinal matrix–subependymal region (less than 10 percent of the ventricle); intraventricular bleeding (10 to 50 percent filling of the ventricle) is seen in grade II; grade III is more than 50 percent involvement with dilated ventricles; and in addition to 50 percent involvement, grade IV includes intraparenchymal extension (Behrman et al. 1996).

The majority of infants with intraventricular hemorrhage will bleed within the first 72 hours after birth; 50 percent occur within the first 24 hours (Volpe 1994). The clinical signs vary. Some infants are asymptomatic; others exhibit catastrophic deterioration with stupor progressing to coma, respiratory distress progressing to apnea, generalized tonic seizures, decerebrate posturing, fixation of pupils to light, and flaccid quadriparesis (Blackburn 1993). Clinical signs of the infants with the catastrophic course include a falling hematocrit, a tight and bulging anterior fontanelle within hours, seizures, and difficulty maintaining a normal body temperature. Prognosis varies with the extent of the bleed. Infants with mild bleeds generally survive and have a low rate of major neurologic sequelae. Infants who experience a severe bleed have a higher mortality rate and tend to have significant motor and cognitive deficits.

Management. Nursing care starts with an awareness of factors that may increase the infant's chance for intraventricular hemorrhage. Monitor vital signs closely, watching for fluctuations in arterial blood pressure. Body tone, activity, and level of consciousness are also monitored frequently. Provide physiologic support to maintain oxygenation, perfusion, normothermia, and normoglycemia. The infant should be handled as little as possible to reduce the risk for hypoxia and fluctuations in arterial blood pressure. The infant should be placed in the prone or side-lying position with the head in midline or to the side without flexing the neck. The head of the bed should be slightly elevated.

Necrotizing Enterocolitis

Description. Necrotizing enterocolitis (NEC) is an acquired disease mainly of preterm infants, although term infants have been affected. The cause of NEC remains unclear, but it is accepted that there are three major mechanisms—the selective ischemia of the bowel, the establishment of bacterial flora, and the effect of feeding.

Ischemia of the bowel occurs during episodes of hypoxia. In the asphyxiated infant or the infant experiencing RDS or apneic episodes, blood is shunted away from the intestines, kidney, and muscles to protect the brain and cardiac system.

The gastrointestinal tract of the preterm infant is immunologically immature and unable to resist bacteria. Although the majority of infants developing NEC have been fed artificial milk, it is unclear whether it is the artificial milk itself, the volume of the feeding, or the effect of bacteria on the artificial milk (Fanaroff and Kliegman 1993). In a multicenter feeding trial, it was found that the occurrence of NEC in human milk–fed infants was significantly less than in infants fed artificial milk (Lucas and Cole 1990).

Human milk provides numerous advantages for the preterm infant. It has been determined that breast milk from mothers who deliver preterm infants differs in composition from breast milk of mothers who deliver at term. Preterm breast milk contains higher concentrations of protein, sodium, calcium, lipids, and selected antiinfective properties (Meier and Mangurten 1993). This provides the preterm infant with milk that has unique nutritional and immunologic properties not available in artificial milk formulas. Additional benefits to the preterm infant who receives mother's milk include prevention of NEC (Lucus and Cole 1990) and higher intelligence scores measured at 18 months and 7½ to 8 years of age (Lucus et al. 1992).

If the infant is unable to feed at breast after birth, the mother should be assisted to pump her breasts on a regular schedule to stimulate her milk production and maintain her supply. An electric pump allows her to pump bilaterally. A lactation consultant should work with the mother (see Chapter 33 for techniques to breastfeed the preterm infant).

Average onset of symptoms of NEC occurs at 3 to 12 days of age. Early signs include decreased bowel sounds, abdominal distention, gastric residuals, vomiting, and bloody stools. Nonspecific signs of infection are lethargy, temperature instability, apnea, and bradycardia.

▼ **Management.** Nursing care involves assessing the infant for any of the signs of NEC. Early signs of NEC may be detected during the physical examination or with routine assessment of vital signs. Feeding intolerance may be exhibited by delayed gastric emptying. Gastric residual can be measured by gently aspirating on a syringe attached to a gastric feeding tube. A pattern of increasing intolerance to the volume of liquid given to the infant often precedes other signs of NEC (Kanto et al. 1994). If there are no findings to suggest NEC, aspirated residual should be placed back into the stomach (Hodges and Vincent 1993). If NEC is suspected, feedings should be discontinued immediately.

Treatment may be medical management or surgical intervention. Aggressive medical management includes bowel rest with parenteral nutrition, decompression of the gastrointestinal tract, and control of sepsis. The gastrointestinal tract is decompressed with a gastric tube placed to intermittent suction. Venous access is obtained for antibiotic therapy and total parenteral nutrition. The infants are monitored closely for signs of perforation of the bowel. Monitoring of urinary output and stools as well as of vital signs including blood pressure is done frequently. The abdomen is carefully examined every 2 hours. Surgical intervention may be necessary to remove necrotic tissue. The bowel ends are brought to the surface to create an ostomy.

Special Considerations of the Preterm Infant

RENAL PROBLEMS

▼ **Description.** In the preterm infant, kidney structure and function are incomplete. The preterm infant has decreased ability to concentrate urine and an increased likelihood of retaining fluids.

▼ **Management.** Fluid management must be monitored carefully to avoid fluid overload or retention. Weight should be obtained and recorded daily or twice a day along with accurate intake and output measurement (Kenner and Brueggemeyer 1993). Imbalance in electrolytes is another problem in the preterm neonate. Electrolytes should be monitored closely, and restrictions may be necessary.

Because of the immature renal system of the preterm infant, there is an alteration in the elimination of drugs through the kidneys. Medication administration should be adjusted according to measurements of drug concentrations in the blood.

RETINOPATHY OF PREMATURITY

▼ **Description.** Retinopathy of prematurity (ROP) is due to the immaturity of the developing retinal blood vessels. It generally occurs in the preterm infant with a very low birth weight. Excessive oxygen appears to disrupt retinal vascular development, especially with prolonged exposure to oxygen. Other factors associated with the development of ROP include the volume of replacement blood transfusions and multiple birth (Martin et al. 1993). Infants with ROP frequently develop myopia. Severe cases of ROP may lead to retinal detachment and blindness.

▼ **Management.** The key to treatment of ROP is prevention and early detection. The arterial Po_2 of all infants receiving supplemental oxygen and those infants at risk for development of ROP should be monitored. Infants at risk for ROP should receive an initial ophthalmologic evaluation at 4 to 6 weeks followed by weekly examinations until vascularization of the retinal tissues is complete (Martin et al. 1993). Abnormal blood vessels can be obliterated by freezing or laser therapy. This decreases the risk for retinal detachment.

SKIN

Description. The skin of a newborn plays a significant role in thermoregulation and as a barrier against infection. The skin of the preterm infant is immature in contrast to the skin of a term infant. The skin of the term infant has a well-developed epidermis. The skin of the preterm infant is thin and gelatinous. There are decreased amounts of subcutaneous fat, brown fat, and glycogen stores. In addition, preterm infants lose heat because of a high body surface area in relation to their body weight and because their posture is more relaxed with less flexion. For these same reasons, preterm infants are less able to generate heat. This places the preterm infant at risk for increased evaporative heat loss, increased fluid requirements, and toxic effects from topically applied substances. The barrier function improves significantly by 10 to 14 days of life (Lefrak-Okikawa and Lund 1993).

In the preterm infant, the epidermis is connected to the dermis with fewer and more widely spaced fibrils than in a term infant. Thus, the preterm infant is vulnerable to blistering and stripping of the epidermis with the removal of adhesives. The adhesives may be more firmly attached to the epidermis than the epidermis is attached to the dermis (Harpin and Rutter 1983). Within 2 or 3 weeks of age, the epidermis resembles that of a term infant (Evans et al. 1986).

Management. The goal of maintaining skin integrity of the preterm infant is to protect and preserve the skin. Skin care practices that may be performed in the NICU include bathing, lubricating with moisturizers, decontaminating the skin before invasive procedures, and affixing adhesives for life support and monitoring devices (Lefrak-Okikawa and Lund 1993). Table 36–2 outlines skin care guidelines for the preterm infant.

In the preterm infant, maintenance of the body temperature within a normal range is necessary to ensure that there is minimal calorie expenditure and oxygen consumption (Fig. 36–5). Care should be taken to maintain skin integrity to prevent evaporative heat loss. Furthermore, maintaining the infant in a neutral thermal environment minimizes heat production, oxygen consumption, and nutritional requirements for growth (Klaus et al. 1993). Equipment used to maintain a neutral thermal environment includes incubators and radiant heaters. A servomotor control may be used to maintain the infant in a thermoneutral zone. In this case, the warming device (incubator or radiant heater) is used to maintain the infant's abdominal skin temperature. If the infant starts to become febrile, the incubator's temperature drops, but there is no change in the infant's temperature. When the nurse evaluates the infant's condition, the temperature of the infant and incubator must be compared to assess the infant's true condition.

Heat loss can be decreased by the use of head coverings. A double-layered hat is recommended for infants requiring a controlled thermal environment (Klaus et al. 1993).

NEUROBEHAVIORAL DEVELOPMENT

Until recently, the focus of the NICU has been on meeting the physiologic needs of the infants (Blackburn and VandenBerg 1993). With the improved outcomes of high-risk infants, there has been increasing concern about the infant's neurobehavioral function. The environment of the NICU may lack sensory input geared to meet the

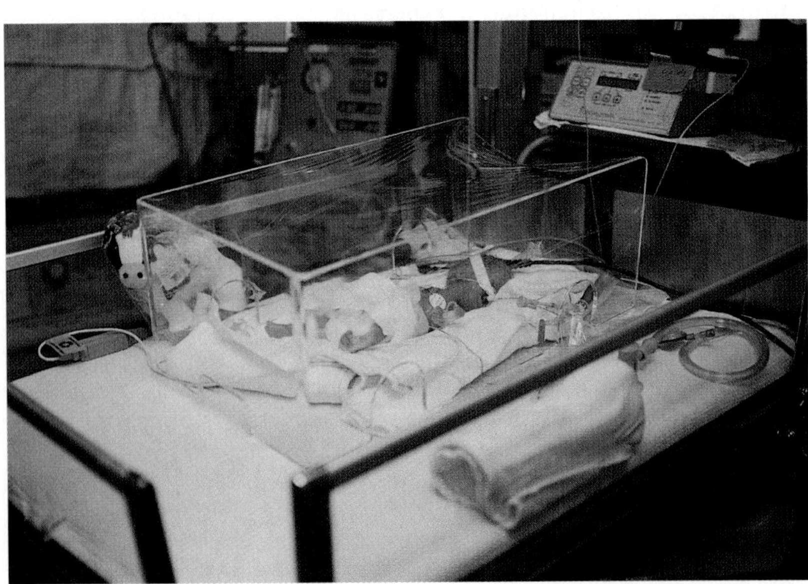

Figure 36–5
A Plexiglas shield for infants in radiant warmers prevents evaporative and convective heat loss. (Courtesy of Wesley Medical Center, Wichita, KS.)

Table 36–2

SKIN CARE GUIDELINES FOR THE PRETERM INFANT

SKIN CARE PRACTICE	TECHNIQUE	FREQUENCY	COMMENTS
Bathing	Use neutral soaps and warm water baths.	2–3 times/wk; if needed between soap baths.	All soaps are irritants; frequent soaping increases the irritant effect. Very-low-birth-weight infants may not be bathed because of the high risk for hypothermia.
Lubrication	Use products free of perfumes and dyes that may be absorbed and may result in sensitization or toxic effects.	Use only when skin is overly dry or looks prone to cracking or fissures.	Lubricants can alter skin pH and allow bacterial and fungal colonization.
Diaper dermatitis	Prevention includes frequent diaper changes to keep the skin dry or the use of a high-absorbent diaper.	Keep skin dry.	If the source of the irritant is fecal, use a thick layer of zinc oxide to provide a protective skin barrier. If *Candida* infection develops, initiate antifungal therapy.
Antimicrobial skin preparation	Use povidone-iodine solution; allow to dry 60 seconds before puncture. After the puncture, remove completely with sterile water.	Use before any invasive procedure that penetrates the skin surface.	Remove povidone-iodine solution with sterile water immediately after the procedure to minimize exposure to povidone-iodine. Avoid use of isopropyl alcohol in very premature infants.
Adhesives: application and removal	Remove tape with water-soaked cotton balls. Consider use of pectin-based barriers between the tape and skin (Hollihesive).	Limit amount of tapes and adhesives used.	Tincture of benzoin should not be used because of its toxicity. Avoid use of solvents to remove tape.
Transparent adhesive dressings	Use as dressing over intravenous catheters.	In very preterm infants, these may be used the first few weeks of life to prevent large evaporative heat and fluid loss by covering large areas of the skin.	With coverage of large areas of skin, there is a potential to increase infection if the skin is colonized before application. It is uncertain whether there is impairment of normal skin maturation that occurs in the first 10–14 days.

Adapted from Lefrak-Okikawa, L., and Lund, C. H. (1993). Nursing practice in the neonatal intensive care unit. In M. H. Klaus and A. A. Fanaroff (Eds.), *Care of the high-risk neonate* (4th ed., pp. 212–227). Philadelphia: W. B. Saunders.

Table 36–3

INTERACTIVE SYSTEMS OF THE NEONATE

STATE	BEHAVIOR
Autonomic system	*Observe:* pattern of respiration, color changes *Visceral signals:* bowel movements, gagging, hiccuping
Motor system	The motor system unfolds from very early embryonic stages with flexor posture and specific limb and trunk movements. With maturity, the movements become differentiated. *Observe:* posture, tone, and movement
State organizational system	As the infant matures, the system develops distinct states of consciousness from a diffuse quasi sleep to increasingly differentiated sleep, wake, and alert states of consciousness. *Observe:* Range, pattern, and clarity of the awake states
Attention and interacting system	As the infant matures, the awake state becomes more differentiated. The infant becomes more selective of social, affective, and cognitive information received. Increasingly, the infant is able to elicit and modify input from the environment.
Self-regulatory system	*Observe:* Strategies the infant uses to maintain an integrated balanced subsystem state; i.e., positioning self when stressed to enhance well-being

individual infant's needs and current level of developmental function. Also, there is concern about the effects of stress and overstimulation on the development of the infant (Blackburn and VandenBerg 1993).

Tools have been developed to assess newborn behavior and adaptation. Brazelton's Neonatal Behavioral Assessment Scale (NBAS) evaluates the neonate's response to environmental events and capacity for self-organization. These reflect the range of behavioral capacities of the normal neonate (Brazelton 1986). See Chapter 31 for more details.

Als and colleagues (1982) developed the Assessment of Preterm Infant Behavior (APIB) tool as a refinement and extension of the NBAS. This tool is most beneficial for the preterm or high-risk infant. The APIB is based on synactive developmental theory. Assessment of the infant's neurologic development is possible by observing the infant's behavior. As infants mature, they are able to organize and regulate their responses, that is, their behavior. Infants can communicate their levels of stress through their behavior. The infant is in continual interaction with the environment through five subsystems (Table 36–3).

By using the APIB, the nurse can identify the infant's current functioning. The tool identifies signs of stress or stability in the infant's autonomic, motor, and state organizational systems. This information is used to adjust the infant's environment to reduce stress behaviors and increase self-regulation by the infant (Fig. 36–6). The infant's care is individualized so that the infant is not continually stressed or underchallenged.

The APIB has been used for research and clinical purposes. It is beneficial to use the tool in the presence of parents. It enables parents to see their infant as a unique and competent individual, thus enhancing their attachment. Before using the APIB to perform assessments, the examiner must complete training in the use of the tool to establish reliability. The training program is available at various locations.

Nursing Process

Using the nursing process helps the nurse devise a plan of care that will enhance the growth and development of the preterm newborn. Beginning on page 1387, Nursing Care Planning Guide: Healthy Preterm Newborn shows how nursing process is applied in creating a plan of care designed to meet an individual's needs.

▼ Assessment

Nursing assessment of the preterm infant includes antepartum or intrapartum identification of a preterm birth. The nurse begins assessment of the preterm infant immediately at birth. The nurse uses tools such as the Newborn Admission Record (p. 1172) and the Newborn Nursery Flow Record (pp. 1173–1174) to record the assessment data collected. As soon as the infant is stabilized, a gestational age assessment is performed. Vital signs, including cardiac status, respiratory status, and temperature, are monitored frequently. Oxygen saturation levels may be monitored by the use of pulse oximetry. The blood glucose level is screened. Intake and output are monitored. Feeding residuals may be measured once the infant is being fed. The infant is weighed routinely, and

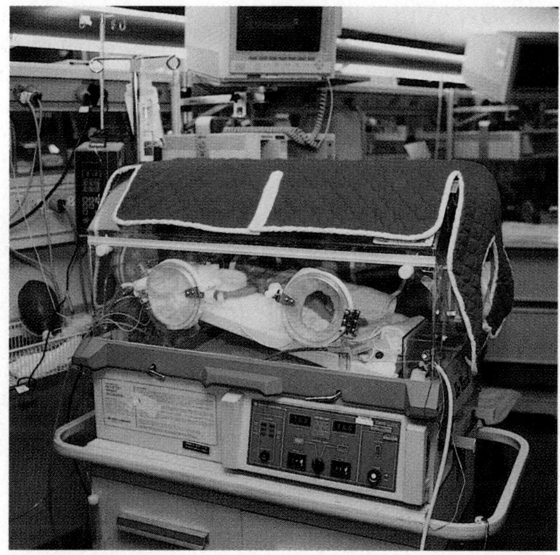

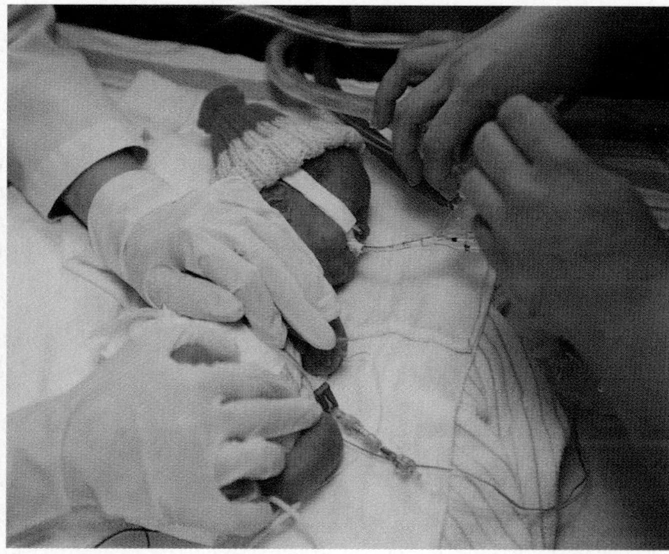

Figure 36–6

Developmental supportive care can be provided in the NICU in a number of ways • *Left,* shielding the isolette provides a barrier to light in the nursery environment • *Right,* containment during procedures such as endotracheal suctioning can support organizational stability. (Courtesy of Wesley Medical Center, Wichita, KS.)

routine measurements include head and abdominal circumferences. It is the nurse's responsibility to monitor laboratory test results as they become available and to notify the physician of any variation from normal.

▼ Diagnosis

Nursing diagnoses for the preterm infant might include

- Ineffective breathing pattern related to respiratory immaturity
- Ineffective thermoregulation related to hypothermia due to large body surface/weight ratio and lack of fat stores
- Impaired skin integrity related to skin immaturity
- Risk for infection related to immature immune system
- Altered nutrition: less than body requirements related to diminished sucking reflex due to gestational immaturity
- Knowledge deficit: parental lack of information related to infant's condition

▼ Planning

The plan of care for the preterm infant might include the following goals:

- The infant will maintain adequate respiratory function as evidenced by normal color, optimal oxygenation, and normal respiratory rate.
- The infant will maintain an axillary temperature between 36.4 and 36.9°C.
- Skin integrity will be maintained as evidenced by intact skin and absence of injury to skin.
- The infant will demonstrate absence of infection as evidenced by normal vital signs and laboratory values and the absence of symptoms of infection.
- The infant will demonstrate adequate nutrition as evidenced by appropriate weight gain (gains 20 to 30 g per day).
- Parents will demonstrate ability to care for their infant.

▼ Intervention

Nursing care of the preterm infant is challenging. The plan of care is continually changing as the nursing assessments provide feedback on the infant's condition. As the nurse provides the highly skilled technical care to the infant, it is imperative to provide the parents with the emotional support they need. The preterm infant's growth and development needs also cannot be neglected.

▼ Evaluation

Evaluation of the effectiveness of the plan of care for the preterm infant is continual. Assessment of the infant's behavior and monitoring of equipment provide the feedback needed to update the plan of care. Thorough documentation of all data provides the basis for ongoing care. Directly observing the parents' behavior, as well as asking them questions, can provide information regarding their knowledge about care of their infant as well as their attachment to their infant.

LARGE-FOR-GESTATIONAL-AGE INFANT

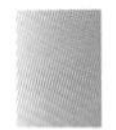

Description

An infant who falls above the 90th percentile on the intrauterine growth curve is LGA. The LGA infant is an infant who grew at an accelerated rate in utero and may be preterm, term, or postterm. The categorization of an infant as LGA may result from a miscalculation of dates. LGA infants often have parents who are large. The mothers of LGA infants tend to be heavier, taller, older, and of greater parity. The LGA infant is heavier and longer with a larger head.

Several specific diseases account for a small proportion of LGA infants:

- Transposition of the great vessels—Among infants with congenital transposition of the great vessels, there is an increased frequency of LGA infants. The reason is unknown.
- Beckwith syndrome—Beckwith syndrome is characterized by infants who are large in body weight and body length. This syndrome is associated with umbilical abnormalities, macroglossia, renal enlargement, and neonatal hypoglycemia.
- Infants of a diabetic mother—Infants of a diabetic mother have increased total body fat resulting in an increased weight/length ratio.

Management

Fetal macrosomia may first be recognized during ultrasonography or from measurements of uterine size larger than normal for gestational date. Prenatal identification of the oversized infant can prevent an abnormal or traumatic labor and birth. The LGA infant has an increased risk for birth trauma from shoulder dystocia, fractured clavicle, depressed skull fracture, brachial plexus palsy, and facial paralysis. Cesarean delivery may be necessary because of cephalopelvic disproportion.

The LGA infant should be assessed for birth injuries. The LGA infant may present with caput succedaneum or cephalhematoma. Asymmetric movement of the mouth or a drooping mouth or eyelid indicates facial nerve damage. A clavicle fracture should be suspected if the infant displays decreased movement of the arm or distress with arm movement. A radiograph will confirm the diagnosis of a fractured clavicle. The LGA infant may have ecchymosis from birth trauma. The LGA infant with cephalhematoma or ecchymosis is at increased risk for hyperbilirubinemia.

Diagnostic testing may include determination of the serum glucose level and radiography, ultrasonography, or CT scan for possible birth injuries.

Nursing Process

▼ Assessment

Nursing care for the LGA infant begins with the nurse's review of the prenatal and intrapartum maternal history. After birth, the infant is identified as LGA during the gestational age assessment. As the nurse performs a physical assessment of the infant, special care is taken to identify any birth injuries. As with all infants, the assessment includes any signs of respiratory distress, such as labored breathing, tachypnea, retractions, nasal flaring, or grunting. The LGA infant should be monitored for hypoglycemia. Symptoms include jitteriness and lethargy with a poor suck reflex. Screening for serum glucose should be performed.

▼ Diagnosis

Nursing diagnoses for the LGA infant might include

- Risk for injury related to birth trauma associated with macrosomatia
- Altered nutrition: less than body requirements related to hypoglycemia
- Impaired gas exchange related to birth asphyxia
- Knowledge deficit: parental lack of information related to infant's condition and care

▼ Planning

The plan of care for the LGA infant might include the following goals:

- Birth injuries will be identified promptly to minimize the effects of the trauma.
- Serum glucose level will be maintained above 40 mg/dL.
- The infant will be without any signs of respiratory distress as noted in the assessment.
- Parents will demonstrate ability to care for their infant.

▼ Intervention

During the initial assessment, the nurse should be aware of any signs of birth trauma. It is the responsibility of the nurse to report any signs of suspected birth injury. If the clavicle is fractured, the affected arm and shoulder will be immobilized. Parents will need help with holding and positioning the infant. Further responsibilities include assessment of vital signs and monitoring for respiratory distress or hypoglycemia.

The parents should be kept aware of the infant's condition. Teaching will include the routine home discharge teaching as well as any special care.

▼ Evaluation

The evaluation of the nursing care plan is based on the stated goals and outcomes. The assessments are continual, and nursing interventions will reflect the findings. For example, if the glucose level on screening is less than 40 mg/dL, a blood sample is drawn for serum glucose determination. The infant will be fed immediately. If the infant is unable to feed, the feeding may be delivered by gavage, or intravenous glucose may be administered.

POSTTERM INFANT

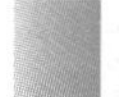

Description

The postterm infant is the infant born at the onset of week 42 of gestation. The postterm infant may be born AGA, SGA, or LGA. Perinatal mortality is higher in postterm infants than in term infants. The mortality rate is two to three times higher for postterm infants than for term infants. This is particularly true of pregnancies that progress into 43 weeks. Placental aging occurs after 38 weeks, resulting in reduced placental functioning that impairs nutrient and oxygen transport. These infants are less able to tolerate the stresses of labor and birth. If the placenta continues to function adequately, then the infant continues to grow and may become LGA.

The postterm infant is at risk for fetal distress during labor because of the reduction in utero of nutrients and oxygen. In response to hypoxia, the fetus may pass meconium and then is at risk for meconium aspiration. Furthermore, amniotic fluid is often decreased in the postterm pregnancy. With decreased amniotic fluid, the meconium is less dilute, which places the infant at an increased risk for meconium aspiration. The decreased amniotic fluid also places the infant at risk during labor for cord compression.

Management

The management of the postterm infant begins during the antepartum and intrapartum period. The infant is monitored carefully during labor for any signs of fetal distress. If meconium is present, precautions are taken to prevent meconium aspiration. These precautions are outlined in the discussion of the SGA infant (p. 1333).

Management of the postterm infant depends on whether the infant is AGA, SGA, or LGA. See the earlier discussions on care of the SGA and LGA infant for management of the postterm infant who is SGA or LGA. The postterm infant is born with decreased protective vernix caseosa. The skin is dry and may be cracked and peeling. Keep the skin dry and clean to maintain skin integrity. Diagnostic procedures for the postterm infant may include determination of serum glucose levels for hypoglycemia and chest radiographs if respiratory distress is present.

Nursing Process

▼ Assessment

Nursing assessment of the postterm infant begins with the maternal antepartum and intrapartum history. Once the infant is born, prompt assessment of the infant guides the nursing care.

The postterm infant may have the physical signs of wasting. There are apparent differences in the appearance of the skin, nails, hair, subcutaneous tissue, and body contour. Characteristically, vernix caseosa is absent in postterm infants except in the deepest skinfolds at the axillae and groin. Shortly after birth, the skin becomes dry and cracked with a parchment-like texture. The nails are often long. The hair is thick. The body appears long and thin. Because the wasting involves depletion of subcutaneous tissue, the skin is loose. The skin, nails, and cord are frequently stained a yellow to green color from meconium passed in utero. The postterm infant may have a wide-eyed, alert appearance. This may indicate chronic intrauterine hypoxia.

▼ Diagnosis

Nursing diagnoses for the postterm infant might include

- Impaired gas exchange related to meconium aspiration
- Altered nutrition: less than body requirements related to hypoglycemia
- Impaired skin integrity related to absence of vernix caseosa
- Knowledge deficit: parental lack of information related to infant's condition

▼ Planning

The planned goals for the postterm infant might include the following:

- The infant will not aspirate meconium.
- Serum glucose levels will remain at or above 40 mg/dL.
- Skin integrity will be maintained.
- Infection will be prevented.
- Parents will demonstrate ability to care for their infant.

▼ Intervention

During birth and immediately after birth, the nurse assists with maintaining a patent airway in the infant. In the presence of meconium in the amniotic fluid, suctioning of the infant begins with the delivery of the head. Detailed care of the infant with meconium in the amniotic fluid is explained in the discussion of the SGA infant (p. 1333).

The nurse is responsible for reporting any suspected birth trauma. The findings are documented in the infant's record. It is the responsibility of the nurse to monitor vital signs and to watch for signs of respiratory distress and hypoglycemia. As soon as the infant is stable, the parents should be given the infant to hold. If the mother is breastfeeding, she should be assisted with the first feeding as soon as possible to prevent hypoglycemia.

As with care of all infants, the nurse should practice good hand washing before handling the infant. Lotions and powders are avoided on the dry, cracked skin to prevent irritation to the skin. The fingernails should be trimmed carefully with blunt-end nail scissors. Parents should be taught how to pull down on the skin behind the nail to prevent cutting the infant's finger. It is easier to trim the fingernails when the infant is sleeping. The nurse should be available to the parents to answer questions and to discuss any concerns they have about their infant's condition. The parents should be kept aware of their infant's progress. Discharge teaching includes the routine newborn care and any special needs of the infant.

▼ Evaluation

The evaluation of the nursing care plan for the postterm infant is directly related to the stated outcomes and goals. Nursing interventions depend on the outcome of assessments.

SPECIAL CLINICAL CONCERNS

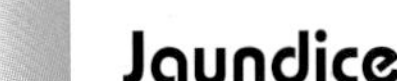

Jaundice

Description. Jaundice is a yellowing of the skin due to the presence of indirect bilirubin in the blood. Bilirubin is produced mainly from the breakdown of hemoglobin. It is processed in the liver and excreted in urine and stools. In the newborn, the body cannot eliminate bilirubin as fast as it is produced. The infant may have decreased bowel motility and delayed meconium passage. In addition, the newborn lacks intestinal flora required for bilirubin reduction. The result is reabsorption of bilirubin from the intestinal tract. The plasma level of bilirubin begins to rise when the production of bilirubin exceeds the newborn liver's capacity to conjugate and eliminate it. Although the conjugating mechanism in the neonatal liver is reduced in the first few days of life, it has the ability to metabolize and excrete two thirds to three quarters of the bilirubin circulating throughout the body (Shaw 1993).

Excessive bilirubin in the system is cause for concern. Free, unbound, unconjugated bilirubin easily crosses the blood-brain barrier and is deposited into the brain cells, causing obvious yellow staining of the brain tissue. The result is kernicterus, necrosis of brain cells. The necrotic brain cells do not regenerate; thus, kernicterus is associated with neurologic damage.

Several factors can increase the risk for kernicterus at lower bilirubin levels. These factors include acidosis, anoxia, asphyxia, hypothermia, hypoglycemia, infection, and prematurity. The most important factor is prematurity because of its effect on both liver and brain metabolism (Lawrence 1994). The severity of jaundice is directly correlated to gestational age (Shaw 1993).

In the full-term infant, serum bilirubin concentration rises within the first 3 days of life to an average of 6.5 to 7.0 mg/dL, which is barely in the visible range, and declines to less than 0.5 mg/dL by the tenth day of life (Poland and Ostrea 1993). This rise and fall in serum bilirubin levels causing the transient hyperbilirubinemia is called physiologic jaundice. Physiologic jaundice never occurs before the second day. Table 36–4 summarizes characteristics of physiologic, breast milk, and pathologic jaundice.

Nonphysiologic jaundice may be suspected if the infant becomes jaundiced before 36 hours of age; if there are maternal-infant ABO or Rh blood group incompatibilities; if the serum bilirubin level rises by greater than 5 mg/dL per day; if the serum bilirubin level is greater than 17 mg/dL in a term breastfeeding infant; or if jaundice persists after 8 days in a term infant or 14 days in a preterm infant.

Infrequently, jaundice develops or progresses after the third day. Bilirubin levels peak from the seventh to the tenth day. This has been called breast milk jaundice or late-onset jaundice. It is thought that the mother's breast milk contains a substance inhibiting the conjugation of bilirubin (Arias et al. 1964). Although the bilirubin may remain elevated for several weeks, breastfeeding may continue uninterrupted (Gutherie and Auerbach 1993). To determine a diagnosis, breastfeeding may be stopped for a period of 12 hours if the bilirubin level rises above 16 mg/dL for more than 24 hours (Lawrence 1994). The infant's mother should be assisted with pumping of her breasts during this period to maintain her supply.

▼ **Management.** The goal of management of jaundice is to prevent kernicterus. Treatment depends on the cause and associated factors. No particular bilirubin concentration has been identified as a threshold for the necessity of treatment. Safe levels of bilirubin depend on the associated factors noted earlier.

Bilirubin levels of 20 mg/dL or more have been associated with kernicterus in the healthy term infant and warrant consideration of treatment. For the preterm infant or the infant with the associated factors, treatment is indicated at much lower levels.

Table 36–4

CHARACTERISTICS OF PHYSIOLOGIC, BREAST MILK, AND PATHOLOGIC JAUNDICE

	PHYSIOLOGIC JAUNDICE	BREAST MILK JAUNDICE	PATHOLOGIC JAUNDICE
Bilirubin concentration	6.5–7.0 mg/dL by third day of life <1.5 mg/dL by tenth day of life	May exceed 20 mg/dL	Visible jaundice within 24 hr >12.5 mg/dL any time
Onset	2–5 days of life	3–4 days of life	Within first 36 hr of life
Etiology	Increased destruction of red blood cells Decreased conjugation Decreased albumin binding Reabsorption of bilirubin from gastrointestinal tract (meconium)	Uncertain Excessive lipase level in breast milk	Excessive production of bilirubin Hemolytic disease Blood incompatibilities Inherited metabolic disorders Birth asphyxia
Treatment	Frequent feeding to promote elimination of direct, water-soluble bilirubin	Discontinue breast feeding for 12 hr Phototherapy	Phototherapy Exchange blood transfusion

Nursing care of the infant with pathologic jaundice includes maintaining a neutral thermal environment to prevent hypothermia and reduce energy expenditures. Encourage frequent feedings to ensure adequate calorie intake, to facilitate excretion of wastes, and to maintain hydration.

Phototherapy may be effective to treat moderate hyperbilirubinemia and to prevent the need for an exchange transfusion after 12 hours of age. Phototherapy may be provided by blue lights overhead or through the use of blue lights in a blanket-like device (Wallaby) that is wrapped around the infant (see Fig. 32–2). The infant undergoing phototherapy requires eye protection to prevent possible retinal damage. Throughout the day, the phototherapy and eye protection should be removed to allow the parents to interact with the infant and to provide visual stimulation. Adequate fluid intake is needed to prevent dehydration in the infant undergoing phototherapy. Insensible water loss is increased in these infants. Serum bilirubin levels must be monitored to evaluate the effectiveness of phototherapy. The phototherapy lights should be turned off during blood sampling for bilirubin levels because the lights can alter the results.

Some healthy infants receive phototherapy in the home setting. The infant must be able to remain normothermic while undressed. The parents must be given home instructions to provide adequate fluid intake and to use the protective eye covering. Blood can be drawn for the serum bilirubin level determinations either in the home by a home health caregiver or in the physician's office.

Exchange transfusion may become necessary to prevent neurologic damage to the infant if the serum bilirubin level is rising rapidly with or without the use of phototherapy or if the infant has significant hemolytic disease, such as hydrops fetalis. Exchange transfusion is indicated if the bilirubin level is 20 to 25 mg/dL in the healthy term infant or as low as 10 mg/dL in the preterm infant or the infant with any of the associated factors. During an exchange transfusion, the newborn's blood is removed and replaced by donor blood, lowering the serum bilirubin level. The umbilical vein is the preferred site for the exchange transfusion (see Nursing Care Guidelines).

Nursing Care Guidelines for the Infant Receiving an Exchange Transfusion

- Parents need to give informed consent.
- Type and crossmatch one unit of whole blood.
- Follow institutional blood transfusion policies for identification and verification of patient and blood before transfusion.
- Obtain a blood warmer to use during the procedure.
- Place the infant in an open warmer.
- Restrain the infant's arms and legs.
- Assess vital signs before the procedure and every 15 minutes throughout the procedure.
- Monitor cardiopulmonary status and blood pressure continuously throughout the procedure.
- Watch the infant carefully for any signs of congestive failure, respiratory or circulatory deterioration, or adverse blood reactions.
- Measure accurately the amount of blood withdrawn and the amount of blood transfused.
- After the procedure, monitor vital signs every 15 minutes for the first 2 to 3 hours or until the infant is stable.
- Monitor blood glucose levels for the first 2 hours after the procedure.
- Resume phototherapy.

Nursing Process

▼ Assessment

Assessment of the infant with jaundice begins with a review of the maternal prenatal and intrapartum history and of the infant's birth record to investigate the presence of any risk factors. The color of the infant's skin and progression of any jaundice should be assessed every shift. If phototherapy is initiated, vital signs including temperature are monitored every 4 hours or more often for temperature instability. Feedings and output are monitored carefully. During an exchange transfusion, vital signs are assessed every 15 minutes; cardiopulmonary status and blood pressure are monitored continuously throughout the exchange transfusion. After completion of an exchange transfusion, vital signs are monitored every 15 minutes for the first 2 to 3 hours or until the infant is stable. Monitor laboratory test results, such as bilirubin level, serum glucose level, and others as ordered.

▼ Diagnosis

Nursing diagnoses for the infant with jaundice may include the following:

- Risk for injury related to toxic bilirubin blood levels and complications associated with phototherapy
- Risk for fluid volume deficit related to insensible water loss and dehydration from phototherapy
- Risk for altered parent-infant attachment related to disruption in parent-infant interaction because of phototherapy

▼ Planning

Goals for positive outcomes for the infant with jaundice may include the following:

- The infant will not develop neurologic sequelae or sustain any complications of phototherapy.
- The infant will maintain adequate hydration.
- Parents will perform infant care activities as they are able.

▼ Intervention

Nursing care of the infant with jaundice requires careful assessment and documentation to track any changes in the infant's condition. In differentiating physiologic jaundice from nonphysiologic jaundice, review of the infant's record to determine onset and severity is of utmost importance. Nursing care of the infant undergoing phototherapy should include the following interventions.

- Monitor temperature every 4 hours; if the infant is in a warmer, shield the probe from the light.
- Increase fluid intake to compensate for increased insensible water loss.
- Shield the eyes from the light source.
- Monitor serum bilirubin levels regularly; turn off lights when drawing blood for serum bilirubin determination because phototherapy lights can alter serum bilirubin results.
- Continue to monitor bilirubin levels for 1 day after phototherapy is discontinued to detect any rebound rise in serum bilirubin levels.
- Remove phototherapy equipment periodically throughout the day to provide visual stimulation to the infant and to facilitate interaction between the infant and parents.

The parents should be informed of all procedures that are being performed on their infant as well as of the infant's condition. Parents may feel intimidated by the equipment; or because of their concern for their infant, they may be reluctant to care for their infant. The nurse should encourage the parents' involvement in the infant's care as much as possible. During feedings, the infant should be held, and the eye shields used during phototherapy should be removed.

▼ Evaluation

The evaluation of the plan of care is based on the stated goals and outcomes. The assessments are made by the nurse before dismissal. Final assessments may be made by the nurse in the clinic or physician's office or by the home health nurse.

Infant of the Diabetic Mother

▼ **Description.** The infant of the diabetic mother (IDM) has higher morbidity and mortality risks (Hollingsworth and Moore 1989). Whatever the severity of the maternal diabetes, all IDMs are at risk for many problems (Table 36–5).

Excess glucose from the maternal circulation during episodes of maternal hyperglycemia crosses the placenta freely and is stored in the placenta. In response to the excessive glucose in the placenta, the fetal pancreas produces increased amounts of insulin. The increased fetal insulin causes a high rate of fetal growth with deposits of increased amounts of adipose tissue. These infants have a smaller head circumference to weight ratio and a larger weight to length ratio.

In the first few hours after birth, the neonate can become hypoglycemic as a result of the hyperinsulinism and loss of maternal glucose. In addition, the IDM is at risk for hypocalcemia and hypomagnesemia. The symptoms are similar to those seen with hypoglycemia.

The IDM is at risk for respiratory distress. Fetal hyperinsulinemia may inhibit surfactant production; as a result, lung maturation may be delayed.

▼ **Management.** Management of the IDM begins in the prenatal period. Careful monitoring and treatment of the diabetic mother are imperative to prevent problems in the infant.

Because the clinical manifestations of hypoglycemia may be subtle and the neurologic sequelae devastating, all IDMs should be monitored closely. The serum glucose level should be screened immediately after birth and frequently thereafter until it has stabilized. Symptoms of hypoglycemia include tremors or jitteriness; abnor-

Table 36–5

NEONATAL EFFECTS FROM DIABETES IN PREGNANCY

NEONATAL EFFECTS	ETIOLOGY
Hypoglycemia	High fetal insulin production and loss of maternal glucose
Hyperbilirubinemia	Impairment of glucuronidation system, or reduction in albumin binding sites
Increased frequency of cesarean birth	Increased fetal insulin acts as a growth promotor, resulting in macrosomatia
Increased frequency of traumatic vaginal birth	Shoulder dystocia secondary to macrosomatia
Neonatal respiratory distress syndrome	High maternal blood glucose level, high placental glucose storage, high placental production of cortisol, low fetal production of cortisol, and low surfactant production lead to decreased lung maturity
Congenital anomalies	Cardiac defects Neural tube defects Gastrointestinal defects

mal cry (high-pitched or weak); apnea, irregular respirations, and cyanosis; lethargy, apathy, and refusal to feed; hypotonia; and eye rolling or seizures. Laboratory tests may include blood glucose, serum calcium, and serum magnesium determinations and venous hematocrit. If the delivery was traumatic, radiographs may be ordered to check for fractures.

Nursing Process

▼ Assessment

The IDM should be assessed for gestational age. Typically, IDMs are LGA. However, diabetes can be associated with intrauterine growth retardation. Early assessment of the IDM by the nurse includes a blood glucose screen. If the glucose level on screening is below 40 mg/dL, a laboratory serum glucose determination is made. The glucose level should be monitored regularly for several hours or until it is stable. The infant should be assessed frequently for any signs of hypoglycemia. If the infant is showing signs of hypoglycemia but the blood glucose level is normal, the calcium level should be evaluated. Feedings are closely monitored by the nurse. Early feedings or intravenous fluids may be necessary to maintain a proper glucose level. It is the responsibility of the nurse to monitor and document vital signs and signs of respiratory distress.

▼ Diagnosis

Nursing diagnoses for the IDM might include

- Risk for injury related to hypoglycemia, hypocalcemia, and hypomagnesemia
- Impaired gas exchange related to delayed lung maturation
- Knowledge deficit: parental lack of information related to care for the IDM

▼ Planning

Goals for positive outcomes for the IDM may include the following:

- The infant will maintain serum glucose, calcium, and magnesium levels at a normal range.
- The infant will be without respiratory distress.
- Parents will be able to verbalize symptoms of hypoglycemia and demonstrate that they are able to care for the special needs of their infant.

▼ Intervention

The mother should be given the infant to feed as soon as the infant is stable. If the mother is breastfeeding, the nurse should assist the mother with positioning and latch-on. Early breastfeeding stabilizes the blood glucose level to prevent hypoglycemia. If the early feeding is dextrose water, a rebound hypoglycemia may occur. A dextrose water feeding should be followed with breast milk or formula within an hour. Many institutions give breast milk or formula feedings immediately when hypoglycemia is present to prevent the rebound hypoglycemia. If the infant does not suck well, gavage feeding may be used. Some infants may require glucose intravenously to prevent hypoglycemia and to maintain a balance to prevent neurologic damage.

The nurse monitors the infant for signs of hypoglycemia and the serum glucose level as described before. The infant should be provided a neutral thermal environment to prevent additional stress on the glycogen stores. The IDM should be monitored for any signs of respiratory distress. It is the responsibility of the nurse to monitor laboratory results and to notify the physician of any abnormal values.

The nurse should apprise the parents of the IDM of the purpose and results of the tests and procedures that are performed on their infant. Their teaching plan should include symptoms of hypoglycemia and the importance of regular feedings in the care of their infant. The nurse should be available to answer questions and to discuss any anxieties of the parents.

▼ Evaluation

The evaluation of the nursing care plan for the IDM is ongoing throughout the infant's hospitalization. The outcome is partially based on the condition of the infant at dismissal time. The final evaluation may occur in the home after dismissal.

Infant Exposed to Human Immunodeficiency Virus

Description. The number of infants exposed to human immunodeficiency virus (HIV) is rapidly increasing. HIV is a retrovirus that leaves the infant vulnerable to bacterial and other types of opportunistic infections. The majority of infants with HIV contracted the infection from their mothers. The most common route of infection is in utero by transplacental passage of the virus. In addition, the infant is at risk during birth from exposure to blood and vaginal secretions and in the postpartum period through breastfeeding.

Management. Care of the HIV-exposed newborn immediately after birth does not differ from care of non–HIV-exposed infants. During invasive procedures, care should be taken to avoid the introduction of any microorganisms. In the early postpartum period, it is impossible to determine whether the infant is HIV-positive. All infants born to HIV-positive mothers will test HIV-positive because of the presence of maternal antibodies. Approximately 33 percent of all infants exposed to HIV will become HIV-positive. The latency period for the infant is much shorter than for the adult. Common clinical manifestations of HIV infection in the infant include failure to thrive, persistent oral candidiasis, generalized lymphadenopathy, hepatosplenomegaly, recurrent diarrhea, recurrent bacterial infections, opportunistic infections, encephalopathy, cardiomyopathy, hepatitis, and nephrotic syndrome. The majority of infants experience opportunistic infections before their first birthday. Prompt intervention is important during any bacterial or opportunistic infections. The infant may be treated with antiretroviral medications. The prognosis for the HIV-positive infant is poor.

Infant Exposed to Substance Abuse

Description. The number of infants with prenatal exposure to cocaine and heroin is increasing. These infants tend to be low birth weight related to prematurity or SGA. Drug-induced vasoconstriction is believed to cause placental blood vessels to constrict, resulting in decreased uteroplacental exchange and low birth weight. Other factors may also have an impact on the decreased intrauterine growth in these infants. These factors include poor maternal nutrition, no or late prenatal care, stresses from a transient lifestyle, and frequent infections. However, a number of women do not fit the picture of the typical drug abuser. Cocaine users come from all socioeconomic classes. Women who use cocaine are often from middle to upper socioeconomic classes.

Infants born to drug-addicted mothers have an increased frequency of aspiration pneumonia. They are more likely to be meconium stained and suffer from meconium aspiration.

Infants born to women abusing drugs are irritable. They are easily overloaded by sensory stimulation. They may cry incessantly and be difficult to console. They hyperextend and posture rather than cuddle when held. Because of this lack of ability to interact with the caretaker, there is decreased caretaker satisfaction.

Moreover, the infant born to a mother addicted to heroin may undergo withdrawal. Withdrawal can occur up to day 6 of life, and the symptoms may last for 8 to 16 weeks. Central nervous system symptoms include hyperactivity, irritability, tremors, high-pitched cry, hypertonicity, and convulsions. Gastrointestinal symptoms may not appear until day 4 to 6 of life and may include regurgitation, vomiting, poor feeding, and diarrhea.

Alcohol Abuse. There is no known safe level of maternal alcohol consumption during pregnancy. However, infants born to women who chronically abuse alcohol are at a higher risk for fetal alcohol syndrome (FAS) than are infants born to women who consume an occasional social drink.

Infants with FAS display characteristic neonatal anomalies, growth patterns, and behavioral manifestations. Neonatal anomalies of the FAS infant include facial anomalies; abnormal palmar creases; and congenital heart disease, primarily septal defects. Facial anomalies include short palpebral fissures, flat midface, thin upper lip, low nasal bridge, short nose, indistinct philtrum, and micrognathia.

Newborns with FAS are smaller at birth and as infants present with failure to thrive. Head circumference and weight are most affected.

Characteristic behaviors of the FAS newborn are not unlike behaviors common to the drug-exposed infant. These behaviors include irritability, tremors, poor feeding, and hypersensitivity to stimuli.

Management. Management of the infant born to a substance-abusing mother is largely supportive care. Because of their intolerance to stimuli, the amount of sensory input should be minimal.

Intake and output should be monitored. If the infant is unable to feed because of an uncoordinated suck and swallow reflex, a nasogastric tube may need to be inserted for gavage feedings. Daily weights and head circumference measurements are necessary to monitor growth. Pharmacologic intervention may be necessary if the infant is experiencing withdrawal from opiates.

In the United States, a positive result of urine toxicologic analysis of an infant is reported to the state's division of children and family services. A social service consultation is initiated. The family may then be observed by a case worker and referred to various community programs.

Nursing Process

Assessment

Assessment of the infant exposed to maternal drugs begins with the prenatal maternal history. However, maternal drug use may not be documented. The infant needs careful ongoing assessment for the behaviors discussed before. Feedings should be monitored closely.

The nurse should assess the maternal-infant attachment and the mother's reaction to the infant's behavior.

Diagnosis

Nursing diagnoses for the infant of a substance-abusing mother might include

- Altered nutrition: less than body requirements related to decreased food intake, hyperirritability, vomiting, diarrhea, or an uncoordinated suck and swallow reflex
- Altered parenting related to hyperirritable behavior of the infant
- Sleep pattern disturbance related to hypersensitivity to stimuli

Planning

The plan of care that is identified for the infant of the substance-abusing mother might include the following goals:

- The infant will receive adequate nutritional intake and gain weight.
- The mother will interact appropriately with the infant by touching and holding and develop confidence in her ability to care for the infant.
- The infant will calm and establish a rest/sleep pattern.

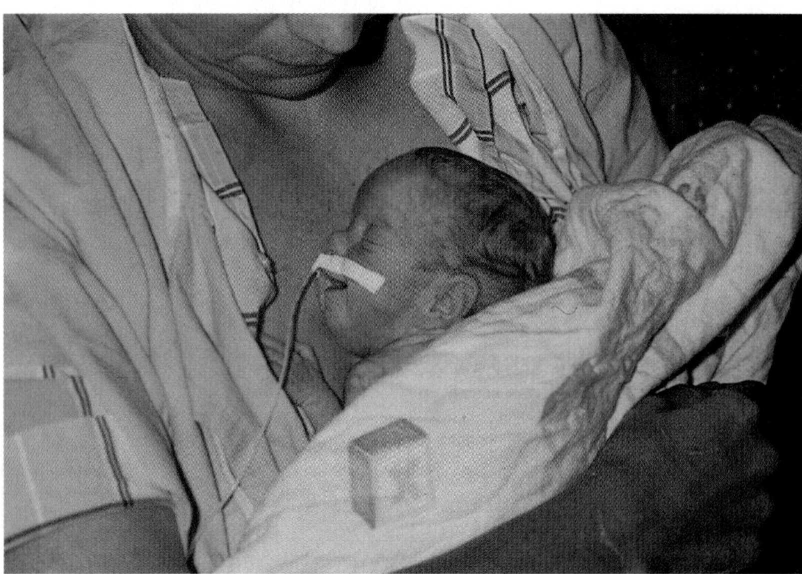

Figure 36–7

This very small preterm infant is obviously enjoying kangaroo care (skin-to-skin contact) with her mother. She was born at 25 weeks of gestation and weighed 1 pound 6 ounces. In this picture, taken by Nedra Smoker, the baby's grandmother, the baby is 2 months old. (Courtesy of Rainbow Babies and Children's Hospital and Dr. Gene C. Anderson, Bolton School of Nursing, Case Western Reserve University, Cleveland, OH.)

Table 36–6

STRATEGIES FOR REDUCING EXCESS NOISE IN THE NICU

Strategies for Reducing Excess Noise

- Gently lower the head on the isolette mattress tray.
- Close portholes and isolette cabinets quietly.
- Set feeding bottles in places other than the top of isolettes.
- Eliminate finger tapping on isolettes.
- Move loud machinery such as computer printers out of the NICU.
- Encourage staff to silence alarms as soon as possible and to silence the ventilator alarm before suctioning.
- Discontinue the audible heart rate beeps.
- Reduce talking over the isolette or across rooms.
- Eliminate radios or reduce their use to designated periods and confine music to calm, soothing music.

Strategies for Reducing Bright Lighting

- Cover isolettes with blankets to reduce the amount of bright light that filters into individual isolettes.
- Dim the lights on a regular schedule, especially in transitional units, to reduce light levels as well as to promote normal day-night cycles.
- Cover infant's eyes with patches during procedures with the heat and bilirubin lamps and shield infants in adjoining isolettes.

Strategies for Reducing Excess Activity

- Move less acute infants to a quieter area.
- Establish quiet times in the nursery when activity as well as light and noise is reduced.

From Katz, K. S., Pokorni, J. L., Long, T. M. (1989). *Chronically ill and at risk infants* (p. 21). Palo Alto, CA: VORT Corporation.

Kangaroo Care

Kangaroo care was originated in Bogotá, Colombia, in 1979 by two pediatricians. They initiated the skin-to-skin approach to reduce the overcrowding in the nursery. Using the kangaroo method, mothers provided care for their premature infants in the home. Only stable premature infants were enrolled in the home care program.

By the mid-1980s, kangaroo care began in Western Europe and now is becoming widespread (Anderson 1991). Kangaroo care began in the United States in 1986. Clinical trials are in progress.

Kangaroo care may begin early with an easily stabilized infant, or it may begin later when the infant is weeks old after the infant has completed the intensive care phase. Infants requiring oxygen or stable infants on a respirator may participate in kangaroo care.

During kangaroo care, the mother holds her stable infant beneath her clothing, skin to skin, between her breasts or on one breast. Fathers can also participate in kangaroo care by holding their infant skin to skin. The infant wears only a diaper. The mother wears a loose blouse, dress, or gown that opens in the front and can be easily wrapped around the infant. The infant is kept warm from heat generated by the mother's body. The infant's temperature should be monitored during kangaroo care to avoid hyperthermia. Benefits to the infant include improved lactation and promotion of parent-infant attachment. Ludington (1990) studied preterm infants during kangaroo care and found that the skin-to-skin contact promotes energy conservation by reducing activity and promoting sleep.

▼ Intervention

The nurse will provide the assessments discussed before. To control sensory stimuli, nursery lights can be dimmed, or a blanket can be placed over the top of the infant's incubator. Reduce noise by not talking loudly at the bedside, turning the radio and intercom volumes low, quickly silencing alarms, and closing incubator doors quietly. These infants benefit from being placed in isolation or a private room or in a quieter area of the nursery (Table 36–6). Minimize the frequency of nursing interventions by grouping nursing care activities. Avoid unnecessary handling. Swaddle the infant to minimize motor activity and soothe the infant. Other soothing techniques include hand holding, vertical rocking, and the use of a pacifier. Kangaroo care (Fig. 36–7) may soothe the infant and promote maternal-infant attachment (see Kangaroo Care, above). To be tolerated, feedings may need to be frequent small amounts. If the mother wishes to breastfeed, a lactation consultant should be called. The mother must be aware of the risks to her infant from the substance abuse while breastfeeding. Breastfeeding is contraindicated with the use of some substances.

Care should be taken to facilitate parent-infant attachment. The nurse should educate the parents about expected infant behavior. Explain matter of factly that the infant experiences drug withdrawal. Help parents learn appropriate times to interact with their infant and how to read the infant's cues.

Finally, health care professionals working with substance-abusing mothers must identify their own feelings about substance-abusing mothers. To work with the mother in a nonjudgmental, empathetic manner, nurses must first acknowledge their feelings and prejudices.

Evaluation

Evaluation of the plan of care for the infant of the substance-abusing mother is based on the stated plan of care. The evaluation is ongoing during hospitalization with necessary adjustments to the plan of care. After dismissal the family should be followed closely. The final assessments may be completed in the home setting.

CONGENITAL ANOMALIES

The birth of an infant with congenital anomalies is an emotional event for both the parents and the care providers. Nurses can become so caught up in providing lifesaving interventions for the infant that they forget about tending to the emotional and spiritual needs of the parents and extended family. As soon as possible, care providers must focus on the family as a unit and pave the way for healing to begin. Responsibilities of the nurse interacting with an infant who has congenital anomalies and the family include (1) recognizing the congenital anomaly, (2) providing nursing interventions that prevent potential complications associated with the anomaly, (3) providing education and emotional support for the family, and (4) facilitating a smooth transition from hospital to home by ensuring appropriate referral to community agencies.

The following section describes some congenital disorders that can be recognized in the newborn period. An attempt is made to identify the cause of the disorder if one is known, to provide a brief description of the disorder and its potential outcome, and to identify nursing implications unique to the disorder.

Congenital anomalies can be classified into three categories: malformations, deformations, and disruptions. Each of these categories can be further defined as a major or minor condition. Major anomalies are potentially life threatening, require complex medical management or detailed cosmetic repair, or carry with them a risk for permanent disability. Conversely, minor anomalies place the infant at relatively small medical risk. These types of anomalies are often viewed as normal variants or as characteristics that "run in the family." The presence of several minor anomalies in one individual may indicate a more serious problem (Jones 1988).

Malformations are caused by the abnormal development of an organ or structure. They can occur in isolation, or there may be multiple conditions present in one individual. Malformations are viewed as intrinsic if the abnormality can be traced to genetic material or extrinsic if the abnormality is associated with environmental or maternal factors.

Deformation is the alteration in the normal shape of the fetus as the result of external pressure. Oligohydramnios, abnormal uterine shape, multiple gestation, and breech presentation may all cause deformation. Once external pressure is removed, the deformation usually begins to resolve.

Disruption is a defect caused by the destruction of a previously normal structure. This results from amniotic bands constricting a body part (Fig. 36–8) or from an abnormality in blood supply that inhibits normal development.

Gastrointestinal Disorders

OMPHALOCELE AND GASTROSCHISIS

Description. An omphalocele results from a defect in the return of the midgut from the yolk sac to the abdomen before 10 weeks' gestation. It occurs in approximately 1 in 5000 to 6000 live births (Robinson and Linden 1993). Boys are more often affected than girls, and 25 to 40 percent of these infants have associated anomalies. The defect is closed by surgical repair, and approximately 70 percent of the infants survive. The major cause of mortality is related to any associated anomalies. If diagnosed prenatally, these infants are usually delivered by cesarean section.

Inspection of the abdomen reveals a midline protruding mass whose size varies from 2 to 12 cm. Small sacs may contain only intestine; larger ones may contain intestines, liver, and spleen. A transparent membrane covers the abdominal contents and is usually intact, but it can rupture in utero or during delivery (Fig. 36–9).

Gastroschisis is a full-thickness, centrally occurring abdominal wall defect. Reported frequency

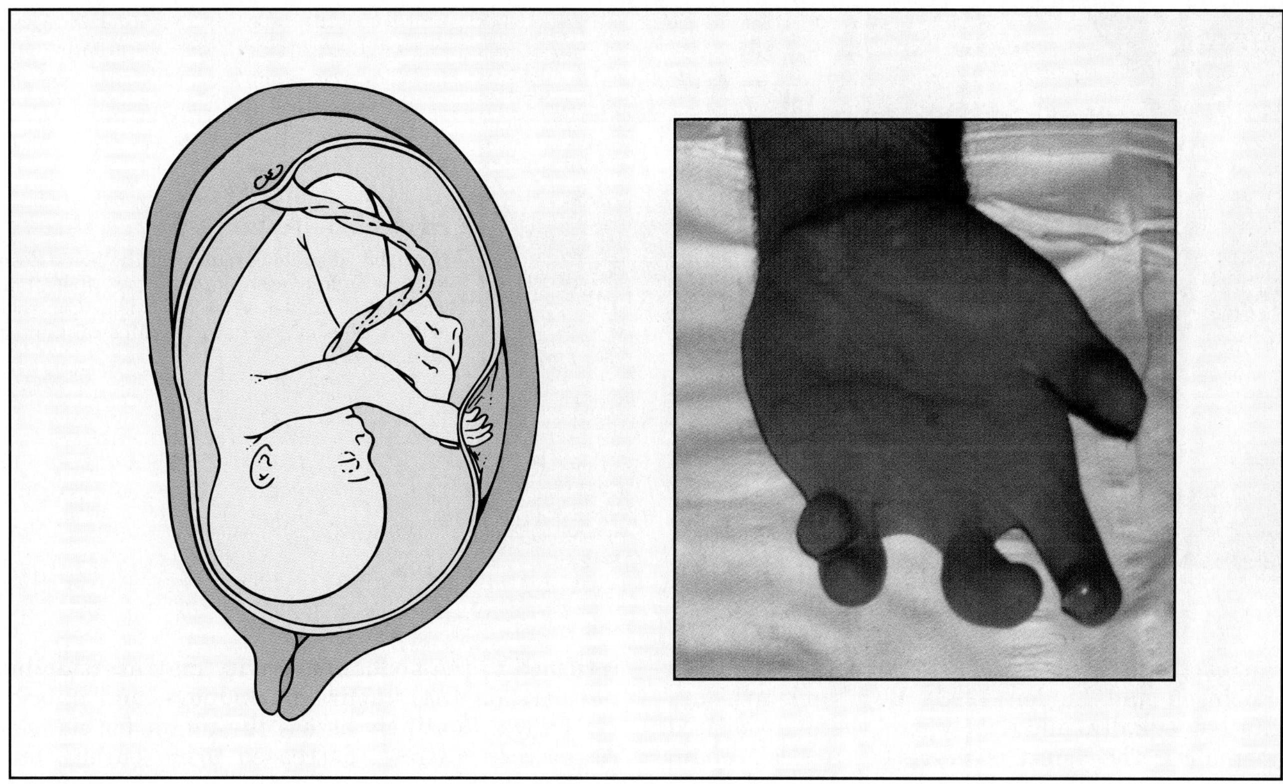

Figure 36–8

Fingers, or other limbs, entrapped in amnion bands produce disruption to the growing limb and result in amniotic band syndrome. (Illustration adapted from Turner, B. S. (1985). Amniotic band syndrome: A nursing perspective. *Journal of Obstetric, Gynecologic, and Neonatal Nursing,* 14 (4), 299; photograph courtesy of R. A. Nelson, M.D., Wesley Medical Center, Wichita, KS.)

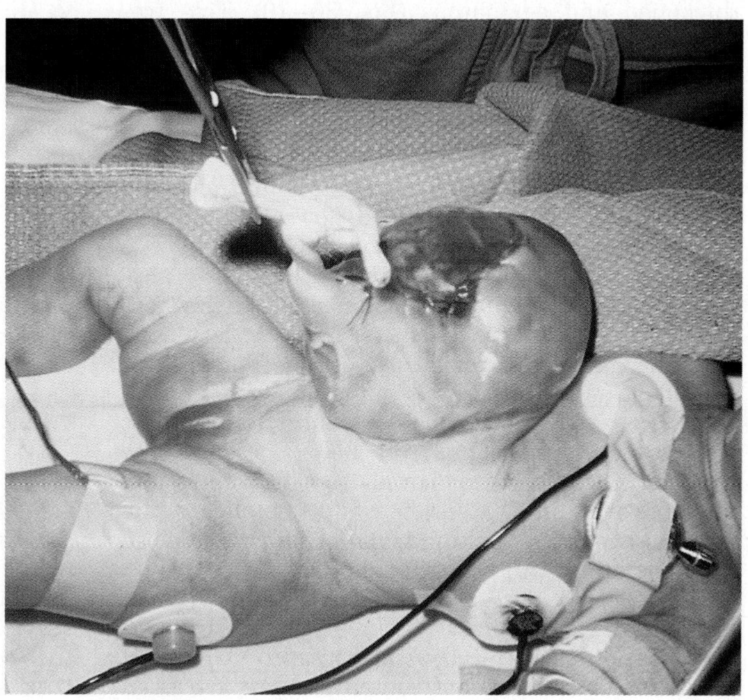

Figure 36–9

A median defect of the abdominal muscles, fascia, and skin at the umbilicus resulted in the large omphalocele seen in this neonate • A membrane of peritoneum and amnion covers the herniation. (Courtesy of Dr. N. E. Wiseman, Pediatric Surgeon, Children's Hospital, Winnipeg, Manitoba, Canada.)

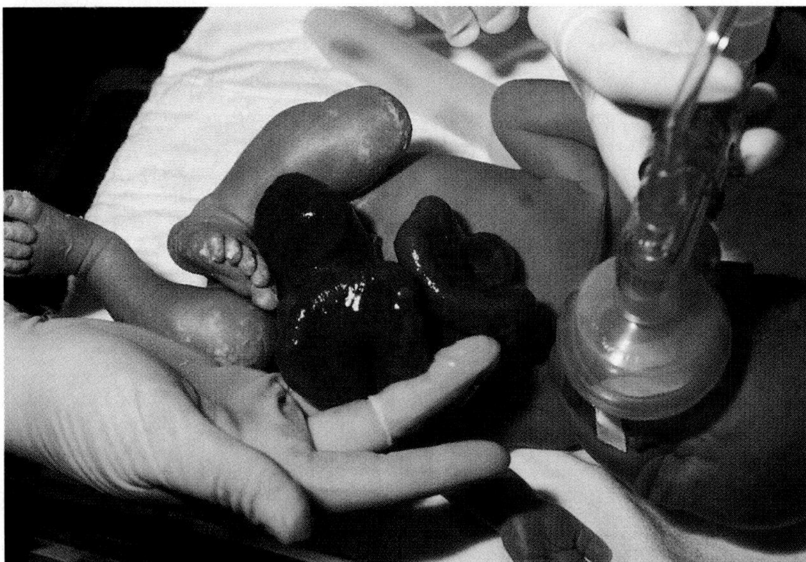

Figure 36–10
Note the edematous nature of the bowel seen in this infant with an anterior abdominal wall defect known as gastroschisis. (Courtesy of R. A. Nelson, M.D., Wesley Medical Center, Wichita, KS.)

ranges from 1 in 20,000 to 30,000 live births (Robinson and Linden 1993). Boys and girls are affected equally, and rarely are there associated anomalies. The defect is closed by surgical repair, and survival is estimated to be above 80 percent. The major causes of mortality are sepsis or complications arising from the inability to establish enteral feedings.

At first inspection, gastroschisis may appear similar to an omphalocele. Gastroschisis is unique in that it never has a membranous covering, and the umbilical cord remains intact and lies just to the left of the defect. In general, no organs other than the bowel are affected. Because of long-term exposure to amniotic fluid, the bowel becomes thickened and edematous (Fig. 36–10). This frequently results in feeding intolerance and a prolonged need for intravenous nutritional support.

▼ **Management.** Immediate preoperative care must include supporting thermoregulation. The exposed abdominal contents place the infant at great risk for hypothermia. As blood flows through the highly vascular bowel, it is rapidly cooled by the air temperature. The defect should be loosely covered with sterile gauze moistened with warmed, sterile, normal saline. A plastic covering is placed over the gauze to provide protection from loss of body heat as well as from trauma and infection.

An orogastric tube should be inserted to allow gastric decompression. This helps prevent the stomach and the distal bowel from becoming distended with air. Distention could complicate the surgical repair by making it more difficult to close the abdominal wall over the defect.

Postoperative care specific to the infant with an abdominal wall defect includes monitoring for complications associated with increased abdominal pressure. The abdominal contents that have been returned to the abdominal cavity may exert undue pressure on the diaphragm, kidneys, and inferior vena cava. Routinely assess the infant for signs of respiratory distress, decreased urine output, and edema of the lower extremities. Also assess the lower extremities for decreased peripheral pulses, decreased perfusion, blanching or cyanosis, and cool skin temperature. Tension on the surgical site can result in wound dehiscence.

Routine assessment should also include observation for behavioral and physiologic responses to pain, including pained crying; grimaced facial expression; excessive gross motor movements; and changes in heart rate, respiratory rate, or blood pressure (Table 36–7). The nurse should attempt to differentiate pain from agitation but not be fooled by infants who do not withdraw from noxious stimuli. The response to pain may be delayed, or infants may be so overstressed that they can no longer respond. Administer pain medications as indicated and observe for the desired effect as well as for any untoward side effects. Provide nonpharmacologic measures to control pain, such as swaddling or containment during painful procedures, decreasing light and environmental noises, and handling the infant as little as possible to promote rest (Broome and Tanzillo 1990; Bell 1994).

ESOPHAGEAL ATRESIA AND TRACHEOESOPHAGEAL FISTULA

▼ **Description.** Esophageal atresia and tracheoesophageal fistula occur in 1 in 3000 live births (Robinson and Linden 1993). Although each malformation may occur in isolation, they are observed together 80 percent of the time. Location of the communication between the esophagus and trachea can vary from proximal to distal (Fig.

Table 36–7

PAIN AND AGITATION BEHAVIORS OF PREMATURE NEONATES

MODE OF EXPRESSION	PAIN BEHAVIORS	IRRITABLE BEHAVIORS
Verbal	Crying, often sudden and loud	Whining cry
Nonverbal	Decreased activity Grimace Flexing extremities Tensing muscles Rigid posture Flushed face Decreased period of alertness	Flailing of extremities Frown Random movements of head and body Rigid posture Altered feeding patterns
Physiologic	Sudden heart rate increase, up to 40% (may follow temporary initial decrease) Blood pressure increase Duskiness Oxygen saturation decrease	Heart rate and blood pressure increase only with activity No diaphoresis No color change unless prolonged No oxygen saturation decrease unless prolonged

From Broome, M. E., and Tanzillo, H. (1990). Differentiating between pain and agitation in premature neonates. *Journal of Perinatal and Neonatal Nursing,* 4 (1), 55. © 1990, Aspen Publishers, Inc.

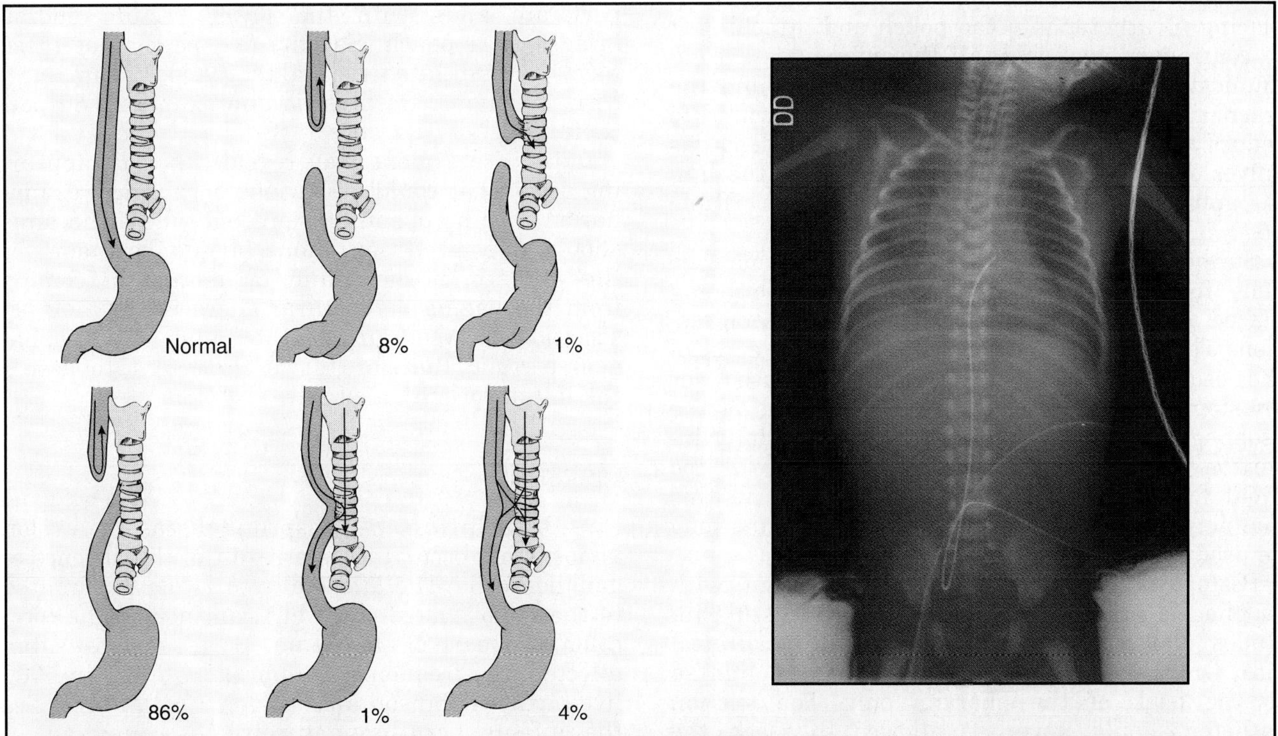

Figure 36–11

There are variations in type and frequency of the disorders esophageal atresia and tracheoesophageal fistula • Note the gasless abdomen, and the tip of the orogastric tube in the esophageal pouch in the photograph of an esophageal atresia. (Photograph courtesy of R. A. Nelson, M.D., Wesley Center, Wichita, KS).

36–11). Associated malformations are common; congenital heart defect occurs 30 percent of the time. Survival in the term infant who has no other complications or associated malformations can be as high as 97 percent. Prematurity and associated malformations reduce survival. Infants who survive are at risk for stricture of the anastomosis, esophageal dysmotility, and gastroesophageal reflux.

In the presence of esophageal atresia, the fetus is unable to swallow amniotic fluid. This may be identified in the maternal history by polyhydramnios. After birth, the infant is unable to handle its own secretions, and the clinical findings are copious oral secretions accompanied by the inability to pass a catheter through the esophagus into the stomach. If there is no fistula between the esophagus and the trachea, a radiograph shows a gasless abdomen.

If communication occurs between the proximal esophagus and the trachea, oral feedings induce coughing, choking, and cyanosis as the fluid enters the pulmonary system. Communication at the distal end may result in abdominal distention from crying or aspiration pneumonia as gastric contents are refluxed from the stomach into the lungs.

Management. Maintaining the airway is of prime importance in infants with esophageal atresia. It is necessary to withhold all oral feedings and keep the esophageal pouch clear of secretions. Oropharyngeal suctioning can be augmented by placing a catheter into the pouch and attaching it to continuous suctioning. If the infant has a communication between the distal esophagus and the trachea, the head of the bed should be elevated to reduce the risk of gastric reflux. Arterial blood gas valves should be monitored and be within the limits appropriate for the infant's condition (Table 36–8).

Surgical repair of esophageal atresia may be done in stages, with a gastrostomy tube being placed initially to accomplish gastric decompression. The distance between the opposing ends of the esophagus dictates the technique used for anastomosis. If necessary, the proximal end of the esophagus can be stretched over time by daily insertion of a weighted tube. If the distance is too great for anastomosis to be accomplished in this manner, a segment of small or large intestine may be used as a replacement tissue.

Postoperative care specific to the infant with esophageal atresia or tracheoesophageal fistula includes maintaining the integrity of the surgical site. Oropharyngeal suctioning should be limited to the back of the pharynx only. The suction catheter should never be allowed to reach the level of the anastomosis. Likewise, if the infant has an endotracheal tube in place and a fistula has been repaired, the tip of the suction catheter should not pass below the length of the tube.

Table 36–8

ARTERIAL BLOOD GAS VALUES FOR NEONATES

VALUE	RANGE
pH	7.35–7.45
Arterial oxygen pressure (Pao_2)	50–80 mm Hg
Arterial carbon dioxide pressure ($Paco_2$)	35–45 mm Hg
Bicarbonate (HCO_3^-)	20–24 mEq/L
Oxygen saturation	>90%

ANORECTAL AGENESIS

Description. Anorectal agenesis or imperforate anus occurs in 1 in approximately 5000 live births (Robinson and Linden 1993). Boys are more often affected than girls. The severity of the anomaly ranges from stenosis of the anus or lower rectum to complete separation of the upper and lower rectum (Fig. 36–12). The most common type is imperforate anus with the lower rectum ending blindly as a pouch. Seventy-five percent of these have an associated fistula to the perineum, urethra, or vagina. Survival is approximately 80 percent.

Initial assessment may reveal a normal-appearing anus, or it could be obvious on physical examination that no opening is present where the anus should appear. Observations should be made for the absence of meconium or meconium coming from the vagina or urethra. There is a strong association between imperforate anus and esophageal atresia; therefore, it is important to assess the infant for that anomaly.

HIRSCHSPRUNG DISEASE

Description. Hirschsprung disease is a colon abnormality occurring as a result of the absence of ganglion cells. The affected area is usually limited to the rectosigmoid colon but can include the total colon and part of the ileum. Boys are most often affected; the frequency is approximately 1 in 5000 live births (Robinson and Linden 1993). Rarely are the infants born prematurely. Associated anomalies are uncommon, but a family history of the disease is present in 30 percent of the cases.

Clinical findings include delayed passage of meconium and abdominal distention with bilious

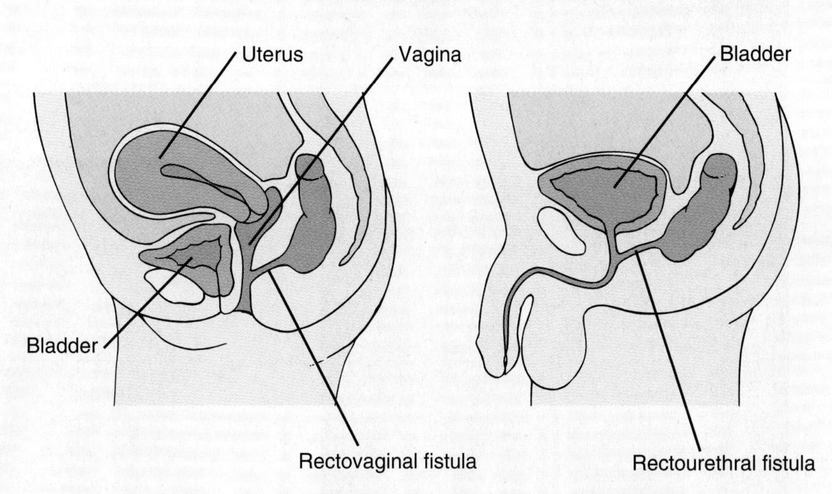

Figure 36–12
A low anorectal agenesis in which the bowel ends as a blind pouch below the pubococcygeal line is most common in girls • A high agenesis in which the bowel ends as a blind pouch above the pubococcygeal line is most common in boys.

vomiting. Ineffective peristalsis leads to abnormal bowel movements and persistent constipation. Obstruction may lead to perforation or peritonitis. Enterocolitis is the major cause of death in these infants.

A radiograph may be suggestive of Hirschsprung disease if a barium enema examination reveals a narrowed segment of colon leading to a dilated proximal segment of colon (Fig. 36–13). A rectal biopsy is required to confirm the diagnosis.

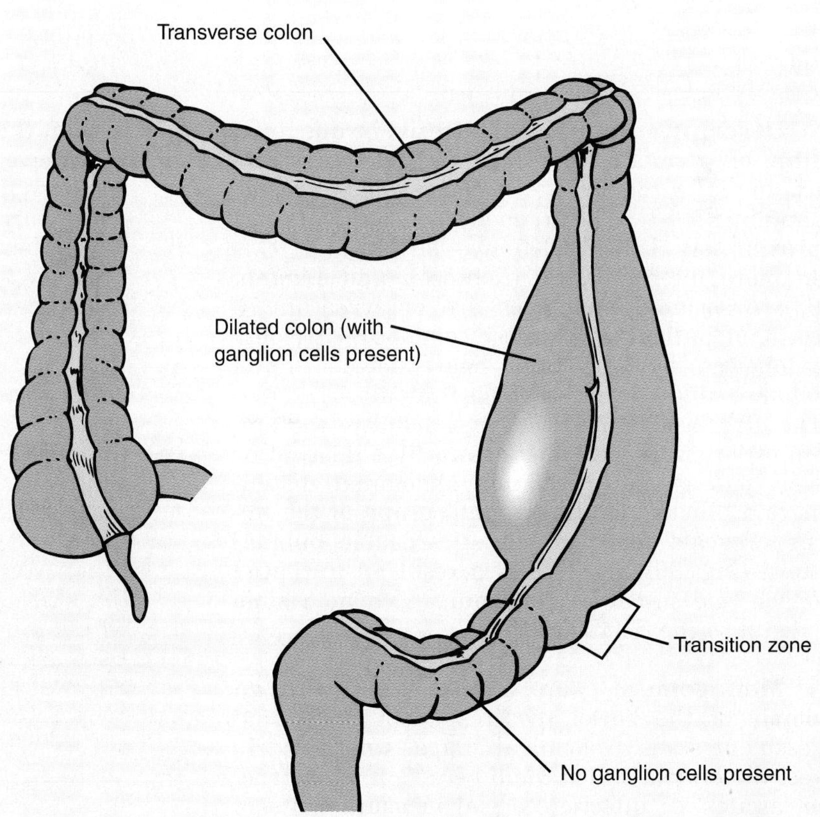

Figure 36–13
The affected bowel in Hirschsprung disease.

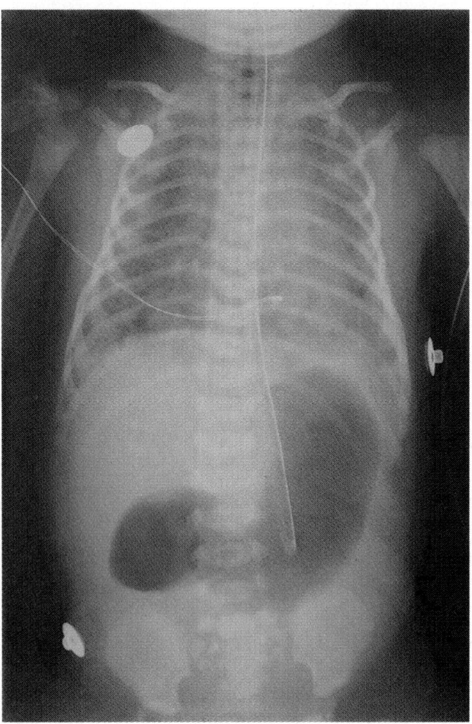

Figure 36–14

Note the "double-bubble" pattern in the abdomen in this example of duodenal atresia. (Courtesy of R. A. Nelson, M.D., Wesley Medical Center, Wichita, KS).

DUODENAL ATRESIA

Description. Duodenal atresia is due to a failure of recanalization of the gastrointestinal tract or is secondary to vascular insufficiency (Shandling 1987). The frequency of occurrence is approximately 1 in 10,000 live births, and it is seen more often in girls (Robinson and Linden, 1993). Associated anomalies are observed in 70 percent of patients. The most common is trisomy 21, followed by congenital heart defects, renal anomalies, and tracheoesophageal fistula.

The atresia usually occurs just distal to the ampulla of Vater. Clinical findings include delayed or absent passage of meconium, abdominal distention, and bilious vomiting. A radiograph of the abdomen reveals the characteristic "double bubble" pattern (Fig. 36–14). This is a result of a dilated stomach and proximal duodenum with no visible air distal to the duodenum.

Management. Care of the infant with an anomaly of the bowel requires adept abdominal assessment skills. Abdominal shape is observed to detect distention, which could be a sign of obstruction, ascites, or infection. Serial measurements of the abdomen should be done to monitor for changes in girth. It is best to take the abdominal measurement directly over the umbilicus when the infant is in the state of full expiration. If nec-

Nursing Care Guidelines for the Infant with a Colostomy

- The goal of pouching a stoma is to maintain skin integrity, contain bowel contents, and minimize odor.
- The infant's size, the size of the stoma, and the location of the stoma on the abdomen should be considered during pouch selection.
- Pouches can be a single-unit appliance, which has the bag permanently attached to the barrier piece (perhaps Stomahesive), or a two-piece system that has a barrier piece and a separate drainage pouch.
- Regardless of the bag type:
    - Adhere to Standard Precautions by using gloves and a gown if appropriate.
    - Clean the area around the stoma with oil-free soap and pat dry.
    - Measure the stoma with a measuring guide or on a piece of paper towel.
    - Trace the size of the stoma onto the barrier.
    - Cut a hole in the barrier slightly bigger than the tracing.
    - Remove the backing from the skin barrier, trying not to touch the sticky side of the barrier with your fingers.
    - Position the barrier over the stoma and gently apply to the infant's skin.
    - The barrier should fit so that no skin is exposed.
- Once placed, routinely check the appliance for leaking. *Do not* tape a leaking barrier—this will lead to skin breakdown.
- Empty the pouch when it is half full. Assess the stool for amount, consistency, color, and odor.
- When replacing the appliance, cleanse the skin and assess for redness and odor, which might be indicative of infection.

Data from Brown, K. C., Harper, S. L., Pettitt, B. J., Ricketts, R. R. (1992). *A parent's guide to ostomy care for children.* Princeton, NJ: ConvaTec.

essary, small markings can be made on the abdomen to ensure proper tape measure placement for subsequent evaluations.

Auscultation for bowel sounds should be made in all four quadrants. Bowel sounds are absent immediately after birth; but as soon as air begins to enter the bowel from crying or sucking, sounds can usually be heard in the upper quadrants (Coen and Koffler 1987).

Any infant with a potential bowel or rectal anomaly should be given nothing by mouth. Nursing care is aimed at decompressing the stomach with an orogastric tube. Nutrition will need to be provided by intravenous therapy.

Surgical repair of duodenal atresia involves removing the affected portion of the bowel. Postsurgical care requires attention to pain management and maintaining security and integrity of the gastrostomy site. The gastrostomy remains in place until bowel function is restored and the anastomosis is healed. Without complications, this usually occurs within 7 to 10 days.

Infants who have either Hirschsprung disease or imperforate anus return from the operating room with a colostomy. The stoma may not be pouched with an ostomy bag initially. The stoma should be dark pink in color without signs of ischemia or excessive bleeding (see Nursing Care Guidelines). Pain management and routine assessments of abdominal stability by measuring girth and assessing stool output are necessary postoperatively (Embon 1990). The management for Hirschsprung disease and imperforate anus is usually more complex than for duodenal atresia. Repeated surgical intervention is usually required, with treatment lasting perhaps until the first birthday.

DIAPHRAGMATIC HERNIA

▼ **Description.** Congenital diaphragmatic hernia (CDH) is a defect in the diaphragm that allows abdominal contents to herniate into the thoracic cavity (Fig. 36–15). The most common site of herniation is on the left side through the foramen of Bochdalek (Guzzetta et al. 1994). Although herniation can occur on the right side, the liver serves as a barrier to block the pleuroperitoneal canal and limits the amount of bowel that can herniate into the chest.

When the abdominal contents invade the thoracic cavity, it impedes normal lung development. The severity of the pulmonary compromise is related to the timing in gestation during which the herniation occurred. The earlier the defect occurs, and the more abdominal contents that are herniated, the more severe the consequence.

Infants born with CDH usually have severe respiratory distress and possibly cardiac compromise

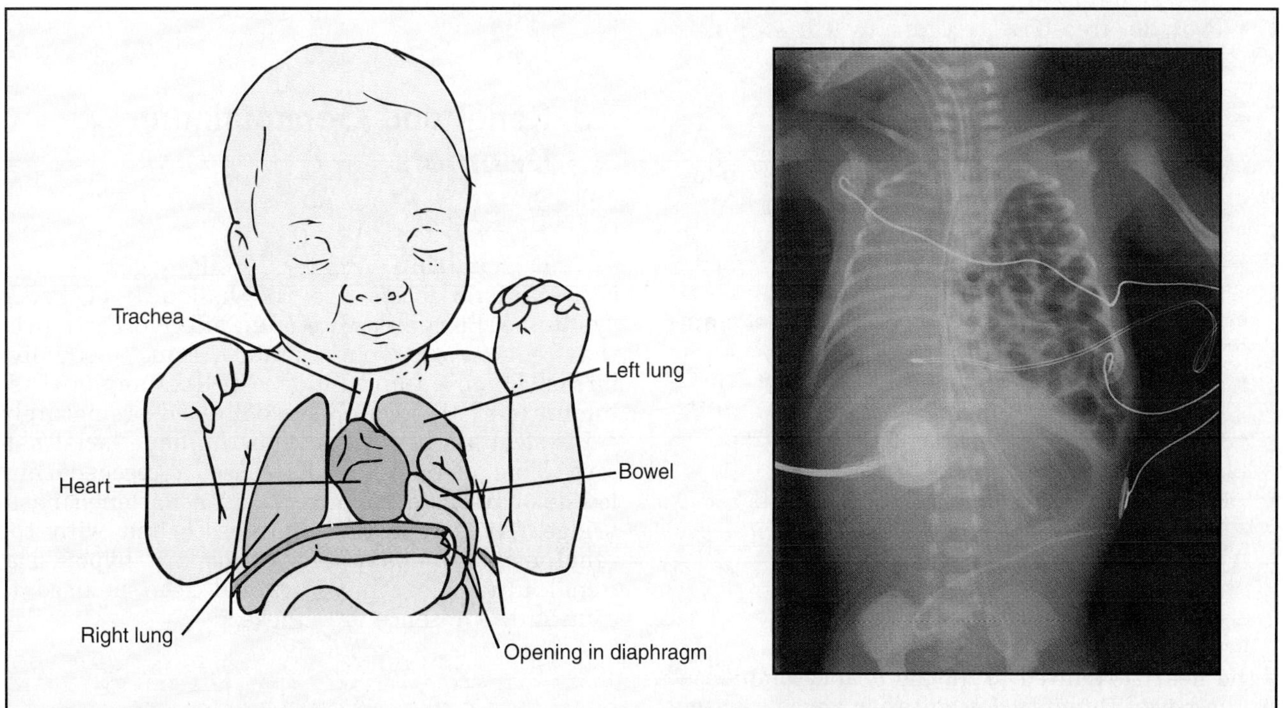

Figure 36–15

A diaphragmatic hernia is caused by a break in the diaphragm that allows a section of bowel to protrude into the chest cavity • In the radiograph, note the bowel in the left thorax, and the cardiac shift to the right caused by this displacement. (Photograph courtesy of R. A. Nelson, M.D., Wesley Medical Center, Wichita, KS.)

Assisting with Endotracheal Intubation

- Assemble the necessary supplies and equipment:
  - Laryngoscope and blade:

    Number 0 for preterm infants
    Number 1 for full-term infants
  - Endotracheal tube that has an internal diameter of appropriate size for the infant's weight:

2.5 mm	less than 1000 g
3.0 mm	1000–2000 g
3.5 mm	2000–3000 g
3.5–4.0 mm	above 3000 g
  - Ventilation and suctioning equipment
  - Scissors and ½- or ¾-inch adhesive tape for securing the tube after placement
- Shorten the endotracheal tube to 13 cm to make it easier for handling.
- Provide a stylet if requested.
- Position the infant flat with the neck slightly extended; a shoulder roll may be used if necessary.
- Provide free-flow oxygen to the infant during the procedure.
- Apply laryngeal pressure if requested.
- Be prepared to provide bag and mask ventilation if intubation cannot be accomplished in 20 seconds.
- Confirm tube placement by auscultating for equal breath sounds and chest rise.
- Secure the endotracheal tube to the face and call for a radiograph.
- Shorten the tube to no more than 4 cm past the lip.
- Document the infant's tolerance of the procedure in the medical record.
- Continue to monitor respiratory status.

Data from Bloom, R. S., and Cropley, C. C. (1994). *Textbook of neonatal resuscitation.* Elk Grove Village, IL: American Heart Association.

if the heart is shifted to the right and compressed by the bowel contents. Auscultation reveals absent or limited breath sounds on the affected side. The abdomen may have a scaphoid appearance.

Stabilization of the newborn is desirable before surgical repair is attempted (Composto 1992). Infants who do not respond to aggressive therapy may be candidates for extracorporeal membrane oxygenation (ECMO).

▼ **Management.** Nursing intervention for the infant with CDH includes measures to assist with cardiopulmonary stabilization. Ventilation should be provided by an endotracheal tube rather than by bag and mask ventilation. This prevents air from entering the bowel. An orogastric tube should be placed to maintain decompression of the stomach. The nurse can assist with the procedure of intubation by gathering the appropriate equipment, supplying equipment to the physician, and monitoring the infant's response to the procedure (see Assisting with Endotracheal Intubation).

Frequent measurement of arterial blood gases is essential for management of the patient. Sedation is often ordered in an attempt to produce relaxation of the chest wall. This allows controlled ventilation and reduces the risk for pulmonary air leaks.

Infants with CDH are at risk for hypoglycemia and need to be monitored with blood glucose analysis. Clinical signs of hypoglycemia in the very sick neonate are often nonspecific and difficult to assess; therefore, routine measurement of blood glucose is the most accurate method of detecting low blood glucose levels. Infants with CDH usually have an arterial line in place for administration of dextrose solutions. It is important to monitor infusion pumps to ensure accurate delivery of prescribed intake.

Renal and Genitourinary Disorders

POTTER SYNDROME

▼ **Description.** Bilateral renal agenesis and characteristic facies are the hallmark of Potter syndrome. Boys are more often affected than girls; the frequency is approximately 1 in 10,000 live births (Robinson and Linden 1993). Many of these infants are stillborn or are delivered prematurely.

Physical assessment reveals a unique facial pattern. This includes a beak nose, a receded chin, low-set ears, hypertelorism, and a flattened nasal bridge. The oligohydramnios associated with the renal agenesis results in pulmonary hypoplasia. Renal ultrasonography or renal scan is used to confirm the absence of kidneys.

POLYCYSTIC AND MULTICYSTIC DYSPLASTIC KIDNEY DISEASE

▼ **Description.** Abdominal masses palpated in the newborn are commonly related to a renal malformation. Infantile polycystic kidney disease is an inherited autosomal recessive disease; cysts replace normal kidney tissue primarily in the collecting tubules. Unfortunately, the disease is usually bilateral, and infants with severe disease rarely survive the neonatal period.

Clinical indicators of the disease include abdominal masses, abdominal distention, oliguria, increased serum creatinine, and hypertension. Diagnosis is confirmed by renal ultrasonography and pyelography. These tests help differentiate polycystic kidney disease from multicystic dysplastic kidney.

Multicystic dysplastic kidney disease is a developmental anomaly occurring in approximately 1 in 4000 live births. The disease is usually unilateral, and this allows a good prognosis.

▼ **Management.** Once a confirmative diagnosis has been made, the primary nursing intervention for an infant with Potter syndrome is the provision of supportive care. The condition is lethal, and death occurs in the first few days. The infant should be kept warm and comfortable while attempts are made to optimize ventilation and oxygenation. Pulmonary hypoplasia inhibits adequate ventilation, and these infants are at risk for PIE and pneumothorax. Auscultate breath sounds frequently and report any changes immediately to the physician.

Emotional and spiritual support of the parents and extended family composes much of the nursing care plan. As the parents prepare for the infant's death, it is important to identify their needs, values, and support systems. Every attempt should be made to accommodate clergy, extended family, or whomever the parents feel offers them support.

Care of the infant with a nonlethal renal condition requires close attention to fluid and electrolyte balance. The goal is to provide adequate hydration without fluid overload. Any fluid given to the infant needs to be counted as intake; even the most minute amounts of saline flush for medication administration should be recorded.

AMBIGUOUS GENITALIA

▼ **Description.** Ambiguous genitalia is defined as the inability to identify the sex of an infant after examination of the external genitalia. Common causes of ambiguity include congenital adrenal hyperplasia, inborn errors of metabolism involving cortisol synthesis, and chromosome abnormalities. Disorders of sexual differentiation are usually classified into four types: male pseudohermaphroditism, true hermaphroditism, gonadal dysgenesis, and female pseudohermaphroditism (Page 1994). Diagnostic evaluation includes measurement of hormones, karyotype, visualization of internal organs, and measurement of external organs.

▼ **Management.** The gender announcement of a newborn infant is an integral part of the birth process. The announcement to family and friends is a source of pride and legacy for the family. Parents can be coached to inform family and friends that the infant has a malformation of the external genitalia. Parents may wish to choose a name for the infant that is gender neutral. Sexual determination can usually be done within a few weeks. Gender assignment for the infant should be based on functional anatomy, and the sooner this can be done, the better.

Families with infants having ambiguous genitalia require intense psychological and emotional support. Genetic counseling is encouraged for future family planning.

Neurologic Disorders

ANENCEPHALY AND MYELOMENINGOCELE

▼ **Description.** Anencephaly occurs as a result of a disturbance in the dorsal inductive process. The neural tube fails to close in the anterior area (Volpe 1994). The upper skull bones are usually absent, exposing minimal brain tissue above the brain stem. The infant appears normal except for the absent skull, which gives the infant a froglike appearance when viewed from the front. Brain tissue that is present lacks definition because of its long-term exposure to amniotic fluid. Although most infants are stillborn, some are delivered alive at term. Death usually occurs in the first few days; however, some infants have been known to survive for months.

Myelomeningocele is a neural tube defect caused by failure of the posterior neural tube to close. Girls are slightly more affected than boys; the frequency ranges from 1 in 1000 to 5 in 1000 live births. The cause is unknown but has been linked to environmental factors, maternal nutrition, genetics, and teratogens. Most of the lesions occur in the lumbar region of the spine and affect the spinal cord segments L2-S1. The meninges are exposed through the surface of the skin in a herniated sac that may be either sealed or leaking. There may also be abnormality of the vasculature, dermal layers, and bone structures (Fig. 36–16). Associated malformations include hydrocephalus, lower extremity deformities, and urologic abnormalities. If diagnosed prenatally, a cesarean delivery may be done to prevent further damage to the spine (Luthy 1991).

Surgical closure of the spinal defect is usually done within the first 24 to 48 hours (Volpe 1994). Long-term outcome for bowel and bladder control and functioning of the lower extremities is dependent on the level and severity of the defect. Infants with a lesion below S-1 may be able to walk

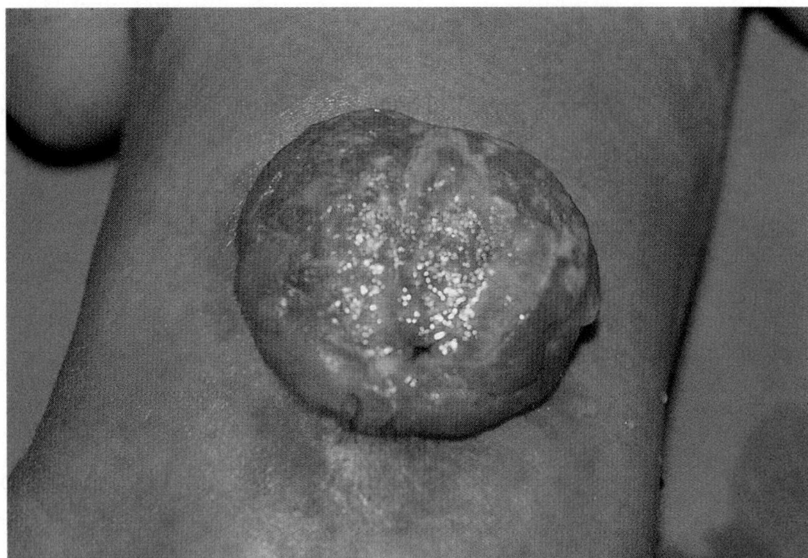

Figure 36–16

This large lumbar meningomyelocele, a type of neural tube defect, is seen on the back of a newborn and is covered with a thin membrane • A warmed, sterile, saline-soaked dressing is often used for protection. (Courtesy of A. E. Chudley, Professor of Pediatrics and Child Health, Children's Hospital, Winnipeg, Manitoba, Canada.)

without any support. Those with lesions above L-2 are usually wheelchair dependent (Volpe 1994).

▼ **Management.** Supportive care is the only thing that can be done for an infant with anencephaly. Parents should be encouraged to see and hold their infant. Any defect they imagine is usually much worse than reality. A small cap can be placed over the exposed brain to contain leaking cerebrospinal fluid and to serve as a barrier for the defect. Organ donation and transplantation are performed at some institutions. With this new technology comes a multitude of ethical issues, and nursing personnel need to play a patient advocate role for the infant as well as a supporting role for the parents.

Neural tube defects on the spine should be protected with a sterile dressing moistened with warmed, sterile saline. To keep the lesion free from feces and urine, a plastic drape over the buttocks may serve as a barrier to contamination.

The infant should be positioned prone and every attempt made to keep proper body alignment. Diaper rolls can be used to keep feet in a neutral position. Passive range of motion may be performed if it is ordered by the physician.

Bowel and bladder function requires close monitoring before and after surgical repair of the defect. Bladder function should be assessed by observing urine color and volume. Make note of constant urine "dribbling" or the presence of bladder distention after spontaneous voiding. Intermittent bladder catheterization may be ordered if urinary retention is diagnosed.

Bowel function is assessed by monitoring stooling patterns for the frequency and consistency of stool. An increasing abdominal girth may be indicative of constipation. Suppositories may be given to promote stool softening.

Infants with myelomeningocele benefit from a multidisciplinary team approach to their care, including medical, nursing, orthopedic, renal, neural, dietary, genetic, and social service consultation.

HYDROCEPHALUS

▼ **Description.** Hydrocephalus is caused by excess cerebrospinal fluid in the ventricles of the brain as a result of either a congenital malformation or an acquired disorder. Congenital hydrocephalus may result from stenosis of the aqueduct of Sylvius (Fig. 36–17), a Dandy-Walker cyst, or an Arnold-Chiari malformation, or it may be an associated malformation with spina bifida or encephalocele.

Physical assessment of congenital hydrocephalus reveals a large head with open sutures, full fontanelles, and sunset eyes. A CT scan or magnetic resonance imaging may be done to evaluate the thickness of the cerebral mantle. This assessment helps predict outcome and the risk for developmental delay (Volpe 1994).

Acquired hydrocephalus is usually a complication of intraventricular hemorrhage. Up to 50 percent of infants with severe intraventricular hemorrhage will have some degree of hydrocephalus (Volpe 1994). If the hydrocephalus does not resolve on its own, a shunt may be surgically placed, which will carry cerebrospinal fluid to an extracranial site where it will then be resorbed. In the infant or young child, the distal end of the shunt is usually positioned in the peritoneal cavity.

▼ **Management.** Nursing care of the infant with hydrocephalus includes obtaining a daily occipital-frontal head circumference and biparietal

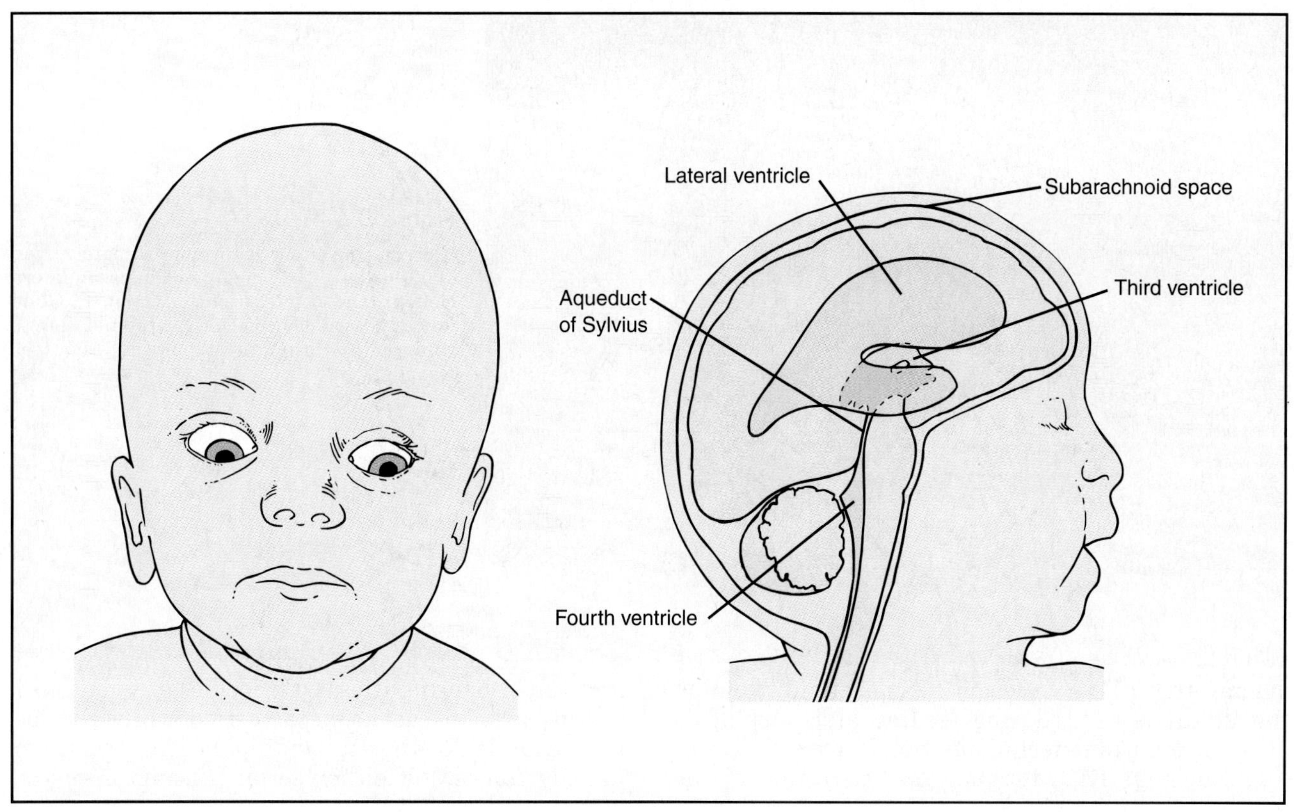

Figure 36–17

In an infant born with hydrocephalus there is an enlargement of the ventricles due to stenosis of the aqueduct of Sylvius.

measurement. This is done by measuring from one ear over the anterior fontanelle to the other ear. Increased cranial pressure may be exhibited by alterations in consciousness and responsiveness, vomiting, bradycardia, or seizures. Any of these requires prompt notification to the physician.

Intervention that can minimize the potential for skin breakdown of the scalp includes frequent position changes with stimulation of the circulation to obvious pressure points, use of a foam pad or water bed, and maintenance of adequate nutrition. Many of these interventions can be done by the parents. Participating in the care of their infant can help decrease stress and promote bonding. These early interactions with the infant increase the comfort level and foster confidence as they deal with more complicated home care instructions.

Craniofacial Disorders

CLEFT LIP AND PALATE

Description. Diagnosis of a cleft lip-palate can be made immediately after birth by observation of the face and inspection of the integrity of the soft and hard palate. Cleft lip is defined as a congenital fissure in the upper lip. The defect can be unilateral or bilateral. If a cleft palate is present, the fissure may be in the soft palate alone or in both the hard and soft palate (Fig. 36–18). Cleft palate can occur as an isolated defect.

Cleft lip-palate can be categorized as associated with another chromosome anomaly, as a result of an environmental insult (FAS, maternal drug use, or amniotic band syndrome), as a familial form, or as a nonfamilial isolated defect. Surgical repair of the lip is usually done at 3 months of age. Repair of the palate is delayed until the child is about 1½ years; however, some institutions are repairing the palate at an earlier age.

Management. Providing adequate oral intake is the primary focus for the infant with a cleft lip-palate. The presence of a cleft lip may make it difficult for the infant to create a seal around a nipple and produce a strong enough suck to obtain formula from the bottle. If there is only a cleft lip, the mother can usually breastfeed with success. If a cleft palate is present, the nipple cannot be compressed effectively, and breastfeeding may be difficult or impossible. Holding the infant's cheeks and making a slightly larger hole in the nipple of the bottle may be of some assistance. If there is a cleft in the palate, special nipples can be used that have a shield to cover the palate, re-

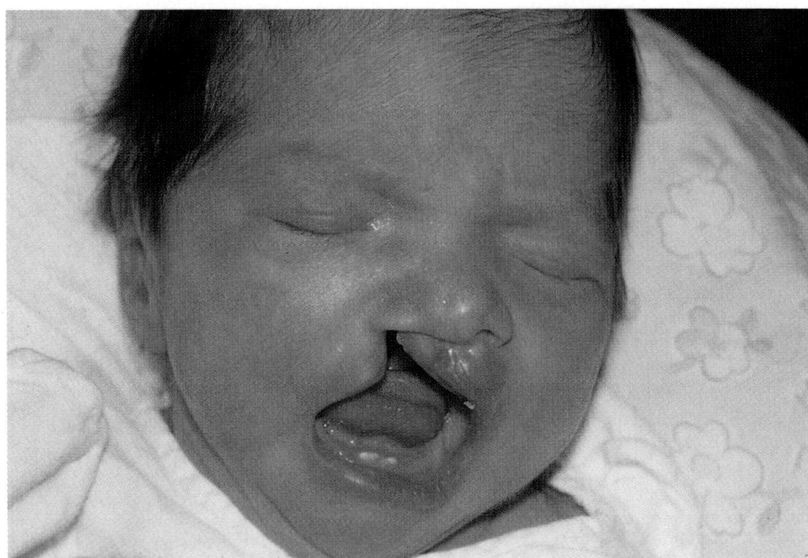

Figure 36–18

Clefts of the lip occur in approximately every 1000 births • This infant has a unilateral cleft lip and palate. (Courtesy of A. E. Chudley, Professor of Pediatrics and Child Health, Children's Hospital, Winnipeg, Manitoba, Canada.)

ducing the risk for formula aspiration. Holding the infant upright during feeding and burping is also an important technique. Small, frequent feedings can help avoid fatigue and frustration in the infant.

The skin integrity of the cleft may be maintained by attention to cleanliness. Washing the area with warm normal saline after feedings can help decrease the amount of secretions that can cause irritation. Offering a small amount of water after formula feeding is also helpful.

Parental support and education are important aspects of the infant's care. The parents need to be shown how to feed their infant and how to cleanse the cleft area. It will be some time before the defect is repaired, and it is imperative that the infant obtain adequate nutrition. Support groups are available that can offer suggestions on how to care for these infants at home. Infants with cleft lip-palate benefit from a multidisciplinary team approach to their care, including medical, nursing, orthodontic, speech, genetic, and social service consultation.

Musculoskeletal Disorders

TALIPES EQUINOVARUS

Talipes equinovarus, also called clubfoot, is one of the most common developmental abnormalities of the foot. It occurs most often in boys, and although it is believed to be related to intrauterine malposition, it does tend to run in families. The foot is turned downward and inward and may be smaller in size than the opposite foot.

Initial assessment must include observation for any bone abnormalities. Orthopedic intervention is begun early in the neonatal period while the foot is amenable to physical manipulation. Treatment usually consists of either serial bracing or casting to return the foot to normal alignment.

SYNDACTYLY

Syndactyly is the abnormal fusion of either the fingers or toes caused by a failure of the webbing between the digits to degenerate. Feet are more often affected than hands, and the disorder is more common in boys. The degree in which the fusion occurs ranges from the base of the digit all the way to the tip. In simple cases, only the skin and soft tissues are affected. Complex cases may involve bone structures, nerves, and blood vessels. Treatment is aimed at promoting function and normalizing appearance. Surgical repair may be done in stages and is dependent on the degree of involvement.

POLYDACTYLY

Polydactyly is defined as extra digits. The extra digit may contain only soft tissue or may be a more complex duplication involving the bone structures. An extra little finger is more commonly seen in the black population and is usually an isolated incident. An extra thumb is more common in the white population and is usually associated with other malformations (Fig. 36–19). Removal of those digits containing only tissue can be done simply and as early as desired. Those that contain bone structures require a more thorough assessment to delineate prominence in use, thereby directing which digit should be removed. Treatment

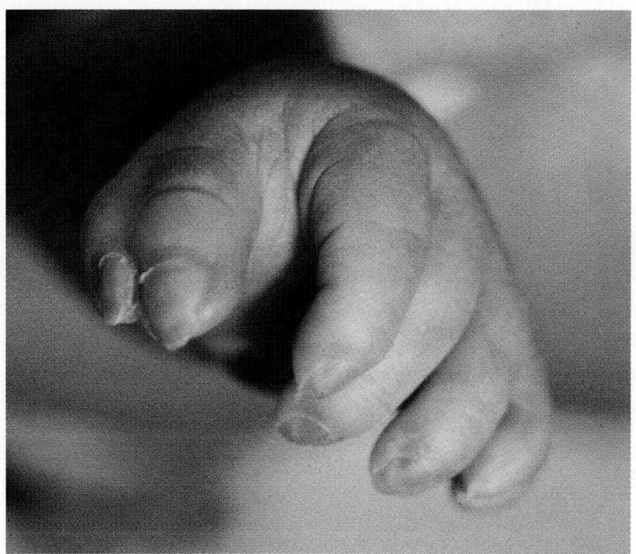

Figure 36–19

This infant with polydactyly shows an extra thumb. (Courtesy of R. A. Nelson, M.D., Wesley Medical Center, Wichita, KS.)

is aimed at promoting function and normalizing appearance.

Chromosome Disorders

Chromosome aberrations may be caused by problems in number or structure. The normal number of human chromosomes is 46 with 23 pairs. Alteration in the normal number of chromosomes usually occurs during gamete formation as a result of abnormal or delayed disjunction during meiosis I or meiosis II. The aberration may be in translocation or mosaicism. Nondisjunction is more common in older mothers, but it can occur at any age. When a chromosome set contains three copies of a chromosome, the aberration is called a trisomy. If only one copy is present, it is called a monosomy. Whenever there is an abnormal number of chromosomes, a malformation of varying degree is expressed. Any time multiple congenital anomalies are present, a chromosome evaluation should be done for proper diagnosis, determination of etiology, and estimation of recurrence risk (see Chapter 13 for a detailed discussion of chromosome disorders and genetics).

TRISOMY 13

Trisomy 13 is the third most common autosomal trisomy condition; its frequency is approximately 1 in 5000 live births. It is often referred to as Patau syndrome. It occurs primarily as a result of nondisjunction and appears to be associated with advanced maternal age. Although many of the features that appear with trisomy 18 may be present in trisomy 13, three specific characteristics often occur in unison: microphthalmos, cleft lip and palate, and polydactyly (Jones 1988).

Outcome is grim; 50 percent die in the first month of life. Those who survive the first year have severe mental retardation. Rarely does life expectancy extend past 3 years of age.

TRISOMY 18

Trisomy 18 is the second most common autosomal trisomy condition; its frequency of occurrence is approximately 1 in 3500 live births. It is often referred to as Edwards syndrome. It occurs primarily as a result of nondisjunction, but translocation or mosaicism does occur. The most common clinical findings include low birth weight, micrognathia, short sternum, congenital heart disease (primarily ventricular septal defect), rocker bottom feet, hypertonia, overlapping of the second finger on the third, and a unique high-pitched cry (Jones 1988).

Mortality is high; only 10 percent survive until 1 year of age (Robinson and Linden 1993). The primary cause of death is related to the cardiac disease. Those who do survive have profound mental retardation and do not learn to walk or talk. They usually succumb to complications from apnea, aspiration, or congenital heart disease.

TRISOMY 21

Trisomy 21 is the most common autosomal trisomy condition and occurs as a result of an extra or part of an extra chromosome 21 (Robinson and Linden 1993). It is often referred to as Down syndrome. Overall rate is approximately 1 in 800 live births; the frequency increases to 1 in 55 for women 45 years and older. The most common physical findings include flattened facial features, oblique palpebral fissures, loose skin on the nape of the neck, pelvic dysplasia, hyperflexibility of joints, folded or dysplastic ears, hypotonia, and poor Moro reflex. Only 40 percent of infants with trisomy 21 have the classic simian crease.

The condition of these infants may be complicated; as many as half have a ventricular septal defect or other congenital heart disease. There is also an increased risk for duodenal atresia. Long-term survival for these infants depends on the severity of any associated anomaly. Without complications, infants with trisomy 21 may live until middle age. They are all developmentally delayed, with an IQ range of 25 to 70. Early intervention is strongly encouraged to maximize the infant's potential.

TURNER SYNDROME

Turner syndrome results from complete or partial absence of the complementary sex chromosome. The paternal X chromosome is more typically missing. The frequency of occurrence is approximately 1 in 10,000 female live births. There does not appear to be any relationship of the syndrome to advanced maternal age.

Because of minimal expression of the syndrome in the neonatal period, many of these infants can escape early diagnosis. Early signs of the syndrome may consist of lymphedema of the dorsum of the hands and feet, webbing of the neck, and a low posterior hairline. Congenital heart defects are present in 20 percent of the cases. Later signs include short stature, amenorrhea, and infertility. Long-term outcome is good, with life expectancy reaching normal rates. Intelligence is rarely impaired in Turner syndrome.

Management. Many infants with trisomy 13 or trisomy 18 expire during the first few hours after birth. The infant should be kept warm and oxygenated. Nutrition may be provided through intravenous lines. As soon as a confirming diagnosis can be made, the parents need to participate in the decisions about the care of their child.

Initial care of an infant with trisomy 21 includes the assessment and treatment of associated anomalies. Providing adequate nutrition may be difficult because of poor bottling or breastfeeding skills related to decreased tone and perhaps a protruding tongue that has a forward moving motion. With time and patience, this can be overcome, and oral nutrition can be given without the need for surgical intervention.

Early detection of Turner syndrome is important so that growth hormone may be offered before fusion of the epiphysis; estrogen replacement therapy is started after fusion. Psychosexual counseling may be important for young women during adolescence and the childbearing years.

Any time a family experiences the birth of a child with an anomaly, genetic consultation and counseling will be an important piece of the care of the family. Genetic counseling allows families to comprehend medical facts and understand the hereditary nature of the disorder as well as the risk for recurrence in future pregnancies. Treatment plans congruent with the family's goals, values, and religious beliefs can also be discussed. Identification of community support groups can aid in making the best possible adjustment to the situation (Robinson and Linden 1993). Not only does it provide biomedical information, it provides empathetic and emotional support as well. Most of the care provided to these infants takes place after discharge with assistance from physicians, community health nurses, school nurses, social workers, and occupational and physical therapists.

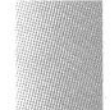

Metabolic Disorders

Screening for inborn errors of metabolism in the newborn period is the best measure for preventing conditions that carry major morbidity and mortality (University of Colorado Health Sciences Center 1988). It enhances the opportunity for early detection and treatment. Because of the importance of these evaluations, many states now require screening for every newborn before hospital discharge.

The challenge for nurses is related to the short length of stay for many newborns and their mothers. It is important that parents be given information about the serious nature of these disorders and the importance of the screening process. If parents are properly informed, they will be more compliant with returning for an outpatient appointment.

PHENYLKETONURIA

The enzyme that normally mediates the transformation of phenylalanine to tyrosine is called phenylalanine hydroxylase. The absence of this enzyme blocks the conversion of phenylalanine and results in an accumulation of the amino acid in the blood. Elevated levels are usually defined as greater than 20 mg/dL.

Early detection of the disorder is possible by using the Guthrie test for phenylketonuria, a bacterial inhibition assay that measures blood phenylalanine. Once the disorder is detected, treatment can begin by offering a diet that is low in protein. A milk substitute that contains a small amount of phenylalanine but normal amounts of other amino acids, carbohydrate, and fat can be given instead of standard infant formula (Rezevani and Auerbach 1987). This prevents the profound mental retardation associated with the disorder. If the disorder remains untreated, in addition to retardation, the infant may develop seizures, psychotic behavior, eczema, and decreased pigmentation.

GALACTOSEMIA

Galactosemia is an autosomal recessive metabolic abnormality of carbohydrate metabolism involving the conversion of galactose to glucose. Lactose, a milk sugar, is composed of galactose and glucose. The frequency of galactosemia is approximately 1 in 50,000 live births.

Before feeding, infants appear normal. Once galactose accumulates in the blood, clinical signs quickly appear. The most common signs include jaundice, irritability, vomiting, hepatomegaly, and failure to thrive during the first week after birth.

Untreated infants develop cataracts and mental retardation. Treatment consists of a diet restricting galactose. Early detection during screening can eliminate the morbidity associated with the disorder.

CONGENITAL HYPOTHYROIDISM

Congenital hypothyroidism is a deficiency of thyroid hormone due to a transient decrease related to prematurity or maternal antithyroid use, a congenital deficiency of the thyroid tissue, an enzymatic impairment, or a deficiency of thyroid-stimulating hormones. The frequency is approximately 1 in 5000 live births.

Clinical findings include large posterior fontanelle, umbilical hernia, protruding tongue, poor feeding, hypothermia, and hyperactivity. Mental retardation occurs if it is left untreated. Treatment consists of thyroid supplementation.

MAPLE SYRUP URINE DISEASE

Maple syrup urine disease (MSUD) is an inborn error of metabolism arising from a deficiency of the enzyme branched-chain keto acid decarboxylase. The frequency is approximately 1 in 175,000 live births.

Infants appear normal at birth; but within 5 days, signs of the disease begin to appear. Initial signs are nonspecific and may include only poor feeding, vomitng, and lethargy. The classic sign of MSDU is a characteristic odor of the urine that resembles burnt sugar or maple syrup. This odor may be present as early as the fifth day after birth.

Oral feeding must be stopped immediately if MSDU is suspected. Without immediate intervention, the infant may lapse into a coma and die. In addition to stopping feedings, peritoneal dialysis or exchange transfusion may be done during the acute phase. Those infants who do survive are at risk for mental retardation and must remain on a diet free of branched-chain amino acids.

Cardiac Disorders

Description. Congenital heart disease (CHD) of the newborn occurs in approximately 1 in 8000 live births. The cause may be related to chromosome abnormalities or a teratogenic effect of drugs such as phenytoin, warfarin, lithium, antineoplastic agents, or alcohol.

Defects are divided into two categories, acyanotic and cyanotic. Because of sufficient oxygenation of the blood, acyanotic defects do not usually result in cyanosis (Fig. 36–20). Cyanotic defects, on the other hand, result in central cyanosis, or that which affects mucous membranes (Fig. 36–21). This type of cyanosis generally worsens when the infant is agitated or is crying. It results from desaturated blood leaving the heart. Complete cardiac assessment consists of auscultation, inspection, and palpation. The overall appearance of the infant needs to be observed. Respiratory patterns should be observed for distress; skin should be evaluated for pallor and sweating. All of these may be indicative of congestive failure. Special attention must be given to differentiation between peripheral (affecting the extremities) cyanosis, which is usually gone within the first few days, and central (affecting the mucous membranes) cyanosis.

The precordium and peripheral pulses should be palpated and assessed for rate, regularity, and equality of pulses in the extremities. The heart sounds should be auscultated with a stethoscope for the presence of a murmur and its placement in the heart sounds. It may be systolic, diastolic, or

Signs of Congestive Heart Failure

Decreased cardiac output

- Restlessness
- Pale, mottled skin color with cool extremities
- Decreased urine output
- Tires easily with oral feedings

Increased respiratory distress

- Tachypnea, nasal flaring, grunting, and retractions
- Cyanosis
- Rales associated with pulmonary edema

Systemic venous congestion

- Rapid weight gain
- Periorbital edema
- Hepatosplenomegaly

Text continued on page 1381

ACYANOTIC HEART LESIONS	PATHOPHYSIOLOGY	CLINICAL FINDINGS	TREATMENT
Patent ductus arteriosus (PDA) 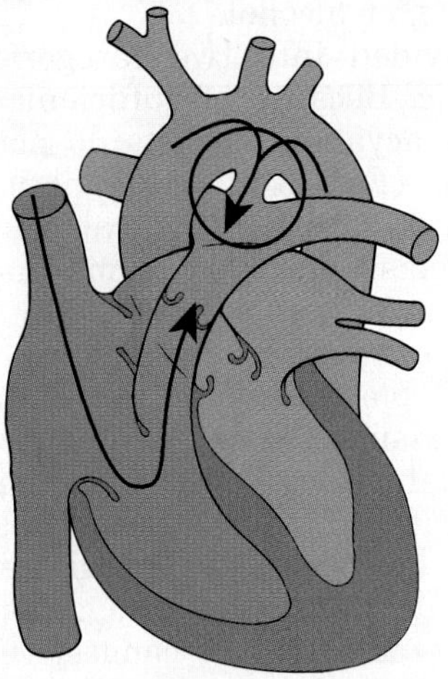	• Blood reenters pulmonary circuit through patent ductus and increases pulmonary blood flow	• Related to gestational age: 40% <1000 g • Bounding peripheral pulses • Murmur • Hepatomagaly • Hyperactive precordium • Widened pulse pressures • Congestive heart failure (CHF)	• Usually closes in 1st 24 hours • Fluid restriction/ diuretics for CHF • Positive end-expiratory pressure to reduce left-to-right shunt • Indomethacin as a prostaglandin inhibitor to close ductus • Surgical closure if pharmacologic management is unsuccessful
Ventricular septal defect (VSD) 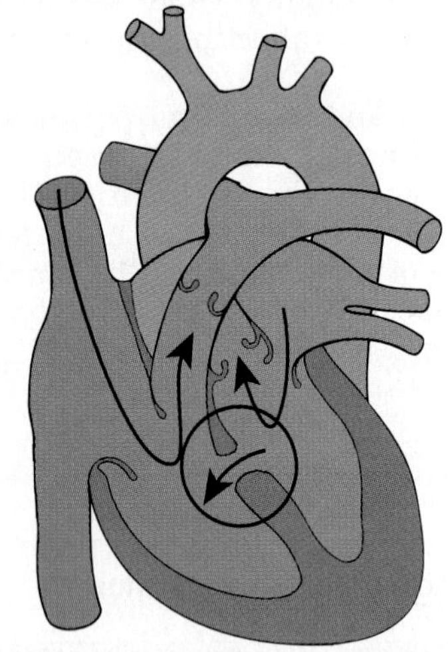	• Abnormal opening in septum between right and left ventricle	• Most common congenital heart defect (CHD) • Small VSD: Asymptomatic, murmur at left sternal border (LSB) • Large VSD: CHF, murmur at lower left sternal border (LLSB)	• Small defects may close without treatment • Fluid restriction/ diuretics for CHF • Digoxin • Surgical repair by either suturing or patching defect
Atrial septal defect (ASD) 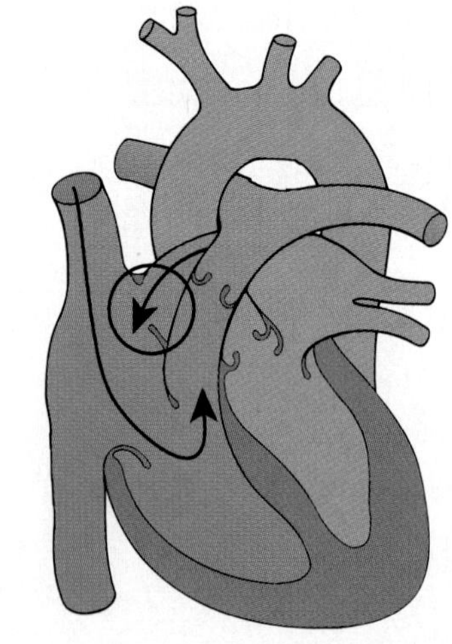	• Abnormal opening in septum between right and left atria • May be an ostium secundum, ostium primum, or sinus venosus defect	• Small ASD: Asymptomatic • Moderate or large ASD: CHF from left-to-right shunting, enlarged right atrium and ventricle on radiograph, systolic murmur at 2nd left intercostal space, diastolic murmur at LLSB, failure to thrive	• Small defects may close without treatment • Fluid restriction/ diuretics for CHF • Surgical repair by either suturing or patching defect

Figure 36–20

Acyanotic heart lesions.

ACYANOTIC HEART LESIONS	PATHOPHYSIOLOGY	CLINICAL FINDINGS	TREATMENT
Aortic stenosis (AS) 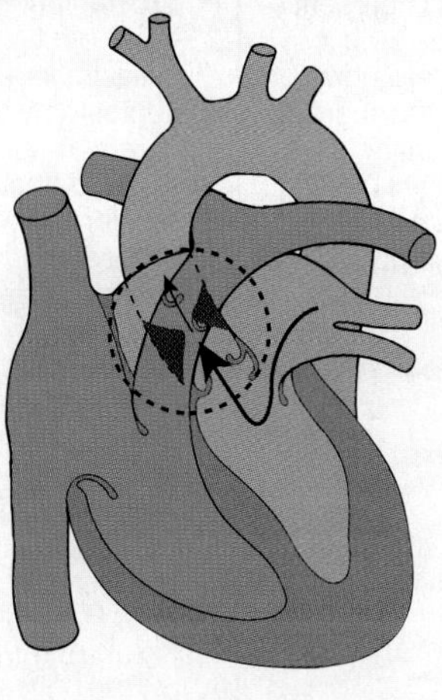	• Valvular stenosis with cusps thickened or deformed • Myocardial hypertrophy	• Asymptomatic at birth • Murmur at LSB • Cardiomegaly on radiography • CHF at later date	• Fluid restriction/ diuretics for CHF • Surgical repair with aortic valvotomy
Coarctation of the aorta (COA) 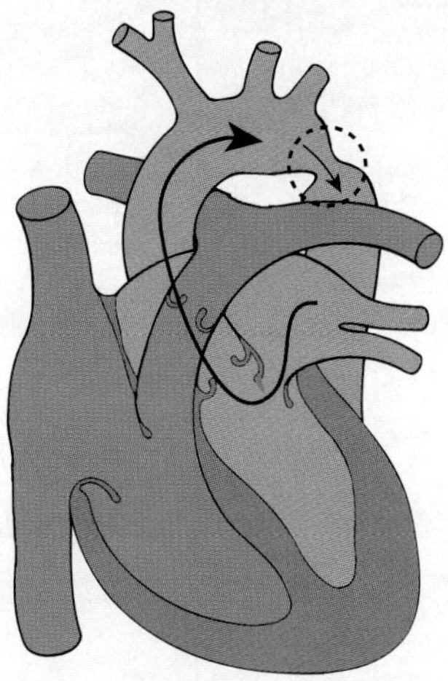	• Narrowing of aorta distal to left subclavian artery • Occurs most commonly at insertion site of ductus arteriosus • If preductal, increased risk for hypoplastic aortic arch and associated cardiac defects	• CHF • Hepatomegaly • Decreased pulses in lower extremities • Decreased pressure in left arm; coarctation at site of left subclavian artery • Decreased pressure in right arm; coarctation below right subclavian artery • Enlarged heart and left ventricular hypertrophy on radiograph	• Fluid restriction/ diuretics for CHF • Prostaglandin E to dilate ductus • Surgical repair by either reanastomosis of abnormal section or patch area across obstruction
Hypoplastic left heart (HLHS) 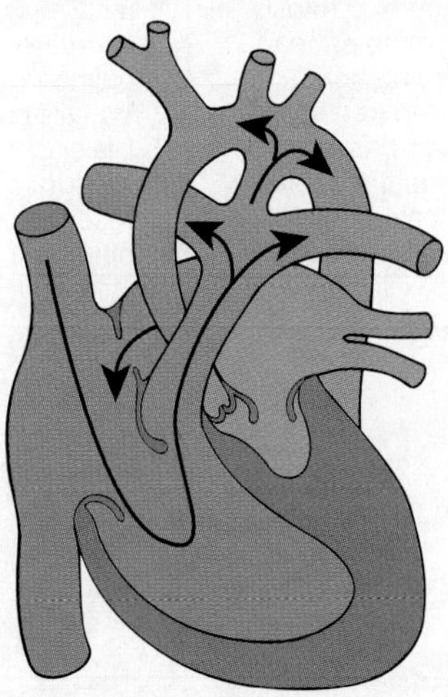	• Hypoplastic left ventricle and ascending aorta • Hypoplastic mitral and aortic valves	• Asymptomatic at birth • Respiratory distress with increasing pulmonary blood flow • CHF • As PDA closes: Mottling and gray pallor, decreased pulses • Cardiomegaly and pulmonary congestion on radiograph	• Prostaglandin E to dilate ductus • Surgical correction by Norwood procedure or heart transplant

Figure 36–20 *Continued*

CYANOTIC HEART LESIONS	PATHOPHYSIOLOGY	CLINICAL FINDINGS	TREATMENT
Transposition of the great vessels (TGV) 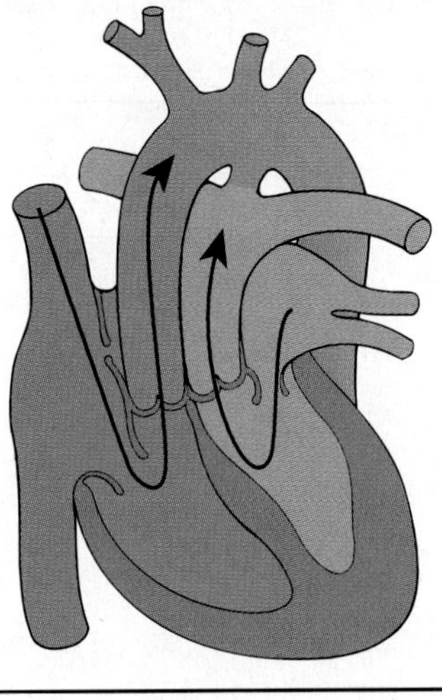	• Position of great arteries is reversed • Pulmonary artery arises from left ventricle • Aorta comes from right ventricle	• Cyanosis is present as early as birth • Murmurs are not heard unless there is a ventricular septal defect (VSD) • Egg–shaped heart on radiograph	• Prostaglandin E to dilate ductus • Initial balloon septostomy to create an atrial septal defect (ASD) • Mustard or Sanning procedure diverts systemic venous blood to left ventricle and pulmonary venous blood to right ventricle • Arterial switch procedure detaches vessels and reconnects to normal ventricle
Truncus arteriosus 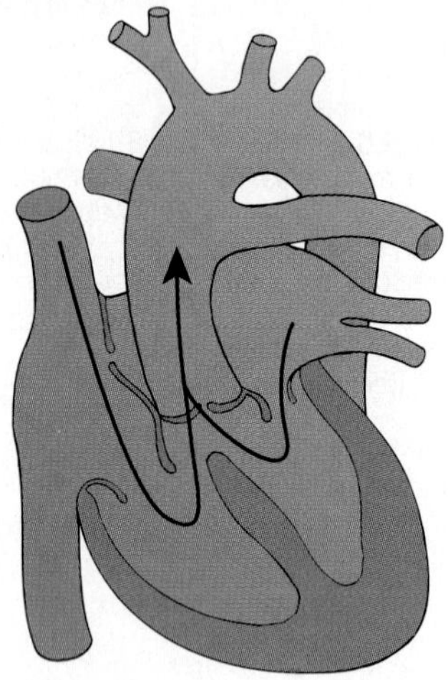	• Single large great vessel arises from both ventricles, with an accompanying VSD	• Cyanosis • Congestive heart failure (CHF) with bounding peripheral pulses • Systolic ejection click with a single S_2 sound • Enlarged heart on radiograph	• Fluid restrictions/ diuretics for CHF • Surgical correction: Homograft between right ventricle and pulmonary artery, patching of VSD
Tetralogy of Fallot (TOF) 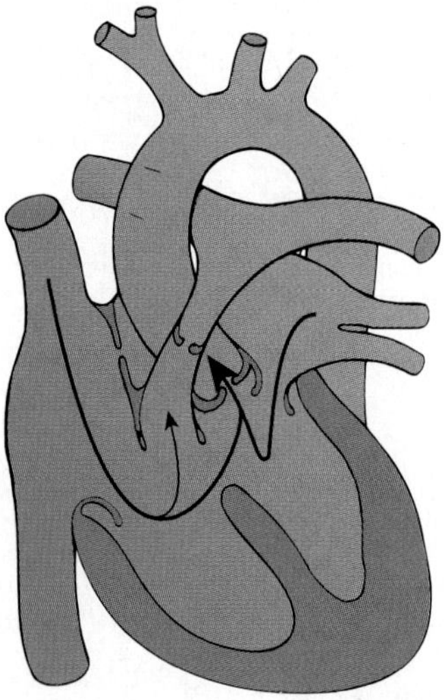	• Combination of four defects: Pulmonary stenosis, VSD, overriding aorta, and right ventricular hypertrophy	• Severity of pulmonary stenosis dictates degree of cyanosis • Boot-shaped heart on radiograph • Hypoxic (tet) spells include paroxysmal dyspnea and severe cyanosis	• Prostaglandin E to dilate ductus • Initial surgical repair to create systemic-pulmonary shunts: Waterston, Potts, Blalock–Taussig • Closure of VSD with resection of pulmonary stenosis

Figure 36–21

Cyanotic heart lesions.

CYANOTIC HEART LESIONS	PATHOPHYSIOLOGY	CLINICAL FINDINGS	TREATMENT
Total anomalous pulmonary venous connection (TAPVC) 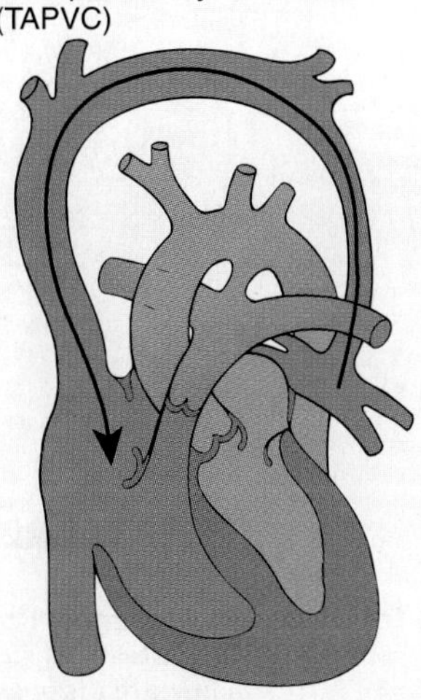	• Pulmonary veins do not connect to left atrium but into right atrium	• Patent foramen ovale or ASD is needed for survival • Cyanosis when there is an obstruction to pulmonary venous return • CHF • Ventricular dilatation on radiograph	• Surgical repair to reattach veins to correct position
Pulmonary stenosis (PS) 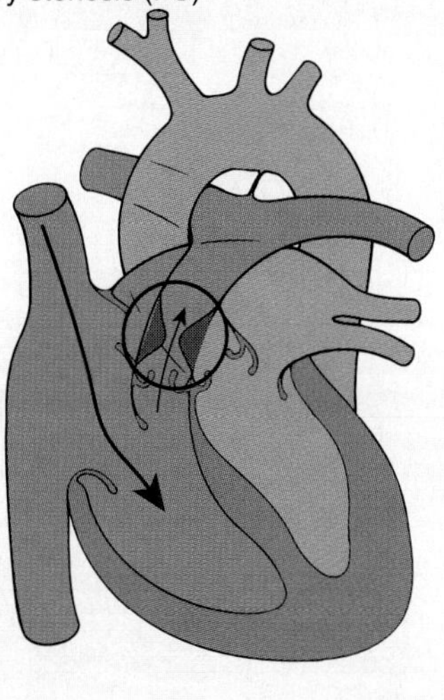	• Pulmonary valve cusps resulting in narrowed opening in pulmonary valve	• Loud murmur at upper left sternal border with mild stenosis • Less of a murmur with moderate stenosis • Cardiomegaly on radiograph	• Prostaglandin E to dilate ductus • Surgical repair with valvotomy

Figure 36–21 *Continued*

continuous. Murmurs are the result of turbulence of blood flow and are caused by abnormal valves, septal defects, regurgitated flow through incompetent valves, and high blood flow across normal structures (Fig. 36–22). The intensity of the murmur is affected by cardiac output. In general, the higher the cardiac output, the more intense the murmur. Murmurs may be graded by use of the following system:

Grade I Barely heard

Grade II Soft but easily heard

Grade III Moderately loud but no thrill

Grade IV Loud with a thrill present

Grade V Loud and heard with a stethoscope barely on the chest wall

Grade VI Loud and heard with a stethoscope near the chest wall

Management. Nursing interventions specific to the infant with CHD involve assessment of cardiac status, monitoring for signs of congestive failure (see Signs of Congestive Heart Failure), maintaining an adequate but balanced fluid and electrolyte status, and maintaining adequate oxygenation.

Postsurgical care is aimed at monitoring hemodynamic stability. Vital signs need to be observed every 5 to 15 minutes immediately after surgery.

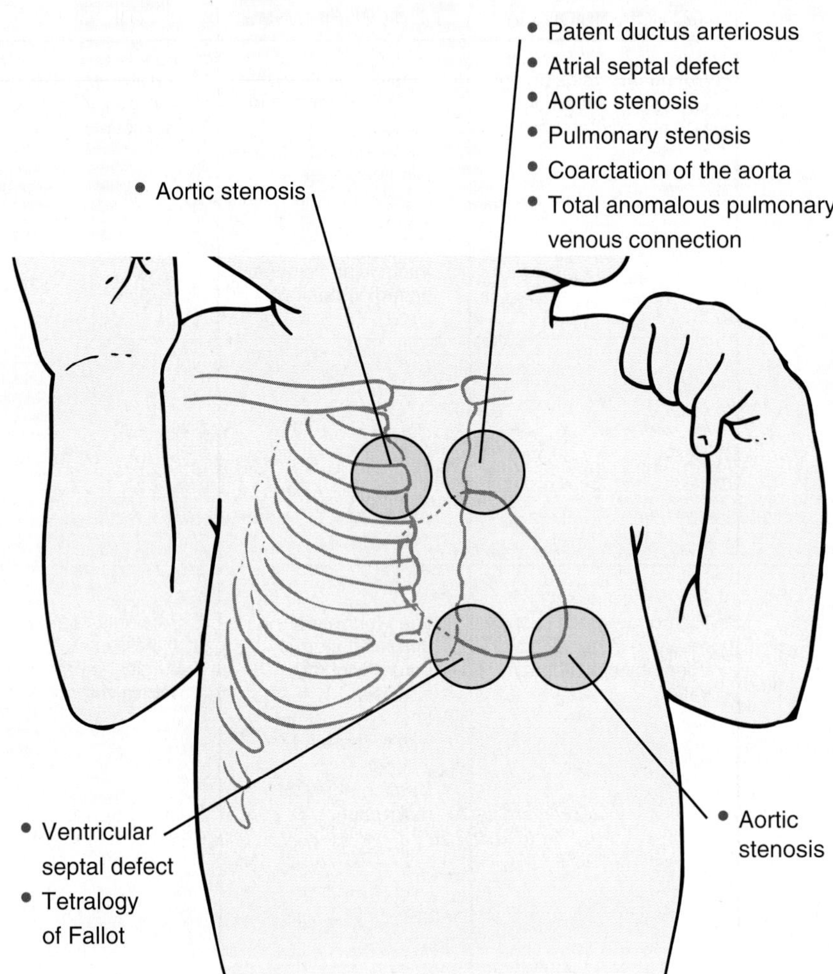

Figure 36–22

The sites at which cardiac murmurs may be heard include the aortic area (*upper left*), pulmonic area (*upper right*), mitral area (*lower right*), and tricuspid area (*lower left*).

Perfusion should be monitored by assessing blood pressure, cardiac output, or cardiac index (Macrae and LeBoeuf 1988). Cardiac tamponade is a postoperative emergency that requires adept nursing assessment skills. Signs of tamponade include increased right atrial or left atrial pressures, narrowing pulse pressure, muffled heart sounds, and decreased perfusion. Prompt diagnosis and reporting allow medical intervention. These infants will return from surgery with a chest tube. It is important to maintain security of the tube by taping it to the chest wall. The tube should remain patent, and no blood should be allowed to clot the tube. Report any abrupt cessation or dramatic increase in chest drainage immediately.

Astute observation of other body systems is also important in caring for these infants. Assessments need to be made of the respiratory status, renal function, fluid and electrolyte status, and neurologic behavior. The nurse must work closely with the cardiovascular surgeon to develop a pain management plan that will not compromise the cardiac status.

Risk Management

The nurse involved in the care of the high-risk infant is at risk for lawsuits, but those risks may be lowered by the nurse. It is the responsibility of the nurse to provide quality care to the infant. The nurse needs to be well prepared educationally to provide quality care. Skills and education can be updated by consultation with other experienced staff nurses, clinical nurse specialists, and nurse practitioners in the field as well as through the attendance of continuing education offerings. Professional organizations provide a wealth of information as well as current standards and practice guidelines.

The use of high-technology equipment provides

benefits to the patient and nurse. It is the responsibility of the nurse to operate the equipment properly and to check for malfunctions according to the manufacturer's guidelines. The equipment must be set accurately, checked, and rechecked to ensure that there is no human error and the patient is receiving the proper treatment. Finally, it is the patient, not the equipment, that is to be assessed.

Another aspect of risk management for the nurse involved in the care of the high-risk infant is frequent and accurate documentation. The medical record is evidence of the activities of assessment, planning, implementation, and evaluation of the infant's care. The charting should be clear, concise, and complete. Communication with other members of the health care team and parents should be part of the record.

Development of a trusting relationship with the neonate's family is an important component of risk management. Frequent open communication with the family builds a rapport that prevents misunderstandings. That rapport leads to a trust in the nurse's judgments and actions.

KEEPING NICU SKILLS SHARP

- PARTICIPATE IN MULTIDISCIPLINARY ROUNDS. Much can be learned from other health care team members. Not only does this widen your knowledge base, it increases your ability to provide holistic patient care.
- CRITICALLY REVIEW RESEARCH ARTICLES IN YOUR AREA OF CLINICAL PRACTICE. This review allows you to discriminate between nursing interventions that are based on research and those based on habit or old ways.
- OBTAIN CERTIFICATION in your area of clinical practice.
- ATTEND LOCAL AND NATIONAL CONFERENCES related to your area of clinical practice.
- VOLUNTEER TO MENTOR/TEACH ANOTHER NURSE. The best way to solidify your knowledge is to share it with others.
- ALWAYS REMEMBER THAT THE INFANT IS PART OF A BIGGER UNIT—THE FAMILY. Your responsibilities for care extend past the infant and include promoting parent-child attachment and facilitating a smooth transition from hospital to home.
- PARTICIPATE IN LEGISLATIVE ACTIVITIES that affect health policy.

Support for the NICU Nurse

The demanding pace of the NICU is challenging for nurses. Although the work is stimulating and rewarding, if nurses fail to care for themselves, they may become stressed and unable to provide their patients and families with quality care. Nurses who are unhappy or have inability coping give less effective nursing care. Coping is enhanced by a person's perception of support. The most effective support involves human interchange and bolsters a person's feelings of self-worth.

Nurses can enhance their perception of support by involvement in their practice. Seek out opportunities to be involved in making decisions about the daily operations of the NICU. Become an active member of influential committees. This involvement provides the staff nurse with decision-making opportunities. Build relationships with other staff nurses in the NICU. It is through the give and take and sharing of ideas and feelings that support networks are built and nurtured (Brooks et al. 1994).

Implications for Research

The NICU provides myriad opportunities for research. This area of neonatal nursing grew rapidly, and many interventions are not research based and need to be scientifically validated (Franck et al. 1993). In their practice, neonatal nurses daily encounter problems that need to be examined and nursing care practices that require validation through research. It is through research that neonatal nurses can improve the nursing care and outcomes for preterm babies. Franck and associates (1993) have identified a number of current neonatal nursing research questions focusing on skin care, nutrition, instruments and procedures, effect of the environment, training, endotracheal tube stabilization and management, pain, thermoregulation, positioning, effects of cocaine, parent teaching techniques, nursing care, and retention of nurses in the critical care setting.

- How can the barrier properties of the skin be improved to prevent infection and water loss?
- How can intravenous access be improved and complications minimized?

- What is the best method for collecting urine? Which scale provides the most accurate weight? Which device provides the most accurate measure of temperature?
- What is the appropriate level of stimulation for preterm infants?
- Is the initial training and ongoing education of ECMO specialists sufficient to maintain emergency management skills?
- How can neonatal pain be assessed? Are there long-term consequences of unrelieved pain experienced in the neonatal period?
- What are the most effective teaching methods for instructing parents in the care of their newborns?
- How do NICU nurses cope with stress?

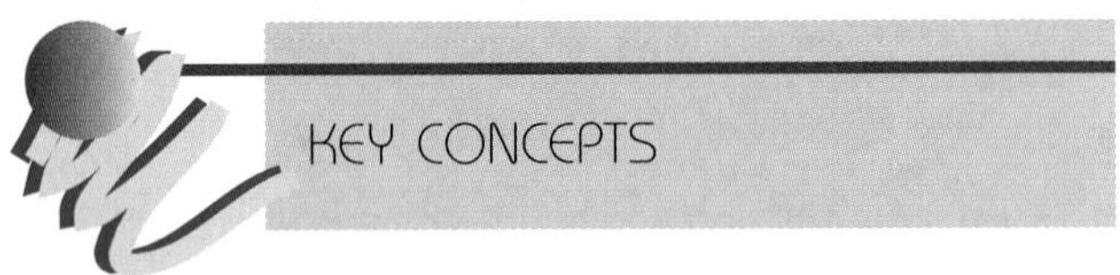

▼ Newborns are classified by gestational age as preterm, term, or postterm. According to weight and age, newborns are classified as small for gestational age, large for gestational age, and appropriate for gestational age.

▼ Early recognition of increased risk, increased awareness, and observation enable the nurse to direct nursing interventions that may minimize poor outcomes.

▼ To meet neurodevelopmental needs of the high-risk infant, modify the high-tech environment of the NICU by reducing excess noise, bright lighting, and excess activity.

▼ Despite technologic advances, the risk for morbidity and mortality remains high in the preterm infant.

▼ Care of the preterm infant is complex. The preterm infant requires extreme vigilance for the development of any complications.

▼ Nurses must develop assessment skills with the normal newborn so that they can readily note any deviation from normal.

▼ The nurse interacting with an infant who has a congenital anomaly and the infant's family has several key responsibilities: (1) recognizing the congenital anomaly; (2) providing nursing interventions that prevent potential complications associated with the anomaly; (3) providing education and emotional support for the family; and (4) facilitating a smooth transition from hospital to home by ensuring appropriate referral to community agencies.

▼ Congenital anomalies can be classified into three categories: malformations, deformations, and disruptions.

▼ Many congenital anomalies require only supportive care to the infants as they die. The nursing care plan will be to provide emotional and spiritual support to the parents and extended family. As the parents prepare for the infant's death, it is important to identify their needs, values, and support systems. Every attempt should be made to accommodate clergy, extended family, or whomever the parents feel offers them support.

References

Als, H., Lester, T. E., Brazelton, T. B. (1982). Assessment of preterm infant behavior (APIB). In H. E. Fitzgerald and M. Yogman (Eds.), *Theory and research in behavioral pediatrics* (Vol. 1, pp. 64–133). New York: Plenum Publishing.

Anderson, G. C. (1991). Current knowledge about skin-to-skin (kangaroo) care for preterm infants. *Journal of Perinatology,* 11 (3), 216–226.

Arias, I. M., Gartner, L. M., Seifter, S., et al. (1964). Prolonged neonatal unconjugated hyperbilirubinemia associated with breast feeding and steroid pregnane-3(alpha), 20(beta)-diol in maternal milk that inhibits glucuronide formation in vitro. *Journal of Clinical Investigation,* 43, 2037–2047.

Behrman, R. E., Kliegman, R. M., Arvin, A. M. (1996). *Nelson textbook of pediatrics* (15th ed.). Philadelphia: W. B. Saunders.

Bell, S. G. (1994). The national pain management guideline: Implications for neonatal intensive care. *Neonatal Network,* 13 (3), 9–17.

Blackburn, S. T. (1993). Assessment and management of neurologic dysfunction. In C. Kenner, A. Brueggemeyer, L. P. Gunderson (Eds.), *Comprehensive neonatal nursing: A physiologic perspective* (pp. 635–689). Philadelphia: W. B. Saunders.

Blackburn, S. T., and Loper, D. L. (1992). *Maternal, fetal, and neonatal physiology.* Philadelphia: W. B. Saunders.

Blackburn, S. T., and VandenBerg, K. A. (1993). Assessment and management of neonatal neurobehavioral development. In C. Kenner, A. Brueggemeyer, L. P. Gunderson (Eds.), *Comprehensive neonatal nursing: A physiologic perspective* (pp. 1094–1129). Philadelphia: W. B. Saunders.

Bloom, R. S., and Cropley, C. C. (1990). *Textbook of neonatal resuscitation.* Elk Grove Village, IL: American Heart Association.

Boeckling, A. C. (1992). Exogenous surfactant therapy for premature infants. *Journal of Perinatal and Neonatal Nursing,* 6 (2), 59–66.

Brazelton, T. B. (1973). Neonatal behavioral assessment scale. *Clinical and Developmental Medicine,* 50.

Brazelton, T. B. (1986). Development of newborn behavior. In F. Falkner and J. M. Tanner (Eds.), *Human growth* (Vol. 2, pp. 519–540). New York: Plenum Publishing.

Brooks, E., Wilkinson, J. M., Popkess-Vawter, S. (1994). Promoting situational support for nurses in practice. *Image,* 26 (4), 305–308.

Broome, M. E., and Tanzillo, H. (1990). Differentiating between pain and agitation in premature neonates. *Journal of Perinatal and Neonatal Nursing,* 4 (1), 53–62.

Brown, K. C., Harper, S. L., Pettitt, B. J., Ricketts, R. R. (1992). *A parent's guide to ostomy care for children.* Princeton, NJ: ConvaTec.

Coen, R. W., and Koffler, H. (1987). *Primary care of the newborn.* Boston: Little, Brown.

Composto, R. (1992). Congenital diaphragmatic hernia: Pathophysiology and nursing care. *Neonatal Network,* 11 (6), 57–61.

Embon, C. M. (1990). Ostomy care for the infant with necrotizing enterocolitis: Nursing considerations. *Journal of Perinatal and Neonatal Nursing,* 4 (3), 56–63.

Evans, N., and Rutter, N. (1986). Development of the epidermis in the newborn. *Biology of the Neonate,* 49, 74–80.

Fanaroff, A. A., and Kliegman, R. M. (1993). Necrotizing enterocolitis. In M. H. Klaus and A. A. Fanaroff (Eds.), *Care of the high-risk neonate* (4th ed., pp. 182–188). Philadelphia: W. B. Saunders.

Franck, L. S., Gunderson, L. P., Kenner, C. (1993). Collaborative research in neonatal nursing. In C. Kenner, A. Brueggemeyer, L. P. Gunderson (Eds.), *Comprehensive neonatal nursing: A physiologic perspective* (pp. 52–66). Philadelphia: W. B. Saunders.

Guthrie, R. A., and Auerbach, K. G. (1993). Jaundice and the breastfeeding baby. In J. Riordan and K. G. Auerbach (Eds.), *Breastfeeding and human lactation* (pp. 333–346). Boston: Jones & Bartlett.

Guzzetta, P. C., Anderson, K. D., Newman, K. D., Rouse, T. M., Schnitzer, J. J., Boyajian, M., Tomaski, S. M. (1994). General surgery. In G. B. Avery, M. A. Fletcher, M. G. MacDonald (Eds.), *Neonatology: Pathophysiology and management of the newborn* (4th ed., [pp. 36–105]). Philadelphia: J. B. Lippincott.

Harpin, V., and Rutter, N. (1983). Barrier properties of the newborn infant's skin. *Journal of Pediatrics,* 102 (3), 419.

Haywood, J. L. Coghill, C. H., Waldemar, A. C., Ross, M. (1993). Assessment and management of respiratory dysfunction. In C. Kenner, A. Brueggemeyer, L. P. Gunderson (Eds.), *Comprehensive neonatal nursing: A physiologic perspective* (pp. 294–312). Philadelphia: W. B. Saunders.

Heymann, M. A. (1989). Fetal and neonatal circulations. In F. H. Adams, G. C. Emmanouilides, T. A. Riemenschneider (Eds.), *Moss' heart disease in infants, children and adolescents* (4th ed., pp. 24–34). Baltimore: Williams & Wilkins.

Heymann, M. A., Teitel, D. F., Liebman, J. (1993). The heart. In M. H. Klaus and A. A. Fanaroff (Eds.), *Care of the high-risk neonate* (4th ed., pp. 345–373). Philadelphia: W. B. Saunders.

Hodges, C., and Vincent, P. A. (1993). Why do NICU nurses not refeed gastric residuals prior to feeding by gavage? *Neonatal Network,* 12 (8), 37–40.

Hollingsworth, D. R., and Moore, T. R. (1989). Diabetes and pregnancy. In R. K. Creasy and R. Resnik (Eds.), *Maternal-fetal medicine* (2nd ed., pp. 925–988). Philadelphia: W. B. Saunders.

Jason, J., and van der Meer, A. (1989). *Parenting your premature baby.* New York: Henry Holt & Co.

Jobe, A. (1986). Surfactant and the developing lung. In D. W. Thibeault and G. A. Gregory (Eds.), *Neonatal pulmonary care* (2nd ed., pp. 75–99). Norwalk, CT: Appleton-Century-Crofts.

Jones, K. (1988). *Smith's recognizable patterns of human malformation.* Philadelphia: W. B. Saunders.

Kanto, W. P., Hunter, J. E., Stoll, B. J. (1994). Recognition and medical management of necrotizing enterocolitis. In B. J. Stoll and R. M. Kliegman (Eds.), *Clinics in perinatology: Necrotizing enterocolitis* (pp. 335–346). Philadelphia: W. B. Saunders.

Katz, K. S., Pokorni, J. L., Long, T. M. (1989). *Chronically ill and at risk infants.* Palo Alto, CA: VORT Corporation.

Kenner, C., and Brueggemeyer, A. (1993). Assessment and management of genitourinary dysfunction. In C. Kenner, A. Brueggemeyer, L. P. Gunderson (Eds.), *Comprehensive neonatal nursing: A physiologic perspective* (pp. 706–741). Philadelphia: W. B. Saunders.

Kenner, C., Brueggemeyer, A., Gunderson, L. P. (1993). *Comprehensive neonatal nursing: A physiologic perspective.* Philadelphia: W. B. Saunders.

Klaus, M. H., Martin, R. J., Fanaroff, A. A. (1993). The physical environment. In M. H. Klaus, and A. A. Fanaroff (Eds.), *The high-risk neonate* (4th ed., pp. 114–129). Philadelphia: W. B. Saunders.

Korones, S. B. (1986). *High risk newborn infants* (4th ed.). St. Louis: C. V. Mosby.

Krause, K. D., and Youngner, V. J. (1992). Nursing diagnoses as guidelines in the care of the neonatal ECMO patient. *Journal of Obstetric, Gynecologic, and Neonatal Nursing,* 21 (3), 169–176.

Lawrence, R. A. (1994). *Breastfeeding: A guide for the medical profession* (2nd ed.). St. Louis: C. V. Mosby.

Lefrak-Okikawa, L., and Lund, C. H. (1993). Nursing practice in the neonatal intensive care unit. In M. H. Klaus and A. A. Fanaroff (Eds.), *Care of the high-risk neonate* (4th ed., pp. 212–227). Philadelphia: W. B. Saunders.

Lucus, A., and Cole, T. J. (1990). Breast milk and neonatal necrotizing enterocolitis. *Lancet,* 336, 1519–1523.

Lucus, A., Morley R., Cole, T. J., et al. (1992). Breast milk and subsequent intelligence quotient in children born premature. *Lancet,* 339, 261.

Ludington, S. M. (1990). Energy conservation during skin-to-skin contact between premature infants and their mothers. *Heart and Lung,* 19 (5), 445–450.

Luthy, D. A., Wardinsky, T., Shurtleff, D. B., Hollenhbach, D. A., Hickok, D. E., Nyberg, D. A., Benedetti, T. J. (1991). Cesarean section before the onset of labor and subsequent motor function in infants with meningomyelocele diagnosed antenatally. *New England Journal of Medicine,* 324 (10), 662–666.

Macrae, M. M., and LeBoeuf, M. B. (1988). Standardized nursing care plan for the open-heart surgery neonate. *Neonatal Network,* 7 (2), 49–56.

Mammel, M. C., and Boros, S. J. (1996). High frequency ventilation. In J. P. Goldsmith and E. H. Korotkin (Eds.), *Assisted ventilation of the neonate* (p. 206). Philadelphia: W. B. Saunders.

Martin, R. J., Fanaroff, A. A., Klaus, M. H. (1993). Respiratory problems. In M. H. Klaus and A. A. Fanaroff (Eds.), *Care of the high-risk neonate* (4th ed., pp. 228–259). Philadelphia: W. B. Saunders.

Meier, P. P., and Mangurten, H. H. (1993). Breastfeeding the preterm infant. In J. Riordan and K. G. Auerbach (Eds.), *Breastfeeding and human lactation* (pp. 253–278). Boston: Jones & Bartlett.

Page, J. (1994). The newborn with ambiguous genitalia. *Neonatal Network,* 13 (5), 15–21.

Park, M. K. (1988). *Pediatric cardiology for practitioners.* Chicago: Mosby–Year Book.

Poland, R. L., and Ostrea, E. M. (1993). Neonatal hyperbilirubinemia. In M. H. Klaus and A. A. Fanaroff (Eds.), *Care of the high-risk neonate* (4th ed., pp. 302–322). Philadelphia: W. B. Saunders.

Rezevani, I., and Auerbach, V. H. (1987). Defects in metabolism of amino acids. In R. E. Behrman and V. C. Vaughn, III (Eds.), *Nelson textbook of pediatrics* (13th ed., pp. 280–306). Philadelphia: W. B. Saunders.

Robinson, A., and Linden, M. G. (1993). *Clinical genetics handbook* (2nd ed). Boston: Blackwell Scientific Publications.

Rushton, C. H. (1991). Humanism in critical care: A blueprint for change. *Pediatric Nursing,* 17 (4), 399–402.

Shandling, B. (1987). Congenital and perinatal anomalies of the gastrointestinal tract and intestinal obstruction. In R. E. Behrman, V. C. Vaughn III, W. E. Nelson (Eds.), *Nelson textbook of pediatrics* (13th ed., pp. 778–791.) Philadelphia: W. B. Saunders.

Shaw, N. (1993). Assessment and management of hematologic dysfunction. In C. Kenner, A. Brueggemeyer, L. P. Gunderson (Eds.), *Comprehensive neonatal nursing: A physiologic perspective* (pp. 582–634). Philadelphia: W. B. Saunders.

Silverman, W., and Anderson, D. (1956). A controlled clinical trial of effects of water mist on obstructive respiratory signs, death rate and necropsy findings among premature infants. *Pediatrics,* 17, 4.

Thibeault, D. W. (1986). Pulmonary barotrauma: Interstitial emphysema, pneumomediastinum, and pneumothorax. In D. W. Thibeault and G. A. Gregory (Eds.), *Neonatal pulmonary care* (2nd ed., pp. 499–517). Norwalk, CT: Appleton-Century-Crofts.

Turner, B. S. (1985). Amniotic band syndrome: A nursing perspective. *Journal of Obstetric, Gynecologic and Neonatal Nursing,* 14 (4), 299.

University of Colorado Health Sciences Center. (1988). *Genetic applications: A health perspective.* Lawrence, KS: Learner Managed Designs.

Urrutia, N. L. (1991). Sorting the complexities of respiratory distress syndrome. *MCN: American Journal of Maternal-Child Nursing,* 16, 308–311.

Volpe, J. J. (1994). *Neurology of the newborn* (3rd ed). Philadelphia: W. B. Saunders.

Weibley, T. T., Adamson, M. Clinkscales, N., Curran, J., Bramson, R. (1987). Gavage tube insertion in the premature infant. *MCN: American Journal of Maternal-Child Nursing,* 12, 24–27.

Whitsett, J. A., Pryhuber, G. S., Rice, W. R., Warner, B. B., Wert, S. E. (1994). Acute respiratory disorders. In G. B. Avery, M. A. Fletcher, M. G. MacDonald (Eds.), *Neonatology: Pathophysiology and management of the newborn* (4th ed., pp. 429–452). Philadelphia: J. B. Lippincott.

NURSING CARE PLANNING GUIDE

Healthy Preterm Newborn

This Nursing Care Planning Guide was developed to be used as a planning tool. You will need to modify and adapt it to individual clients as appropriate.

Performing a complete and thorough assessment is the first step in providing effective nursing care for a client. Major nursing diagnoses used in the care of the healthy preterm newborn include

1 Risk for impaired gas exchange
2 Risk for fluid volume deficit or excess
3 Risk for hypothermia or hyperthermia
4 Risk for central nervous system injury
5 Altered nutrition: less than body requirements
6 Risk for infection
7 Risk for bowel injury
8 Risk for impaired skin integrity
9 Risk for disorganized infant behavior

ASSESSMENT

Assessment of the healthy preterm newborn plays a critical role in facilitating adjustment to extrauterine life and in enhancing growth and development. To collect data, use the following Assessment Tools: Newborn Admission Record (p. 1172) and Newborn Nursery Flow Record (pp. 1173–1174). In the data collected, identify defining characteristics to use as a basis for formulating nursing diagnoses that are appropriate for your client. Areas requiring special attention in the care of the healthy preterm newborn include thermoregulation, nutrition, and respiratory and circulatory status.

Continued on following page

NURSING CARE PLANNING GUIDE Continued

1

Analysis: ▼ **NURSING DIAGNOSIS**

***Risk for impaired gas exchange,* related to**

- Inadequate surfactant
- Immaturity of pulmonary vessel musculature, which restricts vasoconstriction
- Immaturity of central nervous system (CNS)
- Ineffective breathing patterns
- Ineffective airway clearance
- Anemia
- Cold stress

Defining Characteristics

SUBJECTIVE	*OBJECTIVE*
Grunting	Abnormal Po_2
	Abnormal Pco_2
	Symptoms of respiratory distress (tachypnea, nasal flaring, grunting, retractions, rales)
	Diminished or absent breath sounds
	Central cyanosis
	Cardiac arrhythmia

Client Goal/ ▼ **EVALUATION CRITERIA**

Client will demonstrate adequate gas exchange. / ▼ **Client will evidence minimal respiratory distress symptoms, absence of bronchopulmonary dysplasia, normal Po_2/Pco_2 levels.**

▼ **NURSING INTERVENTIONS**	**Rationale**
• Note data placing infant at high risk for impaired gas exchange or respiratory distress. These include gestational age, length of labor, type of delivery, Apgar score, maternal medications during labor, and need for resuscitation.	• Surfactant is necessary for normal lung expansion. It is not produced in sufficient amounts until 32 to 33 weeks' gestation. When there is a long labor, there is a higher degree of hypoxemia associated with a greater number of contractions, which decreases oxygenation. Depressant medications given during labor, such as Demerol, are circulated to the fetus and may depress fetal respirations if

Continued on facing page

NURSING CARE PLANNING GUIDE Continued

	they are not entirely excreted by the time of delivery. The Apgar score incorporates assessment of respiratory effort. Resuscitation at delivery would indicate inadequate gas exchange at that time.
• Assess respiratory rate. Note apnea.	• The normal respiratory rate is 40 to 60 breaths per minute. Normally, respirations are abdominal and periodic but without apnea. Tachypnea indicates respiratory distress. An abnormally low rate indicates respiratory depression. Both are associated with impaired gas exchange.
• Assess for symptoms of respiratory distress. These include tachypnea, nasal flaring, grunting, retractions, and rales.	• The premature newborn may lack sufficient surfactant, which aids lung expansion. In addition, the CNS, which helps regulate respirations, is immature. Immature vascular musculature inhibits vasoconstriction that occurs in response to in creased Po_2 levels. This increases the likelihood of left-to-right shunting through the ductus arteriosus. It also contributes to pulmonary congestion with backup of blood flow in the lungs. All of these predispose the premature to respiratory distress. Tachypnea (>60 breaths per minute) occurs with respiratory distress. Expiratory grunting occurs to maintain expansion of alveoli. Nasal flaring is a mechanism to increase the diameter of the nares to increase oxygen intake. The lung arterioles normally constrict when there is an increased oxygen level; when this is inhibited, there is congestion in the lungs. Rales may be associated with pulmonary vasocongestion.
• Assess for cyanosis.	• Central cyanosis occurs with a low Pao_2 and reduced oxygen saturation.
• Suction nares and oropharynx as needed. Note transcutaneous oxygen monitor or pulse oximeter before suctioning. Limit time of airway obstruction to 10 to 15 seconds. Administer additional oxygen as needed.	• Cilia may not be developed and therefore do not assist in clearing inspired air as effectively. In respiratory distress syndrome, a respiratory exudate develops that can obstruct the airway. Suctioning that is longer than 10 to 15 seconds may stimulate the vagus nerve, causing bradycardia or bronchospasm.
• Assess and record oxygen levels as noted on the transcutaneous oxygen monitor or pulse oximeter. Assess skin under transcutaneous probe site at each probe change.	• These devices provide mechanisms to monitor oxygen levels in a noninvasive way. Transcutaneous electrodes can burn premature skin.
• Assess arterial blood gas values.	• If there is hypoxia, cold stress, or hypercapnia, surfactant production is reduced. Normal values are Pao_2, 50–80 mm Hg or higher; $Paco_2$, 35–45 mm Hg; oxygen saturation, 92%–94%.
• Assess hemoglobin level and hematocrit.	• The preterm newborn is at greater risk for anemia because of decreased iron stores at birth and repeated blood sampling. Anemia is noted by hemoglobin and hematocrit values and indicates lower oxygenation and gas exchange at the tissue level.
• Administer oxygen as needed by mask, hood, endotracheal tube, or mechanical ventilation. Mechanical ventilation includes constant positive airway pressure and intermittent mandatory ventilation	• Hypoxemia and acidemia can decrease surfactant production, increase resistance in pulmonary vasculature, and restrict closing of the ductus arteriosus. Immaturity of the hypothalamus may necessi-

Continued on following page

NURSING CARE PLANNING GUIDE Continued

or intermittent positive-pressure breathing (IPPB) and positive end-expiratory pressure (PEEP).	tate assistance to maintain respiration. PEEP may prevent alveoli collapse, thereby enhancing gas exchange and reducing the amount of oxygen needed. Prolonged high levels of oxygen by IPPB and PEEP predispose to bronchopulmonary dysplasia.
• Note and record oxygen in inspired air (FIO_2) every hour.	• Prolonged high levels of oxygen place the preterm infant at risk for retinal damage (retinopathy of prematurity). The amount of oxygen that is administered is based on arterial oxygen concentration or capillary blood samples and is called FIO_2 (fraction of inspired oxygen).
• Provide for, and note results of, chest radiographs.	• Chest radiographs note atelectasis, or pulmonary congestion.
• Position infant on side with rolled diaper behind back or in supine position with rolled diaper beneath shoulders to produce slight hyperextension.	• Such positions facilitate respirations.
• Perform postural drainage, chest physiotherapy, or lobe vibration as ordered.	• These procedures facilitate removal of respiratory secretions, thereby aiding gas exchange.
• Maintain body temperature (see ineffective thermoregulation).	• Slight changes in environmental temperature can lead to apnea. Oxygen is necessary for metabolism, which helps maintain temperature when there is reduced oxygen or impaired gas exchange.
• Provide feedings by nasogastric or orogastric tubes, not by nipple, until infant is able to suck.	• These feedings require less use of energy and reduce the risk for aspiration that can occur because of an immature suck-swallow reflex.
• Provide tactile stimulation if apnea occurs.	• Touch stimulates the sympathetic nervous system, which stimulates respirations.
• Administer medications ordered to facilitate respirations and gas exchange. These may include sodium bicarbonate, calcium gluconate, and aminophylline.	• Sodium bicarbonate corrects acidosis that occurs with respiratory distress and impaired gas exchange. Apnea may be associated with hypocalcemia; administration of calcium gluconate may, therefore, reduce apnea. Aminophylline stimulates the respiratory center.

2

Analysis: ▼ NURSING DIAGNOSIS

***Risk for fluid deficit or excess,* related to**

Fluid Volume Deficit	Fluid Volume Excess
• Insensible fluid losses in lungs and skin	• Excessive amount of fluids
• Altered intake	• Electrolyte instability

Continued on facing page

NURSING CARE PLANNING GUIDE Continued

- Immature kidney function with inability to conserve fluids
- Electrolyte instability
- Reduced glomerular filtration rate

Defining Characteristics

SUBJECTIVE	*OBJECTIVE*
Fluid Volume Deficit	Fluid Volume Deficit
	Poor skin turgor
	Dry mucous membranes; dry skin
	Depressed anterior fontanelle
	Increased urine output
	Urine specific gravity >1.013; dilute urine
	Glycosuria
	Elevated pulse
Fluid Volume Excess	Fluid Volume Excess
	Weight gain in excess of 20–30 g/day
	Rales, dyspnea, or tachypnea
	Edema
	Elevated blood urea nitrogen and creatinine levels
	Elevated uric acid level
	Acidic pH
	Oliguria

Client Goal/ ▼ EVALUATION CRITERIA

Client will demonstrate adequate fluid volume. / ▼ **Client will evidence adequate hydration, similar intake and output; absence of glycosuria; normal urine specific gravity; normal hematocrit; normal pH; weight gain of 20–30 g/day; normal blood urea nitrogen, creatinine, uric acid levels.**

▼ NURSING INTERVENTIONS	Rationale
Fluid Volume Deficit	
• Assess dehydration. This includes assessing 1. skin turgor 2. anterior fontanelle for depression 3. urine output (amount, frequency, color) 4. specific gravity of urine	• The premature newborn's immature kidneys are often unable to concentrate urine or reabsorb adequate fluids, thereby predisposing the infant to dehydration.
• Weigh daily and record weight at same time of day with the same scale.	• Weight loss may be related to water imbalance or inadequate calorie intake. The premature newborn loses fluid through the lungs and skin. Weight loss should not exceed 1%–2% of total body weight per day.

Continued on following page

NURSING CARE PLANNING GUIDE Continued

• Monitor intake and output and compare. Monitor intravenous (IV) fluids hourly. Monitor output by collection bag or by weighing diapers. Record amount of blood taken in laboratory specimens.	• The output should be 1–3 mL/kg per hour. Fluid needs are 80–100 mL/kg per day and then 120–140 mL/kg per day on the third day of life. A radiant warmer or phototherapy increases insensible water losses by 50%. Blood taken for laboratory tests reduces the fluid volume.
• Assess hemoglobin, hematocrit, and electrolyte values.	• Blood taken for laboratory tests reduces the hemoglobin level and the hematocrit. Dehydration increases the hematocrit (normal hematocrit is 45%–53%) and the sodium level.
• Do a urine specific gravity assay from urine in collection bag or aspirate urine from diaper.	• Renal immaturity and inability to concentrate urine lead to low specific gravity (normal is 1.006–1.013). A low specific gravity indicates excessive fluid volume; a high specific gravity (>1.013) indicates insufficient intake and dehydration.
• Test urine for glucose.	• Glycosuria often occurs as the result of immature kidneys. This may lead to osmotic diuresis and dehydration.
• Assess blood pressure, pulse, and mean arterial pressure.	• A loss in circulating volume may result in shock, lowered mean arterial pressure, and hypotension.
• Minimize loss of water through the skin by using clothing, warming and humidifying oxygen, and monitoring a neutral thermal environment.	• The preterm newborn loses water through the skin because blood vessels are close to the surface and there is little insulating fat.
• Administer IV fluids as ordered.	• Fluid replacement increases the circulating volume.
• Assess calcium, potassium, and serum magnesium levels.	• The preterm infant is at risk for hypocalcemia (calcium <7 mg/dL) because of low stores, depressed parathyroid, stress associated with hypoxia, sepsis, or hypoglycemia. A lowered magnesium level typically accompanies this. Hypokalemia often occurs because of losses with nasogastric tube, diarrhea, and vomiting. Hyperkalemia may occur because of shifts from intracellular to extracellular area, acidosis, or renal failure.
• Assess for symptoms of hypocalcemia. These include lethargy, high-pitched cry, abdominal distention, twitching, hypotonia, convulsions, and apnea.	• The preterm infant is at risk for hypocalcemia as noted before.
• Administer electrolytes as ordered.	• Electrolytes are administered to correct imbalances.
• Assess IV site every hour. Assess for edema or swelling. Do not lower IV fluids below needle level to check needle position.	• Swelling may indicate infiltration or that tape is too tight. When IV fluids are lowered below the needle level to check for needle position, blood backs up. This may clog the needle.
• Assess skin turgor.	• With fluid volume deficit and dehydration, fluid leaves the skin and turgor is poor.
<u>Fluid Volume Excess</u>	
• Weigh daily.	• Weight gain >20–30 g/day indicate edema from excess fluids. Approximately 1 pound weight gain correlates with 1 liter fluid excess.
• Monitor intake and output. Monitor IV fluids, oral feedings, and output by collection bag or by weighing diapers.	• The output should be 1–3 mL/kg per hour. Recording intake and output provides information about fluid balance.

Continued on facing page

NURSING CARE PLANNING GUIDE Continued

• Monitor hemodynamic status.	• With fluid volume excess, blood values are altered.
• Monitor serum electrolytes values.	• Sodium levels decrease with overhydration as a result of dilution.
• Monitor arterial blood gas values.	• Fluid overload in the lungs may lead to decreased oxygen levels in the blood.
• Auscultate breath sounds.	• Fluid volume excess may lead to pulmonary congestion and rales.
• Assess for edema.	• With fluid volume excess, fluid may accumulate, causing edema.

3

Analysis: ▼ NURSING DIAGNOSIS

***Risk for hypothermia or hyperthermia,* related to**

Hypothermia

- Decreased ratio of body mass and body surface area
- Decreased subcutaneous fat; minimal fat
- Limited brown fat
- Exposure to a cold environment

Hyperthermia

- Excessive clothing
- Overwarming
- Inability to sweat
- Inadequate fluids
- Inability to shiver
- Inadequate glycogen stores
- Anaerobic metabolism
- Very thin epidermis with proximity of blood vessels to skin

Defining Characteristics

SUBJECTIVE

Hypothermia

Restlessness

OBJECTIVE

Hypothermia

Skin temperature <97°F

Axillary temperature <97.7°F

Increased activity, restlessness, hyperactive

Poor feeder

Cool, pale skin

Continued on following page

NURSING CARE PLANNING GUIDE Continued

	Cool hands and feet
	Symptoms of respiratory distress
Hyperthermia	Hyperthermia
Restlessness	Axillary temperature >99.5°F
	Perspiration on face, head
	Apnea, seizures
	Increased respiratory rate
	Flushed skin, becoming dry

Client Goal/ ▼ EVALUATION CRITERIA

Client will not have hypothermia or hyperthermia. / ▼ **Client will evidence axillary temperature of 97.7 to 98.6°F; absence of increased activity; absence of perspiration, apnea, seizures, symptoms of respiratory distress; normal heart rate.**

▼ NURSING INTERVENTIONS	Rationale
• Maintain neutral thermal environment. The premature newborn may require radiant warmer, isolette, incubator, or open crib with appropriate clothing.	• A neutral thermal environment is one that assists in maintaining temperature by minimizing heat loss through convection, conduction, radiation, and evaporation. An incubator or isolette provides greater control of environmental temperature.
• Warm humidified oxygen to 88 to 93°F.	• Humidified oxygen that is warmed reduces contact of respiratory tract with cooler air.
• Monitor radiant warmer, and isolette, for temperature and humidity. Environmental temperature should be 98.6°F, relative humidity of 50%–80%.	• Monitoring helps ensure a neutral thermal environment that aids temperature regulation. Monitoring will decrease the risk for hyperthermia. Hyperthermia causes increased metabolic rate, with associated increased need for oxygen and glucose. There is also increased insensible water loss. Hypothermia results in vasoconstriction and increased metabolism, which requires oxygen and increased metabolism, which requires oxygen and calories. If oxygen is not readily available, anaerobic metabolism occurs, which leads to acidosis. There is also depression of respirations caused by inability to respond appropriately to hypoxia. Premature infants have minimal glycogen stores in the liver. Glycogen is converted to glucose for use in metabolism.
• Provide gradual warming after cold stress.	• Rapid increases in temperature can lead to excessive oxygen consumption and apnea.
• Feed regularly by whatever method is appropriate (nasogastric tube, premie nipple). Monitor blood glucose levels.	• Poor feeding is common with thermal instability. Feeding with nipples requires extra energy. Blood glucose level <45 mg/dL indicates hypoglycemia.
• Weigh infant; monitor weight. If there is inadequate weight gain, assess temperature of the environment.	• If the intake consists of sufficient calories and the infant does not gain weight, it may be that the extra calories are used to maintain temperature. Therefore, the environmental temperature should be evaluated and adjusted if needed.

Continued on facing page

NURSING CARE PLANNING GUIDE Continued

- Assess ability to adapt to decreased temperature in isolette or to room temperature.
- Assessment of temperature and for symptoms of hyperthermia and hypothermia will provide information about ability to maintain temperature.
- Monitor laboratory results of studies that may be done for hyperthermia and hypothermia. These may include serum glucose and bilirubin determinations.
- There is an increased need for glucose and oxygen for metabolism that helps maintain temperature. If oxygen needs are not adequate, anaerobic metabolism may result in acidosis. Metabolic acidosis can also occur with hyperthermia. When brown fat is metabolized to maintain temperature, fatty acids are released. They compete with bilirubin for binding sites on albumin, often leading to elevated indirect bilirubin levels.
- Administer intravenous glucose if ordered.
- Dextrose may be given to correct hypoglycemia.

For additional applicable care planning information, see Nursing Diagnosis 3, Risk for hypothermia or hyperthermia, in the Healthy Full-Term Newborn Nursing Care Planning Guide.

4

Analysis: ▼ NURSING DIAGNOSIS

***Risk for central nervous system injury*, related to**

- Hypoxia
- Hypoglycemia
- Birth trauma
- Hyperbilirubinemia (the preterm infant is at greater risk for kernicterus at lower serum bilirubin levels than is the term infant)

Defining Characteristics

SUBJECTIVE

OBJECTIVE

Respiratory distress

Hypoglycemia (twitching, jerking, eye rolling, convulsions)

Tense or bulging fontanelle

Hypotonia

Lethargy

Continued on following page

NURSING CARE PLANNING GUIDE Continued

Large head circumference
Low hemoglobin level and hematocrit
Elevated bilirubin level
High-pitched cry
Opisthotonos
Convulsions
Anemia

Client Goal/ ▼ EVALUATION CRITERIA

Client will remain free from CNS injury. / ▼ **Client will evidence absence of hypoxia, hypoglycemia, hyperbilirubinemia, anemia.**

▼ NURSING INTERVENTIONS	Rationale
• Assess for symptoms of CNS damage. These include 1. lethargy 2. hypotonia 3. tense, bulging fontanelle 4. seizures 5. high-pitched cry 6. labored respirations, cyanosis, apnea 7. flaccid quadriparesis 8. unresponsiveness 9. hypotension 10. tonic posturing	• With increased intracranial pressure, the anterior fontanelle often becomes tense or bulges. Lethargy and hypotonia may occur in preterm infants when there is CNS damage. As the CNS damage increases, symptoms progress to include seizures, respiratory problems, hypotension, and unresponsiveness. CNS damage can occur in the preterm newborn as a result of birth trauma, hypoxia during labor or birth, hypoglycemia, hyperbilirubinemia with kernicterus, subdural hemorrhage, or anemia.
• Assess respirations and apnea. Support respiratory function. Provide supplemental oxygen as needed.	• The preterm infant is at risk for respiratory distress associated with immature lungs. There is diminished gas exchange with respiratory distress as well as lower oxygen levels. As a result, CNS damage may occur.
• Assess for hypoglycemia. This includes observing symptoms of hypoglycemia (twitching, jitteriness, convulsions, eye rolling) and monitoring blood glucose levels. Maintain blood glucose levels by maintaining feeding or administering glucose.	• When blood serum glucose levels are lower than 30–40 mg/dL, the brain can suffer irreparable damage. The preterm infant is at risk for hypoglycemia because glycogen stores are inadequate and the preterm newborn has difficulty in feeding. Therefore, calorie and glucose requirements are often not met. Feeding provides glucose to maintain blood glucose levels.
• Assess for hypocalcemia (twitching, eye rolling, convulsions). Administer calcium as ordered.	• Hypocalcemia often accompanies hypoglycemia. It can lead to apnea and seizures.
• Measure head circumference.	• When increased intracranial pressure occurs as a result of hydrocephalus or subdural hemorrhage, the head circumference may increase.
• Assess for hyperbilirubinemia/kernicterus. This includes assessment of 1. color for jaundice 2. lethargy	• The preterm newborn is at risk for kernicterus at lower bilirubin levels because unconjugated circulating bilirubin can cross the blood-brain barrier more easily. With rising levels, bilirubin may cross

Continued on facing page

NURSING CARE PLANNING GUIDE Continued

3. hyperreflexia
4. opisthotonos
5. convulsions
6. bilirubin levels

the blood-brain barrier and can cause kernicterus, or brain damage.

- Assess for anemia. This includes monitoring hemoglobin levels.

- With low iron stores, hemoglobin levels are decreased. In addition, oxygen levels are lower as a result of respiratory distress. Consequently, the oxygen-carrying capacity is impaired. Lower oxygen levels can cause CNS damage.

- Assist with an exchange transfusion, if needed.

- An exchange transfusion removes blood with high bilirubin levels, replacing it with O-negative blood to prevent further hemolysis of red blood cells, which produce bilirubin.

- Administer medications to control seizures, if necessary. These may include phenobarbital or phenytoin.

- These medications help to control seizures.

5

Analysis: ▼ NURSING DIAGNOSIS

***Altered nutrition: less than body requirements,* related to**

- Inadequate iron stores
- Minimal glycogen stores
- Cold stress that depletes glucose
- Hypoxia that depletes glucose
- Inability of kidney to concentrate and reabsorb substances
- Immature enzyme production that impairs metabolism
- Reduced hydrochloric acid that hampers absorption of fat and fat-soluble vitamins
- Immaturity of cardiac sphincter
- Weak, absent reflexes needed for feeding

Defining Characteristics

SUBJECTIVE

OBJECTIVE

Respiratory distress; unable to nurse

Gags when bottle fed

Dribbles when bottle fed

Tires easily when bottle fed

Requires nipple for premature infants

Unable to maintain adequate suction around nipple

Continued on following page

NURSING CARE PLANNING GUIDE Continued

Loses more than 10%–15% of birth weight

Gains weight slowly

Client Goal/ ▼ EVALUATION CRITERIA

Client will demonstrate adequate nutrition. / ▼ **Client will evidence appropriate weight gain (gains 20–30 g/day).**

▼ NURSING INTERVENTIONS	Rationale
• Assess to determine readiness and ability for feeding. This includes assessment of 1. sucking 2. swallowing 3. gag reflex	• The preterm infant's immature development may result in difficulty with sucking, swallowing, and gagging.
• Assess respirations and respiratory rate.	• When respiratory distress with high respiratory rates occurs (>60 per minute), sucking and feeding are difficult or impossible. Oral fluids cannot be given when there is respiratory distress.
• Assess energy available and degree of fatigue with feeding.	• Energy is expended with feeding. Excessive use of energy to feed leads to fewer calories available for metabolism and growth. If the preterm newborn becomes too fatigued during feedings, tube feedings may be necessary.
• Reduce situations that increase metabolism and need for calories. This includes maintaining the temperature and respirations and handling as little as possible.	• Cold stress results in increased metabolism to maintain the temperature, which uses calories. Respiratory distress results in lower oxygen levels, which alters metabolism. Handling of the infant results in increased activity and energy use. All of these situations require metabolic increases that use calories for these processes rather than for growth and weight gain.
• Weigh daily. Measure head circumference and length weekly.	• Growth is documented by weight gain, growth in head size, and length.
• Auscultate bowel sounds.	• If bowel sounds are present, it is assumed that peristalsis is occurring and feedings can be initiated.
• Observe tolerance of feedings. This includes observation for 1. vomiting 2. regurgitation 3. diarrhea 4. positive guaiac test result 5. excessive gastric residual with tube feedings	• These conditions indicate impaired gastrointestinal functioning with difficulty tolerating feedings. If the gastric residual is >2 mL before a tube feeding, the amount of feeding may need to be decreased.
• Use pacifier during tube feedings.	• Non-nutritive sucking accelerates the development of the sucking reflex and can promote weight gain.

Continued on facing page

NURSING CARE PLANNING GUIDE Continued

• Administer parenteral fluids as needed for total parenteral nutrition (TPN). Assess for reactions. These include 1. elevated temperature 2. dyspnea 3. vomiting 4. cyanosis	• One common complication of TPN is sepsis. Fluid overload, obstruction of the catheter, and dislodgement of the catheter can also occur. The TPN feedings are administered with an infusion pump with an indwelling catheter placed into the vena cava or in a peripheral line. The TPN infusion, which consists of protein hydrolysate, glucose, electrolytes, minerals, and vitamins, is given when there is chronic diarrhea or malabsorption syndrome; after surgical repair of gastrointestinal anomalies; and with obstruction, necrotizing enterocolitis, or extreme prematurity. A TPN infusion of intralipids provides essential fatty acids. It is administered into a peripheral line.
• Administer tube feedings as needed. Ensure proper placement of tube, prevention of air entry to stomach, and slow administration during 20 minutes (1 mL/per minute).	• The nasogastric tube could be improperly placed into the trachea, causing respiratory distress. If the formula is administered too rapidly into the stomach, regurgitation, aspiration, or abdominal distention can occur. Instilling air fills the stomach with air rather than formula.
• Initiate oral feedings when possible. Many start with sterile water, then glucose, then formula. Use a nipple for premature infants at first.	• Oral feeding should be initiated as soon as possible. Calorie intake should provide sufficient calories to prevent catabolism. Formula should provide 120–150 calories per kilogram per day and 3–4 g protein per kilogram per day. Concentrated formulas are used to supply more calories in less volume.
• Initiate intermittent tube feedings as indicated.	• If the infant becomes too fatigued with oral feedings, intermittent tube feeding may be needed.
• Do not perform postural drainage for at least 1 hour after a feeding.	• An hour allows time for absorption of feedings and helps prevent regurgitation, which could occur with handling.

6

Analysis: ▼ NURSING DIAGNOSIS

***Risk for infection,* related to**

- Immature white blood cells (WBCs)
- Reduced transfer of immunoglobulin G (IgG)
- Lack of transfer of immunoglobulin A (IgA) if not breastfed
- Impaired skin integrity
- Ruptured membranes
- Transplacentally acquired infection
- Ascending infection
- Exposure to diagnostic, therapeutic, and monitoring procedures

Continued on following page

NURSING CARE PLANNING GUIDE Continued

Defining Characteristics

SUBJECTIVE	*OBJECTIVE*
Listless	Active infection of parents, visitors, or staff
Poor feeding	Inadequate cord care
	Injection and IV insertion sites not wiped with alcohol
	Equipment not cleaned properly
	Symptoms of sepsis, eye infection, cord infection, or skin infection
	Sudden increase or decrease in WBC count
	Low platelet count (<60,000)
	Temperature instability
	Hypoglycemia
	Hyperglycemia
	Metabolic acidosis
	Culture indicating infection

Client Goal/ ▼ EVALUATION CRITERIA

Client will demonstrate absence of infection. / ▼ **Client will evidence cord drying, absence of phlebitis at IV site, normal WBC count, normal platelet count, normal blood glucose level, normal temperature, normal pH, normal culture, absence of symptoms of infection.**

▼ NURSING INTERVENTIONS	Rationale
• Review labor and delivery records for length of time membranes were ruptured and whether resuscitation was required.	• Resuscitation and other procedures alter skin integrity and expose the premature newborn to pathogens. When membranes are ruptured, pathogens can ascend the maternal reproductive tract and infect the preterm infant. The longer the membranes are ruptured, the greater the risk for infection.
• Note estimated date of confinement. Assess gestational age by the New Ballard Score.	• In the third trimester, IgG is transported across the placenta to the fetus. If the preterm infant is born before 28 to 30 weeks' gestation, IgG transport has been minimal. Therefore, the preterm newborn lacks these protective immunoglobulins.
• Wash hands according to protocol. Have parents wash hands before handling the preterm infant.	• Improper hand washing has been found to be related to increased occurrence of infection in the infant. Hand washing has been found to be the most important infection control practice.
• Ensure proper space between infants, cribs, and isolettes.	• Most agree that 4 to 6 feet of space between infants is advantageous to reduce the spread of droplet and airborne infections.

Continued on facing page

NURSING CARE PLANNING GUIDE Continued

• Isolate infected infants in isolettes or in separate isolation rooms.	• Isolation of infected and potentially infected infants in isolettes or in separate isolation rooms reduces the spread of infection.
• Establish cohorts of infants.	• Grouping of infants born on the same day or within several days limits contact of infants with potential pathogens.
• Follow appropriate medical aseptic practices in handling infant's equipment, linens, and clothing.	• It is advised that each infant's equipment, linens, and clothing be contained within that infant's crib so that pathogens are not transported.
• Assess staff and visitors for infections. This includes skin lesions, draining wounds, respiratory infections, fever, gastroenteritis, active oral herpes simplex, and herpes zoster.	• Visitors and staff who have active infections expose the preterm newborn to pathogens.
• Provide cord care according to hospital protocol.	• Application of various microbials helps prevent infection. Typical agents applied to the cord to prevent infection include triple dye and alcohol.
• Wipe injection site (such as with vitamin K1 injection) or IV site with alcohol (70%) before insertion.	• Wiping the skin with alcohol helps remove pathogens from the skin to reduce exposure to pathogens.
• Use aseptic technique with suctioning. Date solutions used for humidification or nebulization and discard after 24 hours. Clean equipment according to protocol. Replace equipment according to protocol.	• Cleaning and replacing equipment reduces the possibility of contamination.
• Observe for signs of infection. These include 1. hypotonia or hyperthermia 2. lethargy 3. respiratory distress (tachypnea, apnea, cyanosis) 4. petechiae 5. nasal congestion 6. drainage from eyes 7. moist umbilical cord; discharge from umbilical cord 8. rash	• Elevation of temperature, or fever, does not necessarily accompany an infection in the preterm newborn; either hypothermia or hyperthermia can occur. Respiratory distress and nasal congestion could be symptoms of a respiratory infection. Discharge from the eyes could be a symptom of an eye infection. A moist umbilical cord, with drainage, is a symptom of a cord infection. A rash that is differentiated from normal newborn rash could indicate a skin infection.
• Observe for signs of late-onset infection (after the first week).	• Late-onset infections are typically caused by exposure to maternal pathogens in the genital tract or by contaminated equipment or supplies.
• Obtain specimens and assess results of laboratory tests done to diagnose an infection. These could include serial WBC counts with differential, platelet, count, serum glucose determination, pH, urine culture, blood culture, cerebrospinal fluid culture, and sputum culture.	• Specimens from the potentially infected area allow cultures to identify the pathogen and diagnose whether an infection is present; culture also directs appropriate treatment. The preterm newborn has reduced immune responses; the WBC count is lower. A WBC count that suddenly increases or decreases may indicate an infection. Sepsis results in a lower platelet count. The normal platelet count for a preterm is 60,000 to 100,000. Hypoglycemia, hyperglycemia, or metabolic acidosis is often associated with an infection.
• Assist with lumbar puncture.	• If meningitis is suspected, a lumbar puncture is done to obtain cerebrospinal fluid that is examined to identify pathogens and the presence of an infection.

Continued on following page

NURSING CARE PLANNING GUIDE Continued

- Administer antibiotics as ordered.
- Administration of the appropriate antibiotic treats the infection.
- Assess for signs of shock or disseminated intravascular coagulation (DIC). These include
  1. bradycardia
  2. decreasing blood pressure
  3. temperature instability
  4. listlessness
  5. edema of abdominal wall
- DIC may occur with septicemia caused by gram-negative microorganisms.
- Encourage breastfeeding or use of breast milk for feedings.
- Breast milk contains IgA, microphages, lymphocytes, and neutrophils.

7

Analysis: ▼ NURSING DIAGNOSIS

Risk of bowel injury, related to

- Inactivity
- Decreased gastrointestinal motility
- Necrotizing enterocolitis (NEC)
- Altered nutritional intake

Defining Characteristics

SUBJECTIVE

OBJECTIVE

NEC

Distended abdomen

Absent bowel sounds

Bloody diarrhea

Regurgitation

Bile-stained emesis

Excessive gastric residual

Reduced fluid and feeding intake

Dehydration

Diminished bowel sounds

Abnormal stools, constipation or diarrhea

Continued on facing page

NURSING CARE PLANNING GUIDE Continued

Client Goal/ ▼ EVALUATION CRITERIA

Client will demonstrate normal bowel elimination. / ▼ **Client will evidence soft abdomen, active bowel sounds, normal consistency and frequency of stools for breastfed or formula-fed neonate, absence of symptoms of NEC.**

▼ NURSING INTERVENTIONS	Rationale
• Assess stools. This includes assessment of frequency and characteristics.	• The preterm newborn's decreased gastrointestinal motility, inactivity, and altered nutritional intake often result in infrequent stools and abdominal distention.
• Assess bowel sounds.	• The preterm newborn has decreased gastrointestinal motility, which may result in diminished bowel sounds.
• Assess for abdominal distention. This includes measuring abdominal circumference and percussion the abdomen.	• If abdominal distention is occurring, the abdominal circumference will increase and percussion will change (to tympanic sound).
• Assess history for risk factors predisposing the preterm newborn to NEC.	• Various factors have been found to be related to higher risk for NEC. These include hypoxia, sepsis, or patent ductus arteriosus. Other studies indicate that NEC is related to gestational age.
• Ensure adequate fluid intake. This includes 1. supplying sufficient IV, tube, or oral fluids 2. assessing intake and urine output 3. assessing for dehydration	• IV lines, tube feedings, and oral intake supply fluids. Assessment of intake and urine output allows determination of adequacy of fluid intake. Inadequate fluid intake contributes to dry, constipated stools. If fluid intake is inadequate, symptoms of dehydration may occur.
• Reduce trauma and pressure to abdomen. This includes 1. avoiding use of diapers 2. avoiding rectal thermometer 3. touching and stroking extremities, head, and face while talking to infant, rather than handling	• Diapers result in pressure to the abdomen. Rectal thermometers may damage the rectal mucosa. Handling increases the possibility of abdominal pressure. Talking to the infant while stroking the head, face, and extremities provides for nurturing and meeting emotional needs.
• Assess for symptoms of NEC. These include 1. abdominal distention, rigidity, tenderness 2. taut abdominal skin 3. visible bowel loops 4. excessive regurgitation, spitting up 5. bile-stained emesis 6. all of gavage feeding not absorbed; excessive gastric residual 7. absence of bowel sounds	• NEC can lead to bowel perforation and peritonitis; 3%–8% of preterm infants develop NEC.
• Assess for symptoms of sepsis, shock, or DIC. These include 1. bradycardia 2. decreasing blood pressure 3. temperature instability 4. edema of abdominal wall 5. listlessness	• NEC can lead to bowel perforation and peritonitis. Bowel perforation and peritonitis can result in sepsis, shock, and DIC.

Continued on following page

NURSING CARE PLANNING GUIDE Continued

- Assist with, and monitor results of, laboratory tests and radiographs. These may include
  1. WBC count with differential
  2. platelet count
  3. prothrombin time
  4. partial thromboplastin time
  5. abdominal radiographs
  6. stool tested for blood
  7. bloody stool to laboratory for analysis with APT test
- An increased or decreased WBC count with a shift to the left indicates sepsis. Thrombocytopenia or prolonged clotting times may indicate DIC. If NEC is present, the abdominal radiograph would show distended loops of bowel, thickened walls, and ascites. Bloody stools are characteristic of NEC. An Apt test (alum precipitated toxoid) is needed to differentiate maternal from infant blood.
- If NEC develops or is suspected, stop oral or nasogastric feedings for 7 to 10 days and provide TPN feedings.
- Discontinuing oral or nasogastric feedings allows the bowel to rest. This promotes healing. The TPN feedings provide fluids and nutrients to meet nutritional needs.
- If NEC develops, insert orogastric or nasogastric tube and connect to low suction.
- This allows gastric decompression.
- Administer antibiotics as ordered.
- Antibiotics treat enteric infection.
- If NEC requires surgery, prepare for surgery.
- In NEC, surgery may be needed to remove segments of the bowel.

8

Analysis: ▼ NURSING DIAGNOSIS

***Risk for impaired skin integrity,* related to**

- Thin skin, minimal subcutaneous fat
- Fragile capillaries near skin surface
- Invasive procedures

Defining Characteristics

SUBJECTIVE

OBJECTIVE

Redness of areas of skin

Cracking areas of skin

Dry skin

Client Goal/ ▼ EVALUATION CRITERIA

Client will demonstrate skin integrity. / ▼ **Client will evidence intact skin, absence of injury to skin.**

Continued on facing page

NURSING CARE PLANNING GUIDE Continued

▼ NURSING INTERVENTIONS	Rationale
• Observe skin for redness and irritation.	• Redness or irritation of skin indicates areas that are most vulnerable for breakdown.
• Change infant's position routinely.	• Change of position ensures that the same areas of the body and skin are not continuously exposed to pressure, which encourages breakdown of skin.
• Place on fleece or flotation pad.	• The preterm infant's lack of subcutaneous fat predisposes the infant to greater likelihood of skin breakdown over bone prominences. The fleece or flotation pad helps to spread the point of pressure.
• Minimize use of tapes for equipment, such as IV lines and nasogastric tubes, or for urine collection bags.	• Removing tape may remove the epidermis.
• Avoid harsh agents on the skin. Cleanse and bathe gently, mainly with sterile water and mild soap.	• The preterm infant's skin is even more sensitive to cleansing agents than is the full-term infant's skin. Areas that are dry or irritated are more likely to break down.
• Minimize manipulation of infant's skin. Handle gently.	• Frequent use of water dries the skin. Soaps dry the skin and can alter the protective pH of the skin. Gentle handling minimizes trauma.
• Apply petroleum jelly to lips.	• Lips often become dry with reduced fluid intake, absence of oral feedings, and drying effects of oxygen. Application of petroleum jelly helps prevent drying and cracking of lips.
• Apply antibiotic ointment to nares and lips if there is irritation or cracking.	• Applications of an antibiotic ointment may help prevent infection. It also promotes healing of irritated and dry areas.

9

Analysis: ▼ NURSING DIAGNOSIS

***Risk for disorganized infant behavior,* related to**

- Longer hospitalization than for full-term infant
- Immaturity of sensory-perceptual systems
- Restrictive environment of the hospital that limits stimulation
- Reduced interactive handling
- Reduced interaction with parents
- Handling involved with procedures

Continued on following page

NURSING CARE PLANNING GUIDE Continued

Defining Characteristics

SUBJECTIVE	*OBJECTIVE*
Uninterpretable cues	Irritability
	Restlessness
	Apnea
	Color changes
	Bradycardia
	Inability to "alert" and "attend"
	Does not quiet down, does not attend to parental or staff talking
	Unable to follow objects
	Inadequate weight gain

Client Goal/ ▼ EVALUATION CRITERIA

Client will demonstrate organized infant behaviors. / ▼ **Client will evidence normal weight gain, appropriate responses to visual and auditory stimulation.**

▼ NURSING INTERVENTIONS	Rationale
• Assign a primary caregiver for each shift.	• A primary caregiver provides consistent care and follow-through. The caregiver is better able to recognize subtle changes in the infant's behavior. A planned teaching program can be developed for parents.
• Change position frequently. Place rolled diapers at the back for side-lying position or at sides for prone position.	• Changing the preterm newborn's position not only alters areas of pressure to help maintain skin integrity but also provides kinetic stimulation. The preterm newborn is less able to reposition self because of neuromuscular immobility. The rolled diapers provide a sense of security as well as help maintain the position.
• Talk softly to infant. Play soft music.	• Talking provides auditory stimulation. A soft tone is soothing. Music provides auditory stimulation and is soothing.
• Create uterine-like atmosphere at times. Cover isolette or cover top of radiant warmer. Reduce noise, play recordings of placental or maternal heart sounds.	• A dark, quiet environment is soothing and nonstressful. It has been found to be related to weight gain and provides an atmosphere similar to the one the infant would have experienced in utero at this time.
• Place infant in the en face position when infant is held.	• The en face position allows eye contact and provides visual stimulation. The infant is interested in the patterns and movement of eyes.
• Provide designs and pictures in the isolette or crib.	• Visual objects need to be 7 to 9 inches from the face. Infants prefer colors and patterns and attend to them.

Continued on facing page

NURSING CARE PLANNING GUIDE Continued

Intervention	Rationale
• Hold the infant in the over-the-shoulder position for burping.	• This position fosters visual stimulation. This position should be used only if the infant is taking oral feedings without difficulty.
• If infant is receiving phototherapy, uncover eyes periodically.	• Removal of eye patches allows visual stimulation.
• Assess for signs of sensory overload or stress. These include 1. apnea 2. color change 3. bradycardia 4. changes in behavior 5. inability to alert and attend	• If factors associated with sensory overload or stress can be identified, they can be reduced or eliminated. Familiarity with the infant's typical behavior allows identification of subtle behavior changes that may indicate stress. Overstimulation can result in physiologic changes.
• Help parents become aware of the infant's behavioral cues. Encourage parents to interact with the infant and provide appropriate stimulation.	• Parents must learn to recognize the infant's cues, especially those that indicate sensory overload or stress, so that they can reduce stress. If stress is minimized, growth and development is enhanced. Parent-infant interaction fosters attachment and the development of trust in the infant.

Chapter 37

Parenting the High-Risk Neonate

Lynda L. Harrison

> . . . the attachments a parent forms with a high-risk baby may be as important to the child's eventual outcome as all of the hospital's sophisticated medical technology. Even when a baby is very small or very sick at birth, the single most important factor in predicting that child's later development is the quality of the home environment in which he will grow up.
>
> Helen Harrison (1983)

HIGHLIGHTS

- ▼ Parental Reactions to a High-Risk Pregnancy
- ▼ Parental Reactions to the Birth of a High-Risk Infant
- ▼ Parent-Infant Separation
- ▼ Hospitalization-Related Stresses
- ▼ Physical and Behavioral Characteristics of the Infant
- ▼ The Crisis and the Family
- ▼ Parent-Infant Attachment
- ▼ Parents' Relationship with One Another
- ▼ Nursing Practice
- ▼ Implications for Research

Any condition that threatens the health or well-being of the mother, father, or neonate may result in a high-risk pregnancy or delivery and can adversely influence the development of parent-infant attachment. An understanding of the stressors that accompany high-risk parenting can help nurses provide supportive care, promote family coping and adaptation, and promote optimal attachment relationships between physically compromised high-risk infants and parents. The term high-risk infant refers to physically compromised infants, including those born prematurely, those with congenital defects, and those who experience medical problems in the neonatal period.

DEFINITIONS

Anticipatory grief—Expectation of a future loss, frequently precipitated by the crisis of an unexpected illness or by the birth of a high-risk infant. Parents who have high-risk infants and experience anticipatory grief may be hesitant to become involved with their infant's care.

Anticipatory guidance—Counseling or education about what to expect in the future and how to cope with future events.

Crisis—A situation that affects multiple dimensions of an individual, has an uncertain outcome, and may not be resolved with one's usual methods of coping with problems.

High-risk infant—An infant who has an increased likelihood of dying in the neonatal period or an infant who has physiologic problems that threaten health, growth, and development.

Infant social behaviors—Actions of the infant that stimulate and encourage interaction with the caregiver. These behaviors include smiling, gazing, maintaining a quiet and alert state, and grasping.

Interdisciplinary team approach—A method in which members of different disciplines collaborate together in providing services to individuals and families.

Physiologically fragile infant—An infant whose physical condition is unstable and who requires specialized nursing, medical care, and technologic support.

PARENTAL REACTIONS TO A HIGH-RISK PREGNANCY

Family members' reactions to a high-risk pregnancy and birth are influenced by multiple factors including the severity of the mother's or infant's health problem, available support, individual personality variables, and coping styles. Sources of family stress include fear about the pregnancy outcome as well as diagnostic and therapeutic measures needed for treatment of the high-risk condition (Kemp and Page 1986). Parents may be fearful of unfamiliar diagnostic procedures, such as amniocentesis or chorionic villus sampling. Other diagnostic tests may provide helpful reassurance. In a study of 20 women who had normal ultrasound examinations during the second and third trimesters of pregnancy, researchers found that "in most cases, sonography appeared to increase the women's feelings of attachment to and identification with their babies" (Milne and Rich 1981, p. 36). Further research is needed to examine emotional consequences of abnormal sonographic findings (e.g., congenital anomalies or abnormal fetal size).

If the mother is hospitalized for prolonged periods during the pregnancy or after delivery, the family experiences stress related to separation, disruption of familiar routines, and financial strain. High-risk pregnancies often result in limited choices related to childbirth that may lead to further disappointment and frustration. Parents may also have unmet educational needs if they are unable to attend childbirth education classes as planned or if they have not obtained needed information from other sources.

PARENTAL REACTIONS TO THE BIRTH OF A HIGH-RISK INFANT

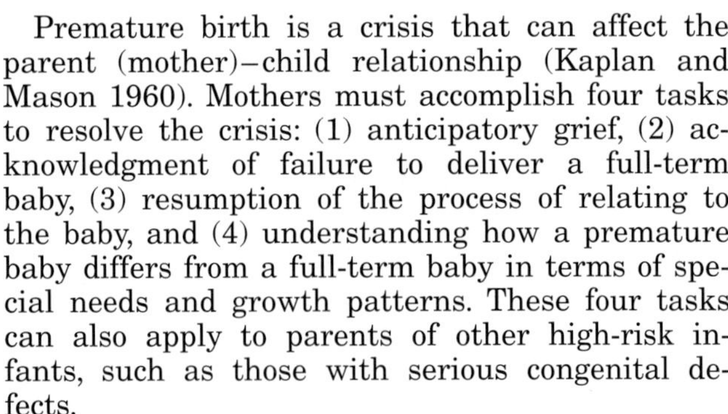

Premature birth is a crisis that can affect the parent (mother)–child relationship (Kaplan and Mason 1960). Mothers must accomplish four tasks to resolve the crisis: (1) anticipatory grief, (2) acknowledgment of failure to deliver a full-term baby, (3) resumption of the process of relating to the baby, and (4) understanding how a premature baby differs from a full-term baby in terms of special needs and growth patterns. These four tasks can also apply to parents of other high-risk infants, such as those with serious congenital defects.

The multiple stresses that result from the birth of a high-risk infant can be grouped into four major categories: unexpected pregnancy outcome, separation of parents and infant during the early neonatal period, hospitalization-related stresses, and physical and behavioral characteristics of the infant.

Unexpected Pregnancy Outcome

Most parents fantasize about their hoped-for, expected infant throughout pregnancy. When an in-

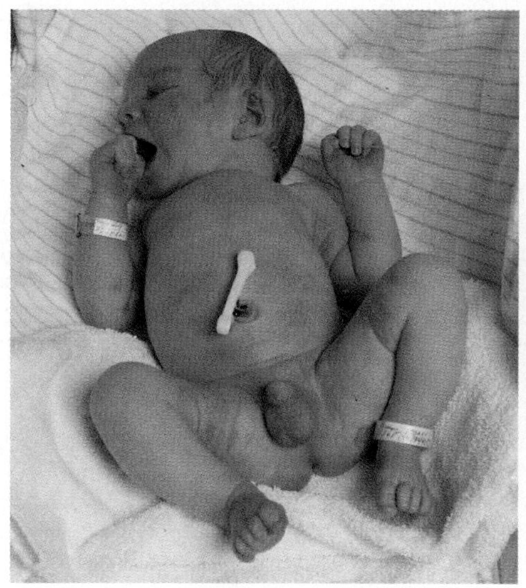

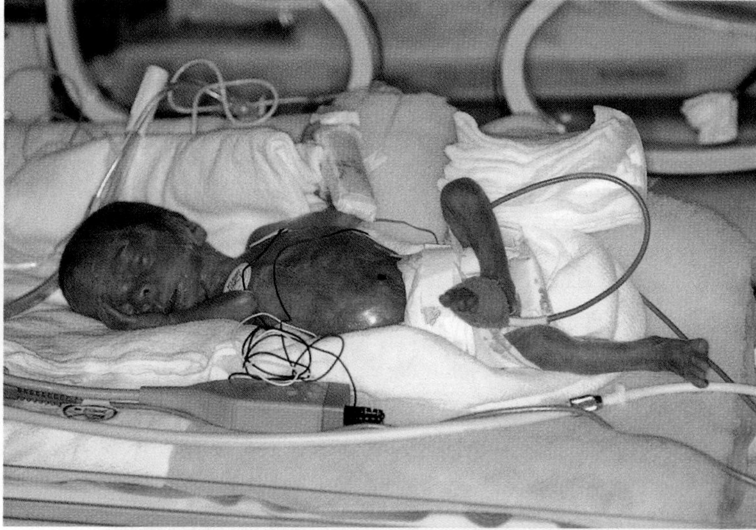

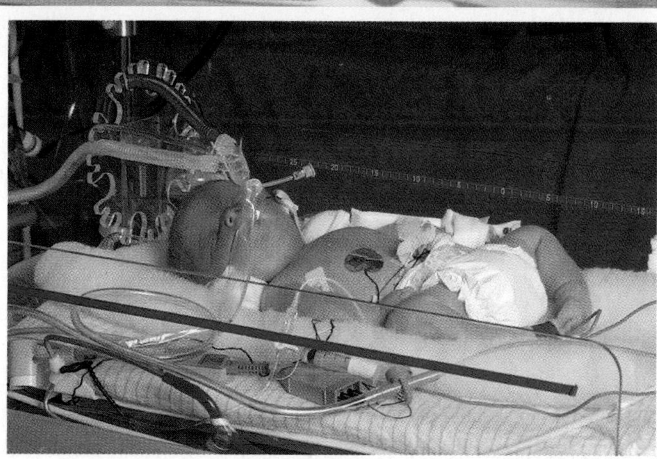

Figure 37–1

Mothers and fathers of high-risk infants experience anguish, fear, and uncertainty in contrast to the joy and excitement they would have felt at the birth of the healthy, full-term newborn they expected. The three photos contrast a healthy, full-term newborn *(upper left),* a preterm infant *(upper right),* and a sick full-term newborn *(lower left).* (Photograph of preterm infant courtesy of Wesley Medical Center, Wichita, KS.)

fant is born prematurely or with a serious health problem, parents are faced with the difficult psychological task of reconciling their real infant with their fantasized ideal infant (Taylor and Hall 1979) (Fig. 37–1). Health problems or stressors of the mother or father may have precipitated the preterm delivery and may still be present after delivery to cause additional problems in parenting (e.g., hypertension, diabetes, alcoholism, sickle cell anemia, drug abuse, or nutritional problems). Table 37–1 illustrates the contrasting emotional reactions and adjustments that may follow the birth of a healthy full-term infant and of a premature infant.

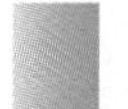

Parent-Infant Separation

Even though the hypothesis of a sensitive period for the development of human parent-infant attachment has not yet been supported, prolonged separation of parents and infants during the newborn period is a major source of family stress. In most neonatal intensive care units (NICUs), parents are encouraged to visit their infants as often as they like. Many parents, however, are able to spend relatively little time with their infants during this period, particularly if they live far from the hospital, have other children to care for at home, or are exhausted from dealing with a stressful pregnancy and childbirth experience. Parents may also experience stress related to coping with preexisting problems that may have contributed to preterm birth or congenital defects (e.g., drug abuse, alcoholism, diabetes). The equipment that is used in caring for the infant often limits parent-infant contact when the parents do visit the nursery and thus imposes a type of mechanical separation (Johnson 1986) (Fig. 37–2). In addition, parental fears of interacting with their child may result in a type of emotional distancing or separation from the child (Johnson 1986). The effects of this type of separation are compounded when parents lack confidence in their parenting abilities and perceive the nursery staff as more efficient caretakers of their infants.

Table 37–1

PARENTS' USUAL EMOTIONAL REACTIONS AND ADJUSTMENT TO FULL-TERM AND PREMATURE BIRTHS

	FULL-TERM BIRTH	PREMATURE BIRTH
Perceptions of event	Gain, success	Loss, failure
Reactions to birth	Joy, relief	Grief, concern
Emotional preparation	Complete	Incomplete
Expectation confirmed	"Wished-for" baby	"Feared" baby
Self-esteem	Increased	Decreased
Baby's primary caregivers	Mother, father	Nurses, physicians
Parents and infants	Together	Separated
Baby's social responsiveness	Well-developed	Decreased or absent
Mother goes home with	Baby	Empty arms
Major psychological tasks remaining	Reconciling real baby and fantasized baby	Grieving for expected baby; anticipatory grieving for baby; individualizing and accepting baby

From Taylor, P. M., and Hall, B. L. (1979). Parent-infant bonding: Problems and opportunities in a perinatal center. *Seminars in Perinatology,* 3 (1), 73–84.

Hospitalization-Related Stresses

Parents whose infants were hospitalized in an NICU have reported that their most stressful experiences were seeing the infant turn blue or pale, seeing the infant stop breathing, being separated for long periods, observing the infant in pain, not knowing how to help the infant, being unable to hold or protect the baby from pain, and feeling that the staff were not communicating openly

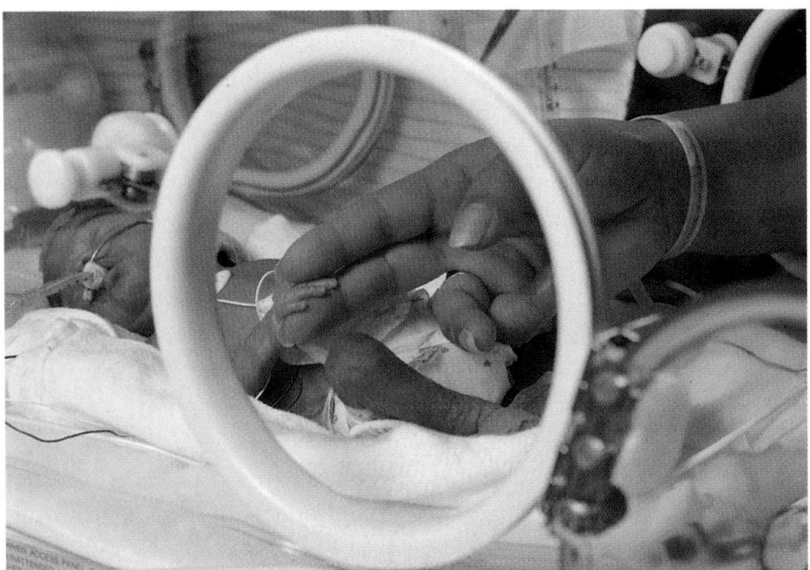

Figure 37–2

The technology and equipment used in the neonatal intensive care unit (NICU) to support the physical needs of premature and sick neonates places additional stress on parental-infant attachment as well as care and comfort of the newborn.

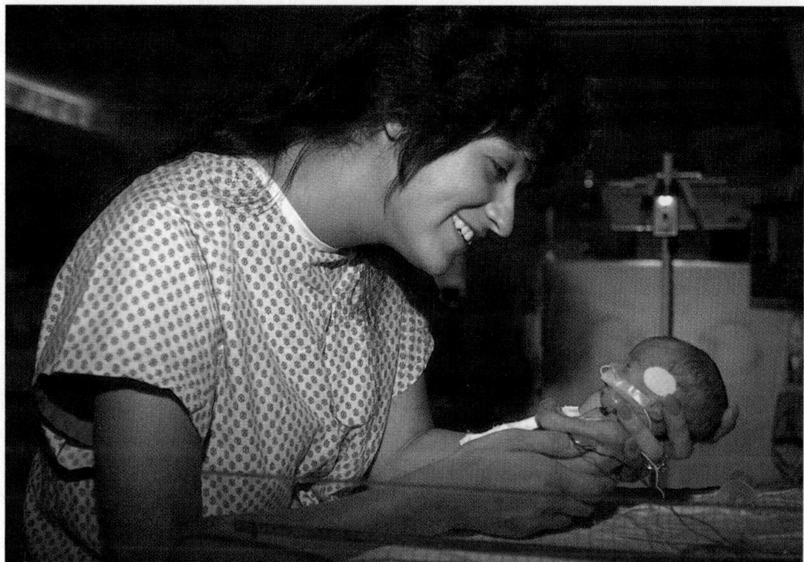

Figure 37–3

Both parents may benefit by spending time alone with their infant. Each parent and baby is unique, and mutual love between a parent and baby develops in its own distinctive way and at its own pace.

about the infant's condition (Miles 1989). Parents also reported being stressed when NICU staff members acted cold, distant, or uncaring. The aspects of the physical environment that were most stressful to parents were malfunctioning equipment and the sounds of monitor alarms.

Another stress imposed by the infant's hospitalization is the tremendous financial burden that is incurred by the family (Brooten 1983). The lack of privacy in the busy nursery environment is also stressful for some parents and interferes with the normal progression of the acquaintance process. In a study examining the behavior of mothers and fathers toward their infants during NICU visits, Thurman and Korteland (1989) found that both mothers and fathers demonstrated more intimate behaviors (e.g., touch, stroke, kiss, and hold) when they visited their infants alone than when they visited together (Fig. 37–3). These investigators suggested that parents may feel the need to support one another, and thus be less focused on the infant, when they visit together. Parents may need opportunities to visit their infants individually to begin to develop an attachment with the infant.

Other aspects of the NICU environment that may affect early parent-infant interactions include the constant stimulation provided by lighting and equipment sounds, the continuous and often unpredictable interventions provided by caregivers, the acute and rapidly changing nature of the infant's medical status, and the intimidating presence of the medical apparatus needed to maintain the infant's stability (Gottwald and Thurman 1990, p. 2). Fathers are often stressed by the extra demands on their time as they attempt to support their wives and other children, establish a relationship with the new infant, and continue their work responsibilities.

Physical and Behavioral Characteristics of the Infant

The physical appearance and behaviors of premature and other high-risk infants may be a source of stress for the parents whose infants were hospitalized in an NICU (Miles 1989). Some parents of premature infants, for example, have been bothered by the infants' large and elongated heads, thin extremities, and transparent skin. Parents of a child with obvious congenital defects, such as cleft lip or palate, ambiguous genitalia, or myelomeningocele, may also be distressed by their infant's appearance.

The care-soliciting and social behaviors of high-risk infants, particularly premature infants, may be less effective than those of full-term or healthy newborns. Preterm infants, for example, sleep more and are usually less active when they are awake than full-term healthy infants are (Brown and Bakeman 1980). Their cry is usually high pitched and weak. The cries of premature infants are perceived by parents as more aversive than the cries of full-term babies (Frodi et al. 1978). Other high-risk infants, such as those with congenital heart defects, also tend to be relatively inactive. As a result of these characteristics, early parent-infant interactions may be frustrating and stressful for the parents. Some parents respond to the decreased attentiveness of their infants by becoming more active and providing their infants with additional stimulation, although such activity often results in decreased interaction from the infant because it is too stressful for the infant. Thus, the parent's increased stimulation may be counterproductive in promoting satisfying parent-infant interactions (Field 1977).

Text continued on page 1420

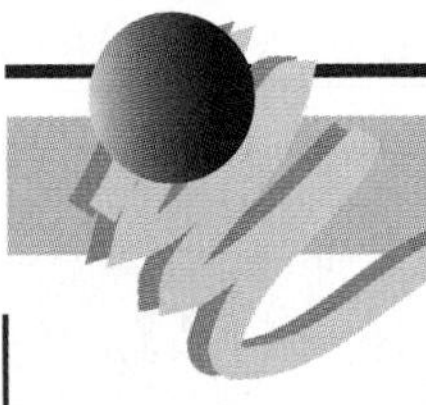

TEACHING GUIDE

HELPING PARENTS UNDERSTAND THEIR PREMATURE INFANT'S BEHAVIORS AND PROVIDE APPROPRIATE DEVELOPMENTAL STIMULATION

TOPIC	*MAJOR CONCEPTS*
Stages of behavioral development in the preterm infant	Preterm infants move through three stages of neurosocial behavioral development at individual rates. These stages influence the infant's behaviors and responses to stimulation from parents and from the environment (Gorski et al. 1979). • The first stage, the physiologic or in-turning stage, lasts until about 32 weeks of conceptional age. The length of this stage is influenced by factors such as postconceptional age at birth and medical-physiologic complications during the neonatal period. • During this stage, the infant's energies are focused on maintaining physiologic homeostasis, and there is little energy available for social interactions. Infants at this stage often become overwhelmed and distressed with supplemental stimulation. During this stage, infants are able to maintain an alert state for 5 to 10 minutes and are often better able to recover from agitation when they are left alone than when they are actively consoled (Luddington 1983). • During the second coming-out stage, the infant begins to show signs of behavioral organization in response to environmental stimuli. • This coming-out stage begins when the baby is no longer acutely ill and lasts until the baby is able to be discharged home. • During the third stage (which generally begins at around 34 to 35 weeks of conceptional age), the infant is able to maintain basic physiologic homeostasis and begins to seek social interaction.
Reflex behaviors	• Preterm infants may have an exaggerated Moro reflex and startle easily when parents touch or talk to them. Approaching the infant slowly may limit this response. • Initially, the preterm infant's grasp may be weak. • Until 32 to 34 weeks' gestational age, preterm infants may have difficulty coordinating sucking and swallowing. • As the baby matures, all of these reflexes will develop.

Continued on facing page

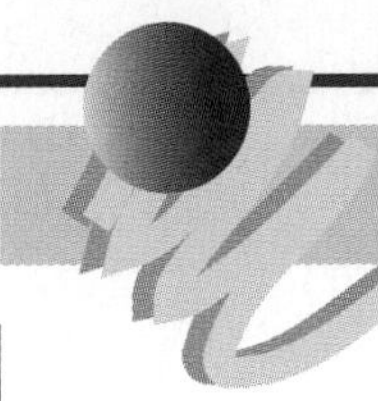

HELPING PARENTS UNDERSTAND THEIR PREMATURE INFANT'S BEHAVIORS AND PROVIDE APPROPRIATE DEVELOPMENTAL STIMULATION

TOPIC	*MAJOR CONCEPTS*
Behavioral states	Infants' behavioral states represent different degrees of arousal and have a significant influence on their interactions and behavioral responses. Blackburn (1983) identified caregiving implications of the six major behavioral states as follows: • Quiet sleep: Infants in this state have occasional startles, but no facial or eye movements, and are difficult to arouse. Parents should not try to feed babies in this state. • Active sleep (light sleep or rapid eye movement [REM] sleep): This state is characterized by rapid eye movements beneath closed eyelids, irregular respirations, and occasional smiles. Babies spend most of their sleep time in light sleep and may make fussy or crying sounds during this state before they are ready to awaken or feed. • Drowsy: In this state, the baby's eyes may be open or closed, and responses to stimulation are delayed. Caregivers can arouse drowsy infants to a more alert state by providing visual or auditory stimulation (Blackburn 1983). • Quiet alert: During this state, infants' eyes are open and bright, and they are receptive to environmental stimuli and to interactions from their caregivers. • Active alert: Infants in this stage have high levels of body activity and may be fussy and sensitive to disturbing stimuli such as "hunger, noise, fatigue or excessive handling" (Blackburn 1983, p. 81s). Babies in this stage may need calming and consoling by their caregivers. • Crying: Crying is the means by which infants communicate their needs. Babies can sometimes return to lower states by using consoling behaviors such as hand-to-mouth movements, sucking, changing position, or attending to the environment (Brazelton 1984).
Behavioral differences in infants	• Each baby is a unique person and has individual patterns of behavior that influence parent-infant interactions.

Continued on following page

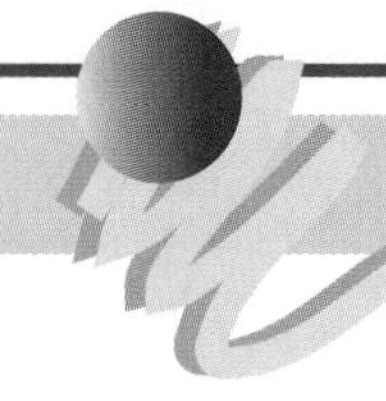

HELPING PARENTS UNDERSTAND THEIR PREMATURE INFANT'S BEHAVIORS AND PROVIDE APPROPRIATE DEVELOPMENTAL STIMULATION

TOPIC	*MAJOR CONCEPTS*
	• Understanding the behavioral patterns of their infants can help parents develop more satisfying early interactions. • Parents can identify the unique behavioral patterns of their infants in these areas by periodically completing an Infant Behavior Assessment Record (Blackburn 1991). Blackburn (1991) identified caregiving implications for eight aspects of infant behavioral patterns. 1a. Visual response: Babies vary in their abilities to follow and focus on an object. Parents can encourage visual responses by holding the baby in a semi-upright position and talking to the infant while moving slowly from one side to the other. 1b. Auditory response: As preterm infants mature, they are increasingly able to turn their heads to an auditory stimulus. 2. Habituation: Infants differ in their abilities to decrease their responses to repeated stimuli. Babies who have difficulty with habituation may need a less stimulating environment. 3. Cuddliness: Although most infants enjoy being cuddled, some babies become agitated when they are held too closely. Parents may misinterpret an infant's resistance to cuddling as indicating lack of attachment. 4. Consolability: Infants also differ in the ease with which they can console themselves or be consoled by others. Infants respond differently to various consoling measures, such as touching, swaddling, holding, rocking, holding arms, or sucking on a pacifier. Parents can try various methods to learn what works best for their infant. 5. Motor behavior and activity: During the early weeks, preterm infants' movements may be jerky, and the infant may have frequent startles or chin tremors. As the infants mature, their movements will become smoother and more coordinated.

Continued on facing page

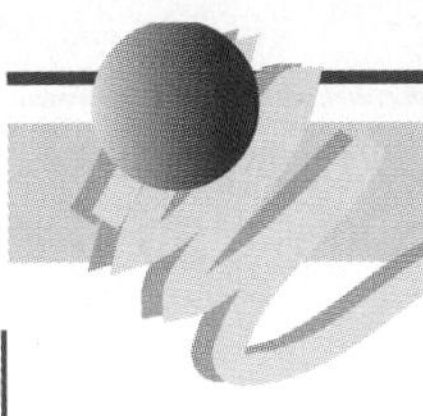

HELPING PARENTS UNDERSTAND THEIR PREMATURE INFANT'S BEHAVIORS AND PROVIDE APPROPRIATE DEVELOPMENTAL STIMULATION

TOPIC	*MAJOR CONCEPTS*
	6. Irritability: Some infants are more sensitive to internal and external stimuli and have frequent periods of fussing and crying. These babies need frequent consoling and predictable routines. Parents need to learn that the infant's irritability is related to his or her temperament and not to the parent's caregiving. 7a. Readability: "Infants differ in the clarity with which they make their needs known and in the consistency of their sleeping, waking, and eating cycles" (Blackburn 1991). 7b. "By observing and understanding an infant's characteristic patterns, parents can respond more appropriately to their infant as an individual" (Blackburn 1991). 8. Smiling: During the first few weeks of life, most smiles are reflexive. Social smiles develop by the age of 40 to 43 weeks after conception and are reinforced by parents' responses to the smile.
Signs of attention	Parents should base their interactions and stimulation on the infant's responses. Signs of attentiveness include decreased motor activity and turning toward or looking at the stimulus (Blackburn 1983, p. 83s).
Behaviors indicating distress	Young preterm infants may become easily overwhelmed with too much stimulation. Blackburn (1983) described signs of sensory overload or distress, including • Blank, dazed appearance or gaze aversion • Color changes (pale, mottled, dusky, cyanotic, or red) • Increased, decreased, or irregular respiratory or heart rate • Jerky limb movements • Hiccups • Spitting • Vomiting • Decreased muscle tone Such signs suggest the need for decreased or more soothing stimulation.

Continued on following page

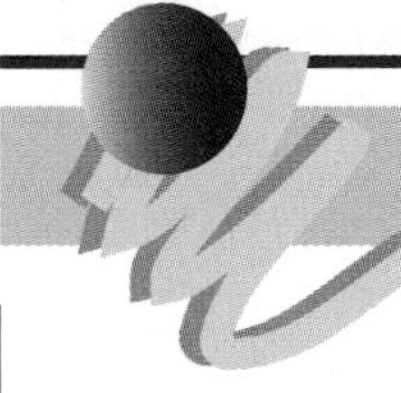

HELPING PARENTS UNDERSTAND THEIR PREMATURE INFANT'S BEHAVIORS AND PROVIDE APPROPRIATE DEVELOPMENTAL STIMULATION

TOPIC	*MAJOR CONCEPTS*
Providing appropriate stimulation to promote infant development	• Infants are most receptive to stimulation when they are in the quiet alert state and when their basic physiologic needs have been satisfied. • The quality and quantity of stimulation should be based on the infant's individual interests and responses. • Appropriate timing of stimulation is important. "The stimulus needs to be available long enough to arouse the infant's interest. However, if the infant receives a constant, unphased barrage of stimuli with no pauses for response, he/she may become fussy or turn away or decompensate physiologically" (Blackburn 1983, p. 82s). • Because preterm infants may become easily "overstimulated," it may be best initially to stimulate only one sensory modality at a time (Blackburn 1983, p. 85s).
Auditory stimulation	• Infants prefer sounds of the human voice; rhythmic, continuous sounds (e.g., a heartbeat) have a soothing effect. • Many preterm infants become responsive to auditory stimuli before they develop the ability to respond to visual stimuli (Blackburn 1983, p. 82s).
Visual stimulation	• Preterm infants may not exhibit visual alertness until they reach 36 to 40 weeks of conception age. • Infants are best able to see objects placed 6 to 8 inches away from their eyes. • Parents can stimulate visual alertness when the infant is in a drowsy, quiet alert, or active alert state by holding him or her in an upright or en face position, talking to the infant, and shading the baby's eyes from bright lights (Blackburn 1983, p. 82s).
Tactile stimulation	In the NICU, infants who are in the physiologic state of behavioral development (e.g., less than 32 weeks' gestational age) may not be able to tolerate vigorous tactile stimulation such as stroking. Parents should observe the infant's responses to determine the best ways to touch

Continued on facing page

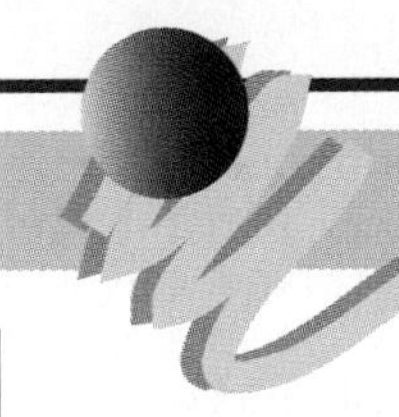

HELPING PARENTS UNDERSTAND THEIR PREMATURE INFANT'S BEHAVIORS AND PROVIDE APPROPRIATE DEVELOPMENTAL STIMULATION

TOPIC

MAJOR CONCEPTS

their infants. Simply placing a hand on the baby's head or hand may be the most appropriate type of tactile stimulation for very small, medically fragile infants.

Luddington (1983) identified the following principles of stimulation with the high-risk premature infant:

1. Observe for behaviors indicating distress to identify optimal levels of stimulation.
2. Contain limbs when moving infants to prevent cardiac or respiratory distress.
3. Be aware that neuromuscular development occurs in spurts, with occasional regressions.
4. Limit the amount of supplemental stimulation provided to infants during the physiologic and coming-out stages.
5. Do not present auditory, visual, or tactile stimulation to infants in the coming-out phase during light sleep or fussy states. Begin sensory stimulation when these infants are in an active alert state.

Teaching Aids

1. *Baby Behavior—How Your Baby Expresses Personal Style.* A pamphlet for parents written by Judi Withers, C.R.N. M.N. Available from The Childbirth Center at Northwest Hospital, 1550 N. 115th Street, Seattle, WA 98133, (206) 364–0500.
2. *Getting to Know Your Premature Baby.* Written by Lynda Harrison, R.N., Ph.D., and available from Children's Hospital Child Health Education Center, P.O. Box 15010, Knoxville, TN 37901.
3. *My Special Signals—A Guide to Parents of Premature Infants.* Pamphlet illustrating preterm infants' behavioral cues and suggestions for interactions. Available from the Patient Education Office, Division of Education and Research, North Carolina Memorial Hospital Department of Nursing, Chapel Hill, NC 27514.
4. *Nursing Systems Toward Effective Parenting—Preterm* (NSTEP-P). A continuing education program that teaches home visitors how to implement protocols designed to help parents provide optimal care for their preterm infants after hospital discharge. For further information, contact Nursing Child Assessment Satellite Training, University of Washington, WJ–10, Seattle, WA 98195, (206) 543–8528.
5. *The Premature Baby.* (1987). Videotape developed by Judi Withers, R.N., demonstrating a preterm infant's behavioral responses and performance on Brazelton's Neonatal Behavioral Assessment Scale. Available from Telemation, 1200 Stewart Street, Seattle, WA 98101.
6. *The Premature Infant.* Videotape MD261653, available from 55 Inverness Drive East, Englewood, CO 80112–5498. Describes physical and behavioral characteristics of preterm infants.
7. *Touch—The Language of Love.* Pamphlet available from Johnson & Johnson Baby Products Company, Grandview Road, Skillman, NJ 08558 (1-800-526-3967). Includes a section on touch and the preterm infant.

Another characteristic of premature infants that may affect early parent-infant interactions is the immaturity of their reflex behaviors. Parents are often disappointed in not being able to feed their infants from the breast or bottle because of the infant's weak suck and swallow reflexes that necessitate gavage feeding (Johnson and Grubbs 1975). Immaturity of the reflexes controlling respirations in preterm infants often results in apneic episodes that are extremely frightening to parents. The exaggerated Moro reflex may cause parents to fear touching their infants. Finally, parents may be disappointed if their infants are not able to hold on to their fingers because of an immature or weak grasp reflex.

EFFECTS OF THE BIRTH OF A HIGH-RISK INFANT

The Crisis and the Family

Most parents of high-risk infants experience grief over the loss of their expected infant and some degree of anxiety regarding the infant's prognosis (Gennaro 1986). Many factors influence the parents' reactions to the crisis, including age, socioeconomic status, culture, previous experiences, and existing support system. Their grief reactions may be manifested by feelings of shock, anger, fear, depression, helplessness, and guilt or a sense of inadequacy (Johnson 1986; Klaus and Kennell 1982; Taylor and Hall 1979). A model to describe parental adaptation to the birth of a child with a congenital malformation was developed by Drotar and coworkers (1975). According to this model, family members progress through five stages after the birth of a child with a congenital defect: shock; denial; sadness, anger, and anxiety; adaptation reflected by increased ability to care for the infant; and reorganization, reflected by increased satisfaction with the infant. If family members move through these stages at different times, as they often do, conflict may result.

Parent-Infant Attachment

The birth of a high-risk infant poses risks for the development of optimal parent-infant attachments. The rate of child abuse is higher among children who were born prematurely than among children born at term (Hunter et al. 1978; Lynch and Roberts 1977). Leonard and associates (1990) observed 129 very-low-birth-weight infants from birth to school age and found that 15 percent had referrals for abuse or neglect. Siefert and coworkers (1983) found that lack of family closeness was a better predictor of parenting problems in parents of high-risk infants than were factors such as infant morbidity or the parents' experiences in the NICU.

When parents expect that their child may die prematurely, they may be reluctant to develop a close attachment to the child (Moore 1983). Green and Solnit (1964) reported that parents who worry that their child may die prematurely often have difficulty in developing a secure attachment relationship with the child and in providing appropriate discipline as the child grows. Children who are perceived by their parents as "vulnerable" may be aware of their parents' perceptions and as a result have unusual difficulties with separation, frequent psychosomatic complaints, and problems with academic achievement (Green and Solnit 1964). Parents of all high-risk infants must resolve their grief before they can develop a close attachment to the infant.

Despite the increased frequency of problems in parent-infant attachment, most parents of high-risk infants who receive adequate support do eventually develop satisfying attachment relationships with their babies. Herzog (1979), for example, interviewed 100 families of premature infants and found that 80 percent of the mothers eventually became attached to their infants. Those who had experienced prolonged postpartum depression or had unsupportive husbands were most likely to have problems with attachment.

Parents' Relationship with One Another

The relationship between the mother and father before the infant's birth has a great impact on how the family copes with the crisis and how the crisis affects the couple's subsequent relationship. Parents who are mutually supportive and who maintain open lines of communication often experience increased closeness as a result of the crisis. Those who are unable to be mutually supportive or who tend to blame one another for the infant's problems often experience marital conflict as a result of the crisis. Nursing interventions that foster open communication and support between the mother and father have a great impact on prevention of future conflict and family disunity. It is also important to use an interdisciplinary team approach and make referrals to other professionals (such as social workers, psychologists, or chaplains as appropriate).

Siblings and Members of the Extended Family

It is easy for siblings and extended family members to feel neglected during the early weeks after the birth of a high-risk infant. The parents' attention is frequently centered on the infant, and most of their time is spent at the hospital. If hospital policies do not allow siblings and grandparents to visit the infant in the NICU, their feelings of isolation are compounded.

Siblings' reactions to the birth of a high-risk infant vary with the developmental stage of the sibling and with the particular family situation. Aspects of the infant's hospitalization that may be stressful for the siblings include frequent changes in caretaking arrangements, decreased financial resources available for family activities, difficulty in understanding behavioral changes in the parents, and difficulty in explaining the baby's condition to peers (Sammons and Lewis 1985). After the preterm infant returns home, siblings face stressors related to jealousy over the amount of time parents spend with the infant and difficulty accepting protective restrictions on their interactions with the infant or on visits from friends (Sammons and Lewis 1985).

Grandparents' reactions to a preterm birth are similar to the parents' reactions. In addition, they grieve because the parents are exposed to a difficult situation. Grandparents need help resolving their own reactions to the high-risk infant before they can support the parents (Blackburn and Lowen 1986). Major sources of stress for grandparents after the birth of a preterm infant include the atmosphere in the NICU, which serves as a reminder to the grandparents of their own mortality, and difficulty in knowing how to be helpful but not overbearing to the infant's parents (Sammons and Lewis 1985). Many times, both the grandparents and friends feel helpless and frustrated (Nance 1982). If the grandparents and parents have a mutually supportive relationship, the wisdom and experience of the grandparents can be a tremendous source of support to both the parents and the other siblings (Sammons and Lewis 1985).

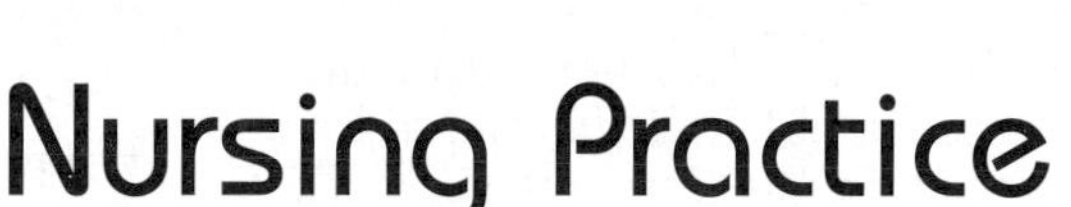

Nursing Practice

Nursing Process

▼ Assessment

To plan appropriate nursing interventions to promote attachment between high-risk infants and parents, nurses must first assess the parents' reactions to the high-risk pregnancy and the infant after delivery. During the prenatal period, nurses should assess behaviors that reflect accomplishment of the developmental tasks of pregnancy (see Chapter 17). The following behaviors may indicate problems in task accomplishment and potential problems with parent-infant attachment (Moore 1983):

- Delay in seeking prenatal care
- Consideration of abortion or relinquishment of the baby
- Missed appointments or lack of cooperation with the treatment plan
- Verbal statements indicating a lack of acceptance of the pregnancy by either the mother or her significant others

- Lack of interest in the fetus or in fetal movement
- Failure to prepare for the birth

If the infant is born prematurely or with significant health problems, nursing assessment should be focused on behaviors that reflect the normal grieving process. The strategies outlined in Chapter 34 for assessing early parent-infant relationships can also be used to assess the early interactions between high-risk parents and infants.

▼ Diagnosis

As soon as the possibility of a high-risk pregnancy or birth is suspected, nursing interventions should be initiated to help parents cope with their probable crisis and to promote optimal parent-child relationships. Interventions should be based on nursing assessment and diagnosis. In addition, the diagnoses related to parenting of healthy infants that were outlined in Chapter 34 may also apply to parents of high-risk infants. In this chapter, intervention strategies for high-risk parents at four different periods are reviewed: during the prenatal and intrapartum experience, during the early days of the infant's hospitalization in the NICU, during the infant's prolonged hospital stay, and after the infant's discharge from the hospital.

Diagnoses that are applicable to these periods include

- Altered family processes related to a family that normally functions effectively experiencing dysfunction
- Anticipatory grieving related to individual/family grieving before an actual loss
- Dysfunctional grieving related to extended, unsuccessful use of intellectual and emotional responses by which individuals attempt to work through the process of modifying self-concept based on the perception of loss
- Fatigue related to an overwhelming sustained sense of exhaustion and decreased capacity for physical and mental work
- Fear related to the feeling of dread identified by a source that the person validates
- Ineffective family coping: compromised, related to insufficient, ineffective, or compromised family support systems that may alter the family member's or family's competence in adaptive tasks concerning the present health challenge
- Ineffective family coping: disabling, related to the behavior of one or more family members that incapacitates the family (or individual members) to therapeutically adapt to the existing health challenge
- Ineffective individual coping related to impairment of adaptive behaviors and problem-solving abilities of a person in meeting life's demands and roles
- Situational low self-esteem related to a negative self-evaluation or feelings about self that develop in response to a loss or change in an individual who previously had a positive self-evaluation

▼ Planning

The goals for the nursing care of each family will depend on the needs of that family and the health status of their infant(s). Goals will be unique to each family and change continuously depending on the condition of the infant and the parents' level of involvement in caring for the infant. General goals for nursing care that are usually applicable to all parents with high-risk infants are as follows:

- Promote each parent's ability to cope effectively with the situation
- Facilitate each parent's ability to grieve in relation to the loss of the expected infant
- Promote parent-infant attachment by teaching parents how to nurture and care for their high-risk infant
- Enable parents to increase competence and attachment to the infant by encouraging them to participate in the care of their infant
- Foster effective family coping through the identification of support systems and provision of needed resources

▼ Intervention

When the mother is ill or at risk for illness during pregnancy, nurses can promote attachment to the fetus and newborn by facilitating the mother's accomplishment of prenatal developmental tasks. The following nursing interventions can be used to facilitate attachment (Moore 1983):

- Provide opportunities for the parents to talk about the meaning of the pregnancy for themselves.
- Establish a supportive, nonjudgmental, and trusting relationship with the parents.
- Communicate openly and honestly with parents about the health status of the mother and baby.
- Encourage realistic hope about the pregnancy outcome.

▼ ANTICIPATORY GUIDANCE

If it appears that the infant will be at physical risk after delivery, parents will benefit from anticipatory guidance about what to expect during and after the birth. Miles (1989) interviewed 53 parents whose infants were hospitalized in an NICU and found that half of the parents felt they had not been prepared adequately for the experience. In another study, many parents of premature infants recommended including more information about high-risk infants in prenatal education classes (Harrison 1982). Montgomery and Williams-Judge (1986) described an anticipatory support program for high-risk parents that included weekly high-risk perinatal rounds with representatives from the inpatient and outpatient antepartum, labor and delivery, postpartum, and neonatal units. Nursery clinicians meet with all clients identified as high risk to provide anticipatory guidance as needed. The meetings occur in the clinic, the inpatient antepartum unit, or the labor and delivery unit. During the meetings, the nurse explains admission criteria for the NICU and the types of care that are likely to be provided for the infant. When the mother's condition permits, the parents are accompanied on a tour of the NICU. A number of hospitals have established high-risk antenatal ambulatory units, providing an excellent opportunity for nurses to initiate assessment and educational interventions during the prenatal period. Nurses working in these units can maintain contact with families after delivery to provide ongoing support.

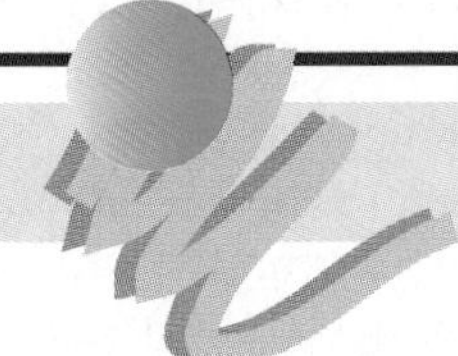

HISTORICAL PERSPECTIVES

TRENDS IN CARING FOR PHYSICALLY COMPROMISED HIGH-RISK INFANTS AND THEIR FAMILIES

1900–1940 Preterm infants were not expected to live. Martin Courney exhibited many preterm infants in major fairs between 1902 and 1940.

1923 The first hospital center for premature care in the United States was established at the Sarah Morris Hospital in Chicago. Mothers were encouraged to express breast milk at home but were not encouraged to participate in their infant's care.

1945–1947 Miller and Spence conducted a study in England comparing home care with hospital care for preterm infants weighing more than 3½ pounds at birth. The researchers concluded that "home care was safer from the standpoint of infection, more economical, and it served the essential purpose of unifying the infant's family" (Kennell and Klaus 1982, p. 154). The practice of providing home care for preterm infants remained confined to England and Europe and did not extend to the United States.

1945–1960 Textbooks recommended isolating preterm infants from visitors, including parents, and recommended limited handling of the infants.

1953 Prugh described emotional reactions of mothers of preterm infants during the time when mothers were generally excluded from preterm nurseries, noting that anxiety and guilt were common reactions.

1960 Kaplan and Mason identified four psychological tasks that mothers of preterm infants must accomplish to establish positive mother-infant relationships.

1970s Klaus and Kennell's study on the essential nature of early mother-infant contact dramatically altered hospital practices, and parents were encouraged to visit their infants in the NICU.

1970–present Numerous studies were conducted to examine stresses experienced by parents of preterm infants and evaluate intervention programs to promote parent-infant attachment. Parents, grandparents, and siblings are now encouraged to visit the high-risk infant in the NICU, and parents are encouraged to participate in the infant's care.

Adapted from Kennell, J. H., and Klaus, M. H. (1982). Caring for the parents of premature or sick infants. In M. H. Klaus and J. H. Kennell (Eds.), *Parent-infant bonding* (pp. 151–226). St. Louis: C. V. Mosby.

▼ THE CHILDBIRTH EXPERIENCE

The labor and birth experience for parents of high-risk infants is often accompanied by a sense of danger and emergency. A member of the neonatal team should be present at delivery to provide immediate care for the newborn so that the maternal-newborn nurse is free to support the parents (Johnson 1986). Parents will need an opportunity later to review the labor and delivery experience in order to express their feelings about any stresses they encountered. Allowing parents to see and touch their infant before transporting the baby to the NICU helps initiate the bonding process and may alleviate the anxiety that accompanies uncertainty about the infant's appearance and condition. If the infant is to be transferred to another hospital, it is helpful to take a Polaroid photograph for the parents to keep. Huckabay (1987) provided 20 mothers with Polaroid pictures of their preterm infants and compared their bonding behaviors with those of a randomly assigned control group of mothers who did not receive photographs. Mothers in the experimental group had significantly more bonding behaviors when the infants were 4 weeks old than mothers who did not receive a photograph. Photographs can promote mother-infant attachment by serving as constant reminders of the infant and enhancing the amount of time the mothers thought about their babies (Huckabay 1987).

Conferences about the baby's medical condition should include both parents together whenever possible to avoid communication problems. Information should be honest, but it is important for physicians and nurses to maintain an optimistic attitude if the infant is likely to survive (Klaus and Kennell 1982). It is also vital to ascertain what the parents already know or expect in relation to their infant's condition to identify their learning needs.

▼ NEONATAL TRANSPORT

If the infant must be transferred to an NICU in another hospital, it is helpful for the father (or another family member if the father is unavailable) to follow the transport team and spend at least several hours in the nursery. This allows him to become familiar with the nursery staff, equipment, and plans for the infant's care so he can provide the mother with first-hand information about their baby's status. Providing parents with photographs or videotapes of their infants in the NICU can decrease the stress imposed by early parent-infant separation. Mussell and associates (1990) described a live closed-circuit television and videotaping service that allows families to watch their infants in the NICU on a television screen in the mother's room in another hospital. Parents reported that the live videotaping helped them to understand their infant's health status. Copies of the videotapes can also be mailed to families who live far from the NICU or are unable to visit frequently.

Many fathers may experience conflict between the desire to accompany the baby to the NICU and their desire to remain with the mother to provide her with needed support. The nurse can be helpful by encouraging the parents to share their feelings and decide together on the best course of action.

Regularly scheduled telephone calls to parents by the infant's primary nurse are also extremely helpful, particularly for parents who are unable to visit the NICU frequently or for mothers who must remain hospitalized after delivery.

▼ PARENT VISITS TO NICU

A parent's first visit to the NICU is extremely stressful. Ideally, a nurse or social worker should meet with the parents before they enter the NICU for the first time to prepare them for the experience. Discussing the infant's condition and the equipment being used is an important component of this preparation. Nurses should focus on helping parents understand and cope with their infant's appearance (Miles 1989). Many nurseries have developed booklets with photographs of infants and equipment in the NICU as well as information about the nursery policies and routines. Such booklets can also help to prepare siblings and grandparents for their first nursery visit. The nurse should provide parents with comfortable chairs or stools beside their baby's bed and give them guidelines about how to interact with their infants.

Many studies have confirmed that physiologically stable preterm infants benefit from supplemental tactile, auditory, and kinesthetic stimulation (see Harrison 1985 for a review of these studies). Infants who are physiologically fragile (e.g., those who require supplemental oxygen or are critically ill), however, may not be able to cope with any extra stimulation.

Preterm infants with fewer medical complications were found to respond to tactile and auditory stimuli with more smiles and hand-to-mouth activity than did ill infants. Ill infants demonstrated more avoidance signals when they were stroked and talked to simultaneously, "suggesting that stimulation in two sensory modalities was the most aversive" (Oehler 1985, p. 31). Oehler (1985) reported that there was no significant change in heart rate after the stimuli among either the well or ill infants. Among infants who had transcutaneous oxygen monitors in place, the oxygen level remained the same or increased during auditory stimulation; however, the level tended to decrease during touching or simultaneous touching and talking. There is a need for further research to determine "whether ways of providing

WORKING WITH PARENTS OF PHYSIOLOGICALLY COMPROMISED HIGH-RISK INFANTS

The nurse in the NICU is in a key position to develop a supportive relationship with families as they cope with their infant's illness. Primary nursing goals should promote positive parent-infant attachment and help parents become competent in meeting the special needs of their infants. The following principles can help enhance the nurse's effectiveness in achieving these goals.

- PROVIDE PARENTS WITH ANTICIPATORY GUIDANCE. Preparing parents for what they might experience helps them to develop successful coping strategies. The nurse can provide anticipatory guidance before the parents first enter the NICU so that they will be less frightened and intimidated during their initial visit. Throughout the hospital stay, the nurse can teach parents about expected changes and progress in the infant's status. Discharge teaching should include anticipatory guidance about what to expect during the early weeks at home.

- ENCOURAGE PARENTS TO PARTICIPATE IN CARING FOR THEIR INFANTS, and help them develop confidence in their parenting abilities. Parents sometimes feel intimidated by the skill and competence of NICU nurses and lack confidence in their own parenting skills. By showing parents how to identify and respond to their infant's physiologic and behavioral cues, the nurse can promote parental competence and facilitate the development of positive parent-infant attachment.

- ASSESS FAMILY RESPONSES TO THE INFANT'S ILLNESS. By assessing the reactions of parents, siblings, and extended family members, the nurse can identify families who may need additional support and make appropriate referrals to other members of the health care team.

tactile stimulation other than stroking may prove to be enriching for the infants and not cause avoidance behaviors or hypoxia" (Oehler 1985, p. 32). Providing stimulation should be based on the infant's individual behavioral cues.

The effects of touch provided by parents to 36 preterm infants who were 27 to 33 weeks of gestational age at birth were studied by Harrison and colleagues (1990). Infants were videotaped during parents' visits to the NICU during the first 4 weeks after birth. Parents were instructed to interact with their infants as they normally would. There was considerable variability in the types and amounts of touch provided to the infants. The mean percentage of time during the visits when mothers touched their infants was 43 percent, and the mean duration of touch during each visit was 17.5 minutes. The most frequently touched locations were the infant's hands, back, and head. The touch actions used most frequently were hold, stroke, and skin-to-skin contact (Harrison and Woods 1991). There were no differences in mean heart rate or oxygen saturation during episodes of a parent's touch compared with levels at baseline assessment or after the visit, but there was more variability in both of these parameters during episodes of a parent's touch. Although there were more abnormally low oxygen saturation levels during episodes of a parent's touch compared with levels at baseline assessment and after the visit, there were wide individual differences in the infants' physiologic responses to touch. For example, mean oxygen levels decreased during touch for 60 percent of the infants but increased for 31 percent of the infants.

These researchers concluded that blanket policies limiting touch during the early weeks of life for preterm infants are inappropriate. Rather, decisions about supplemental touch should be based on the individual needs and responses of each baby. Until further research is available to provide guidelines about the most appropriate ways for parents to interact with medically fragile infants, parents can be advised to modify their interactions on the basis of the baby's responses. For example, if the baby becomes agitated or has a decreased oxygen level when stroked, parents might be encouraged to simply hold the baby's hand or to speak to the infant in a slow, soft voice.

Because the parent-infant acquaintance process may be impeded in the tense NICU environment, the effect of transporting healthy premature infants to their mother's hospital rooms for the first parent-infant contact was examined by Klaus and Kennell (1982). In the study, an NICU nurse brought the baby to the mother's room in a transport incubator. During the hour-long visit, the nurse remained seated at the head of the mother's bed and the baby was placed on the bed under a radiant heat panel. Mothers in this study touched their infants 80 percent of the time and spoke to them 40 percent of the time during the visit. Klaus and Kennell (1982) reported that in an earlier study, mothers having their first contact with their preterm infants in the NICU touched their infants only 20 percent of the time and rarely spoke to them. If staffing patterns are adequate and the baby's condition is stable, transporting the baby to the mother's hospital room (or to a parent visiting room away from the tense NICU environment) for the first visit may promote the bonding process.

Levin (1994) described a mother-baby unit at Tallinn Children's Hospital in Estonia where mothers room-in and provide most of the care for their preterm or sick full-term infants. Benefits of this approach to care include reduced maternal-infant separation, increased maternal confidence, and reduced exposure of the infants to stressors and pathogens associated with having multiple caregivers. This unit was originally established to provide care to the infants with a limited number of professional nurses in the former Soviet Republic. The benefits of this approach have important implications for neonatal units both in developing countries and in countries that have more access to technology and professional health care workers. Further research is needed to discern the long-term effects of maternal transport and maternal rooming-in.

Parents need to feel free to visit their infants or call the NICU as often as they wish. It is helpful if one staff member assumes primary responsibility for relating to the parents to avoid problems with inconsistent information and to foster the development of a supportive relationship with the family. A primary nurse can fulfill this role nicely.

Encouraging parents to express their feelings of helplessness in not knowing how to aid their infant can help them cope with their feelings of failure, anger, and guilt (Miles 1989). Parents should be encouraged to express these feelings with their primary nurse and with each other. Infrequent parental visiting may be an indicator of problems in the development of parent-infant attachment (Fanaroff et al. 1972). Parents of an infant with a chronic illness are likely to experience chronic sorrow or episodes of grief throughout their child's life (Olshansky 1962). If parents deny the seriousness of their infant's condition, the nurse needs to accept their response but gradually help them to face reality. Parents must begin to resolve their initial grief before they can develop an attachment to their infant.

The infant's prolonged stay in the NICU provides the nurse with an opportunity for ongoing assessment of the developing parent-infant relationship. Interventions to promote parent-infant attachment discussed in Chapter 34 can be adapted for parents of high-risk infants. In addition, parents of high-risk infants have special needs for open communication, education, support, and preparation for the infant's hospital discharge.

▼ COMMUNICATION

Frequent, open communication between parents and hospital staff is essential so that the parents will have realistic perceptions of their infant's condition and care. It is also essential that the NICU staff keep each other informed about the parents' status and the information they have received. When parents live far from the NICU and are unable to visit frequently, the NICU nurse or social worker should make a point to telephone the family on a regular basis. Parents greatly appreciate

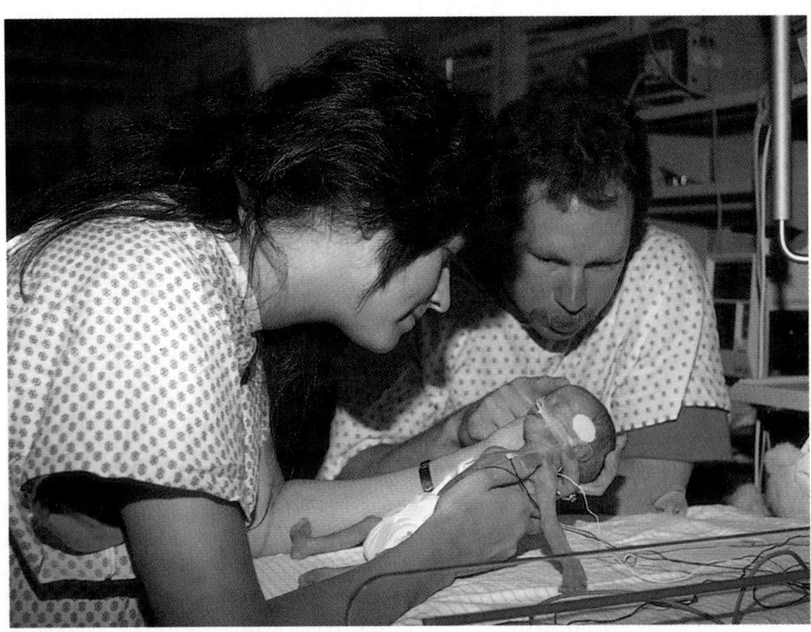

Figure 37–4
A mother and father hold and caress their tiny preterm infant in the NICU. The bond between parents and infant becomes stronger as parents are more comfortable with their baby. Once parents learn that their baby will not break when touched, they are able to participate and assume more and more control over their baby's care.

receiving photographs or videotapes of their infant accompanied by letters from the NICU nurses describing the baby's progress. Open communication between the parents themselves is also important to prevent stress on the couple's relationship with one another. Nurses can facilitate this communication by encouraging the parents to spend time alone together and talk about their feelings.

Parents also need information about the normal characteristics and behaviors of premature or older high-risk infants; the individual characteristics of their infants; and ways to care for, stimulate, and interact with their infants. One strategy that has been used to help parents understand and respond to their preterm infant's unique behaviors is demonstrating the infant's performance on Brazelton's Neonatal Behavioral Assessment Scale (BNBAS) or having mothers assess their infants on the Mother's Assessment of the Behavior of Her Infant (MABI) scale (Harrison et al. 1991). Demonstrating the BNBAS to teenage mothers of preterm infants in the hospital was found to enhance mother-infant interaction and the development of the infants (Widmayer and Field 1981). Demonstrating the Assessment of Premature Infant Behavior (APIB) scale to parents of preterm infants was shown to decrease their anxiety and promote more realistic perceptions of their babies (Culp et al. 1989). Harrison and associates (1991) found that mothers of preterm infants were able to assess their infant's behaviors accurately using the MABI scale. These findings suggest that parents can learn how to understand and respond to their infant's behaviors by observing a BNBAS or APIB examination as it is performed by a trained examiner or by assessing their infants at regular intervals (e.g., weekly) by use of the MABI scale. Because administration of the BNBAS takes about 30 minutes and may be stressful to physiologically compromised infants, nurses should not administer the entire examination until the infant is physically stable. It may be best to administer only selected parts of the examination (e.g., orientation items or habituation items) at one time when teaching parents about their baby's behaviors.

It is important for nurses to avoid overwhelming parents with too much information at once and to proceed at a pace the parents are able to handle. Some parents may benefit from reading books and articles about their infant's condition, but the nurse should ensure that the parents also have an opportunity for individual teaching and discussion.

Parents of children with congenital defects that may be hereditary need referral for genetic counseling. The American Society of Human Genetics has identified the following five objectives of genetic counseling (Wilson 1983):

1. To understand the diagnosis, cause, and treatment of the disorder
2. To understand the risk of recurrence of the disorder
3. To understand alternative choices of dealing with the risk of recurrence
4. To choose an appropriate plan of action
5. To adjust to the disorder or risk of recurrence

In some perinatal centers, nurses with advanced training provide genetic counseling services. In other centers, the primary role of the nurse is to initiate the referral, prepare the family for what to expect, and then reinforce or clarify the information the family receives.

Parents also need support as they cope with the many stressors associated with the prolonged hospitalization of their infant. Such assistance might include ongoing grief counseling or help in finding appropriate community resources. Support from other parents who have had similar experiences is extremely useful. Many hospitals have initiated organized parent-to-parent support programs (Erdman 1977; Garrand et al. 1978). Mothers who participated in a parent support group were found to have more positive interactions with their infants than did mothers who were not invited to participate in the support group (Minde et al. 1980).

▼ DISCHARGE OF INFANT FROM HOSPITAL

Preparation for the infant's hospital discharge involves ensuring that the parents are comfortable and competent in caring for their infant, identifying appropriate community resources, and making plans for family follow-up. Allowing parents to room-in with their babies in a private hospital room for one or two nights before the infant's hospital discharge helps parents feel more comfortable in making the transition from hospital to home (Klaus and Kennell 1982). In Harrison's (1982) study, one mother of a premature infant confided that she actually worried that she might kill her infant during the baby's first week at home. After all the skilled nursing care the baby required in the hospital, this mother felt extremely insecure about her ability to care for her infant adequately. Parents need ample opportunity to prepare for assuming responsibility for their infant's care while the baby is still in the hospital setting.

The predischarge and postdischarge teaching needs of parents whose very-low-birth-weight infants were discharged early from the hospital and observed at home by a perinatal clinical specialist have been described by Brooten and colleagues (1989). Before hospital discharge, the main teaching needs identified by the clinical specialists were related to infant caretaking (feeding, bathing, handling, sleeping, and clothing), infant health (preventing and recognizing infection), and growth and development (infant stimulation). Teaching in the postdischarge period focused on infant caretaking and health and also on managing within the health care system and maintaining a safe home environment.

Parents of severely handicapped children may need help in making decisions about whether to place their child in an institution or to try to care for him or her at home.

▼ FOLLOW-UP AFTER DISCHARGE

After the infant is discharged from the hospital, parents continue to need support and guidance. Mothers who have experienced prenatal or postpartum health problems may need time to recuperate and regain their strength. Parents may benefit from help with housekeeping responsibilities so that they can focus their energy and attention on the infant. Parents of high-risk infants often need help learning to provide for the baby's health and safety needs without overprotecting the infant. Community health nurses have an excellent opportunity to provide this type of follow-up support. Other community resources that can offer support for home care of the high-risk infant include parent education and support groups (such as Premature, Incorporated), infant stimulation programs, physicians, social workers, and services such as physical therapy or rehabilitation programs when the child has special needs in these areas. Brooten and coworkers (1989) found that perinatal clinical specialists were able to provide much of their postdischarge follow-up by telephone consultation.

After a review of 19 studies evaluating interventions to promote positive relationships between preterm infants and parents, Patteson and Barnard (1990) concluded that key components of successful programs were multiple parental contacts with the same intervener and active involvement of the parent in the intervention and in interacting with the infant. All studies that involved home-based interventions had positive outcomes. Field and coworkers (1980), for example, evaluated the effects of an 8-month home-based intervention program for teenage low-income black mothers and their preterm infants. The intervention consisted of home visits during which the mothers were taught about developmental milestones, infant stimulation techniques, and ways to interact with their infants. Follow-up assessments at 4 and 8 months revealed a number of significant differences in favor of the mothers and infants who participated in the program compared with a control group.

Bromwich and Parmalee (1979) also evaluated a home-based support program designed to help parents become more sensitive and responsive to their high-risk infants. At the end of the program, mothers in the intervention group received higher scores on a measure of maternal attentiveness and reciprocity than did mothers in a control group.

▼ Evaluation

Evaluating the effects of interventions designed to promote positive parenting should be an ongoing process. Nurses can base their evaluations on observational assessments of parent-infant interactions as described in Chapter 34. It is also important to ask parents about their perceptions of their infants and of their developing relationships. Patteson and Barnard (1990) noted that most parent intervention programs have been based on the conceptualizations and value systems of the investigators evaluating the programs and that most evaluations of these programs have failed to include feedback from participating parents. Nurses can encourage parents to verbalize their feelings and concerns and modify intervention strategies accordingly.

Implications for Research

Even though there have been many studies focusing on preterm infants and parents during the past 20 years, there are still many unanswered questions. Some areas of focus for future research include the following. Nurse researchers can make a significant contribution by designing studies that will address these questions and provide a scientific base for nursing practice with high-risk families.

- There is a great need for research to identify prenatal nursing interventions that could decrease the frequency of high-risk births and thereby reduce stressors that may threaten the development of positive parent-infant relationships. The results of the descriptive study by Milne and Rich (1981) suggested that ultrasonography may enhance mother-fetal attachment. Further research is needed to confirm this preliminary finding using more controlled, experimental designs. Future studies should also evaluate the effects of ultrasound examinations on father-infant attachment and assess parents' emotional responses to the ultrasound diagnosis of fetal abnormalities.
- Several researchers reported a higher rate of child abuse among preterm infants; however, most parents develop positive relationships with their high-risk infants. Further research is needed to identify those infants at greatest risk for abuse or neglect so that appropriate intervention can be initiated.

- There is a need for research to identify the most appropriate ways for parents to interact with medically fragile infants during the early weeks of life. Although many studies have found that premature infants benefit from extra tactile and kinesthetic stimulation once they are medically stable, the results of studies by Harrison and coworkers (1990) and Oehler (1985) suggested that some types of interactions (e.g., touching or simultaneously touching and talking) may be stressful for medically fragile preterm infants.
- Further research is needed to determine whether certain types of early interactions (e.g., providing gentle touch rather than stroking) have beneficial effects on both preterm infants and their parents. Studies should examine differences in interaction patterns when parents visit the NICU alone and when they visit as a couple (Thurman and Korteland 1989).
- Patteson and Barnard (1990) identified the need for research to define the specific ingredients of effective intervention programs for high-risk families. In the present era of cost containment, there is a great need to identify cost-effective hospital-based programs that can promote attachment.
- Studies are also needed to identify which families should receive home-based intervention and to evaluate whether telephone follow-up is as effective as home visiting in promoting positive interactions between high-risk infants and parents.
- Patteson and Barnard (1990) identified the need for research evaluating the long-term effects of interventions for parents and their high-risk infants, since most studies to date have observed families for less than 3 years after the infant's birth.

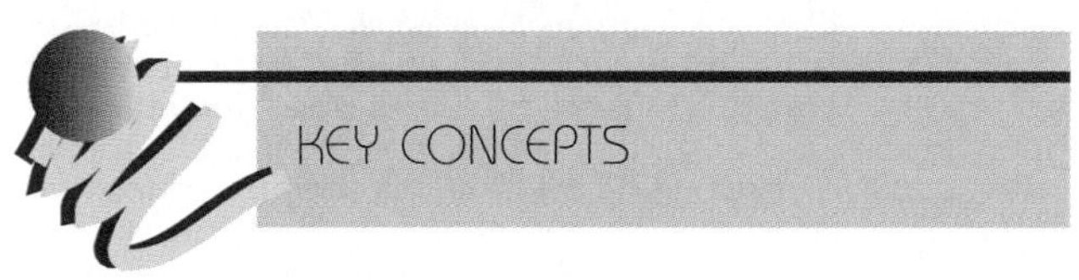

KEY CONCEPTS

- ▼ Family members' reactions to a high-risk pregnancy and birth are influenced by multiple factors including the severity of the mother's or infant's health problem, available support, individual personality variables, coping styles, age of parents, socioeconomic status, and cultural variables.
- ▼ Parents must accomplish four tasks to resolve the crisis associated with the birth of a high-risk premature infant: anticipatory grief, acknowledgment of failure to deliver a full-term baby, resumption of the process of relating to the baby, and understanding how a premature baby differs from a full-term baby in terms of special needs and growth patterns.
- ▼ The stresses that result from the birth of a high-risk infant are related to unexpected pregnancy outcome, separation of parents and infant during the early neonatal period, stresses associated with hospitalization, and physical and behavioral characteristics of the infant.
- ▼ The birth of a high-risk infant poses risks for the development of optimal parent-infant attachments, although with adequate support, most parents develop satisfying attachments with their high-risk infants.
- ▼ When parents expect that their child may die prematurely, they may be reluctant to develop a close attachment to the child.
- ▼ Nursing interventions that foster open communication and support between the mother and father can help prevent future conflict related to the birth of a high-risk infant.
- ▼ Siblings and extended family members may feel neglected and isolated because the parents' attention is focused on the high-risk infant.
- ▼ Sibling reactions to the birth of a high-risk infant vary with the developmental stage of the sibling and with the particular family situation.
- ▼ During the prenatal period, nurses should assess parental behaviors that reflect accomplishment of the developmental tasks of pregnancy.
- ▼ If it appears that the infant will be at physical risk after delivery, parents need anticipatory guidance about what to expect during and after the birth.
- ▼ Conferences about the baby's medical condition should include both parents together whenever possible to avoid communication problems.
- ▼ Strategies to decrease the stress associated with early parent-infant separation include providing parents with photographs or videotapes of their infants in the NICU, encouraging parents' visits and phone calls, transporting stable infants to their mothers' hospital rooms, and allowing mothers to room-in or help care for their hospitalized infants.
- ▼ Parents need anticipatory guidance before their first NICU visit to prepare them for what to expect in terms of equipment and the infant's appearance.

- ▼ Preterm infants who are physiologically stable benefit from supplemental tactile, auditory, and kinesthetic stimulation. However, preterm infants who are physiologically fragile may not be able to cope with any extra stimulation.
- ▼ Frequent, open communication between parents and hospital staff is essential so that parents will have realistic perceptions of their infant's condition and care.
- ▼ Preparation for the infant's hospital discharge involves ensuring that the parents are comfortable and competent in caring for their infant, identifying appropriate community resources, and making plans for family follow-up.
- ▼ Key components of successful intervention programs for parents of preterm infants include multiple contacts with the same intervener and active parental involvement in interacting with the infant.

References

Blackburn, S. (1983). Fostering behavioral development of high-risk infants. *Journal of Obstetric, Gynecologic, and Neonatal Nursing,* 12, 76s–85s.

Blackburn, S. (1991). State-related behaviors and individual differences. In S. Blackburn and R. Kang, *Early parent-infant relationships* (2nd ed.). White Plains, NY: March of Dimes Birth Defects Foundation.

Blackburn, S., and Lowen, L. (1986). Impact of an infant's premature birth on the grandparents and parents. *Journal of Obstetric, Gynecologic, and Neonatal Nursing,* 15, 173–178.

Brazelton, T. B. (1984). *Neonatal behavioral assessment scale* (2nd ed.). Philadelphia: J. B. Lippincott.

Bromwich, R. M., and Parmalee, A. H. (1979). An intervention program for pre-term infants. In T. M. Field, A. M. Sostek, S. Goldberg, H. H. Shuman (Eds.), *Infants born at risk—behavior and development.* New York: Spectrum.

Brooten, D. (1983). Issues for research on alternative patterns of care for low birthweight infants. *Image: The Journal of Nursing Scholarship,* 15 (3), 80–83.

Brooten, D., Gennaro, S., Knapp, H., Brown, L., York, R. (1989). Clinical specialist pre- and postdischarge teaching of parents of very low birth weight infants. *Journal of Obstetric, Gynecologic, and Neonatal Nursing,* 18, 316–322.

Brown, J. V., and Bakeman, R. (1980). Relationships of human mothers during the first year of life: Effects of prematurity. In R. W. Bell and W. P. Smotherman (Eds.), *Maternal influences and early behavior.* Jamaica, NY: Spectrum.

Culp, R. E., Culp, A. M., Harmon, R. J. (1989). A tool for educating parents about their premature infants. *Birth,* 16 (1), 23–26.

Drotar, D., Baskiewicz, A., Irvin, N., Kennell, J. H., Klaus, M. H. (1975). The adaptation of parents to the birth of an infant with a congenital malformation: A hypothetical model. *Pediatrics,* 56, 710–717.

Erdman, D. (1977). Parent-to-parent support: The best for those with sick newborns. *MCN: American Journal of Maternal-Child Nursing,* 2, 291–292.

Fanaroff, A. A., Kennell, J. H., Klaus, M. H. (1972). Follow-up of low birthweight infants: The predictive value of maternal visiting patterns. *Pediatrics,* 49, 288–290.

Field, T. (1977). Effects of early separation, interaction deficits, and experimental manipulations on infant-mother face-to-face interactions. *Child Development,* 48, 763–772.

Field, T. M., Widmayer, S. M., Stringer, S., Ignatoff, E. (1980). Teenage, lower-class, black mothers and their preterm infants: An intervention and developmental follow-up. *Child Development,* 51, 426–436.

Frodi, A. M., Lamb, M. E., Leavitt, L. A., Donovan, W. L., Sherry, D. (1978). Fathers' and mothers' responses to the faces and cries of normal and premature infants. *Developmental Psychology,* 14, 490–498.

Garrand, S., Sherman, N., Rentchler, D., Jung, A. L. (1978). A parent-to-parent program. *Family and Community Health,* 1, 103–113.

Gennaro, S. (1986). Anxiety and problem-solving ability in mothers of premature infants. *Journal of Obstetric, Gynecologic, and Neonatal Nursing,* 15, 160–164.

Gorski, P. A., Davison, M. F., Brazelton, T. B. (1979). Stages of behavioral organization in the high-risk neonate: Theoretical and clinical considerations. *Seminars in Perinatology,* 3 (1), 61–72.

Gottwald, S. R., and Thurman, S. K. (1990). Parent-infant interaction in neonatal intensive care units: Implications for research and service delivery. *Infants and Young Children,* 2 (3), 1–9.

Green, M., and Solnit, A. J. (1964). Reactions to the threatened loss of a child: A vulnerable child syndrome: Pediatric management of the dying child, Part III. *Pediatrics,* 34, 58–66.

Harrison, H. (1983). *The premature baby book: A parent's guide to coping and caring in the first years* (pp. 29–30). New York: St. Martin's Press.

Harrison, L. (1982). *Teaching mothers about their premature infants: Effects on perceptions and attachment.* Unpublished doctoral dissertation, University of Tennessee, Knoxville.

Harrison, L. L. (1985). Effects of early supplemental stimulation on preterm infants: Review of the literature. *Maternal-Child Nursing Journal,* 14 (2), 69–90.

Harrison, L. L., and Woods, S. (1991). Characteristics of early parent touch provided to hospitalized preterm infants. *Journal of Obstetric, Gynecologic, and Neonatal Nursing,* 20 (4), 299–306.

Harrison, L. L., Leeper, J., Yoon, M. (1990). Effects of early parent touch on preterm infants' heart rates and arterial oxygen saturation levels. *Journal of Advanced Nursing,* 15, 877–885.

Harrison, L. L., Sherrod, R. A., Dunn, L., Olivet, L., Jeon, J. (1991). Effects of hospital-based instruction on interactions between parents and preterm infants. *Neonatal Network,* 9 (7), 27–33.

Herzog, J. M. (1979). Disturbances in parenting high-risk infants: Clinical impressions and hypotheses. In T. M. Field, A. M. Sostek, S. Goldberg, H. H. Shuman (Eds.), *Infants born at risk—behavior and development.* New York: Spectrum.

Huckabay, L. M. D. (1987). The effect on bonding behavior of giving a mother her premature baby's picture. *Scholarly Inquiry for Nursing Practice,* 1 (2), 115–129.

Hunter, R. S., Kilstrom, N., Kraybill, E. N., Loda, F. (1978). Antecedents of child abuse and neglect in premature infants: A prospective study in a newborn intensive care unit. *Pediatrics,* 61 (4), 629–635.

Johnson, S. H. (1986). The premature infant. In S. H. Johnson (Ed.), *High-risk parenting: Nursing assessment and strategies for the family at risk* (2nd ed.). Philadelphia: J. B. Lippincott.

Johnson, S. H., and Grubbs, J. B. (1975). The premature infant's reflex behaviors: Effect on the maternal-child relationship. *Journal of Obstetric, Gynecologic, and Neonatal Nursing,* 4, 15–21.

Kaplan, D. M., and Mason, E. A. (1960). Maternal reactions to premature birth viewed as an acute emotional disorder. *American Journal of Orthopsychiatry,* 30, 539–546.

Kemp, V. H., and Page, C. K. (1986). The psychosocial impact of a high-risk pregnancy on the family. *Journal of Obstetric, Gynecologic, and Neonatal Nursing,* 14, 232–236.

Kennell, J. H., and Klaus, M. H. (1982). Caring for the parents of premature or sick infants. In M. H. Klaus and J. H. Kennell (Eds.), *Parent-infant bonding* (2nd ed., pp. 151–226). St. Louis: C. V. Mosby.

Klaus, M. H., and Kennell, J. H. (1982). *Parent-infant bonding* (2nd ed.). St. Louis: C. V. Mosby.

Leonard, C. H., Clyman, R. S., Piecuch, R. E., Juster, R. B., Ballard, R. A., Behle, M. B. (1990). Effect of medical and social risk factors on outcome of prematurity and very low birth weight. *Journal of Pediatrics,* 116 (4), 620–626.

Levin, A. (1994). The mother-infant unit at Tallinn Children's Hospital in Estonia: A truly baby-friendly unit. *Birth: Issues in Perinatal Care,* 21 (1), 39–44.

Luddington, S. M. (1983). *Infant stimulation: New concepts in neonatal growth and development.* Conference held in Dallas, TX, June 21–24, 1983.

Lynch, M. A., and Roberts, J. (1977). Predicting child abuse: Signs of bonding failure in the maternity hospital. *British Medical Journal,* 1, 624–626.

McFarland, G. K., and McFarlane, E. A. (1989). *Nursing diagnosis and intervention: Planning for patient care.* St. Louis: C. V. Mosby.

Miles, M. S. (1989). Parents of critically ill premature infants: Sources of stress. *Critical Care Nursing Quarterly,* 12 (3), 69–74.

Milne, L. S., and Rich, O. J. (1981). Cognitive and effective aspects of the responses of pregnant women to sonography. *Maternal-Child Nursing Journal,* 10 (1), 15–39.

Minde, K., Shosenberg, N., Marton, P., Thompson, J., Ripley, J., Burns, S. (1980). Self-help groups in the premature nursery—controlled evaluation. *Journal of Pediatrics,* 96 (5), 933–940.

Montgomery, L. V., and Williams-Judge, S. (1986). An anticipatory support program for high-risk parents. *Neonatal Network,* 4, 33–35.

Moore, M. L. (1983). Potential alterations in attachment: Maternal and/or neonatal illness. *NAACOG Update Series, Lesson 7, Volume 1.*

Mussell, G., Galke, K., Block, D., Connors, R. (1990). Use of live video transmission in the NICU. *Neonatal Network,* 3 (4), 37–38, 51–52.

Nance, S. (1982). *Premature babies: A handbook for parents.* New York: Priam Books.

Oehler, J. M. (1985). Examining the issue of tactile stimulation for preterm infants. *Neonatal Network,* 4 (3), 25–33.

Olshansky, S. (1962). Chronic sorrow: A response to having a mentally defective child. *Social Casework,* 43, 190–193.

Patteson, D. M., and Barnard, K. E. (1990). Parenting of low-birthweight infants: A review of issues and interventions. *Infant Mental Health Journal,* 11 (1), 37–56.

Sammons, W. A., and Lewis, J. M. (1985). *Premature babies: A different beginning.* St. Louis: C. V. Mosby.

Siefert, K., Thompson, T., Ten Bensel, R. W., Hunt, C. (1983). Perinatal stress: A study of factors linked to the risk of parenting problems. *Health and Social Work,* 8, 107–121.

Taylor, P. M., and Hall, B. L. (1979). Parent-infant bonding: Problems and opportunities in a perinatal center. *Seminars in Perinatology,* 3 (1), 73–84.

Thurman, S. K., and Korteland, C. (1989). The behavior of mothers and fathers toward their infants during neonatal intensive care visits. *Children's Health Care,* 18 (4), 247–251.

Widmayer, S. M., and Field, T. M. (1981). Effects of Brazelton demonstrations for mothers on the development of preterm infants. *Pediatrics,* 67 (5), 711–714.

Wilson, G. N. (1983). Counseling parents of children with genetic problems. *Ross Timesaver: Feelings and Their Medical Significance,* 25 (4), 13–16.

38 Chapter

> Sit down and tell us the truth. . . . Take us in to see the baby. . . . Suggest to us what has helped other people.
>
> A Grieving Father (Page-Lieberman and Hughes, 1990)

Perinatal Loss and Grief

Mary Lou Moore

HIGHLIGHTS

- The Scope of Perinatal Loss
- Characteristics of the Mourner and Relationship to the Fetus or Infant
- Anticipatory Grieving, Normal Grieving, Pathologic Grieving
- Phases of Mourning
- Immediate Support Through Environment, Validation of Loss, and Anticipatory Guidance
- The Timing of Subsequent Pregnancy
- Continuing Support as Parents Cope with Other Family Members and Adjustment
- Special Circumstances and Needs
- Caring for the Caregiver
- Implications for Research

Expectant mothers and fathers, nurses, and other health care professionals have an expectation of a healthy, joyous outcome as the culmination of pregnancy and birth. This is particularly true in those nations where maternal and infant mortality rates are relatively low in comparison with the mortality rates in developing nations of the world. For most families, healthy pregnancy and birth and a healthy baby are the realities of their childbearing experience; but for a significant number of others, the reality is loss, grief, and mourning.

Our society prepares prospective and practicing nurses as well as parents and their extended families and friends to expect a healthy baby. There is little preparation for death or severe illness in the childbearing years, either for expectant parents or for the nurses who care for them.

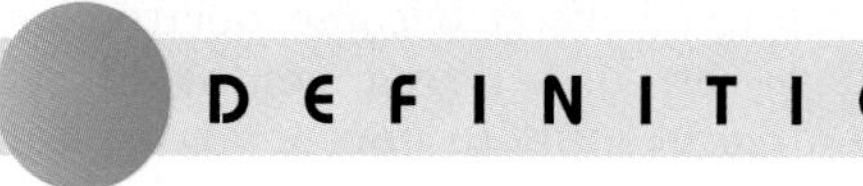

DEFINITIONS

Mourning—The process of grieving that involves accepting the loss, experiencing the pain in response to the loss, adjusting to life after the loss, and redirecting the energy from grieving to reconstructing one's life.

Pathologic grieving—Mourning that includes severe psychiatric symptoms at any time during mourning as well as prolonged mourning; has also been called disordered mourning.

Perinatal grief—The emotional reactions to a significant loss related to childbearing that can occur from the preconceptional period through early infancy.

Perinatal loss—Feelings of loss related to childbearing and the need to grieve (mourn) at any time from the preconceptional period through early infancy.

Replacement-child syndrome—An individual's obsession about having another child as soon as possible after the death of a baby.

THE SCOPE OF PERINATAL LOSS

Feelings of loss and the need to grieve (mourn) may occur at any time in the childbearing year from the preconceptional period through early infancy. Grieving related to infertility is described in Chapter 12. In the first and second trimesters, spontaneous and induced abortions and ectopic pregnancies are losses for which parents may grieve. Late second-trimester and third-trimester losses include intrauterine fetal death, induced abortion, death of a newborn infant, premature birth, birth of an infant with a congenital anomaly, and relinquishment of an infant for adoption. A preterm infant may live days or weeks and then die. For some parents who strongly desire an infant of a particular gender, disappointment over the gender of their new baby may bring a sense of loss and resultant grief. Beyond the loss of the baby, maternal death or illness is a source of grief for other family members.

How often does perinatal loss occur after conception? If 100 women conceive, it is estimated that 15 to 30 will have a spontaneous abortion (miscarriage, i.e., death of an embryo or fetus who weighs less than 500 g before 20 weeks of gestation). In some instances, these spontaneous abortions occur so early in pregnancy that the pregnancy itself will not have been recognized, and a sense of loss will not be present. Other early losses, however, may bring as profound a sense of loss and grief as death at term or in the neonatal period (Peppers and Knapp 1980, 1985). Mothers who choose elective abortion or relinquishment through adoption also mourn their infants.

Stillbirth refers to death of a fetus weighing more than 500 g before birth. The frequency of stillbirth in the United States is 1 in 80 births (1.2 percent). Neonatal death (death in the first 28 days of life) occurs on the average of 1 in 60 deliveries, although the risk for neonatal death varies greatly within population groups; African-American women experience rates far higher than those of other groups. Approximately 5 percent of infants are born prematurely; 1 percent of those infants weigh less than 1500 g and thereby face prolonged hospitalization and a risk for neonatal death. Four infants in every 100 will have a congenital anomaly; some of these anomalies may be minor from the perspective of health care providers but not necessarily minor to the newborn infant's parents. Once in every 100 births, the anomaly will be sufficiently severe to threaten life or require a lifetime of specialized care (Pettit 1987).

WHY IS PERINATAL GRIEF DIFFERENT?

Parkes (1985) identified four factors that are important in adjustment to the death of a loved one: the circumstances surrounding the death, the relationship of the individual to the deceased, individual characteristics of the mourner, and social support. These factors are considered in relationship to all perinatal losses, not only death.

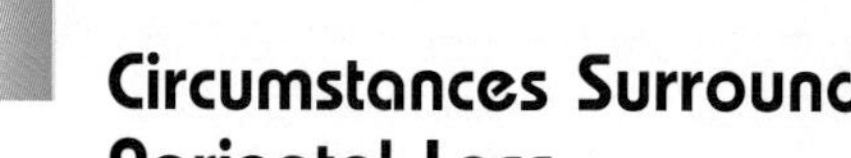

Circumstances Surrounding Perinatal Loss

Most parents expect a healthy baby as the outcome of pregnancy; indeed, most parents have a healthy baby. For those parents who experience an outcome of pregnancy different from their expectation and from the experience of most of the people they know, feelings of loss are intense. A traumatic event has been substituted for what was expected to be a joyous event. These circumstances are markedly different from those surrounding the death of persons who have been ill for some time or who are elderly. When a congenital anomaly or intrauterine fetal demise is diagnosed before the onset of labor, there may be a few hours or even days of anticipation. In many instances, perinatal loss follows a period of maternal illness or labor at birth, which leaves parents physically and emotionally stressed.

When death occurs later in life, the cause of death is frequently clear—heart disease, cancer, or perhaps an accident. In perinatal loss, the cause is often unknown. A seemingly perfect fetus is stillborn. Even when the immediate cause is clear, as in extreme prematurity, the underlying cause is not. This unknowing can aggravate both guilt and anger, which may result in comments such as "I must have done something wrong" or "The nurse (the doctor, my partner) must have done something wrong." Another difference surrounding certain types of perinatal loss is the absence of a visible object of mourning. For example, when loss occurs in the first trimester, there is no visible baby to grieve.

Relationship of the Individual to the Fetus or Infant

The relationship of parents and other family members to a fetus, newborn, or infant who dies is unique in that it is an attachment based on fantasy and hope rather than on actual knowledge of the lost person (Johannsen 1989).

When a person one has known dies, even if the person was known for a relatively brief period, there are memories of that person. When an infant is lost to early miscarriage, to stillbirth, or to loss in the immediate period after birth, there are limited memories—perhaps an ultrasound image, sometimes a single photograph, or remembering the feel of a fetal kick. The relationship of a mother to the fetus within her is clearly unique. She may feel betrayed by her own body and experience a sense of vulnerability and lack of control (Herz 1984).

Characteristics of the Mourner

Mourners who suffer perinatal loss are often young. For some, the death or illness of their infant may be the first occurrence of such a loss in their lives. Many parents have ambivalent feelings when they first become pregnant. Pregnancies that are unplanned often become desired as they progress; however, underlying conflicted feelings may be a source of guilt to one or both parents if there is a loss. A perinatal loss may be one of a series of losses perpetuating a chronic sorrow, such as multiple miscarriages, stillbirths, therapeutic abortion, or infertility.

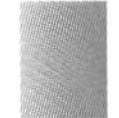

Social Support

Social support from family and community is embodied in rituals that accompany death. These rituals include wakes, funerals, the bringing of food, and talking about the deceased. When there is a perinatal loss, those who might provide social support under other circumstances may be reluctant to discuss the loss itself or the deceased infant (when the loss involves death). Close family members, such as grandparents, are also grieving; conversely, friends and family may not recognize the significance of the loss to the parents and may, therefore, not provide social support. The parents experiencing the loss may feel the need to be strong for each other; this need diminishes the ability of each to talk about their feelings with the other.

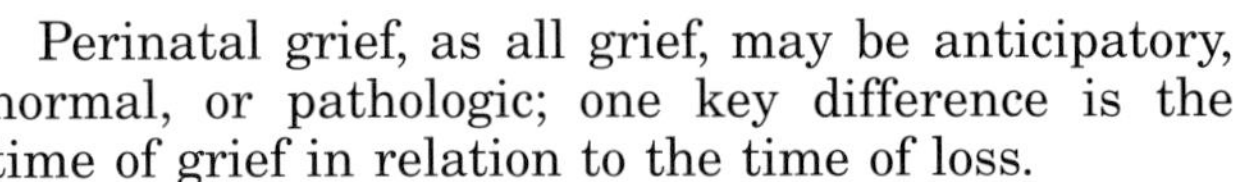

CATEGORIZING GRIEF

Perinatal grief, as all grief, may be anticipatory, normal, or pathologic; one key difference is the time of grief in relation to the time of loss.

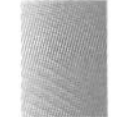

Anticipatory Grieving

Anticipatory grieving occurs in advance of and in anticipation of the actual loss. In the perinatal period, the parents of a sick infant in the intensive care nursery or of a fetus with an intrauterine diagnosis of a congenital anomaly may experience anticipatory grief. Anticipatory grief is normal and includes behaviors similar to those of grief after loss.

Does grieving in anticipation of loss alleviate grief after the loss? Johnson (1987), focusing on anticipatory grief in relation to death, noted that when there is time to prepare for loss, the total period of grief may be shorter, although there will be a resurgence of grief symptoms at the time of death.

Normal Grieving

Normal grieving refers to behaviors after loss, such as those described in this chapter. The period of normal grief begins at the time of loss and can last for many months. It is not unusual for parents to mourn their dead infant for 12 to 18 months, although the intensity of their grief will vary during this period.

Pathologic Grieving

Pathologic grieving, also called disordered mourning, includes severe psychiatric symptoms at any time during mourning as well as prolonged mourning, often defined as mourning beyond a year after the loss of the baby. Although a variety of studies have addressed the issue of pathologic grief, there has been little consistency of definition. As a whole, research data suggest that 20 to 30 percent of women who experience perinatal death will have some psychiatric symptoms during the first year after the loss (serious depression, anxiety attacks, phobias, psychosis). Not all of these women would be considered to have pathologic grief, however. Inhibited, delayed, or absent grief may also be pathologic; nurses must clearly differentiate the absence of overt expression of grieving, which can be related to both cultural and individual mourning styles, from the failure to experience symptoms of grief (Lindemann 1944).

Lack of social support, particularly from one's partner, and significant life stress during pregnancy have been identified as two factors most frequently associated with pathologic grief (Forrest et al. 1982; Nichols and Lewin 1986; Leon 1986). Supportive intervention may reduce the occurrence of pathologic grief (Forrest et al. 1982; Parkes 1985). In studies in which bereaved parents were interviewed on several occasions, a lower frequency of pathologic grieving was reported (Rowe et al. 1978; Park et al. 1979; Kirkby-Best and Kellner 1982). Could the opportunity to speak with an interviewer on more than one occasion have served as a supportive intervention?

FACTORS INFLUENCING MOURNING

A number of factors may influence mourning in both positive and negative ways. These factors may be divided into individual and family characteristics and the effect of circumstances and interventions surrounding the loss (Graham et al. 1987).

Age at the time of loss may affect mourning. Adolescents may have special needs as they mourn (see Special Circumstances and Needs). Loss later in reproductive years may also have special meaning for parents who may have viewed this pregnancy as their last opportunity for a child. Gender has been shown to affect both the meaning of a loss and the way in which grief is expressed (Tudehope et al. 1986; Null 1989). For example, in pregnancy, a mother may have developed a closer attachment to her baby than the father has and may feel the loss more acutely. This incongruent bonding results in incongruent grieving, which in turn may lead to a perception by the woman that her partner is uncaring. Since the perception of support from partner or family is important, parents need to be helped to express their own feelings and to accept the feelings of their partners (Nichols and Lewin 1986; Tudehope et al. 1986).

Littlefield and Rushton (1986) found that the mean grief intensity for mothers was higher than for fathers, according to both male and female estimates. Incongruent grieving, in which male and female partners are at different stages of grieving and grieve in different ways, is a common source of marital misunderstanding (Wallerstedt and Higgins 1996). No relationship between grief and the number of other living children was found by Littlefield and Rushton (1986).

Cultural differences, which include economic, ethnic, and spiritual factors, affect practices at the time of death and in subsequent weeks and months. Cultural differences also affect expressions of grief. Unfortunately, limited research has been done with minority populations, and thus our knowledge about cultural influences related to perinatal grieving is inadequate.

The attitude toward this pregnancy is a part of the relationship with the fetus and infant. Attitude toward pregnancy was found to be positively correlated with intensity of grief in mothers by Kennell and coworkers (1970) but not by Benfield and colleagues (1978), who found a positive association only in fathers. The importance of gestational age in mourning varies from one study to another. Individual differences (cognitive versus affective style; extrovert versus introvert) are also important. When these differences are not taken into account, there may be a lack of synchrony among family members as well as a lack of synchrony between nurses and other health care providers and parents.

Not all parents grieve after a perinatal loss. If the pregnancy and the baby were not yet real to the parents, then the loss, especially loss through early spontaneous abortion, may be viewed as vaginal bleeding and will not be accompanied by grief.

PHASES OF MOURNING

Mourning is frequently described as a series of phases or stages. These include initial shock and disbelief, a phase of anxiety and searching, a phase of disorganization, and finally, a phase of reorganization (Kubler-Ross 1969). Each phase is characterized by physical symptoms, behaviors, and feelings. While this concept of a sequence of phases may be helpful in understanding mourning, it is necessary to recognize that individuals mourn in different ways. Rarely (if ever) does mourning proceed in an orderly or linear fashion. Feelings such as anger or guilt may appear to be resolved, only to resurface at a later time. Feelings, behaviors, and physical symptoms may intensify at some times and wane at other times. The following phases and time periods provide broad guidance for understanding loss and helping parents and others through this painful period of their lives.

Shock and Disbelief

Shock is almost always the initial response to loss. Responses associated with shock include disbelief, crying, wanting to escape, and becoming numb or incoherent. The feeling of shock may protect parents from the full impact of their loss in the period immediately after the loss (Parkes 1985; Stierman 1987). Giles (1970) reported that of 40 women interviewed immediately after the death of a baby, 22 expressed feelings of emptiness and numbness. Two reported that they had no feeling, and one was worried about how she would react. Feelings of shock may last from a few hours to 1 to 2 weeks and may recur weeks or months after the loss.

During this period, parents and others may verbalize statements of denial, such as "There must be a mistake." Other characteristics of this phase include apathy; inappropriate behavior, such as giggling or unexpected calm; impaired concentration; difficulty in decision making; and physical detachment. These feelings may last from several days to several weeks.

Nurses who care for parents during this period may be puzzled by what seems to be inappropriate behavior, without expression of sadness. It is important for nurses to recognize that denial is a defense mechanism that serves a useful purpose of giving the person time to mobilize coping resources. Questions may need to be answered on numerous occasions during this phase, because the mourner is unable to comprehend answers. Unfortunately, during this time when decision-making is particularly difficult, parents may be asked to make difficult decisions about their child if the baby is alive but critically ill or requiring surgery as well as decisions about funeral arrangements. If these decisions cannot be postponed, nurses can help parents by clearly explaining alternatives as frequently as necessary.

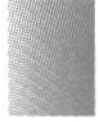

Yearning, Searching, and Anxiety

A second phase of mourning, which is commonly intense from the second week to the fourth or fifth month after a loss, has been described as a time of yearning, searching, and anxiety (Davidson 1979). Blaming is characteristic of this time as parents search for cause and meaning and repeatedly review events surrounding their loss. Blaming may be directed outward and manifested as anger or be directed inward as guilt and self-reproach.

Anger in many forms is a frequent characteristic of this period. Anger can be directed at the most readily available target, which may be a nurse or other health care provider, or at seemingly insignificant incidents. Anxiety and fear may result in restlessness, disorganized thoughts, uncontrolled crying, and insomnia. Some mothers report phantom crying of an infant (Davidson 1979) or the feeling of fetal movements (Klingbeil 1986). Physical symptoms of anxiety may include diarrhea, vomiting, tachycardia, urinary frequency, and palmar sweating.

Disorganization, Despair, and Depression

Disorganization, despair, and depression frequently follow the full realization of the reality of loss. At a time when the rest of the world may expect parents to have resolved their grief, a mother and father may be experiencing an intense period of mourning 4 to 6 months after the loss and for several months thereafter. Parents often find it difficult to accomplish their normal tasks during this period. Physical symptoms (such as aching arms or aching of the entire body, restlessness, malaise, anorexia), feelings of sadness and futility, lowered self-esteem, social withdrawal, and preoccupation with the lost infant are some characteristics of this period (Forrest et al. 1982; Parkes 1985). Some parents may use alcohol or other drugs in an attempt to ease their pain. Others seeks medical remedies for their physical symptoms. Marital problems may be common during this stressful time.

Reorganization

The restoration of the capacity to interact with others and to plan for the future signals a resolution of the grief process. Parents no longer carry out daily activities by merely going through the motions. Preoccupation with what might have been wanes; sadness is only occasionally acute. These changes do not mean that the loss of the infant is forgotten; research suggests that this will not happen. Parents are able, however, to look toward the future. Family relations stabilize, and the capacity to interact is restored (Zeanah 1989). Families find joy in other aspects of their lives.

HELPING GRIEVING PARENTS AND OTHER FAMILY MEMBERS

Nursing intervention to assist parents and other family members through the process of mourning requires a consideration of all the variables described in this chapter (see Strategies for Helping Families Cope with Perinatal Loss). Nurses can encourage emotionally healthy activities after perinatal loss.

Immediate Support

Issues to be considered in planning nursing support include providing an environment most comfortable for an individual family; validating the family's feelings about their loss; encouraging the acknowledgment of the baby's existence, which in-

Strategies for Helping Families Cope with Perinatal Loss

VALIDATING THE LOSS

- Be sensitive to funeral rituals and methods of disposing of the infant's body that are in keeping with the family's cultural values.
- Support and encourage the father to participate in the mother's care and in sharing the grief process.
- Recognize that each fetus or infant is significant and special. Do not rationalize the loss with comments such as "You can have other babies" or "You have other children at home, so don't worry about this one."
- Encourage parents to verbalize their feelings of loss; give them verbal and tactile permission to grieve.
- Do not be afraid to touch or hold parents when they cry.
- Be real; share feelings of distress and sadness with the parents. These are not unprofessional behaviors. Do not wear professional armor.
- Acknowledge that attachment begins long before birth and that feelings of loss are normal.
- Do not deny the loss to the parents by avoiding or sedating the mother.
- Be willing and available to talk with the parents about the loss.
- Reassure the parents that their expression of grief and the intense feelings associated with grief are normal.
- Discuss what and how to tell surviving children about the death; encourage the parents to allow their other children to grieve.
- Refer parents to perinatal bereavement support groups.

MAKING THE LOSS REAL

- Allow the parents to see and hold the dead baby if they wish.
- Prepare parents for what they will see, if they choose to see and hold the dead baby. Give

Continued on following page

Strategies for Helping Families Cope with Perinatal Loss Continued

them a description that includes body temperature, color, size, bruises, and deformities. Stay with them unless they request time alone with the baby.

- Point out characteristics of the baby that are familial and those that are unique (e.g., "He has your nose") to promote the attachment-termination process.
- Wrap the baby in a clean, warm baby blanket. The care taken with the baby demonstrates respect.
- Encourage the parents to name the baby and use this name when talking about the baby. Otherwise, be careful to refer to the baby by the correct sex.
- Take a photograph of the dead baby and keep it on file if it is not immediately wanted by the parents.
- Encourage the parents to have a funeral or a memorial service; allow both parents to be active in planning for the service.
- Help parents create memories by asking them about the loss and their dreams and aspirations for this child.
- Discuss medical findings and autopsy results in a frank and sensitive manner.
- Give extra grief counseling and support when a subsequent pregnancy occurs; the parents' levels of fear and anxiety will be high.
- Encourage family members and friends to allow the parents to disassemble the nursery at home; advise against doing it for them.

TEACHING PARENTS ABOUT THE GRIEF PROCESS

- Give the parents anticipatory guidance regarding what they might experience during the period of acute grief: somatic complaints, feelings of unreality, loneliness, depression, guilt, anger, irritability, loss of routine patterns, preoccupation with an image of the infant, insomnia, and difficulties with friends and relatives.
- Talk with the parents about possible differences in grief style and length of grieving between the mother and the father.
- Discuss subsequent pregnancy and the replacement-child syndrome. Some questions you can have the family ask themselves before another pregnancy: "Does the loss consume my every thought?" "Am I obsessed with becoming pregnant?" "Can I think about the loss without being torn apart?" "Am I expecting this next child to make me feel better?"
- Warn the parents about "roller coaster" emotional shifts. Warn them that even when life seems to be back to normal, there might still be some unexpected painful reminders, such as the anniversary of the due date or the anniversary of the loss.

HELPING THE WOMAN WHO IS BEING SEEN IN A PHYSICIAN'S OFFICE

- Do not make the woman and her family experiencing a pregnancy loss wait in the waiting room.
- Do not leave the woman and her family alone for long periods.
- Allow the woman and her family to leave by an exit that is comfortable for them.
- Make sure the woman has a ride home and is not going home alone.
- Set up a system to flag charts so that on return visits, everyone is aware of the situation.
- Follow-up for these women and their families is essential and should be done at the time of death; 2 to 3 days after discharge; 2 to 4 months after the death—this is a critical time because support has dropped off, the shock has worn off, and the reality of the infant's death has set in; 1 year after the loss.
- If follow-up throughout the year is not possible, a call at about 3 weeks after the death is most helpful.

Continued on facing page

Strategies for Helping Families Cope with Perinatal Loss Continued

PROVIDING EFFECTIVE FOLLOW-UP

- Provide information about the possible cause of death.
- Provide needed medical information.
- Give an opportunity to review and discuss what happened, somatic complaints, mourning reactions, and relationship difficulties.
- Reduce the families' feelings of isolation or abandonment.
- Formulate and ask questions during follow-up phone calls, such as "How did it feel to go home?" "What was the hardest part for you once you returned home?" "Is there anyone you can talk with about the death of your baby?" "How do your friends act? How are your coworkers responding?" "What is the response of your family members?" "How are the siblings reacting? How did you tell them about what happened?" "What questions do you have for me?"

USING OTHER APPROACHES TO HELP GRIEVING FAMILIES

- Use a checklist that is a guide to teaching and steps to take that can be helpful to the parents. This helps increase consistency of care for all families and increases communication among health care providers.
- Use a special magnet or card on the patient's door frame that all employees, including housekeeping, dietary, and those in other ancillary departments, have been trained to recognize as indicating that the patient's baby died.
- Take a photograph of the baby who has died. This is done with self-developing film using a camera kept in the labor and delivery area so that the parents will have photos immediately.
- Give a disposable camera to each family who has experienced a perinatal loss. The nurse also takes photos with that camera, and the camera is given to the family to develop the film in their own time. These photos will be of better quality and will last longer than the instant photos.
- Give a memory box to each of these families. This box should include a condolence card from the staff, a card for baby information, a card for a footprint, a small seal-top plastic bag for a lock of hair, clothes for burial or as a keepsake, and a card with resource information.

From Lowe, M., and Neumann, M. (1995). Perinatal loss: How to deal with a difficult situation. *NCC News,* May, 5–7.

cludes identifying and including the infant as a part of their family; and providing anticipatory guidance about the process of mourning. Immediate support may include calling a support person, such as a close friend, family, or clergy, and ensuring that the mother is not left by herself (Benkendorf 1987; Davis et al. 1988).

ENVIRONMENT

Are grieving mothers who are hospitalized best served on a maternity unit or in another area of the hospital? Wolff and colleagues (1970) reported that 54 percent would have preferred the maternity unit, while 32 percent would have chosen a medical-surgical unit. Some preferred the company of others, while 30 percent preferred a private room. These data suggest that women have different needs and should be asked about their preferences.

The creation of a supportive environment frequently involves some way of identifying the mother as one who has experienced a loss. Some institutions use a colored dot or a tear that is placed on the door of the mother's room and on the Kardex or chart. Many mothers have had the unfortunate experience of being asked "Did you have a boy or a girl?" by a friendly laboratory technician or housekeeper who did not know of their loss. A system of identification helps to protect the mother from this kind of situation (Fig. 38–1).

Providing a consistent caregiver and eliminating unnecessary interactions and procedures are help-

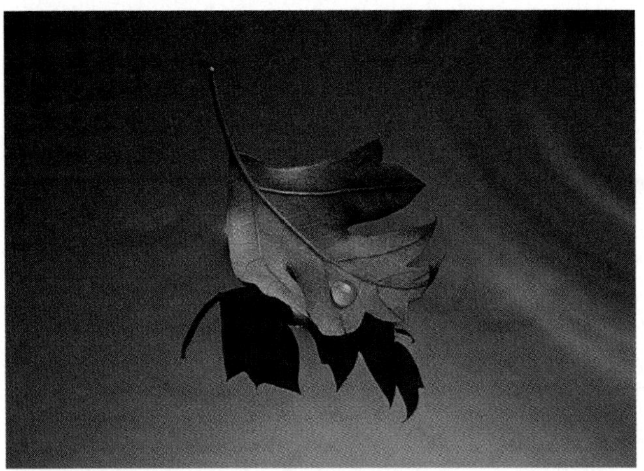

Figure 38–1

A door card placed on the hospital room door of grieving parents is a gentle visual alert to staff of the need for sensitivity when entering the room. (Photo courtesy of © RTS Bereavement Services, Gundersen Lutheran Medical Center, LaCrosse, WI.)

ful. The primary nurse should be available to spend time with parents, to listen, and to answer questions—sometimes answering the same questions on more than one occasion. The checklist shown in Table 38–1 defines the standard of care that all families who experience perinatal loss should receive. Using a comprehensive checklist also facilitates consistency and continuity of care, serves as a central location for essential documentation, and provides an organizer and reminder of the nursing care that should be provided for women and their families (Ryan et al. 1991).

VALIDATING FEELINGS OF LOSS

Of all that nurses do for parents, being present with them, listening, holding a hand as they cry, and accepting their anger even when it is directed toward the nurse are examples of behaviors that communicate the message that their grief is real

Table 38–1

A COMPREHENSIVE CHECKLIST FOR PERINATAL LOSS

Parents' names ____________________
Address ____________________
Phone ____________________
Description of loss ____________________
____
Description of previous loss(es) ____________________
____

L.M.P. __________ E.D.C. __________
Weeks of gestation __________
Sex of baby (if known) __________
Religious affiliation __________

	Office Staff	E.R. Staff	Labor/Delivery	Postpartum	Neonatal ICU	O.R. Staff	GYN/Post Op	Community Health	Date(s)
Received pregnancy confirmation									____
Lab/amnio results	☐	☐	☐			☐			____
Sonogram photo	☐		☐			☐			____
Acknowledgment of loss/impaired fertility	☐	☐	☐	☐	☐	☐	☐	☐	____
Bring up the subject									
Refer to the baby/expected child									
Call the baby by name									
Anticipatory guidance about normal grief									____
Mother	☐	☐	☐	☐	☐	☐	☐	☐	____
Father	☐	☐	☐	☐	☐	☐	☐	☐	____
Family members	☐	☐	☐	☐	☐	☐	☐	☐	____
Postloss options given									
To go home/maternity floor/alternate floor	☐	☐	☐			☐			____
Father to remain with mother/private room			☐	☐			☐		____

Table continued on facing page

Table 38–1

A COMPREHENSIVE CHECKLIST FOR PERINATAL LOSS *Continued*

	Office Staff	E.R. Staff	Labor/Delivery	Postpartum	Neonatal ICU	O.R. Staff	GYN/Post Op	Community Health	Date(s)
Saw/touched/held baby or products of conception	☐	☐	☐		☐	☐	☐		____
If refused, later offers made			☐	☐	☐		☐		____
Family members included in offer	☐	☐	☐	☐	☐	☐	☐		____
Received mementos									
Footprints			☐	☐	☐				____
Bracelet			☐	☐	☐				____
Lock of hair			☐	☐	☐				____
Crib card			☐	☐	☐				____
Blanket			☐	☐	☐				____
Tape measure			☐	☐	☐				____
Certificate of life/remembrance	☐	☐	☐	☐	☐	☐	☐	☐	____
Photographs taken									
Given to parents			☐		☐				____
Filed with chart			☐		☐				____
Bathed/dressed baby			☐		☐				____
Postdeath options discussed	☐	☐	☐	☐	☐		☐		____
Need/desire for funeral director									
Type/location/timing of service									
Burial/cremation/hospital disposal									
Parent involvement									
Choosing burial outfit/mementos									
Announcements—public/personal									
Religious options									
Baby baptized	☐	☐	☐		☐	☐	☐		____
Clergy notified	☐	☐	☐	☐	☐	☐	☐	☐	____
Received information about									
Birth/death certificates	☐	☐		☐	☐		☐	☐	____
Autopsy option discussed	☐	☐	☐	☐	☐		☐		____
Marked chart/room with identifying symbol (e.g., butterfly, rainbow, rose)	☐	☐	☐	☐	☐	☐	☐	☐	____
Received literature/suggested readings	☐	☐	☐	☐	☐	☐	☐	☐	____
Hospital admitting office notified	☐	☐							____
SHARE/support group referral made	☐	☐	☐	☐	☐	☐	☐	☐	____

From Family Nursing Associates, Manlius, N.Y., as adapted in Ryan, P. F., Cote-Arsenault, D., Sugarman, L. L. (1991). Facilitating care after perinatal loss: A comprehensive checklist. *Journal of Obstetric, Gynecologic, and Neonatal Nursing,* 20 (5), 387.

and appropriate. Shakespeare wrote, "Give sorrow words; the grief that does not speak knits up the overwrought heart and bids it break" *(Macbeth)*. Brice (1991), a clinical psychologist, noted that "a bereaved mother accomplishes her mourning by engaging in dialogue with others." She "must find at least one person, a listening mother, to whom she may mourn." The listener needs to present a "nonintrusive, inclusive presence."

Nurses often worry about what they can say to parents experiencing perinatal loss. "I'm sorry" both acknowledges the baby's death and expresses feelings of caring. Among the phrases that parents report as distressing are "You can have another baby," "It was God's will," and, in the case of an early-trimester loss, "It's nature's way of getting rid of a defective baby."

ENCOURAGING THE ACKNOWLEDGMENT OF THE BABY'S EXISTENCE

Contact with their baby has been identified as helpful to parents' mourning (Benfield et al. 1978; Kirkby-Best and Kellner 1982; Nicol et al. 1986). Whitaker (1986), a perinatal nurse and mother of

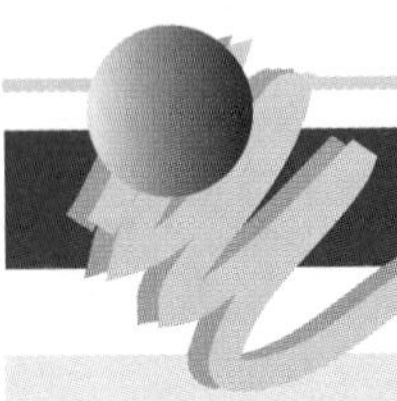

IMPROVING YOUR PRACTICE

CARING FOR GRIEVING PARENTS

Knowing what to say to grieving parents and what to do for them is one of the most difficult situations the nurse faces. This is especially true because we expect birth to be a happy and joyous time. Interventions and statements based on the research of grief and loss that are helpful to grieving parents and that can be devastating are listed here. The hurtful practices are usually made by caring family members and nurses, who just do not know what to say or do. Practice using the helpful approaches by role playing a situation in which you are the nurse caring for grieving parents. This can be done in clinical conferences or classroom settings.

Do

- Say "I'm sorry."
- Take some time to stay with me and listen to me if I want to talk about my pregnancy, labor, birth, or baby.
- Allow me to cry or be angry.
- Ask me how I'm doing and what you can do for me.
- Ask me whom I would like you to notify, including clergy, and let them know what has happened.
- Understand that you may have to repeat explanations more than one time; I can't take all of this in at once.
- Let me see and hold my dead baby if I want to.
- Call my baby by name, if I have chosen a name, and know if my baby is a boy or a girl.
- Take pictures and save them with other mementos of my baby, even if I don't want them right now.
- Let me know what to expect in the coming weeks.
- Assure me that my feelings and behavior are not strange.
- Let me know about options for a funeral or memorial service.
- Tell me about sources of support in the community.

Don't

- Avoid me.
- Tell me my loss was "God's will" or that we have "an angel in heaven."
- Tell me I can have another baby or that I'm lucky because I have other children.
- Tell me that "this happened for the best," "it's very common," or "there was something wrong with the baby anyway."
- Tell me to try and forget.
- Try to protect me by keeping information about my baby's death from me.
- Be afraid to show caring and compassion.

a stillborn infant, wrote, "I don't believe that I fully accepted the death of my baby until I saw him for myself. I consider the few moments that I had with my son very important. The memories of those moments are all that I have left of my second child."

What if parents choose not to see the baby? Krone and Harris (1988) have described a series of steps in which the nurse first explains to the parents why it could be important to see and touch their infant. Subsequently, at a later time, the nurse brings the infant's footprints for the parents to see. Still later, the nurse brings a picture of their infant and talks about the baby while they look at the picture. Finally, the nurse brings the wrapped infant to their room but does not insist that they hold the baby. Throughout the process, the nurse constantly monitors the parents' behavior and expression for clues about a potential next step. The result may be several hours of holding the infant by both parents and grandparents.

This sequence is described not as a plan for all parents but as an example of a creative nursing approach that combines a theoretic understanding of parental bereavement with an individualized plan based on clues provided during interaction of nurse and parents. Some parents may go no further than looking at footprints, baby bracelet, or photographs (ultrasound image or photograph taken after birth). Some may not take these mementos when they first leave the hospital but may ask for them at a later time (Fig. 38–2). In 20 families studied by Krone and Harris (1988), every parent wanted a memento of their baby, even if they were unwilling to view the baby initially. In my experience as an interviewer in a postneonatal mortality study more than 20 years ago, every mother was eager to show me a picture of her infant. In each instance, at least 3 months had passed since the baby's death (by study design).

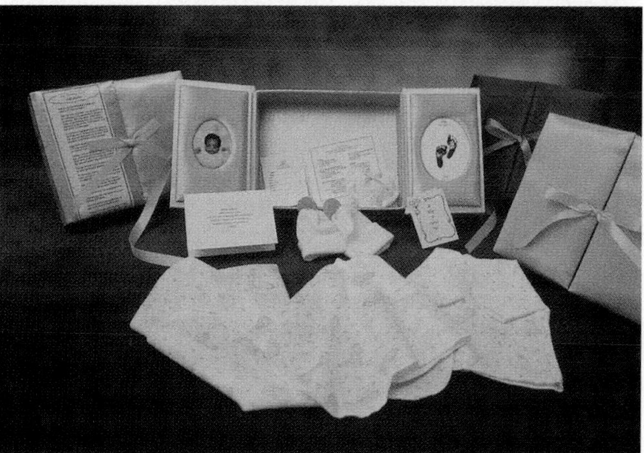

Figure 38–2

A Memory Box is a special place to hold mementos of the baby. This satin-covered box includes a card from the staff, a card for baby information, a photograph, a card for footprints, a small seal-top bag for a lock of hair, clothes for burial or as a keepsake, and a card with resource information. (Photo courtesy of Memories Unlimited, 1994; 1740 Redwood Way, Upland, CA.)

A significant way in which parents acknowledge their baby is through naming their infant. If the baby has been named, it is important to use that name whenever the nurse refers to the baby. Some families will want to name the baby in a service of baptism. Not all religious groups believe in infant baptism; however, it is important to identify parents' wishes.

AUTOPSY REQUESTS

Obtaining permission for an autopsy is the responsibility of a physician in most care settings. Yet families may choose to discuss the decision with nurses. A mother may see the autopsy as a disfiguring surgical procedure and not understand that an autopsy may clarify the cause of death. Reassurance that an autopsy will not interfere with whatever funeral arrangement the family desires may help families make the decision. In some instances, an autopsy may help relieve parents' guilt about the baby's death or answer questions about the possibility of recurrence. Information may assist in the management of a future pregnancy, should the parents choose to have another child.

PROVIDING ANTICIPATORY GUIDANCE

While no one can predict what grief will be like for an individual family, some general information about the course of grief, without timetables, can help parents realize that their reactions are not a sign of craziness (which many fear) and that the pain will get better (Drill 1987). Parents need to know that certain days may be particularly difficult, such as the anniversary of their baby's death, Mother's Day and Father's Day, Christmas, or the expected date of birth in the case of a loss early in pregnancy.

Anticipatory guidance can also help prepare parents for what others, both family and friends, may say to them. Well-intended but painful statements include "At least you didn't know her very long," "You can always have another baby," "Don't talk about it," "Be thankful for your other blessings (children)," and "Try to forget." Unfortunately, these or similar statements sometimes come from the health care team, from whom they are equally or more distressing.

Packing away clothes and furnishings prepared for the baby is also difficult. Mothers can be encouraged to wait until they feel ready. Sometimes friends or relatives will plan to do this before the mother returns from the hospital, but many mothers and counselors believe that this is not as helpful as it is intended to be. The process, when the mother is ready, can emphasize the reality that must be accepted as a part of normal grieving.

Information about physiologic changes is also a part of anticipatory guidance (Brice 1989, 1991). A mother whose baby has died will still experience breast engorgement and the contractions of involution, which serve as painful reminders of her loss. Measures for patient comfort that are taught to all postpartum mothers must not be overlooked for grieving mothers. Special attention to postpartum care is necessary when the mother chooses to be on a nursing unit where postpartum care is rare, such as a medical-surgical unit.

Helping Parents Cope with the Reaction of the Infant's Siblings

When an expected baby dies, siblings also need solace, comforting, and help in understanding the death. The way in which these needs will be met varies with the age of the child. Small children may not understand about the baby's death at all but will be affected by their parents' grief. Death is not a permanent state to a child younger than 3 years, but separation, particularly separation from parents, is a major source of anxiety. Children between the ages of 3 and 5 years may have some ideas about death but still may not view death as permanent. The "magical thinking" of preschoolers may make them feel responsible for the death if they had felt ambivalent about a new sibling. Gradually, after 6 years of age, children begin to understand the permanency of death. Children between the ages of 5 and 8 years seem to be more afraid of death than younger or older children are.

Parents who are grieving themselves often have great difficulty talking about the baby's death with their other children. A number of books about death written for children may help both parents and children verbalize their feelings of sadness. Parents can be helped to acknowledge their feelings and to reassure their other children with such statements as "Mommy is sad because our baby died, but she is happy that you are here."

Parents frequently ask if siblings should attend the baby's funeral. There is no single answer to this question. Many variables, including the child's age and his or her wish to attend or not, must be considered. Some children would feel isolated if they were not a part of this ritual. If children do attend a funeral, a family friend or relative should assume the responsibility for their care and support. If children are unable to sit throughout the service, they should be able to leave with the adults who are caring for them.

Continuing Support

DURING THE FIRST MONTH

Within the first 1 to 2 weeks after a mother's discharge, a phone call from a member of the hospital nursing staff can provide support and comfort. The call has several purposes. The nurse can encourage both questions and the verbalization of feelings. If a follow-up conference has not been previously arranged, this is an appropriate time to do so. Inquiry into the effects of the loss on the marriage and on other members of the family is a part of this assessment. If the availability of a support group was previously discussed, the nurse can ask whether contact has been made and what that was like for the mother. Follow-up using these principles results in decreased problems for the family (Klingbeil 1986).

AFTER THE FIRST MONTH

At approximately 4 to 6 weeks after the death, a grief conference provides an opportunity for assessment and for sharing information with the family. If there has been an autopsy or pathology report, the information can be discussed. Anticipatory guidance about the coming weeks and months is helpful. Specific issues, including sexual relations and future pregnancies, are usually discussed at this time. Many couples report that they have neither the desire nor the energy for sex; others find sex a comfort; and still others desire sex to conceive another child.

The significance of anniversaries for parents who have experienced perinatal loss should be explored. The anniversary may be the date of the loss, the expected date of birth, the actual date of the baby's birth, or some other time of special significance. Many parents dread this reminder of a devastating day in their life and may have both physical and emotional symptoms as early as 2 to 4 weeks before the anniversary date itself. Knowing that what feels like a regression in their mourning is common may be helpful. Some parents cope by choosing to do something for another child or some altruistic cause on the anniversary. For many, the goal is to get through that day.

EXPECTED OUTCOMES

The process of mourning occurs during many months; nurses frequently do not have the opportunity to observe long-term adaptation and acceptance of a perinatal loss. In the initial period after the loss, expected outcomes include expression of grief such as crying (within the context of family cultural norms) and beginning communication about the loss within the family and between family members and staff.

When contact occurs at later periods (e.g., a month, 6 months), expected outcomes include further adaptation to loss, evidenced by the ability to discuss their loss realistically without expressions of guilt; evidence of interfamily support and understanding; and eventually, evidence of looking forward to the future.

The Timing of Subsequent Pregnancy

Should subsequent pregnancy be postponed until sufficient time for mourning has occurred, or does subsequent pregnancy contribute to the resolution of grief through a replacement child? The emotional drive for another child appears strong in many parents; increased fertility rates after perinatal loss have been noted in both developed and developing countries (Vogel and Knox 1975; Park et al. 1979). While Rowe and coworkers (1978) found that mothers who became pregnant within 5 months after a loss were at risk for prolonged grieving, LaRoche and colleagues (1984) found no significant difference between women conceiving in the first 6 months and those conceiving after the first 6 months.

In past generations, parents who experienced perinatal death were frequently advised to conceive another baby quickly to hasten recovery from the pain of their loss. As more attention has been given to understanding the process of mourning, there has been concern that a subsequent pregnancy too soon may both prolong grief (Rowe et al. 1978) and also affect a subsequent mother-baby relationship (Poznanski 1972).

An additional concern is allowing time for physical recovery. Pregnancies less than a year apart have been shown to be one risk factor for a low-birth-weight baby (Ernest et al. 1988). In a study of 24 mothers, Davis and colleagues (1989) found that mothers made their own decisions about the timing of subsequent pregnancies, regardless of the advice given by nurses or physicians. Helping the mother identify factors in her own life that are important in the decision for a subsequent pregnancy and explaining both advantages and disadvantages of postponing pregnancy may be more useful and effective than giving specific advice.

During a subsequent pregnancy, nurses must watch for heightened anxiety, particularly at the gestational age of a previous loss or when medical procedures (ultrasonography or amniocentesis, for example) are undertaken. Parents need anticipatory guidance about the feelings that may occur at these times and also during childbirth education classes and at the time of labor and birth. Memories of their previous loss may be strong at this time. As during their initial grief, the opportunity to talk with an understanding nurse, as well as with each other, can help them accept these feelings.

SPECIAL CIRCUMSTANCES AND NEEDS

The unique characteristics of parents who are part of certain specific groups require additional consideration. Adolescent parents, a mother who is single, parents of multiple gestations in which one or more infants live while one or more die or are severely handicapped, mothers who relinquish their infants for adoption, and mothers with loss in the early trimesters (spontaneous abortion) are examples of parents who have special needs.

When Parents Are Adolescents

The special needs of adolescents who are bereaved parents have received limited attention. Studies examining loss and mourning have rarely examined the effects of parental age, yet rates of perinatal loss are higher in adolescence than among parents older than 20 years.

Experience with bereaved adolescent parents suggests that while many reactions are similar to those of adults, adolescents may also have special needs (Barnickol et al. 1986). Adolescents may have had no previous experience with death; members of their peer group, to whom they may turn for support, may be equally inexperienced. The level of cognitive development and education in teens may limit their understanding of medical terminology. Some adolescents may be reluctant to appear dumb by asking questions.

Both immediate and extended family relationships may differ for teens. Fathers may no longer be involved, yet may grieve. A teen mother may lack support from the baby's father, and her parents may feel and perhaps articulate that death of the infant was a blessing that will allow the young parents to resume their teenage lives. If the loss is a matter of congenital malformation, the resources to care for an infant with special needs is likely to be more limited among teen parents.

The counseling and support given to all parents who mourn a perinatal loss may need to be augmented for teen parents. Modification will be based on the nurse's assessment of (1) previous experience with death, (2) relationship between the infant's mother and father, (3) support system, and (4) level of cognitive understanding.

Nurses may need to spend more time with teen parents for both information and support. If family members or others appear to minimize the loss by statements that suggest it is best for the teen, nurses may need to help teen parents understand and become advocates for themselves. In many instances, grandparents may also be grieving. For those teens attending school, involvement of schoolteachers or counselors as support persons may facilitate this on an ongoing basis.

When the Mother Is a Single Woman

Pregnant single women are a diverse group that includes teens, women who are widowed or divorced during pregnancy, and women who choose to become single parents. Because of the diversity, the feelings of single women about their loss vary considerably, yet there may be some common needs. While not all single women lack a supportive partner, the relationship usually differs from that of marriage. Other family members, perhaps disapproving of the pregnancy, may see the loss as a welcome solution. Nurses, too, may sometimes view the loss as a blessing in disguise and feel less supportive than when loss occurs in a two-parent family. Support groups for bereaved parents may consist primarily of couples, and the single mother, especially if she is young, may not feel comfortable.

Guilt, which is a common emotion of mourning, may be particularly strong for some single women because of ambivalence about the pregnancy or guilt engendered by social disapproval.

Spontaneous Abortion and Miscarriage

Spontaneous abortions occur approximately 800,000 times a year in the United States alone, affecting 15 to 30 percent of all conceptions. Classification and etiology of spontaneous abortion are discussed in Chapter 21. Although nurses and other health care providers frequently use the term abortion rather than miscarriage, this term has a different meaning to the general public and should rarely be used in talking with parents (Borg and Lasker 1981).

After miscarriage, parents may feel a sense of loss and bereavement as intense as in losses later in pregnancy. They mourn their fantasized baby, but friends, families, and many health care providers may act as though the loss is a minor event. Particularly when the loss occurs early in pregnancy, the rituals that accompany other losses may be absent, such as a funeral, flowers, or messages of condolence.

Recurrent spontaneous abortion presents a special kind of grief. Each loss may cause parents to regrieve previous losses. Moreover, with each additional loss, the possibility of future successful pregnancies may seem less likely and may indeed be less likely.

A remark frequently made to parents at the time of spontaneous abortion is that it was nature's way of getting rid of an imperfect fetus. Aside from the fact that this is not the only cause and may not be applicable in a particular situation, it is a distressing comment for parents, particularly at the time of loss. Parents also report a conspiracy of silence, the avoidance of the topic of their pregnancy loss by professionals.

Women's feelings associated with spontaneous abortion may include the sense of a loss of a part of themselves, sadness over loss of both the baby and the pregnancy, and guilt if there was ambivalence about the pregnancy or activities in which they may have engaged or failed to engage. For men, if the loss occurred early in pregnancy, the baby may not yet seem real; their major concern may be the mother's physical and emotional health rather than the loss of the baby. Men may also experience guilt.

Death of an Infant in a Hospital Nursery

An infant may live beyond the immediate period after birth and subsequently die days or weeks later. During the time between birth and death, parents should be encouraged to spend as much time as possible with their baby. Some parents resist becoming attached to their baby, particularly if loss is expected, because they fear it will "hurt too much." The experience of families who have lost infants suggests quite the opposite. Loss is painful under any circumstances, but knowing their baby and thus grieving for someone they know is ultimately helpful for most parents. Providing opportunities to care for their infant and, in the final period before death, to hold their infant and say goodbye is a part of nursing care.

In many nurseries, the provision of privacy for families is difficult. Unlike units for adults, nurseries are not usually designed with private rooms or even curtains to screen one patient from another. Each nursery should identify a place where families can comfortably spend private time with their dying infant.

Although some time for the family to be together by themselves may be desired, a nurse should be with the family or immediately available most of the time. The nurse may sit quietly, saying little or nothing, but the nurse's presence indicates that support is available. Other professionals, such as the hospital chaplain, family clergyman, nursery social worker, or physician, may also provide support. No family should feel alone and abandoned during this difficult time.

Many families have religious beliefs and practices that are important at the time of death. For example, Roman Catholic and Episcopal families as well as some others will desire infant baptism. Some families will have a brief prayer service at the infant's bedside, in which they affirm their belief that their baby is returning to God. When families are away from their home community because the baby has been transferred to a regional center, nurses need to assess the parents' religious desires and help the family contact their own clergyman or a clergyman of their denomination if they wish to do so.

Group meetings for parents of infants who are dying or have died are helpful to some families. Other families may not feel that these will be helpful to them. Informal support of one family by parents of other babies in the nursery may also occur. Each family will deal with grief in a manner unique to them. Nurses must assess family needs individually, provide information about the resources available, and allow families to decide whether a particular resource will be helpful.

Intrauterine Fetal Death

As pregnancy proceeds, a mother develops a unique and special relationship to her fetus that is both physical and psychological and that is different from her relationship to any other person, even the baby's father—and so, when the baby dies before birth, the mother's experience of loss is also different from that of any other person (Grubb-Phillips 1988).

Intrauterine fetal death may occur before or during the course of labor. If the death is before labor, a period of days may elapse before labor either begins spontaneously or is induced. During this period, a mother is at some physical risk herself (disseminated intravascular coagulation, emboli, sepsis). Moreover, the presence of the dead fetus within her may conjure an image of a dead, decomposing thing within her. She continues to look pregnant so she must either tell those who inquire about her pregnancy that her baby has died or pretend her baby is still alive. During the period between death and the stillbirth, a mother may continue to hope that the diagnosis is wrong. Because of this, mourning usually will not begin until after the infant's death.

Death in a Multiple Gestation

In multiple gestation pregnancies, when one or more infants die as a result of miscarriage, stillbirth, or neonatal death, parents experience the stress of coping with conflicting emotions: joy for the birth and grief for the death. For some families, the sense of loss may extend to the loss of the fantasy of being the parents of twins or other multiples, fear of the loss of friendship with other parents of multiples they may have met during the pregnancy, and loss of the special attention or prestige they received as prospective parents of multiples. If the surviving infant is ill, anticipatory grief may coexist with grief for the child who has died (Johnson 1987; Swanson-Kauffman 1988).

While it is hard to grieve fully for one child in the presence of a living twin, it is essential both for the parents' well-being and for the future healthy development of the survivor. When grief is unresolved, the survivor must compete with an idealized sibling and may grow to feel guilty about survival (Wilson et al. 1982). Parents may also be overprotective toward the survivor, fearful that they will lose this child as well.

Helping parents recognize the reality of the infant who has died through holding, touching, naming, and planning memorial services will serve to separate the two children in the parents' minds and facilitate grieving. Conversely, attempts to lessen grief by denying the existence of the child who died can only be counterproductive. Comments such as "You're lucky to have a living child" are frequently made and are highly detrimental (Wilson et al. 1982). Birthdays can be particularly bittersweet; the life of one child is celebrated at the same time the loss of another is remembered with sorrow.

The Relinquishing Mother

As attitudes toward single mothers and abortion have changed and knowledge about contraception has increased, the number of mothers who relinquish infants for adoption has decreased. Nevertheless, relinquishment of an infant for adoption is and will continue to be a source of perinatal grief.

Mothers may feel forced to make the only choice

that seems an option for them, even when professionals try hard not to influence that choice. Anger, associated with original feelings of lack of options, may continue for years if a mother's attempt to gather information about her child is frustrated (Condon 1986). Because the child remains alive, mothers may not say good-bye, but they may nurture a fantasy of being reunited at some time and thereby exist in a state of chronic grief for years afterward. Lack of information about the child's well-being may contribute to fantasies.

Although less research is focused on relinquishment than on other aspects of perinatal grieving, some direction for caring is suggested by available data. The mother's wishes about seeing and caring for her child should be respected. It can help to validate that it takes a great deal of love to let her baby go to another home.

CARING FOR THE CAREGIVER

The sense of loss and the grief that accompanies loss are not limited to family members. Nurses and their professional colleagues grieve as well.

Table 38–2

MANIFESTATIONS OF THE GRIEF PROCESS IN NURSES AND FAMILIES

EMOTION	NURSES	FAMILIES
Shock and disbelief	Particularly acute when baby who appeared to be doing well worsens—Why this baby?	Why me? Why us? Why our baby?
Shame, loss of self-esteem	Inability to prevent death seen as threat to self-esteem	Why could we not produce a healthy child?
Guilt	Guilt about care given or not given	Guilt about preterm birth or anomaly Guilt about not wanting to attach to baby
Anxiety	Fear of helplessness Coping with anxiety by remaining detached, enforcing "rules"	Fear of attaching to baby, growing to love baby Fear of loss of baby
Denial	Denial of severity of illness to self and parents	Denial of severity of infant's illness
Anger	Anger at baby Anger at parents Anger at other team members Blaming parents and team members	Anger at baby Anger at staff Anger at other family members
Bargaining	Promises to God and others	Promises to God and others
Acceptance	Need opportunities to express feelings and ask questions Require acceptance of colleagues' expressions in nonjudgmental fashion	Need opportunities to express feelings and ask questions

From Moore, M. L. (1983). *Realities in childbearing* (2nd ed.). Philadelphia: W. B. Saunders.

Before nurses can be helpful to parents and families, they must recognize their own potential for grief (Weiss et al. 1989). It is difficult not to identify with young parents who are grieving. Many nurses are in their own childbearing years; some have experienced a perinatal loss themselves or may fear such a loss in the future. Mothers tell us that they often feel that nurses (and other health care providers) avoid talking with them about their baby who has died or been relinquished for adoption or who is in intensive care. Because parents may be feeling angry and guilty, they are frequently sensitive to the behavior of others toward themselves and their infant. Table 38–2 suggests some of the behaviors through which nurses may manifest grief in comparison with the ways families manifest grief.

Implications for Research

Many important questions concerning parents' responses to perinatal loss remain partially or completely unanswered. Longitudinal studies that track the process of mourning in varying population groups will help understand the mourning process over time. Most studies have involved middle-class white parents. We need to know whether physical symptoms, behaviors, and feelings vary in other populations. Other areas for investigation include

- How do grief reactions to different types of perinatal loss vary? How do the needs of fathers differ from those of mothers?
- What are the factors related to, and interventions helpful in, incongruent mourning and the strain of perinatal loss on marital relationships?
- Can the potential for pathologic grief be identified and modified?
- What are the effects of individual personal characteristics on grieving? How can guilt be alleviated?
- What specific interventions are most valuable for particular parents?
- What are the differences between the effects of specific programs of varying institutions?
- What interventions are most helpful for siblings? for grandparents?
- What effects do the circumstances surrounding the death have?
- Which parents are vulnerable to replacement-child syndrome? What strategies are effective for helping these parents?

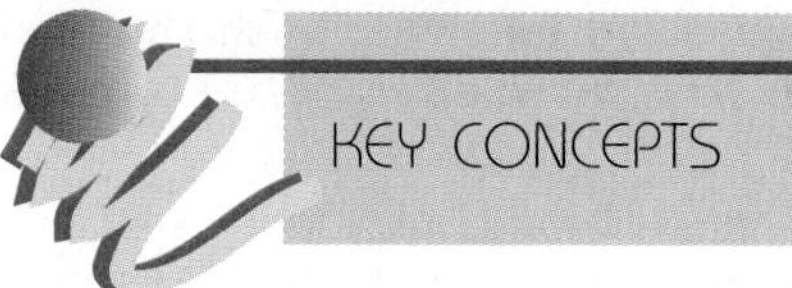

KEY CONCEPTS

- ▼ Expectant mothers and fathers, nurses, and other health care professionals expect pregnancy to have a healthy, joyous outcome.
- ▼ Expectant parents and the nurses who care for them usually have little preparation for death or severe illness in the childbearing year.
- ▼ Feelings of loss and the need to grieve (mourn) may occur at any time in the childbearing year from the preconceptional period through early infancy.
- ▼ Perinatal grief is different from other types of grief because most parents expect a healthy outcome; the relationship of the parents and other family members to the loss (fetus, newborn, or infant) is based on fantasy and hope rather than on actual knowledge; expectant parents are often young, and this may be their first experience with such a loss; and individuals who are in the position to most likely provide social support during the grieving period to the individuals who suffered a loss are often reluctant or unable to do so.
- ▼ Perinatal grief, as all grief, may be anticipatory, normal, or pathologic.
- ▼ A number of factors may influence mourning in both positive and negative ways. These factors are individual and family characteristics, the effect of circumstances surrounding the loss, and interventions that assist parents and other family members through the process of mourning.
- ▼ Mourning is a series of phases or stages through which the mourner moves from initial shock and disbelief, through a phase of anxiety and searching, through a phase of disorganization, to a phase of reorganization.
- ▼ Nurses can use specific strategies to help parents validate the loss, help parents make the loss real, teach parents about the grief process, help a grieving woman and her family who are being seen in a physician's office, and provide effective follow-up to parents during the time after a perinatal loss.
- ▼ Using a comprehensive checklist for caring for individuals who have suffered perinatal loss facilitates consistency and continuity of care, serves as a central location for essential documentation, and provides an organizer and reminder of the nursing care that should be provided for women and their families.

- ▼ Continuing support and follow-up with the parents during the first year after perinatal loss are essential.
- ▼ Adolescent parents, single mothers, parents who have multiple births in which one infant dies, mothers who relinquish their babies for adoption, and mothers who have early-trimester losses compose groups that have special needs after a perinatal loss and require additional assistance.

References

Barnickol, C., Fuller, H., Shinners, B. (1986). Helping bereaved adolescent parents. In C. Corr and J McNeil (Eds), *Adolescence and death.* New York: Springer.

Benfield, D. G., Leib, S., Vollman, J. (1978). Grief response of parents to neonatal death and parent participation in deciding care. *Pediatrics,* 62 (2), 171–177.

Benkendorf, J. (1987). Grieving and believing: Helping parents through imperfect beginnings. *Birth Defects Original Article Series,* 23 (6), 25–36.

Borg, S., and Lasker, J. (1981). *When pregnancy fails: Families coping with miscarriage, stillbirth and infant death.* Boston: Beacon Press.

Brice, C. (1989). The relational essence of maternal mourning: An existential-psychoanalytic perspective. *Humanistic Psychologist,* 17, 22–40.

Brice, C. (1991). Paradoxes of maternal mourning. *Psychiatry,* 54, 1–12.

Condon, J. (1986). Psychological disability in women who relinquish a baby for adoption. *Medical Journal of Australia,* 144 (3), 117–119.

Davis, D., Stewart, M., Harmon, R. (1988). Perinatal loss: Providing emotional support for bereaved parents. *Birth,* 15 (4), 242–246.

Davis, D., Stewart, M., Harmon, R. (1989). Postponing pregnancy after perinatal death: Perspectives on doctor advice. *Journal of the American Academy of Child and Adolescent Psychiatry,* 28 (3), 481–487.

Davidson, G. (1979). *Understanding the death of the wished-for child.* Springfield, IL: Order of the Golden Rule Publishing Corp., 1979.

Drill, M. (1987). The call: Anticipatory guidance for the death of a family's newborn. *Pediatrics in Review,* 8 (7), 196–199.

Ernest, J. M., Michielutte, R., Meis, P., Moore, M. L., Sharp, P. (1988). Identification of women at high risk for preterm low birthweight births. *Preventive Medicine,* 17, 60–72.

Forrest, G., Standish, E., Baum, J. (1982). Support after perinatal death: A study of support and counseling after perinatal bereavement. *British Medical Journal,* 285, 1475–1479.

Giles, P. (1970). Reactions of women to perinatal death. *Australia and New Zealand Journal of Obstetrics and Gynaecology,* 10, 207–210.

Graham, M., Thompson, S., Estrada, M., Yonekura, M. (1987). Factors affecting psychological adjustment to a fetal death. *American Journal of Obstetrics and Gynecology,* 157, 254–257.

Grubb-Phillips, C. (1988). Intrauterine fetal death: The maternal bereavement experience. *Journal of Perinatal and Neonatal Nursing,* 2 (2), 34–44.

Herz, E. (1984). Psychological repercussions of pregnancy loss. *Psychiatric Annals,* 14, 454–457.

Johannsen, L. (1989). As birth and death coincide. *MCN: American Journal of Maternal Child Nursing,* 14 (2), 89–92.

Johnson, S. (1987). *After a child dies. Counseling bereaved families.* New York: Springer.

Kennell, J., Slyter, H., Klaus, M. (1970). The mourning response of parents to the death of a newborn infant. *New England Journal of Medicine,* 283, 344–349.

Kirkby-Best, E., and Kellner, K. (1982). The forgotten grief: A review of the psychology of stillbirth. *American Journal of Orthopsychiatry,* 52, 420–429.

Klingbeil, C. (1986). Extended nursing care after a perinatal loss: Theoretical implications. *Neonatal Network,* December, 21–28.

Krone, C., and Harris, C. (1988). The importance of infant gender and family resemblance within parents' perinatal bereavement process: Establishing parenthood. *Journal of Perinatal and Neonatal Nursing,* 2 (2), 1–11.

Kubler-Ross, E. (1969). *On death and dying.* New York: Macmillan.

LaRoche, C., Lainec-Michaud, M., Engelsmann, F., et al. (1984). Grief reactions to perinatal death. *Canadian Journal of Psychiatry,* 29, 14–19.

Leon, J. (1986). Psychodynamics of perinatal loss. *Psychiatry,* 49, 312–323.

Lindemann, E. (1944). Symptomatology and management of acute grief. *American Journal of Psychiatry,* 101, 141.

Littlefield, C., and Rushton, J. P. (1986). When a child dies: The sociobiology of bereavement. *Journal of Personality and Social Psychology,* 51 (4), 797–802.

Nichols, A., and Lewin, T. (1986). Grief reactions of parental couples: Congenital handicap and cot death. *Medical Journal of Australia,* 144 (6), 292–295.

Nicol, M., Tompkins, J., Campbell, N., Syme, G. (1986). Maternal grieving response after perinatal death. *Medical Journal of Australia,* 144, 287–289.

Null, S. (1989). Nursing care to ease parents' grief. *MCN: American Journal of Maternal Child Nursing,* 14 (2), 84–89.

Page-Lieberman, J., and Hughes, C. B. (1990). How fathers perceive perinatal death. *MCN: American Journal of Maternal Child Nursing,* 15 (5), 321.

Park, C., Han, S., Choe, M. (1979). The effect of infant death on subsequent fertility in Korea and the role of family planning. *American Journal of Public Health,* 69, 557–565.

Parkes, C. (1985). Bereavement. *British Journal of Psychiatry,* 146, 11–17.

Peppers, L., and Knapp, R. (1980). *Motherhood and mourning: Perinatal death.* New York: Praeger.

Peppers, L., and Knapp, R. (1985). *How to go on living after the death of a baby.* Atlanta: Peachtree Publishers.

Pettit, D. B. (1987). The epidemiology of fetal death. *Clinical Obstetrics and Gynecology,* 30, 253–258.

Poznanski, E. (1972). The "replacement child": A saga of unresolved parental grief. *Behavioral Pediatrics,* 81 (6), 1190–1193.

Rowe, J., Clyman, R., Green, C., et al. (1978). Follow-up of families who experience a perinatal death. *Pediatrics,* 62, 166–170.

Ryan, P. A., Cote-Arsenault, D., Sugarman, L. L. (1991). Facilitating care after perinatal loss: A comprehensive checklist. *Journal of Obstetric, Gynecologic, and Neonatal Nursing,* 20 (5), 385–389.

Stierman, E. (1987). Emotional aspects of perinatal death. *Clinical Obstetrics and Gynecology,* 30 (2), 352–361.

Swanson-Kauffman, K. (1988). There should have been two: Nursing care of parents experiencing the perinatal death of a twin. *Journal of Perinatal and Neonatal Nursing,* 2 (2), 78–86.

Tudehope, D., Iredell, J., Rodgers, D., Gunn, A. (1986). Neonatal death: Grieving families. *Medical Journal of Australia,* 144 (6), 290–292.

Vogel, H., and Knox, E. (1975). Reproductive patterns after stillbirth and early infant death. *Journal of Biosocial Science,* 7, 103–111.

Wallerstedt, C., and Higgins, P. (1996). Facilitating perinatal grieving between the mother and the father. *Journal of Obstetric, Gynecologic, and Neonatal Nursing,* 25 (5), 389–394.

Weiss, L., Frescher, L., Richman, J. (1989). Parental adjustment to intrapartum and delivery room loss: The role of a hospital-based support program. *Clinics in Perinatology,* 16 (4), 1009–1019.

Whitaker, C. (1986). Death before birth. *American Journal of Nursing,* 86 (2), 157–158.

Wilson, A., Fenton, L., Stevens, D., Soule, D. (1982). The death of a newborn twin: An analysis of parental bereavement. *Pediatrics,* 70 (4), 587–591.

Wolff, J., Nelson, P., Schiller, P. (1970). The emotional reaction to a stillbirth. *American Journal of Obstetrics and Gynecology,* 108, 73–76.

Zeanah, C. (1989). Adaptation following perinatal loss: A critical review. *Journal of the American Academy of Child and Adolescent Psychiatry,* 28 (3), 467–480.

39 Chapter

Teen pregnancy is less about young women and their sex lives than it is about restricted horizons and the boundaries of hope. It is about race and class and how those realities limit opportunities for young people. More centrally, however, it is typically about being young, female, poor, and nonwhite and about how having a child seems to be one of the few avenues of satisfaction, fulfillment, and self-esteem.

K. Luker (1991)

Adolescent Pregnancy and Parenthood

Francine H. Nichols
Mary Jo Podgurski

HIGHLIGHTS

- The Problem of Adolescent Pregnancy
- Statistics Concerning Adolescent Pregnancy
- Cultural Influences on Adolescent Pregnancy
- Adolescent Sexual Activity
- The Consequences of Adolescent Pregnancy and Parenthood
- Types of Adolescent Pregnancy Prevention Programs
- Issues and Approaches Related to the Problem of Adolescent Pregnancy
- Nursing Implications
- Risk Management
- Implications for Research

Adolescent pregnancy is a poignant human experience that is painfully private yet starkly public at the same time. Pregnancy dramatically signals to the world that reproductive maturity has been achieved. The difficult decisions that the often frightened and uncertain pregnant adolescent has to make have serious implications for her future, and society, and require a maturity beyond her years. Society is struggling with the economic burden of adolescent pregnancy. In 1990, the federal government spent more than $25 billion for Aid to Families with Dependent Children (AFDC), food stamps, and Medicaid to support women who first gave birth as teenagers (Center for Population Options 1992). Adolescent pregnancy with its financial and social problems has as much significance for the future of our nation as do the budget deficit, the trade deficit, interest rates, and unemployment. All individuals are affected by adolescent pregnancy and childbearing in some manner—financially, socially, or personally.

DEFINITIONS

Abstinence-based/postpone sexuality education—An approach that focuses on the strategy of delaying intercourse on the basis of the belief that coitus in early adolescence is particularly risky and that it is either unrealistic or inappropriate to advocate abstinence by all persons in late adolescence. These programs typically stress abstinence, postponing intercourse, and skill building while discussing contraception.

Abstinence-only sexuality education—A curriculum that presents abstinence as the only solution to teenage pregnancy and sexually transmitted diseases. Other preventive methods, such as condoms, are not discussed.

Adolescence—The transition years between puberty and adulthood; the teenage years.

Comprehensive sexuality education—A comprehensive approach that involves a broad range of topics focusing on the belief that sexuality education should prepare adolescents for the healthy expression of their sexuality instead of only preventing negative consequences. This curriculum deals with traditional areas, such as reproductive biology and puberty, marriage, and sexually transmitted diseases, but also covers many controversial topics, such as sexual pleasure, noncoital sexual expression, and homosexuality.

Early adolescence—Ages ranging from 11 to 13 years.

Late adolescence—Ages 17 to 19 years.

Middle adolescence—Ages ranging from 14 to 16 years.

Traditional sexuality education—An educational approach that basically includes instruction on reproductive biology and sexually transmitted diseases with an emphasis on preventing adolescent sexual activity.

Every aspect of adolescent pregnancy—teens becoming sexually active, their decision to take contraceptives, providing contraceptives to teens, the dilemmas of abortion and adoption, the decision of an immature teen to keep her baby—is enmeshed in moral and ethical issues. There is heated controversy about which approaches should be used to resolve the problem of adolescent pregnancy.

DIMENSIONS OF THE PROBLEM

Adolescent pregnancy is not a new phenomenon in the United States; however, its dimensions are changing. In the past, marriage was the usual approach taken to resolve an adolescent's premarital pregnancy. Today, if the pregnancy is carried to term, 96 percent of all teenage mothers remain single and choose to keep and care for their children (Alan Guttmacher Institute 1994). Increasingly, young women today choose to remain single and have a child rather than have an early unwanted marriage. There is a high probability that these adolescent mothers will require public assistance to support their families.

Two dimensions of adolescent pregnancy that have received recent attention are the relationship between prior sexual abuse and conception and the difference in age between adolescent mothers and their partners. Research indicates that sexual abuse as well as other forms of maltreatment may affect children in all areas of development and may be a contributing factor in early childbearing (Butler and Burton 1990; Boyer and Fine 1992). Collaborative efforts to combine sexual assault services with teen pregnancy programs have been initiated in some areas and hold promise (Podgurski 1996a). Research indicates that the younger a sexually experienced teenager is, the more likely she is to have had involuntary sex (Alan Guttmacher Institute 1994). Age of the female teen's sexual partner is another factor in adolescent pregnancy. A survey conducted of more than 10,000 pregnant teens, ages 15 to 19 years, showed that slightly more than half the babies conceived by young mothers in the 15- to 17-year age bracket were fathered by men older than 20 years (Landry and Forrest 1995; Alan Guttmacher Institute 1994).

THE STATISTICS

The statistics on adolescent pregnancy in the United States are grim. More than 1 million adolescent females become pregnant in the United States every year. Approximately three fourths of these pregnancies are unintended. One in four fe-

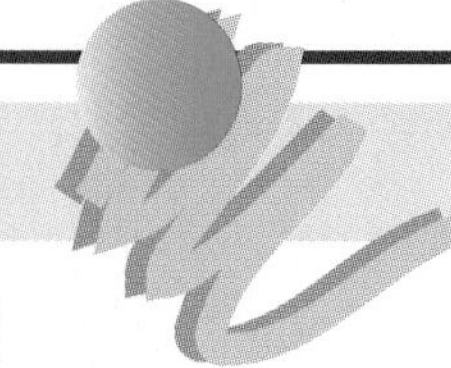

HISTORICAL PERSPECTIVES

DECREASING THE INCIDENCE OF EARLY ADOLESCENT SEXUAL ACTIVITY AND ADOLESCENT PREGNANCIES

In 1978, Joseph Califano, the United States Secretary of Health, Education, and Welfare, proclaimed adolescent pregnancy the top domestic priority of the Carter Administration. During the debates on adolescent pregnancy in the United States Congress that followed in 1978, and again in 1981, legislators disagreed about whether the incidence of adolescent sexual activity and pregnancy could be decreased and, if so, what approaches should be used to accomplish that goal. Some policymakers, appearing to believe that the trend could not be reduced once a society reached high levels of early premarital sexual activity, fervently supported approaches that would improve contraceptive use among teens. Others who thought that efforts should be directed toward reducing adolescent sexual activity vehemently opposed this approach and ardently espoused educational approaches directed toward encouraging sexual abstinence among adolescents. These two views still reflect the prevailing philosophies of legislators and citizens today.

A historical examination of variations in premarital sexual activity and pregnancy and the causes of those variations during the past 350 years can provide information that is useful as a basis for determining public policy and developing adolescent health care programs today. In early America, early sexual activity was viewed as a serious problem. Direct measurement of teenage sexual activity at the time is not possible because the data are not available. Since modern contraceptives were not available, premarital sexual behavior *trends* can be estimated by calculating the percentage of first births born 6 or 8½ months after marriage. Only a small proportion of premarital sexual activity results in pregnancy and the birth of a child; however, this *index* of premarital pregnancies can be useful for *approximating shifts* in premarital sexual activity in early America.

To consider trends in adolescent premarital pregnancies over time, the data should be separated by a female's age at the time of marriage. Unfortunately, such historical data are available only from two Massachusetts communities, Andover and Hingham. The data from those communities from the early 1700s to the late 1800s indicate that adolescents 15 to 19 years old had a significantly higher rate of premarital pregnancies than did older women.

The data from 5665 marriages in the United States in the seventeenth, eighteenth, and nineteenth centuries indicate a wide fluctuation in the number of premarital pregnancies. Premarital pregnancies range from a low of less than 10 percent of first births in the seventeenth century to a high of almost 30 percent in the second half of the eighteenth century.

The Seventeenth and Eighteenth Centuries

The Puritan influence in early America greatly contributed to the low rate of premarital pregnancies in the seventeenth century. While sexual activity before marriage was common in the fifteenth and sixteenth centuries in England, the seventeenth century Puritans in both England and the New World strongly opposed premarital and extramarital sexual activity and were effective in greatly reducing the occurrence of sexual behavior before marriage. As late as the 1670s, more than half of the couples in Essex County, Massachusetts, who had premarital pregnancies were publicly chastised, convicted, and punished as sexual offenders. The value of sexual abstinence outside of marriage became routinely accepted by seventeenth century citizens.

Toward the end of the seventeenth century, church, government, and community opposition to premarital sexual behavior decreased. Church leaders found that when they tried to punish parishioners for "lax moral standards," they could no longer count on the support of their

Continued on facing page

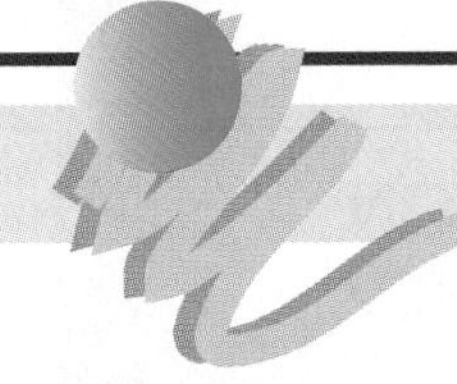

HISTORICAL PERSPECTIVES Continued

congregations or the community. Premarital sexual activity became more tolerated, and sexual intimacy returned as a normal part of courtship behavior. The promise to marry often led to sexual intercourse between couples. Premarital pregnancies were tolerated, as long as the community did not have to assume the financial burden for illegitimate children. The result was a rapid rise in premarital pregnancies in the late seventeenth and early eighteenth centuries.

The Nineteenth and Twentieth Centuries

In the early 1800s, the incidence of premarital pregnancies decreased, partly in response to the social attitude strongly condemning sexual activity outside of marriage. While the Puritans in the 1600s emphasized public censure of deviants, reformers in the early 1800s focused on instilling values of self-control and self-discipline. Religious leaders preached the gospel of sexual abstinence. Medical writings of the time reinforced the importance of sexual abstinence by pointing out to adolescents that sexual activity and masturbation would decrease their strength and vitality.

Perhaps the most important deterrent to sexual activity was the societal standard of what was respectable behavior for women during this time. Any sexual experience before marriage was thought to contaminate a woman and make her a less desirable marriage partner. Early sexual activity was also linked with female delinquency. Any unmarried female who participated in sexual activity or who became pregnant was socially ostracized. The stigma attached to out-of-wedlock births led to an increase in elective abortions among single women and a decline in premarital sexual activity.

During the twentieth century, the incidence of adolescent pregnancy has increased again, most likely as a result of a permissive climate that tolerates, condones, and, some say, even fosters sexual intercourse among teenagers. Because of the enormous cost of adolescent pregnancy to society, the federal government began to take an active role in resolving the problem. Because of heated controversy over which approaches should be used, there has been limited success.

History Indicates that Reducing Adolescent Sexual Activity and Pregnancy Is Possible

A look at the incidence of premarital pregnancy in America during the last 350 years indicates that it is possible to reduce adolescent sexual activity and pregnancy. The prevailing societal sexual norms that did not condone premarital sexual activity appear to be the most plausible cause for the low incidence of premarital sexual activity in the seventeenth century and the decrease in premarital sexual activity in the nineteenth century.

On the basis of a careful examination of the history of adolescent sexual activity and pregnancy and attempts taken to resolve them, Vinovskis (1988) proposed two major approaches that are most likely to reduce adolescent sexual activity and adolescent pregnancy. First, society should *convey in strong and unambiguous terms that early sexual activity is inappropriate and unacceptable for adolescents.* It is unlikely that this would be totally successful. Thus, a second approach, *teaching sexual responsibility and improving contraceptive use by sexually active teens,* is also needed. Rather than a singular approach, either emphasizing postponing early sexual activity (the abstinence approach) or increasing the availability of contraceptives to adolescents (the planned parenthood approach), it appears that both approaches are needed if we are to decrease the incidence of early adolescent sexual activity and pregnancy.

Data from Vinovskis, M. A. (1988). *An epidemic of adolescent pregnancy? Some historical and policy considerations.* New York: Oxford University Press.

male teens will experience a pregnancy before completing high school. One of every ten female teens will become a mother while still a teenager (Alan Guttmacher Institute 1994).

Each year, approximately 50 percent of teens who get pregnant will give birth, approximately 40 percent will choose to have an abortion, and approximately 10 percent will spontaneously abort or have a fetal death. Within 2 years after a first pregnancy, 40 to 50 percent of teenagers who have been pregnant once will be pregnant again (Alan Guttmacher Institute 1994).

The rates of sexual activity and the age of initiation of sexual activity in the United States are similar to those of other Western developed countries; yet American teens have significantly higher rates of adolescent pregnancy, abortion, and childbearing than their counterparts in virtually every other industrialized nation (Fig. 39–1).

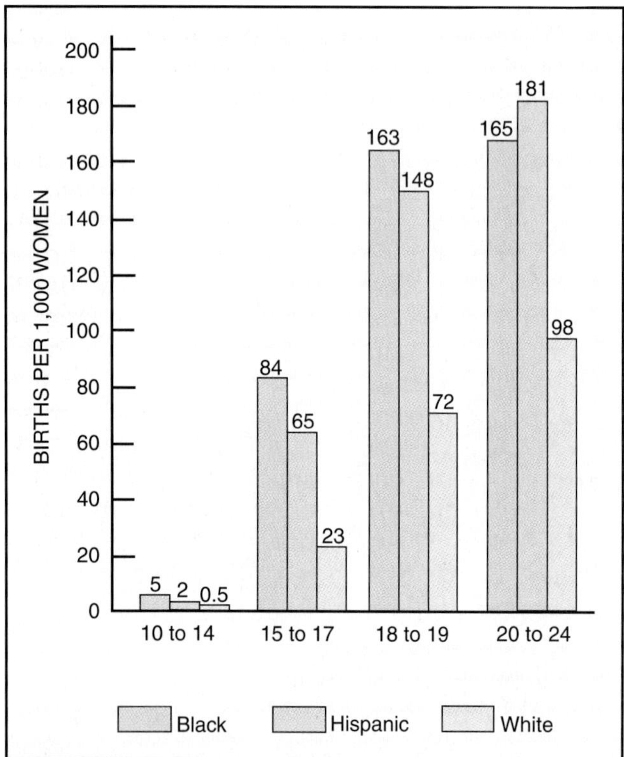

Figure 39–1

Racial differences are seen in birth rates at every age • Statistics show that black and Hispanic women are more likely than white women to give birth as adolescents. (Reproduced with the permission of The Alan Guttmacher Institute from *Sex and America's Teenagers.* The Alan Guttmacher Institute, 1994, New York.)

CULTURAL INFLUENCES ON ADOLESCENT PREGNANCY

Societal influences, family influences, and ethnic influences determine the meaning of pregnancy to the adolescent as well as the responses of others to her situation and the amount of support that she will receive. The societal influences, family influences, and ethnic influences of the culture of the pregnant adolescent require careful assessment in terms of their implications for providing nursing care for her.

Societal Influences

Every society has cultural rules that influence premarital sexual behavior. While these rules vary widely among societies, there are four major categories of societal rules for premarital sexual behavior. In some societies, both modern and primitive, premarital sexual activity is strictly taboo, and adolescent pregnancy is considered "shameful" and results in the condemnation of the adolescent. Other societies are more concerned with premarital pregnancy than with premarital sexual intercourse and permit or even encourage sexual intimacy if proper contraceptives are used; adolescents are expected to take responsibility for their sexual behavior and use appropriate contraceptive measures, and adolescent pregnancy is not condoned. Still other societies, while not approving premarital sexual behavior in general or adolescent pregnancy, ignore the sexual behavior of adolescents if it is done discreetly, or they permit sexual intercourse under some circumstances while forbidding it in others. Finally, in a few primitive societies, promiscuous premarital sexual activity is encouraged as a necessary part of courtship (Lancaster and Hamburg 1986, p. 278).

Societies vary in the clarity of the message that they give to adolescents regarding proper sexual behavior. Some societies provide clear guidance regarding expected sexual norms and practices, while other societies provide confusing and sometimes conflicting messages about accepted behavior.

Societal expectations also determine the impact of pregnancy on the adolescent. In nonindustrial societies, children and adolescents often have many opportunities to learn mothering through communal task sharing of caring for children and role modeling from adult women. Adolescents are expected to marry and have children, often at an early age. Childbirth typically may occur a few years after puberty, usually within the context of marriage, and the adolescent is supported to function competently in her roles as wife and mother through the strong institutions of marriage and family. Positive outcomes for the pregnant adolescent are far less likely in a modern industrial culture, such as the United States, that is much more complex and in which education and vocational skills are more highly valued. To be a productive member of society in an industrial culture requires advanced education and specialized skills. Pregnancy hinders adolescents in obtaining these essential basic skills because it usually leads to an interruption of school, work goals, and career plans (Alan Guttmacher Institute 1994).

Family Influences

Each family is governed by their own rules and expectations, which are often unspoken and may sometimes be in conflict with the verbal instructions given to members. Roles are assigned to various family members, and patterns of expected behavior are based on established family rules. These patterns of behavior are often passed down from generation to generation; for example, the role of an unwed mother is often passed down from mother to daughter through several generations (Rich 1991). Family rules, expectations, and patterns of behavior are often not readily apparent to the nurse. Yet, they have a most significant influence on the impact of the pregnancy for the adolescent, how the adolescent will resolve the pregnancy, the problems that will be encountered, and which interventions will be most effective. An understanding of the principles of family dynamics (see Chapter 4) is essential to work effectively with the pregnant adolescent and her family. The adolescent will bring her family with her when she seeks health care—if not in person, then as a part of her perception of herself and her situation, her learned pattern of response, and her framework for decision making. Parents play an important role in decisions that the adolescent has to make related to the pregnancy (Rich 1991).

Most teens are living with their families when they initiate sexual activity and when the pregnancy occurs. Approximately 80 percent of the unmarried teens who give birth will remain living with their families (Alan Guttmacher Institute 1994). It is the adolescents' families who are their primary source of financial and emotional support. The unmarried pregnant adolescent is in a unique dilemma in regard to her family of origin. As a part of the normal developmental processes of adolescence, she is struggling to establish her own identity and to achieve independence and separate from her family. Yet, the pregnancy forces her to become increasingly dependent on her family for help and support. This dilemma heightens the crisis of an unintended pregnancy during adolescence.

The family system in which the adolescent is functioning will be an influential or even a determining factor in the adolescent's resolution of the pregnancy. In turn, the adolescent's decisions will affect her family and the functioning of her family system. The problem of adolescent pregnancy is a family crisis as well as an individual crisis and must be approached as such.

Ethnic Influences

The impact of pregnancy on family relationships and hence the adolescent herself differs among different ethnic groups. These patterns produce different psychosocial profiles and indicate that teens from different cultures have different problems and needs. The studies on adolescent pregnancy and parenthood have included mostly black and Hispanic teens, undoubtedly because nonwhite teens have a higher birthrate than do white teens; the younger the teen, the greater the proportion of nonwhite births. While there are probably multiple reasons, poverty accounts for some racial difference, and the earlier sexual maturation of black adolescents is another contributing variable (Mercer 1979). Earlier sexual maturity is associated with earlier sexual activity (Abrahamse et al. 1988) (Fig. 39–2).

In the Hispanic culture, marriage usually follows shortly after the pregnancy is confirmed. If the teen remains single, the infant will usually be accepted into the family and the daughter will continue to live with her family. Pregnant Hispanic teens are more likely to come from large intact families, choose to drop out of school, and marry men who are usually several years older with steady jobs. They usually do not smoke cigarettes during pregnancy and are likely to breastfeed their baby (McAnarney 1983). Hispanic adolescents often do not use birth control after childbirth, so they have an increased risk for a second pregnancy. The young Hispanic mother typically receives a great deal of support from her mother, siblings, and other family members. The birth of her child usually establishes the Hispanic adolescent as a mother and woman in her own right, in the eyes of her partner and family, and she usually finds fulfillment in remaining at home with her infant (Humenick et al. 1991).

The profile of the black pregnant teen is much different from that of the pregnant Hispanic teen. The black adolescent is more likely to come from a

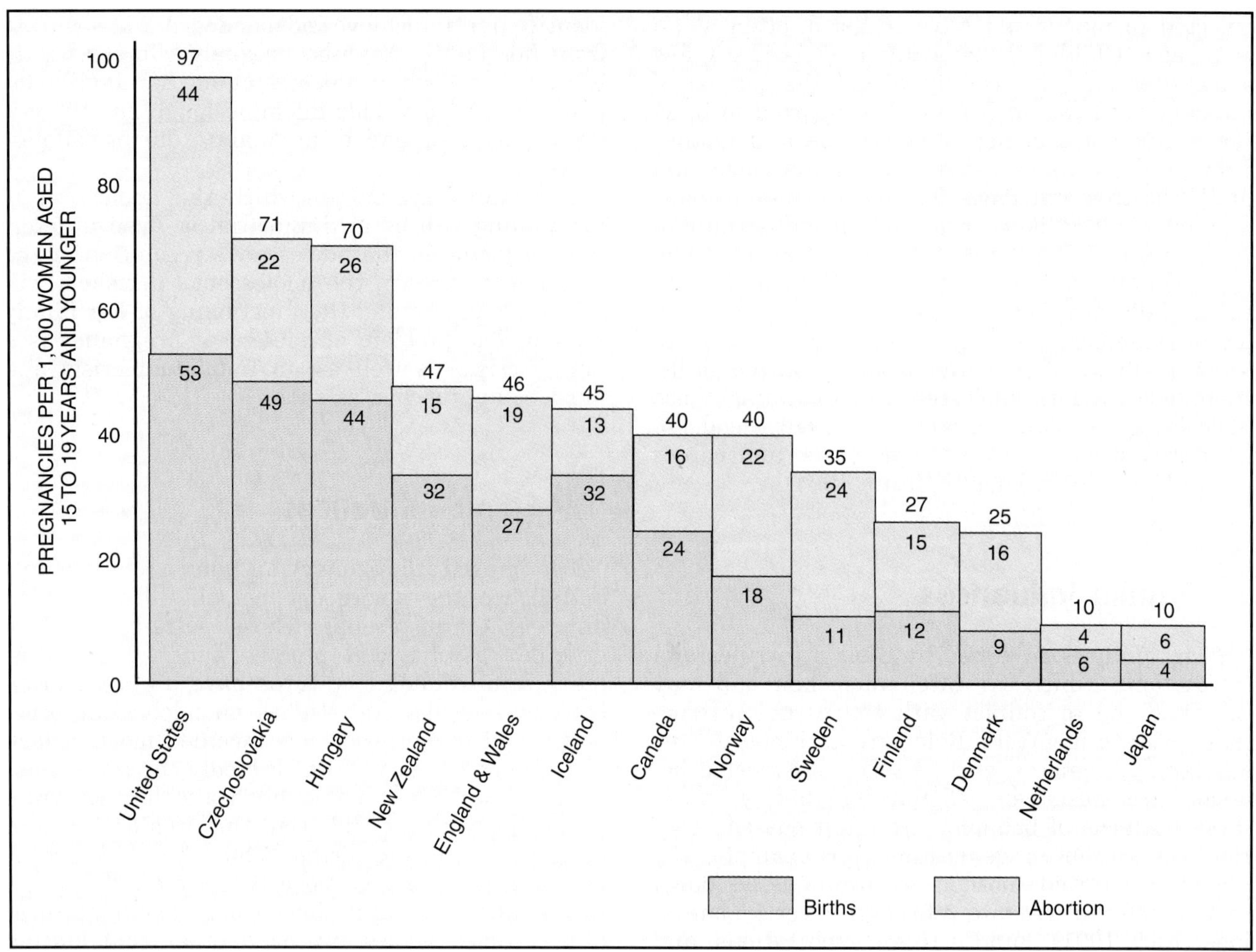

Figure 39–2

Data provide an international perspective on teenage pregnancy • The United States has higher adolescent pregnancy rates than many other industrialized countries. (Reproduced with the permission of The Alan Guttmacher Institute from *Sex and America's Teenagers.* The Alan Guttmacher Institute, 1994, New York.)

one-parent family in which the mother is the main provider and where there is a family history of out-of-wedlock births. Black families, although not approving of out-of-wedlock pregnancy, are accepting, and the infant is usually readily accepted into the family (McAnarney 1983). Black teens generally have a good mother-daughter relationship and usually continue to live with their family during pregnancy. They are least likely to marry the father of the baby. Black teens are more likely to remain in school than Hispanic teens are; however, their academic success in school as well as how long they continue will be determined by the amount of support they receive from their families.

There is solid evidence to support that white teens who become pregnant are more likely to come from troubled families and exhibit problem behaviors such as drug, alcohol, and tobacco use and problem behaviors in school (Abrahamse et al. 1988).

ADOLESCENT SEXUAL ACTIVITY

Seventy percent of never-married American women and 80 percent of never-married men become sexually active during their teens (Alan

IMPROVING YOUR PRACTICE

WORKING EFFECTIVELY WITH PREGNANT ADOLESCENTS

Working with pregnant teens can be challenging and rewarding, difficult and frustrating. Adolescents' enthusiasm, energy, resiliency, and capacity for fun are their biggest assets and characteristics that you can use to achieve health care goals. In contrast, adolescents' ever-changing moods and erratic and often contradictory behavior hinder the achievement of health care goals and require a sensitive, flexible, objective, and creative caregiver. Pregnancy does not change that teens are struggling with the physical and psychological changes of adolescence, and they are usually not ready to assume an adult role. Yet, society's typical response to pregnant teens is to expect them to perform as adults and assume all responsibilities associated with pregnancy—and parenting if that is their choice. Most adolescents will have difficulty fulfilling these expectations.

A self-assessment to determine your strengths and areas that need improvement is the first step in improving your skills with pregnant teens. You should assess four primary areas: your expectations of pregnant teens, your knowledge of adolescent development, your approaches to teaching, and your ability to establish a relationship with pregnant teens.

- EVALUATE YOUR EXPECTATIONS AND THE EFFECT THEY MIGHT HAVE ON YOUR INTERACTIONS WITH TEENS. While you probably would not expect a teen to do household chores without a reminder and occasional prodding, do you expect her to keep her prenatal appointments faithfully, to be punctual, and to follow your recommendations carefully and consistently? If so, you can expect to be disappointed, frustrated, and angry. Examine how objective and tolerant you can be when typical adolescent behaviors conflict with essential health care behaviors. Consider various ways in which you can motivate teens to participate in needed health care and education. What is most important to them? What is most important to you? How can you satisfy their needs and meet your objectives as well?
- EVALUATE YOUR UNDERSTANDING OF ADOLESCENT DEVELOPMENT. Consider the typical developmental behaviors that you would expect. How are they likely to conflict with behaviors related to pregnancy and parenting? Think about approaches that you can use that will match the teen's phase of development. For example, since teens are self-centered (because of their developmental stage), if you present information in terms of how it will make life easier for them, they will be more likely to use it. Your knowledge and use of principles of adolescent development are critical to the success of your interventions.
- THINK ABOUT THE CHARACTERISTICS OF TEENS AND TEACHING STRATEGIES THAT ARE MOST EFFECTIVE WITH THEM. What approaches do you use when teaching? Do the teaching strategies you have selected match the developmental phase of the teens? A fundamental principle in teaching teens is that the younger the teen, the more concrete and experiential the teaching strategy has to be in order to be effective. Information "taught" is not always information "learned." Clarify the teen's understanding of the material and reinforce the information by using different approaches. In general, you need to determine your strengths in the area of teaching and those areas that you need to refine or change.
- REFLECT ON YOUR RELATIONSHIP AND INTERACTIONS WITH PREGNANT TEENS. Do you genuinely like working with them? Do you respect them as individuals? Are you sensitive to their needs? Can you set limits on their behavior in a firm yet warm and caring manner? How would you describe your relationship with them? Is it warm, empathic, and genuine, or is it mechanical, uninvolved, and distant? Your ability to develop rapport and trust with a pregnant adolescent is an important determinant of whether she continues to seek health care and makes needed lifestyle changes.

If you carefully evaluate your ability to work with pregnant teens and make a conscious, planned effort to strengthen your skills (even competency can be improved), you will find that both you and the pregnant teens with whom you work will benefit. You will become a more skilled practitioner. They will be more likely to continue prenatal care and be more responsive to your teaching, thus improving outcomes for them and their babies.

Guttmacher Institute 1994). Factors that influence the initiation of sexual intercourse are biologic, social, and environmental (Abrahamse et al. 1988).

The biologic influences are

- Early sexual maturation is associated with early sexual activity; pubertal development happens earlier in black girls than in white girls, and black girls often initiate sexual activity at an earlier age.
- Increasing hormone levels directly influence and increase sexual motivation and sexual behavior among adolescent men.

The social influences are

- Different racial groups have distinctive patterns of precoital heterosexual behaviors in early adolescence.
- The pattern of sexual activity commences earlier and progresses faster among black teens than among white teens; for white teenagers, an extended period of noncoital petting behavior usually precedes the first act of intercourse.
- Strong religious beliefs are capable of inhibiting sexual intercourse among adolescents.
- High educational expectations and career aspirations are associated with postponing sexual activity.
- Family structure, with earlier onset of sexual activity among adolescents from disrupted families, influences teenagers; teens who have a sister who is a teenage mother are more likely to be sexually active.

The environmental influences are

- Neighborhoods in which the adolescent lives; young women living in poverty face substantially increased risk for early sexual activity.
- Peers who accept unwed childbearing can influence each other at school and in the community at large and increase the risk for single parenthood.

CONSEQUENCES OF ADOLESCENT PREGNANCY AND PARENTHOOD

The pregnant adolescent is considered a high-risk client. She is more likely to have (1) obstetric complications, such as hypertension, third-trimester bleeding, preeclampsia, eclampsia, amnionitis, abruptio placentae, and labor dysfunctions (Alan Guttmacher Institute 1994); (2) neonatal morbidity and mortality, primarily based on increased prematurity and low birth weight; and (3) multiple socioeconomic factors (Corbett and Meyer 1987).

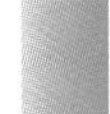

Maternal Factors

Research has shown that a comprehensive health care program can improve outcomes for both adolescent mothers and their infants (O'Sullivan and Jacobsen 1992). Obstetric complications may well be as much a result of poor socioeconomic circumstances as of maternal age (Schauberger 1986). Certainly preexisting biologic conditions (e.g., diabetes, a congenital cardiac condition, or asthma) can create difficulties that require management by a high-risk team, regardless of the age of the mother. The maternal mortality rate for adolescents younger than 15 years has been reported to be 2.5 times that of pregnant woman aged 20 to 24 years (Alan Guttmacher Institute 1994).

Other factors that can contribute to increased maternal morbidity and mortality include poor health habits, response to peer influence, inadequate prenatal care, and noncompliance with clinical management.

POOR HEALTH HABITS

Nurses working with teens should try to instill an awareness of proper eating habits during the pregnancy. Teenagers tend to choose fast food and carbonated beverages over balanced meals and milk or juice. Adolescents are often confused about the impact of proper nutrition on their diet. For example, one teen said "but the chips were cheese flavored" in response to the nurse's statement about the lack of protein in her diet. Malnutrition is a risk for adolescents during pregnancy. Societal pressures to be slim and slender may make it difficult for the adolescent to accept her blossoming figure. The adolescent may have intense concerns about body weight and appearance. Crash dieting and poor maternal weight gain, as well as poor eating habits and low prepregnancy weight, may contribute to low birth weight and prematurity in adolescents' infants. The youngest adolescent is at the highest risk. Those young women who conceive within 2 years of their menarche are still growing rapidly themselves. A competition exists, therefore, for nutrients for the mother and the fetus. Young teens need to gain more weight than do older teens and adults to produce appropriately grown infants (Peterson and Crockett 1986).

RESPONSE TO PEER INFLUENCE

Adolescents have an increased need for acceptance and support from others. While this is a normal developmental milestone, it can also adversely affect a teen who overly conforms to group standards. Peterson and Crockett (1986) suggested that along with increased libido and the need for emotional intimacy, the tendency to go along with the crowd is likely to result in early sexual experimentation and pregnancy. This experimentation may add multiple risk behaviors to the lifestyle of the pregnant adolescent. Fetal and maternal outcome can be affected by teen substance abuse, cigarette smoking, third-trimester coitus (especially with multiple partners), and the acquisition of sexually transmitted diseases (STDs). Fully 25 percent of the STDs in the United States occur in the adolescent age group. Human immunodeficiency virus (HIV) infection is also a concern (Shafer 1988).

INADEQUATE PRENATAL CARE

Adolescents seek prenatal care later than adult women do. More than half of all pregnant adolescents receive no first-trimester care, and nearly 20 percent receive their first obstetric contact during the last trimester or at delivery. Factors in this inadequate prenatal care may be denial of pregnancy, fear of revealing the pregnancy to parents or other adults, uncertainty about abortion, lack of access to health care through transportation, lack of knowledge of available programs, or fear of medical procedures or personnel (Zuckerman et al. 1984).

NONCOMPLIANCE WITH CLINICAL MANAGEMENT

Adolescents may not follow health care recommendations, and this is a factor in healthy outcomes for both the adolescent mother and her infant. Adolescents react negatively to meeting different clinicians at every visit, a long wait before seeing the caregiver, and times for appointments that conflict with their lifestyle. Pregnant adolescents tend to perceive these short-term problems as of greater consequence than the long-term one of promoting a healthy pregnancy. Living in the "now," her compliance with detailed instructions that bear no immediate gratification may be pushed to the bottom of her priorities. Support from her parents, in particular from her mother, and from the father of the baby can reinforce the health teaching a teen receives. The adolescent who has a support person, whether it is the nurse at her caregiver's office, a nurse or educator at her school, or a big sister or community worker, will be more likely to take the actions that will benefit her infant. Like all expectant mothers, the adolescent responds to affirmative information. She may react with awe at the sight of an ultrasound picture and should be given an opportunity to hear the fetal heart sounds. Visual aids that are colorful, clear, and easy to read can provide identification of the growing bulge in her stomach as an infant in need of her care. Since many adolescents may have low literacy skills, information should be geared to the fifth- or sixth-grade reading level, and posters or visual aids should be simple and clear (Doak et al. 1985).

Neonatal Factors

The neonatal mortality rate in the United States is highest for the youngest (younger than 15 years) and oldest (older than 40 years) mothers. The neonatal mortality rate for these young adolescents is nearly double that of the older teens (Lawrence and Marritt 1981). Statistically, nonwhite infants have greater mortality rates than white infants do.

Morbidity in babies of adolescents may be attributed to two common causes: prematurity (less than 38 weeks' gestation) and low birth weight (2500 g or less at birth). The young adolescent is at even greater risk than are those older than 15 years. Among adolescents below the age of 15 years, the majority receive late or no prenatal care. The infants born to these young adolescents are at a greater risk for low birth weight. Factors contributing to low birth weight and prematurity in adolescents include child spacing, poor nutrition, chronic illness, lack of prenatal care, low prepregnancy weight, previous premature birth or fetal death, placental abnormalities, drug use, smoking, anemia, and socioeconomic status such as unmarried status and ethnic origin (James et al. 1994).

The incidence of STD in adolescents has increased rapidly with increased sexual activity and multiple partners. Each year, approximately 25 percent of all reported cases of STDs occur in persons 15 to 19 years old. About 2.5 million teenagers (one of seven) are infected with an STD annually. There is significant risk for infants exposed to STDs both in utero and during vaginal delivery. The presence of two STDs together has a strong effect on prematurity and low birth weight. Chlamydial infection and trichomoniasis together, or trichomoniasis alone, shortens gestation. Infants whose mothers had third-trimester chlamydial infection have a higher frequency of upper respiratory infections, conjunctivitis, and pneumonia in the first months of life (Mercer 1986). Chlamydial infection is the most prevalent STD today, affecting one in seven sexually active female adolescents and one in ten sexually active men. Syphilis accounts for 0.5 percent of all STDs in the heterosexual adolescent and is rising. Syphilis and gonorrhea cases in teens have increased markedly since 1956. The potential for congenital syphilis exists. Infants born to HIV-infected women are at risk for HIV infection. The number of HIV-positive adolescents is steadily on the rise, although many of these young people are asymptomatic and not readily identifiable during prenatal care (Centers for Disease Control 1989).

Psychosocial Consequences

Adolescent pregnancy often creates a cycle of low education and poverty for the new family unit created by the infant's birth. Adolescent parenthood tends to recur with each new generation. It is likely that adolescent mothers and fathers had adolescent parents themselves. Pregnancy and parenthood often result in the adolescent mother's leaving the educational system entirely (Children's Defense Fund 1989). Approximately 51 percent of unmarried teens with children and 75 percent of married adolescent mothers across the nation leave school before graduation. An alternative to the high-school diploma is the GED, or General Equivalency Diploma Program. Although many adolescents who drop out of school state their intention to complete their GED, the reality is that only 18 percent of 15- to 17-year-olds actually do so by the age of 26 (Children's Defense Fund 1988). The teenage father has many vocational and educational issues to consider (Elster and Panzarine 1983; Rivara-Casale et al. 1986). Eighteen months after the birth of the baby, more fathers were heads of households, and more of them had dropped out of school than had young male teens who were not fathers. Unfinished education, coupled with the low employment rate for young men and women regardless of educational status, decreases the socioeconomic status of the family with the addition of an infant.

Adolescent mothers are 2.6 times more likely to receive AFDC benefits than are those who bear children after 20 years of age (Simkins 1984). The public cost is substantial. In 1985, nearly $17 billion was paid through three programs—AFDC, food stamps, and Medicaid—to women who first gave birth as adolescents. The government will pay an average of $13,902 in the next 20 years for each family begun by a first birth to an adolescent in 1985. If all births were delayed until the mother was 20 years old, the potential savings would be an aggregate $2.06 billion (Hatcher 1996).

Adolescent mothers typically choose to keep and try to raise their babies. Often the maternal grandmother becomes a primary caretaker if the adolescent mother is trying to remain in school. Adolescents rarely select adoption anymore. About 96 percent of pregnant adolescents keep their babies (Barr and Monserret 1992). This creates strain on the adolescent mother's family. In many cases, the infant initiates conflict between the young mother and her own mother, now forced into both a child care and early grandparent role. The mother-daughter relationship is a volatile one in any case during adolescence; the challenge of living in close quarters with three generations in an unexpected situation frays those fragile relationship bonds even more.

One of the most difficult psychosocial aspects of adolescent pregnancy is the possibility that some young women are planning their pregnancies (Dash 1990). Whether from a general feeling of wanting someone to love or to increase the possibility of their holding on to a boyfriend, the planned adolescent pregnancy is both difficult to predict and prevent. Young women who picture a romantic lifestyle similar to the ones they have witnessed on television or at the movies may imagine motherhood unrealistically. One teen mother expressed her confusion about the real infant she had brought home from the hospital, sharing this sentiment: "The babies on the soap operas just went down for a nap and the mothers' lives stayed the same. But my baby doesn't sleep much at all." Making this realism a part of an adolescent's knowledge base before conception is difficult.

When adolescents attempt to set up a family structure of their own by entering marriage, the resultant family unit is often unstable. Divorce rates are high. The divorce rate for parents younger than 18 years is three times greater than that for parents who have their first child after the age of 20 years, and it is greater for couples with premarital pregnancies than for those who conceive after marriage (Furstenberg and Talvitie 1980. Twenty-three percent of married 15- to 17-year-olds separate within 5 years (Children's Defense Fund 1988), and the cycle perpetuates itself. Approximately 37 percent of teen mothers have a second pregnancy within 24 months (Children's Defense Fund 1988).

The consequences for children of adolescent parents are long reaching. The adolescent is rarely prepared to parent a child. Prepubertal, early, and middle adolescents typically do not think in terms of long-term consequences of their behavior (Reedy 1991). The issues of adequate infant nutrition and child safety may not seem of grave importance to a young mother. Classes on parenting and infant care, using hands-on techniques and role play for education, are essential in encouraging good parenting skills. Some schools may permit the young mothers to bring their infants to class with them. Observing the interaction between infant and mother is an invaluable tool for evaluating babies at risk. A nutritional session could include lunch

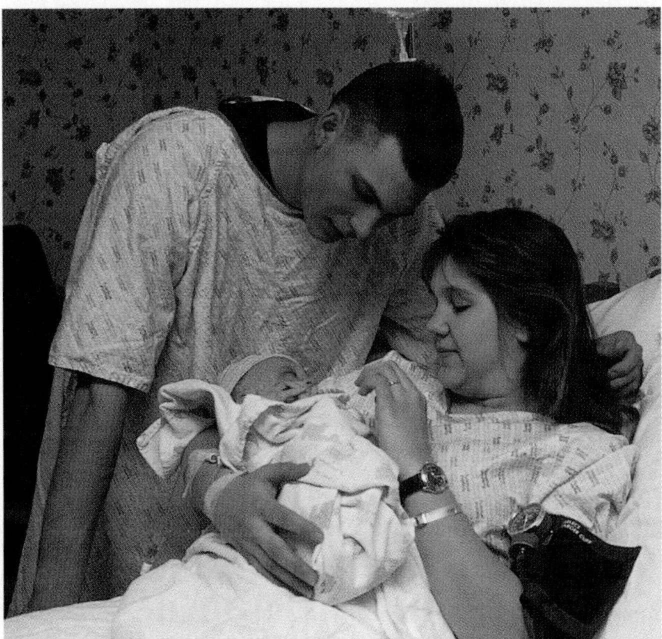
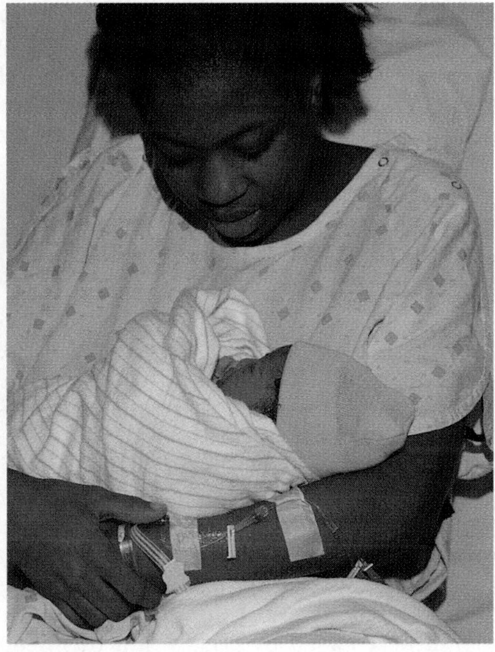

Figure 39–3
The needs of the adolescent mother vary, depending on her age, her specific circumstances, and her support system. *Left,* A late adolescent couple share a moment with their newborn son. *Right,* A midadolescent single mother cradles her daughter.

for both mother and an older baby. An astute caregiver can easily evaluate the mother's understanding of her infant's needs as she observes her feeding her infant. Young mothers need instruction, with practice, in handling crisis situations. Role playing *What should you do next?* for a variety of scenarios is a useful learning tool.

The cycle of child abuse and neglect is often ongoing as well. Many adolescent parents were never exposed to positive role models as children themselves. Many of them were emotionally or physically abused. Parents tend to parent as they themselves were parented. The importance of touching, of interaction, and of eye contact to young infants should be stressed before discharge from the hospital. The teen mother needs to direct positive messages toward her infant long before the baby can speak. Infant stimulation classes are an integral part of any teen parenting program. Since both emotional and physical abuse may be a part of the teen's background, the issues of expressing anger and the possibility of potentially abusing their infants should be discussed. As parents, they will tend to perpetuate the roles that were scripted on them, by verbally and by acting out their own parents' behavior. The real possibility of injury to a baby physically by acting-out behavior, such as shaking the baby to try to stop a crying jag, needs to be discussed.

TYPES OF ADOLESCENT PREGNANCY PREVENTION PROGRAMS

There are four primary types of educational programs for prevention of teen pregnancy: traditional sexuality education, abstinence-only sexuality education, abstinence-based/postpone programs, and comprehensive sexuality education. All approaches to adolescent sexuality, although different, have been brought sharply into focus by the emerging HIV/AIDS epidemic.

Traditional Sexuality Education

This is the "nuts and bolts" approach, and is the most common sexuality education in America today. Reproductive anatomy and physiology is taught, as well as an emphasis on sexually transmitted diseases with a goal of preventing adolescent sex. This type of program supports a traditional family unit and heterosexual sex only during marriage (Sears 1992).

The major criticism of this approach is that it rarely includes a discussion of social and psychological issues involved in adolescent sexuality.

Abstinence-Only Sexuality Education

Many abstinence-only curricula were developed with federal grants from the Office of Adolescent Pregnancy Program. In most cases, contraception and abortion are not mentioned, while chastity and abstinence are stressed as the only safe and viable choices for young people. Examples are *Sex respect: the option of true sexual freedom and teen aid* (Mast 1986) and *Sexuality, commitment and family* (Potter and Roach 1989).

The major criticism of this approach is that it is considered fear based by critics and has been seen to promote the agenda of the political and religious far right. Withdrawal of such a curriculum has occurred in several school districts owing to allegations that the curriculum violates laws excluding the teaching of religious beliefs in public schools (Huberman 1993) (Coleman v. Caddo Parish School Board).

Abstinence-Based/Postpone Sexuality Education

In this approach, abstinence is discussed, but disease and pregnancy prevention methods are included as well, and the primary strategy is to promote the delay of intercourse. The acquisition of decision-making and refusal skills is often stressed. Examples of this category include *Postponing sexual involvement* (Howard 1984), *Reducing the risk: building skills to prevent teen pregnancy* (Barth 1993), and *Values and choices* (Search Institute 1991). These programs have demonstrated positive outcomes including decreased intercourse and higher use of prevention methods.

The major criticism of this approach is that concern has been expressed that the introduction of prevention information in a curriculum stressing postponing sexual involvement is a double message.

Comprehensive Sexuality Education

This approach seeks to educate teens about their sexuality in a broad-based manner. Not only does it deal with reproduction, dating, sexually transmitted diseases, and marriage, but it also covers sexual pleasure, noncoital sexual expression, and homosexuality. Two examples of guides for the comprehensive approach that come from prominent national organizations are *Sexuality education within comprehensive school health education* (Neutens et al. 1991) and *Guidelines for comprehensive sexuality education—kindergarten–12th grade* (National Guidelines Task Force 1991). The major criticism of this approach is of the introduction of the concepts of "outercourse" (nonsexual intercourse) and the discussion of homosexuality.

ISSUES AND APPROACHES RELATED TO THE PROBLEM OF ADOLESCENT PREGNANCY

Two complex issues of teen contraceptive use and abortion prevent many communities from developing comprehensive services for pregnant and parenting adolescents. Some communities deny that there is a need for adolescent pregnancy and parenting programs. Other communities refuse to allow teens access to complete information on contraception or abortion.

Contraception information for adolescents is controversial and often nonexistent. Even though some studies estimate that 45 percent of all 16-year-olds and 33 percent of all 15-year-olds in this country have had sexual intercourse (Howard 1988), few sex education courses exist in schools in the United States. In Sweden, the Netherlands, England, Wales, and France, adolescent contraceptive services are well established and publicly funded (Jones et al. 1986). Data from these countries show regular contraceptive use among their adolescents and low rates of adolescent pregnancy.

Of the more than 1 million pregnancies among American adolescents, more than 400,000 choose to terminate the pregnancy (Alan Guttmacher Institute 1994). Because of the issues surrounding abortion, counseling adolescents about abortion services is a sensitive and difficult task. The developmental status of the adolescent further compounds the problem of decision making. The majority of adolescents have never made a major adult development decision, such as the selection of a career, a mate, or an educational path (Brown 1983). The full ramifications of an abortion, as well as the reality of childbearing, need to be addressed with use of a framework for decision making.

Pregnancy Decision Making

While the decisions involved in facing an unplanned pregnancy are challenging ones for any woman, the decision-making process is intensified in an adolescent. Situations that may complicate the decision-making process include the developmental readiness of the adolescent to make decisions; the relationship of the expectant teen with the father of the baby; the relationship of the expectant teen with her parent or guardian; the developmental tendency of youth to live in the present, thus avoiding the need for a decision until some choices are no longer available; peer influences; substance abuse; lack of knowledge of options and choices; denial of the problem—in this case, pregnancy, until visible evidence of gestation occurs; lack of maturity to enable the formation of a plan of action; and lack of finances to permit implementation of decisions once they have been formulated.

The earlier the pregnancy is discovered, the more options that are available. Using a model to teach decision-making and problem-solving skills

Do You Have a Decision to Make? Problem: Possible Unintended Pregnancy

PROBLEM SOLVING

Examine the Facts

Know the truth about the problem—don't minimize (make it smaller than it is) or exaggerate (make it bigger).

- What are the signs of possible pregnancy you are experiencing?
- Have you taken a pregnancy test?
- Have you arranged for a clinic visit?

Own the Problem

Reframe it in relationship to *you,* not someone else. This isn't your friend's problem, or even your family's. It's your problem. Although it may help to listen to what other people did in a similar situation, you need to understand what's happening to you and go from there.

- Advice given by friends may be given with good intentions, but this is *your* life and your body.
- Will your friends be there for you throughout this situation? Even if they are, the final decision must be *yours*.

Be Open to Help

Seek assistance from others and communicate your needs. Help may come from an area where you least expect to receive it. Don't close doors.

- Have you considered all possible sources of help: parents, family, teachers, guidance personnel, nurses, clinic staff, church workers?

List Possible Options

Think through your choices. Be honest, and real.

- Abortion, married parenting, single parenting, adoption.

Evaluate Outcomes

Pros and cons of your decision should be thought through.

- Abortion—How will it affect you long term?
- Married parenting—Are you ready for this commitment?
- Single parenting—Do you have support as the baby grows?
- Adoption—Have you considered open adoption?

Make It Happen

Act on your decision.

Review and Rethink Your Decision

What did you learn from this experience?

---

ensures consistency and completeness (see Do You Have a Decision To Make?). An unmarried expectant adolescent faces several options on confirmation of her pregnancy. Ideally, her partner is a part of the decision-making process; but in reality, he may be absent, or there may be a conflict between him and the mother-to-be. Possible options in early pregnancy include married parenting, single parenting, adoption, and abortion.

MARRIED OR SINGLE PARENTING

The majority of teenagers bearing children do so out of wedlock. Nationally, out-of-wedlock births have increased in general, while societal sanction against them has decreased. Most births to teenagers do occur outside marriage; however, adolescents account for only 30 percent of all out-of-wedlock births—a decrease from 50 percent in 1970 (Moore et al 1995). The younger the mother, the more likely it is that she conceived and gave birth outside of marriage. A disproportionate number of nonmarital teen births occur to black women (Alan Guttmacher Institute 1994).

Single parenting leaves a young, inexperienced parent with little potential support in charge of rearing a child. Programs to provide training for teens vary widely. Once a young woman has chosen to bear her child and keep the baby, the following four priorities should be the focus of any program: (1) ensuring a safe pregnancy and birth; (2) remaining in school, with the ultimate goal of graduation and increased employability; (3) mentoring for positive parenting skills; and (4) avoiding additional unintentional pregnancies (Hatcher 1996; Podgurski 1996b).

ADOPTION

Like older mothers, adolescent mothers face formidable odds if they are considering adoption as a choice. There is a lack of understanding about adoption as an option among adolescents. Support for this choice is difficult to find, with the resulting statistic of 96 percent of teen mothers keeping their babies virtually unchanged in decades.

Open adoption presents an option that provides both the birth mother and the adoptive parents with an empathetic means to deal with this difficult situation. A closed adoption denies all parties involved in the process access to information about each other. A common theme among birth mothers in a closed adoption has been shown to be the mother's inability to deal effectively with her loss and unresolved grief. More birth mothers in closed adoptions were found to be "reluctant givers" than "grateful givers" (Fig. 39–4). In contrast, open adoption provides birth mothers participation, control, and support. Their loss may be just as painful as the loss of a relinquisher in a closed adoption, but the active participation in the decision-making process permits acceptance of the

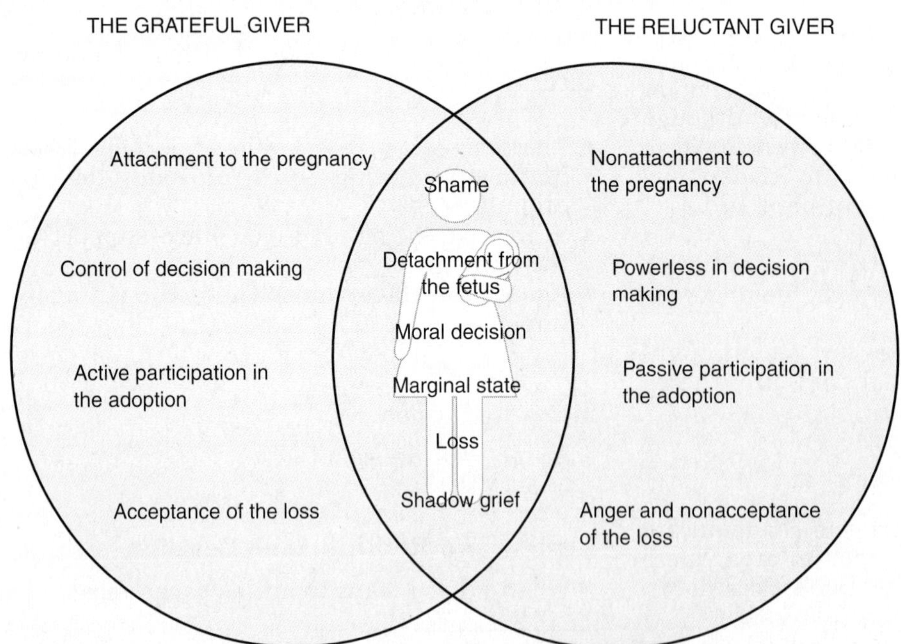

Figure 39–4

The circumstances surrounding the decision to relinquish a baby influence the birth mother's participation in the process and the feelings she experiences • While those mothers who have come to terms with relinquishing their babies and those mothers who reluctantly relinquish their babies have many feelings in common, their acceptance of the loss and the related feelings vary.

Guidelines for Helping Teens Breastfeed

- **Avoid "turn-offs."** Extend the same courtesy to the teen as you would to an adult. Treat the teen with respect. Do not invade the teen's territorial boundaries and space. Ask permission before touching the teen, especially the breast area. Avoid overfamiliar touching and be sensitive to whether the teen is pulling back emotionally.
- **Do not assume that the teen understands.** Gear handouts and visual aids to the teen's developmental level. Handouts should be at a fifth- or sixth-grade reading level and posters should be clear and concise to avoid confusion. Have a question box available to permit teens to anonymously ask questions in a nonthreatening manner. Teens are often afraid to admit they do not understand and fear ridicule if they ask questions.
- **Be sensitive to the teen's culture.** Include the nuances of the adolescent's culture that are particularly important to the young mother. Issues of peer approval and modesty will be uppermost in her mind if she is considering breastfeeding. Encourage the teen to choose music she likes to play while breastfeeding her baby. Help her choose shirts and tops that are attractive and promote modesty while breastfeeding. Provide opportunities for the teen mother to talk with other teen mothers who are breastfeeding. Invite a successful breastfeeding teen to talk about her experience at class or clinic. Choose videos carefully with the teen's culture uppermost in mind. If possible, use videos that show teens breastfeeding.
- **Ask permission before setting up postpartum support calls.** Postpartum support calls are essential in helping teens breastfeed successfully. However, to be successful, teens must be able to accept or refuse them. The nurse should explain the reasons for the visits to the teen—to answer questions and to support her in breastfeeding and parenting. The nurse must be viewed by the teen as a support system instead of an authority figure if follow-up calls are to be successful.
- **Develop the teen's support system.** The teen's support system often decreases the first few weeks after the birth of the baby, leaving her feeling alone and isolated. Assist her in identifying sources of support, first within her family and among friends and then within the community. The stronger the teen's support system, the better her chances are of successful breastfeeding.
- **Involve the teen father.** Encourage the teen father if he shows even the smallest interest to become involved in breastfeeding. Like female adolescents, he will most likely perceive his partner's breasts only in a sexual way. If he understands the benefits of breastfeeding and how it can be accomplished modestly and easily, his support for the teen mother in breastfeeding will increase the potential for success.
- **Encourage support within the school system.** Seek support for the breastfeeding teen within the school system. Find an individual who will support the teen at school and find privacy for her to pump during the school day. Have that individual draw up a contract regarding breastfeeding with the teen. Follow up with the individual by phone or a visit to determine how things are going. Always send a note thanking the individual for helping the teen and her baby.
- **Give the teen permission to change her mind about breastfeeding.** While the benefits of breastfeeding are many, if the teen is unhappy with breastfeeding, she needs to be free to change to bottle feeding.
- **Use teachable moments to reinforce contraception information.** A clear understanding of conception and contraception is critical for the sexually active teen. Clarifying the teen's misconceptions about contraception can be integrated easily with breastfeeding education.
- **Be real!** An honest, nonjudgmental, sincere approach is essential for nurses counseling teen breastfeeding mothers. Teens are quick to identify attitudes other than that and will retreat rapidly. Regardless of the situation, to be an effective teen breastfeeding counselor, the nurse must have empathy for the teen mother.

From Podgurski, M. J. (1995). Supporting the breastfeeding teen. *Journal of Perinatal Education,* 4 (2), 11–14.

loss at a different level. Teen mothers who make the choice to relinquish without parental or partner influence are rare. Repeated pregnancy is common in a young woman who is forced or coerced to relinquish her baby for adoption. With proper counseling, however, an open adoption can be a caring option for both the teen mother and her child.

ABORTION

What prompts a teenager to make the difficult decision to end a pregnancy? Studies show that financially well off teens are more likely than those from poorer homes to choose abortion. Some factors found to increase the likelihood of abortion among pregnant teens are higher income and insurance coverage. Medicaid patients are considerably less likely to have abortions, in part because most states do not pay for abortion services, yet all states currently pay for prenatal care and childbirth. Higher parental level of education in family of origin, future goals, race and ethnic background, and age of the male partner are also contributing factors (Alan Guttmacher Institute 1994).

ROLE OF THE NURSE

Nursing care begins with a complete and comprehensive assessment of the adolescent and her specific situation (Fig. 39–5). For adolescents to make good decisions during this stressful time, they need support from the nurse, the clinic staff, and their parents, teachers, and peers. The possibility of sexual abuse and alienation from their family further intensifies the isolation a pregnant teenager feels. The nurse may be the teen's primary source of support during this time. Teens' access to a nurse on a 24-hour basis through either a pager or an answering service will increase the potential for available support when it is needed and for ongoing communications to occur. After the assessment is completed, nursing diagnoses are formulated and a plan of care is developed for the teenager on the basis of her specific needs.

Interventions focus on decision making regarding the pregnancy, referral to health care providers, support, prenatal care, contraceptive counseling, and participation in the appropriate adolescent pregnancy or parenthood program. Research has shown that teens are more likely to continue health care and identify with one caregiver (Brown 1983). Thus, it is most effective when one nurse assumes the primary responsibility for the pregnant adolescent or teen mother. Evaluation of the outcomes of nursing care is conducted on an ongoing basis, and the plan of care is modified as needed.

Risk Management

The stress of adolescent pregnancy and parenthood increases the potential risk of teenagers' misunderstanding or having incomplete or inaccurate information about the situation and what needs to be done. Teens may not follow health care recommendations because other things seem more important to them. The key to decreasing risk is excellent, ongoing communication between the nurse and the adolescent that encourages and guides the teen to follow through on needed behaviors. Close, continued follow-up is needed to promote the desired actions. Easy-to-read information, such as a checklist, about what needs to be done increases the potential that the desired outcomes will be achieved.

Implications for Research

There is a wealth of descriptive information about adolescent pregnancy and parenthood. There has been little formal evaluation on the effectiveness of adolescent pregnancy and parenting programs. Programs have been established in response to a specific need. Although clinical evidence indicates some are effective, the research data to support this effectiveness do not exist. There is a critical need for research on all aspects of interventions that are used in caring for the pregnant adolescent and the adolescent mother. Especially important is the need to determine the effectiveness of each program element and their relationship so that programs can be replicated. A comprehensive effectiveness approach for addressing the problem of adolescent pregnancy and parenthood will not be achieved until we know what is effective, for whom, and in what situations. Research questions that need to be answered are

- What is the effectiveness of adolescent pregnancy and parenting programs?
- What program elements are most effective and for whom?
- What types of adolescent pregnancy and parenting programs are most effective for specific ethnic and cultural groups of adolescents?

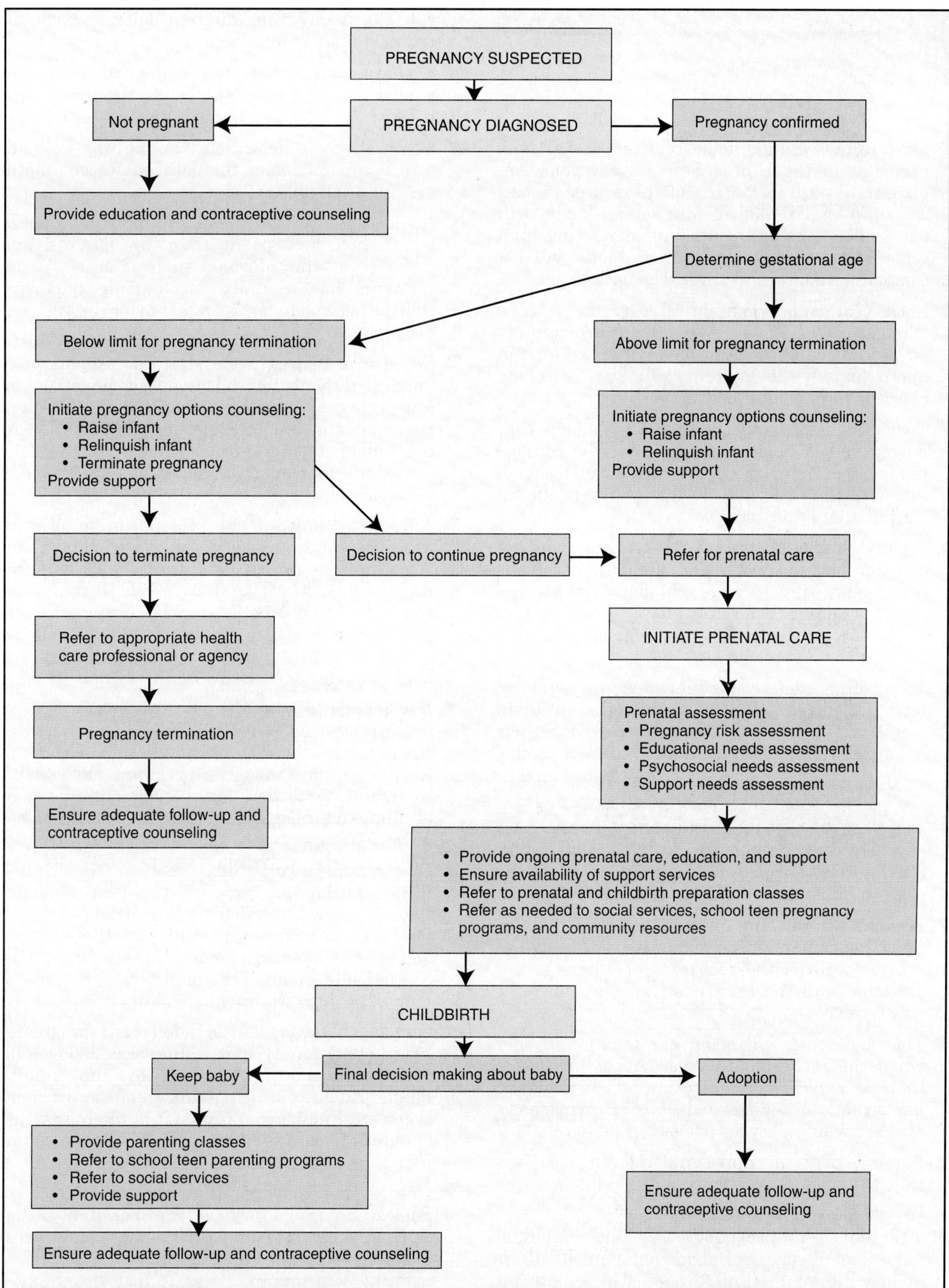

Figure 39–5

Decision tree to aid in planning the care for pregnant adolescents (maternal age of 19 years or younger).

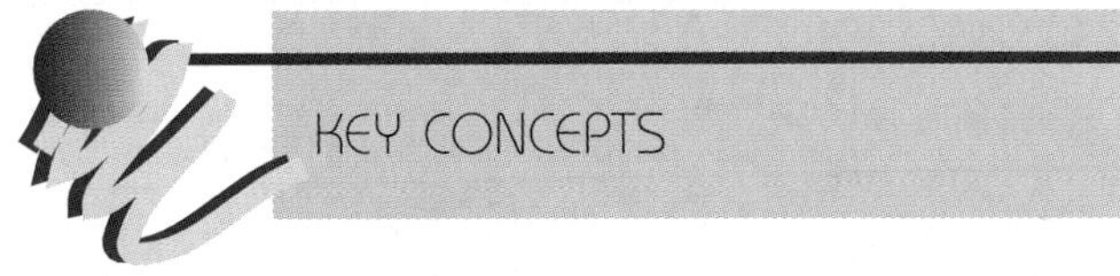

- More than 1 million adolescent females become pregnant in the United States every year. Approximately three fourths of these pregnancies are unintended. One in four female teens will experience a pregnancy before completing high school. One of every ten female teens will become a mother while still a teenager.
- Each year, approximately 50 percent of teens who get pregnant will give birth, approximately 40 percent will choose to have an abortion, and approximately 10 percent will spontaneously abort or have a fetal death.
- Two dimensions of adolescent pregnancy that have received recent attention are the connections between prior sexual abuse and conception and the difference in age between adolescent mothers and their partners.
- Society is struggling with the economic and social burden of adolescent pregnancy. It has been said that teenage childbearing has as much significance for the future of our nation as do the budget deficit, trade deficit, interest rates, and unemployment.
- Today, if an adolescent's pregnancy is carried to term, 96 percent of all teenage mothers remain single and choose to keep and care for their children. Increasingly, young women today choose to have a child out of wedlock rather than an early unwanted marriage.
- American teens have significantly higher rates of adolescent pregnancy, abortion, and childbearing than their counterparts in virtually every other industrialized nation.
- Societal, family, and ethnic influences determine the meaning of pregnancy to the adolescent as well as the responses of others to her situation and the amount of support that she will receive.
- The adolescent will bring her family with her when she seeks health care—if not in person, then as a part of her perception of herself and her situation, her learned pattern of response, and her framework for decision making.
- Parents play an important role in decisions that the adolescent has to make related to the pregnancy.
- The impact of pregnancy on family relationships and hence the adolescent herself differs among different ethnic groups. These patterns produce different psychosocial profiles and indicate that teens from different cultures have different problems and needs.
- Seventy percent of never-married American women and 80 percent of never-married men become sexually active during their teens.
- Comprehensive health care is one way to facilitate better outcomes for both adolescent mothers and their infants.
- Adolescents are increasingly more influenced by friends and peers than by parents and teachers as they develop their identity. Media influence has assumed a far more pervasive role as a model for teen behavior in the last decade.
- Societal pressures to be slim and slender may make it difficult for the pregnant adolescent to accept her blossoming figure. Crash diets and poor maternal weight gain, as well as poor eating habits and low prepregnancy weight, may contribute to low birth weight and prematurity in adolescents' infants.
- Adolescent patterns of seeking prenatal care are different from those seen with older mothers. Multiple studies show that adolescents initiate prenatal care later, so much so that more than half of all pregnant adolescents receive no first-trimester care, and nearly 20 percent receive their first obstetric contact during the last trimester or at delivery.
- Developmentally, pregnant adolescents tend to perceive the short-term problem as of greater consequence than a long-term one. Living in the "now" may push the pregnant adolescent's compliance with detailed instructions that bear no immediate gratification to the bottom of her priorities.
- The maternal mortality rate in the United States is highest for the youngest (younger than 15 years) and oldest (older than 40 years) mothers. The mortality rate for these young adolescents is nearly double that of older teens. Statistically, nonwhite infants have greater mortality rates than white infants do.
- One of the tragedies of adolescent pregnancy for the new family unit is the cycle of low education and poverty created by the infant's birth. Adolescent pregnancy often becomes cyclic with new generations; it is likely that the adolescent mother and father had adolescent parents themselves.
- One of the most difficult psychosocial aspects of adolescent pregnancy is the possibility that some young women are planning their pregnancies. Whether from a general feeling of wanting someone to love or to increase the possibility of their holding on to a boyfriend, the

planned adolescent pregnancy is both difficult to predict and prevent.

- ▼ Classes on parenting and infant care, using hands-on techniques and role play for education, are essential in encouraging good parenting skills.
- ▼ Adolescent pregnancy programs most often focus on prevention of adolescent pregnancy and the support of the adolescent family. There is much debate regarding that approach.
- ▼ There are four primary types of educational programs for prevention of teen pregnancy: traditional sexuality education, abstinence-only sexuality education, abstinence-based/postpone sexuality education, and comprehensive sexuality education. All approaches to adolescent sexuality, although different, have been brought sharply into focus by the emerging HIV/AIDS epidemic.
- ▼ As the numbers of pregnant adolescents began to rise in the 1960s, hospitals and eventually schools began to develop specialized programs to address the twin issues of the teenage mother and her infant's health. Although each program varied widely, they typically included social services, nutritional services, pediatric services, and family planning services.
- ▼ The issues of teen contraception use and abortion have deterred many communities from developing comprehensive services for pregnant adolescents.
- ▼ Contraception information for adolescents is controversial and often nonexistent in most parts of the United States.

References

Abrahamse, A. F., Morrison, P. A., Waite, L. J. (1988). *Beyond stereotypes: Who becomes a single mother?* Santa Monica, CA: The Rand Corporation.

Alan Guttmacher Institute. (1994). *Sex and America's teenagers.* New York: Author.

Barr, L., and Monserret, C. (1992). *Working with pregnant and parenting teens.* Albuquerque, NM: New Futures.

Barth, R. (1993). *Reducing the risk—building skills to prevent pregnancy, STD & HIV.* California: ETR Associates.

Boyer, D., and Fine, D. (1992). Sexual abuse as a factor in adolescent pregnancy and child maltreatment. *Family Planning Perspectives, 24,* 4–11, 19.

Brown, A. (1983). Adolescents and abortion: A theoretical framework for decision making. *Journal of Obstetric and Gynecological Nursing,* 241–247.

Burt, M. R., and Levy, F. (1987). *Risking the future: adolescent sexuality, pregnancy and childbearing.* Washington, D.C.: National Academy Press.

Butler, J., and Burton, L. (1990). Rethinking teenage childbearing: Is sexual abuse a missing link? *Family Relations, 39,* 73–80.

Center for Population Options. (1992). *Cost of teenage childbearing.* Washington, D.C.: Author.

Centers for Disease Control. (1989). Sexually transmitted diseases treatment guidelines. *MMWR* 38(Suppl.) 8, 1–43.

Children's Defense Fund. (1988). *Teenage pregnancy: An advocate's guide to the numbers.* Washington, DC: Author.

Coleman et al. v. Caddo Parish School Board. (1993). First Judicial District Court, Caddo Parish, Louisiana, 385, 230, Section C.

Corbett, M., and Meyer, J. (1987). *The adolescent and pregnancy.* Boston: Blackwell Scientific Publications.

Dash, L. (1990). *When children want children: An insider's look at the crisis of teenage parenthood.* New York: Viking Press.

Doak, C., Doak, L., Root, J. (1985). *Teaching patients with low literacy skills.* Philadelphia: J. B. Lippincott.

Elster, A. B., and Panzarine, S. (1983). *Adolescent fathers.* New York: Grune & Stratton.

Furstenberg, E. F., and Talvitie, K. G. (1980). Children's names and paternal claims; bonds between unmarried fathers and their children. *Journal of Family Issues,* 1, 31–37.

Hatcher, R. A. (1996). *Contraceptive technology, 1994–1996.* New York: Irvinton Publishers.

Howard, M. (1988). *How to help your teenager postpone sexual involvement.* New York: The Continuum Publishing Company.

Huberman, B. (1993). Winning one in North Carolina, *SIECUS Report* 21 (2): 9.

Humenick, S. S., Wilkerson, N. N., Paul, N. W. (1991). *Adolescent pregnancy: Nursing perspectives on prevention.* White Plains, NY: March of Dimes Birth Defects Foundation.

James, D. K., Steer, P. J., Weiner, C. P., Gonik, B. (1994). *High risk pregnancy: management options.* Philadelphia: W. B. Saunders.

Jones, E. F., et al. (1986). *Teenage pregnancy in industrialized countries.* New Haven: Yale University Press.

Lancaster, J. B., and Hamburg, B. A. (1986). *School-age pregnancy and parenthood: Biosocial dimensions.* New York: Aldine de Gruyter.

Landry, D., and Forrest, J. (1995). How old are U.S. fathers? *Family Planning Perspectives, 27,* 159–161, 165.

Lawrence, R. A., and Marritt, T. A. (1981). Infants of adolescent mothers: Perinatal, neonatal and infancy outcome. *Seminars in Perinatology,* 5 (1), 19–32.

Luger, K. (1991). Dubious conceptions, the controversy over teen pregnancy. *American Prospects, 5*: 75–83.

Mast, C. K. (1986). *Sex respect: the option of true sexual freedom.* Gold, II Project Respect.

McAnarney, E. (Ed.). (1983). *Premature adolescent pregnancy and parenthood.* New York: Grune & Straton.

Mercer, R. T. (1979). *Perspectives on adolescent health care.* Philadelphia: J. B. Lippincott.

Mercer, R. T. (1986). *First time motherhood: Experience from teens to forties.* New York: Springer Publishing.

Moore, K., Miller, B., Glei, D., Morrison, D. (1995). *Adolescent sex, contraception and childbearing: A review of recent research.* Washington, D. C.: Child Trends, Inc.

National Guidelines Task Force. (1991). *Guidelines for comprehensive sexuality education—kindergarten–12th grade.* New York: Sex Information Education Council of the United States.

Neutens, J. J., Drolet, C., DuShaw, M., Jubb, W. H. (Eds.). (1991). *Sexuality education within comprehensive school health education.* Kent, OH: American School Health Association.

O'Sullivan, A., and Jacobsen, B. (1992). A randomized trial of a health care program for first time adolescent mothers and their infants. *Nursing Research,* 41, (4), 210–215.

Peterson, A. C., and Crockett, C. (1986). Pubertal development and its relation to cognitive and psychosocial development in adolescent girls: Implications for parenting. *School Age Pregnancy and Parenthood.* New York: Aldine de Gruyter.

Podgurski, M. J. (1996a). *Taking charge: fire and sex.* Pennsylvania Coalition for Teen Pregnancy Prevention Newsletter, Volume 4.

Podgurski, M. J. (1996b). *Teen pregnancy: what we can do. Childbirth Instructor,* 2nd Quarter, 18–21.

Potter, S., and Roach, N. (1989). *Sexuality, commitment and family.* Spokane, WA: Teen-Aid, Inc.

Reedy, N. J. (1991). The very young pregnant adolescent. *NAACOG's Clinical Issues in Perinatal and Women's Health Nursing,* 2 (2), 209–228.

Rich, O. (1991). Family-focused tertiary prevention with the adolescent mother and her child. In S. S. Humenick, N. N. Wilkerson, N. W. Paul (Eds.), *Adolescent pregnancy: Nursing perspectives on prevention* (pp. 137–154). White Plains, NY: March of Dimes Birth Defects Foundation.

Rivera-Casale, C., Dlerman, L. V., Manela, R. (1986). The relevance of child-support enforcement to school-age parents. *Child Welfare,* 63 (6), 521–532.

Schauberger, C. (1986). Adolescent obstetrics. *Seminars in Adolescent Medicine,* 2 (3), 197–205.

Search Institute. *Values and Choices.* (1991). Minneapolis, MN.

Sears, J. T. (1992). *Dilemmas and possibilities of sexuality education.* New York: Teachers College Press.

Shafer, M. (1988). *High risk behavior among adolescents.* New York: Elsevier.

Shaw, R. D., and Hirsch, N. J. (1984). Infants of teenage mothers: The Blank Children's Hospital experience. *Seminars in Adolescent Medicine,* 2 (3), 243–250.

Simkins, L. (1984). Consequences of teenage pregnancy and motherhood. *Adolescence,* 19, 39–54.

Vinovskis, M. A. (1988). *An epidemic of adolescent pregnancy? Some historical and policy considerations.* New York: Oxford University Press.

Zuckerman, B. S., et al. (1984). Adolescent pregnancy: Biobehavioral determinants of outcome. *Journal of Pediatrics,* 105 (6), 857–863.

Chapter 40

Perinatal Infections

Donna Frede Vinal
Susan Gothard Huffman

The pregnant woman and her fetus are susceptible to many infections and infectious diseases. Some of these may be quite serious and life-threatening for the mother, whereas others may have a profound impact on fetal outcome. . . . Infections pose unique problems during a coexisting pregnancy.

F. Gary Cunningham, Paul MacDonald, Norman Gant, Kenneth Leveno, and Larry Gilstrap

HIGHLIGHTS

- Infectious Disorders That May Affect the Pregnant Woman, the Fetus, or the Neonate
- Classification of Disorders: Bacterial, Parasitic, Viral, and Other
- Description of the Organism and Mode of Transmission
- Risks to the Mother
- Risks to the Fetus/Neonate
- How the Organism or Disorder Is Identified
- Treatment and Prevention
- Nursing Considerations

Maternal infection with pathogenic organisms continues to cause problems for both mothers and babies. The advent of antibiotics led to a significant reduction in maternal morbidity and perinatal mortality due to infections. Today, although maternal deaths from infections are rare, infection is the leading cause of fetal and neonatal morbidity and mortality (Faix 1991). There are new strains of pathogens that demonstrate resistance to antibiotics or are incurable, such as penicillinase-producing *Neisseria gonorrhoeae* and human immunodeficiency virus (HIV).

Organisms that lead to serious disease during the peripartum period include bacteria, parasites, viruses, fungi, and protozoa. The identification of organisms such as HIV, *Borrelia burgdorferi* (the causative agent of Lyme disease), and chlamydiae as agents of disease in pregnancy along with the persistence of such age-old diseases as syphilis and tuberculosis demands a depth and breadth of knowledge for the nurse working in the field of obstetrics. Pregnant women are subject to these and all other acute and chronic infections that affect the nonpregnant population.

Table 40–1

PERINATAL INFECTIONS

Bacterial Infections
Chlamydial infection
Gonorrhea
Group B streptococcus infection
Listeriosis
Lyme disease
Infections caused by mycoplasmas
Syphilis
Tuberculosis
Parasitic Disease
Trichomoniasis
Toxoplasmosis
Viral Diseases
Cytomegalovirus
Viral hepatitis (A; B; C; delta; non-A, non-B)
Human immunodeficiency virus
Herpes simplex types 1 and 2
Human papillomavirus
Influenza
Measles
Mumps
Parvovirus
Rubella
Varicella-zoster/herpes zoster
Other Infections
Candidiasis (yeast infection)
Bacterial vaginosis (*Gardnerella* vaginosis)
Urinary tract infections
Scabies/lice

These infections may be acquired through a variety of modes, from sexual contact to occupational exposure. The woman of reproductive age is at risk for acquiring a range of infections from varicella (chickenpox) as a daycare center employee to HIV infection resulting from sexual contact or contact with infected blood. Many of these infections are classified as sexually transmitted diseases (STDs).

STDs are infections spread by intimate contact. This contact includes sexual intercourse and close body contact, such as kissing, cunnilingus, anilingus, fellatio, mouth-breast contact, and anal intercourse. Many of these infections can be transferred to the fetus and neonate through the placenta, by ascending infections, or during birth.

The risks involved in these infections range from maternal cervical cancer and infertility to conjunctivitis, pneumonia, neurologic disease, and death for the fetus or neonate. Acquiring these infections during pregnancy puts two lives in jeopardy. More newborns eventually die of congenitally acquired infections than of all other causes of infant mortality combined (Minkoff 1991).

In this chapter, infectious diseases most frequently occurring and of particular importance to nurses caring for pregnant women and their newborns are described (Table 40–1). The organisms chosen are divided into three categories: bacteria, viruses, and protozoa. The description includes the organism, its mode of transmission, the risks of infections for both mother and fetus/neonate, signs/symptoms, diagnosis and treatment of the infection, prevention approaches, and nursing considerations.

ROLE OF THE NURSE

Infection is still a major cause of morbidity and mortality during the perinatal period. The goal of nursing care is twofold: the prevention of infection in the woman, her fetus, and her newborn infant (Fig. 40–1); and early identification of signs and symtoms of infection so that appropriate treatment can be initiated. Nurses are often the first to recognize that something is "wrong" with the woman or infant. Their astute detection of signs and symptoms of infection, and prompt reporting to the health care provider, are critical in giving the woman and infant the proper medical treatment.

Nursing diagnoses that may be applicable to the woman and fetus with a perinatal infection include

Infection, actual or risk for

Noncompliance, risk for

Respiratory function, alterations in

Coping, ineffective individual/family

Parenting, alterations in

Skin integrity, impairment of

Fear (related to effects of infection on self, pregnancy, and infant)

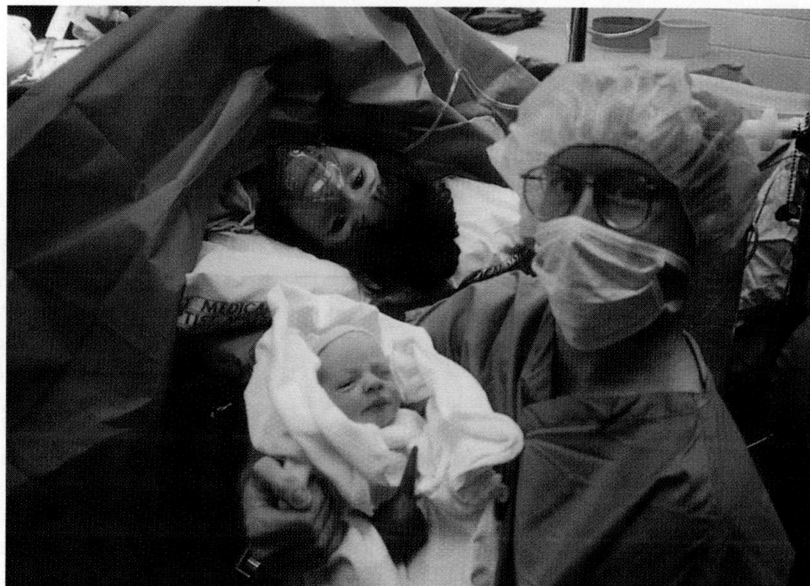

Figure 40–1

A critical role of the nurse is to promote the health of the new family unit. This is accomplished by protecting the woman and her infant from infection through the use of Standard Precautions to prevent the spread of infection (see Appendix VI) and by early detection of signs and symptoms of infection so that prompt treatment can be initiated.

Fear (related to subsequent or future pregnancy complications)

Comfort, alterations in

Fetal injury, potential for

BACTERIAL INFECTIONS

Bacteria are single-celled potentially pathogenic microscopic organisms with the ability to invade cells as intracellular pathogens or cause problems as extracellular pathogens. Infections due to bacteria can range from minor to fatal and be caused by normally occurring body flora or microbes of particular virulence to humans. Fighting against a bacterial pathogen depends on many factors, including normal host defenses (such as intact skin, cilia in the respiratory mucosa, and gastric acids) and immune factors (such as specific antibodies, phagocytes, and polymorphonuclear leukocytes) (Wang and Smaill 1989; Sweet 1990).

The manifestations of infection are not due to any direct action of the infecting organism but primarily reflect the responses of the infected host. Signs such as inflammation (due to polymorphonuclear leukocytes) and systemic symptoms such as fever (caused by direct action on the thermoregulatory center in the hypothalamus by a protein released by leukocytes after contact with bacteria), chills (caused by a hypothalamic response to raise the temperature to a new level), and fatigue (systemic absorption of toxic material along the lymphatic system and into the bloodstream) are caused not by the bacteria but by human defense mechanisms. The immune system works specifically on intracellular bacteria with cell-mediated immunity (interferon-gamma, macrophages, and T cells). Extracellular pathogens cause humoral immunity reactions (antibodies and complement proteins) and polymorphonuclear leukocytes, which arise to defend against such invasion (Hammill and Gilstrap 1990).

The defense mechanisms from within the immune system are altered during pregnancy (pregnancy-induced immunodeficiency syndrome/immunosuppression). This places the pregnant woman at an increased risk for becoming infected by certain bacteria. Those bacteria most commonly causing problems during pregnancy are discussed.

Chlamydial Infection

▼ **Organism.** *Chlamydia trachomatis* is a nonmotile obligate intracellular parasite and is classified as a bacterium since it contains both DNA and RNA, has a cell wall and ribosomes, and is susceptible to erythromycin and tetracycline. *Chlamydia* is found in the genitourinary tract of 20 to 25 percent of U.S. women. It is currently the most commonly occurring STD (Hammill and Gilstrap 1990; Merkatz and Thompson 1990). The primary sites of infection in women are the cervix, endocervix, and anus. During pregnancy, if colonized within the genital tract, it can be transmitted to the neonate. *C. trachomatis* is responsible for trachoma, lymphogranuloma venereum, conjunctivitis, and nonspecific genitourinary diseases such as urethritis. Its prevalence rate has been found to be as high as 25 percent in young, low socioeconomic status persons with concurrent STDs. The prevalence of infection in pregnant women is equal to or greater than 5 percent (Centers for Disease Control [CDC] 1993, p. 93).

▼ **Mode of Transmission.** *C. trachomatis* is transmitted by sexual intimacy. Close body contact can cause the spread of the organism. It may be transmitted during the intrapartum period from the birth canal. It is most commonly spread during the birth process (60 to 70 percent frequency). Chlamydial infection can also be spread by infected particles in water (inadequately chlorinated swimming pools) (Burrow and Ferris 1995; Sever et al. 1989).

Predisposing factors that increase the likelihood for chlamydial infection are single status, concurrent gonorrhea, oral contraceptive use, young age, absence of pelvic pain, and complaints of vaginal discharge (Gleicher 1992).

▼ **Risks to Mother.** The major risks to women include pelvic inflammatory disease and salpingitis. The organism is also the cause of infertility and ectopic pregnancy (due to scarring of the fallopian tubes after infection). During pregnancy, the infection has been known to induce premature onset of labor and premature rupture of membranes (Lee 1988). The organism has been found as a causative agent in chorioamnionitis cultures, having ascended the birth canal and infected amniotic fluid. *Chlamydia* is also a cause of postpartum endometritis and "sterile" pyuria. Blood-borne disease in the mother is expressed as fetal wastage or neonatal sepsis.

▼ **Risks to Fetus/Neonate.** Chlamydial infection is the leading cause of conjunctivitis, known as ophthalmia neonatorum (30 to 50 percent), and afebrile pneumonia (10 to 20 percent) in infants younger than 6 months of age (Freeman and Poland 1992). Prematurity due to premature onset of labor and premature rupture of membranes in the mother is also a problem.

▼ **Signs/Symptoms.** Most infections are asymptomatic but can present as mucopurulent cervicitis with associated vaginal discharge and lower abdominal pain. Urinary tract infection symptoms and symptoms such as fever, lower abdominal pain, and cramping are indicative of chlamydial infection.

▼ **Identification/Diagnosis.** Diagnosis is confirmed by an enzyme-linked immunosorbent assay (ELISA). Any other technique that identifies chlamydial antigens must be confirmed by culture of the organism itself. Newer, rapid tests that are now available are enzyme immunoassay (Chlamydiazyme) and direct fluorescent antibody staining (Micro Trak). These are inexpensive, have good sensitivity and specificity (70 to 99 percent), and require no expertise for interpretation (Gleicher 1992). ELISA is preferred for office or clinic diagnosis because it is easy to perform during a pelvic examination and involves no special equipment or medium.

The CDC recommends presumptive treatment of women at sufficient risk for genital chlamydial infection with the following: male sexual partner with urethritis or epididymitis; cervicitis, especially with mucopurulent discharge; pelvic inflammatory disease; infant with chlamydial infection; any two of the following: age younger than 20 years, multiple sexual partners, oral contraceptive use, sexually active women of lower socioeconomic status; late postpartum endometritis; postabortal endometritis; sterile pyuria; any newly acquired STD; pelvic pain; infertility; ectopic pregnancy; prepubertal vaginitis; and cervical neoplasia (American College of Obstetricians and Gynecologists [ACOG] 1985; CDC 1989).

▼ **Treatment.** Topical antibiotics are ineffective for prophylaxis or treatment of *C. trachomatis* conjunctivitis (CDC 1993, pp. 53–54). The recommended treatment of pregnant women is erythromycin for 7 days. Doxycycline is the treatment of choice for nonpregnant women. Drainage/secretion precautions are necessary for infected infants, and isolation is recommended for infants with chlamydial pneumonia. Orally administered erythromycin is the drug of choice for neonates with chlamydial infections (Freeman and Poland 1992).

▼ **Prevention.** Prenatal screening for chlamydiae in priority high-risk groups is necessary according to the CDC. High-risk groups include the following clients: pregnant, single, adolescents, women with multiple sex partners, those from low socioeconomic status groups, and those with a history of other STDs. Barrier contraceptives are strongly encouraged to stem the rise in infection rates.

NURSING CONSIDERATIONS

Explain the infectious nature of the disease and the need to refrain from infecting others (abstinence).

Assist with screening/identification of the organism.

Identify/treat all of the woman's sexual partners.

Teach about personal hygiene.

Teach about medication compliance.

Encourage use of barrier contraceptives for protection (nonoxynal 9) (sponges or condoms).

Treat infected infants—drainage/secretion precautions, isolation of infants with pneumonia.

Provide psychological support (accepting, nonjudgmental attitude).

Gonorrhea (Gonococcus, GC, "Clap")

▼ **Organism.** Gonorrhea is an acute infectious disease of the urethra, cervix, rectum, and other areas of the body that may give rise to bacteremia and organ complications. *Neisseria gonorrhoeae* is an anaerobic, gram-negative, kidney-shaped diplococcus that does not survive in the presence of oxygen or in the cold. The disease is usually spread by sexual contact and is considered an STD. The incidence of the disease is stated to range from 10 to 30 percent. The prevalence of gonorrhea in most prenatal patient populations is less than 1 percent, although it may be higher in some settings (CDC 1993, p. 62). The organism is found most commonly in the cervix, vulva, perineum, and anus. Of note, there are new strains of penicillinase-producing gonococci and chromosome-mediated resistant *N. gonorrhoeae* that necessitate newer antibiotics (cephalosporins and beta-lactamase drugs.) The organism is killed rapidly by drying, sunlight, heat, and most disinfectants (Gleicher 1992).

▼ **Mode of Transmission.** The disease is spread by sexual contact. The bacteria can be spread as an ascending vaginal tract infection, especially during prolonged rupture of fetal membranes. The bacteria have been isolated from amniotic fluid. The pathogen can also be transmitted to the newborn during birth.

▼ **Risks to Mother.** In women, pelvic inflammatory disease is an important clinical problem. The ascending nature of the infection is also a cause of chorioamnionitis. Premature rupture of membranes and prematurity have been linked to gonorrheal infections (Gilstrap and Cox 1989; Gleicher 1992; Hammill and Gilstrap 1990; Lee 1988). Prolonged rupture of membranes promotes the ascent of the pathogen into the uterine cavity. Gonorrhea is also a cause of puerperal fever (endometritis). Complications of untreated gonorrhea include septic joint arthritis, septicemia with polyarthralgia, dermatitis, tenosynovitis, meningitis, and subacute bacterial endocarditis (Gleicher 1992).

▼ **Risks to Fetus/Neonate.** Risks of gonorrhea to the fetus include intrauterine growth restriction, prematurity, and stillbirth. Risks to the neonate include *ophthalmia neonatorum,* which is a severe infection of the conjunctiva. Conjunctivitis caused by *N. gonorrhoeae* is seen as purulent discharge from the eyes by the third to fourth day of life. (Conjunctivitis caused by chlamydial infection tends to appear later.) The gastrointestinal tract of the neonate is also a common site of gonococcal infection and may result in septic arthritis, meningitis, and septicemia (Freeman and Poland 1992; Gleicher 1992; Hammill and Gilstrap 1990).

▼ **Signs/Symptoms.** Most women are asymptomatic with gonorrheal infections. Women may be symptomless carriers of the pathogen for months and be identified only through sexual contact tracing. Symptoms can be any of the following: a purulent yellowish vaginal discharge, urinary frequency, or painful urination. After exposure, symptoms may take up to 21 days to appear, if at all. Rectal or oropharyngeal infection is often symptomless, but a discharge or complaints of a sore throat may occur.

▼ **Identification/Diagnosis.** The diagnosis of gonorrhea is most commonly done by culture. A new nonculture rapid screening test is in the testing phase.

Gram stain is a preliminary test done while awaiting culture results. The presence of gram-negative diplococci on a gram-stained smear is suggestive of a diagnosis of infection with *N. gonorrhoeae*. The endocervix is swabbed, and the swab is then streaked onto the culture medium (Thayer-Martin or Transgrow). Other sites for culture are the rectum, urethra, and oropharynx. Presumptive treatment may be started on the basis of these findings while confirmatory culture results are pending (CDC 1993, pp. 57–60, 62–65). Other laboratory tests include a serologic coagulation test and a monoclonal antibody immunofluorescent test.

▼ **Treatment.** Instillation of 1 percent silver nitrate solution or erythromycin ophthalmic ointment to the eyes of all newborns is recommended and even mandated by many states. Blindness may occur without treatment (CDC 1993, p. 63). Antibiotic therapy is instituted. Pregnant women should not be treated with doxycycline or tetracyclines. Those infected with *N. gonorrhoeae* should be treated with a recommended or alternative cephalosporin (CDC 1993, p. 60). Spectinomycin may be used if the client cannot tolerate a cephalosporin.

▼ **Prevention.** All pregnant women should be screened at least once during pregnancy (Merkatz and Thompson 1990; Wang and Smaill 1989). It has been recommended that all pregnant women be screened in both the first and third trimester of pregnancy. Prenatal cervical culture screening at the initial visit and again in the third trimester with appropriate treatment is recommended. The use of condoms for protection against *N. gonorrhoeae* is highly recommended. Reexamination after antibiotic treatment has been completed is recommended (Gleicher 1992).

NURSING CONSIDERATIONS

Explain the infectious nature of the organism and the need to refrain from infecting others.

Identify/treat all sexual partners of the woman.

Teach about medication administration and the need for compliance with medical regimen.

Encourage condom use or abstinence until infection is cured.

Emphasize the need for follow-up for reculture to determine if infection is cured.

Provide psychological support (accepting, nonjudgmental attitude).

Group B Streptococcus Disease

Streptococcal infections can be classified according to their characteristics microbially and classified clinically by the type of infection. When grown on blood agar plates, Group B beta-hemolytic streptococci produce zones of clear hemolysis. Clinically, streptococcal infections are divided into two types: (1) carrier state, in which a person harbors the organism without apparent infection; and (2) acute illness. Group B streptococcal infection is the most common cause of neonatal sepsis. In the mother, Group B streptococcus (GBS) is a significant cause of postpartum infection, most commonly endometritis, aminionitis, and urinary tract infection (CDC 1996a).

▼ **Mode of Transmission.** Women are select carriers of the organism within the cervix, vagina, anus, and urethra. They may be transient, intermittent, or chronic carriers of GBS. The organism can be transmitted through sexual contact and can spread through the lymphatic system and into the bloodstream easily. It is estimated that approximately 15 to 35 percent of pregnant women are colonized with the organism. The reservoir for the bacteria and the source of infection for the neomate is the gastrointestinal or genitourinary tract of the woman. Transmission rates from colonized women to babies at birth are as high as 70 percent (Kircher et al. 1996). Infection of the neonate occurs through ascending genital tract infection (blood-borne to amniotic fluid) or during birth. Neonatal colonization can occur with a carrier mother regardless of whether the route of delivery is vaginal or abdominal. Nosocomial neonatal infection can occur from neonate to neonate by way of the hands of nursery personnel (CDC 1996a).

▼ **Risks to Mothers.** GBS disease can cause any or all of the following maternal complications: (CDC 1996a):

- Urinary tract infection
- Abortion
- Endometritis
- Chorioamnionitis
- Fetal death
- Puerperal sepsis
- Episiotomy site fasciitis
- Preterm labor and premature birth

▼ **Risks to Fetus/Neonate.** Infants born to women who were identified prenatally as GBS carriers have been shown to have 29 times the risk of early-onset disease. Neonatal colonization results in early-onset disease (1 to 7 days) or late-onset disease (>7 days to 3 months). The risk of early-onset cases is increased by prolonged rupture of membranes (>12 to 18 hours), prematurity, prolonged labor, low birth weight, and/or maternal fever. Early-onset neonatal sepsis occurs within 7 days and has a 6 percent mortality rate (CDC 1996a). The infant displays acute respiratory distress and pneumonia. Heart failure and death occur rapidly. Mortality rates are inversely proportional to birth weight. Late-onset GBS disease most commonly presents as meningitis. Mortality rates for GBS meningitis range from 10 to 20 percent, with 15 to 30 percent of survivors developing neurologic impairment (CDC 1996a).

▼ **Identification/Diagnosis.** Diagnosis is confirmed by a culture from the urine, cervix, vagina, or rectum of the woman. Cultures from the newborn are taken from the external ear, umbilicus, throat, or anus. In the neonate the signs of acute respiratory distress and meningitis appear rapidly.

▼ **Signs/Symptoms.** The signs and symptoms of streptococcal infection depend on the category into which the infection falls. Carrier states are identified only through cultures taken from the site (which usually shows no evidence of inflammation and no clue that GBS is present). Group B streptococci can normally be found in the pharynx, urine, and vagina of carrier individuals (gastrointestinal or genitourinary colonization). Acute infections can manifest as bacteremia, endocarditis, urinary tract infections, pneumonia, or meningitis. Symptoms of neonatal infection are respiratory in nature. With early-onset disease, the neonate displays symptoms of severe respiratory distress, apneic periods, or pneumonia. Meningitis is the classic manifestation of late-onset GBS infection.

▼ **Treatment.** Administration of antimicrobial agents before the onset of labor or before the rupture of membranes is not likely to prevent GBS disease, although in some studies maternal colonization with GBS was reduced by this means. Intrapartum chemoprophylaxis (penicillin is usually the drug of choice) after the onset of labor or after membranes rupture is the most likely method of preventing both early-onset neonatal GBS disease and maternal illness (CDC 1996a).

The CDC has developed prevention and treatment guidlines in collaboration with the American College of Obstetricians and Gynecologists, the American Academy of Pediatrics, and other professional organizations. The use of one of two prevention strategies is recommended. In the first stategy, intrapartum antibiotic prophylaxis is offered to women identified as GBS carriers through prenatal screening cultures collected at 35 to 37 weeks' gestation and also to women who develop premature onset of labor or rupture of membranes at less than 37 weeks' gestation. In the second strategy, intrapartum antibiotic prophylaxis is provided to women who develop one or more risk conditions at the time of labor or membrane rupture (CDC 1996a).

Education of prenatal patients about GBS disease is also an integral aspect of prevention. Early identification of risk factors for perinatal GBS disease is critical so that prompt treatment can be initiated. These risk factors include preterm labor and birth, longer duration of ruptured membranes, intrapartum fever, age under 20 years, and black race (CDC 1996a).

▼ **Prevention.** It has been documented that premature labor and premature rupture of membranes in women who are GBS carriers can be prevented with the use of penicillin (Siegel and Cushion 1996). The routine screening of health care providers in newborn nursery settings to identify GBS carriers (asymptomatic carriers) is recommended.

Prenatal screening is recommended by the CDC, as is intrapartum treatment of high-risk mothers (prolonged rupture of membranes, fevers, premature rupture of membranes, and prolonged labor) (CDC 1996a). Nosocomial infection can be limited by meticulous handwashing.

NURSING CONSIDERATIONS

Assist with assessment and identification of the organism through prenatal screening.

Recognize risk factors that are associated with the possibility of GBS neonatal infection:

- Maternal carrier/colonized
- Premature onset of labor
- Premature rupture of membranes
- Prolonged rupture of membranes (>12 to 18 hours)
- Prolonged labor
- High number (more than four) of vaginal (cervix) examinations during labor
- Low-birth-weight infant

Nurses are accountable for the number of vaginal examinations conducted during labor with ruptured membranes. The least number of vaginal examinations possible should be done during labor, to protect the mother and infant from infection.

Give, if ordered, intrapartum intravenous ampicillin to women if expecting premature infant (<2500 gm); or with PROM or ROM >20 hours; or if maternal fever >37.5°C.

Use meticulous handwashing and consistently apply Standard Precautions in caring for the woman and the neonate.

Carry out client education concerning the organism, its mode of transmission, its risks, and the need for compliance with the medication regimen.

Listeriosis

▼ **Organism.** *Listeria monocytogenes* is a motile, gram-positive, aerobic, intracellular coccobacillus that is found worldwide; it is a well-known perinatal pathogen. The organism accounts for 20 percent of all cases of neonatal meningitis and is the cause of the neonatal syndrome known as granulomatosis infantiseptica. Listeriosis manifests itself differently according to the site of infection and the age of the patient. The frequency of occurrence is highest in neonates and persons older than 50 years, and it peaks in July and August. Among persons of all ages, an estimated 1850 serious cases occur in the United States annually, of which 425 are fatal.

L. monocytogenes is found in soil, water, sewage, and nearly every type of animal including asymptomatic humans (Gleicher 1992). Dairy cattle are the chief reservoir for human infection. Human carrier rates range from 29 percent of poultry workers to 77 percent of public health laboratory workers involved in *Listeria* isolation. Vaginal and cervical carrier rates among women are reported to be 1 to 2 percent (Gleicher 1992). Contamination is by way of the oral-fecal route and by food in epidemic disease. Animals are infected with *L. monocytogenes* by eating contaminated feed. Human outbreaks are attributed to contaminated food and animal products (cheese, milk). Humans can act as carriers of the bacteria (saprophyte) or become infected (pathogen) by the organism. The bacteria may be carried within the gastrointestinal or genitourinary tract as a saprophyte. Venereal spread has been known in animals and is suspected in humans. Pregnant women, persons younger than 1 year and older than 55 years, persons with chronic illnesses, and immunocompromised persons are at high risk for infection. Neonates have an unusual sensitivity to the organism. Half of all listeriosis in humans occurs in pregnant women and neonates. Listeriosis causes meningitis and sepsis in humans and host carriers.

▼ **Mode of Transmission.** Proven transmission occurs in the antepartum and intrapartum periods from mother to child. All other cases are infected from animal carriers. Food-borne and oral-fecal contamination have been documented. As a saprophyte or pathogen in the mother, *L. monocytogenes* can be asymptomatic or appear as an influenza-like syndrome. The organism is transmitted to the fetus transplacentally (hematogenous transmission), as an ascending maternal genital tract infection, or during birth (aspiration or swallowing of infected amniotic fluid or vaginal secretions). Nosocomial transmission may also occur (Burrow and Ferris 1995; Sever et al. 1989).

▼ **Risks to Mother.** The risks to the mother from infection involve influenza-like symptoms and sepsis. With antepartum infection, abortion, premature birth, or stillbirth can result. Intrapartum infection can result in chorioamnionitis. Recurrent habitual abortions have been linked to listeriosis.

Only two maternal deaths due to listeriosis have been reported; one woman had AIDS and the other had systemic lupus erythematosus (Burrow and Ferris 1995).

▼ **Risks to Fetus/Neonate.** Congenitally acquired listeriosis can result in prematurity, diffuse granulomatous skin papules, diffuse sepsis, meningitis, congenital pneumonia, or the syndrome known as granulomatosis infantiseptica. Granulomatosis infantiseptica occurring early in neonatal life has a 90 percent mortality rate; the late-onset syndrome (within the second week of life) exhibits a 40 percent mortality rate. The syndrome results in granuloma formation in organs such as the liver, adrenals, lungs, and brain. Major sequelae to surviving the infection include hydrocephalus and mental retardation.

▼ **Signs/Symptoms.** If the disease is nonspecific in the mother, an influenza-like syndrome or meningitis may lead to diagnosis. In the neonate, the disease appears to cause respiratory distress, sepsis, heart failure, or meningitis. It is difficult to differentiate from GBS sepsis.

▼ **Identification/Diagnosis.** The diagnosis must be confirmed by positive blood culture since clinical diagnosis is extremely difficult. A Gram stain of the cervix or fecal matter will reveal whether the organism is gram-negative or gram-positive. Fecal smears, cord blood, or cerebrospinal fluid is commonly used for diagnosis in the neonate. The organism can be confused with several other bacterial pathogens, so the laboratory should be informed that *L. monocytogenes* is suspected.

▼ **Treatment.** Treatment consists of antibiotic therapy. Ampicillin or erythromycin is prescribed (on the basis of body weight). Antibiotic susceptibility testing is recommended before therapy; however, initiation of therapy should not be delayed pending results. Therapy is continued for 2 to 3 weeks. Prognosis remains poor when diagnosis and treatment are delayed (50 percent mortality) (Gleicher 1992; Sever et al. 1989).

▼ **Prevention.** Prevention resides in identification of contaminated herds (dairy farms) and identification of contaminated food products (dairy products). Screening for asymptomatic maternal carriers (gastrointestinal or genitourinary tract) in endemic or epidemic regions is recommended for prevention of neonatal listeriosis.

NURSING CONSIDERATIONS

Provide screening for disease in endemic and epidemic regions.

Educate client about the organism, its mode of transmission, and the risks associated with the disease (avoid undercooked meat and unpasteurized dairy products).

Educate client regarding medication regimen and the importance of medication compliance.

Use drainage/secretion precautions for infected neonates.

Provide psychological support.

Lyme Disease

Lyme disease et al. is currently the most common vector-borne infection in the United States (Smith et al. 1990). Lyme disease is also known as Lyme borreliosis. It was discovered in Lyme, Connecticut, after an epidemic increase of juvenile arthritis. It is an inflammatory disorder characterized by early skin lesions (erythema migrans) that may be followed weeks to months later by neurologic, cardiac, or joint abnormalities.

Organism. The disease is caused by the spirochete *Borrelia burgdorferi* and is most commonly transmitted by the deer tick (*Ixodes scapularis*). In 1990, a review documented it in more than 50 pregnancies in a 5-year period (Smith et al. 1990). It usually occurs in epidemic proportions during spring and early summer and early fall (May to November) and makes no discrimination among sex or age, as the tick shows no favorites. Cases have been documented in residents of 47 states, Europe, and Asia.

The disease is characterized by a distinct bull's-eye skin lesion (erythema migrans) followed by neurologic, cardiac, and arthritic manifestations. The spirochete invades many organs and progresses in typical stages. Early infection includes localized disease and symptoms of infection such as fever, myalgia, and fatigue. Late infection begins a year or more after the time of initial tick bite and includes multiple organ system involvement of varying degrees.

Mode of Transmission. Transmission of the spirochete is caused by ticks (deer ticks) with tick attachment of more than 24 hours. There is evidence of maternal-fetal transplacental transmission. No other form of person-to-person transmission has been documented.

Risks to Mother. The risks of Lyme borreliosis remain largely undefined. There have been some reports of effects including fetal loss, abortion, and premature labor and birth.

Risks to Fetus/Neonate. The risk to the fetus and neonate is largely unknown. No mention of fetal infection or maternal infection as a contraindication to breastfeeding is found in the *1994 Red Book: Report of the Committee on Infectious Diseases* (American Academy of Pediatrics [AAP] 1994). The reported but unproven risks to the neonate are numerous and include prematurity and congenital malformations of the heart, spleen, and bone marrow. Syndactyly has also been attributed to the infection.

Signs/Symptoms. The bull's-eye (tick attachment) skin lesion known as erythema migrans occurs in 80 percent of patients. Early infection can include rash and influenza-like symptoms. Late infection involves neurologic manifestations such as headaches and mild meningitis. Musculoskeletal pains are typical and occur in muscle, joints, bone, and tendons. Cardiac symptoms include atrioventricular block. There may be prolonged fatigue. The most common late manifestation is arthritis, usually in the knee and large joints. There is no evidence that the infection is more severe during pregnancy.

Identification/Diagnosis. Laboratory testing and interpretation of results can be difficult at times. A two-test approach for active Lyme disease and for previous infection using a sensitive enzyme immunoassay (EIA) or immunofluorescent assay (IFA) followed by a Western immunoblot is the procedure of choice. All specimens positive or equivocal by a sensitive EIA or IFA should be tested by a standardized Western immunoblot. Specimens negative by a sensitive EIA or IFA need not be tested further (CDC 1995b).

Treatment. Antibiotic therapy during the early stages of Lyme disease is the most effective treatment, especially in preventing the major manifestations of late disease. Tetracyclines are contraindicated during pregnancy. Most experts recommend the same therapy as for nonpregnant persons (AAP 1994).

Prevention. Avoidance of thickly wooded areas and wearing long pants tucked in at the ankle and long-sleeved shirts in wooded areas will help prevent tick attachment. Shower after each exposure (Check body carefully for ticks). Vaccines are now being evaluated in trials but are not commercially available in 1996. Preconceptional vaccination is likely to be recommended when it is available.

NURSING CONSIDERATIONS

Educate client concerning the disease and its modes of transmission.

Instruct client in when and how to perform tick checks in endemic areas.

Instruct client concerning medication administration and compliance.

Provide psychological support.

Infections Caused by Mycoplasmas

Organism. The organisms that relate to perinatal infections from this group are *Mycoplasma hominis* and *Ureaplasma urealyticum.* Mycoplasmas are the smallest of free-living bacteria. The organism was first recognized as the causative agent of genitourinary infections in cattle by veterinarians. These organisms are components of the normal gastrointestinal and genitourinary flora of healthy, sexually active men and women. The colonization rate for women is estimated at 50 to 80 percent. It is unknown why and how the organisms become virulent and cause disease and infection.

▼ **Mode of Transmission.** The organisms are sexually transmitted during intimate contact. The organisms are also spread during birth. They have been implicated in ascending infection during prolonged labor and premature rupture of membranes (Gleicher 1992; Smeltzer and Whipple 1991).

▼ **Risks to Mother.** Mycoplasmas have been implicated as causative or associated agents in the following conditions: nongonococcal urethritis, pelvic inflammatory disease, asymptomatic bacteriuria, urinary tract infections, pyelonephritis, infertility, abortion, prematurity, neonatal infection, puerperal infection, chorioamnionitis, and bacterial vaginosis.

▼ **Risks to Fetus/Neonate.** Risks to the fetus and neonate include prematurity, low birth weight, pneumonia, and central nervous system (CNS) disease.

▼ **Identification/Diagnosis.** Diagnosis is based on isolation of the organism by laboratory analysis. Not all laboratories have this routinely available.

▼ **Treatment.** Erythromycin is the preferred antibiotic. Concurrent therapies are sometimes necessary when the client is infected with other STDs simultaneously.

▼ **Prevention.** Screening at this time is not feasible or recommended (Merkatz and Thompson 1990; Sever et al. 1989).

NURSING CONSIDERATIONS

Explain the infectious nature of the organism and the need to refrain from infecting others.

Identify/treat all sexual partners of the woman.

Teach the client about medication administration and the need for compliance with medical regimen.

Encourage condom use or abstinence until cure.

Teach about antibiotics contraindicated in pregnancy.

Provide follow-up for reculture to determine if disease is cured.

Provide psychological support (accepting, nonjudgmental attitude).

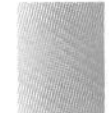

Syphilis

▼ **Organism.** Syphilis is an acute and chronic, complex STD caused by *Treponema pallidum,* a motile spirochete. The organism is capable of invading all tissues and organs, and the disease has active manifestations followed by years of symptomless latent disease. The organism cannot survive long outside the human body. The spirochete invades the body through the mucous membranes or skin abrasions and disseminates rapidly throughout the entire body.

Between 1985 and 1990, the incidence doubled; however, since 1990, there has been a decline (CDC 1995a). In 1991, the CDC established a new surveillance definition of syphilis and guidelines for congenital syphilis infections. It is estimated to affect 1 percent of the maternal population, and 20 percent of their infants will have acquired congenital syphilis (Crane 1992).

▼ **Mode of Transmission.** Syphilis is an STD and as such can be spread by urogenital and anorectal contact, kissing, or close body contact. Without treatment, the host is contagious for a period of years, until the latent and tertiary stages are reached. With adequate treatment, infectivity is usually eliminated within 24 to 48 hours (CDC 1993). The spirochete can be acquired transplacentally (hematogenous transmission), during birth, or through neonatal exposure to infected material such as maternal secretions or blood. Congenital syphilis causes death in 40 to 50 percent of affected infants (CDC 1989). Transplacental infection can occur throughout pregnancy and at any stage of maternal infection (Freeman and Poland 1992). Congenital syphilis is usually transmitted to the fetus in utero, but the neonate can become infected during vaginal birth (Mandell et al. 1995, p. 2119).

▼ **Signs/Symptoms.** The spirochete is transmitted by direct contact with an infectious moist lesion. The organism passes through intact mucous membranes and forms a primary lesion (chancre). The chancre heals within 2 to 6 weeks and is followed by the rash of secondary syphilis (on palms and soles), which appears approximately 6 to 8 weeks later. The rash heals spontaneously within 2 to 6 weeks after it appears. With congenitally acquired syphilis, the neonate displays lymphadenitis, hepatosplenomegaly, and bone irregularities. Symptoms may take weeks or months to develop. Risk to the fetus is directly proportional to the quantity of spirochetes in the maternal bloodstream.

Clinical symptoms of congenital syphilis may be absent until after the first month of life. Symptoms in the neonate include hepatosplenomegaly, joint swellings, rash, anemia, jaundice, snuffles, ascites, pneumonitis, and cerebrospinal fluid changes.

Syphilis is divided into progressive stages of disease.

Primary Syphilis. The primary lesion of syphilis (chancre) appears within 4 weeks of infection and heals within 2 to 6 weeks in untreated persons. There is painless swelling of the regional lymph nodes. Chancres (painless ulcer with indurated, hard base) can be found on the genitalia, anus, rectum, lips, tongue, buccal mucosa, tonsils, and fingers. Chancres are not diagnosed in women as frequently as in men because the cervix is a frequent site of the painless ulcer.

Secondary Syphilis. Secondary syphilis appears as a diffuse macular rash on the trunk and extremities within 6 to 8 weeks after infection. There are characteristic lesions manifested as a rash on the palms and soles. The rash frequently heals but may recur within weeks to months. Symptoms also include headache, anorexia, nausea, fatigue, aching bone pain, and neck stiffness. Condylomata lata papules can develop during this phase. These papules are dull pink to gray in color and flattened. Patchy hair loss may also occur during this stage.

Latent Syphilis. Latent syphilis occurs 3 to 12 weeks after the onset of secondary syphilis. The infected person enters an asymptomatic latency period.

Late/Tertiary Syphilis. After the latency period, usually more than 1 year to as many as 20 years, the infected person develops tertiary syphilis characterized by destructive lesions (gummas) of the skin, bone, and organs. Cardiovascular and neurologic lesions are also involved. The infected person appears normal without development of contagious lesions. This stage of the disease can result in liver failure, pneumonitis, CNS disease, and eventual death (Tillman 1992).

▼ **Risks to Mother.** Death can occur (10 percent mortality rate) if the disease is undetected or left untreated. Stillbirth or fetal death has been reported in infected women. Preterm labor and birth are highly supported as directly related to maternal infection (Crane 1992; Gleicher 1992).

▼ **Risks to Fetus/Neonate.** Risk to the fetus and neonate are directly proportional to the degree of maternal spirochetemia and the duration of untreated maternal infection. These risks include preterm birth, stillbirth, and low birth weight (MacLean 1990; Minkoff 1991). Congenital effects are irreversible and may include CNS damage and hearing loss. There is a 10 to 30 percent mortality, if untreated, due to pneumonitis or liver failure in the neonate.

▼ **Identification/Diagnosis.** Several categories of tests are used for identification. The VDRL (Venereal Disease Research Laboratory) and the RPR (rapid plasma reagin) tests are commonly used "nontreponemal" tests. The results of these tests are based on titers; those high enough are reactive or show positive results, and those with low titers are nonreactive or have negative results. The RPR has a false-positive rate of up to 30 percent. The second type of test detects antibody specifically directed against *T. pallidum* and is called a treponemal test. Commonly used tests of this type are the microhemagglutination assay for antibodies to *T. pallidum* (MHA-TP) and the fluorescent treponemal antibody absorption test (FTA-ABS). These test results are reported as positive or negative and are used to confirm true-positive nontreponemal test results. Treponema tests remain reactive for life, giving the person permanent seropositivity, thus negating differentiation of present infection from past infection. The spirochete can also be identified through darkfield microscopic examination (Gleicher 1992; Sever et al. 1989).

In diagnosis of congenital syphilis, a combination of maternal and neonatal serologic tests, neonatal examination, and other neonatal laboratory evaluations (including lumbar puncture) is necessary to determine such a diagnosis with any certainty.

▼ **Treatment.** Penicillin is the best treatment available for syphilis for both adults and neonates with any stage of syphilis. In pregnancy, allergy testing to confirm penicillin allergy is recommended, and desensitization to penicillin followed by penicillin treatment is considered the best option. If a true allergy to penicillin exists, erythromycin or doxycycline is prescribed. Penicillin is effective for preventing transmission to fetuses and for treating established infection among fetuses (CDC 1995a, p. 39).

▼ **Prevention.** All women should be screened serologically for syphilis during the early stages of pregnancy. In populations in which use of prenatal care is not optimal, RPR-card test screening (and treatment if that test is reactive) should be performed at the time a pregnancy is diagnosed. In communities and populations with high syphilis prevalence or for patients at high risk, serologic testing should be repeated during the third trimester and again at delivery. (Some states mandate screening at delivery for all women.) Any woman who delivers a stillborn infant after 20 weeks' gestation should be tested for syphilis. No infant should leave the hospital without the serologic status of the infant's mother having been determined at least once during pregnancy. Treatment before 20 weeks' gestation rarely results in acquired congenital syphilis, barring reinfection of the mother. Improved access to prenatal care, screening in emergency departments for obstetric patients, and screening whenever or wherever pregnant women are seen would greatly decrease the rate of congenital syphilis (Tillman 1992).

NURSING CONSIDERATIONS

Educate client concerning the disease and its stages, risks, and mode of transmission.

Provide close follow-up care.

Assist with identification and treatment of all sexual partners of the woman.

Encourage client's medication administration compliance.

Teach client concerning use of condoms for protection.

Observe newborns for palmar rash and snuffles.

Use drainage/secretion precautions with suspected congenital syphilis (wear gloves when handling neonate until after 24 hours of antibiotic therapy).

Provide anticipatory guidance for treated persons regarding the Jarisch-Herxheimer reaction after treatment of early syphilis. This reaction follows penicillin treatment of active syphilis and is probably related to the killing of a large number of spirochetes. The signs of the reaction include fever, tachycardia, mild hypotension, vasodilation, headaches, and erythematous painful lesions. The reaction occurs several hours after treatment and abates by 24 hours. Pregnant women may experience transient uterine contractions, decreased fetal movement, and late fetal heart rate decelerations. Women must be warned of this reaction and educated accordingly.

Assist with obtaining postpartum follow-up serologic tests to determine status of infection (Crane 1992).

Provide psychological support.

Tuberculosis

Tuberculosis (TB) steadily decreased in the United States from the 1950s through 1984. From 1985 to 1992, rates increased, but the trend has been reversed. During 1995, the number of cases in U.S.-born persons decreased in all age groups; the decrease was largest (17.0 percent) among persons aged 25 to 44 years. In comparison, the number of cases in foreign-born persons reported in 1995 increased in all age groups except for children younger than 15 years (decreased 7.4 percent) and persons aged 15 to 24 years (CDC 1996b). (TB is endemic in Southeast Asia, Central America, and South America.) The frequency of positive skin testing in pregnant women ranges from 1 to 5 percent. The occurrence of TB in the newborn is uncommon today in the United States (Merkatz and Thompson 1990).

▼ **Organism.** TB is an acute or chronic infection caused by *Mycobacterium tuberculosis,* a nonmotile, aerobic, intracellular bacterium (rod bacillus). It is characterized clinically by a lifelong balance between the host and the infection. Pulmonary or extrapulmonary sites of infection may reactivate at any time, often after long periods of latency. TB is characterized by the formation of tubercles made up of giant cells and possesses the tendency toward either fibrosis or caseation (a form of nonliquefying necrosis).

▼ **Mode of Transmission.** The infection is spread primarily by inhalation. Prolonged exposure is usually required for infection to occur. Infectious droplets are inhaled by the individual, and infection begins in the lung. The infection usually occurs first in the apical segments of the lung and moves to the lower lobes as the infection progresses. Coughing is the most common source of aerosolized contamination. The droplets can dry while they are suspended in the air and contaminate the space for a long time. The infection can be spread transplacentally (hematogenous transmission), but this is rare. The infant can become infected during birth through aspiration of infected amniotic fluid. The neonate can also become infected during the neonatal period from contact with infected individuals (Maccato 1989).

A vaccine is available. BCG (bacille Calmette-Guérin) is an attenuated strain of the bacteria. Neonates born to infected mothers with active disease can be vaccinated with BCG. Pregnancy and immunosuppression are contraindications to BCG administration.

▼ **Risks to Mother.** The risks of acquiring TB include active pulmonary disease (with weight loss, cough) and reactivation of disease at any point in later life. Active disease during pregnancy has been associated with an increase in hypertensive disorders of pregnancy. There have been an increased number of spontaneous abortions seen in pregnancies with active TB disease (Maccato 1989).

▼ **Risks to Fetus/Neonate.** Although there is a risk for fetal/neonatal infection transplacentally, congenital tuberculosis is rare. Congenital tuberculosis can result in pneumonia and death.

Signs/Symptoms. Maternal infection may be asymptomatic. The disease becomes apparent only when the lesion is large enough to be visible radiographically. Active pulmonary disease or reactivation can occur during pregnancy. There may be a history of fever and chills, night sweats, weight loss, fatigue, and cough (consumption). The cough is due to irritative secretions draining from sloughing areas of lung tissue. Hemoptysis, green or yellow sputum, dyspnea, and pleural pain may also be symptomatic of TB.

In the neonate, symptoms of active TB include fever, lethargy, poor feeding (failure to thrive), hepatosplenomegaly, and respiratory distress. Meningitis can result from lesions in the brain. The disease can spread to all major organs (CNS, heart, liver, bones, joints, gastrointestinal tract, and genitourinary tract).

Identification/Diagnosis. Pulmonary TB is often diagnosed on the basis of chest x-ray findings. Microscopic identification of acid-fast bacilli on culture of sputum is diagnostic of TB. The tuberculin skin test (PPD) is used as an adjunct diagnostic aid. It is used to identify most infected individuals. A chest radiograph is not routinely done during pregnancy but may aid in confirmation of the diagnosis. The radiograph is done with lead shielding of the abdomen and fetus (Maccato 1989). TB skin testing is safe during pregnancy (Maccato 1989; Merkatz and Thompson 1990).

Treatment

Mother. Administration of isoniazid (INH), ethambutol, and rifampin for 6 to 12 months has been used successfully during and after pregnancy. The infected individual should receive a combination of two of these drugs. Pyridoxine should be administered along with INH to pregnant women to prevent the development of peripheral neuropathy due to INH. Ethambutol may be used instead of rifampin because of the unknown teratogenicity of rifampin.

Breastfeeding is not contraindicated with the use of these medications. They do not cross over to the infant in quantities sufficient to achieve effective treatment or prophylaxis in the neonate.

Neonate. The neonate born to a mother with active TB should be treated with INH for 3 months. Isolation and separation of mother and infant during active disease is required until the mother is known to be noninfectious (a minimum of 3 weeks of drug therapy). Administer BCG vaccine to infant if ordered. Mantoux test turns positive after BCG vaccine is given.

Prevention. Preventive therapy with INH for household members or other close contacts of infectious persons is recommended. Although no adverse effects of INH to the fetus have been observed, preventive therapy for exposed pregnant women should be delayed until after delivery. Health care providers should wear masks when they are involved with active disease and use good handwashing techniques to prevent the spread of the organism. It has been recommended that skin test screening be performed only in women at high risk or in high-risk populations or endemic areas (Merkatz 1990).

NURSING CONSIDERATIONS

Check skin test site at 48 to 72 hours for induration of 10 mm or more.

Separate mother-infant dyad during active disease for at least 3 weeks of treatment.

Teach client regarding contamination/infection separation.

Teach client about medication regimen and importance of compliance.

Isolate women with active disease from others during labor.

Ensure that supplemental vitamin B_6 (pyridoxine) is given with therapy because of the tendency of INH to induce neuritis and peripheral neuropathy (lack of vitamin B_6).

Promote breastfeeding *if* mother is noninfectious.

Provide follow-up care for sputum cultures and chest films as necessary.

Provide psychological support.

PARASITIC DISEASE

Trichomoniasis

Organism. Trichomoniasis is a commonly occurring STD found during pregnancy. It is reported that *Trichomonas* can be recovered from 25 to 30 percent of all pregnant patients (Gleicher 1992). *Trichomonas vaginalis* is a motile, flagellated, protozoan parasite. The protozoa thrive in less acid vaginal secretions. The parasite commonly exists as normal flora in vaginal and cervical secretions and in the seminal fluid in men. Men tend to be asymptomatic and, as such, the vector for transmission. The human is the only known host of *T. vaginalis.* Trichomoniasis accounts for up to 30 percent of female genital tract infections. The infection is acquired through sexual intimacy or contact with infected, shared wet towels, swimsuits, or bath facilities (CDC 1989). The organism promotes growth of bacteria (anaerobic), resulting in bacterial vaginosis.

▼ **Mode of Transmission.** The organism is transmitted through sexual intimacy. During pregnancy, the organism can be spread through an ascending infection from the maternal genitourinary tract. The neonate can acquire the parasite during birth. It has also been proved to be a water-borne (bath and swimming pools) infection.

▼ **Risks to Mother.** Concurrent infections with *N. gonorrhoeae* and chlamydiae are highly likely, and screening should be done for these organisms. There is an increased occurrence of premature rupture of membranes and premature onset of labor in infected women (Gleicher 1992; Merkatz and Thompson 1990).

▼ **Risks to Fetus/Neonate.** The frequency of actual adverse fetal effects from maternal infection is unknown. It appears to be a rare phenomenon. Pneumonia has been associated with neonatal infection.

▼ **Signs/Symptoms.** The symptoms depend on the severity of inflammation and the presence of secondary infections. The vaginal discharge associated with the infection is greenish yellow and may vary from frothy and thick to watery in consistency; it is often malodorous. Perineal itching also signals the disease. Urinary tract infection symptoms are also associated with the disease because of the excoriation of the area (dysuria).

▼ **Identification/Diagnosis.** Identification of the organism is characteristically achieved through a vaginal "wet mount" preparation (vaginal smear on a microscope slide with a drop of saline). Diagnosis consists of identification of the organism under the microscope as a motile flagellate. Clinical diagnosis is made on the basis of persistent leukorrhea with a frothy greenish appearance and foul smell. Inflammation of the labia, perineum, and vagina are common. Vaginal mucosa (through speculum examination) reveals multiple petechiae (strawberry spots).

▼ **Treatment.** All partners are treated simultaneously with metronidazole. Metronidazole is contraindicated in early pregnancy (organogenesis) and during lactation. Metronidazole may be given after the first trimester of pregnancy (CDC 1989).

▼ **Prevention.** Prevention is related to preconceptional screening and treatment with avoidance of intercourse until cure is achieved. The use of barrier contraceptives is preventive in nature. Recontamination and reinfection are avoided by treatment and cure of all sexual partners.

NURSING CONSIDERATIONS

Identify all of the woman's sexual partners (trace contacts).

Treat all sexual partners simultaneously.

Teach client about:

- Avoidance of sexual intimacy until after treatment is completed
- Avoidance of alcohol ingestion while taking metronidazole (reacts with cramping, flushing, vomiting, and tremors)

Observe women with premature rupture of membranes, prolonged rupture of membranes, and a high number of vaginal examinations during labor for signs and symptoms of chorioamnionitis.

Assist with assessment and identification of organism.

Educate client concerning the disease, its risks, and its mode of transmission.

Provide psychological support.

Toxoplasmosis

▼ **Organism.** Toxoplasmosis is a generalized parasitic infection caused by *Toxoplasma gondii.* The disease occurs worldwide and has a frequency of up to 5 to 95 percent among adults living in different geographic areas. *T. gondii* is a protozoan parasite found in nature and is in evidence wherever domestic animals and humans are found. The protozoan infects any warm-blooded animal. Sexual multiplication occurs in the intestinal tract of cats (the definitive host), and oocysts are formed and shed in the stool.

Evidence of infection with *T. gondii* among pregnant women in the United States varies from 12 to 41 percent, based on serologic testing (Gleicher 1992). The frequency of maternal *Toxoplasma* infection during pregnancy is approximately 0.2 to 1 percent. An estimated 500 to 4000 infants with congenital toxoplasmosis are born annually in the United States (Wong and Remington 1994, p. 854).

T. gondii is usually innocuous and asymptomatic in the mother, but it is harmful to the fetus when infection occurs during pregnancy. The incidence in the United States is 2 to 8 per 1000 pregnant women with primary disease, and 2 in 10,000 neonates contract the disease. The timing of maternal infection has been shown to increase from 25 percent during the first trimester to 65 percent during the third trimester. None of the infants exposed in the third trimester has shown congenitally acquired problems; 75 percent of the infants exposed in the first trimester are severely affected (Gleicher 1992).

▼ **Mode of Transmission.** Transmission occurs transplacentally after ingestion of raw meat or undercooked meat containing cysts or by exposure to oocysts in infected cat feces. Transplacental transfer of the parasite occurs only when the protozoan is acquired during pregnancy (primary infection at conception or during pregnancy). Infection rate increases with increase in gestational age at time of maternal infection (Burrow and Ferris 1995; Sever et al. 1989).

▼ **Risks to Mother.** Although asymptomatic infections are most common, abortion may ensue if infection occurs early in pregnancy. Infection later in pregnancy may result in stillbirth or the birth of a child with clinical disease. If the disease is symptomatic, influenza-like symptoms may be followed by swollen cervical lymph nodes. The disease is similar to mononucleosis or Epstein-Barr virus infection in symptoms. Premature onset of labor and premature birth have been associated with the disease. An increased frequency of thrombophlebitis and asthma during pregnancy with active disease can occur.

▼ **Risks to Fetus/Neonate.** Congenitally acquired toxoplasmosis can be severe and rapidly fatal or asymptomatic at birth. The severity of the disease appears dependent on the gestational age at which the primary infection occurred in the mother. Congenital infection ending in convulsions and coma has a frequency of 40 percent of those infected with the disease. Initial signs include intrauterine growth retardation, jaundice, hepatosplenomegaly, and rash. Other risks of congenital toxoplasmosis include encephalitis, microcephaly, mental retardation, and chorioretinitis. The disease is worse the earlier it is contracted during pregnancy. Only women acutely infected with *T. gondii* during pregnancy can have a child with congenital toxoplasmosis.

▼ **Signs/Symptoms.** Although the disease is mostly asymptomatic in the mother, she may experience fatigue, muscle pain, or lymphadenopathy. The symptoms are mostly subclinical and mimic mononucleosis or Epstein-Barr virus infection. In the neonate, the infection can be asymptomatic or present with a rash, microcephaly, jaundice, hepatosplenomegaly, chorioretinitis, hydrocephalus, or meningitis. The prognosis for the neonate is poor. Most survivors develop severe neurologic and ocular sequelae.

▼ **Identification/Diagnosis.** Diagnosis of a primary infection in pregnancy is usually based on serial antibody titers. Pregnant women can be screened with an antibody titer at the initial visit, and the tests are repeated monthly if necessary to detect seroconversion. Indirect fluorescent antibody testing or the Sabin-Feldman dye test is the most frequently used test to determine immunoglobulin G (IgG) titers. ELISA is also widely accepted as diagnostic of IgM antibodies (which occur only with acute infection, usually within 5 days of infection, but may persist for up to 12 months, complicating the diagnosis of acute infection). The IgM antibody titer is considered the best indicator of primary infection during pregnancy. Other tests include establishing a rising titer of neonatal IgG antibodies or the finding of cysts on placental histologic examination.

▼ **Treatment.** Treatment is not necessary if the serologic test result is positive before pregnancy. The fetus is protected by maternal immunity when maternal infection predates pregnancy. Antibiotics used in the treatment of toxoplasmosis include sulfadiazine (a sulfonamide), pyrimethamine, and spiramycin (available in the United States only by special application to the Food and Drug Administration) for 28 days. Pyrimethamine cannot be used during the first trimester because it is a folic acid antagonist. When it is prescribed, folic acid should be given concurrently for 4 to 6 weeks (Burrow and Ferris 1995). The sulfonamide should not be given in the third trimester because of binding bilirubin sites and predisposing the neonate to kernicterus. Isolation is not necessary. Termination of the pregnancy may be offered to those who have a well-diagnosed acute infection during the first trimester of pregnancy.

▼ **Prevention.** Ideally, all women contemplating pregnancy should be screened preconceptionally for antibody titers for toxoplasmosis. If the mother is seropositive, no harm will come to a conceptus. If the woman is seronegative, then intense educational preparation can prevent the occurrence of the infection. Education must include the following: feed cats only commercially prepared cat foods; keep cats inside during the pregnancy to avoid ingestion of wild game or animals; mode of transmission; source of disease; thoroughly cooking meats; no sampling of uncooked meats or sampling while cooking; washing hands thoroughly when contacting raw meat, cats, catbox litter, or soil; do not clean or have contact with the litter box or dispose of feces and/or do not garden where cats have access. Identifying all at-risk women before pregnancy would also assist in the decline of the disease. A vaccine is being attempted, primarily one to immunize cats.

NURSING CONSIDERATIONS

Provide preconceptional education and screening.

Educate client to

- Use good hygienic measures
- Thoroughly cook meats to kill organisms
- Use good handwashing

Provide all teaching noted in the Prevention section.

Provide psychological support.

VIRAL DISEASES

Viral disease in pregnancy can cause significant mortality and morbidity in the pregnant woman and her fetus or newborn. Viral disease as a teratogen was first mentioned in 1941 by Norman Gregg, an ophthalmologist in Sydney, Australia. He clinically noted congenital cataracts related to prenatal exposure to rubella (part of the rubella triad of congenital cataract, hearing impairment, and cardiac defects). Since that time, more than 400 viruses have been identified that infect humans.

A virus is a particle or virion classified according to property characteristics. Categories of classification are morphologic, genetic, physical, and chemical. Viruses share characteristics. They have a nucleic acid or genome surrounded by a protein shell and can multiply only within a living cell. They have no synthetic or energy-producing systems.

A virus has an effect or causes disease by adsorption, penetration and coating, synthetic reproduction, release, and lysis. Adsorption occurs with cell entry. Penetration and uncoating are necessary to reproduce within the cell. Synthetic reproduction occurs in the cell nucleus or cytoplasm. A release of viral progeny occurs in the cell, which is associated with lysis or cell death.

Chronic or persistent viral infection occurs when cell growth and viral multiplication occur together. Latent phases of several viruses cause recurrent lytic infection in another cell. Viral host disease includes inflammation, tissue destruction, and an immunologically mediated cellular and tissue destruction. Viral identification involves serologic and tissue testing for the virus, antigen, and antibody.

A viral teratogen acts between conception and birth, causing a developmental deviation of structure, function, or biochemical nature. Damage to an embryo or fetus is related to a threshold phenomenon involving timing, amount, and vulnerability of multicellular response. The greatest risk time in the gestational age sequence is the time of maximal tissue differentiation. A virus may persist postnatally in neonatal organs.

Direct viral control involves antiviral therapy, removing the vector of transmission, and immunization. Antiviral pharmacology was developed in the 1960s. It involves chemically inhibiting a viral reproductive phase. Vector control is contact and environment related and is accomplished by techniques such as isolation, cohorting, hygiene, universal precautions, and avoiding crowds (especially at peak infection times and during outbreaks). Active immunization began with Jenner and smallpox in the eighteenth century. Pasteur is credited with development of a live attenuated rabies vaccine in the early twentieth century. A live and attenuated poliovirus vaccine is a product of the 1950s, followed in the 1960s by an attenuated measles vaccine and killed influenza virus vaccine. Contemporary work has provided an improved rabies vaccine and killed hepatitis B vaccine. Immune globulins are used for antiviral passive immunization for hepatitis B, varicella-zoster, and rabies. Viral control depends on the prevention of vector transmission, the use of antiviral drugs, and active and passive immunization.

Cytomegalovirus

"CMV is the most common congenitally and perinatally acquired virus disease known in humans and the single most important infectious cause of mental retardation and congenital deafness in the United States" (Gleicher 1992, p. 633). Cytomegalovirus (CMV) is unique to humans, primarily asymptomatic, and infection is more common than disease. The virus becomes latent with periodic reactivation and viral shedding despite production of antibodies. Cell rather than antibody immunity seems to be the body's mechanism of control, which places the fetus and infant at high risk for sequelae (Cunningham et al. 1993). Almost everyone (80 to 90 percent) is exposed to the virus in a lifetime (Gleicher 1992). The incidence of seroconversion and congenital infection is 1 to 3 percent yearly. Up to 60 percent of beginning school-age children have antibodies to CMV (Sever et al. 1989).

▼ **Organism.** Morphologically, CMV is a member of the herpesvirus family. It is an enveloped virus that produces large cell size (cytomegaly) in host cells by causing intranuclear inclusion bodies (Gleicher 1992; Urang 1990).

▼ **Mode of Transmission.** Modes of transmission are contact (mucous membrane contact with infected body fluids or tissue), respiratory, sexual, and transplacental. Vehicles of transmission include urine, cervical excretion, semen, saliva, blood, transplant tissue, amniocentesis, intrauterine transfusion, and breast milk. The incubation period from exposure to symptoms or excretion is 4 to 12 weeks. CMV may manifest as a latent infection that is activated by a blood transfusion or as an immunosuppressed state that some authors associate with a physiologic mechanism of normal pregnancy (Cunningham et al. 1989; Urang 1990). General spread of a CMV infection is facilitated by asymptomatic primary and recurrent infections, multiple sites of excretion, prolonged excretion despite antibody formation, and no cross-reactive immunity with similar herpesviruses (Gleicher 1992).

There is a relatively constant percentage (5 to 15 percent) of infected individuals excreting CMV virus from the genitourinary tract. CMV infection in a neonate is defined as viral excretion or serologic evidence demonstrated within 2 weeks of delivery (Gleicher 1992). All infected infants excrete CMV at birth and may for years. The CMV virus readily crosses the placenta and genitourinary tract and is transmitted in breast milk.

▼ **Risks to Mother.** A primary CMV infection in pregnancy is defined as seroconversion during pregnancy. The risk for primary seroconversion in each pregnancy is 0.5 to 1 percent. Pregnancy does not increase the risk of contracting CMV or the consequences of CMV infection. Viral excretion during pregnancy tends to increase with gestation. Identified risk factors for primary infection include age younger than 25 years, poverty, overcrowding, early age of first intercourse (sexual promiscuity), and exposure to young children at home or in the workplace (Gleicher 1992; Urang 1990).

▼ **Risks to Fetus/Neonate.** The risk for fetal congenital CMV infection is 1 to 3 percent of all births (Gleicher 1992). Severe CMV infection in a newborn is relatively rare and is almost exclusively the result of a primary maternal infection (Urang 1990). Approximately 40 to 50 percent of mothers with a primary infection during pregnancy vertically transmit the infection to their fetus (Urang 1990; Gleicher 1992; Freeman and Poland 1992). Although the excretion of CMV virus is represented as increasing with gestation, the risk for neonatal disease with complication is greater if the maternal infection occurs during the first half of pregnancy (Gleicher 1992; Freeman and Poland 1992). Five to 10 percent of congenitally infected infants have clinically apparent infection with a subsequent 20 to 30 percent mortality. Ninety percent of the survivors of congenital infection develop significant morbidity. Ten percent of the asymptomatic congenitally infected infants (90 percent of incidence) develop late complications, primarily sensorineural hearing loss (Freeman and Poland 1992; Gleicher 1992). Symptoms in addition to sensorineural hearing loss include intrauterine growth restriction, small-for-gestational age infant, bilateral diffuse pneumonitis, microcephaly, cerebral calcification, seizures, cerebral palsy or mental retardation, developmental delay, chorioretinitis, petechiae ("blueberry muffin baby"), hepatosplenomegaly, jaundice, and dental enamel abnormality (Freeman and Poland 1992; Gleicher 1992; Urang 1990). Neonates of seronegative mothers who become infected are at risk for severe morbidity and mortality (Freeman and Poland 1992).

▼ **Identification/Diagnosis.** Almost all maternal infections are asymptomatic; cases of mononucleosis-like illness are rare (Sever et al. 1989). If symptoms are present, they may include fever (high, spiking, and prolonged 3 to 5 weeks), malaise, myalgia, arthralgia, hepatosplenomegaly, pharyngitis, lymphadenopathy, pneumonitis, rubella-like rash, hemolytic anemia, thrombocytopenia, myocarditis, pericarditis, cholestatic hepatitis, intestinal ulceration, aseptic meningitis, encephalitis, and Guillain-Barré syndrome (Gleicher 1992). Symptomatic neonatal common abnormalities include characteristic petechiae, hepatosplenomegaly, jaundice, microcephaly, dental enamel abnormality, and chorioretinitis. Laboratory identification includes viral isolation and serology. Diagnosis is confirmed by microscopic identification of cells in tissue, tissue culture, or serum. Serologic studies include IgM and IgG antibody identification. IgM does not cross the placenta. Identification of IgM in the fetus confirms congenital infection (Urang 1990; Sever et al. 1989). Placentas are smaller or large, hydropic, and pale with opaque membranes. There may be acute vasculitis with thrombi, calcification, and hemosiderin deposition (Baker 1990; Urang 1990).

▼ **Treatment.** Treatment during pregnancy is symptom related and includes rest. Breastfeeding the healthy term infant is not contraindicated. Acquisition through breast milk in a healthy term infant is of little consequence. A premature or immunocompromised neonate of a seropositive mother should not be breastfed and should not receive donor milk from a milk bank even if it is pasteurized or frozen (Lawrence 1989; Gleicher 1992; Urang 1990). A seropositive mother who desires to breastfeed may be advised to discard her milk until infant cord and urine cultures are available. If the infant is seronegative, a referral to neonatology or pediatric infectious disease services will provide counsel and guidance (Urang 1990).

An identified congenitally infected infant may require psychological, speech, and hearing rehabilitation. An antiviral drug, dihydroxypropoxymethylguanine, is being evaluated in preliminary safety and tolerance studies for use in infected symptomatic infants.

▼ **Prevention.** No specific recommendations have been made related to the prevention of CMV infection of a pregnant woman (Freeman and Poland 1992; Gleicher 1992; Merkatz and Thompson 1990). Routine screening is not generally practical but might be considered in women of childbearing age working in daycare centers, intensive care nurseries, dialysis units, and institutions for the mentally handicapped.

Studies with attenuated CMV vaccines are under investigation using normal patients and selected transplant recipients.

NURSING CONSIDERATIONS

Identify high-risk pregnant women for screening.

- Symptoms include low-grade fevers, sore throat, swollen glands, influenza-like illness, myalgias

Refer known seronegative patients who convert during pregnancy to a perinatologist.

Actively participate in education and prevention.

- Provide preconceptional and prenatal counseling for known seronegative patients (staff).
- Consider seronegative and pregnancy status in assignments with known CMV excreters.
- Use universal precautions, hand washing, appropriate hygiene.
- Wash infants infected or at known high risk before transport to the postpartum area.
- Consider single-room, rooming-in care. (*Red Book* [AAP 1994] states that "no special precautions are recommended. Hospitalized patients do not need separate rooms." However, since CMV is spread by intimate contact with infectious secretions, hand washing after exposure to secretions is particularly important for pregnant personnel.)
- Discuss the high rate of transfer to seronegative mothers from young children in daycare.
- Counsel that fetal diagnostic procedures are used to confirm diagnosis but not to alter the situation in risk/benefit discussions, including risk of infection with procedure. Therapeutic abortions are not recommended without unequivocal evidence of fetal disease.
- Provide guidance related to appropriate follow-up of known or suspected infection. Facilitate pediatric follow-up.
- Encourage and support breastfeeding with seropositive mothers of seropositive, otherwise healthy term infants. Support counseling related to the risk/benefit of seropositive mothers breastfeeding healthy term seronegative infants.

Viral Hepatitis

Viral hepatitis has a number of known forms: hepatitis B; hepatitis A; delta hepatitis; and non-A, non-B hepatitis, composed of blood-borne hepatitis C and enteric hepatitis E. Each has similar and specific characteristics. Hepatitis is a major cause of worldwide morbidity and the most common cause of jaundice in pregnancy. It can be anicteric and subclinical. Hepatitis B is the focus of this section because of its potential impact on the maternal-fetal unit. The other types are briefly discussed to define, distinguish, and describe obstetric implications.

Hepatitis B Virus

Hepatitis B virus (HBV) infection, formerly called serum hepatitis and Australian antigen hepatitis, is a common (second most common after gonorrhea), reportable, occasionally fatal infectious disease in the United States. Hepatitis B is a common endemic disease worldwide (Asia, Africa, Central America, and South America). It was identified in 1965, and a safe, effective vaccine has been available since 1982. Hepatitis B occurs primarily in young adults, and its incidence increased by 100,000 in the 1980s. Three hundred thousand new cases occur annually in the United States, and approximately 1 million individuals are HBV carriers. The frequency of HBV infection is estimated at 1 to 2 per 1000 adults in the United States. Adolescent and adult prevalence of HBV infection is threefold to fourfold greater for blacks than for whites and is associated with previous syphilis infection (CDC 1991a). There is currently a 5 percent lifetime risk for HBV infection in the United States and a 1 to 5 percent risk for chronic infection with persistent viremia. The most serious consequence of HBV infection is a chronic carrier state with a subsequent risk for chronic persistent hepatitis, chronic active hepatitis, cirrhosis, or primary hepatocellular carcinoma. In an estimated 6 to 10 percent of infected adults and a higher proportion of infected children (25 percent of perinatally transmitted untreated), infection leads to a chronic carrier state.

▼ **Organism.** HBV is an enveloped, double-shelled, spherical DNA virus. It is hepatotropic but can infect pancreatic cells as well as leukocytes. Infected blood has about 1 million viral particles per milliliter. There are three distinct viral particles associated with HBV: a surface particle, a core particle, and a core derivative (e). The sur-

Table 40–2

HEPATITIS B VIRUS–RELATED NOMENCLATURE

HBV	Hepatitis B virus	Etiologic agent of serum hepatitis, Dane particle
HBsAg	HBV surface antigen	Identified in serum 30–60 days after exposure Persists for variable time
Anti-HBs	Antibody to HBsAg	Last antibody to appear Develops after a resolved infection Is responsible for long-term immunity Lifelong marker of prior infection May also indicate immunity from hepatitis B immune globulin (temporary) or immune response to hepatitis B vaccine
HBcAG	HBV core antigen	No commercial test available Identified only in liver cells, not serum
Anti-HBc	Antibody to HBcAg	Develops in all HBV infections and persists indefinitely Lifelong marker of prior infection
IgM	IgM class specific	Appears early in infection (usually with symptoms), and anti-HBc persists 4 to 6 months Marker of acute or recent HBV infection
HBeAg	HBV e antigen	Derivative of HBcAg Correlates with viral replication and high infectivity
Anti-HBeAg		Antibody to HBeAg Develops in most HBV infections Correlates with loss of replication and lower infectivity

face of the outer envelope generates hepatitis B surface antigen (HBsAg). The surface of the core harbors core antigen (HBcAg) and e antigen (HBeAg), its derivative (Table 40–2).

If anti-HBsAg does not develop and HBsAg persists beyond 6 months after acute infection, the following may be expected: 60 percent develop chronic persistent hepatitis; 30 percent develop chronic active hepatitis; and 10 percent develop an asymptomatic carrier state. All of these can potentially infect others. Chronic active hepatitis is associated with HBeAg and the greatest risk for transmission (to 90 percent vertical perinatal). The asymptomatic carrier state is the most common form of HBV infection and the predominant reservoir for transmission. The carrier is central to the epidemiology of HBV transmission. A carrier is defined by the CDC as a person who is either HBsAG-positive on at least two occasions, at least 6 months apart, or who is HBsAg-positive and IgM anti-HBc–negative on one occasion (CDC 1991b).

▼ **Mode of Transmission.** There are two epidemiologic patterns of transmission: an endemic pattern characterized by transmission through intimate contact; and a nonendemic pattern common to the United States characterized by transmission through blood and blood products, predominantly intravenous drug use. Today, about half of new hepatitis B cases are sexually transmitted (CDC 1993, p. 91). HBV infection causes a viremia that lasts weeks to months (years) and is transmitted horizontally and vertically. Horizontal transmission occurs primarily by sexual contact and parenteral exposure. Vertical transmission occurs as a result of perinatal transmission and can be transplacental; intrapartum exposure to infected blood, amniotic fluid, or vaginal secretions; postpartum exposure; and through breastfeeding.

Individuals or groups at high risk include intravenous drug users, homosexuals with multiple partners, heterosexuals with a bisexual partner, health care workers with blood or needle stick exposure, recipients of multiple blood transfusions (antihemophilic factor), dialysis patients, household contacts of HBV carriers, male prisoners, patients in custodial institutions for the developmentally disabled, and infants born to infected mothers.

The incubation period for HBV infection is long and ranges from 45 to 160 days (15 to 210 days) with an average of 120 days (60 to 90 days) (CDC 1991b; Gleicher 1992).

▼ **Risks to Mother.** The maternal risk parallels the risk to the general population with about a 10 percent chance of progression to chronic disease. Maternal-fetal risk in uncomplicated hepatitis B is not generally increased unless infection occurs in the third trimester or in the immediate postpartum period. Intrapartum risk includes increased risk for prematurity, premature delivery, and vertical fetal transmission. A chromosome abnormality with no chromosomal syndrome has been identified in the leukocytes of newborns of chronic HBV carriers. Postpartum risk for transmission is by horizontal contact (oral-oral transmission through saliva exchange in kissing, food preparation, and utensil/fomite). Breastfeeding has been implicated and is addressed with treatment strategies.

Fulminant hepatitis is a rare major complication of viral hepatitis characterized by progressive hepatic failure leading to coma and death in 70 to 95 percent of cases. Therapy is supportive.

▼ **Risks to Fetus/Neonate.** The risk of vertical perinatal transmission from an HBsAg-positive woman in the United States is 10 to 20 percent. If the acute infection occurs early in pregnancy, 10 percent of infants will be HBsAg-positive; if the acute infection occurs in the third trimester or early postpartum period, 80 to 90 percent of infants will be HBsAg-positive. If maternal serum is positive for HBeAg at delivery, 90 percent of infants will become infected, and 85 to 90 percent of them will become chronic carriers for years if they are not immunized. The infected newborn has a high probability of chronic disease. The likelihood of becoming chronically infected with HBV varies inversely with the age at which infection occurs: vertical (perinatal), 90 percent; children younger than 5 years, 25 to 50 percent.

The infected newborn's risks include prolonged infectivity and chronic hepatitis. Infections in early life are usually asymptomatic and anicteric but may persist for years. This infant is identified as an HBsAg carrier. Chronic hepatitis is demonstrated by elevation in serum aminotransferase activity and carries the subsequent risk for chronic acute hepatitis, postnecrotic cirrhosis, and primary hepatocellular carcinoma. Carcinoma can occur as early as 3 to 4 years, but the latent period is estimated to be 20 to 50 years. A chronic infection in an infant is also associated with membranous glomerulonephritis and nephrosis.

▼ **Identification/Diagnosis.** Clinical manifestation ranges from asymptomatic to fulminant disease. HBV infection is associated with a variety of nonspecific influenza-like symptoms and gastrointestinal symptoms similar to pregnancy complaints. Phases include incubation, preicteric, icteric, and convalescent. After the incubation phase with an average range of medians from 60 to 120 days (88+), the preicteric phase lasts approximately 3 to 10 days (CDC 1990a). Symptoms during this phase may include pharyngitis, cough, coryza, photophobia, headache, myalgia, fatigue, malaise, anorexia, nausea, vomiting, emesis, and right upper quadrant pain. The icteric phase lasts 1 to 3 weeks with jaundice occurring in 25 percent of cases. Pruritus of mild, short duration may accompany jaundice. Fever is uncommon in hepatitis B. Physical examination may reveal a mildly enlarged, easily palpated, slightly tender liver uncommon in normal pregnancy. Diagnosis is related to antigen-antibody and immunoglobulin serologic markers, enzyme levels, and histologic findings.

▼ **Treatment.** Acute hepatitis B can run a course of 3 to 6 months with complete recovery. The 1 to 5 percent of infected adults who become chronically infected have circulating antigen for months to years. Unless hepatitis B is severe, the management is symptomatic with maintenance of calorie and fluid intake. Food may be better tolerated early in the day. Activity including rest is determined by fatigue and malaise. Alcohol and nonessential drugs are contraindicated as in any pregnancy. Conservative obstetric management is indicated. Breastfeeding is not contraindicated if an infected (HBsAg-positive) mother and infant are treated (Lawrence 1989; Ross and Dickason 1992; Gleicher 1992; Sever et al. 1989).

▼ **Prevention.** Prevention is accomplished by vaccination and the use of universal precautions. In the past, prevention has been difficult because historical information identified only a portion of infected individuals, and there is no treatment to eliminate chronic HBV infection. New infections are only eliminated by vaccinating susceptible persons. Therefore, the CDC (1991c) has identified a comprehensive prevention strategy to include

1. Prenatal testing of pregnant women for HBsAg to identify newborns who require immunoprophylaxis for the prevention of perinatal infection and to identify household contacts who should be vaccinated
2. Universal, routine vaccination of children born to HBsAg-negative mothers
3. Vaccination of certain adolescents
4. Vaccination of adults at high risk for infection, including health care workers if tasks include contact with blood and blood products

Two recombinant yeast-derived vaccines providing long-term protection and an immune globulin providing temporary protection (3 to 6 months) are available for preexposure and postexposure HBV infection prophylaxis. HBV vaccine is not effective if an individual is already infected. The vaccine contains noninfectious HBsAg particles, so pregnancy and lactation are not contraindications for administration. The vaccines are 80 to 95 percent effective in preventing HBV infection and clinical hepatitis, 100 percent effective if antibody response occurs. Infant vaccination can be accomplished with the routine immunization schedule, with the first dose given before discharge from the hospital. HBV vaccine is administered intramuscularly in the anterolateral thigh of neonates and infants and the deltoid muscle of adults and children. The immunogenicity of the vaccine for adults and children is substantially lower when injections are administered in the buttock (CDC 1991c). The recommended vaccine schedule is three injections, the second and third administered 1 and 6 months, respectively, after the first.

Hepatitis B immune globulin containing HBsAg antibodies for postexposure prophylaxis is prepared from human plasma screened for HIV antibodies. The preparation process inactivates and eliminates HIV from the final product.

Immune globulin and vaccine are given to all HBsAg-positive newborns within 2 to 12 hours of delivery, at least before 24 hours and not more than 7 days after birth. Two subsequent doses of HBV vaccine are administered at 1 and 6 months. If a mother is identified positive more than 1 month after delivery, her HBsAg-negative infant should be treated.

NURSING CONSIDERATIONS

Be aware of your HBsAg (HBeAg) or vaccination/conversion status.

Encourage participation in the vaccination program.

Do not participate in invasive procedures with known HBeAg-positive status. Seek counsel from an expert review panel as defined by the CDC.

Participate in education and prevention.

- Screening, vaccination, immune globulin administration, universal precautions
- Discourage shared razors, toothbrushes, unprotected intercourse

Provide supportive patient care.

Encourage adequate rest and diet.

- Anorexia, nausea, and vomiting increase during the day; provide ample breakfast
- Activities of daily living are regulated by fatigue; plan and cluster care

Minimize intrapartum ascending infection.

- Be aware of rupture time and potential infection source.
- Maintain perineal hygiene.
- Minimize vaginal examinations, assess vital signs and laboratory results, and monitor signs of infection (increased fetal heart rate, decreased variability, late decelerations).
- Facilitate least traumatic delivery.
- Observe universal precautions, double glove for extended periods of blood contact.

Prevent newborn infection.

- Protect scalp integrity when possible (scalp electrode, pH monitoring, forceps use).
- Careful use of pressure catheters.
- Remove maternal blood from the newborn immediately.
- Suction the nasopharynx on the perineum with wall suction. Stabilize and suction nasopharynx and gastric secretions to minimize swallowed maternal fluid.
- Cut cord with new sterile scissors not used on the perineum.
- Hold invasive procedures until bathed, if appropriate.
- Instill eye prophylaxis after face is clean and dry (prevent tracking blood into the conjunctiva).
- Let alcohol dry on the skin for a full minute before injection.
- Encourage hand washing and gloving with diapering until determination of status.
- Monitor vital signs and glucose level if indicated.
- Administer immune globulin and vaccine if indicated, as ordered.
- Guard from maternal blood and body fluid on the bed or peripad. Discourage kissing, nuzzling until mother and infant have been treated.
- Encourage and support breastfeeding, after maternal and newborn treatment, if indicated.
- Facilitate pediatric, health department, or clinic follow-up vaccination awareness and scheduling.
- Include patient in assessment information for home evaluation and follow-up.

Hepatitis A Virus

Hepatitis A virus (HAV) infection, formerly called infectious hepatitis, is an acute, self-limited viral infection. HAV is an enterovirus with single-stranded RNA. It causes no chronic liver injury or carrier state. The mode of transmission of HAV is fecal-oral. Sources include fecal contamination of the fingers, eating utensils, crockery, and food sources including bivalve mollusks and water. The virus is excreted in the stools of infected persons. Hepatitis A has a short-lived viremic phase. Incubation is 15 to 50 days with a mean of 30 days. Hepatitis A causes increased maternal risk for fulminant hepatitis. Generalized signs and symptoms are similar to hepatitis B, except a low-grade fever is common. Abdominal discomfort may be accompanied by dark urine and jaundice. Immune globulin given before exposure or during incubation is protective against clinical illness. IgM anti-HAV is diagnostic of acute infection. IgG anti-HAV is representative of convalescence and immunity. Prevention is related to hygiene and decreasing contact with known infected individuals. Frequency of occurrence is increased in daycare settings for preschool children and institutions for the mentally retarded. In traveling to developing countries, avoid potentially contaminated food and water. Also avoid beverages with ice, uncooked shellfish, or uncooked fruits and vegetables. Immune globulin may be recommended for living in or visiting rural areas, eating or drinking in poor/uncertain sanitation, or having close contact with local persons. If you plan to reside in a high-risk area, you may need immune globulin regularly (unnecessary with anti-HAV status). Postexposure prophylaxis has to be given within 2 weeks of the last exposure to be effective. See CDC recommendations for specific postexposure prophylaxis. Hepatitis A vaccine has been available in the United States since 1995.

Delta Hepatitis

Delta hepatitis (HDV) infection occurs as a coinfection with acute hepatitis B or is a superinfection of a hepatitis carrier. HDV is a single-stranded RNA virus and has an internal protein antigen (HDAg) coated with HBsAg. Transmission is the same as for HBV. A coinfection usually resolves. A superinfection frequently causes chronic hepatitis D and chronic active hepatitis B. Both infections may lead to the more serious fulminant hepatitis. Diagnosis is made by identifying HDV or anti-HDV (IgM antibody) during or after infection. The treatment is the same as for hepatitis B. Because it is dependent on HBV for replication, prevention of hepatitis B prevents both.

Non-A, non-B Hepatitis

Non-A, non-B acute infectious hepatitis is responsible for 20 to 40 percent of viral hepatitis in the United States. This category includes two distinct viruses, hepatitis E (endemic, water-borne, fecal-oral) and hepatitis C (parenteral, associated with transfusion).

Hepatitis E is not endemic in the United States. It is not a chronic infection. However, hepatitis E is associated with a high mortality and susceptibility to fatal fulminant hepatitis and is increased in pregnancy. There is no commercial laboratory test for hepatitis E. It is diagnosed by epidemic clustering. Hepatitis E causes malaise, anorexia, fever, vomiting, and diarrhea. It can also cause jaundice, transaminase elevation, and hyperbilirubinemia. There is no evidence that immune globulin will prevent hepatitis E. The only prevention known is to avoid contaminated food and water.

Hepatitis C is responsible for 90 percent of post-transfusion hepatitis (5 percent of all hepatitis). The frequency of hepatitis C is 7.1 per 100,000, 1.2 percent of health care workers. Hepatitis C virus is a single-stranded RNA virus. It is blood-borne and transmitted transcutaneously by intravenous drug use, transfusion, and needle stick or nonpercutaneously by sexual and perinatal contact. It can also be transmitted through organ transplantation and human bites. The incubation period is 15 to 160 days with a major peak at 50 days and an earlier peak at 2 to 4 weeks. Seroconversion occurs at a mean of 21.9 weeks. Seventy-five percent of infected individuals are symptomatic. There is no known effect on the course of pregnancy. The risk for chronic carrier state is higher than with HBV (Gleicher 1992). The risk for chronic liver disease, failure, and carcinoma is unknown (Lynch-Salamon and Combs 1992). There is vertical transmission to the fetus in two thirds of cases when there is acute infection in the third trimester. One third of the infected newborns may develop chronic liver disease. The only symptom may be an increase in transaminase level. Symptoms include malaise, fever, abdominal pain, jaundice, and elevated transaminase activity. With chronic infection, the elevation of transaminase activity lasts for more than 6 months. Diagnosis is made by ELISA screen followed by recombinant blot antibody identification. Cure is associated with seronegative response after positive serologic response. Universal screening is not justified at this time. A screen may be offered to high-risk groups: intravenous drug users, prostitutes, HIV-positive individuals, patients with acute hepatitis of unknown origin, patients who received transfusions before 1989, seropositive partners, and individuals with multiple STDs or multiple sex partners. Breastfeeding is discouraged in seropositive women. Patients are advised not to donate blood, even if they become seronegative.

Herpes (Perinatal Herpes Simplex Infections)

Herpes, from the Greek "to creep," is a major venereal infection with the potential for significant short- and long-term sequelae for infected mothers and newborns. It is estimated that 1 percent of all pregnant women excrete herpes simplex virus (HSV) during gestation (Merkatz and Thompson 1990). Frequency is thought to be 1 to 2 per 5000 deliveries in the United States, which produces approximately 1000 cases of neonatal

HSV infection per year. Seventy to 90 percent of childbearing-age individuals are serologic-positive with evidence of prior exposure. The age range for peak occurrence is 14 to 39 years. Caucasian middle-class women are showing the highest rate of new disease. Original high prevalence was reported in lower socioeconomic groups. Patients delivering vaginally with primary active genital infection (lesion) have a 50 percent risk of vertical transmission to the neonate, and risk to the neonate if the mother has recurrent HSV infection is 3 to 5 percent. Most infected newborns (60 to 70 percent) have a mother with no lesions or history of lesions (Freeman and Poland 1992; Sever et al. 1989).

▼ **Organism.** HSV is an enveloped linear double-stranded DNA virus. HSV-1 and HSV-2 share 50 percent of their DNA sequences. Humans are the natural host of HSV. HSV is neurotropic. It associates with nerve cell endings in the epithelium, which it ascends to the local ganglia. Most commonly, HSV-1 is at the trigeminal ganglion and HSV-2 at the sacral dorsal root ganglia. On macroscopic examination, the fluid-filled vesicles are on an erythematous base, cutaneous or mucosal. Ulcerative necrotic cervical lesions are associated with a profuse watery discharge.

▼ **Mode of Transmission.** HSV is transmitted by intimate contact: oral-oral, genital-genital, and oral-genital. It is possible but rare that infection is associated with fomites freshly contaminated with body fluid. Eighty percent of infections above the waist are HSV-1, and 80 percent of infections below the waist are HSV-2. Transmission mechanisms include local hematogenous (viremia, infected leukocytes) and ascension (peripheral nerves to ganglia). Ganglia harbor the virus in a latent state. The latent virus is periodically reactivated. Factors associated with reactivation are exposure to ultraviolet light, fever, fever therapy, trauma, nerve stimulation, menstruation, stress, and immunosuppressive therapy.

Incubation from exposure to onset for primary genital herpes is 3 to 9 days. Prodromal tingling, itching, and burning may occur 1 to 2 days before vesicle eruption. New lesions occur for approximately 3 to 6 weeks. Individual ulcers persist for up to 2 weeks. Symptoms, including pain (external lesions), dysuria, lymphadenopathy, and pharyngitis, worsen for the first 7 to 10 days. Primary infection is also associated with increased urinary tract infection and increased viral excretion at delivery. Because of the increased viral excretion, vertical transmission to the exposed newborn is a major concern and is estimated at 50 percent.

The course of recurrent genital herpes is different with less fetal risk (approximately 3 to 5 percent) if infection is active at delivery. Fifty percent of infections recur within 6 months and then at regular intervals. Fifty percent of individuals have prodromal tingling or itching for 1 to 2 days before outbreak. Vesicles form discrete patches that ulcerate in 24 to 48 hours. Complete resolution usually occurs in 7 to 10 days.

Neonatal incubation is 4 to 12 days with an increased risk for up to 1 month.

▼ **Risks to Mother.** Maternal risks in addition to the infection course as described include the chronicity of infection and rare dissemination on the skin or viremic dissemination with potential hepatitis, thrombocytopenia, leukopenia, coagulopathy, and encephalitis. It is suggested that the hormonal and immunologic events of pregnancy enhance the virulence of the virus or alter the immune response to the virus with primary HSV infection (Burrow and Ferris 1995).

Congenital infection early in gestation can cause fetal demise and spontaneous abortion rather than congenital anomalies. Infection later in gestation causes mortality with major multiorgan morbidity, intrauterine growth retardation, and premature labor and delivery.

▼ **Risks to Fetus/Neonate.** Fifty percent of infected newborns will die in 6 to 10 days, and half of the survivors will have permanent ocular or neurologic sequelae. Forty to 50 percent of the newborns with apparently localized lesions will have the same odds. According to the AAP (1994, p. 243), risk to the infant whose mother has recurrent HSV infection is 3 to 5 percent.

▼ **Identification/Diagnosis.** Maternal clinical diagnosis includes a history of exposure and vesicle identification (extragenital mucocutaneous sites include buttocks, groin, thighs, eyes, mouth [cold sore, herpes labialis], and finger [whitlow]). Infection is associated with regional and generalized lymphadenopathy, chills, fever, malaise, headache, myalgia, splenomegaly, and lymphocytosis. Genital herpes can cause pruritus, dysuria, retention, dyspareunia, dysesthesia, and unusual vaginal discharge.

Signs in the newborn may be nonspecific and subtle. With a history of exposure, a newborn is observed for vesicular lesions (eyes, skin, oral cavity) and unexplained illness, respiratory distress, convulsions, irritability, lethargy, temperature instability, hepatosplenomegaly, poor feeding, and sepsis. Up to 70 percent of infected newborns will have no history of exposure.

Laboratory diagnosis is by viral isolation, direct detection of virus, and serology. The virus is present for 1 to 3 weeks to isolate. Newborn culture sites include vesicle fluid, ulcerating lesions, nasopharynx, urine, and cerebrospinal fluid. Serology includes IgM-specific antibody titer evaluation and other less specific tests.

Treatment. The Infectious Disease Society for Obstetrics-Gynecology (1988d) endorsed the following recommendations.

A positive history for either partner or for a woman with a history of genital herpes, but without lesions:

1. Weekly prenatal cultures should be abandoned.
2. In the absence of genital lesions, vaginal delivery (unless other indication for cesarean delivery).
3. To identify potentially exposed neonate, maternal or neonatal viral culture should be done on delivery day.
4. Maternal isolation is not necessary.
5. Recognized neonatal risk for HSV infection; 1 per 3000 to 1 per 20,000 (APA 1994, p. 243).

With herpetic genital tract lesion in labor or with membrane rupture:

1. Cesarean delivery can reduce neonatal infection risk.
2. Cesarean delivery within 4 to 6 hours of rupture is ideal but should be performed regardless of time duration.

Merkatz and Thompson (1990) recommended (because 70 percent of infected newborns have no maternal history) if lesions occur prenatally:

1. Perform a single culture to confirm diagnosis.
2. Visually observe the labia, vagina, and cervix when presenting for delivery: no lesion, vaginal delivery; lesion, cesarean delivery as soon as possible, supporting culture.

There is no specific treatment available for use during pregnancy. Good hygiene is recommended along with loose-fitting undergarments. Symptomatic treatment includes Burow solution topically, warm sitz baths, cool compresses, plain soap and water wash, dry heat from a hair dryer on cool or a heat lamp, and other pregnancy-appropriate symptom-related strategies (pain relief, fever management, and catheterization). Use local analgesics with caution because they may cause contact dermatitis (Pernoll 1991). Topical anesthetics, antibiotics, and corticosteroids are not indicated. Phenazopyridine may be ordered for dysuria (Burrow and Ferris 1995). Treatment of secondary yeast infection has been recommended as supportive care (Sweet and Gibbs 1990).

The safety of systemic acyclovir therapy among pregnant women has not been established. Burroughs Wellcome Co., in cooperation with the CDC, maintains a registry to assess the effects of the use of acyclovir during pregnancy. Women who receive acyclovir during pregnancy should be reported to this registry (1-800-722-9292, ext. 58465).

Current registry findings do not indicate an increase in the number of birth defects identified among the prospective reports compared with those expected in the general population. Moreover, no consistent pattern of abnormalities emerges among retrospective reports. These findings provide some assurance in counseling women who have had inadvertent prenatal exposure to acyclovir. However, accumulated case histories compose a sample of insufficient size for reaching reliable and definitive conclusions regarding the risks of acyclovir treatment to pregnant women and to their fetuses (CDC 1993, p. 25). Acyclovir, although not approved for use during pregnancy, selectively inhibits HSV DNA. It is being used for uncomplicated primary genital herpes and recurrent genital herpes near term. Modality (oral, intravenous) is directed by gestational age, primary versus recurrent infection, and dissemination. Intravenous therapy is usually reserved for gestation greater than 10 weeks (Brown and Baker 1989).

Procedures such as amniocentesis (contraindicated by ACOG 1988a), vaginal examinations, internal monitoring, fetal scalp sampling, and forceps delivery must be considered carefully (ACOG 1988d; Gleicher 1992; Burrow and Ferris 1995). Maternal management with active infection includes Standard Precautions, blood and body fluid, in all obstetric areas. Primary lesions require contact isolation with private room. The patient should use gloves for direct contact with an infected area or contaminated material from an infected area. Meticulous hand washing is essential. Recommendations include washing after removing gloves and changing wet clothes.

A newborn with exposure history is carefully observed for 4 weeks. Physically separate care in the nursery with contact isolation (isolation room is desirable), gown and glove with potential lesion contact, is recommended (Freeman and Poland 1992; Sever et al. 1989). Viral cultures are obtained from the nasopharynx or mouth, conjunctiva, and skin. Consultation and management in a level III facility is suggested by Perinatal Guidelines for infected infants with treatment with acyclovir. If the infection is disseminated, intravenous vidarabine is indicated and is approved for all forms of systemic herpes in newborns (Sever et al. 1989). Circumcision of HSV-exposed newborns should be delayed for up to a month in cases of vaginal birth with active lesions.

Breastfeeding is not contraindicated if there are no herpetic lesions on the breast and cutaneous lesions are adequately covered (ACOG 1988d; Freeman and Poland 1992; Lawrence 1989).

Prevention. Prevention includes evolving delivery guidelines, antiviral therapy, and education. Patient education includes information about the natural history of HSV genital infection and advice to abstain from sexual contact if either partner has a lesion. Asymptomatic infected individuals should use condoms. Pregnant women should avoid sexual contact during the last several months of gestation if their partner is actively infected. Avoid oral-genital sex if a partner has a lesion. A mother, father, family member, staff, or others with herpes labialis (cold sore) or stomatitis should avoid kissing, nuzzling, or direct exposure with a newborn until lesions have cleared. Infected health care workers may care for mothers and newborns with appropriate precautions because of the low risk for transmission (ACOG 1988b). A surgical mask or direct lesion cover may be used until a lesion is crusted and dried or cleared. Hygiene including handwashing is important. A clean gown or barrier should be used to prevent contact with lesions or potentially infectious material.

NURSING CONSIDERATIONS

Educate the client about

- Hygiene, universal and contact isolation, including sexual practice

Provide home follow-up for the mother and newborn.

Provide supportive patient care.

Facilitate pediatric follow-up.

Encourage and support breastfeeding mothers.

- Counsel regarding delaying breastfeeding with breast lesions and covering cutaneous lesions

Human Immunodeficiency Virus (HIV/AIDS)*

Although it was first recognized clinically in the United States only in 1981, the virus now known as HIV (human immunodeficiency virus), and the clinical manifestations known as AIDS, have most likely been an unrecognized human pathogen and disease for at least several decades.

Only the late stage of HIV infection (AIDS) is reportable in the United States, and estimated projections are made about the number of persons who are well, but infected. The World Health Organization (WHO) estimates the prevalence of existing infection and the rising incidence of new cases in developing countries to be at catastrophic levels. Women, in particular poor women and women in poor countries, are extraordinarily vulnerable to this deadly infection. In 1990, the WHO estimated that there were 3 million women infected worldwide, representing 30% of total cases (Ickovics and Rodin 1992). HIV is a leading cause of morbidity and mortality among women, particularly those of childbearing age.

The medical management of HIV/AIDS in the adult and the child can change rapidly and frequently, particularly the pharmacologic interventions. Nurses are encouraged to rely on the periodical literature and other sources of continuing education to stay abreast of current recommendations and to be aware that because of this evolution, physicians may differ among themselves in their medical approach. The goals of nursing care and the principles of patient education are less subject to variation.

▼ **Organism.** HIV is a retrovirus that has an affinity for CD4 lymphocytes. It binds to the surface of the cell, integrates itself into the nucleus, and by "reverse transcriptase" uses the nucleus to reproduce. The very cells that would "fight" such a virus are converted into "factories" for the virus and then die in 1.6 days. Therefore, HIV infection impairs cellular and humoral immune function by decreasing the number of CD4 lymphocytes, and also impairs related macrophage response to microbes. The virus is lymphophilic and neurophilic; that is, it has an affinity for the lymphatic and neurologic systems and has a high capacity for mutation and variation. It is now known that HIV is rapidly reproducing from acute infection onward. (It was previously thought that there was a "latent" period.) With new laboratory techniques that can "amplify" HIV RNA, it has been learned that 10 billion new HIV virions are produced each day. This information has altered the direction of medical and pharmacologic management of persons with HIV for the first time in a decade (Saag 1996).

▼ **Mode of Transmission.** HIV is less highly contagious than hepatitis B (HBV) and is transmitted in the same manner. For transmission to occur, there must be body fluids infected with virus from a host and contact with a "portal of entry" in the recipient. All body fluids of an infected host except perspiration have been shown to contain virus. Blood, semen, and breast milk have higher concentrations of virus than urine, saliva, vomitus, and stool. It is also known that HIV can cross some membranes such as the placental barrier, the blood-brain barrier, and vaginal mucosa and (in the neonate) the walls of the gastrointestinal tract. Modes of transmission are: sexual contact, transfusion with blood or blood products, occupational exposure (health care workers), sharing needles or using "dirty" needles (drug use), and vertical transmission from mother to infant.

▼ **Prevention.** HIV is preventable. There are several levels on which nurses can work to pre-

*This section was written by Margaret Lynch.

vent the further spread of HIV. The first is the social level. HIV prevention requires effective community and government intervention to address the precursor conditions for HIV: the economic and social disenfranchisement of women, drug abuse, sexual abuse, and the exploitation of women and children (Paris Declaration 1990). Barriers for sexual contact (male and female condoms, dental dams) must be readily available and substance abuse treatment must be easily accessible. The second level is that of individual patient care. Nurses must learn to be effective, compassionate individuals. Sexual and social histories are gathered more effectively by teaching prevention to patients at all age levels and of all sexual orientations (Andrist 1988). Women are at particularly high risk for HIV. We know that male-to-female sexual transmission is two to four times easier than female to male. Women need help at all points of contact in the health care system to overcome the social and personal barriers necessary to incorporate safer sex into their relationship(s) or to abstain from unprotected sex. (See Chapter 10 for safer sex information.)

Third, nurses also have a responsibility to protect themselves and their patients. *Standard Precautions,* which now supersede *Universal Precautions,* are an important part of nursing practice education to patients and families. (See Appendix VI.)

Exposure of health care workers to HIV-infected body fluids via percutaneous injury carries an average of 0.3 percent risk of transmission. Of 1000 health care workers exposed to HIV from needlestick or some other break in the skin, three will become infected. (Just as not all sex partners or all infants exposed to HIV will contract the infection, neither will all health care workers.) This is probably relative to the strain of the virus, the quantity of the virus, and perhaps the immune factors of the recipient host. Recent recommendations have been issued on postexposure prophylaxis (PEP) for health care workers (MMWR 1996). Currently, a regimen of a combination of antiretroviral medications, commencing within hours of exposure and continuing for 4 weeks, is recommended. Since these protocols can change, nurses are advised to refer to the current literature and to their institution's occupational exposure policy if they experience an exposure.

▼ **Identification/Diagnosis.** For pregnancy, current recommendations endorsed by the Centers for Disease Control (CDC), the American Academy of Pediatrics (AAP), The American College of Nurse Midwives (ACNM), The American College of Obstetricians and Gynecologists (ACOG), and the American Medical Association (AMA) are *universal, mandatory HIV counseling and education and voluntary HIV antibody screening.* The goals of HIV education and counseling are to

- educate women on HIV, their own or their partner(s)' risk behaviors, and methods of risk reduction
- educate women on the risk and means of preventing HIV transmission to infants, and their reproductive options (in one survey, 85% of HIV infected women elected to continue their pregnancies; Stratton et al. 1992)
- offer women HIV antibody testing when they are ready and if they are able to make informed consent
- permit the early identification of infants affected by HIV

Some states have ordinances governing the standards of HIV counseling and testing, and nurses must be aware of what the statutes are in their practice area. However, all institutions and practices should be following the federal guidelines published in 1994 and 1995. Owing to the social climate of stigma that has surrounded HIV infection for the past 16 years, HIV testing is unlike any other diagnostic test that health care providers may administer (Task Force on AIDS 1992).

In an adult, a serum ELISA test is performed for purposes of screening for HIV antibody. This test is very sensitive but not highly specific. If an ELISA is positive, a Western blot test is done. Western blot is more specific and more expensive. Results may be read as positive, negative, or "indeterminate." All HIV test results must be given to the patient *in person.* Giving any HIV test result is another opportunity for assessment and educational intervention. The patient who is negative and who seems to be at "low risk" should be counseled to have her partner tested as well, and her plans for future prevention and use of appropriate approaches should be discussed; the patient whose test results are indeterminate needs education and counseling about the meaning of such a result, prevention of further infection, and encouraging her partner to be tested; and the patient who tests HIV antibody positive needs a great deal of support.

An indeterminate reading may indicate recent infection of a patient who is only beginning to make antibody. An indeterminate result during pregnancy warrants consultation with an HIV specialist, who may recommend a different test to determine whether any actual virus can be detected. A positive HIV result by polymerase chain reaction (PCR) would indicate certain infection; the level of virus could determine the stage of infection; and medical intervention both for the mother and to prevent transmission to the fetus could be instituted with the patient's consent (Cotton and Watts 1995).

A negative HIV antibody result for a woman who, by history, appears to be at risk for possible HIV (a patient or partner who uses substances, particularly crack, or injects drugs; a health care worker with a history of recent exposure) warrants further risk reduction education. The patient should be retested; it usually takes 6 to 12 weeks for a host to manufacture detectable HIV antibody.

A prenatal patient with a positive HIV antibody test requires medical, nursing, and social service intervention. Receiving the news of a positive test for HIV is a shocking experience; and patients usually react as much to the stigma that surrounds HIV as to the medical implications of such a diagnosis (Lester et al. 1995). Many women report being unaware of their risk for HIV until they learn that they have a positive HIV antibody test (Lindsay et al. 1991). It is important for health care providers to recognize that patients may cease to hear anything else said to them after they have received such test results (Witt et al. 1992). It is wise to prepare at the pretest session for the post-test session. All patients should be encouraged to bring someone whom they trust with them. Failing that, the provider should help patients plan what they are going to do for the next few hours and the next day and help them find one person whom they can tell. Although the actual test results may be given by a physician, the nurse usually participates in the assessment and planning for the patient's well-being. Positive HIV antibody tests should always be confirmed by a second test. A positive HIV test is not a medical emergency; the immediate goal is to provide a supportive relationship and take actions to promote the safety of the client.

When the patient is able to cope with additional information, acknowledging her grief and counseling the patient on her obstetric and medical options is the next step. A referral to an HIV care team, including psychotherapeutic and social services is important. However, much of the patient's medical needs can be met in the setting of the obstetric practice.

Some patients choose to terminate their pregnancy. If the woman does not choose to terminate her pregnancy, she needs information on the prevention of transmission to the fetus and on her own self-care. It is now recommended that women with HIV infection take AZT (zidovudine), 200 mg po tid starting in the 14th week of the pregnancy to prevent transmission to the fetus. If the mother also has a high viral load, indicator illnesses, or a low CD4 count, she should be taking a second drug for her own health and to further decrease the risk of transmission to the fetus. The goal of medical management of HIV infection is to keep the viral load as low as possible for as long as possible (Saag 1996).

▼ **Signs/Symptoms.** HIV infection develops slowly over years. Initial viremia or primary infection results in what is described as a "flulike" illness or mononucleosis-like picture. This includes fever, myalgia, lymphadenopathy, and headache. In most cases an illness like this, which can be caused by many viruses, goes undetected as primary HIV infection. Some clinicians advise treating known primary HIV infection with antiretroviral medication, but this practice is not widespread at this time. In pregnancy the use of antiretrovirals is initiated after the 14th week of pregnancy to minimize teratogenicity. The decision whether to use combination antiretroviral medication for primary HIV infection in a pregnant patient will continue to be addressed by providers and researchers in the future.

The second stage of HIV infection was initially thought to be "latent" but is now considered "active" but asymptomatic. This stage can last for many years. Patients can have normal, decreasing, and even low CD4 counts and widely variant viral loads (e.g., a positive HIV result by PCR) and yet not be symptomatic. In some cases, patients have one unusual event such as an outbreak of herpes zoster (shingles) or a transient thrombocytopenia, and then remain asymptomatic for many years. Providers are divided about when and whether to begin antiretroviral medication during this stage. Most feel that a rising viral level warrants intervention with at least two drugs.

The third stage is symptomatic HIV infection. Usually, patients show some evidence of immune dysfunction by their laboratory parameters: a CD4 count below 500, a low CD4:CD8 ratio, and perhaps elevation in CD8 cells and rising viral loads. Because HIV is protean and because host immune function differs, until there is advanced immune dysfunction, HIV can be variable in its course and presentation from patient to patient. All body systems can present with signs of mild or early immune dysfunction. Integument and gynecologic problems are common. Patients may have increased vulnerability to common fungi, worsening of preexisting conditions such as psoriasis, and advent of molluscum contagiosum or human papillomavirus (warts). They may experience reemergence of old infections such as PID, recurrent and refractory vaginal candidiasis, cervical dysplasia, and HPV.

The fourth stage is advanced HIV infection, or AIDS, which is usually marked by a drop below 200 in CD4 cells and a recurrent vulnerability to common bacterial infections or unusual "opportunistic" infections (IOs). The medical management of HIV with chemoprophylaxis against OIs, and the earlier and increased use of combination antiretroviral therapy, have served to delay the onset of this stage in patient or have decreased the morbidity of opportunistic infections.

The diagnosis of AIDS is made on the basis of selected criteria determined by the CDC. Patients can reach advanced stages and show evidence of serious immune compromise without yet "qualifying" for a diagnosis of AIDS. Additionally, some patients can have one "qualifying" illness early in the course of their illness and then be well for a long time. While a diagnosis of AIDS (most simply a CD4 count below 200 cells/mm^3) holds important meaning to the patient and to service providers, it is the clinical picture of the individual patient that is most important.

Risks to Mother. The obstetric patient with HIV is regarded as and managed as "high risk," although there are few untoward events that HIV causes during pregnancy, and it is thought that pregnancy does not have a deleterious effect on HIV disease (Hocke et al. 1995; Cotton 1995, p. 46). However, "Most pregnant women, regardless of serostatus, have frequent complaints of fatigue, shortness of breath, nausea, back pain, urinary frequency and headaches" (Deneberg 1995). It therefore behooves the nurse and other providers to investigate these symptoms more thoroughly in the HIV-positive pregnant woman, as these "common complaints" may be the hallmark of serious illness, particularly in the patient with an already compromised immune system. Patients with HIV may need longer courses of antibiotics to eradicate common infections such as UTIs, may be more vulnerable to postpartum infections, and may have difficulty tolerating medications prescribed because of the common symptoms of pregnancy.

Obstetric and Medical Management. Caring for an obstetric patient with HIV has several goals:

- Prevention of maternal opportunistic infections, which involves patient education and pharmacologic prophylaxis when indicated by the patient's CD4 count. Patients should be taught about good handwashing; should avoid persons who are ill; should not care for fish tanks or in any way come into contact with cat feces or litter; and should avoid undercooked meat, raw eggs, and unpasteurized dairy products. In a way that does not alarm them, patients should be taught information about avoiding microbes to which they might be more vulnerable.
- Prevention of further exposure to HIV either through sexual contact or through the use of needles.
- Initiating recovery from substance abuse; crack cocaine in particular has been shown to have more of a deleterious effect on pregnancy than does HIV disease (Mauri 1995).
- Helping the patient and family plan for the birth.
- A safe delivery of a healthy child without maternal complications.

During the intrapartal period, some caveats in obstetric care must be observed to reduce transmission to the neonate. If the fetus has not been exposed to HIV in utero, the most risky time is its journey through the birth canal. Scalp electrodes should never be used, as they would create a portal of entry to the neonate; episiotomy is to be judiciously avoided to decrease the amount of maternal blood in and around the birth canal (lubricating to soften the perineum decreases the possibility of tears). To that end, unless the mother has another condition that warrants induction, such as premature rupture of membranes, pharmacologic (oxytocin) induction should be avoided. Oxytocin contractions can be very strong, and sometimes the infant arrives so quickly that the floor of the pelvis cannot stretch, necessitating an episiotomy or inducing tears (Fekety 1989). Also, some think that the extra hard contractions may expose the infant to maternal fluids under positive pressure. Placing heavy absorbent pads under the mother's hips can control some of the body's amniotic and blood exposure. Although the impact of the events of delivery and birth on rates of transmission of HIV are not yet fully known, Standard Precautions dictate minimizing the infant's exposure to maternal blood and body fluids (Gliden 1996); (Cotton 1995, p. 49). A common misunderstanding parents may not voice is that their baby, if it has HIV, will be born *ill.* Parents need to know that their baby will not look sick from HIV at birth and that there will be a period of uncertainty before it is known whether the baby has acquired the infection.

During labor, women should receive zidovudine intravenously (2 mg/kg over 1 hour and then 1 mg/kg/hr until delivery). This regimen, combined with oral zidovudine during the second and third trimesters of pregnancy, followed by PEP in the infant for the first 6 weeks of life, is advised as a result of data collected during a trial conducted between 1991 and 1993. Of the 400 subjects who had "mildly symptomatic" HIV disease in this placebo-controlled study, the infants born to women who received zidovudine, not placebo, had a lower incidence of HIV infection by 60% (Connor et al. 1994). As more antiretroviral medications appear to be safe, at least in the second and third trimesters, and as combination therapy has become accepted treatment for lowering the viral load, more clinical trials will determine the direction of antiretroviral HIV treatment during pregnancy. The long-term effects, particularly on the fetus and neonate, of being exposed to zidovudine and other medications are not yet known.

During the postpartum period, women need normal postpartum care; birth control planning and education on the care of the infant; administration of the medication; and evaluation of coping, fatigue, depression and other common occurrences. Depending on the stage of HIV infection, the postpartum woman may be at a higher risk for infections and should be observed for this and taught how to take her temperature and what symptoms to look for. It is usual practice to advise HIV-positive women living in areas with a safe water supply and sanitation system not to breastfeed to avoid postnatal transmission to a child who may not have been infected in utero.

HIV Disease and the Neonate

In the United States, 1.7 of 1000 pregnant women are estimated to be HIV positive. In 1993, HIV infection was the fourth leading cause of death among women of childbearing age. As of 1995, more than 5500 cases of AIDS in children below the age of 13 had been reported in the United States and it is estimated that between 1000 and 2000 U.S. infants are born every year infected with HIV either in utero or during labor (CDC 1995d). Before the use of zidovudine during pregnancy, labor, and infancy, the rate of transmission from infected mother to infant was between 20 and 30 percent in the United States. Theoretically, the use of antiviral medication, the careful reduction of infant exposure to maternal blood and body fluids, and the early identification of HIV disease in pregnancy will reduce this by half or more. However, many barriers exist that prevent all these measures from being implemented: provider awareness and implementation of care standards, patient adherence, and coexisting medical conditions may impede optimal care (Ferri 1996).

▼ **Mode of Transmission.** Infants and neonates are vulnerable to HIV infection at three junctures: across the placental barrier, during labor and delivery, and from breast milk. All infants acquire maternal antibody to HIV infection, but not all acquire infection. It is not understood why not all infants acquire infection across the placenta. It is thought that the quantity of maternal viremia, coexisting infections, and viral strain are factors. It is also thought that more than 50% of HIV transmission to infants take place during the intrapartal period. (Kuhn and Stein 1995).

▼ **Prevention.** The prevention of transmission of HIV to infants begins with the prevention of transmission to women before they are pregnant. HIV antibody testing and administration of zidovudine in pregnancy and labor is a *late-stage* intervention in the prevention of neonatal HIV disease.

In addition to the prevention of transmission during the intrapartal period, the neonate should be suctioned promptly using wall suction or bulb syringe. The infant should be bathed carefully and thoroughly before any procedure such as administration of vitamin K, heel sticks, or venipunctures. The use of Standard Precautions apply in all care procedures. Infants can room with their mothers.

Additionally, PEP is recommended. Parent(s) should have been informed before the birth about the recommendations for giving zidovudine to newborns for the first 6 weeks of life. They may be understandably concerned about the potential for short- and long-term side effects. Zidovudine is a strong drug; in its action to "kill" virus, it also suppresses the bone marrow of the recipient, and some patients experience more unpleasant side effects than others. However, research data to date have not demonstrated untoward effects on neonates except for a mild anemia. Because the long-term side effects of zidovudine on the neonate are unknown, some institutions require that patients sign a consent form.

The dose of zidovudine for infants is 2 mg/kg/dose of suspension PO every 6 hours for the first 6 weeks of life. Mothers can use a tuberculin syringe for measuring and administering the medication. The pediatric provider can adjust the dose as the baby gains weight.

▼ **Identification/Diagnosis.** The early diagnosis of infants has become easier since 1995. In the past, it was not known definitively whether a child had acquired HIV infection until he or she could be tested for HIV antibody without the interference of maternal antibody, usually between 15 and 18 months of age. As in the adult HIV population, the use of PCR testing for HIV infection has begun to change HIV diagnosis and care of the infant. It is now believed that HIV infection "can be reasonably excluded with two negative HIV cultures or PCR viral load tests, one obtained at or after 1 month of age and the other at or after 4 months" (Grubman 1995). PCR testing for HIV can also take up to 4 weeks to obtain results.

The other recommended prophylaxis is for *Pneumocystis carinii* infection. In the immune-compromised adult, illness as a result of *Pneumocystis* is almost always from an "old" infection that the individual can no longer contain, much as previous tuberculosis infection can emerge after the immune suppression of chemotherapy in the cancer patient. In the neonate, however, *Pneumocystis* infection is a primary infection that has high morbidity and, if untreated, 100% mortality. Therefore, in 1995 guidelines were published recommending that *all* HIV-exposed infants be treated with medication to prevent infection by *P. carinii.* Trimethoprim-sulfamethoxazole begun at 1 month of age is the drug of choice. It is considered a "safe" drug for the short course that it is given until HIV infection can be ruled out (the majority of infants) or if HIV is "ruled in" until 1 year of age and thereafter based on CD4 counts.

▼ **Signs/Symptoms.** An infant who has contracted HIV infection may have no outward signs for the first several months of life. Without intervention and treatment, more than half of children with HIV infection will be symptomatic by their first birthday. They should be observed and examined for early signs of immune deficiency, including enlarged spleen and/or liver, lymphadenopathy, and any impairment in growth and development.

NURSING CONSIDERATIONS

Ensure that children at risk for HIV are seen by their primary pediatric provider at birth and at 1 week, 2 weeks, 1 month, and then 2 months of life. This is twice the number of visits required of a family without HIV infection. Some families need transportation services to make such frequent office visits.

Assess, at each visit, the family's stage of grieving and coping, and review medication teaching and the meaning of diagnostic tests.

Refer all infants at risk for HIV for Early Intervention services.

Ensure that parents have clear access to a health care provider whom they can trust after hours and on weekends.

See that infants with or at risk for HIV infection receive all recommended immunizations at the regular schedule. These infants should receive inactivated polio vaccine by injection instead of oral polio vaccine. Oral polio vaccine causes a shedding of polio virus in the stool, which may be a risk to the immunocompromised family members.

Provide support. Because of the need for testing requiring phlebotomy and the increased injections on the immunization schedule, infants at risk for HIV and their parents can be very traumatized by primary care visits. The baby should be bundled or swaddled and at least one other person should be present to comfort the infant, support the parents if they wish to stay, and assist the phlebotomist.

Many children now survive to go to daycare and primary school, but the long-term prognosis of HIV disease in adults and children is still poor. Families need support and encouragement to plan for the future and to grieve in anticipation. More children will be orphaned by HIV than will become ill from HIV. Because of the psychological trauma involved with HIV infection/AIDS, individuals and families will benefit from a multidisciplinary treatment approach that includes psychological support and counseling.

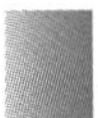

Human Papillomavirus

Human papillomavirus (HPV) is a common, multifocal STD that infects both partners, causing symptomatic and asymptomatic common warts and genital warts (condylomata acuminata) of the cervix and vagina and the skin of the vulva, perineum, and perianal areas; laryngeal papillomas; and cervical neoplasia (ACOG 1987; Baker 1990; Pernoll 1991). The resultant warts are benign epithelial or fibroepithelial tumors of the skin or contiguous mucous membranes with growth and host immunity-related response (Baker 1990; Gleicher 1992). Approximately 20 percent of the population is infected (Baker 1990; Gleicher 1992). The frequency of HPV infection has increased dramatically in the last 10 years and is much higher in teens than in adults (Gleicher 1992). Seventy-five percent of all adults have antibodies suggestive of prior HPV infection. Two to 10 percent of all women of childbearing age are estimated to have genital warts (Sever 1989). The total estimated infectivity in the United States is approximately 12 million, with 75,000 new infections yearly (Fletcher 1991).

No therapy has been shown to eradicate HPV. Therefore, the goal of treatment is removal of exophytic warts and the amelioration of signs and symptoms, not eradication (CDC 1989).

There is growing concern regarding genital warts caused by HPV because

1. They are becoming more common in clinical practice.
2. They account for a large majority of abnormal Pap smears.
3. They may be related to the later development of genital neoplasms.
4. They are difficult to treat.

▼ **Organism.** HPV is a supercoiled, covalent, closed, circular double-stranded DNA molecule of the Papovaviridae family found in human and animal hosts (Gleicher 1992). There are 60 subtypes of HPV, which appear to be associated with different disease manifestations (ACOG 1987; Burrow and Ferris 1995). HPV-1 and HPV-2 are present in common and plantar warts. HPV-6 and HPV-11 are present in genital warts and laryngeal papillomas of children. HPV types 6, 11, 16, and 18 are found in flat and papillomatous condylomata acuminata. HPV types 16, 18, 31, 33, and 35 are found in advanced cervical lesions (ACOG 1987; Burrow and Ferris 1995; Cunningham et al. 1989). A mature virus forms in the nuclei of superficial cells, sheds, and infects other cells. A latency period that lasts many years may follow (Fletcher 1991).

▼ **Mode of Transmission.** HPV is transmitted sexually and perinatally by contact after direct inoculation through abrasions in the skin. The virus may also be transmitted transplacentally (Sever 1989). Single cells are infected, which are stimulated to divide (Lee 1988). Warts occur at genital sites and nongenital sites (oral cavity, larynx, respiratory tract). HPV growth and host response are immunity mediated; therefore, the process may be exacerbated with larger, more extensive lesions in diabetes, pregnancy, and immunocompromised states (ACOG 1987; Baker 1990; Gleicher 1992). Vaginal warts classically involve the upper and lower third of the vaginal vault, sparing the middle. HPV infection tends to occur first at the posterior introitus and adjacent labia with perineal and anal extension in 20 percent of cases (Fletcher 1991). Anal warts occur in association with genital warts more frequently in women. Penile warts are more common in circumcised men (Fletcher 1991). The incubation period for HPV is 1 to 6 months, with an average of 3 to 4 months, but it may persist for years or life (ACOG 1987; Fletcher 1991; Gleicher 1992; Osborne and Adelson 1990). Approximately one third of warts disappear spontaneously in a 6-month period owing to a host immune system alteration or a limited life span of infected cells (Gleicher 1992).

▼ **Risks to Mother.** Maternal risks include proliferation causing soft tissue dystocia, increasing friability, and development of cervical carcinoma (ACOG 1987; Schwartz 1987; Sever et al. 1989). A permissive immune status and increased vascularity during pregnancy favor HPV replication, with enlargement and proliferation of lesions causing distress and mechanical obstruction. HPV growth is stimulated by estrogen (glucocorticoids and cellular factors). A shift in T-cell population occurs in pregnancy, which favors viral replication. The ratio of T-helper to T-suppressor cells decreases as gestational age progresses. Unsuspected warts may become visible, and existing lesions may enlarge and proliferate. Mechanical obstruction may occur as the lesions cover the perineum and impede or occlude the vagina and cervix. The lesions may cause extreme discomfort, limit mobility, and impede urination and defecation. In addition, as lesions become friable, there is increased risk for hemorrhage, hemostasis, laceration, poor healing, dehiscence, and fistula (Osborne and Adelson 1990; Schwartz et al. 1987). Maternal risk is compounded by a medical history of immunocompromise due to genetic, infectious, or medically induced causes. Diabetes is associated with severe HPV infection (ACOG 1987).

▼ **Risks to Fetus/Neonate.** The rare but greatest and increasing risk to the fetus is intractable, recurrent juvenile- and adult-onset laryngeal papillomatosis caused by HPV types 6 and 11 (most frequently found HPV types in the genital tract of men and women). The infection is caused by transplacental or transvaginal viral inoculation of the respiratory tract (larynx, trachea, and pulmonary tree), causing hoarseness, respiratory distress, obstruction, and death. There is no curative treatment for a laryngeal papilloma. Recurrence is the rule with repeated treatment and lifelong morbidity. The peak age of onset is 2 to 5 years with a latency period of 5 years to adulthood. Approximately 40 to 50 percent of cases are adult onset.

▼ **Identification/Diagnosis.** HPV warts are usually diagnosed by history, clinical symptoms, clinical examination, or Pap smear (ACOG 1987). Symptoms include itching, burning, pain, tenderness, bleeding, and visible proliferation. At colposcopic examination using acetic acid (3 percent), lesions appear as white epithelium with prominent surface capillaries. A Pap smear shows the cellular change of koilocytosis (halo cells), which is diagnostic of HPV infection (ACOG 1987; Fletcher 1991). Identification in the child is by clinical appearance and respiratory obstruction (Sever et al. 1989). In addition to the Pap smear, other laboratory diagnostic modalities include histologic examination, serologic antibody identification, and Vira-Pap.

▼ **Treatment.** At best, treatment is difficult, prolonged, and marginally effective (Fletcher 1991). The goal of treatment therefore becomes removal of lesions, not eradication (CDC 1989; Fletcher 1991). Indications for treatment during pregnancy fall into three categories:

1. Maternal pain and bleeding and potential for infection
2. Possible obstruction of labor
3. Concern related to antepartum or birth-related HPV infection with inoculation of the fetal or neonatal respiratory tract (Baker 1990).

Cesarean birth is recommended for soft tissue dystocia, mechanical obstruction, or other legitimate obstetric indications, not the potential risk for laryngeal papillomatosis (ACOG 1987; Baker 1990; Sever et al. 1989). Treatment includes cytotoxic, cryosurgical, electrocautery, and surgical modalities.

Of the two cytotoxic agents commonly used to treat HPV infection (podophyllin and trichloroacetic acid), only trichloroacetic acid is indicated for use during pregnancy. Podophyllin, derived from the mayapple plant, in 10 to 25 percent tincture of benzoin is used biweekly for 4 weeks in nonpregnant patients with small, external genital and perianal warts. It is not used in pregnancy because its local and systemic effects have been associated with maternal flaccid paralysis, hypokalemia, coma with fetal death and abortion, premature rupture of the membranes, fetal death, and teratogenicity in rats (Fletcher 1991; Gleicher 1992; Osborne and Adelson 1990; Schwartz 1987).

Trichloroacetic acid (80 to 85 percent) is a caustic topical astringent agent that acts by precipitating proteins at the site of local application with a 20 to 30 percent effectiveness. Trichloroacetic acid does not cause inflammation but produces a white slough that peels off in a few days. Depending on efficacy, it may be repeated every 7 to 10 days. It is recommended for safe use in pregnancy (ACOG 1987; Fletcher 1991).

Cryosurgery during pregnancy is limited to liquid nitrogen applied for 30 to 60 seconds to cervical warts. A cryoprobe may cause vaginal perforation and fistula formation (Fletcher 1991). Carbon dioxide laser therapy used with skill during pregnancy has many advantages over other treatments, including precision, rapid healing, reduced pain, reduced scarring, technical advantage for larger lesions, and facility for use in the upper vagina. Laser ablation or photovaporization has been more effective than other treatment modalities but is not without risk. The operator has to fully understand and apply the physical and surgical principles essential to its safe use (Schwartz et al. 1987).

Surgical excision risks hemorrhage, tissue denudation, trauma, cellulitis, and infection. Risk is greater during pregnancy with increased proliferation and vascularity. Intrapartum radical therapy should be avoided if possible because spontaneous resolution frequently occurs post partum. An autologous vaccine has been used on a limited scale with favorable results.

Treatment of laryngeal papillomas involves difficult surgery with a high recurrence rate (Sweet and Gibbs 1990). Neonates born to mothers with active HPV infection are not managed with special precautions in the nursery (Freeman and Poland 1992).

▼ **Prevention.** The epidemiology of HPV infection precludes a plan until we are more knowledgeable about transmission and detection. It is advisable to avoid contact with known infected individuals.

NURSING CONSIDERATIONS

Advise client to use condom/barrier methods of birth control appropriate to site with active infection.

Advise client to use appropriate precautions with oral lesions.

Encourage client to practice good personal hygiene related to warm, moist skinfolds of perineum.

Advise client to wash external genitalia plus cleansing of the vagina by gentle douching, followed by thorough drying once a day to inhibit proliferation and minimize discomfort. This should be done under medical advisement during pregnancy and post partum with the following precautions: For douching the client should not use hand bulb syringes because of the danger of air embolism. The douche bag should be no more than 2 feet above the level of the hips to prevent high fluid pressure. The nozzle should not be inserted more than 3 inches through the vulva (Cunningham et al. 1989).

Provide supportive care.

Facilitate pediatric follow-up.

Influenza

Influenza is an acute self-limiting febrile respiratory illness characterized by myalgias and laryngotracheobronchitis with a brassy nonproductive cough. Influenza is associated with acute and chronic debilitation and periodic epidemics (2 to 4 years). Pandemics have occurred four times in the twentieth century: 1918–19, 1957, 1968, and 1977. The longer the periodic interval between epidemics, the more susceptible the population. Epidemics of shorter periodic interval find children the most susceptible group (spare adults).

▼ **Organism.** Influenza is caused by an enveloped RNA capsid. There are three antigenically distinct types of influenza virus—A, B, and C. Type A causes most epidemics and severe illness. It has antigen-altering capability to elude previous humoral immunity. Type B causes a milder disease. Type C is the least significant and of little clinical importance.

▼ **Mode of Transmission.** Influenza is a respiratory virus spread by aerosol and direct contact. A contributing factor to spread is crowding and close contact as occurs in classrooms, barracks, dorms, and nursing homes and on aircraft or ships. The incubation period for influenza is less than 5 days. Viral shedding follows for about 3 to 5 days, with recovery in several days.

▼ **Risks to Mother.** The maternal risks include pneumonia and exacerbation of chronic cardiovascular or other disorders. Additional studies are needed to assess the maternal and fetal risks during pregnancy. Case reports and limited studies suggest that women in the third trimester of pregnancy and early puerperium, including those women without underlying risk factors, might be at increased risk for serious complications following influenza infection (CDC 1996d).

▼ **Risks to Fetus/Neonate.** Symptoms in a newborn may be generalized and indistinguishable from sepsis. Infection in the first trimester has been associated with neural tube defects; influenza-like illness has been associated with cleft lip and palate, limb reduction, neoplasms, and cardiac lesions. There is no convincing evidence that influenza is a teratogen or carcinogen (Gleicher 1992).

▼ **Identification/Diagnosis.** Generalized influenza symptoms include chills, fever, malaise, myalgias, conjunctivitis, and extraocular muscle pain with photophobia, headache, sore throat, brassy nonproductive cough, and scattered pulmonary rales and rhonchi. Complications include bacterial superinfections and problems related to viral dissemination, including primary influenzal pneumonia, myositis, myocarditis, encephalitis, and transplacental infection. Fetal infection occurs with recovery if the mother eliminates the virus. Laboratory identification can be made by viral isolation and serology. Complement fixation and hemagglutination inhibition are the most commonly used serologic methods, requiring acute and convalescent specimens.

▼ **Treatment.** Treatment is symptomatic and includes bed rest, fluids, humidity, cough relief, acetaminophen, and frequent support and reassurance. Amantadine and rimantadine are antiviral replication blocking agents effective for treatment or prophylaxis of type A influenza. They dampen and shorten the clinical course of infection but are embryotoxic and teratogenic in rodents; therefore, they are contraindicated during pregnancy.

▼ **Prevention.** Primary prevention is immunization with inactivated multivalent influenza vaccine before conception. Influenza vaccine is administered intramuscularly in the deltoid muscle of adults and older children and in the anterolateral thigh muscle of infants and young children. Persons known to have anaphylactic hypersensitivity to eggs and persons with acute febrile illnesses should not be vaccinated. Persons who have had no exposure to the influenza virus antigens may experience fever, malaise, myalgia, and other systemic symptoms from the vaccine that begin in 6 to 12 hours and may last 1 or 2 days.

Influenza vaccine can inhibit the clearance of warfarin and theophylline. Influenza vaccine must be given yearly (unlike pneumococcal vaccine, which can be given concomitantly at a different site and should be given only once). October and November is the best time for vaccination campaigns because influenza generally peaks between late December and early March (CDC 1996d, p. 9). Vaccine is year antigen–specific, and the same batch should not be reused the following year. Pregnant women who have other medical conditions that increase their risk for complications from influenza should be vaccinated. The vaccine is considered safe for pregnant women. The vaccine should ideally be given after the first trimester, but it should not be withheld from a pregnant woman who will be in the first trimester when the influenza season begins.

Influenza vaccine is strongly recommended for any person 6 months of age and older who, because of age or underlying medical condition, is at increased risk for complications of influenza. Health care workers and others (including household members) in close contact with high-risk persons should also be vaccinated (CDC 1991b). Unreported studies have indicated that influenza vaccine is no problem and perhaps a benefit for breastfeeding infants, especially those younger than 6 months (Lawrence 1989).

NURSING CONSIDERATIONS

Nursing actions include activities related to prevention, education, assessment, and supportive treatment.

Mumps

Mumps is an acute, generally self-limiting, complication-free, benign infection characterized by parotitis (salivary gland) inflammation. A presenting adult complication may be meningoencephalitis. Mastitis is a rare complication in any mature woman. Adults may be more susceptible because the disease is less contagious than measles or chickenpox. It is more common in the spring. Incidence is related to state immunization laws; 1692 cases were reported in 1993, the lowest number ever and a 99 percent decrease from the 152,209 cases reported in 1968 (CDC 1995b).

▼ **Organism.** Mumps is an RNA virus with a protein core and lipid-containing outer membrane.

▼ **Mode of Transmission.** Mumps is spread by an aerosol droplet respiratory route (saliva). The virus replicates in the respiratory tract and disseminates to regional lymph nodes. Subsequent viremia lasting up to 5 days seeds target organs:

meninges, pancreas, breasts, thyroid, heart, liver, and gonads. The incubation period is 2 to 3 weeks (16 to 18 days).

▼ **Risks to Mother.** Mumps occurs in 0.8 to 10 per 10,000 deliveries. It enters the placental-fetal unit through maternal viremia with seeding. The infection has been associated with increased frequency of spontaneous abortion in the first trimester. The general risk to a woman is unilateral sensorineural deafness, meningitis, pancreatitis, oophoritis, and death.

▼ **Risks to Fetus/Neonate.** There is no significant proof of any fetal anomaly directly related to mumps. Association has been made to the CNS (aqueductal stenosis with hydrocephalus, corneal opacity, chorioretinitis), cardiac abnormalities (endocardial), fibroelastosis, parotitis, and pneumonia.

▼ **Identification/Diagnosis.** Clinical identification is related to history of exposure 2 to 3 weeks before symptoms of fever, unilateral or bilateral enlargement of the parotid glands, CNS deficit (especially eighth cranial nerve, acoustic, vestibulocochlear), or mastitis. There is a potential for meningitis, meningoencephalitis, encephalitis, and residual hearing loss. The virus can be isolated from urine, blood, throat, and cerebrospinal fluid. Fetal diagnosis can be verified by viral isolation and identification of IgM antibodies in cord blood.

▼ **Treatment.** Mumps is treated symptomatically. Respiratory isolation is indicated for the first week after symptoms appear. Maternal counseling is indicated with infection during pregnancy. Infection is not represented as an indication for termination. An exposed or infected mother or infant should be isolated from other patients and infants but not from each other. Lawrence (1989, p. 390) does not present mumps as a major hazard in the newborn nursery: "Should mumps occur, breastfeeding should continue because the exposure has already occurred during the prodromata and the IgA in the breast milk may help to mitigate the symptoms in the infant."

▼ **Prevention.** Since the mid-1970s, a live attenuated vaccine has been available without serious side effects that affords 95 percent long-term protection. It is given as a combined measles-mumps-rubella (MMR) vaccine. The virus can infect the placenta, and therefore the MMR vaccine should not be given during pregnancy. Pregnancy should be avoided for 3 months after MMR vaccination. MMR vaccine can be safely given to the children of pregnant women because viral shedding does not result from immunization (Mandell et al. 1995, p. 1500).

NURSING CONSIDERATIONS

Encourage active participation in education and prevention.

- Subcutaneous injection route to nonpregnant patient
- Appropriate isolation/cohorting

Provide supportive patient care.

Encourage and support breastfeeding.

Measles

Measles (rubeola) is a common, highly communicable, worldwide human infection characterized by a generalized rash and fever. Measles has been documented since the seventh century AD. It occurs primarily in children and is generally more severe when it occurs in adults and newborns. The frequency of occurrence in adults is low because most adults are immune, but adult infection can lead to death from pneumonia or encephalitis. A vaccine has been available since 1963. The number of yearly cases in the United States dropped from 27,786 in 1990 to 301 in 1995 (CDC 1996e).

▼ **Organism.** Measles (rubeola) is caused by a paramyxovirus capable of isolation and growth in chick embryo cells.

▼ **Mode of Transmission.** Rubeola is transmitted by contaminated aerosol droplet infecting the respiratory mucosa. The incubation period is 10 to 14 days, with viremia (including the placenta) followed by symptoms of an upper respiratory infection lasting approximately 8 days. The infection is contagious from 1 to 4 days before coryza to four days after the appearance of the rash.

▼ **Risks to Mother.** The incidence in pregnancy before the availability of immunization was low (6 to 40 per 100,000). Since vaccination has been available, children younger than 5 years represent most measles cases. Infection in pregnancy follows the same course as in nonpregnant women, although epidemiologic study has shown increased mortality related to pneumonia in pregnancy. Abortion, stillbirth, prematurity, and low birth weight have been associated with the infection by some authors.

▼ **Risks to Fetus/Neonate.** Thirty percent of infants born to mothers with infection 7 days before or within 7 days of delivery will become transplacentally infected, with 27 percent mortality from pneumonia and increased occurrence of otitis media. Extrauterine infection (from exposure after birth) occurs by definition 14 days after birth, and its course is usually mild. A premature or low-birth-weight infant presents with factors potentially complicating active infection. All reviewed sources negate an association of infection with specific congenital anomaly.

▼ **Identification/Diagnosis.** A high fever with reddened mucous membranes and conjunctivae including pharyngeal Koplik spots to the buccal mucosa appears before a rash. Inflammatory lesions of the submucosal glands cause a concentrated characteristic maculopapular rash beginning on the face and neck and concentrated at its peak on the face and trunk. Pneumonia manifests as bronchiolitis and interstitial bronchopneumonia.

Rubeola is reportable to the health department. For that purpose, it is defined as fever (temperature above 101°F), with rash for more than 3 days, and cough, coryza, or conjunctivitis (Gleicher 1992). This is clinically diagnostic until proven otherwise.

Serologic tests are used for confirmation of diagnosis. A fourfold rise in antititers or complement fixation between acute serum (within 3 days of rash) and convalescent serum (10 to 20 days later) or IgM-I specific antibody (2 to 3 days after rash) is diagnostic. IgG antibody remains for years to mark immunity.

▼ **Treatment.** No specific treatment is recommended for rubeola. Immune globulin is recommended after known or suspected nonimmune maternal exposure in the hope of modifying fetal disease. It is further recommended that an infant be treated with immune globulin if there is maternal infection the last week of pregnancy or the first week post partum. An infected infant can breastfeed because specific antibodies are present in the milk in 48 hours, which outweighs any other theoretic risk (Lawrence 1989). A clinically uninfected infant and infected mother are isolated separately pending maternal resolution of infectivity or development of symptoms in the neonate.

▼ **Prevention.** A 95 percent effective live attenuated vaccine has been available for subcutaneous administration to nonpregnant individuals since 1963. Pregnancy is not recommended for 3 months after vaccination with MMR or 30 days with monovalent measles vaccine, and its occurrence is reported to the CDC for follow-up. Immune globulin is recommended after exposure (preferably within 72 hours, but up to 7 days) in nonvaccinated, nonimmune women and infants as outlined before.

Vaccine is recommended for children at 12 to 15 months of age. Newborns exposed before that time should be given a modifying dose of immune globulin. Routine vaccination is not recommended for up to 11 months after administration of immune globulin (CDC 1994).

Nurses should be aware of their immune status, if possible. Routine screening for health workers is recommended as a part of preemployment evaluation. Rubeola, rubella, and varicella status should be documented.

NURSING CONSIDERATIONS

Provide education and information on prevention.

- Assist with vaccination programs for women and children.
- Isolate clients with infection as required. If maternal status is positive, isolation is required until the mother is no longer infectious, unless the newborn is infected.

Provide supportive patient care.

Facilitate pediatric follow-up.

Encourage and support breastfeeding with maternal infection and known noninfectious or infected newborns. Unknown or unvaccinated status in an exposed woman within 2 weeks before delivery precludes breastfeeding (and requires isolation from the newborn unless the newborn is infected) until maternal status is definitive. Pediatric infectious disease consultation may be a resource before active breastfeeding is discounted. An infectious mother may be encouraged to pump and discard breast milk until she is noninfectious or until the newborn's status is infectious as well.

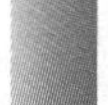

Parvovirus

Human parvovirus (B19, erythema infectiosum, fifth disease, "slapped face disease") was recognized in 1975 and is a common childhood viral infection shown to be associated with increased rates of abortion and stillbirth. Parvovirus has been shown to be the primary etiologic agent of transient aplastic crisis in patients with chronic hemolytic anemias (Gilstrap and Cox 1989; Gleicher 1992; Sever et al. 1989). At-risk groups identified for more severe consequences of parvovirus infection include patients with chronic hemolytic anemias, patients with congenital or acquired immunodeficiencies, and pregnant women as a consequence of fetal effects (Patsner et al. 1990). Parvovirus infection has pregnancy-related consequences and may cause hydrops fetalis and death (Patsner et al. 1990; Sever et al. 1989). Fifty percent of women in an average American city will demonstrate immunity to parvovirus infection (Freeman and Poland 1992). Twenty to twenty-five percent of infections are asymptomatic (Gilstrap and Cox 1989; Gleicher 1992; Patsner et al. 1990). Symmetric peripheral arthritis (hands, wrists, and knees) as a late manifestation that can persist for months occurs in 60 percent of infected adults and 3 percent of infected children (Patsner et al. 1990).

▼ **Organism.** The parvovirus is an autonomous (requires no helper virus), coated, nonenveloped, single-stranded DNA virus that infects humans only.

▼ **Mode of Transmission.** The parvovirus is transmitted by respiratory secretions, by transfusion, and transplacentally. The primary site of replication is the red blood cell precursor in the bone marrow. The incubation period for the parvovirus is 4 to 21 days. The virus is infectious only before the rash unless the infection is related to an aplastic crisis. An aplastic crisis develops approximately 1 week after onset of acute illness, extending the infectious process for approximately 7 days. The normal course is that of a febrile illness of approximately 7 days with reticulocytopenia.

Transmissibility of the virus is 50 to 90 percent among susceptible household contacts, 10 to 60 percent among susceptible school contacts, and 20 to 30 percent among susceptible staff contacts (Gilstrap and Cox 1989). Peak occurrence is in late winter and spring, lasting 2 to 6 months and persisting into the summer months (Gleicher 1992; Patsner et al. 1990).

▼ **Risks to Mother.** Maternal risk is for increased spontaneous abortion in the first half of pregnancy and increased stillbirth in the second half of pregnancy (Patsner et al. 1990; Sever et al. 1989). The risk of fetal death after maternal infection is 3 to 9 percent, with spontaneous abortion occurring 4 to 6 weeks after infection in the first half of pregnancy.

▼ **Risks to Fetus/Neonate.** The parvovirus has a propensity for infecting rapidly dividing cells, particularly erythroblasts, which are the precursors of red blood cells in the fetus. Fetal death occurs as a result of aplastic crisis and nonimmune hydrops. The process is probably a combination of shortened red blood cell life span, increased hematopoiesis, and decreased hepatic function leading to high-output cardiac failure, hypoalbuminemia or hepatitis, edema, and death. The process is related to viremia and is transient. Identification and fetal transfusion in utero may enable an infected fetus to survive (Gleicher 1992; Patsner et al. 1990). Congenital anomalies have not been associated with B19 infection (AAP 1994, p. 346).

▼ **Identification/Diagnosis.** In addition to arthritis and arthralgias, parvovirus infection causes malaise, sore throat, coryza, and a low-grade fever. There may be a characteristic "slapped face" maculopapular rash on the face and a lacelike reticulated rash on the trunk, buttocks, and extensor surfaces of the extremities. The rash can be papular, vesicular, and purpuric and usually lasts less than 10 days (Gleicher 1992; Sever et al. 1992; Sweet and Gibbs 1990). The rash sometimes waxes and wanes for several weeks to months (AAP 1994, p. 345).

Fetal diagnosis is facilitated by determination of maternal alpha-fetoprotein, which is elevated as early as 4 weeks before hydrops. Ultrasonography is also used for diagnosis of fetal damage (Patsner et al. 1990; AAP 1994, p. 347). Parvovirus IgM serum antibodies may be identified after the third day of the rash and decline after 30 to 60 days (Gleicher 1992).

▼ **Treatment.** Maternal treatment is symptomatic. Fetal treatment is maternal serum alpha-fetoprotein determination and intrauterine transfusion if the determination and ultrasound examination indicate impending nonimmune hydrops fetalis.

▼ **Prevention.** The following are recommendations of the American Academy of Pediatrics Committee on Infectious Diseases (AAP 1994, p. 347):

1. Children with erythema infectiosum do not need to be isolated during hospitalization and may attend school or daycare, because they are unlikely to be infectious after the rash appears and the diagnosis is made.
2. Hospitalized children with aplastic crises or immunosuppressed patients with chronic aplastic anemia must receive contact isolation, including use of gowns and gloves for the duration of the illness. Masks should also be worn for close contact. Acute and convalescent sera should be obtained for parvovirus antigen and antibody testing, if available.
3. Pregnant women who subsequently find that they have been in contact with children who are in the incubation period of erythema infectiosum or children who are in aplastic crisis should have the relatively low potential risk explained to them, and the option of having serologic tests performed should be offered if possible. Testing for parvovirus B19 IgM antibody is available for selected patients from the CDC through state health departments and commercial laboratories. Fetal ultrasound examination and alpha-fetoprotein determinations are useful in assessing damage to the fetus.
4. Women who are exposed to children at work (such as teachers or daycare workers) or at home are at increased risk for infection with parvovirus B19. However, because of widespread inapparent infection in both adults and

children, all women are at some risk of exposure, particularly those women with school-age children. In view of the high prevalence of parvovirus B19, the low risk of ill effect to the fetus, and the fact that avoidance of child care or teaching can only reduce but not eliminate the risk for infection, a routine policy of exclusion of pregnant women from the workplace where erythema infectiosum is occurring is not recommended. However, pregnant health care workers should not care for patients with aplastic crises, who may be highly contagious. Eventually, when IgG testing for parvovirus is more widely available, women at increased risk may be able to have their susceptibility determined. (IgG testing is available through commercial laboratories as well as some health department laboratories and research settings.)

5. Transmission of infection can be lessened by routine hygienic practices for control of respiratory secretions, which include hand washing and the disposal of facial tissues containing secretions.
6. Pregnant health care workers without antibodies to B19 should not be assigned to B19-infected patients in aplastic crisis.

NURSING CONSIDERATIONS

Maintain isolation of B19 patients in aplastic crisis.

Provide education.

Provide supportive care.

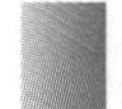

Rubella

Rubella (German measles, 3-day measles) is a mild exanthematous viral infection primarily affecting children. The name German measles probably comes from the early nineteenth century German investigators who differentiated the infection from rubeola and scarlet fever. Historically, before the viral isolation in 1962 and the availability of an effective vaccine in 1968, rubella cycled as a 6- to 9-year epidemic. Twenty thousand infants were infected in the 1964–65 epidemic. Norman Gregg, an ophthalmologist in Sydney, Australia, in 1941 associated maternal rubella infection with increased cataracts in children and defects of the heart, deafness, and other manifestations of congenital rubella syndrome. An estimated 15 to 20 percent of the young adult population in the United States, including women of childbearing age, are not vaccinated or are seronegative after vaccination (5 percent) and susceptible to infection, with subsequent infant mortality and morbidity. In pregnancy, maternal viremia can lead to placental infection with cell destruction and chronic fetal infection, resulting in cellular viral shedding for weeks to years.

The United States, Canada, and a few European countries are examples of the few countries that immunize for rubella. Silent, asymptomatic infection occurs in 25 to 50 percent of infections (AAP 1994, p. 406).

▼ **Organism.** The rubella virus is a small RNA virus. Infected cells produce complement-fixing and hemagglutinating antigens. Isolation of the virus takes 4 to 6 weeks and is available only in a few laboratories in the country.

▼ **Mode of Transmission.** Rubella virus is spread by aerosol droplet through the upper respiratory tract followed by viremia with dissemination. The incubation period is 14 to 21 days, usually 16 to 18 days. The most contagious period is the few days before the rash and up to 5 to 10 days after the rash (AAP 1994, p. 406).

▼ **Risks to Mother.** Rubella, which can be asymptomatic in up to 50 percent of cases, is neither more severe in pregnancy nor a cause of maternal complications in pregnancy. Complications associated with the infection include arthralgia, neuritis, thrombocytopenic purpura, and meningoencephalitis. Placental infection from maternal viremia can lead to spontaneous abortion, stillbirth, congenital defects, or a normal-appearing infant.

▼ **Risks to Fetus/Neonate.** The risk of maternal and subsequent fetal infection or congenital infection is related to trimester of placental infection. Maternal infection the first 8 weeks of gestation carries an approximate 85 percent placental infection rate and 50 percent fetal infection rate. After 8 to 10 weeks, the rates drop to 30 percent placental infection rate and 5 to 10 percent (as high as 25 percent) fetal infection rate. Second-trimester maternal infection is associated with fetal hearing loss and congenital anomalies. An embryo or fetus can be infected with an asymptomatic maternal infection. Not all infected infants have congenital rubella syndrome, but all infected infants shed the rubella virus.

Abnormalities associated with congenital rubella infection can be transient (persist up to 6 months), permanent, or late. Congenital rubella syndrome has permanent sequelae and involves growth restriction and chronic cellular infection. The syndrome includes one or more of the following (Cunningham 1989):

1. Eye lesions, including cataracts, glaucoma, microphthalmia, and various other abnormalities

2. Heart disease, including patent ductus arteriosus, septal defects, and pulmonary artery stenosis
3. Auditory defects
4. CNS defects including meningoencephalitis
5. Restricted fetal growth
6. Thrombocytopenia and anemia
7. Hepatosplenomegaly and jaundice
8. Chronic diffuse interstitial pneumonitis
9. Osseous changes
10. Chromosome abnormalities

Delayed fetal response to infection can manifest in the second to third decade of life and can include endocrinopathies (diabetes, thyroid disease, growth hormone deficiency), sensorineural hearing loss, ocular damage, and vascular abnormalities (sclerosis, hypertension, and panencephalitis) (Burrow and Ferris 1995).

▼ **Identification/Diagnosis.** Maternal identification is based on a history of exposure 2 or 3 weeks before and clinical manifestations (occurring two thirds of the time). Signs include a pink-red maculopapular rash that begins on the face/thorax and extends distally to the extremities. It may coalesce into a red blush and an enanthem of red spots fading centrally before extending to the extremities, lasting close to 3 days. Suboccipital, postauricular, and cervical lymph nodes may enlarge even before the rash appears. A slight fever may occur before or during the rash. Arthralgia occurs more commonly in older women with symptomatic rubella.

Laboratory diagnosis is made by viral isolation and serologic testing. The virus can be isolated from 7 days before to 14 days after rash onset from the oropharynx. It has also been recovered from stool, urine, conjunctiva, blood leukocytes, skin lesions, and cervical secretion. Isolation in the laboratory takes 4 to 6 weeks. Serology includes documentation of IgM and IgG antibodies.

Recent infection is identified by an IgM-specific rubella antibody present about 1 week after onset and persisting for about a month. The presence of IgG-specific antibody with absence of IgM indicates immunity from past illness or effective rubella immunization.

Newborn infection manifests as no symptoms, multiorgan symptoms, or congenital rubella syndrome. The most important predetermining factor is the gestational age at maternal infection. Laboratory confirmation in the newborn is based on the same principle as in the mother. Viral shedding decreases with age, and virus can be isolated from infected infants for months (50 percent from oropharynx at 6 months, 10 percent at 8 months, rarely by 1 year). Other sources are urine and cerebrospinal fluid. Serologic testing for rubella-specific IgM antibody can begin with cord blood. IgM does not cross the placenta. It can be detected for 1 to 6 months. An elevated rubella-specific IgG antibody titer that persists past 6 months and before immunization is also diagnostic of infection.

▼ **Treatment.** The administration of immune globulin after rubella exposure may modify clinical rubella but will not prevent infection or viremia. If a woman chooses to carry her pregnancy after counseling regarding neonatal risk, it is recommended by the American Academy of Pediatrics (AAP 1994) that immune globulin be considered as soon as possible after exposure. It is important to document the infection by viral isolation or serologic testing for appropriate reporting and follow-up.

Symptomatic treatment with a mild analgesic and rest may be recommended to offset fever, malaise, and arthralgia. Women should be seen and handled in a way that minimizes the risk of contact with other susceptible women and children. Symptomatic or exposed neonates are managed with contact isolation, preferably in a private room. The virus should be isolated to document infection. With documentation, the infant should have appropriate follow-up and, without negative cultures, be considered contagious for up to a year.

Breastfeeding is not contraindicated. According to Lawrence (1989, p. 385), "Rubella infection in the mother post partum will be spread to the neonate long before it is identified. If there is breastfeeding, it should be continued. A sick breastfed infant does better when breastfeeding is maintained."

Cases of congenital rubella syndrome or birth defects believed to be caused by rubella infection should be reported to the state health department (Freeman and Poland 1992). Vaccination within 3 months of conception (before or after) should be reported to the state health department or to the CDC.

▼ **Prevention.** A live attenuated vaccine that evokes an antibody response that confers immunity from natural infection for more than 15 years and probably a lifetime has been available since 1968. Indications and recommendations for vaccination include

1. Vaccinate all children 12 to 15 months of age.
   Vaccinate older seronegative or unvaccinated nonpregnant children.
   Vaccinate postpubertal seronegative or unvaccinated nonpregnant women.
   Vaccinate seronegative women after childbirth or abortion.
   Vaccinate all seronegative or unvaccinated personnel who might have contact with pregnant women.

2. Serologically screen all pregnant women for rubella status the first trimester of pregnancy. Rescreen for known exposure or symptoms. Counsel a woman who seroconverts the first trimester regarding potential fetal risk and choice related to pregnancy termination.
3. Protect pregnant women from contact with a potentially infected newborn until rubella status is determined (until negative if infected).

There is no danger to a pregnant woman related to the immunization of another child or individual regardless of her immune status. The vaccine virus is not transmissible (Gleicher 1992; Merkatz and Thompson 1990). Vaccination may be contraindicated with allergy to egg or neomycin because of culture/growth medium. Postponement of vaccination may be considered with recent (within 3 months) administration of immune globulins or antibody blood products. Vaccine can be given to an individual who is also receiving Rh immune globulin post partum. The vaccine may be more effective given 48 to 72 hours post partum because of the influence of falling titers of progesterone. Rubella vaccine can be administered at the same time as other immunizations. No harm can be done vaccinating an immune individual.

Adverse reactions to vaccine include symptoms 7 to 21 days after administration lasting 1 to 3 days. Symptoms may include arthralgia. Transmission has not been demonstrated during this time.

All health care personnel should be aware of rubella status. Neonatal care should be provided only by known rubella-immune staff.

NURSING CONSIDERATIONS

Actively participate in education and prevention.

- Screening, vaccination, isolation
- Subcutaneous vaccination route for nonpregnant women
- Advise no pregnancy for 3 months after immunization (use contraception)

Provide supportive patient care.

Facilitate pediatric follow-up.

Encourage and support breastfeeding mothers.

Varicella-Zoster/Herpes Zoster

Varicella-zoster virus (VZV) causes the primary (no previous infection or antiviral antibodies) infection varicella-zoster (chickenpox) and the secondary (reactivation of latent virus) infection herpes zoster (shingles). Varicella is Latin for tiny spot. Zoster is Greek for belt or girdle. Varicella-zoster or chickenpox is a highly contagious, generally benign, childhood infection. Infection during pregnancy with varicella-zoster has been associated with congenital defects or fetal damage in 2 percent of cases in the first trimester (Benenson 1995, p. 88; AAP 1994, p. 511). Ninety percent of the population has chickenpox by 15 years of age, 95 percent by young adulthood (Russell 1992). Severity is inversely related to incidence, with a 2 per 100,000 mortality in children and a 30 per 100,000 mortality in individuals older than 20 years (Russell 1992). Seventy to 80 percent of women who report a negative history are seropositive for antibody (Merkatz and Thompson 1990; Russell 1992). The antibody correlation with a positive history is high (Gleicher 1992). The incidence of shingles is low, 1.3 per 1000 population with a 10 to 20 percent lifetime risk that increases with age. Half of cases occur past childbearing age (older than 50 years) (Russell 1992).

▼ **Organism.** VZV is a large enveloped herpes family DNA particle. Its only natural host is human. The virus has the ability to remain latent in nerve roots for years. It becomes activated, travels down the nerve, and causes herpes zoster or shingles.

▼ **Mode of Transmission.** Varicella-zoster is transmitted by respiratory secretions and droplets, by contact, by fomites, and transplacentally. After local replication, the virus is disseminated rapidly by viremia. The incubation period is 10 to 20 days. Varicella is contagious from about 1 to 2 days before rash until the lesions scab and crust (5 days) (Benenson 1995, p. 89). Antibody formation begins on the fourth day after skin lesions appear and infection subsides. Transplacental transmission is congenital in early pregnancy and infective within 3 weeks of delivery (Burrow and Ferris 1995). The virus invades sensory nerves and ganglia and becomes latent. Reactivation, which may occur years later, causes a less contagious secondary infection, herpes zoster or shingles. Herpes zoster is not communicable per se; VZV is infectious, so a person susceptible to chickenpox can be exposed to chickenpox from a person who has shingles. However, the virus is not as easily transmitted from a person with shingles as it is from a person with chickenpox. Transmission of herpes zoster is by contact with the vesicular fluid of the lesion. The lesions are infective for a week after they appear or until dry and crusted (Russell 1992).

▼ **Risks to Mother.** A varicella-zoster infection in pregnancy is rare but may be severe. Incidence is estimated at 0.01 to 0.7 per 1000 to 1 to 5 per 10,000 pregnancies. (Incidence of herpes zoster is less, 0.5 per 10,000 pregnancies*) (Burrow and Ferris 1995; Russell 1992). As stated, adults in general have increased morbidity and mortality related to a varicella-zoster infection. The consequences and course of the infection in pregnancy are similar to those in the general population; however, varicella pneumonia, especially in the third trimester, is more severe with increased mortality (Gleicher 1992).

▼ **Risks to Fetus/Neonate.** Infection during pregnancy may lead to

1. Intrauterine infection, very rarely leading to congenital anomalies (congenital varicella syndrome)
2. Postnatal newborn disease (varicella of the newborn), ranging from varicella with a benign course to fatal disseminated infection
3. Zoster (shingles) appearing months or years later (Burrow and Ferris 1995; Merkatz and Thompson 1990)

A perinatal infection is acquired transplacentally or postnatally. The infection is congenital if it occurs within 10 days of delivery. The greatest risk for congenital infection associated with malformations, congenital varicella syndrome, occurs in the first half of pregnancy. Maternal infection 5 to 21 days before delivery may result in newborn infection. A rash develops, and the course is generally mild (Sever et al. 1989). The neonate at greatest risk from infection is the neonate exposed to a maternal rash 4 days before or 2 days after delivery. This neonate will be exposed to maternal viremia without benefit of maternal antibody cushion. Infectivity rate is 20 to 50 percent with 20 to 30 percent mortality (Freeman and Poland 1992; Gleicher 1992; Prober et al. 1990; Sever et al. 1989). If maternal rash occurs 3 days or more after delivery, newborn infection will be from respiratory rather than blood-borne transmission, and the infection may be less severe because of the chance of a smaller systemic inoculum (Prober et al. 1990). Postnatally acquired infection carries a slightly higher case fatality than does infection in an older child and should be avoided (Russell 1992).

Congenital varicella syndrome is associated with low birth weight, failure to thrive, and repeated infections as well as the following: scarred skin lesions in dermatome distribution, CNS effects (seizures, paralysis, mental retardation), limb deformity (hypoplasia of one or more extremities and malformed digits), muscle atrophy, clubfeet, microphthalmia, chorioretinitis, cataracts, and nystagmus.

*Cases of varicella-zoster (chickenpox) in the United States per year are approximately 3.5 million. Cases of herpes zoster infections per year in the United States are estimated at a half-million (Mandell et al. 1995).

▼ **Identification/Diagnosis.** Varicella-zoster has a 2- to 3-day prodrome with systemic symptoms including fever, chills, myalgia, and arthralgia. The prodrome is followed by malaise and a rash that progresses from macule to papule to discrete pruritic vesicles beginning on the head and neck and progressing to the trunk and extremities. New lesions appear for 3 to 5 days. Lesions scab in 3 to 4 days. Pneumonia is the most common secondary infection in adults (15 percent). Symptoms of pneumonia include a nonproductive cough, dyspnea, fever, and pleuritic chest pain 1 to 6 days after varicella-zoster rash.

Common secondary infections in children are encephalitis and Reye syndrome (Russell 1992). Herpes zoster lesions involve one sensory ganglion with pain, paresthesia, and moderate to severe neuralgia. Lesions are localized, grouped vesicles in a pattern over one to three dermatomes (thoracic and lumbar most common). The lesions erupt from an erythematous base and become pustular by 3 to 4 days. Crusts are formed by 7 to 10 days with resolution in 2 to 3 weeks (Gleicher 1992; Russell 1992). The pain and neuralgia may persist for weeks to months but have been known to persist as long as 15 to 20 years in older adults (Gleicher 1992; Russell 1992).

Diagnosis is generally by history and symptoms. Laboratory diagnosis is by virus isolation and serology. Vesicular fluid viral analysis is submitted the first 3 to 4 days of the rash. Results may be expected in 3 to 14 days. Serologic antibody markers (IgG, IgM, IgA) are detectable within 5 days of rash onset (Russell 1992; Sever et al. 1989).

▼ **Treatment.** No therapy for VZV infection is definitive (Merkatz and Thompson 1990). Passive immunity is expected to modify the severity of VZV infection. If a pregnant woman has a negative history of prior infection and is exposed to VZV, she should be tested for immunity (antibody status). If she is not immune or testing is not available within 96 hours, she should be given varicella-zoster immune globulin (VZIG) within 5 days of exposure. If the onset of clinical maternal infection occurs within 4 to 5 days before delivery or 2 days after delivery (before maternal antibody response), VZIG should be given to the neonate within 72 hours of delivery (Freeman and Poland 1992; Merkatz and Thompson 1990; Prober et al. 1990; Sever et al. 1989). The value of VZIG remains to be established, but it is believed to have an ameliorative effect on the severity of the infection (Freeman and Poland 1992; Merkatz and

Thompson 1990). VZIG is also recommended for premature infants (less than 28 weeks) postnatally exposed to VZV because of poor placental antibody transfer early in gestation; it should be considered on an individual basis in the immunocompromised infant (Freeman and Poland 1992; Prober et al. 1990). VZIG is available through the American Red Cross Blood Services.

Pregnancy termination is not recommended because the risk for congenital varicella syndrome is small. Tocolysis may be used to delay labor and delivery of an infected mother to allow time for antibody production and transfer (Russell 1992). A newborn and mother may be together after the administration of VZIG, if indicated (Freeman and Poland 1992). Antibodies appear in breast milk within 48 hours of disease onset, making it theoretically appropriate for breastfeeding as soon as it is appropriate for the mother and newborn to be together (Lawrence 1989).

▼ **Prevention.** A vaccine is now available.* Passive immunization was licensed in the United States in 1981. VZIG has not prevented transmission in utero, but it is thought to be 50 percent effective in preventing or modifying VZV infection (MacLean 1990; Russell 1992). VZIG is prepared from plasma of healthy screened (for HBV and HIV) donors with high VZV antibody titers. In addition to Standard Precautions in routine care, contact and respiratory isolation are indicated with active infectivity (Sever et al. 1989). Isolation of women with VZV infection is recommended because of the highly contagious nature of the virus. (Freeman and Poland 1992). Neonates with congenital VZV infection from early in gestation do not need special management. Neonates exposed late in utero or postnatally to VZV should be isolated and managed expectantly during the incubation period. Neonates with VZV infection should be isolated in a private room until they are no longer infective (Freeman and Poland 1992).

Pregnant health care workers should not be assigned to infectious cases. Using cohort care and assigning the same staff each day as much as possible will minimize the spreading infection.

NURSING CONSIDERATIONS

Participate in education and prevention.

- Provide information, maintain precautions including isolation as appropriate.
- Provide counseling with appropriate current information.

Provide supportive care.

Involve pediatric infectious disease service, infection control nurse; facilitate pediatric follow-up.

Encourage and support active breastfeeding as soon as it is appropriate for mother and neonate to be together. Support pumping and discarding milk until that time.

*Recommendations for immunization were scheduled for release in the summer of 1996. AAP Advisory Committee Draft Recommendations were issued in 1995.

OTHER INFECTIONS

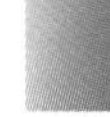

Candidiasis

▼ **Organism.** Candidiasis is a yeast infection of the genital tract (vulvovaginal candidiasis) generally caused by *Candida albicans.* It is one of the three most common types of vaginitis seen during pregnancy. *Candida* is a widely spread microorganism located in the oropharynx, gut, vagina, and skin. The organism can be cultured in 30 to 50 percent of all pregnant women. The increased frequency (10 to 20 times more common during pregnancy) of this infection is attributed to the high levels of estrogen and progesterone, which provide a higher glycogen content in the vagina and thus feed the yeast in abundance. The organism thrives in a warm, acid environment. The yeast is normally occurring in some women and is not pathogenic. The reason for this is not clearly understood.

▼ **Risks to Mother.** Predisposing factors to the increased occurrence of candidiasis during pregnancy include the following: high levels of glycogen in the vagina promoting growth of the organism; use of the oral contraceptive pill; use of broad-spectrum antibiotic therapy; diabetes mellitus; use of corticosteroids; use of immunosuppressive drugs; and HIV infection. Risks to the mother also include vaginitis/pruritus of perineum and vagina.

▼ **Risks to Fetus/Neonate.** Severe cases of candidal chorioamnionitis have been documented (Gleicher 1992). Severe systemic infection with the yeast has been seen, as has intrauterine fetal death. Predisposing factors include the use of an intrauterine device prior to pregnancy, which functions as a "ladder" (ladder for vaginal *Candida* organisms to reach the uterine lining and later infect the placenta and fetus) and premature rupture of membranes. Infection in the first trimester may result in abortion. Neonatal thrush is a complication of vaginal delivery through an infected birth canal.

Signs/Symptoms. Candidiasis may remain asymptomatic in some pregnant women. Women develop a vulval irritation with itching and vaginal discharge. Discharge can be scant or profuse in amount and white in color. There may be a "cottage cheese" appearance to the discharge. The vagina may be coated with a curdlike white substance that adheres to the vaginal mucosa (thrushlike).

Candidiasis is seen more frequently in conditions of elevated blood glucose levels and in cases of decreased cellular immunity, both of which occur during pregnancy. The normal flora of lactobacilli and corynebacteria that inhabit the vagina is altered in pregnancy because of fluctuations in estrogen and progesterone.

Identification/Diagnosis. Immediate diagnosis can be made on the basis of a smear from the vagina on a microscope slide. The slide is fixed with a 10 percent potassium hydroxide solution that displays oval, budding cells with elongated filamented pseudohyphae (mycelia). The organism can be cultured on Nickerson medium for confirmation.

Treatment. Antifungal therapy is suggested for all cases. Local application of an antifungal agent is prescribed. A variety of preparations are available over the counter. These preparations are safe to use during pregnancy. The antifungal may be prepared as a cream or a vaginal suppository, and 7-day therapy is preferred. Preparations containing imidazoles have been proved more effective than the traditional nystatin preparation for candidiasis. The drug butoconazole may be even more effective in that it has a proven cure rate after 3 days of therapy, compared with 7 days for the other therapeutic agents (Wang and Smaill 1989).

Vulvovaginal candidiasis is not acquired through sexual intercourse; treatment of sex partners has not been demonstrated to reduce the frequency of recurrences. Therefore, routine notification or treatment of sex partners is not warranted. A minority of male sex partners may have balanitis, which is characterized by erythematous areas on the glans in conjunction with pruritus or irritation. These partners may benefit from treatment with topical antifungal agents to relieve symptoms (CDC 1993, p. 74).

Prevention. Avoidance of constrictive or poorly ventilated underclothing is recommended, as is avoidance of nylon, nonbreathable material (pantyhose) for underclothing. Prevention of sequelae and neonatal sepsis is related to detection and treatment of maternal infection.

NURSING CONSIDERATIONS

Observe client for symptoms of the disease.

Educate client concerning prevention of the disease and good perineal hygiene.

Provide dietary counseling of clients concerning yogurt products containing active cultures of lactobacilli as a palliative and possibly curative therapy (eating it or using it as a douche).

Educate client concerning medication regimen and compliance.

Educate client concerning the use of vaginal suppositories or creams for the duration of treatment (usually 7 days).

Educate client concerning avoidance of douching and use of vaginal perfumes, deodorant sprays, or perfumed lubricants.

Provide psychological support.

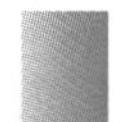

Bacterial Vaginosis (*Gardnerella* Vaginosis)

Organism. Bacterial vaginosis (BV) was previously known as nonspecific vaginitis or *Gardnerella* vaginitis. The disease is characterized by a replacement of the normal flora (lactobacilli) of the vagina with other bacteria, especially with the gram-negative coccobacilli known as *Gardnerella vaginalis* (formerly *Haemophilus vaginalis*). BV can be sexually transmitted or occur normally within the vagina of some women (carriers). The name was changed because the disease is neither inflammatory nor nonspecific in nature.

Risks. BV has been associated with increasing virulence as gestation progresses. BV is more troublesome in the second and third trimesters. There has been an association between BV and premature rupture of membranes and premature labor (Gleicher 1992; Merkatz and Thompson 1990). The organism *G. vaginalis* has been demonstrated in these findings. Postpartum fever, salpingitis, and endometritis are associated with BV (Mandell et al. 1995, p. 1080).

Signs/Symptoms. *G. vaginalis* is seen as the marker for the overgrowth of many different anaerobic bacteria. BV is not categorized as an actual infection (Gleicher 1992). There are often no clinical signs of an infection, merely the replacement of lactobacilli with many different types of anaerobic bacteria. Estimates of the prevalence of *G. vaginalis* during pregnancy vary from 32 to 44 percent of pregnant women experiencing symptomatic vaginal disease (Gleicher 1992).

▼ **Identification/Diagnosis.** The diagnosis of BV is based on clinical findings and culture of the organism. The clinical symptoms include a fishy odor to the vaginal secretions, clue cells seen on a wet prepared microscope slide, and a vaginal pH greater than 4.5. The "positive whiff test" occurs when a small drop of 10 percent potassium hydroxide is added to the vaginal secretions and a characteristic "fishy" odor is released.

▼ **Treatment.** Treatment of BV consists of a course of metronidazole. The reestablishment of normal vaginal flora (lactobacilli) is also instrumental in effecting a cure for BV. The use of metronidazole during pregnancy remains controversial. Many experts recommend treatment with the drug because the risk for BV-associated prematurity outweighs the potential risk for teratogenic effects during the last two trimesters of pregnancy (Gleicher 1992). Alternative therapy is clindamycin (CDC 1993).

Some health care providers remain concerned about the possibility of metronidazole mutagenecity, which has been suggested by experiments on animals using extremely high and prolonged doses. However, there is no evidence for mutagenecity in humans. Some health care providers prefer the intravaginal route because of lack of systemic side effects, such as mild to moderate gastrointestinal upset and unpleasant taste (mean peak serum concentrations of metronidazole after intravaginal administration are less than 2 percent of those of standard 500-mg oral doses, and mean bioavailability of clindamycin cream is about 4 percent) (CDC 1995a, p. 69).

▼ **Prevention.** Prevention of BV during pregnancy is difficult, since the organism may be normal vaginal flora. The use of condoms is encouraged for protection and prevention.

NURSING CONSIDERATIONS

Treat all partners simultaneously.

Teach client re:

- Avoidance of sexual intimacy until after treatment is completed
- Avoidance of alcohol ingestion while taking metronidazole (reacts with cramping, flushing, vomiting, and tremors)

Observe women with premature rupture of membranes, prolonged rupture of membranes, and a high number of vaginal examinations during labor for signs and symptoms of chorioamnionitis.

Assist with the assessment and identification of organism.

Educate client concerning the disease, its risks, and its mode of transmission.

Provide psychological support.

Urinary Tract Infections

Urinary tract infections are one of the most common medical complications of pregnancy. These infections can cause considerable problems for both mother and fetus if they are not detected and managed properly. Three patterns of infection are seen during pregnancy: asymptomatic bacteriuria, acute symptomatic cystitis, and acute pyelonephritis. It is estimated that 2 to 10 percent of pregnant women harbor significant colonizations of bacteria in their urine without showing any symptoms (Sever et al. 1989). Only half of these women will develop symptomatic urinary tract infections (Wang and Smaill 1989).

▼ **Risks to Mother.** Pyelonephritis can progress to endotoxic shock, acute renal failure, pulmonary disorders, and bleeding disorders. The disease is serious and can have long-term sequelae. The recurrence rate is 20 percent among pregnant patients.

▼ **Risks to Fetus/Neonate.** Neonatal effects of pyelonephritis include prematurity, a small-for-gestational-age neonate, and sepsis. Low birth weight and premature rupture of membranes have also been associated with maternal urinary tract infections (Burrow and Ferris 1995). Infection during pregnancy has been linked to possibly causing defects of dorsal midline fusion in the fetus (Sever et al. 1989).

▼ **Signs/Symptoms.** Urinary tract infections are more common during pregnancy because of the lack of muscle tone in the urethra, bladder, and ureters due to progesterone. The cardinal symptoms of acute cystitis are urinary frequency, dysuria, and suprapubic discomfort. Pyelonephritis presents with fever and chills, flank pain (costovertebral angle tenderness), dysuria, and a positive urine culture. Infected persons are hospitalized for intravenous antibiotic therapy (ampicillin or an aminoglycoside). *Escherichia coli* is the most common pathogen found on culture (90 percent). Increasingly, group B streptococcus is found, along with *Klebsiella* and *Enterobacter* organisms.

▼ **Identification/Diagnosis.** Screening for infection is done with a clean-catch urine sample. Colony counts are observed microscopically (100 to 1000 colony-forming units per milliliter) and cultured for pathogen identification. Care must be taken to minimize contamination of the specimen. Microscopic analysis of clean-catch spun urine is often used as a rapid detection screening alternative and can be done in the office or at the bedside. Catheterization is not recommended for diagnostic purposes because of the great possibility of ascending contamination.

▼ **Treatment.** Single-dose antibiotic therapy has proved effective in nonpregnant women and has obvious advantages in terms of compliance, low cost, and minimal side effects. Trials suggest that this therapy should be afforded during pregnancy, but longer term antibiotic treatment is preferred. Traditional treatment remains a choice of sulfonamides, nitrofurantoin, ampicillin, or a cephalosporin prescription for 7 to 14 days. Sulfonamides are avoided during the last half of pregnancy (after age of viability) because of binding sites for bilirubin, thus predisposing the neonate to kernicterus.

If the bacteriuria progresses to pyelonephritis (30 percent of asymptomatic cases and 1 to 2 percent of all pregnant women), antibiotic therapy with second- and third-generation cephalosporins is recommended. Pyelonephritis and symptomatic cystitis occur most frequently during the second trimester.

▼ **Prevention.** All pregnant women should be screened for bacteriuria at initial visits by culture and colony count from a clean-catch urine specimen. A series of cultures (one each trimester) is highly recommended by some experts (Gleicher 1988; Sever et al. 1989).

NURSING CONSIDERATIONS

Instruct client concerning how to obtain a clean-catch urine sample.

Instruct client about proper fluid intake (8 glasses of water per day, cranberry juice).

Instruct client about medication administration and compliance.

Observation for signs and symptoms of infection in all patients, with special attention to those with sickle cell anemia (routine culture each month because of the high frequency of urinary tract infections), those with diabetes, and those with complaints of suprapubic discomfort/cramping.

Obtain medical history from client of previous urinary tract infections, symptomatic or asymptomatic; this is a predisposing factor during pregnancy.

Repeat clean-catch urinalysis within 4 days of completion of antibiotic therapy for cure or recurrence.

Repeat clean-catch urinalysis every 4 to 6 weeks until delivery, then post partum on day 3 and 6 weeks for recurrence.

Educate client regarding avoidance of douching, vaginal deodorants, bubble bath, perfumed lubricant preparations.

Educate client regarding the necessity of frequent urination during pregnancy (every 2 hours).

Teach client to:

- Avoid bladder irritants such as caffeine, alcohol, and carbonated beverages
- Use good perineal hygiene (front to back)
- Urinate before and after intercourse
- Wear cotton underwear, avoid pantyhose

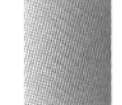

Scabies/Lice

Scabies *(Sarcoptes scabiei)* and lice are transmissible parasitic skin infections characterized by superficial burrows, intense itching, and secondary infection. Infestation by lice may involve the head *(Pediculus humanus capitis),* body *(Pediculus humanus corporis),* or genital area *(Phthirus pubis).* Infestations are widespread in conditions of overcrowding, inadequate personal hygiene, or inability to clean clothing. The prevalence rate varies between 6 and 27 percent (Gleicher 1992).

SCABIES

Scabies is caused by the itch mite *Sarcoptes scabiei,* an obligate parasite in humans. The parasite is a white, translucent, eyeless mite with eight legs. The male remains on the surface of the skin. The pregnant female mite tunnels under the superficial skin layer of the human host and deposits her eggs along a line (burrow). The eggs hatch within a few days and congregate around hair follicles. Within 2 weeks, the larvae mature into adults and start the process of mating (tunneling) once again. The mites can survive up to 2 days away from the skin. The itching results from hypersensitivity to the parasites. Scabies is transmitted readily by skin-to-skin contact. Is is also acquired through sexual intimacy.

The mite causes intense itching. The most severe pruritus occurs at night. Likely sites for infestation are the finger webs, elbows, wrists, and axillary folds; along the belt line; the lower buttocks; and the genital area. The face may be involved in infants.

Diagnosis is confirmed by scrapings from a site, fixed with any clear solution, that demonstrate the parasite.

Treatment with lindane (gamma benzene hexachloride) is contraindicated in pregnancy and lactation. Crotamiton lotion or permethrin 1 percent cream rinse is used during pregnancy (CDC 1993, p. 96).

LICE

Lice are wingless, flat parasites with three pairs of legs and claws. The adults anchor themselves onto the skin with their mouth and live off the blood of the host. The head louse and crab (pubic) louse live directly on the host; the body louse can live in clothing. These parasites are transmitted by personal contact or sexual intimacy. Head lice can be acquired through sharing objects such as combs and hats. The infestation is predominantly located on the scalp but can involve the eyebrows, eyelashes, and beard. Diagnosis involves inspection of the scalp with nits seen fixed on the hair shafts that cannot be dislodged. Body lice are uncommon under good hygienic conditions. Nits can be found on the body hairs, in underclothing, and in the seams of clothing. Crab lice infest the anogenital hairs. Itching occurs in the anogenital region. Parasites can be demonstrated on close observation.

Treatment for nonpregnant and nonlactating women is application of 1 percent gamma benzene hexachloride (lindane, Kwell) applied as a shampoo, cream, or lotion. Application is repeated in 10 days to destroy nits. All sources of transmission such as combs, hats, clothing, and bedding should be decontaminated by boiling, thorough laundering, or dry cleaning; washing or drying at a temperature higher than 131°F (55°C) for 20 minutes is sufficient to destroy lice (Berenson 1994, p. 346). If articles are difficult to clean, storage for 2 weeks will ensure no living lice or eggs. For pubic lice, all sexual contacts should be treated.

Pregnancy does not have any effect on the infestation of lice or scabies or its manifestations. The major concern about scabies and lice in pregnancy is the potential toxic effect of the therapeutic agents on the fetus. Many experts recommend refraining from use during pregnancy. Therapeutic agents have not been shown to be teratogenic, but there are documented cases of CNS toxic effects. Alternative choices for use during pregnancy include 10 percent crotamiton cream or lotion (Eurax) applied from the neck down every 24 hours for two to three applications or 6 percent sulfur precipitate in petroleum nightly for 3 nights (Gleicher 1992). The CDC recommends that lindane not be used in pregnant or lactating women.

Alternative treatment for lice includes the over-the-counter preparation of 0.3 percent pyrethrins and 3 percent piperonyl butoxide (RID) applied to affected areas for 10 minutes. This treatment should be repeated in 10 days.

It is essential to find and treat all sexual partners. Also, knowledge of the contraindicated medications for use on lice/scabies during pregnancy and lactation is critical.

NURSING CONSIDERATIONS

Assess for the presence of parasites from observation/clinical signs.

Educate client about

- how to kill the parasites
- medication treatment
- laundering of clothing and bedding; dry cleaning or storage of articles for 2 weeks to rid the material of lice/nits
- the necessity of reapplication of the treatment in 10 days

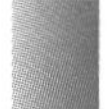

References

American Academy of Pediatrics. (1994). *1994 Red Book: Report of the Committee on Infectious Diseases* (23rd ed.). Elk Grove Village, IL: American Academy of Pediatrics.

American College of Obstetricians and Gynecologists. (1985). *Gonorrhea and chlamydial infections* (Technical Bulletin 89). Washington, DC: Author.

American College of Obstetricians and Gynecologists. (1987). *Genital human papillomavirus infections* (Technical Bulletin 105). Washington, DC: Author.

American College of Obstetricians and Gynecologists. (1988a). Editorial: Management of genital herpes infection in pregnancy. *Obstetrics and Gynecology,* 71 (5), 779–780.

American College of Obstetricians and Gynecologists. (1988d). *Perinatal herpes simplex virus infections* (Technical Bulletin 122). Washington, DC: Author.

Andrist, L. (1988). Sexual history taking and safer sex education. *Nursing Clinics of North America,* 23(4), 959–973.

Baker, D. A. (1990). Viral diseases in pregnancy. *Clinical Obstetrics and Gynecology,* 33 (2).

Benenson, A. S. (Ed.). (1995). *Control of communicable diseases manual* (16th ed.). Washington, DC: American Public Health Association.

Brown, Z., and Baker, D. (1989). Review: Acyclovir therapy during pregnancy. *Obstetrics and Gynecology,* 73 (3, pt 2), 526–531.

Burrow, G. N., and Ferris, T. F. (Eds.). (1995). *Medical complications during pregnancy* (4th ed.). Philadelphia: W. B. Saunders.

Centers for Disease Control. (1988). Prevention of perinatal transmission of hepatitis B virus: Prenatal screening of all women for hepatitis B surface antigen. *Morbidity and Mortality Weekly Report,* 37 (22).

Centers for Disease Control. (1989). Sexually transmitted diseases treatment guidelines. *Morbidity and Mortality Weekly Report,* 38 (8 Suppl.).

Centers for Disease Control. (1990a). Protection against viral hepatitis: Recommendations of the Immunization Practices Advisory Committee. *Morbidity and Mortality Weekly Report,* 39 (S-2).

Centers for Disease Control. (1990b). Rubella prevention: Recommendations of the Immunization Practices Advisory Committee. *Morbidity and Mortality Weekly Report,* 39 (RR-15), 1–18.

Centers for Disease Control. (1991a). Hepatitis B virus: A comprehensive strategy for eliminating transmission in the United States through universal childhood vaccination: Recommendations of the Immunization Practices Advisory Committee. *Morbidity and Mortality Weekly Report,* 40 (RR-13).

Centers for Disease Control. (1991b). Prevention and control of influenza: Recommendations of the Immunization Practices Advisory Committee. *Morbidity and Mortality Weekly Report,* 40 (RR-6).

Centers for Disease Control. (1991c). Recommendations for preventing transmission of HIV and hepatitis B virus to patients during exposure-prone invasive procedures. *Morbidity and Mortality Weekly Report,* 40 (RR-8).

Centers for Disease Control. (1992a). Current trends: Update: Serologic testing for human T-lymphotropic virus type I—United States, 1989 and 1990. *Morbidity and Mortality Weekly Report,* 41 (15).

Centers for Disease Control. (1992b). Measles surveillance—United States, 1991. *Morbidity and Mortality Weekly Report,* 41 (SS-6).

Centers for Disease Control. (1993). Sexually transmitted diseases treatment guidelines, 1993. *Morbidity and Mortality Weekly Report,* 42 (RR-14).

Centers for Disease Control. (1994). Rubella prevention: Recommendations of the Immunization Practices Advisory Committee. *Morbidity and Mortality Weekly Report,*

Centers for Disease Control, Division of STD Prevention. (1995a). *Sexually transmitted disease surveillance, 1994.* U.S. Department of Health and Human Services, Public Health Service. Atlanta: Centers for Disease Control and Prevention.

Centers for Disease Control (1995b). Recommendations for Test Performance and Interpretation from the Second National Conference on Serologic diagnosis of Lyme Disease. *Morbidity and Mortality Weekly Report,* 44 (31), 590.

Centers for Disease Control. (1995c). Mumps surveillance—United States, 1988–1993. *Morbidity and Mortality Weekly Report,* 44 (SS-3).

Centers for Disease Control. (1995d). U.S. Public Health Service recommendations for human immunodeficiency virus counseling and voluntary testing for pregnant women. *Morbidity and Mortality Weekly Report,* 44 (RR-7).

Centers for Disease Control. (1996a). Prevention of perinatal group B streptococcal disease: A public health perspective. *Morbidity and Mortality Weekly Report,* 45 (RR-7).

Centers for Disease Control. (1996b). Tuberculosis morbidity—United States, 1995. *Morbidity and Mortality Weekly Report,* 45 (18).

Centers for Disease Control. (1996c). The role of BCG vaccine in the prevention and control of tuberculosis in the United States. *Morbidity and Mortality Weekly Report,* 45 (RR-4).

Centers for Disease Control. (1996d). Prevention and control of influenza: Recommendations of the Advisory Committee on Immunization Practices. *Morbidity and Mortality Weekly Report,* 45(RR-5).

Centers for Disease Control. (1996e). Measles—United States, 1995. *Morbidity and Mortality Weekly Report,* 45 (15).

Connor, E., Sperling, R., Gelber, R., Kiselev, P., et al. (1994). Reduction of maternal-infant transmission of human immunodeficiency virus type 1 with zidovudine treatment. *New England Journal of Medicine* 331 (18), 1173–1180.

Cotton, D., and Watts H. Management of HIV infection during pregnancy: new options, new questions. *AIDS Clinical Care* 7(6), 45–49.

Crane, M. J. (1992). The diagnosis and management of maternal and congenital syphilis. *Journal of Nurse-Midwifery*, 37 (1), 4–15.

Cunningham, F. G., MacDonald, P., Gant, N., Leveno, K., Gilstrap, L. (1993). *Williams obstetrics* (19th ed.). East Norwalk, CT: Appleton & Lange.

Deneberg, R. (1995). Pregnancy and HIV. *Treatment Issues* 5(6), 6–10.

Faix, R. (1991). Maternal immunization to prevent fetal and neonatal infection. *Clinical Obstetrics and Gynecology,* 34 (2), 277–287.

Falloon, J., Eddy, J., Wiener, L., Pizzo, P. A. (1989). Human immunodeficiency virus infection in children. *Journal of Pediatrics,* 114 (1), 1–23.

Fekety, S. (1989). Managing the HIV-positive patient and her newborn in a CNM service. *Journal of Nurse-Midwifery,* 34 (5) 253–257.

Ferri R. (1996). Roadblocks seen in preventing vertical transmission. *Clinician Reviews,* 6 (7), 122–126.

Fletcher, J. L. (1991). Perinatal transmission of HPV. *American Journal of Family Practice,* 43 (1), 143–148.

Freeman, R. K., and Poland, R. L. (1992). *Guidelines for perinatal care* (3rd ed., pp. 117–140). Washington, DC: American Academy of Pediatrics/American College of Obstetricians and Gynecologists.

Gibbs, R. S., Amstey, M. S., Sweet, R. L., Mead, P. B., Sever, J. L. (Infectious Disease Society for OB/GYN). (1988). Editorial: Management of genital herpes infection in pregnancy. *Obstetrics and Gynecology,* 71 (5), 779–780.

Gilstrap, L., and Cox, S. (1989). Acute amnionitis. *Obstetrics and Gynecology Clinics of North America,* 16 (2), 373–379.

Gleicher, N. (ed.). (1992). *Principles and practice of medical therapy in pregnancy* (2nd ed.). New York: Appleton & Lange.

Gliden, D. (1996). The viral burden of motherhood. *Treatment Issues,* 10 (4), 5–6.

Grubman, R. (1995) Pediatric treatment update. *Treatment Issues,* 10 (3), 7–9.

Hammill, H. A., and Gilstrap, L. C. (Eds.). (1990). *Infections in pregnancy.* New York: Alan R. Liss.

Hocke, C., Morlat, P., Chene, G., Dequae, L., et al. Prospective cohort study of the effect of pregnancy on the progression of human immunodeficiency virus infection. *Obstetrics and Gynecology,* 86 (6), 886–891.

Kircher, S. M., Meyer, M. P., Jordan, J. A. (1996). Comparison of a modified DNA hybridization assay with standard culture enrichment for detecting group B streptococci in obstetric patients. *Journal of Clinical Microbiology,* 33 (2), 258–267.

Kuhn, L., and Stein, Z. A. (1995). Mother to infant HIV transmission: timing, risk factors and prevention. *Paediatric Perinatal Epidemiology,* 9 (1), 1–29.

Lawrence, R. A. (1989). *Breastfeeding: A guide for health care professionals* (3rd ed.). St. Louis: C. V. Mosby.

Lederman, S. A. (1992). From the Center for Population and Family Health, School of Public Health and Institute for Human Nutrition. Estimating infant mortality from HIV and other causes in breast-feeding and bottle-feeding populations. *Pediatrics.*

Lee, M. (1988). Infections and prematurity: Is there a relationship? *Journal of Perinatal and Neonatal Nursing,* 2 (1), 10–20.

Lester, P., Partridge, J. C., Chesney, M.A., Cooke, M. (1995). The consequences of a positive prenatal HIV antibody test for women. *Journal of Acquired Immune Deficiency Syndrome Human Retrovirology,* 10 (3), 341–349.

Lindsay M., Peterson, H., Willis S., Slade, B. (1991). Incidence and prevalence of human immunodeficiency virus infection in a prenatal population undergoing routine voluntary human immunodeficiency virus screening, July 1987–June 1990. Part 1. *American Journal of Obstetrics and Gynecology,* 165(4) 961–964.

Lynch-Salamon, D. I., and Combs, C. A. (1992). Hepatitis C in obstetrics and gynecology. *Obstetrics and Gynecology,* 79 (4), 621–629.

Maccato, M. (1989). Pneumonia and pulmonary tuberculosis in pregnancy. *Obstetric and Gynecology Clinics of North America,* 16 (2), 417–430.

MacLean, A. B. (Ed.). (1990). *Clinical infection in obstetrics and gynecology.* Cambridge: Blackwell Scientific Publications.

Mandell, G. L., Bennett, J. E., Dolin, R. (1995). *Mandell, Douglas and Bennett's principles and practice of infectious diseases* (4th ed.). New York: Churchill Livingstone.

Mauri, A., Piccione, E., Deiana, P., Volpe, A. (1995). Obstetric and perinatal outcome in human immunodeficiency virus–infected pregnant women with and without opiate addiction.

European Journal of Obstetrics, Gynecology, and Reproductive Biology, 58 (2) 135–140.

Merkatz, I. R., and Thompson, J. E. (Eds.). (1990). *New perspectives on prenatal care.* New York: Elsevier Science Publishing.

Minkoff, H. (1991). Preventing fetal damage from sexually transmitted diseases. *Clinical Obstetrics and Gynecology,* 34 (2), 336–344.

Minkoff, H. L. (1990). HIV disease in pregnancy. *Obstetrics and Gynecology Clinics of North America,* 17 (3).

Minkoff, H. L., and Feinkind, L. (1989). Management of pregnancies of HIV-infected women. *Clinical Obstetrics and Gynecology,* 32 (3), 467–476.

MMWR. (1996). Update: Provisional Public Health Service recommendations for chemoprophylaxis after occupational exposure to HIV. 45(22), 468–472.

Nanda, D., and Minkoff, H. L. (1989). HIV in pregnancy—transmission and immune effects. *Clinical Obstetrics and Gynecology,* 32 (3), 456–466.

Nolan, K. (1990). HIV infection, women, and pregnancy. *Obstetrics and Gynecology Clinics of North America,* 17 (3), 651–668.

Osborne, N. G., and Adelson, M. D. (1990). Herpes simplex and HPV genital infections: Controversy over obstetric management. *Clinical Obstetrics and Gynecology,* 33 (4), 801–811.

Paris Declaration. (1990). *World Health,* November-December 1990, 16–17.

Patsner, B. P., Baker, D. A., Orr, J. W. (1990). Human papillomavirus genital tract infections during pregnancy. *Clinical Obstetrics and Gynecology,* 33 (2), 258–267.

Pernoll, M. L. (Ed.). (1991). *Current obstetric and gynecologic diagnosis and treatment* (7th ed.). East Norwalk, CT: Appleton & Lange.

Prober, C. G., Gershon, A. A., Grose, C., McCracken, G. H., Nelson, J. D. (1990). Consensus: Varicella-zoster infections in pregnancy and the perinatal period. *Pediatric Infectious Disease Journal,* 9 (12), 865–869.

Ross, T., and Dickason, E. J. (1992). Nursing alert: Vertical transmission of HIV and HPV *MCN: American Journal of Maternal-Newborn Nursing,* 17, 193–195.

Russell, L. K. (1992). Management of varicella-zoster virus infections during pregnancy and the peripartum. *Journal of Nurse-Midwifery,* 37 (1), 17–24.

Saag, M., Holodniy, M., Kuritzkes, D., et al. (1996) HIV viral load markers in clinical practice. *Nature* 2(6), 625–629.

Schwartz, D. B., Greenberg, M. D., Daoud, Y., Reid, R. (1987). The management of genital condylomas in pregnant women. *Obstetrics and Gynecology Clinics of North America,* 14 (2), 589–599.

Sever, J. L., Larsen, J. W., Grossman, J. H. (1989). *Handbook of perinatal infections.* Boston: Little, Brown.

Smeltzer, S. C., and Whipple, B. (1991). Women and HIV infection. *Image: Journal of Nursing Scholarship,* 23 (4), 249–255.

Smith, L., Pearlman, M., Smith, L., Faro, S. (1990). Lyme disease: A review with emphasis on the pregnant woman. *Obstetrical and Gynecological Survey,* 46 (3), 125–130.

Stratton, P., Mofenson, L., Willoughby, A. (1992). Human immunodeficiency virus infection in pregnant women under the care of AIDS clinical trials centers in the United States. *Obstetrics and Gynecology,* 79(3), 364–368.

Sweet, R. L. (1990). Hepatitis B infection in pregnancy. *Obstetrics/Gynecology Report,* 2 (2), 128–139.

Sweet, R. L., and Gibbs, R. S. (1990). *Infectious diseases of the female genital tract.* Baltimore: Williams & Wilkins.

Task Force on Pediatric AIDS. (1992). Perinatal human immunodeficiency virus (HIV) testing. *Pediatrics* 89(4), 791–794.

Tillman, J. (1992). An old disease, a contemporary perinatal problem. *Journal of Obstetric, Gynecologic, and Neonatal Nursing,* 21 (3), 209–213.

Urang, S. (1990). Cytomegalovirus infection in pregnancy. *Journal of Nurse-Midwifery,* 35 (5), 299–306.

Wang, E., and Smaill, F. (1989). Infection in pregnancy. In I. Chalmers, M. Enkin, M. Keirse (Eds.): *Effective care in pregnancy and childbirth* (pp. 534–564). Oxford, UK: Oxford University Press.

Witt, R., Silvestre, A. J., Rinaldo, C. R., Lyter, D. W. (1992). Guidelines for disclosing HIV antibody test results to clients. *Nurse Practitioner,* (1), 55, 59, 63.

Wong, S. Y., and Remington, J. S. (1994). Toxoplasmosis in pregnancy. *Clinical Infectious Disease,* 18, 853–862.

World Health Organization. (1993). Women and AIDS: Women face avoidable risk of AIDS. Press release, August 23, 1993, Geneva, Switzerland.

Appendices

I Appendix

Collaborative Care Paths

Collaborative care paths are being developed under many names, some generic and some specific to particular institutions: clinical paths, care maps, Care Trac, clinical pathways. Care paths differ in format, amount of detail, and method of recording. Some are preprinted by the institution, others are computer generated. Most have four characteristics in common (Ignatavicius and Hausman 1995)*:

1. *Patient outcomes* to be achieved by the time of discharge from the health care setting.
2. *Timeline* for sequencing interventions. In maternity settings, time guidelines may be by the day or by shorter periods.
3. *Collaboration* is a key element in the development of a care path. Interventions provided by physicians, nurse-midwives, and nursing and other disciplines are included.
4. *Comprehensive aspects of care.* Care paths provide guidelines for and track the various aspects of care, including laboratory tests, direct care, client teaching, referrals to social services, and referrals to specialists.

Included in this Appendix are samples of care paths, courtesy of the originating agencies:

St. John's Mercy Medical Center, St. Louis, Missouri

CARE PATH: Clinic Obstetric Prenatal

Women's East Pavilion, Chattanooga, Tennessee

CARE TRAC. DRG #391-C Normal Newborn

CARE TRAC. DRG #371 Cesarean Birth Without Complications

John Muir Medical Center, Walnut Creek, California

Normal Vaginal Delivery—Clinical Path

Preterm Labor (PTL)—Magnesium Sulfate ($MgSO_4$) → Oral Terbutaline

Preterm Labor → Oral Terbutaline—(Length of Stay 2 Days)

Variance Report. Note that a Variance Report can be used with any clinical path.

Documentation by variance means that each intervention on the clinical path is not documented separately. Rather, if a client deviates from the guidelines ("falls off the path"), the variance and the reason for the variance are documented.

Fairfax Hospital, INOVA Health System, Falls Church, Virginia

Clinical Pathway for Preterm Labor

Clinical Pathway—Premature Rupture of Membranes

Clinical Pathway—Placenta Previa

NICU Clinical Path: Growing Preemie—Uncomplicated

NICU Clinical Path: Growing Preemie—Complicated

NICU Clinical Pathway: Term Infant, Suspect Sepsis—Simple and Complex

INOVA Home Infusion Clinical Pathways for Pediatric Home IV Therapy Term

Infant: Suspect Sepsis—Uncomplicated

Loyola University Medical Center, Maywood, Illinois

Collaborative Carepath: Acutely Ill Neonatal Transport

Collaborative Carepath: Neonatal Return Transport

*Ignatavicius, D. D., and Hausman, K. A.: *Clinical pathways for collaborative practice.* Philadelphia: W. B. Saunders, 1995.

St.John's Mercy Medical Center

Name: ______________________________

This care path is a guideline and is not intended to create a standard of care. This guideline may be modified based on individual patient's needs.

	Consults Date	Proced/Tests Date	Pt/Family Ed Date	Routine visits	Meds Date	Other Date	Initials
Pre-conception	MD RD, prn RN, prn MSW, prn	PAP, breast exam Hx/family hx screen for Sickle cell, TaySach prn	Wellness ed. Nutrition Self br. exam Abstain from Tob, ETOH, etc	Yearly and prn	PNV FeSO-4 Folic acid		
Week 1-8	MD RD RN MSW	Preg test, prn Initial labs HIV, prn Sickle cell, prn	Given prenatal handbook Additional info:	1/Mo. First 32 Weeks, and prn ↓	PNV, FeSO-4 ↓		
Week 8-12	MD RD, prn RN, prn MSW, prn	PAP, breast exam DNA probe Urine tox.					
Week 12-16	MD RD, prn RN, prn MSW, prn	Order MSAFP to be done in weeks 15-17					
Week 16-20	MD RD, prn RN, prn MSW, prn	Order U/S to be done in weeks 18-22	Refer to childbirth/ VBAC class				
Week 20-24	MD RD, prn RN, prn MSW, prn	Order 1 hr GTT, H&H ~ 24 weeks	Epidural class Breastfeed or bottle				
Week 24-28	MD RD, prn RN, prn MSW, prn	GBS 28 weeks, prn	Additional info.		(Rhogam 28 wks prn)		
Weeks 28-32	MD RD, prn RN, prn MSW, prn		S/Sx PTL				
Weeks 32-36	MD RD, prn RN, prn MSW, prn	Vag exam at 36 wks if ctx	S/Sx labor	Bi-monthly		NST, prn Fetal/pelvic index, prn	
Weeks 36-40	MD RD, prn RN, prn MSW, prn			Weekly til del.			
Week 40-del.	MD RD, prn RN, prn MSW, prn						
Postpartum	MD RD, prn RN, prn MSW, prn	PAP, breast exam	Care of self PP (care of infant) Family planning Wellness	(2 wks for C/S) 6 weeks	(Rhogam prn) (Rubella prn)		

Patient Problems Identified:

____
____
____
____

PATIENT IDENTIFICATION

CARE PATH: Clinic Obstetric Prenatal
Care Path Code: 080

ST. JOHN'S MERCY MEDICAL CENTER, ST. LOUIS, MO

Rev. 9/95

Courtesy of St. John's Mercy Medical Center, St. Louis, MO.

WOMEN'S E♦A♦S♦T PAVILION
1751 Gunbarrel Road
Chattanooga
Tennessee 37421

C A R E T R A C

DRG#: **391-C NORMAL NEWBORN**

I have reviewed and will participate in my plan of care.
Patient Signature: ____________________
Nurse's Signature: ____________________
Birth Date: ____________________ Time:__________
Expected LOS: **48-72 hrs.** Physician: ____________________
Discharge Date: ____________________ Time:__________

PHASE / SOURCE ▶	DISCHARGE OUTCOMES		**A** 0-4 Hrs/______	**B** 4-12 Hrs/______
1 CONSULTS			__ Physical exam between 1-24 hrs by MD ········	········▶
2 TESTS		LABS	__ Maternal Hepatitis B status confirmed ❑ Cord blood for type/coombs (Rh negative mother only) ❑ Capillary hematocrit ❑ Admission BBGT (blood glucose test) for SGA or LGA	
3 NURSING ACTIVITIES/ TREATMENTS	The newborn will be afebrile with no complications.	VITAL SIGNS	__ Admission TPR within 30 min. __ TPR q 30 x 2 then q 1 hr x 2 __ Q 6 hrs when stable __ Weight/length/head circumference __ Physical assessment __ Gestational age assessment	__ TPR every 6 hrs __ Breastfeeding assessment every 8 hrs
		TREAT-MENTS	__ ID bands on __ ID band sheet checked/signed X 2 RN's	__ Bath after 4 hrs
		GU/GI	__ Document voiding and stooling ····	········▶
4 MEDICATIONS	The newborn's pain may be controlled with oral analgesics.	PAIN MGMT	__ Erythromycin ointment, OU within 1 hr __ Aquamephyton 1.0 mg, IM within 1 hr	
	The newborn will receive required medications		❑ Engerix-B 0.5 ml, IM within 12 hrs (newborn of Hepatitis B positive mother) ····	········▶
5 DIET	The newborn will demonstrate effective suck/swallow and ability to tolerate feedings ❑ BREAST ❑ FORMULA		__ Breastfeeding within 1 hr __ Formula feeding within 4 hrs ······▶	__ 5-7 breastfeedings within 12 hrs __ 3 formula feedings within 12 hrs ······▶
6 PATIENT/ FAMILY TEACHING **DISCHARGE PLANNING**	NEWBORN AT MOTHER'S BEDSIDE TO FACILITATE TEACHING OPPORTUNITIES			

SRMC 210 *Care Tracs do not represent a standard of care. They are designed to serve as guidelines and may be modified to meet individual patient needs.*

Continued on facing page

Newborn: ______________________ ❑ M ❑ F
Weight: ______________
Risks/Problems/Nursing Considerations: ______________

ADDRESSOGRAPH

C 12-24 Hrs/________	D 24-48 Hrs/________	E 48-72 Hrs/________
....................► ❑ Circumcision by MD ....► ❑ Dorsal penile nerve block by MD		__ One pre-discharge exam by MD/NP
	__ Metabolic screening prior to discharge (preferably after 24 hrs of age) ....►	
__ TPR every 6 hrs __ Breastfeeding assessment every 8 hrs	__ TPR every 6 hrs __ Breastfeeding assessment every 8 hrs	__ Discharge weight __ TPR every 6 hrs __ Breastfeeding assessment every 8 hrs
	__ Cord clamp removed	__ ID band checked/removed __ ID band sheet signed by parent and RN/LPN
....►		
__ Alcohol to cord every 8 hrs ....►	__ Alcohol to cord every 8 hrs	__ Alcohol to cord every 8 hrs
__ 5-7 breastfeedings within 12 hrs .....► __ 3 formula feedings within 12 hrs	__ 9-12 breastfeedings within 24 hrs .....► __ 6 formula feedings within 24 hrs	__ 9-12 breastfeedings within 24 hrs __ 6 formula feedings within 24 hrs

CARE TRAC C-NORMAL NEWBORN (03/96)

Courtesy of Women's East Pavilion, Chattanooga, TN.

WOMEN'S E♦A♦S♦T PAVILION
1751 Gunbarrel Road
Chattanooga
Tennessee 37421

CARE TRAC

DRG#: **371 CESAREAN BIRTH WITHOUT COMPLICATIONS**

I have reviewed and will participate in my plan of care.
Patient Signature: ____________________
Nurse's Signature: ____________________
Birth Date: ____________ Time: ________
Expected LOS: **48-72 hrs.** Physician: ____________
Discharge Date: ____________ Time: ________

PHASE ▶ / SOURCE ▼	DISCHARGE OUTCOMES		A PRENATAL	B PRE-OPERATIVE	C 0-4 Hrs PP/________
1 CONSULTS			__ Pre-registration __ Prenatal care __ Prenatal history available	__ One pre-operative visit by MD (surgeon) __ One pre-operative visit by MDA/CRNA	
2 TESTS		LABS	Results Confirmed: __ Blood type, Rh __ Hemoglobin __ Serology __ Rubella __ Hepatitis B	__ Hemoglobin __ Blood type and screen ❑ Urinalysis ❑ Serum Postassium ❑ Blood crossmatch	
3 NURSING ACTIVITIES/ TREATMENTS	The mother will be afebrile with wound healing and no complications.	VITAL SIGNS		__ TPR/BP __ Fetal heart rate	BP, P fundus, flow ________ every 15 x 4 ________ every 30 x 2 ________ every 1 hr x 2 ________ Temperature x 1 ❑ RR every 15 x 2 hrs with intrathecal narcotics ❑ RR every 30 x 2 hrs with intrathecal narcotics
		TREAT-MENTS		__ IV fluids started · · · · __ TED hose applied __ Abdomen shaved	· · · · · · · · · · · · ▶ __ Perineal care
		GU/GI		__ Foley catheter inserted ·	__ Intake and output · ▶ · · · · · · · · · · · · ▶
4 MEDICATIONS	The mother's pain will be controlled with oral analgesics.	PAIN MGMT	__ Prenatal vitamins	__ Bicitra, 30 cc, PO	❑ Aleve 2 tabs PO q 3-4 hrs PRN ❑ Percocet 1 tab PO q 3-4 hrs PRN ❑ Percodan 1 tab PO q 3-4 hrs PRN ❑ Mepergan Fortis 1 tab PO q 3-4 hrs PRN
5 DIET				__ Nothing by mouth	__ Diet as tolerated · · ▶
6 ACTIVITY					
7 PATIENT/ FAMILY TEACHING **DISCHARGE PLANNING**	The mother will verbalize and/or demonstrate ability to: • care for self • care for newborn • observe for maternal/ newborn complications NEWBORN AT MOTHER'S BEDSIDE TO FACILITATE TEACHING OPPORTUNITIES		__ Prenatal classes	__ Pre-operative teaching to include: Recovery Room, pain medications, coughing, deep breathing and activity.	__ Orient to unit __ Orient to unit routines __ Self medication admin. __ Intravenous fluids, intake and output, Foley catheter __ Incision/dressing/drains __ TED hose, coughing, deep breathing and activity __ Perineal care __ Newborn safety/security __ Newborn airway safety __ Newborn positioning

SRMC 204 *Care Tracs do not represent a standard of care. They are designed to serve as guidelines and may be modified to meet individual patient needs.*

Continued on facing page

Room # ________ Mother: ______________________
Significant Other: ______________________
Grav________ Para________ Epis________
Blood Type/Rh:______ Needs Rhogam: Y N Needs Rubella: Y N
Allergies: ______________________
Risks/Problems/Nursing Considerations: ______________________

ADDRESSOGRAPH

D 4-12 Hrs PP/________	**E** 12-24 Hrs PP/________	**F** 24-48 Hrs PP/________	**G** 48-72 Hrs PP/________
		__ First post-operative day visit by MD ❑ Any necessary consults: • Specialty MD • Social Service • Lactation • Homecare	__ One pre-discharge visit by MD
		__ Hemoglobin	
__ TPR/BP every 4 hrs ❑ RR every 1 hr x 10 hrs with intrathecal narcotics __ Postpartum assessment every 8 hrs	__ TPR/BP every 4 hrs ❑ RR every 1 hr x 2 hrs with intrathecal narcotics __ Postpartum assessment every 8 hrs	__ TPR/BP every 8 hrs __ Postpartum assessment every 8 hrs	__ TPR/BP every 8 hrs __ Postpartum assessment every 8 hrs
__ Shower/bath as tolerated 8 to 48 hours after surgery		__ Discontinue IV fluids 24 hrs after surgery	__ Staples removed from incision __ Steri-strips applied to incision
__ Discontinue Foley catheter 8 to 24 hrs after surgery __ Assess voiding	__ Assess voiding	__ Discontinue intake and output __ Assess voiding	
		❑ Rubella immunization ❑ Rhogam	
__ Up with assistance as ordered by MD	__ Up with assistance as needed	__ Ambulate without assistance	
❑ BREASTFEEDING __ Frequency __ Cues of readiness __ Positioning __ Latching on, suck/swallow __ Duration __ Removal from nipple __ Burping __ Breast/nipple care __ Preventing engorgement	❑ FORMULA FEEDING __ Type of formula __ Frequency, amount, technique __ Burping ❑ CIRCUMCISION CARE __ Basic sponge bath/skin care __ Cord care __ Taking an axillary temperature __ Diapering/clothing __ Newborn voiding and stooling	DISCHARGE MATERNAL __ Review discharge instructions __ Self care/activity/diet next 24-48 hours __ Need for birth control information ❑ Medications DISCHARGE NEWBORN __ Review discharge instructions __ Bunch/stretch feeding cycles, night time management __ Review breastfeeding techniques __ Formula prep/storage for formula fed infants __ Behavior/activity next 24-48 hours	

CARE TRAC CESAREAN BIRTH WITHOUT COMPLICATIONS (03/96)

Courtesy of Women's East Pavilion, Chattanooga, TN.

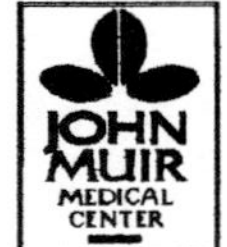

Normal Vaginal Delivery- Clinical Path

	LABOR & DELIVERY	1ST HOUR POST DELIVERY	4 HOURS POST DELIVERY	12 HOURS POST DELIVERY	1ST DAY POST PARTUM	POST PARTUM HOME VISIT
• DIAGNOSTICS ◊ Lab ◊ X-Ray ◊ Other	• CBC, U/A with C&S, prn [1]				• Hematocrit and Hemoglobin if increased blood loss after delivery	
TREATMENTS	• Fetal Monitoring • Vital Signs • Assess per Standard	• Offer pain Medication, prn • Monitor Vital Signs • Assess per Labor and Delivery Standards	• Ice to perineum • Perineal spray, Tucks, Anusol HC™ , prn. • Catheterize if unable to void. • Assess VS per standard • Assess fundus and lochia • Breast Care • Assess bonding	• Assess vital signs per standard. • Ice to perineum for 8 hours.	• Assess vital signs per standard. • Assess for adequate bowel function	• Assess vital signs of infant and mother.
IV's & MEDICATIONS	• Continuous IV • Pain medication, prn	• Oxytocin per protocol • Breast feeding, prn.	• IV discontinued when completed. Saline/Heparin Lock, prn. • Pain medication, prn	• Pain medication, prn	• Pain medication, prn • Rhogam, as indicated	
DIET	• Sips & chips	• As tolerated.	• Regular-as tolerated.	• Regular-as tolerated.	• Regular-as tolerated.	
ACTIVITY	• Bed rest if spontaneous (SROM) or artificial (AROM) rupture of membranes if presenting part unengaged. • Ambulatory, if presenting part engaged.	• Bed rest • Bonding activity • Breast Feeding	• Ambulate with assist	• Ambulate as tolerated; with assist, if epidural or spinal anesthesia	• Up, as desired	• Assess activity of infant and mother.
CONSULTATIONS	• Anesthesia • Screen for Social Services		• Lactation consultant, prn, if infant in Intensive Care Nursery; if inverted nipples; primipara.		• Public Health Nurse • Women-Infant-Children (WIC) program, prn.	• Lactation consultant, prn, for breast-feeding difficulties • Public Health Nurse, prn. • Pediatrician, • Obstetrician

[1] Culture & Sensitivity

	LABOR & DELIVERY	1ST HOUR POST DELIVERY	4 HOURS POST DELIVERY	12 HOURS POST DELIVERY	1ST DAY POST PARTUM	POST PARTUM HOME VISIT
TEACHING	• Comfort measures • Understanding of equipment • Support during labor	• Self-care instructions • Initial breast feeding instruction. • Use of bulb syringe. • Infant Security	• Reinforce teaching already done. • Identify need for assistance when ambulating • Explain security system for newborn	• Continue to reinforce teaching.	• Reinforce teaching. • Evidence of bonding. • Mom demonstrates competency in self and infant care.	• Reinforce teaching. • Evidence of bonding. • Mom demonstrates competency in self and infant care.
DISCHARGE PLANNING				• Assess home discharge needs. ◊ Car seat ◊ Layette ◊ Help status ◊ Nutrition	• Coordinate discharge date with attending physician and insurance. • Discharge home.	
COLLABORATIVE DIAGNOSIS	• Standard of Care of patient in labor per hospital policy					
QUALITY INDICATORS	• Delivery of viable infant • Spontaneous delivery of the placenta	• BP <140/90 or consistent with prenatal course. • Fundus firm without excessive bleeding. • Absence of bladder distention. • Perineum/stitches-intact.	• Able to verbalize newborn nursery phone number. • Voiding without difficulty.	• Able to empty bladder.	• Fundus firm without excessive bleeding. • Able to breast or bottle feed infant. • Bowel movement before discharge. • Verbalizes and/or demonstrates knowledge about self-care. • Breast care. • Activity/Exercise. • Elimination • Diet/Vitamins • Warning signs of illness. • Verbalizes and/or demonstrates knowledge of infant care.	• Fundus firm without excessive bleeding. • Able to breast or bottle feed infant. • Bowel movement before discharge. • Verbalizes and/or demonstrates knowledge about self-care. • Breast care. • Activity/Exercise. • Elimination • Diet/Vitamins • Warning signs of illness. • Verbalizes and/or demonstrates knowledge of infant care.

[i] Developed by Meredith Pence, RNC, MBA, CNAA @ John Muir Medical Center.
[ii] This material is intended for use as a guideline only. It is not intended to define the standard of care.

Courtesy of John Muir Medical Center, Walnut Creek, CA.

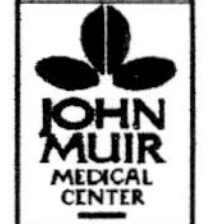

Preterm Labor (PTL) - Magnesium Sulfate ($MgSO_4$)→ Oral Terbutaline

i ii

	Admission→ 24°	24° to 48°	48° to 72°	72° to Discharge
CONSULTS	• Investigate need for special consults.	• Neonatal, prn. • Perinatal, prn. • Social Services, prn • Clinical Nurse Specialist (CNS)-Perinatal/Neonatal, prn.	• Neonatal, prn. • Perinatal, prn. • Social Services, prn • CNS-Perinatal/Neonatal, prn.	• Neonatal, prn. • Perinatal, prn. • Social Services, prn • CNS-Perinatal/Neonatal, prn.
TESTS	• U/A with C & S • Cervical Cultures (Herpes, GC[1], ß Strep, Chlamydia), prn. • Electrolytes, prn. • CBC, prn. • Ultrasound/Amniocentesis, prn. • Magnesium (Mg) levels: 2° after completion of bolus and q 6° for 1st 24 hours.	• Mg levels q day, if stable infusion rate..	• EKG-prior to Terbutaline administration, if indicated. • DC Mg levels	
TREATMENTS	• Evaluate cervix (Vaginal exam, speculum exam) R/O spontaneous rupture of membranes (SROM) • Electronic Fetal monitoring (EFM) continuous uterine & fetal. • Vital Signs: • Temp - Admission and q 4 hours thereafter • BP, P = Admission q 1 h hour x 3, then q 4 hours until stable. • R &/or DTR's q 1° • Daily weight • Positioning/Comfort (Side-lying, "egg-crate" mattress) • Strict I&O. • Fluid restriction (IV & PO) 3000 cc's/24°	• Continuous uterine monitoring, Fetal heart rate [FHR] monitoring q shift (continuous FHR if UC's resume.) • Vital Signs: • BP, T-P q 4 hours while on stable infusion rate. • R &/or DTR's q 1° W/A (if infusion rate stable. • Daily weight • Positioning/Comfort • Strict I&O. • Fluid restriction (IV & PO) 3000 cc's/24	• Continuous UC monitoring, FHR monitoring q shift (continuous FHR if UC's resume.) • Vital Signs • BP, TPR q 4 hours W/A • DC daily weight • Add sitting positions. • DC I&O • DC fluid restriction.	• Continuous UC, FHR monitoring q shift continuous FHR if UC's resume.) • Vital Signs • BP, TPR q 4 hours W/A
MEDICATIONS	• IV-Main line per order. • Secondary line-Mg • $MgSO_4$ bolus = 6 GMs over 20 to 30 minutes. • $MgSO_4$ Maintenance dose = 2 to 3 GMs and hour, titered to UC's. • Prenatal Vitamins • Other medications as required by individual patient (i.e. antibiotics, stool softener)	• IV-Main line per order. • Secondary line-Mg • $MgSO_4$ Maintenance dose = 2 to 3 GMs and hour, titered to UC's. • Prenatal Vitamins • Other medications as required by individual patient (i.e. antibiotics, stool softener)	• IV-Main line per order. • Secondary line-Mg • Wean Mg infusion over 12°, then DC. • Begin PO Terbutaline 5 mg, q 4°.	• DC IV per physician order • PO Terbutaline 5 mg, q 4°.
DIET	• Clear liquids until stable. Advance to regular (high fiber) when stable. • Assess nutrition status. Nutrition consult, prn.	• Regular-high fiber. ◊ Assess nutrition status. Nutrition consult, prn.	• Regular-high fiber. ◊ Assess nutrition status. Nutrition consult, prn.	• Regular-high fiber. ◊ Assess nutrition status. Nutrition consult, prn.

[1] GC indicates a test for Gonorrhea

	Admission→ 24°	24° to 48°	48° to 72°	72° to Discharge
ACTIVITY	• Bedrest with bathroom privileges (BRP). • Trendelenburg if advanced cervical dilation, PROM or bulging bag.	• Bedrest with BRP. • Trendelenberg if advanced cervical dilation, PROM or bulging bag. • Bed bath or bathing assist.	• DC Trendelenberg • Bathing assist	• Shower
TEACHING	• Side effects of medication. • Keep informed	• Side effects of medication. • Keep informed • Signs and symptoms of preterm labor. • Signs and symptoms of SROM • Review & discuss plan of care.	• Keep informed • Signs and symptoms of PTL. • Signs and symptoms of SROM • Review & discuss plan of care. • Taking pulse • Tachycardia and its relationship to Terbutaline. • Importance of compliance with treatment. • Tour of Intensive Care Nursery (ICN), prn..	• Keep informed • Signs and symptoms of PTL. • Signs and symptoms of SROM • Review & discuss plan of care. • Taking pulse • Tachycardia and its relationship to Terbutaline. • Importance of compliance with treatment. • Tour of ICN, prn.. • When to call the doctor. • Written information related to PTL and Terbutaline medication administration. • Provide reading material related to importance of avoiding preterm delivery, managing bedrest at home, family role changes, feelings, nutrition etc.
DISCHARGE PLANNING	• Discuss home situation (number of young children at home, availability of transportation, support systems). • Social Services consult, prn. (Community References) • Discuss need for maintaining muscle tone while on bedrest. • Investigate need for home care support (Home uterine activity monitoring, home visits by RN.). If home care agency care ordered, begin insurance eligibility review. If eligible contact Home care agency	• Review plans for care at home after discharge. • Social Services consult, prn. (Community References) • Physical Therapy: (isotonic exercises for PTL patients on bedrest, prn.) • Establish interface with home care agency, prn.	• Review plans for care at home after discharge. • Social Services consult, prn. (Community References) • Physical Therapy: (isotonic exercises for PTL patients on bedrest, prn.) • Establish interface with home care agency, prn.	• Review plans for care at home after discharge. • Social Services consult, prn. (Community References) • Physical Therapy: (isotonic exercises for PTL patients on bedrest, prn.) • Give discharge report to home care agency, prn. • Discharge

[i] Developed by Meredith Pence, RNC, MBA, CNAA & Carol Kelly, RNC, MSN @ John Muir Medical Center.
[ii] This material is intended for use as a guideline only. It is not intended to define the standard of care.

Courtesy of John Muir Medical Center, Walnut Creek, CA.

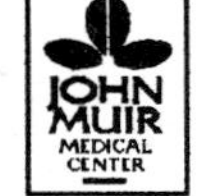

Preterm Labor → Oral Terbutaline - (Length of Stay 2 Days)[i][ii]

	• Day 1 - Admission	• Day 2
CONSULTS	• Investigate need for special consults. • Neonatal/Perinatal, prn. • Social Services, prn • Clinical Nurse Specialist-Perinatal/Neonatal, prn.	• Investigate need for special consults. • Neonatal/Perinatal, prn. • Social Services, prn • Clinical Nurse Specialist-Perinatal/Neonatal, prn.
TESTS	• U/A with C & S • Cervical Cultures (Herpes, GC[1], ß Strep, Chlamydia), prn. • CBC, Electrolytes, prn. • Ultrasound/Amniocentesis, prn.	• If mature-consider no intervention.
TREATMENTS	• Evaluate cervix (Vaginal exam, speculum exam) • R/O spontaneous rupture of membranes (SROM) • Electronic Fetal monitoring (EFM) continuous uterine & fetal. • Vital Signs (BP, Temp., Pulse, Resps [BP, TPR], initially and q 4 hours while awake) • Pulse prior to each Terbutaline medication. Hold medication and notify physician if pulse ≅ 120 bpm • Daily weight • Hydration (Oral/ IV, measure intake & output [I&O]) • Positioning/Comfort (Side-lying, "egg-crate" mattress)	• Continuous uterine (UC) monitoring, Fetal heart rate [FHR] monitoring each shift (continuous FHR if contractions resume) • Vital Signs (BP, TPR) initially and q 4 hours while awake. • Pulse prior to each Terbutaline medication. Hold medication and notify physician if pulse ≅ 120 bpm • DC I&O. DC IV per physician order. • Add sitting positions.
MEDICATIONS	• Sub-cutaneous (SQ)/oral (po) Terbutaline (if sub-cutaneous, follow 1st dose with oral Terbutaline • Prenatal Vitamins • Other medications as required by individual patient.	• Terbutaline po • Prenatal Vitamins • Other medications as required by individual patient.
DIET	• Clear liquids. Advance to regular (high fiber) when stable. • Assess nutrition status. Nutrition consult, prn.	• Advance to regular (high fiber) when stable. • Assess nutrition status. Nutrition consult, prn.
ACTIVITY	• Bedrest with bathroom privileges (BRP).	• Bedrest with bathroom privileges (BRP).
TEACHING	• Side effects of medication. • Signs and symptoms of preterm labor, Spontaneous Rupture of Membranes(SROM) • When to call the doctor. • Importance of compliance with treatment. • Keep informed	• Review • Review • Review • Review • Keep informed • Tour of Intensive Care Nursery, prn. • Provide written information related to Preterm labor and Terbutaline medication administration (include show to take pulse; reading material related to importance of avoiding preterm delivery, managing bedrest at home, family role changes, feelings, nutrition etc.
DISCHARGE PLANNING	• Discuss home situation (young children at home, availability of transportation, support systems). • Physical Therapy: (isotonic exercises for PTL patients on bedrest, prn.) • Contact Home care agency, if ordered. Begin insurance eligibility review.	• Review plans for self care after discharge. Social Services consult, prn. (Community References) • Physical Therapy: (isotonic exercises for PTL patients on bedrest, prn.) • Establish interface with home care agency, prn. • Discharge.

[i] Developed by Meredith Pence, RNC, MBA, CNAA & Carol Kelly, RNC, MSN @ John Muir Medical Center
[ii] This material is intended for use as a guideline only. It is not intended to define the standard of care.

[1] GC indicates a test for Gonorrhea

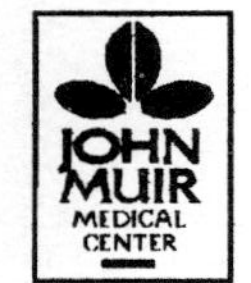

Variance Report[1 2]

Admit Date:________________ **Discharge Date:**________________ **Length of Stay:**________________

Hospital Day	Path Day	Problem #/ Pathway Category	Specify Variance	Source	Reason	Action Plan /Comments	Initials

Problem #
0 = Problem not on path
1,2,3 = as on path

Pathway Category
A = Diagnostic Studies
B = Treatments
C = Medications
D = Diet
E = Consults
F = Activity
G = Teaching
H = Discharge Planning

Variance Sources
A = Patient/Family
B = Clinician
C = Hospital
D = Community

Variance Reason
1 = Pt. condition
2 = Pt./family decision
3 = Pt./family availability
4 = Pt./family other
5 = MD order
6 = Caregiver decision
7 = Caregiver response
8 = Caregiver other
9 = Bed/appt. availability
10 = Information availability
11 = Supplies/equip availability
12 = Dept. overbooked, etc.
13 = Hospital other
14 = Placement/Homecare
15 = Transportation availability
16 = Community other

1 Developed by Kris Andreason, RN @ John Muir Medical Center
2 Variance Report may be used for any Clinical Path.

Courtesy of John Muir Medical Center, Walnut Creek, CA.

Fairfax Hospital, Falls Church, Virginia

CLINICAL PATHWAY FOR PRETERM LABOR

This care path is a guideline and is not intended to create a standard of care. This guideline may be modified based on individual patient's needs.

	LDR/TRIAGE	HRP DAY 1	HRP DAY 2	HRP DAY 3
CONSULTS	SW IF HOMELESS, <19 YEARS OLD, + DRUG SCREEN, VERBALIZED CONCERNS RE:IMPACT OF PTL	----------> NEONATOLOGY	-----------> NOTIFY HOME HEALTH IF INDICATED	------------> ------------>
TESTS/ DIAGNOSTICS	CBC W/DIFF CHEM 6 WITH CREATININE UA, C & S VIA CLEAN CATCH CERVICAL CULT FOR UREAPLASMA, CTM, STREP SCREEN AND CULTURE SONO FOR EFW, AFI, PRESENTATION IF INDICATED ELECTRONIC FETAL MONITORING (EFM)	REPEAT ANY ABNORMAL LABS PRN AFI QOD IF ON INDOCIN BPP IF NST NR OR AS ORDERED EFM/NST (TOCO AND FHR) Q AM AND PRN WITH CONTRACTIONS	-----------→ -----------→ -----------→ -----------→	------------→ ------------→ ------------→ ------------→
ACTIVITY/ SAFETY	BEDREST W/BRP NOTIFY MD FOR >4 CTX/1 HR, VAG BLEEDING OR LEAKAGE OF FLUID	----------> MAY SHOWER FETAL KICK COUNT QD ---------->	UP TO CHAIR ------------→ ------------→ ----------->	AMBULATION FOR PERSONAL ADL'S - SHOWER, BATHROOM, ----------------→ -----------------→
TREATMENTS/ CARE	I & O VS PER PROTOCOL - ESTABLISH BASELINE PULSE	----------> VS W/FHTT PER TOCOLYTIC PROTOCOL	D/C I & O VS W/FHT PER TOCOLYTIC PROTOCOL	 ----------->
DIET/FLUID BALANCE	0.2 NS @125/HR CLEAR LIQUIDS	SALINE LOK IV 2500 CC PO/24 H REG DIET W/ ↑FIBER	------------> ------------> ------------>	D/C IV -----------> ----------->

Continued on facing page

CLINICAL PATHWAY FOR PRETERM LABOR

This care path is a guideline and is not intended to create a standard of care. This guideline may be modified based on individual patient's needs.

	LDR/TRIAGE	HRP DAY 1	HRP DAY 2	HRP DAY 3
MEDICATION	TOCOLYTIC OF CHOICE PER PROTOCOL NOTIFY MD IF TCOLYTIC NOT WORK BETAMETHASONE 12.5 MG IM. REPEAT 12.5 MG IM IN 12 - 24 H PNV 1 PO QD COLACE 100 MG PO BID IF TWINS: FOLATE 1 MG PO QD FESO4 325 MG PO BID	TOCOLYTIC PER PROTOCOL REPEAT BETAMETHASONE 12.5 MG IM IF 2ND DOSE NOT GIVEN IN LDR ------------→ ------------→ ------------→ ------------→	------------> ------------> ------------> ------------> ------------>	-----------> REPEAT BETAMETHASONE 12.5 MG IM X TWO DOSES 12 - 24 HOURS APART Q WEEK UNTIL COMPLETES 34 WKS GESTATION -----------> -----------> -----------> ----------->
D/C PLANNING	EVAL FOR CONCERNS RE: HOSPITALIZATION - FINANCIAL, EMOTIONAL, SOCIAL	-----------> MANAGEMENT OF FINANCES, OTHER CHILDREN, JOB. FAMILY'S PREVIOUS EXPERIENCES W/PTL	------------> ------------>	-----------> -----------> AMBULATION FOR PERSONAL ADL'S - SHOWER, BATHROOM, PREPARE **OWN** MEALS
TEACHING	S & S OF PTL SIDE EFFECTS OF MEDS PALPATION OF CONTRACTIONS	INSTRUCT PT RE: PULSE, FETAL MOVEMENT RECORD (KICK COUNT), BOWEL FUNCTION - R/T FLUID INTAKE, ACTIVITY, MEDS. REVIEW PREVIOUS DAY'S INFO	INSTRUCT PT RE: WHEN TO TAKE TERB PRN, WHEN TO CALL MD, S & S OF ROM. REVIEW, RETURN DEMOS OF PREVIOUS DAY'S INFO	-----------> -----------> IMPORTANCE OF LATERAL SIDE LYING POSITION, ACTIVITY LEVEL

Courtesy of Fairfax Hospital, INOVA Health System, Falls Church, VA.

Fairfax Hospital, Falls Church, Virginia

CLINICAL PATHWAY - PREMATURE RUPTURE OF MEMBRANES

This care path is a guideline and is not intended to create a standard of care. This guideline may be modified based on individual patient's needs.

	LDR/TRIAGE	HRP DAY 1 → 7	HRP DAY 7 → DEL
CONSULTS		NEONATOLOGY	
TESTS/ DIAGNOSTICS	CBC W/DIFF CERVICAL CX FOR UREAPLASMA, CTM, GBS UA/C & S - CATH NITRAZINE/FERN ON AF EFM SONO/AFI, EFW PER ORDERS	DAILY CBC W/DIFF AFI,BPP 3 X WEEK IF $\geq$ 24 WKS NST QD $\geq$ 25 WKS OR IF < 25 WKS AND INITIAL NST REACTIVE **IF RECEIVES BETAMETHASONE AND NST NR**, DAILY BPP X 3 OR UNTIL REACTIVE	-----------→ -----------→ -----------→ -----------→
ACTIVITY/SAFETY	BEDREST NOTIFY MD FOR •$\geq$ 4 CTX/H, •T > 99.5, •S/S OF INFECTION	BEDREST W/BRP, SHOWER -------------→	PERSONAL ADL'S TO A MINIMUM -------------→
TREATMENTS/CARE	VS PER PROTOCOL	-------------→	-------------→
DIET/FLUID BALANCE	NPO IV O.2 NS OR D5/0.2 NS @ 125/H I & O	REGULAR DIET IV TO SALINE LOK (CHG Q 3 D) D/C I & O	-------------→ -------------→
MEDICATION	CLINDAMYCIN 900 MG IV Q 8H	-------------→ TIL COMPLETED 3 DAYS IV THEN TO CLEOCIN 300 MG PO QID TIL COMPLETED 5 DAYS OF PO TREATMENT	-------------→ CONTINUE CLEOCIN TIL COMPLETED 5 DAYS OF PO TREATMENT
D/C PLANNING		EVALUATE FOR CONCERNS RE: HOSPITALIZATION, EMOTIONAL, SOCIAL	-------------→
TEACHING	TEACH S & S OF INFECTION	-------------→ •HANDWASHING •PERICARE •NOTIFY NURSE RE: $\downarrow$ FM, CTX, CHANGE IN COLOR, ODOR, AMT OF AF, VAGINAL BLDING, UTERINE CRAMPING	-------------→ -------------→ -------------→ •DEMONSTRATE TAKING TEMP QID WHEN AWAKE •COMPLIANT W/TAKING MEDS •WEAR MINIPAD, CHANGE AT LEAST Q 4 H

 Fairfax Hospital, Falls Church, Virginia

CLINICAL PATHWAY - PLACENTA PREVIA

This care path is a guideline and is not intended to create a standard of care. This guideline may be modified based on individual patient's needs.

	LDR/TRIAGE	HRP DAYS 1 - 3
CONSULTS	•ANESTHESIA IF ACTIVELY BLEEDING •PERINATOLOGY IF EARLY GESTATION •NEONATOLOGY IF DELIVERY IS IMMINENT •SOCIAL WORK PER PATIENT CONCERNS	•IV THERAPY FOR MIDLINE CATHETER PLACEMENT •NEONATOLOGY IF DELIVERY POSSIBLE THIS ADMISSION
TESTS/ DIAGNOSTICS	CBC (IF NEW ADMIT) TYPE AND CROSS MATCH FOR 2 UNITS EFM DIAGNOSTIC U/S	TYPE AND CROSS Q 3 DAYS EFM IF CONTRACTIONS OR BLEEDING
ACTIVITY/SAFETY	STRICT BEDREST NOTIFY MD IF BLEEDING, CONTRACTIONS	BRP IF NO BLEEDING FOR 24 HOURS --------------------→
TREATMENTS/CARE	VS/ASSESSMENT PER PROTOCOL	--------------------→
DIET/FLUID BALANCE	NPO IV (18 GAUGE) AS ORDERED I & O	CLEAR LIQUID IF BRIGHT RED SPOTTING REGULAR DIET IF NO BLEEDING ▲ IV TO SALINE LOK DAY 1 IF NO ACTIVE BLEEDING
MEDICATION	BETAMETHASONE 12.5 MG IM (1ST DOSE)	--------------------→ (2ND DOSE) REPEAT BETAMETHASONE 12.5 MG IM IN SPLIT DOSES 12 - 24 HOURS APART Q WEEK UNTIL COMPLETES 34 WEEKS GESTATION PRENATAL VITAMIN 1 PO QD COLACE 100 MG PO BID FeSO4 325 MG PO AS ORDERED
D/C PLANNING	EVALUATE FOR CONCERNS RE: HOSPITALIZATION, EMOTIONAL, SOCIAL, FINANCIAL	----------------------→
TEACHING	IF PATIENT CONTRACTING, INSTRUCT PATIENT RE: PALPATION AND IDENTIFICATION OF CONTRACTIONS	NOTIFY NURSE FOR BRIGHT RED VAG BLEEDING, CRAMPING OR CONTRACTIONS, DECREASED FETAL MOVEMENT, ABD PAIN DIET RE: CONSTIPATION, KICK COUNT

Courtesy of Fairfax Hospital, INOVA Health System, Falls Church, VA.

Fairfax Hospital, Falls Church, Virginia

NICU CLINICAL PATH: GROWING PREEMIE - UNCOMPLICATED

Patient Name________________ M.R. Number____________
Date Clinical Path Initiated____________ Anticipated Length of Stay: ________
Admission Date__________ Discharge Date__________ Actual LOS________

This care path is a guideline and is not intended to create a standard of care. This guideline may be modified based on individual patient's needs.

	1500-1600 gms.__wks Zone 1	1600-1700 gms.__wks Zone 2	1700-1800 gms.__wks Zone 3	1800-1900 gms.__wks Zone 4	1900+ gms.___ __wks Zone 5
Tests/ Procedures	Metabolic screen per MD order Hct (q Monday)	------------------------>	------------------------>	Alk phos 5-7 days prior to discharge if ≥1500gms. birthweight Hct 5-7 days prior to d/c Outcome: HCT ≥25 If <25, needs serial assessments after discharge	------------------------>
	Ophthalmology exam at 4-6 weeks of age if ≤31 weeks or ≤1500gms. F/U exams per ophthalmologist	------------------------>	------------------------>	Outcome: noncritical exams done prior to day of d/c or scheduled outpatient	------------------------>
			HUS at 1800gms. if birth-weight <1750 or no medical reason earlier in hospitalization Circumcision permit___	Schedule circ prior to day of discharge OB called___ done___ Outcome: circ healing without complications	------------------------>
				BAER: weight >1800gms. and ≥34 weeks gestation	

	1500-1600 gms.__wks Zone 1	1600-1700 gms.__wks Zone 2	1700-1800 gms.__wks Zone 3	1800-1900 gms.__wks Zone 4	1900+ gms.___ __wks Zone 5
Treatments	CR monitor	------------------------------>	------------------------------>	Start home monitor when appropriate	--------------------------> Outcome: if home monitor required, pt should be free of alarms requiring intervention 48-72° prior to discharge. If no home monitor required, pt should be alarm free >2 weeks.
	O_2 sat monitor Bath q 3 days Weight q day HC & length q Monday VS with feedings BP as needed I&O as needed	------------------------------>	------------------------------>	------------------------------>	Outcomes: - gaining weight consistently - normal head & length growth - VS WNL
Nutrition	Nipple/gavage q 3° Nipple/breast 1-2x/day	------------------------------>	Increase frequency of nipple/ breastfeed q 3°. Decrease frequency of gavage.	Nipple feed all feedings	Advance volume and frequency of feedings to q3-4°. Change to 20 cal milk. Order special formulas for home use 1 day prior to discharge. Outcomes: - Tolerates formula/ breastmilk - Nipplefeeds well with minimal support

Continued on following page

NICU CLINICAL PATH: GROWING PREEMIE - UNCOMPLICATED (continued)

Patient Name____________________ M.R. Number_______________
Date Clinical Path Initiated_______________ Anticipated Length of Stay: __________
Admission Date____________ Discharge Date____________ Actual LOS__________

	1500-1600 gms.__wks Zone 1	1600-1700 gms.__wks Zone 2	1700-1800 gms.__wks Zone 3	1800-1900 gms.__wks Zone 4	1900+ gms.__ __wks Zone 5
Thermo-regulation	Isolette change every 7 days. Remove sheepskin, eggcrate mattress, water pillows at 1500gms. Discontinue skin probe at 1500gms. Out of isolette to feed.	Begin to decrease isolette temp (not less than 28°C) Bundle baby.	Assess readiness for weaning to open crib ----------------------->	Wean to open crib when: - all nipple feeding - consistent weight gain - stable body temperature ---------------------------->	Outcome: maintains normal temperature in open crib ---------------------->
Patient Teaching	Implement discharge teaching program. Begin demonstrations. Parents begin return demos.	----------------------------> ---------------------------->	------------------------------> Demonstrate tub bath Home monitor training if appropriate - CPR class___ - monitor class___	----------------------------> Parents continue to return demos and participate in care. Reinforce monitor training if needed___ Schedule care by parent prior to day of discharge Demonstrate med administration prior to day of d/c	Outcome: teaching completed prior to day of discharge. -------------------------> Outcome: - parent responds appropriately to monitor alarms - exhibits understanding of d/c instructions related to home monitoring Parent accurately administers meds

	1500-1600 gms.__wks Zone 1	1600-1700 gms.__wks Zone 2	1700-1800 gms.__wks Zone 3	1800-1900 gms.__wks Zone 4	1900+ gms.___ __wks Zone 5
Discharge Planning	Evaluate possibility of back transport. Assess discharge needs including social and community supports.	------------------------------> ------------------------------>	Schedule discharge planning conference___. Identify pediatrician. Medicaid/self pay patients: - refer to peds clinic - give list of PMDs	Write prescriptions prior to day of discharge. ID other F/U prior to d/c: - public health/WIC___ - home health___ - OT/PT___ - other MD F/U	----------------------------> Day of discharge: - discharge summary to family for pediatrician - make clinic appointment
Consults	Evaluate need for: - lactation consult___ - social services___ - OT/PT___ - speech if ≥34 weeks for evaluation of nippling status if needed	------------------------------>	------------------------------> Infant apnea program for home monitoring if appropriate	------------------------------>	Outcomes: need for consults done at appropriate time

Courtesy of Fairfax Hospital, INOVA Health System, Falls Church, VA.

Fairfax Hospital, Falls Church, Virginia

NICU CLINICAL PATH: GROWING PREEMIE - COMPLICATED

Patient Name__________ M.R. Number__________
Date Clinical Path Initiated__________ Anticipated Length of Stay__________
Admission Date__________ Discharge Date__________ Actual LOS__________

This care path is a guideline and is not intended to create a standard of care. This guideline may be modified based on individual patient's needs.

	Zone 1	Zone 2	Zone 3	Zone 4	Zone 5
Tests/ Procedures	Metabolic screen per MD order				
	HUS 3-5 days after admission if <1750gm birthweight, then as needed	------------------------>	------------------------>	------------------------>	------------------------>
	Hct (q Monday)	------------------------>	------------------------>	------------------------>	Hct 1 day prior to d/c Outcome: Hct $\geq$25 If <25, needs serial assessment after d/c
	Alk phos (q Monday or at 1800gm)	------------------------>	------------------------>	Outcome: alk phos level <400 on regular formula	Make decision regarding special formula
	CXR after Corpak insertion & before feeding started to check for proper placement in stomach.		Circumcision permit___	Schedule circumcision prior to day of discharge. OB called___ Done___ Outcome: circ healing without complications	------------------------>
			BAER - weight >1800gm - tolerating feedings - $\geq$34 weeks gestation - off Decadron or tolerating weaning dose		
	Ophthalmology exam at 4-6 weeks of age if $\leq$31 weeks or $\leq$1500gms. F/U exams per ophthalmologist	------------------------>	------------------------>	Outcome: noncritical exams done prior to day of d/c or scheduled outpatient	------------------------>

	Zone 1	Zone 2	Zone 3	Zone 4	Zone 5
Treatments	CR monitor	--------------------------->	--------------------------->	Start home monitor when appropriate.	--------------------------- > Outcomes: patient should be free of alarms requiring intervention 48-72° prior to discharge
	O_2 sat monitor Bath q 3 days Weight q day HC and length q Monday VS with feedings BP as needed I&O as needed	--------------------------->	--------------------------->	--------------------------->	Outcomes: - gaining weight consistently - normal head and length growth - VS WNL
	Convert to nasal canula O_2 when appropriate	--------------------------->	--------------------------->	Make decision regarding home O_2	Outcome: O_2 sats >88

Continued on following page

NICU CLINICAL PATH: GROWING PREEMIE - COMPLICATED (continued)

Patient Name__________ M.R. Number__________
Date Clinical Path Initiated__________ Anticipated Length of Stay__________
Admission Date__________ Discharge Date__________ Actual LOS__________

	Zone 1	Zone 2	Zone 3	Zone 4	Zone 5
Nutrition	Continuous nasogastric feedings	- Wean to bolus gavage q 2-3 hours - Begin skin-to-skin contact with mother - D/C Corpak when bolus feeds tolerated	Nipple/gavage q 3° Nipple/breastfeed 1-2x/day Decrease frequency of gavage Increase frequency of nipple	Nipple feeds all feedings q 3°	Advance volume & frequency of feedings to 3-4° Change to 20 cal milk Order special formulas for home use 1 day prior to discharge Outcomes: - nipple feeds well with minimal support - tolerates formula/ breastmilk - Nipple feeds with coordinated suck, swallow, breath

	Zone 1	Zone 2	Zone 3	Zone 4	Zone 5
Thermo- regulation	Isolette change q 7 days Remove sheepskin, eggcrate mattress, water pillows at 1500gms discontinue skin probe at 1500gms Out of isolette for holding	Begin to decrease isolette temperature (not less than 28°C) Bundle baby	Assess readiness for weaning to open crib ----------------------------->	Wean to open crib: - consistently gaining weight - stable body temperature ----------------------------->	Outcome: maintains normal temperature in open crib -------------------------->
Patient Teaching	Implement discharge teaching program Begin demonstrations Parents begin return demos	---------------------------> --------------------------->	-----------------------------> Demonstrate tub bath after 1500gms Home monitor training: - CPR___ - Monitor___	-----------------------------> Parents continue to return demonstrations and participate in care Reinforce monitor training if needed___ Schedule care by parent prior to day of d/c___ Demonstrate med administration prior to day of d/c If home O_2 required, teach principles of O_2 admin. Speech discharge teaching OT/PT discharge teaching	Outcome: teaching completed prior to day of discharge --------------------------> Outcome: - parent responds appropriately to monitor alarms - exhibits understanding of d/c instructions related to home monitoring - parent accurately administers meds Outcome: parents will exhibit understanding of O_2 administration principles prior to day of discharge

Continued on following page

NICU CLINICAL PATH: GROWING PREEMIE - COMPLICATED (continued)

Patient Name________________ M.R. Number________
Date Clinical Path Initiated________ Anticipated Length of Stay_____
Admission Date_______ Discharge Date_______ Actual LOS_____

	Zone 1	Zone 2	Zone 3	Zone 4	Zone 5
D/C Planning	Evaluate possibility of back transport. Assess discharge needs including social and community supports.	------------------------>	Schedule discharge planning conference Identify pediatrician. Medicaid/self pay patients: - refer to peds clinic - give list of PMDs	ID other F/U prior to day of discharge: - public health/WIC___ - home health___ - OT/PT___ - other MD F/U Write prescriptions prior to day of discharge Arrange for home O_2 if needed	Day of discharge: - discharge summary to family for pediatrician - make clinic appointment - discharge instructions to family Outcome: parents will have filled prescriptions prior to discharge Outcome: parents will have O_2 at home day of d/c
Consults	Social Services OT/PT Public Health	------------------------> Lactation consultant Speech therapy evaluation of non-nutritive suck	------------------------> ------------------------> If $\geq$34 weeks, speech evaluation of nippling status Infant apnea program for home monitor evaluation	------------------------> ------------------------> ------------------------> Ophthalmology exam prior to day of d/c unless critical exam	------------------------> ------------------------> ------------------------>

Courtesy of Fairfax Hospital, INOVA Health System, Falls Church, VA.

Fairfax Hospital, Falls Church, Virginia

NICU CLINICAL PATHWAY
TERM INFANT, SUSPECT SEPSIS - SIMPLE AND COMPLEX

Patient Name__________ M.R. Number__________
Date Clinical Path Initiated__________ Anticipated LOS__________
Admission Date__________ Discharge Date__________ Actual LOS__________

This care path is a guideline and is not intended to create a standard of care. This guideline may be modified based on individual patient's needs.

	Day 1	Day 2	Day 3	Day 4 - Discharge
Tests/ Procedures	Blood C&S CBC on adm & repeat as ordered Urine GBS Ag - collect per order Metabolic screen per order If mild RDS: Blood gas Chest x-ray AP Lytes, Ca, BUN if IV fluids If LP done: CSF for gram stain, cell count, differential, protein, glucose Blood glucose for any CBGD <45	CBC If IV fluids: Lytes, Ca, BUN qam D/C when off fluids If stable, no IV & no O_2 Schedule circ Gentamicin trough/peak levels with 3rd dose	Obtain culture results CBC & bilirubin ------------------------->	Expected outcome: Cultures negative CBC WNL ------------------------->

Continued on following page

	Day 1	Day 2	Day 3	Day 4 - Discharge
Treatments	CR monitor, pulse oximeter HC & length q week Daily weights If simple R/O sepsis & no IV fluids: Admit to isolette/warmer; wean to open crib when temp 97^8 - 99 VS on adm & at 1°, then q3-4° AC Assessment q8-12° BP on adm & at 1°, then q 8-12° if stable & mean ≥40 Heplock, neonatal flush q3-6° CBGD on adm & AC x1 CBGD at 1° if <4° old If complex R/O sepsis with mild RDS +/- O_2: Admit to warmer; move to isolette when stable VS on adm & at 1°, then as ordered Assessment q3-6° until stable, then q8-12° BP q1° until stable & mean ≥40, then as ordered CBGD on adm, then q6-8° if stable CBGD at 1° if <4° old O_2 orders pr Resp. flowsheet Adjust O_2 to maintain Sats at 92-96%	D/C monitors when transferred to FCC --------------------------> --------------------------> VS q6-8° if stable in open crib --------------------------> D/C BP if stable & mean ≥40 --------------------------> Move to open crib when stable; no IV & no IV fluids --------------------------> BP QD if stable & mean ≥40 CBGD QD until IV fluids D/C'd -------------------------->	--------------------------> --------------------------> --------------------------> --------------------------> --------------------------> D/C Heplock when antibiotics D/C'd --------------------------> --------------------------> D/C BP's if stable & mean ≥40 --------------------------> -------------------------->	--------------------------> --------------------------> --------------------------> Expected outcome: VS, BP and assessment WNL --------------------------> --------------------------> --------------------------> --------------------------> -------------------------->
Medications	Erythromycin to eyes (if not done) Vit K 1mgm IM (if not done) Ampicillin IV q12° per order Gentamicin IV q12° per order	Day 2 antibiotics	Day 3 antibiotics Assess need for longer course ABx If home ABx Rx: Adjust adm times If q8°: 7-3-10 IF q12°: 8, 9 or 10	Day 4 antibiotics If home ABx Rx: Change heplock site Expected outcome: Well functioning heplock
Nutrition	If simple R/O sepsis & no IV fluids: Start po feedings when awake, hungry & bowel sounds present Brfeed/mother's choice formula q3-4° ad lib NPO no longer than 6° If complex R/O sepsis with mild RDS, IV fluids, +/- O_2: NPO, strict I&O, SG & dipstick urine q12° PIV - $D_{10}W$ (80cc/Kg) per order if <24° old - $D_{10}E_{48}$ (100cc/Kg) per order if >24° old	Advance feedings as tolerated q3-4° Begin feedings when stable per order	--------------------------> Advance feedings as tolerated q3-4° D/C IV fluids per order when tolerating full feeds	Expected outcomes: Nipple feeds well with minimal support Tolerates brmilk/formula
Consults	Notify pediatrician & OB of admission Social work evaluation for possible home ABx Rx Lactation consultant as needed	--------------------------> -------------------------->	--------------------------> -------------------------->	--------------------------> -------------------------->

Fairfax Hospital, Falls Church, Virginia

NICU CLINICAL PATHWAY

TERM INFANT, SUSPECT SEPSIS - SIMPLE AND COMPLEX **(continued)**

Patient Name____________________ M.R. Number____________

Date Clinical Path Initiated____________________ Anticipated LOS____________

Admission Date____________ Discharge Date____________ Actual LOS____________

This care path is a guideline and is not intended to create a standard of care. This guideline may be modified based on individual patient's needs.

	Day 1	**Day 2**	**Day 3**	**Day 4 - Discharge**
Patient Teaching	Orient family to unit Begin instruction of disease process Begin family involvement in baby care when possible Implement discharge teaching	Begin return demos of baby care Review circ care	Complete D/C teaching	Outcome: Teaching completed by day of discharge
Discharge Planning	Notify pediatrician & OB of admission Screen for pediatric clinic eligibility Assess readiness for transfer to FCC Begin home/financial assessment for possible home ABx Rx	If no ped, discuss need with family & assist as appropriate -------------------------> Transfer to FCC when: Feedings tolerated No IV fluids No apnea/bradycardia Temp 97^{8} - 99 Resp rate <70 Stabilized CBC Discuss anticipated d/c with family Refer to public health liaison nurse if appropriate Make referral to appropriate home health agency as soon as possible Advise agency IV RN of need for pre-discharge assessment	Identify home follow-up appointments needed -------------------------> If home ABx Rx: Write d/c orders Arrange for a.m. d/c time with family	Expected outcomes: Pediatrician identified If pediatric clinic eligible, 1st appointment made and given to family -------------------------> Expected outcomes: D/C on home ABx Rx with appropraiate home followup If no ABx Rx: D/C to home when: Feedings tolerated No IV fluids No apnea/bradycardia Temp stable in open crib Resp rate <70 Stabilized CBC No signs/symptoms of sepsis

Courtesy of Fairfax Hospital, INOVA Health System, Falls Church, VA.

Fairfax Hospital, Falls Church, Virginia

INOVA HOME INFUSION
CLINICAL PATHWAYS FOR PEDIATRIC HOME IV THERAPY
TERM INFANT: SUSPECT SEPSIS - UNCOMPLICATED

Patient Name: ____________ Admission Date:__________ Anticipated LOS_____ Days
See Problem List:

	VISIT DAY 0 (PREDISCHARGE VISIT)__________	ADMISSION VISIT DATE _____	VISIT 2 DATE ________	VISIT 3 DATE ___ ___	D/C VISIT DATE __ _____
CONSULTS/ COORDINA-TION OF CARE	• ASSESSMENT AND EVALUATION FOR HOME IV CARE PRIOR TO HOSPITAL DISCHARGE. • OBTAIN CULTURE RESULTS. • AUTHORIZATION AND CONSENT. • COMMUNICATE TO FIELD OFFICE RE: FREQUENCE OF VISITS AND DURATION. • COMPLETION OF ADMISSION PACKET. • IDENTIFY LABS TO BE DRAWN AT HOME. INITIAL _____	• LABS IF ORDERED. • F/U W/RESULTS TO PMD AND/OR NEONATOLOGIST. • CONSULT WITH PHARMACY FOR DRUG INTER-ACTION AND REVIEW ALLERGY HISTORY. INITIAL _____	• CONSULT WITH PMD PRIOR TO INSERTING SCALP IV. • CONSULT WITH PEDIATRIC SUPERVISOR IF UNABLE TO RESTART IV PRIOR TO GIVING IM. INITIAL _____	• DISCUSS WITH FAMILY ANY CHANGES IN IV HOME THERAPY. • NOTIFY CLINICAL COORDIN-ATOR AND CASE MANAGER OF CHANGES. INITIAL _____	• F/U WITH HOME PHOTO-THERAPY IF NEEDED. • NOTIFY IHI CLINICAL COORDINA-TOR, PHARMACY, REFERRING PHYSICIAN, PMD AND INSURANCE COMPANY OF DISCHARGE. INITIAL _____

Care Tracs do not represent a standard of care. They are designed to serve as guidelines and may be modified to meet individual patient needs.

	VISIT DAY 0 (PREDISCHARGE VISIT)__________	ADMISSION VISIT DATE ______	VISIT 2 DATE ________ -	VISIT 3 DATE ___ ___	D/C VISIT DATE __ ______
TREATMENT/ CARE	• ADMISSION PHYSICAL ASSESSMENT COMPLETE. • IDENTIFY LABS TO TO BE DRAWN AT HOME • ASSESS IV ACCESS. INITIAL ______	• VITAL SIGNS AND ASSESSMENT OF VISIT. • BP A DAY. • LABS AS ORDERED. • INITIATE HOME PHOTOTHERAPY PRN. INITIAL ______	• ASSESS IV PATENCY Q VISIT. • ASSESS COMPLIANCE WITH HOME PHOTOTHERAPY REGIME IF INITIATED. INITIAL ______	INITIAL ______	• DISCONTINUE IV HEPARIN LOCK AFTER LAST DOSE OF ANTIBIOTIC. INITIAL ______
DIET	• OBTAIN BIRTHWEIGHT AND D/C WEIGHT • ASSESS FEEDING ROUTINE INITIAL ____	• OBTAIN WEIGHT QD • ASSESS I&O • ASSESS BREAST FEEDING OR BOTTLE FEEDING ABILITIES. INITIAL ______	------------------------->$ ------------------------->$ ------------------------->$ INITIAL ______	--------------------->$ --------------------->$ INITIAL ______	• REFER TO COMMUNITY LACTATION CONSULTANT FOR UNRESOLVED ISSUES. INITIAL ______

Continued on following page

INOVA HOME INFUSION
CLINICAL PATHWAYS FOR PEDIATRIC HOME IV THERAPY
TERM INFANT: SUSPECT SEPSIS - UNCOMPLICATED (continued)

Patient Name: ____________ Admission Date:________ Anticipated LOS_____ Days
See Problem List:

	VISIT DAY 0 (PREDISCHARGE VISIT)__________	ADMISSION VISIT DATE ______	VISIT 2 DATE ________ -	VISIT 3 DATE ___ ___	D/C VISIT DATE __ _____
MEDICATIONS	• ASSESS FEASIBILITY OF MEDICATION TIME FOR HOME THERAPY. • CALCULATE APPROPRIATE DOSE BASED ON WEIGHT AND INDICATION. • REVIEW PHARMACY CARE PLAN. • VERIFY DRUG MONOGRAPH RECEIPT. • OBTAIN ONE X ORDER FOR IM IF IV OUT. INITIAL _____	• AMPICILLIN_____ MG IV Q 12 • GENTAMICIN_____ MG IV Q 12 • ROCEPHIN______ MG IV Q____ • CLAFORAN______ MG IV Q____ • ASSESS FOR ADVERSITY/ INTERACTION/EF FICACY. • EDUCATE PARENT/CAREGIV ER ABOUT ANTIBIOTIC S/E. INITIAL _____	• ASSESS COMPLI-ANCE WITH MEDICATION REGIME. • REPORT TO PHARMACIST AND IVT COORDINATOR DEVIATIONS FROM PHARMACY CARE PLAN. INITIAL _____	• EVALUATE ONGOING LAB RESULTS AND THERA-PEUTIC RESPONSE TO ANTIBIOTIC THERAPY. INITIAL _____	→ → INITIAL _____
DISCHARGE PLANNING PSYCHO-SOCIAL	• DISCUSS WITH LIAISONS COMMUNITY REFERRALS MADE AND NEEDED. • ASCERTAIN FAMILY PLANS FOR PMD F/U. • IF APPROPRIATE, F/U WITH DR. KELLY AT FAIRFAX HOSPITAL PEDIATRIC CLINIC. INITIAL _____	• DISCUSS PLAN FOR LENGTH OF HOME CARE. • REFER PRN TO PERINATAL OUTREACH/COM MUNITY SERVICES F/U WITH FAMILY. • PMD APPOINT-MENT WITHIN 7-10 DAYS OF DISCHARGE. INITIAL _____	----------------------------> INITIAL _____	---------------------> INITIAL _____	• DISCHARGE SUMMARY TO MD. • FOLLOW UP APPT. ESTABLISHED WITH PMD. INITIAL _____

	VISIT DAY 0 (PREDISCHARGE VISIT)___________	ADMISSION VISIT DATE ______	VISIT 2 DATE ________ -	VISIT 3 DATE ___ ___	D/C VISIT DATE __ ______
TEACHING	• DISCUSS WITH THE FAMILY THE ROLE OF THE HOME RN AND FAMILY RESPONSIBILITIES • INQUIRE IF PATIENT HAS QUESTIONS REGARDING MEDICATION MONOGRAPH • REVIEW CARE PLAN WITH FAMILY/ CAREGIVER. INITIAL _____	• ORIENT FAMILY TO INOVA HOME INFUSION. • ASSESS PARENTS' ABILITY TO CARE FOR CIRCUM-CISION/WELL BABY/PHOTO THERAPY INITIAL _____	INITIAL _____	--------------------- > --------------------- > INITIAL ______	• PARENTS VERBALIZE D/C INSTRUCTIONS RE: 1. EDUCATION LITERATURE. 2. EMERGENCY ASSISTANCE. 3. POST D/C HOME ISSUES. INITIAL ______

Courtesy of Fairfax Hospital, INOVA Health System, Falls Church, VA.

Fairfax Hospital, Falls Church, Virginia

INOVA HOME HEALTH INFUSION
PEDIATRIC HOME IV THERAPY TERM INFANT, SUSPECT SEPSIS - UNCOMPLICATED OUTCOMES

Patient:____________________ **ID #** ____________________

OUTCOME	DATE	SIGNATURE
DISCHARGE FROM INOVA HOME INFUSION WITHOUT IV COMPLICATIONS		
NO SIGNS/SYMPTOMS OF SEPSIS		
APPROPRIATE HOME ENVIRONMENT FOR WELL BABY		
NO ADVERSE REACTIONS TO ANTIBIOTIC THERAPY		
FOLLOW UP APPOINTMENT WITH PEDIATRICIAN ESTABLISHED AT D/C		

Courtesy of Fairfax Hospital, INOVA Health System, Falls Church, VA.

LUMC PERINATAL NETWORK
REFERRAL HOSPITAL: ________________

COLLABORATIVE CAREPATH: **ACUTELY ILL NEONATAL TRANSPORT**

LOYOLA
UNIVERSITY
MEDICAL CENTER
AD · MAJOREM · DEI · GLORIAM 1870
Loyola University Chicago

Patient: ________________ Date/Time of Birth: ________________

Neonatologist/Pediatrician: ________________ Infant Apgars: ________________

Referring Obstetrician: ________________ Gestational Age: ________________

Referral Hospital Phone #: ________________ Maternal Gravida/Parity: ________________

Date: Time:	TRANSFER **ACCEPTED** (TIME_____) UNTIL TEAM ARRIVES	TEAM **ARRIVAL** (TIME_______)	TEAM **DEPARTURE** (TIME_______)	DISCHARGE OUTCOMES
Care Unit:	LEVEL II NURSERY			Safe transport.
Consults/Physicians:	Neonatology/Pediatrician Written transfer order			Follow-up for return transport criteria.
Tests: **(Check all that were done)**	_CBC _Blood Cultures _Blood Type/Coomb _Blood Gases _Glucose (serum) _Newborn Screen (PKU, etc.) _Mother's Maiden Name:__________ _Mother's Social Security #:__________ _Urine CIE _Urine Toxicology _Surface Cultures _CXR _X-ray post tube/line placement **OTHER:** ________________			Values available at time of transfer, except cultures.
Treatment/ Procedures: **(Check all that were done)**	_Resuscitation: _O2 _Bag/ Mask _Compressions _Medications _Intubation Tube size ____ Cm at lip line ____ _Surfactant Time________ Type__________ _Umbilical Line _Chest Tube _Lumbar Puncture		Complete newborn identification verification.	Infant stable for transport post treatment intervention and identification.
Activity:	**Skin Care:** Utilize pectin based barriers under any/all tape (i.e. E.T., Umbilical lines, NG, etc.). Use of bowel bag (Vi-drape) for abdominal defects.			Skin integrity will be maintained.
Nutrition:	Intake: IV fluid______________ Rate__________ enteric (type)______________ Output: Urine: Mother desires: _ Breast/ _ Bottle Stool: Blood: Other:		TOTALS: Intake: Output:	Promote optimal maintenance of hydration/ nutrition.

Continued on following page

Nutrition:	**Intake:** IV fluid__________ Rate________ IV lock in place, Last flushed:__________ Milk used:________ Route: _CNG _intermittent _ng _po/ng _po _ad lib Feeding amount:________ Feeding frequency: q______ Last feeding time:________ Feeding issues: Emesis Reflux Residuals Other:______ Breast: _Mom pumping _Attempted at breast _Breastfeeding well _Breastmilk supply brought with patient **Output:** Last Void: __________ Last Stool:__________ Problems:__________ Other:__________		Promote optimal maintenance of hydration/ nutrition.
Assessment & Monitoring:	Head circumference:______ Abdominal circumference:____ Chest circumference:______ Length:________ V/S frequency:______ Last V/S: T___ P___ R___ B/P___ Pulse oximeter: _None _Continuous _Intermittent Pulse oximetry 02 Saturation range: ____ to ____ Other:__________		Stabilization for a safe transport.
Expected Outcomes:	Transfer Summary (history) prepared. _Brought with infant _To be faxed	Transfer Summary endorsed. Level II admission documentation initiated.	Hospitalization history endorsed for safe transition of care.
Psychosocial & Educational Needs: Patient & Family <u>(Check those applicable)</u>	Parent contact history endorsed. Parent competencies achieved: _bath _temperature taking _diapering _feeding _CPR _Other:________	Parent involvement and competencies endorsed to Level II. Personal belongings accepted by Level II.	Patient and family needs are met. Orientate parents to unit.
Discharge Plan:	Pediatrician identified ________ Neonatal Follow-up Clinic Appointment ________ Ophthalmology Follow-up Appointment ________ Other Follow-up needs: ________	Infant admitted to Level II for ongoing care and discharge planning.	Safe transport and appropriate documentation completed.

REFERRAL HOSPITAL R.N. (INITIALS) __________ (____) TRANSFER HOSPITAL R.N. (INITIALS) __________ (____)

REFERRAL HOSPITAL R.N. (INITIALS) __________ (____) TRANSFER HOSPITAL R.N. (INITIALS) __________ (____)

REFERRAL HOSPITAL M.D. ______________

This care path is a guideline and is not intended to create a standard of care. This guideline may be modified based on individual patient's needs.

Courtesy of Loyola University Medical Center, Maywood, IL.

LUMC PERINATAL NETWORK
LOYOLA UNIVERSITY MEDICAL CENTER
Maywood, Illinois

AD · MAJOREM · DEI · GLORIAM 1870
LOYOLA UNIVERSITY MEDICAL CENTER
Loyola University Chicago

COLLABORATIVE CAREPATH: NEONATAL RETURN TRANSPORT

Patient: ____________ Gestational age @ Birth:________ DOL:________ Date: ____________

Birthweight:____________ Current Weight:____________ Diagnosis:____________ Current Condition:____________

Accepting Neonatologist/Pediatrician: ____________ Referring Neonatologist:____________

Accepting Hospital:____________ Accepting Hospital Phone #: ____________

Date: Time:	TRANSFER TIME AGREED UPON (TIME_____)	TIME TEAM ARRIVED AT LEVEL II (TIME____)	DISCHARGE OUTCOMES
Care Unit:	LEVEL III NURSERY	LEVEL II NURSERY	Safe transport.
Communication:	Nurse verifies consent for transfer. Nurse to Nurse report. Parent notification of tentative transfer time. Parent given Level II phone number.	Infant identification process completed.	Return transport and infant identification safely completed.
Tests: (Check all that are done)	_Newborn Screen (PKU, etc.) Date:________ _Hearing Screen Date:________ _Pass/_Fail _Eye Exam Date:________ Follow-up:__________ _Last Hematocrit Date:________ Result:__________ _Drug Levels ____________ _Other pertinent Labs (i.e. toxicology screen, blood cultures, blood gases, etc.) ____________ ____________		Values available and endorsed at time of transfer, except newborn screen.
Treatment/ Procedures: (Check those applicable)	Environment: _Open Crib _Isolette (bed temperature ___) _Warmer Respiratory Support: _None _02____% _NC____L flow _Hood _CPAP +___ _Other: (Circumcision,etc.)__________ ____________		Infant stable for transport post treatment intervention and identification.
Medications: (list current medications)	MEDICATION DOSE ROUTE FREQUENCY LAST DOSE ________ ____ ______ ________ ________ ________ ____ ______ ________ ________ ________ ____ ______ ________ ________ ________ ____ ______ ________ ________ If antibiotic, list day of treatment_____/anticipated length of treatment______ _Immunization card provided to referral hospital		Endorsement of medication plan.
Activity: (Check those applicable)	_Reflux precautions. _Kangaroo care. _Apnea and bradycardia status. _Other:____________ ____________		Outlined activities will be maintained.

Continued on following page

Nutrition:	**Intake:** IV fluid__________ Rate________ IV lock in place, Last flushed:__________ Milk used:________ Route: _CNG _intermittent _ng _po/ng _po _ad lib Feeding amount:________ Feeding frequency: q______ Last feeding time:________ Feeding issues: Emesis Reflux Residuals Other:________ Breast: _Mom pumping _Attempted at breast _Breastfeeding well _Breastmilk supply brought with patient **Output:** Last Void: __________ Last Stool:__________ Problems:__________ Other:__________		Promote optimal maintenance of hydration/ nutrition.
Assessment & Monitoring:	Head circumference:______ Abdominal circumference:______ Chest circumference:______ Length:________ V/S frequency:________ Last V/S: T___ P___ R___ B/P___ Pulse oximeter: _None _Continuous _Intermittent Pulse oximetry 02 Saturation range: _____ to _____ Other:__________		Stabilization for a safe transport.
Expected Outcomes:	Transfer Summary (history) prepared. _Brought with infant _To be faxed	Transfer Summary endorsed. Level II admission documentation initiated.	Hospitalization history endorsed for safe transition of care.
Psychosocial & Educational Needs: Patient & Family <u>(Check those applicable)</u>	Parent contact history endorsed. Parent competencies achieved: _bath _temperature taking _diapering _feeding _CPR _Other:________ ________	Parent involvement and competencies endorsed to Level II. Personal belongings accepted by Level II.	Patient and family needs are met. Orientate parents to unit.
Discharge Plan:	Pediatrician identified ________ Neonatal Follow-up Clinic Appointment ________ Ophthalmology Follow-up Appointment ________ Other Follow-up needs: ________ ________	Infant admitted to Level II for ongoing care and discharge planning.	Safe transport and appropriate documentation completed.

REFERRAL HOSPITAL R.N. (INITIALS) __________ (____) **TRANSFER HOSPITAL R.N. (INITIALS)** __________ (____)

REFERRAL HOSPITAL R.N. (INITIALS) __________ (____) **TRANSFER HOSPITAL R.N. (INITIALS)** __________ (____)

REFERRAL HOSPITAL M.D. ______________

This care path is a guideline and is not intended to create a standard of care. This guideline may be modified based on individual patient's needs.

Courtesy of Loyola University Medical Center, Maywood, IL.

Appendix II

AWHONN's Standards for the Nursing Care of Women and Newborns

UNIVERSAL NURSING PRACTICE STANDARDS

STANDARD I NURSING PRACTICE

Comprehensive nursing care for women and newborns focuses on helping individuals, families, and communities achieve their optimum health potential. This is best achieved within the framework of the nursing process.

The nurse is responsible for decisions and actions within the domain of nursing practice, which may include

- integration of the nursing process components of assessment, planning, implementation, and evaluation in all areas of nursing practice;
- individualization and prioritization of nursing care to meet the physical, psychological, spiritual, and social needs of patients;
- collaboration with the individual, family, and other members of the health-care team;
- promotion of a safe and therapeutic environment for both the recipients and providers of nursing care;
- demonstration and validation of competence in nursing practice;
- acquisition of specialized knowledge and skills and additional formal education to provide specialized care; and
- provision for complete and accurate documentation of care.

The written or computerized patient record is the documented means of communication among all members of the health-care team. It also promotes continuity of care and provides a mechanism for evaluating care. The record should contain accurate and complete recordings of the patient's history and physical examination as well as the nursing plan of care, including goals, interventions, health education, and evaluation of patient and family responses. Additional documentation may include planned follow-up and appropriate referrals. All information contained in the patient record and related to the care of the patient and family is confidential and should be released only according to institutional policy.

Note: To apply this universal standard to a specific area of gynecologic, obstetric, or neonatal nursing practice, refer directly to the specialty-specific nursing practice standards section.

STANDARD II HEALTH EDUCATION AND COUNSELING

Health education for the individual, family, and community is an integral part of comprehensive nursing care. Such education encourages participation in, and shared responsibility for, health promotion, maintenance, and restoration.

Comprehensive health education includes

- identification of the needs and abilities of the learner;
- collaboration with the patient and other health-care providers in design, content, and follow-up of the educational plan;
- provision of accurate and current information;
- provision of information based on educationally sound principles of teaching and learning;
- recognition of patient rights, responsibilities, and alternative choices;
- utilization of available educational resources in the practice environment;
- utilization of available educational resources to provide health education information to individuals/families in the community; and
- documentation and evaluation of health education including patient response.

The nurse participates in and/or coordinates the health education and counseling process. It begins with the initial patient contact or admission to the unit or service and is an ongoing, continuous process.

Note: To apply this universal standard to a specific area of gynecologic, obstetric, or neonatal nursing practice, refer directly to the specialty-specific nursing practice standards section.

STANDARD III
POLICIES, PROCEDURES, AND PROTOCOLS

Written policies, procedures, and protocols clarify the scope of nursing practice and delineate the qualifications of personnel authorized to provide care to women and newborns within the health-care setting.

The components of policies, procedures, and protocols are based on

- recognition of the organization's philosophy;
- recognition of the unit's philosophy;
- coordination with the overall mission of the organization;
- assessment of the practice setting and determination of types of services to be provided;
- incorporation of a multidisciplinary approach in their development;
- identification of specific areas of practice to be addressed;
- reflection of current practice, standards, and local regulations; and
- anticipated use as references for health-care providers, orientation of new personnel and students, quality assurance activities, and/or guiding nursing actions in emergency situations.

The development of policies, procedures, and protocols should include consideration of staff availability, skill, and licensure; the physical plant and equipment; effects on other departments; and fiscal impact. Policies, procedures, and protocols should be reviewed and revised at least on an annual basis or more frequently as science/technology changes.

Note: To apply this universal standard to a specific area of gynecologic, obstetric, or neonatal nursing practice, refer directly to the specialty-specific nursing practice standards section.

STANDARD IV
PROFESSIONAL RESPONSIBILITY AND ACCOUNTABILITY

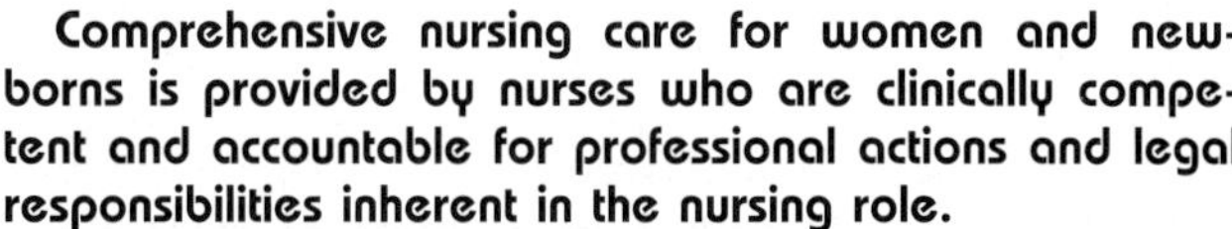

Comprehensive nursing care for women and newborns is provided by nurses who are clinically competent and accountable for professional actions and legal responsibilities inherent in the nursing role.

Responsibility and accountability for knowledge and competence in nursing practice for women and newborns include

- awareness of changing practices and professional and ethical issues;
- knowledge and clinical skills gained through inservice education, professional continuing education, research data, and professional literature;
- implementation of newly acquired knowledge and skills;
- collaboration through networking and sharing with other professionals;
- participation in the development of standards and policies, procedures, and protocols;
- participation with professional committees within the institution;
- participation in periodic peer- and self-evaluations; and
- recognition of certification as one mechanism for the demonstration of special knowledge within a specialty area of practice.

Legal accountability extends to the

- nurse practice acts;
- parameters of professional practice established by professional organizations;
- institutional standards;
- legislative changes that affect practice; and
- policies, procedures, and protocols within the practice environment.

STANDARD V UTILIZATION OF NURSING PERSONNEL

Nursing care for women and newborns is conducted in practice settings that have qualified nursing staff in sufficient numbers to meet patient-care needs.

Each practice setting should have sufficient nursing personnel to meet patient-care requirements. Nursing staff who provide direct care to women and newborns should be supervised by registered nurses who are clinically proficient in the specialty area of practice. The patient-care unit or service is managed by a professional nurse who is prepared educationally and clinically to assume a leadership position. In all practice settings, the nurse may practice independently or collaboratively with other health-care team members. It is essential that nurses know both the responsibilities and the limitations of professional nursing practice specific to the practice setting.

Many variables are considered in determining both the number and type of nursing staff needed for a practice setting. Among these variables are those related to the patient, practice, organization, and personnel.

Patient-related variables may include

- patient demographics and acuity of patients served;
- length of stay;
- educational needs;
- cultural factors and level of comprehension;
- communication barriers; and
- discharge or home-care needs.

Practice-related variables may include

- difference in educational and experiential level of nursing staff;
- nursing philosophy;
- type of nursing-care delivery system;
- use of assistive personnel;
- use of nurses in expanded roles; and
- participation in teaching programs.

Organizational variables may include

- scope of services provided;
- availability of support services;
- patient volume;
- mission or philosophy of the organization;
- risk-management concerns;
- quality assurance programs;
- policies, procedures, and protocols;
- physical plant;
- marketing strategies; and
- fiscal considerations.

Personnel variables relate to the type and number of professional and nonprofessional staff and may include

- education, skill, and experience of the nursing leadership;
- educational preparation, skill, and experience of staff;
- types and mix of nursing staff;
- availability of qualified alternative staff to deal with emergencies or unanticipated volumes;
- distribution of staff, e.g., temporary reassignment, floating, on-call, cross-training, and supplemental staffing;
- responsibilities for orientation, precepting, or students;
- turnover rates; and
- clerical and technical support.

Competency-based job descriptions should be available for each level of nursing staff. Orientation for all personnel should include a general overview of the organization and specific information about the individual practice setting. Performance evaluations for all personnel should be conducted, documented, and discussed on a regular basis with input from the individual, colleagues, and supervisory staff.

STANDARD VI ETHICS

Ethical principles guide the process of decision making for nurses caring for women and newborns at all times and especially when personal or professional values conflict with those of the patient, family, colleagues, or practice setting.

The nurse should have the opportunity to participate in the ethical decision-making process. To participate actively, nurses should

- clarify their own personal and professional values;
- recognize the difficulty in selecting a course of action that is morally and ethically acceptable to all parties;
- communicate openly and assertively;
- identify options; and
- seek consultations.

Nurses must carefully examine their own value systems since values influence the decision-making process. Opportunities should be provided in the practice setting for discussion of potential ethical issues. Each practice setting should have a framework for decision making regarding bioethical dilemmas. Ethical dilemmas generally arise when there is a conflict between loyalties, rights, duties, or values.

For nurses, most ethical dilemmas occur when there is a real or perceived requirement to act in a manner contrary to personal values or when care ordered or provided does not seem compatible with the best interest of the patient. Common areas of concern may include

- nursing autonomy and decision making;
- maternal interests versus fetal interests;
- issues of duty, obligation, and loyalty (for example, employer to employee, professional to public, professional to professional);
- patients' rights to resources, privacy, confidentiality, information, participation in decision making, and refusal of therapy;
- the right to live or die;
- life cycle concerns, including contraception, sterilization, pregnancy termination, genetic manipulation, infanticide, sexuality and choices of life style, and euthanasia;
- fetal or neonatal conditions incompatible with life;
- fetal tissue use; and
- biomedical intervention.

The bioethics literature can provide nurses with strategies to cope with or resolve decisions in situations when conflicts of values occur. For ethical decision-making frameworks to be applied to practice situations, working relationships must be established in which individuals may express their own points of view. All persons potentially affected by an ethical decision have the right to participate in the decision-making process.

STANDARD VII RESEARCH

Nurses caring for women and newborns utilize research findings, conduct nursing research, and evaluate nursing practice to improve the outcomes of care.

Knowledge of the research process and participation in scientific inquiry are necessary to

- conduct or participate in the conduct of research according to ethical guidelines;
- use research findings to provide appropriate and safe nursing care;
- use research findings as a basis for validating standards of nursing care;
- evaluate the relevance and application of research findings from nursing and related disciplines; and
- validate the effect of nursing practice on patient outcomes.

STANDARD VIII QUALITY ASSURANCE

Quality and appropriateness of patient care are evaluated through a planned assessment program using specific, identified clinical indicators.

Each unit or service should have a written quality assurance plan that reflects a philosophy that is coordinated with the organization's mission and overall quality assurance program. Objectives of the unit-based or service-based quality assurance plan should include

- assurance of consistent quality patient outcomes;
- identification and correction of potential nursing practice deficiencies;
- promotion of professional nursing practice based on appropriate nursing standards; and
- education and participation of staff in quality assurance activities.

The unit nurse manager is responsible for developing and implementing the unit-based quality assurance plan. The plan should include

- responsibilities of all personnel in the quality assurance process;
- the scope of service provided;
- important aspects of care or service involving high-risk, high-volume, and problem-prone patients or activities;
- clinical indicators or measurable standards that affect the aspects of care and service that have been identified as important;
- specific criteria and thresholds for use in monitoring clinical indicators;
- methods for the collection and analysis of data, including reference to collection tools, sample size, time frame, and staff responsibility;
- determination of appropriate corrective action, when indicated, that will fall into one of three categories: educational, organizational, or behavioral change;
- follow-up assessment of identified problems;
- documentation of all aspects of the quality assurance program, including results; and
- a process for communication related to quality assurance activities within the total organization.

From *NAACOG standards for the nursing care of women and newborns* (4th ed.). Washington, DC: NAACOG, 1991.

Appendix III

NANDA Approved Nursing Diagnoses

NORTH AMERICAN NURSING DIAGNOSIS ASSOCIATION (NANDA) 1994 APPROVED NURSING DIAGNOSES FOR CLINICAL USE AND TESTING

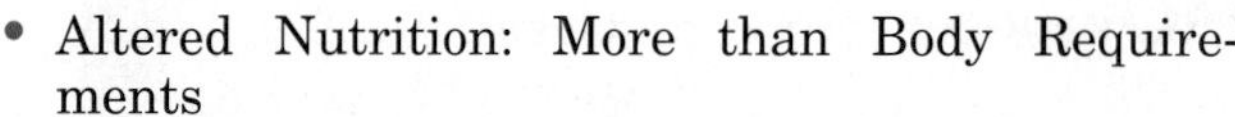

PATTERN 1 EXCHANGING

- Altered Nutrition: More than Body Requirements
- Altered Nutrition: Less than Body Requirements
- Altered Nutrition: Potential for More than Body Requirements
- Risk for Infection
- Risk for Altered Body Temperature
- Hypothermia
- Hyperthermia
- Ineffective Thermoregulation
- Dysreflexia
- Constipation
- Perceived Constipation
- Colonic Constipation
- Diarrhea
- Bowel Incontinence
- Altered Urinary Elimination
- Stress Incontinence
- Reflex Incontinence
- Urge Incontinence
- Functional Incontinence
- Total Incontinence
- Urinary Retention
- Altered (Specify Type) Tissue Perfusion (Renal, Cerebral, Cardiopulmonary, Gastrointestinal, Peripheral)
- Fluid Volume Excess
- Fluid Volume Deficit
- Risk for Fluid Volume Deficit
- Decreased Cardiac Output
- Impaired Gas Exchange
- Ineffective Airway Clearance
- Ineffective Breathing Pattern
- Inability to Sustain Spontaneous Ventilation
- Dysfunctional Ventilatory Weaning Response
- Risk for Injury
- Risk for Suffocation
- Risk for Poisoning
- Risk for Trauma
- Risk for Aspiration
- Risk for Disuse Syndrome
- Altered Protection
- Impaired Tissue Integrity
- Altered Oral Mucous Membrane
- Impaired Skin Integrity
- Risk for Impaired Skin Integrity
- Decreased Adaptive Capacity: Intracranial
- Energy Field Disturbance

PATTERN 2 COMMUNICATING

- Impaired Verbal Communication

PATTERN 3 RELATING

- Impaired Social Interaction
- Social Isolation
- Risk for Loneliness
- Altered Role Performance
- Altered Parenting
- Risk for Altered Parenting
- Risk for Altered Parent/Infant/Child Attachment
- Sexual Dysfunction
- Altered Family Processes
- Caregiver Role Strain
- Risk for Caregiver Role Strain
- Altered Family Process: Alcoholism
- Parental Role Conflict
- Altered Sexuality Patterns

PATTERN 4 VALUING

- Spiritual Distress (Distress of the Human Spirit)
- Potential for Enhanced Spiritual Well-Being

PATTERN 5 CHOOSING

- Ineffective Individual Coping
- Impaired Adjustment
- Defensive Coping
- Ineffective Denial
- Ineffective Family Coping: Disabling
- Ineffective Family Coping: Compromised
- Family Coping: Potential for Growth
- Potential for Enhanced Community Coping
- Ineffective Community Coping
- Ineffective Management of Therapeutic Regimen: Individuals
- Noncompliance (Specify)
- Ineffective Management of Therapeutic Regimen: Families
- Ineffective Management of Therapeutic Regimen: Community
- Ineffective Management of Therapeutic Regimen: Individual
- Decisional Conflict (Specify)
- Health Seeking Behaviors (Specify)

PATTERN 6 MOVING

- Impaired Physical Mobility
- Risk for Peripheral Neurovascular Dysfunction
- Risk for Perioperative Positioning Injury
- Activity Intolerance
- Fatigue
- Risk for Activity Intolerance
- Sleep Pattern Disturbance
- Diversional Activity Deficit
- Impaired Home Maintenance Management
- Altered Health Maintenance
- Feeding Self-Care Deficit
- Impaired Swallowing
- Ineffective Breastfeeding
- Interrupted Breastfeeding
- Effective Breastfeeding
- Ineffective Infant Feeding Pattern
- Bathing/Hygiene Self-Care Deficit
- Dressing/Grooming Self-Care Deficit
- Toileting Self-Care Deficit
- Altered Growth and Development

- Relocation Stress Syndrome
- Risk for Disorganized Infant Behavior
- Disorganized Infant Behavior
- Potential for Enhanced Organized Infant Behavior

PATTERN 7 PERCEIVING

- Body Image Disturbance
- Self-Esteem Disturbance
- Chronic Low Self-Esteem
- Situational Low Self-Esteem
- Personal Identity Disturbance
- Sensory/Perceptual Alterations (Specify) (Visual, Auditory, Kinesthetic, Gustatory, Tactile, Olfactory)
- Unilateral Neglect
- Hopelessness
- Powerlessness

PATTERN 8 KNOWING

- Knowledge Deficit (Specify)
- Impaired Environmental Interpretation Syndrome
- Acute Confusion
- Chronic Confusion
- Altered Thought Process
- Impaired Memory

PATTERN 9 FEELING

- Pain
- Chronic Pain
- Dysfunctional Grieving
- Anticipatory Grieving
- Risk for Violence: Self-Directed or Directed at Others
- Risk for Self-Mutilation
- Post-Trauma Response
- Rape-Trauma Syndrome
- Rape-Trauma Syndrome: Compound Reaction
- Rape-Trauma Syndrome: Silent Reaction
- Anxiety
- Fear

From NANDA. (1994). *Nursing diagnoses: Definitions and classification 1995–1996.* Philadelphia: Author. Reprinted with permission.

IV Appendix

The Pregnant Patient's Bill of Rights and the Pregnant Patient's Responsibilities

THE PREGNANT PATIENT'S BILL OF RIGHTS

The pregnant patient has the right to participate in decisions involving her well-being and that of her unborn child, unless there is a clear-cut medical emergency that prevents her participation. In addition to the rights set forth in the American Hospital Association's "Patient's Bill of Rights" (which has also been adopted by the New York City Department of Health), the pregnant patient, because she represents *two* patients rather than one, should be recognized as having the additional rights listed below.

1. *The pregnant patient has the right,* prior to the administration of any drug or procedure, to be informed by the health professional caring for her of any potential direct or indirect effects, risks, or hazards to herself or her unborn or newborn infant that may result from the use of a drug or procedure prescribed for or administered to her during pregnancy, labor, birth, or lactation.
2. *The pregnant patient has the right,* prior to the proposed therapy, to be informed not only of the benefits, risks, and hazards of the proposed therapy but also of known alternative therapy, such as available childbirth education classes, that could help to prepare the pregnant patient physically and mentally to cope with the discomfort or stress of pregnancy and the experience of childbirth, thereby reducing or eliminating her need for drugs and obstetric intervention. She should be offered such information early in her pregnancy in order that she may make a reasoned decision.
3. *The pregnant patient has the right,* prior to the administration of any drug, to be informed by the health professional who is prescribing or administering the drug to her that any drug she receives during pregnancy, labor, and birth, no matter how or when the drug is taken or administered, may adversely affect her unborn baby, directly or indirectly, and that no drug or chemical has been proved safe for the unborn child.
4. *The pregnant patient has the right,* if cesarean birth is anticipated, to be informed prior to the administration of any drug, and preferably prior to her hospitalization, that minimizing her and, in turn, her baby's intake of nonessential preoperative medicine will benefit her baby.
5. *The pregnant patient has the right,* prior to the administration of a drug or procedure, to be informed of the areas of uncertainty if there is *no* properly controlled follow-up research that has established the safety of the drug or procedure with regard to its direct or indirect effects on the physiologic, mental, and neurologic development of the child exposed, via the mother, to the drug or procedure during pregnancy, labor, birth, or lactation (this would apply to virtually all drugs and the vast majority of obstetric procedures).

6. *The pregnant patient has the right,* prior to the administration of any drug, to be informed of the brand name and generic name of the drug in order that she may advise the health professional of any past adverse reaction to the drug.
7. *The pregnant patient has the right* to determine for herself, without pressure from her attendant, whether she will accept the risks inherent in the proposed therapy or refuse a drug or procedure.
8. *The pregnant patient has the right* to know the name and qualifications of the individual administering a medication or procedure to her during labor or birth.
9. *The pregnant patient has the right* to be informed, prior to the administration of any procedure, whether that procedure is being administered to her for her or her baby's benefit (medically indicated) or as an elective procedure (for convenience, teaching purposes, or research).
10. *The pregnant patient has the right* to be accompanied during the stress of labor and birth by someone she cares for and to whom she looks for emotional comfort and encouragement.
11. *The pregnant patient has the right* after appropriate medical consultation to choose a position for labor and for birth that is least stressful to her baby and to herself.
12. *The obstetric patient has the right* to have her baby cared for at her bedside if her baby is normal and to feed her baby according to her baby's needs rather than according to the hospital regimen.
13. *The obstetric patient has the right* to be informed in writing of the name of the person who actually delivered her baby and the professional qualifications of that person. This information should also be on the birth certificate.
14. *The obstetric patient has the right* to be informed if there is any known or indicated aspect of her or her baby's care or condition that may cause her or her baby later difficulty or problems.
15. *The obstetric patient has the right* to have her and her baby's hospital medical records complete, accurate, and legible and to have their records, including nurses' notes, retained by the hospital until the child reaches at least the age of majority or, alternatively, to have the records offered to her before they are destroyed.
16. *The obstetric patient,* both during and after her hospital stay, has the right to have access to her complete hospital medical records, including nurses' notes, and to receive a copy on payment of a reasonable fee and without incurring the expense of retaining an attorney.

It is the obstetric patient and her baby, not the health professional, who must sustain any trauma or injury resulting from the use of a drug or obstetric procedure. The observation of the rights listed above will not only permit the obstetric patient to participate in the decisions involving her and her baby's health care but will help to protect the health professional and the hospital against litigation arising from resentment or misunderstanding on the part of the mother.

THE PREGNANT PATIENT'S RESPONSIBILITIES

In addition to understanding her rights, the pregnant patient should also understand that she too has certain responsibilities. The pregnant patient's responsibilities include the following:

1. The pregnant patient is responsible for learning about the physical and psychological process of labor, birth, and postpartum recovery. The better informed expectant parents are, the better they will be able to participate in decisions concerning the planning of their care.
2. The pregnant patient is responsible for learning what comprises good prenatal and intranatal care and for making an effort to obtain the best care possible.
3. Expectant parents are responsible for knowing about those hospital policies and regulations that will affect their birth and postpartum experience.
4. The pregnant patient is responsible for arranging for a companion or support person (husband, mother, sister, friend) who will share in her plans for birth and who will accompany her during her labor and birth experience.
5. The pregnant patient is responsible for making her preferences known clearly to the health professionals involved in her case in a courteous and cooperative manner and for making mutually agreed-on arrangements regarding maternity care alternatives with her physician and hospital in advance of labor.
6. Expectant parents are responsible for listening to their chosen physician or midwife with an open mind, just as they expect him or her to listen openly to them.
7. Once they have agreed to a course of health care, expectant parents are responsible, to the best of their ability, for seeing that the pro-

gram is carried out in consultation with others with whom they have made the agreement.

8. The pregnant patient is responsible for obtaining information in advance regarding the approximate cost of her obstetric and hospital care.
9. The pregnant patient who intends to change her physician or hospital is responsible for notifying all concerned, well in advance of the birth if possible, and for informing both of her reasons for changing.
10. In all their interactions with medical and nursing personnel, the expectant parents should behave toward those caring for them with the same respect and consideration they themselves would like.
11. During the mother's hospital stay, the mother is responsible for learning about her and her baby's continuing care after discharge from the hospital.
12. After birth, the parents should put into writing constructive comments and feelings of satisfaction or dissatisfaction with the care (nursing, medical, and personal) they received. Good service to families in the future will be facilitated by those parents who take the time and responsibility to write letters expressing their feelings about the maternity care they received.

All the previous statements assume a normal birth and postpartum experience. Expectant parents should realize that if complications develop in their cases, there will be an increased need to trust the expertise of the physician and hospital staff they have chosen. However, if problems occur, the childbearing woman still retains her responsibility for making informed decisions about her care or treatment and that of her baby. If she is incapable of assuming that responsibility because of her physical condition, her previously authorized companion or support person should assume responsibility for making informed decisions on her behalf.

The Pregnant Patient's Bill of Rights was prepared by Doris Haire, Chair, Committee on Health Law and Regulation, International Childbirth Education Association, Inc., Rochester, NY. *The Pregnant Patient's Responsibilities* was prepared by members of International Childbirth Education Association, Inc.

Appendix V

Transfer of Drugs and Other Chemicals Into Human Milk

Table 1

DRUGS THAT ARE CONTRAINDICATED DURING BREASTFEEDING

DRUG	REASON FOR CONCERN, REPORTED SIGN OR SYMPTOM IN INFANT, OR EFFECT ON LACTATION
Bromocriptine	Suppresses lactation; may be hazardous to the mother
Cocaine	Cocaine intoxication
Cyclophosphamide	Possible immune suppression; unknown effect on growth or association with carcinogenesis; neutropenia
Cyclosporine	Possible immune suppression; unknown effect on growth or association with carcinogenesis
Doxorubicin*	Possible immune suppression; unknown effect on growth or association with carcinogenesis
Ergotamine	Vomiting, diarrhea, convulsions (doses used in migraine medications)
Lithium	One-third to one-half therapeutic blood concentration in infants
Methotrexate	Possible immune suppression; unknown effect on growth or association with carcinogenesis; neutropenia
Phencyclidine (PCP)	Potent hallucinogen
Phenindione	Anticoagulant; increased prothrombin and partial thromboplastin time in one infant; not used in United States

*Drug is concentrated in human milk.

Table 2

DRUGS OF ABUSE: CONTRAINDICATED DURING BREASTFEEDING*

DRUG REFERENCE	REPORTED EFFECT OR REASON FOR CONCERN
Amphetamine†	Irritability, poor sleeping pattern
Cocaine	Cocaine intoxication

Table continued on following page

Table 2

DRUGS OF ABUSE: CONTRAINDICATED DURING BREASTFEEDING* Continued

DRUG REFERENCE	REPORTED EFFECT OR REASON FOR CONCERN
Heroin	Tremors, restlessness, vomiting, poor feeding
Marijuana	Only one report in literature; no effect mentioned
Nicotine (smoking)	Shock, vomiting, diarrhea, rapid heart rate, restlessness; decreased milk production
Phencyclidine	Potent hallucinogen

*The Committee on Drugs strongly believes that nursing mothers should not ingest any compounds listed in Table 2. Not only are they hazardous to the nursing infant, but they are also detrimental to the physical and emotional health of the mother. This list is obviously not complete; no drug of abuse should be ingested by nursing mothers even though adverse reports are not in the literature.
†Drug is concentrated in human milk.

Table 3

RADIOACTIVE COMPOUNDS THAT REQUIRE TEMPORARY CESSATION OF BREASTFEEDING*

DRUG	RECOMMENDED TIME FOR CESSATION OF BREASTFEEDING
Copper 64 (^{64}Cu)	Radioactivity in milk present at 50 h
Gallium 67 (^{67}Ga)	Radioactivity in milk present for 2 wk
Indium 111 (^{111}In)	Very small amount present at 20 h
Iodine 123 (^{123}I)	Radioactivity in milk present up to 36 h
Iodine 125 (^{125}I)	Radioactivity in milk present for 12 d
Iodine 131 (^{131}I)	Radioactivity in milk present 2–14 d, depending on study
Radioactive sodium	Radioactivity in milk present 96 h
Technetium-99m (^{99m}Tc), ^{99m}Rc macroaggregates, ^{99m}Tc O4	Radioactivity in milk present 15 h to 3 d

*Consult nuclear medicine physician before performing diagnostic study so that radionuclide that has shortest excretion time in breast milk can be used. Before study, the mother should pump her breast and store enough milk in freezer for feeding the infant; after study, the mother should pump her breast to maintain milk production but discard all milk pumped for the required time that radioactivity is present in milk. Milk samples can be screened by radiology department for radioactivity before resumption of nursing.

Table 4

Psychotropic drugs, the compounds listed under antianxiety, antidepressant, and antipsychotic categories, are of special concern when given to nursing mothers for long periods. Although there are no case reports of adverse effects in breastfeeding infants, these drugs do appear in human milk and thus could conceivably alter short-term and long-term central nervous system function.

DRUG	REPORTED OR POSSIBLE EFFECT
Antianxiety	
Diazepam	None
Lorazepam	None
Midazolam	—
Perphenazine	None
Prazepam*	None
Quazepam	None
Temazepam	—
Antidepressants	
Amitriptyline	None
Amoxapine	None
Desipramine	None
Dothiepin	None
Doxepin	None
Fluoxetine	—
Fluvoxamine	—
Imipramine	None
Trazodone	None
Antipsychotic	
Chlorpromazine	Galactorrhea in adult; drowsiness and lethargy in infant
Chlorprothixene	None
Haloperidol	None
Mesoridazine	None
Chloramphenicol	Possible idiosyncratic bone marrow suppression
Metoclopramide*	None described; dopaminergic blocking agent
Metronidazole	In vitro mutagen; may discontinue breastfeeding 12–24 h to allow excretion of dose when single-dose therapy given to mother
Tinidazole	See metronidazole

*Drug is concentrated in human milk.

Table 5

DRUGS THAT HAVE BEEN ASSOCIATED WITH SIGNIFICANT EFFECTS ON SOME NURSING INFANTS AND SHOULD BE GIVEN TO NURSING MOTHERS WITH CAUTION*

DRUG	REPORTED EFFECT
5-Aminosalicylic acid	Diarrhea (1 case)
Aspirin (salicylates)	Metabolic acidosis (1 case)
Clemastine	Drowsiness, irritability, refusal to feed, high-pitched cry, neck stiffness (1 case)

Table continued on following page

Table 5

DRUGS THAT HAVE BEEN ASSOCIATED WITH SIGNIFICANT EFFECTS ON SOME NURSING INFANTS AND SHOULD BE GIVEN TO NURSING MOTHERS WITH CAUTION* Continued

DRUG	REPORTED EFFECT
Phenobarbital	Sedation; infantile spasms after weaning from milk containing phenobarbital, methemoglobinemia (1 case)
Primidone	Sedation, feeding problems
Sulfasalazine (salicylazosulfapyridine)	Bloody diarrhea (1 case)

*Measure blood concentration in the infant when possible.

Table 6

MATERNAL MEDICATION USUALLY COMPATIBLE WITH BREASTFEEDING*

DRUG	REPORTED SIGN OR SYMPTOM IN INFANT OR EFFECT ON LACTATION
Acebutolol	None
Acetaminophen	None
Acetazolamide	None
Acitretin	—
Acyclovir†	None
Alcohol (ethanol)	With large amounts drowsiness, diaphoresis, deep sleep, weakness, decrease in linear growth, abnormal weight gain; maternal ingestion of 1 g/kg daily decreases milk ejection reflex
Allopurinol	—
Amoxicillin	None
Antimony	—
Atenolol	None
Atropine	None
Azapropazone (apazone)	—
B_1 (thiamin)	None
B_6 (pyridoxine)	None
B_{12}	None
Baclofen	None
Barbiturate	See Table 5
Bendroflumethiazide	Suppresses lactation
Bishydroxycoumarin (dicumarol)	None
Bromide	Rash, weakness, absence of cry with maternal intake of 5.4 g/d
Butorphanol	None
Caffeine	Irritability, poor sleeping pattern, excreted slowly; no effect with usual amount of caffeine beverages
Captopril	None
Carbamazepine	None
Carbimazole	Goiter
Cascara	None
Cefadroxil	None

Table continued on facing page

Table 6

MATERNAL MEDICATION USUALLY COMPATIBLE WITH BREASTFEEDING* Continued

DRUG	REPORTED SIGN OR SYMPTOM IN INFANT OR EFFECT ON LACTATION
Cefazolin	None
Cefotaxime	None
Cefoxitin	None
Cefprozil	—
Ceftazidime	None
Ceftriaxone	None
Chloral hydrate	Sleepiness
Chloroform	None
Chloroquine	None
Chlorothiazide	None
Chlorthalidone	Excreted slowly
Cimetidine†	None
Cisapride	None
Cisplatin	Not found in milk
Clindamycin	None
Clogestone	None
Clomipramine	—
Codeine	None
Colchicine	—
Contraceptive pill with estrogen/progesterone	Rare breast enlargement; decrease in milk production and protein content (not confirmed in several studies)
Cycloserine	None
D (Vitamin)	None; follow up infant's serum calcium level if mother receives pharmacologic doses
Danthron	Increased bowel activity
Dapsone	None; sulfonamide detected in infant's urine
Dexbrompheniramine malcate with *d*-isoephedrine	Crying, poor sleeping patterns, irritability
Digoxin	None
Diltiazem	None
Dipyrone	None
Disopyramide	None
Damperidone	None
Dyphylline†	None
Enalapril	—
Erythromycin†	None
Estradiol	Withdrawal, vaginal bleeding
Ethambutol	None
Ethanol (cf. alcohol)	—
Ethosuximide	None, drug appears in infant serum
Fentanyl	—
Flecainide	—
Flufenamic acid	None
Fluorescein	—
Folic acid	None
Gold salts	None
Halothane	None
Hydralazine	None
Hydrochlorothiazide	—
Hydroxychloroquine†	None
Ibuprofen	None
Indomethacin	Seizure (1 case)

Table continued on following page

Table 6

MATERNAL MEDICATION USUALLY COMPATIBLE WITH BREASTFEEDING* Continued

DRUG	REPORTED SIGN OR SYMPTOM IN INFANT OR EFFECT ON LACTATION
Iodides	May affect thyroid activity
Iodine (povidone-iodine/vaginal douche)	Elevated iodine levels in breast milk, odor of iodine on infant's skin
Iodine	Goiter
Iopanoic acid	None
Isoniazid	None; acetyl metabolite also secreted; ? hepatotoxic
K_1 (vitamin)	None
Kanamycin	None
Ketorolac	—
Labetalol	None
Levonorgestrel	—
Lidocaine	None
Loperamide	—
Magnesium sulfate	None
Medroxyprogesterone	None
Mefenamic acid	None
Methadone	None if mother receiving ≤20 mg/24 h
Methimazole (active metabolite of carbimazole)	None
Methocarbamol	None
Methyldopa	None
Methyprylon	Drowsiness
Metoprolol†	None
Metrizamide	None
Mexiletine	None
Minoxidil	None
Morphine	None; infant may have significant blood concentration
Moxalactam	None
Nadolol†	None
Nalidixic acid	Hemolysis in infant with glucose-6-phosphate dehydrogenase (G-6-PD) deficiency
Naproxen	—
Nefopam	None
Nifedipine	—
Nitrofurantoin	Hemolysis in infant with G-6-PD deficiency
Norethynodrel	None
Norsteroids	None
Noscapine	None
Oxprenolol	None
Phenylbutazone	None
Phenytoin	Methemoglobinemia (1 case)
Piroxicam	None
Prednisone	None
Procainamide	None
Progesterone	None
Propoxyphene	None
Propranolol	None
Propylthiouracil	None
Pseudoephedrine†	None
Pyridostigmine	None
Pyrimethamine	None

Table continued on facing page

Table 6

MATERNAL MEDICATION USUALLY COMPATIBLE WITH BREASTFEEDING* Continued

DRUG	REPORTED SIGN OR SYMPTOM IN INFANT OR EFFECT ON LACTATION
Quinidine	None
Quinine	None
Riboflavin	None
Rifampin	None
Scopolamine	—
Secobarbital	None
Senna	None
Sotalol	—
Spironolactone	None
Streptomycin	None
Sulbactam	None
Sulfapyridine	Caution in infant with jaundice or G-6-PD deficiency, and ill, stressed, or premature infant; appears in infant's milk
Sulfisoxazole	Caution in infant with jaundice or G-6-PD deficiency, and ill, stressed, or premature infant; appears in infant's milk
Suprofen	None
Terbutaline	None
Tetracycline	None; negligible absorption by infant
Theophylline	Irritability
Thiopental	None
Thiouracil	None mentioned; drug not used in United States
Ticarcillin	None
Timolol	None
Tolbutamide	Possible jaundice
Tolmetin	None
Trimethoprim/sulfamethoxazole	None
Triprolidine	None
Valproic acid	None
Verapamil	None
Warfarin	None
Zolpidem	None

*Drugs listed have been reported in the literature as having the effects listed or no effect. The word "none" means that no observable change was seen in the nursing infant while the mother was ingesting the compound. It is emphasized that most of the literature citations concern single case reports or small series of infants.
†Drug is concentrated in human milk.

Table 7

FOOD AND ENVIRONMENTAL AGENTS: EFFECT ON BREASTFEEDING

AGENT	REPORTED SIGN OR SYMPTOM IN INFANT OR EFFECT ON LACTATION
Aflatoxin	None
Aspartame	Caution if mother or infant has phenylketonuria
Bromide (photographic laboratory)	Potential absorption and bromide transfer into milk; see Table 6

Table continued on following page

Table 7

FOOD AND ENVIRONMENTAL AGENTS: EFFECT ON BREASTFEEDING Continued

AGENT	REPORTED SIGN OR SYMPTOM IN INFANT OR EFFECT ON LACTATION
Cadmium	None reported
Chlordane	None reported
Chocolate (theobromine)	Irritability or increased bowel activity if excess amounts (16 oz/d) consumed by mother
DDT, benzenehexachlorides, dieldrin, aldrin, hepatachlorepoxide	None
Fava beans	Hemolysis in patient with glucose-6-phosphate dehydrogenase (G-6-PD) deficiency
Fluorides	None
Hexachlorobenzene	Skin rash, diarrhea, vomiting, dark urine, neurotoxicity, death
Hexachlorophene	None; possible contamination of milk from nipple washing
Lead	Possible neurotoxicity
Methyl mercury, mercury	May affect neurodevelopment
Monosodium glutamate	None
Polychlorinated biphenyls and polybrominated biphenyls	Lack of endurance, hypotonia, sullen expressionless facies
Tetrachlorethylene-cleaning fluid (perchloroethylene)	Obstructive jaundice, dark urine
Vegetarian diet	Signs of B_{12} deficiency

Appendix V is modified from Committee on Drugs (1994). The transfer of drugs and other chemicals into human milk. *Pediatrics,* 93 (1), 137–150. Used with permission of the American Academy of Pediatrics.

Appendix VI

Guideline for Isolation Precautions in Hospitals

The following is a condensation of the Centers for Disease Control (CDC) and the Hospital Infection Control Practices Advisory Committee (HICPAC). (1996). Special communication: Guideline for isolation precautions in hospitals. Part I. Evolution of isolation practices. Part II. Recommendations for isolation precautions in hospitals. *American Journal of Infection Control,* 24 (1), 24–52.

PART I EVOLUTION OF ISOLATION PRACTICES

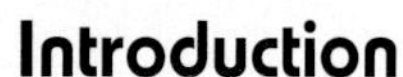

Introduction

To assist hospitals in maintaining up-to-date isolation practices, the CDC and the HICPAC have revised the *CDC Guideline for Isolation Precautions in Hospitals.* HICPAC was established in 1991 to provide advice and guidance to the Secretary, Department of Health and Human Services (DHHS); the Assistant Secretary for Health, DHHS; the Director, CDC; and the Director, National Center for Infectious Diseases regarding the practice of hospital infection control and strategies for surveillance, prevention, and control of nosocomial infection in U.S. hospitals.

The guideline supersedes previous CDC recommendations for isolation precautions in hospitals and is based on the latest epidemiologic information on transmission of infection in hospitals. The recommendations are intended primarily for use in the care of patients in acute-care hospitals, although some of the recommendations may be applicable for some patients receiving care in subacute-care or extended-care facilities. The recommendations are not intended for use in day care, well care, or domiciliary care programs.

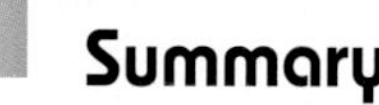

Summary

The *Guideline for Isolation Precautions in Hospitals* was revised to meet the following objectives: (1) to be epidemiologically sound, (2) to recognize the importance of all body fluids, secretions, and excretions in the transmission of nosocomial pathogens, (3) to contain adequate precautions for infections transmitted by the airborne, droplet, and contact routes of transmission, (4) to be as simple and user-friendly as possible, and (5) to use new terms to avoid confusion with existing infection control and isolation systems.

The revised guideline contains two tiers of precautions. In the first and most important tier are those precautions designed for the care of all patients in hospitals regardless of their diagnosis or presumed infection status. Implementation of these "Standard Precautions" is the primary strategy for successful nosocomial infection control. In the second tier are precautions designed only for the care of specified patients. These additional "Transmission-based Precautions" are used for patients known to be or suspected of being infected or colonized with epidemiologically important pathogens that can be transmitted by airborne or droplet transmission or by contact with dry skin or contaminated surfaces.

Standard Precautions synthesize the major features of Universal (Blood and Body Fluid) Precautions (1985, designed to reduce the risk of transmission of blood-borne pathogens) and Body Substance Isolation (1987, designed to reduce the risk of transmission of pathogens from moist body substances). Standard Precautions apply to (1) blood, (2) all body fluids, secretions, and excretions *except sweat* regardless of whether they contain visible blood, (3) nonintact skin, and (4) mucous membranes. Standard Precautions are designed to reduce the risk of transmission of microorganisms from both recognized and unrecognized sources of infection in hospitals.

Transmission-based Precautions are designed for patients known to be or suspected of being infected or colonized with highly transmissible or epidemiologically important pathogens for which additional precautions beyond Standard Precautions are needed to interrupt transmission in hospitals. There are three types of Transmission-based Precautions: Airborne Precautions, Droplet Precautions, and Contact Precautions. They may be combined together for diseases that have multiple routes of transmission. When used either singularly or in combination, they are to be used in addition to Standard Precautions.

The revised guideline also lists specific clinical syndromes or conditions in both adult and pediatric patients that are highly suspicious for infection and identifies appropriate Transmission-based Precautions to use on an empirical, temporary basis until a diagnosis can be made; these empirical, temporary precautions are also to be used in addition to Standard Precautions (see Chapter 40).

PART II RECOMMENDATIONS FOR ISOLATION PRECAUTIONS IN HOSPITALS

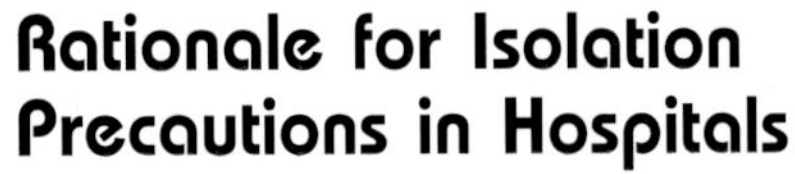

Rationale for Isolation Precautions in Hospitals

Transmission of infection within a hospital requires three elements: a source of infecting microorganisms, a susceptible host, and a means of transmission for the microorganism.

SOURCE

Human sources of the infecting microorganisms in hospitals may be patients, personnel, or, on occasion, visitors and may include persons with acute disease, persons in the incubation period of a disease, persons who are colonized by an infectious agent but have no apparent disease, or persons who are chronic carriers of an infectious agent. Other sources of infecting microorganisms can be the patient's own endogenous flora, which may be difficult to control, and inanimate environmental objects that have become contaminated, including equipment and medications.

HOST

Resistance among persons to pathogenic microorganisms varies greatly. Some persons may be immune to infections or be able to resist colonization by an infectious agent; others exposed to the same agent may establish a commensal relationship with the infecting microorganism and become symptom-free carriers; still others may have development of clinical disease. Host factors such as age; underlying diseases; certain treatments with antimicrobials, corticosteroids, or other immunosuppressive agents; irradiation; and breaks in the first line of defense mechanisms caused by such factors as surgical operations, anesthesia, and indwelling catheters may render patients more susceptible to infection.

TRANSMISSION

Microorganisms are transmitted in hospitals by several routes, and the same microorganism may be transmitted by more than one route. There are five main routes of transmission—contact, droplet, airborne, common vehicle, and vector-borne. For the purpose of this guideline, common vehicle and vector-borne transmission will be discussed only briefly because neither plays a significant role in typical nosocomial infections.

Fundamentals of Isolation Precautions

A variety of infection control measures are used for decreasing the risk of transmission of microorganisms in hospitals. These measures make up the fundamentals of isolation precautions.

HAND WASHING AND GLOVING

Hand washing is frequently called the single most important measure to reduce the risks of transmitting microorganisms from one person to another or from one site to another on the same patient. The scientific rationale, indications, methods, and products for hand washing have been delineated in other publications.

Washing hands as promptly and thoroughly as possible between patient contacts and after contact with blood, body fluids, secretions, excretions, and equipment or articles contaminated by them is an important component of infection control and isolation precautions. In addition to hand washing, gloves play an important role in reducing the risks of transmission of microorganisms.

Gloves are worn for three important reasons in hospitals. First, gloves are worn to provide a protective barrier and prevent gross contamination of the hands when touching blood, body fluids, secretions, excretions, mucous membranes, and nonintact skin. Second, gloves are worn to reduce the likelihood that microorganisms present on the hands of personnel will be transmitted to patients during invasive or other patient care procedures that involve touching a patient's mucous membranes and nonintact skin. Third, gloves are worn to reduce the likelihood that hands of personnel contaminated with microorganisms from a patient or a fomite can transmit these microorganisms to another patient; in this situation, gloves must be changed between patient contacts and hands washed after gloves are removed.

Wearing gloves does not replace the need for hand washing because (1) gloves may have small inapparent defects or be torn during use and (2) hands can become contaminated during removal of gloves. Failure to change gloves between patient contacts is an infection control hazard.

PATIENT PLACEMENT

Appropriate patient placement is a significant component of isolation precautions. A private room is important to prevent direct- or indirect-contact transmission when the source patient has poor hygienic habits, contaminates the environment, or cannot be expected to assist in maintaining infection control precautions to limit transmission of microorganisms (i.e., infants, children, and patients with altered mental status). When possible, a patient with highly transmissible or epidemiologically important microorganisms is placed in a private room with hand washing and toilet facilities to reduce opportunities for transmission of microorganisms.

TRANSPORT OF INFECTED PATIENTS

Limiting the movement and transport of patients infected with virulent or epidemiologically important microorganisms and ensuring that such patients leave their own rooms only for essential purposes reduce opportunities for transmission of microorganisms in hospitals.

MASKS, RESPIRATORY PROTECTION, EYE PROTECTION, FACE SHIELDS

Various types of masks, goggles, and face shields are worn alone or in combination to provide barrier protection. A mask that covers both the nose and mouth and goggles or a face shield is worn by hospital personnel during procedures and patient-care activities that are likely to generate splashes or sprays of blood, body fluids, secretions, or excretions, to provide protection of the mucous membranes of the eyes, nose, and mouth from contact transmission of pathogens.

GOWNS AND PROTECTIVE APPAREL

Various types of gowns and protective apparel are worn to provide barrier protection and reduce opportunities for transmission of microorganisms in hospitals. Gowns are worn to prevent contamination of clothing and protect the skin of personnel from blood and body fluid exposure. Gowns specially treated to make them impermeable to liquids, leg coverings, boots, or shoe covers provide greater protection to the skin when splashes or large quantities of infective material are present or anticipated.

PATIENT-CARE EQUIPMENT AND ARTICLES

Many factors determine whether special handling and disposal of used patient-care equipment and articles are prudent or required, including the likelihood of contamination with infective material; the ability to cut, stick, or otherwise cause injury (needles, scalpels, and other sharp instruments [sharps]); the severity of the associated disease; and the environmental stability of the pathogens involved. Some used articles are enclosed in containers or bags to prevent inadvertent exposure to patients, personnel, and visitors and to prevent contamination of the environment. Used sharps are placed in puncture-resistant containers; other articles are placed in a bag. One bag is adequate if the bag is sturdy and the article can be placed in the bag without contaminating the outside of the bag; otherwise, two bags are used.

LINENS AND LAUNDRY

Although soiled linen may be contaminated with pathogenic microorganisms, the risk of disease transmission is negligible if it is handled, transported, and laundered in a manner that avoids transfer of microorganisms to patients, personnel, and environments. Rather than rigid rules and regulations, hygienic and commonsense storage and processing of clean and soiled linen are recommended.

DISHES, GLASSES AND CUPS, AND EATING UTENSILS

No special precautions are needed for dishes, glasses and cups, or eating utensils. Either disposable or reusable dishes and utensils can be used for patients on isolation precautions. The combination of hot water and detergents used in hospital dishwashers is sufficient to decontaminate dishes, glasses and cups, and eating utensils.

ROUTINE AND TERMINAL CLEANING

The room or cubicle and bedside equipment of patients on Transmission-based Precautions are cleaned with the same procedures used for patients on Standard Precautions, unless the infecting microorganisms and the amount of environmental contamination indicate special cleaning. In addition to thorough cleaning, adequate disinfection of bedside equipment and environmental surfaces (e.g., bedrails, bedside tables, carts, commodes, doorknobs, faucet handles) is indicated for certain pathogens, especially enterococci, that can survive in the inanimate environment for prolonged periods of time.

Immunocompromised Patients

Immunocompromised patients vary in their susceptibility to nosocomial infections depending on the severity and duration of immunosuppression. They are generally at increased risk for bacterial, fungal, parasitic, and viral infections from both endogenous and exogenous sources. The use of Standard Precautions for all patients and Transmission-based Precautions for specified patients should reduce the acquisition by these patients of institutionally acquired bacteria from other patients and environments.

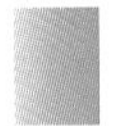

Recommendations

The recommendations presented below are categorized as follows:

Category IA. Strongly recommended for all hospitals and strongly supported by well-designed experimental or epidemiologic studies.

Category IB. Strongly recommended for all hospitals and reviewed as effective by experts in the field and a consensus of HICPAC on the basis of strong rationale and suggestive evidence, even though definitive scientific studies have not been done.

Category II. Suggested for implementation in many hospitals. Recommendations may be supported by suggestive clinical or epidemiologic studies, a strong theoretical rationale, or definitive studies applicable to some but not all hospitals.

No recommendation; unresolved issue. Practices for which insufficient evidence or consensus regarding efficacy exists.

The recommendations are limited to the topic of isolation precautions. Therefore, they must be supplemented by hospital policies and procedures for other aspects of infection and environmental control, occupational health, administrative and legal issues, and other issues beyond the scope of this guideline.

I. Administrative Controls

A. Education

Develop a system to ensure that hospital patients, personnel, and visitors are educated about use of precautions and their responsibility for adherence to them. *Category IB*

B. Adherence to precautions

Periodically evaluate adherence to precautions, and use findings to direct improvements. *Category IB*

II. Standard Precautions

Use Standard Precautions, or the equivalent, for the care of all patients. *Category IB*

A. Handwashing

1. Wash hands after touching blood, body fluids, secretions, excretions, and contaminated items, regardless of whether gloves are worn. Wash hands immediately after gloves are removed, between patient contacts, and when otherwise indicated to avoid transfer of microorganisms to other patients or environments. It may be necessary to wash hands between tasks and procedures on the same patient to prevent cross-contamination of different body sites. *Category IB*
2. Use a plain (nonantimicrobial) soap for routine hand washing. *Category IB*
3. Use an antimicrobial agent or waterless antiseptic agent for specific circumstances (e.g., control of outbreaks or hyperendemic infections) as defined by the infection control program. *Category IB* (See Contact Precautions for additional recommendations on use of antimicrobial and antiseptic agents.)

B. Gloves

Wear gloves (clean nonsterile gloves are adequate) when touching blood, body fluids, secretions, excretions, and contaminated items; put on clean gloves just before touching mucous membranes and nonintact skin. Change gloves between tasks and procedures on the same patient after contact with material that may contain a high concentration of microorganisms. Remove gloves promptly after use, before touching noncontaminated items and environmental surfaces, and before going to another patient, and wash hands immediately to avoid transfer of microorganisms to other patients or environments. *Category IB*

C. Mask, eye protection, face shield
Wear a mask and eye protection or a face shield to protect mucous membranes of the eyes, nose, and mouth during procedures and patient-care activities that are likely to generate splashes or sprays of blood, body fluids, secretions, and excretions. *Category IB*

D. Gown
Wear a gown (a clean nonsterile gown is adequate) to protect skin and prevent soiling of clothing during procedures and patient-care activities that are likely to generate splashes or sprays of blood, body fluids, secretions, or excretions or cause soiling of clothing. Select a gown that is appropriate for the activity and amount of fluid likely to be encountered. Remove a soiled gown as promptly as possible and wash hands to avoid transfer of microorganisms to other patients or environments. *Category IB*

E. Patient-care equipment
Handle used patient-care equipment soiled with blood, body fluids, secretions, and excretions in a manner that prevents skin and mucous membrane exposures, contamination of clothing, and transfer of microorganisms to other patients and environments. Ensure that reusable equipment is not used for the care of another patient until it has been appropriately cleaned and reprocessed and single-use items are properly discarded. *Category IB*

F. Environmental control
Ensure that the hospital has adequate procedures for the routine care, cleaning, and disinfection of environmental surfaces, beds, bedrails, bedside equipment, and other frequently touched surfaces and that these procedures are being followed. *Category IB*

G. Linen
Handle, transport, and process used linen soiled with blood, body fluids, secretions, and excretions in a manner that prevents skin and mucous membrane exposures, contamination of clothing, and transfer of microorganisms to other patients and environments. *Category IB*

H. Occupational health and blood-borne pathogens
   1. Take care to prevent injuries when using needles, scalpels, and other sharp instruments or devices; when handling sharp instruments after procedures; when cleaning used instruments; and when disposing of used needles. Never recap used needles or otherwise manipulate them using both hands, or any other technique that involves directing the point of a needle toward any part of the body; rather, use either a one-handed "scoop" technique or a mechanical device designed for holding the needle sheath. Do not remove used needles from disposable syringes by hand, and do not bend, break, or otherwise manipulate used needles by hand. Place used disposable syringes and needles, scalpel blades, and other sharp items in appropriate puncture-resistant containers located as close as practical to the area in which the items were used, and place reusable syringes and needles in a puncture-resistant container for transport to the reprocessing area. *Category IB*
   2. Use mouthpieces, resuscitation bags, or other ventilation devices as an alternative to mouth-to-mouth resuscitation methods in areas where the need for resuscitation is predictable. *Category IB*

I. Patient placement
Place a patient who contaminates the environment or who does not (or cannot be expected to) assist in maintaining appropriate hygiene or environmental control in a private room. If a private room is not available, consult with ICPs regarding patient placement or other alternatives. *Category IB*

III. Airborne Precautions

In addition to Standard Precautions, use Airborne Precautions, or the equivalent, for patients known to be or suspected of being infected with microorganisms transmitted by airborne droplet nuclei (small-particle residue [5 μm or smaller in size] of evaporated droplets containing microorganisms that remain suspended in the air and can be widely dispersed by air currents within a room or over a long distance). *Category IB*

A. Patient placement
Place the patient in a private room that has (1) monitored negative air pressure in relation to the surrounding areas, (2) 6 to 12 air changes per hour, and (3) appropriate discharge of air outdoors or monitored high-efficiency filtration of room air before the air is circulated to other areas in the hospital. Keep the room door closed and the patient in the room. When a private room is not available, place the patient in a room with a patient who has active infection with the same microorganism, unless otherwise recommended, but with no other infection. When a private room is not available and cohorting is not desir-

able, consultation with ICPs is advised before patient placement. *Category IB*

B. Respiratory protection
Wear respiratory protection when entering the room of a patient with known or suspected infectious pulmonary tuberculosis. Susceptible persons should not enter the room of patients known or suspected to have measles (rubeola) or varicella (chickenpox) if other immune caregivers are available. If susceptible persons must enter the room of a patient known or suspected to have measles (rubeola) or varicella, they should wear respiratory protection. Persons immune to measles (rubeola) or varicella need not wear respiratory protection. *Category IB*

C. Patient transport
Limit the movement and transport of the patient from the room to essential purposes only. If transport or movement is necessary, minimize patient dispersal of droplet nuclei by placing a surgical mask on the patient, if possible. *Category IB*

D. Additional precautions for preventing transmission of tuberculosis
Consult CDC *Guidelines for Preventing the Transmission of Tuberculosis in Health-Care Facilities* for additional prevention strategies.

IV. Droplet Precautions

In addition to Standard Precautions, use Droplet Precautions, or the equivalent, for a patient known to be or suspected of being infected with microorganisms transmitted by droplets (large-particle droplets [larger than 5 μm in size] that can be generated by the patient during coughing, sneezing, talking, or the performance of procedures). *Category IB*

A. Patient placement
Place the patient in a private room. When a private room is not available, place the patient in a room with a patient who has active infection with the same microorganism, but with no other infection (cohorting). When a private room is not available and cohorting is not achievable, maintain spatial separation of at least 3 feet between the infected patient and other patients and visitors. Special air handling and ventilation are not necessary, and the door may remain open. *Category IB*

B. Mask
In addition to Standard Precautions, wear a mask when working within 3 feet of the patient. (Logistically, some hospitals may want to implement the wearing of a mask to enter the room.) *Category IB*

C. Patient transport
Limit the movement and transport of the patient from the room to essential purposes only. If transport or movement is necessary, minimize patient dispersal of droplets by masking the patient, if possible. *Category IB*

V. Contact Precautions

In addition to Standard Precautions, use Contact Precautions, or the equivalent, for specified patients known to be or suspected of being infected or colonized with epidemiologically important microorganisms that can be transmitted by direct contact with the patient (hand or skin-to-skin contact that occurs when performing patient-care activities that require touching the patient's dry skin) or indirect contact (touching) with environmental surfaces or patient-care items in the patient's environment. *Category IB*

A. Patient placement
Place the patient in a private room. When a private room is not available, place the patient in a room with a patient who has active infection with the same microorganism, but with no other infection (cohorting). When a private room is not available and cohorting is not achievable, consider the epidemiologic pattern of the microorganism and the patient population when determining patient placement; consultation with ICPs is advised before patient placement. *Category IB*

B. Gloves and hand washing
In addition to wearing gloves as outlined under Standard Precautions, wear gloves (clean nonsterile gloves are adequate) when entering the room. During the course of providing care for a patient, change gloves after having contact with infective material that may contain high concentrations of microorganisms (fecal material and wound drainage). Remove gloves before leaving the patient's environment and wash hands immediately with an antimicrobial agent or a waterless antiseptic agent. After glove removal and hand washing, ensure that hands do not touch potentially contaminated environmental surfaces or items in the patient's room to avoid transfer of microorganisms to other patients or environments. *Category IB*

C. Gown
In addition to wearing a gown as outlined under Standard Precautions, wear a gown (a clean nonsterile gown is adequate) when entering the room if you anticipate that your clothing will have substantial contact with the patient, environmental surfaces, or items in the patient's room, or if the patient is incontinent or has diarrhea, an ileostomy, a colostomy, or wound drainage not contained by a dressing. Re-

move the gown before leaving the patient's environment. After gown removal, ensure that clothing does not contact potentially contaminated environmental surfaces to avoid transfer of microorganisms to other patients or environments. *Category IB*

D. Patient transport
Limit the movement and transport of the patient from the room to essential purposes only. If the patient is transported out of the room, ensure that precautions are maintained to minimize the risk of transmission of microorganisms to other patients and contamination of environmental surfaces or equipment. *Category IB*

E. Patient-care equipment
When possible, dedicate the use of noncritical patient-care equipment to a single patient (or cohort of patients infected or colonized with the pathogen requiring precautions) to avoid sharing between patients. If use of common equipment or items is unavoidable, then adequately clean and disinfect them before use for another patient. *Category IB*

F. Additional precautions for preventing the spread of vancomycin resistance
Consult the HICPAC report on preventing the spread of vancomycin resistance for additional prevention strategies.

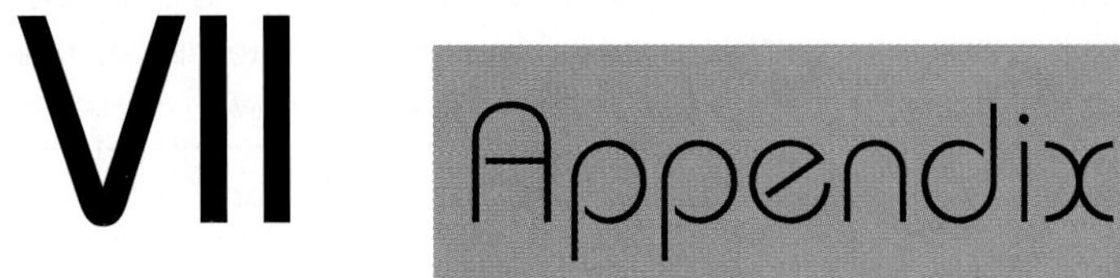

VII Appendix

Recommended Childhood Immunization Schedule

United States, July–December 1996

Vaccines are listed under the routinely recommended ages. Bars indicate range of acceptable ages for vaccination. Shaded bars indicate catch-up vaccination: at 11-12 years of age, hepatitis B vaccine should be administered to children not previously vaccinated, and Varicella Zoster Virus vaccine should be administered to children not previously vaccinated who lack a reliable history of chickenpox.

Age ► / Vaccine ▼	Birth	1 mo	2 mos	4 mos	6 mos	12 mos	15 mos	18 mos	4-6 yrs	11-12 yrs	14-16 yrs
Hepatitis B[1,2]	Hep B-1										
			Hep B-2		Hep B-3					Hep B[2]	
Diphtheria, Tetanus, Pertussis[3]			DTP	DTP	DTP	DTP[3] (DTaP at 15+ m)			DTP or DTaP	Td	
H. influenzae type b[4]			Hib	Hib	Hib[4]	Hib[4]					
Polio[5]			OPV[5]	OPV	OPV				OPV		
Measles, Mumps, Rubella[6]						MMR			MMR[6] or	MMR[6]	
Varicella Zoster Virus Vaccine[7]							Var			Var[7]	

Approved by the Advisory Committee on Immunization Practices (ACIP), the American Academy of Pediatrics (AAP), and the American Academy of Family Physicians (AAFP).

IS 5081

(For **necessary footnotes** and important information, see facing page.)

[1] **Infants born to HBsAg-negative mothers** should receive 2.5 μg of Merck vaccine (Recombivax HB) or 10 μg of SmithKline Beecham (SB) vaccine (Engerix-B). The 2nd dose should be administered ≥1 mo after the 1st dose.
Infants born to HBsAg-positive mothers should receive 0.5 mL Hepatitis B Immune Globulin (HBIG) within 12 hr of birth, and either 5 μg of Merck vaccine (Recombivax HB) or 10 μg of SB vaccine (Engerix-B) at a separate site. The 2nd dose is recommended at 1-2 mos of age and the 3rd dose at 6 mos of age.
Infants born to mothers whose HBsAg status is unknown should receive either 5 μg of Merck vaccine (Recombivax HB) or 10 μg of SB vaccine (Engerix-B) within 12 hr of birth. The 2nd dose of vaccine is recommended at 1 mo of age and the 3rd dose at 6 mos of age.

[2] Adolescents who have not previously received 3 doses of hepatitis B vaccine should initiate or complete the series at the 11-12 year-old visit. The 2nd dose should be administered at least 1 mo after the 1st dose, and the 3rd dose should be administered at least 4 mos after the 1st dose and at least 2 mos after the 2nd dose.

[3] DTP4 may be administered at 12 mos of age, if at least 6 mos have elapsed since DTP3. DTaP (diphtheria and tetanus toxoids and acellular pertussis vaccine) is licensed for the 4th and/or 5th vaccine dose(s) for children aged ≥15 mos and may be preferred for these doses in this age group. Td (tetanus and diphtheria toxoids, adsorbed, for adult use) is recommended at 11-12 years of age if at least 5 years have elapsed since the last dose of DTP, DTaP, or DT.

[4] Three *H. influenzae* type b (Hib) conjugate vaccines are licensed for infant use. If PRP-OMP (PedvaxHIB [Merck]) is administered at 2 and 4 mos of age, a dose at 6 mos is not required. After completing the primary series, any Hib conjugate vaccine may be used as a booster.

[5] Oral poliovirus vaccine (OPV) is recommended for routine infant vaccination. Inactivated poliovirus vaccine (IPV) is recommended for persons with a congenital or acquired immune deficiency disease or an altered immune status as a result of disease or immunosuppressive therapy, as well as their household contacts, and is an acceptable alternative for other persons. The primary 3-dose series for IPV should be given with a minimum interval of 4 wks between the 1st and 2nd doses and 6 mos between the 2nd and 3rd doses.

[6] The 2nd dose of MMR is routinely recommended at 4-6 yrs of age or at 11-12 yrs of age, but may be administered at any visit, provided at least 1 mo has elapsed since receipt of the 1st dose.

[7] Varicella zoster virus vaccine (Var) can be administered to susceptible children any time after 12 months of age. Unvaccinated children who lack a reliable history of chickenpox should be vaccinated at the 11-12 year-old visit.

Immunization Protects Children

Regular checkups at your pediatrician's office or local health clinic are an important way to keep children healthy.

By making sure that your child gets immunized on time, you can provide the best available defense against many dangerous childhood diseases. Immunizations protect children against: hepatitis B, polio, measles, mumps, rubella (German measles), pertussis (whooping cough), diphtheria, tetanus (lockjaw), *Haemophilus influenzae* type b, and chickenpox. All of these immunizations need to be given before children are 2 years old in order for them to be protected during their most vulnerable period. Are your child's immunizations up-to-date?

The chart on the other side of this fact sheet includes immunization recommendations from the American Academy of Pediatrics. Remember to keep track of your child's immunizations—it's the only way you can be sure your child is up-to-date. Also, check with your pediatrician or health clinic at each visit to find out if your child needs any booster shots or if any new vaccines have been recommended since this schedule was prepared.

If you don't have a pediatrician, call your local health department. Public health clinics usually have supplies of vaccine and may give shots free.

American Academy of Pediatrics

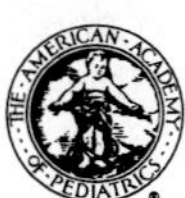

The information contained in this publication should not be used as a substitute for the medical care and advice of your pediatrician. There may be variations in treatment that your pediatrician may recommend based on individual facts and circumstances.

VIII Appendix

Resources

AMERICAN ACADEMY OF HUSBAND-COACHED CHILDBIRTH (BRADLEY METHOD)
P.O. Box 5224
Sherman Oaks, CA 91413-5224
800-4-A-BIRTH

AMERICAN COLLEGE OF NURSE-MIDWIVES (ACNM)
818 Connecticut Avenue NW, Suite 900
Washington, DC 20006
202-728-9860

AMERICAN COLLEGE OF OBSTETRICIANS AND GYNECOLOGISTS (ACOG)
409 12th Street SW
Washington, DC 20024
202-638-5577

AMERICAN SOCIETY FOR PSYCHOPROPHYLAXIS IN OBSTETRICS (ASPO/LAMAZE)
1200 19th Street NW, Suite 300
Washington, DC 20036
202-857-1128; 800-368-4404; FAX 202-223-4579

ASSOCIATION OF WOMEN'S HEALTH, OBSTETRIC AND NEONATAL NURSES (AWHONN)
[In 1993, The Nurses Association of the American College of Obstetricians and Gynecologists (NAACOG) became AWHONN; citations and references in the literature before 1993 will be to NAACOG.]

700 14th Street NW, Suite 600
Washington, DC 20005
202-662-1600; FAX 202-737-0578

HEALTH RESOURCES AND SERVICES ADMINISTRATION–MATERNAL AND CHILD HEALTH BUREAU
Office of the Director
Parklawn Building, Room 18-05
5600 Fishers Lane
Rockville, MD 20857
301-443-2170

INTERNATIONAL BOARD OF LACTATION CONSULTANT EXAMINERS (IBLCE)
P.O. Box 2348
Falls Church, VA 22042
703-560-7330; FAX 703-560-7332

INTERNATIONAL CHILDBIRTH EDUCATION ASSOCIATION (ICEA)
8060 26th Avenue South
Bloomington, MN 55425
612-854-8660; 800-624-4934

LA LECHE LEAGUE INTERNATIONAL
1400 N Meacham Road
Schaumburg, IL 60173
847-519-7730

MARCH OF DIMES BIRTH DEFECTS FOUNDATION
1275 Mamaroneck Avenue
White Plains, NY 10605
914-428-7100

MATERNITY CENTER ASSOCIATION
281 Park Avenue South, 5th Floor
New York, NY 10010
212-777-5000

NATIONAL ASSOCIATION OF NEONATAL NURSES (NANN)
1304 Southpoint Blvd., Suite 280
Petaluma, CA 94954
707-762-5588

NATIONAL ASSOCIATION OF PEDIATRIC NURSE ASSOCIATES AND PRACTITIONERS, INC. (NAPNAP)
1101 Kings Highway North, Suite 206
Cherry Hill, NJ 08034
609-667-1773

NATIONAL CERTIFICATION CORPORATION FOR THE OBSTETRIC, GYNECOLOGIC, AND NEONATAL NURSING SPECIALTIES (NCC)
P.O. Box 11082
Chicago, IL 60611-0082
800-367-5613

NATIONAL INSTITUTE OF CHILD HEALTH AND HUMAN DEVELOPMENT (NICHD)
National Institutes of Health
Center for Research on Mothers and Children
Building 6100, Room 4B05
Bethesda, MD 20892
301-496-5097

NATIONAL INSTITUTE OF NURSING RESEARCH (NINR)
National Institutes of Health
31 Center Drive, MSC 2178
Bethesda, MD 20892
301-496-0207

RTS BEREAVEMENT SERVICES (PERINATAL LOSS)
1910 South Avenue
LaCrosse, WI 54601
800-362-9564

RESOLVE (INFERTILITY EDUCATION)
1310 Broadway
Somerville, MA 02144
617-623-0744

SOCIETY FOR ASSISTED REPRODUCTIVE TECHNOLOGY (SART)
1209 Montgomery Highway
Birmingham, AL 35216
205-978-5000

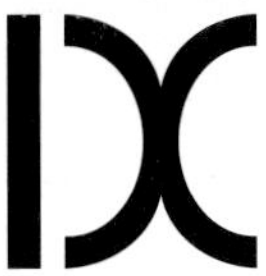

IX Appendix

Effective Care in Pregnancy and Childbirth: A Review of the Research Literature

Enkin and colleagues have created a comprehensive, systematic review of all randomized, controlled research trials relevant to the care of the woman during pregnancy and childbirth and of newborn infants. The authors of *Maternal-Newborn Nursing: Theory and Practice* encourage all nurses to carefully review the summary of that work, *A Guide to Effective Care in Pregnancy and Childbirth.* In Enkin and colleagues' text, Tables 1 to 6, which have been reproduced here, are cross-referenced to the specific chapters in which each is discussed.

BOOKS

- Enkin, M. W., Keirse, M. J. N. C., Renfrew, M., Neilson, J. (1995). *Effective care in pregnancy and childbirth* (2nd ed., 1500 pp.). Oxford, UK: Oxford University Press (two large volumes with detailed reviews and findings from the study).
- Enkin, M. W., Keirse, M. J. N. C., Renfrew, M., Neilson, J. (1995). *A guide to effective care in pregnancy and childbirth* (2nd ed., 300 pp.). Oxford, UK: Oxford University Press (summary of *Effective care in pregnancy and childbirth*).

DATABASE

- The Cochrane Pregnancy and Childbirth Database, based on Enkin and colleagues' work, is published twice yearly by UPDATE SOFTWARE. For information, contact: UPDATE SOFTWARE, Summertown Pavilion, Middle Way, Oxford, OX2 7LG, UK; telephone/FAX 44 1865 513902 (UK 01865 513902); e-mail: update@cochrane.co.uk.

Table 1

BENEFICIAL FORMS OF CARE: EFFECTIVENESS DEMONSTRATED BY CLEAR EVIDENCE FROM CONTROLLED TRIALS
BASIC CARE
Support for socially disadvantaged mothers to improve child care
Women carrying their case notes during pregnancy to enhance their feeling of being in control
Pre- and periconceptional folic acid supplementation to prevent recurrent neural tube defects
Folic acid supplementation (or high-folate diet) for all women contemplating pregnancy
Programs (particularly behavioral strategies) to assist stopping smoking during pregnancy
Balanced energy and protein supplementation of diet when supplementation is required

Table continued on facing page

Table 1

BENEFICIAL FORMS OF CARE: EFFECTIVENESS DEMONSTRATED BY CLEAR EVIDENCE FROM CONTROLLED TRIALS Continued

Vitamin D supplementation for women with inadequate exposure to sunlight
Iodine supplementation in populations with a high incidence of endemic cretinism

SCREENING
Doppler ultrasound in pregnancies at high risk of fetal compromise

PREGNANCY PROBLEMS
Antihistamines for nausea and vomiting of pregnancy if simple measures are ineffective
Local imidazoles for vaginal candida infection (thrush)
Local imidazoles instead of nystatin for vaginal candida infection (thrush)
Postpartum administration of anti-D immunoglobulin to rhesus-negative women with a rhesus-positive fetus
Administration of anti-D immunoglobulin to rhesus-negative women at 28 weeks of pregnancy
Antibiotic treatment of asymptomatic bacteriuria
Antibiotics during labor for women colonized with group B streptococcus
Tight as opposed to too strict or moderate control of blood sugar levels in diabetic women
External cephalic version at term to avoid breech presentation at birth
Corticosteroids to promote fetal maturation before preterm delivery
Offering induction of labor at 41+ weeks gestation

CHILDBIRTH
Emotional and psychological support during labor and birth
Maternal mobility and choice of position in labor
Agents to reduce acidity of stomach contents before general anesthesia
Fetal acid-base assessment as an adjunct to fetal heart monitoring in labor

PROBLEMS DURING CHILDBIRTH
Free mobility during labor to augment slow labor
Absorbable instead of nonabsorbable sutures for skin repair of perineal trauma
Polyglycolic acid sutures instead of chromic catgut for repair of perineal trauma

TECHNIQUES OF INDUCTION AND OPERATIVE DELIVERY
Prostaglandins to increase cervical readiness for induction of labor
Amniotomy plus oxytocin for induction of labor instead of either amniotomy or oxytocin alone
Vaginal prostaglandin E_2 for induction of labor
Vaginal prostaglandin E_2 instead of $PGF_{2\alpha}$ for induction of labor
Vacuum extraction instead of forceps when operative vaginal delivery is required
Antibiotic prophylaxis (short course or intraperitoneal lavage) with cesarean section

CARE AFTER CHILDBIRTH
Use of surfactant for very preterm infants to prevent respiratory distress syndrome
Consistent support for breastfeeding mothers
Personal support from a knowledgeable individual for breastfeeding mothers
Unrestricted breastfeeding
Local anesthetic sprays for relief of perineal pain postpartum
Cabergoline instead of bromocriptine for relief of breast symptoms in nonbreastfeeding mothers

Table 2

FORMS OF CARE LIKELY TO BE BENEFICIAL: THE EVIDENCE IN FAVOR OF THESE FORMS OF CARE IS NOT AS FIRMLY ESTABLISHED AS FOR THOSE IN TABLE 1

BASIC CARE

Adequate access to care for all childbearing women
Social support for childbearing women
Financial support for childbearing women in need
Legislation on paid leave and income maintenance during maternity or parental leave
Midwifery care for women with no serious risk factors
Continuity of care for childbearing women
Antenatal classes for women and their partners who want them
Advice to avoid excessive alcohol consumption during pregnancy
Avoidance of heavy physical work during pregnancy

SCREENING

Selective use of ultrasound to answer specific questions about fetal size, structure, or position
Selective use of ultrasound to assess amniotic fluid volume
Selective use of ultrasound to estimate gestational age in first and early second trimester
Ultrasound to facilitate intrauterine interventions
Ultrasound to determine whether the embyro is alive in threatened miscarriage
Ultrasound to confirm suspected multiple pregnancy
Ultrasound for placental location in suspected placenta previa
Early second trimester amniocentesis to identify chromosomal abnormalities in pregnancies at risk
Genetic counseling before prenatal diagnosis
Transabdominal instead of transcervical chorion villus sampling
Regular monitoring of blood pressure during pregnancy
Testing for proteinuria during pregnancy
Uric acid levels for following the course of pre-eclampsia
Fundal height measurements during pregnancy

PREGNANCY PROBLEMS

Antacids for heartburn of pregnancy if simple measures are ineffective
Bulking agents for constipation if simple measures are ineffective
Local metronidazole for symptomatic trichomonal vaginitis after first trimester
Antihypertensive agents to control moderate to severe hypertension in pregnancy
Antithrombotic and antiplatelet agents to prevent pre-eclampsia
Anticonvulsant agents for eclampsia
Screening all pregnant women for blood group isoimmunization
Anti-D immunoglobulin to rhesus-negative women after any bleeding episode during pregnancy
Anti-D immunoglobulin to rhesus-negative women after any intrauterine procedure
Anti-D immunoglobulin to rhesus-negative women sustaining abdominal trauma
Intrauterine transfusion for a severely affected isoimmunized fetus
Routine screening for and treatment of syphilis in pregnancy
Rubella vaccination of seronegative women postpartum
Screening for and treatment of chlamydia in high prevalence populations
Cesarean section for active herpes (with visible lesion) in labor with intact membranes
Prepregnancy counseling for women with diabetes
Specialist care for pregnant women with diabetes
Home instead of hospital glucose monitoring for pregnant women with diabetes
Ultrasound surveillance of fetal growth for pregnant women with diabetes
Allowing pregnancy to continue to term in otherwise uncomplicated diabetic pregnancies
Careful attention to insulin requirements postpartum
Encouraging diabetic women to breastfeed
Tests for blood clotting defect with severe placental abruption
Vaginal instead of cesarean delivery for placental abruption in the absence of fetal distress
Vaginal instead of cesarean delivery of a dead fetus after placental abruption
Repeat scanning at about 32 weeks for low-lying placenta
Delaying planned cesarean section for placenta previa until term
Cesarean section for placenta previa covering any portion of the cervical os
Ultrasound examination for vaginal bleeding of undetermined origin

Table continued on facing page

Table 2

FORMS OF CARE LIKELY TO BE BENEFICIAL: THE EVIDENCE IN FAVOR OF THESE FORMS OF CARE IS NOT AS FIRMLY ESTABLISHED AS FOR THOSE IN TABLE 1 Continued

External cephalic version for transverse lie at term
External cephalic version for breech in early labor if membranes are intact
Corticosteroid administration after prelabor rupture of membranes preterm
Vaginal culture after prelabor rupture of membranes preterm
Antibiotics for prelabor rupture of membranes with suspected intrauterine infection
Allowing labor to progress after spontaneous onset in prelabor rupture of membranes preterm
Elective delivery for prelabor rupture of membranes preterm with signs of infection
Amnioinfusion for fetal distress thought to be due to oligohydramnios in labor
Short-term indomethacin to stop preterm labor
Offering induction of labor as an option after fetal death
Vaginal prostaglandin $E_{2\alpha}$ for induction of labor after fetal death
Prostaglandin analogues for induction of labor after fetal death

CHILDBIRTH

Respecting women's choice of companions during labor and birth
Respecting women's choice of place of birth
Presence of a companion on admission to hospital
Giving women as much information as they desire
Change of mother's position for fetal distress in labor
Intravenous betamimetics for fetal distress in labor to "buy time"
Woman's choice of position for the second stage of labor or giving birth
Oxytocics to treat postpartum hemorrhage
Intramyometrial prostaglandins for severe postpartum hemorrhage

PROBLEMS DURING CHILDBIRTH

Regular top-ups of epidural analgesia instead of top-ups on maternal demand
Maternal movement and position changes to relieve pain in labor
Counterpressure to relieve pain in labor
Superficial heat or cold to relieve pain in labor
Touch and massage to relieve pain in labor
Attention focusing and distraction to relieve pain in labor
Music and audioanalgesia to relive pain in labor
Epidural instead of narcotic analgesia for preterm labor and birth
Amniotomy to augment slow or prolonged labor
Continuous subcuticular suture for perineal skin repair
Primary repair of episiotomy breakdown
Delivery of a very preterm baby in a center with adequate facilities to care for immature babies
Presence of a pediatrician at a very preterm birth
Trial of labor after previous lower segment cesarean section
Trial of labor after more than one previous lower segment cesarean section
Use of oxytocin when indicated after previous cesarean section
Use of epidural analgesia in labor when needed after previous cesarean section

TECHNIQUES OF INDUCTION AND OPERATIVE DELIVERY

Assessing the state of the cervix before induction of labor
Transverse instead of vertical skin incision for cesarean section
Low-dose heparin with cesarean section to prevent thromboembolism
Transverse lower segment uterine incision for cesarean section

CARE AFTER CHILDBIRTH

Keeping babies warm immediately after birth
Prophylactic vitamin K to the baby to prevent hemorrhagic disease of the newborn
Nasopharyngeal suctioning of infants who have passed meconium before birth
Presence of someone skilled in neonatal resuscitation at birth of all infants likely to be at risk
Oxygen for resuscitation of distressed newborn infants
Cardiac massage for infants born with absent heart beat
Naloxone for infants with respiratory depression due to narcotic administration before birth

Table continued on following page

Table 2

FORMS OF CARE LIKELY TO BE BENEFICIAL: THE EVIDENCE IN FAVOR OF THESE FORMS OF CARE IS NOT AS FIRMLY ESTABLISHED AS FOR THOSE IN TABLE 1 Continued

Encouraging early mother-infant contact
Allowing mothers access to their own supply of symptom-relieving drugs in hospital
Consistent advice to new mothers
Allowing women choice of length of postpartum stay in hospital
Telephone service of advice and information after women go home from hospital after birth
Psychological support for women depressed after childbirth
Encouraging early breastfeeding when mother and baby are ready
Skilled help with first breastfeed
Correct positioning of baby at breast for breastfeeding
Flexibility in breastfeeding practices
Antibiotics for infectious mastitis in breastfeeding women
Hospital support programs of care for bereaved parents
Encouraging parental contact with a dying or dead baby
Providing parents with prompt, accurate information about a severely ill baby
Encouraging autopsy for a dead baby and imparting results to parents
Help with funeral arrangements for a dead baby
Self-help groups for bereaved parents
Specialist counselors for parents with prolonged grief reactions

Table 3

FORMS OF CARE WITH A TRADE-OFF BETWEEN BENEFICIAL AND ADVERSE EFFECTS: WOMEN AND CAREGIVERS SHOULD WEIGH THESE EFFECTS ACCORDING TO INDIVIDUAL CIRCUMSTANCES AND PRIORITIES

BASIC CARE
Continuity of caregiver for childbearing women
Legislation restricting type of employment for childbearing women

SCREENING
Formal systems of risk scoring
Routine early ultrasound
Chorion villus sampling versus amniocentesis for diagnosis of chromosomal abnormalities
Serum alpha-fetoprotein screening for neural tube defects
Routine fetal movement counting to improve perinatal outcome

PREGNANCY PROBLEMS
Screening for toxoplasmosis during pregnancy
Corticosteroids to promote fetal maturation before preterm delivery in diabetic women
Induction of labor for prelabor rupture of membranes at term
Betamimetic drugs to delay preterm delivery for implementation of effective measures
Oral betamimetics to maintain labor inhibition
Cervical cerclage for women at risk of preterm birth
Betamimetic drugs to stop preterm labor
Expectant care versus induction of labor after fetal death

CHILDBIRTH
Continuous electronic fetal monitoring plus scalp sampling versus intermittent auscultation during labor
Midline versus mediolateral episiotomy, when episiotomy is necessary

Table continued on facing page

Table 3

FORMS OF CARE WITH A TRADE-OFF BETWEEN BENEFICIAL AND ADVERSE EFFECTS: WOMEN AND CAREGIVERS SHOULD WEIGH THESE EFFECTS ACCORDING TO INDIVIDUAL CIRCUMSTANCES AND PRIORITIES Continued

Prophylactic oxytocics in the third stage of labor
Active versus expectant management of third stage of labor

PROBLEMS DURING CHILDBIRTH
Routine preloading with intravenous fluids before epidural analgesia
Narcotics to relieve pain in labor
Inhalation analgesia to relieve pain in labor
Epidural analgesia to relieve pain in labor
Epidural administration of opiates to relieve pain in labor
Early amniotomy in spontaneous labor

TECHNIQUES OF INDUCTION AND OPERATIVE DELIVERY
Endocervical versus vaginal prostaglandin for cervical ripening before induction of labor
Oral prostaglandins for induction of labor with a ripe cervix
Prostaglandins versus oxytocin for induction of labor
Regional versus general anesthesia for cesarean section
Epidural versus spinal anesthesia for cesarean section
Ampicillin versus broader-spectrum antibiotics for cesarean section

CARE AFTER CHILDBIRTH
Prophylactic antibiotic eye ointments to prevent eye infection in the newborn
Prophylactic versus "rescue" surfactant for very preterm infants

Table 4

FORMS OF CARE OF UNKNOWN EFFECTIVENESS: THERE ARE INSUFFICIENT OR INADEQUATE QUALITY DATA UPON WHICH TO BASE A RECOMMENDATION FOR PRACTICE

BASIC CARE
Social support for high-risk women to prevent preterm birth
Formal preconceptional care for all women
Fish oil supplementation to improve pregnancy outcome
Prostaglandin precursors to improve pregnancy outcome
Changes in salt intake to prevent pre-eclampsia
Calcium supplementation to improve pregnancy outcome
Magnesium supplementation to improve pregnancy outcome
Zinc supplementation to improve pregnancy outcome
Antigen avoidance diets to reduce risk of an atopic child

SCREENING
Placental grading by ultrasound to improve perinatal outcome
Fetal biophysical profile for fetal surveillance

PREGNANCY PROBLEMS
Acupressure for nausea and vomiting of pregnancy if simple measures are ineffective
Vitamin B_6 for nausea and vomiting of pregnancy if simple measure are inefffective

Table continued on following page

Table 4

FORMS OF CARE OF UNKNOWN EFFECTIVENESS: THERE ARE INSUFFICIENT OR INADEQUATE QUALITY DATA UPON WHICH TO BASE A RECOMMENDATION FOR PRACTICE Continued

Ginger for nausea and vomiting of pregnancy
Prostigmine for heartburn of pregnancy if simple measures are ineffective
Dilute acid or lemon juice for heartburn of pregnancy if antacids do not provide relief
Increased salt intake for leg cramps
Progestogens for threatened miscarriage with a live fetus
Human chorionic gonadotropin for threatened miscarriage with a live fetus
Immunotherapy for recurrent miscarriage
Bed-rest for women with pre-eclampsia
Plasma volume expansion for pre-eclampsia
Choice among magnesium sulphate, benzodiazepines, and phenytoin for eclampsia
Hospitalization and bed-rest for impaired fetal growth
Abdominal decompression for impaired fetal growth
Betamimetics for impaired fetal growth
Oxygen therapy for impaired fetal growth
Hormone therapy for impaired fetal growth
Calcium-channel blockers for impaired fetal growth
Plasma volume expanders for impaired fetal growth
Prophylactic betamimetics for multiple pregnancy
Hospitalization and bed-rest for triplet and higher-order pregnancy
Treatment of group B streptococcus colonization during pregnancy
Antiviral agents for women with a history of recurrent genital herpes
Routine elective cesarean for breech presentation
Postural techniques for cephalic version of breech presentation
Prophylactic antibiotics for prelabor rupture of membranes at term or preterm
Postpartum prophylactic antibiotics after prelabor rupture of membranes
Home uterine activity monitoring for prevention of preterm birth
Bed-rest to prevent preterm birth
Magnesium supplementation to prevent preterm birth
Calcium supplementation to prevent preterm birth
Progestogens to prevent preterm birth
Magnesium sulphate to stop preterm labor
Calcium antagonists to stop preterm labor
Routine cervical assessment for prevention of preterm birth
Antibiotic therapy in preterm labor
Oxytocin antagonists to stop preterm labor
Adding thyrotropin-releasing hormone to corticosteroids to promote fetal maturation
Sweeping of membranes to prevent post-term pregnancy
Nipple stimulation to prevent post-term pregnancy
Induction instead of surveillance for pregnancy at 41+ weeks gestation

CHILDBIRTH

Routine amnioscopy to detect meconium in labor
Routine artificial rupture of membranes to detect meconium in labor
Short periods of electronic fetal monitoring as an admission screening test in labor
Fetal stimulation tests for fetal assessment in labor
Maternal oxygen administration for fetal distress in labor
Routinely repeated blood pressure measurements in labor
Guarding the perineum versus watchful waiting during birth
Prophylactic ergometrine + oxytocin versus oxytocin alone in third stage of labor
Early versus late clamping of the umbilical cord
Controlled cord traction in third stage of labor
Intraumbilical vein oxytocin for retained placenta

PROBLEMS DURING CHILDBIRTH

Abdominal decompression to relieve pain in labor
Immersion in water to relieve pain in labor

Table continued on facing page

Table 4

FORMS OF CARE OF UNKNOWN EFFECTIVENESS: THERE ARE INSUFFICIENT OR INADEQUATE QUALITY DATA UPON WHICH TO BASE A RECOMMENDATION FOR PRACTICE Continued

Acupuncture to relieve pain in labor
Acupressure to relieve pain in labor
Transcutaneous electrical nerve stimulation to relieve pain in labor
Intradermal injection of sterile water to relieve pain in labor
Aromatherapy to relieve pain in labor
Hypnosis to relieve pain in labor
Continuous infusion versus intermittent top-ups for epidural analgesia
Early use of oxytocin to augment slow or prolonged labor
"Active management" of labor
Cervical vibration for slow or prolonged labor
Histoacryl tissue adhesive for perineal skin repair
Phenobarbitone to the mother to prevent intraventricular hemorrhage in the very preterm infant
Vitamin K to the mother to prevent intraventricular hemorrhage in the very preterm infant
Cesarean section for very preterm delivery
Cesarean section for preterm breech delivery
Immediate versus delayed cord clamping at preterm birth

TECHNIQUES OF INDUCTION AND OPERATIVE DELIVERY

Oxytocin by automatic infusion systems versus 'standard regimens' for induction of labor
Use of hemostatic stapler for the uterine incision at cesarean section
Single-layer versus two-layer closure of the uterine incision at cesarean section
Systemic versus intraperitoneal prophylactic antibiotics at cesarean section

CARE AFTER CHILDBIRTH

Tracheal suctioning for meconium in babies without respiratory depression
Routine use of antiseptics for the cord
Oral proteolytic enzymes for breast engorgement in breastfeeding mothers
Cabbage leaves for breast engorgement in breastfeeding mothers
Dopamine agonists to improve milk supply in breastfeeding mothers
Oxytocin nasal spray to improve milk supply in breastfeeding mothers
Oral proteolytic enzymes for perineal pain postpartum
Ultrasound and pulsed electromagnetic energy for perineal pain
Rubber rings and similar devices to prevent pressure for perineal pain
Cabergoline versus physical methods of suppressing lactation

Table 5

FORMS OF CARE UNLIKELY TO BE BENEFICIAL: THE EVIDENCE AGAINST THESE FORMS OF CARE IS NOT AS FIRMLY ESTABLISHED AS FOR THOSE IN TABLE 6

BASIC CARE

Reliance on expert opinion instead of on good evidence for decisions about care
Routinely involving doctors in the care of all women during pregnancy and childbirth
Routinely involving obstetricians in the care of all women during pregnancy and childbirth
Not involving obstetricians in the care of women with serious risk factors
Fragmentation of care during pregnancy and childbirth
Advice to restrict sexual activity during pregnancy
Prohibition of all alcohol intake during pregnancy
Imposing dietary restrictions during pregnancy

Table continued on following page

Table 5

FORMS OF CARE UNLIKELY TO BE BENEFICIAL: THE EVIDENCE AGAINST THESE FORMS OF CARE IS NOT AS FIRMLY ESTABLISHED AS FOR THOSE IN TABLE 6 Continued

Routine vitamin supplementation in late pregnancy in well-nourished populations
Routine hematinic supplementation in pregnancy in well-nourished populations
High-protein dietary supplementation

SCREENING

Routine use of ultrasound for fetal anthropometry in late pregnancy
Using edema to screen for pre-eclampsia
Cold pressor test to screen for pre-eclampsia
Roll-over test to screen for pre-eclampsia
Isometric exercise test to screen for pre-eclampsia
Measuring uric acid as a diagnostic test for pre-eclampsia
Screening for "gestational diabetes"
Routine glucose challenge test during pregnancy
Routine measurement of blood glucose during pregnancy
Insulin plus diet therapy for "gestational diabetes"
Diet therapy for "gestational diabetes"
Routine use of Doppler ultrasound screening in all pregnancies
Measurement of placental proteins or hormones (including estriol and HPL)

PREGNANCY PROBLEMS

Calcium supplementation for leg cramps
Screening for and treatment of candidal colonization without symptoms
Screening for and treatment of *Trichomonas* colonization without symptoms
Bed-rest for threatened miscarriage
Diazoxide for pre-eclampsia or hypertension in pregnancy
Diuretics for pregnancy-induced hypertension
Hospitalization and bed-rest in twin pregnancy
Cervical cerclage for multiple pregnancy
Routine cesarean section for multiple pregnancy
Routine screening for mycoplasmas during pregnancy
Cesarean section for nonactive herpes simplex before or at the onset of labor
Elective delivery before term in women with otherwise uncomplicated diabetes
Elective cesarean section for pregnant women with diabetes
Discouraging breastfeeding in women with diabetes
Prohibition of oral contraceptives for diabetic women
Vaginal or rectal examination when placenta previa is suspected
X-ray pelvimetry to diagnose cephalopelvic disproportion
Computer tomographic pelvimetry to predict cephalopelvic disproportion
Liberal use (pretrial of labor) of cesarean section for macrosomia
Amniocentesis for prelabor rupture of membranes preterm
Prophylactic tocolytics with prelabor rupture of membranes preterm
Regular leukocyte counts for surveillance in prelabor rupture of membranes
Betamimetics for preterm labor in women with heart disease or diabetes
Hydration to arrest preterm labor
Diazoxide to stop preterm labor

CHILDBIRTH

Withholding food and drink from women in labor
Routine intravenous infusion in labor
Routine measurement of intrauterine pressure with oxytocin administration
Face masks during vaginal examinations
Frequent scheduled vaginal examinations in labor
Routine directed pushing during the second stage of labor
Pushing by sustained bearing down during second stage of labor
Breath-holding during the second stage of labor
Early bearing down during the second stage of labor
Arbitrary limitation of the duration of the second stage of labor

Table continued on facing page

Table 5

FORMS OF CARE UNLIKELY TO BE BENEFICIAL: THE EVIDENCE AGAINST THESE FORMS OF CARE IS NOT AS FIRMLY ESTABLISHED AS FOR THOSE IN TABLE 6 Continued

"Ironing out" or massaging the perineum during the second stage of labor
Routine manual exploration of uterus after vaginal delivery

PROBLEMS DURING CHILDBIRTH
Biofeedback to relieve pain in labor
Sedatives and tranquilizers to relieve pain in labor
Caudal block to relieve pain in labor
Paracervical block to relieve pain in labor
Intrapartum x-ray to diagnose cephalopelvic disproportion
Diagnosing cephalopelvic disproportion without ensuring adequate uterine contractions
Relaxin for slow or prolonged labor
Hyaluronidase for slow or prolonged labor
Delivery of a very preterm infant without adequate facilities to care for an immature baby
Elective forceps for preterm delivery
Routine use of episiotomy for preterm birth
Trial of labor after previous classical cesarean section
Manual exploration of the uterus to assess previous cesarean section scar

TECHNIQUES OF INDUCTION AND OPERATIVE DELIVERY
Mechanical methods for cervical ripening before induction of labor
Relaxin for cervical ripening before induction of labor
Nipple stimulation for cervical ripening before induction of labor
Extra-amniotic instead of other prostaglandin regimens for cervical ripening
Instrumental vaginal delivery to shorten second stage of labor
Routine exteriorization of the uterus for repair of uterine incision at cesarean section

CARE AFTER CHILDBIRTH
Silver nitrate to prevent eye infection in newborn babies
Elective tracheal intubation for very low birthweight infants who are not depressed
Routine suctioning of newborn babies
Medicated bathing of babies to reduce infection
Wearing hospital gowns in newborn nurseries
Restriction of sibling visits to babies in hospital
Routine measurements of temperature, pulse, blood pressure, and fundal height postpartum
Limiting use of women's own nonprescription drugs postpartum in hospital
Administering nonprescription symptom-relieving drugs at regularly set intervals
Antenatal breast or nipple care for women who plan to breastfeed
Nipple shields for breastfeeding mothers
Switching breasts before babies spontaneously terminate the feed
Oxytocin for breast engorgement in breastfeeding mothers
Antibiotics for localized breast engorgement (milk stasis)
Discontinuing breastfeeding for localized breast engorgement (milk stasis)
Combinations of local anesthetics and topical steroids for relief of perineal pain
Relying on these tables without referring to the rest of the book

Table 6

FORMS OF CARE LIKELY TO BE INEFFECTIVE OR HARMFUL: INEFFECTIVENESS OR HARM DEMONSTRATED BY CLEAR EVIDENCE

BASIC CARE
Dietary restriction to prevent pre-eclampsia

SCREENING
Contraction stress cardiotocography to improve perinatal outcome
Nipple-stimulation test cardiotocography to improve perinatal outcome
Nonstress cardiotocography to improve perinatal outcome

PREGNANCY PROBLEMS
ACTH for severe vomiting of pregnancy
Diethylstillbestrol during pregnancy
External cephalic version preterm to avoid breech presentation at birth
Elective delivery for prelabor rupture of membranes preterm
Ethanol to stop preterm labor
Progestogens to stop preterm labor

CHILDBIRTH
Routine enema in labor
Routine pubic shaving in preparation for delivery
Electronic fetal monitoring without access to fetal scalp sampling during labor
Prophylactic intrapartum amnioinfusion for oligohydramnios
Rectal examinations to assess labor progress
Requiring a supine (flat or back) position for second stage of labor
Routine use of the lithotomy position for the second stage of labor
Routine or liberal episiotomy for birth
Ergometrine instead of oxytocin in third stage of labor

PROBLEMS IN CHILDBIRTH
Glycerol-impregnated catgut for repair of perineal trauma

TECHNIQUES OF INDUCTION AND OPERATIVE DELIVERY
Oral prostaglandins for cervical ripening
Estrogens for cervical ripening or for induction of labor
Oxytocin for cervical ripening before induction of labor

CARE AFTER CHILDBIRTH
Sodium bicarbonate for asphyxiated babies
Routine restriction of mother-infant contact
Routine nursery care for babies in hospital
Antenatal Hoffman exercises for inverted or flat nipples
Antenatal breast shells for inverted or flat nipples
Limitation of suckling time for breastfeeding
Nipple creams or ointments for breastfeeding mothers
Routine supplements of water or formula for breastfed babies
Samples of formula for breastfeeding mothers
Encouraging fluid intake beyond demands of thirst for breastfeeding mothers
Combined estrogen-progesterone oral contraceptives for breastfeeding mothers
Test weighing of breastfed infants
Witch hazel for relief of perineal pain
Adding salt to bath water for perineal pain
Antiseptic solutions added to bath water for perineal pain
Hormones for relief of breast symptoms in nonbreastfeeding mothers
Bromocriptine for relief of breast symptoms in nonbreastfeeding mothers

From Enkin, M. W., Keirse, M. J. N. C., Renfrew, M., Neilson, J. (1995). *A Guide to Effective Care in Pregnancy and Childbirth* (2d ed.). Oxford, UK: Oxford University Press. Used with permission.

Glossary

abdominal pregnancy—Implantation of the fertilized ovum in the peritoneal cavity; usually the result of a tubal pregnancy that has ruptured into the abdomen.

abortion—The termination of a pregnancy prior to fetal viability; can be spontaneous (miscarriage), elective (planned), or therapeutic (medical).

abortion rate—The number of legal abortions per 1000 women aged 15 to 44 years.

abortion ratio—The number of legal abortions per 1000 live births.

abortion-related death—A death that results from a direct complication of an abortion, from an indirect complication caused by the chain of events initiated by an abortion, or from the aggravation of a preexisting condition by the physiologic or psychological effects of an abortion.

abruptio placentae—Premature separation of the placenta from the uterine wall; usually results in maternal hemorrhage and fetal compromise.

abstinence—Refraining from sexual intercourse completely for a period of time; can be used as a method of birth control.

abstinence-based sexuality education—An approach that focuses on the strategy of delaying intercourse on the basis of the belief that coitus in early adolescence is particularly risky and that it is either unrealistic or inappropriate to advocate abstinence by all persons in late adolescence. These programs typically stress abstinence, postponing intercourse, and skill building while discussing contraception.

abstinence-only education—Curricula that present abstinence as the only solution to teenage pregnancy and sexually transmitted diseases. Other preventive methods, such as condoms, are not discussed.

acceleration—An increase of at least 15 bpm over baseline fetal heart rate that lasts at least 15 seconds and is often associated with fetal movement and a sign of fetal well-being.

Accu-Check II—Device for determining blood glucose level by analyzing blood placed on a Chemstrip.

acini cells—Cells in the breast that secrete milk during lactation.

acme—Peak of a contraction.

acrocyanosis—Bluish discoloration of the hands and feet in the newborn; also termed peripheral cyanosis. Considered normal immediately after birth but should not persist for longer than 24 hours.

active phase—The second phase of first-stage labor; dilatation from 4 to 7 cm.

acupressure—The application of pressure with the thumb, index finger, or palm of the hand to an acupuncture point to relieve pain.

acupuncture—A nonpharmacologic pain relief method whereby needles are inserted at the site of acupuncture points to correct an imbalance in energy (chi) and thus reduce pain.

acute care—Health care services provided within the hospital setting.

adaptive parenting behaviors—Behaviors that facilitate the development of positive parent-infant attachment.

adnexa—Adjoining parts of the uterus; the ovaries and fallopian tubes.

adolescence—The transition years between puberty and adulthood; the teenage years.

adoptive family—The family to which the individual belongs through adoption, usually by legal means.

advanced practice—Nurses with advanced education in specialty areas within maternal-newborn nursing; nurse-midwife, nurse practitioner, and clinical nurse specialist.

afterbirth—The placenta and membranes; expelled after the birth of the baby during the third stage of labor.

afterpains—Painful uterine cramps during the first few postpartum days that result from normal uterine contractions.

agency adoption—An adoption handled through either public or private agencies that provide various services, usually including both pre-adoption and postadoption counseling.

agenesis—Absence or failure of development of any organ or part.

aggressive treatment—Using all means of treatment available when the outcome of the individual appears hopeless.

agonist-antagonist drugs—Narcotic analgesic drugs that have the property of both providing pain relief (agonist) and blocking respiratory depression (antagonist).

AIDS—Acquired immunodeficiency syndrome; caused by the HIV virus.

air embolism—Air blown into the vagina during orogenital sexual activity that can be rapidly absorbed by the uterine lining, transported to all areas of the body through the maternal bloodstream, and result in sudden death of the pregnant woman.

alleles—Alternative forms of a gene that may occupy a given locus.

alternate massage—A technique to sustain the infant's sucking at breast that increases the volume and fat content per feed. The breast is massaged and compressed during each pause between sucking bursts.

alveoli—The milk-producing cells in the breast.

ambivalence—Mixed feelings regarding pregnancy; feeling happy and excited at one moment and then unhappy or depressed the next.

ambulatory care—Health care services provided within clinics and outpatient settings.

amenorrhea—Absence or suppression of menses.

amicus brief—A concise written statement from some person or group not a party to the case presented to the court with the court's permission that presents argument of information relevant to the case.

amnesic drugs—Drugs that block memory.

amniocentesis—The process in which amniotic fluid is removed through a needle inserted into the amniotic sac. The fluid can be used to determine fetal maturity and fetal health.

amnion—The inner layer of the two membranes that comprise the amniotic sac.

amnionitis—Inflammation (infection) of the amnion and amniotic fluid.

amniotic fluid—The clear, colorless, odorless fluid contained within the amniotic sac that surrounds the fetus in utero; protects the fetus from injury and maintains constant body temperature.

amniotic fluid embolism—Infusion of a large amount of amniotic fluid into the maternal circulation; can culminate in respiratory arrest and maternal death.

amniotomy—Artificial rupture of the membranes (AROM) using an instrument called an amnihook.

anal atresia—Absence of the anal canal or orifice.

anal stage—The stage of development identified by Freud during which the young child's interest revolves around the processes of elimination.

analgesics—Drugs that decrease the perception of pain.

anencephalic—The condition of having no encephalon or brain.

anencephaly—A congenital defect in the newborn's skull resulting from failed closure of the anterior neural tube.

anesthetics—Pain relief modalities that have the ability to totally block the sensation of pain; local, regional, or general anesthetics.

aneuploidy—Any chromosome number that is not an exact multiple of the haploid number (23), as in trisomy and monosomy.

anomaly—A deviation from the normal, usually from a congenital or hereditary origin.

anorexia—Eating disorder reflective of a distorted body image, characterized by strict control of diet and exercise regimens.

antenatal—Prior to birth.

antepartum—The period of pregnancy from conception to the onset of labor.

anthropometric measurements—Measurements of size, weight, and proportions of the human body.

anticipatory grief—Expectation of a future loss, frequently precipitated by the crisis of an unexpected illness or by the birth of a high-risk infant. Parents who have high-risk infants and experience anticipatory grief may be hesitant to become involved with their infant's care.

anticipatory guidance—Counseling or education about what to expect in the future and how to cope with future events.

antrum—Fluid-filled space in the follicle that marks the maturation of the ovum.

Apgar score—The immediate assessment of the newborn at 1 and 5 minutes after birth; evaluates heart rate, respiratory effort, muscle tone, reflex irritability, and color.

apnea—Respiratory pause greater than or equal to 20 seconds in length, associated with bradycardia and cyanosis.

applied research—The scientific investigation of techniques to directly improve patient care.

appraisal support—A type of social support in which information is shared to help people evaluate themselves or a given situation.

appropriate for gestational age (AGA)—An infant whose weight, length, and head circumference fall between the 10th and 90th percentiles for gestational age when plotted on a standard growth curve.

areola—Dark pigmented area around the nipple of the breast.

artificial insemination—Placement of one or more semen samples, produced by the husband or a donor, in the vagina, cervical canal, or uterus of a woman by artificial means such as a syringe.

artificial rupture of membranes (AROM)—Breaking the amniotic sac with the use of an Amnihook to facilitate labor progress.

atony of the uterus—Most common cause of postpartum hemorrhage; caused by inability of the uterus to contract efficiently after birth.

attachment—The affectionate relationship that develops between parents and the infant during the first year of life.

augmentation of labor—Use of amniotomy or oxytocin (Pitocin) to stimulate uterine contractions in an already established but dysfunctional labor.

auscultation—Listening directly to the fetal heart rate with the use of a fetoscope or stethoscope.

autosomal dominant—A trait affecting either sex, caused by an allele on an autosome that exerts an observable effect when present in one copy.

autosomal recessive—A trait affecting either sex, caused by an allele on an autosome that must be present in two copies to exert an observable effect.

autosome—Any chromosome other than the sex chromosomes; 22 pairs in the human karyotype.

Ballard—Simplified version of the Dubowitz tool for evaluation of newborn gestational age.

ballottement—A maneuver done with palpation to test for a floating object in the body; in pregnancy, done during vaginal or abdominal examination to detect the rebound movement of the fetus; light tapping or pushing of the fingers causes the fetus to move away and then return to touch the examiner's fingers.

bands—Alternating dark and light areas visible on chromosomes after certain types of stains are used.

barbiturate drugs—Sedative or hypnotic drugs that produce sleep.

Barr body—The inactive X chromosome, visible as a densely stained chromatin mass in the somatic cells of normal females. Also known as sex chromatin.

Bartholin glands—Greater vestibular glands located on either side of the vaginal orifice that secrete mucus during intercourse.

basal body temperature (BBT)—A method of natural family planning based on identification of the shift in the woman's body temperature that takes place after ovulation.

baseline fetal heart rate—The most typical fetal heart rate over a 10-minute period or between uterine contractions in labor. The normal baseline rate is 120 to 160 bpm.

basic research—The scientific investigation of fundamental processes that are usually not directly observable. Such processes, when explained, provide understanding of observed events.

beta-adrenergic agonist—A drug that has as one of its actions an effect on the myometrial cell through a membrane-mediated mechanism; theorized to act as a tocolytic; examples are terbutaline (Brethine) and ritodrine (Yutopar).

bicornuate uterus—Uterus that develops abnormally with a septum dividing.

bimanual examination—An examination in which one hand is placed on the abdomen while two fingers of the other hand are placed in the vagina to palpate the pelvic organs.

binding-in—The commitment that the pregnant woman forms to her baby by the end of pregnancy; similar to prenatal attachment.

biofeedback—The use of monitoring instruments to recognize and alter physiologic processes within the body.

biophysical profile (BPP)—A group of fetal well-being tests that include a nonstress test, ultrasound examination of the fetus to assess fetal activities (fetal movements, fetal breathing movements, and fetal tone), amniotic fluid volume, and the grade of the placenta.

birth centers—A maternity unit that provides low-technology care in a homelike setting from which women return home shortly after giving birth.

birth partner—The person (husband, father of baby, mother, family member, friend, or other person) who accompanies the woman during her labor and birth; also called labor companion, coach, or support person.

birth rate—The number of births per 1000 population.

birthing room—A single-room concept seen in many hospitals for labor, delivery, and recovery (LDR); in some settings, the room may also be used for the postpartum stay (LDRP).

Bishop score—A system for rating the readiness of the cervix for labor based on the assessment of cervical position, consistency, effacement, dilatation, and fetal station.

blastocyst—Stage of growth and development that follows a morula; at this point, approximately 100 cells exist.

blastomere—Stage of growth and development that follows the zygote; at this point, approximately two to eight cells exist.

blended family—A family that includes a child who is biologically related to only one of the adult partners.

blocking polyspermy—Normal physiologic changes that make more than one sperm unable to fertilize the same ovum.

bloody show—Bloody vaginal discharge, often mixed with mucus, caused by the rupture of capillaries in the cervix as it begins to efface and dilate; often is present during latent labor.

body image—The subjective mental picture of her body that the woman develops in her mind during pregnancy.

body mechanics—Safe movements of the body when rising from a lying position, bending, or lifting to protect abdominal and low back muscles during pregnancy.

bonding—A parent's feeling of closeness toward the newborn infant that is facilitated by early physical contact between parent and infant.

bonding theory—A theory by Klaus and Kennell that used the concept of a "sensitive period" to explain mothers' attachment to their infants as well as disruptions in attachment.

boundary—Filters both the kind and rate of inputs and outputs to and from the system.

brachial palsy—Paralysis (partial or complete) of the infant's arm due to trauma to the brachial plexus during birth.

Bradley husband-coached childbirth—A method of prepared childbirth developed by Robert Bradley and published in 1965 in *Husband-Coached Childbirth.* This method advocates deep relaxation techniques and slow abdominal breathing to promote comfort. The woman's spouse is viewed as the most effective support person for her during labor.

bradycardia—A heart rate less than 80 to 100 beats per minute in the newborn.

Braxton Hicks contractions—The normal painless contractions of the uterus that occur throughout pregnancy; caused by increased estrogen and uterine distention. These contractions are often associated with false labor; contractions occur but progressive cervical changes are not apparent.

Brazelton Neonatal Behavioral Assessment Scale (BNBAS)—An assessment tool that can be used to measure certain aspects of infant behavior and identify individual differences in infant behavior. It can be used as a diagnostic tool for neurologic impairment or to teach parents the unique social and interactive capabilities of their newborn. The scale is designed for infants from birth to 1 month of age.

breast shells—Plastic devices worn during pregnancy or between breastfeedings to revert flat or retracted nipples.

breech presentation—A presentation of the fetus in which the bottom (breech) of the fetus is coming first; the breech presentation can be complete, frank, footling, or kneeling.

bregma—The area of the fetal head that includes the anterior fontanelle.

bronchopulmonary dysplasia (BPD)—Chronic lung condition characterized by obstructive bronchiolitis, hyperinfiltration, and pulmonary fibrosis.

brow presentation—A presentation of the fetus in which the brow, the area between the orbital ridges and the bregma, is presenting as a result of the failure of the head to flex; results in a difficult labor because of a larger diameter of the head moving through the pelvis.

brown adipose tissue—Often called brown fat, this substance provides the energy for thermogenesis in the newborn.

bulimia—Eating disorder characterized by binging and purging.

calcium channel blockers—A group of organic compounds used for tocolysis to manage preterm labor; inhibit the influx of extracellular calcium across the cell membrane, leading to a decrease of myometrial contractions.

calendar method—A method of natural family planning, also known as the rhythm method, based on mathematical calculations to predict the time of ovulation.

capacitation—Penetration of the zona pellucida by a mature sperm.

captain-of-the-ship doctrine—The concept that as "captain," the physician was held responsible for the "crew," including nurses.

caput succedaneum—Edema in the tissues of the presenting part that may cross the suture lines of the skull bones.

cardinal movements—The movements the fetus must accomplish to negotiate passage through the maternal pelvis and be born; engagement, descent, flexion, internal rotation, extension, restitution, external rotation, and expulsion (birth).

carrier—An individual who has a copy of a disease-causing gene but does not express the disease. The term is used to denote heterozygotes for a recessive disease gene.

case management—Health care management that uses individuals to determine the necessity of services for clients and then to authorize necessary services.

central cyanosis—Overall cyanosis, including the central or trunk area of the neonate.

centromere—The primary constriction of a chromosome that separates the short arms from the long arms of the chromosome. Centromeres are the sites of attachment of spindle fibers during cell division.

cephalhematoma—A collection of blood between the cranial bone and the periosteum that does not cross the suture lines of the skull bones.

cephalic presentation—A presentation of the fetus in which the head is coming first.

cephalocaudal—Growth and development from the head down the body to the lower extremities.

cephalopelvic disproportion (CPD)—A relationship between the fetal head and the maternal pelvis in which either the fetus is too large for the pelvis or the pelvis is too small to allow passage of the fetal head.

certified nurse-midwife (CNM)—A registered nurse who has specialized training to care for women during pregnancy and childbirth and who is certified by the American College of Nurse-Midwives.

cervical cap—A barrier method of contraception; a small, thimble-shaped cup that fits over the cervix to block sperm from entering the uterus; used with a spermicidal agent.

cervical mucus method—A method of natural family planning that uses the recognition of changes in cervical mucus to identify fertile and infertile periods of the menstrual cycle; also known as the ovulation method.

cervical ripening—The softening of the cervix before the beginning of active labor.

cervix—Lowermost portion of uterus that extends into the vagina; the opening of the uterus that dilates during labor.

cesarean birth—The delivery of the fetus through an abdominal and uterine incision; a primary cesarean is the first cesarean a woman experiences; all following cesarean deliveries are called repeat cesareans.

Chadwick sign—Bluish coloration of the vaginal mucosa caused by increased vascularity of pregnancy; observed at about 4 weeks' gestation.

change agent—An individual or a group who initiates change or assists others to initiate change within a system.

charitable immunity—The concept that hospitals as charitable organizations should not be sued for negligence.

child abuse—The physical abuse or neglect, emotional abuse or mistreatment, or sexual abuse of a child.

child health assessment model—A model developed by Barnard that explains how perinatal, parental, and child characteristics and parent-child interaction factors may interact in complex ways to shape development of children.

childbearing family—An intimate social unit of persons living together in a household, going through the development processes of conceiving, bearing, and raising children.

childhood sexual abuse—The use, persuasion, or coercion of a child to engage in sexually explicit conduct or any simulation of such conduct.

chlamydial infection—A sexually transmitted infectious disease caused by the organism *Chlamydia trachomatis.*

chloasma—A "mask of pregnancy" exhibited as brown pigmentation over the bridge of the nose and cheeks in some women.

chorioamnionitis—Infection of the chorion, amnion, and amniotic fluid.

chorion—The outer layer of the two membranes that comprise the amniotic sac.

chorionic villus—Tissue is formed into projections; part of the placenta.

chorionic villus sampling (CVS)—A technique for the diagnosis of genetic disorders in which chorionic villi from the placenta are aspirated and examined.

chromosomes—Microscopic structures present in the cell nucleus composed of chromatin. Chromosomes contain genetic information and are constant in number in a species; humans have 46 chromosomes, 22 autosome pairs and 2 sex chromosomes.

circumcision—Surgical procedure that removes the foreskin (prepuce) from the penis.

claims made insurance—Insurance coverage occurs only when a policy is currently in force.

cleavage—Cell division.

cleft lip—A congenital defect in the upper lip.

clitoris—Female organ composed of erectile tissue located at the top of the vulva; the homolog of the male penis.

clonus—Spasmodic contraction and relaxation of a muscle.

closed family system—A family system with strong boundaries that is mostly resistant to inputs from the environment. There is minimal processing of information by the family and minimal feedback to the environment.

closed or confidential adoption—An adoption in which there is no contact between the adoptive parents and birth parents.

closing phase—The final portion of a home visit, in which the content of the visit is summarized, goal accomplishment is evaluated, and plans are made for future visits.

clubfoot—Congenital deformity of the foot in which the forefoot is adducted and turns medially; also called talipes equinovarus. There is varus of the heel, and the foot and toes point downward.

coccyx—Terminal portion of vertebral column consisting of four rudimentary vertebrae.

code of ethics—An ethical document that contains general principles of appropriate behavior.

codominance—Alleles that are both expressed when they occur together in the heterozygous state. An example is the A and B alleles of the ABO blood group system.

codon—A group of three bases in a DNA or RNA molecule, specifying a single amino acid.

cognitive control theory—Steven's psychological pain management strategy, which proposes that mental activities can alter the awareness of pain sensation.

cognitive dissonance—A difference between what is expected and what is actually experienced.

coitus—Sexual intercourse.

coitus interruptus—The practice of the male withdrawing the penis when ejaculation seems imminent to prevent the deposit of sperm in the vaginal tract.

cold stress—Excessive loss of heat in a newborn, leading to increased respirations and nonshivering thermogenesis.

collaborative care map—A multidisciplinary plan of care for a client that includes the key interventions necessary to promote desired client outcomes and efficient use of resources according to a timeline. A collaborative care map may also be called a case management plan, critical pathway, or care map.

colostrum—The first food the infant receives from the breast. The yellowish fluid is present in the breasts from the fourth month of pregnancy and contains immunoglobulins for disease protection.

community—Variously defined to mean the group of persons with whom the client interacts or shares common characteristics, or more commonly, a geographic area, from a neighborhood to a large city, consisting of persons, organizations, and services for independent and interdependent living.

community resources—Organizations or services available in the community to meet a variety of client needs.

competency motivation—An intrinsic motive to cope effectively with the environment.

complete abortion—Expulsion of the entire conceptus; before 10 weeks' gestation, complete emptying of the uterus is the norm and is evidenced by cessation of pain and bleeding.

compound presentation—When a fetal extremity presents along with the primary presenting part, such as an arm along with the head.

comprehensive sexuality education—A comprehensive approach that involves a broad range of topics focusing on the belief that sexuality education should prepare adolescents for the healthy expression of their sexuality instead of focusing only on the prevention of negative consequences. These curricula deal with traditional areas of reproductive biology, puberty, marriage, and sexually transmitted diseases but also cover many controversial topics, such as sexual pleasure, noncoital sexual expression, and homosexuality.

concept—A mental picture of an event or object.

conception—Fertilization resulting from the union of the female ovum and male sperm.

condom—A rubber or animal skin sheath placed on the erect penis before sexual intercourse to prevent deposition of semen in the vagina.

conduction—The mechanism of heat loss through direct skin contact with a cool surface.

congenital—Condition present at birth.

congenital heart disease—A spectrum of cardiac anomalies present at birth.

consanguinity—The mating of related individals.

consultant—An individual with expertise in a specialized area who provides advice and recommendations.

consumer advocacy—Informing, supporting, and encouraging clients to participate in making decisions that affect their well-being and that of their unborn child.

contraception—Prevention of conception.

contraction—Intermittent tightening of the uterine muscle during labor; accomplishes the effacement and dilatation of the cervix and facilitates fetal descent through the pelvis.

contraction stress test (CST)—A test of fetal well-being in which an electronic fetal monitor is applied and the woman is stimulated to have uterine contractions by receiving intravenous oxytocin (Pitocin). The woman may also use nipple stimulation to induce contractions. The fetal heart rate response to the contractions is assessed. Also known as an oxytocin challenge test.

convection—The mechanism of heat loss into the atmosphere, usually as air blows over the infant.

Coombs test—A test to determine the presence of Rh-positive antibodies in maternal blood (indirect) or maternal Rh-positive antibodies in fetal cord blood (direct).

cord presentation or prolapse—Presentation in which the cord lies below the fetus and thus presents first; also known as funic presentation.

corpus—The body of the uterus, comprising the upper two thirds of the organ.

corpus luteum—Remnant of the ruptured ovarian follicle that facilitates production of progesterone in second half of menstrual cycle.

cotyledon—A segment of the uterine surface of the placenta.

couvade—Physical symptoms of pregnancy or birth experienced by some expectant fathers during their partner's pregnancy.

crisis—A critical life event that results in the disruption of one's normal equilibrium and requires some form of coping effort; caused by normal maturational experiences in the life cycle (developmental crises) or by unexpected life situations (situational crises).

critical thinking—The examination and analysis of ideas, assumptions, beliefs, arguments, conclusions, and actions to determine their validity and credibility using scientific reasoning, problem-solving, and decision-making skills.

crowning—When the biparietal diameter of the fetal head is encircled by the vulvar ring just before birth; if the fetus is in a cephalic presentation, the crown of the head is visualized.

cryopreserved embryo transfer (CPE)—Frozen embryos that are preserved after a previous assisted reproductive technology and then thawed for transfer to the uterus for another attempt at implantation.

cryotherapy—Procedure to treat retinopathy of prematurity. A probe cooled with liquid nitrogen is applied to the external sclera over the area of abnormal blood vessels resulting in scarring that causes regression of the disease process.

cultural proscriptions—Behaviors that are taboo or prohibited in a culture, as in the case of new mothers.

culture—The ideas, customs, skills, and arts of a given people in a given period of history.

cumulus—Term used to describe several layers of granulosa cells in ovum.

cunnilingus—Oral sexual stimulation of the female genitals.

curettage—Suction and sharp curettage procedures performed at 12 weeks or less of gestation.

cyanosis, central—Bluish discoloration of the skin and mucous membranes related to hypoxia.

cyanosis, circumoral—Bluish discoloration of the lips and the area surrounding the mouth.

de novo—Arising anew. Refers to a new mutation.

decidua—Endometrium during pregnancy; subdivided into basal, capsular, and parietal sections.

decrement—Diminution of a contraction.

DeLee catheter—A plastic catheter used to suction the respiratory tract of the neonate; suction is supplied by the operator or the catheter is adapted to mechanical wall suction, and fluids are collected in a plastic reservoir.

deletion—The loss of chromosome material.

denominator—Point chosen by convention to allow standardization regarding fetal presentation or position; for example, the occiput is used for a vertex presentation, the sacrum for a breech.

deoxyribonucleic acid (DNA)—A double-helix molecule that consists of a sugar-phosphate backbone and four nitrogenous bases (adenine, cytosine, guanine, and thymine). DNA bases encode messenger RNA (mRNA), which in turn encodes amino acid sequences.

Depo-Provera—A long-acting injectable progestin contraceptive.

dermatoglyphics—The patterns of the ridged skin of the digits, palms, and soles, which are useful in the diagnosis of certain disorders.

developmental tasks of pregnancy—Necessary adaptations that need to be accomplished to prepare the woman and her partner for the birth of the baby and the role of parenting.

Dextrostix—Glucose strips used to assess the neonate's blood sugar level by comparing the color strip with a color chart after the strip is saturated with blood.

diagonal conjugate—An anterior-posterior pelvic measurement estimated with the examiner's hand from the lower margin of the symphysis pubis to the sacral promontory.

diaphragm—A barrier method of birth control; a shallow, dome-shaped device with a flexible metal rim that fits into the vagina against the cervix to block sperm from entering the uterus; used with a spermicidal agent.

diaphragmatic hernia—Congenital defect whereby the abdominal contents enter the thoracic cavity through an opening in the diaphragm.

diastasis recti—Separation of the abdominal rectus muscles that may occur in pregnancy.

Dick-Read prepared childbirth—A method of prepared childbirth developed by Dr. Grantly Dick-Read and published in 1933 in *Natural Childbirth.* Information, muscular relaxation techniques, and slow abdominal breathing strategies were advocated to interrupt the fear-tension-pain cycle.

dilatation—The opening of the cervical os, also called dilation; measured from 0 to 10 cm.

dilatation and curettage (D & C)—When used in referring to abortion, D & C is the termination of pregnancy during the first trimester by either suction (the most commonly used) or sharp (the oldest method) curettage.

dilatation and evacuation (D & E)—The termination of pregnancy during the second trimester by presurgical dilatation of the cervix followed by suction curettage.

diploid—Having two copies of each chromosome. In humans, the diploid number is 46.

disseminated intravascular coagulation (DIC)—A hypocoagulation syndrome resulting from inappropriate activation of the clotting process; the underlying disease process causes intravascular consumption of plasma clotting factors and platelets such that hemorrhage occurs.

distress/disengagement cues—Behavioral cues that indicate the infant's lack of organization and signal a need for a time-out period of rest and recuperation.

dizygous twins—Two separate ova are fertilized and two separate embryos develop.

DNA fingerprinting—A method used to distinguish individuals on the basis of differences in DNA sequence.

dominant—A trait expressed when the gene is present in a single dose or copy.

doula—Labor support persons.

drug therapy—To regulate and stimulate ovulation, fertility drugs (clomiphene [Clomid] and renotropins [Pergonal]) are given to women as the first step in assisted reproductive technology.

Down syndrome—A congenital abnormality caused by the presence of an extra number 21 chromosome (trisomy 21); results in a characteristic physical appearance and mental retardation.

Duncan presentation—Expulsion of the placenta with the maternal side presenting first; because of the dark, irregular appearance of the maternal side, this presentation is often called "dirty Duncan."

ductus arteriosus—A channel between the fetal aorta and main pulmonary artery that closes after birth as a result of normal respiratory function.

ductus venosus—A fetal blood vessel that connects the umbilical vein and the inferior vena cava.

duration—The length of a labor contraction, measured from the beginning to the end of the contraction; recorded in seconds.

dyspareunia—Painful intercourse.

dystocia—Abnormal or difficult labor; caused by problems related to the maternal pelvis, maternal soft tissues, or fetus; can refer to abnormal labor pattern when compared with the Friedman curve.

early adolescence—Developmental ages ranging from 11 to 13 years.

early contact—Interaction between parent and newborn infant during the first few days after birth.

early decelerations—A decrease in the fetal heart rate that begins and ends at the same time as the uterine contraction, causing a consistent U-shaped waveform that mirrors the contraction on an electronic fetal monitor; thought to be caused by head compression during labor.

early prenatal care—The first prenatal care visit to a health provider is within 3 months of conception (first trimester).

eclampsia—A hypertensive disorder of pregnancy in which maternal convulsions occur along with the hypertension, edema, and proteinuria associated with preeclampsia.

ectopic pregnancy—Implantation of a fertilized ovum outside the endometrium/decidua of the uterine cavity; often, but not exclusively, implantation is in the fallopian tubes.

effacement—The thinning or flattening of the edge of the cervical os; measured from 0 to 100 percent.

effleurage—Light fingertip massage of the abdomen used along with controlled breathing techniques to provide comfort during labor contractions.

egg donation—Eggs are removed from the ovaries of a donor (who meets certain age and health requirements and is usually paid) and transferred after fertilization in a laboratory Petri dish to the uterus of an infertile woman.

ejaculation—The release of seminal fluid from the penis during the orgasmic phase of sexual intercourse or masturbation.

Electra complex—The jealousy experienced by a young girl of her mother's relationship with her father.

electronic fetal monitoring (EFM)—Continuous recording of the fetal heart rate and uterine contractions by an electronic fetal monitor using external or internal modes.

embryo—Stage of growth and development from implantation to the end of the seventh postconceptional week.

emotional lability—Frequency and/or extremes in emotional changes experienced by a woman during pregnancy.

emotional support—A type of social support in which communication of empathy, caring, love, and trust are given to an individual.

endogenous biochemical pain theory—Pain theory based on the existence of morphine-like substances within the body that can alter pain perception.

endometriosis—A condition in which tissue containing typical endometrial elements grows outside of the uterus in the pelvic cavity or some other area of the body.

endometritis—Inflammation of the endometrial lining of the uterus.

endometrium—Mucous membrane lining of the uterus.

endorphins—Morphine-like polypeptides produced in the pituitary gland that are released in response to pain, exercise, or cutaneous stimulation and serve to decrease pain perception.

engagement—The entrance of the presenting part of the fetus into the pelvic inlet and the beginning of the mechanism of descent.

engorgement—Swelling and distention of the breast, usually in the early days after delivery, due to edema, vascular congestion, and the increased production of milk.

entrepreneur—An individual who undertakes a business venture.

epidural block—A regional anesthetic given in active first-stage labor by injection of the agent through an indwelling plastic catheter into the epidural (peridural) space of the spinal column; provides pain relief of the contractions of labor and for delivery.

episiotomy—The surgical incision made in the perineum to enlarge the vaginal opening for delivery. There are two types of incisions: mediolateral, an incision at a 45-degree angle from the midline; and midline or median, an incision straight in the midline toward the rectum.

epistaxis—Nosebleeds that can occur in pregnancy as a result of elevated estrogen and edema of the nasal mucosa.

epulis—Swelling and bleeding of the gums caused by increased vascularity and proliferation of connective tissue due to increased estrogen levels in pregnancy.

erythema toxicum—Normal papular rash of the newborn, appearing within 1 to 2 days after birth.

erythroblastosis fetalis—Hemolytic disease of the fetus and newborn resulting from isoimmunization; caused by Rh or ABO incompatibility with maternal blood.

esophageal atresia—Lack of continuity of the esophagus.

estrogen—Female hormone secreted by the ovary; has an effect on the development of secondary sexual characteristics, the menstrual cycle, and pregnancy.

ethical decision making—The process of resolving an ethical dilemma through critical and systematic analyses, using the principles of ethics to reach a decision about what it is morally right to do in the situation.

ethical dilemma—A difficult situation in which there are conflicting values, obligations, or principles about resolution.

ethics—A philosophy of moral behavior that deals with basic questions of meaning and value.

ethnicity—Affiliation with a homogeneous population as distinguished by customs, characteristics, language, or common history.

euploidy—Having a complete correct chromosome set.

eutocia—Normal labor; usually refers to labor progress, often in comparison to a Friedman curve.

evaporation—The mechanism of heat loss when water is lost through the skin to the environment.

exchange transfusion—Replacement of 75 to 85 percent of the circulating blood volume.

excitement phase—The first phase of the sexual response cycle during which the initiation of the physiologic processes of vasocongestion and myotonia results from sexual excitement.

executive—A manager or administrator.

executive subsystem—The governing family members, usually the parents.

exon—Portions of genes that encode amino acids and are retained after the primary mRNA transcript is spliced.

expressivity—Variation in the clinical expression of a trait ranging from mild to severe.

extended family—A family group that includes at least three generations of individuals related by blood or marriage.

extension—An attitude of the fetus in which the head is in a straight alignment or tilted back and the extremities are extended.

external cephalic version—Manual turning of the fetus in a noncephalic presentation into a cephalic presentation.

external ultrasound transducer—A disk that is attached by a belt around the woman's abdomen to record the fetal heart rate through sound waves on an electronic fetal monitor.

face presentation—A presentation of the fetus in which the fetal head is hyperextended so that the face is the presenting part.

fallopian tubes—Oviduct.

false labor—A period of regular or irregular Braxton Hicks contractions that occur toward the end of the pregnancy but do not result in progressive cervical dilatation.

false pelvis—The portion of the maternal bony pelvis above the linea terminalis (brim) and between the iliac crests.

family—A group of individuals related by blood, marriage, or mutual goals.

family-centered maternity care (FCMC)—Maternity care that is family oriented and views childbirth as a vital, natural life event rather than an illness.

family developmental tasks—Skills or competencies acquired by a family at a particular stage of development.

family of origin—The family into which the individual was born, also called biologic family.

fantasy—A stage in the process of maternal role development in which the woman engages in a form of daydreaming about how she will behave as a mother.

fear-tension-pain theory—Dick-Read's theory that fear of childbirth causes uterine tension, which then increases perceived pain.

fecundity—Fertility.

feeding cues—Signs of feeding readiness in the infant demonstrated by rapid eye movements under the eyelids, sucking movements of the mouth and tongue, hand-to-mouth movements, body movements, and small sounds.

female condom—A female method of birth control consisting of a polyurethane sheath with a flexible ring at each end that is placed inside the vagina to prevent sperm from entering the cervix.

Ferguson reflex—A circular process in which the stretching of the cervix from pressure of the fetal presenting part causes the release of oxytocin, resulting in increased myometrial activity.

ferning test—Microscopic evaluation of vaginal secretions for a ferning pattern; such a pattern is present after rupture of membranes due to salt in amniotic fluid.

fertility rate—The number of live births per 1000 women aged 15 to 44 years.

fertilization—Uniting of mature ovum and sperm.

fetal admission test—A fetal heart rate tracing obtained by an external fetal monitor for 20 to 30 minutes on admission to the hospital; also called a baseline tracing.

fetal age—The age of the fetus as calculated in weeks from the time of conception.

fetal alcohol syndrome (FAS)—A group of physical and mental alterations in the newborn caused by the ingestion of alcohol during pregnancy.

fetal attitude—The relation of fetal parts to one another; a state of either flexion or extension.

fetal bradycardia—A baseline fetal heart rate that is less than 120 beats per minute.

fetal distress—Decreased oxygenation to the fetus in utero resulting from a general decrease of maternal oxygen content of the blood, decreased oxygen-carrying capacity, or diminished blood flow.

fetal embodiment—Recognition of the developing fetus as part of the woman's body image.

fetal heart rate (FHR)—The number of fetal heart beats per minute; traditionally, the normal range is 120 to 160 bpm. The normal range for the mature fetus is 110 to 160 bpm.

fetal lie—The relationship of the long axis of the fetus to the long axis of the mother; can be horizontal or longitudinal.

fetal movement counts—A test of fetal well-being in which the woman is asked to count and record the number of movements she feels in a specified time.

fetal position—The relationship of the presenting part of the fetus to the front, back, or side of the maternal pelvis.

fetal presentation—The part of the fetal body that appears at the pelvic outlet first; also called the presenting part.

fetal scalp blood pH sampling (FSBS)—A test of fetal well-being in which a sample of fetal blood is obtained from the scalp during labor to assess the acid-base condition of the central circulation.

fetal scalp electrode—A spiral of stainless steel wire that inserts under the skin of the fetal presenting part to record the fetal heart rate.

fetal scalp stimulation—A test of fetal well-being in which the fetal scalp is stimulated by doing a vaginal examination to look for a reassuring response of a fetal heart rate acceleration.

fetal tachycardia—A fetal heart rate that is greater than 160 beats per minute.

fetoscope—A specialized stethoscope used to listen to the fetal heart tones.

fetus—Stage of growth and development from the embryo period until birth.

fimbriae—Projections on terminus of fallopian tube that facilitate capture of ovum into tube.

first-stage labor—The period of labor from the onset of regular contractions to 10 cm of dilatation; divided into the latent, active, and transition phases.

flat or retracted nipple—Identified when the nipple fails to protrude when it is compressed for breastfeeding.

flexion—An attitude of the fetus in which the head is bent forward on the chest, the back is rounded, and the extremities are tucked in against the body.

flush-back effect—Rapid return of blood flow to the uterus and placenta after a period of exercise during pregnancy.

follicle-stimulating hormone (FSH)—The hormone produced by the anterior pituitary during the first phase of the menstrual cycle; stimulates development of the graafian follicle.

fontanelles—Soft spots at the top (anterior) and back (posterior) of the fetal head, covered with strong connective tissue, that result from the junction of the suture lines between the unfused bones of the fetal head; allow the bones to override one another and the head to mold during the birth process.

football hold—A position for holding a newborn in which the baby's back is supported on the nurse's or parent's forearm, the head is held securely in the hand, and the lower extremities are tucked between the upper arm and side of the caregiver.

foramen ovale—An opening between the atria of the fetal heart that normally closes shortly after birth.

forceps—Spoonlike instruments designed to assist in the delivery of the fetal head.

foremilk—The milk obtained at the beginning of a breastfeed. The high water content serves to hydrate the baby and supply water-soluble vitamins.

fourchette—Junction between vaginal vestibule and perineum.

fourth-stage labor—The first hour of recovery after the birth of the baby.

frequency—Measurement of the interval of labor contractions, from the beginning of one contraction to the beginning of the next; recorded in minutes.

Friedman curve—Partograph based on Emanuel Friedman's work documenting the progress of labor.

fundal dominance—Importance of the fundus in determining rhythmicity of contractions. It is assumed that the pacemaker for the regularity of contractions is located in the fundus. Also reflects the fact that contractions begin in the fundus.

fundus—The upper portion of the uterus.

funic presentation—Presentation in which the cord lies below the fetus and thus presents first; also known as cord presentation.

funic souffle—A swooshing sound that can be heard with a fetoscope during pregnancy that is the blood pumping through the umbilical artery; the rate is synchronous with the fetal heart rate.

gamete—A reproductive cell (sperm and ovum) with the haploid chromosome number, or 23 chromosomes.

gamete intrafallopian transfer (GIFT)—A variation of the IVF procedure in which oocytes are removed, identified, and then placed with sperm into the end of a fallopian tube by laparoscopic surgery. Fertilization is allowed to occur naturally within the body.

gametogenesis—Process of development of mature spermatozoa (for the male) or ova (for the female).

gastroschisis—Protrusion of abdominal contents and other organs through an abdominal wall defect lateral to the midline.

gate control theory—Pain theory proposed by Melzack and Wall, which proposes the presence of a gating mechanism along the nervous system that can block pain through stimulation of large-diameter nerve fibers, sensory and cognitive stimulation, and affective modulation.

gene mapping—The assignment of genes to specific locations on specific chromosomes.

general anesthesia—An anesthetic given just before the delivery by use of a combination of intravenous and inhalation agents and oxygen; loss of consciousness and complete pain relief are provided for the delivery and episiotomy repair.

genes—The fundamental units of heredity. Genes are segments of DNA that direct the process of protein synthesis.

genetic code—The base triplets that specify the 20 amino acids found in proteins.

genetic counseling—The provision of information to affected individuals or family members at risk for a disorder that may be genetic, concerning the consequences of the disorder, the probability of developing or transmitting it, and ways it may be prevented or ameliorated.

genetic screening—Testing of a specific population to identify individuals at risk for having or transmitting a specific disorder.

genital stage—The adolescent stage of development identified by Freud during which the oral, anal, and genital sexual urges fuse together.

genome—The total genetic complement of an organism; the complete DNA sequence, containing the entire genetic information of an organism.

genotype—The genetic constitution of an individual; more specifically, the alleles present at a locus.

gestation—The period of fetal development from the time of fertilization of the ovum to birth.

gestational age—The length of time between fertilization of the egg and birth of the infant.

gestational age assessment—An evaluation of the infant that includes assessment of 11 external physical characteristics and 10 neurologic signs and is used to estimate gestational age of the infant.

gestational diabetes—Carbohydrate intolerance that is diagnosed during pregnancy and disappears after delivery; can be insulin-dependent (IDDM) or diet-controlled (NIDDM).

gestational trophoblastic disease—The spectrum of diseases resulting from abnormal proliferation of the placental trophoblast; it includes hydatidiform mole and both metastatic and nonmetastatic trophoblastic neoplasias.

glabella—The bridge of the nose of the fetal head.

Goodell sign—The softening of the cervix and vagina that occurs around the second month of pregnancy.

graafian follicles—Mature ovarian follicles that contain the ripe ovum and secrete estrogen.

gravida—A woman who is pregnant.

grief work—A stage in the process of maternal role development in which the woman must let go of her former identities that are not congruent with mothering.

gynecoid—One of the four classic types of pelves, the gynecoid pelvis is considered the normal female pelvis. The others—android, anthropoid, and platypellpoid—vary in shape, inlet, and diameter of the midpelvis.

habitual (recurrent) abortion—Three or more consecutive first-trimester spontaneous abortions.

habituation—The ability of the infant to "tune out" an incoming stimulus and not respond to it after prolonged exposure to it.

haploid—The chromosome number of a normal gamete, with only one member of each chromosome pair. In humans, the haploid number is 23.

harlequin sign—A color change observed in the neonate in which one side of the body is a deep color while the other side is light and pale, thus resembling a clown suit; caused by vasomotor disturbances, which are usually transient.

health behavior—Behavior directed at maintenance of health or prevention of illness.

health promotion—Education and counseling to maintain and enhance health, support healthful behaviors, and facilitate decision making regarding health care.

Hegar sign—The softening of the lower uterine segment that occurs around the second month of pregnancy.

HELLP syndrome—A unique syndrome that appears in some women with preeclampsia; includes intravascular hemolysis, elevated liver enzymes, and low platelets.

hematoma—A tumor-like mass produced by bleeding from an injured blood vessel into the surrounding tissue.

hemizygous—A gene present in only a single copy. Most commonly refers to genes on the X chromosome in males.

hemorrhage—Blood loss in excess of 500 mL.

hernia, inguinal—Muscle wall defect in the inguinal area through which bowel loops or gonads enter the male scrotal sac or the female soft tissues.

herpesvirus—A family of viruses causing herpes simplex, herpes zoster, and varicella (chickenpox).

heterozygote (heterozygous)—An individual or genotype with two different alleles at a given locus on a pair of homologous chromosomes.

high-risk childbirth—Maternal or fetal factors that increase the likelihood that complications will develop during labor or birth.

high-risk infant—An infant who has an increased likelihood of dying in the neonatal period or an infant who has physiologic problems that threaten health, growth, and development.

hindmilk—The milk obtained after the milk ejection reflex has occurred and nearer to the end of a feeding. Fat content is two to three times that of foremilk.

HIV—Human immunodeficiency virus; causes the collapse of the body's immune system and eventual death due to opportunistic infections; can lead to AIDS.

Homan sign—Pain in the calf occurring with dorsiflexion of the foot; indication of thrombophlebitis or thrombosis.

home care—Health care services that are provided within the client's home.

home health agency—An organization through which nurses work under physicians' orders to provide direct skilled nursing care to clients in their homes.

home visit—A goal-directed nurse-client interaction that takes place in the client's residence.

homologous chromosomes—A pair of chromosomes of one type, one inherited from each parent, having the same sequence of genes.

homozygote (homozygous)—An individual or genotype with identical alleles at a given locus on a pair of homologous chromosomes.

human chorionic gonadotropin (hCG)—Hormone produced by cells of the cytotrophoblast layer; the measurement of hCG levels is the basis of pregnancy tests.

Human Genome Project—A major current research project, international in scope, that aims to map and sequence the entire human genome.

human papillomavirus (HPV)—A sexually transmitted virus that can lead to the development of cervical cancer.

human placental lactogen (hPL)—Also known as human chorionic somatomammotropin; stimulates metabolic changes during pregnancy to ensure that increased amounts of protein, glucose, and minerals are available for the fetus.

hydatidiform mole—Abnormal development of the placenta in which the fetal part of the pregnancy fails to develop; the chorionic villi of the placenta become a mass of cystlike clear vesicles that hang in clusters, resembling a bunch of grapes.

hydramnios—Excessive amniotic fluid.

hydrocephalus—Excessive cerebrospinal fluid within the ventricular and subarachnoid spaces.

hymen—Membrane that completely or partially covers the vaginal opening.

hyperbilirubinemia—An abnormally large amount of bilirubin circulating in the blood.

hyperemesis gravidarum—Intractable, excessive vomiting during pregnancy.

hyperplasia—Increase in number of normal cells due to growth in tissue or an organ.

hypertensive disorders of pregnancy—Disorders characterized by hypertension and classified as preeclampsia-eclampsia, chronic hypertension, and transient hypertension. Preeclampsia is characterized by hypertension with edema or proteinuria; preeclampsia becomes eclampsia in the presence of maternal convulsions; transient hypertension is elevated blood pressure without edema or proteinuria.

hypertonic uterine dysfunction—An incoordinate uterine dysfunction characterized by an elevated basal tonus or a distorted pressure gradient; seen in the latent phase of labor.

hypertrophy—Increase in the size of existing cells.

hypoglycemia—Blood glucose level less than 40 mg/dL.

hypospadias—Location of the urethral meatus on the ventral surface of the penis.

hypothermia—Neonate's temperature below normal levels.

hypotonic uterine dysfunction—Inadequate uterine pressure with each contraction that is insufficient to dilate the cervix at an adequate rate; seen in the active phase of labor.

hypoxia—Decreased amount of oxygen in the organs and tissues.

identified adoption—Situation in which adoptive parents and birth parents find each other and go to an agency or attorney to complete the adoption.

identity—The final stage in the process of maternal role development in which the woman comfortably takes on the behaviors associated with the maternal role.

illness behavior—Adoption of the sick role, resulting in exemption from normal role responsibilities and increased dependence on others.

imagery—The conscious use of mental images to promote relaxation or decrease pain.

implantation—Nidation or the embedding of the fertilized ovum, usually in the uterine decidua.

in vitro fertilization (IVF)—A procedure in which mature oocytes are removed from the ovaries and placed together with sperm in a Petri dish to aid fertilization. After fertilization occurs, embryos are transferred by a small catheter into the uterus, where they may implant.

incident—An event outside that expected in the ordinary course of business of health care.

incomplete abortion—Incomplete expulsion of the products of conception; usually occurs after 10 weeks' gestation, when the placenta may be retained after the fetus has been expelled.

increment—The building up of a contraction and the longest time during a contraction.

indemnity—An assurance by one person to another that the other will be free from loss or damage.

independent assortment—One of Mendel's fundamental principles; dictates that alleles at different loci are transmitted independently of one another.

independent or private adoption—The adoptive parents work to find a birth parent or child directly through a physician, lawyer, or nonagency adoption source.

induction of labor—Interventions designed to initiate labor; such interventions include nipple stimulation, acupressure, prostaglandin E_2 gel, amniotomy, and oxytocin.

inevitable abortion—The presence of cervical dilatation and/or spontaneous rupture of membranes in addition to vaginal bleeding.

infant—A baby born alive; also from 28 days of age until the first birthday.

infant mortality rate—Number of deaths of infants under 1 year of age per 1000 live births.

infant-parent attachment—A behavioral system that develops during the first year of life by which the infant develops a trusting relationship with his or her caregiver.

infant social behaviors—Actions of the infant that stimulate and encourage interaction with the caregiver. These behaviors include smiling, gazing, maintaining a quiet and alert state, and grasping.

infant temperament—A characteristic style by which an infant responds to the animate and inanimate environment.

infertility—The inability to conceive a child after a year or more of regular unprotected intercourse or the inability to carry a pregnancy to live birth (recurrent miscarriages).

informational support—A type of social support in which information is shared with an individual to help in his or her coping with problems.

initial period of reactivity—A period lasting 15 to 30 minutes up to as long as 1½ hours after birth in which the infant is in a state of alertness and responsiveness.

input—Products, events, or series of events that are brought into the system.

instrumental support—A type of social support in which direct aid is given to assist an individual.

intensity—Increase in uterine pressure during a contraction; measured in mm Hg on a fetal monitor (see tonus).

interdisciplinary team approach—A method in which members of different disciplines collaborate in providing services to individuals and families.

internal rotation—The mechanism of labor in which the fetus turns during descent to align the presenting part for birth; also known as cardinal movements.

internal version—A procedure in which the physician inserts a hand into the uterus to grasp the feet of the infant to turn it from a transverse to a breech presentation; used for the delivery of a second twin.

international or intercountry adoption—Situations in which parents adopt a child from another country.

intra-amniotic instillation—The instillation of a hyperosmotic fluid into the amniotic sac that causes fetal death and induces labor.

intracytoplasmic sperm injection (ICSI)—A micromanipulation procedure in which a single sperm is directly inserted into a single egg to increase the likelihood of fertilization in couples when the sperm shows poor mobility. The embryo is then transferred to the uterus.

intrapartum—The period of labor and birth.

intrauterine device—A small plastic device inserted into the uterus for an extended period to prevent pregnancy by causing cellular and biochemical changes in the endometrium.

intrauterine fetal demise (IUFD)—The death of the fetus in utero before it is born.

intrauterine growth restriction (IUGR)—Fetal growth restriction; can be caused by many factors, including malnutrition during pregnancy.

intrauterine insemination—This procedure is one of the simplest fertility treatments and is often performed in conjunction with drug therapy. Sperm from the partner or a donor is shuttled with a catheter into the uterus, where fertilization may occur.

intrauterine pressure catheter (IUPC)—A polyethylene tube inserted into the uterus after rupture of membranes to measure and record pressure from uterine contractions on the electronic fetal monitor.

introitus—The vaginal opening.

introjection-projection-rejection—A stage in the process of maternal role development in which the woman evaluates the type of behaviors she has observed to see what would fit for herself.

intron—DNA sequence found between two exons, transcribed into primary mRNA but spliced out in the formation of the mature mRNA transcript.

inversion of the uterus—A condition in which the uterus turns partially or completely inside out.

involution—The return of the reproductive organs to a nonpregnant state.

iron deficiency anemia—A nutritional deficiency of iron that is reflected in a hematocrit of less than 30 percent or a hemoglobin concentration of less than 10 g/dL.

isochromosome—An abnormal chromosome in which there is loss of one arm and two identical copies of the other arm, formed when the centromere splits in the wrong plane.

isthmus—The narrow portion of the uterus between the body (corpus) and the cervix.

jaundice—Yellow coloration of neonate's skin as a result of bilirubin breakdown or bile pigments.

karyotype—A photomicrograph of the chromosomes of an individual arranged in a standard classification.

Kegel exercises—Alternate contraction and release of the pubococcygeal muscle to strengthen the pelvic floor muscles; done during pregnancy to promote elasticity for birth; done throughout life to maintain tone for support of abdominal organs and to enhance sexuality.

kernicterus—Free bilirubin crosses the blood-brain barrier, causing yellow staining of the brain cells. This condition is associated with neurologic damage.

labia majora—The larger folds of skin that form the overall architecture of the vulva.

labia minora—Thin folds of skin under the labia majora; contain sebaceous and sweat glands.

labor—Regular uterine contractions associated with effacement and dilatation of the cervix, resulting in the birth of the baby.

labor support—Activities that include both affective and psychomotor behaviors that enhance the woman's participation in childbirth and that foster activity enabling her to cope more effectively.

lactation—The process of milk production in a postpartum woman.

lactose intolerance—Sensitivity to milk products containing lactose, resulting in gastrointestinal disturbances.

Lamaze prepared childbirth—A method of prepared childbirth that includes information about pregnancy and childbirth, the use of a relaxation and paced breathing strategy, and other nonpharmacologic pain management techniques. This method was adapted from the Russian psychoprophylaxis model by French obstetrician Fernand Lamaze.

lanugo—The soft, downy hair that covers the body of a fetus in utero to protect the skin.

laparoscopy—The insertion of a telescope-like instrument through a small umbilical incision. A second incision at the pubic hairline is made to allow the insertion of a probe for manipulation of the pelvic organs.

large for gestational age (LGA)—An infant whose weight, length, and head circumfer-ence fall above the 90th percentile for gestational age when plotted on a standard growth curve.

latch-on—The act of attaching to the breast by drawing the nipple and part of the areola into the baby's mouth.

late deceleration—A decrease in the fetal heart rate that begins after the onset of the contraction and ends after the contraction has ended; caused by compromised uteroplacental perfusion.

latent phase—The first phase of first-stage labor; dilatation from 0 to 3 cm; also called early phase.

latent stage—The stage of development identified by Freud during which the school-age child experiences decreased interest in sexuality.

later adolescence—Proceeding from age 17 to 19 years.

law of segregation—One of Mendel's fundamental principles: alleles separate and pass to different gametes during meiosis.

lecithin/sphingomyelin (L/S) ratio—The phospholipid components of surfactant; the L/S ratio should be 2:1 for fetal lungs to be mature.

legal abortion—An abortion performed by a licensed physician or by someone acting under the supervision of a licensed physician. Also referred to as induced or elective abortion.

Leopold maneuvers—A series of abdominal palpation maneuvers that give information regarding fetal presentation, position, presenting part, attitude, and descent.

lesbian or gay family—Families having the same-sex couples or those single-parent families headed by a lesbian woman or gay man.

letdown or milk ejection reflex—A reflex initiated by sucking at the breast, which triggers the pituitary gland to release oxytocin into the bloodstream. When oxytocin reaches the myoepithelial cells surrounding the milk-making glands and collecting ducts, it causes them to contract and eject milk from the breast.

leukorrhea—A white or yellowish vaginal mucous discharge.

lie—Relationship of the long axis of the fetus to the long axis of the mother; can be longitudinal, transverse, or oblique.

lightening—Engagement of the fetal presenting part into the maternal pelvis.

linea nigra—The dark pigmented line from the umbilicus to the symphysis pubis seen on the abdomen of some pregnant women.

litogen—An agent, although not associated with teratogenic effects, that increases the risk of litigation.

live birth—An infant who after birth demonstrates evidence of life, including heartbeat, pulsation of the umbilical cord, and movement of voluntary muscles.

living ligature—Smooth muscle fibers of the uterus that contract to close off blood vessels.

LMP—The date of the first day of the last menstrual period.

local anesthesia—The injection of an anesthetic agent directly into the muscles and tissue of the perineum for the delivery and episiotomy repair; provides pain relief for the tissues of the perineum.

lochia—Postpartum bleeding; can be rubra, serosa, or alba.

locus—The location of a gene on a chromosome.

long-term variability (LTV)—The number of oscillations or undulations in the fetal heart rate baseline over 1 minute; usually two to six per minute.

low birth weight (LBW)—Weight less than 2500 g at birth; very low birth weight is less than 1500 g at birth.

luteal phase defect—Failure of endometrial development, a factor in as many as a third of first-trimester spontaneous abortions.

luteinizing hormone (LH)—Hormone released from the anterior pituitary that stimulates ovulation and the development of the corpus luteum.

Lyon hypothesis—The well-accepted principle that one of the two X chromosomes is randomly inactivated in each somatic cell of the normal female embryo, and the same X chromosome remains inactivated in all subsequent generations of that cell.

macrosomatia—In the infant, a birth weight of more than 4000 g.

magnesium sulfate—A drug used to decrease the risk for seizures in pregnancy-induced hypertension and for tocolysis in the management of preterm labor; thought to decrease the net calcium available for the light-chain phosphorylation of myosin, thus interfering with muscle contractility.

maladaptation—Failure to adapt to the normal developmental or psychological tasks of pregnancy, resulting in potential alterations in parenting.

maladaptive parenting behaviors—Behaviors that interfere with the development of positive parent-infant attachment.

malposition—A position of the fetus that does not allow the best passage of the fetal head through the maternal pelvis, such as an occiput posterior position.

malpractice—A specialized form of negligence based on breach of a standard of care known to a person because of education in a professional field.

malpresentation—Fetal presentation that is noncephalic; examples include transverse lie, breech, brow, and face presentations.

manifesting heterozygote—A female carrier of an X-linked trait who has clinical manifestations of the trait.

Marfan syndrome—A genetic disorder of connective tissue marked by joint deformities, dislocation of the ocular lens, and cardiac abnormalities.

mastitis—Inflammation or an infective process in the breast.

masturbation—Self-stimulation of the genitals or other body parts to achieve sexual excitement or orgasm.

maternal mortality rate—The number of deaths of women from complications of pregnancy, childbirth, and the postpartum period per 100,000 live births.

maternal-newborn nursing science—An organization of tested theories and research findings related to the field of maternal-newborn nursing.

maternal-newborn theories—Abstract descriptions and explanations of phenomena that pertain to pregnancy, childbirth, and parenting.

maternal role—Behaviors learned by a woman either indirectly or directly for the nurturing of a child.

maternal-role attainment theory—A theory that describes the psychological aspects that accompany pregnancy and the postpartum period and the factors that hinder or facilitate women's successful development of the maternal role. Rubin and Mercer have both contributed to the development of maternal-role attainment theory.

McDonald sign—The ease with which the body of the uterus can be flexed against the cervix; a physical change that can be diagnostic of pregnancy.

meconium—A sticky green or black substance that is present in the fetal intestine. It forms the first neonatal stool but may be passed before birth into the amniotic fluid.

meconium aspiration syndrome—As a result of fetal hypoxia, meconium is passed; with gasping respiration, meconium is aspirated into the lungs.

medical abortion—An abortion induced through the means of a drug such as RU 486 (mifepristone).

megaloblastic anemia—A folic acid deficiency that causes a low hematocrit and low hemoglobin level; in rare cases, it is due to vitamin B_{12} deficiency.

meiosis—Cell division process in which gametes containing the haploid chromosome number are produced from diploid germ cells.

menarche—The beginning of the menstrual cycle and reproductive function in the female.

mendelian—Referring to Gregor Mendel, describes a trait that is attributable to a single gene.

menstrual cycle—The female cycle occurring every 28 days in response to hormonal influence resulting in the buildup of the endometrium, ovulation, and then sloughing of the endometrium as menstrual bleeding.

mentum—The fetal chin.

messenger RNA (mRNA)—RNA molecules that copy the genetic information coded within the DNA and migrate to the cytoplasm, where they form a template for the formation of proteins as directed by the original DNA.

microcephaly—A head circumference below the 10th percentile for gestational age.

micromanipulation—Techniques that can be performed in a Petri dish in the laboratory under a microscope in which an embryologist manipulates egg and sperm to improve the chances of pregnancy.

middle adolescence—Developmental ages ranging from 14 to 16 years.

milia—Temporary, tiny white papules located on the bridge of the nose, chin, and cheeks of a newborn and caused by blocked sebaceous glands.

mimicry—A stage in the process of maternal role development in which the woman copies behaviors that manifest the mothering role.

minipill—A progestin-only hormonal contraceptive that prevents pregnancy by changing the cervical mucus, altering ovum transport, and inhibiting endometrial lining development.

miscarriage—The lay term for a spontaneous abortion.

missed abortion—Prolonged retention of the products of conception after embryonic or fetal demise, before 20 weeks' gestation.

mitosis—The process of somatic cell division, resulting in the formation of two cells genetically identical to the parent cell.

mitral regurgitation—As a consequence of prolapse of the mitral valve during diastole, blood is allowed to flow back into the left atrium.

mitral stenosis—A form of rheumatic heart disease, usually a sequela of rheumatic fever, that reduces cardiac output because of the stenotic mitral valve.

mittelschmerz—Ovulatory pain that is usually attributed to intra-abdominal irritation.

molding—The elongated shaping of the fetal head as it moves through the bony pelvis during labor and birth; caused by the normal overriding of the unfused bones of the fetal skull.

mongolian spot—An area of dark pigmentation, often mistaken for a bruise, common in black and other dark-skinned babies. Mongolian spots are typically found on the sacrum or buttocks; they disappear by early childhood.

monoamniotic twins—Embryos who share a common amniotic sac.

monosomy—A state in which one member of a chromosome pair is missing, resulting in 45 chromosomes.

monozygous twins—A single fertilized egg that divides into two separate and identical embryos.

mons pubis—Hair-covered fat pad overlying the symphysis pubis.

Montgomery's glands—Sebaceous glands located around the areola of the breast that secrete a lubricant to protect the nipple during breastfeeding.

morals—A code of behavior established by traditions or societal norms.

morning-after pill—A postcoital oral contraceptive that can be taken within 72 hours after sexual intercourse to prevent implantation; still experimental in the United States.

morning sickness—Nausea and vomiting of early pregnancy; most commonly occurs in the morning but may occur at any time of day.

Moro reflex—The startle response of a newborn to a stimulus whereby the arms are extended and then drawn in with an embracing gesture.

morula—Stage of growth and development when conceptus is approximately 16 cells in size.

mosaicism—A condition in which there are two or more genetically different cell lines in an individual that are derived from a single zygote.

mourning—The process of grieving that involves accepting the loss, experiencing the pain in response to the loss, adjusting to life after the loss, and redirecting the energy from grieving to reconstructing one's life.

mucous plug—Protective mucus that plugs the cervical os during pregnancy.

multifactorial—Describes traits or diseases that are the product of the interaction of multiple genetic and environmental factors; also known as nonmendelian inheritance.

multifetal pregnancy reduction (MFPR)—A procedure in which the number of fetuses in a multifetal pregnancy is decreased during the first trimester to improve the outcome of pregnancy.

multigravida—Woman who is pregnant and has been pregnant previously.

multipara—Woman who has carried two or more pregnancies to viability.

murmur—A prolonged heart sound caused by turbulent blood flow.

mutant—A gene that has been altered by mutation.

mutation—A change in the genetic material.

myometrium—Muscular middle layer of the uterus.

myotonia—Increase in muscle tension experienced during sexual excitement.

Nagele rule—A formula for calculating the EDC; LMP − 3 months ± 7 days.

narcotic antagonist drugs—Drugs that counteract central nervous system depression in the fetus or neonate.

natural family planning—A fertility awareness form of birth control that consists of a group of methods based on an understanding and awareness of the woman's reproductive cycle and its associated symptoms; includes the calendar method, basal body temperature method, cervical mucus method, and symptothermal method.

necrotizing enterocolitis (NEC)—Ischemia of the intestinal tract and invasion of the mucosa with enteric pathogens.

negligence—An unintentional action or inaction that breaches a duty of care owed another person and foreseeably causes harm to that person.

neonatal—The period from birth to 28 days of life.

neonatal assessment—An evaluation of the health status of the infant that includes maternal, obstetric, and perinatal history; physical assessment; gestational age assessment; and behavioral assessment.

neonatal mortality rate—The number of deaths for infants under 28 days per 1000 live births.

nesting behavior—The psychological need experienced by some pregnant women at the end of pregnancy to prepare the home for the baby.

neutral thermal environment—An environment that minimizes the neonate's need to expend calories to maintain heat; an environment that provides for minimal heat loss.

nidation—Alternative term for implantation.

nipple shields—Rubber, silicone, or latex coverings for the nipple-areola with a firm nipple sometimes used for latch-on difficulties or sore nipples.

Nitrazine test—Test for rupture of membranes based on the fact that amniotic fluid is more basic than vaginal secretions; thus, pH-type Nitrazine paper will change to a blue shade in the presence of amniotic fluid.

nondisjunction—The failure of two members of a chromosome pair to separate appropriately during cell division, resulting in abnormal chromosome numbers in gametes or cells.

nonnutritive sucking—Characterized by two sucks per second, drawing in no milk.

nonpharmacologic pain relief—Pain relief based on a variety of methods other than analgesics or anesthetics.

nonstress test (NST)—A test of fetal well-being in which the external fetal monitor is used to measure the accelerations of the fetal heart rate; usually in response to fetal movement.

Norplant—A long-acting progestin contraceptive that is implanted subdermally in a woman's upper arm.

nuchal cord—An umbilical cord that is wrapped around the neck of the fetus.

nuclear family—A family created by marriage or an ongoing relationship of two individuals and their children by birth.

nucleotide—A molecule composed of a nitrogenous base, a 5-carbon sugar, and a phosphate group.

nulligravida—Woman who has never been pregnant.

nullipara—Woman who has never carried a pregnancy to viability.

nursing care planning guide—A written form of the nursing process that specifies the nursing care needed for an individual client.

nursing process—A critical decision-making tool used to plan individualized, theory-based nursing care.

nutritive sucking—Characterized by one suck per second, a drawing in of the nipple-areola, and milk transfer from the breast to the baby's mouth.

occiput—The posterior portion of the fetal head located over the occipital bone and below the posterior fontanelle.

occiput anterior (OA)—A position of the fetal head that occurs when the occiput of the head and posterior fontanelle are in the anterior portions of the maternal pelvis and the brow and bregma are in the posterior portion.

occiput posterior (OP)—A position of the fetal head that occurs when the occiput of the head and posterior fontanelle are in the posterior portions of the maternal pelvis and the brow and bregma are in the anterior portion; can be a cause of back labor.

occupational health hazards—Workplace exposure to potential reproductive toxins, physical hazards (e.g., ionizing radiation), chemical agents, and biologic hazards.

occurrence insurance—Coverage by a carrier if a policy was in force at the time of occurrence of the events leading to a lawsuit.

Oedipus complex—The jealousy experienced by a young boy of his father's relationship with his mother.

oligohydramnios—Abnormal decrease in the amount of amniotic fluid.

omphalocele—Protrusion of abdominal contents through a large defect at the umbilicus.

oocyte—Early primitive ovum prior to complete development.

oogenesis—Female process of gametogenesis.

open adoption—An adoption in which there is open communication between the adoptive family and birth family.

open family system—A family system with permeable boundaries that allows information to enter the system; the family is open to information from the environment. The information is processed (throughput) by the family and then provided as feedback (output) to the environment.

ophthalmia neonatorum—Purulent conjunctivitis of the newborn, usually caused by gonococci.

oral contraceptive—"The pill"; a hormonal contraceptive that combines estrogen and progestin to prevent pregnancy by suppressing ovulation and altering cervical mucus production, tubal mobility, and endometrial lining development.

oral stage—The stage of development identified by Freud during which the infant receives pleasure and gratification through sucking.

orgasmic phase—The third phase of the sexual response cycle during which rhythmic contractions of the pelvic floor muscles result from the peaking of sexual arousal.

output—The product of throughput, given off the system; feedback.

ovulation—Release of ovum in response to complex endocrinologic/physiologic events.

ovulation method—A method of natural family planning that uses the recognition of changes in cervical mucus to identify the fertile and infertile periods of the menstrual cycle; also known as the cervical mucus method.

ovum—Female egg produced by the ovaries.

oxytocin—Steroid that is either endogenous from the posterior pituitary or exogenous from a synthetic creation. As an exogenous pharmaceutical agent, it can be used for uterine stimulation as for induction or augmentation of labor or to facilitate uterine contractions postpartally; most commonly used agent is Pitocin.

oxytocin challenge test (OCT)—*See* contraction stress test.

paracervical block—Regional anesthesia given in first-stage labor by injection of the agent into the cervical tissue; provides pain relief for the contractions of labor but must be followed by another anesthetic for the delivery.

paradigm—An abstract pattern, example, or model of a family of related theories.

parametritis—Pelvic cellulitis, when the infection process extends beyond the endometrium into the broad ligaments.

parent-infant attachment—A reciprocal process by which parents develop synchronous and loving relationships with their infants.

parental role attainment—Process of acquiring the parenting role.

parity—The number of pregnancies that have been carried to viability.

partograph—Plotting of cervical dilatation and pelvic station against time to document labor progress; the most commonly used partograph for labor is the Friedman curve.

parturition—The act or process of giving birth.

patent ductus arteriosus (PDA)—Failure of the ductus arteriosus to close after birth, allowing blood to flow from the aorta to the pulmonary artery.

pathologic grieving—Mourning that includes severe psychiatric symptoms at any time during mourning as well as prolonged mourning; has also been called disordered mourning.

patient's rights—The rights of the patient to informed, safe, competent, confidential, and considerate care.

pedigree—A diagram of the family history that shows family relationships, gender, disease status, and other attributes.

pelvic inflammatory disease (PID)—A general term for inflammation of the female genital tract. PID is caused by a number of microorganisms, most often gonococcal or chlamydial infections, and can produce irreparable damage to fallopian tubes, resulting in infertility and ectopic (tubal) pregnancies.

pelvic inlet—The upper border of the true pelvis; also called the linea terminalis or brim.

pelvic outlet—The lower border of the true pelvis.

pelvic rock—An exercise done during pregnancy to prevent or relieve low backache and tone abdominal muscles.

penetrance—Concept referring to whether a mutant gene is clinically expressed; the frequency of expression of the genotype.

penis—Male external reproductive organ composed of erectile tissue; the homolog of the female clitoris.

percutaneous umbilical blood sampling (PUBS)—A procedure to obtain fetal blood from the umbilical cord in utero; also called cordocentesis.

perinatal education—Health education for the family unit during pregnancy, childbirth, and the early parenting period.

perinatal grief—The emotional reactions to a significant loss related to childbearing that can occur from the preconceptional period through early infancy.

perinatal loss—Feelings of loss related to childbearing and the need to grieve (mourn) at any time from the preconceptional period through early infancy.

perinatal period—From the 28th week of gestation through the 28th day after birth.

perineum—Tissues posterior to the labia and anterior to the anus.

period of relative inactivity—A period after the initial active period in which the infant is sleepy, drowsy, and relatively insensitive to both external and internal stimuli.

periods of reactivity—Predictable patterns of neonatal behavior in the initial stabilization after birth.

peripartum cardiomyopathy—Congestive heart failure with myocardial disease that occurs either late in pregnancy or in the first 5 months post partum.

peritonitis—An extension of the infectious process into the peritoneum by gradual progression or the rupture of a pelvic abscess.

phallic stage—The stage of development identified by Freud during which the preschool child demonstrates an increased focus on sex play and masturbation.

pharmacologic pain relief—Pain relief based on the use of analgesics or anesthetics.

phenomenon—An event that actually occurs and can be observed.

phenotype—The observable characteristics of an individual.

phenylketonuria (PKU)—A metabolic disease caused by an inborn error in the metabolism of the amino acid phenylalanine; if not treated, causes mental retardation.

phototherapy—A process by which blue light therapy decomposes bilirubin by photoisomerization.

physiologic anemia of pregnancy—A normal decrease in hematocrit, which peaks at 28 to 32 weeks' gestation; caused by a larger proportional increase in blood plasma than in red blood cell mass.

physiologic jaundice—Normal jaundice of the newborn.

physiologically fragile infant—An infant whose physical condition is unstable and who requires specialized nursing, medical care, and technologic support.

pica—The practice of ingesting substances that have no nutritive value.

placenta—Organ of exchange between the pregnant woman and her fetus.

placenta accreta—An abnormal adherence of the placenta to the endometrium in which the chorionic villi attach to the myometrium.

placenta increta—An abnormal adherence of the placenta to the endometrium in which the chorionic villi attach to the myometrium.

placenta percreta—An abnormal adherence of the placenta to the endometrium in which the chorionic villi attach through the myometrium.

placenta previa—Abnormal placement of placenta so that it partially covers the cervix; dilatation results in bleeding, which can be of hemorrhagic proportions.

plateau phase—The second phase of the sexual response cycle during which vasocongestion and myotonia increase as excitement builds to orgasm.

pneumothorax—Accumulation of air in the pleural space.

polar body—Small daughter cell produced as a result of maturation of the ovum during oogenesis.

political activism—Acting as a maternal-newborn advocate through the political process, support for candidate's campaigns for public office, recruitment of voters, work for change through political parties and nonpartisan groups, and involvement in advocacy activities of professional nursing associations.

polycythemia—A peripheral venous hematocrit of more than 65 percent.

polydactyly—One or more extra digits on the hands or feet.

polygenic—Describes a trait determined by many genes at different loci, with small additive effects.

polyhydramnios—Abnormal increase in the amount of amniotic fluid.

polyploidy—An abnormal chromosome complement that exceeds the diploid number and is an exact multiple of the haploid set; an example is 69 chromosomes with 3 copies of each chromosome.

postcoital test—A microscopic examination of mucus taken from the cervix within 24 hours of intercourse to evaluate sperm-mucus interaction.

postpartum blues—A common transient mood change in the early postpartum period characterized by insomnia, tearfulness, anxiety, poor concentration, and a mild depressive affect.

postpartum depression—A psychological disorder that is nonpsychotic in nature. Although the symptoms are similar to postpartum blues, they remain more persistent, lasting 2 weeks to 1 year or more.

postpartum hemorrhage—Blood loss greater than 500 mL during the postpartum period.

postpartum (or puerperal) infection—Maternal temperature elevation to 100.4°F (38°C) or higher on two successive postpartum days, not including the 24 hours after birth.

postpartum period—Also termed the puerperium, the postpartum period is the 6-week period after childbirth during which the woman's body is returning to its nonpregnant state.

postpartum psychosis—Psychotic mood disorder occurring within 3 weeks post partum. It is characterized by delusions, hallucinations, and debilitating confusion.

postterm—An infant born after the end of week 42 of gestation.

postterm pregnancy—A pregnancy that continues for 42 weeks or more from the first day of the last menses in a 28-day cycle.

poverty—The lack of money and material goods (visible poverty) and/or social and cultural deprivation (invisible poverty).

precipitate labor—A rapid labor, lasting less than 3 hours.

preeclampsia—Hypertensive disorder of pregnancy characterized by increased blood pressure, albuminuria, and edema.

premature labor and birth—Labor and birth before completion of week 37 of gestation.

premature rupture of membranes (PROM)—Spontaneous rupture of membranes before onset of labor but after 37 weeks' gestation.

prenatal attachment—The beginning development of affiliation, love, or bonding to the fetus that begins during pregnancy.

prenatal care—Prenatal care consists of health promotion, risk assessment, and intervention activities carried out by prenatal health care providers, women, and families during pregnancy to promote healthy outcomes for women and their infants.

presenting part—The portion of the fetus that is coming first through the dilating cervix.

preterm—An infant born at less than 38 weeks' gestation.

preterm birth—Birth of less than 37 completed weeks of gestation.

preterm labor—Labor that begins before 37 completed weeks of gestation.

preterm premature rupture of membranes (PPROM)—Spontaneous rupture of membranes before 37 weeks' gestation.

primary health care provider—The physician or other health care professional who assumes basic responsibility for the client's health care.

primary infertility—Occurs when the female partner has no history of pregnancy.

primigravida—Woman who is pregnant for the first time.

primipara—Woman who has carried one pregnancy to viability.

principles of ethics—A set of rules that can be universally applied to all situations. They provide a framework by which values, morals, beliefs, and attitudes may be identified, ethical dilemmas examined and clarified, and obligations ordered in terms of their precedence.

progesterone—The female hormone secreted by the corpus luteum that stimulates proliferation of the endometrium.

prolactin—The hormone secreted by the anterior pituitary that promotes breast development and milk production.

prolapsed cord—The loop of umbilical cord that falls below the presenting part of the fetus and becomes trapped as the fetus descends.

prophylaxis—Prevention.

prostaglandin (PG)—Fatty acid found in many tissues of the body; stimulates uterine contractions.

prostaglandin synthesis inhibitor—A drug used for tocolysis in the management of preterm labor by inactivating the enzyme cyclooxygenase that is required for synthesis of prostaglandin, a substance required for uterine contractility; also known as nonsteroidal antiinflammatory drugs (NSAIDs); an example of this drug is indomethacin (Indocin).

psychoeducational intervention—An intervention that uses educational and psychological strategies to decrease pain, enhance recovery, promote psychological well-being, and increase satisfaction with health care. Psychoeducational interventions include three areas of content: information about events, procedures, sensations, or self-care activities; skills to reduce discomfort and complications; and psychological support to reduce anxieties and enhance coping.

psychoprophylaxis—A method of childbirth preparation known in North America as the Lamaze method.

ptyalism—The production of excessive, sometimes bitter saliva during pregnancy caused by increased estrogen or nausea.

pubis—Bony part of the innominate pelvic bone found where the rami merge.

pudendal block—Regional anesthesia given immediately prior to birth by injection of the agent transvaginally to the pudendal nerves; provides pain relief for the upper two thirds of the vagina and the perineum.

pudendal nerves—Nerves located bilaterally and proximate to the sacrospinous ligaments on either side of the uterus.

puerperium—The time after birth, approximately 6 weeks, during which anatomic and physiologic changes of pregnancy resolve.

pulse pressure—The difference between the systolic and the diastolic blood pressure.

quickening—The first maternal perception of fetal movement, usually between the 16th and 20th weeks of pregnancy.

race—A population of people that differs from others according to genetic traits, geographic location, ancestry, lineage, habits, and ideas.

radiant warmer—Overhead device that warms the baby by radiant heat.

radiation—The mechanism of heat loss when an infant loses heat to cooler objects in the environment.

random or weak family system—A family system with diffuse boundaries. Any and all information enters into this system. The family fails to process the information adequately, and the information may easily or may not at all influence the family system.

rape—A sexual act with a nonconsenting victim, including the use of physical force, intimidation, deception, threat, and coitus or vaginal penetration.

recessive—A trait expressed when two copies of the gene are present.

reciprocity—Rhythmic cycles of attention and nonattention during synchronous mother-infant interactions.

recommended dietary allowances (RDAs)—Guidelines for daily intake of essential food nutrients.

referral—The process of connecting a client with another professional, organization, or service for the purpose of meeting client needs.

regional anesthesia—A nerve block that provides analgesia or anesthesia to one particular area or region of the body; includes paracervical, epidural, spinal, pudendal, and local blocks.

replacement-child syndrome—An individual's obsession about having another child as soon as possible after the death of a baby.

research-based nursing intervention—A scientifically tested method or approach to a health-related need of mothers or infants that has been shown to be effective.

resolution phase—The final phase of the sexual response cycle during which the body returns to its unaroused state.

respiratory distress syndrome (RDS)—Disease of the newborn caused by immaturity of the lungs; characteristics include grunting, retractions, and cyanosis.

respondeat superior—The concept that the employer is responsible for the actions of the employees.

restitution—Rotational movement of the infant's head immediately after it is born, which causes it to rotate back to the direction it faced when labor began.

retained placenta—A placenta that does not spontaneously separate from the uterine wall after the expulsion of the infant.

retinopathy of prematurity (ROP)—Formation of fibrotic tissue behind the lens of the eye or retinal detachment; seen with hypoxemia in preterm infants.

retraction—Shortening of muscle fibers in response to a stimulus. Myometrial cells in the fundus retract, and during labor the upper segment becomes shorter and thicker while the lower uterine segment thins. Retraction is sometimes also termed brachystasis.

retractions—A drawing in of the chest during inspiration. Often associated with respiratory distress.

reverse genetics—The molecular approach to identifying genes on the basis of their location in the genome, without knowledge of the gene product.

rhythm method—A form of natural family planning also known as the calendar method.

ribonucleic acid (RNA)—A single-stranded molecule that consists of a sugar (ribose), phosphate group, and nitrogenous bases (adenine, cytosine, guanine, and uracil).

risk assessment—The identification of the presence or absence of medical, obstetric, or psychosocial risks throughout pregnancy through history taking, physical examination, or laboratory tests.

risk management—Activities undertaken by any organization to identify, prevent, provide for risk coverage for, and respond to adverse events that do occur.

role—Pattern of socially accepted behaviors that guide the functions of an individual in a given social situation.

role conflict—Stress resulting from two or more competing roles assumed by an individual at the same time.

role dimensions—The components of a role. Core dimensions are those components that are always present in the maternal-newborn nursing role. Functional dimensions may be present, depending on a specific role of the maternal-newborn nurse.

role partner—A person who assumes a role that is reciprocal to the role of another person; a mother and her baby are role partners.

role play—A stage in the process of maternal role development in which behaviors are acted out or tried on for size.

role stress—A situation in which an individual encounters role overload (excessive demands), role conflict (contradictory role expectations), role ambiguity (norms for the role are vague or ill-defined), and/or role incongruity (role expectations are different from individual's self-perception, attitudes, or values).

rooting reflex—A reflexive response seen in a newborn in which the head turns and the mouth opens in the direction of stroking of the cheek.

sacral promontory—The bony projection of the upper portion of the sacrum into the pelvic cavity that serves as a landmark in determining pelvic measurements.

sacrum—Five fused vertebrae linking the fifth lumbar vertebra to the bony pelvis and terminating at the coccyx.

salpingitis—Inflammation of the fallopian tubes.

scarf sign—The position of the elbow of a newborn when the hand is drawn across the body to the opposite shoulder; part of a gestational age assessment.

Schultz presentation—Expulsion of the placenta with the fetal side presenting first; because of the glistening appearance of the fetal side, this is often called "shiny Schultz."

scrotum—Sac of tissue posterior to the penis containing the male testes.

second period of reactivity—The third stage of the transitional period that begins at approximately 2 hours and lasts up to 6 hours. During this time, the baby becomes more active, heart rate and respiration fluctuate with activity, the first meconium stool is often passed, and the infant may experience abrupt color changes and have oral mucus.

second-stage labor—The period of labor from 10 cm of cervical dilatation to the birth of the baby; the period of expulsion.

secondary infertility—A condition when previous pregnancy has occurred regardless of the outcome.

selective reduction—A procedure sometimes used during pregnancy when there are multiple fetuses to reduce the number of fetuses.

semen—The fluid containing sperm that is ejaculated by the male in the orgasmic phase of the sexual response cycle.

sensitive period—The period in the early weeks after birth when parents develop close attachments to their infants.

sensory transformation—A pain management strategy that teaches individuals to mentally transform a pain stimulus into a pleasant feeling.

servomechanism-controlled incubator—Enclosed device that helps maintain a baby's temperature by maintaining constant environmental air temperature.

sex chromosomes—The X and Y chromosomes in the human karyotype that are responsible for sex determination.

sexually transmitted disease (STD)—An infection passed from one individual to another through direct sexual contact.

short-term variability (STV)—The beat-to-beat interval changes in the fetal heart rate. STV can be measured only by internal/direct fetal monitoring.

shoulder dystocia—Failure to deliver the fetal shoulders by the usual methods after the fetal head has emerged.

sibling subsystems—Usually the children.

sinciput—The anterior portion of the fetal head known as the brow.

single-parent family—A single parent and the individual's children.

single-room maternity care (SRMC)—A birthing environment in which women labor, give birth, and remain during the immediate or entire postpartum period.

Skene glands—Paraurethral glands; secretions help lubricate the vagina during intercourse.

skin temperature—Temperature of the neonate's skin, recorded by a probe device placed on the baby's skin.

small for gestational age (SGA)—An infant whose weight, length, and head circumference fall below the 10th percentile for gestational age when plotted on a standard growth curve.

social context—The environment or situation in which an event takes place.

social exchange theory—This theory is derived from economic theories and is based on the premise that the interaction between persons in the family is an exchange of goods, material and nonmaterial.

social phase—The brief, opening portion of a home visit, in which friendly conversation paves the way for the concentrated work of the visit.

social support—Activities and information leading to the belief that one is cared for, loved, esteemed, valued, and part of a network of communication and mutual obligation.

special-needs adoption—An adoption that involves children with severe medical or emotional problems, or a number of children who must be placed together.

specific informed consent—The person understands (1) the nature and purpose of the treatment or procedure; (2) the alternatives including no treatment or procedure; and (3) the expected outcomes, that is, the material risks, benefits, and probabilities of success.

spermatogenesis—Male process of gametogeny.

spermicide—An agent that is destructive to spermatazoa; includes creams, foams, jellies, and vaginal suppositories.

spinal block—Regional anesthesia given just prior to birth by injection of the agent through the dura into the cerebrospinal fluid of the subarachnoid space of the spinal column; provides pain relief for the delivery and perineal repair.

spinnbarkeit—The characteristic viscosity or elasticity of cervical mucus seen as ovulation approaches.

spontaneous abortion—The naturally occurring termination of a pregnancy before viability, which is usually defined as either before 20 weeks' gestation or weight less than 500 g.

spontaneous rupture of membranes (SROM)—The natural breaking of the amniotic sac, either before the onset of labor or during the process of labor.

stability/engagement cues—Behavioral cues indicating that an infant has good organization and is ready to participate in an interaction.

standards of care—A written description of a competent level of nursing care.

station—Relationship between the presenting part of the fetus and the midpoint of the pelvis at the level of the ischial spines; measurement of fetal descent.

sterilization—Permanent birth control methods, including tubal ligation for the female and vasectomy for the male.

stillbirth—The birth of a dead fetus.

stork bites—Telangiectatic nevi; temporary, dark pink discolorations that may appear on the skin of a newborn, particularly on the eyelids or nape of the neck.

stress reduction techniques—Physical and mental relaxation skills used to counter tension and stress; examples include progressive relaxation, massage, visual imagery, biofeedback, and controlled breathing.

striae gravidarum—Red or white lines that appear on the breasts, abdomen, or thighs during pregnancy as a result of stretching of the skin; also called "stretch marks."

subconjunctival hemorrhage—Tiny hemorrhages seen on the sclera of the newborn's eyes resulting from changes in vascular tension during the birth process.

subinvolution—Slower than expected return of the uterus to its prepregnancy status after childbirth.

substance abuse—The use of any mind-altering drug or agent in such a way that it interferes with the individual's ability to function, either physiologically, emotionally, or socioculturally.

subsystem—Each family member belongs to a subsystem within the family system.

sucking reflex—The normal reflex that enables a newborn to respond to the stimulus of a nipple or finger placed in the mouth with strong rhythmic sucking.

supplemental feeding devices—Devices other than bottles with artificial nipples. These may include dropper, spoon, cup, feeding tube attached to a syringe, or commercial feeding tube devices.

surfactant—Lipoproteins secreted by the alveoli of the lungs that reduce surface tension and contribute to the elasticity of pulmonary tissue.

surgical abortion—An abortion induced by surgical means of curettage, D & E, intra-amniotic instillation, hysterotomy, or hysterectomy.

surrogacy—A woman is implanted with an embryo and is paid, or volunteers, to carry the child to term. The egg may come from the legal or surrogate mother, the sperm from the legal father or a donor.

surrogate parenthood—The contractual hiring of a woman by a couple to bear their child for a fee.

suture lines—The areas between the unfused bones of the fetal skull, covered by strong connective tissue, that allow the unfused bones of the fetal head to override one another during the birth process.

symbolic interaction theory—A family theory based on the broader interactionist perspective that uses concepts to illustrate the internal processes that occur within individuals and families. The basic concepts include mind, self, and society.

symphysis pubis—Fibrocartilaginous joint found in the midline of the bony pelvis that lacks a capsule or synovial membranes.

symptothermal method—A method of natural family planning that uses multiple indicators of cervical mucus patterns, basal body temperature patterns, and additional secondary physical symptoms of ovulation.

syndactyly—Congenital webbing of the fingers or toes.

system—A set of elements (family members) interacting with each other within a boundary.

systems theory—Within this theory, the family is viewed as an open, ongoing interaction system in which every member influences the family system and is influenced by it.

tachycardia—A heart rate greater than 180 to 200 beats per minute in the newborn.

tachypnea—Respirations of greater than 60 breaths per minute in the newborn.

tail policy—Negligence and malpractice insurance coverage for persons who have stopped working or retired and who previously carried claims made insurance.

taking-hold phase—The phase in the process of maternal role attainment during which mothers attempt to master their new maternal roles.

taking-in phase—The first few days after delivery during which mothers focus primarily on meeting their own needs.

teratogens—Environmental substances that can cause alterations in fetal growth and development during pregnancy.

teratology—Study of congenital malformations or of agents producing such malformations.

testes—Male gonads containing seminiferous tubules and Leydig cells, where sperm and testosterone are produced.

testosterone—The male hormone responsible for the development of secondary sexual characteristics.

tetralogy of Fallot—A congenital cardiac anomaly consisting of right ventricular outflow obstruction, ventricular septal defect, right ventricular hypertrophy, and an overriding aorta.

theca—Outer layer of maturing follicle.

theory—An interrelated set of abstract concepts and statements that gives a systematic picture of phenomena in a field of study. A theory can describe, explain, predict, provide the potential for control, or give a sense of understanding about what is happening.

therapeutic donor insemination—Insemination with donor semen.

thermal shift—The rise in basal body temperature that occurs after a woman has ovulated.

thermoregulation—Processes of the neonate to "regulate" or attempt to maintain body temperature in the normal range.

third-party payer—An entity other than the client or the health care provider that assumes responsibility for the cost of the health care; most commonly a health insurance company, the client's employer, Medicare, or Medicaid.

third-stage labor—The period of labor when the placenta is expelled.

threatened abortion—Occurrence of vaginal bleeding or spotting before 20 weeks' gestation, with or without cramping, in the presence of a live fetus.

thromboembolism—Inflammation of a vein, often accompanied by a clot resulting from venous stasis, infection, vessel wall trauma, or hypercoagulability.

thrombophlebitis—Inflammation of the wall of a vein; precedes the formation of a clot.

thrombosis—An abnormal clot occurring within a blood vessel.

throughput—Input is processed, organized, and transformed.

thrush—White plaques seen in the mouth of some newborn infants caused by the fungus *Candida albicans.*

tocodynamometer (toco)—A pressure-sensitive transducer that is placed over the maternal uterine fundus to record uterine activity. It is held in place by a belt around the abdomen.

tocolytic—Agent designed to promote uterine quiescence.

tonic neck reflex—A characteristic posture observed in newborns; when the supine infant's head is turned to one side, the arm and leg on that side extend while the opposite arm and leg flex.

tonus—Degree of pressure on the uterus. Tonus is measured in millimeters of mercury and may also be referred to as torr. Normal baseline tonus is 8 to 12 mm Hg, with tonus at an acme of a contraction rising to 40 to 75 mm Hg.

TORCH infections—Refers to several agents that can infect the fetus (T = toxoplasmosis, O = other, R = rubella, C = cytomegalovirus, H = herpesvirus).

TPAL—Method of summarizing the woman's obstetric history (T = term pregnancies; P = preterm infants; A = abortions; and L = living children).

tracheoesophageal fistula—Congenital defect in which there is a connection of the esophagus with the trachea by way of a fistula.

traditional sexuality education—An educational approach that basically includes instruction on reproductive biology and sexually transmitted diseases with an emphasis on preventing adolescent sexual activity.

tranquilizers—Ataractic or relaxant drugs that decrease apprehension, provide mild sedation, and have an antiemetic effect.

transcutaneous electrical nerve stimulation (TENS)—Use of a device that emits low-voltage electricity to the body through electrodes placed on the skin to alter pain perception.

transition phase—The third phase of first-stage labor; dilatation from 8 to 10 cm.

transitional period—The period from birth to 6 hours after birth in which the newborn exhibits a typical pattern of physiologic and behavioral changes.

translocation—A chromosome, or a piece of a chromosome, becomes attached to another chromosome. Translocation is balanced when no chromosome material is lost or gained in the rearrangement.

transracial domestic adoption—An adoption in which the adoptive parents and the adoptive child are from the same country but are of different racial or ethnic backgrounds.

transverse lie—A position of the fetus in utero in which the long axis of the fetus and the long axis of the mother are at right angles; the shoulder of the fetus is the presenting part.

trimester—One of three 3-month periods into which pregnancy is divided.

trisomy—The presence of an extra member of a chromosome pair, producing 47 chromosomes.

trophoblast—Specialized cells in blastocyst that provide nutrients.

true pelvis—The portion of the maternal bony pelvis below the linea terminalis (brim).

tubal ligation—A sterilization procedure for females in which the fallopian tubes are cut, tied, cauterized, plugged, capped, coagulated, or clipped to prevent the passage of the ovum through the tubes.

twin-to-twin transfusion (twin transfusion syndrome)—A vascular connection that exists between the two fetal circulations in a twin pregnancy with blood flowing in one direction such that one twin is donor and one is recipient.

ultrasonography—The use of high-frequency sound waves directed through the maternal abdomen by a transducer to produce an image of the fetus and fetal body structures.

ultrasound transducer—A sending and receiving device that is attached by a belt around the woman's abdomen to obtain and record the fetal heart rate by ultrasound waves.

umbilical artery catheter—A radiopaque catheter placed in one of the umbilical arteries through which parenteral fluids may be delivered or blood samples withdrawn.

umbilical cord—The structure connecting the fetus from the umbilicus to the placenta; contains two arteries and one vein that allow exchange of maternal nutrients and fetal wastes.

umbilical cord blood pH—A test of fetal well-being in which blood is collected from the cord at the time of delivery to check for acidosis.

unexplained infertility—Prolonged infertility in the absence of a known pathologic process.

unlicensed assistive personnel—Persons trained to perform nursing tasks under the supervision of a licensed nurse.

uterine atony—Failure of the uterine muscle to contract after birth.

uterine dysfunction—Uterine force insufficiently strong or inappropriately coordinated to efface and dilate the cervix.

uterine inversion—A turning inside out of the uterus.

uterine involution—The normal process whereby the uterus contracts to its original size.

uterine rupture—Abrupt tearing of the uterus that can be an obstetric catastrophe.

uterine souffle—A swooshing sound that can be heard with a fetoscope during pregnancy that is the maternal blood pumping through the uterine vessels and placenta; the rate is synchronous with the maternal heart rate.

uterotropins—Agents that facilitate the body's readiness for labor, including softening such tissue as the cervix.

uterus—Female reproductive organ composed of inner lining (endometrium) that sheds during menstruation; composed of the fundus, corpus (body), isthmus, and cervix.

vacuum extractor—An instrument used to assist in the delivery of the fetus that consists of a cup connected by tubing to a vacuum pump; the cup is placed on the fetal occiput and negative pressure is exerted with the pump, as gentle traction assists in the delivery of the head.

vagina—Fibromuscular canal linking the female external genitalia and the internal reproductive organs.

vaginal birth after cesarean (VBAC)—The vaginal delivery of a woman who has had a previous cesarean birth; a VBAC is possible if the woman's previous cesarean was done with a lower uterine segment incision and no other complications exist that make vaginal birth a risk.

vaginal spermicidal agent—A compound that is inserted in the vagina before sexual intercourse to destroy sperm; can be in the form of a cream, jelly, foam, or vaginal suppository.

values clarification—The process of examining and clarifying one's values.

variable deceleration—A rapid decrease in the fetal heart rate and a rapid return to baseline that may occur during or between contractions and has a characteristic V shape; caused by cord compression.

vasectomy—A sterilization procedure for males in which the vasa deferentia are severed, tied, clipped, or coagulated to prevent the passage of sperm.

vasocongestion—Primary response to sexual stimulation, in which veins in genital area fill with blood.

vena caval syndrome—The phenomena that can occur when a pregnant woman lies supine with the weight of the uterus on the vena cava; results in symptoms of dizziness, clamminess, and nausea due to decreased blood pressure.

vernix caseosa—The protective white cheeselike substance that covers the fetal skin in utero.

version—Manipulation to change the presentation of the fetus in utero.

vertex—The top portion of the fetal head, between the anterior and posterior fontanelles.

viability—The period of gestation at which the fetus is capable of sustaining life outside the uterus; now considered to be between 20 and 24 weeks' gestation.

vibroacoustic stimulation—A test of fetal well-being in which vibration or noise is applied to the maternal abdomen for 3 to 5 seconds to assess for a reactive fetal response of acceleration in the fetal heart rate.

violence—The use of physical force to injure or harm, which is a major social problem threatening the physical health as well as spiritual and emotional well-being of women and children.

warning signs—Symptoms in pregnancy that are not normal discomforts but may signal the development of a complication.

weaning—The process of terminating breastfeeding and introducing other foods to an infant.

Women, Infants, and Children (WIC) Program—Federal- and state-funded food supplementation program.

100 women years—The effectiveness of a contraceptive for 1 year's use in a group of 100 women.

working phase—The goal-directed portion of a home visit, in which the nursing process is employed to meet the client's needs.

X-linked—Refers to genes that are located on the X chromosome.

zona pellucida—Thick membrane lining the ovum.

zygote—The diploid cell formed by fusion of a haploid egg and haploid sperm during fertilization that develops into the embryo.

zygote intrafallopian transfer (ZIFT)—A variation of the IVF or GIFT procedure in which eggs fertilized in a Petri dish (zygotes) are placed in the woman's fallopian tubes, where they may move on their own to the uterus.

Index

Note: Page numbers in *italics* refer to illustrations; page numbers followed by the letter t refer to tables.

C

E

F

I

J

N

O

T

V

Y

Z